Scott-Brown's Otorhinolaryngology, Head and Neck Surgery

Scott–Brown's Otorhinolaryngology, Head and Neck Surgery
7th edition

Lead editor: Michael Gleeson

Volume 1

Part 1 Cell biology, edited by Nicholas S Jones
Part 2 Wound healing, edited by Nicholas S Jones
Part 3 Immunology, edited by Nicholas S Jones
Part 4 Microbiology, edited by Nicholas S Jones
Part 5 Haematology, edited by Nicholas S Jones
Part 6 Endocrinology, edited by Nicholas S Jones
Part 7 Pharmacotherapeutics, edited by Martin J Burton
Part 8 Perioperative management, edited by Martin J Burton
Part 9 Safe and effective practice, edited by Martin J Burton
Part 10 Interpretation and management of data, edited by Martin J Burton
Part 11 Recent advances in technology, edited by Martin J Burton
Part 12 Paediatric otorhinolaryngology, edited by Ray Clarke

Volume 2

Part 13 The nose and paranasal sinuses, edited by Valerie J Lund
Part 14 The neck, edited by John Hibbert
Part 15 The upper digestive tract, edited by John Hibbert
Part 16 The upper airway, edited by John Hibbert
Part 17 Head and neck tumours, edited by John Hibbert

Volume 3

Part 18 Plastic surgery of the head and neck, edited by John C Watkinson
Part 19 The ear, hearing and balance, edited by George G Browning and Linda M Luxon
Part 20 Skull base, edited by Michael Gleeson
Index
CD-ROM

George G Browning MD FRCS
Professor of Otorhinolaryngology, MRC Institute of Hearing Research, Glasgow Royal Infirmary, Glasgow, UK

Martin J Burton MA DM FRCS
Senior Clinical Lecturer, University of Oxford; and Consultant Otolaryngologist, Oxford Radcliffe NHS Trust Oxford, UK

Ray Clarke BSc DCH FRCS FRCS (ORL)
Consultant Paediatric Otolaryngologist, Royal Liverpool University Children's Hospital, Alder Hey, Liverpool, UK

Michael Gleeson MD FRCS
Professor of Otolaryngology and Skull Base Surgery, Institute of Neurology, University College London; and Consultant, Guy's, Kings and St Thomas' and the National Hospital for Neurology and Neurosurgery, London UK; and Honorary Consultant Skull Base Surgeon, Great Ormond Street Hospital for Sick Children, London, UK

John Hibbert ChM FRCS
Formerly Consultant Otolaryngologist, Department of Otolaryngology, Guy's Hospital, London, UK

Nicholas S Jones MD FRCS FRCS (ORL)
Professor of Otorhinolaryngology, Queen's Medical Centre, University of Nottingham, Nottingham UK

Valerie J Lund MS FRCS FRCS (Ed)
Professor of Rhinology, The Ear Institute, University College London, London, UK

Linda M Luxon BSc MBBS FRCP
Professor of Audiovestibular Medicine, University of London at University College London, Academic Unit of Audiovestibular Medicine; and Consultant Physician, National Hospital for Neurology and Neurosurgery; and Honorary Consultant Physician, Great Ormond Street Hospital for Children, London, UK

John C Watkinson MSc MS FRCS (Ed, Glas, Land) DLO
Consultant Head and Neck and Thyroid Surgeon, Department of Otorhinolaryngology/Head and Neck Surgery, Queen Elizabeth Hospital, University of Birmingham NHS Trust, Birmingham, UK

Scott-Brown's Otorhinolaryngology, Head and Neck Surgery

7th edition

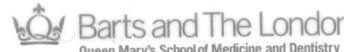
Volume

Edited by

Michael Gl

George G Brow

Ray Clarke, Joh

Valerie J Lund,

John C Watkin

Hodder Arnold

www.hoddereducation.com

First published in Great Britain in 1952 by Butterworth & Co.

Second edition 1965
Third edition 1971
Fourth edition 1979
Fifth edition 1987
Sixth edition 1997

This seventh edition published in Great Britain in 2008 by Hodder Arnold
An imprint of Hodder Education, a part of Hachette Livre UK, 338 Euston Road, London NW1 3BH

http://www.hoddereducation.com

© 2008 Edward Arnold (Publishers) Ltd

Whilst the advice and information in this book are believed to be true and accurate at the date of going to press, neither the author[s] nor the publisher can accept any legal responsibility or liability for any errors or omissions that may be made. In particular (but without limiting the generality of the preceding disclaimer) every effort has been made to check drug dosages; however it is still possible that errors have been missed. Furthermore, dosage schedules are constantly being revised and new side-effects recognized. For these reasons the reader is strongly urged to consult the drug companies' printed instructions before administering any of the drugs recommended in this book.

British Library Cataloguing in Publication Data
A catalogue record for this book is available from the British Library

Library of Congress Cataloging-in-Publication Data
A catalog record for this book is available from the Library of Congress

ISBN   978 0 340 808 931

1 2 3 4 5 6 7 8 9 10

Commissioning Editor: Joanna Koster
Project Editor: Zelah Pengilley
Production Controller: Lindsay Smith / Andre Sim
Text and Cover Designer: Amina Dudhia

Cover photograph © MEHAU KULYK/SCIENCE PHOTO LIBRARY

Typeset in 10 pt Minion by Macmillan India
Printed and bound in India.

What do you think about this book? Or any other Hodder Arnold title?
Please send your comments to www.hoddereducation.com

Contents

Contributors xi

Preface xxix

How to use this book xxxi

Abbreviations xxxiii

PART 1 CELL BIOLOGY – EDITED BY NICHOLAS S JONES 1

3
1   Molecular biology
    Michael Kuo and Richard Irving

15
2   Genetics
    Karen P Steel

23
3   Gene therapy
    Scott M Graham and John H Lee

34
4   Mechanisms of anticancer drugs
    Sarah Payne and David Miles

47
5   Radiotherapy and radiosensitizers
    Stewart G Martin and David AL Morgan

56
6   Apoptosis and cell death
    Michael Saunders

66
7   Stem cells
    A John Harris and Archana Vats

PART 2 WOUND HEALING – EDITED BY NICHOLAS S JONES 85

87
8   Soft and hard tissue repair
    Stephen R Young and Melissa Calvin

110
9   Skin flap physiology
    A Graeme B Perks

118
10 Biomaterials, tissue engineering and their applications
    Colin A Scotchford, Matthew Evans and Archana Vats

PART 3 IMMUNOLOGY – EDITED BY NICHOLAS S JONES 131

133
11 Defence mechanisms
    Ian Todd and Richard J Powell

144
12 Allergy: basic mechanisms and tests
    Stephen R Durham and Graham Banfield

13 Evaluation of the immune system   167
    Elizabeth Drewe and Richard J Powell

14 Primary immunodeficiencies   174
    Elizabeth Drewe and Richard J Powell

15 Rheumatological diseases   183
    Adrian Drake-Lee

PART 4 MICROBIOLOGY – EDITED BY NICHOLAS S JONES   **193**

16 Microorganisms   195
    Vivienne Weston

17 Viruses and antiviral agents   204
    Paul Simons and Karl G Nicholson

18 Fungi   213
    Juliette Morgan and David W Warnock

19 Antimicrobial therapy   228
    Vivienne Weston

20 HIV and otolaryngology   238
    Thomas A Tami and Jahmal A Hairston

PART 5 HAEMATOLOGY – EDITED BY NICHOLAS S JONES   **251**

21 Blood groups, blood components and alternatives to transfusion   253
    Fiona Regan and Ian Gabriel

22 Haemato-oncology   265
    Clare Wykes and Fiona Regan

23 Haemostasis: normal physiology, disorders of haemostasis and thrombosis and their management   278
    Fiona Regan

PART 6 ENDOCRINOLOGY – EDITED BY NICHOLAS S JONES   **293**

24 The pituitary gland: anatomy and physiology   295
    John Hill

25 The pituitary: imaging and tests of function   303
    Alan P Johnson, Swarupsinh Chavda and Paul Stewart

26 The thyroid gland: anatomy and physiology   314
    Julian A McGlashan

27 The thyroid gland: function tests and imaging   327
    Susan Clarke

28 The thyroid: nonmalignant disease   338
    Lorraine M Albon and Jayne A Franklyn

29 The parathyroid glands: anatomy and physiology   367
    Mateen H Arastu and William J Owen†

30 Parathyroid function tests and imaging   379
    David Hosking

31 Parathyroid dysfunction: medical and surgical therapy   387
    E Dinakara Babu, Bill Fleming and JA Lynn

32 Head and neck manifestations of endocrine disease   398
    Jonathan M Morgan and Thomas McCaffrey

PART 7 PHARMACOTHERAPEUTICS – EDITED BY MARTIN J BURTON   405

33   Drug administration and monitoring   407
Geraldine Gallagher

34   Corticosteroids in otolaryngology   418
Niels Mygind and Jens Thomsen

35   Drug therapy in otology   429
Wendy Smith and Martin Burton

36   Drug therapy in rhinology   436
Wendy Smith and Grant Bates

37   Drug therapy in laryngology and head and neck surgery   446
Wendy Smith and Rogan Corbridge

PART 8 PERIOPERATIVE MANAGEMENT – EDITED BY MARTIN J BURTON   455

38   Preparation of the patient for surgery   457
Adrian Pearce

39   Recognition and management of the difficult airway   467
Adrian Pearce

40   Adult anaesthesia   488
Andrew D Farmery and Jaideep J Pandit

41   Paediatric anaesthesia   507
Alistair Cranston

42   Adult critical care   526
Gavin G Lavery

43   Paediatric intensive care   542
Helen Allen and Rob Ross Russell

PART 9 SAFE AND EFFECTIVE PRACTICE – EDITED BY MARTIN J BURTON   549

44   Training, accreditation and the maintenance of skills   551
Paul O'Flynn

45   Communication and the medical consultation   559
Damian Gardner-Thorpe and Richard Canter

46   Clinical governance: Improving the quality of patient care   568
Debbie Wall, Patrick J Bradley and Aidan Halligan

47   Medical ethics   581
Katherine Wasson

48   Medical jurisprudence and otorhinolaryngology   594
Maurice Hawthorne and Desmond Watson

PART 10 INTERPRETATION AND MANAGEMENT OF DATA – EDITED BY MARTIN J BURTON   613

49   Epidemiology   615
Jan HP van der Meulen and David A Lowe

50   Outcomes research   633
Iain RC Swan

51   Evidence-based medicine   645
Martin J Burton

52   Critical appraisal skills   649
Martin Dawes

PART 11 RECENT ADVANCES IN TECHNOLOGY – EDITED BY MARTIN J BURTON   673

53 Functional magnetic resonance imaging: Principles and illustrative applications for otolaryngology   675
    Paul M Matthews

54 Positron emission tomography and integrated PET/computed tomography   684
    Wai Lup Wong

55 Image-guided surgery, 3D planning and reconstruction   701
    Ghassan Alusi and Michael Gleeson

56 Ultrasound in ear, nose and throat practice   711
    Keshthra Satchithananda and Paul S Sidhu

57 Interventional techniques   731
    James V Byrne

58 Laser principles in otolaryngology, head and neck surgery   742
    Brian JG Bingham

59 Electrophysiology and monitoring   748
    Patrick R Axon and David M Baguley

60 Optical coherence tomography   755
    Mariah Hahn and Brett E Bouma

61 Contact endoscopy   762
    Mario Andrea and Oscar Dias

PART 12 PAEDIATRIC OTORHINOLARYNGOLOGY – EDITED BY RAY CLARKE   769

62 Introduction   771
    Ray Clarke

63 The paediatric consultation   776
    Ray Clarke and Ken Pearman

64 ENT input for children with special needs   783
    Francis Lannigan

65 Head and neck embryology   792
    T Clive Lee

66 Molecular otology, development of the auditory system and recent advances in genetic manipulation   811
    Henry Pau

67 Hearing loss in preschool children: screening and surveillance   821
    Kai Uus and John Bamford

68 Hearing tests in children   834
    Glynnis Parker

69 Investigation and management of the deaf child   844
    Sujata De, Sue Archbold and Ray Clarke

70 Paediatric cochlear implantation   860
    Joseph G Toner

71 Congenital middle ear abnormalities in children   869
    Jonathan P Harcourt

72 Otitis media with effusion   877
    George Browning

73 Acute otitis media in children   912
    Peter Rea and John Graham

74 Chronic otitis media in childhood   928
    John Hamilton

75 Management of congenital deformities of the external and middle ear   965
    David Gault and Mike Rothera

76 Disorders of speech and language in paediatric otolaryngology   990
    Ray Clarke and Siobhan McMahon

77 Cleft lip and palate   996
    Chris Penfold

78 Craniofacial anomalies: genetics and management   1019
    Dean Kissun, David Richardson, Elizabeth Sweeney and Paul May

79 Vertigo in children   1040
    Gavin AJ Morrison

80 Facial paralysis in childhood   1052
    SS Musheer Hussain

81 Epistaxis in children   1063
    Ray Clarke

82 Nasal obstruction in children   1070
    Michelle Wyatt

83 Paediatric rhinosinusitis   1079
    Glenis Scadding and Helen Caulfield

84 The adenoid and adenoidectomy   1094
    Peter J Robb

85 Obstructive sleep apnoea in childhood   1102
    Helen M Caulfield

86 Stridor   1114
    David Albert

87 Acute laryngeal infections   1127
    Susanna Leighton†

88 Congenital disorders of the larynx, trachea and bronchi   1135
    Martin Bailey

89 Laryngeal stenosis   1150
    Michael J Rutter and Robin T Cotton

90 Paediatric voice disorders   1167
    Ben Hartley

91 Juvenile-onset recurrent respiratory papillomatosis   1174
    Michael Kuo and William J Primrose

92 Foreign bodies in the ear and the aerodigestive tract in children   1184
    A Simon Carney, Nimesh Patel and Ray Clarke

93 Tracheostomy and home care   1194
    Michael Saunders

94 Cervicofacial infections in children   1210
    Ben Hartley

95 Diseases of the tonsil   1219
    William S McKerrow

96 Tonsillectomy   1229
    William S McKerrow and Ray Clarke

97 Salivary gland disorders in childhood   1242
    Peter D Bull

98 Tumours of the head and neck in childhood   1251
    Fiona B MacGregor

99   Branchial arch fistulae, thyroglossal duct anomalies and lymphangioma   1264
     Peter D Bull

100 Gastro-oesophageal reflux and aspiration   1272
     Haytham Kubba

101 Diseases of the oesophagus, swallowing disorders and caustic ingestion   1282
     Lewis Spitz

102 Imaging in paediatric ENT   1295
     Neville Wright

103 Medical negligence in paediatric otolaryngology   1305
     Maurice Hawthorne

Please note: The table of contents for all three volumes can be found on the *Scott-Brown* website at: www.scottbrownENT.com. The index for all three volumes is included in Volume 3.

Contributors

Victor J Abdullah MBBS FRCS (Eng) FRCS (Edin)
Consultant, Department of ENT
United Christian Hospital; and
Chief of Service in ENT
Kowloon East Cluster, Hospital Authority; and
Honorary Clinical Associate Professor
Department of Otorhinolaryngology, Head and Neck Surgery
The Chinese University of Hong Kong
Shatin, Hong Kong

Jose M Acuin MD MSc
Professor in Otolaryngology–Head and Neck Surgery
De La Salle Health Sciences Campus
Dasmarinas, Cavite, Philippines

Richard Adamson MB BS FRCS
Consultant Otolaryngologist/Head and Neck Surgeon
Fife Hospitals NHS Trust
Scotland, UK

David Albert FRCS
Lead clinician
Department of Otolaryngology
Hospital for Sick Children
Great Ormond Street
London, UK

Lorraine M Albon MSc MRCP
Consultant Endocrinologist and Acute Physician
Queen Alexandra Hospital
Portsmouth, UK

Helen Allen MBChB MRCP MRCPCH
Specialist Registrar in Paediatrics
Addenbrookes Hospital
Cambridge, UK

Ghassan Alusi PhD FRCS (ORL-HNS)
Consultant Otolaryngologist
ENT Department
Barts and the London NHS Trust
London, UK

Mario Andrea MD PhD
Professor and Chairman
Department of Otolaryngology, Voice and Communication
Disorders
Faculty of Medicine of Lisbon
Lisbon, Portugal

Jawaher Ansari MBBS MRCP FRCR
Specialist Registrar in Clinical Oncology
Queen Elizabeth Hospital
Birmingham, UK

Mateen H Arastu MBBS BSc MRCS (Eng)
Specialist Registrar in Trauma and Orthopaedic Surgery
South West Thamas Region, UK

Sue Archbold MPhil
Education Co-ordinator
The Ear Foundation
Nottingham, UK

Stig Arlinger PhD
Professor of Technical Andiology
Department of Clinical and Experimental Medicine
Division of Technical Audiology
Linköping University
Linköping, Sweden

Marcus Atlas
Professor of Otolaryngology
University of Western Australia; and
Director, Ear Science Institute Australia
Sir Charles Gairdner Hospital
Nedlands, Western Australia

Patrick R Axon MD FRCS (ORL-HNS)
Consultant Otologist and Skull Base Surgeon
Department of Otolaryngology
Cambridge University Hospitals
Cambridge, UK

E Dinakara Babu MS FRCS (Eng) FRCS (Ire) FRCS (Glas) FRCS (Inter collegiate) Diploma
in Laparoscopy (France)
Consultant and Clinical Head
Breast and Endocrine Surgery
Hillingdon Hospital
Uxbridge, UK

Claus Bachert MD PhD
Department of Oto-Rhino-Laryngology
Ghent University Hospital
Ghent, Belgium

Lydia Badia FRCS (ORL-HNS)
Consultant ENT Surgeon
Rhinology and Facial Plastics
Royal National Throat, Nose and Ear Hospital
London, UK

Jose V Sebastian Bagan MD DDS PhD
Hospital General Universitario de Valencia
Valencia, Spain

Dan Bagger-Sjöbäck MD PhD
Professor in Ear, Nose and Throat Diseases
Karolinska Institute
Stockholm, Sweden

David M Baguley BSc MSc MBA PhD
Consultant Audiological Scientist
Cambridge University Hospitals NHS Foundation Trust
Cambridge, UK

S Bahadur MS FAMS PhD
Professor of Otolaryngology and Head/Neck Surgery
All India Institute of Medical Sciences
New Delhi, India

Martin Bailey BSc FRCS
Consultant Paediatric Otolaryngologist
Great Ormond Street Hospital for Children
London, UK

John Bamford BA PhD
Ellis Llywd Jones Professor of Audiology and Deaf Education
School of Psychological Sciences
Faculty of Medical and Human Sciences
University of Manchester
Manchester, UK

Doris-Eva Bamiou MD MSc PhD
Consultant in Audiological Medicine
Department of Neuro-otology
National Hospital for Neurology and Neurosurgery; and
Honorary Senior Lecturer
Academic Unit of Audiological Medicine
University College London Institute of Child Health
Great Ormond Street Hospital
London, UK

Dev Banerjee BSc MBChB MD MRCP
Consultant Respiratory and Sleep Physician
Sleep and Ventilation Unit
Department of Respiratory Medicine
Birmingham Heartlands Hospital
Birmingham, UK

Graham Banfield MD DLO FRCS Ed (ORL-HNS)
Consultant ENT Surgeon
The Great Western Hospital
Swindon, UK

Jane A Baran PhD
Professor and Chair
Department of Communication Disorders
University of Massachusetts Amherst
Amherst, MA, USA

Michael E Baser†
Formerly of Department of Environmental Health Sciences
Johns Hopkins School of Hygiene and Public Health
Baltimore, MD, USA

Grant Bates BSc (Hons) BM Bch FRCS
Consultant ENT Surgeon
John Radcliffe Hospital
Oxford, UK

Nigel Beasley FRCS (ORL-HNS)
Consultant in Otolaryngology
Queen's Medical Centre
Nottingham, UK

Michael S Benninger MD
Chairman Department of Otolaryngology-Head and Neck Surgery
Henry Ford Hospital
Detroit, USA

Barry KB Berkovitz MSc PhD BDS FDSRCS (Eng)
Department of Anatomy and Human Sciences
School of Biomedical and Health Sciences
King's College
London, UK

Thanos Bibas MSc (Lond) DrMed FRCSI (Otol)
Consultant and Lecturer in Otolaryngology
Hippokrateion Hospital University of Athens
Athens, Greece

Carsten Bindslev-Jensen MD PhD DSc
Head, Allergy Center
Department of Dermatology
Odense University Hospital
Odense, Denmark

Brian JG Bingham MBChB FRCS Ed Glas
Consultant ENT Surgeon
Department of Otolaryngology
Victoria Infirmary; and
Honorary Senior Lecturer in Otorhinolaryngology
University of Glasgow
Glasgow, UK

† Deceased

Martin A Birchall MD (Cantab) FRCS FRCS (Oto) FRCS (ORL)
Professor of Laryngology
University of Bristol
Bristol, UK; and
Consultant in Otolaryngology Head and Neck Surgery
Royal United Hospital Bath NHS Trust
Bath, UK

Ian D Bottrill BM FRCS (ORL)
Consultant Otolaryngologist; and
Honorary Senior Lecturer
ENT Department
University of Oxford
John Radcliffe Hospital
Oxford, UK

An Boudewyns MD PhD
Professor of Otorhinolaryngology
Department of Otorhinolaryngology, Head and Neck Surgery
University of Antwerp Hospital – University of Antwerp
Antwerp, Belgium

Brett E Bouma PhD
Associate Professor, Department of Dermatology
Member of the Faculty of the Harvard-MIT Division of Health
Science and Technology
Harvard Medical School
Boston, MA, USA

Jean Bousquet MD
Service des Maladies Respiratoires
Hôpital Arnaud de Villeneuve
Montpellier, France

Patrick J Bradley MBA FRCS FRACS (Hon) FRCSLT (Hon)
Professor of Head and Neck Oncologic Surgery
Department of ORL-HNS
Nottingham University Hospitals
Queen's Medical Centre Campus
Nottingham, UK

Stefan Brew MB ChB MHB (Hons) MSc FRANZCR
Consultant Neuroradiologist
The National Hospital for Neurology and Neurosurgery
London, UK

Steven M Bromley MD
Clinical Assistant Professor of Neurology (Medicine)
and Attending Neurologist
University of Medicine and Dentistry of New Jersey
Robert Wood Johnson Medical School
Cooper University Hospital, Camden, NJ; and
Bromley Neurology PC, Audubon, NJ; and
Smell and Taste Center
University of Pennsylvania Medical Center
Philadelphia, PA
USA

Adolfo M Bronstein MD PhD FRCP
Professor of Clinical Neuro-otology; and
Head, Neuro-otology Unit
Division of Neuroscience and Mental Health
Charing Cross Hospital, Imperial College London; and
Honorary Consultant Neurologist
Charing Cross Hospital; and
National Hospital for Neurology and Neurosurgery
Queen Square, London, UK

Gerald Brookes FRCS
Consultant Otologist and Neuro-Otologist
The National Hospital for Neurology and Neurosurgery; and
The Royal National Throat, Nose and Ear Hospital
London, UK

George G Browning MD FRCS
Professor of Otorhinolaryngology
MRC Institute of Hearing Research
Glasgow Royal Infirmary
Glasgow, UK

Peter D Bull MB FRCS
Consultant Otolaryngologist
Royal Hallamshire Hospital and Sheffield Children's Hospital; and
Honorary Senior Clinical Lecturer
University of Sheffield
Sheffield, UK

Martin J Burton MA DM FRCS
Senior Clinical Lecturer
University of Oxford; and
Consultant Otolaryngologist
Oxford Radcliffe NHS Trust
Oxford, UK

James V Byrne MD FRCS FRCR
Professor of Neuroradiology
University of Oxford; and
Consultant Neuroradiologist
John Radcliffe Hospital
Oxford, UK

Melissa Calvin MRCOG PhD BSc (Hons)
Department of Obstetrics and Gynaecology
Lister Hospital
Stevenage, UK

Richard Canter PhD FRCS FRCS (Otol) Hon FRCS (Edin)
Consultant Otolaryngologist
Royal United Hospital; and
Honorary Senior Lecturer
University of Bath
Bath, UK

Paul Carding FRCSLT
Professor of Voice Pathology
The Medical School, Newcastle University; and
Head of Speech, Voice and Swallowing Department
Otolarygology Directorate, Freeman Hospital
Newcastle on Tyne, UK

A Simon Carney BSc (Hons) MBChB FRCS FRACS MD
Associate Professor and Head of ENT Unit
Flinders University and Flinders Medical Centre
Adelaide, South Australia

Anna Cassoni BSc FRCP FRCR
Consultant in Clinical Oncology
University College Hospitals NHS Foundation Trust
London, UK

Helen Caulfield MBBS FRCS (ORL-HNS)
Consultant ENT Surgeon
Department of Otolaryngology
The Royal Free Hospital
London, UK

Roderick Cawson† MD FRCPath
Formerly Emeritus Professor of Oral Medicine
Guy's Hospital
London, UK

Borka Ceranic MD ENTspec PhD
Consultant in Audiological Medicine
Department of Audiology
St George's Hospital
London, UK

Swarupsinh V Chavda MBChB DMRD FRCR
Consultant Neuroradiologist and Honorary Senior Lecturer
Queen Elizabeth Hospital
University Hospital Birmingham Foundation Trust
Birmingham, UK

Elfy B Chevretton BSc MBBS FRCS MS
Consultant Otolaryngologist
Department of ENT Surgery
Guy's and St Thomas' NHS Trust
London, UK

Peter Clarke BSc FRCS
Consultant ENT Surgeon
Charing Cross Hospital
London, UK

Ray Clarke BSc DCH FRCS FRCS (ORL)
Consultant Paediatric Otolaryngologist
Royal Liverpool University Children's Hospital
Alder Hey, Liverpool, UK

Susan Clarke MSc FRCP FRCR
Senior Lecturer and Consultant Physician
Department of Nuclear Medicine
Guy's and St Thomas' Hospital
London, UK

Rogan Corbridge MBBS BSc FRCS FRCS (ORL)
Consultant ENT Surgeon
Oxford Centre for Head and Neck Oncology
John Radcliffe Hospital
Oxford, UK

Robin T Cotton MD
Director, Pediatric Otolaryngology–Head and Neck Surgery
Children's Hospital Medical Center; and
Professor of Pediatric Otolaryngology
Department of Otolaryngology, Head and Neck Surgery
University of Cincinnati College of Medicine
Cincinnati, OH, USA

Graham J Cox BDS FRCS
Consultant ENT Surgeon; and
Macmillan Head and Neck Surgical Oncologist
John Radcliffe Hospital
Oxford, UK

Alistair Cranston MBBS FRCA
Consultant Anaesthetist
Birmingham Children's Hospital
Birmingham, UK

Cor WRJ Cremers
Department of Otorhinolaryngology
University Medical Center
St Radboud
Nijmegen, The Netherlands

Ian S Curthoys PhD
Emeritus Professor
School of Psychology
University of Sydney
Sydney, Australia

Rosalyn A Davies FRCP PhD
Consultant in Audiovestibular Medicine
Department of Neuro-Otology
The National Hospital for Neurology and Neurosurgery; and
Honorary Senior Lecturer
Institute of Neurology
Queen Square, London, UK

Martin Dawes MB BS MD (Lond) FRCGP
Chair, Family Medicine
McGill University
Quebec, Canada

Ranit De MPhil FRCS (ORL-HNS)
Consultant ENT Surgeon
University Hospital North Staffordshire NHS Trust; and
Stoke-on-Trent and Mid-Staffordshire NHS Trust
Stafford, UK

† Deceased

Sujata De MBBS FRCS (ORL-HNS)
Consultant Paediatric Otorhinolaryngologist
Alder Hey Children's Hospital
Liverpool, UK

Charles Diamond FRCS (Glas) Dip Pall Med
Honorary Consultant Otolaryngologist
Freeman Hospital and St. Oswald's Hospice
Newcastle upon Tyne, UK

Oscar Dias MD PhD
Associate Professor
Department of Otolaryngology, Voice and Communication
Disorders
Faculty of Medicine of Lisbon
Lisbon, Portugal

Harvey Dillon B Eng (Hons I) PhD
Director of Research
National Acoustic Laboratories
Chatswood, Australia

Richard L Doty PhD
Smell and Taste Center
University of Pennsylvania Medical Center
Philadelphia, PA, USA

M Stephen Dover FDSRCS FRCS
Consultant Oral and Maxillofacial Surgeon, and
Honorary Senior Lecturer
Department of Maxillofacial Surgery
University Hospital Birmingham NHS Foundation Trust
Birmingham, UK

Wolfgang Draf Prof Dr Med Dr HC FRCS
Director, Department of Ear, Nose and
Throat Diseases, Head and Neck Surgery
International Neuroscience Institute
Hanover, Germany

Adrian Drake-Lee MMEd PhD FRCS
Consultant ENT Surgeon
Queen Elizabeth Hospital
University Hospital, NHS Trust
Birmingham, UK

Elizabeth Drewe MBBS PhD MRCP MRCPath
Consultant Clinical Immunologist
Nottingham University Hospitals NHS Trust
Nottingham, UK

Stephen R Durham MA MD FRCP
Professor of Allergy and Respiratory Medicine
Imperial College School of Medicine
National Heart and Lung Institute
London, UK

Sunil Narayan Dutt MS DNB PhD FRCS Ed (ORL-HNS) DLO (Eng) DORL
Senior Consultant and Clinical Coordinator
Department of Otolaryngology and Head and Neck Surgery
Apollo Group of Hospitals
Bangalore, India

Charles East FRCS
Consultant Otolaryngologist, Head and Neck Surgeon
The Royal Free Hampstead NHS Trust
London, UK

Ronald Eccles BSc PhD DSc
Director, Common Cold Centre and
Healthcare Clinical Trials
Cardiff School of Biosciences
Cardiff University
Cardiff, Wales, UK

D Gareth R Evans MD FRCP
Professor, Department of Medical Genetics
St Mary's Hospital
Manchester, UK

Matthew Evans PhD
Editorial Manager
Caudex Medical
Oxford, UK

Johannes J Fagan MBChB, FCS (SA) MMed (Otol)
Professor and Chairman
Division of Otolaryngology
University of Cape Town and Groote Schuur Hospital
Cape Town, South Africa

Andrew D Farmery BSc MA MD FRCA
Senior Lecturer in Anaesthetics
Nuffield Department of Anaesthetics
University of Oxford
Oxford, UK

Neil Fergie FRCS MD
Consultant in Otorhinolaryngology Head and Neck Surgery
Kings Mill Hospital, Mansfield; and
Queens Medical Centre
Nottingham, UK

John Fleetham MB BS FRCP(C)
Professor of Medicine
Respiratory Division
University of British Columbia and Vancouver Hospital
Vancouver, BC, Canada

Bill Fleming FRACS FRCS
Consultant Endocrine Surgeon
Hammersmith Hospital
Imperial Healthcare NHS Trust
London, UK

Liam M Flood MB BS FRCS
ENT Consultant
James Cook University Hospital
Middlesbrough, UK

Adrian Fourcin PhD FIoA
Emeritus Professor, Department of Phonetics and Linguistics
University College London
London, UK

Jayne A Franklyn MD PhD FRCP FMedSci
Professor of Medicine
Division of Medical Sciences
University of Birmingham
Queen Elizabeth Hospital
Birmingham, UK

Nicole JM Freling MD PhD
Department of Radiology
Academic Medical Centre
Amsterdam, The Netherlands

David N Furness BSc PhD
School of Life Sciences
Keele University
Staffordshire, UK

Ian Gabriel MBBS BSc (Hons) MRCP (UK) DipRCPath
Department of Haematology
St Mary's Hospital Campus
Imperial College School of Medicine
London, UK

Geraldine Gallagher FRCSI
Antrim Area Hospital
Belfast, Northern Ireland

Damian Gardner-Thorpe MRCP (UK) MRCS (Eng) MRCGP (UK)
General Practitioner
The Pulteney Practice
Bath, UK

David Gault MB ChB FRCS
Consultant Plastic Surgeon
London Centre for Ear Reconstruction
The Portland Hospital
London, UK

Garrick A Georgeu MB ChB FRCS (Ed) FRCS PLAS MSc
Plastic Surgery Department
Selly Oak Hospital
University Hospital Birmingham
Birmingham, UK

Kevin P Gibbin
Consultant Otolaryngologist
University Hospital
Nottingham, UK

Ralph W Gilbert MD FRCS (C)
Professor of Otolaryngology/Head and Neck Surgery
University of Toronto
University Health Network
Princess Margaret Hospital
Toronto, Ontario, Canada

John Glaholm BSc FRCP FRCR (Clin Oncol)
Consultant Clinical Oncologist
Cancer Centre, Queen Elizabeth Hospital
Birmingham, UK

Michael Gleeson MD FRCS
Professor of Otolaryngology and Skull Base Surgery
Institute of Neurology
University College London; and
Consultant
Guy's, Kings and St Thomas' and the National Hospital for
Neurology and Neurosurgery
London UK; and
Honorary Consultant Skull Base Surgeon
Great Ormond Street Hospital for Sick Children
London, UK

Kees Graamans MD PhD
Professor and Chairman
Department of Otorhinolaryngology
University Medical Centre Nijmegen
Nijmegen, The Netherlands

John Graham MA BM BCh FRCS
Consultant Otolaryngologist
The Royal National Throat, Nose, and Ear Hospital
Gray's Inn Road
London, UK

Scott M Graham MD
Professor
Department of Otolaryngology – Head and Neck Surgery
The University of Iowa; and
Director of Rhinology, University of Iowa Hospital and Clinics
Iowa City, IA, USA

Luisa F Grymer MD
Grymer Private Hospital
Aarhus, Denmark

Carole M Hackney BSc PhD
Department of Physiology, Development and Neuroscience
University of Cambridge
Cambridge, UK

Mariah Hahn PhD
Assistant Professor
Department of Chemical Engineering
Texas A&M University
Texas, USA

Jahmal A Hairston MD
Department of Otolaryngology
University of Cincinnati College of Medicine
Cincinnati, OH, USA

Aidan Halligan FRCP FRCOG MA MD MRCPI FFPHM
Chief Executive, Elision Health Ltd; and
Deputy Chief Medical Officer, England (2003–2005); and
Director of Clinical Governance for the NHS (1999–2006)
Leicester, UK

G Michael Halmagyi MD FRACP
Clinical Professor
Department of Neurology
Royal Prince Alfred Hospital
Sydney, Australia

John Hamilton FRCS
Department of Otolaryngology
Gloucestershire Royal Hospital
Gloucester, UK

Ravinder PS Harar FRCS (ORL-HNS)
Specialist Registrar Otolaryngology, Head and Neck Surgery
The National Hospital for Neurology and Neurosurgery; and
The Royal National Throat, Nose and Ear Hospital
London, UK

Jonathan P Harcourt MA FRCS
Consultant ENT Surgeon
Charing Cross Hospital
London, UK

Meredydd Harries FRCS MSc (Voice)
Consultant ENT Surgeon
The Royal Sussex County Hospital
Brighton, UK

A John Harris PhD
Developmental Biology Laboratory
Department of Physiology
University of Otago
Dunedin, New Zealand

Douglas Harrison FRCS
Consultant Plastic Surgeon
The Wellington Hospital
London, UK

Ben Hartley MBBS BSc FRCS
Consultant Paediatric Otolaryngologist
Great Ormond Street Hospital for Children
London, UK

Richard J Harvey BScMed MB BS FRACS
Nuffield Fellow, University of Oxford, UK; and
Rhinologist and Endoscopic Skull Base Surgeon
St Vincent's Hospital
Sydney, Australia

Peter Haughton BSc PhD
Formerly Clinical Scientist and Head of Audiology
Department of Medical Physics
Royal Hull Hospitals
Kingston upon Hull, UK

Maurice Hawthorne FRCS
Consultant Otolaryngologist, Head and Neck Surgeon
James Cook University Hospital
Middlesbrough, UK

John Hibbert ChM FRCS
Formerly Consultant Otolaryngologist
Department of Otolaryngology
Guy's Hospital
London, UK

John M Hilinski MD
Facial Plastic and Reconstructive Surgery
San Diego Face and Neck Specialties
University of California, San Diego Medical Center
San Diego, CA, USA

John Hill FRCS FRCSEd
Department of ORL-HNS
The Freeman Hospital
Newcastle upon Tyne, UK

Malcolm P Hilton MA BM BCh FRCS (ENG) FRCS (ORL-HNS)
Consultant Otolaryngologist
Royal Devon and Exeter Hospital; and
Honorary Clinical Lecturer
Peninsula Medical School
University of Exeter
Exeter, UK

Lisa J Hirst BSc PhD Cert MCRSLT
Head of Service
Speech and Language Therapist
Salisbury District Hospital
Wiltshire, UK

Simon Holmes BDS MBBS (Hons) FDS RCS Eng FRCS (OMFS)
Consultant Oral and Maxillofacial Surgeon
Barts and The London NHS Trust
London, UK

David Hosking MD FRCP
Consultant Physician
Division of Mineral Metabolism
City Hospital
Nottingham, UK

David J Howard BSc FRCS FRCS (Ed)
Emeritus Senior Lecturer
University College London; and
Consultant Head and Neck Surgeon
Royal Throat, Nose and Ear Hospital; and
Charing Cross Hospital
London, UK

SS Musheer Hussain MB MSc (Manc) FRCS (ORL)
Consultant Otolaryngologist and Head
ENT and Audiology Services
Ninewells Hospital and Medical School; and
Honorary Senior Lecturer and Director
Temporal Bone Laboratory; and
Licenced Teacher of Anatomy
Department of Otolaryngology
University of Dundee
Dundee, UK

Richard M Irving MD FRCS (ORL-HNS)
Consultant in Neurotology
University Hospital Birmingham NHS Trust and
Diana Princess of Wales (Birmingham Childrens) Hospital; and
Honorary Senior Lecturer
University of Birmingham
Birmingham, UK

Mark E Izzard MB BS FRACS
Senior Lecturer in Otolaryngology
University of Auckland; and
Consultant Head and Neck Surgeon
Auckland District Health Board
Auckland, New Zealand

Jean-Pierre Jeannon MB ChB FRCS (OTO) FRCS (ORL)
Consultant Ear Nose and Throat/Head and Neck Surgeon
Guy's and St Thomas' Hospital
London, UK

Chris R Jennings
Department of Otolaryngology
The Queen Elizabeth Hospital
Birmingham, UK

Dan Jiang PhD FRCSI (Otol) FRCS (ORL-HNS)
Consultant Otolaryngologist
Department of Otolaryngology, Head and Neck Surgery
Guy's, St Thomas' and Evelina Children's Hospitals
London, UK

Alan P Johnson FRCS
Department of Otolaryngology
Queen Elizabeth Hospital
Birmingham, UK

Andrew S Jones MB BCh MD FRCSE FRCS
Professor, School of Cancer Studies
Division of Surgery and Oncology
Royal Liverpool University Hospital
Liverpool, UK

Nicholas S Jones MD FRCS FRCS (ORL)
Professor of Otorhinolaryngology
Queens Medical Centre
University of Nottingham
Nottingham, UK

Petros D Karkos MPhil AFRCSI
Specialist Registrar in Otolaryngology
Mersey Deanery
Chester, UK

Gerard Kelly MD FRCS (ORL-HNS)
Consultant Ear, Nose and Throat and Skull Base Surgeon; and
Clinical Director of Otolaryngology
The Leeds Teaching Hospitals NHS Trust
Leeds, UK

Andras Armand Kemeny MD FRCS
The National Centre for Stereotactic Radiosurgery
Royal Hallamshire Hospital
Sheffield, UK

David W Kennedy MD FACS FRCSI
Department of Otorhinolaryngology-Head and Neck Surgery
University of Pennsylvania
Philadelphia, PA, USA

Richard SC Kerr BSc MS MBBS FRCS
Consultant Neurosurgeon
Oxford Skull Base Unit
Oxford Radcliffe NHS Trust; and
Honorary Senior Lecturer, University of Oxford
Oxford, UK

Dean Kissun FRCS (OMFS)
Consultant Maxillofacial Surgeon
NHS Lothian
Edinburgh, UK

Jean Michel Klossek MD
ENT Professor, University of Poitiers; and
ENT and Head and Neck Surgery Department
University Hospital Jean Bernard
Poitiers, France

Gary Kroukamp MBChB FCORL (SA)
Faculty of Health Sciences
University of Stellenbosch, Tygerberg Hospital
Tygerberg, South Africa

Haytham Kubba MPhil MD FRCS (ORL-HNS)
Consultant Paediatric Otolaryngologist, Head and Neck Surgeon
The Royal Hospital for Sick Children
Glasgow, UK

Michael Kuo PhD FRCS (Eng) FRCS (ORL-HNS) DCH
Consultant Otolaryngologist – Head and Neck Surgeon
Birmingham Children's Hospital
Birmingham, UK

Francis Lannigan MB ChB MD FRCS (Eng) Ed (ORL) FRACS
Department of Otolaryngology – Head and Neck Surgery
Princess Margaret Hospital for Children; and
Clinical Professor, The University of Western Australia
Perth, Western Australia

Gavin G Lavery MB BCh BAO FCARCSI MD
Director of Critical Care Services
Royal Hospitals, Belfast, UK; and
Visiting Professor, Faculty of Life and Health Sciences
University of Ulster
Northern Ireland

Brian Leatherbarrow BSc MBChB DO FRCS FRCOphth
Consultant Ophthalmic, Oculoplastic and Orbital Surgeon
Manchester Royal Eye Hospital
Manchester, UK

John H Lee MD
Assistant Professor
Department of Otolaryngology – Head and Neck Surgery
University of Iowa
Iowa City, IA, USA

T Clive Lee MA MSc MD PhD FRCSI FRCSEd CEng FIEI
Professor of Anatomy
Royal College of Surgeons in Ireland
Dublin, Ireland

Susanna Leighton† BSc FRCS (ORL-HNS)
Formerly Consultant Paediatric Otolaryngologist
Great Ormond Street Hospital for Children
London, UK

Paula Leslie PhD Cert MRCSLT
Associate Professor
Communication Science and Disorders
University of Pittsburgh
Pittsburgh, PA, USA

Tristram HJ Lesser AKC FRCSEd MS
Otolaryngology/Head and Neck Surgery
University Hospital
Liverpool, UK

James W Loock MB ChB (UCT) FCS (SA) ORL
Professor and Head
Department of Otorhinolaryngology
University of Stellenbosch
Tygerberg Hospital
Cape Town, South Africa

David A Lowe BSc FRCSEd FRCS
Research Fellow
Clinical Effectiveness Unit
The Royal College of Surgeons of England
London, UK

Valerie J Lund MS FRCS FRCS (Ed)
Professor of Rhinology
The Ear Institute
University College London
London, UK

Linda M Luxon BSc MBBS FRCP
Professor of Audiovestibular Medicine
University of London at University College London
Academic Unit of Audiovestibular Medicine; and
Consultant Physician, National Hospital for
Neurology and Neurosurgery; and
Honorary Consultant Physician
Great Ormond Street Hospital for Children
London, UK

JA Lynn MS FRCS
Consultant Surgeon
Cromwell Hospital
London, UK

Fiona B MacGregor MBChB FRCS (ORL HNS)
Consultant Otolaryngologist
Royal Hospital for Sick Children
Glasgow, UK

Ian S Mackay FRCS
Consultant ENT Surgeon
Royal Brompton Hospital and Charing Cross Hospital
London, UK

Kenneth MacKenzie MB ChB FRCS (Ed)
Consultant Otorhinolaryngologist and Honorary Senior Lecturer
Glasgow Royal Infirmary
University of Glasgow
Glasgow, UK

Marcelle Macnamara MA MBBS FRCS MPhil FRCS (ORL-HNS)
Retired Consultant Otolaryngologist, Head and Neck Surgeon
Heart of England Foundation Trust
Birmingham, UK

Arnold GD Maran MD DSc FRCS (Ed, Eng, Glasg) FRCP FDS
Emeritus Professor of Otolaryngology
University of Edinburgh
Edinburgh, UK

Andrew H Marshall Bsc MBBS FRCS
Consultant Otolaryngologist
Department of Otorhinolaryngology and Head and Neck Surgery
University Hospital
Nottingham, UK

Stewart G Martin BSc (Hons) MSc PhD
Associate Professor of Oncology
MSc Course Director and Head of Translational Radiation
Biology Research Group
University of Nottingham
Nottingham, UK

Robert C Mason BSc ChM MD FRCS
Consultant Upper GI Surgeon
Guy's and St Thomas' Hospitals
London, UK

† Deceased

Lesley Mathieson FRCSLT
Visiting Lecturer in Voice Pathology
The Ear Institute
University College London; and
Honorary Research Adviser
Speech and Language Therapy Department
Royal National Throat Nose and Ear Hospital
London, UK

Paul M Matthews MA (Oxon) MD DPhil FRCP
Vice-President for Imaging Genetics and for Neurology; and
Head, GSK Clinical Imaging Center
Clinical Pharmacology and Discovery Medicine GlaxoSmithKline;
and Professor of Clinical Neurosciences
Department of Clinical Neurosciences
Imperial College, London; and
(Hon.) MRC Clinical Research Professor
Department of Clinical Neurology
University of Oxford
Oxford, UK

Paul May MBBS FRCS FRCPCH
Consultant Paediatric Neurosurgeon
Craniofacial Unit, Alder Hey Children's Hospital
Liverpool, UK

Thomas McCaffrey MD PhD
Professor and Chair
Department of Otolaryngology Head and Neck Surgery
University of South Florida
Tampa, FL, USA

Leo McClymont MBChB MD FRCSEd FRCSGlas
Raigmore Hospital
Highland Acute Hospitals NHS Trust Inverness
Inverness, UK

Andrew McCombe MD FRCS (ORL)
Consultant ENT Surgeon
Frimley Park Hospital
Camberley, UK

Gerald W McGarry MD FRCS (RCPSGlasg) FRCS(Ed) FRCS (ORL-HNS)
Consultant Otorhinolaryngologist
Glasgow Royal Infirmary; and
Honorary Senior Lecturer
University of Glasgow
Glasgow, UK

Julian A McGlashan MBBS FRCS (ORL)
Special Lecturer and Consultant
Department of Otorhinolaryngology
Queen's Medical Centre Campus
Nottingham University Hospitals
Nottingham, UK

Mark McGurk MD BDS FRCS FDSRCS DLO
Consultant in Oral and Maxillofacial Surgery
Guy's Hospital
London, UK

Stephen McHanwell BSC PhD MIBiol CBiol
Professor of Anatomical Sciences; and
National Teaching Fellow 2007; and
Director of Stage 1 & 2 BDS
School of Dental Sciences
Dental School
Newcastle upon Tyne, UK

Michael J McKenna MD
Professor, Department of Otology and Laryngology
Harvard Medical School; and
Surgeon, Department of Otolaryngology
Massachusetts Eye and Ear Infirmary
Boston, MA, USA

William S McKerrow MB ChB MRCGP (exam) FRCSEd & Glasg
Consultant Otolaryngologist
Department of ENT/Head and Neck Surgery
Raigmore Hospital
Inverness, UK

Siobhan McMahon BSc MRCSLT
Speech and Language Therapy
Department Alder Hey Hospital
Liverpool, UK

Brent A McMonagle MBBS FRACS
Department of Otolaryngology
Guy's Hospital
London, UK

Hisham Mehanna BmedSc (Hons) MBChB (Hons) FRCS (ORL-HNS)
Consultant ENT – Head and Neck and Thyroid Surgeon; and
Honorary Senior Lecturer
University Hospitals Coventry and Warwickshire
Walsgrave Hospital
Coventry, UK

Saumil N Merchant MD
Gudrun Larsen Eliasen and Nels Kristian Eliasen
Professor of Otology and Laryngology
Harvard Medical School; and
Surgeon in Otolaryngology and
Director of Otopathology Laboratory
Department of Otolaryngology
Massachusetts Eye and Ear Infirmary
Boston; and
Affiliate Faculty Member
Harvard University-Massachusetts Institute of Technology
Division of Health Sciences and Technology
Cambridge, MA, USA

David Miles FRCP MD
Consultant in Medical Oncology
Mount Vernon Cancer Centre
Middlesex, UK

Christopher A Milford FRCS
Consultant Otolaryngologist
Oxford Skull Base Unit
John Radcliffe Hospital
Oxford, UK

Robert Mills MS MPhil FRCS (Eng) FRCS (Ed)
Otolaryngology Unit
University of Edinburgh
Royal Infirmary of Edinburgh
Edinburgh, UK

Steven Ross Mobley MD
Director of Facial Plastic and Reconstructive Surgery
Division of Otolaryngology-HNS
University of Utah School of Medicine
Salt Lake City, UT, USA

David Moffat BSc MA FRCS
Consultant Neuro-Otologist
Department of Otoneurotological and Skull Base Surgery
Addenbrookes
Cambridge University Teaching Hospital NHS Foundation Trust;
and Associate Lecturer, Cambridge University
Cambridge, UK

Brian CJ Moore MA PhD FMedSci FRS
Professor of Auditory Perception
Department of Experimental Psychology
University of Cambridge
Cambridge, UK

David AL Morgan FRCR
Consultant Clinical Oncologist
Department of Clinical Oncology
Nottingham University Hospitals
Nottingham, UK

Jonathan M Morgan MD
Instructor
Department of Otolaryngology Head and Neck Surgery
University of South Florida
Tampa, FL, USA

Juliette Morgan MD
Division of Foodborne Bacterial and Mycotic Diseases
National Center for Zoonotic, Vector-Borne and Enteric Diseases
Centers for Disease Control and Prevention
Atlanta, GA, USA

Gavin AJ Morrison MA MBBS FRCS
Consultant ENT Surgeon
Guy's, St Thomas' and Evelina Hospitals
London, UK

Randall P Morton MB MSc FRACS
Professor of Otolaryngology
University of Auckland; and
Consultant Otolaryngologist–Head and Neck Surgeon
Counties Manukau and Auckland District Health Boards
Auckland, New Zealand

Frank E Musiek PhD
Professor and Director of Auditory Research
Department of Communication Sciences; and
Professor of Otolaryngology
School of Medicine University of Connecticut
Storrs, CT, USA

Niels Mygind MD
Formerly Consultant in Lung Medicine
Department of Respiratory Medicine
University Hospital of Aarhus
Aarhus, Denmark

Karl G Nicholson MBBS MRCS FRCP
Professor of Infectious Diseases
Department of Infectious Diseases and Tropical Medicine
Leicester Royal Infirmary
Leicester, UK

Andrew J Nicol MBChB, FCS (SA)
Associate Professor
General Surgery; and
Head of Trauma Unit
Groote Schuur Hospital
Cape Town, South Africa

Gilbert J Nolst Trenité MD PhD
Professor of Otorhinolaryngology
Academic Medical Center
University of Amsterdam
The Netherlands

Desmond A Nunez FRCS (ORL) MD
Director, Department of Otolaryngology
North Bristol NHS Trust; and
Honorary Senior Lecturer
University of Bristol
Bristol, UK

Michael O'Connell BSc, MPhil, FRCS
Consultant Otorhinolaryngologist,
Facial Plastic Surgeon and Honorary Senior Lecturer
Brighton and Sussex University Hospitals NHS Trust
Brighton, UK

Alec Fitzgerald O'Connor FRCS
Consultant Otolaryngologist
St Thomas Hospital
London, UK

Paul O'Flynn FRCS
Consultant ENT/Head and Neck Surgeon
University College Hospitals; and
Honorary Consultant
The Royal National Throat, Nose and Ear Hospital
London, UK

Stephen O'Leary MB BS BMedSc PhD FRACS
The Department of Otolaryngology
Royal Victorian Eye and Ear Hospital
East Melbourne, Australia

Morten Osterballe MD
Allergy Center, Odense University Hospital
Odense, Denmark

Peter O'Sullivan Bsc MPhil FRCSI (ORL–HNS)
Clinical Fellow, Neurotology
Department of Otolaryngology
Sir Charles Gairdner Hospital
Nedlands, Western Australia

William J Owen† MS FRCS
Formerly Oesophageal Investigation Unit
Department of Surgery, St Thomas' Hospital
London, UK

Jaideep J Pandit MA BM DPhil FRCA
Consultant Anaesthetist
Nuffield Department of Anaesthetics
University of Oxford
Oxford, UK

Andrew J Parker MBChB (hons) DLO ChM FRCS
Consultant ENT Surgeon
Department of Otolaryngology
Royal Hallamshire Hospital
Sheffield, UK

Glynnis Parker MB ChB FRCP DCH MSc
Audiovestibular Physician
Sheffield Children's Hospital
Sheffield, UK

Nimesh Patel MBChB FRCS FRCS (ORL–HNS)
Consultant Otolaryngologist
Southampton General Hospital
Liverpool, UK

John P Patten BSc MB FRCP
Consultant Neurologist (retired)
South West Thames Regional Health Authority
London, UK

Henry Pau MD MBChB FRCSEd FRCS Ed (ORL–HNS) FRCS
Consultant Otorhinolaryngologist; and
Honorary Senior Lecturer
University Hospitals of Leicester
Leicester, UK

Santdeep H Paun FRCS (ORL–HNS)
Consultant Nasal and Facial Plastic Surgeon
St Bartholomew's Hospital
London, UK

Sarah Payne BSc (Hons) MRCP
SpR in Medical Oncology
Centre for Tumour Biology
Institute of Cancer and the CR-UK Clinical Centre
Barts and the London
Queen Mary's School of Medicine and Dentistry
London, UK

Adrian Pearce FRCA
Consultant Anaesthetist
Department of Anaesthesia
Guy's and St Thomas' Hospital
London, UK

Ken Pearman FRCS
Consultant Paediatric Otolaryngologist
Children's Hospital
Birmingham, UK

Chris Penfold FDSRCS FRCS
Consultant Oral and Maxillofacial Surgeon
Alder Hey Childen's Hospital
Liverpool, UK

A Graeme B Perks FRCS FRCS (Plast) FRACS
Consultant Plastic Surgeon
The City Hospital
Nottingham, UK

Alison Perry PhD FRCSLT
Chair, School of Human Communication Sciences
Faculty of Health Sciences
La Trobe University
Melbourne, Australia

James O Pickles MA MSc PhD DSc
Head of Hearing Unit
Vision, Touch and Hearing Research Centre
Department of Physiology and Pharmacology
University of Queensland
Brisbane, Australia

Lisa Pitkin BSc MSc FRCS ORL–HNS
Specialist Registrar in Otolaryngology
South (West) Thames Otolaryngology Training Region
Royal Marsden NHS Foundation Trust
London, UK

Laysan Pope BSc MB BS MRCS
Specialist Registrar in Otolaryngology, Head and Neck Surgery
John Radcliffe Hospital
Oxford, UK

Stephen R Porter BSc MD PhD FDS RCS FDS RCSE
Professor of Oral Medicine
UCL Eastman Dental Institute
London, UK

Richard J Powell MBBS DM FRCP FRCPath
Consultant and Professor in Clinical Immunology
University of Nottingham
Nottingham, UK

Paul Pracy BSc MBBS FRCS (Glas) FRCS (ORL–HNS)
Consultant Head and Neck Surgeon
Department of Otorhinolaryngology/Head and Neck Surgery
Queen Elizabeth Hospital
University Hospital Birmingham NHS Trust
Birmingham, UK

† Deceased

Hillel Pratt PhD
Evoked Potentials Laboratory
Technion – Israel Institute of Technology
Haifa, Israel

Tim Price Bsc MBChB MRCS DLO FRCS (ORL-HNS)
Consultant Otolaryngologist, Head and Neck Surgeon
Dorset County Hospital
Dorchester, UK

William J Primrose MB FRCS
Consultant Otolarnyngologist/Head and Neck Surgeon
Royal Victoria Hospital, Belfast
Northern Ireland, UK

Matthias Radatz MD FRCS
The National Centre for Stereotactic Radiosurgery
Royal Hallamshire Hospital
Sheffield, UK

Ullas Raghavan FRCS (ORL-HNS)
Consultant Ear Nose and Throat and Facial Plastic Surgeon
Doncaster Royal Infirmary
Doncaster, UK

Gunesh P Rajan MD FMH (Ch) FRACS
Senior Lecturer of Otolaryngology, Head and Neck Surgery
Department of Otolaryngology, Head and Neck Surgery
University of Western Australia
Fremantle, Australia

James Ramsden PhD FRCS
Specialist Registrar in Otolaryngology/Head and Neck Surgery
John Radcliffe Hospital
Oxford, UK

Richard Ramsden FRCS
Manchester Royal Infirmary
Manchester, UK

Sheila C Rankin FRCR
Consultant Radiologist
Guy's and St Thomas' Hospital NHS Trust
London, UK

Helge Rask-Andersen MD PhD
Professor in Experimental Otology
Department of Otolaryngology
Uppsala University Hospital
Uppsala, Sweden

Peter Rea MA FRCS (Eng) FRCS (ORL-HNS)
Consultant Otolaryngologist
Leicester Royal Infirmary
Leicester, UK

Fiona Regan MBBS FRCP FRCPath
Consultant Haematologist
Department of Haematology
Imperial College School of Medicine; and
Honorary Senior Lecturer and Consultant Haematologist
National Blood Service
London, UK

Claud Regnard FRCP (Lon)
Consultant in Palliative Care Medicine
St. Oswald's Hospice, Newcastle-upon-Tyne; and
Freeman Hospital (Newcastle Hospitals NHS Trust)
Newcastle-upon-Tyne and
Northumberland Tyne and Wear NHS Trust
Northumberland, UK

Evan Reid BSc MB ChB PhD FRCP
Wellcome Trust Senior Research Fellow in Clinical Science; and
Honorary Consultant in Medical Genetics
Department of Medical Genetics and
Cambridge Institute for Medical Research
Addenbrooke's Campus, University of Cambridge
Cambridge, UK

Gerhard Rettinger Prof Dr Med
Head ENT-University-Department
Ulm, Germany

David Richardson FRCS FDSRCS
Consultant Maxillofacial Surgeon
Supra Regional Paediatric Craniofacial Unit
Royal Liverpool Childrens Hospital; and
Maxillofacial Unit
University Hospital Aintree
Liverpool, UK

Peter J Robb BSc (Hons) MB BS FRCS FRCSEd
Epsom and St Helier University Hospitals NHS Trust
Surrey, UK

David Roberts FRCS
St Thomas and Guy's Hospital NHS Trust
London, UK

Philip J Robinson MB ChB FRCS FRCS (Otolaryngology)
Consultant Otolaryngologist
ENT Department, Southmead Hospital
Bristol, UK

Nicholas J Roland MBChB MD FRCS
Consultant ENT/Head and Neck Surgeon
University Hospital Aintree
Liverpool, UK

Geoffrey E Rose DSc MS MRCP FRCS FRCOphth
Consultant Orbital Surgeon
Moorfields Eye Hospital
London, UK

Rob Ross Russell MD FRCPCH
Consultant in Paediatric Intensive Care and Respiratory Medicine
Addenbrooke's Hospital
Cambridge, UK

Mike Rothera MBBS FRCS
Consultant Paediatric ENT Surgeon
Royal Manchester Childrens' Hospital
Manchester, UK

Jeremy Rowe MA DM FRCS (SN)
The National Centre for Stereotactic Radiosurgery
Royal Hallamshire Hospital
Sheffield, UK

Julian Rowe-Jones MB BS FRCS (ORL)
Consultant Rhinologist and Nasal Plastic Surgeon
Department of Otorhinolaryngology – Head and Neck/
Facial Plastic Surgery
Royal Surrey County Hospital
Guildford, UK

Claudia Rudack PD Dr Med
ENT-University-Department
Münster, Germany

Michael J Rutter FRACS
Division of Pediatric Otolaryngology/Head and Neck Surgery,
Cincinnati Children's Hospital Medical Center; and
Associate Professor of Pediatric Otolaryngology
Department of Otolaryngology, Head and Neck Surgery
University of Cincinnati College of Medicine
Cincinnati, OH, USA

Shakeel R Saeed MBBS (Lon) FRCS (Ed) FRCS (Eng) FRCS (Orl) MD (Man)
Consultant ENT and Skull Base Surgeon
University Department of Otolaryngology–
Head and Neck Surgery
Manchester Royal Infirmary and Hope Hospital
Manchester, UK

Hesham Saleh MBBCh FRCS FRCS (ORL-HNS)
Consultant Rhinologist/Facial Plastic Surgeon
Charing Cross Hospital and the Royal Brompton Hospital; and
Honorary Senior Lecturer
Imperial College of Medicine
London, UK

Robert J Sanderson† MB ChB FRCS (Ed) FRCS (Eng) FRCS (ORL-HNS)
Formerly Consultant Otolaryngologist/Head and Neck Surgeon
Western General Hospital
Edinburg, UK

Keshthra Satchithananda BDS FDSRCS MB BS FRCS FRCR
Consultant Radiodogist
Department of Radiology
Charing Cross Hospital
London, UK

Michael Saunders MD FRCS
Consultant Otolaryngologist
Department of Otorhinolaryngology, Head and Neck Surgery
St Michael's Hospital
Bristol, UK

Glenis Scadding MA MD FRCP
Consultant Immunologist, Rhinologist and Allergy Specialist
Royal National Throat Nose and Ear Hospital
London, UK

Jochen Schacht PhD
Professor and Director
Kresge Hearing Research Institute
Department of Otolaryngology
University of Michigan
Ann Arbor, MI, USA

Rodney J Schlosser MD
Department of Otolaryngology
Medical University of South Carolina
Charleston, SC, USA

Stephan Schmid MD
Professor of Otolaryngology
Department of Otorhinolaryngology, Head and Neck Surgery
Universitatsspital Zurich
Zurich, Switzerland

Colin A Scotchford PhD
Associate Professor
School of Mechanical, Materials and Manufacturing Engineering
University of Nottingham
Nottingham, UK

Andrew Scott FRCS (ORL-HNS) MPhil
The Royal Shrewsbury Hospital
Shrewsbury, UK

Crispian Scully CBE MD PhD MDS MRCS FDSRCS FDSRCPS FFDRCSI FDSRCSE FRCPath FMedSci DSc
Professor of Oral Medicine, Pathology and Microbiology
University of London; and
Professor of Special Care Dentistry
UCL-Eastman Dental Institute
London, UK

Su-Hua Sha MD
Research Investigator
Kresge Hearing Research Institute
Department of Otolaryngology
University of Michigan
Ann Arbor, MI, USA

Naomi Sibtain MBBS MRCP FRCR
Consultant Neuroradiologist
King's College Hospital
London, UK

Paul S Sidhu BSc MB BS MRCP FRCR DTM&H
Senior Lecturer and Consultant Radiologist
Department of Radiology
King's College Hospital
London, UK

Richard Sim MD FRCS (Oro)
Department of Ear, Nose and Throat
Royal United Hospital
Bath, UK

Paul Simons MBBS BSc MRCP MRCGP DCH DRCOG DFFP
Marcham Road Health Centre
Abingdon, UK

Robert Slack BSc MB ChB FRCS (Ed) FRCS (Eng)
Department of Ear, Nose and Throat
Royal United Hospital
Bath, UK

Wendy Smith BPharm MBBS DLO FRCS (ORL-HNS)
Locum Consultant Otorhinolaryngology
The Leeds Teaching Hospitals NHS Trust
Leeds, UK

Lewis Spitz PhD FRCS
Institute of Child Health (University College London) and
Great Ormond Street Hospital for Children
London, UK

Jacob Bertram Springborg MD PhD
University Clinic of Neurosurgery
The Neuroscience Centre
Copenhagen University Hospital
Copenhagen, Denmark

Nicholas D Stafford MB FRCS
Director, Postgraduate Medical Institute
University of Hull
Hull, UK

H Stammberger MD Hon FRCS (Ed) Hon FRCS (Engl)
Professor and Head
Department of General ORL, H & NS
Medical University
Graz, Austria

Michael Stearns BDS MB BS FRCS
The Royal Free Hospital
London, UK

Karen P Steel Phd FMedSci
The Wellcome Trust Sanger Institute
Hinxton, UK

Paul Stewart FRCP
Department of Medicine
Queen Elizabeth Hospital
Birmingham, UK

Iain RC Swan MB ChB MD FRCS (Ed)
Department of Otolaryngology
North Glasgow University NHS Trust
Glasgow, UK

Elizabeth Sweeney FRCP DRGOC MD
Consultant Clinical Geneticist
Craniofacial Unit
Alder Hey Children's Hospital
Liverpool, UK

Andrew C Swift ChM FRCS FRCS (Ed)
Consultant in Otorhinolaryngology
University Hospital Aintree
Liverpool, UK

Andra E Talaska BS
Kresge Hearing Research Institute
Department of Otolaryngology
University of Michigan
Ann Arbor, MI, USA

Thomas A Tami MD
Professor of Otolaryngology
Department of Otolaryngology
University of Cincinnati College of Medicine
Cincinnati, OH, USA

Rinze A Tange MD PhD UHD
Associate Professor of Otology
Department of ORL, Head and Neck Surgery
Academic Medical Centre
University of Amsterdam
Amsterdam, The Netherlands

A Thakar MS FRCS
Associate Professor of Otolaryngology and Head/Neck Surgery
All India Institute of Medical Sciences
New Delhi, India

J Regan Thomas MD
Francis L. Lederer Professor and Head
University of Illinois at Chicago
Department of Otolaryngology – Head and Neck Surgery
Chicago, IL, USA

Jens Thomsen MD DMSc FRCS
Professor of Otolaryngology
Department of Otorhinolaryngology, Head and Neck Surgery
Gentofte Hospital, University of Copenhagen
Hellerup, Denmark

Matthew J Thurtell MSc (Med) MBBS FRACP
Neuro-Opthalmology Fellow
Department of Neurology
University Hospitals of Cleveland
Cleveland, OH, USA

Bo Tideholm MD PhD
ENT Specialist
Department of Otorhinolaryngology
University Hospital
Malmö, Sweden

Paul Tierney BA BM BCh (Oxon) FRCS (Eng.) FRCS (ORL-HNS)
Consultant Otolaryngologist – Head and Neck Surgeon
North Bristol NHS Trust; and
Honorary Senior Lecturer
Bristol University
Bristol, UK

Ian Todd PhD
Associate Professor and Reader in Cellular Immunopathology
University of Nottingham
Nottingham, UK

Joseph G Toner MB MA FRCS
Consultant/Honorary Senior Lecturer, Otolaryngology
Belfast HSC Trust
Queens University
Belfast, UK

Michael Chi Fai Tong MBChB (CUHK) MD (CUHK) FRCS (Ed) FHKAM (ORL)
Professor and Head of Academic Divisions
Department of Otorhinolaryngology, Head and Neck Surgery
The Chinese University of Hong Kong
Hong Kong

Dean M Toriumi MD
Division of Facial Plastic and Reconstructive Surgery
Department of Otolaryngology – Head and Neck Surgery
University of Illinois at Chicago
Chicago, IL, USA

Mirko Tos Prof MD DMSc Dr Hc
Emeritus Professor, Ear, Nose and Throat Department
Gentofte Hospital
University of Copenhagen
Hellerup, Denmark; and
Professor of Otolaryngology
University of Maribor
Maribor, Slovenia

Stephen C Toynton MB FRCS (ORL)
Consultant Otorhinolaryngologist
Derriford Hospital, Plymouth Hospitals NHS Trust; and
Otology Advisor to Diving Diseases Research Centre and
Hyperbaric Medical Unit
Plymouth, UK

Kai Uus MD PhD
Lecturer in Audiology
School of Psychological Sciences
Faculty of Medical and Human Sciences
University of Manchester
Manchester, UK

Peter Valentine BSc FRCS (ORL-HNS)
Consultant Otologist and ENT Surgeon
Royal Surrey County Hospital NHS Trust
Guildford; and
Ashford and St Peter's Hospitals NHS Trust
Chertsey, UK

Jan HP van der Meulen PhD FFPH
Reader in Clinical Epidemiology
Health Services Research Unit
London School of Hygiene and Tropical Medicine
London, UK

C Andrew van Hasselt MBChB FRCS FRCS (Edin) FCS (SA)
Chairman, Department of Surgery; and
Professor of Surgery (Otorhinolaryngology)
Department of Otorhinolaryngology, Head and Neck Surgery
The Chinese University of Hong Kong
Shatin, Hong Kong

Adriaan F van Olphen MD PhD
ENT Surgeon
University Medical Centre Utrecht
Utrecht, The Netherlands

Archana Vats MA (Cantab) FRCS (Eng) FRCS (Oto) PhD
Imperial College and St. Mary's NHS Trust
London, UK

Antonio M Vignola†
Formerly of Istituto di Fisiopatologia Respiratoria
Università Palermo
Palermo, Italy

Alexander C Vlantis MBBCh FCS (SA) FCSHK
Associate Professor
Department of Otorhinolaryngology, Head and Neck Surgery
The Chinese University of Hong Kong
Shatin, Hong Kong

Sherryl Wagstaff FRACS
Consultant Otologist
Royal Victorian Eye and Ear Hospital
Melbourne University Teaching Hospital
East Melbourne, Australia

Debbie Wall BEd (Hons) MA
Senior Researcher
NHS Clinical Governance Support Team
Leicester, UK

David Ward MBBS FRCS FRCS (Ed)
Consultant Plastic Surgeon
Leicester Royal Infirmary
Leicester, UK

David W Warnock PhD FRCPath
Division of Foodborne Bacterial and Mycotic Diseases
National Center for Zoonotic, Vector-Borne and Enteric Diseases
Centers for Disease Control and Prevention
Atlanta, GA, USA

Katherine Wasson BA PhD MPH
Chief, Clinical Ethics Service; and
Assistant Professor, Critical Care
The University of Texas M.D. Andersson Cancer Center
Houston, Texas, USA

John C Watkinson MSc MS FRCS (Ed, Glas, Lond) DLO
Consultant Head and Neck and Thyroid Surgeon
Department of Otorhinolaryngology/Head and Neck Surgery
Queen Elizabeth Hospital
University of Birmingham NHS Trust
Birmingham, UK

† Deceased

Desmond Watson BM BCh MA FRCS
Former Consultant Ear Nose and Throat Surgeon and Advisor
Medical Protection Society
Leeds, UK

Keith Webster MMedSci FRCS FRCS (OMFS) FDSRCS
Consultant Oral and Maxillofacial Surgeon
University Hospital Birmingham NHS Foundation Trust; and
Honorary Senior Lecturer
Faculty of Dentistry and Medicine
University of Birmingham
Birmingham, UK

Vivienne Weston MBBS FRCP MSc FRCPath
Consultant Medical Microbiologist
Nottingham University Hospitals NHS Trust
Nottingham, UK

Richard Wight MB BS FRCS Eng (Otol) FRCS Ed (Otol)
Consultant Head and Neck Surgeon
James Cook University Hospital
Middlesbrough, UK

Janet A Wilson BSc MD FRCSEd FRCS Eng
Professor of Otolaryngology, Head and Neck Surgery
Newcastle University Freeman Hospital
Newcastle Upon Tyne, UK

Wai Lup Wong BA (Hons) MRCP FRCR
Paul Strickland Scanner Centre
Mount Vernon Hospital
Northwood, UK

John Kong Sang Woo MBBS FCSHK FRCSEd FHKAM (Otorhinolaryngology)
Consultant, Department of ENT, Prince of Wales Hospital; and
Chief of Service in ENT
New Territories East Cluster, Hospital Authority; and
Honorary Clinical Associate Professor
Department of Otorhinolaryngology, Head and Neck Surgery
The Chinese University of Hong Kong
Hong Kong

Tim J Woolford MD FRCS (ORL)
Consultant in Otorhinolaryngology
Manchester Royal Infirmary
University of Manchester
Manchester, UK

Peter-John Wormald MD FRACS FRCS (Ed) FCS (SA) MBChB
Department of Otolarnyngology, Head and Neck Surgery
Adelaide and Flinders Universities
Adelaide, Australia

Steve Worrollo FIMPT
Consultant Maxillofacial Prosthetist
Department of Maxillofacial Surgery
University Hospital Birmingham NHS Trust
Birmingham, UK

Neville Wright DMRD FRCR
Consultant Paediatric Radiologist
Central Manchester and
Manchester Children's Hospitals NHS Trust
Department of Radiology
Royal Manchester Children's Hospital
Manchester, UK

Tony Wright LLM DM FRCS Tech RMS
Professor of Otolaryngology
UCL Ear Institute
London, UK

Floris L Wuyts PhD
Professor of Medical Physics
University of Antwerp; and
Head of AUREA (Antwerp University Research Centre for
Equilibrium and Aerospace)
Department of ENT
University Hospital of Antwerp
Antwerp, Belgium

Michelle Wyatt MA FRCS (ORL-HNS)
Consultant Paediatric Otolaryngologist
Great Ormond Street Hospital
London, UK

Clare Wykes BSc MRCP DipRCPath
Haematology SpR
Hammersmith Hospitals NHS Trust
London, UK

Stephen R Young BSc (Hons) PhD
Faculty of Science
The American International University in London
Surrey, UK

Preface

Fifty-five years have passed since the first edition of *Scott-Brown's Otorhinolaryngology: Head and Neck Surgery* was published. Many otorhinolaryngologists have read at least one edition, committed it to memory and passed their specialist examinations because of it. All will have kept referring to it throughout their careers and remember it with affection. Looking back it is apparent that a radical change in structure and format has taken place every 15 to 20 years. It is 20 years since Alan Kerr made the last radical change with the publication of the 5th edition, 20 years that have seen an information technology explosion. The internet, on-line libraries, e-delivery of journals and increasingly books, computerised search engines, CD-ROMs, DVDs, digital photography; the list goes on. These technological advances have transformed medical education, influenced significantly the way the current generation learns and the methods by which their competencies and knowledge are assessed. Certainly sufficient time has elapsed for *Scott-Brown* to evolve dramatically once more. This edition has been completely re-written. It bears little resemblance to its predecessors other than by title, and in its philosophy to provide a complete resume of the knowledge base that underpins modern ORL practice and which will guide clinicians in their everyday patient care for years to come. The number of chapters has almost doubled, with large topics dissected into more digestible parts. This reflects the expansion of our specialty such that it is now a group of subspecialties linked by the common thread, each concerned with, and committed to, the care of patients with disorders of the head and neck.

Our authors are the leading experts in their respective fields of interest and have been selected from all over the world. Almost all the text is illustrated in colour and it comes with its own CD-ROM, containing all the text and illustrations in an accessible and searchable form, with references linked to PubMed.

So what else could the trainee or practising otorhinolaryngologist want from the definitive reference to the field at the beginning of the new millennium? Quite simply, the level of evidence for the advice we offer and the practice we undertake. Nowadays specialties need to define best clinical practice, if only to guide and remind health care providers of their duty to their patients to practice in accordance with accepted evidence and to strive for excellence in clinical standards at all times. Surgeons also need to know how their actions might be viewed by the courts and the areas of practice that are currently exercising the legal profession. This edition has tried to provide that information.

It has not been an easy task for our contributors, some of whom were not writing in their mother tongue. That they were able to write to a structured format was much to their credit. I was fortunate to recruit, and am extremely grateful to, my team of section editors all of whom worked tirelessly with a common purpose. George G Browning, Martin J Burton, Ray Clarke, John Hibbert, Nicholas S Jones, Valerie J Lund, Linda M Luxon and John C Watkinson represent some of the very best and most respected clinicians in the United Kingdom, each one an international authority, each one with a heavy professional commitment. Alan Kerr's advice and encouragement throughout was always welcome and extremely useful. Marcelle McNamara came to my aid and assistance numerous times during the project. She gave tirelessly of her time and energy during a very serious illness, writing chapters and putting others into format and a more readable form. She was an example and inspiration throughout.

The creation of this edition has also been an interesting experience for the publishing staff. During a lengthy period of gestation, this text has changed ownership several times as the publishing houses traded and re-aligned their lists. Without the drive and perseverance of Zelah Pengilley and Jo Koster from Hodder Education it would surely have fallen by the wayside. Words cannot express my gratitude to them adequately. Understanding when clinical work overwhelmed me, they hid their frustrations over slow progress or irritatingly incomplete manuscripts. They buoyed us all up when the end seemed so far away.

Sadly, some of our contributors will never see their chapters in print as they have died during the preparation of this text. Some had long, unpleasant illnesses but wrote despite them. Others were cut down unexpectedly in their prime but have now left a legacy, and a few were my close friends and colleagues. I am proud to have my name linked permanently through this publication with Michael Baser, Roderick Cawson, Susanna Leighton,

William Owen, Robert Sanderson and Antonio Vignola. We hope that their families will draw some comfort also by seeing their loved ones live on in this book.

Finally, there are four very special people whose constant love and affection drives me on through life. They are of course my wife, Ann, and our children, Andrew, Clare and Mark. They too will breathe a deep sigh of relief with the publication of this text and I thank them with all my heart.

Michael Gleeson
September 2007

How to use this book

This new edition of *Scott-Brown's Otorhinolaryngology, Head and Neck Surgery* incorporates some special features to aid the readers' understanding and navigation of the text. These are described below.

SEARCH STRATEGY

The majority of the chapters feature a search strategy indicating the key words used by the author when conducting their literature review in order to prepare the chapter, so that the reader can repeat and develop the search.

EVIDENCE SCORING

For the major sections in each chapter, the authors have used a hierarchical system to indicate the level of evidence supporting their statements. This is shown in the text in the form [***], with the number of stars indicating the level of evidence. The key to this system is shown in the table below.

Level	Category of evidence
****	Systematic reviews, meta-analyses of randomized controlled trials and randomized controlled trials
***	Non-randomised studies
**	Observational or non-experimental studies
*	Expert opinion

Where no level is shown, the quality of supporting evidence, if any exists, is of low grade only (for example, case reports, clinical experience etc.). For more information on evidence scoring, please refer to Chapter 304, Evidence-based medicine; and 305 Critical appraisal skills.

CLINICAL RECOMMENDATIONS

The authors have indicated the basis on which they have made clinical recommendations by grading them according to the level of the supporting evidence. This is shown in the text in the form [Grade A], with the grade indicating the level of evidence supporting the recommendation. The key to this system is shown in the table below.

Grade	Nature of supporting evidence
A	Recommendation based on evidence from meta-analyses of randomized controlled trails
B	Recommendation based on evidence from high quality case-controlled or cohort studies
C	Recommendation based on evidence from low quality case-controlled or cohort studies
D	Recommendation based on evidence from clinical series or expert opinion

Recommendations are graded where the author is satisfied that the literature supports such a grading; otherwise a grading may not be given.

REFERENCE ANNOTATION

The reference lists are annotated with an asterisk, where appropriate, to guide readers to key primary papers and major review articles. We hope that this feature will render the lists of references more useful to the reader and will encourage self-directed learning among both trainees and practicing physicians.

Abbreviations

2,3DPG	2,3-diphosphoglycerate
2D	two-dimensional
3,4-DAP	3,4-diaminopyridine
3D	three-dimensional
5-FdUMP	5-fluoro-2 deoxyuridine monophophate
5-FU	5-fluorouracil
5-FUMP	5-fluorouridine monophosphate
5-HT	5-hydroxytryptamine
6MP	6-Mercaptopurine
18-FDG	2-18-fluoro-2-deoxy-D-glucose
A	adenine; or anterior
AABR	automated auditory brainstem response
AAHL	age-associated hearing loss
AAOHNS	American Academy of Otolaryngologists/ Head and Neck Surgeons
AAV	adeno-associated virus
ABC	aspiration biopsy cytology
ABEP	auditory nerve and brainstem evoked potential
ABG	air–bone gap
ABI	auditory brainstem implant
ABLB	alternate binaural loudness balance
ABPA	allergic bronchopulmonary aspergillosis
ABR	auditory brainstem response; or acoustic brainstem evoked response
ABRS	acute bacterial rhinosinusitis
AC	air conduction; or alternating coupled
ACC	adenoid cystic carcinoma; or American College of Cardiology
ACE	angiotensin-converting enzyme
ACF	anterior cranial fossa
ACh	Acetylcholine
AchR	acetyl choline receptor
ACT	Aid for Children with Tracheostomies
ACTH	adrenocorticotropic hormone
A/D	analogue-to-digital
AD	Alzheimer's disease
ADA	adenosine deaminase
ADAM-33	A disintegrin and metalloprotease 33κ
ADCC	antibody-dependent cellular cytotoxicity
ADH	antidiuretic hormone
ADHD	attention deficit hyperactivity disorder
ADR	adverse drug reaction

Ad-VEGF	adenovirus-encoding vascular endothelial growth factor
AECRS	acute exacerbation of chronic rhinosinusitis
AED	aerodynamic equivalent diameter
AEDS	atopic eczema dermatitis syndrome
AEF	auditory-evoked cortical magnetic field
AF	atrial fibrillation; or anterior fontanelle
AFB	acid-fast bacilli
AFRS	allergic fungal rhinosinusitis
AgNOR	silver staining nucleolar organizer region
AHA	American Heart Association
AHCPR	Agency for Health Care Policy and Research (USA)
AHI	apnoea/hypopnoea index
AI	apoptotic index
AICA	anterior inferior cerebellar artery
AIDS	acquired immunodeficiency syndrome
AIRE	autoimmune regulator gene
AJCC	American Joint Committee on Cancer
ALD	assistive listening device
ALEP	auditory long-latency (or late) evoked potential
ALL	acute lymphoblastic leukaemia
$\alpha2\beta2$	two α and two β globin chains
$\alpha2\delta2$	HbA2
$\alpha2\gamma2$	foetal haemoglobin
ALPS	autoimmune lymphoproliferative syndrome
ALS	amyotrophic lateral sclerosis
ALT	alternative lengthening of telomere; or alternating chemoradiotherapy
ALTB	acute laryngotracheobronchitis
ALTE	apparent life-threatening event
AML	acute myeloid leukaemia
AN	acoustic neuroma; or auditory neuropathy; or audiovestibular nerve
ANA	anti-nuclear antibody
AN/AD	auditory neuropathy/auditory dyssynchrony
ANCA	antineutrophil cytoplasmic antibody
AND	allow a natural death
ANUG	acute necrotizing ulcerative gingivitis
AOAE	automated otoacoustic emission
AoCD	anaemia of chronic disease
AOM	acute otitis media

AON	anterior olfactory nucleus	
AP	anterior–posterior; or action potential	
APB	ALT-associated promyelocytic leukaemia body	
APC	antigen presenting cell; or activated protein C; or argon plasma coagulation; or adenomatous polyposis coli	
APD	auditory processing disorder	
APECED	autoimmune polyendocrinopathy–candidiasis–ectodermal dystrophy	
APHAB	Abbreviated Profile of Hearing Aid Benefit	
APL	anti-phospholipid	
APMET	aggressive papillary middle ear tumour	
APQ	amplitude perturbation quotient	
APTT	activated partial thromboplastin time	
APUD	amine precursor uptake and decarboxylation	
ARF	acute renal failure	
ARIA	allergic rhinitis and its impact on asthma	
ARR	absolute risk reduction	
ARS	acute rhinosinusitis	
ART	advanced rotating tomograph; or antiretroviral therapy	
ARTA	age-related typical audiogram	
ASA	aspirin-induced asthma; or aspirin-sensitive asthma; or American Society of Anesthesiologists	
a-SCC	anterior semicircular canal	
ASIC	application specific integrated circuit	
ASL	American sign language; or arterial spin labelling	
ASPO	American Society of Pediatric Otolaryngologists	
ASSR	auditory steady state response	
AST	arterial spin tagging	
AT	ataxia telangiectasia; or auditory therapy or training	
ATD	ascending tract of Deiters	
ATIII	antithrombin III	
ATN	auriculotemporal nerve	
ATP	adenosine triphosphate	
ATRA	all-trans retinoic acid	
AUC	area under the curve	
AV	apical vesicles; or arteriovenous	
AVCN	anteroventral cochlear nuclei	
AVM	arteriovenous malformation	
aVOR	angular VOR	
AZT	3′azido3′deoxythymidone zidovudine; or azothiaprine	
BAC	bacterial artificial chromosome	
BACDA	British Association of Community Doctors in Audiology	
BADS	British Association of Day Surgery	
BAES	British Association of Endocrine Surgeons	
BAHA	bone-anchored hearing aid	

BAHNO	British Association of Head and Neck Oncologists
BAO-HNS	British Association of Otorhinolaryngologists – Head and Neck Surgeons
BAPO	British Association for Paediatric Otolaryngology
BCC	basal cell carcinoma
BCG	Bacillus Calmette–Guérin
BCHA	bone conductor hearing aid
BCSH	British Committee for Standards in Haematology
BDP	beclomethasone dipropionate
BE	bulla ethmoidalis
BF	biofeedback
BFU-E	burst-forming unit erythroid
BiPAP	bilevel positive airway pressure
BIPP	bismuth and iodoform paraffin paste
BL	Burkitt's lymphoma
BMA	British Medical Association
BMI	body mass index
BMP	bone morphogenetic protein; or bone morphogenic protein
BMS	burning mouth syndrome
BMT/SCT	bone marrow stem cell transplantation
BOA	behavioural observation audiometry
BOLD	blood oxygenation level-dependent
BOR	brachio-oto-renal
BP	blood pressure
BPD	bronchopulmonary dysplasia
BPPV	benign positional paroxysmal vertigo
BPV	benign paroxysmal vertigo; or benign positional vertigo
BS	Behçet's syndrome
BSE	bedside swallowing examination; or bovine spongiform encephalopathy
BSL	British sign language
BTE	behind the ear
BVF	bilateral vestibular failure
C	cytosine
CAD	caspase-activated DNase
CADCAM	computer-aided design, computer-aided manufacture
CAGE	cerebral air gas embolism
cAMP	3′,5′-monophosphate
CANS	central auditory nervous system
CAP	compound action potential; or category of auditory performance
CAPD	central auditory processing disorder
CaR	calcium sensing receptor
CAS	computer-assisted surgery
CATCH-22	cardiac defects, abnormal facies, thymic hypoplasia, cleft palate and hypocalcaemia-22
CB	concha bullosa; or critical bandwidth
CBF	ciliary beat frequency

CBT	cognitive-behavioural therapy	CNO	chronic nasal obstruction
CCA	common carotid artery	CNS	central nervous system
CCDU	colour-coded duplex ultrasonography	CO_2	carbon dioxide
CCR	chemokine receptor	COAD	chronic obstructive airway disease
CCW	counter-clockwise	COM	chronic otitis media
CD	cluster of differentiation; or colloid droplets; or compact disk	COPD	chronic obstructive pulmonary disease
		COR	conditioned orientation reflex
CDA	cold dry air	COSI	Client Oriented Scale of Improvement
CDC	Centers for Disease Control and Prevention	COX-2	cyclo-oxygenase 2
CDK	cyclin-dependent kinase	CP	cleft palate
CDP	computerized dynamic posturography	CPA	cerebellopontine angle
CE-CT	contrast-enhanced computed tomography	CPAP	continuous positive airway pressure
CEA	carcinoembryonic antigen	CPD	citrate phosphate dextrose; or continuing professional development
CEPOD	Confidential Enquiry into Perioperative Deaths		
		CPG	central pattern generator
CER	control event rate	CPO	cleft palate only
CERA	cortical evoked response audiometry	CPPIH	Commission for Patient and Public Involvement in Health (UK)
CEVMP	click-evoked vestibular myogenic potential		
CF	cystic fibrosis; or characteristic frequency	CPR	cardiopulmonary resuscitation
CFD	colour-flow duplex Doppler	CQI	continuous quality improvement
CFR	craniofacial resection	CREST	calcinosis, Raynaud's, oesophageal involvement, sclerodactyly, telangiectasis
CFTR	cystic fibrosis transmembrane conductance regulator		
		CRF	corticotrophin-releasing factor
CFU	colony-forming unit	CRH	corticotropin-releasing hormone
CFU-GM	colony-forming unit, granulocyte-macrophage	CROS	contralateral routing of signal or sound
		CRP	C-reactive protein; or canalith repositioning procedure
CFU-Mk	colony-forming unit, megakaryocyte		
CG	clinical governance	CRRT	continous renal replacement therapy
CGD	chronic granulomatous disease	CRS	chronic rhinosinusitis; or congenital rubella syndrome
CGH	comparative genomic hybridization		
CGRP	calcitonin gene-related peptide	CRSS	chronic rhinosinusitis
CGST	Clinical Governance Support Team	CS	corticosteroid
CHARGE	coloboma, heart defects, atresia choanae, retardation of growth, genital anomalies and ear abnormalities	CSCI	Commission for Social Care Inspection (UK)
		CSF	cerebrospinal fluid
CHART	continuous, hyperfractionated, accelerated radiotherapy	CSM	Committee on Safety of Medicines
		CSOM	chronic suppurative otitis media
CHI	Commission for Healthcare Improvement (UK)	CT	computed tomography
		CTA	composite tissue allograft
CI	cochlear implant; or cardiac index; or confidence interval; or concha inferior	CTL	cytotoxic T-lymphocyte
		CTLA	cytotoxic T-lymphocyte-associated antigen
CID	Central Institute for the Deaf	CTLL	cytotoxic T-lymphocyte leukaemic
CJD	Creutzfeldt–Jakob disease	CTM	cricothyroid membrane
CL	cleft lip	cTNM	clinical tumour, nodes, metastases
CL/P	cleft lip with or without cleft palate	CTR	cricotracheal resection
CLL	chronic lymphatic leukaemia; or chronic lymphocytic leukaemia	CTZ	chemoreceptor trigger zone
		Cu-ATSM	Cu(II)-diacetyl-bis-N4-methylthiosemicarbozone
CM	concha media; or cochlear microphonic; or cricothyroid muscle		
		CUP	carcinoma of unknown primary origin
CMAP	compound muscle action potential	CUSA	cavitational ultrasonic surgical aspirator
CME	continuing medical education	CVA	cerebrovascular accident
CMI	cell-mediated immunity	CVD	central vestibular disorder
CML	chronic myeloid leukaemia	CVI	common variable immunodeficiency
CMT	Charcot-Marie-Tooth	CVP	central venous pressure
CMV	*Cytomegalovirus*	CW	clockwise
CN	cranial nerve; or cochlear nuclei; or cochlear nerve	CXR	chest x-ray
		CYP	cytochrome P450

DACH	diaminocyclohexane	EAC	external auditory canal; or external acoustic canal
DAHANCA	Danish Head and Neck Cancer Study		
DAHNO	Data for Head and Neck Oncology (UK)	EAL	ethmoidal artery ligation
dB	decibel	EAM	external auditory meatus
dB SPL	decibel sound pressure level	EB	epidermolysis bullosa
DBPCFC	double-blind placebo-controlled food challenge	EBM	evidence-based medicine
		EBNA	Epstein–Barr virus-associated nuclear antigen
DCIA	deep circumflex iliac artery		
DCN	dorsal cochlear nucleus	EBP	evidence-based practice
DCR	dacryocystorhinostomy	EBV	Epstein–Barr virus
DD	death domain	EC	embryonic carcinoma
DDHS	Direct Drive Hearing System	ECA	external carotid artery
DFF	DNA fragmentation factor	ECAL	external carotid artery ligation
DFN3	deafness type 3	ECAP	electrically evoked compound action potential
DFO-H	deferoxamine-hespan		
DHA-S	dehydroepiandrosterone sulphate	ECC	extracorporeal circuit
DHE	dihaematoporphyrinether	ECG	electrocardiogram
DHI	dizziness handicap inventory	ECM	extracellular matrix
DHTR	delayed haemolytic transfusion reaction	ECMO	extracorporeal membrane oxygenation
DIC	disseminated intravascular coagulation	EcochG	electrocochleography
DIEP	deep inferior epigastric perforator	ECog	electrocochleogram
DILS	diffuse infiltrated lymphocytosis syndrome	ECOG	Eastern Cooperative Oncology Group (USA)
DIT	diiodotyrosine	ECP	eosinophil cationic protein
DLE	discoid lupus erythematosus	ECR	extracapsular rupture
DM	diabetes mellitus	EDGT	early goal-directed therapy
DMD	Duchenne muscular dystrophy	EDN	eosinophil-derived neurotoxin
DMSA	dimercapto succinic acid	EDS	excessive daytime sleepiness
DMSO	dimethylsulfoxide	EDTA	ethylenediaminetetraacetic acid
DNA	deoxyribonucleic acid	EDV	end diastolic velocity
DNAR	do not attempt resuscitation	EE	external frontoethmoidectomy
DNL	nasolacrimal duct	EEG	electroencephalography; or electroencephalogram
DNR	do not resuscitate		
dNTP	deoxynucleoside triphosphate	EER	experimental event rate
DP	directional preponderance	EFS	event-free survival
DPA	Data Protection Act (UK)	EG	embryonic germ
DPOAE	distortion product otoacoustic emission	EGF	epidermal growth factor
DR	death receptor; or drug resistance	EGFR	epidermal growth factor receptor
DRS	Dysphagia Research Society	EIA	enzyme immunoassay
DSA	digital subtraction angiography	ELDCR	endonasal laser dacryocystorhinostomy
DSI	Dysphonia Symptom Index	ELG	electrolaryngography
DSL	desired sensation level	ELISA	enzyme-linked immunosorbent assay
DTD	DT-diaphorase	ELST	endolymphatic sac tumour
DTIC	dimethyl triazeno imidazole carboxamide	EM	erythema multiforme
dTMP	deoxythymidine monophosphate	EMEA	European Agency for the Evaluation of Medicinal Products
DTPA	diethylene triamine pentacetic acid		
dUMP	deoxyuridine monophophase	EMG	electromyography
DVB	degree of voice break	EMI	elective mucosal irradiation
DVLA	Driver and Vehicle Licensing Authority (UK)	EN	enteral nutrition
		ENA	extra nuclear antigen
DVN	descending vestibular nuclei	ENG	electronystagmography
DVT	deep vein thrombosis	ENoG	electroneurography
DWI	diffusion weighted image	ENT	ear, nose and throat
		EOG	electroolfactogram; or electrooculography
EA	episodic ataxia; or early antigen	EORTC	European Organisation for Research and Treatment of Cancer
EAACI	European Academy of Allergology and Clinical Immunology		
		EP	endolymphatic potential

EPO	erythropoietin
EQ-5D	EuroQol
ER	enhancement ratio; or endoplasmic reticulum
ERB	equivalent rectangular bandwidth
ERM	ezrin, radixin, moesin
ERP	event-related potential
ERT	external radiotherapy
Er:YAG	erbium:yttrium-aluminium-garnet
ES	embryonic stem; or endolymphatic sac
ESPAL	endonasal ligation of the sphenopalatine artery
ESR	erythrocyte sedimentation rate
ESS	endoscopic sinus surgery; or Epworth Sleepiness Scale
ET	essential thrombocytosis; or endotracheal tube
ET-1	endothelin-1
ETT	endotracheal tube
EU	European Union
EUA	examination under anaesthesia
EVAS	enlarged vestibular aqueduct syndrome
EXIT	extrauterine intrapartum treatment
F_0	fundamental frequency
FAAF	four alternative auditory feature
Fab	fragment antigen binding
FACS	fluorescence-activated cell sorter
FACT	functional assessment of cancer therapy
FAMM	facial artery myomucosal flap
Fas-L	Fas ligand
FBC	full blood count
Fc	fragment crystallizable
FD	fibrous dysplasia
FDA	Food and Drug Administration (USA)
FDG	fluorodeoxyglucose; or 2-[^{18}F] fluoro-2-deoxy-D-glucose; or F18-fluoro-2-deoxy-D-glucose
FDG-PET	2-[^{18}F] fluoro-2-deoxy-D-glucose–positron emission tomography; or fluorine-18-labelled deoxyglucose positron emission tomography
FEES	fibreoptic endoscopic evaluation of swallowing
FEESST	fibreoptic endoscopic evaluation of swallowing with sensory testing
FESS	functional endoscopic sinus surgery
FETNIM	fluorine-18 fluoroerythronitroimidazone
FFP	fresh frozen plasma
FFT	fast Fourier transform
FGF	fibroblast growth factor
FHH	familial hypocalciuric hypercalcaemia
FISH	fluorescence in situ hybridization
FIV	feline immunodeficiency virus
FLAIR	fluid attenuated inversion recovery
FMISO	fluorine-18 fluoromisonidazole
fMRI	functional magnetic resonance imaging
FN	facial nerve
FNA	fine-needle aspiration
FNAB	fine-needle aspiration biopsy
FNAC	fine-needle aspiration cytology
FOAR	fronto-orbital advancement and remodelling
FOI	fibreoptic orotracheal intubation
FPANS	fluticasone propionate aqueous nasal spray
FS	folliculostellate
FSH	follicle-stimulating hormone
FT	fibrous tissue
FTA	fluorescent treponemal antibody
FTA-ABS	fluorescent treponemal antibody test
FTC	frequency threshold curve
FTP	Fitness to Practise
G	guanine
G6PD	glucose-6-phosphate deficiency
Ga-67	gallium
GABA	gamma-aminobutyric acid
GABHS	group A beta-haemolytic streptococcus
GAG	glycosaminoglycan
GALT	gut-associated lymphoid tissue
GAS	Goal Attainment Scaling
G&S	group and screen
GBI	Glasgow Benefit Inventory
GBLC	geometric broken line closure
GCS	Glasgow Coma Score
G-CSF	granulocyte-colony stimulating factor
GD	Graves' disease
GERD	gastrooesophageal reflux disease
GH	growth hormone
GHABP	Glasgow Hearing Aid Benefit Profile
GHRH	growth hormone-releasing hormone
GI	gastrointestinal
GIA	gravitoinertial acceleration
GIC	glass ionomer cement
GIST	gastrointestinal stromal tumour
GLM	ground lamella of middle turbinate, middle (frontal) portion
GMC	ganglion mother cell; or General Medical Council (UK)
GM-CSF	granulocyte-macrophage colony-stimulating factor
GN	glossopharyngeal nerve
GNE	glottal-to-noise excitation
GnRH	gonadotropin-releasing hormone
GOR	gastro-oesophageal reflux
GORD	gastro-oesophageal reflux disease
GOSH	Great Ormond Street Hospital (UK)
gp	glycoprotein
GP	general practitioner
GPN	glossopharyngeal neuralgia
GPP	gingivo-periosteoplasty
G protein	guanine nucleotide-binding regulatory protein
GRB2	growth factor receptor binding protein 2

GSH	glutathione	HMWC	high molecular weight compound
GSPN	greater superficial petrosal nerve	HNC	head and neck cancer
GST	glutathione S-transferase	HNR	harmonics-to-noise ratio
GSW	gun shot wound	HNRQ	Head and Neck Radiotherapy Questionnaire
GTN	nitroglycerin	HNSCC	head and neck squamous cell carcinoma
GTR	guided tissue regeneration	HPA	hypothalamic–pituitary–adrenal
GVHD	graft-versus-host disease	HPC	haemangiopericytoma
		HPD	haematoporphyrin derivative
H&E	haematoxylin and eosin	HPL	horizontal partial laryngectomy
H&N	head and neck	HPT	hyperparathyroidism
H2	histamine receptor type 2	HPV	human papillomavirus; or human herpes virus 8
HA	hydroxyapatite		
HAART	highly active antiretroviral therapy	HRA	Human Rights Act
HAE	hereditary angioedema	HRCT	high-resolution computed tomography
HAEM	HSV-associated erythema multiforme	HRM	high-resolution manometry
HAPI	Hearing Aid Performance Inventory	HRQOL	health-related quality of life
HB	House–Brackmann	HRT	hormone replacement therapy
Hb	haemoglobin	HS	hiatus semilunaris
HbA	adult haemoglobin	h-SCC	horizontal semicircular canal
HBO	hyperbaric oxygen	HSCT	haemopoietic stem cell transplant
HBOT	hyperbaric oxygen therapy	HSMN	hereditary sensory-motor neuropathy
HBsAg	hepatitis B surface antigen	HSPG	heparin sulphate proteoglycan
HC	Healthcare Commission (UK)	HSV	herpes simplex virus
HCA	hydroxycarbonate apatite	HSV-1	herpes simplex virus type 1
HCG	human chorionic gonadotrophin	HSV-2	herpes simplex virus type 2
HCSU	Health Care Standards Unit (UK)	HSV-TK	herpes simplex thymidine kinase
Hct	haematocrit	HT	hydroxytryptamine
HCV	hepatitis C virus; or human T-lymphocytic virus 1	hTERT	human telomerase reverse transcriptase
		hTR	human telomerase RNA
HD	haemodialysis	HU	Hounsfield unit
HDL	high-density lipoprotein	HUI	Health Utilities Index
HDM	house dust mite	HUS	haemolytic uraemic syndrome
HDPE	high-density polyethylene	Hz	hertz
HDU	high dependency unit	HZV	herpes zoster virus
He-Ne	helium-neon		
HEp-2	human epithelial type 2	IAC	internal auditory canal
HFT	hereditary familial telangiectasia	IAM	internal auditory meatus
HGF	hepatocyte growth factor	IBP	invasive monitoring of blood pressure
HHI	Hearing Handicap Inventory	IC	inferior colliculus; or immunochemistry
HHIE	Hearing Handicap Inventory for the Elderly	ICA	internal carotid artery
HHT	hereditary haemorrhagic telangiectasia	ICAM	intercellular adhesion molecule
HHV-6	human herpesvirus 6	ICAM-1	intercellular adhesion molecule 1
HHV-8	human herpesvirus 8	ICD	International Classification of Disease
HI	hearing impaired	ICM	intensive care medicine
HiB	*Haemophilus influenzae* B	ICP	intracranial pressure
HIT	heparin-induced thrombocytopenia	ICRA	International Collegium of Rehabilitative Audiology
HITT	heparin-induced thrombocytopenia with thrombosis		
		ICU	intensive care unit
HIV	human immunodeficiency virus	ID	inferior dental
HIV-SGD	HIV-associated salivary gland disease	IDA	iron deficiency anaemia
HJB	high jugular bulb	IDT	infant distraction test
HL	hearing loss; or hearing level; or hairy leukoplakia	IDU	intravenous drug user
		IF	intrinsic factor
HLA	human leukocyte antigen	IFN	interferon
HM	history of migraine; or hemifacial microsomia	IFN-α	interferon-alpha
		IFN-β	inteferon-beta
HMW	high molecular weight	IFN-γ	interferon gamma

IFNP	idiopathic facial nerve paralysis		K	Kirschner
Ig	immunoglobulin		KAR	killer activating receptor
IgE	immunoglobulin E		keV	kilo electron volt
IGF	insulin-like growth factor		KIR	killer inhibitory receptor
IGFI	insulin-like growth factor I		KS	Kaposi's sarcoma
IGFII	insulin-like growth factor II		KSS	Kearns–Sayre syndrome
IgG	immunoglobulin G		KTP	potassium titanyl phosphate
IGS	image-guided surgery			
IHAFF	International Hearing Aid Fitting Forum		LA	lymphangioma
IHC	immunohistochemistry; or inner hair cell		LAD	leukocyte adhesion defect
			LAP	left anteroposterior
IHS	International Headache Society		LARP	left anterior–right posterior
IL	interleukin		LAUP	laser-assisted uvulopalatoplasty
IL-1	interleukin-1		LB	lateral bundle
IL-2	interleukin-2		LCH	Langerhans' cell histiocytosis
IL-3	interleukin-3		LCM	laser capture microdissection
IL-6	interleukin-6		LD	lymphocytic depleted
ILMA	intubating laryngeal mask airway		LDH	lactate dehydrogenase
IMA	internal maxillary artery		LDL	low-density lipoprotein; or loudness discomfort level
IMAL	internal maxillary artery ligation			
IMF	intermaxillary fixation		LDUH	low-dose unfractionated heparin
IMRT	intensity-modulated radiation therapy		LED	light-emitting diode
IMSPAC	imitative test of speech pattern contrast perception		LFA	lymphocyte-function associated antigen
			LGOB	loudness growth in octave bands
INC	immunonuclear chemistry		LH	luteinizing hormone
INE	intranasal ethmoidectomy		LHRH	leuteinizing hormone-releasing hormone
INO	internuclear ophthalmoplegia		LIF	leukaemia-inhibitory factor
iNOS	inducible nitric oxide synthase		LINks	Local Involvement Networks (UK)
INR	international normalized ratio; or interventional neuroradiology		LL	lateral lemniscus
			LM	laryngeal mask
IOC	Interim Orders Committee (UK)		LMA	laryngeal mask airway
IOPI	Iowa Oral Performance Instrument		LMN	lower motor neuron
IP$_3$	1,4,5-inositol triphosphate		LMW	low molecular weight
IPSS	inferior petrosal sinus sampling		LMWC	low molecular weight compound
IRMA	immunoradiometric assay		LMWH	low molecular weight heparin
IRS	Intergroup Rhabdomyosarcoma Study		LOD	logarithm to the base 10 of the odds that the markers are linked at a recombination distance of N centimorgans
ISAAC	International Study of Asthma and Allergies in Childhood			
ISEL	*in situ* end labeling		LOH	loss of heterozygosity
ISJ	incudostapedial joint		LOS	length of stay; or lower oesophageal sphincter
ISO	International Standards Organization			
ISS	immunostimulatory DNA sequence		LP	lamina papyracea; or lichen planus; or lymphocyte predominant
ISSNHL	idiopathic sudden sensorineural hearing loss			
			LPC	linear predictive coding
IT	inferior turbinate		LPR	laryngopharyngeal reflux
ITA	inferior thyroid artery		LR	likelihood ratio
ITE	in the ear		LREC	local research ethics committee
ITP	idiopathic thrombocytopenic purpura		LSCC	lateral semicircular canal
ITU	intensive therapy unit		LT	leukotriene
IUCC	International Union against Cancer		LTAS	long-term average spectrum
i.v.	intravenous		LTASS	long-term average speech spectrum
IVIg	intravenous immunoglobulin		LTB	laryngotracheobronchitis; or laryngotracheobronchoscopy
JFC	just-follow-conversation		LTC4-S	leukotriene C4 synthase
JNA	juvenile nasopharyngeal angiofibroma		LTR	laryngotracheal reconstruction
JORPP	juvenile-onset recurrent respiratory papillomatosis		LTRA	leukotriene receptor antagonists
			LVA	large vestibular aqueduct

LVAS	large vestibular aqueduct syndrome	MIDD	maternally inherited diabetes and deafness
LVN	lateral vestibular nuclei	MIP	minimally invasive open parathyroidectomy; or maximum intensity projection; or macrophage inflammatory protein
LVOR	linear vestibulo–ocular reflex		
M	metastases		
MAb	monoclonal antibodies	MIP-1α	macrophage inflammatory protein-1α
MABP	mean arterial blood pressure	MISS	minimally invasive sinus surgery
MAC	membrane attack complex; or *Mycobacterium avium* complex	MIT	monoiodotyrosine
		MIVAP	minimally invasive video-assisted parathoidectomy
MACS	magnetic-activated cell sorter; or minimal access cranial suspension	ML	mixed cellularity
MAF	minimum audible field	MLD	masking level difference
MALT	mucosa-associated lymphoid tissue	MLF	medial longitudinal fascicle or fasciculus
MAOI	monoamine oxidase inhibitor	MLR	middle latency response
MAP	minimum audible pressure	MLTB	microlaryngotracheobronchoscopy
MAPK	mitogen-activated protein kinase	MM	malignant melanoma
MAS	mandibular advancement splint	MMC	mitomycin C
MB	medial bundle	MMN	mismatch negativity
MBL	mannose-binding lectin	MMP	mucous membrane pemphigoid; or matrix-metalloprotease
MBP	major basic protein		
MBS	modified barium swallow	MMR	measles, mumps and rubella
MCP	monocyte chemotactic protein	MMS	Moh's micrographic surgery
MCP-1	monocyte chemotactic protein-1	MND	motor neurone disease
MCS	mental component summary	MNG	multinodular goitre
M-CSF	macrophage-colony stimulating factor	MOC	medial olivocochlear
MCV	mean corpuscular volume	MODS	multiple organ dysfunction syndrome
MDC	macrophage derived chemokine	MOT	malignant odontogenic tumour
MDR	multiple drug resistance	MPA	microscopic polyangiitis
MDRTB	multidrug resistant tuberculosis	MPL	monophosphoryl lipid A
MDS	myelodysplastic syndrome	MPO	myeloperoxidase
MDT	multidisciplinary team	MPT	maximum phonation time
MDVP	Multidimensional Voice Program	MPTP	1-methyl-4-phenyl-1,2,3,6-tetrahydropyridine
ME	middle ear		
MEE	medial edge epithelium	MR	magnetic resonance
MEG	magnetoencephalography	MRA	magnetic resonance angiography
MEK	MAPK/extracellular signal related kinase	MRC	Medical Research Council (UK)
MELAS	mitochondrial encephalopathy, lactic acidosis and stroke-like episode	MREC	multicentre regional ethics committee
		MRI	magnetic resonance imaging
MEMS	microelectromechanical system	MRL	minimal response level
MEN	multiple endocrine neoplasia	mRNA	messenger ribonucleic acid
MERRF	myoclonic epilepsy and ragged red fibre	MRND	modified radical neck dissection
MeSH	medical subject heading	MRS	Melkersson–Rosenthal syndrome; or magnetic resonance sialography
MESS	microscopic endonasal sinus surgery		
MET	middle ear transducer	MRSA	methicillin-resistant *Staphylococcus aureus*
MF	middle fossa	MRV	migraine-related vestibulopathy
M-FISH	multifluor FISH	MS	multiple sclerosis
MFR	mean airflow rate	MSA	multiple systems atrophy
MGB	medial geniculate body	MSBOS	maximum surgical blood ordering schedule
MGSA	melanoma growth stimulating activity	MSG	monosodium glutamate
MGUS	monoclonal gammopathy of uncertain significance	MST	maximal stimulation test
		MT	maxilloturbinal; or middle turbinate
MHC	major histocompatibility complex	MTC	medullary thyroid carcinoma
MI	myocardial infarction	MTD	muscle tension dysphonia
MIBG	metaiodobenzylguanidine; or iodine-123-metaiodobenzylguanidine	mtDNA	mitochondrial DNA
		MTHFR	methylenetetrahydrofolate reductase
MIBI	sestamibi; or technetium-99m	mTHPC	meso-tetra (hydroxyphenyl) chlorin
MIC	minimum inhibitory concentration	MUS	medically unexplained symptom

MV	mechanical ventilation
MVN	medial vestibular nuclei
N	nodal
NA	noradrenaline
NADP	nicotinamide adenine dinucleotide phosphate
NADPH	reduced form of nicotinamide adenine dinucleotide phosphate
NAL	National Acoustic Laboratories (Australia)
NAMCS	National Ambulatory Medical Care Survey (USA)
NANIPER	nonallergic noninfectious perennial rhinitis
NARES	nonallergic rhinitis with eosinophilia syndrome
NATA	National Anonymous Tonsil Archive
NBCA	n-butyl-2-cyanoacrylate; or N-butyl-cyanoacrylate
NBT	nitro blue tetrazolium
NCAA	National Clinical Assessment Authority (UK)
NCAS	National Clinical Assessment Service (UK)
NCASP	National Clinical Audit Support Programme (UK)
NCCG	non-consultant career-grade
NCCN	National Comprehensive Cancer Network
NCDB	National Cancer Data Base (USA)
NCEPOD	National Confidential Enquiry into Patient Outcome Death (UK)
NCIC	National Cancer Institute of Canada
NEET	nose, ear, eye and temple
NESSTAC	North of England and Scotland Study on Tonsillectomy and Adenoidectomy in Children
NET	nerve excitability test
NFκB	nuclear factor kappa B
NF1	neurofibromatosis type 1
NF2	neurofibromatosis type 2
NFA	nonfunctioning pituitary adenomas; or nasofrontal approach
NG	nasogastric
NH	normal hearing
NHL	non-Hodgkin's lymphoma
NHS	National Health Service (UK)
NHSP	Newborn Hearing Screening Programme
NIBP	automatic noninvasive blood pressure
NICE	National Institute for Health and Clinical Excellence (UK)
NICU	nonimmunological contact urticaria; or neonatal intensive care unit
NIDDM	noninsulin dependent diabetes mellitus
NIH	National Institutes of Health (USA)
NIHL	noise-induced hearing loss
NIPF	nasal inspiratory peak flow
NIS	Na+/I– symporter
NK	natural killer
N/m^2	Newtons/square metre

NMCC	nasal mucociliary clearance
NMDA	N-methyl-d-aspartate; or National Minimum Data Set (UK)
NNE	normalized noise energy
NNT	number needed to treat
NO	nitric oxide
NO_2	nitric dioxide
NOE	naso-orbito-ethmoid
non-REM	nonrapid eye movement sleep
NOS	not otherwise specified
NP	nasopharynx; or nasopharyngeal
NPC	nasopharyngeal cancer; or nasopharyngeal carcinoma
NPSA	National Patient Safety Agency (UK)
NPTA	National Prospective Tonsillectomy Audit (UK)
NPV	negative predictive value
NPY	neuropeptide Y
NRA	nucleus retroambigualis
NRLS	National Reporting and Learning System (UK)
NRT	neural response telemetry
NS	nodular sclerosing
NSAID	nonsteroidal antiinflammatory drug
NSCAG	National Specialist Commissioning Advisory Group (UK)
NSF	national service framework
NSHPT	neonatal severe hyperparathyroidism
NSRAN	nonsyndromic recessive auditory neuropathy
NT	nasoturbinal
NTD	neural tube defect
NTM	non-tuberculous mycobacteria
NTS	nucleus tractus solitarius
NYHA	New York Heart Association
O_3	ozone
OAE	otoacoustic emission
OAN	olfactory neuroblastoma
OAS	oral allergy syndrome
OB	olfactory bulb
OCB	olivocochlear bundle
OCFC	open controlled food challenge
OCT	optical coherence tomography
ODI	oxygen desaturation index
ODT	olfactory detection threshold
OEC	olfactory ensheathing cell
OFG	orofacial granulomatosis
OGTT	oral glucose tolerance test
OHC	outer hair cell
OHL	oral hairy leukoplakia
OHS	obesity hypoventilation syndrome
OKN	optokinetic nystagmus
OM	occipitomental
OMC	ostiomeatal complex
OME	otitis media with effusion
OMENS	orbit, mandible, ears, nerves and soft-tissue

OMIM	Online Mendelian Inheritance in Man
OPCS	Office for Population Censuses and Surveys (UK)
OPG	orthopantomogram
OR	occupational rhinitis
OREP	olfactory event-related potential
ORL	otorhinolaryngology
OS	osteosarcoma
OSA	obstructive sleep apnoea
OSAH	obstructive sleep apnoea/hypopnoea
OSAHS	obstructive sleep apnoea/hypopnoea syndrome
OSAS	obstructive sleep apnoea syndrome
OSC	overview and scrutiny committee
OSPH	ostium of sphenoid sinus
OSPL	output sound pressure level
OTOF	otoferlin
OVAR	off-vertical axis rotation
P	phosphate; or posterior
PA	pernicious anaemia
PAC	P1 artificial chromosome; or pulmonary artery catheter
PAD	preoperative autologous deposit
PAF	platelet-activating factor
PAG	periaqueductal grey matter
PAI-1	plasminogen activator inhibitor type 1
PALS	Patient Advice and Liaison Service (UK)
PA-RT	partly accelerated radiotherapy
PAS	periodic acid–Schiff
PBP	progressive bulbar palsy
PCA	patient-controlled analgesia
PCC	prothrombin complex concentrate; or Professional Conduct Committee (UK)
PCD	primary ciliary dyskinesia
PCHI	permanent childhood hearing impairment
PCNA	proliferating cell nuclear antigen
PCR	polymerase chain reaction
Pcrit	critical pressure
PCS	physical component summary
PCT	primary care trust
PCTR	partial cricotracheal resection
PD	Parkinson's disease
PD-ECGF	platelet-derived endothelial cell growth factor
PDGF	platelet-derived growth factor
PDGFR	platelet-derived growth factor receptor
PDL	pulsed dye laser
PDR	*Physicians' Desk Reference*
PDS	polydimethylsiloxane
PDT	photodynamic therapy
PE	polyethylene; or pulmonary embolism; or pharyngo–oesophageal
PEEP	positive-end expiratory pressure
PEG	percutaneous endoscopic gastrostomy
PEMA/THFMA	poly (ethylmethacrylate)/tetrahydrofurfuryl methacrylate

PET	polyethylene terephthalate; or positron emission tomography
PET-CT	positron emission tomography/computed tomography
PF	posterior fontanelle; or cisplatinum/5-fluorouracil
PF4	platelet factor 4
PFAPA	periodic fever, aphthous stomatitis, pharyngitis and cervical adenitis
PFC	perfluorocarbon
PFG	percutaneous fluoroscopic gastrostomy
PGA	polyglycolic acid
PGE$_1$	prostaglandin-E$_1$
PGI$_2$	prostacycline; or prostaglandin I$_2$
PGL	persistent generalized lymphadenopathy
pHPT	primary hyperparathyroidism
PI	pulsatility index
PI3-K	phosphotidyinositol 3
PICA	posterior inferior cerebellar artery
PICU	paediatric intensive care unit
PIF	prolactin release inhibiting factor
PIFR	peak inspiratory flow
PIHA	partially implantable hearing aid
PIII	parathyroid III
PIV	parainfluenza virus; or parathyroid IV
PIVC	parietoinsular vestibular cortex
PLA	polylactic acid
PLD	potentially lethal damage
PLF	congenital perilymphatic fistula
PLG	polylactide-coglycolide
PLMD	periodic limb movement disorder
PLS	primary lateral sclerosis
PM	particulate matter
PMS	pharyngeal mucosal space
PNP	purine nucleoside phosphorylase; or paraneoplastic pemphigus
PNS	peripheral nervous system; or postnasal space
POGO	prescription of gain and output
PONV	postoperative nausea/vomiting
PORP	partial ossicular replacement prosthesis
PP	pyrophosphate
PPC	Preliminary Proceedings Committee (UK)
PPD	purified protein derivative
PPI	proton pump inhibitor; or patient and public involvement
PPRF	parapontine reticular formation; or paramedian pontine reticular formation
PPS	parapharyngeal space
PPV	positive predictive value
PR3	proteinase 3
PRCT	prospective randomized controlled trial
PRL	prolactin
PRP	platelet-rich plasma
PRPP	5-phospho-alpha-D-ribose 1-diphosphate
PRS	persistent rhinosinusitis
PRV	polycythaemia rubra vera

PSA	prostate-specific antigen; or pleomorphic salivary adenoma; or persistent stapedial artery
p-SCC	posterior semicircular canal
PSG	polysomnography
PS-OCT	polarization-sensitive OCT
PSP	progressive supranuclear palsy
PSV	peak systolic velocity
PT	prothrombin time
PTA	pure tone average; or peritonsillar abscess
PTC	psychophysical tuning curve
PTFE	polytetrafluoroethylene
PTH	parathyroid hormone
PTHrP	parathyroid hormone-related protein; or parathyroid hormone-related peptide
pTNM	pathological tumour, nodes, metastases
PTP	post-transfusion purpura
PTS	permanent threshold shift
PTU	propylthiouracil
PU	uncinate process
PV	pemphigus vulgaris
PVA	polyvinyl alcohol
PVC	polyvinyl chloride
PVCN	posteroventral cochlear nuclei
PVP	pause vestibular position; or position vestibular pause
PVS	persistent vegetative state
PZT	lead zirconate titanate
QALY	quality adjusted life year
QOL	quality of life
QTL	quantitative trait loci
RA	retinoic acid
RAE	Ring, Adair, Elwyn
RAI	radioactive iodine
RALP	right anterior–left posterior
RAM	Rahmonic amplitude
RANTES	regulated on activation, normal T-cell expressed and secreted
RAP	right anteroposterior
RARα	retinoic acid receptor α gene
RARS	recurrent acute rhinosinusitis
RAS	recurrent aphthous stomatitis
RAST	radioallergosorbent test
RAT	rapid antigen testing
RB	retinoblastoma
RBC	red blood cell
rCBF	regional cerebral blood flow
RCPCH	Royal College of Paediatrics and Child Health
RCT	randomized controlled trial
RDI	respiratory disturbance index
REAG	real-ear aided gain
REAL	Revised European American Lymphoma
RECD	real ear to coupler difference
REIG	real-ear insertion gain

REM	rapid eye movement
rEPO	recombinant erythropoietin
RET	rearranged during transfection
RFS	rhinofrontal sinuseptotomy
RFTVR	radiofrequency tissue volume reduction
RFVR	radiofrequency volumetric reduction
RHD	Reported Hearing Disability
RI	resistance index
RIA	radioimmuno assay
riMLF	rostral interstitial nucleus of the medial longitudinal faciculus
RLN	recurrent laryngeal nerve
RLS	restless leg syndrome
RMS	root mean square; or rhabdomyosarcoma
RNA	ribonucleic acid
RND	radical neck dissection
RNID	Royal National Institute for Deaf and Hard of Hearing People (UK)
RNP	ribonucleoprotein
ROC	receiver operating characteristic
ROI	region of interest; or reactive oxygen intermediate
ROM	range of motion
ROOF	retro-orbicularis orbital fat
ROS	reactive oxygen species
RP	rapid prototyping
RPA	retropharyngeal abscess
RPT	rapid pull through
RR	relative risk
RRP	recurrent respiratory papillomatosis
RRR	relative risk reduction
RS	retrosigmoid
RSDI	Rhinosinusitis Disability Index
RSOM	rhinosinusitis outcome measure
RSTL	relaxed skin tension line
RSV	respiratory syncytial virus
RT	radiotherapy
rT3	reverse triiodothyronine
RTK	receptor tyrosine kinase
RTL	right thyroid artery
rTMS	repetitive low-frequency transcranial magnetic stimulation
RT-PCR	reverse transcriptase-polymerase chain reaction
RUDS	reactive upper airways dysfunction syndrome
SACE	serum angiotensin converting enzyme
SAD	supraglottic airway device
SAGM	saline-adenine-glucose-mannitol
SALT	speech and language therapist
SANS	subacute necrotizing sialadenitis
SAP	signalling lymphocyte activation molecule associated protein
SAPALDIA	Swiss Study on Air Pollution and Lung Diseases in Adults
SBS	sick building syndrome

s.c.	subcutaneous
SCBU	special care baby unit
SCC	squamous cell carcinoma or cancer; or semicircular canal
SCCA	squamous cell carcinoma antigen
SCCHN	squamous cell carcinoma of the head and neck
SCD	sickle cell disease
SCF	stem cell factor
SCID	severe combined immunodeficiency
SCN	severe congenital neutropenia
SCUBA	self-contained underwater breathing apparatus
$ScvO_2$	central venous oxygen saturation
SEAC	Spongiform Encephalopathy Advisory Committee
SEM	scanning electron microscopy
sEMG	surface electromyography
SF-36	Medical Outcome Study Short-Form 36-Item Health Survey
SfBH	Standards for Better Health (UK)
SFF	speaking fundamental frequency
SFOAE	stimulus frequency otoacoustic emission
SGC	spiral ganglion cell
Shh	sonic hedgehog
SHO	senior house officer
SHOT	serious hazards of transfusion
SIADH	syndrome of inappropriate antidiuretic hormone
SIDS	sudden infant death syndrome
sIg	surface immunoglobulin
SIGN	Scottish Intercollegiate Guidelines Network
SIMEHD	semi-implantable middle ear electromagnetic hearing device
SIP	sickness impact profile
SIR	speech intelligibility rating; or standardized incidence ratio
SIRS	systemic inflammatory response syndrome
SL	sensation level
SLD	sublethal damage
SLE	systemic lupus erythematosus
SLIT	sublingual immunotherapy
SLN	superior laryngeal nerve
SLNB	sentinel lymph node biopsy
SLP	superficial lamina propria
SLT	speech and language therapist
SMAS	superficial or subcutaneous muscloaponeurotic system
SMOFIT	submucous resection of the turbinate
SMR	submucosal resection
SMS	short message service; or indium-111 pentetreotide
S/N	speech-to-noise
SNC	sinonasal cancer
SNHL	sensorineural hearing loss
SNOMED	Systematized nomenclature of medicine
SNOMED CT	Systematized Nomenclature of Medicine – Clinical Terms
SNOT	sino-nasal outcome test
SNR	signal-to-noise ratio
SNUC	sinonasal undifferentiated carcinoma
SO_2	sulphur dioxide
SOAE	spontaneous otoacoustic emission
SOC	superior olivary complex
SOM	secretory otitis media
SOOF	suborbicularis oculi fat
SOS	guanine nucleotide exchange factor (son of sevenless)
SP	substance P; or summating potential
SPECT	single photon emission computed tomography
SPET	single photon emission tomography
SPF	sphenopalatine foramen
SPI	soft phonation index
SPIO	superparamagnetic iron oxide
SPL	sound pressure level
SPT	skin prick test; or station pull through
SRS	subacute rhinosinusitis
SRS-A	slow reacting substance of anaphylaxis
SRT	speech recognition threshold; or speech reception threshold
SSC	superior semicircular canal
SSEP	steady-state potential
SSG	split skin graft
SSLP	simple sequence length polymorphism
SSNHL	sudden sensorineural hearing loss
SSPE	subacute sclerosing panencephalitis
SSPL	saturation sound pressure level
SSR	steady-state response
SSRI	selective serotonin reuptake inhibitor
ST	superior turbinate
STAT	signal transducer and activator of transcription
STD	standard deviation
STIR	short time inversion recovery
STRP	short tandem repeat polymorphism
SUV	standardized uptake value
SVCO	superior vena caval obstruction
SVL	strobovideolaryngoscopy
SVN	superior vestibular nuclei; or superior vestibular nerve
SVV	subjective visual vertical
SVZ	subventricular zone
SWS	slow wave sleep
T	thymine; or tumour
T1WI	T1-weighted images
T2WI	T2-weighted images
T3	triiodothyronine
T4	thyroxine
T/A	tonsillectomy and/or adenoidectomy
TAGVHD	transfusion-associated graft-versus-host disease

TARC	thymus and activation-regulated chemokine
TARGET	Trial of Alternative Regimens in Glue Ear Treatment
TB	tuberculosis; or *Mycobacterium tuberculosis*
TBG	thyroxine-binding globulin
Tc	T cytotoxic
Tc-99m	technetium
Tc-99m (v) DMSA	pentavalent dimercaptosuccinic acid
TC	thyroid cartilage
TCF	tracheocutaneous fistula
TCI	target-controlled infusion
TCP	tricalcium phosphate
TCR	T cell receptor
TdT	terminal deoxynucleotidyl transferase
TEC	Tissue Engineering and Regenerative Medicine Centre
TENS	transcutaneous electrical nerve stimulation
TEOAE	transient evoked otoacoustic emission
TEP	tracheo-oesophageal puncture
TFG	temporalis fascia graft
TFT	thyroid function test
TG	thyroglobulin
TGF	transforming growth factor
TGF-α	transforming growth factor alpha
TGF-β	transforming growth factor beta
TGF-β1	transforming growth factor beta 1
Th	T helper
TIA	transient ischaemic attack
TIBC	total iron binding capacity
TICA	totally implantable cochlear amplifier
TKI	tyrosine kinase inhibitor
TM	tympanic membrane
TMC1	transmembrane channel-like gene 1
TMD	temporomandibular disorder
TMJ	temporomandibular joint
TMTF	temporal modulation transfer function
TN	trigeminal neuralgia; or trigeminal nerve
TNF	tumour necrosis factor
TNF-α	tumour necrosis factor alpha
TNM	tumour, node, metastasis
TOAE	transient evoked otoacoustic emission
TOE	transoesophageal echocardiography; or *Trichophyton, Oidiomycetes* and *Epidermophyton*
TOF	tracheo-oesophageal fistula
TOF-o-gram	tracheo-oesophageal fistulogram
TORP	total ossicular replacement prosthesis
TPA	tissue polypeptide antigen
TPF	docetaxel/cisplatinum/5-fluorouracil; or temporoparietal fascia
TPHA	*T. pallidum* haemagglutination test; or treponemal haemagglutination
TPI	*T. pallidum* immobilization
TPN	total parenteral nutrition
TPO	thyroid peroxidase; or thyroperoxidase
Tpot	potential doubling times
TQM	total quality management

TRALI	transfusion-related acute lung injury
TRAM	transverse rectus abdominis myocutaneous
TRH	thyrotropin-releasing hormone
tRNA	transfer ribonucleic acid
TRP	transient receptor potential
TRT	tinnitus retraining therapy
TSG	tumour suppressor gene
TSH	thyroid-stimulating hormone; or thyrotropin
TSHoma	TSH-secreting adenoma
TSS	transitional space surgery
TT	thrombin time
TTN	thalamic taste nucleus
TTP	thrombotic thrombocytopeniac purpura
TTR	transthyretin
TTS	temporary threshold shift
TUNEL	TdT-mediated nick end labelling
TXA$_2$	thromboxane A$_2$
U	uracil
UADT	upper aerodigestive tract
UARS	upper airway resistance syndrome
UCL	uncomfortable loudness level
UICC	International Union Against Cancer
UK-CCSG	United Kingdom Children with Cancer Study Group
UKCISG	UK Cochlear Implant Study Group
UMN	upper motor neuron
UMP	uridine monophosphate
UNICEF	United Nations Children's Fund
UOS	upper oesophageal sphincter
UP	uncinate process
UPP	uvulopalatopharyngoplasty
UPPP	uvulopalatopharyngoplasty
UPSIT	University of Pennsylvania Smell Identification Test
URT	upper respiratory tract
URTI	upper respiratory tract infection
US	ultrasound; or ultrasonography
USH	Usher syndrome
USH1B	Usher syndrome type 1B
USPIO	ultra-small super paramagnetic iron oxide
UV	ultraviolet
uVD	unilateral vestibular deafferentiation
UVPP	uvulopalatopharyngoplasty
UWQOL	University of Washington Quality of Life Questionnaire
VA	Veterans' Affairs; or vestibular aqueduct
VAAP	voice activity and participation
VAC	vacuum-assisted closure
VAM	variation of amplitude
VAS	visual analogue scale; or visual analogue score
VATER	vertebral, anal, tracheooesophageal and radial
VCA	viral capsid antigen

VCAM-1	vascular cell adhesion molecule-1	VPQ	patient questionnaire of vocal performance
vCJD	variant Creutzfeldt-Jakob disease		
VCR	vestibulocollic reflex	VRA	visual reinforcement audiometry
VDRL	Venereal Disease Research Laboratory	VRE	vancomycin-resistant enterococci
VEES	video endoscopic evaluation of swallowing	V-RQOL	voice-related quality of life
VEGF	vascular endothelial growth factor	VS	vestibular schwannoma
VEMP	vestibular-evoked myogenic potential	VSM	velocity storage mechanism
VEP	vestibular evoked potential	VSR	vestibulospinal reflex
VFSS	videofluoroscopic swallowing study	VTE	venous thromboembolism
VHI	Voice Handicap Index	VVI	vocal velocity index
VHI-10	Voice Handicap Index-10	vWD	von Willebrand disease
VHL	Von Hippel–Lindau	vWF	von Willebrand factor
VHQ	Vertigo Handicap Questionnaire	VZV	varicella zoster virus
VHT	vestibular habituation training		
VILI	ventilator induced lung injury	WAS	Wiskott Aldrich syndrome
VIP	vasoactive intestinal polypeptide	WBC	white blood cell
VLA	very late activation antigen	WHO	World Health Organization
VLA4	very late activation antigen 4	WMD	weighted mean difference
VLDL	very low-density lipoprotein	WOB	work of breathing
VMA	vanillylmandelic acid	WP	Woodruff's plexus
VN	vestibular nuclei; or vagus nerve	WPC	WARN, PAUSE, CHECK
VOC	volatile organic compound		
VOG	video-oculography	XHIM	X-linked hyper immunoglobin M
VoiSS	voice symptom scale	XLA	X-linked agammaglobulinaemia
VOR	vestibulo-ocular reflex	XLP	X-linked lymphoproliferative syndrome
VORP	vibrating ossicular prosthesis		
VORS	vestibulo-ocular reflex suppression	YAC	yeast artificial chromosome
VPI	velopharyngeal insufficiency	YAG	yttrium aluminium garnate

PART **1**

CELL BIOLOGY

EDITED BY NICHOLAS S JONES

1 Molecular biology
  Michael Kuo and Richard Irving   3

2 Genetics
  Karen P Steel   15

3 Gene therapy
  Scott M Graham and John H Lee   23

4 Mechanisms of anticancer drugs
  Sarah Payne and David Miles   34

5 Radiotherapy and radiosensitizers
  Stewart G Martin and David AL Morgan   47

6 Apoptosis and cell death
  Michael Saunders   56

7 Stem cells
  A John Harris and Archana Vats   66

Molecular biology

MICHAEL KUO AND RICHARD IRVING

Introduction	3	Mapping and identification of genes associated with disease	11
Molecular genetics: DNA structure and function	3	Key point	11
Key points	5	Deficiencies in current knowledge and areas for future research	11
Methods in molecular biology	5	References	13
Key points	8	Further reading	14
Molecular aberrations of cellular biology	8		
Key points	10		

SEARCH STRATEGY

The data in this chapter are supported by a Medline search using the key words molecular biology, genetics, and cell biology.

INTRODUCTION

Molecular biology describes the study of the biochemical processes that govern the behaviour of cells. These processes form the fundamental mechanisms by which cell function, cell–cell interactions and cell turnover are regulated. Disruption of this regulation may lead to disease, whilst an understanding of these mechanisms allows the physician to attempt to predict disease behaviour and to explore methods of restoring this regulation at a molecular level. This chapter reviews the principles of molecular genetics and outlines aspects of the molecular biology of the cell in the context of otolaryngological disease processes and describes some of the techniques that form the backbone of current molecular biology. It should give the reader sufficient background knowledge of molecular biology to understand subsequent chapters discussing the molecular biology of specific otolaryngological conditions.

MOLECULAR GENETICS: DNA STRUCTURE AND FUNCTION

Hereditary information in eukaryotes is stored in the form of double-stranded deoxyribonucleic acid (DNA) and is referred to as the genome. DNA forms a double-helix structure as a result of hydrogen bonds between complementary pairs of nucleotides, adenine (A) with thymine (T) and cytosine (C) with guanine (G). The nucleotides on each strand are organized linearly in triplets, known as codons. Each specific sequence determines a single specific amino acid, for example ACU specifies threonine. However, as there are more triplet combinations (64) than commonly encountered amino acids (20), some proteins may be represented by different codons (e.g. lysine by AAA as well as AAG) and some codons (UAA, UGA and UAG) are 'stop' codons, constituting a signal for arrest of translation. The overwhelming majority of this DNA (99.9 percent) exists in the cell nucleus as the nuclear genome, which, in the human, is estimated to be 3000 megabase pairs in physical size and encodes 30,000–35,000 genes. The remaining DNA (16.6 kilobase pairs) forms the mitochondrial genome, encoding 37 genes. The mitochondrial genome and its potential role in cancer diagnostics will be discussed later.

Each DNA molecule is packaged into a chromosome by complex folding of the DNA around proteins. Diploid human cells contain 22 pairs of autosomes (1 to 22) and a pair of sex chromosomes (XX or XY) which determines the sex of the organism. One of each pair of chromosomes is maternally inherited and the other is paternally inherited. Each chromosome has a distinctive shape, size and banding pattern, but have the common appearance of two arms apparently separated by a constriction. The centromere is microscopically recognizable as the central constriction separating the chromosome into a long arm (q for queue) and a short arm (p for petit), but its biological role lies in anchoring the chromosome to the mitotic spindle for segregation during cell division. The ends of the chromosomes are capped by telomeres, which are specialized structures containing unique simple repetitive sequences. They maintain the structural integrity of the chromosome and provide a solution for complete replication of the extreme ends of the chromosome. The conventional nomenclature for chromosomal locus assignment is given by the chromosome number, followed by the arm and finally the position on the arm, for example, 3p21 indicates position 21(two-one) on the short arm of chromosome three.

During normal cell division, DNA replication is achieved by the separation of the two strands by DNA helicase. Each separated single strand then acts as a template for polymerization, catalyzed by DNA polymerase, of nucleotides forming a new complementary strand and thus double-stranded DNA identical to the original dsDNA. As each daughter DNA consists of one original and one newly synthesized DNA strand, the process is known as semi-conservative replication. The specificity of the complementary relationship between the nucleotides on each strand forms the basis for many techniques of modern molecular biology and molecular cytogenetics.[1] The accuracy with which DNA replication takes place is remarkable with an estimated error rate of less than one in 10^9 nucleotide additions. Such accuracy is of vital importance to the individual as a permanent change in DNA, or mutation may cause inactivation of a gene essential to cell survival or cell cycle control. The high fidelity of DNA sequence replication is achieved by unidirectional 5'-to-3' direction of DNA replication, a rigorous DNA proofreading mechanism which detects mismatched DNA and efficient DNA repair pathways which excise and repair DNA damage. Failure of these mechanisms, such as is encountered in xeroderma pigmentosum, Fanconi's anaemia and ataxia telangiectasia, leads to accumulation of DNA replication errors and a high incidence of malignancies.

Although the human nuclear genome is 3×10^9 base pairs in size, about 90 percent of it is noncoding, with all the genes being coded by the remaining 10 percent of the DNA. Within the noncoding DNA are dispersed short arrays of repeat units of pairs or triplets of nucleotides (di-/trinucleotides). The exact function of these microsatellite repeats is not entirely clear, but their existence and frequency of dispersion throughout the genome have greatly facilitated study of the genetics of

tumours and many inherited disorders, which will be discussed later.

A gene is a region of the chromosomal DNA that produces a functional ribonucleic acid molecule (RNA). It comprises regulatory DNA sequences which determine when and in which cell types that gene is expressed, exons which are coding sequences and interspersed introns which are noncoding DNA sequences. These regulatory sequences often consist of CpG islands, short stretches of DNA rich in dinucleotides of cytosine and guanine. The methylation status of these CpG islands determines whether that gene is expressed in a particular cell or tissue, being unmethylated in tissues where the genes are expressed. As will be discussed later, aberration of this control is one of the mechanisms of tumour suppressor gene inactivation. Transcription is the intranuclear process driven by RNA polymerase whereby one of the two DNA strands acts as a template for the synthesis of a single RNA strand which is complementary to the DNA, except that uracil replaces thymine in RNA. This primary RNA transcript then undergoes post-transcriptional processing, or splicing.[2] Traditional dogma held that one gene produces one protein and therefore splicing was considered to occur simply in order to remove the noncoding intronic sequences, producing messenger RNA (mRNA). It is now known that by 'alternative splicing', one gene can result in the production of several different but often related proteins in different tissues.[3]

The mature mRNA then migrates into the cytoplasm where it acts as a template for the synthesis of a polypeptide during translation, a process regulated and catalyzed by cytoplasmic ribosomes. Successive amino acids are added to the polypeptide chain according to the triplet code on the mRNA, which is recognized by the transfer RNA (tRNA), to which each corresponding amino acid is covalently bound. Translation is commenced upon recognition of an initiation codon (usually but not exclusively AUG/methionine) and terminated upon recognition of a stop codon. The polypeptide subsequently undergoes a variable degree of post-translational modification and/or cleavage to produce the mature protein product, which may have an intracellular role or may be exported to the endoplasmic reticulum and hence to the extracellular space to execute its function.

The mitochondrial genome is considerably smaller than the nuclear genome, but it deserves mention here because of the increasing recognition of the role of mitochondrial DNA (mtDNA) mutations in human disease. The mitochondrial genome is only 16.6 kb in size, comprising 37 genes, which encode polypeptides which are principally involved in the respiratory chain. mtDNA is double-stranded but does not form a double-helix nor does it form chromosomes, but instead it takes the form of a circular double-stranded DNA structure with a heavy and a light strand. Unlike the nuclear genome, which is inherited from mother and father, the mitochondrial genome of an individual is entirely maternally inherited.

KEY POINTS

- The double-stranded alpha helical structure of DNA, mainly located in the nucleus, consists of nucleotide triplets called codons which code for specific amino acids and stop signals, and forms the substrate for hereditary information in eukaryotes.
- The 22 pairs of autosomes and one pair of sex chromosomes, each with their distinctive shape, size and banding pattern, represent a complex folding of DNA around proteins to give the characteristic shape of a central constriction (centromere) separating the chromosome into a long arm (q) and a short arm (p) with a telomere cap at each end to maintain structural integrity.
- Chromosome locus nomenclature: chromosome number – 3p21 – position on chromosome arm.
- Semiconservative replication of DNA during normal cell division results in the separation of two strands of DNA by DNA helicase, each strand then acting as a template for polymerization by DNA polymerase. High fidelity is vital to prevent permanent change or mutations.
- A gene is a region of chromosomal DNA which produces functional RNA consisting of:
  - regulatory DNA sequences;
  - exons, which are coding sequences;
  - introns, which are noncoding sequences.
- Transcription is the intranuclear process driven by RNA polymerase whereby one of the two DNA strands acts as a template for single-stranded RNA synthesis complementary to the DNA, except that in RNA U is replaced by T. Splicing refers to post-transcriptional processing of RNA.
- Translation is the cytoplasmic process in which mRNA acts as a template for the synthesis of polypeptide by adding successive amino acids to the polypeptide chain, according to the triplet codon of the mRNA which is recognized by the tRNA to which the corresponding amino acid is covalently bonded. This process is regulated and catalyzed by cytoplasmic ribosomes. Post-translational modification produces mature proteins.

METHODS IN MOLECULAR BIOLOGY

Basic techniques of DNA fragmentation and identification

Unlike RNA, DNA is extremely stable, which is understandable from the function that each has in the cell. For purposes of studying the DNA and in order to clone specific DNA, the DNA molecule needs to be divided into manageable fragments. Although the ability to cut (and also to join up) DNA molecules now appears to be a very straightforward process, it was only 1970 when the first restriction endonuclease was identified in a strain of *Haemophilus influenzae*, hence its name *Hind*II (pronounced Hin-dee-two). It is believed that this restriction endonucleases act *in vivo* in bacteria as an immune or host-defence system, recognizing non-self DNA in bacteriophages and cleaving them. By surveying many different bacteria, a wide range of restriction endonucleases is now available, each of which recognize specific target sites based on sequences of four to eight nucleotides. As a specific, seven nucleotide sequence (heptanucleotide) will occur less frequently than a four nucleotide sequence (tetranucleotide), statistically, endonucleases recognizing heptanucleotide targets will cut less frequently thereby yielding larger fragments than those recognizing tetranucleotides. As the DNA is double-stranded, the resultant fragments may have blunt ends or cohesive ('sticky') ends (**Figure 1.1**). The nature of the ends of DNA fragments thus generated impact upon the way in which they can be ligated (joined) into recombinant molecules. Ligation of DNA fragments with cohesive ends is more efficient than joining of blunt-ended fragments.

ELECTROPHORESIS

Negatively charged phosphate groups on the DNA backbone confer a net negative charge on linear DNA. This allows fragments of different sizes to be resolved within a suitable gel matrix by the application of an electric current across the matrix. The DNA will migrate toward the positive electrode with the smaller fragments travelling faster than the larger fragments.[4] The size of the fragment can be estimated by the use of a graduated DNA

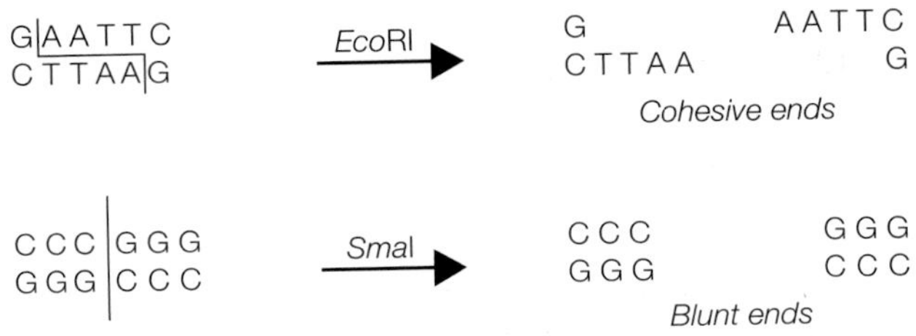

Figure 1.1 DNA cleavage by restriction endonucleases. Derived from Ref. 11, with permission.

ladder containing fragments of known molecular weight. The choice of the particular matrix depends on the fragment sizes that one is trying to resolve. Polyacrylamide gels can resolve differences of just one base pair between fragments of several hundred base pairs in size by virtue of a small pore size in the gel matrix. These gels can be used for DNA sequencing and resolution of alleles varying in only one dinucleotide repeat. Agarose gels can resolve fragment sizes from around 100 bp to 20 kb. Beyond that size, electrophoretic mobility is no longer proportional to fragment size. Resolution of fragments sizes in excess of 50 kb, such as larger bacterial artificial chromosomes (BAC) or yeast artificial chromosomes (YAC) require the use of pulsed field electrophoresis.

HYBRIDIZATION

Hybridization is the specific annealing of single DNA (or RNA) strands, the probe, to a DNA sample, the target. It serves to detect the presence of a specific sequence of DNA either in the cell or on a hybridization membrane and recognition that hybridization has occurred is achieved either by radioactively labelling the probe and localizing the radioactivity by autoradiography or by labelling the probe with fluorochromes which fluoresce when excited by light of specific wavelengths (**Figure 1.2**). Hybridization on a membrane requires the initial transfer of DNA on to a nitrocellulose membrane from an agarose gel. This elegantly simple process is eponymously known as Southern blotting after the scientist who described the process in 1975. Two other commonly used transfer techniques have their names derived from Southern blotting as jargon terms. Northern blotting is essentially the same process used for transfer of RNA to a membrane. Western blotting is one of the mainstays of protein analysis and involves the transfer of electrophoresed protein bands from a polyacrylamide gel on to a nitrocellulose or nylon membrane to which they bind strongly. Detection of the protein is usually achieved by the use of antibodies to specific antigens presented by the protein with the antibody being labelled radioactively, enzymatically or fluorescently.

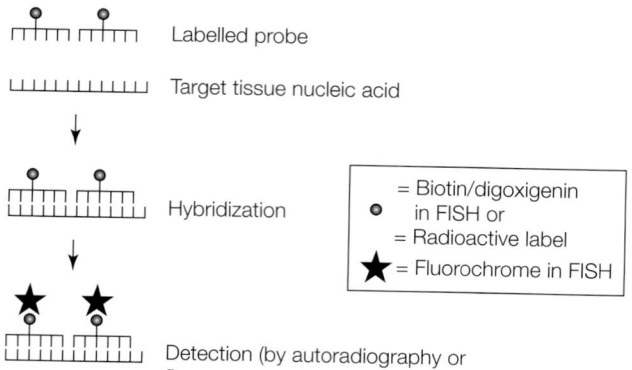

Labelled probe

Target tissue nucleic acid

Hybridization

= Biotin/digoxigenin in FISH or
= Radioactive label
★ = Fluorochrome in FISH

Detection (by autoradiography or fluorescence microscopy)

Figure 1.2 *In situ* hybridization.

CYTOGENETICS AND MOLECULAR CYTOGENETICS

Although microscopy had already reached high levels of resolution in the early 1930s, the correct number of human chromosomes was not determined until 1958. The era of classical cytogenetics was thus begun. Cytogenetics is the study of chromosomal abnormalities and rearrangements. It currently has a major role to play in prenatal diagnosis of Downs syndrome and other congenital syndromes characterized by numerical chromosomal abnormalities. In the early part of this century, Theodore Boveri proposed that cancer arose from chromosomal alterations. This hypothesis was not proven until the consistent chromosomal translocation, t(9;22), was demonstrated in chronic myeloid leukaemia. Since that time, cytogenetic analysis has been the mainstay of genetic analysis in reticuloendothelial malignancies, being responsible for the identification of consistent translocations in different leukaemias. Its use in solid tumours has been hampered by the difficulties of establishing short-term primary cultures from head and neck cancers for chromosomal analysis and the erratically acquired chromosomal changes in long-term cell lines, which may have occurred *in vitro*, influenced by culture conditions. Nevertheless, some studies have identified chromosomal areas consistently showing frequent breakpoints suggesting the location of putative tumour suppressor genes (including 3p21, 5p14, 8p11, 17p21, 18q21) and gain or amplification implying the presence of putative proto-oncogenes at other sites (including 3q, 5p, 8q, 11q13). Although the refinement of karyotyping has been radically enhanced by the introduction of 24-colour combinatorial multifluor FISH (M-FISH), the resolution and therefore utility of solid tumour karyotyping remains limited.[5]

Hybridization to target DNA in cells, using fluorescence detection, is known as fluorescence *in situ* hybridization (FISH). Fluorescence *in situ* hybridization allows the analysis of copy number of a known specific DNA sequence within intact nuclei. In reticuloendothelial malignancies and solid tumour-derived cell lines, the use of both single-copy probes and centromere alpha-satellite repeat probes on metaphase preparations has enhanced and refined classical karyotyping. Interphase FISH has been applied to solid tumour sections to assess the copy number of a known sequence in breast, prostate, bladder, brain, lung and head and neck tumours.

Fluorescence-labelled hybridization has also been combined with cytogenetics to produce the powerful technique of comparative genomic hybridization (CGH).[6] Comparative genomic hybridization permits the rapid medium resolution screening of the entire genome by comparatively hybridizing matched tumour and normal DNA from a patient, which are labelled with different fluorochromes, on to normal metaphase chromosome preparations. Under red-green dual filter fluorescence microscopy and computer-aided image analysis, areas of genetic 'neutrality' appear yellow, under-representation appears green, and over-representation appears red. Areas of genetic under-representation suggest the possibility of a tumour suppressor gene lying within that region while areas of over-representation may indicate the location of a putative oncogene. This technique has been applied to the rapid genetic analysis of many tumour types including squamous cell carcinomas of the head and neck. The advent of molecular cytogenetics has obviated the need for primary short-term cultures and refined the location of chromosomal aberrations in solid tumours.

POLYMERASE CHAIN REACTION

Perhaps the single molecular technique which has had the most dramatic impact on molecular biology has been the polymerase chain reaction (PCR). The original problem lay in obtaining sufficient quantities of a particular DNA sequence such that DNA profiling (e.g. sequencing) and DNA manipulation (e.g. cloning) could be achieved. The only 'requirement' is that the sequences flanking the stretch of DNA of interest is known. With that proviso, PCR achieves faithful and exponential amplification of a specific sequence of DNA by repeated cycles each consisting of dsDNA denaturation, hybridization of specific oligonucleotides (primers) and extension of the polynucleotide by rapidly altering the reaction temperature between segments of each cycle. dsDNA denaturation is achieved by raising the temperature of the reaction to 94°C for 30 seconds, thus disrupting the hydrogen bonds between the strands and exposing the hydrogen bond donor and acceptor groups to allow base pairing. The oligonucleotide primers are then allowed to hybridize to the denatured DNA (annealing) at around 55–65°C for 90 seconds before the reaction temperature is raised to 72°C to permit extension of the DNA strand by DNA polymerase in the presence of deoxynucleoside triphosphates (dNTPs). With each cycle resulting in the

doubling of the copies of the DNA sequence, a 30-cycle PCR taking approximately two hours would amplify a single copy of a DNA sequence 268 million-fold (**Figure 1.3**). Although the PCR was originally described by Mullis and Faloona in 1987, one practical problem prevented its instant exploitation.[7] The DNA polymerase used in the original reaction was denatured during the DNA denaturation segment and therefore had to be added after each and every cycle. The solution came in 1989 when Lawyer isolated and characterized the DNA polymerase, Taq polymerase, from the thermophilic bacterium *Thermus aquaticus* which normally resided in temperatures above 95°C.[8] This polymerase was therefore 'heat resistant' and did not need to be replenished between cycles.

The PCR holds a central position in many molecular biological techniques as well as clinical diagnostic methods. The fundamental principle of DNA amplification has been adapted to amplify messenger RNA and to amplify areas where the initial flanking oligonucleotide sequences are not known. It is often described as a sensitive and powerful technique, but with great power comes the potential for corruption! In theory, a single copy of DNA can be amplified. Therefore, careless experimental technique may lead to contamination of the DNA sample with other DNA (e.g. from the skin of the investigator) and consequently to an artefactual result. The Taq polymerase originally described in the technique does not have proofreading properties, but newer cloned enzymes such as Pfu polymerase incorporates a proofreading function to increase amplification fidelity for sequencing reactions.

The sensitivity of PCR also presented a problem for the analysis of genetic alterations in certain solid tumours. Squamous cell carcinomas of the head and neck are histologically often characterized by a large stromal element within the tumour. The genetic alterations in the tumour may not be present in the stromal

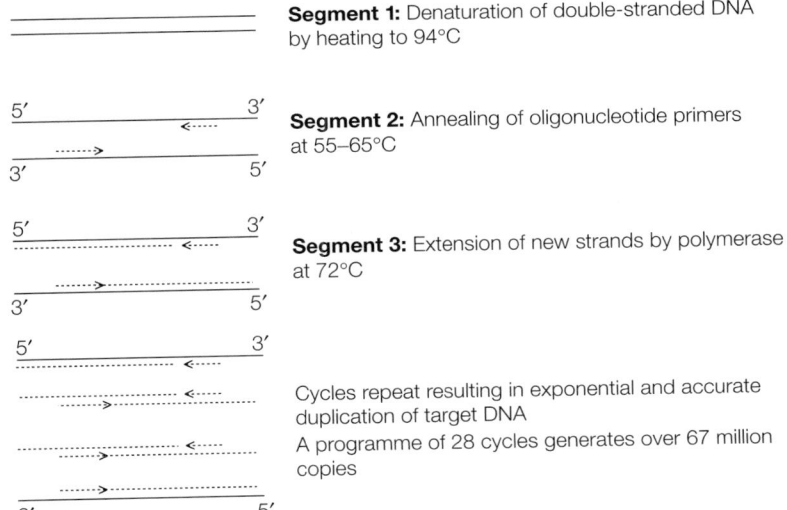

Segment 1: Denaturation of double-stranded DNA by heating to 94°C

Segment 2: Annealing of oligonucleotide primers at 55–65°C

Segment 3: Extension of new strands by polymerase at 72°C

Cycles repeat resulting in exponential and accurate duplication of target DNA
A programme of 28 cycles generates over 67 million copies

Figure 1.3 The polymerase chain reaction.

tissue and thus total DNA extracted from the tumour will contain DNA from both benign and malignant tissue. This *in situ* contamination can now be eliminated by the use of laser capture microdissection (LCM) of tumours. LCM involves the placement of a laser-activated film over a tissue specimen. When areas of 'pure' tumour cells are identified, a focal laser pulse lifts the tissue on to the film in specimens down to 30 μm in diameter.[9]

KEY POINTS

- Restriction endonucleases are enzymes that were initially identified in bacteria that can cut and join up DNA. They recognize specific target sites based on sequences of four and eight nucleotides.
- Electrophoresis is a technique for resolving the size of DNA fragments, which carry a negative charge from the phosphate groups on their backbone. Using a gel matrix with an electric current applied across it, the DNA will migrate to the positive electrode at a rate inversely proportional to its size.
- Hybridization is the specific annealing of single DNA or RNA strands (probe) to a DNA sample (target) to detect the presence of a specific sequence of DNA in the cell or hybridization membrane. Variants include the eponomously named Southern, Northern and Western blotting techniques.
- Cytogenetics is the study of chromosomal abnormalities and rearrangements important in the diagnosis of congenital syndromes characterized by numerical chromosomal abnormalities, e.g. Downs syndrome and leukaemia types.
- FISH refers to fluorescence *in situ* hybridization which involves hybridization to target DNA cells using fluorescence detection and allows the analysis of copy number of a known specific DNA sequence within intact nuclei.
- PCR achieves faithful and exponential amplification of a specific sequence of DNA by repeated cycles each consisting of:
  - DNA denaturation by heating to 94°C to denature hydrogen bonds between strands;
  - annealing (hybridization) of oligonucleotide primers to denatured DNA at 55–65°C;
  - extension of DNA strand by DNA polymerase.

MOLECULAR ABERRATIONS OF CELLULAR BIOLOGY

Loss of heterozygosity and the expression of recessive mutant alleles

Retinoblastoma is a childhood cancer, which exhibits both hereditary and sporadic occurrence, with the inherited form transmitted as a highly penetrant autosomal dominant trait. The proposition by Alfred Knudson in 1971, based upon a statistical analysis of the occurrence of retinoblastoma in children, that two genetic events were required to inactivate the gene mitigating against development of the cancer, was a major landmark in the understanding of tumour suppressor genetics.[10] In hereditary retinoblastomas, a single additional somatic event in a cell that carried the inherited mutation was sufficient to give rise to the disease while two somatic events were required to produce a sporadic retinoblastoma. This became known as Knudson's 'two-hit' hypothesis. The subsequent study on matched tumour and blood DNA from patients with sporadic retinoblastoma by Webster Cavenee not only proved Knudson's hypothesis but also established the paradigm for all subsequent investigations of tumour suppressor genes.[11] For the first time, the now widely accepted mechanisms of tumourigenesis were reconciled, viz. that neoplasms can arise in a multistep manner, that chromosomal events can lead to tumour formation and that chromosome loss with or without reduplication can lead to expression of recessive mutations. Perhaps even more strikingly, the authors presciently suggested that development of homozygosity for recessive mutant alleles at the *Rb-1* locus may give rise to the development of other tumours and that other additional dominant mutations may be involved in the development of retinoblastoma. Cavenee proposed the various chromosomal mechanisms that could reveal recessive mutations and these are summarized for a putative tumour suppressor gene in **Figure 1.4**, adapted from the figure in his original paper. To these can now be added hypermethylation of the 5′ CpG island resulting in transcriptional inactivation of the gene, discussed below.[12] The simplest way of revealing a recessive mutant allele is by deletion of the wild-type allele, resulting in hemizygosity at the particular locus on the remaining chromosome. It is inferred from this that areas of frequent allelic loss in tumours may represent the location of putative tumour suppressor genes and this hypothesis underpins the commonly employed method of molecular detection of allelic losses, loss of heterozygosity (LOH).

The practical exploitation of the concepts outlined above hinges on the presence of the previously described microsatellites, highly polymorphic noncoding DNA sequences, also referred to as simple sequence length polymorphisms (SSLP) or short tandem repeat

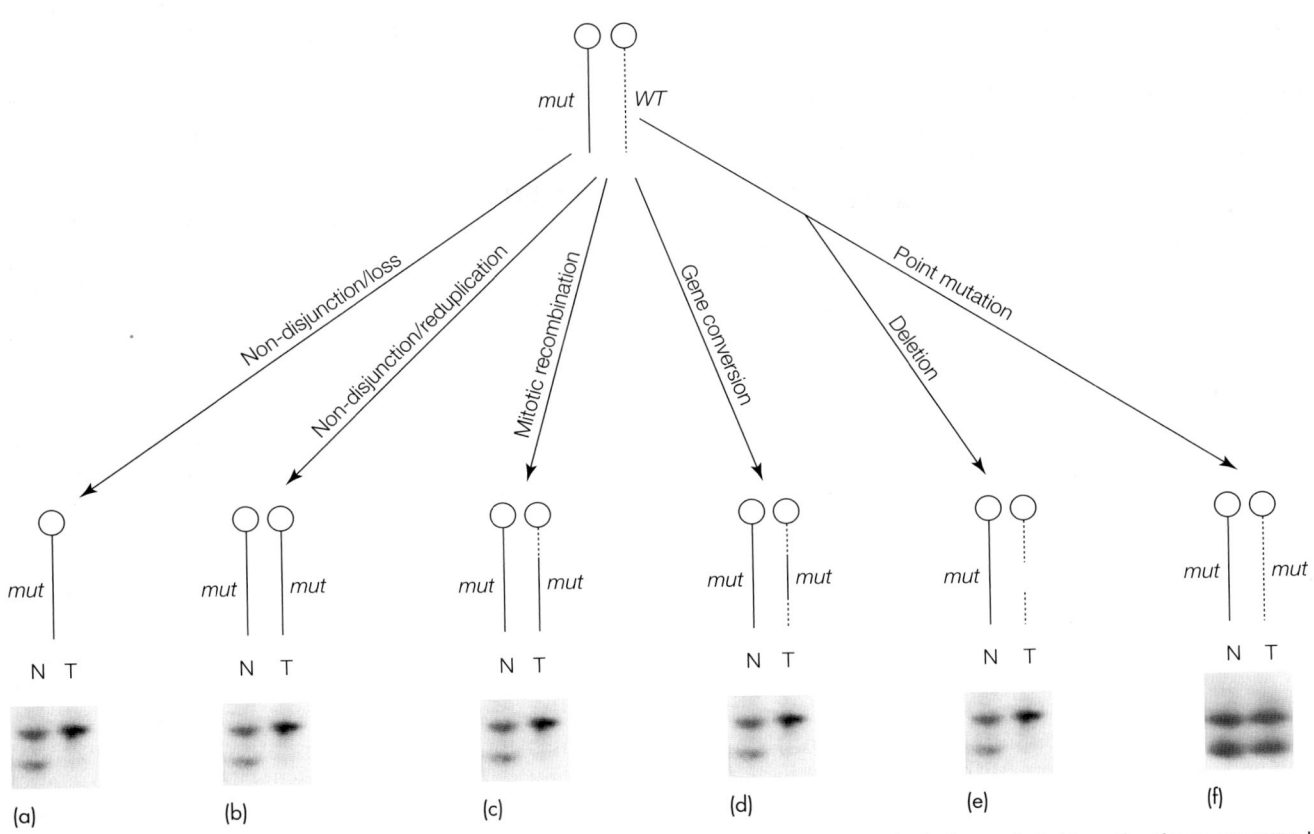

Figure 1.4 Chromosomal mechanisms that could reveal recessive mutations. In this example, before cell division, the tissue concerned carries a mutation in one copy of the hypothetical tumour suppressor gene. In each of the scenarios (a–f), the recessive mutation is revealed. If the individual is heterozygous for a microsatellite marker within or very close to the mutated gene, the hypothetical PCR results are given below each ideotype. The only mechanism which escapes observed loss of heterozygosity is F. *mut*, mutated; N, normal; T, tumour; *WT*. wildtype. After Ref. 11, with permission.

polymorphisms (STRP), which are distributed approximately every 100,000 bp throughout the human genome. These microsatellites contain small dinucleotide or trinucleotide repeat units, the number of which may differ between the two alleles in a particular person. Microsatellite markers are now available which map thousands of these sequences to chromosomal loci. When DNA sequences containing these microsatellite markers are amplified by PCR in a person heterozygous for that particular microsatellite, the PCR will yield two products of different lengths, which can be resolved on an electrophoretic gel. Where amplification of tumour DNA from such a subject yields only one product, the tumour is said to show LOH, implying allelic loss. Persons who are homozygous for a particular marker are said to be noninformative for that marker. The concept of examining the variation and extent of allelic deletion in tumours was introduced by Vogelstein in an analysis of colorectal carcinomas and termed allelotyping.[13] Allelotypes generated in this fashion have identified several areas of frequent allelic deletion from which some of the responsible tumour suppressor genes have been cloned or identified. The most common areas of loss in HNSCC are at chromosome 9p21, 17p21, 13q14, 4p, 5q21 and several discrete regions on 3p and 8p.[14, 15]

Inactivation of genes and oncogenic transformation

Allelic deletion is only one mechanism by which a copy of a gene can be inactivated. As there are two copies of each gene, inactivation of the gene requires inactivation of both copies of the gene, 'the second hit'. This may occur as a result of a genetic mutation or transcriptional silencing. Conversely, a protooncogene may be converted into an oncogene by a simple increase in the copy number of the gene (gene amplification) resulting in an overproduction of protein or by point mutations that affect the control of protein activity.

Not all mutations result in alteration in function of a gene. DNA mutation may occur as a result of base substitutions, as well as nucleotide insertions and deletions. Insertions and deletions of nucleotides are very rare in coding DNA, but if they occur they may produce a shift in the 'reading frame' which dramatically alters the coding downstream from the mutation. Base substitution is a more common form of mutation in coding DNA which may have a range of consequences on the function of the gene; a loss of function (e.g. *p53*, *Rb*), a gain in function, often due to stabilization of the active protein (e.g. *c-erbB2*, *K-ras*) or no net functional effect. Since an amino acid may be encoded by different codons with a 'third base wobble', e.g. GU**A**, GA**C**, GU**G** and GU**U** all encode valine, a substitution of the third base would result in no change to the amino acid. This is known as a silent substitution. At the other extreme is the nonsense mutation, whereby base substitution results in a stop codon which leads to truncation of the polypeptide and a dramatic reduction in function.

Loss of function in the presence of a normal (wildtype) allele may occur as a result of transcription silencing. The methylation status of CpG islands surrounding the promoter regions of genes determines whether a particular gene is expressed within a cell such that methylation of a CpG island 'switches off' the gene that it is regulating. CpG islands regulating housekeeping genes, i.e. genes encoding proteins essential for cell survival, are unmethylated in all cell types whereas those regulating cell-specific genes, e.g. muscle-specific actin gene in muscle cells, are only unmethylated in the relevant cell. Many tumour suppressor genes (e.g. *p16*, *APC*, *RASSF1A*) are now recognized to be inactivated by hypermethylation of the promoter region in malignant tumours.

Proteomics

As the Human Genome Mapping Project powers its way towards a high-resolution sequence of the entire genome, the natural progression of research has been towards the elucidation of the repertoire of proteins that control cell signalling and cell growth. Proteomics, the profiling of proteins in cells and serum by two-dimensional gel analysis separating proteins by charge and mass, by x-ray crystallography and by examination of protein interactions (e.g. with the yeast two-hybrid system) remains a young but rapidly expanding field in both basic and translational research.[16] Proteomics has the ability to identify post-translational modifications, some of which are cancer cell-specific, which would not be detected by genetic or expression profiling. The power of this approach is particularly evident in cancer studies as it has the ability to compare the entire protein pattern of tumour tissue and normal tissue in a manner analogous to comparative genomic hybridization.

Telomerase

Aberration of telomere biology has a now well-recognized role to play in cancer development. The length of the telomere is maintained in germline cells by the enzyme telomerase that is absent in normal somatic cells.[17] This observation led to the theory that progressive shortening of telomeres with each cell division leads to cell senescence and ageing of the organism. Several mechanisms for this have been proposed. A critical shortening of the telomere may leave a nontelomere free DNA end which signals cell cycle arrest. Telomere loss could also extend to the deletion or inactivation of genes located subtelomerically, again leading to cell-cycle arrest. Two important consequences of critical telomere shortening in cells which survive the cell crisis are genomic rearrangements and chromosomal loss which may in turn lead to malignant transformation. This is particularly relevant to rapidly dividing and regenerating tissues, such as skin and mucosa. Paradoxically, while some of these survivors will subsequently go into cell cycle arrest due to critical telomere length shortening, a proportion will then express telomerase activity. Such activity is capable of cell immortalization by maintaining telomere length indefinitely and its role in cancer is now unquestionable. Telomerase activity has been demonstrated in 80 percent of oral cancers and around 50 percent of oral leukoplakia lesions.[18] Even among premalignant lesions, telomerase activity was associated with degree of dysplasia, suggesting that telomerase activation occurs during the late stage of oral premalignancy. The potential for anti-telomerase drugs as a novel treatment remains promising.

KEY POINTS

- Practical techniques based on loss of heterozygosity of tumour DNA are based on Knudson's two-hit hypothesis which states that two genetic events are required to inactivate the gene mitigating against developing a condition.
- The number of microsatellite repeats, i.e. noncoding base pairs dispersed throughout the genome, may differ between two alleles in the same person making that person heterozygous for that particular allele. If tumour DNA from such a subject when amplified by PCR yields only one product, the tumour is said to show loss of heterozygosity implying allelic loss.
- Inactivation of genes can occur by
  - allelic deletion;
  - genetic mutation;
  - transcriptional silencing;
  - conversion of protooncogene to oncogene due to gene amplification.
- Some mutations do not result in change of function. They can be silent or nonsense mutations.

- Proteomics refers to the profiling of proteins in cells and serum by 2D gel analysis, x-ray crystallography and by examination of protein interactions. This can be used to identify post-translational modifications, some of which are cancer cell specific and are not detected by genetic profiling.
- Critical telomere shortening can lead to both cell cycle arrest and cell immortalization due to expression of telomerase which, for example, has been demonstrated in 80 percent of oral cancers.

MAPPING AND IDENTIFICATION OF GENES ASSOCIATED WITH DISEASE

The traditional approach to understanding the molecular biology of disease was to look for and characterize the abnormal protein. Diabetes mellitus and sickle cell anaemia are two conditions that were elucidated at the molecular level in this way. Finding the protein when present in minute quantities, in an inaccessible site such as the inner ear, or when nothing is known of its mode of action, is however virtually impossible. This is the case with most of the genes involved in cellular growth control and also in inner ear function. Our approach to understanding such conditions relies on determining the chromosomal location, isolating and sequencing the gene so that the structure of the protein can be determined. This is known as the reverse genetic or positional cloning technique.

Strategies employed in determining the sites of these disease genes include cytogenetic analysis, molecular genetic analysis (typically LOH studies) and linkage analysis. Where a clearcut inheritance of a disease can be demonstrated, then linkage analysis can be useful in determining the location of the responsible gene. The key advance that has made this approach increasingly successful has been the construction of a high-resolution linkage map of the entire human genome. This map consists of genetic markers spaced less than 1 centimorgan apart and the process of linkage involves determining which of these the disease gene is close to. Analysis of the coinheritance of the genetic marker and the disease trait in families allows one to determine the probability of their physical proximity or linkage to each other. The statistical probability of linkage is expressed in terms of LOD scores. LOD is short for logarithm to the base 10 of the odds that the markers are linked at a recombination distance of N centimorgans. An LOD score of 3.0 favours linkage while a score of -2.0 effectively rules out linkage.

Successful linkage analysis typically requires large pedigrees with many individuals known to have the disease trait and likewise many confirmed to be free of the disease. The process involves initial family analysis with clinical evaluation and accurate diagnosis. DNA samples are then obtained from each individual and genotyping and linkage analysis can then be carried out. Linkage and molecular deletion analysis generate genetic markers either side of the disease gene location. These genetic markers can be used to identify 'chunks of genomic DNA' cloned into yeast (yeast artificial chromosomes (YAC)) or bacteria (bacterial artificial chromosomes/P1 artificial chromosomes (BAC/PAC)) and organized into libraries. By a number of methods, these 'chunks' of genomic DNA can be directionally organized to produce a physical map of the region of interest from which candidate disease genes can be identified. The Human Genome Mapping Project has, to a great extent, physically mapped the human genome such that in some cases, when the region of interest is sufficiently small, all genes known to be between the markers can be considered positional candidates. The candidates are then analysed in disease families until one is found that demonstrates mutations in affected individuals.

To facilitate the identification of the disease gene from a number of candidates within a particular region, several strategies are available. One such approach exploits our knowledge of animal models of the diseases that parallel human inherited disorders. Another potential source of candidate genes is to identify and characterize genes that are expressed within a particular tissue. Genes expressed within the cochlea, for example, represent the genes critical for cochlear function and thus are excellent candidates genes for hereditary hearing loss.

KEY POINT

- Strategies employed in determining the sites of disease genes which code for the abnormal proteins include cytogenetic, molecular genetic and linkage analysis.

Deficiencies in current knowledge and areas for future research

Although giant strides have already been made in the delineation of molecular events underlying disease processes, the knowledge of these events is far from comprehensive. A clearly identifiable adenoma–carcinoma sequence facilitated the correlation between genetic and histopathological progression models in colorectal cancer.[13] Several similar progression models have been proposed in head and neck squamous cell carcinoma evolution from epithelial dysplasia through to frank carcinoma, but the heterogeneity of carcinomas in different subsites precludes a molecular genetic progression model of equal rigour to that in colorectal cancer. Nevertheless, *p16* and *p53* inactivation have been identified as the two most frequent and critical events in head and neck carcinogenesis. An understanding of the sequence of genetic aberrations that occur in pathogenesis of tumours can assist in the prediction of progression from premalignant conditions to frank malignancy. An example of this is seen in the accumulation of genetic abnormalities in oral epithelium leading to the progression of oral dysplasia to oral squamous cell carcinoma. By analysing for loss of heterozygosity at 19 microsatellite loci in a series of oral dysplastic lesions and oral malignancies, Rosin *et al.*[19] showed that LOH at 3p and/or 9p occurred in virtually all cases of oral dysplasia which progressed to frank malignancy implying a 'gatekeeper' role of genes at those loci in the development of oral cancer, in themselves imparting a 3.8-fold increased relative risk of progression to squamous carcinoma. Furthermore, additional LOH at 4q, 8p, 11q or 17p imparted a 33-fold increased relative risk for developing cancer.[19] In certain cases, molecular genetic profiling has added a new dimension to age-old debates. For example, discordant genetic anomalies in inverted sinonasal papillomas and sinonasal carcinomas lend weight to the opinion that the former does not undergo malignant degeneration into the latter.[20]

Traditional methods of allelotyping and mutational analysis remain extremely time-consuming and labour-intensive. Recent years have seen the development of gene arrays (or 'gene chips') which allow the rapid assessment of the genetic profile of tumours or cell lines.[21] cDNA of up to 30,000 genes can be placed in arrays on glass slides on to which DNA and RNA samples can be allowed to hybridize using an automated two-colour fluorescence method for detection.[22] Hybridization with DNA can yield extensive genomic information, while hybridization with RNA takes genetic profiling a step further by semiquantitatively analysing the expression of genes rather than simply the presence or absence of the DNA. As the genetic aberrations and pathways associated with specific tumour development become better dissected, 'designer' chips can be produced which allow for screening for known mutations of those involved genes.[23] Array technology has also been married with molecular cytogenetics to produce array-based comparative genomic hybridization, which obviates the need for metaphase chromosome spreads for CGH.

The clinician might be forgiven for an expression of cynicism regarding the 'molecular revolution', feeling that little has changed despite ambitious predictions. The translation of molecular biology research into clinical practice – 'from laboratory to bedside' is without doubt the greatest challenge facing the clinician scientist. Progress so far has been largely at the level of disease classification, premorbid diagnosis and patient

counselling. However, several discrete arms to translational research have hinted at the future role of genetic analysis determining the likely effectiveness of existing anti-cancer treatments. There are also isolated examples of effective novel therapeutic interventions.

Molecular analysis played a vital role in differentiating neurofibromatosis type I from neurofibromatosis type II, and it now seems difficult to understand how we ever confused the two in the first place. Such clarity of diagnosis is also anticipated for many syndromic and nonsyndromic causes of sensorineural hearing loss as the genes are characterized and the clinical features analysed in more detail. This may enable clinicians to determine in which cases hearing loss will be progressive and target monitoring more appropriately. Diagnostic genetic testing will also become increasingly available to families with hereditary hearing loss and clinicians will need to be conversant with the ethical issues of testing and the implications of the results. By characterizing hearing loss at the molecular level we are also developing a greater understanding of inner ear physiology as the critical proteins involved in hearing become elucidated. This may lead to the development of agents able to repair and regenerate the diseased inner ear. The administration of these agents is already being evaluated using miniature infusion pumps.

It is hoped that in the future molecular characterization of tumour tissue will provide for a more accurate diagnosis and prognosis than conventional histopathological analysis. This may lead to a more rational treatment plan based on molecular features. Some genotype–phenotype correlations have already been made, particularly with respect to radio- and chemoresistance in tumours, but which need confirmation with larger sample sizes as to their applicability into clinical practice. Refinement of the staging of tumours by probing of resection margins and the detection of histological subclinical metastatic disease in regional lymph nodes have been elegantly demonstrated by Brennan *et al.*[24] at Johns Hopkins. However, the technical complexity of the methodology has precluded its widespread application in the clinical arena. The development of technically simpler but equally sensitive techniques will inevitably render molecular staging routine in oncological practice. Although surveillance for tumour recurrence is less of a problem in the upper aerodigestive tract when compared with intraabdominal malignancies, the emergence of molecular markers in saliva and serum will have a role in follow-up protocols for head and neck cancers.[25]

A comprehensive understanding of the molecular mechanisms underlying disease processes gives the potential of therapeutic restoration of DNA or protein function, as well as exploitation of the genetic abnormality for targetting of therapy. An example of the latter is the use of ONYX-015. ONYX-015 is an E1B

55-kDa gene-deleted adenovirus engineered to selectively replicate in and lyse *p53*-deficient cells while sparing normal cells. This tumour-targetting property has led to a successful phase II trial of concomitant ONYX-015 and cisplatin/5-FU in the treatment of recurrent HNSCC which indicated substantial objective responses, as well as a high proportion of complete responses.[26] Post-treatment biopsies of tumour masses confirmed the replication selectivity of the virus *in vivo*.

A consideration of some of the landmarks in molecular biology, e.g. enzymatic DNA cleavage (1970) and PCR (1987), readily indicates that molecular biology is a relatively young science. However, the rapid development of molecular techniques of such power and diversity as comparative genomic hybridization and gene array technology has permitted the dissection of molecular pathways and the identification of their disruption in disease processes. Some of these processes in specific diseases will be discussed in subsequent chapters. The future in the laboratory lies in the extension of our understanding of these molecular processes and the future in the clinic lies in the exploitation of these molecular techniques in better informing disease classification, staging and treatment:

➤ Development of a molecular genetic progression model for head and neck squamous cell carcinoma of similar rigour to that for colorectal carcinoma.
➤ Development of gene arrays or gene chips which allow the rapid assessment of the genetic profile of tumours and can allow semiquantitative analysis of gene expression.
➤ Designer chips may be produced which allow for screening for unknown mutations of involved genes.
➤ Potential role for genetic analysis in determining the likely effectiveness of existing anticancer treatments.
➤ Providing more accurate diagnosis and prognosis than conventional histopathological techniques.
➤ Potential therapeutic restoration of DNA or protein function, as well as exploitation of a genetic abnormality for targeting therapy, e.g. use of ONYX-015.

REFERENCES

1. Hampson K, Bourn D. Principles of molecular genetics. *Journal of Laryngology and Otology*. 1998; **112**: 128–31.
2. Sharp PA. Splicing of messenger RNA precursors. *Science*. 1987; **235**: 766–71.
3. McKeown M. Alternative mRNA splicing. *Annual Review of Cell Biology*. 1992; **8**: 133–55.
4. Broomfield A, Bourn D. Basic techniques in molecular genetics. *Journal of Laryngology and Otology*. 1998; **112**: 230–4.
5. Speicher MR, Gwyn Ballard S, Ward DC. Karyotyping human chromosomes by combinatorial multi-fluor FISH. *Nature Genetics*. 1996; **12**: 368–75.
6. Kallioniemi A, Kallioniemi OP, Sudar D, Rutovitz D, Gray JW, Waldman F et al. Comparative genomic hybridization for molecular cytogenetic analysis of solid tumors. *Science*. 1992; **258**: 818–21.
7. Mullis KB, Faloona FA. Specific synthesis of DNA in vitro via a polymerase-catalyzed chain reaction. *Methods in Enzymology*. 1987; **155**: 335–50.
8. Lawyer FC, Stoffel S, Saiki RK, Myambo K, Drummond R, Gelfand DH. Isolation, characterization, and expression in *Escherichia coli* of the DNA polymerase gene from *Thermus aquaticus*. *Journal of Biological Chemistry*. 1989; **264**: 6427–37.
9. Emmert-Buck MR, Bonner RF, Smith PD, Chuaqui RF, Zhuang Z, Goldstein SR et al. Laser capture microdissection. *Science*. 1996; **274**: 998–1001.
10. Knudson Jr. AG. Mutation and cancer: statistical study of retinoblastoma. *Proceedings of the National Academy of Sciences of the United States of America*. 1971; **68**: 820–3.
11. Cavenee WK, Dryja TP, Phillips RA, Benedict WF, Godbout R, Gallie BL et al. Expression of recessive alleles by chromosomal mechanisms in retinoblastoma. *Nature*. 1983; **305**: 779–84.
12. Merlo A, Herman JG, Mao L, Lee DJ, Gabrielson E, Burger PC et al. 5′ CpG island methylation is associated with transcriptional silencing of the tumour suppressor p16/CDKN2/MTS1 in human cancers. *Nature Medicine*. 1995; **1**: 686–92.
13. Vogelstein B, Fearon ER, Kern SE, Hamilton SR, Preisinger AC, Nakamura Y et al. Allelotype of colorectal carcinomas. *Science*. 1989; **244**: 207–11.
14. Ah-See KW, Cooke TG, Pickford IR, Soutar D, Balmain A. An allelotype of squamous carcinoma of the head and neck using microsatellite markers. *Cancer Research*. 1994; **54**: 1617–21.
15. Nawroz H, van der Riet P, Hruban RH, Koch W, Ruppert JM, Sidransky D. Allelotype of head and neck squamous cell carcinoma. *Cancer Research*. 1994; **54**: 1152–5.
16. Pandey A, Mann M. Proteomics to study genes and genomes. *Nature*. 2000; **405**: 837–46.
17. Greider CW. Telomeres, telomerase and senescence. *Bioessays*. 1990; **12**: 363–9.
18. Mutirangura A, Supiyaphun P, Trirekapan S, Sriuranpong V, Sakuntabhai A, Yenrudi S et al. Telomerase activity in oral leukoplakia and head and neck squamous cell carcinoma. *Cancer Research*. 1996; **56**: 3530–3.
19. Rosin MP, Cheng X, Poh C, Lam WL, Huang Y, Lovas J et al. Use of allelic loss to predict malignant risk for low-grade oral epithelial dysplasia. *Clinical Cancer Research*. 2000; **6**: 357–62.
20. Califano J, Koch W, Sidransky D, Westra WH. Inverted sinonasal papilloma: a molecular genetic appraisal of its putative status as a precursor to squamous cell carcinoma. *American Journal of Pathology*. 2000; **156**: 333–7.

21. Lakhani SR, Ashworth A. Microarray and histopathological analysis of tumours: the future and the past? Nature Reviews. *Cancer*. 2001; **1**: 151–7.

22. Schena M, Shalon D, Davis RW, Brown PO. Quantitative monitoring of gene expression patterns with a complementary DNA microarray. *Science*. 1995; **270**: 467–70.

23. Perou CM, Sorlie T, Eisen MB, van de Rijn M, Jeffrey SS, Rees CA *et al.* Molecular portraits of human breast tumours. *Nature*. 2000; **406**: 747–52.

24. Brennan JA, Mao L, Hruban RH, Boyle JO, Eby YJ, Koch WM *et al.* Molecular assessment of histopathological staging in squamous-cell carcinoma of the head and neck. *New England Journal of Medicine*. 1995; **332**: 429–35.

25. Boyle JO, Mao L, Brennan JA, Koch WM, Eisele DW, Saunders JR *et al.* Gene mutations in saliva as molecular markers for head and neck squamous cell carcinomas. *American Journal of Surgery*. 1994; **168**: 429–32.

26. Khuri FR, Nemunaitis J, Ganly I, Arseneau J, Tannock IF, Romel L *et al.* A controlled trial of intratumoral ONYX-015, a selectively-replicating adenovirus, in combination with cisplatin and 5-fluorouracil in patients with recurrent head and neck cancer. *Nature Medicine*. 2000; **6**: 879–85.

FURTHER READING

Alberts B, Johnson A, Lewis J, Raff M, Roberts K, Walter P. *Molecular biology of the cell*, 4th edn. Oxford: Garland Science, 2002.

Latchman D (ed.). *Basic molecular and cell biology*, 3rd edn. London: BMJ Publishing Group, 1997.

Primrose SB, Twyman RM, Old RW. *Principles of Gene Manipulation*, 6th edn. Oxford: Blackwell Science, 2002.

Strachan T, Read AP. *Human molecular genetics*, 2nd edn. Oxford: BIOS Scientific Publishers, 2001.

2

Genetics

KAREN P STEEL

Introduction to DNA and its use	15	The mouse as a model	20
Variation	16	Other otorhinolaryngological disorders	20
Gene interactions	16	What lessons have we learned from genetic research so far?	20
Genes and environment	16		
What is the contribution of genetics to hearing impairment?	17	Key points	21
		Deficiencies in current knowledge and areas for future research	21
How many genes are involved?	18		
Inheritance	18	References	21
Mapping and cloning genes	19		

SEARCH STRATEGY

The data in this chapter are supported by a large number of PubMed searches using a wide variety of relevant key words, including names of authors, names of syndromes and general terms such as hearing impairment. Key words included genetics, DNA, inheritance, hearing impairment, deafness and balance.

INTRODUCTION TO DNA AND ITS USE

Our genome has a pervasive influence upon all aspects of our lives, including hearing and balance. Each cell in our body contains 23 pairs of chromosomes, one of each pair inherited from our mother and the other of the pair from our father, and each complete set consists of a total of 3,000,000,000 bases (3000 Mb) of deoxyribonucleic acid (DNA). The sequence of these DNA bases has been established to a high degree of certainty and is freely available through the world wide web.[1] Much of the sequence has no known function (yet), but using a variety of techniques it has been estimated that there are probably up to 30,000 genes scattered throughout the genome. A gene can be defined simply as a functional unit, a sequence that can be used by the cell to produce a useful molecule, most frequently a protein. The gene is used to make a copy (transcription into messenger RNA or mRNA) which is then used for translation by the cellular machinery into a string of amino acids to form a protein.

Each run of three bases in the mRNA copy of the gene is called a codon. As there are four different types of base available and three bases per codon, there are a total of 64 different combinations that each determine the addition of a specific amino acid to the end of the growing chain or alternatively will stop the translation at the end of the protein (a stop codon). This specification of a particular amino acid by a string of three bases is called the genetic code.

Genes are sometimes present in the genome as a single contiguous sequence of DNA, but most often they are broken up into smaller stretches (exons) that are separated by stretches of noncoding DNA (introns). The number of exons varies between genes; for example, the GJB2 gene commonly involved in childhood deafness has only two exons, while the MYO7A gene which underlies one form of Usher syndrome has 49 exons, and some very large genes can have over 100 exons. After transcription of the mRNA from the gene, the introns are removed from the copy by splicing. Many genes show alternative splicing, which means that some mRNA copies (and presumably the proteins constructed using these mRNAs) are made with some exons excluded, or with exons used in different combinations. These variant splice forms may produce proteins that serve different functions in the cell, so the phenomenon of alternative splicing can lead to an enormous diversity of functional molecules from the relatively small number of 30,000 genes.

As a cell differentiates to serve a specific purpose in the body, such as a sensory hair cell or a neuron, it requires a specific set of proteins to carry out its function. Furthermore, the process of development into a specific cell type is driven by the expression (use of a gene to produce a protein by the cell) of particular genes. Thus, it is clear that control of transcription and translation of genes is critical to normal development and function. Many of the genes we study encode transcription factors, which are proteins that influence the transcription and translation (expression) of other genes. We know that some of the noncoding stretches of DNA in the genome have a critical role in this process of control of expression. Therefore, when we search for variations (mutations) in DNA sequences that lead to hearing or balance problems, we need to consider noncoding sequences that may influence gene expression as well as looking for changes in the coding sequences of genes. For example, the *POU3F4* gene is involved in X-linked mixed conductive and sensorineural hearing impairment with gusher, but some of the mutations affecting expression of this gene lie far upstream (900 kb away) of the coding sequence.[2] Variants in noncoding sequences may control the amount of expression of a gene, the location (which cell types) of expression, or the timing of expression during development.

VARIATION

DNA sequence from different individuals differs at around one base per thousand. This variation is called polymorphism. We are a long way from understanding the consequences of all variations in sequence, but it is reasonable to assume that some of these polymorphisms will influence the development and function of the person. The polymorphisms may consist of a substitution of one base by another, the deletion or addition of one or more bases or of large stretches of DNA, or rearrangements of large chromosomal regions such as inversions. As there are so many variations in DNA sequence between individuals, it is difficult to establish conclusively which of the many differences is responsible for a particular feature, such as hearing impairment. The term mutation is often used to describe a change in DNA that has a deleterious effect, but strictly speaking it can also be used to describe a polymorphism with a beneficial influence.

GENE INTERACTIONS

Genes do not work in isolation. They work in the context of the variations in all the other genes carried by that individual and the environment to which the individual is exposed. Thus, a person may have a hearing impairment because of a mutation in a single gene, or because they carry two or more variations in genes that together contribute towards poor auditory function, or because they carry a variation that makes the individual more susceptible to adverse environmental conditions. We know most about the role of single gene mutations in deafness because these are the simplest causes to study as there is only one gene to track down and the mutations often have a clearcut, categorical effect that is easy to ascertain, such as severe or profound deafness.[3, 4, 5] Interactions between two or more gene variants are more difficult to study. Phenotypic features associated with variants in several genes are referred to as polygenic features, and the locations (loci) of these variations in the genome are often called quantitative trait loci (QTL) because they each make a contribution to a trait that can be measured (such as auditory thresholds). Finding the causative variations in these situations is usually very difficult because each variant may account for only a small fraction of the measurable trait, such as 10 percent or less. Furthermore, it is thought that many diseases may be influenced by a number of variant genes dispersed amongst the population, so a group of people with the same measurable deficit (for example, the same degree of hearing impairment) may carry different combinations of variant genes making it even more difficult to find each one.

Even in cases where a single gene defect is the primary cause of a hearing impairment, the clinical phenotype may be influenced by variants in other genes, called modifiers, carried in the genetic background of an individual. Modifiers are variants of genes that can either ameliorate or exacerbate the effects of a single gene mutation and they may account for differences in the degree or time of onset of a hearing impairment in two people who carry the same primary deleterious mutation.[6] We presume the modifiers act in the same molecular pathway as the primary gene. For example, modifiers may lead to increased expression of alternative genes that might be able to compensate to some extent for the abnormal function of the primary gene. A modifier would not necessarily have any obvious effect on hearing in the absence of a primary deleterious mutation.

GENES AND ENVIRONMENT

It is well known that environmental factors, such as excessive noise exposure, drugs like aminoglycosides or diuretics, or infections including meningitis can lead to hearing loss. However, not all people working in the same noisy environment develop the same degree of hearing loss, and not all children who contract meningitis end up deaf. Why should this be? It has long been suspected that individuals may have a genetic predisposition to damaging environmental factors, and we are now beginning to accumulate evidence for genetic variations that can make a carrier more or less sensitive to damage. The clearest example in humans is the A1555G mutation of the mitochondrial genome, in which the normal base A at position 1555 in the sequence is changed to a G. People carrying this mutation show a greatly increased sensitivity to hearing loss after treatment with aminoglycoside antibiotics.[7] In mice, we now know of variants in at least four different genes that make the carriers more sensitive to noise-induced hearing loss.[8] It is clear that we are only just beginning to reveal the role of specific gene variants in making us more or less susceptible to hearing loss triggered by environmental factors, and that there are many more such variants awaiting discovery.

WHAT IS THE CONTRIBUTION OF GENETICS TO HEARING IMPAIRMENT?

Hearing impairment affects all age groups. Around one in 850 children is born with a significant, permanent hearing impairment, and this proportion doubles during the first decade or so of life as further children develop progressive hearing loss.[9] The number of hearing-impaired individuals increases with each additional decade, until as many as 60 percent of the over 70 age group show a 25 dB or worse permanent threshold loss.[10] Thus, a very large proportion of the population suffers some degree of hearing impairment at some stage of their life.

It is often difficult to give an accurate diagnosis of the cause of hearing impairment in an individual, so any estimates of the relative contributions of genetics and environment in the population must be viewed with caution. Most estimates suggest about half the cases of severe or profound permanent childhood deafness are due primarily to genetic causes.[11, 12] However, this is likely to be an underestimate of the true contribution of genetics because, as discussed above, it is difficult to disentangle the effects of damaging environmental factors from genetic predispositions. It is likely that all cases of hearing impairment have a genetic contribution of some sort, varying from a major contribution from a deleterious mutation in a single gene that is essential for auditory function to a minor contribution from a genetic variant that makes an individual slightly more sensitive to environmental damage.

What is the contribution of genetics to hearing impairment in older age groups? Often genetics is not considered as a potential major contributor to age-related hearing impairment (presbyacusis) and it is true that we currently know very little about the exact causes of later onset progressive deafness in the population. However, there are a number of observations that indicate that genetics does play a significant role in progressive hearing loss. Firstly, a surprisingly large number of single gene mutations have been found to be associated with late-onset progressive hearing loss.[3, 13] Some of these mutations have been identified and some only localized to a specific region of the genome. These single genes have been discovered, though the study of large pedigrees in which it is clear that hearing loss is inherited as a single gene defect, mostly as dominantly-inherited mutations (see below under Inheritance). It is a simple and logical step to suggest that a gene shown to be involved in progressive hearing impairment with onset in the 20–50-year age range in some families may have a mutation with a milder effect leading to later onset hearing loss in other families. Thus, the genes already identified as being involved with progressive hearing loss are good candidates to search for milder mutations associated with presbyacusis. Secondly, we know from studies of the mouse that there is a strong genetic influence on late-onset hearing loss, and we are starting to identify some of the genes involved in these mice. This is a useful approach because it is much easier to identify a mutated gene in the mouse than in humans because it is possible to generate large numbers of genetically well-defined mice carrying the same mutation for linkage analysis (the method used to localize a mutation to a specific region of a chromosome). Any genes contributing to late-onset hearing loss identified in the mouse represent further good candidates to screen for their involvement in human presbyacusis. Mice represent excellent models for human deafness and just about every gene discovered to be involved in deafness in the mouse has later been found to underlie a form of human deafness. Thirdly, there have been several studies published that measure the heritability (the proportion of the variance due to genetics) of auditory function in middle-aged and older human populations, using either twins, siblings or other family groups.[14, 15, 16] All these studies found relatively large estimates of heritability, from around 30 to 50 percent or more, with the higher frequencies and younger age groups (for example, 40–60 years old) showing greater degrees of heritability than lower frequencies and older age groups. These findings suggest that genetics plays an important role in presbyacusis, although it is not yet clear whether each person develops progressive hearing loss because of a single gene mutation, because of the polygenic effects of several genes summed together, or because affected people carry mutations that make them especially sensitive to environmental damage. Indeed, it seems likely that all three mechanisms will contribute to presbyacusis in the human population, even if one mechanism is the predominant cause in each individual.

The recognition that genes play a key role in progressive hearing loss is important because it changes the way we view the problem. Having a genetic basis to hearing loss is equivalent to holding a key to the molecular basis of the pathology, because we can use genetics as a tool to identify the molecules that are involved, a first step to thinking about medical strategies for treatments.

HOW MANY GENES ARE INVOLVED?

It seems likely that hundreds of genes may be involved in hearing impairment. In the case of nonsyndromic deafness (deafness alone, with no other distinguishing feature), we know at least 86 different genes can underlie deafness because we have found this number of different chromosomal locations of mutations associated with deafness.[3] Thirty-six of these genes have been identified, so we know the gene involved and the mutations of that gene that lead to hearing impairment, while in the remainder we know only a defined region of a chromosome that must contain the mutated gene, but have not yet identified the mutation that causes the deafness.[3] In the case of syndromic deafness (deafness as part of a group of features), over 400 different syndromes that include deafness are listed in Online Mendelian Inheritance in Man (OMIM), the main clinical database of genetic diseases.[17] Although the mutations leading to many of these syndromes have not yet been identified or even mapped to a specific chromosome, the fact that there are so many distinct, inherited syndromes with deafness does suggest that many further genes may be involved in hearing impairment in these cases. An excellent, up-to-date compendium of deafness genes with links to primary references and other useful databases is available on the internet.[3]

Some genes are involved only rarely in human deafness, while others have a larger role in the human population. For example, mutations in the GJB2 gene, encoding the gap junction protein connexin 26, are a relatively common cause of severe or profound childhood deafness, accounting for between 25 and 50 percent of children with recessively inherited congenital deafness in some populations.[18, 19, 20, 21] As we identify more of the genes associated with deafness, it will be important to assess their involvement in the hearing-impaired population at large, in order to develop a rational strategy for diagnosis, looking for the most common mutations first and to prioritize genes for further research.

INHERITANCE

Single gene mutations leading to a clearcut phenotype (like deafness) that is either present or absent may be inherited in several different ways. These patterns are referred to as Mendelian (after Mendel) and a Mendelian pattern of inheritance is usually a good indication that a single gene is involved rather than several genes or a complex interaction between genome and environment. The mutated gene may be located on the X chromosome or on one of the other 22 chromosomes, referred to as autosomes, or may be part of the mitochondrial genome.

The majority of genes are located on an autosome. If only a single copy of the mutation is required to have an effect on the phenotype (for example, a mutation causing Waardenburg syndrome), and the effect of this mutation overrides the action of the normal copy of the gene on the other one of the pair of chromosomes, then the mutation is said to be inherited in a dominant manner. If two copies of a mutant gene are needed to have an effect on the phenotype, one on each of the pair of chromosomes, then the inheritance is termed recessive. People carrying just one copy of a recessively inherited mutant gene will show no obvious effect. If individuals carrying just one copy of a mutant gene (heterozygotes) show a phenotype that is intermediate between those carrying two copies of the normal gene and those carrying two copies of the mutant gene (homozygotes), then the inheritance is called codominant (or semidominant). It may be the case that many mutations that are thought of as dominant are in fact codominant, but individuals with two copies of the mutant gene are rarely, if ever, seen. Autosomal recessive inheritance appears to be the most common pattern of inheritance involved in childhood deafness, while autosomal dominant inheritance often seems to be found in families with later-onset progressive hearing loss.[3, 13] A typical family with known recessive inheritance will have unaffected parents but one or more affected children, while in typical families with dominantly inherited deafness, one of the parents will have hearing impairment as well as half the children.

Mutations located on the X chromosome are called X-linked. They may be recessive or dominant in their action. However, X-linked mutations show a distinctive pattern of inheritance because males have only one X chromosome and the other of the pair is a Y chromosome containing very few genes. Therefore, males carrying a recessive mutation on their X chromosome will have no normal copy of the gene to compensate, so will show the phenotype. Females have two X chromosomes, so if they carry one copy of the mutant gene, they will usually appear normal because they have a normal copy on their other X chromosome. This leads to an unusual pattern of inheritance: only males will be affected in a family, but the mutation can only be passed on to offspring through a carrier female because males always inherit their X chromosome from their mother and their Y from their father.

Finally, mutations of the mitochondrial genome have been associated with deafness, particularly progressive hearing loss. Mitochondria are intracellular organelles that carry their own small stretch of DNA, with many copies in each cell rather than just two as for the chromosomes. Mitochondrial DNA is inherited only through the mother, not through the father, by being passed on in the cytoplasm of the oocyte. Thus, any mitochondrial mutations will show maternal inheritance, but male and female offspring can be affected equally.

Mendelian patterns of inheritance can be very useful in attributing a phenotype like deafness to a single gene defect, but they will not pick out all cases in any clinical sample. There are many reasons for this. Firstly, human families are usually relatively small and may be geographically dispersed, making it difficult to draw up and assess a pedigree and the phenotypes accurately. For recessive inheritance, the effect of small family size is that the majority of cases will probably be the first to be affected in the family, as the parents will be carriers and have a normal appearance and more distant relatives are also unlikely to be affected. One important clue to recessive inheritance in a single deaf child in some families is the relationship between the parents: if they are blood relatives, such as cousins, then it is highly likely that a recessive mutation is the cause of hearing impairment in their child. There are many different genes involved in deafness, and each is relatively rare, so any degree of common ancestry of the parents increases the likelihood that two copies of the same mutant gene will come together by chance in a child, causing deafness. Secondly, even in dominantly inherited deafness in which each generation should be affected, the hearing impairment in older relatives may have been attributed to other causes, like presbyacusis, infection or excessive noise exposure. Many cases of dominant hearing loss show progressive loss, which is often (mistakenly) not thought of as likely to be due to a single gene defect, leading to such misdiagnosis. Dominantly inherited conditions often appear to be quite variable in phenotype, showing variable expression characterized by differing degrees of impairment in affected individuals, or reduced penetrance, in which some carriers of the mutation may not show the impairment at all. Furthermore, some genes seem to be relatively mutable, so that new dominantly inherited mutations can arise *de novo* in a family causing deafness, and these can be passed on to successive generations. These features will all complicate interpretation of the pedigree and make diagnosis of a genetic cause for hearing impairment in an individual difficult.

MAPPING AND CLONING GENES

There has been considerable effort worldwide over the past few years to identify genes involved in deafness,[3, 4, 5, 22] because an understanding of the molecular basis of hearing impairment is an essential first step in devising treatment strategies using a medical approach. Development of new treatments as an alternative to the imperfect approaches of amplification with hearing aids or cochlear implantation is the primary goal of this genetic research.[23, 24] Having a mutation in a single gene associated with deafness is an extremely valuable tool, because it gives us a means to identify a molecule that is essential for normal hearing. Furthermore, the understanding gained from studying genes involved in deafness will be useful for developing generic treatments for many types of hearing impairment, not just types caused by single gene defects.

How do we go about identifying genes involved in deafness? One approach might be to guess which gene is a likely candidate based upon what we know of the molecules involved in auditory function, and search for mutations in that gene in DNA samples from affected individuals. This is not a useful strategy at the moment, because it is constrained by the very limited knowledge we have of the molecular basis of hearing. There are 30,000 genes to search through, and guessing the right one is too great a gamble for funding agencies to consider. Our experience to date has been that many different classes of genes have been shown to underlie deafness and that few if any of them would have been thought of as a good candidate *a priori*. Even if genomic changes are found in a favourite gene, proving a causal link with deafness is very difficult. Thus, we need to limit the search using additional criteria. Expression is increasingly used as a means of reducing the list of candidate genes, by looking at which genes are transcribed and/or translated into proteins by the cell. However, as each cell type probably will express several thousand genes at different stages in its development, this approach may not reduce the list by very much.

Positional cloning is the usual method used for identifying genes associated with diseases like deafness.[25] The term positional simply means using the position of a mutation on a chromosome as a clue, while cloning refers to a way of copying the stretch of DNA of interest which is no longer an essential part of the process but is still a term in common usage; identification is a more accurate term to use for finding the causative mutation. The first stage of positional cloning is mapping, or localizing, the mutation to a region of a particular chromosome by linkage analysis. Mapping mutations involves collecting DNA from families showing mendelian inheritance of a phenotype and typing polymorphic markers that span the entire genome (a genome scan) to find chromosomal markers that tend to be inherited with the mutation. This will suggest that these markers are located close to the mutation (linked to the mutation), as the further any marker is from the mutation, the more likely it is to be physically separated from the mutation by crossing over during meiosis. Mapping requires large numbers of family members, some with and some without the phenotype, so most deafness genes that have been identified to date have been mapped first in families from cultures where large numbers of children are common, or in geographically isolated communities. When a restricted region of a chromosome has been defined as containing the mutation, the next step is to look at the genes within that region and prioritize them for detailed mutation screening, usually by sequencing the exons (coding parts) of the genes. There may still be hundreds of genes within the region defined by mapping, so usually researchers look carefully to try to pick out the best candidates for involvement in deafness, and expression in the ear can be useful in suggesting good candidates. When a genomic change is discovered, further evidence is needed to determine whether it is indeed the mutation causing the pathology, as there are likely to be many genomic variants within the target chromosomal region. If the putative mutation is not found in the unaffected population, it is predicted to have a severe effect on protein structure and the gene is known to be expressed in the ear, this would argue in favour of the mutation being causative. If other mutations in the same gene can be found in affected members of other families or in an animal model like the mouse showing the same phenotype, this would further strengthen the claim.

THE MOUSE AS A MODEL

An animal model is vital for understanding the molecular and developmental basis of deafness, and the mouse is the model of choice.[26, 27] The mouse is a mammal, with middle and inner ears very similar to human ears, and the many deaf mouse mutants available show similar types of pathological features as their human counterparts. Furthermore, genes found to be associated with deafness in the mouse are with only very few exceptions also found to underlie human deafness, and *vice versa*. Many basic studies such as early developmental analysis, genetic manipulation, damaging noise exposure and so forth are only possible in an animal model, and mice can be bred to provide thousands of individuals for high resolution mapping of deafness genes, making the mouse a valuable model for studying the genetics of deafness.

OTHER OTORHINOLARYNGOLOGICAL DISORDERS

Although this chapter has focussed on hearing impairment in illustrating the basic principles of genetics, other disorders will also be influenced to some degree by genetics. For example, allergic rhinitis shows a strong genetic influence, but it appears that several genes are involved, each contributing to the risk of the carrier developing rhinitis.[28, 29] No doubt environmental factors play a role in the development of rhinitis as well as the genetic predisposition.

WHAT LESSONS HAVE WE LEARNED FROM GENETIC RESEARCH SO FAR?

Complexity and heterogeneity are the main features. There are many different single genes that can be involved in deafness, probably hundreds of them, and genetic variants contribute to all forms of hearing impairment including sensitivity to environmental damage and age-related progressive hearing loss. Some genes can harbour

different mutations giving either dominant or recessive hearing impairment, others can involve either childhood deafness or progressive, later-onset loss, and yet other genes can underlie both syndromic and nonsyndromic deafness.[3] A good example of this level of complication is the *MYO7A* gene and Usher syndrome (USH). Usher syndrome type 1 is characterized by a set of common features: profound childhood deafness, balance dysfunction and progressive retinitis pigmentosa. However, at least seven genes can be involved in this syndrome, four of which have been identified and the others only localized to date.[3] The most common cause of USH1 is mutation of the *MYO7A* gene, defined as USH1B. *MYO7A* mutations can also be associated with two forms of nonsyndromic deafness, with no evidence of retinitis pigmentosa: the dominantly inherited DFNA11 with later-onset progressive hearing loss and the recessive childhood deafness, DFNB2.[3]

Other lessons we have learnt include the finding that some genes are involved in only a small number of cases of deafness, while others (such as *GJB2*) account for a much greater proportion of deafness in the population. The majority of cases of deafness in the population still have no clear diagnosis, suggesting that there are many deafness-associated genes remaining to be found.

Work on mouse models has given us further indications of general features of genetic deafness. Firstly, almost all single gene defects leading to hearing impairment have a primary effect in the middle or inner ears, with very few examples in which a central auditory system defect is the primary cause of the deafness.[27] Secondly, although it is commonly thought that hair cell degeneration is a major cause of hearing impairment, work with many mouse mutants suggests that hair cell degeneration is either a correlate or a consequence of a primary dysfunction either of hair cells or another part of the auditory system, rather than a primary cause. Even in cases of noise-induced damage, it seems that auditory dysfunction is more closely associated with stereocilia disruption than with hair cell degeneration.[8, 30] Hair cells may die later, making the hearing impairment essentially irreversible with current technologies, but it is important to appreciate that hair cell death is secondary to a primary dysfunction when developing new treatment strategies. For example, there is no point in attempting to regenerate hair cells that will not function because of an inherent abnormality. Thirdly, supporting cells are critical to cochlear function, so any approach involving regeneration of hair cells as a treatment must also include regeneration of support cells. Fourthly, many genes involved in deafness are expressed in structures other than hair cells. The *GJB2* gene is a good example of this, as it is expressed in the supporting cell network and spiral ligament of the cochlear duct and not in hair cells. Therefore, any attempts to treat deafness will need to be targeted to the appropriate structures, making accurate diagnosis a critical part of the process.

KEY POINTS

- There are 3,000,000,000 bases of DNA in each set of 23 human chromosomes, including approximately 30,000 genes.
- Variation is very common with sequences differing between individuals at around one base per thousand. This makes it difficult to establish which DNA variant might be the cause of a particular inherited feature, such as deafness.
- Genes interact with the environment; some variants of genes will make us more or less susceptible to environmental insults, such as noise damage.
- Genes also interact with each other in shaping our phenotype.
- Genetic variation makes a major contribution to hearing impairment, including age-related hearing loss which shows a heritability of around 50 percent.
- There are hundreds of genes involved in hearing and balance and any one can be involved in deafness in an individual. In other cases, problems can arise from variants in several genes acting together.
- Many genes involved in deafness are inherited in a Mendelian fashion: dominant, recessive, X-linked or mitochondrial. The collection of large families with affected individuals has allowed us to map the causative mutation to specific chromosomes and then identify the gene and the mutation by a process called positional cloning.
- The mouse is an excellent and very useful model for understanding the genetics and pathology of human deafness.
- Complexity and heterogeneity are the hallmarks of the aetiology of deafness and balance problems.

Deficiencies in current knowledge and areas for future research

Genetics will have an increasing impact on day-to-day clinical practice in the future. Genetic research will lead to new treatment possibilities and improved diagnostic tools over the next 10–15 years. Exactly how this might develop has been discussed in detail elsewhere,[23, 24] but it is clear that clinicians must be at the heart of the process, having genetics at the top of their list when considering causes of hearing impairment and developing close communication with the research community.

REFERENCES

1. International Human Genome Sequencing Consortium. Initial sequencing and analysis of the human genome. *Nature*. 2001; **409**: 860–921.
2. de Kok YJ, Vossenaar ER, Cremers CW, Dahl N, Laporte J, Hu LJ et al. Identification of a hot spot for microdeletions in patients with X-linked deafness type 3 (DFN3) 900 kb proximal to the DFN3 gene *POU3F4*. *Human Molecular Genetics*. 1996; **5**: 1229–35.
* 3. Van Camp G, Smith RJH. Hereditary hearing loss homepage; last accessed 11 December 2003. Available from: http://webhost.ua.ac.be/hhh/.
* 4. Petit C, Levilliers J, Hardelin JP. Molecular genetics of hearing loss. *Annual Review of Genetics*. 2001; **35**: 589–646.
* 5. Bitner-Glindzicz M. Hereditary deafness and phenotyping in humans. *British Medical Bulletin*. 2002; **63**: 73–94.
6. Riazuddin S, Castelein CM, Ahmed ZM, Lalwani AK, Mastroianni MA, Naz S et al. Dominant modifier DFNM1 suppresses recessive deafness DFNB26. *Nature Genetics*. 2000; **26**: 431–4.
7. Estivill X, Govea N, Barcelo E, Badenas C, Romero E, Moral L et al. Familial progressive sensorineural deafness is mainly due to the mtDNA A1555G mutation and is enhanced by treatment of aminoglycosides. *American Journal of Human Genetics*. 1998; **62**: 27–35.
8. Holme RH, Steel KP. Progressive hearing loss and increased susceptibility to noise-induced hearing loss in mice carrying a *Cdh23*, but not a *Myo7a* mutation. *Journal of the Association for Research in Otolaryngology*. 2004; **5**: 66–79.
* 9. Fortnum HM, Summerfield AQ, Marshall DH. Prevalence of childhood hearing impairment in the United Kingdom and implications for universal neonatal hearing screening: questionnaire based ascertainment study. *British Medical Journal*. 2001; **323**: 536–40.
10. Davis AC. *Hearing in adults*. London: Whurr, 1995.
11. Cohen MM, Gorlin RJ. Epidemiology, etiology, and genetic patterns. In: Gorlin RJ, Toriello HV, Cohen MM (eds). *Hereditary hearing loss and its syndromes. Oxford monographs on medical genetics. No. 28*. New York: Oxford University Press, 1995: 9–21.
12. Morton NE. Genetic epidemiology of hearing impairment. *Annals of the New York Academy of Sciences*. 1991; **630**: 16–31.
13. Van Camp G, Willems PJ, Smith RJH. Nonsyndromic hearing impairment: unparalleled heterogeneity. *American Journal of Human Genetics*. 1997; **60**: 758–64.
14. DeStefano AL, Gates GA, Heard-Costa N, Myers RH, Baldwin CT. Genomewide linkage analysis to presbyacusis in the Framingham heart study. *Archives of Otolaryngology – Head and Neck Surgery*. 2003; **129**: 285–9.
15. Gates GA, Couropmitree NN, Myers RH. Genetic associations in age-related hearing thresholds. *Archives of Otolaryngology – Head and Neck Surgery*. 1999; **125**: 654–9.

16. Karlsson KK, Harris JR, Svartengren M. Description and primary results from an audiometric study of male twins. *Ear and Hearing*. 1997; **18**: 114–20.

17. OMIM, Online Mendelian Inheritance in Man. Bethesda, MD: Center for Medical Genetics, Johns Hopkins University (Baltimore, MD) and National Center for Biotechnology Information, National Library of Medicine (Bethesda, MD); last accessed 11 December 2003. Available from: http://www.ncbi.nlm.nih.gov/omim/.

18. del Castillo I, Moreno-Pelayo MA, del Castillo FJ, Brownstein Z, Marlin S, Adina Q *et al.* Prevalence and evolutionary origins of the del(GJB6-D13S1830) mutation in the DFNB1 locus in hearing-impaired subjects: a multicenter study. *American Journal of Human Genetics*. 2003; **73**: 1452–8.

∗ 19. Hutchin T, Coy NN, Conlon H, Telford E, Bromelow K, Blaydon D *et al.* Assessment of the genetic causes of recessive childhood non-syndromic deafness in the UK – implications for genetic testing. *Clinical Genetics*. 2005; **68**: 506–12.

20. Estivill X, Fortina P, Surrey S, Rabionet R, Melchionda S, D'Agruma L *et al.* Connexin-26 mutations in sporadic and inherited sensorineural deafness. *Lancet*. 1998; **351**: 394–8.

21. Denoyelle F, Marlin S, Weil D, Moatti L, Chauvin P, Garabedian EN *et al.* Clinical features of the prevalent form of childhood deafness, DFNB1, due to a connexion-26 gene defect: implications for genetic counselling. *Lancet*. 1999; **353**: 1298–1303.

22. Steel KP, Kros CJ. A genetic approach to understanding auditory function. *Nature Genetics*. 2001; **27**: 143–9.

23. Avraham KB, Raphael Y. Prospects for gene therapy in hearing loss. *Journal of Basic and Clinical Physiology and Pharmacology*. 2003; **14**: 77–83.

∗ 24. Steel KP. New interventions in hearing impairment. *British Medical Journal*. 2000; **320**: 622–5.

25. Steel KP, Kimberling WJ. Approaches to understanding the molecular genetics of hearing and deafness. In: Van de Water TR, Fay RR, Popper AN (eds). *Springer handbook of auditory research*, Vol VII. New York: Springer, 1996: 10–40.

26. Steel KP. Using mouse mutants to understand the genetics of deafness. In: Tranebjærg L, Christensen-Dalsgaard J, Andersen T, Poulsen T (eds). *Genetics and the function of the auditory system*. Kolding, Denmark: Danavox, 2001: 109–29.

27. Steel KP, Erven A, Kiernan AE. Mice as models for human hereditary deafness. In: Keats BJ, Popper AN, Fay RR (eds). *Springer handbook of auditory research, genetics and auditory disorders*. New York: Springer, 2002: 247–96.

28. Daniels SE, Bhattacharrya S, James A, Leaves NI, Young A, Hill RH *et al.* A genome-wide search for quantitative trait loci underlying asthma. *Nature*. 1996; **383**: 247–51.

29. Cookson WO, Sharp PA, Faux JA, Hopkin JM. Linkage between immunoglobulin E responses underlying asthma and rhinitis and chromosome 11q. *Lancet*. 1989; **8650**: 1293–4.

30. Liberman MC, Dodds LW. Single-neuron labelling and chronic cochlear pathology. III. Stereocilia damage and alterations of threshold tuning curves. *Hearing Research*. 1984; **16**: 55–74.

3

Gene therapy

SCOTT M GRAHAM AND JOHN H LEE

Introduction	23	Key points	29
Cystic fibrosis	24	Deficiencies in current knowledge and areas for future	
Key points	26	research	29
Head and neck cancer	26	References	30

SEARCH STRATEGY

The data in this chapter are supported by a Medline search using the key words gene therapy, cystic fibrosis, head and neck cancer, gene transfer, adenoviral vectors, adeno-associated vectors, ballistic gene delivery, chemosensitization and retroviral vectors.

INTRODUCTION

Few new treatment protocols seem to reflect the allure of modern science quite as elegantly as gene therapy. The promise of gene therapy in treating a variety of diseases is, simply put, incredible. This promise has captured the hopes and enthusiasm of the scientific and lay communities alike. Notable initial success in treating severe combined immune deficiency (SCID) seemed to herald imminent success in treating a whole variety of other conditions. In reality, however, progress in bringing the allure of the science to a useful clinical application has been quite limited. Even in the group of SCID subjects[1] – an apparent 'cure' – a patient has died from an unusual lymphoproliferative disease. This has led to a reassessment of the risks of retroviral therapy trials. While great strides have been made in understanding the complexities of disease states and vectors, the barriers to clinical utility continue to be formidable.

Today, some 63 human clinical trials of gene therapy exist. The disease processes involved can be broadly divided into three groups: infectious disease trials, which entirely comprise human immunodeficiency virus (HIV); secondly, monogenetic diseases such as cystic fibrosis (CF) and hemophilia B and thirdly diseases that are polygenic such as rheumatoid arthritis or cancer. These studies deliver genetic material to target cells via vectors, which act as delivery vehicles to bypass host defences. In the very select circumstances of the skin or eye, a 'gene gun' can be used. The treatment aims to replace or repair the defective gene causing a given disease or to provide a new or altered function in a cell. The most common vectors are a variety of replication-deficient viruses although nonviral vectors, such as liposomes, are also used.

In reviewing progress to date in gene therapy, two diseases of interest to otolaryngologists encapsulate the potential and difficulties of this technique. We will review an apparently attractive candidate for gene therapy, a disease caused by a single mutation inherited in an autosomal recessive fashion – cystic fibrosis.[2] We will also review progress in a condition with a variety of causalities and a disparate genetic basis, head and neck cancer[3] – a superficially unattractive candidate for gene therapy. These two diverse diseases serve to illustrate many of the principles, advances and frustrations of gene therapy. In both these examples, human trials are in their infancy. Trial sample size is small and results so far do not readily lend themselves to the categorization of levels of evidence, as displayed in other chapters in this text.

CYSTIC FIBROSIS

Cystic fibrosis represents a seemingly ideal disease for gene therapy. It is the most common lethal genetic disease of one of the wealthiest racial subgroups in the world. There are perhaps 30,000 people with CF in the United States and a similar number in Europe. It is inherited with an autosomal recessive pattern with carrier rates of 5 percent in some Caucasian populations.[4] Remarkably, the median survival for CF patients is now 31 years. Unfortunately, the disease remains almost uniformly fatal, invariably from its pulmonary sequelae.[4] Despite dramatic improvements in the understanding of the molecular basis of CF, there has as yet been no clinically useful breakthrough in its treatment. Clearly, new treatments are needed. Conceptually, gene therapy offers the promise of a dramatic and new treatment.

Genetic basis

The discovery of the gene for CF in 1989[5] set in motion a remarkable series of events, often covered by the lay press with the hyperbole of popular culture, which have culminated in attempts at gene therapy. CF is caused by mutations in a gene on the long arm of chromosome 7. This gene encodes a protein, cystic fibrosis transmembrane conductance regulator (CFTR), which has been shown to be a cAMP-dependent chloride channel.[6] Abnormalities of CFTR produce abnormalities of salt and water transport across a variety of epithelia. This produces the various manifestations of the disease. The deletion of a single phenylalanine residue at position 508 of CFTR, designated ΔF508, is the most common mutation in cystic fibrosis comprising some 70 percent of cases. Other mutations, now numbering nearly 1000, are uncommon, occurring in less than 1 percent of screened populations.[7]

The nasal model for gene transfer in cystic fibrosis

Most interest in CF amongst otolaryngologists has centred around CF sinus disease. Recent reports have claimed benefit from aggressive treatment of CF sinus disease[8] and have also suggested that the rhinologic sequelae of CF are important in production of the eventually life-threatening pulmonary complications. Not as widely reported has been the utility of the nose and sinuses in CF as a model for pulmonary disease.[9] While the eventual goal of CF gene therapy will clearly be intrapulmonary administration, there are clearly some difficulties with the lungs for routine experimentation. Chief amongst these concerns is safety. The prospect of an adverse reaction to vector administration in the lungs of a patient with pre-existing pulmonary compromise is

real. In a dose-escalating trial reported by Crystal et al.[10] in 1994 of intrapulmonary adenoviral vector administration, the patient who received the largest dose developed a significant adverse reaction with opacities on chest x-ray. The risk of a significant adverse reaction in a localized area of the nose or sinuses is clearly less.[11] The lungs are also more inaccessible than the nose and the nose and sinuses offer ease of access for vector administration and experimental manipulation. For a variety of reasons, CF clinical trials are performed on adults. These patients invariably have severe pre-existing pulmonary compromise and any incremental benefits in pulmonary function afforded by gene therapy would be difficult to measure.

The nasal potential in CF provides a measurable endpoint for gene transfer experimentation. Nasal mucosa maintains and generates a potential difference across its surface and a characteristic voltage trace can be obtained in normal patients. In CF, the nasal mucosa, like the lung mucosa, exhibits the characteristic chloride transport abnormality. CF patients, because of their abnormal ion transport, produce a nasal potential that is different from normal both in its absolute negativity and in its response to certain pharmacologic influences.[12] This trace is so characteristic for CF that it is referred to as its bio-electric phenotype. This potential can be readily and reproducibly measured, in contrast to a number of bronchopulmonary indices and has been a target of gene therapy strategies in the nose.

In vitro and animal studies

Initially, the feasibility of gene transfer to airway cells was demonstrated *in vitro* and then in a variety of animal experiments. Only one year after the identification of the gene, Rich et al.[13] showed that expression of cDNA for wildtype CFTR corrected the Cl^- channel defect in cultured CF airway epithelia. Zabner et al.[14] demonstrated that recombinant adenoviral vectors could deliver CFTR cDNA safely in both cotton rats and rhesus monkeys. Transgenic CF mice provided a means to perform functional testing of CFTR gene expression and have even allowed reversal of the CF phenotype by gene therapy *in utero*.[15] Unfortunately, however, the mice do not produce a disease state comparable to the effects of CF on human lungs.[16] Encouraging *in vitro* and animal studies were the basis for progression to trials to address questions that could only be answered in humans.

Human adenovirus studies – viral vectors

Most of the early human cystic fibrosis gene therapy trials in the United States employed adenoviral vectors. Adenovirus has a degree of tropism for respiratory mucosa and a substantial body of knowledge already existed about adenoviruses as respiratory pathogens.

Recombinant viruses are produced by replacing the DNA sequence responsible for replication with CFTR cDNA. The viruses are thus replication-deficient, but still remain sufficiently active to transport genetic material into the target cell. In 1993, Zabner et al.[17] reported correction of the CF bioelectric potential in a single-dose study where an escalating dose of vector encoding CFTR was applied to the nasal epithelium of three CF patients. Two CF patients underwent a sham procedure using saline and served as controls. No change was noted in the bioelectric phenotype in these two patients. One year later Crystal et al.[10] published a study in which an adenovirus containing CFTR cDNA was applied to both the upper and lower respiratory tracts of four patients. No statement was made about the nasal potential, but CFTR was detected by immunohistochemistry. This report was notable for the widely publicized event of pulmonary toxicity in one of the participants following vector delivery to the lungs. This toxicity was thought to be due to vector-induced inflammation and a reduction of viral vector dose has largely overcome the problem of acute inflammation in subsequent studies. Hay et al.[18] produced a further study revealing improvement in the nasal potential in a single escalating-dose protocol the following year.

Knowles et al.[19] found molecular evidence of low efficiency gene transfer, but no correction of the nasal potential in a 1995 report. Their experiment involved administration of logarithmically increasing vector doses to four cohorts of three patients. A further study by Zabner et al.[20] in 1996 addressed the likely need for repeat vector administration. Six patients in two centers in the United States received four or five applications of sequentially escalating concentrations of recombinant adenovirus encoding CFTR. In this series, the correction of the nasal potential was more subtle and, importantly, evidence of immunologic response to repeat administration was noted.

Studies involving intrapulmonary vector administration have scarcely fared better. Zuckerman et al.[21] delivered adenovirus encoding CFTR to a segmental bronchus in a dose-escalating study. There was evidence of low level gene expression, as well as evidence of immune and inflammatory responses. In contrast, a single-escalating dose trial from France revealed gene transfer and no detectable immune or inflammatory response after administration of Ad/CFTR.[22]

Adenovirus vectors, while efficient delivery vehicles in the laboratory setting, clearly have difficulties in human trials. The human respiratory tract has evolved to efficiently repel a variety of microbial attacks, including of course adenoviruses. Adenovirus does not integrate into the genome and thus repeat administration is required. With repeat administration come concerns of inflammation and immunogenicity. All viral vectors aimed at the epithelial surface suffer from the limitation of the viral receptors being located in the basolateral membrane, away from the cell surface. This may be in part overcome by the use of calcium chelators[23] that briefly disrupt tight epithelial functions, allowing the vector access to the basolateral membrane.

Adeno–associated virus

Serotypes 5 and 6 of the adeno-associated virus (AAV) enter airway cells from the apical surface.[16] Furthermore, adeno-associated viruses offer the potential for integration into the host genome. In practical terms, however, adeno-associated viruses are also associated with inefficient expression. Using the maxillary sinus model, ten CF patients who had undergone prior maxillary antrostomy had AAV vector encoding CFTR applied to their maxillary sinus.[24] Molecular evidence of gene transfer was detected as late as 41 days. A functional endpoint of maxillary sinus voltage measurement was also employed. Some evidence of functional improvement was detected at day 14. There appeared to be no effect on maxillary sinusitis, as assessed endoscopically. Importantly, the utility of this model has been called into question by other studies.[25]

Lentivirus

Lentiviruses are an apparently attractive addition to the list of possible vectors. They have the ability to integrate into and consequently persist in the host genome. They can transduce nondividing cells – an advantage in airway epithelium where cell turnover is generally low. While a variety of lentiviral options exists, most work has been carried out with the feline immunodeficiency virus (FIV).[16]

Nonviral vectors

The shortcomings of viral vectors have led to the investigation of nonviral delivery systems. These have included purified or naked DNA in plasmid form or ballistic gene delivery, the so-called gene gun. Only exposed surfaces accessible to a microcarrier coated with DNA are candidates for the gene gun. Most interest in nonviral gene delivery has centred on liposomes. Liposomes bind to DNA, spontaneously forming complexes that have high affinity for plasma cell membranes. DNA containing liposomes are incorporated into the cell by endocytosis. The advantages of nonviral vectors mainly revolve around safety. They are nonimmunogenic and there is no potential for insertional mutagenesis. The main difficulties with nonviral vectors relate to inefficient gene transfer and transient expression.

A 20 percent correction of nasal potential in nine patients, peaking at three days and disappearing by seven days, was reported by Caplen et al.[26] employing a cationic liposome vector. The vector was applied by a nasal pump spray, a practical method for likely repeat administration should clinical gene therapy become a reality. In 1997, Gill et al.[27] showed functional CFTR gene transfer in six of eight subjects in a further nasal mucosal/liposome study. Alton et al.[28] reported a placebo-controlled study of liposome-mediated CFTR transfer to the lungs and nasal mucosa of CF patients. The treatment group displayed some improvement in airway potential not seen in the liposome-only group. Interestingly, some aspects of toxicity were only seen with pulmonary administration leading the authors to question the value of the nasal model, at least from a safety viewpoint.

KEY POINTS

- Remarkable progress has been made in understanding the molecular basis of cystic fibrosis.
- Equally dramatic progress has been made in examining the basic science of vector production and vector interaction with airway cells.
- The challenge remains to apply this new knowledge and in vitro gene therapy success to a clinically relevant and measurable endpoint.

HEAD AND NECK CANCER

In 2000, an estimated 130,000 cases of new head and neck cancer were diagnosed in developed countries.[29] Advances in surgical techniques, radiation treatment strategies and chemotherapy medications have improved the survival and quality of life for many of these patients. Unfortunately, despite these innovations, treatment strategies for advanced stage cancer squamous cancer and certain other head and neck cancer subtypes have not increased survival over the last 40 years.[30, 31] In order to offer therapy in these advanced cases and to potentially augment current successful therapies, alternative treatment strategies have been examined. Many of these therapies have evolved as a result of our appreciation of the biological basis of oncogenesis. Specifically, this increased understanding has given us gene targets to potentially correct by either replacing or blocking the effect of the mutated gene. The various strategies used in gene therapy fall into four major categories: immune modulation, restorative gene replacement, selective oncolysis and chemosensitization. To accomplish these strategies, it is now possible to deliver genes by several different vectors. The following discussion will review both the methods to deliver the genes and the various strategies used with these vectors.

Delivery

The common goal of all gene therapy is to achieve expression of the gene of interest in the targeted cancer cell. To accomplish this goal several barriers must be overcome: (1) targeting – ideally only cells which require the gene would be affected; (2) binding and internalization – once a gene reaches the cells it must bind and become internalized; (3) cellular trafficing to the nucleus – most methods of internalization require the gene to escape from endosomal degradation and traffic through the cell to the nucleus; and (4) nuclear expression – once in the nucleus the quantity of gene expression and stability of expression for a given strategy also need to be determined. Each method of delivering a gene to a cell varies in its ability to overcome these barriers.

Plasmid DNA

Naked DNA is one of the most extensively studied methods of gene therapy. This nonviral method of gene therapy has several advantages. These include simplicity, ease of large scale production, minimal immune response and safety.[32] The major obstacle for plasmid gene therapy is efficiency. When DNA is placed in an organism, most of the DNA is not internalized. Even if internalization does occur, endosomal degradation destroys nearly all of the remaining plasmid prior to nuclear membrane transit and expression of the desired gene does not occur. In addition, since plasmid uptake is not receptor-mediated, targeting of the plasmid to a specific cell also remains a major obstacle. In the past 15 years, substantial progress has been made in overcoming these obstacles to nonviral gene transfer.

Rapid degradation by serum nuclei and the mononuclear cell system occurs when naked DNA is injected systemically (e.g. intravascularly).[32] Several strategies have been designed to overcome this barrier.[33, 34, 35] If expression is only needed at a specific site, a gene gun, hydrodynamic injection, ultrasound, electroporation and blood flow restriction have shown promise.[36, 37, 38, 39] Electroporation has been shown to increase interleukin (IL)-12 and interferon (IFN)-alpha expression intratumourally.[40, 41] It may be possible to accomplish this increased electroporation by using an electrode attached to a syringe needle.[42] If more than local expression is needed, significant advances have also been made in systemic delivery. Complexing DNA with lipids, peptides, polymers or various cationic compounds has been shown to greatly increase expression. These complexes can help with almost every component of plasmid delivery.[43, 44] Cationic lipids and dendrimers have been shown to increase expression by increasing cell binding/internalization and decreasing endosomal degradation.[45, 46] Targeting a specific cell type has also been shown to be possible by linking a ligand to these DNA complexes.[47]

Lastly, plasmid-mediated transfer results in transient expression because the plasmid is lost with cell division. Several methods using site-specific integration or expression of viral proteins have shown promise as a means to overcome this difficulty.[48, 49] Many of the past therapeutic attempts to utilize plasmid-mediated gene transfer have shown only modest potential. However, as all aspects of plasmid effeciency increase, this should directly correlate with the ability to utillize this technology in therapeutic interventions.

Adenovirus

Adenovirus is a human pathogenic, nonencapsulated, DNA virus. It has been extensively studied both as a means to deliver a gene both *in vitro* and in human trials. Adenovirus has several characteristics which make it suitable as a therapeutic vector in gene therapy. Relatively simple amplification methods have been developed to propagate high titer replication defective vectors.[50] Adenovirus efficiently infects both dividing and non-dividing cells by binding to the cox-adenovirus receptor.[51] Once a cell binds the viral vector, adenovirus is internalized, escapes from the endosome and is trafficked to the nucleus very effeciently. Even if a specific cell is lacking viral receptors, the virus can be combined with complexes to be internalized via nonreceptor-mediated mechanisms. In this alternative pathway of entry, the other components of viral gene delivery remain intact, and therefore efficiency is maintained.[52, 53] This relative versatility, the ease of construction, efficiency of infection and the efficient expression of transgene make adenovirus an attractive vector for gene therapy.

Adenovirus does have some drawbacks compared to other vectors and nonviral systems. It is immunogenic which limits its ability to reinfect.[54] Multiple studies have shown that both cell- and humoral-mediated immune systems are activated after viral delivery, especially if greater than 10^{10} particles are delivered.[55] This toxicity led to the well-publicized death of a subject in a University of Pennsylvania trial.[1] Besides limiting redelivery, this immune response also results in the clearance of cells expressing the transgene.[56] Several strategies have shown promise in overcoming this immune-stimulatory problem. 'Gutted' vectors, missing almost all of the viral genes, have been shown to be less immunogenic and are expressed for longer periods *in vivo*.[57, 58] Immune modulation at the time of delivery may decrease the initial imflammatory reaction to the virus.[57, 58] A further difficulty of adenovirus is that gene expression is transient. The viral genome does not integrate or persist with cell division and gene expression is lost as the cells divide. As demonstrated by over 50 current open protocols, the adenoviral vector is a very versatile means of gene delivery. As the obstacle of immune stimulation and persistence are addressed, this vector should only become more useful.

Retrovirus

Retroviral vectors have the substantial advantage of persistent gene expression. A discussion of retroviral vectors requires a basic understanding of the viral genome and replication. Retroviruses are small, encapsulating vectors with a genome composed of two identical single strands of RNA. The virus binds and is internalized into the cell via interactions between the cell membrane and viral capsule. Once internalized the RNA genome is reverse-transcribed and transported to the nucleus where it integrates as a provirus into the host chromosome. In a normal infectious process, this provirus would then produce viral proteins and RNA genomes for viral packaging. In all retroviral gene therapy vectors, the genome of the virus has been made replication-incompetent by removing the components of the viral gene required for packaging. Thus, these vectors integrated and express the desired gene but will not produce infectious particles.

Several retroviral systems for gene therapy are currently available. Murine oncogenic retroviruses have been the most extensively analyzed and used in preclinical studies.[59] Because murine retroviruses only infect dividing cells, the clinical utility of these initial retroviral vectors has been significantly limited.[59] To circumvent this obstacle, newer retroviral systems have been developed based on the lentivirus genus of retroviruses. This group of viral vectors which contains the human immunodeficiency virus offer the advantage of infecting dividing and nondividing cells. They have shown significant promise in preclinical *in vivo* studies.[60] A further biosafety-related issue of retroviruses is that insertion of the provirus is not controlled. It is possible that insertion of the virus next to a protooncogene may lead to therapy-induced cancer. Initial evidence from the first successful therapy in patients with severe combined immune defiency using retroviral gene replacement suggests that a minority of the patients may have developed a nontypable lymphoproliferative disorder as a result of therapy.[1] In addition to controlling insertion, chromosomal silencing of inserted genes has also been reported. In chromosomal silencing, methylation or acetylation of the promotor leads to significant downregulation of transgene expression.[61, 62, 63] For both of these obstacles, current research has suggested potential solutions. These include controllable chromosomal insertion, chromosomal buffers and methods to controllably excise the provirus.

Adeno–associated virus

The AAV vector has more recently emerged as a vector with significant therapeutic promise. AAV is a single-stranded encapsulated virus that belongs to the group of human parvoviruses. Several features of this virus make it attractive as a potential therapeutic tool. Firstly, although it infects human cells this virus has not been associated with a pathologic human disease. It may, therefore, be a safer alternative than other viral vectors. Secondly, because recombinant AAV vectors do not encode viral proteins, delivery of this vector results in very little immunogenicity.[64, 65] AAV also persists and infects dividing and nondividing cells. Although the mechanisms are not fully clear, it appears that in quiescent cells AAV integrates into the host chromosome and in rapidly dividing cells it persists as an extrachromosal episome.[66] These factors have made this vector a popular delivery vehicle for many preclinical and human trials.

Other viral vectors

Many other viruses, including herpes and vaccinia, are currently under investigation as potential means to deliver genes. As more is understood about viral biology, it may be possible to match a particular vector with the needs of a given therapy and cell type. For instance, if long-term expression is required with low immunogenicity in muscle, it would be ideal to put the gene to be delivered in AAV. In future years, the choice of a virus for a particular cancer may be as evidence based as the choice of an antibiotic for a particular bacterial infection.

Therapy strategies

Gene therapy offers a novel paradigm that leads to the destruction of tumour cells in cancer patients. To date, the approaches to target specific cancer cells fall into four basic categories: (1) chemosensitization; (2) cytokine gene transfer; (3) inactivation of protooncogene production; and (4) selective oncolytic viruses. In the discussion to follow, the rationale and specific results from preliminary gene therapy trials will be presented.

CHEMOSENSITIZATION

Selective sensitization of cancer cells using gene therapy would be an ideal way to kill cancer cells. Using this approach, the expected gene is delivered only to cancer cells and then a second therapy (e.g. radiotherapy or chemotherapy) is used to induce killing in the cells which express the transgene. The best example of this model is delivery of herpes simplex thymidine kinase (HSV-TK).[67, 68] In this strategy, HSV-TK is delivered to cancer cells. Once expressed, this enzyme changes the prodrug gancyclovir to its toxic nucleoside analogue, which induces cell death. Using this system one would expect that 100 percent infection of the cancer cell would be required in order to be effective. In reality, a phenomenon termed the bystander effect increases the efficiency of such therapies. In the bystander effect, the infected cell spreads the expressed genes to the cells surrounding it via cell–cell contacts. Using mixing experiments, it has been shown

that because of this effect, only half of the cells need to initially express the toxic gene to have the desired affect.[68, 69] Transfer of *p53* is another example of chemosensitization, as inclusion of this cellular gene sensitizes a cancer cell to apoptosis after treatment with either radition therapy or chemotherapy.[70] Initial laboratory studies showed great promise for these types of therapies. Preclinical animal studies, however, showed only modest *in vivo* results.[67, 71] Efficiency and targeting have been shown to be difficult *in vivo*. Methods to increase cancer targeting may make these strategies more amenable for human trials in the future. These strategies include redesigning the adenovirus binding site to increase cancer cell selectivity.[72, 73]

IMMUNE MODULATION

The host immune response has been shown to play a role in cancer eradication. Immune suppression increases the risk of cancer development. In addition to generalized suppression, it has been shown that individuals with head and neck cancer lack an effective local immune response even early in the disease.[74] This immune dysfunction begins at the site of the tumour and progresses systemically with disease progression. This dysfunction occurs as a result of the normal immune system not recognizing the tumour cells. Causes of this include immunological ignorance,[75] downregulation of major histocompatibility complexes and loss of costimulatory receptor and pathways.[76, 77] In some tumours, the cytokine stimulatory pathways (interleukin-2 (IL-2), interferon-gamma and IL-12) which normally upregulate the normal tumour immune response are depressed. One method to break this immune dysregulation is to overexpress the downregulated cytokines. The basis of the first cytokine-based trial for locoregional disease was compelling data from preclinical studies in mice.[78] A subsequent phase I trial using soluble proteins showed three complete responses and three partial responses in 10 patients.[79] All these response were transient. A subsequent phase II trial showed similar transient responses which did not correlate with dose escalation.[80, 81, 82] However, when IL-2 is administered systemically, significant toxicity develops, including capillary leak syndrome. Gene therapy offers the ability to increase local expression and possibly improve tumour response while limiting systemic toxicity. Phase I trials using nonviral plasmids expressing IL-2 are currently under way.[83] Even if such single agent cytokines do not prove useful, it may be possible to deliver combinations, which activate the immune pathway in a synergistic manner. Many such costimulatory questions are currently being examined in preclinical studies.[84, 85, 86, 87] As our understanding of tumour immunity increases, better therapies aimed at reactivating the dysfunctional immune response will develop. Gene therapy may likely play a role in the delivery of such therapies.

RESTORATIVE GENE THERAPY

Restoring the function of a key cellular gene whose dysfunction has resulted in cancer progression can be a major goal of gene therapy. Several strategies to replace dysfunctional genes are currently being tested.[88, 89] The majority of these involve the disrupted apoptotic pathway found in cancer cells. The most common mutations of these genes in squamous cell cancer of the head and neck are *p53* and *p16*. The most extensively studied of these genes in head and neck cancer is *p53*. This gene plays a role in triggering cell death in many different pathways involving apoptosis. Using an adenoviral vector, placed intralesionally, this mutated gene was delivered to 33 patients with locally recurrent squamous cell cancer in a phase I trial.[90] The study had two arms, surgical and nonsurgical. In the surgical arm, patients received treatment preoperatively, intraoperatively and postoperatively. Of these patients, four patients were alive and disease free at one year, nine died of their disease and two died of unrelated causes. In the nonsurgical arm, two of 17 had a partial response, six had stable disease and nine had progressive disease. The responses seen were most likely not due to effective replacement of mutated genes because *p53* status did not correlate with response.[90] Phase II trials with adenovirus expressing *p53* are currently being completed, as well as studies which combine this therapy with chemotherapy.[91] The safety of replacing another gene, *p16*, is also currently being investigated.

SELECTIVE ONCOLYTIC VIRUS

Infection with wildtype adenovirus results in viral replication and eventual cell lysis. A therapy which harnesses this virus by only allowing replication in cancer cells would offer a self-propagating therapy which continues to produce virus and lyze cancer cells until a tumour is completely destroyed. Using replication-selective viruses to treat cancer is not entirely new. Initial reports as early as 1912 have used this approach in cancer therapy.[92] With the advent of increased knowledge of the genetic defects in cancer, we have been able to design vectors aimed at only replicating in cancer cells.[93, 94] The ONYX-015 is an adenovirus therapy design to accomplish this goal. ONYX-015 is missing the adenovirus E1B gene which normally inhibits the cellular *p53* genes. p53 cellular expression allows only minimal viral expression. Aproximately 60 percent of squamous cell carcinoma (SCCA) do not express functional p53. The ONYX-015 virus will selectively replicate only in SCCA cancers with p53 mutations. Phase I and II clinical trials have shown significant promise with this stategy.[95, 96, 97] The initial phase I trial showed the virus was safe even when given in high doses.[98] Fever and injection site pain were the most common adverse effects. Phase II and III clinical trials are currently enrolling patients. In addition to developing this therapy as a single agent treatment, its role in combined therapies is also being examined. Phase II studies have shown this combined approach increases response rates from 33 percent for chemotherapy (5-fluorouracil (5-FU) and cisplatin) to a 65 percent response rate when intratumoural injections of ONYX-015 are added to the regimen.[97] Another potential advantage of the ONYX-015 vector is that if it is given intravenously it may circulate and offer potential therapy for distant metastasis. The safety of an intravenous delivery approach has been confirmed in phase I trials revealing safe delivery of high titers of viral vectors. The most common side effects were fever, rigors and elevated liver enzymes.[96] To more fully evaluate the potential of this strategy, more work has to be completed in areas of safety and delivery. Overall, however, this self-propagating tumour selective approach offers significant therapeutic promise.

KEY POINTS

- Our increased understanding of cellular oncogenesis will lead to the development of novel cancer therapies in the years to come.
- Gene therapy is likely be a part of these therapies.
- A head and neck oncologist will need to understand both the viral vectors and their strategies of implementation to offer a full range of treatment to the cancer patient.

Deficiencies in current knowledge and areas for future research

The death of an 18-year-old man in a 1999 adenoviral gene therapy trial in Philadelphia caused scientists around the world to examine more critically the risks of human gene therapy experimentation. Three years later, a three-year-old boy died in France from a leukaemia-like condition, probably a result of insertional mutagenesis in a retroviral gene therapy trial for SCID. Both of these tragic events have resulted in increased scrutiny for human gene therapy trials. These events have also brought into sharper focus the balance between risks and the incredible promise of this treatment. Remarkable progress has been made in the last decade in improving the understanding of the basic science and the complexities of host–vector interaction. The challenge for the next decade is to translate this new expertise into clinical situations in a safe and effective manner.

REFERENCES

1. Check E. A tragic setback. *Nature.* 2002; **420**: 116–8.
2. Goebel EA, Davidson BL, Zabner J, Graham SM, Kern JA. Adenovirus-mediated gene therapy for head and neck squamous cell carcinomas. *Annals of Otology, Rhinology, and Laryngology.* 1996; **105**: 562–7.
3. Graham SM. Gene therapy for cystic fibrosis: perspectives for the otolaryngologist. *Clinical Otolaryngology.* 1998; **23**: 481–3.
4. Welsh MJ, Tsui LC, Boat TF, Beaudet AL. Cystic fibrosis. In: Scribner CR, Beaudet AL, Sly WS, Valle D (eds). *The Metabolic and molecular basis of inherited disease*, 7th edn. New York: McGraw-Hill, 1995: 3799–876.
* 5. Rommens JM, Iannuzzi MC, Kerem B, Drumm ML, Melmer G, Dean M et al. Identification of the cystic fibrosis gene: chromosome walking and jumping. *Science.* 1989; **245**: 1059–65.
6. Welsh MJ, Anderson MP, Rich DP, Berger HA, Denning GM, Ostedgaard LS et al. Cystic fibrosis transmembrane conductance regulator: a chloride channel with novel regulation. *Neuron.* 1992; **8**: 821–9.
7. Cystic Fibrosis Genetic Analysis Consortium. Cystic Fibrosis Mutation Database. Last updated 02/03/2007. Cited April 2007. Available from: www.genet.sickkids.on.ca/cftr/Home.html
8. Davidson TM, Murphy C, Mitchell M, Smith C, Light M. Management of chronic sinusitis in cystic fibrosis. *Laryngoscope.* 1995; **105**: 354–8.
9. Graham SM, Launspach JL. Utility of the nasal model in gene transfer studies in cystic fibrosis. *Rhinology.* 1997; **35**: 149–53.
10. Crystal RG, McElvaney NG, Rosenfeld MA, Chu CS, Mastrangeli A, Hay JG et al. Administration of an adenovirus containing the human CFTR cDNA to the respiratory tract of individuals with cystic fibrosis. *Nature Genetics.* 1994; **8**: 42–51.
11. Welsh MJ, Smith AE, Zabner J, Rich DP, Graham SM, Gregory RJ et al. Cystic fibrosis gene therapy using an adenovirus vector: in vivo safety and efficacy in nasal epithelium. *Human Gene Therapy.* 1994; **5**: 209–19.
12. Welsh MJ, Zabner J, Graham SM, Smith AE, Moscicki R, Wadsworth S. Adenovirus-mediated gene transfer for cystic fibrosis: Part A. Safety of dose and repeat administration in the nasal epithelium. Part B. Clinical efficacy in the maxillary sinus. *Human Gene Therapy.* 1995; **6**: 205–18.
13. Rich DP, Anderson MP, Gregory RJ, Cheng SH, Paul S, Jefferson DM et al. Expression of cystic fibrosis transmembrane conductance regulator corrects defective chloride channel regulation in cystic fibrosis airway epithelial cells. *Nature.* 1990; **347**: 358–63.
14. Zabner J, Petersen DM, Puga AP, Graham SM, Couture LA, Keyes LD et al. Safety and efficacy of repetitive adenovirus-mediated transfer of CFTR cDNA to airway epithelia of primates and cotton rats. *Nature Genetics.* 1994; **6**: 75–83.
15. Larson JE, Morrow SL, Happel L, Sharp JF, Cohen JC. Reversal of cystic fibrosis phenotype in mice by gene therapy in utero. *Lancet.* 1997; **349**: 619–20.
* 16. McCray Jr. PB. Cystic fibrosis. Difficulties of gene therapy. *Lancet.* 2001; **358**: S19.
17. Zabner J, Couture LA, Gregory RJ, Graham SM, Smith AE, Welsh MJ. Adenovirus-mediated gene transfer transiently corrects the chloride transport defect in nasal epithelia of patients with cystic fibrosis. *Cell.* 1993; **75**: 207–16.
18. Hay JG, McElvaney NG, Herena J, Crystal RG. Modification of nasal epithelial potential differences of individuals with cystic fibrosis consequent to local administration of a normal CFTR cDNA adenovirus gene transfer vector. *Human Gene Therapy.* 1995; **6**: 1487–96.
19. Knowles MR, Hohneker KW, Zhou Z, Olsen JC, Noah TL, Hu PC et al. A controlled study of adenoviral-vector-mediated gene transfer in the nasal epithelium of patients with cystic fibrosis. *New England Journal of Medicine.* 1995; **333**: 823–31.
20. Zabner J, Ramsey BW, Meeker DP, Aitken ML, Balfour RP, Gibson RL et al. Repeat administration of an adenovirus vector encoding cystic fibrosis transmembrane conductance regulator to the nasal epithelium of patients with cystic fibrosis. *Journal of Clinical Investigation.* 1996; **97**: 1504–11.
21. Zuckerman JB, Robinson CB, McCoy KS, Shell R, Sferra TJ, Chirmule N et al. A phase I study of adenovirus-mediated transfer of the human cystic fibrosis transmembrane conductance regulator gene to a lung segment of individuals with cystic fibrosis. *Human Gene Therapy.* 1999; **10**: 2973–85.
22. Bellon G, Michel-Calemard L, Thouvenot D, Jagneaux V, Poitevin F, Malcus C et al. Aerosol administration of a recombinant adenovirus expressing CFTR to cystic fibrosis patients: a phase I clinical trial. *Human Gene Therapy.* 1997; **8**: 15–25.
23. Yi SM, Lee JH, Graham S, Zabner J, Welsh MJ. Adenovirus calcium phosphate coprecipitates enhance squamous cell carcinoma gene transfer. *Laryngoscope.* 2001; **111**: 1290–6.
24. Wagner JA, Reynolds T, Moran ML, Moss RB, Wine JJ, Flotte TR et al. Efficient and persistent gene transfer of AAV-CFTR in maxillary sinus. *Lancet.* 1998; **351**: 1702–3.
25. Graham SM, Launspach JL, Welsh MJ, Zabner J. Sequential magnetic resonance imaging analysis of the maxillary sinuses: implications for a model of gene therapy in cystic fibrosis. *Journal of Laryngology and Otology.* 1999; **113**: 329–35.
* 26. Caplen NJ, Alton EW, Middleton PG, Dorin JR, Stevenson BJ, Gao X et al. Liposome-mediated CFTR gene transfer to the nasal epithelium of patients with cystic fibrosis. *Nature Medicine.* 1995; **1**: 39–46.
27. Gill DR, Southern KW, Mofford KA, Seddon T, Huang L, Sorgi F et al. A placebo-controlled study of liposome-mediated gene transfer to the nasal epithelium of patients with cystic fibrosis. *Gene Therapy.* 1997; **4**: 199–209.
28. Alton EW, Stern M, Farley R, Jaffe A, Chadwick SL, Phillips J et al. Cationic lipid-mediated CFTR gene transfer to the

lungs and nose of patients with cystic fibrosis: A double-blind placebo-controlled trial. *Lancet.* 1999; **353**: 947–54.

29. Greenlee RT, Hill-Harmon MB, Murray T, Thun M. Cancer statistics, 2001. *CA: A Cancer Journal for Clinicians.* 2001; **51**: 15–36.
30. Ganly I, Soutar DS, Kaye SB. Current role of Gene Therapy in head and neck cancer. *European Journal of Surgical Oncology.* 2000; **26**: 338–43.
31. American Cancer Society Facts and Figures. Publication No 93-400. Washington, DC: American Cancer Society, 1993.
32. Niidome T, Huang L. Gene therapy progress and prospects: nonviral vectors. *Gene Therapy.* 2002; **9**: 1647–52.
33. Harada-Shiba M, Yamauchi K, Harada A, Takamisawa I, Shimokado K, Kataoka K. Polyion complex micelles as vectors in gene therapy – pharmacokinetics and *in vivo* gene transfer. *Gene Therapy.* 2002; **9**: 407–14.
34. Ahn CH, Chae SY, Bae YH, Kim SW. Biodegradable poly(ethylenimine) for plasmid DNA delivery. *Journal of Controlled Release.* 2002; **80**: 273–82.
35. Wang J, Mao HQ, Leong KW. A novel biodegradable gene carrier based on polyphosphoester. *Journal of the American Chemical Society.* 2001; **123**: 9480–1.
36. Li S, Ma Z. Nonviral gene therapy. *Current Gene Therapy.* 2001; **1**: 201–26.
37. Somiari S, Glasspool-Malone J, Drabick JJ, Gilbert RA, Heller R, Jaroszeski MJ *et al.* Theory and in vivo application of electroporative gene delivery. *Molecular Therapy.* 2000; **2**: 178–87.
38. Drabick JJ, Glasspool-Malone J, King A, Malone RW. Cutaneous transfection and immune responses to intradermal nucleic acid vaccination are significantly enhanced by *in vivo* electropermeabilization. *Molecular Therapy.* 2001; **3**: 249–55.
39. Maruyama H, Ataka K, Higuchi N, Sakamoto F, Gejyo F, Miyazaki J. Skin-targeted gene transfer using in vivo electroporation. *Gene Therapy.* 2001; **8**: 1808–12.
40. Li S, Zhang X, Xia X, Zhou L, Breau R, Suen J *et al.* Intramuscular electroporation delivery of IFN-alpha gene therapy for inhibition of tumor growth located at a distant site. *Gene Therapy.* 2001; **8**: 400–7.
41. Tamura T, Nishi T, Goto T, Takeshima H, Dev SB, Ushio Y *et al.* Intratumoral delivery of interleukin 12 expression plasmids with in vivo electroporation is effective for colon and renal cancer. *Human Gene Therapy.* 2001; **12**: 1265–76.
42. Liu F, Huang L. A syringe electrode device for simultaneous injection of DNA and electrotransfer. *Molecular Therapy.* 2002; **5**: 323–8.
43. Koh JJ, Ko KS, Lee M, Han S, Park JS, Kim SW. Degradable polymeric carrier for the delivery of IL-10 plasmid DNA to prevent autoimmune insulitis of NOD mice. *Gene Therapy.* 2000; **7**: 2099–104.
44. Wightman L, Kircheis R, Rossler V, Carotta S, Ruzicka R, Kursa M *et al.* Different behavior of branched and linear polyethylenimine for gene delivery *in vitro* and *in vivo.* *Journal of Gene Medicine.* 2001; **3**: 362–72.

45. Lee H, Jeong JH, Park TG. A new gene delivery formulation of polyethylenimine/DNA complexes coated with PEG conjugated fusogenic peptide. *Journal of Controlled Release.* 2001; **76**: 183–92.
46. Tousignant JD, Gates AL, Ingram LA, Johnson CL, Nietupski JB, Cheng SH *et al.* Comprehensive analysis of the acute toxicities induced by systemic administration of cationic lipid:plasmid DNA complexes in mice. *Human Gene Therapy.* 2000; **11**: 2493–513.
47. Miao CH, Ohashi K, Patijn GA, Meuse L, Ye X, Thompson AR *et al.* Inclusion of the hepatic locus control region, an intron, and untranslated region increases and stabilizes hepatic factor IX gene expression *in vivo* but not *in vitro.* *Molecular Therapy.* 2000; **1**: 522–32.
48. Cui FD, Kishida T, Ohashi S, Asada H, Yasutomi K, Satoh E *et al.* Highly efficient gene transfer into murine liver achieved by intravenous administration of naked Epstein-Barr virus (EBV)-based plasmid vectors. *Gene Therapy.* 2001; **8**: 1508–13.
49. Stoll SM, Sclimenti CR, Baba EJ, Meuse L, Kay MA, Calos MP. Epstein-Barr virus/human vector provides high-level, long-term expression of alpha1-antitrypsin in mice. *Molecular Therapy.* 2001; **4**: 122–9.
50. Anderson RD, Haskell RE, Xia H, Roessler BJ, Davidson BL. A simple method for the rapid generation of recombinant adenovirus vectors. *Gene Therapy.* 2000; **7**: 1034–8.
51. Bergelson JM, Cunningham JA, Droguett G, Kurt-Jones EA, Krithivas A, Hong JS *et al.* Isolation of a common receptor for Coxsackie B viruses and adenoviruses 2 and 5. *Science.* 1997; **275**: 1320–3.
52. Fasbender A, Lee JH, Walters RW, Moninger TO, Zabner J, Welsh MJ. Incorporation of adenovirus in calcium phosphate precipitates enhances gene transfer to airway epithelia *in vitro* and *in vivo.* *Journal of Clinical Investigation.* 1998; **102**: 184–93.
53. Chillon M, Lee JH, Fasbender A, Welsh MJ. Adenovirus complexed with polyethylene glycol and cationic lipid is shielded from neutralizing antibodies in vitro. *Gene Therapy.* 1998; **5**: 995–1002.
54. Harvey BG, Hackett NR, Ely S, Crystal RG. Host responses and persistence of vector genome following intrabronchial administration of an E1(–)E3(–) adenovirus gene transfer vector to normal individuals. *Molecular Therapy.* 2001; **3**: 206–15.
* 55. Zaiss AK, Liu Q, Bowen GP, Wong NC, Bartlett JS, Muruve DA. Differential activation of innate immune responses by adenovirus and adeno-associated virus vectors. *Journal of Virology.* 2002; **76**: 4580–90.
56. Bristol JA, Gallo-Penn A, Andrews J, Idamakanti N, Kaleko M, Connelly S. Adenovirus-mediated factor VIII gene expression results in attenuated anti-factor VIII-specific immunity in hemophilia A mice compared with factor VIII protein infusion. *Human Gene Therapy.* 2001; **12**: 1651–61.
* 57. DelloRusso C, Scott JM, Hartigan-O'Connor D, Salvatori G, Barjot C, Robinson AS *et al.* Functional correction of adult mdx mouse muscle using gutted adenoviral vectors

expressing full-length dystrophin. *Proceedings of the National Academy of Sciences of the United States of America.* 2002; **99**: 12979–84.

58. Hartigan-O'Connor D, Barjot C, Salvatori G, Chamberlain JS. Generation and growth of gutted adenoviral vectors. *Methods in Enzymology.* 2002; **346**: 224–46.

59. Buchschacher Jr. GL, Wong-Staal F. Development of lentiviral vectors for gene therapy for human diseases. *Blood.* 2000; **95**: 2499–504.

60. Lewis PF, Emerman M. Passage through mitosis is required for oncoretroviruses but not for the human immunodeficiency virus. *Journal of Virology.* 1994; **68**: 510–6.

61. Rosenqvist N, Hard Af Segerstad C, Samuelsson C, Johansen J, Lundberg C. Activation of silenced transgene expression in neural precursor cell lines by inhibitors of histone deacetylation. *Journal of Gene Medicine.* 2002; **4**: 248–57.

62. Hanlon L, Barr NI, Blyth K, Stewart M, Haviernik P, Wolff L et al. Long-range effects of retroviral insertion on c-myb: overexpression may be obscured by silencing during tumor growth *in vitro. Journal of Virology.* 2003; **77**: 1059–68.

63. Lorincz MC, Schubeler D, Groudine M. Methylation-mediated proviral silencing is associated with MeCP2 recruitment and localized histone H3 deacetylation. *Molecular and Cellular Biology.* 2001; **21**: 7913–22.

64. Samulski RJ, Chang LS, Shenk T. Helper-free stocks of recombinant adeno-associated viruses: Normal integration does not require viral gene expression. *Journal of Virology.* 1989; **63**: 3822–8.

65. Jooss K, Yang Y, Fisher KJ, Wilson JM. Transduction of dendritic cells by DNA viral vectors directs the immune response to transgene products in muscle fibers. *Journal of Virology.* 1998; **72**: 4212–23.

* 66. Ponnazhagan S, Curiel DT, Shaw DR, Alvarez RD, Siegal GP. Adeno-associated virus for cancer gene therapy. *Cancer Res.* 2001; **61**: 6313–21.

67. Goebel EA, Davidson BL, Graham SM, Kern JA. Tumor reduction *in vivo* after adenoviral mediated gene transfer of the herpes simplex virus thymidine kinase gene and ganciclovir treatment in human head and neck squamous cell carcinoma. *Otolaryngology and Head and Neck Surgery.* 1998; **119**: 331–6.

68. Bi W, Kim YG, Feliciano ES, Pavelic L, Wilson KM, Pavelic ZP et al. An HSVtk-mediated local and distant antitumor bystander effect in tumors of head and neck origin in athymic mice. *Cancer Gene Therapy.* 1997; **4**: 246–52.

* 69. Frank DK, Frederick MJ, Liu TJ, Clayman GL. Bystander effect in the adenovirus-mediated wild-type p53 gene therapy model of human squamous cell carcinoma of the head and neck. *Clinical Cancer Research.* 1998; **4**: 2521–8.

70. Thomas SM, Naresh KN, Wagle AS, Mulherkar R. Preclinical studies on suicide Gene Therapy for head/neck cancer: a novel method for evaluation of treatment efficacy. *Anticancer Research.* 1998; **18**: 4393–8.

71. Sewell DA, Li D, Duan L, Westra WH, O'Malley Jr. BW. Safety of *in vivo* adenovirus-mediated thymidine kinase

treatment of oral cancer. *Archives of Otolaryngology – Head and Neck Surgery.* 1997; **123**: 1298–1302.

72. Kasono K, Blackwell JL, Douglas JT, Dmitriev I, Strong TV, Reynolds P et al. Selective gene delivery to head and neck cancer cells via an integrin targeted adenoviral vector. *Clinical Cancer Research.* 1999; **5**: 2571–9.

73. Lang S, Zeidler R, Mayer A, Reiman V, Wollenberg B, Kastenbauer E. Targeting head and neck cancer by GM-CSF-mediated gene therapy *in vitro. Anticancer Research.* 1999; **19**: 5335–9.

74. Finke J, Ferrone S, Frey A, Mufson A, Ochoa A. Where have all the T cells gone? Mechanisms of immune evasion by tumors. *Immunology Today.* 1999; **20**: 158–60.

75. Melero I, Bach N, Chen L. Costimulation, tolerance and ignorance of cytolytic T lymphocytes in immune responses to tumor antigens. *Life Sciences.* 1997; **60**: 2035–41.

76. Seliger B, Maeurer MJ, Ferrone S. TAP off–tumors on. *Immunology Today.* 1997; **18**: 292–9.

* 77. Petersson M, Charo J, Salazar-Onfray F, Noffz G, Mohaupt M, Qin Z et al. Constitutive IL-10 production accounts for the high NK sensitivity, low MHC class I expression, and poor transporter associated with antigen processing (TAP)-1/2 function in the prototype NK target YAC-1. *Journal of Immunology.* 1998; **161**: 2099–105.

* 78. Forni G, Giovarelli M, Santoni A. Lymphokine-activated tumor inhibition *in vivo*. I. The local administration of interleukin 2 triggers nonreactive lymphocytes from tumor-bearing mice to inhibit tumor growth. *Journal of Immunology.* 1985; **134**: 1305–11.

* 79. Cortesina G, De Stefani A, Giovarelli M, Barioglio MG, Cavallo GP, Jemma C et al. Treatment of recurrent squamous cell carcinoma of the head and neck with low doses of interleukin-2 injected perilymphatically. *Cancer.* 1988; **62**: 2482–5.

80. Cortesina G, De Stefani A, Galeazzi E, Cavallo GP, Jemma C, Giovarelli M et al. Interleukin-2 injected around tumor-draining lymph nodes in head and neck cancer. *Head and Neck.* 1991; **13**: 125–31.

81. Mattijssen V, De Mulder PH, Schornagel JH, Verweij J, Van den Broek P, Galazka A et al. Clinical and immunopathological results of a phase II study of perilymphatically injected recombinant interleukin-2 in locally far advanced, nonpretreated head and neck squamous cell carcinoma. *Journal of Immunotherapy.* 1991; **10**: 63–8.

82. Vlock DR, Snyderman CH, Johnson JT, Myers EN, Eibling DE, Rubin JS et al. Phase Ib trial of the effect of peritumoral and intranodal injections of interleukin-2 in patients with advanced squamous cell carcinoma of the head and neck: an Eastern Cooperative Oncology Group trial. *Journal of Immunotherapy with Emphasis on Tumor Immunology.* 1994; **15**: 134–9.

83. Wollenberg B, Kastenbauer, Mundl H, Schaumberg J, Mayer A, Andratschke M et al. Gene therapy – phase I trial for primary untreated head and neck squamous cell cancer (HNSCC) UICC stage II-IV with a single intratumoral

injection of hIL-2 plasmids formulated in DOTMA/Chol. *Human Gene Therapy*. 1999; **10**: 141–7.

84. Endo S, Zeng Q, Burke NA, He Y, Melhem MF, Watkins SF *et al.* TGF-alpha antisense gene therapy inhibits head and neck squamous cell carcinoma growth *in vivo*. *Gene Therapy*. 2000; **7**: 1906–14.

85. Li D, Jiang W, Bishop JS, Ralston R, O'Malley Jr. BW. Combination surgery and nonviral interleukin 2 Gene Therapy for head and neck cancer. *Clinical Cancer Research*. 1999; **5**: 1551–6.

86. Day KV, Li D, Liu S, Guo M, O'Malley Jr. BW. Granulocyte–macrophage colony-stimulating factor in a combination gene therapy strategy for head and neck cancer. *Laryngoscope*. 2001; **111**: 801–6.

87. Li D, Zeiders JW, Liu S, Guo M, Xu Y, Bishop JS *et al.* Combination nonviral cytokine gene therapy for head and neck cancer. *Laryngoscope*. 2001; **111**: 815–20.

88. Mobley SR, Liu TJ, Hudson JM, Clayman GL. *In vitro* growth suppression by adenoviral transduction of p21 and p16 in squamous cell carcinoma of the head and neck: a research model for combination gene therapy. *Archives of Otolaryngology – Head and Neck Surgery*. 1998; **124**: 88–92.

∗ 89. Clayman GL, Frank DK, Bruso PA, Goepfert H. Adenovirus-mediated wild-type p53 gene transfer as a surgical adjuvant in advanced head and neck cancers. *Clinical Cancer Research*. 1999; **5**: 1715–22.

90. Clayman GL. The current status of gene therapy. *Seminars in Oncology*. 2000; **27**: 39–43.

91. Fujiwara T, Grimm EA, Mukhopadhyay T, Zhang WW, Owen-Schaub LB, Roth JA. Induction of chemosensitivity in human lung cancer cells *in vivo* by adenovirus-mediated transfer of the wild-type p53 gene. *Cancer Research*. 1994; **54**: 2287–91.

92. De Pace NG. Case report: Cervical cancer regression following rabies vaccination. *Ginnecologia*. 1912; **9**: 82.

93. Heise CC, Williams A, Olesch J, Kirn DH. Efficacy of a replication-competent adenovirus (ONYX-015) following intratumoral injection: intratumoral spread and distribution effects. *Cancer Gene Therapy*. 1999; **6**: 499–504.

∗ 94. Heise C, Sampson-Johannes A, Williams A, McCormick F, Von Hoff DD, Kirn DH. ONYX-015, an E1B gene-attenuated adenovirus, causes tumor-specific cytolysis and antitumoral efficacy that can be augmented by standard chemotherapeutic agents. *Nature Medicine*. 1997; **3**: 639–45.

∗ 95. Nemunaitis J, Khuri F, Ganly I, Arseneau J, Posner M, Vokes E *et al.* Phase II trial of intratumoral administration of ONYX-015, a replication-selective adenovirus, in patients with refractory head and neck cancer. *Journal of Clinical Oncology*. 2001; **19**: 289–98.

96. Nemunaitis J, Cunningham C, Buchanan A, Blackburn A, Edelman G, Maples P *et al.* Intravenous infusion of a replication-selective adenovirus (ONYX-015) in cancer patients: safety, feasibility and biological activity. *Gene Therapy*. 2001; **8**: 746–59.

97. Lamont JP, Nemunaitis J, Kuhn JA, Landers SA, McCarty TM. A prospective phase II trial of ONYX-015 adenovirus and chemotherapy in recurrent squamous cell carcinoma of the head and neck (the Baylor experience). *Annals of Surgical Oncology*. 2000; **7**: 588–92.

98. Ganly I, Kirn D, Eckhardt G, Rodriguez GI, Soutar DS, Otto R *et al.* A phase I study of Onyx-015, an E1B attenuated adenovirus, administered intratumorally to patients with recurrent head and neck cancer. *Clinical Cancer Research*. 2000; **6**: 798–806.

4

Mechanisms of anticancer drugs

SARAH PAYNE AND DAVID MILES

Introduction	34	Novel therapies for the future	41
Principles of chemotherapy	34	Other novel treatments	44
Principles of tumour biology	34	Conclusion	44
Classification of chemotherapeutic agents	37	Key points	45
Limitations of cytotoxic agents	40	Deficiencies in current knowledge and areas for future	
Chemotherapy in head and neck cancer	40	research	45
Choice of chemotherapy in head and neck cancer	40	References	45
Chemotherapy strategies	40	Further reading	46

SEARCH STRATEGY

The data in this chapter are supported by a Medline search using the key words chemotherapy and head and neck neoplasms, and focus on mechanisms of action of current and experimental drugs.

INTRODUCTION

The discovery of the toxic action of nitrogen mustards on cells of the haematopoietic system more than 50 years ago initially triggered research into the development of cytotoxic agents. The initial promise of these drugs in the management of haematological and other rare malignancies has not been sustained and cure of the more common epithelial malignancies when metastatic, remains an elusive goal.

Many of the current chemotherapeutic agents have been discovered as a result of screening compounds for cytotoxic potency *in vitro* against murine and/or human cancer cells or *in vivo* against rodent tumour models. With our better understanding of the molecular basis of cancer there is now interest in target-directed drug therapies. The aim being to develop agents that can modulate or inhibit specific molecular targets identified as being essential for tumour growth.

PRINCIPLES OF CHEMOTHERAPY

Many forms of chemotherapy are targeted at the process of cell division. The rationale being that cancer cells are more likely to be replicating than normal cells. Unfortunately as their action is not specific, they are associated with significant toxicity. An understanding of the principles of tumour biology and cellular kinetics is helpful to appreciate the mechanisms of action of cancer chemotherapy.

PRINCIPLES OF TUMOUR BIOLOGY

Cellular kinetics

CELL CYCLE

Uncontrolled cell division is a result of interference in the normal balance of the cell cycle. The cell cycle is divided into a number of phases governed by an elaborate set of molecular switches (**Figure 4.1**). Normal nondividing cells are in G0. When actively recruited into the cell cycle they then pass through four phases:

1. **G1**: the growth phase in which the cell increases in size and prepares to copy its DNA;
2. **S (synthesis)**: which allows doubling of the chromosomal material;

3. **G2**: a further growth phase before cell division;
4. **M (mitosis)**: where the chromosomes separate and the cell divides.

At the end of a cycle the daughter cells can either continue through the cycle, leave and enter the resting phase (G0) or become terminally differentiated.

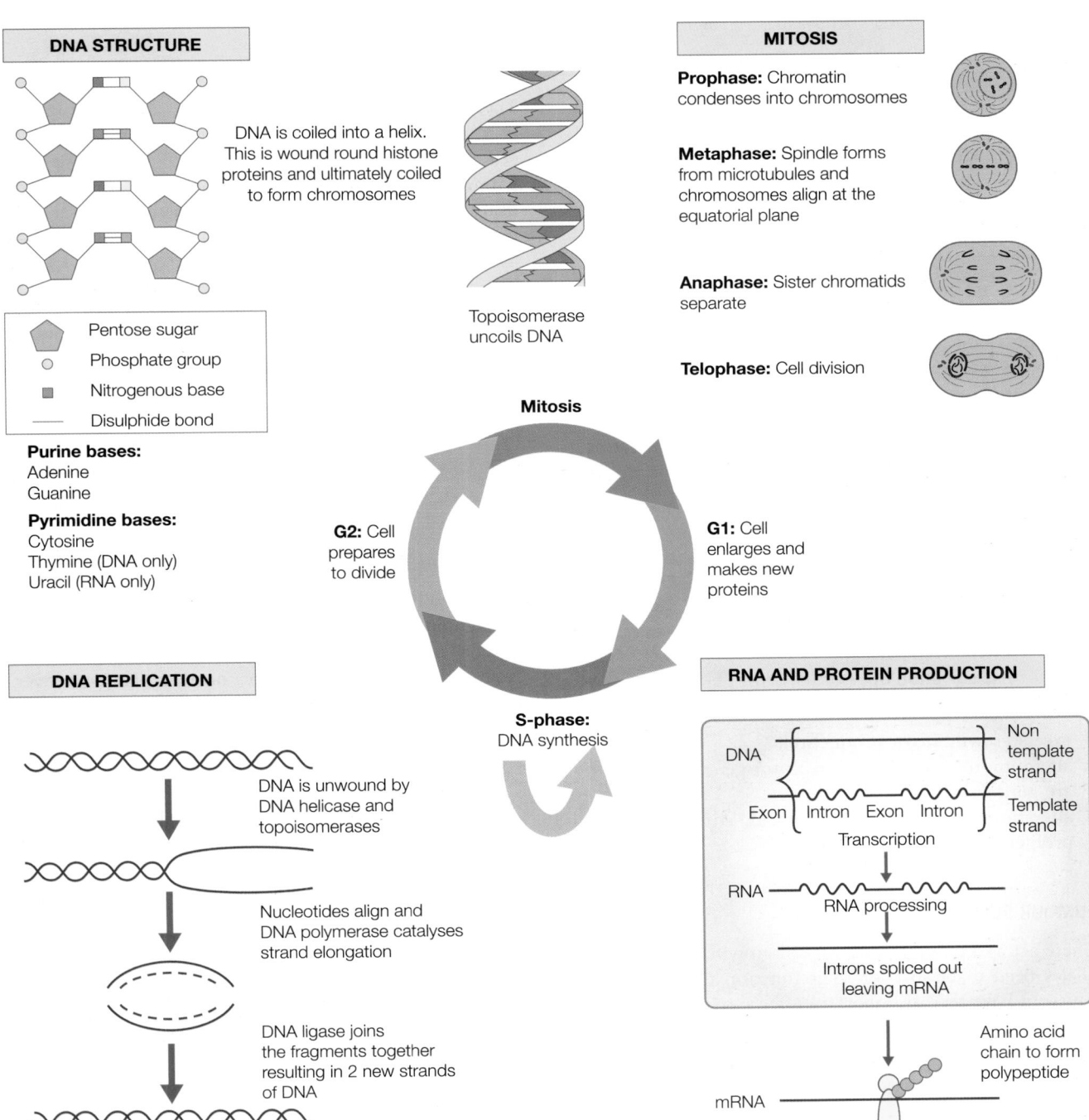

DNA STRUCTURE

DNA is coiled into a helix. This is wound round histone proteins and ultimately coiled to form chromosomes

- Pentose sugar
- Phosphate group
- Nitrogenous base
- Disulphide bond

Purine bases:
Adenine
Guanine

Pyrimidine bases:
Cytosine
Thymine (DNA only)
Uracil (RNA only)

Topoisomerase uncoils DNA

MITOSIS

Prophase: Chromatin condenses into chromosomes

Metaphase: Spindle forms from microtubules and chromosomes align at the equatorial plane

Anaphase: Sister chromatids separate

Telophase: Cell division

Mitosis

G2: Cell prepares to divide

G1: Cell enlarges and makes new proteins

S-phase: DNA synthesis

DNA REPLICATION

DNA is unwound by DNA helicase and topoisomerases

Nucleotides align and DNA polymerase catalyses strand elongation

DNA ligase joins the fragments together resulting in 2 new strands of DNA

RNA AND PROTEIN PRODUCTION

DNA

Non template strand

Exon | Intron | Exon | Intron

Template strand

Transcription

RNA

RNA processing

Introns spliced out leaving mRNA

Amino acid chain to form polypeptide

mRNA

Ribosome

Figure 4.1 Cell cycle: possible targets for chemotherapy.

TUMOUR GROWTH

The kinetics of any population of tumour cells is regulated by the following:

- **doubling time**: the cell cycle time, which varies considerably between tissue types;
- **growth fraction**: the percentage of cells passing through the cell cycle at a given point in time which is greatest in the early stages;
- **cell loss**: which can result from unsuccessful division, death, desquamation, metastasis and migration.

Tumours characteristically follow a sigmoid-shaped growth curve, in which tumour doubling size varies with tumour size. Tumours grow most rapidly at small volumes. As they become larger, growth is influenced by the rate of cell death and the availability of blood supply.

Cell signalling

Cells respond to their environment via external signals called growth factors. These interact with cell surface receptors that activate an internal signalling cascade. This ultimately acts at the DNA level through transcription factors that bind to the promoter regions of relevant genes, stimulating the cell cycle and influencing many important processes including cell division, migration, programmed cell death (apoptosis).

ONCOGENES

Protooncogenes are involved in controlling normal cell growth. Mutated forms, known as oncogenes, can lead to inappropriate stimulation of the cell cycle and excessive cell growth. Alternatively, malignancy can also arise secondary to abnormal activation of a normal gene. The consequences of gene activation associated with tumour growth include:

- excess growth factor production;
- alteration of growth factor receptor genes so that they are permanently switched on;
- alteration of the intracellular cascade stimulating proliferation.

TUMOUR SUPPRESSOR GENES

These act as a natural brake on cell growth. Usually both alleles need to be lost for their function to be affected. This can have several important effects, which include:

- impairment of the inhibitory signals influencing receptor genes or intracellular signalling;
- loss of the counter signals controlling protooncogene function;
- inhibition of apoptosis, often as a consequence of a mutation of p53, the protein associated with DNA repair.

Metastatic spread

A tumour is considered malignant when it has the capacity to spread beyond its original site and invade surrounding tissue. Normally cells are anchored to the extracellular matrix by cell adhesion molecules, including the integrins. Abnormalities of the factors maintaining tissue integrity will allow local invasion and ultimately metastases of the tumour cells.

Mechanism of cell death

There are two main types of cell death: apoptosis and necrosis. Necrotic cell death is caused by gross cell injury and results in the death of groups of cells within a tissue. Apoptosis is a regulated form of cell death that may be induced or is preprogrammed into the cell (e.g. during development) and is characterized by specific DNA changes and no accompanying inflammatory response. It can be triggered if mistakes in DNA replication are identified. Loss of this protective mechanism would allow mutant cells to continue to divide and grow, thereby conserving mutations in subsequent cell divisions.

Many cytotoxic anticancer drugs and radiotherapy act by inducing mutations in cancer cells which are not sufficient to cause cell death, but which can be recognized by the cell, triggering apoptosis.

FRACTIONAL CELL KILL HYPOTHESIS AND DRUG DOSING

Theoretically the administration of successive doses of chemotherapy will result in a fixed reduction in the number of cancer cells with each cycle.[1] A gap between cycles is necessary to allow normal tissue recover. Unfortunately, these first-order dynamics are not observed in clinical practice. Factors such as variation in tumour sensitivity and effective drug delivery with each course result in an unpredictable cell response.

Clinical responses to antitumour therapies are defined by arbitrary criteria that have been used as part of the evaluation process in assessing the potential utility of novel agents.

- **Tumour size:**
  - complete response is defined as the apparent disappearance of the tumour;
  - partial response represents a reduction of more than 50 percent;
  - progression is defined as an increase in tumour size by more than 25 percent;
  - stable disease is an intermediate between partial response and tumour progression.
- **Tumour products:**
  - biochemical or other tests can be used to assess response, including circulating tumour markers.

CLASSIFICATION OF CHEMOTHERAPEUTIC AGENTS

Classification according to phase-specific toxicity

Cytotoxic drugs can be classified according to whether they are more likely to target cells in a particular phase of their growth cycle. More crudely, they can also be divided into whether they are more toxic to cells that are actively dividing rather than cells in both the proliferating and resting phases.

PHASE-SPECIFIC CHEMOTHERAPY

These drugs, such as methotrexate and vinca alkaloids, kill proliferating cells only during a specific part or parts of the cell cycle. Antimetabolites, such as methotrexate, are more active against S-phase cells (inhibiting DNA synthesis) whereas vinca alkaloids are more M-phase specific (inhibiting spindle formation and alignment of chromosomes).

Attempts have been made to time drug administration in such a way that the cells are synchronized into a phase of the cell cycle that renders them especially sensitive to the cytotoxic agent. For example, vinblastine can arrest cells in mitosis. These synchronized cells enter the S-phase together and can be killed by a phase-specific agent, such as cytosine arabinoside. Most current drug schedules, however, have not been devised on the basis of cell kinetics.

CELL CYCLE-SPECIFIC CHEMOTHERAPY

Most chemotherapy agents are cell cycle-specific, meaning that they act predominantly on cells that are actively dividing. They have a dose-related plateau in their cell killing ability because only a subset of proliferating cells remain fully sensitive to drug-induced cytotoxicity at any one time. The way to increase cell kill is therefore to increase the duration of exposure rather than increasing the drug dose.

CELL CYCLE-NONSPECIFIC CHEMOTHERAPY

These drugs, for example alkylating agents and platinum derivatives, have an equal effect on tumour and normal cells whether they are in the proliferating or resting phase. They have a linear dose–response curve; that is, the greater the dose of the drug, the greater the fractional cell kill.

Classification according to mechanism

Classifying cytotoxic drugs according to their mechanism of action is the preferred system in use between clinicians.

ALKYLATING AGENTS

These highly reactive compounds produce their effects by covalently linking an alkyl group (R-CH2) to a chemical species in nucleic acids or proteins. The site at which the cross-links are formed and the number of cross-links formed is drug specific. Most alkylating agents are bipolar, i.e. they contain two groups capable of reacting with DNA. They can thus form bridges between a single strand or two separate strands of DNA, interfering with the action of the enzymes involved in DNA replication. The cell then either dies or is physically unable to divide or triggers apoptosis. The damage is most serious during the S-phase, as the cell has less time to remove the damaged fragments. Examples include:

- nitrogen mustards (e.g. melphalan and chlorambucil);
- oxazaphosphorenes (e.g. cyclophosphamide, ifosfamide);
- alkyl alkane sulphonates (busulphan);
- nitrosureas (e.g. carmustine (BCNU), lomustine (CCNU));
- tetrazines (e.g. dacarbazine, mitozolomide and temozolomide);
- aziridines (thiopeta, mitomycin C);
- procarbazine.

HEAVY METALS

Platinum agents

These include carboplatin, cisplatin and oxaliplatin. Cisplatin is an organic heavy metal complex. Chloride ions are lost from the molecule after it diffuses into a cell allowing the compound to cross-link with the DNA strands, mostly to guanine groups. This causes intra- and interstrand DNA cross-links, resulting in inhibition of DNA, RNA and protein synthesis.

Carboplatin has the same platinum moiety as cisplatin, but is bonded to an organic carboxylate group. This leads to increased water solubility and slower hydrolysis that has an influence on its toxicity profile. It is less nephrotoxic and neurotoxic, but causes more marked myelosuppression.

Oxaliplatin belongs to a new class of platinum agent. It contains a platinum atom complexed with oxalate and a bulky diaminocyclohexane (DACH) group. It forms reactive platinum complexes that are believed to inhibit DNA synthesis by forming interstrand and intra-strand cross-linking of DNA molecules. Oxaliplatin is not generally cross-resistant to cisplatin or carboplatin, possibly due to the DACH group.

ANTIMETABOLITES

Antimetabolites are compounds that bear a structural similarity to naturally occurring substances such as vitamins, nucleosides or amino acids. They compete with the natural substrate for the active site on an essential enzyme or receptor. Some are incorporated directly into DNA or RNA. Most are phase-specific, acting during the S-phase of the cell cycle. Their efficacy is usually greater over a prolonged period of time, so they are usually given continuously. There are three main classes.

Folic acid antagonists

Methotrexate competitively inhibits dihydrofolate reductase, which is responsible for the formation of tetrahydrofolate from dihydrofolate. This is essential for the generation of a variety of coenzymes that are involved in the synthesis of purines, thymidylate, methionine and glycine. A critical influence on cell division also appears to be inhibition of the production of thymidine monophosphate, which is essential for DNA and RNA synthesis. The block in activity of dihydrofolate reductase can be bypassed by supplying an intermediary metabolite, most commonly folinic acid. This is converted to tetrahydrofolate that is required for thymidylate synthetase function (**Figure 4.2**).

Pyrimidine analogues

These drugs resemble pyrimidine molecules and work by either inhibiting the synthesis of nucleic acids (e.g. fluorouracil (**Figure 4.3**)), inhibiting enzymes involved in DNA synthesis (e.g. cytarabine, which inhibits DNA polymerase) or by becoming incorporated into DNA (e.g. gemcitabine), interfering with DNA synthesis and resulting in cell death.

Purine analogues

These are analogues of the natural purine bases and nucleotides. 6-Mercaptopurine (6MP) and thioguanine are derivatives of adenine and guanine, respectively. A sulphur group replaces the keto group on carbon-6 in these compounds. In many cases, the drugs require initial activation. They are then able to inhibit nucleotide biosynthesis by direct incorporation into DNA.

CYTOTOXIC ANTIBIOTICS

Most antitumour antibiotics have been produced from bacterial and fungal cultures (often *Streptomyces* species). They affect the function and synthesis of nucleic acids in different ways.

- **Anthracyclines** (e.g. doxorubicin, daunorubicin, epirubicin) intercalate with DNA and affect the topoiosmerase II enzyme. This DNA gyrase splits the DNA helix and reconnects it to overcome the torsional forces that would interfere with replication. The anthracyclines stabilize the DNA tomoisomerase II complex and thus prevent reconnection of the strands.
- **Actinomycin D** intercalates between guanine and cytosine base pairs. This interferes with the transcription of DNA at high doses. At low doses DNA-directed RNA synthesis is blocked.
- **Bleomycin** consists of a mixture of glycopeptides that cause DNA fragmentation.
- **Mitomycin C** inhibits DNA synthesis by cross-linking DNA, acting like an alkylating agent.

SPINDLE POISONS

Vinca alkaloids

The two prominent agents in this group are vincristine and vinblastine that are extracted from the periwinkle

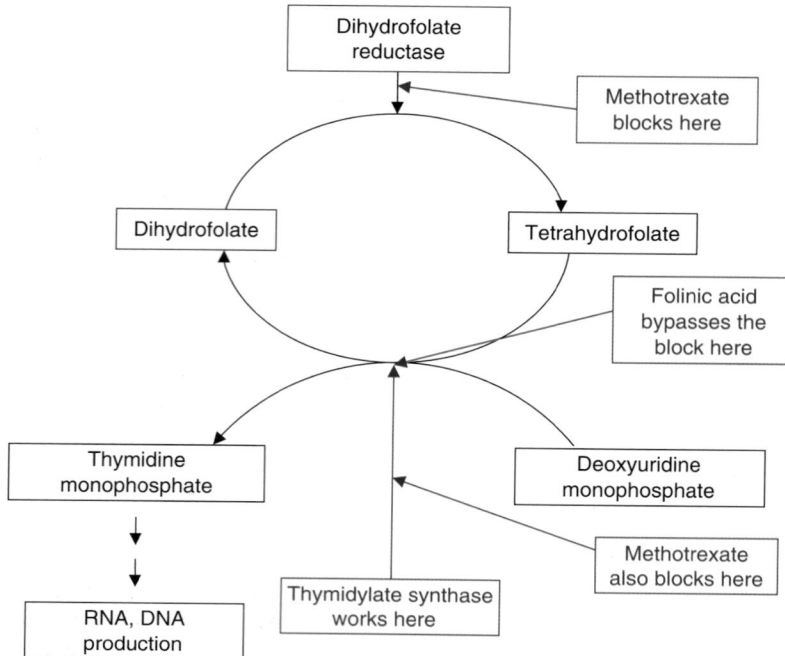

Figure 4.2 Mechanism of action of cytotoxic drugs: methotrexate.

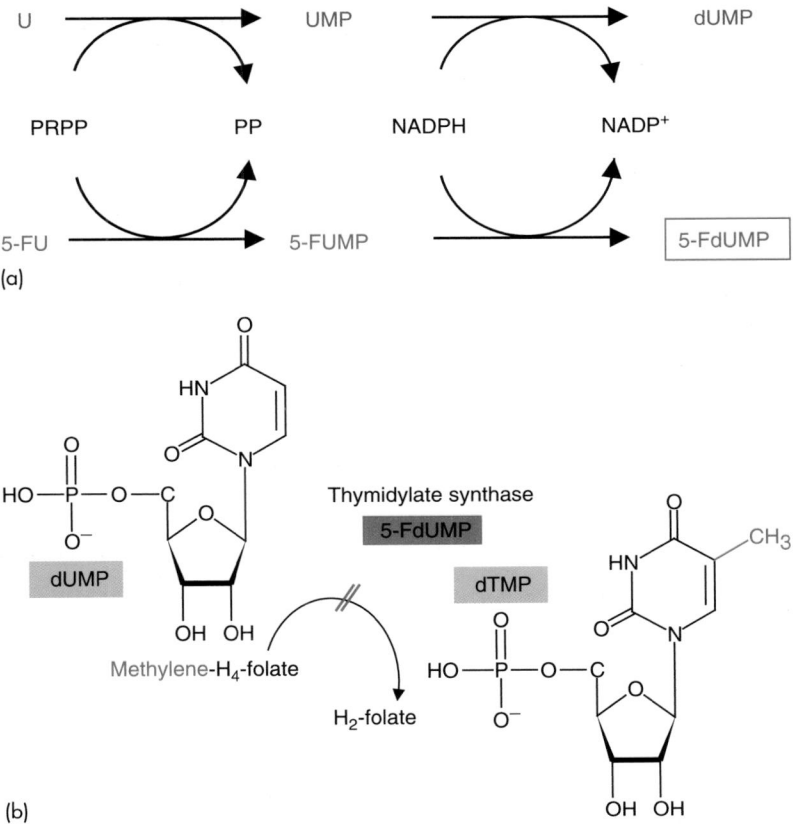

Figure 4.3 Mechanism of action of cytotoxic drugs: Fluorouracil. 5-Fluorouracil (5FU) can participate in many reactions in which uracil would normally be involved. Firstly, it has to be converted to its active form, 5-fluoro-2 deoxyuridine monophophate (5-FdUMP) (a). This then interferes with DNA synthesis by binding to the enzyme thymidylate synthetase, causing it to be inactivated (b). The binding can be stabilized by the addition of folinic acid. 5FdUMP, 5-fluorodeoxyuridine monophosphate; 5FU, 5-fluorouracil; 5FUMP, 5-fluorouridine monophosphate; dTMP, deoxythymidine monophosphate; dUMP, deoxyuridine monophophase; NADP, nicotinamide adenine dinucleotide phosphate; NADPH, reduced form of nicotinamide adenine dinucleotide phosphate; PP, pyrophosphate; PRPP, 5-phospho-alpha-D-ribose 1-diphosphate; U, uracil; UMP, uridine monophosphate.

plant. They are mitotic spindle poisons that act by binding to tubulin, the building block of the microtubules. This inhibits further assembly of the spindle during metaphase, thus inhibiting mitosis. Although microtubules are important in other cell functions (hormone secretion, axonal transport and cell motility), it is likely that the influence of this group of drugs on DNA repair contributes most significantly to their toxicity. Other newer examples include vindesine and vinorelbine.

Taxoids

Paclitaxel (Taxol) is a drug derived from the bark of the pacific yew, *Taxus brevifolia*. It promotes assembly of microtubules and inhibits their disassembly. Direct activation of apoptotic pathways has also been suggested to be critical to the cytotoxicity of this drug.[2] Docetaxel (Taxotere) is a semisynthetic derivative.

TOPOISOMERASE INHIBITORS

Topoisomerases are responsible for altering the 3D structure of DNA by a cleaving/unwinding/rejoining

reaction. They are involved in DNA replication, chromatid segregation and transcription. It has previously been considered that the efficacy of topoisomerase inhibitors in the treatment of cancer was based solely on their ability to inhibit DNA replication. It has now been suggested that drug efficacy may also depend on the simultaneous manipulation of other cellular pathways within tumour cells.[3] The drugs are phase-specific and prevent cells from entering mitosis from G2. There are two broad classes:

Topoisomerase I inhibitors

Camptothecin, derived from *Camptotheca acuminata* (a Chinese tree), binds to the enzyme–DNA complex, stabilizing it and preventing DNA replication. Irinotecan and topetecan have been derived from this prototype.

Topoisomerase II inhibitors

Epipodophyllotoxin derivatives (e.g. etoposide, vespid) are semisynthetic derivatives of *Podophyllum peltatum*, the American mandrake. They stabilize the complex between topoisomerase II and DNA that causes strand breaks and ultimately inhibits DNA replication.

LIMITATIONS OF CYTOTOXIC AGENTS

There are a number of problems with the safety profile and efficacy of chemotherapeutic agents. Cytotoxics predominantly affect rapidly dividing cells so do not specifically target cancer cells in the resting phase. They also only influence a cell's ability to divide and have little effect on other aspects of tumour progression such as tissue invasion, metastases or progressive loss of differentiation. Finally, cytotoxics are associated with a high incidence of adverse effects. The most notable examples include bone marrow suppression, alopecia, mucositis, nausea and vomiting.

CHEMOTHERAPY IN HEAD AND NECK CANCER

Worldwide, squamous cell cancer of the head and neck accounts for an estimated 500,000 new cancer cases per year. One-third of these patients present with early stage disease that is amenable to cure with surgery or radiotherapy alone. The remaining patients usually present with locally advanced disease. Unfortunately, this group exhibit high recurrence rates of approximately 65 percent despite radical surgery and radiotherapy. To date, the addition of chemotherapy has not changed this. It has, however, allowed improved organ preservation when combined with radiotherapy and has led to a reduction in rates of distant metastases. Chemotherapy also has a role in the palliative treatment of advanced disease.

Currently, surgery or radiotherapy are the standard curative options for early stage head and neck cancer. Chemotherapy in combination with surgery, radiotherapy or both is employed for locoregionally advanced disease. Stage IV disease is managed with palliative chemotherapy (see also Chapter 200, Developments in radiotherapy for head and neck cancer).

CHOICE OF CHEMOTHERAPY IN HEAD AND NECK CANCER

The single agents active in head and neck cancer, with response rates between 15 and 40 percent, include methotrexate, cisplatin, carboplatin, fluorouracil, ifosfamide, bleomycin, paclitaxel and docetaxel. Cisplatin is particularly popular for use either as a single agent or in combination with other drugs because for a long time it was viewed as one of the most active drugs in squamous head and neck cancer.[4] Taxoids and gemcitabine are now gaining favour and are being incorporated into many current drug trials. [***]

CHEMOTHERAPY STRATEGIES

Combination chemotherapy

Combinations of cytotoxic agents are widely used for many cancers and may be more effective than single agents. Possible explanations for this include:

- exposure to agents with different mechanisms of action and nonoverlapping toxicities;
- reduction in the development of drug resistance;
- the ability to use combinations of drugs that may be synergistic.

In practice, the predominant dose-limiting toxicity of many cytotoxic drugs is myelosuppression and this limits the doses of individual drugs when used in combination.

Adjuvant chemotherapy

This is the use of chemotherapy in patients known to be at risk of relapse by virtue of features determined at the time of definitive local treatment (e.g. tumour grade, lymph node status, etc.). The intention of adjuvant chemotherapy is therefore the eradication of micrometastatic disease.

Randomized trials assessing the use of adjuvant chemotherapy for the patients with head and neck squamous carcinoma do not suggest a significant benefit.[5] [****]

Neoadjuvant chemotherapy

Neoadjuvant, or induction chemotherapy, is the use of chemotherapy before definitive surgery or radiotherapy in patients with locally advanced disease. The intention of this strategy is to improve local and distant control of the disease in order to achieve greater organ preservation and overall survival.

Numerous phase III trials have considered the benefit of neoadjuvant chemotherapy followed by definitive surgery, by surgery and radiotherapy, or by radiotherapy alone as compared to definitive management without chemotherapy. Unfortunately, these studies have not demonstrated a survival advantage. To date, only subset analyses of trials using neoadjuvant cisplatin and 5-fluorouracil combination chemotherapy compared with locoregional treatment alone have shown a small survival gain.[5] In addition, neoadjuvant chemotherapy has been shown to have little impact on reducing locoregional failure. This is perhaps surprising given the consistently observed high initial tumour response rates of up to 70–85 percent.

The role of neoadjuvant chemotherapy therefore continues to remain controversial and further studies are planned, particularly looking at more effective drug combinations. [****]

Concurrent chemoradiation

This involves the synchronous use of chemotherapy and radiotherapy. Multiple randomized trials comparing concurrent radiotherapy and chemotherapy with radiotherapy alone have shown significant improvement in locoregional control, relapse-free survival and overall survival rates in patients with locally advanced, unresectable disease.[6] These results may reflect the influence of chemotherapy on micrometastatic disease or its ability to enhance tumour radiosensitivity.[7] Some chemotherapy agents are recognized to be more active in certain radioresistant cell types. Other drugs may act synergistically with radiotherapy by hindering the repair of radiation-induced DNA damage (cisplatin), by synchronizing or arresting cells during radiosensitive phases (hydroxyurea, paclitaxel) or by hindering regrowth between fractions of treatment.

Many different drug combinations and radiation schedules have been evaluated. Each combination clearly has unique toxicities, risks and benefits. At present, there is still debate regarding the optimum chemoradiotherapy regimen that should become the standard of care. [****/**]

High-dose chemotherapy

Many chemotherapy drugs have a linear dose–response curve, but their use at high doses is limited by myelosuppression. This may be overcome by using bone marrow or peripheral stem cell infusions. While high-dose chemotherapy appears to have a role in the management of leukaemias, myeloma and certain lymphomas, little benefit has been demonstrated in common solid tumours. [****]

Chemoprevention

This is a novel approach with the aim of reversing or halting carcinogenesis with the use of pharmacologic or natural agents. Retinoids have been tested in head and neck carcinogenesis both in animal models and against oral premalignant lesions and in the prevention of secondary tumours in humans, with initial encouraging results.[8, 9] Studies are also looking at the benefit of using cyclo-oxygenase 2 (COX-2) inhibitors in a similar role.[10] [**]

NOVEL THERAPIES FOR THE FUTURE

Despite the introduction of new cytotoxic drugs, such as antimetabolites (capecitabine) and topoisomerase I inhibitors, the management of advanced head and neck cancer remains challenging. Over the last years interest has focussed more on novel agents with a more targeted mechanisms of action.

Targeted therapy aims to specifically act on a well-defined target or biologic pathway that, when inactivated, causes regression or destruction of the malignant process. The main strategies of research have looked at the use of monoclonal antibodies or targeted small molecules.

Monoclonal antibodies

In the early 1980s, it became apparent that targetted therapy using monoclonal antibodies (MAb) might be useful in the detection and treatment of cancer. Monoclonal antibodies can be derived from a variety of sources:

- murine: mouse antibodies;
- chimeric: part mouse/part human antibodies;
- humanized: engineered to be mostly human;
- human: fully human antibodies.

Murine monoclonal antibodies may themselves induce an immune response that may limit repeated administration. Humanized and, to a lesser extent, chimeric antibodies are less immunogenic and can be given repeatedly.

There are several proposed mechanisms of action of monoclonal antibodies.[11] These include:

- direct effects:
  - induction of apoptosis;
  - inhibition of signalling through the receptors needed for cell proliferation/function;
  - anti-idiotype antibody formation, determinants amplifying an immune response to the tumour cell;
- indirect effects:
  - antibody-dependent cellular cytotoxicity (ADCC, conjugating the 'killer cell' to the tumour cell);
  - complement-mediated cellular cytotoxicity (fixation of complement leading to cytotoxicity).

A desirable target for MAbs would have the following properties:

- wide distribution on tumour cells;
- high level of expression;
- bound to tumour, allowing cell lysis;
- absent from normal tissues;
- trigger activation of complement on MAb binding;
- limited antigenic modulation of target.

Antibodies have also been used as vectors for the delivery of drugs and radiopharmaceuticals to a target of tumour cells.

The earliest and most successful clinical use of antibodies in oncology has been for the treatment of haematological malignancies. Interest in the development of antibodies for solid tumours has become increasingly popular, especially with respect to the epidermal and vascular endothelial growth factor receptors.

Epidermal growth factor receptor biology

Epidermal growth factor receptor (EGFR) biology is a 170-kDa transmembrane protein composed of an extracellular ligand-binding domain, a transmembrane lipophilic region and an intracellular protein tyrosine kinase domain (**Figure 4.4**). When a substrate binds to the receptor, the ligand–receptor complex dimerizes and is internalized by the host cell. This activates an intracellular protein kinase by autophosphorylation, which in

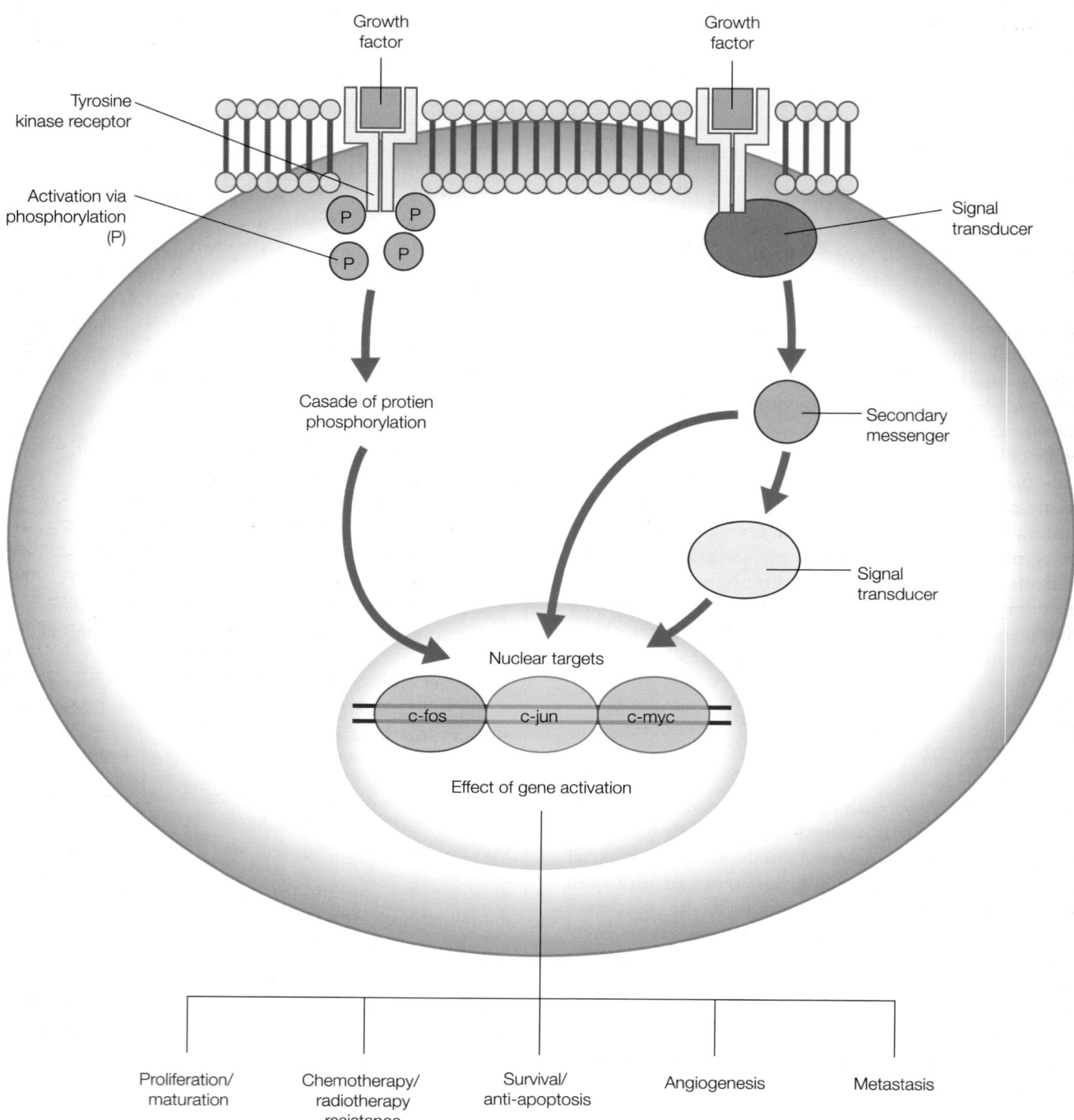

Figure 4.4 Simplified epidermal growth factor receptor signal transduction pathways and opportunities for intervention. GRB2, growth factor receptor binding protein 2; MAPK, mitogen-activated protein kinase; MEK, MAPK/extracellular signal related kinase; SOS, guanine nucleotide exchange factor (son of sevenless); c-fos, c-jun and c-myc, nuclear targets involved in gene transcription/cell cycle progression; P, phosphate; TGFα, transformation growth factor α; PI3-K, phosphotidyinositol 3; AKT, serine/threonine kinase, prosurvival protein; STAT, signal transducing activation of transcription.

turn activates signal transduction pathways, influencing cell function. This can lead to cell proliferation, as well as invasion and metastasis.

Several investigators have described amplification of the EGFR gene and overexpression of the EGFR surface membrane protein in a large number of human cancers, including squamous cell carcinoma of the head and neck.[12]

Overexpression is associated with increased proliferative capacity and metastatic potential and is an independent indicator of poor prognosis.[13] Blockade of the EGFR pathway has been shown to inhibit the proliferation of malignant cells and also appears to influence angiogenesis, cell motility and invasion.[14] Various strategies have been investigated to manipulate EGFR.

Monoclonal antibodies against epidermal growth factor receptor

MAb technology has been directed against EGFR. The chimeric IgG antibody cetuximab (C225) has the binding affinity equal to that of the natural ligand and can effectively block the effect of epidermal growth factor and transforming growth factor α.[6] It has been shown to enhance the antitumour effects of chemotherapy and radiotherapy in preclinical models.[15, 16, 17] More recently, cetuximab has been evaluated alone and in combination with radiotherapy and various cytotoxic chemotherapeutic agents in a series of phase II and III studies involving patients with head and neck cancers.[15, 18] The studies are encouraging, but it is still too early to determine the exact role the antibody will play in treatment regimens.

Targeted small molecules against epidermal growth factor receptor

Gefitinib (Iressa) and erlotinib (Tarceva) are orally active epidermal growth factor receptor tyrosine kinase inhibitors (EGFR-TKI) that block the EGFR signalling cascade, thereby inhibiting the growth, proliferation and survival of many solid tumours. They have single agent activity in patients with recurrent or metastatic head and neck cancer, and have an acceptable safety profile compared with conventional chemotherapy.[19, 20] Results of phase III trials are awaited and will help determine their optimal use in head and neck cancers.

Interestingly, one of the noted side effects of the drugs is an acneiform rash. Analysis of phase II trials of erlotinib in nonsmall-cell lung cancer, head and neck cancer and ovarian cancer shows a significant association between the rash severity and objective tumour response and overall survival.[21] Similar findings have been made with cetuximab and gefitinib. This association suggests that the rash may serve as a marker of response to treatment and could be used to guide treatment to obtain optimal dose.

Despite these successes, these agents have modest activity when used as single agents in unselected patients. It is clear that the clinical development of these agents is far from simple. It is important that we try to understand better the biological and clinical criteria for patient selection and also how best to use the different available agents. The recent discovery of EGFR mutations and the potential identification of other markers that might predict patient response could help to optimize the use of these agents in the future.

Inhibitors of angiogenesis

Angiogenesis is the process of new blood vessel formation, triggered by hypoxia and regulated by numerous stimulators and inhibitors (**Figure 4.5**). It is vital for cancer development. A tumour cannot extend beyond 2–3 mm without inducing a vascular supply. New vessels develop on the edge of the tumour and then migrate into the tumour. This process relies on degradation of the extracellular matrix surrounding the tumour by matrix metalloproteinases, such as collagenase, that are expressed at high levels in some tumour and stromal cells. Angiogenesis is then dependent on the migration and proliferation of endothelial cells.

It has been found that antiangiogenic agents tend to be cytostatic rather than cytotoxic, hence stabilizing the tumour and preventing spread. As a consequence, they may be valuable for use in combination with cytotoxic drugs, as maintenance therapy in early-stage cancers or as adjuvant treatment after definitive radiotherapy or surgery. There is evidence to support the fact that suppressing angiogenesis can maintain metastases in a state of dormancy.[22] Interestingly, development of resistance does not appear to be a feature of these drugs.[23] [**]

Vascular endothelial growth factor receptor

Vascular endothelial growth factor is a multifunctional cytokine released in response to hypoxia and is an important stimulator of angiogenesis. It binds to two structurally related trans-membrane receptors present on endothelial cells, called Flt-1 and KDR. High VEGF protein and receptor expression has been demonstrated in certain head and neck cancers and is associated with a higher tumour proliferation rate and worse survival.[24]

Monoclonal antibodies against vascular endothelial growth factor receptor

Bevacizumab (Avastin) is a humanized murine monoclonal antibody targeting VEGF. It is the first antiangiogenic drug to have induced a survival advantage in cancer therapy, within a randomized trial of irinotecan,

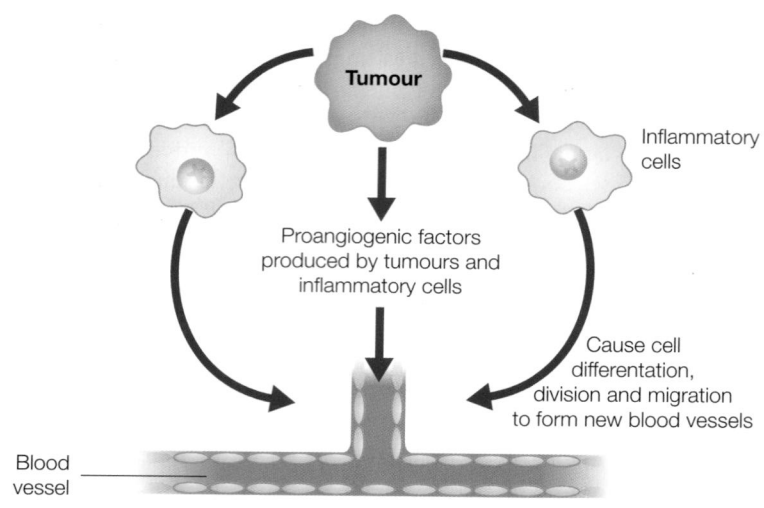

Pro-angiogenic factors	Anti-angiogenic factors
Fibroblast growth factor	Thrombospondin I
Placental growth factor	Angiostatin
Vascular endothelial growth factor	Interferon alpha
Transforming growth factors	Prolactin
Angiogenin	Metallo-proteinase inhibitors
Interleukin-8	Endostatin
Hepatocyte growth factor	Platelet factor 4
Platelet derived enthothelial cell growth factor	Placental profliferin-related protein

Figure 4.5 Schematic representation of possible anti-angiogenesis targets, including natural stimulators and inhibitors.

5-fluorouracil, leucovorin combined with bevacizumab or placebo in metastatic colorectal cancer.[25] The use of bevacizumab in head and neck cancer is supported by data from preclinical studies.[26] Currently, clinical trials are exploring the feasibility and the therapeutic potential of a combination of bevacizumab and EGFR-targeted drugs.[27]

OTHER NOVEL TREATMENTS

There are now a large number of new types of agents entering all phases of clinical trials. To date, they have met with variable success. It is important to mention a few drugs which have really made an impact on treatment of specific cancers in the last few years.

- **Trastuzumab (Herceptin):** A humanized monoclonal antibody against the HER-2 receptor which is now becoming increasingly important in the treatment of both locally advanced and metastatic breast cancer.
- **Imatinib mesylate (Gleevec):** An adenosine triphosphate binding selective inhibitor of bcr-abl that has been shown to produce durable complete haematologic and cytogenetic remissions in early chronic phase CML. It also has remarkable activity against relapsed and metastatic gastrointestinal stromal tumours (GIST) that characteristically feature a mutation in the c-kit receptor tyrosine kinase gene.

- **Ritiximab (Mabthera):** The rituximab antibody is a genetically engineered chimeric murine/human monoclonal antibody directed against the CD20 antigen found on the surface of normal and malignant B lymphocytes. It is being increasingly used in combination with chemotherapy to manage many different types of indolent and aggressive B-cell lymphomas.
- **Bortezomib (Velcade):** Velcade is the first of a new class of agents called proteasome inhibitors and the first treatment in more than a decade to be approved for patients with multiple myeloma.

The proteasome is an enzyme complex that exists in all cells and plays an important role in degrading proteins fundamental to all cellular processes, in particular those involved in cell growth and survival. Velcade is a potent but reversible inhibitor of the proteasome. By disrupting normal cellular processes, proteasome inhibition promotes apoptosis. Cancer cells appear to be more susceptible to this effect than normal cells. Due to the reversibility of proteasome inhibition with Velcade, normal cells are more readily able to recover, whereas cancer cells are more likely to undergo apoptosis.

CONCLUSION

The majority of conventional chemotherapeutic agents cause cell death by directly inhibiting the synthesis of

DNA or interfering with its function. This means that they are often not tumour-specific and are associated with considerable morbidity. Trials have demonstrated that combination chemotherapy regimens can cause dramatic regression of head and neck tumours, especially when used concomitantly with radiotherapy. Unfortunately, this has not been associated with an increase in survival rates.

There is considerable excitement over the development of new target-directed cytotoxic agents. These have been developed to modulate or inhibit specific molecular targets critical to the development of or control of cancer cells. Particular interest has focussed on the field of monoclonal antibody development, particularly in relation to the epidermal growth factor. Other drugs affecting signal transduction, programmed cell death, transcription regulation, matrix invasion and angiogenesis are currently involved in clinical trials. The results of these are obviously eagerly awaited and will potentially radically change current therapeutic strategies.

KEY POINTS

- Traditional chemotherapy agents interfere with DNA synthesis and function and are classified according to their mechanism of action.
- Many agents are associated with significant side-effect profiles.
- The role of chemotherapy in head and neck cancer is still being defined, but there is increasing popularity of concurrent chemotherapy and radiotherapy regimens.
- Current research is focussing on molecular targeted therapy.
- Recent strategies have looked at the use of monoclonal antibodies.
- Drugs are being designed that influence signal transduction, specifically cell cycle regulation, apoptosis, matrix invasion and angiogenesis.
- Results of clinical trials are eagerly awaited.

Deficiencies in current knowledge and areas for future research

The effect of chemotherapy on nonmetastatic head and neck cancers is still being elucidated. The optimum combination of chemotherapeutic agents and the timing of their use in relation to surgery have not been defined, especially in combination with radiotherapy. As this continues to be assessed, significant advances are being made in relation to more specific targeted therapies. The results of clinical trials with these new agents and their incorporation into management regimens are eagerly awaited.

- ➤ The optimum regimen of chemotherapy agents for use in head and neck cancers needs to be defined aiming to improve survival, quality of life and organ function.
- ➤ The role of molecular target-specific chemotherapy agents in the management of head and neck cancers needs to become more familiar.

REFERENCES

1. Skipper HE, Schabel FM, Wilcox WS. Experimental evaluation of potential anti-cancer agents. XIII On the criteria and kinetics associated with 'curability' of experimental leukaemia. *Cancer Chemotherapy Reports.* 1964; **35**: 1–111.
2. Herscher LL, Cook J. Taxanes as radiosensitizers for head and neck cancer. *Current Opinion in Oncology.* 1999; **11**: 183–6.
3. Guichard SM, Danks MK. Topoisomerase enzymes as drug targets. *Current Opinion in oncology.* 1999; **11**: 482–9.
* 4. Henk JM. Concomitant chemotherapy for head and neck cancer: saving lives or grays? *Clinical Oncology (Royal College of Radiologists (Great Britain)).* 2001; **13**: 333–5. *Brief summary of important issues and trials with respect to the role of chemotherapy and radiotherapy in head and neck cancers.*
* 5. Pignon JP, Bourhis J, Domenge C, Designe L. Chemotherapy added to locoregional treatment for head and neck squamous-cell carcinoma: three meta-analyses of updated individual data. *Lancet.* 2000; **355**: 949–55. *Main meta-analysis on the effect of chemotherapy on nonmetastatic head and neck squamous-cell carcinoma.*
* 6. Forastiere A, Koch W, Trotti A, Sidransky D. Head and Neck Cancer. *New England Journal of Medicine.* 2001; **345**: 1890–1900. *Very good summary of the important advances in the treatment of patients with head and neck cancer and the future importance of molecular biology.*
7. Haffty BG. Concurrent chemoradiation in the treatment of head and neck cancer. *Hematology/Oncology Clinics of North America.* 1999; **13**: 719–42.
8. Hong WK, Endicott J, Itri LM, Doos W, Batsakis JG, Bell R et al. 13-Cis retinoic acid in the treatment of oral leukoplakia. *New England Journal of Medicine.* 1986; **315**: 1501–5.
9. Hong WK, Lippman SM, Itri LM, Karp DD, Lee JS, Byers RM et al. Prevention of second primary tumours with isotretinoin in squamous-cell carcinoma of the head and neck. *New England Journal of Medicine.* 1990; **323**: 795–801.

10. Chan G, Boyle JO, Yang EK, Zhang F, Sacks PG, Shah JP et al. Cyclooxygenase-2 expression is up-regulated in squamous cell carcinoma of the head and neck. *Cancer Research*. 1999; 59: 991–4.

11. Green MC, Murray JL, Hortobagyi GN. Monoclonal antibody therapy for solid tumours. *Cancer Treatment Reviews*. 2000; 26: 269–86.

12. Ke LD, Adler-Storthz K, Clayman GL, Yung AW, Chen Z. Differential expression of epidermal growth factor receptor in human head and neck cancers. *Head and Neck*. 1998; 20: 320–7.

13. Mauizi M, Almadori G, Ferrandina G, Distefano M, Romanini M, Cadoni G et al. Prognostic significance of epidermal growth factor receptor in laryngeal squamous cell carcinoma. *British Journal of Cancer*. 1996; 74: 1253–7.

14. Perrotte P, Matsumoto T, Inoue K, Kuniyasu H, Eve BY, Hicklin DJ et al. Anti-epidermal growth factor receptor antibody C225 inhibits angiogenesis in human transitional cell carcinoma growing orthotopically in nude mice. *Clinical Cancer Research*. 1999; 5: 257–64.

15. Baselga J. The EGFR as a target for anticancer therapy: focus on cetuximab. *European Journal of Cancer*. 2001; 37: S16–22.

16. Wheeler RH, Spencer S, Buchsbaum D, Robert F. Monoclonal antibodies as potentiators of radiotherapy and chemotherapy in the management of head and neck cancer. *Current Opinion in Oncology*. 1999; 11: 187–190.

17. Saleh M, Buchsbaum D, Meredith R, Lalison D, Wheeler R. *In vitro* and *in vivo* evaluation of the cytotoxicity of radiation combined with chimeric monoclonal antibody to the epidermal growth factor receptor. *Proceedings for the American Association for Cancer Research*. 1996; 37: 612 (Abstr. 4197).

18. Herbst RS, Langer CJ. Epidermal growth factor receptors as a target for cancer treatment: the emerging role of IMC-C225 in the treatment of lung and head and neck cancers. *Seminars in Oncology*. 2002; 29: 27–36.

19. Cohen EE, Rosen F, Stadler WM, Recant WM, Stenson K, Huo D et al. Phase II trial of ZD1839 in recurrent or metastatic squamous cell carcinoma of the head and neck. *Journal of Clinical Oncology*. May 15, 2003; 21: 1980–7.

20. Caponigro F. Rationale and clinical validation of epidermal growth factor receptor as a target in the treatment of head and neck cancer. *Anticancer Drugs*. April, 2004; 15: 311–20.

21. Perez-Soler R. Can rash associated with HER1/EGFR inhibition be used as a marker of treatment outcome? *Oncology* (Williston Park, NY). 2003; 17: 23–8.

22. Folkman J. Seminars in Medicine of Beth Israel Hospital, Boston. Clinical application of research on angiogenesis. *New England Journal of Medicine*. 1995; 333: 1757–63.

23. Boehm T, Folkman J, Browder T, O'Reilly MS. Antiangiogenic treatment of experimental cancer does not induce acquired drug resistance. *Nature*. 1997; 390: 404–7.

24. Kyzas PA, Stefanou D, Batistatou A, Agnantis NJ. Potential autocrine function of vascular endothelial growth factor in head and neck cancer via vascular endothelial growth factor receptor-2. *Modern Pathology*. 2005; 18: 485–94.

25. Hurwitz H, Fehrenbacker L, Novotny W, Cartwright T, Hainsworth J, Heim W et al. Bevacizumab plus irinotecan, fluorouracil, and leucovorin for metastatic colorectal cancer. *New England Journal of Medicine*. 2004; 350: 2335–42.

26. Caponigro F, Formato R, Caraglia M, Normanno N, Iaffaioli RV. Monoclonal antibodies targeting epidermal growth factor receptor and vascular endothelial growth factor with a focus on head and neck tumors. *Current Opinion in Oncology*. 2005; 17: 212–7.

27. Caponigro F, Basile M, de Rosa V, Normanno N. New drugs in cancer therapy, National Tumor Institute, Naples, 17–18 June 2004. *Anticancer Drugs*. 2005; 16: 211–21.

FURTHER READING

Dancey J, Arbuck S. Cancer Drugs and Cancer Drug Development for the New Millennium. In: Khayat D, Hortobagyi GN (eds). *Progress in anti-cancer chemotherapy*, Volume IV. 2000: 91–107. *Detailed discussion of the mechanism of novel chemotherapeutic agents, particularly molecular targeted therapies.*

5

Radiotherapy and radiosensitizers

STEWART G MARTIN AND DAVID AL MORGAN

Introduction	47	Adjuvant chemotherapy	51
Fractionation	48	Targeted therapies	52
Radiosensitizers	49	Key points	53
Bioreductive drugs	50	References	54

SEARCH STRATEGY

The data in this chapter are supported by a Medline search using the key words neoplasms, radiotherapy, radiation-sensitizing agents, drug therapy and antineoplastic agents

INTRODUCTION

Radiotherapy is the therapeutic use of ionizing radiation, usually high-energy x-rays (photons), although gamma rays, high-energy electron beams and other particle beams (hadrons) have all been employed clinically. As the name implies, the radiation interacts with matter by ejecting electrons from their orbits, resulting in ionization. The ejected particles interact with further atoms, ejecting further electrons and causing a cascade of ionizations after each initial interaction. In biological material, the free radicals that result, primarily from interactions with water molecules, are highly reactive and are particularly damaging to the cell when they interact with DNA (hydrated electrons are rapidly deactivated by oxygen, see under Bioreductive drugs). In total, about 100 distinct lesions have been identified amongst which strand breaks (i.e. sugar-phosphate backbone damage) predominate in terms of importance at the cellular level. Traditionally, the main cause of cell death following radiation was thought to result from direct damage to the DNA. This has gradually been modified over the last few years as an increasing number of studies have shown that ionizing radiation also targets the plasma membrane where it can initiate multiple signal transduction pathways, many of which lead to radiation-induced apoptosis (e.g. hydrolysis of the membrane phospholipid sphingomyelin by the enzyme sphingomyelinase resulting in the generation of ceramide). DNA damage in mammalian cells triggers three pathways: cell cycle arrest, DNA repair and apoptosis. Historically, three types of damage have been recognized: sublethal damage (SLD), potentially lethal damage (PLD) and irreparable or lethal damage. These categories may not reflect different types of damage, but instead reflect the category of repair processes that act to modify the radiation-induced lesions. If the DNA damage is particularly severe then cell death may result, usually when the cell attempts to divide.

The fact that cell death occurs at a time after the actual exposure to irradiation, depending on the time of cell division (and also upon the tissue structure and life span of the mature functional cells), explains one of the most important clinical observations about radiotherapy, that tissues that are dividing rapidly manifest the effects of radiation sooner than those where cell division is slow. Tissues such as bone marrow, skin and the mucosa of the upper aerodigestive tract manifest the effects of radiation within days. Connective tissue, bone and neural tissue may only show the effect years later. Squamous head and neck cancers, as might be expected, behave as an acute-reacting tissue, like the squamous mucosa from which they originate. In addition to the kinetics (turnover rate) of the population as a whole, the response of tissues and organs is also dependent upon inherent cellular radiosensitivity. The sensitivity of the cell to radiation is determined to some degree by its state of maturity and its functional role. Generally speaking, immature cells are considerably more sensitive to radiation than mature cells and as mitotic activity increases (metabolic activity, proliferation), sensitivity also increases. There is general agreement as to which of the target cells is responsible for acute effects (stem cells of rapidly dividing tissues), but the target cells that determine the late effects have not been defined clearly. In general, if any clonogens from acute responding normal tissues survive they can rapidly repopulate and replace lost cells. Late-reacting tissues do not have this ability to repopulate rapidly and therefore whilst most acute reactions heal, most late reactions, if anything, continue to progress with time. It is the severity of predicted late effects that can limit the delivered dose of radiation.

FRACTIONATION

The differences between 'acute-reacting' and 'late-reacting' tissues are very important to the science of fractionation in radiotherapy. At low single doses, tumour and early-responding tissues are more sensitive than late-responding tissues (more cells are in cycle). At high doses, the nondividing late responding cell response that compensates for tissue loss is slow and therefore organs appear more radiosensitive than rapidly dividing tumour and early-responding tissues.

A fraction is the individual dose of radiation delivered at a single session of radiotherapy; in the treatment of head and neck cancer a total course of radiotherapy will take several weeks and consist of numerous fractions. The fraction size, measured in physical dose, is traditionally and almost invariably constant throughout a course of radiotherapy. In conventional radiotherapy, fractions are given once a day, five days per week. This accords with normal working practices, rather than being founded on a sound scientific basis, and alternative fractionation schedules have been much studied in recent years (see below).

In general, the relationship between the dose of radiation in a single fraction and the number of cells killed approximates closely to a straight line on a semilogarithmic graph, conventionally drawing dose arithmetically on the x-axis and surviving fraction of cells on a declining logarithmic scale on the negative y-axis. This is shown in **Figure 5.1**. It should be noted though that while the general relationship is linear, at the lowest doses this is not so, and the line is curved (has a shoulder). For most cells, the range in which this curve applies is close to most widely used fraction sizes (in other words around 2 Gy) and this has important implications for clinical practice.

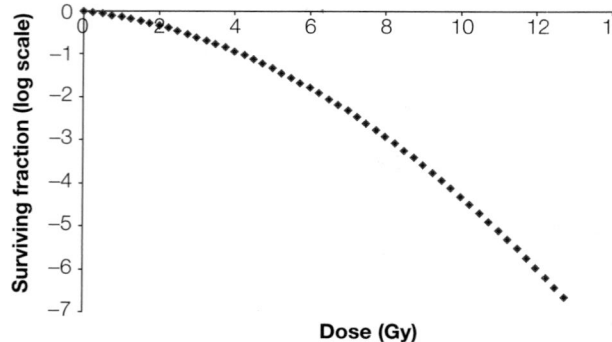

Figure 5.1 Typical radiation dose-response curve following a single radiation exposure. Note that the radiation dose (x-axis) is a linear scale, while surviving fraction (y-axis) is logarithmic. The effect for small doses is relatively 'curvy' compared to that for higher. The consequences of this are explained in the text.

The extent of the 'curviness' of the graph varies with many factors. Most importantly for day-to-day routine radiotherapy, late-reacting tissues generally have a more 'curvy' graph than do acute-reacting ones and therefore increasing the fraction size tends to have a greater effect (altered severity) on late-reacting as opposed to early-reacting tissues. Graphs for exposure to neutrons or other heavy particles tend to be less curvy than do those for x-rays. Cells from patients with ataxia-telangiectasia show almost no curve. This is because these patients are deficient in certain mechanisms that act to repair DNA. The shoulder on the graph is a reflection of the capacity for DNA to repair damaged cells.

The importance of this shoulder region to radiotherapy relates to the fact that as long as sufficient time elapses between fractions, a subsequent dose of radiation has the same shaped survival curve as an initial dose, including the shoulder, i.e. full repair of the initial damage has occurred. Thus, if the shoulder is considerable, the net effect of two doses is very much less than if the same total physical dose was given as a single fraction. The general shape of the cell survival curves, including the shoulder, is probably best described by the linear quadratic equation:

$$SF = N/No = e^{-}(\alpha D + \beta D^2) \quad \text{or} \quad -\ln SF = \alpha D + \beta D^2$$

In this equation, No is the number of cells in the population originally and N is the number surviving after irradiation with dose D, with N/No representing the surviving fraction (SF). Only two parameters, α (the initial slope) and β (the terminal slope) are required to describe the dose–response curve. Absolute values of alpha and beta are not well known, but the alpha/beta ratio (i.e. the dose at which the contribution to killing from the α component or nonreparable damage, is equal to that of the β component or reparable damage) has been identified with a reasonable degree of approximation for numerous tissues. In general, the α/β ratio tends to be low for late-reacting tissues, and for these the shoulder on the graph is considerable, whereas it is high for acute-reacting tissues, where the shoulder is less marked. As mentioned above, when this is translated into practice, the total effect is more fraction size-dependent for late-reacting tissues than for acute-reacting tissues. Thus, for example, the effect achieved with a dose of 70 Gy in 2 Gy fractions will differ less from the effect of the same total dose in fractions of 1 Gy for acute-reacting tissues than it will be for late-reacting tissues. There will be more 'sparing' of late-reacting tissues by breaking the same total dose up into a greater number of smaller fractions. Having said this, because of the ability of early-reacting tissue (notably head and neck squamous cell carcinomas (SCC)) to repopulate rapidly, these comparisons are only valid if the overall treatment time is the same for the different schedules. This necessitates a shorter interfraction interval for the schedule of many small fractions. This interval still needs to be long enough for adequate repair of sublethal damage to occur if the full sparing effect on late reactions by reducing factor size is to be seen.

The corollary of this is that by using many small fractions it will be possible to give a higher total dose, but without increasing the amount of late damage, whereas a greater effect will be seen on acute-reacting tissues, notably squamous head and neck cancers. This is the theory of 'hyperfractionation'.

The theoretical benefits of hyperfractionation were confirmed in clinical practice in a randomized trial comparing a 'conventional' schedule of 70 Gy in seven weeks with a hyperfractionated schedule, in which two fractions of 1.15 Gy were given daily, also over seven weeks, so that the total dose was 80.5 Gy.[1] [****] Better local control was achieved in the experimental hyperfractionation arm, with no observed increase in late side effects.

Other ways of modifying radiotherapy fractionation schedules have also been explored in head and neck cancer. The problem of tumour clonogen proliferation during a prolonged course of radiotherapy has already been alluded to. The consequence of this is that if radiotherapy schedules are prolonged for reasons such as holidays, machine breakdowns and so on, tumour control is adversely affected. A number of retrospective series have confirmed this (it cannot, of course, be ethically tested in a prospective randomized trial). The evidence has been strong enough for the Royal College of Radiologists in the UK to publish guidelines on how to minimize the harm done by such interruptions.[2] [*] Of course, if prolongation of schedules is detrimental in terms of control of tumours, it might well be expected that to shorten the overall time (acceleration) would result in better control. A number of trials have also been set up to test this hypothesis. The evidence is convincing that shortening overall time is beneficial in terms of tumour control. One problem that all the trials of accelerated treatments have

faced is that increasing the effect on the tumour by shortening the overall time also increases the effect on the adjacent normal mucosa, and severe acute reactions are to some extent unavoidable. The problem is compounded by the fact that very severe acute reactions sometimes lead, rather more than might be expected, to an increase in the extent of late reactions, and this has rather limited the extent to which improvements in outcomes can be achieved by shortening radiotherapy schedules. Even so, the many studies published in this area leave little doubt that it is indeed possible to employ the strategy of acceleration without incurring too high a penalty in terms of normal tissue effects, although the optimum strategy in terms of fraction size, interval, number of fractions per day, number of treatment days per week, total dose and overall time, remains elusive.[3]

RADIOSENSITIZERS

As well as modifying the physical parameters (time, dose, etc.) of radiotherapy, other interesting avenues of exploration have involved using various agents to enhance its effects. It is reasonable to refer to all of these as 'radiosensitizers', although the scientific purists may argue about the appropriate use of this term. Numerous types of agents have been used, with varying degrees of success. The rapid advances that are currently occurring in molecular oncology seem likely to make this an area of fruitful exploration in the near future.

The evidence that emerged from laboratory studies that hypoxic cells were relatively radioresistant to x-rays when compared with fully oxygenated ones prompted the earliest attempts at radiosensitization. As the centre of many tumours are necrotic, it was felt that this was evidence that the proliferation of cells within tumours led to growth outstripping blood supply (i.e. the diffusion distance for oxygen is ~150–200 μm from an adjacent blood vessel) and that therefore it was logical to assume that there would be many chronically hypoxic cells within tumours (hypoxia can also be acute due to the transient opening and closing of tumour blood vessels). It was hypothesized that chronic and acute hypoxia would make the centre of tumours relatively radioresistant. Modern technology has made it possible to precisely measure oxygen levels in tumour and normal tissues, and this hypothesis has indeed been confirmed. If this hypoxic effect could be overcome, radiotherapy would be more likely to be successful. A significant amount of time and effort has been expended over many years testing whether this could be achieved in clinical practice. Many diverse strategies have been employed and new strategies are continually being investigated.

The earliest avenue explored was probably the most direct. In an attempt to ensure greater oxygenation within tumours, patients were placed in hyperbaric oxygen tanks during radiotherapy. Clinical trial results failed to demonstrate that this approach yielded better results than 'standard' radiotherapy. There have been reports that increasing the haemoglobin level could be beneficial as anaemic patients may respond less well to radiotherapy.[4, 5] [***] Initial studies suggested that those patients given transfusions and hyperbaric oxygenation (HBO) did better than those given HBO alone, however, recent results with recombinant erythropoietin have not been very encouraging.[6] [***]

An alternative approach used the agent nicotinamide, which is thought to dilate small vessels to improve blood flow through the vascularized parts of tumours, in combination with patients breathing carbogen (a mixture of oxygen and carbon dioxide) during radiotherapy in an attempt to ensure good oxygenization.[7] Randomized phase III trials are currently underway and the results awaited. A reversal of this approach has met with limited success in certain situations, i.e. tourniquet hypoxia has been used to reduce the radiosensitivity of normal tissues in patients with osteosarcomas of limbs.

A number of pharmaceutical approaches have been used in an attempt to make hypoxic tumour cells more radiosensitive. True sensitizers have little or no cytotoxic action without radiation, but significantly enhance the efficiency of radiation killing when present during radiation. Apparent sensitizers include a variety of compounds, such as antibiotics, alkylating agents and antimetabolites, that act by diverse mechanisms. In general, sensitizers can be regarded as agents that increase the lethal effects of radiation. They should show a gain between tumours and normal tissues. Such a therapeutic gain could result from selective uptake (concentration), a differential absorption rate or biological half-life. Ideally they should be effective at systemically nontoxic dosages, thereby minimizing side effects.

Halogenated pyrimidines (IUdR, BrdUrd) work by being incorporated into actively dividing tumour cells to a greater degree than slowly dividing (cell maintenance) normal tissues. Appreciable quantities need to accumulate for several generations for them to be incorporated to set up stresses in the DNA and make them more susceptible to radiation damage. They therefore seem to be particularly useful with tumours having a high growth fraction and high labelling index. BrdUrd is also a sensitizer to ultraviolet (UV) radiation therefore skin may be the limiting tissue. This is less of a problem with IUdR.

Hypoxic cell sensitizers are electron affinic and act to increase the sensitivity of radioresistant hypoxic cells by mimicking O_2. They are not rapidly metabolized and therefore have time to diffuse into poorly vascularized areas.

Cells are more responsive to sensitizers if they are depleted of their natural radioprotector, glutathione (GSH), a radical scavenger that eliminates reactive radicals before they have the opportunity of causing DNA damage. This may be accomplished by incubation with thiol binding agents, such as diamide and diethylmaleate, or inhibition of GSH synthesis with buthionine sulphoximine before delivering the radiation. The effectiveness of hypoxic cell sensitizers is measured in terms of the enhancement ratio (ER).

The nitroimidazoles have been extensively evaluated as potential radiosensitizers. One of the first compounds investigated was metronidazole, a trichomonacide. At 10 mM, an ER of 1.6 was obtained with no effect on aerated cells. The large concentrations required led to investigations for more effective derivatives and other nitroimidazole drugs appeared more promising in this respect.

Although many hypoxic cell sensitizers have been investigated (including misonidazole, metronidazole, benznidazole, desmethylmisonidazole, etanidazole, pimonidazole, nimorazole, ornidazole and doranidazole), controversy exists regarding the role of these agents in conventional radiotherapy. So far only one major randomized trial of the many that have been performed has shown a therapeutic benefit and in this Danish trial, a benefit for nimorazole use during radiotherapy of pharyngeal and supraglottic laryngeal cancers when combined with conventional therapy was shown.[8] [****] Although nimorazole has been shown to be of potential benefit, these sensitizers generally show greater benefit in situations where large, single doses of radiation are given (e.g. intraoperative radiotherapy, interstitial radiotherapy, radiosurgery). As only this one trial out of many has shown a statistically significant benefit, the international clinical community remains unconvinced that there is a true benefit for the use of nitroimidazoles, and they are still not widely used outside Denmark.

BIOREDUCTIVE DRUGS

Adjuncts to radiation, which are not true radiosensitizers, include bioreductive drugs. These agents are reduced intracellularly to form cytotoxic agents. Bioreduction is favoured under hypoxic conditions (due to cytochrome P450 and DT diaphorase reductases). The efficiency of bioreductive drugs may be increased by inducing increased hypoxia in tumours through the use of vasoactive drugs, such as hydralazine. This induces vasodilation in normal tissues thus diverting blood from the tumour.

Examples of bioreductive drugs include tirapazamine (SR-4233) and mitomycin C. The latter is an antitumour antibiotic that is bioreduced to form products that crosslink DNA. It is cell cycle nonspecific, is more toxic to hypoxic than aerated cells, is usually administered i.v. and is rapidly cleared from plasma (half-life, 10–15 minutes). The drug does not cross the blood–brain barrier and the major toxicity is myelosuppression. Indoloquinone EO9 is a synthetic analogue of mitomycin C (MMC), which was expected to have similar properties to MMC, but fundamental differences have emerged; for example, EO9 is a much better substrate for DT-diaphorase (DTD) and it has the ability to redox cycle more readily than MMC after reduction by purified DTD. In addition, EO9 has the ability to increase the cytotoxicity to hypoxic cells 49-fold over MMC. The overall capacity of the tumour to metabolize EO9 has been suggested to be the most important determinant for EO9 activity. This, along with the rapid clearance of EO9 in humans, has been suggested as one of the reasons for the disappointing results obtained from phase II clinical trials.[9, 10] [****]

Aliphatic amine N-oxides have long been identified as nontoxic metabolites of a large number of tertiary amines drugs. Bioreduction of such N-oxides generate the active parent amine. This principle has been adopted to develop AQ4N, a di-N-oxide anticancer prodrug with little intrinsic cytotoxicity. However, AQ4N is bioreduced in hypoxic regions of solid tumours and micrometastatic deposits to generate a cytotoxic alkylaminoanthraquinone metabolite. The metabolite of AQ4N has high affinity for DNA and is a potent inhibitor of topoisomerase II. Preclinical studies *in vivo* have demonstrated that although AQ4N has little or no intrinsic cytotoxic activity *per se*, it (i) enhances the antitumour effects of radiation and conventional chemotherapeutic agents; (ii) is pharmacokinetically stable; and (iii) is a substrate for cytochrome P450 (CYP). AQ4N is currently in clinical trials.[11, 12] [***]

In general, as with the hypoxic cell sensitizers mentioned above, there is little clinical evidence from large randomized trials of bioreductive agents showing increased efficacy when combined with conventional radiotherapy.

A number of drugs are currently under preclinical evaluation. Synthetic allosteric modifiers of haemoglobin (e.g. RSR13) are designed to effect a conformational change in the haemoglobin (Hb) tetramer that stabilizes deoxyHb, thereby reducing Hb-O_2 binding affinity. It has been hypothesized that the radioresistant hypoxic regions of tumours might be eliminated if improved O_2 delivery to tumours could be accomplished using its reduced haemoglobin-oxygen (Hb-O_2) binding affinity. In preclinical studies, RSR13 has been shown to increase pO_2, decrease intratumoural hypoxia and increase tumour cell killing in animal tumour systems.[13] [**] The drug is currently under clinical evaluation, primarily for the treatment of brain metastases from breast cancer.[14] OFU is a prodrug of 5-FU, under laboratory investigation, which is activated by capturing hydrated electrons that are produced by hypoxic irradiation. As hydrated electrons are rapidly deactivated by oxygen, the 5-FU release occurs specifically upon hypoxic irradiation.

Certain agents that induce vascular damage (and therefore presumably affect the oxygen status), e.g. hyperthermia or photodynamic therapy, have successfully been combined with radiotherapy to increase tumour cell killing (the reasons for combining these modalities were other than their antivascular effects). The rationale for combining therapeutic modalities is based predominately on three concepts: enhanced tumour efficacy, nonoverlapping toxicities, or spatial cooperation. Abnormal tumour microenvironments, tumour progression and metastatic spread of neoplastic cells are all major factors that contribute to radiotherapy failures – all of these may be affected by angiosuppressive or vessel destructive treatments. Antivascular agents eliminate many of the problems in tumours (e.g. aberrant vascular morphology, spatial heterogeneity metabolic microenvironments, etc.) associated with adverse efficacy of radiotherapy by causing extensive haemorrhagic necrosis in the centre of tumours, i.e. the radiation response is improved by impacting the radiation-resistant hypoxic subpopulation of tumours. Cells surviving treatment using antivascular agents tend to be located in areas at the tumour periphery near normal tissues; most likely those areas supplied by normal tissue vessels.[15] [****] Such residual tissue is likely to be well oxygenated and therefore sensitive to radiation. A number of preclinical studies have shown that if such combination therapy is used, the tumour's hypoxic cell population can be dramatically reduced or eliminated and a number of investigations have shown that vascular targeting strategies can effectively enhance radiation treatment.[15] [**] Targeting the growth factors that induce new vessel growth may also be effective.[16, 17] There is also evidence to suggest that certain antiangiogenic agents enhance the effects of radiation by direct effects, i.e. by radiosensitizing endothelial cells.[18] [**] This direct effect, which leads to decreased microvessel density, may have a significant role in enhancing the effect of radiation. The scheduling of such antiangiogenic and antivascular therapies is an area that is under active investigation as are, since side-effects are minimal in comparison to conventional cytotoxics, clinical biomarkers of efficacy.

ADJUVANT CHEMOTHERAPY

Perhaps a clinically more successful (therapeutic) strategy than trying to overcome hypoxia has been the rather more empirical approach of simply combining 'conventional' chemotherapy with radiotherapy. Squamous head and neck cancers show a clinical response to a number of chemotherapeutic agents, so the strategy of combining such drugs with radiotherapy seems justifiable.

Many randomized trials have been conducted in which a combination of chemotherapy and radiotherapy have been compared with radiotherapy alone. Although the majority of these trials have been relatively small, when combined there are vast numbers of patients, and the technique of 'meta-analysis' has been applied. This has convincingly shown that the addition of chemotherapy does give better results than those achieved with radiotherapy alone.[19] [****] The counterargument has been made that the same could be achieved by simply giving more radiotherapy. However, it is known that beyond a certain level the incidence of complications rises rapidly if additional radiotherapy is given, which is why the doses used in common practice are as they are. It has proved feasible to give chemotherapy in combination with such doses, and to date, there is no strong suggestion that this does lead to an unacceptable increase in damage to normal tissue. The same cannot be said of the proposed strategy of simply giving higher doses of radiotherapy (other than in the context of fractionation trials, particularly hyperfractionation, as discussed previously).

Combined chemotherapy and radiotherapy schedules have been tested in randomized controlled trials against a policy of primary surgery for moderately advanced laryngeal and hypopharyngeal cancers. In fact, in these trials the drugs have been given before radiotherapy, so are certainly not acting as 'true' radiosensitizers. They have been shown to be no less effective than radical surgery in terms of survival, but confer the advantage of enabling preservation of a functioning larynx in a substantial number of patients. Such 'organ preservation' represents a significant advance in radiotherapy of head and neck cancer, and continue to attract a great deal of attention, with trials of different drug/radiation schedules, and involving other head and neck sites.

There are many chemotherapeutic agents that are effective for head and neck cancer and the possible scheduling combinations of radiotherapy and chemotherapy are numerous. Because of this the meta-analyses have not been able to identify clearly which of the various options is the best, although a strategy of giving cisplatin concurrently or in rapidly alternating sequences, with radiotherapy (perhaps with other drugs as well) is emerging as a front runner. Even so, confirmation that this is the best way of using chemotherapy agents as radiosensitizers is not strong. Drugs other than cisplatin have also been found to add to the effect of radiotherapy in head and neck cancer. The most widely used is fluorouracil, although it is usually used alongside cisplatin. Again, there is debate as to whether it is a 'true radiosensitizer', but combined radiotherapy/cisplatin/fluorouracil schedules are increasingly widely used. Other agents include methotrexate, bleomycin and the taxanes. Of these, there is certainly some evidence that the taxanes are radiosensitizers. The same can be said for the new agent gemcitabine, although clinical experience of the use of this with radiotherapy in head and neck cancer is minimal.

TARGETED THERAPIES

Our understanding of the molecular mechanisms that drive cancer cells has grown at an accelerating pace within recent years. This has led to the emergence of the first wave of drugs that act against cancer cells in a more targeted way than the cytotoxic agents that have been the mainstay of chemotherapy in the past. Because of their specificity, such agents hold the promise of being much less toxic than conventional chemotherapy.

Among these new classes of agents there are some interesting suggestions of synergy with radiation. In head and neck cancer, one target has so far attracted significant attention, the epidermal growth factor receptor, EGFR (erbB1, HER1). This is one of a family of transmembrane receptor tyrosine kinases, other members being HER2/neu (erbB2), HER3 (erbB3) and HER4 (erbB4). Ligand-binding receptor dimerization occurs, which induces a conformational change in the intracellular kinase domain, thereby inducing a cascade of phosphorylation events or activation of signal transduction (e.g. activation of the MAPK or ras signal transduction pathway). As implied by its name and as might be expected in a tumour arising from squamous epithelium, overexpression of this receptor is a very frequent event in head and neck squamous carcinomas. Its overexpression, with or without gene amplification, is often associated with increased production of EGFR ligands, particularly epidermal growth factor (EGF) and transforming growth factor alpha (TGFα). Two broad classes of agent have been developed to counteract the way in which the epidermal growth factor receptor signals the cell to proliferate. The first of these target the extracellular ligand-binding domain using a monoclonal antibody approach. Cetuximab is a chimeric 'humanized' monoclonal antibody that competitively binds to EGFR (it has a 2-log higher affinity for EGFR than TGFα and EGF). Once bound to the receptor, the complex is internalized and the receptor thereby rendered inactive. Cetuximab has undergone clinical trials in head and neck cancer used both as monotherapy and as combined therapy (radiation, chemotherapy). Results from a large randomized phase III trial were very impressive in that improved locoregional control and reduced mortality have been obtained with little increase in toxicity.[20] [****] Cetuximab may, in addition to exerting antiproliferative effects by inhibiting the MAPK signal transduction pathway, act as an antiangiogenic agent and therefore exert radiosensitizing effects via mechanisms described above.[21] [**]

The second approach available to target receptor tyrosine kinases is via the use of small molecules that compete for the ATP binding site of the kinase domain. The low molecular weight of these molecules may allow them to penetrate tumours better and they can be administered orally making them suitable for chronic therapy. Several agents, including gefitinib and erlotinib, have progressed quite far in clinical trials as monotherapy[22] [***] and in combination with standard chemotherapy, but little is known regarding their combined use with radiotherapy – it is an area of active investigation. As these agents are very well tolerated, one area that is as yet unresolved is the identification of their optimal dose, i.e. the dose that completely inhibits the receptor rather than the maximally tolerated dose that is conventionally used with standard chemotherapy approaches.

A number of other novel 'radiosensitization' studies are under way (e.g. anti-HER2 antibody-induced radiosensitization, targeting the NFκβ pathway (e.g. by proteosome inhibition using PS-341), *ras* inhibitors, cox-2 inhibitors, etc.), but this area is, as yet, even less developed than the EGFR inhibitors mentioned above and are therefore beyond the scope of this review.[23, 24, 25, 26, 27] It does appear, however, that 'radiosensitizers' are with us to stay and that their use is set to increase.

KEY POINTS

- Conventional radiotherapy uses photons that both directly and indirectly damage the DNA, through the production of ions and free radicals. The majority of damage induced by photons is via this 'indirect action'.
- Although the DNA is generally considered to be the most important target for radiation-induced damage, this dogma is gradually being amended to include effects on other cellular constituents, particularly cellular membranes.
- Tissues that are dividing rapidly manifest the effects of radiation sooner than those where cell division is slow. In addition to the kinetics (turnover rate) of the population as a whole, the response of tissues and organs is also dependent upon inherent cellular radiosensitivity. The sensitivity of the cell to radiation is determined to some degree by its state of maturity and its functional role; immature rapidly proliferating cells generally being more radiosensitive than slowly proliferating fully differentiated cells.
- The response of a tumour to radiotherapy is dependent upon inherent **r**adiosensitivity, tumour cell **r**epopulation, **r**edistribution through the cell cycle (G2/M is the most sensitive phase of the cell cycle, late-S phase is the most radioresistant), **r**epair of radiation induced damage and **r**eoxygenation of tumour tissues between fractions. These parameters represent the '5 Rs of radiotherapy'.
- A fraction is the individual dose of radiation delivered at a single session of radiotherapy. In the treatment of head and neck cancer, a total course of radiotherapy will take several weeks and comprise numerous fractions. In conventional radiotherapy, fractions are given once a day, five days per week. The fraction size is, almost invariably, constant throughout a course of radiotherapy. Increasing the fraction size tends to have a greater effect

(altered severity) on late-reacting as opposed to early-reacting tissues.
- Hypoxic cells (those under low O_2 tension) are relatively resistant to x-rays when compared with fully oxygenated ones. Chronic and acute hypoxia make tumours relatively radioresistant. If such hypoxia is overcome, radiotherapy is more likely to be successful.
- Many approaches to overcome tumour hypoxia are currently under clinical evaluation – these include improving blood flow through the vascularized parts of tumours, tourniquet hypoxia to reduce the radiosensitivity of normal tissues and pharmaceutical approaches to make hypoxic tumour cells more radiosensitive (radiosensitizer drugs).
- The nitroimidazoles have been extensively evaluated as potential radiosensitizers; however, controversy exists regarding the role of these agents in conventional radiotherapy. So far, only one major randomized trial, of the many that have been performed, has shown a therapeutic benefit (with nimorazole).
- Adjuncts to radiation, which are not true radiosensitizers, include bioreductive drugs. These agents are reduced intracellularly to form cytotoxic agents. A number are under clinical evaluation in head and neck cancers.
- Perhaps a clinically more successful (therapeutic) strategy than trying to overcome hypoxia has been the rather more empirical approach of simply combining 'conventional' chemotherapy with radiotherapy. Combined chemotherapy and radiotherapy schedules have been tested in randomized controlled trials against a policy of primary surgery for moderately advanced laryngeal and hypopharyngeal cancers. Results have been shown to be no less effective than radical surgery in terms of survival, but confer the advantage of enabling preservation of a functioning larynx in a substantial number of patients. Such 'organ preservation' represents a significant advance in radiotherapy of head and neck cancer.
- Meta-analyses have not been able to clearly identify which of the various adjuvant chemotherapy options is the best, although a strategy of giving cisplatin concurrently or in rapidly alternating sequences, with radiotherapy (perhaps with other drugs as well) is emerging as a 'front runner'.
- Novel, molecularly targeted, agents hold the promise of being much less toxic than

conventional chemotherapy. Of the agents under evaluation, Cetuximab, a humanized monocloncal antibody that competitively binds to EGFR, has undergone clinical trials in head and neck cancer used both as monotherapy and as combined therapy (radiation, chemotherapy). Results from a large randomized trial were very impressive in that improved locoregional control and reduced mortality have been obtained with little increase in toxicity.

REFERENCES

1. Horiot JC, le Fur R, N'Guyen T, Chenal C, Schraub S, Alfonsi S et al. Hyperfractionation versus conventional fractionation in oropharyngeal carcinoma: final result of a randomized trial of the EORTC Cooperative Group of Radiotherapy. *Radiotherapy and Oncology.* 1992; **25**: 231–41.

2. Board of the Faculty of Clinical Oncology, The Royal College of Radiologists. *Guidelines for the management of the unscheduled interruption or prolongation of a radical course of radiotherapy,* 2nd edn. London: The Royal College of Radiologists, 2002.

* 3. Morgan DAL. Fractionation experiments in head and neck cancer: the lessons so far. *Clinical Oncology.* 1997; **9**: 302–7.

4. van Acht MJ, Hermans J, Boks DE, Leer JW. The prognostic value of hemoglobin and a decrease in hemoglobin during radiotherapy in laryngeal carcinoma. *Radiotherapy and Oncology.* 1992; **23**: 229–35.

5. Glaser CM, Millesi W, Kornek GV, Lang S, Schull B, Watzinger F et al. Impact of hemoglobin level and use of recombinant erythropoietin on efficacy of preoperative chemoradiation therapy for squamous cell carcinoma of the oral cavity and oropharynx. *International Journal of Radiation Oncology, Biology, Physics.* 2001; **50**: 705–15.

6. Henke M, Lasziq R, Rube C, Schafer U, Hasse KD, Schilcher B et al. Erythropoietin to treat head and neck cancer patients with anaemia undergoing radiotherapy: randomised, double-blind, placebo-controlled trial. *Lancet.* 2003; **362**: 1255–60.

* 7. Kaanders JHAM, Pop LAM, Marres HAM, Bruaset I, van den Hoogen FJA, Merkx MAW et al. ARCON: Experience in 215 patients with advanced head-and-neck cancer. *International Journal of Radiation Oncology, Biology, Physics.* 2002; **52**: 769–78.

8. Overgaard J, Hansen HS, Overgaard M, Bastholt L, Berthelsen A, Specht L et al. A randomized double-blind phase III study of nimorazole as a hypoxic radiosensitizer of primary radiotherapy in supraglottic larynx and pharynx carcinoma, results of the Danish Head and Neck Cancer Study (DAHANCA) protocol 5-85. *Radiotherapy and Oncology.* 1998; **46**: 135–46.

9. Rauth AM, Melo T, Misra V. Bioreductive therapies: an overview of drugs and their mechanisms of action. *International Journal of Radiation Oncology, Biology, Physics.* 1998; **42**: 755–62.

10. Gutierrez PL. The role of NAD(P)H oxidoreductase (DT-diaphorase) in the bioactivation of quinone-containing antitumor agents: A review. *Free Radical Biology and Medicine.* 2000; **29**: 263–75.

11. Patterson LH, McKeown SR, Ruparella K, Double JA, Bibby MC, Cole S et al. Enhancement of chemotherapy and radiotherapy of murine tumours by AQ4N, a bioreductively activated anti-tumour agent. *British Journal of Cancer.* 2000; **82**: 1984–90.

12. Benghiat A, Steward WP, Loadman PM, Middleton M, Talbot D, Patterson LH et al. Phase 1 dose escalation study of AQ4N, a selective hypoxic cell cytotoxin, with fractionated radiotherapy (RT): First report. *Journal of Clinical Oncology.* 2004; **22**: 2091 Suppl. S.

13. Amorino GP, Lee H, Holburn GE, Paschal CB, Hercules SK, Shyr Y et al. Enhancement of tumor oxygenation and radiation response by the allosteric effector of hemoglobin, RSR13. *Radiation Research.* 2001; **156**: 294–300.

14. Charpentier MM. Efaproxiral: A radiation enhancer used in brain metastases from breast cancer. *Annals of Pharmacotherapy.* 2005; **39**: 2038–45.

15. Siemann DW, Warrington KH, Horsman MR. Targeting tumor blood vessels: an adjuvant strategy for radiation therapy. *Radiotherapy and Oncology.* 2000; **57**: 5–12.

16. Martin SG, Orridge C, Mukherjee A, Morgan DAL. Vascular endothelial growth factor expression predicts outcome after primary radiotherapy for head and neck squamous cell cancer. *Clinical Oncology.* 2007; **19**: 71–6.

17. Lee C-G, Heijn M, di Thomaso E, Griffon-Etienne G, Ancukiewicz M, Koike C et al. Anti-vascular endothelial growth factor treatment augments tumour radiation response under normoxic or hypoxic conditions. *Cancer Research.* 2000; **60**: 5565–70.

18. Gorski DH, Beckett MA, Jaskowiak NT, Calvin DP, Mauceri HJ, Salloum RM et al. Blockade of the vascular endothelial growth factor stress response increases the antitumor effects of ionizing radiation. *Cancer Research.* 1999; **59**: 3374–8.

* 19. Pignon JP, Bourhis J, Domenge C, Designe L. Chemotherapy added to locoregional treatment for head and neck squamous-cell carcinoma: three meta-analyses of updated individual data. MACH-NC Collaborative Group. Meta-Analysis of Chemotherapy on Head and Neck Cancer. *Lancet.* 2000; **355**: 949–55.

* 20. Bonner JA, Harari PM, Giralt J, Azarnia N, Shin DM, Cohen RB et al. Radiotherapy plus cetuximab for squamous cell carcinoma of the head and neck. *New England Journal of Medicine.* 2006; **354**: 567–78.

21. O-chroenrat P, Rhys-Evans P, Modjtahedi H, Eccles S. Vascular endothelial growth factor family members are

differentially regulated by c-erbB signalling in head and neck squamous carcinoma cells. *Clinical and Experimental Metastasis*. 2000; **18**: 155–61.

22. Kirby AM, A'Hern RP, D'Ambrosio C, Tanay M, Syrigos KN, Rogers SJ *et al.* Gefitinib (ZD1839, Iressa^{TM}) as palliative treatment in recurrent or metastatic head and neck cancer. *British Journal of Cancer*. 2006; **94**: 631–6.

23. Uno M, Otsuki T, Kurebayashi J, Sakaguchi H, Isozaki Y, Ueki A *et al.* Anti-HER2-antibody enhances irradiation-induced growth inhibition in head and neck carcinoma. *International Journal of Cancer*. 2001; **94**: 474–9.

24. Jung M, Dritchilo A. NF- KappaB signalling pathway as a target for human tumour radiosensitisation. *Seminars in Radiation Oncology*. 2001; **11**: 346–51.

25. Adams J. Proteosome inhibition in cancer: Development of PS-341. *Seminars in Oncology*. 2001; **28**: 613–9.

26. Jones HA, Hahn SM, Bernhard E, McKenna WG. Ras inhibitors and radiation therapy. *Seminars in Radiation Oncology*. 2001; **11**: 328–37.

27. Milas L. Cyclooxygenase-2 (COX-2) enzyme inhibitors as potential enhancers of tumour radioresponse. *Seminars in Radiation Oncology*. 2001; **11**: 290–9.

6

Apoptosis and cell death

MICHAEL SAUNDERS

Overview of apoptosis	56	Apoptosis in disease	61
Mechanisms of apoptosis	57	Apoptosis and cancer	62
Methods of detecting and measuring apoptosis	60	References	64

SEARCH STRATEGY AND EVIDENCE–BASE

The data in this chapter are supported by a Medline search using the key words apoptosis, cell cycle, cell signalling, cell cycle. The majority of papers referenced are based on strict histopathological studies and whilst some do not have age- and sex-matched controls, the majority represent level 1 evidence. Some papers referenced are observational and represent level 4 evidence and where these are referenced this will be inserted into the text.

OVERVIEW OF APOPTOSIS

Historical perspective

Apoptosis is a mode of cell death. At the time of Kerr's original description of apoptosis as a distinct phenomenon in 1971,[1] much was already known about cell division, but little attention had been paid to the end of a cell's life.

The word 'apoptosis' is derived from the Greek word for 'falling off', in reference to the falling of leaves from trees in autumn. Much of the early understanding of the molecular biology of apoptosis stemmed from 1980's studies on the nematode *Caenorhabditis elegans*. Ellis and Horvitz[2] were able to clone the specific genes (*ced* genes) responsible for cell death during the nematode's development. It was already known that exactly 131 cells die during the development of *C. elegans*, however, these normally doomed cells were allowed to survive to maturity by inducing mutations in genes *ced-3* and *ced-4*.[3] Close similarities between the nematode *ced* genes and human genes were identified (e.g. *ced-9* and the mammalian oncogene *Bcl-2*[4]) suggesting a function for such mammalian genes in apoptotic pathways.

In the last decade, there has been intense research activity into apoptosis (see **Figure 6.1**). The literature and research can be confusing to the reader because of the pace of change in this field. New genes and gene products are regularly discovered. However, a number of genes, gene products and receptors with separate names may eventually prove to be one and the same but the different names remain in use for some time (e.g. Fas/APO-1/CD95).

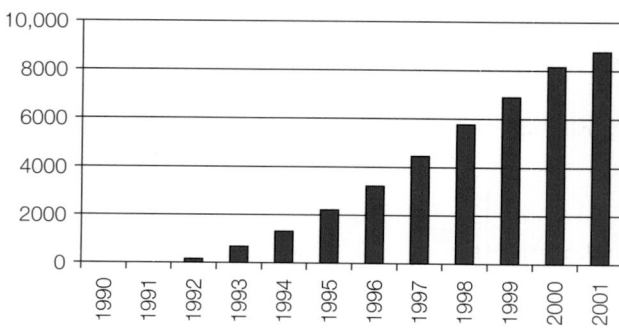

Figure 6.1 Apoptosis related scientific publications per annum (Source: Medline).

Apoptosis in cell populations

It is easy to underestimate the relative importance of apoptosis as a physiological, as well as a pathological, event. Daily in the human body millions of marrow cells undergo apoptosis as part of the function of the immune system. Just as a cell population can be varied by cell production, it can also be varied by cell death; cells can be lost in a number of ways:

1. shedding after terminal differentiation (for example, gut epithelium into the lumen of the bowel);
2. necrosis;
3. apoptosis.

Whereas necrosis is always a pathological event as a result of noxious stimuli, the key importance of apoptosis is that it is the only means of cell loss that can be controlled, both physiologically and genetically. The main differences between apoptosis and necrosis are summarized in **Table 6.1**.

Apoptotic cell loss is now recognized to be fundamental in the regulation of cell populations. This is particularly true in developmental processes and in cell populations with high turnover, such as the intestinal mucosa.

Studies of potential doubling times (Tpot) of tumour cell populations would suggest that the growth rate of tumours should be far greater than observed. This necessary cell loss cannot be accounted for by exfoliation or necrosis, and therefore apoptotic cell loss plays an important part in the rate of tumour growth.[5, 6] In fact, tumour growth is a result of the balance between mitosis and apoptosis. The balance between cell division and cell loss is sometimes referred to as tissue homeostasis.

MECHANISMS OF APOPTOSIS

Executors and triggers of apoptosis

A range of stimuli both physiological and pathological can trigger apoptosis (see **Table 6.2**).

The molecular changes during apoptosis are largely governed by a family of at least 14 separate enzymes referred to as caspases (**c**ysteine **asp**artate specific prote**ases**). Caspases have a variety of actions (both initiator and effector) including cleavage of DNA and cytoplasmic structure. The two most important pathways of caspase activation (death receptor and intracellular/mitochondrial pathways) share a final common irreversible step in the activation of caspase 3.

Extracellular signalling, death receptors, caspase 8

Cells can be directed to self-destruct by intercellular signals mediated by cell surface receptors that are capable or triggering apoptosis when bound by antibody or ligand molecules. These are known as death receptors (DR). These may allow extracellular signals such as cytokines and hormones to effect apoptosis in target tissue. The death receptors currently recognized include Fas, TNFα receptor 1 and the RD4 and DR5 receptors.

Fas is bound by the extracellular antibody Fas ligand (Fas-L) and this pathway is important in the regulation of the immune system and the deletion of unwanted T-lymphocytes.[7] Cytotoxic T cells express Fas-L and cause apoptosis by binding Fas receptors on the target cell. Failure of this system (e.g. by Fas mutation) may be implicated in autoimmune disorders.[8]

Table 6.1 Summary of differences between apoptosis and necrosis.

	Apoptosis	Necrosis
Occurrence	Part of physiological or pathological processes	Always pathological
Initiating factors	Range of extracellular and intracellular factors	Direct result of injury and cellular anoxia
Distribution	Isolated apoptotic cells scattered widely throughout tissues	Occurs in groups/whole areas of tissue
Mechanism	Active process – ATP dependent	Passive
	Regulated mechanism	Regulation lost
Cytoplasmic changes	Cytoplasmic shrinkage	Swelling of cell membrane
	Blebbing of cell membrane into apoptotic bodies	Rupture of cell membrane with loss of contents to extracellular space
	Many organelles preserved and bound into apoptotic bodies	Organelles lost
Nuclear changes	Endonuclease activation, cutting of DNA into oligosomal fragments	Random digestion of DNA
	Chromatin condenses into specific 'crescents' visible on light microscopy	Chromatin flocculates
Effect on surrounding tissue	Little or none	Intense inflammation

Table 6.2 Stimuli capable of triggering apoptosis.

	Stimuli
Physical cell damage	Heat
	Free radicals
	UV light
DNA damage	Ionizing radiation
	Alkylating agents
Cell signalling	Steroid hormones
	Interleukins
	Cytokines

Death receptors are trans-membrane proteins with intracellular and extracellular components. Part of the intracellular component is referred to as the death domain (DD). Binding of the extracelluar component of the receptor protein leads to binding of the death domain to an adaptor molecule (Fas binds to FADD). This in turn changes the inactve procaspase 8 into the active caspase 8, which itself triggers formation of caspase 3 and ensuing cell death. Although other death receptors bind with different adaptor molecules, the common pathway in death receptor signalling remains activation of initiator caspase 8.

Intracellular signalling, mitochondria and Bcl–2, caspase 9

Although the exact mechanisms are unclear, it is believed that certain stimuli (cell damage, withdrawal of growth factors) effect cell death through a mitochondrial pathway of which the *Bcl-2* family is a key component. Although Bcl-2 was originally described as a protooncogene in B-cell lymphomas, the family is now known to contain at least 15 proteins that reside on the mitochondrial outer membrane. The family has both pro-apoptotic (e.g. *Bax*, *Bak*) and anti-apoptotic components (e.g. *Bcl-2*, *Bcl-xL*), the balance between the two being crucial in terms of cell survival.

The action of these molecules in triggering apoptosis is to alter the permeability of the mitochondrial membrane, allowing the escape of mitochondrial cytochrome-c. This then binds to the adapter protein Apaf-1 and inactive procaspase 9 to generate active caspase 9, which (like caspase 8) is an initiator of apoptosis.

The cell cycle and apoptosis, *p53*

Allowing cells with damaged DNA, unreplicated or misaligned chromosomes to replicate by mitosis might lead to daughter cells, which are not only unhealthy or incapable of further division, but potentially neoplastic.

To ensure healthy replication of cells there exist cell cycle checkpoints or restriction points, at which replication can be halted in response to a variety of external signals (stress, growth factors) and internal signals (DNA damage). The first of these occurs between the G1 and S-phase (G1/S checkpoint), the second between G2 and mitosis (G2/M checkpoint).

Progression through the checkpoints is dependent on the expression and function of cyclins (e.g. D1, B1). These can be induced by both extracellular and intracellular stimuli. The upstream pathways leading to cyclin expression are complex and mutations in this system can lead to unregulated passage through the checkpoints.

DNA damage at this point can lead to cell cycle arrest. Two protein kinases, ATM and ATR, are known to be active in the detection of DNA damage. ATM is the protein deficient in the human disease ataxia telangectasia, one of the manifestations of which is increased sensitivity to DNA damage by irradiation.[9]

Expression of ATM and ATR proteins leads to phosphorylation of p53 and hence, through its downstream effector molecules, such as p21, arrest of the cell cycle.

p53 'GUARDIAN OF THE GENOME'

Although a full discussion of the nature and activity of p53 is beyond the scope of this chapter, it occupies a pivotal role in the cell cycle as well as apoptosis induction. Essentially p53 is involved in the detection of abnormal DNA, the decision to cause cell cycle arrest and the decision whether to initiate DNA repair or initiate apoptosis.[10] If DNA damage is irreparable, p53 can, through interactions with the molecules Apaf-1 and Bax , trigger apoptosis by activating caspase 9.

Loss of the ability to express p53 in its native state or the presence of mutated p53 leads to the inability to achieve G1 arrest and the loss of cells' ability to undergo apoptosis in response to DNA damage. The majority of human tumours have inactivation of p53 and *p53* gene mutation is the most common genetic alteration in squamous cell carcinoma of the head and neck (SCCHN).[11] Around 65 percent of SCCHN tumours express abnormal amounts of p53 suggesting the presence of mutation.[12, 13]

Nuclear/biochemical change

As a relatively late event in apoptosis, endonuclease activity cleaves nuclear DNA into fragments of specific length (180 base pairs) known as oligosomal fragments. The specific endonuclease involved in this (caspase-activated DNase or DNA fragmentation factor (CAD/DFF)) is activated by cleavage from its inhibitor, iCAD/DFF45 by caspase 3. The ends of these fragments are specifically 3-OH and 5-P. These oligosomal fragments are an important marker of apoptotic cell death and can be identified by biochemical methods.

Morphological cellular changes

At a nuclear level, widespread DNA fragmentation is associated with the loss of chromatin and its condensation into masses, which form next to the nuclear membrane. This chromatin condensation is regarded as a morphological hallmark of apoptosis and can be seen in light microscopy and electron microscopy as 'crescent' formation within the nucleus. The nuclear membrane itself begins to bleb into nuclear fragments (see **Figures 6.2, 6.3, 6.4** and **6.5**).

At the same time, there is a reduction in cytoplasmic volume. Organelles are preserved but the endoplasmic reticulum vesiculates can become fused with the cell membrane at various points. In addition, specialized structures on the cell surface become lost and the membrane assumes a smooth and featureless appearance. The cell membrane becomes detached from neighbouring cells as a result of loss of volume and structure. From this point, the cell rapidly fragments into membrane-bound apoptotic bodies, which contain cellular components, such as nuclear fragments. These are short-lived and are

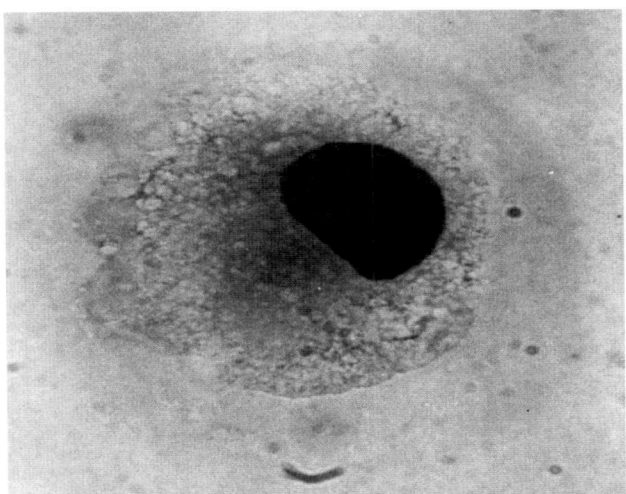

Figure 6.2 Apoptosis in fibroblast cell: Wright stain, light microscopy. Normal appearance, high cytoplasm:nuclear ratio. Acknowledgements to Dr C. Stewart PhD, Department of Surgery, University of Bristol, UK.

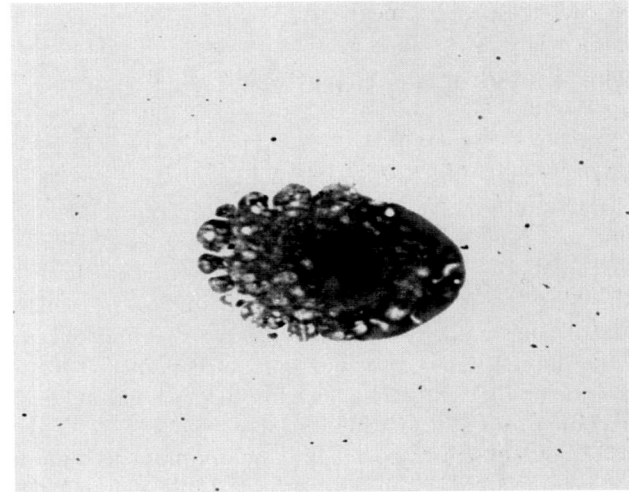

Figure 6.4 Apoptosis in fibroblast cell: Wright stain, light microscopy. Membrane blebbing and apoptotic body formation is shown. Acknowledgements to Dr C. Stewart PhD, Department of Surgery, University of Bristol, UK.

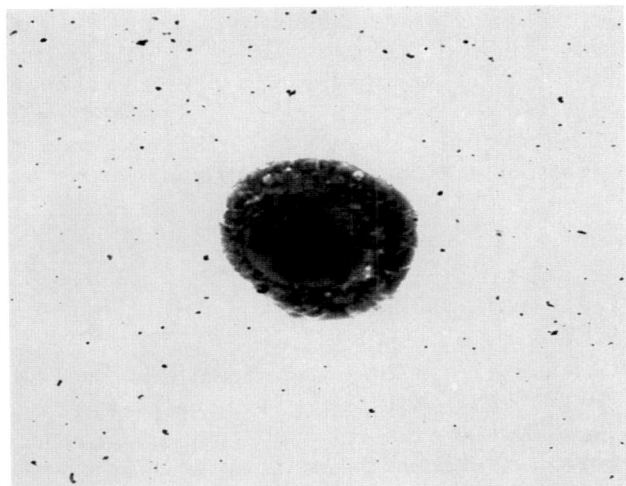

Figure 6.3 Apoptosis in fibroblast cell: Wright stain, light microscopy. Cell shrinkage is shown with nuclear integrity lost as demonstrated by dark staining cytoplasm, decline in cytoplasmic:nuclear ratio. Acknowledgements to Dr C. Stewart PhD, Department of Surgery, University of Bristol, UK.

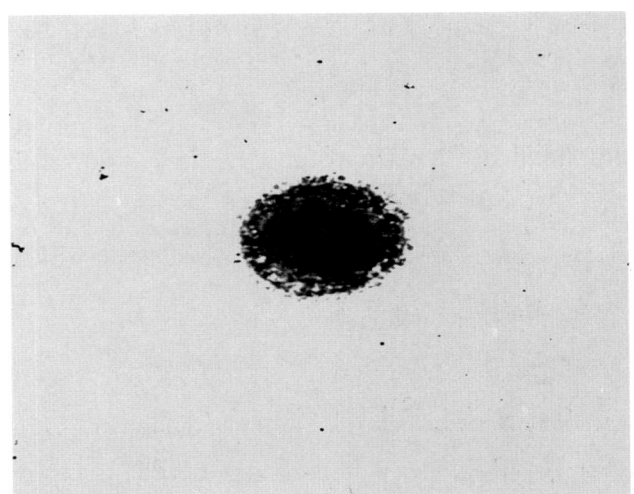

Figure 6.5 Apoptosis in fibroblast cell: Wright stain, light microscopy. Continued shrinkage, cell fragmentation, nuclear pyknosis is shown. Acknowledgements to Dr C. Stewart PhD, Department of Surgery, University of Bristol, UK.

phagocytosed by adjacent cells or macrophages. These changes take place in a matter of hours, although in cell or organ culture it is not clear if the clearance of apoptotic products is as rapid.

METHODS OF DETECTING AND MEASURING APOPTOSIS

Apoptosis may be identified by its morphological or biochemical features (**Table 6.3**). Some techniques are applicable only to single cell suspensions, others may be used to identify cell death in whole tissues such as sections of pathological specimens.

Morphological identification

Light microscopy using a ×100 oil immersion objective lens is sufficiently sensitive to detect morphological changes, such as cytoplasmic shrinkage, nuclear condensation and apoptotic body formation (**Figure 6.6**). Haematoxylin and eosin (H&E) is repeatable and uncomplicated and has been used extensively in studies in which identification and quantification of apoptosis is undertaken. Other more specialized tissue stains, such as methyl-green pyronin and Wright staining (**Figures 6.2**, **6.3**, **6.4** and **6.5**) may offer some advantages over H&E.

Electron microscopy remains the optimum technique for identification of morphological features of apoptosis. Chromatin condensation (**Figure 6.7**) and formation of apoptotic bodies are easily seen. However, electron microscopy only allows relatively small amounts of tissue to be examined and its use in quantifying apoptosis in tissue section is limited.

The fluorescent dye acridine orange can identify apoptosis morphologically or part of flow cytometric analysis. However, as the cells examined need to be living, its use is reserved for cell suspensions derived from experiments with cell culture.

Biochemical identification

Flow cytometry allows a variety of measurements to be made concerning a cell population, including changes in

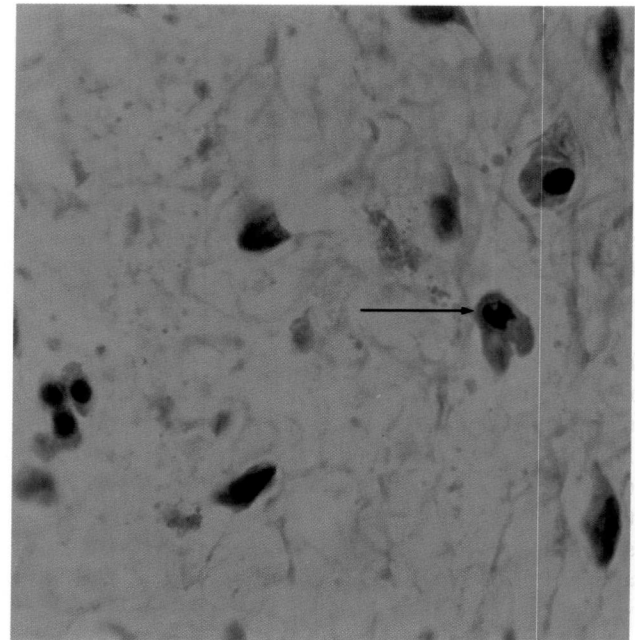

Figure 6.6 Haematoxylin and eosin stain of nasal polyp stromal cells suggesting nuclear condensation.

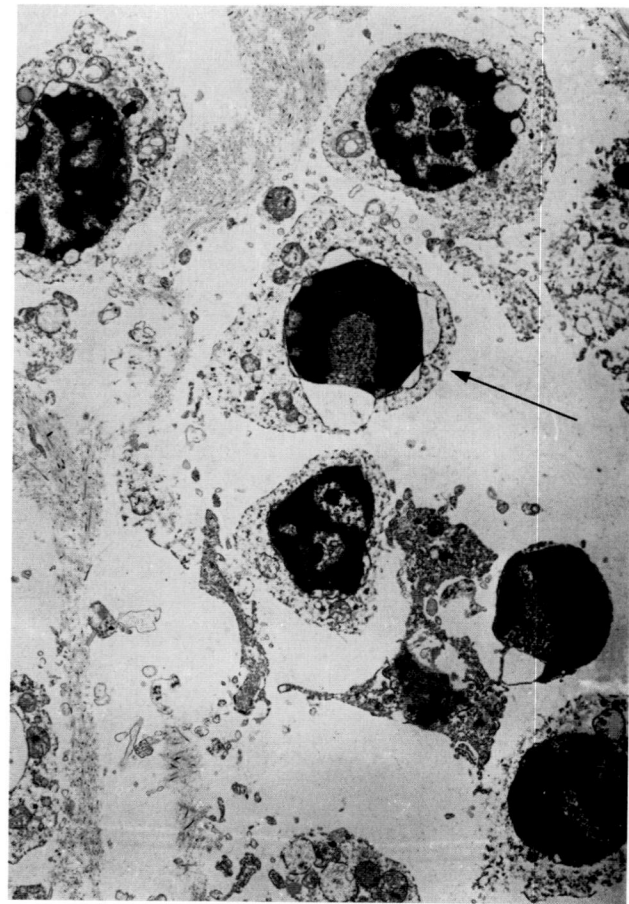

Figure 6.7 Electron micrograph of nasal polyp stroma cells after incubation with dexamethasone, demonstrating margination of chromatin and 'crescent' formation.

Table 6.3   Identifying features of apoptosis.

Morphological	Biochemical
Cytoplasmic shrinkage from surrounding cells	Externalization of phosphatidyl serine
Nuclear condensation and pyknosis	180 base pair oligosomal DNA fragments
Chromatin condensation and crescent formation	3-OH ends of oligosomal fragments
Formation of apoptotic bodies	

cell size, DNA and chromatin structure. A variety of methods of identifying apoptotic cells using flow cytometry have been described, one of the most common techniques is to attempt to identify a pre-G1 peak when the number of cells in each phase of the cell cycle is counted using propidium iodide as a nuclear stain.

Endonuclease-mediated division of DNA into oligosomal fragments is easily identified by the appearance of a ladder of bands in multiples of 180 bp on agarose gel electrophoresis.

Apoptosis can be identified in tissue sections by labelling the characteristic free 3-OH termini of DNA fragments with a modified nucleotide, mediated by the terminal deoxynucletidyl transferase (TdT) enzyme or DNA polymerase. This is referred to as *in situ* end labelling (ISEL) or TdT-mediated nick end labelling (TUNEL). The technique is available in commercially produced reagent sets. However, although end labelling may be used in archived tissue sections, 'staining' problems can arise with varying ages and fixation times of samples.

Annexin-V is a phoshpolipid which binds to phosphatidylserine residues. Early in the apoptotic process these are flipped from the inner to the outer cell membrane. Annexin-V can be identified by immunoassay and detects an earlier stage of apoptosis than end labelling for DNA fragments.

APOPTOSIS IN DISEASE

Much research in the last decade has aimed at identifying apoptosis (or failure of apoptosis) as a part of the pathogenesis of specific diseases. In fact, as apoptosis is such a fundamental part of normal tissue function, it should not be surprising to discover that apoptosis can be identified at some stage in most disease processes. In some diseases, failure of apoptosis regulation (see **Table 6.4**) is more fundamental than others in which apoptosis is merely one step in a larger pathological process.

Apoptosis in non-neoplastic disease

CONGENITAL DEFECTS

Certain cells are destined to die by apoptosis before birth as a part of normal development and maturation, a classical example being the cells in the tail of a tadpole. Failure of apoptotic mechanisms or abnormal apoptotic activity is implicated in a variety of congenital abnormalities, including cardiac defects and cleft palate.

VIRAL INFECTION

A cell's normal response to infection would be to die. However, viral genes may encode proteins, which mimic the host cell's own antiapoptotic proteins to artificially prolong the life of an infected host cell.[15] This allows the virus more time in which to replicate. In other situations, viruses act by inducing apoptosis in host cells, the human immunodeficiency virus (HIV) virus causes apoptosis in infected CD4$^+$ lymphocytes in the acquired immunodeficiency syndrome (AIDS).[16]

SENSORINEURAL DEAFNESS

It seems likely that most sensorineural hearing loss is likely to be mediated by apoptotic loss of hair cells and

Table 6.4 Diseases with dysregulated apoptosis.

Excessive apoptosis	Deficient apoptosis
Degenerative neurological diseases (Alzheimer's, Huntington's, Parkinson's)	Autoimmune lymphoproliferative syndrome (Canale–Smith syndrome)
Aplastic anaemia	Graves' disease
Acquired immunodeficiency syndrome	Hypereosinophilia syndrome
Hashimoto's thyroiditis	Hashimoto's thyroiditis
Lupus erythematosus	Lupus erythematosus
Liver failure	Lymphoma
Multiple sclerosis	Leukemia
Myelodysplastic syndrome	Solid tumors
Type I diabetes mellitus	Type I diabetes mellitus
Ulcerative colitis	Osteoporosis
Wilson's disease	Developmental defects
Chronic neutropenia	
Developmental defects	

Reproduced from Ref. 14, with permission.

inner ear structures. The cochleas of gerbils treated with the ototoxic doses of cisplatin demonstrate apoptosis in the organ of Corti, the spiral ganglion, and the stria vascularis.[17] In the inner ear of the senescence-accelerated mouse, apoptosis has been identified in inner and outer hair cells as well as in the saccules, suggesting that this is the way in which these cells are lost in presbycusis.[18] Apoptosis is also implicated in the differentiation of cells in the developing inner ear.[19]

EOSINOPHIL APOPTOSIS AND NASAL POLYPS

Apoptosis is thought to be an important process in the reduction of inflammatory cell numbers and resolution of inflammatory processes and eosinophil apoptosis is delayed in allergic inflammation. Resolution of asthma attacks after treatment with corticosteroids is accompanied by apoptotic cell death in eosinophils and their subsequent engulfment by macrophages.[20] Although corticosteroid-induced eosinophil apoptosis can be seen *in vitro* in explants of nasal polyp tissue, this effect has not yet been demonstrated in clinical trials.[21]

The potential action of steroids on inflammatory cells in nasal polyps may be indirect, reducing the production of cytokines, such as interleukin (IL)-5. Cytokines IL-3, IL-5 and granulocyte–macrophage colony-stimulating factor (GM-CSF) have an antiapoptotic effect on eosinophils (possibly mediated through Bcl-x) and this effect is inhibited by glucocorticoids. Notably, relative to other cytokines IL-5 is significantly upregulated in nasal polyps.[22]

Fas/FasL mediates a separate pathway for eosinophil apoptosis; stimulation by an anti-Fas monoclonal antibody leads to eosinophil apoptosis and resolution of airway inflammation.[23] Fas expression is greater in nasal polyp tissue and this may have implications in the pathogenesis of the condition.[24]

THYROID DISEASE

The Fas/Fas-L mechanism of apoptosis induction is important in the pathogenesis of autoimmune disease. Immunoprivileged cells, such as thyrocytes, express Fas-L and are able to cause apoptosis by binding to Fas receptors on selfreactive lymphocytes and preventing themselves being killed. Failure of this mechanism can lead to autoimmune disorders. Alternatively, IL-1β (a cytokine produced by infiltrating macrophages) can induce Fas expression in thyrocytes themselves which then causes thyrocytes to kill each other.[25, 26] In this way, an autoimmune process might be triggered by infection. Conversely, the antibody responsible for Grave's disease and the hormone TSH downregulate Fas expression,[27] leading to an increase in thyrocyte numbers and thyroxine production.

APOPTOSIS AND CANCER

Apoptosis and carcinogenesis

As apoptosis is the way in which the body deletes cells with abnormal DNA, then neoplastic change may accompany failure of apoptotic mechanisms.[28] As well as the mutations in p53 already discussed, mutations affecting the genes coding for other components may also be associated with cancer. Many of these components (e.g. Bcl-2, Bax, Apaf-1, p21) can be identified in tissue sections by immunoassay. However, interpretation of the significance of their expression in head and neck cancer is more difficult.

Apoptotic indices in cancer

In studies of head and neck cancers, in the progression from dysplasia through carcinoma *in situ* to invasive carcinoma, there is an increase in mitosis but no change in the apoptotic index.[29] Effectively, the apoptosis/mitosis ratio falls with progression towards increasing malignancy. The relative position of apoptotic and mitotic events in the epithelium also differs in that with increasing malignancy, mitoses tend to shift towards the basal layer, whereas apoptotic events, normally located in the basal or stem cell layer, become more superficial.[30]

Numerous studies investigated the fraction of cells undergoing apoptosis (apoptotic index, AI) in tumours. The relationship between AI and outcome measures, such as recurrence after radiotherapy and survival, varies with different tumours and in different series. Such studies in head and neck cancer are summarized in **Table 6.5**.

The exact mechanism by which the apoptotic index is related to outcome remains unclear. There are a number of potential explanations and these are outlined below.

APOPTOTIC INDEX AS A MEASURE OF CELLULAR TURNOVER IN TUMOURS

Rates of apoptosis and mitosis are generally highly correlated and as such, AI may be regarded as an index of cell turnover in a tumour population. In this case, AI would correlate negatively with survival, as tumours with high proliferative indices generally have a poorer prognosis. Indeed, the frequency of mitotic figures helps to determine the degree of differentiation of a tumour. Poor differentiation is known to be associated with high apoptotic index in head and neck cancer.[36]

LOSS OF APOPTOTIC MECHANISMS WITH INCREASING MALIGNANCY

If one accepts that a cell population's ability to undergo apoptosis is important in the removal of abnormal cells, then a higher frequency of apoptotic bodies might suggest

Table 6.5 Studies of apoptosis and outcome in laryngeal carcinoma.

Study	Site of cancer studied	Treatment modality	Number of patients	Method of identification of apoptosis	Relationship of increasing AI to prognosis
Hotz et al.[31]	All head and neck	Radiotherapy, surgery, chemotherapy	26	TUNEL	Negative
Lera et al.[32]	Larynx	Surgery adjuvant radiotherapy	57	H&E	Negative
Hirvikoski et al.[33]	Larynx	Not stated	172	TUNEL	Negative
Pulkkinen et al.[34]	Larynx	Not stated	66	TUNEL	None
Kraxner et al.[35]	All head and neck	Radiotherapy	15	H&E	?[a]
Saunders and Birchall (unpublished data)	Larynx, hypopharynx	Radiotherapy, surgery	83	H&E	Negative

[a]Investigated induction of apoptosis by radiotherapy.

that the population of tumour cells still has the ability to police itself and highly abnormal cells could be removed. As tumour cell lines become more poorly differentiated and lose normal apoptotic mechanisms, such as normal p53 function, they will become more aggressive and survival will be poorer.

APOPTOSIS IS INCIDENTALLY RELATED TO OUTCOME

Poorly differentiated and aggressive tumours have large areas of poor blood supply and necrosis. Apoptosis is noted to be more common in areas adjacent to necrotic foci[37] and areas of hypoxia are more common in larger tumours, suggesting that any relationship between apoptosis and outcome is an epiphenomenon. Hypoxic and poorly perfused tumours are radioresistant[38] and apoptosis can itself be a reaction to hypoxia rather than a function of malignant change.

Radiotherapy and apoptosis

If apoptosis is induced by nuclear damage, then it might be assumed that the devastating nuclear effects of ionizing radiation at radiotherapy treatment doses would lead to widespread apoptosis. However, the main mode of cell death in irradiated tissues is reproductive or mitotic cell death, in which the cell is unable to complete replication and dies in mid-division.[39] Apoptotic cell death after radiation appears to have greater significance in haemo-poetic cells than in epithelial tissue. In vitro studies with cell lines suggest the dose of radiation required to induce apoptosis varies considerably (2.5–25 Gy). It is of interest that the apoptotic response is related to the rate of regression with treatment[40] and the preirradiation or natural apoptotic index for a tumour is related to the apoptotic response to radiotherapy.[41] The maximum fraction of cells that may be induced into apoptosis is only around 40 percent,[42] suggesting that not only are the

remainder radioresistant, but confirming that there are other modes of cell death involved in the radiotherapy response. Kraxner reported that the greater induction of tumour cell apoptosis after the first 2 Gy of radiotherapy in head and neck cancer patients was associated with increased survival.[35] The fraction of cell death induced by radiotherapy may be of relatively greater importance in 'fractionated' radiotherapy.[43]

Apoptosis is also responsible for some of the side effects of radiotherapy, such as the loss of cells in irradiated lacrimal and salivary glands.[44]

Chemotherapy and apoptosis

It is likely that all chemical agents currently used to kill cancer cells in clinical practice do so by in some way triggering the apoptotic pathway.[45] After a cell recognizes drug-induced damage as irreparable (for example, the detection of DNA damage by p53), apoptotic pathways are activated. In addition, some agents directly activate components of the apoptosis pathway; bleomycin and doxorubicin upregulate expression of Fas and Fas ligand.[46]

To a greater or lesser extent, these mechanisms rely on the presence of normal apoptotic pathways for their execution. It is known that some cells are more resistant to chemotherapy apoptosis than others because of their relatively slow turnover.[47] However, abnormalities in the apoptotic mechanisms in tumour cells may underlie the majority of chemotherapeutic drug resistance. Tumours with *p53* mutations are known to be less chemosensitive. Overexpression of the antiapoptotic BCL-2 in chronic lymphocytic leukaemia leads to relative resistance to fludarabine and mitoxantrone.[48] Breast and prostate cancer cell lines can have their chemosensitivity enhanced by gene transfer of wild type *p53*.[49] Restoration of normal *p53* function to cancer cells is one form of gene therapy, which is discussed in Chapter 3, Gene therapy.

REFERENCES

* 1. Kerr J. Shrinkage necrosis: A distinct mode of cellular death. *Journal of Pathology.* 1971; **105**: 13–20. *The original description of apoptosis as a distinct mode of cell death.*

* 2. Ellis E, Horvitz H. Genetic control of programmed cell death in the nematode. *Caenorhabditis elegans. Cell.* 1986; **4**: 817–29. *First description of the genetics in cell death in the nematode, which led to similar discoveries in mammalian apoptosis.*

3. Metzstein MM, Stanfield GM, Horvitz HR. Genetics of programmed cell death in *C. elegans*: Past present and future. *Trends in Genetics.* 1998; **14**: 410–6.

4. Korsmeyer S. Bcl-2 initiates a new category of oncogenes: Regulators of cell death. *Blood.* 1992; **80**: 879–96.

5. Bertuzzi A, Gandolfi A, Sinisgalli C, Starace G, Ubezio P. Cell loss and the concept of potential doubling time. *Cytometry.* 1997; **29**: 34–40.

6. Tinnemans MM, Schutte B, Lenders MH, Ten Velde GP, Ramaekers FC, Blijham GH. Cytokinetic analysis of lung cancer by *in vivo* bromodeoxyuridine labelling. *British Journal of Cancer.* 1993; **67**: 1217–22.

7. Nagata S. Apoptosis by death factor. *Cell.* 1997; **88**: 355–65.

8. Nagata S. Human autoimmune lymphoproliferative syndrome, a defect in the apoptosis-inducing fas receptor: A lesson from the mouse model. *Journal of Human Genetics.* 1998; **43**: 2–8.

9. Kastan M, Zhan Q, El-Deiry W, Carrier F, Jacks T, Walsh W et al. A mammalian cell cycle checkpoint pathway utilising p53 and gadd45 is defective in ataxia telangectasia. *Cell.* 1992; **71**: 587–97.

* 10. Lane D. P53, guardian of the genome. *Nature.* 1992; **358**: 15–6. *Description of the function of p53 and its importance in regulation of DNA replication, repair and apoptosis.*

11. Somers K, Merrick A, Lopez M, Incognito L, Scheckter G, Casey G. Frequent p53 mutations in head and neck cancer. *Cancer Research.* 1992; **52**: 5997–6000.

12. Field JK, Spandidos DA, Malliri A, Gosney JR, Yiagnisis M, Stell PM. Elevated p53 expression correlates with a history of heavy smoking in squamous cell carcinoma of the head and neck. *British Journal of Cancer.* 1991; **64**: 573–7.

13. Nylander K, Nilsson P, Mehle C, Roos G. P53 mutations, protein expression and cell proliferation in squamous cell carcinomas of the head and neck. *British Journal of Cancer.* 1995; **71**: 826–30.

14. Saikumar P, Dong Z, Mikhailov V, Denton M, Weinberg JM, Venkatachalam MA. Apoptosis: Definition, mechanisms, and relevance to disease. *American Journal of Medicine.* 1999; **107**: 489–506.

15. Young L, Dawson C, Eliopoulos A. Viruses and apoptosis. *British Medical Bulletin.* 1997; **53**: 509–21.

16. Terai C, Kornbluth T, Pauza C, Richman D, Carson A. Apoptosis as a mechanism of cell death in cultured t lymphoblasts acutely infected with HIV-1. *Journal of Clinical Investigation.* 1991; **87**: 1710–5.

17. Alam SA, Ikeda K, Oshima T, Suzuki M, Kawase T, Kikuchi T et al. Cisplatin-induced apoptotic cell death in mongolian gerbil cochlea. *Hearing Research.* 2000; **141**: 28–38.

18. Shaheen Ara Alam KI, Takeshi Oshima, Masaaki Suzuki, Tetsuaki Kawase, Toshihiko Kikuchi, Tomonori Takasaka. Cell death in the inner ear associated with aging is apoptosis? *Hearing Research.* 2000; **141**: 28–38.

19. Nishikazi K, Anniko M, Orita Y, Karita K, Masuda Y, Yoshino T. Programmed cell death in the developing epithelium of the mouse inner ear. *Anatomy Records.* 1998; **118**: 96–100.

20. Woolley KL, Gibson PG, Carty K, Wilson AJ, Twaddell SH, Woolley MJ. Eosinophil apoptosis and the resolution of airway inflammation in asthma. *American Journal of Respiratory and Critical Care Medicine.* 1996; **154**: 237–43.

21. Saunders M, Wheatley A, George S, Lai T, Birchall M. Do corticosteroids induce apoptosis in nasal polyp inflammatory cells? *In vivo* and *in vitro* studies. *Laryngoscope.* 1999; **109**: 785–90.

22. Bachert C, Wagenmann M, Hauser U, Rudack C. IL-5 synthesis is upregulated in human nasal polyp tissue. *Journal of Allergy and Clinical Immunology.* 1997; **99**: 837–42.

23. Tsuyuki S, Bertrand C, Erard F, Trifilieff A, Tsuyuki J, Wesp M et al. Activation of the fas receptor on lung eosinophils leads to apoptosis and the resolution of eosinophilic inflammation of the airways. *Journal of Clinical Investigation.* 1995; **96**: 2924–31.

24. Fang SY, Yang BC. Overexpression of fas-ligand in human nasal polyps. *Annals of Otology, Rhinology and Laryngology.* 2000; **109**: 267–70.

25. Giordano C, Stassi G, Maria RD, Todaro M, Richiusa P, Papoff G et al. Potential involvement of fas and its ligand in the pathogenesis of Hashimoto's thyroiditis. *Science.* 1997; **275**: 960–3.

26. Stassi G, Todaro M, Bucchieri F, Stoppaciaro A, Farina F, Zumo G et al. Fas/fas ligand driven T cell apoptosis as a consequence of ineffective thyroid immunoprivilege in Hashimoto's thyroiditis. *Journal of Immunology.* 1999; **162**: 263–7.

27. Kawakami A, Eguchi K, Matsuoka N, Tsuboi M, Urayama S, Kawabe Y et al. Modulation of fas-mediated apoptosis of human thyroid epithelial cells by igg from patients with Grave's disease (GD) and idiopathic myxoedema. *Clinical and Experimental Immunology.* 1997; **110**: 434–9.

28. Bowen ID, Bowen SM, Jones AH. *Mitosis and apoptosis: Matters of life and death.* London: Chapman & Hall, 1998: 182.

29. Birchall MA, Winterford CM, Allan DJ, Harmon BV. Apoptosis in normal epithelium, premalignant and malignant lesions of the oropharynx and oral cavity: A preliminary study. *European Journal of Cancer. Part B, Oral Oncology.* 1995; **31B**: 380–3.

30. Birchall M, Winterford C, Tripconi L, Gobe G, Harmon B. Apoptosis and mitosis in oral and oropharyngeal epithelia: Evidence for a topographic switch in premalignant lesions. *Cell Proliferation*. 1996; **29**: 447–56.

31. Hotz MA, Bosq J, Zbaeren P, Reed J, Schwab G, Krajewski S *et al*. Spontaneous apoptosis and the expression of p53 and bcl-2 family proteins in locally advanced head and neck cancer. *Archives of Otolaryngology – Head and Neck Surgery*. 1999; **125**: 417–22.

32. Lera J, Lara PC, Perez S, Cabrera JL, Santana C. Tumor proliferation, p53 expression, and apoptosis in laryngeal carcinoma: Relation to the results of radiotherapy. *Cancer*. 1998; **83**: 2493–501.

33. Hirvikoski P, Kumpulainen E, Virtaniemi J, Pirinen R, Salmi L, Halonen P *et al*. Enhanced apoptosis correlates with poor survival in patients with laryngeal cancer but not with cell proliferation, bcl-2 or p53 expression. *European Journal of Cancer*. 1999; **35**: 231–7.

34. Pulkkinen JO, Klemi P, Martikainen P, Grenman R. Apoptosis *in situ*, p53, bcl-2 and agnor counts as prognostic factors in laryngeal carcinoma. *Anticancer Research*. 1999; **19**: 703–7.

35. Kraxner H, Tamas L, Jaray B, Ribari O, Szentirmay Z, Szende B. Search for prognostic factors in head and neck cancer. *Acta Oto-Laryngologica – Supplement*. 1997; **527**: 145–9.

36. Roland NJ, Caslin AW, Nash J, Stell PM. Value of grading squamous cell carcinoma of the head and neck. *Head and Neck*. 1992; **14**: 224–9.

37. Kerr J, Wyllie A, Currie A. Apoptosis: A basic biological phenomenon with wider ranging implication is tissue kinetics. *British Journal of Cancer*. 1972; **24**: 239–57.

38. Guichard M, Lartigau E. New trends for improving radiation sensitivity by counteracting chronic and acute hypoxia. *Advances in Radiation Biology*. 1994; **18**.

39. Puck T. Action of radiation on mammalian cells. Iii. Relationship between reproductive death and induction of chromosome anomalies by x-irradiation of euploid human cells *in vitro*. *Proceedings of the National Academy of Science of the USA*. 1958; **44**: 772–80.

40. Stephens L, Ang K, Schultheiss T, Milas L, Meyn R. Apoptosis in irradiated murine tumours. *Radiation Research*. 1991; **127**: 308–16.

∗ 41. Meyn R, Stephens L, Ang K, Hunter N, Milas L, Peters L. Heterogeneity in apoptosis development in irradiated murine tumours. *International Journal of Radiation, Biology Physics*. 1993; **64**: 583–91. *Basic research in cell lines describing relationship between radiation and apoptosis.*

42. Milas L, Stephens L, Meyn R. Relation of apoptosis to cancer therapy. *In Vivo*. 1994; **8**: 665–74.

43. Olsen D. Calculation of the biological effect of fractionated radiotherapy: The importance of radiation-induced apoptosis. *British Journal of Radiology*. 1995; **68**: 1230–6.

44. Stephens L, Schultheiss T, Price R, Ang K, Peters L. Radiation apoptosis of serous acinar cells of salivary and lacrimal glands. *Cancer*. 1991; **67**: 1539–43.

∗ 45. Bold R, Termuhlen P, McConkey D. Apoptosis, cancer and cancer therapy. *Surgical Oncology*. 1997; **6**: 133–42. *Review of the mechanics of apoptosis with respect to cancer and cancer therapy.*

46. Friesen C, Herr I, Krammer P, Debatin K. Involvment of the cd95 (apo1/fas) receptor/ligand system in drug induced apoptosis in leukaemia cells. *Nature Medicine*. 1996; **2**: 574–7.

47. Hickman J. Apoptosis and chemotherapy resistance. *European Journal of Cancer*. 1996; **32**: 921–6.

48. McConkey D, Chandra J, Wright S, Plunkett W, McDonnell T, Reed J *et al*. Apoptosis sensitivity in chronic lymphocytic leukaemia is determined by exogenous endonuclease content and relative expression of bcl-2 and bax. *Journal of Immunology*. 1996; **156**: 2624–30.

49. Xu L, Pirollo KF, Chang EH. Tumor-targeted p53-gene therapy enhances the efficacy of conventional chemo/radiotherapy. *Journal of Controlled Release*. 2001; **74**: 115–28.

7

Stem cells

A JOHN HARRIS AND ARCHANA VATS

Stem cells	66	Stem cell migration	71
Properties of stem cells	67	Stem cell-released growth factors	71
Stem cell niches	67	Regeneration of human tissues	72
Activation of stem cells in adult tissues	67	Cells for tissue maintenance have two possible origins	72
Asymmetric division	67	Bone marrow has two populations of multipotent cells	72
Specificity of stem cell differentiation	68	Possible therapeutic uses for stem cells	72
Stem cells and expression of connexins	68	Therapeutic use of embryonic stem cells	73
Stem cell hierarchies	68	Potential therapeutic use of cells engineered to support	
Carcinogenetic potential of stem cells	69	regeneration	74
Pluripotent stem cells may be isolated from adult tissues	70	Key points	76
Nerves and stem cell activation	70	Deficiencies in current knowledge and areas for future	
Telomerase activity in stem cells	70	research	78
Embryonic origins of stem cells	71	References	78

SEARCH STRATEGY AND EVIDENCE-BASE

The data in this chapter are supported by a Medline search using the key words stem cells, pluripotent stem cells, regeneration, multipotent cells and differentiation. The majority of papers referenced are based on strict histopathological or immunocytochemical studies that represent level 1 evidence. Some papers referenced are statements that are based on expert opinion and are level 4 evidence and where this occurs this will be inserted into the text.

STEM CELLS

Disease or therapy in otorhinolaryngology-head and neck surgery may both result in the destruction or malformation of tissues and organs such as nasal cartilages, pinna and trachea. Reconstructing an injured face is a prime example of when such damage may occur. The ability to regenerate adult teeth, or cochlear hair cells to restore hearing would offer massive benefits. There is a growing hope that stem cells, derived from either adult and embryonic sources, may have therapeutic potential, but much research is required before their use is commonplace.

Human embryonic stem cells can be maintained in tissue culture as immortal cell lines with the potential to differentiate into any cell in the body, or by incorporation into a blastocyst to give rise to an new individual.[1,2] They offer great potential as therapeutic agents to repair traumatized tissues, regenerate whole organs or to treat diseases such as diabetes, Alzheimer's or Parkinson's disease and congential disorders such as immune deficiencies. Problems and concerns about their use include the question of immune compatibility, worries about their origins from aborted human foetuses and the question of how to regulate their differentiation accurately.

Adult stem cells are present in every tissue and may be manipulated to differentiate into a range of cell types. These cells may be isolated, multiplied in culture and then used as homografts to treat problems in their donor without risk of immune rejection or ethical concerns.

PROPERTIES OF STEM CELLS

Every human tissue includes a population of cells capable of entering the mitotic cycle to produce daughter cells which can differentiate and carry out tissue replacement or growth. These are stem cells, and their essential characteristic is asymmetric division; one of the daughter cells remains undifferentiated and potentially immortal. Stem cells may also undergo proliferative divisions to expand the stem cell population. Recent technical developments permit the isolation of stem cells from any tissue and it has been a surprise to find that even in the central nervous system where neurons are not normally replaced, stem cell lines can be isolated that generate neurons as well as glial cells.

STEM CELL NICHES

Stem cell function depends on maintaining a stable population of stem cells which may be activated when required and whose daughter cells can gain access to appropriate regions of the tissue. This requires a tissue niche where stem cells are grouped for control of their self-renewal and differentiation.[3]

Specificity of the niche environment depends upon paracrine signalling from supporting cells, formation of gap junctions with supporting cells, and on localized extracellular matrix molecules, such as heparin sulphate proteoglycan (HSPG)[4] which bind cytokines, fibroblast growth factors (FGF) and other signalling molecules. In general, experimental activation of stem cells to engineer their multiplication involves removing them from the stabilizing influence of the niche environment, as well as exposing them to stimulating growth factors.

In bone marrow, transplanted labelled haemopoietic stem cells form uniformly sized clusters on the stroma[5] in association with a class of stromal cell which supports human stem cells but does not allow their expansion.[6] In mouse hair follicles, the melanocyte niche has been identified in the lower part of the follicle, occupied by a group of stable, immature, differentiation-competent stem cells.[7] If hepatocyte proliferation is blocked in the liver, regeneration may still occur by multiplication and differentiation of oval cells released from a niche on the biliary ducts.[8] A niche for adult neurogenic stem cells has been identified in the adult subventricular zone (SVZ).[9] Cells of the SVZ express bone morphogenetic protein (BMP) which suppresses neurogenesis and so maintains the undifferentiated stem cells. Nearby ependymal cells, however, express Noggin which antagonizes BMP and so stimulates neurogenesis. Cells from this niche migrate to form interneurons in the olfactory bulb.[10]

ACTIVATION OF STEM CELLS IN ADULT TISSUES

Maintenance of an adult tissue requires a perfect balance between cell death and the production of new replacement cells. The slightest inequality between cell loss and stem cell activation would quickly lead to tissue hypertrophy or atrophy. A further demonstration of the environmental control of stem cell activation is that stem cells transferred to new environments demonstrate a competence to differentiate into other tissue types.

Stem cells are activated under different circumstances for tissue maintenance or for tissue repair. Tissue maintenance in the simplest case employs local feedback systems where differentiated cells signal stem cells to inhibit their proliferation. Activation for tissue repair may reflect the exposure of heparin-binding growth factors such as FGF-2, signals from macrophages as part of the inflammatory reaction and paracrine signals from the damaged cells. In a recent analysis of this question Frye et al.[11] used gene array technology to follow epidermal stem cell activation triggered by c-myc expression. Classes of genes whose expression was upregulated included genes involved in cell proliferation and differentiation, and in RNA and protein synthesis and processing. A large proportion of downregulated genes coded for cell adhesion molecules and cytoskeletal proteins. These findings signify that stem cell quiescence requires stable interactions between stem cells and their supporting cells in the niche, and activation involves release from this stabilization.

An interesting question in stem cell biology is why adult tissues may contain stem cells capable of generating cells which are never seen to be replaced in vivo. For example, stem cells isolated from rat spinal cord can differentiate into motoneurons,[12] but regeneration of mammalian motoneurons has never been described in humans nor in animal models of human regeneration. Similarly, stem cells have been isolated from mouse vestibular organs which differentiate into hair cells when implanted into chick otic vesicles,[13] although hair cells are not known to regenerate naturally in mammals.

ASYMMETRIC DIVISION

Tissues that undergo continuous cell replacement throughout life retain stable numbers of stem cells. Stem cells divide asymmetrically to produce two daughters, one which will undergo many symmetrical divisions to produce a large population of differentiated offspring, and the other another stem cell. It is possible, however, for a stem cell to undergo proliferative division to produce more stem cells, or for surplus stem cells to undergo apoptosis, in order to retain appropriate numbers of stem cells. This can be illustrated by reconstitution of haemopoietic stem cells in bone marrow following x-irradiation to treat lymphoma. The number of stem cells in the regenerated bone marrow is independent of the number injected into the blood stream.

Understanding the genetic mechanisms for this regulation is founded on experiments with *Drosophila*, followed by recognition of homologous genes in mammalian tissues. These experiments demonstrate two principle mechanisms: segregation of proteins into the prospective stem cell during asymmetric cell division; and a system of interactive signalling between prospective stem cells and prospective differentiation-competent daughter cells.

Drosophila neural stem cells divide asymmetrically into another neuroblast, and a ganglion mother cell (GMC) which is cleaved once into two neurons. The neural fate determination proteins *Numb* (which suppresses *Notch* signalling) and *Prospero* (a transcription factor) are localized to the basal surface of the stem cell. To coordinate mitotic spindle orientation with the polarized localization of the neural fate determinants, the apical surface is defined by localization of *Inscutable* and *Bazooka*, and the basal surface by *Lethal giant larvae* and *Lethal discs large*[14] so that when the cell divides, proteins in the basal compartment segregate to the GMC.

Interactive signalling between daughter stem cells and GMC is mediated by the *Notch-Delta* system. Lateral inhibition of stem cells by their surrounding daughter cells maintains them in a nonproliferative state.[15, 16]

SPECIFICITY OF STEM CELL DIFFERENTIATION

Stem cell differentiation within healthy adult tissues is tissue-specific, and new cells are appropriate in type, location and number. This does not, however, mean that adult stem cells are necessarily restricted to a single fate, because under experimental circumstances many examples are known where differentiation into cell types not present in the tissue of origin is determined by a community effect. Isolated stem cells, exposed to a sufficient number of differentiated cells from another tissue, differentiate into cells of the new tissue. Human neural stem cells allowed to aggregate with human myoblasts, differentiated into myoblasts.[17] It was essential to disaggregate the neural cells; as long as they remained in contact with one another, their neural competence was conserved. Similarly, embryonic human endothelial cells cocultured with cardiomyoblasts can differentiate into cardiac myocytes.[18] Rat spinal cord stem cells, which in tissue culture differentiate only into glial cells, when implanted into rat hipppocampus formed granule cells.[19] The concept of community effect was first formulated in relation to embryonic myogenesis.[20] It appears to involve tissue-specific paracrine signalling and in the case of muscle several candidate signalling molecules have been proposed.[21, 22]

A single stem cell population may generate several cell types, as seen in haemopoiesis in bone marrow or in the basal layer of the epidermis. In the epidermis, stem cells may differentiate into sebaceous gland cells, hair follicle cells or keratinocytes. Within a developing hair follicle, cells must migrate to be exposed to determination factors which initiate differentiation into a hair.[11]

Although human embryonic stem (ES) cells are pluripotent, within a developing embryo they differentiate into cell types appropriate for different embryonic tissues in an orderly way. Differentiation specificity is determined by environmental signals. For example, if human ES cells are cocultured with stromal cells from bone marrow, they differentiate into haemopoietic stem cells.[23] If they are treated with FGF-2, a growth factor important in regulation of brain development (reviewed in Haik et al.[24]), a substantial proportion aggregate and differentiate into neural tube-like structures. If these aggregates are later dispersed into single cells and cultured without FGF-2, they differentiate into neurons and glia. Similarly, if they are transplanted into the brain of a newborn mouse they differentiate into neurons and astrocytes within apparently normal brain structures.[25]

STEM CELLS AND EXPRESSION OF CONNEXINS

Connexins are a family of proteins which form gap junctions, permitting the movement of ions and small molecules between the cytoplasm of adjacent cells. The expression of connexins is often used as a marker to define the transition between a stem cell and its differentiated progeny. Lack of expression of connexins is also considered to be evidence of malignancy in neoplastic cells.

The connexin family consists of at least 14 different proteins, making it technically difficult to categorically define their absence. Also, they are expressed by supporting cells within a stem cell niche,[26] leading to the hypothesis that they may be necessary for stem cell activation. Stem cell proliferation was normal in tissue from connexin-43 null-mutant mice, casting doubt on this proposal,[27] although other connexin isoforms are also expressed by these cells.[28]

STEM CELL HIERARCHIES

Stem cells have traditionally been classified in a hierarchy. The fertilized egg and its progeny from the first three cell divisions are totipotent. One of these cells placed in a woman's uterus has the potential to develop into a foetus.

As embryonic development proceeds, the totipotent cells multiply to form the spherical blastocyst, with an outer layer of cells committed to form the placenta and other extra-embryonic tissues and an inner cell mass which forms the embryo. Cells of the inner cell mass are pluripotent embryonic stem cells. They can give rise to any body tissue, but if implanted into a uterus do not form a new individual as they have lost the capacity to form extra-embryonic tissues. Maintenance of pluripotency is associated with expression of the homeobox protein *Nanog*, a transcription factor which drives the expression of other proteins required to maintain the pluripotent state.[29, 30]

Human pluripotent embryonic stem cell lines isolated either from blastocyst inner cell masses[2] or from foetal testes or ovaries[1] appear to have similar properties, including the potential to give rise to a new human being, although for ethical reasons none has yet been permitted to express this potential. One reason for their isolation is their potential for supporting tissue regeneration in adults. This potential is now overtaken by the finding that pluripotent cells may be isolated from adult tissues, a possibility that escapes the ethical problems associated with the embryonic tissues, as well as the problem of immune rejection. Immortal tissue culture cell lines of pluripotent mouse embryonic stem cells have created the thriving industrial production of transgenic mice: a blastocyst is isolated from a normal mouse, genetically modified cultured embryonic stem cells are injected into the inner cell mass, and the blastocyst reimplanted into a surrogate mother. If descendants of one of the modified cells enter the germline to become oocytes or sperm it is then possible to isolate a new strain of mice in which every individual has the genome of the tissue culture cell.

As an embryo develops through the stages of gastrulation and neurulation, pluripotent cells are segregated into ectoderm, mesoderm and endoderm, and then into particular tissues such as brain, muscle, bone or gut. Stem cells in these tissues are multipotent, being committed to generate cells to form each particular tissue in an orderly manner. Finally, multipotent stem cells may give rise to tissue-specific committed stem cells, which generate only one cell type.

This orderly hierarchical classification: totipotent, pluripotent, multipotent and committed, validly describes normal tissue growth and maintenance, but is not absolute. It has become commonplace to discover that stem cells which *in vivo* are multipotent or committed, when isolated from their host tissue and transferred to a different environment express pluripotent characteristics. For example, skeletal muscle has a resident stem cell population known as satellite cells. When these are activated to enter the cell cycle they support muscle growth or regeneration by differentiating into myoblasts which fuse with multinucleated muscle fibres. If a biopsy sample of human muscle is minced and placed in normal tissue culture medium, satellite cells multiply and form multinucleated striated muscle fibres in the tissue culture dish. If, however, an appropriate growth factor is added to the culture, the muscle stem cells differentiate into bone or adipose tissue. Adult muscle tissue also includes a separate population of stem cells which can reconstitute haemopoietic tissue in an x-irradiated host.[31]

Stem cells within different levels of their hierarchy have different levels of competence to respond to growth signals. The currently best understood system is that of haemopoietetic stem cells, capable of generating progeny which may differentiate into any of the cells of the blood, osteoclasts or dendritic cells. These occupy a complex niche environment in bone marrow where they interact with a three-dimensional network of stromal supporting cells and extracellular matrix, bone spicules and blood vessels. Haemopoietic stem cells can be classified as true progenitor cells, intermediate progenitors and mature progenitors, which are acted upon by three corresponding classes of growth factors, classes I, II and III, respectively. In tissue culture assays, class I factors which include stem cell factor (SCF) and interleukin-1 (IL-1) do not support colony formation on their own, but in the presence of class II and III factors support the formation of very large clones which may contain all the classes of haemopoietic cell formed by bone marrow. Class III factors (granulocyte-colony stimulating factor (G-CSF), macrophage-colony stimulating factor (M-CSF), erythropoietin) stimulate mature stem cells to form small colonies, and act on the differentiated cells to enhance their functions, for example increasing the adhesiveness of neutrophils. Class II factors (interleukin-3 (IL-3), granulocyte–macrophage-colony stimulating factor (GM-CSF)) can induce colony formation with fewer mature stem cells, but the addition of class III factors is necessary for stem cells to become fully functional.

CARCINOGENETIC POTENTIAL OF STEM CELLS

Stem cells have the capacity to generate large numbers of progeny cells and share with malignant carcinoma cells properties such as expression of telomerase and lack of expression of connexins. It is important to consider whether their use as therapeutic tools is associated with a concurrent risk of cancer.

The stem cell theory of cancer suggests that many or most cancers arise from defects in stem cell growth control,[32] although this theory does not imply that normal stem cells are malignant. Normal cells respond to growth controls and apoptotic signals, are competent to differentiate and to respond adaptively to environmental conditions and eventually become senescent. Stem cells and their derivatives, after disaggregation and grafting into a new environment, appear generally to behave as normal cells in these regards, but if they are implanted as a cell mass they may be less able to respond to local growth control signals. A commercial cell line of mouse embryonic stem cells transplanted into an embryo as a cell mass may form a mass of undifferentiated cells or even a teratoma.[33] One or a few of the same cells injected into the inner cell mass of a blastocyst can participate in generating a normal mouse, indicating their competence to respond to signals regulating growth. Similarly, the fate of stem cells isolated from adult tissues including human breast, kidney, brain or pancreas can be either neoplastic or committed to normal differentiation, according to how they are manipulated.[34]

There is little evidence for stem cells exhibiting cancer-like properties, and more evidence for the contrary view.[35] Stem cells are exquisitely sensitive to growth regulation from their environment and have several mechanisms to retain the integrity of their genome. Mechanisms to maintain the integrity of a stem cell genome include segregation of template and daughter DNA,[36] incompetence for DNA repair and apoptosis of cells with errors in template strands. Selective retention of template DNA strands following mitosis so that the copied strands are passed to the daughter cell whose progeny will eventually differentiate, greatly reduces the possibility of copying errors entering the stem cell population. A further mechanism to conserve the integrity of the genome is lack of competence to repair random DNA damage, so that the stem cell undergoes apoptosis rather than risking a DNA repair error.[35]

PLURIPOTENT STEM CELLS MAY BE ISOLATED FROM ADULT TISSUES

A small population of bone marrow cells which home to bone marrow in irradiated hosts[37] are not only capable of repopulating the bone marrow stem cell niche, but can also differentiate into cells of the liver, gastrointestinal tract, lungs and skin. A subpopulation of blood monocytes have similar properties.[38] Stem cells isolated from aspirates of human adipose tissue can be induced to form bone by exposure to BMP[39] or myocytes by exposure to 5-azocytidine.[40] The human olfactory bulb contains undifferentiated stem cells and their homologues from rats or mice can be induced to differentiate into many neural and glial cell types, and when mixed with myoblasts may differentiate into muscle.[40] Haemopoietic or neural stem cells, implanted into mouse blastocysts, become incorporated into multiple tissues but with some preference for blood or brain, respectively.[41] Hair follicle cells have the competence to form haemopoietic tissue.[42]

Much remains to be learned of the heirarchy of control mechanisms regulating stem cell competence, but the examples given above typify evidence that apparently committed cells can be induced to become multipotent or even totipotent, offering avenues for therapy with autologous tissues.

NERVES AND STEM CELL ACTIVATION

Many instances are known where denervation results in tissue atrophy or failure to regenerate. A classic example is an amputated urodele amphibian limb which will regenerate only if the nerve is intact.[43] The long-sought neurotrophic factor may be a member of the neuregulin family.[44] Human taste buds are continually shed from the tongue and replaced by proliferation and differentiation of basal cells. This process depends on the integrity of the sensory innervation of the tongue. Following partial hepatectomy, proliferation of hepatocytes is impaired if the vagus nerve is sectioned,[45] an observation which may explain the lower rates of hepatocyte proliferation seen in transplanted livers. If skin is denervated, the epidermis is thinned and keratinocyte proliferation is reduced.[46, 47, 48] Healing of experimental bone fractures in rat hindlimbs is significantly impeded by section of the sciatic nerve.[49] Denervated skeletal muscles suffer profound atrophy and numbers of foetal myoblasts or early postnatal satellite cells are severely reduced following denervation.[50, 51]

The idea that nerves influence regeneration and healing is deeply embedded in medical tradition and was responsible for early theories of neurotrophism. Its true importance and its mechanisms are still obscure. The slowing of wound healing in denervated skin may be the consequence of reduced infiltration by macrophages in the absence of nociceptor-induced tissue inflammation, with a consequent reduction in macrophage-released tissue growth factors.[52] Muscle nerves have a clear neurotrophic influence on post-synaptic receptors,[53, 54] but many other influences of nerve on muscle may simply be activity-dependent. Gustatory nerve terminals signal basal cells in taste buds via a paracrine pathway to upregulate basal cell expression of the mammalian analogue of *Drosophila* achaete-scute proneural gene complex, *Mash 1*, and induce the differentiation of taste receptor cells in the tongue.[55]

Despite its prominence in stem cell activity, the neural dependence of bone marrow function has received little attention. Bone marrow receives both autonomic and sensory innervation. Blood flow to bone marrow is strongly influenced by haemopoietic activity, apparently regulated by cytokines released from bone marrow cells, rather than by autonomic neural control.[56] A recent study[57] showing depression of immune function and of haemopoiesis in patients with complete spinal cord transections supports the idea that bone marrow function is neurally regulated, but details of mechanism are yet to be discovered.

TELOMERASE ACTIVITY IN STEM CELLS

A feature of the mechanics of DNA replication is that DNA sequence at the ends of a chromosome is not fully replicated, so that unless there is some form of repair, chromosomes progressively shorten by 70–90 bp with each mitotic cycle. Chromosome ends are capped with telomeres, specialized structures made up of characteristic DNA repeat sequences and a complex of associated proteins. In most somatic cells, each cell division cycle results in telomere shortening, whereas in germ cells and stem cells, telomere lengths are conserved. The primary mechanism for preventing telomere attrition and hence protecting cells from senescence is activation of telomerase. This is a ribonucleoprotein complex with two major components, human telomerase reverse transcriptase (hTERT) and human telomerase RNA (hTR). The RNA provides a template for telomeric repeat synthesis, allowing telomerase to catalyze the addition of TTAGGG repeats to the chromosome end.

During embryogenesis, telomerase levels typically fall and activity is absent in most adult human somatic cells. Telomerase can be used as a marker to help identify stem cells in adult tissues, but cells with functional competence to act as stem cells do not necessarily express high levels of telomerase.[58] A considerable number of experiments have used viral constructs to express telomerase and hence rescue stem cell function, with varied results. Tissue transplants from aged donors may consist of cells with relatively short telomere lengths and little competence to regenerate in their new host. In some cases, transfection with an expression vector for hTERT resulted in immortalized tissue culture lines with the potential to act as effective tissue transplants. For example, cells in human adrenal cortex proliferate throughout life and adrenals do not have a stem cell or basal cell compartment. Telomere lengths progressively shorten, and cell proliferative capacity is lost. Adrenal cortical cells can be immortalized by transfection with hTERT making them possible effective candidates for transplantation,[59] although the possibility that they might be malignant would need to be checked.

Cells in some tumours have telomeres of normal or greater than normal length, but no telomerase activity. Here, telomere lengths are retained by a separate mechanism (alternative lengthening of telomeres (ALT)) employing homologous recombination.[60] Utilization of ALT is associated with the presence of ALT-associated promyelocytic leukaemia bodies (APB) which contain human telomere repeat sequences and DNA recombination enzymes[61] giving a histological marker for ALT-positive cells. These have not been observed in normal stem cells.

EMBRYONIC ORIGINS OF STEM CELLS

Whether or not stem cells in adult tissues are leftovers from embryonic development or whether they should be considered as having a distinct adult phenotype, is a question which probably does not have a general answer. Muscle satellite cells amplified in tissue culture and reimplanted in place of embryonic myogenic cells cannot recapitulate the process of embryonic development of muscle.[62] Conversely, satellite cells do not form in Pax-7 null-mutant mice, but embryonic and foetal development of muscle appears to be normal.[63] Thus in this case, satellite cells are specialized adult muscle stem cells, not leftover embryonic stem cells. Muscle does, however, include another stem cell population with a larger range of competence and these are possibly endothelial stem

cells which migrated into muscles during the formation of muscle vasculature.[64]

This example from skeletal muscle appears part of a general case. Tissues may have tissue-specific stem cells, often part of a highly organized tissue structure, and may also include stem cells of endothelial or haemopoietic origin which have arrived in the blood circulation. The roles of tissue-specific cells in tissue maintenance are most easily recognized. Activation of blood-borne stem cells may only be evident in the case of severe tissue damage. They have generated great interest with their obvious potential for clinical manipulation to promote healing of tissues which do not normally regenerate.

The developmental origins of primate neural stem cells were investigated by injecting human neural stem cells into the brain ventricles of foetal monkeys.[65] Some of the injected cells were integrated into brain structures, while others populated the subventricular zone, a source of stem cells in the adult brain. The authors suggest that adult stem cells are the end result of a developmental program rather than representing prolonged embryogenesis.

STEM CELL MIGRATION

Many, perhaps most, embryonic precursor cells migrate from their site of origin to their ultimate tissue residence where they will multiply and differentiate. Thus, when considering transplantation into an adult or activation of stem cells resident in adult tissues, it is not surprising to find that these too may migrate and integrate into adult tissues in an orderly and constructive manner. Neural stem cells provide some robust examples. Human neural stem cells injected into the cerebral ventricles of a monkey foetus integrated into the ventricular germinal zone from where they either migrated along radial glia to their appropriate cortical target zone, or remained as an undifferentiated population in the subventricular zone with a potential for later activation.[65] If implanted into adult tissue, neural stem cells were attracted to migrate towards degenerating neural tissue.[66] The attractant molecule was identified as stromal cell-derived factor 1α, an inflammatory chemoattractant molecule common to many pathologies. Imitola et al.[66] propose a general model where tissue injury evokes chemoattractants which activate and attract resident stem cells and direct their migration to the site of injury. These cells would inhabit injury-induced stem cell niches where potentially reparative signals were transiently expressed. Once entered into the injury site, the stem cells express antiinflammatory molecules,[67, 68] leading to stabilization of the injury response.

STEM CELL-RELEASED GROWTH FACTORS

Stem cells not only have the potential to multiply and differentiate to generate new tissue, they also release growth factors which may support healing and regeneration. As an example, dopaminergic neurons were lesioned with a selective neurotoxin (a mouse model for Parkinson's disease) and then mouse neural stem cells were implanted into one side of the midbrain.[69] Dopaminergic neural function was partially restored and most dopaminergic neurons were identified as rescued host neurons, rather than differentiated grafted neurons. Evidently this was due to secretion of a neuroprotective factor or factors by the grafted stem cells. An assay of growth factors and cytokines secreted by bone marrow-derived mesenchymal stem cells[70] revealed a multiplicity of factors including interleukins, leukaemia-inhibitory factor and stem cell factor. If the cells were induced to differentiate into different cell types, such as osteoblasts, adipocytes or endothelial cells, many of these growth factors continued to be expressed. In addition, tissue-specific growth factor secretion was upregulated, for example osteopontin in osteoblasts and vascular epithelial growth factor in endothelial cells.

REGENERATION OF HUMAN TISSUES

The capacity to regenerate organs or appendages is scattered throughout phylogeny and even where regeneration occurs, closely related species may lack this ability.[71] Some coelenterates can regenerate a new organism from a body fragment or even a single cell. Many, but not all urodele amphibia, such as the axolotl, can regenerate a limb; an adult newt can regenerate limbs, tail, upper or lower jaws, neural retina or lens, and even portions of the heart; and humans may regenerate a severed finger-tip.[72]

Mechanisms of tissue or organ regeneration comprise two principle classes. First, differentiated cells may dedifferentiate, multiply and then redifferentiate. Second, the tissue may include a reserve of stem cells which may be activated and produce a population of differentiation-competent daughter cells, as well as retaining a constant reserve population of stem cells.

The spectacular examples of organ regeneration in urodele amphibia depend on the first of these mechanisms. Dedifferentiated cells multiply to form a blastema, an aggregate of undifferentiated cells with the capacity to differentiate into any of the cell types necessary to regenerate the organ. These cells re-express embryonic patterning genes, for example Pax-6 during eye regeneration,[73] and region-specific Hox genes,[74, 75] growth factors important in regulating embryonic tissue development, such as members of the FGF family,[76, 77] and dorsal-ventral patterning genes[78] during limb regeneration.

Mammalian cells are capable of similar dedifferentiation, even if in many tissues this does not normally occur. Identification of mammalian homologues of genes expressed in newt blastemas[79] may help identify targets for therapeutic interventions in people. Transgenic expression

of the homeobox gene msx-1 in tissue-cultured mouse muscle cells triggers them to dedifferentiate and fragment into mononucleated cells with the capacity to proliferate and differentiate into bone, adipose tissue, muscle or cartilage.[80] In humans, liver hepatocytes and vascular smooth muscle cells are examples where dedifferentiation--redifferentiation are part of everyday tissue maintenance and growth. In the liver, every hepatocyte is able to divide and to regenerate liver tissue following hepatectomy.[81]

CELLS FOR TISSUE MAINTENANCE HAVE TWO POSSIBLE ORIGINS

It now appears that every tissue in the body includes a population of stem cells, but the degree to which these are employed in everyday tissue maintenance varies considerably.

Dedifferentiation, cell multiplication and redifferentiation are characteristic of several tissues, notably liver, smooth muscle and peripheral nerve Schwann cells. In a healthy liver, hepatocytes are constantly replaced and at any one moment around 8 percent are in a proliferative state,[82] indicating a half-life of about ten days. Tissues with stem cell niches employed in tissue maintenance include blood, skin and mucosa, olfactory epithelium and bone. The principle function of satellite cells in skeletal muscle is to support post-natal muscle growth,[63] but they can be activated to support adult muscle regeneration.

BONE MARROW HAS TWO POPULATIONS OF MULTIPOTENT CELLS

Bone marrow contains two different types of multipotent cells. Mesenchymal stem cells populate the bone marrow stroma and have the potential to give rise to mesodermal tissues, such as bone, cartilage, adipose tissue and skeletal muscle cells. Haemopoietic stem cells generate cells of the blood and immune system.

Circulating bone marrow cells have been shown to contribute to regeneration in many tissues including heart,[83] skeletal muscle,[84, 85] endothelium,[86, 87] liver[88, 89] and skin.[90] The ease with which they can be isolated and their capacity to home to damaged tissues to promote regeneration make them attractive candidates for therapeutic tools.[85]

POSSIBLE THERAPEUTIC USES FOR STEM CELLS

Stem cell therapy is still largely confined to laboratory models but is rapidly approaching clinical utility. How may these therapies be applied?

First, and perhaps most obvious, endogenous stem cells may be activated to promote tissue regeneration to compensate for trauma, disease or ageing. Some tissues contain stem cells with little potential for natural activation *in vivo*, but which can be activated experimentally; these include articular cartilage, neurons and adult teeth. Activation might involve their removal and isolation, multiplication and replacement *in vivo*, or alternatively may be achieved by local application of specific growth factors. Examples at the research level are isolation and multiplication of neural stem cells,[91] of chondrogenic cells to repair articular cartilage,[92, 93] and of vestibular hair cells to restore balance or hearing.[13, 94]

Second, endogenous stem cells may be removed and cultured on a substrate to generate an organ rudiment, which may then be grafted back into the patient. An example of current application is for skin grafts to treat burns patients, and at the research level, attempts to engineer tooth buds to replace adult teeth.[95] An extension of this approach is to genetically engineer the isolated cells before amplification and replacement, for example with a construct which might express a necessary growth factor. An example is to express BMP in osteogenic stem cells to induce cartilage repair.[96]

A third application is to use stem cell therapy to compensate for genetic disorders. Much effort has been applied to Duchenne muscular dystrophy (DMD) with the hope that skeletal muscle stem cells expressing a normal dystrophin protein might be targetted to degenerating muscles in DMD patients, but technical hurdles have not yet been overcome.

Potential stem cell therapies are being considered for a wide range of pathological conditions and diseases, including neural stem cells to replace neurons lost in ageing or dementia; pancreatic islet cells in diabetics; specialized glial cells to promote regeneration of peripheral nerves or long fibre tracts in the central nervous system (CNS); chondrogenic stem cells to repair cartilage, bones and joints; stem cells to replace cochlear hair cells; tooth germs to regenerate teeth and many others.

THERAPEUTIC USE OF EMBRYONIC STEM CELLS

Embryonic stem cells are isolated from the inner cell mass of the preimplantation blastocyst[2, 97] and have been derived from mice, nonhuman primates and humans. They are pluripotent cells, retaining the capacity to generate any and all foetal and adult cell types *in vivo* and *in vitro*.[98] These cells can be maintained and expanded *in vitro* in an undifferentiated, pluripotent state almost indefinitely in the presence of leukaemia-inhibitory factor (LIF) or embryonic fibroblasts. This provides a potentially unlimited source of stem cells. If LIF is withdrawn, ES cells spontaneously differentiate to form cellular aggregates or embryoid bodies, which contain differentiating cells of ectodermal, endodermal and mesodermal lineage. ES cell differentiation pathways can be controlled and restricted by manipulation of culture conditions to generate cultures enriched for lineage-specific precursors. The generation of a range of distinct phenotypes from mouse ES cells, including haematopoietic precursors,[99] neural cells,[100] adipocytes,[101] muscle cells,[102] myocytes,[103] chondrocytes[104] and osteoblasts[105] has been achieved using this approach.

Other sources of pluripotent stem cells are embryonic germ (EG) cells derived from the gonadal ridge of the early foetus,[106] embryonic carcinoma (EC) cells derived from teratocarcinomas,[107] and mesenchymal stem cells from placental cord blood.[108]

Isolation of human ES cells[1, 2] now makes it possible that human ES cells can be developed for tissue repair and regeneration. Differentiation protocols developed for mouse ES cells are likely to be relevant to human ES cells[109] as even though there are differences in their morphology, propagation and culture requirements, they are broadly similar in their potential to differentiate into specific cell types.

There are a number of ways to control ES cell differentiation and preferentially select a particular phenotype. A relatively simple approach is to culture in media supplemented with cytokines, hormones or other factors that stimulate the cell type of interest. This requires detailed knowledge of the biology of the cell type of interest, but this biochemical selection approach is relatively effective. Osteoblasts can be generated from mouse ES cells and derivation of osteoblasts was demonstrated by simply maintaining dispersed embryoid bodies in a culture medium routinely used to culture explanted mouse osteoblasts. On refining the culture conditions, it was found that whilst the biochemical composition of the medium in which the differentiating ES cells are maintained was an import stimulus for selecting the osteoblast phenotype, the timing of stimulation was also crucial. Thus, by delaying the addition of one particular factor, in this example dexamethasone, for up to 14 days after dispersal and culture of the embryoid bodies, a seven-fold enrichment of cells capable of expressing the osteoblast phenotype was attained.[105] Coculture with mouse osteoblasts is an effective inducer of osteogenic differentiation in ES cells. There are unpublished reports from other workers to show that implantation of human ES cells into mouse organs and tissues, including brain and liver, is an effective method to induce neural or hepatic phenotypes. Such observations are consistent with those on adult stem cells and further emphasize the influence of environment on stem cells and the acquisition of a particular phenotype.

Biochemical selection, although useful for generating cultures enriched with a particular phenotype, does not effectively exclude other phenotypes. Approximately 60–70 percent enrichment of cells with osteoblast lineage was found in experiments at the Tissue Engineering and Regenerative Medicine Centre (TEC), with the remaining cells comprising a mixed population of other phenotypes, such as neural cells. Methods to further purify or select cells of the desired lineage/phenotype need to be developed if ES cells are to be considered for use for transplantation therapy. Methods such as fluorescence-activated cell sorter (FACS) or magnetic-activated cell sorter (MACS) are useful to sort and purify a particular cell type or population. A cell surface marker expressed by the cell type of interest that can be recognized by a fluorescence or magnetic microbead tagged antibody is used to preferentially select that cell. To be effective, the cell surface marker should be restricted to the desired cell lineage and ideally should not be sensitive to activation upon binding of the tagged antibody. FACS and MACS have been used to purify osteoprogenitors from marrow stromal stem cells.

As an alternative, stem cells (both ES cells and adult stem cells) can be transduced with a lineage-specific gene. In this knock-in approach, the gene insert can also carry one of several resistance genes which allow for preferential selection of cell subpopulations that should be restricted to the lineage of interest. This method has been used to select neural[110] and cardiomyocyte phenotypes.[103] In the latter example, the selected cardiomyocytes were subsequently implanted into the damaged hearts of mice and shown to form stable grafts.[111] The potential to use ES cells for tissue repair and regeneration could be enhanced by using nuclear transfer to make the cells autologous and so remove risks of tissue rejection, or by using human ES cell lines with modifications to the major histocompatibility complex.

Human ES cells are derived by growing cleavage-stage embryos into blastocysts and then removing the inner cell mass. The embryos from which the initial human ES cell lines were derived were produced by in vitro fertilization and donated with the informed consent of the parents. The use of such 'spare' embryos was widely held to be acceptable. As they were created for reproductive purposes for which they were no longer required, it was considered ethically superior to use them for medical research rather than destroying them or storing them. Another way to derive human embryonic stem cells is by somatic nuclear transfer or cloning. In nuclear cloning an enucleated oocyte is fused with the nucleus of a somatic cell which can go on to generate an intact embryo and produce a viable organism that is genetically identical to the donor of the somatic nucleus.[112] The factors and mechanisms that induce this remarkable transformation are not known, but it seems likely that a component of the enucleated oocyte can initiate rewinding of the genetic programme of the somatic nucleus to generate a 'totipotent cell'.

Human ES cells show several morphological and behavioural differences from murine ES cells. They grow more slowly and tend to form flat rather than spherical colonies. Differentiating human ES cell cultures include cells with several distinct morphologies including neurons, epithelium and cardiomyocytes. As with murine ES cells, manipulating the culture conditions under which the cells are kept can encourage the differentiation of different cell lineages. Specific local influences, through coculture with mature cells can also encourage the formation of a particular lineage.

The potential use of human ES cells to create cell populations, tissues or organs for implantation through the use of therapeutic nuclear transfer or other methods, could revolutionize medicine by providing unlimited material compatible with the patient's own tissues. The cells might also be used as in vitro systems for studying the differentiation of specific cell types and for evaluating new drugs and identifying new genes as potential therapeutic targets.

POTENTIAL THERAPEUTIC USE OF CELLS ENGINEERED TO SUPPORT REGENERATION

Olfactory ensheathing cells are a class of glial cells which support regeneration of olfactory receptor neurons in the olfactory epithelium. When transplanted to other regions of the brain they may support regeneration of other classes of neurons.[113] They also support axon regeneration and have been successfully employed in rat models of spinal cord regeneration.[114, 115]

Periosteal stem cells and muscle stem cells have been engineered to express BMP, Sonic hedgehog (Shh) or vascular endothelial growth factor (VEGF) and then used in animal models of bone repair.[96, 116] Expression of the growth factors improved the quality of repair.

Examples of stem cell use to promote tissue regeneration

OLFACTORY SYSTEM

The mammalian olfactory system has the distinction of being the only part of the CNS undergoing continuous renewal. Olfactory receptor neurons have half-lives of a few weeks and are renewed by division of stem cells in the olfactory epithelium which give rise both to neurons and to supporting cells.[117, 118] Their number is selfregulated by secretion of inhibitory factors, including GDF-11[119] and FGF and BMP[120] from the olfactory neurons. Newly generated receptor neurons extend axons through the cribriform plate to accurately reinnervate particular olfactory glomeruli specific for each odour receptor type (ca. 400 in humans, ca. 900 in rodents). Their regeneration is promoted by growth factors secreted by olfactory ensheathing cells (OEC) located beneath the olfactory epithelium.[113] OEC are a form of glia and there is much interest in their possible therapeutic use to stimulate axon regeneration in other regions of the brain.[113, 114, 115, 121]

Not only are olfactory receptor neurons continuously renewed, but also their target neurons in the olfactory bulb. These form from neural stem cells in the subventricular zones of the lateral ventricles,[122] and then migrate as a chain of neural precursor cells[10, 123] to form neurons in the olfactory bulb.

USE OF CHONDROCYTES FOR TISSUE REPAIR

Although articular cartilage has a low capacity for repair, mesenchymal stem cells with the capacity to form cartilage, bone or adipose tissue can be extracted from it.[92] Autologous transplantation of amplified stem cells to repair damaged cartilage is reported to have good outcomes,[124, 125] which may in future be enhanced by engineering them to express growth factors[96] and by transplanting them embedded in a matrix rather than in suspension.[126, 127]

Human nasal septum is a good source of chondrogenic cells with the potential to be used to engineer transplants for restorative surgery in otolaryngology.[128]

REGENERATION OF ADULT TEETH

The casting of 'baby' teeth and their replacement with adult teeth is part of normal human development and it is reasonable to speculate that it will be possible to induce a second round of tooth development. Development of teeth depends on an epithelial–mesenchymal interaction which employs highly conserved genetic signalling mechanisms, common to the formation of many other tissues (see http://bite-it.helsinki.fi for an up-to-date summary).

Embryonic tooth morphogenesis critically depends on the migration of cranial neural crest cells into the first branchial arch.[129] Their odontogenic potential is realized in response to signalling molecules from the oral epithelium including Shh, BMP and FGF.

Adult human odontogenic stem cells have been isolated from dental pulp tissue.[130] Tooth morphogenesis can occur in a number of experimental systems *in vitro* giving potential to generate tissue for experimental therapeutic use.[131, 132]

REGENERATION OF SKIN

Autografts of cultured epidermal cells are commonly used to treat burns patients, although several limitations remain to be overcome. In particular, several weeks are required to amplify cells taken from the patient and the grafted skin does not include hair follicles. To create a skin-equivalent tissue suitable for grafting, organotypic coculture of keratinocytes together with skin fibroblasts offers promise.[133] In a model system, rat hair follicle dermal cells acted as stem cells that could reconstitute both dermis and hair follicles, offering promise for clinical use.[134]

COCHLEAR HAIR CELLS

Normal hearing depends on the integrity of around 3500 inner hair cells in each cochlea. These cells are generated early in the embryo, during the first trimester. After that time they are not normally capable of renewal or regeneration, and must survive for an individual's entire life. Hair cell loss is the most common cause of deafness and is currently irreversible. In birds, by contrast, new inner hair cells are generated following loss or injury,[135] giving hope for therapeutic intervention in humans.[136]

In both birds and mammals, the auditory epithelium includes differentiated hair cells with an orderly spacing among supporting cells, similar in many respects to other sensory organs in which receptor cells are regenerated from the supporting cells. This is what occurs in birds, but following loss of a hair cell in mammals the supporting cells form a scar. If, however, the sensory epithelium is disaggregated, stem cells with competence to differentiate into hair cells (and other cell types) can be isolated.[13] Further definition of the signalling systems responsible for their quiescence and activation may allow development of therapies for deafness and loss of balance.

NEURAL STEM CELLS

There have been many efforts to use tissue grafts of dopaminergic cells to treat Parkinson's disease, but these have not yet proved to be clinically useful,[137] although intraventricular injection of neural stem cells in a mouse model offers promise.[69] Many other proposals exist to use neural stem cells to treat degenerative diseases and stroke or to ameliorate the effects of ageing and are currently being trialled in animal models.

Use of stem cells for organ replacement

Examples from urodele amphibia, where multipotent blastemal cells can regenerate limbs, heart or retina, inspire hope that stem cell therapies may be developed to regenerate entire human organs. This goal currently is achieved only with blood, for example reconstituting haemopoietic tissue following whole body irradiation to treat leukaemia.

One approach is to immunoisolate the grafted tissue by confinement in a diffusion chamber, for example in experimental treatment of diabetes.[138] This technique imposes severe restrictions on tissue size as tissues are not directly perfused with blood.

Use of stem cells to treat genetic disorders

Treatment of congenital disorders requires either replacement of an affected cell type or supplementation of the functions of a defective tissue. Replacement of haemopoietic tissue, for example, to treat congenital immune system disorders or anaemias is effective in animal models[139] and is being applied clinically.[140] Stem cell therapies to treat disorders of other tissues have yet to be developed. Considerable effort has been applied to find strategies to treat Duchenne muscular dystrophy, but these are limited by the global distribution of skeletal muscle in the body and the necessity to destroy existing muscle before any successful multiplication of grafted muscle stem cells will occur.

KEY POINTS

- Human embryonic stem cells have the potential to differentiate into any cell in the body.
- Embryonic stem cells have therapeutic potential.
- Difficulties in applying embryonic stem cells therapeutically include tissue rejection, controlling their differentiation and ethical concerns.
- Stem cells are present in every tissue.
- Adult stem cells may be multipotent and offer better therapeutic potential than embryonic stem cells.
- Properties of stem cells:
  - potentially immortal due to asymmetric division;
  - stem cells are found in all tissues;
  - occupy a 'niche' where their numbers are regulated to remain relatively constant throughout life;
  - surplus stem cells may undergo apoptosis so as to retain their appropriate number;
  - may be activated to undergo mitosis to support tissue growth, repair or maintenance;
  - asymmetric division: one daughter cell remains undifferentiated and potentially immortal;
  - differentiated phenotype is strongly influenced by environmental signals;
  - stem cells do not express connexins or form gap junctions.
- Traditional definition of a hierarchy of stem cell potency:
  - totipotent (has the potential to develop into a whole organism);
  - pluripotent (can give rise to any cell in the body);
  - multipotent (committed to generate the cells of a particular tissue);
  - committed (can generate only one cell type).
- Stem cell carcinomas are not a likely outcome of stem cell therapy:
  - stem cell proliferation responds to signals that regulate growth;

- embryonal carcinomas typically are benign: metastases occur only after secondary transformation to malignancy.
- Stem cells possess several mechanisms to preserve the integrity of their genomes:
  - segregation of template and daughter DNA to selectively retain template DNA in the stem cell lineage;
  - inactivation of DNA repair mechanisms;
  - apoptosis of cells with errors in template strands.
- Recently, pluripotent stem cells have been isolated from adult tissues:
  - multipotent or committed stem cells in an appropriate environment or treated with appropriate growth factors behave as pluripotent stem cells.
- Two principle mechanisms underly the regulation of stem cell number:
  - segregation of some classes of protein into the prospective stem cell during asymmetric cell division;
  - interactive signalling between prospective stem cells and prospective differentiation-competent daughter cells.
- Stem cells occupy a tissue niche:
  - stem cells are grouped for control of their self-renewal and differentiation;
  - specificity of the niche environment depends both on paracrine signalling from supporting cells and on local extracellular matrix molecules, such as heparin sulphate proteoglycan, which bind cytokines, FGF and other signalling molecules.
- Stem cell activation may require innervation:
  - denervation may result in tissue atrophy and failure to regenerate;
  - the idea of a neural influence on regeneration and healing is deeply embedded in medical tradition, but its true importance and mechanisms are still obscure.
- Differentiation of intrinsic stem cells is tissue-specific:
  - stem cell fate can be experimentally modulated by disaggregating stem cells (so they no longer contact one another) and exposing them to a different environment.
- Many, but not all, stem cells express telomerase:
  - telomere lengths are conserved during stem cell division;
  - telomerase is a ribonucleoprotein complex with two major components: human telomerase reverse transcriptase and human telomerase RNA;

- telomerase RNA provides a template for
  telomerase repeat synthesis, catalyzing the
  addition of TTAGGG repeats to the
  chromosome end to restore telomere
  lengths after each cell division.
- Tissues may have stem cell populations with
  multiple embryonic origins:
  - tissue-specific adult stem cells distinct from
    embryonic stem cells;
  - endothelial stem cells which have migrated
    into the tissue during the formation of the
    vasculature;
  - stem cells from bone marrow which have
    arrived via circulation of blood.
- Stem cells are capable of migration:
  - most embryonic precursor cells migrate
    from their site of origin to their ultimate
    tissue residence;
  - adult stem cells retain the capacity for
    orderly migration and integration into
    tissues.
- Stem cells release growth factors:
  - their release from grafted stem cells may
    support healing and regeneration in host
    tissues.
- The capacity to regenerate organs or
  appendages is scattered throughout
  phylogeny:
  - some urodele amphibia can regenerate
    whole limbs, jaws, neural retina or
    portions of the heart;
  - closely related species may greatly differ in
    their competence to regenerate;
  - regeneration often depends upon the
    formation of a blastema which may be
    derived from a reserve of stem cells,
    or by dedifferentiation of tissue-specific
    cells;
  - blastemal cells re-express embryonic
    patterning genes.
- Cells for tissue maintenance have two
  possible origins, dedifferentiation,
  multiplication and redifferentiation; or
  activation of tissue-specific stem cells:
  - liver hepatocytes, vascular smooth muscle
    cells and peripheral nerve Schwann cells
    are examples of tissues which regenerate
    via dedifferentiation;
  - blood, skeletal muscle and skin are
    examples of tissues regenerating from
    tissue-specific stem cells.
- Bone marrow has two populations of
  multipotent cells:
  - mesenchymal stem cells occupy the bone
    marrow stroma and give rise to mesodermal
    tissues including bone, cartilage, adipose
    tissue and skeletal muscle cells;

- haemopoietic stem cells generate cells of
  the blood and immune systems;
- circulating bone marrow cells have been
  shown to contribute to regeneration in
  many tissues including heart, skeletal
  muscle, endothelium, liver and skin.
- Possible therapeutic uses for stem cells
  include:
  - regeneration within damaged tissues;
  - organ replacement;
  - compensation for genetic disorders;
  - cells engineered to express growth factors
    or hormones.
- Two major approaches to therapy are: (1)
  activation of stem cells *in situ* and (2)
  isolation, multiplication *in vitro* and grafting
  of amplified stem cells back into the donor
  or into a new host:
  - some tissues contain stem cells with little
    potential for natural activation *in vivo* but
    which can be activated experimentally;
    these include articular cartilage, neurons,
    vestibular hair cells and adult teeth;
  - multiplication *in vitro* is routine in
    production of skin for grafting and is in
    experimental development for other
    tissues.
- Therapeutic use of embryonic stem cells
  isolated from human embryos poses
  immunological and ethical concerns:
  - as with any organ transplant, there is a risk
    of tissue rejection;
  - there is public resistance to using cells or
    tissues from aborted foetuses, or to
    collecting fertilized ova specifically to
    generate cells for transplants;
  - isolation of embryonic stem cells from
    placental cord blood or the use of
    'universal' human embryonic stem cell
    lines may alleviate ethical concerns.
- Examples of potential therapeutic use of cells
  engineered to support regeneration:
  - olfactory ensheathing cells to promote
    axonal regeneration across spinal cord
    lesions;
  - engineered expression of bone
    morphogenetic protein or Sonic hedgehog
    by periosteal stem cells to promote
    cartilage regeneration;
  - use of muscle-derived stem cells engineered
    to express bone morphogenetic protein or
    vascular endothelial growth factor to
    promote bone healing.
- Examples of stem cell use to promote tissue
  regeneration:
  - reconstitution of olfactory epithelium;
  - use of chondrocytes for cartilage repair;

– use of odontogenic adult stem cells to regenerate adult teeth;
– regeneration of dermis using epidermal stem cells expanded in culture;
– restoration of hearing by regeneration of hair cells in the organ of Corti;
– neural stem cells.
• Examples of stem cell use to promote organ replacement:
– reconstitution of haemopoietic tissue;
– endocrine cells in diffusion chambers to treat diabetes and other endocrine dysfunctions.
• Using stem cells to treat genetic disorders:
– dystrophin and Duchenne muscular dystrophy;
– haemopoietic disorders: restoration of immune competence.

Deficiencies in current knowledge and areas for future research

Potentially immortal stem cells can be isolated from every human tissue. Stem cell tissue culture lines can also be created from inner cell masses of human blastocysts or from human foetal gonads. These cells have the competence to differentiate into multiple cell types and the potential to support regeneration of any adult human tissue.

In tissues where stem cells are active in tissue maintenance or can support tissue regeneration following damage, stem cells occupy niche environments where their numbers can be maintained and their activities regulated. Stem cells possess special mechanisms to preserve them from genetic damage and to selectively eliminate cells with mutated DNA. In contrast with malignant cells, stem cells are exquisitely sensitive to multiple growth control mechanisms and preserve the integrity of their genomes. Adult resident stem cell populations derive from developmental programs and are not simply left over from embryonic development of each tissue. Adult tissues may also include stem cells which have arrived in the blood circulation, derived from both embryonic and adult endothelial or bone marrow cells.

Stem cell biology is an extremely active and expanding field of research with annual publications in the thousands. The popular press is replete with articles promising new technology to regenerate tissues, reverse neurodegeneration or produce designer children. These possibilities are not yet applicable to human subjects, although housing designer mice has become a problem for most laboratory animal facilities.

Deeper understanding of the mechanisms of stem cell activation may generate technologies for controlled regeneration of particular tissues, using their intrinsic stem cell populations. The demonstration that bone marrow-derived cells can be activated to differentiate into specific cell types and to home to particular tissues offers the possibility of stimulating tissue regeneration by intravenous infusion of appropriate cell populations. Cultured stem cells may be surgically grafted into sites where regeneration is required. One can only speculate on the speed with which these speculations can become clinical reality.

Possible future directions include:
➤ tissues of special interest to otolaryngology include bone, cartilage, mucosal epithelia, epidermis, vestibular and cochlear hair cells, nerve and brain, skeletal muscle, teeth and vascular tissues;
➤ enhanced activation of intrinsic adult stem cells: teeth, articular cartilage, brain, blood vessels, wound healing;
➤ homografted and heterografted stem cells: skin, hair, blood;
➤ use of embryonic stem cells to regenerate limbs or other body parts.

REFERENCES

* 1. Shamblott MJ, Axelman J, Wang S, Bugg EM, Littlefield JW, Donovan PJ et al. Derivation of pluripotent stem cells from cultured human primordial germ cells. Proceedings of the National Academy of Sciences of the United States of America. 1998; 95: 13726–31.
* 2. Thomson JA, Itskovitz-Eldor J, Shapiro SS, Waknitz MA, Swiergiel JJ, Marshall VS et al. Embryonic stem cell lines derived from human blastocysts. Science. 1998; 282: 1145–7.
3. Schofield R. The relationship between the spleen colony-forming cell and the haemopoietic stem cell. Blood Cells. 1978; 4: 7–25.
4. Gupta P, Oegema Jr. TR, Brazil JJ, Dudek AZ, Slungaard A, Verfaillie CM. Structurally specific heparan sulfates support primitive human hematopoiesis by formation of a multimolecular stem cell niche. Blood. 1998; 92: 4641–51.
5. Askenasy N, Zorina T, Farkas DL, Shalit I. Transplanted hematopoietic cells seed in clusters in recipient bone marrow in vivo. Stem Cells. 2002; 20: 301–10.
6. Hackney JA, Charbord P, Brunk BP, Stoeckert CJ, Lemischka IR, Moore KA. A molecular profile of a hematopoietic stem cell niche. Proceedings of the National Academy of Sciences of the United States of America. 2002; 99: 13061–66.
7. Nishimura EK, Jordan SA, Oshima H, Yoshida H, Osawa M, Moriyama M et al. Dominant role of the niche in melanocyte stem-cell fate determination. Nature. 2002; 416: 854–60.

8. Paku S, Schnur J, Nagy P, Thorgeirsson SS. Origin and structural evolution of the early proliferating oval cells in rat liver. *American Journal of Pathology*. 2001; **158**: 1313–23.

* 9. Lim DA, Tramontin AD, Trevejo JM, Herrera DG, Garcia-Verdugo JM, Alvarez-Buylla A. Noggin antagonizes BMP signaling to create a niche for adult neurogenesis. *Neuron*. 2000; **28**: 713–26.

10. Lois C, Garcia-Verdugo JM, Alvarez-Buylla A. Chain migration of neuronal precursors. *Science*. 1996; **271**: 978–81.

* 11. Frye M, Gardner C, Li ER, Arnold I, Watt FM. Evidence that Myc activation depletes the epidermal stem cell compartment by modulating adhesive interactions with the local microenvironment. *Development*. 2003; **130**: 2793–808.

12. Shihabuddin LS, Ray J, Gage FH. FGF-2 is sufficient to isolate progenitors found in the adult mammalian spinal cord. *Experimental Neurology*. 1997; **148**: 577–86.

13. Li H, Liu H, Heller S. Pluripotent stem cells from the adult mouse inner ear. *Nature Medicine*. 2003; **9**: 1293–99.

14. Ohshiro T, Yagami T, Zhang C, Matsuzaki F. Role of cortical tumour-suppressor proteins in asymmetric division of Drosophila neuroblast. *Nature*. 2000; **408**: 593–96.

* 15. Henrique D, Hirsinger E, Adam J, Le Roux I, Pourquie O, Ish-Horowicz D et al. Maintenance of neuroepithelial progenitor cells by Delta-Notch signalling in the embryonic chick retina. *Current Biology*. 1997; **7**: 661–70.

16. Lowell S, Jones P, Le Roux I, Dunne J, Watt FM. Stimulation of human epidermal differentiation by delta-notch signalling at the boundaries of stem-cell clusters. *Current Biology*. 2000; **10**: 491–500.

17. Galli R, Borello U, Gritti A, Minasi MG, Bjornson C, Coletta M et al. Skeletal myogenic potential of human and mouse neural stem cells. *Nature Neuroscience*. 2000; **3**: 986–91.

18. Condorelli G, Borello U, De Angelis L, Latronico M, Sirabella D, Coletta M et al. Cardiomyocytes induce endothelial cells to trans-differentiate into cardiac muscle: implications for myocardium regeneration. *Proceedings of the National Academy of Sciences of the United States of America*. 2001; **98**: 10733–38.

19. Shihabuddin LS, Horner PJ, Ray J, Gage FH. Adult spinal cord stem cells generate neurons after transplantation in the adult dentate gyrus. *Journal of Neuroscience*. 2000; **20**: 8727–35.

* 20. Gurdon JB. A community effect in animal development. *Nature*. 1988; **336**: 772–4.

21. Kim D, Chi S, Lee KH, Rhee S, Kwon YK, Chung CH et al. Neuregulin stimulates myogenic differentiation in an autocrine manner. *Journal of Biological Chemistry*. 1999; **274**: 15395–400.

22. Standley HJ, Zorn AM, Gurdon JB. eFGF and its mode of action in the community effect during Xenopus myogenesis. *Development*. 2001; **128**: 1347–57.

23. Kaufman DS, Thomson JA. Human ES cells – haematopoiesis and transplantation strategies. *Journal of Anatomy*. 2002; **200**: 243–8.

24. Haik S, Gauthier LR, Granotier C, Peyrin JM, Lages CS, Dormont D et al. Fibroblast growth factor 2 up regulates telomerase activity in neural precursor cells. *Oncogene*. 2000; **19**: 2957–66.

25. Zhang SC, Wernig M, Duncan ID, Brustle O, Thomson JA. In vitro differentiation of transplantable neural precursors from human embryonic stem cells. *Nature Biotechnology*. 2001; **19**: 1129–33.

26. Rosendaal M, Mayen A, de Koning A, Dunina-Barkovskaya T, Krenacs T, Ploemacher R. Does transmembrane communication through gap junctions enable stem cells to overcome stromal inhibition?. *Leukemia*. 1997; **11**: 1281–9.

27. Rosendaal M, Jopling C. Hematopoietic capacity of connexin43 wild-type and knock-out fetal liver cells not different on wild-type stroma. *Blood*. 2003; **101**: 2996–8.

28. Cancelas JA, Koevoet WL, de Koning AE, Mayen AE, Rombouts EJ, Ploemacher RE. Connexin-43 gap junctions are involved in multiconnexin-expressing stromal support of hemopoietic progenitors and stem cells. *Blood*. 2000; **96**: 498–505.

29. Chambers I, Colby D, Robertson M, Nichols J, Lee S, Tweedie S et al. Functional expression cloning of nanog, a pluripotency sustaining factor in embryonic stem cells. *Cell*. 2003; **113**: 643–55.

30. Mitsui K, Tokuzawa Y, Itoh H, Segawa K, Murakami M, Takahashi K et al. The homeoprotein Nanog is required for maintenance of pluripotency in mouse epiblast and ES cells. *Cell*. 2003; **113**: 631–42.

31. McKinney-Freeman SL, Jackson KA, Camargo FD, Ferrari G, Mavilio F, Goodell MA. Muscle-derived hematopoietic stem cells are hematopoietic in origin. *Proceedings of the National Academy of Sciences of the United States of America*. 2002; **99**: 1341–6.

* 32. Trosko JE. The role of stem cells and gap junctional intercellular communication in carcinogenesis. *Journal of Biochemistry and Molecular Biology*. 2003; **36**: 43–8.

33. Wakitani S, Takaoka K, Hattori T, Miyazawa N, Iwanaga T, Takeda S et al. Embryonic stem cells injected into the mouse knee joint form teratomas and subsequently destroy the joint. *Rheumatology (Oxford)*. 2003; **42**: 162–5.

34. Trosko JE, Chang CC. Isolation and characterization of normal adult human epithelial pluripotent stem cells. *Oncology Research*. 2003; **13**: 353–7.

* 35. Cairns J. Somatic stem cells and the kinetics of mutagenesis and carcinogenesis. *Proceedings of the National Academy of Sciences of the United States of America*. 2002; **99**: 10567–70.

* 36. Potten CS, Hume WJ, Reid P, Cairns J. The segregation of DNA in epithelial stem cells. *Cell*. 1978; **15**: 899–906.

* 37. Krause DS, Theise ND, Collector MI, Henegariu O, Hwang S, Gardner R et al. Multi-organ, multi-lineage engraftment by a single bone marrow-derived stem cell. *Cell*. 2001; **105**: 369–77.

38. Zhao Y, Glesne D, Huberman E. A human peripheral blood monocyte-derived subset acts as pluripotent stem cells.

Proceedings of the National Academy of Sciences of the United States of America. 2003; **100**: 2426–31.

39. Dragoo JL, Choi JY, Lieberman JR, Huang J, Zuk PA, Zhang J et al. Bone induction by BMP-2 transduced stem cells derived from human fat. *Journal of Orthopaedic Research.* 2003; **21**: 622–9.

40. Liu Z, Martin LJ. Olfactory bulb core is a rich source of neural progenitor and stem cells in adult rodent and human. *Journal of Comparative Neurology.* 2003; **459**: 368–91.

41. Harder F, Kirchhof N, Petrovic S, Schmittwolf C, Durr M, Muller AM. Developmental potentials of hematopoietic and neural stem cells following injection into pre-implantation blastocysts. *Annals of Hematology.* 2002; **81**: S20–1.

42. Lako M, Armstrong L, Cairns PM, Harris S, Hole N, Jahoda CA. Hair follicle dermal cells repopulate the mouse haematopoietic system. *Journal of Cell Science.* 2002; **115**: 3967–74.

* 43. Endo T, Tamura K, Ide H. Analysis of gene expressions during Xenopus forelimb regeneration. *Developmental Biology.* 2000; **220**: 296–306.

44. Wang L, Marchionni MA, Tassava RA. Cloning and neuronal expression of a type III newt neuregulin and rescue of denervated, nerve-dependent newt limb blastemas by rhGGF2. *Journal of Neurobiology.* 2000; **43**: 150–8.

45. Cassiman D, Libbrecht L, Sinelli N, Desmet V, Denef C, Roskams T. The vagal nerve stimulates activation of the hepatic progenitor cell compartment via muscarinic acetylcholine receptor type 3. *American Journal of Pathology.* 2002; **161**: 521–30.

46. Chiang HY, Huang IT, Chen WP, Chien HF, Shun CT, Chang YC et al. Regional difference in epidermal thinning after skin denervation. *Experimental Neurology.* 1998; **154**: 137–45.

47. Hsieh ST, Lin WM. Modulation of keratinocyte proliferation by skin innervation. *Journal of Investigative Dermatology.* 1999; **113**: 579–86.

48. Huang IT, Lin WM, Shun CT, Hsieh ST. Influence of cutaneous nerves on keratinocyte proliferation and epidermal thickness in mice. *Neuroscience.* 1999; **94**: 965–73.

49. Madsen JE, Hukkanen M, Aune AK, Basran I, Moller JF, Polak JM et al. Fracture healing and callus innervation after peripheral nerve resection in rats. *Clinical Orthopaedics.* 1998: 230–40.

* 50. Ross JJ, Duxson MJ, Harris AJ. Neural determination of muscle fibre numbers in embryonic rat lumbrical muscles. *Development.* 1987; **100**: 395–409.

51. Rodrigues Ade C, Geuna S, Rodrigues SP, Silva MD, Aragon FF. Satellite cells and myonuclei in neonatally denervated rat muscle. *Italian Journal of Anatomy and Embryology.* 2002; **107**: 51–6.

52. Richards AM, Floyd DC, Terenghi G, McGrouther DA. Cellular changes in denervated tissue during wound healing in a rat model. *British Journal of Dermatology.* 1999; **140**: 1093–9.

53. Lin W, Burgess RW, Dominguez B, Pfaff SL, Sanes JR, Lee KF. Distinct roles of nerve and muscle in postsynaptic differentiation of the neuromuscular synapse. *Nature.* 2001; **410**: 1057–64.

54. Herbst R, Burden SJ. The juxtamembrane region of MuSK has a critical role in agrin-mediated signaling. *EMBO Journal.* 2000; **19**: 67–77.

55. Seta Y, Toyono T, Takeda S, Toyoshima K. Expression of Mash1 in basal cells of rat circumvallate taste buds is dependent upon gustatory innervation. *FEBS Letters.* 1999; **444**: 43–6.

56. Iversen PO. Blood flow to the haemopoietic bone marrow. *Acta Physiologica Scandinavica.* 1997; **159**: 269–76.

57. Iversen PO, Hjeltnes N, Holm B, Flatebo T, Strom-Gundersen I, Ronning W et al. Depressed immunity and impaired proliferation of hematopoietic progenitor cells in patients with complete spinal cord injury. *Blood.* 2000; **96**: 2081–83.

* 58. Bickenbach JR, Vormwald-Dogan V, Bachor C, Bleuel K, Schnapp G, Boukamp P. Telomerase is not an epidermal stem cell marker and is downregulated by calcium. *Journal of Investigative Dermatology.* 1998; **111**: 1045–52.

59. Yang L, Suwa T, Wright WE, Shay JW, Hornsby PJ. Telomere shortening and decline in replicative potential as a function of donor age in human adrenocortical cells. *Mechanisms of ageing and development.* 2001; **122**: 1685–94.

* 60. Hakin-Smith V, Jellinek DA, Levy D, Carroll T, Teo M, Timperley WR et al. Alternative lengthening of telomeres and survival in patients with glioblastoma multiforme. *Lancet.* 2003; **361**: 836–8.

61. Yeager TR, Neumann AA, Englezou A, Huschtscha LI, Noble JR, Reddel RR. Telomerase-negative immortalized human cells contain a novel type of promyelocytic leukemia (PML) body. *Cancer Research.* 1999; **59**: 4175–9.

62. Chevallier A, Pautou MP, Harris AJ, Kieny M. On the non-equivalence of skeletal muscle satellite cells and embryonic myoblasts. *Archives d'Anatomie Microscopique et de Morphologie Expérimentale.* 1986; **75**: 161–6.

63. Seale P, Sabourin LA, Girgis-Gabardo A, Mansouri A, Gruss P, Rudnicki MA. Pax7 is required for the specification of myogenic satellite cells. *Cell.* 2000; **102**: 777–86.

* 64. Cossu G, De Angelis L, Borello U, Berarducci B, Buffa V, Sonnino C et al. Determination, diversification and multipotency of mammalian myogenic cells. *International Journal of Developmental Biology.* 2000; **44**: 699–706.

65. Ourednik V, Ourednik J, Flax JD, Zawada WM, Hutt C, Yang C et al. Segregation of human neural stem cells in the developing primate forebrain. *Science.* 2001; **293**: 1820–4.

* 66. Imitola J, Raddassi K, Park KI, Mueller FJ, Nieto M, Teng YD et al. Directed migration of neural stem cells to sites of CNS injury by the stromal cell-derived factor 1alpha/CXC chemokine receptor 4 pathway. *Proceedings of the National Academy of Sciences of the United States of America.* 2004; **101**: 18117–22.

67. Teng YD, Lavik EB, Qu X, Park KI, Ourednik J, Zurakowski D et al. Functional recovery following traumatic spinal cord

injury mediated by a unique polymer scaffold seeded with neural stem cells. *Proceedings of the National Academy of Sciences of the United States of America.* 2002; **99**: 3024–9.

68. Pluchino S, Quattrini A, Brambilla E, Gritti A, Salani G, Dina G *et al.* Injection of adult neurospheres induces recovery in a chronic model of multiple sclerosis. *Nature.* 2003; **422**: 688–94.

69. Ourednik J, Ourednik V, Lynch WP, Schachner M, Snyder EY. Neural stem cells display an inherent mechanism for rescuing dysfunctional neurons. *Nature Biotechnology.* 2002; **20**: 1103–10.

70. Kim DH, Yoo KH, Choi KS, Choi J, Choi SY, Yang SE *et al.* Gene expression profile of cytokine and growth factor during differentiation of bone marrow-derived mesenchymal stem cell. *Cytokine.* 2005; **31**: 119–26.

∗ 71. Brockes JP, Kumar A, Velloso CP. Regeneration as an evolutionary variable. *Journal of Anatomy.* 2001; **199**: 3–11.

72. Singer M, Weckesser EC, Geraudie J, Maier CE, Singer J. Open finger tip healing and replacement after distal amputation in rhesus monkey with comparison to limb regeneration in lower vertebrates. *Anatomy and Embryology.* 1987; **177**: 29–36.

73. Del Rio-Tsonis K, Washabaugh CH, Tsonis PA. Expression of pax-6 during urodele eye development and lens regeneration. *Proceedings of the National Academy of Sciences of the United States of America.* 1995; **92**: 5092–6.

74. Carlson MR, Komine Y, Bryant SV, Gardiner DM. Expression of Hoxb13 and Hoxc10 in developing and regenerating Axolotl limbs and tails. *Developmental Biology.* 2001; **229**: 396–406.

75. Torok MA, Gardiner DM, Shubin NH, Bryant SV. Expression of HoxD genes in developing and regenerating axolotl limbs. *Developmental Biology.* 1998; **200**: 225–33.

76. Yokoyama H, Ide H, Tamura K. FGF-10 stimulates limb regeneration ability in Xenopus laevis. *Developmental Biology.* 2001; **233**: 72–9.

77. Christensen RN, Weinstein M, Tassava RA. Expression of fibroblast growth factors 4, 8, and 10 in limbs, flanks, and blastemas of Ambystoma. *Developmental Dynamics.* 2002; **223**: 193–203.

78. Matsuda H, Yokoyama H, Endo T, Tamura K, Ide H. An epidermal signal regulates Lmx-1 expression and dorsal-ventral pattern during Xenopus limb regeneration. *Developmental Biology.* 2001; **229**: 351–62.

∗ 79. Morais da Silva S, Gates PB, Eib DW, Martens GJ, Brockes JP. The expression pattern of tomoregulin-1 in urodele limb regeneration and mouse limb development. *Mechanisms of Development.* 2001; **104**: 125–8.

80. Odelberg SJ, Kollhoff A, Keating MT. Dedifferentiation of mammalian myotubes induced by msx1. *Cell.* 2000; **103**: 1099–109.

∗ 81. Harada H, Imamura H, Miyagawa S, Kawasaki S. Fate of the human liver after hemihepatic portal vein embolization: cell kinetic and morphometric study. *Hepatology.* 1997; **26**: 1162–70.

82. Chiu JH, Wu LH, Kao HL, Chang HM, Tsay SH, Loong CC *et al.* Can determination of the proliferative capacity of the nontumor portion predict the risk of tumor recurrence in the liver remnant after resection of human hepatocellular carcinoma? *Hepatology.* 1993; **18**: 96–102.

83. Orlic D, Kajstura J, Chimenti S, Limana F, Jakoniuk I, Quaini F *et al.* Mobilized bone marrow cells repair the infarcted heart, improving function and survival. *Proceedings of the National Academy of Sciences of the United States of America.* 2001; **98**: 10344–49.

∗ 84. Ferrari G, Cusella-De Angelis G, Coletta M, Paolucci E, Stornaiuolo A, Cossu G *et al.* Muscle regeneration by bone marrow-derived myogenic progenitors. *Science.* 1998; **279**: 1528–30.

85. Majka SM, Jackson KA, Kienstra KA, Majesky MW, Goodell MA, Hirschi KK. Distinct progenitor populations in skeletal muscle are bone marrow derived and exhibit different cell fates during vascular regeneration. *Journal of Clinical Investigation.* 2003; **111**: 71–9.

86. Hess DC, Hill WD, Martin-Studdard A, Carroll J, Brailer J, Carothers J. Bone marrow as a source of endothelial cells and NeuN-expressing cells After stroke. *Stroke.* 2002; **33**: 1362–8.

87. Reyes M, Dudek A, Jahagirdar B, Koodie L, Marker PH, Verfaillie CM. Origin of endothelial progenitors in human postnatal bone marrow. *Journal of Clinical Investigation.* 2002; **109**: 337–46.

88. Alison MR, Poulsom R, Jeffery R, Dhillon AP, Quaglia A, Jacob J *et al.* Hepatocytes from non-hepatic adult stem cells. *Nature.* 2000; **406**: 257.

89. Theise ND, Nimmakayalu M, Gardner R, Illei PB, Morgan G, Teperman L *et al.* Liver from bone marrow in humans. *Hepatology.* 2000; **32**: 11–6.

90. Korbling M, Katz RL, Khanna A, Ruifrok AC, Rondon G, Albitar M *et al.* Hepatocytes and epithelial cells of donor origin in recipients of peripheral-blood stem cells. *New England Journal of Medicine.* 2002; **346**: 738–46.

91. Fricker RA, Carpenter MK, Winkler C, Greco C, Gates MA, Bjorklund A. Site-specific migration and neuronal differentiation of human neural progenitor cells after transplantation in the adult rat brain. *Journal of Neuroscience.* 1999; **19**: 5990–6005.

92. Tallheden T, Dennis JE, Lennon DP, Sjogren-Jansson E, Caplan AI, Lindahl A. Phenotypic plasticity of human articular chondrocytes. *Journal of Bone and Joint Surgery American volume.* 2003; **85-A**: 93–100.

93. Barry FP. Mesenchymal stem cell therapy in joint disease. *Novartis Foundation Symposium.* 2003; **249**: 86–96; discussion -102, 70-4, 239-41.

94. Kopke RD, Jackson RL, Li G, Rasmussen MD, Hoffer ME, Frenz DA *et al.* Growth factor treatment enhances vestibular hair cell renewal and results in improved vestibular function. *Proceedings of the National Academy of Sciences of the United States of America.* 2001; **98**: 5886–91.

95. Young CS, Terada S, Vacanti JP, Honda M, Bartlett JD, Yelick PC. Tissue engineering of complex tooth structures

on biodegradable polymer scaffolds. *Journal of Dental Research.* 2002; **81**: 695–700.

96. Grande DA, Mason J, Light E, Dines D. Stem cells as platforms for delivery of genes to enhance cartilage repair. *Journal of Bone and Joint Surgery American volume.* 2003; **85-A**: 111–6.

97. Martin GR. Isolation of a pluripotent cell line from early mouse embryos cultured in medium conditioned by teratocarcinoma stem cells. *Proceedings of the National Academy of Sciences of the United States of America.* 1981; **78**: 7634–8.

* 98. Wiles MV, Johansson BM. Embryonic stem cell development in a chemically defined medium. *Experimental Cell Research.* 1999; **247**: 241–8.

99. Wiles MV, Keller G. Multiple hematopoietic lineages develop from embryonic stem (ES) cells in culture. *Development.* 1991; **111**: 259–67.

100. Ying QL, Stavridis M, Griffiths D, Li M, Smith A. Conversion of embryonic stem cells into neuroectodermal precursors in adherent monoculture. *Nature Biotechnology.* 2003; **21**: 183–6.

101. Dani C, Smith AG, Dessolin S, Leroy P, Staccini L, Villageois P *et al.* Differentiation of embryonic stem cells into adipocytes *in vitro. Journal of Cell Science.* 1997; **110**: 1279–85.

102. Rohwedel J, Maltsev V, Bober E, Arnold HH, Hescheler J, Wobus AM. Muscle cell differentiation of embryonic stem cells reflects myogenesis *in vivo*: developmentally regulated expression of myogenic determination genes and functional expression of ionic currents. *Developmental Biology.* 1994; **164**: 87–101.

*103. Klug MG, Soonpaa MH, Koh GY, Field LJ. Genetically selected cardiomyocytes from differentiating embronic stem cells form stable intracardiac grafts. *Journal of Clinical Investigation.* 1996; **98**: 216–24.

104. Hegert C, Kramer J, Hargus G, Muller J, Guan K, Wobus AM *et al.* Differentiation plasticity of chondrocytes derived from mouse embryonic stem cells. *Journal of Cell Science.* 2002; **115**: 4617–28.

105. Buttery LD, Bourne S, Xynos JD, Wood H, Hughes FJ, Hughes SP *et al.* Differentiation of osteoblasts and *in vitro* bone formation from murine embryonic stem cells. *Tissue Eng.* 2001; **7**: 89–99.

106. Shamblott MJ, Axelman J, Littlefield JW, Blumenthal PD, Huggins GR, Cui Y *et al.* Human embryonic germ cell derivatives express a broad range of developmentally distinct markers and proliferate extensively *in vitro. Proceedings of the National Academy of Sciences of the United States of America.* 2001; **98**: 113–8.

107. Andrews PW. From teratocarcinomas to embryonic stem cells. *Philosophical Transactions of the Royal Society of London. Series B, Biological Sciences.* 2002; **357**: 405–17.

108. Romanov YA, Svintsitskaya VA, Smirnov VN. Searching for alternative sources of postnatal human mesenchymal stem cells: candidate MSC-like cells from umbilical cord. *Stem Cells.* 2003; **21**: 105–10.

109. Odorico JS, Kaufman DS, Thomson JA. Multilineage differentiation from human embryonic stem cell lines. *Stem Cells.* 2001; **19**: 193–204.

110. Li M, Pevny L, Lovell-Badge R, Smith A. Generation of purified neural precursors from embryonic stem cells by lineage selection. *Current Biology.* 1998; **8**: 971–4.

111. Kikyo N, Wolffe AP. Reprogramming nuclei: insights from cloning, nuclear transfer and heterokaryons. *Journal of Cell Science.* 2000; **113**: 11–20.

112. Lanza RP, Cibelli JB, West MD. Prospects for the use of nuclear transfer in human transplantation. *Nature Biotechnology.* 1999; **17**: 1171–4.

113. Au E, Roskams AJ. Olfactory ensheathing cells of the lamina propria *in vivo* and *in vitro. Glia.* 2003; **41**: 224–36.

114. DeLucia TA, Conners JJ, Brown TJ, Cronin CM, Khan T, Jones KJ. Use of a cell line to investigate olfactory ensheathing cell-enhanced axonal regeneration. *Anatomical Record.* 2003; **271B**: 61–70.

115. Li Y, Decherchi P, Raisman G. Transplantation of olfactory ensheathing cells into spinal cord lesions restores breathing and climbing. *Journal of Neuroscience.* 2003; **23**: 727–31.

116. Peng H, Wright V, Usas A, Gearhart B, Shen HC, Cummins J *et al.* Synergistic enhancement of bone formation and healing by stem cell-expressed VEGF and bone morphogenetic protein-4. *Journal of Clinical Investigation.* 2002; **110**: 751–9.

117. Murray RC, Navi D, Fesenko J, Lander AD, Calof AL. Widespread defects in the primary olfactory pathway caused by loss of Mash1 function. *Journal of Neuroscience.* 2003; **23**: 1769–80.

118. Jang W, Youngentob SL, Schwob JE. Globose basal cells are required for reconstitution of olfactory epithelium after methyl bromide lesion. *Journal of Comparative Neurology.* 2003; **460**: 123–40.

119. Wu HH, Ivkovic S, Murray RC, Jaramillo S, Lyons KM, Johnson JE *et al.* Autoregulation of neurogenesis by GDF11. *Neuron.* 2003; **37**: 197–207.

120. Calof AL, Bonnin A, Crocker C, Kawauchi S, Murray RC, Shou J *et al.* Progenitor cells of the olfactory receptor neuron lineage. *Microscopy Research and Technique.* 2002; **58**: 176–88.

121. Lipson AC, Widenfalk J, Lindqvist E, Ebendal T, Olson L. Neurotrophic properties of olfactory ensheathing glia. *Experimental Neurology.* 2003; **180**: 167–71.

122. Doetsch F, Caille I, Lim DA, Garcia-Verdugo JM, Alvarez-Buylla A. Subventricular zone astrocytes are neural stem cells in the adult mammalian brain. *Cell.* 1999; **97**: 703–16.

123. Lois C, Alvarez-Buylla A. Long-distance neuronal migration in the adult mammalian brain. *Science.* 1994; **264**: 1145–8.

124. Lindahl A, Brittberg M, Peterson L. Cartilage repair with chondrocytes: clinical and cellular aspects. *Novartis Foundation Symposium.* 2003; **249**: 175–86; discussion 86-9, 234-8, 9-41.

125. Peterson L, Minas T, Brittberg M, Lindahl A. Treatment of osteochondritis dissecans of the knee with autologous chondrocyte transplantation: results at two to ten years.

Journal of Bone and Joint Surgery American volume. 2003; **85-A**: 17–24.

126. Ochi M, Uchio Y, Kawasaki K, Wakitani S, Iwasa J. Transplantation of cartilage-like tissue made by tissue engineering in the treatment of cartilage defects of the knee. *Journal of Bone and Joint Surgery. British volume.* 2002; **84**: 571–8.

127. Kuriwaka M, Ochi M, Uchio Y, Maniwa S, Adachi N, Mori R *et al.* Optimum combination of monolayer and three-dimensional cultures for cartilage-like tissue engineering. *Tissue Engineering.* 2003; **9**: 41–9.

128. Lavezzi A, Mantovani M, della Berta LG, Matturri L. Cell kinetics of human nasal septal chondrocytes in vitro: importance for cartilage grafting in otolaryngology. *Journal of Otolaryngology.* 2002; **31**: 366–70.

129. Zhang Y, Wang S, Song Y, Han J, Chai Y, Chen Y. Timing of odontogenic neural crest cell migration and tooth-forming capability in mice. *Developmental Dynamics.* 2003; **226**: 713–8.

130. Gronthos S, Brahim J, Li W, Fisher LW, Cherman N, Boyde A *et al.* Stem cell properties of human dental pulp stem cells. *Journal of Dental Research.* 2002; **81**: 531–5.

131. Chai Y, Bringas Jr. P, Shuler C, Devaney E, Grosschedl R, Slavkin HC. A mouse mandibular culture model permits the study of neural crest cell migration and tooth development. *International Journal of Developmental Biology.* 1998; **42**: 87–94.

*132. Koyama E, Wu C, Shimo T, Pacifici M. Chick limbs with mouse teeth: An effective in vivo culture system for tooth germ development and analysis. *Developmental Dynamics.* 2003; **226**: 149–54.

133. el-Ghalbzouri A, Gibbs S, Lamme E, Van Blitterswijk CA, Ponec M. Effect of fibroblasts on epidermal regeneration. *British Journal of Dermatology.* 2002; **147**: 230–43.

134. Gharzi A, Reynolds AJ, Jahoda CA. Plasticity of hair follicle dermal cells in wound healing and induction. *Experimental Dermatology.* 2003; **12**: 126–36.

135. Cruz RM, Lambert PR, Rubel EW. Light microscopic evidence of hair cell regeneration after gentamicin toxicity in chick cochlea. *Archives of Otolaryngology – Head and Neck Surgery.* 1987; **113**: 1058–62.

*136. Bermingham-McDonogh O, Rubel EW. Hair cell regeneration: winging our way towards a sound future. *Current Opinion in Neurobiology.* 2003; **13**: 119–26.

137. Mendez I, Dagher A, Hong M, Gaudet P, Weerasinghe S, McAlister V *et al.* Simultaneous intrastriatal and intranigral fetal dopaminergic grafts in patients with Parkinson disease: a pilot study. Report of three cases. *Journal of Neurosurgery.* 2002; **96**: 589–96.

138. Edamura K, Itakura S, Nasu K, Iwami Y, Ogawa H, Sasaki N *et al.* Xenotransplantation of porcine pancreatic endocrine cells to total pancreatectomized dogs. *Journal of Veterinary Medical Science.* 2003; **65**: 549–56.

139. Ikehara S. New Strategies for BMT, Organ transplantation, and regeneration therapy. *Hematology.* 2003; **8**: 77–81.

140. Ayas M, al-Jefri A, Baothman A, al-Mahr M, Mustafa MM, Khalil S *et al.* Transfusion-dependent congenital dyserythropoietic anemia type I successfully treated with allogeneic stem cell transplantation. *Bone Marrow Transplantation.* 2002; **29**: 681–2.

PART 2

WOUND HEALING

EDITED BY NICHOLAS S JONES

8 Soft and hard tissue repair   87
Stephen R Young and Melissa Calvin

9 Skin flap physiology   110
A Graeme B Perks

10 Biomaterials, tissue engineering and their applications   118
Colin A Scotchford, Matthew Evans and Archana Vats

Soft and hard tissue repair

STEPHEN R YOUNG AND MELISSA CALVIN

Introduction	87	Key points	103
Healing by first intention	88	Best clinical practice	104
Healing by second intention	88	Deficiencies in current knowledge and areas for future	
How do we now link this basic knowledge to practice?	94	research	104
Summary	102	References	105

SEARCH STRATEGY AND EVIDENCE-BASE

The data in this chapter are supported by a Medline search using the key words wound healing, tissue repair, wound assessment, chronic wounds and wound dressings. The data are based on levels of evidence 1 and 2 and clinical recommendations are grades B and C.

INTRODUCTION

The term 'wound' can be defined as a bodily injury, in which there is disruption of the normal continuity of structures resulting from physical, chemical or thermal damage, or developing as a result of the presence of an underlying physiological disorder. It is an event associated with a loss of substance, and a corresponding impairment of function.[1] Wound healing is the restoration of tissue continuity after injury[2] and it involves wound closure and restoration of function to the damaged tissue.

Injured tissue heals by either partial or complete regeneration, or by repair. Regeneration implies a complete re-establishment of the original tissue structure. In humans, tissues which have the power to regenerate, include epithelium (including the epidermis, alimentary tract epithelium and tracheobronchial epithelium), liver parenchyma, bone, smooth muscle and some skeletal muscle. Tissues and organs, such as the dermis, which are incapable of responding to injury by regeneration, undergo a process of repair in which the original tissue is replaced with nonspecific connective tissue, which forms a functionally inferior scar. The scar tissue performs few of the specialized functions of the original tissue, but serves to hold together the remaining tissue. However, even in this capacity, scar tissue is less effective than the tissue it replaces, having a reduced tensile strength and energy absorbing capacity, which may be associated with the arrangement of its collagen fibres.[3]

An injury to the skin results in the epidermis being regenerated and the dermis being repaired by replacement with scar tissue. Skin is therefore an interesting structure in which to observe wound healing, because both these processes of regeneration and repair occur upon injury, it is a frequent site of injury, and access to the skin for experimental purposes is relatively easy.

It was a Greek physician, Galen (129–199BC), who identified two forms of wound healing – primary and secondary intention – depending on the physician's aim in treating the wound. The primary intention of the physician was seen as approximating the wound edges so that minimal scar formation would result. With gaping wound edges, loss of tissue had to be compensated by the formation of new connective tissue and wound contraction, often resulting in cosmetically and functionally inferior scar formation.

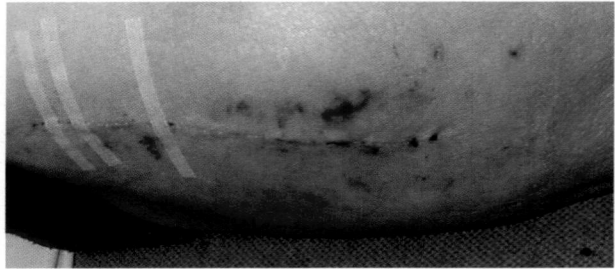

Figure 8.1 A typical surgical incision. Image supplied by the Tissue Viability Unit (TVU), Guy's Nuffield House.

Galen's notions are still valid in modern medicine and healing is still divided into two types – healing by first and second intention.

HEALING BY FIRST INTENTION

Healing by first intention is seen in clean, well-perfused, incised surgical wounds (**Figure 8.1**) and casual wounds inflicted by sharp-edged objects, where there is minimum destruction of tissue, the edges being closely apposed shortly after injury, where healing occurs without complication.

Epithelial proliferation occurs rapidly (within 24 hours) sealing the wound at the level of the basal cells of the epidermis. Apposition of the wound edges decreases the distance that the cells need to migrate. There is also minimal granulation tissue formation, so that the end result is an intact epithelium (regeneration), and a small fibrous scar (repair) – the most satisfactory result following injury.[2, 4]

HEALING BY SECOND INTENTION

Healing by second intention is seen when the wound is large (**Figure 8.2**), where there has been significant loss or destruction of tissue such that the edges cannot be apposed, or when complications such as infection occur.

Thus, secondary healing is indicated in the case of gaping wounds with lacerated edges, large defects that cannot be covered by grafting, extensive trophic disturbances such as leg ulcers, highly suppurative wounds, wounds interspersed with foreign bodies, infected wounds that have undergone primary closure and wounds that heal better cosmetically and functionally as a result of contraction rather than sutures, e.g. fingertip injuries.

In these situations, sealing of the epithelium across the wound does not occur rapidly, since the cells have to grow down and spread progressively across the wound at the junction of viable and nonviable tissue. There is also more granulation tissue formation growing from the base of the wound to fill the defect, accompanied by wound contraction, so that the end result is an intact epithelium

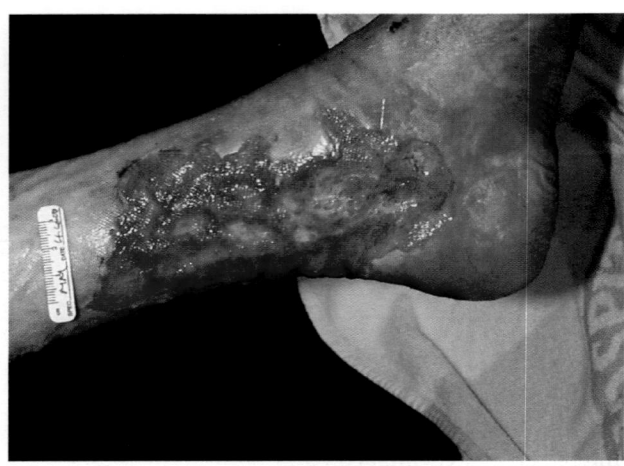

Figure 8.2 A typical venous leg ulcer. Image provided by TVU.

(regeneration), but more tissue distortion and an extensive, cosmetically unsatisfactory scar, which often causes an impairment of function (repair).[2, 4]

In mammalian skin, this type of tissue injury initiates a complex, but orderly, series of biochemical and cellular events which, influenced by a large number of chemical mediators, leads to haemostasis, wound healing and the eventual generation of the scar tissue. The repair process can be arbitrarily divided into three main overlapping and inter-relating phases,[5] namely:

1. inflammation;
2. new tissue formation (proliferation);
3. matrix formation and remodelling.

It should be emphasized that there is no clear demarcation between the phases of wound healing; the process of tissue repair being a continuous phenomenon.

Inflammation

Inflammation can be defined as a localized protective tissue response elicited by injury or destruction of tissues, which serves to destroy, dilute or wall off both the injurious agent and the injured tissues. The acute inflammatory response, which usually extends from the onset of injury to approximately the fourth day of healing, generates an environment conducive to the generation of granulation tissue, and is similar whether the causative agent is a microbial infection (e.g. pyogenic bacteria, viruses), hypersensitivity reaction (e.g. due to parasites, tubercle bacilli), physical agent (e.g. trauma, ionizing irradiation, heat, cold), chemical (e.g. corrosives, acids, alkalis, reducing agents, bacterial toxins) or tissue necrosis (e.g. ischaemic infarction).[2] It must be remembered that some of the above may be iatrogenic in origin.

Tissue injury causes both cell death and vessel disruption. The most obvious results of the inflammatory phase are ridding the injured area of debris and necrotic tissue, and the local reduction of infection. This process of inflammation is an essential part of the reparative process and can be temporally divided into early and late phases.[5]

EARLY INFLAMMATION

This is characterized by clot formation, both within damaged vessels resulting in cessation of haemorrhage and within the wound void, providing a provisional matrix of fibrin, fibronectin, von Willebrand factor (vWF) and thrombospondin,[6, 7, 8] which facilitates the early migration of cells into the wound environment,[9] stimulates fibroblast proliferation (via thrombin), and shields mitogenic and chemotactic factors from inhibitors.[10]

During this process of clotting, haemostasis is enhanced by a five to ten-minute period of vasoconstriction, thought to be initiated by platelet-induced mediators which modulate vascular tone and permeability.[11] Additional activities of platelets are mediated by the release of an array of biologically active substances that stimulate the synthesis of extracellular matrix components (ECM) and consequently initiate the subsequent phases of repair, and also promote cell migration and ingrowth to the site of injury.[12] These substances include platelet-derived growth factor (PDGF),[13, 14] platelet factor 4 (PF4),[15] transforming growth factor alpha (TGFα)[16] and transforming growth factor beta (TGFβ).[17]

In addition to its role in haemostasis, blood clotting is a crucial part of inflammation, because activation of Hageman factor leads to the generation of bradykinin,[18] and to the initiation of the classical and alternative complement cascades,[19] generating the complement-derived anaphylatoxins C3a and C5a.[20] Bradykinin and the anaphylatoxins increase the permeability of the uninjured local blood vessels,[21] resulting in the release of plasma proteins and the generation of an extravascular clot. The mechanism by which bradykinin increases vessel permeability is thought to involve an induction of prostaglandin production.[22]

The anaphylatoxins also stimulate the release of the vasoactive mediators histamine and leukotrienes (LT) C4 and D4 from mast cells,[23] the release of lysosomal granules and oxygen products from neutrophils[24] and macrophages, and are also thought to attract neutrophils and monocytes to the wound;[25] the latter develop into macrophages, which characterize the late inflammatory phase.

Neutrophils (polymorphonuclear leukocytes) and monocytes are both attracted to the wound site at the same time,[26] but neutrophils arrive initially in greater numbers, partly due to their greater abundance in the blood, and thus the early phase of inflammation is classified as being neutrophil-rich. They are attracted by a variety of general leukocyte chemotactic factors,[5] including fibrinopeptides,[27] fibrin lysis products,[28, 29] C5a,[25] LT B4,[30] formyl methionyl peptides,[31] platelet-activating

factor (PAF),[32] tumour necrosis factor alpha (TNFα),[33] PF4[15] and PDGF.[34] Members of the α-chemokine family of low molecular weight chemotactic factors are generally specific for neutrophils[35] and are exemplified by IL-8, growth-related protein and melanoma growth stimulating activity (MGSA).[36] In contrast, the monocyte influx is further stimulated by representatives of the β-chemokine family,[35] including factors such as monocyte chemoattractant protein-1 (MCP 1)[37] and macrophage inflammatory protein-1α (MIP-1α).[38] Other monocyte chemotactic factors implicated as attractants of this cell type *in vivo* are platelet-derived endothelial cell growth factor (PD-ECGF),[39] thrombin,[40] TGFβ[34] and fragments of collagen,[41] elastin,[42, 43] and fibronectin.[44]

The main function of the neutrophils which infiltrate the wound bed is the phagocytosis of pathogenic bacteria and debris.[45] The inflammatory environment stimulates the release of toxic reactive oxygen intermediates from the neutrophil granules, destroying the contaminating bacteria,[46] but also having the capacity to cause significant damage to the surrounding tissues.[47] However, the presence of neutrophils in the wound environment is not critical as neutropenia does not adversely interfere with wound healing.[48]

Neutrophil infiltration ceases within a few days of injury in the absence of bacterial infection, but is lengthened in contaminated wounds.[49] Once bacterial contamination has been controlled, effete neutrophils are entrapped within the clot or phagocytosed by tissue macrophages or fibroblasts[50] and neutrophil infiltration ceases, indicating the end of the early inflammatory phase of repair.

LATE INFLAMMATION

The transition from the early to the late inflammatory phase is made as the neutrophil infiltrate resolves and the accumulation of macrophages continues. Monocytes rapidly differentiate into macrophages after migrating from the vasculature into the wound site. The factors responsible for this differentiation have not been fully identified, but may include the presence of insoluble fibronectin,[51] low oxygen tension,[52] chemotactic agents[53] and the presence of bacterial lipopolysaccharides and interferons.[35] Wound macrophages eliminate deleterious materials, e.g. microorganisms and wound debris, by phagocytosis,[54] generate chemotactic factors, which are responsible for the recruitment of additional inflammatory cells, and release collagenases which are degrading enzymes that lyse necrotic material.[55, 56] Wound macrophages are also thought to synthesize and release growth and regulatory factors, critical to the coordination of granulation tissue formation[57, 58] including PDGF,[59] TGFβ,[60] TGFα,[61] fibroblast growth factor (FGF)[62] and interleukin (IL)-1.[63] Leibovich and Ross[64] researched the role of macrophages in the repair of guinea-pig wounds, and found that macrophage deletion caused severe lack of wound debridement and a delay in fibroblast recruitment and proliferation, and in matrix biosynthesis. This suggests that the growth factors and chemotactic factors released by the macrophage are important in the initiation and propagation of granulation tissue and that the macrophage plays a vital role in the transition from the inflammatory phase to the proliferative phase of wound repair.[35, 65]

New tissue formation (proliferation)

Overlapping with and also following the inflammatory response approximately five days post-injury,[66] there is a proliferation at, and migration into, the wound site of those cells that are responsible for the remainder of the repair process, for the ensuing 10–14 days.[67] This dense population of macrophages, fibroblasts and endothelial cells, etc., embedded in a loose matrix of collagen types I and III, fibrin, fibronectin and proteoglycans rich in hyaluronic acid, is referred to as granulation tissue. The term 'granulation tissue' is derived from the granular surface appearance of the loops of newly formed capillaries in the tissue, before their coverage by epidermal cells (**Figure 8.3**).

The macrophages, fibroblasts and endothelial cells migrate into the wound bed (**Figure 8.4**) as a mutually dependent unit, known as the 'wound module'.[68]

The macrophage as described above, releases chemotactic and growth factors, which attract fibroblasts and endothelial cells into the wound. The fibroblasts respond to these stimuli by constructing a new ECM, through which the macrophages,[69] blood vessels[70] and fibroblasts themselves[71] can migrate. The endothelial cells respond by bud formation, creating the neovasculature which supplies nutrients and oxygen to the wound, enabling the metabolic demands of macrophage and fibroblast ingrowth to be satisfied.

During cutaneous wound repair, the proliferative phase is manifest by re-epithelialization and granulation tissue formation.

RE–EPITHELIALIZATION

Re-epithelialization is the reconstitution of the cells of the epidermis into an organized, keratinized, stratified squamous epithelium, which covers the wound defect and restores the barrier properties of skin, decreasing morbidity and mortality after cutaneous injury.[5]

The process occurs rapidly, beginning within hours of the initial insult to the tissue, and continuing throughout the proliferative phase of repair,[72] with the migration of intact keratinocytes from the free edge of the cut epidermis (**Figure 8.5**) across the defect.[73] The rate of migration is dependent on the tissue oxygen tension, being highest in hyperbaric conditions, where the rate of cell movement is approximately 12–21 μm per hour[67] and

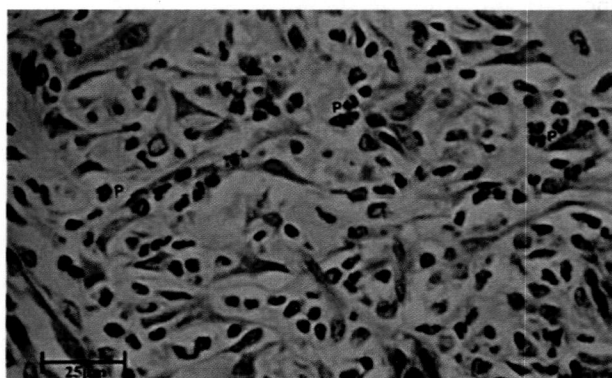

Figure 8.4 Histology section showing a typical diverse cell population during the proliferative phase of repair. Image supplied by M. Calvin.

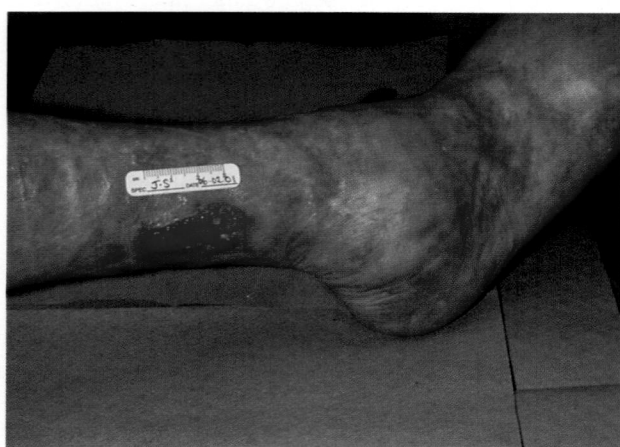

Figure 8.3 A granulating venous leg ulcer. Image provided by TVU.

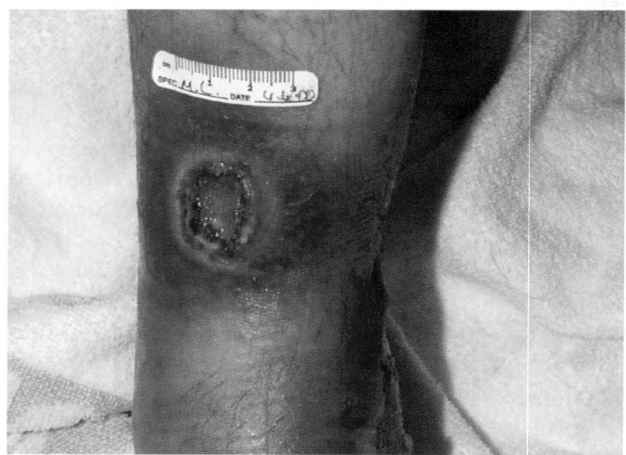

Figure 8.5 Leg ulcer showing migrating epithelium from the wound edges. Image supplied by TVU.

on the humidity of the environment, migration occurring at a faster rate in moist conditions.[74]

In partial thickness wounds, hair follicles and the ducts of sweat glands act as a source of epidermal skin cells, whereas in full thickness wounds the only source is the wound margin.

If, during migration, keratinocytes come across small foreign particles, these are removed by phagocytosis.[75] If larger particles are encountered, the keratinocytes will migrate deep to the particles, dissecting viable tissue from desiccated nonviable tissue that is later sloughed off.[44] This process is thought to involve the secretion of collagenase and plasminogen activator by the migrating cells.[76] The stimuli for the initiation of epidermal migration are not clear, but they may involve contact guidance by matrix components of the clot.

Once the process of re-epithelialization is complete and the migrating edges have united, migration ceases, the rate of epithelial proliferation falls to approximately three to four times the normal rate; the epidermal cells rapidly reassume their original morphology and function and re-establish their desmosomal, and hemidesmosomal attachments.

GRANULATION TISSUE FORMATION

The process of granulation tissue formation consists of fibroplasia and angiogenesis.

Fibroplasia

Fibroplasia may be defined as the process of fibroblast recruitment into the wound site and the ensuing synthesis and secretion of the collagenous and noncollagenous matrix. The colonization of the wound site by fibroblasts, essential for the production and organization of the major extracellular components of the granulation tissue,[77] is thought to involve both fibroblast migration and proliferation. For optimal fibroblastic activity, a mildly acidic medium is necessary, provided by accumulation of lactate from anaerobic metabolism in the wound.[67]

After injury, the fibroblasts undergo an alteration of cell phenotype when they migrate into the wound bed, including sequestration of the endoplasmic reticula and Golgi apparatus at perinuclear locations, and the formation of large actin bundles orientated longitudinally in the peripheral cell cytoplasm.[78] These phenotypically altered fibroblasts have acquired the capacity for contraction and increased motility and are termed myofibroblasts.[79, 80] It is thought these myofibroblasts originate from resting fibrocytes and fibroblasts situated in the wound margins[81] and that the factors which induce this phenotypic alteration, although unknown, probably include the same growth factors[58, 82] and chemoattractants which stimulate fibroblast migration.[83]

Once in the wound, fibroblasts undergo proliferation, thought to be influenced by a plethora of growth factors produced in part by activated macrophages,[61] as well as the hypoxic conditions found in the centre of wounds.[74]

In the wound area, the fibroblasts and myofibroblasts secrete a loose ECM, which initially contains large quantities of the glycoprotein fibronectin.[84] The fibronectin produced affects fibroblast function in wound healing in several ways, including aiding the adhesion of fibroblasts to the ECM, the stimulation of migration of fibroblasts, the provision of a support mechanism for the deposition and orientation of collagen fibrils and the mediation of wound contraction.[7] Hyaluronic acid and collagen type III are also secreted, the peak rate of synthesis occurring five to seven days after injury.[68] Once a collagen-rich matrix is deposited in the wound, the fibroblasts are downregulated and cease collagen production, possibly under the influence of interferon gamma (IFNγ)[85] and the secreted collagen matrix itself.[86]

Wound contraction

Wound contraction is the reduction of part or all of a skin defect, by centripetal movement of the surrounding undamaged skin.[87] It begins approximately seven days after injury, peaking at two weeks post-insult and reduces the need for scar tissue, by reducing the size of the wound. It progresses at a rate of 0.6–0.7 mm per day, independent of the size of the wound.[67]

Wound contraction is a major form of wound closure in mobile-skinned animals such as rats, where the *panniculus carnosus* enables the skin to move easily over the underlying fascia, and therefore contraction rarely leads to loss of function of the involved tissue. In humans, however, where the skin is less mobile due to its attachment to underlying structures, contraction alone rarely closes a wound, the degree of contraction varying with the depth of the wound.[74]

For optimal healing, the degree of contraction needs to be maintained in equilibrium; a diminished level of contraction leads to delayed wound closure, resulting in excess bleeding and possible infection, whereas excessive contraction may lead to tissue contracture, possibly causing deformity and dysfunction (**Figure 8.6**).

There are currently two main theories postulated to explain how fibroblasts may generate and transmit the force necessary to facilitate wound contraction:

1. cell contraction – myofibroblast theory;[88]
2. cell traction – fibroblast theory.[89]

Myofibroblast theory

This theory suggests that myofibroblast cells which have morphological characteristics of both fibroblasts and smooth muscle cells and are aligned within the wound along the lines of contraction[5] are responsible for the process of wound contraction. The myofibroblast displays many cell-to-cell and cell-to-matrix contacts and these contacts provide a means by which cellular contraction

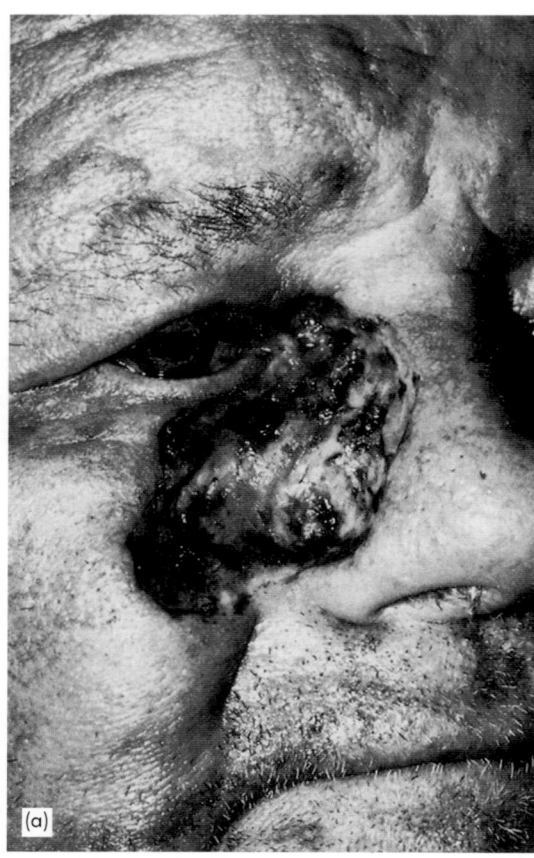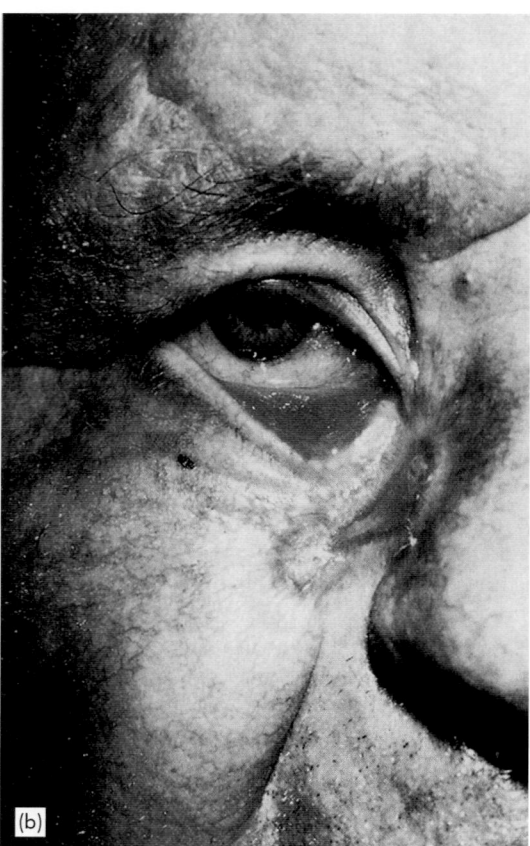

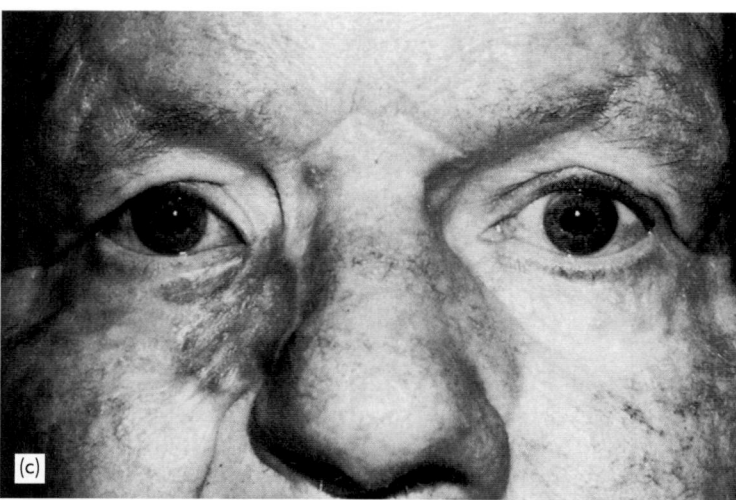

Figure 8.6 (a) Patient has had a skin cancer (basal cell cacinoma) removed from the side of his nose and cheek. The wound was allowed to heal by secondary intention. (b) Appearance of wound four weeks later. Note how the natural forces of wound contraction have produced a severe distortion of the eyelid (ectropion). (c) To repair the ectropion, scar was removed and a full thickness skin graft was applied to the area. Appearance one month following skin grafting. Courtesy of William Panje.

pulls collagen fibrils towards the body of the myofibroblast,[90] causing a reduction in granulation tissue area.

Fibroblast theory

This theory suggests that fibroblasts act as the agents of wound closure by exerting 'tread-like traction forces' on the ECM fibres to which they are attached; the process being analogous to the traction forces exerted by wheels on a surface.[91] This theory proposes that fibroblasts neither shorten in length, nor act in a coordinated multicellular manner, but rather that the traction forces of many individual fibroblasts are responsible for wound contraction.[92]

Wound contraction may be brought about by a combination of both these theories. It is possible that the wound matrix is initially remodelled by the process of fibroblast traction, which is subsequently superseded by the contractile activity of myofibroblastic cells, as traction is known to proceed initially without myofibroblast cells.[93]

Angiogenesis

Angiogenesis (the process of new blood vessel formation) occurs simultaneously with fibroplasia, commencing two to three days after injury,[94] and is a process involving phenotypic alteration, migration, proliferation and synthesis of ECM,[70] whereby capillaries bud from pre-existing functioning small venules in close proximity to the wound, and extend into the wound site.[95] Granulation tissue produced during the proliferative phase of repair, while only transient, is metabolically very active and consequently requires a profuse blood supply. Without such a supply, invasion of the wound bed by macrophages and fibroblasts would cease, partly through lack of oxygen and nutrients.

The process of angiogenesis during dermal repair is thought to result from the actions of various angiogenic stimuli, generated during injury or as a consequence of the initiation of the repair process.[5] Activated macrophages release potent angiogenic stimuli[58] including FGF, which is strongly mitogenic for endothelial cells and stimulates angiogenesis both *in vitro* and *in vivo*,[7] TNFα[96] and IL-8.[97] Endothelial cell proliferation is also stimulated by lactic acid,[98] biogenic amines[99] and low oxygen tension,[100] all of which are generated in the relatively hypoxic wound environment. Various platelet-derived substances, such as PD-ECGF, have been shown to promote endothelial cell migration and proliferation,[101] and TGFβ also influences the migration of endothelial cells.[57, 102] Other platelet-derived substances which indirectly affect angiogenesis by recruiting monocytes or other cells to produce angiogenic factors[103] include PAF,[32] PDGF[104] and PF4.[15] Heparin[105] and fibronectin[7] are also thought to be involved in the process of angiogenic stimulation.

The pericyte–endothelial cell interaction may also play an important role in the formation of new blood vessels, since pericytes have been shown to regulate endothelial proliferation and differentiation, function as progenitor cells and synthesize and release structural constituents of the basement membrane and extracellular matrix.[106]

Angiogenesis is a limited process, but the mechanisms regulating it are not clear. It is thought that the loss of angiogenic stimuli may result in its downregulation. Pericytes may reduce the angiogenic response by inhibiting the growth of adjacent endothelial cells.[106, 107] Other events that may act as a brake to the angiogenic process include the cessation of chemotactic and mitogenic factor generation as the inflammatory response wanes, the inactivation of FGF by heparin-like molecules and a return to the normal, nonmacrophage-activating oxygen tension, thus reducing the availability of angiogenic factors produced by macrophages.[100]

Matrix formation and remodelling

Remodelling of the immature tissue matrix commences simultaneously with granulation tissue formation, although for clarity it is normally regarded as forming the third and final phase of wound healing due to its continuation for many months or years after granulation tissue has been resolved.[44] During this phase, the highly cellular and highly vascular granulation tissue is gradually replaced and remodelled forming scar tissue, which is less cellular and less vascular than the granulation tissue. This decrease in cellularity may be due to the migration of the cells out of the wound site or by programmed cell death (apoptosis).

The scar tissue of the wound remains functionally inferior to the original tissue and serves as a diffusional barrier to nutrients and oxygen.[108] It also never regains its original tensile strength, only reaching 70–80 percent of that of normal skin.[109] Work carried out in rats by Pickett *et al.*[110] demonstrates that the tensile strength of wounds closed under tension exceeds that of tensionless wounds from seven days post-wounding.

The composition and structure of the granulation tissue ECM is constantly changing from the time of its first deposition.[111] The ECM is first deposited at the wound margins at the onset of granulation tissue development, but is later laid down more centrally as the granulation tissue fills the wound space. Therefore, the characteristics of the granulation tissue ECM at a given time within the wound, depend on both the time elapsed since tissue injury and the location within the wound, with regard to its distance from the wound margin.[84]

As the matrix matures, both hyaluronic acid and fibronectin, which play an important role in cellular ingrowth to the wound site, are reduced. There is an accumulation of type I collagen bundles and an alteration in their intermolecular cross-links,[112] which provide increasing tensile strength to the residual scar. Proteoglycans are also deposited and these increase the wound's resilience to deformation.

The increase in tensile strength is caused not only by the increase in collagen deposition, but also by the remodelling and realignment of the collagen into larger fibrillar bundles,[113] and an alteration of intermolecular cross-links.[112] During remodelling, the fibres become less randomly orientated. This may be due to the mechanical forces exerted on the scar during normal usage, improving its mechanical function so it resembles uninjured dermis more closely.[45]

The remodelling of collagen is dependent upon the interplay of continued collagen synthesis and collagen degradation.[44] The degradation is controlled by a variety of collagenase enzymes synthesized by granulocytes, macrophages, epidermal cells and fibroblasts.[114]

The process of collagen remodelling continues for many months or years in the healing wound,[5] but the tensile strength of the scar tissue, a functional assessment of collagen, can only reach 70–80 percent of its pre-injury strength.[74] The mechanical and cosmetic properties of the scar never reach those of the uninjured skin.

REPAIR OF BONE TISSUE

The repair process of bone tissue is essentially the same as that described for soft tissue, with an added osteogenic component. In summary, immediately after injury haemorrhage occurs. The clot is formed, and the acute inflammatory phase of repair begins. As with soft tissues, mast cells, neutrophils and macrophages move into the area releasing factors, which stimulate tissue repair. Wound debris is removed by the action of macrophages and osteoclasts and a gradual formation of granulation tissue occurs to replace the clot. This is completed within several days depending upon the nature and severity of the injury.

Osteoblasts, whether derived from osteocytes, fibroblasts or a number of other sources, are activated. This activation is due to the combined action of a number of factors, including mast-cell factors, anoxic conditions and bone-morphogenic substances. Chondroblasts may also become active under certain conditions, especially when oxygen levels are low. Small groups of cartilaginous cells appear within the new matrix, mainly in the region of the periosteum. Calcium is deposited by the osteoblasts both directly in the tissue matrix and in the islands of cartilage. The fracture site at this stage of repair is referred to as the soft callus, due to its flexible nature.

Following this stage, both subperiosteal and endochondral ossification continues. After approximately two months, the bone ends become united to form the hard callus. Remodelling continues in the callus to form mature lamellar bone, involving the action of both osteoblasts and osteoclasts. The remodelling restores the marrow cavity, and at the same time the contour of the bone becomes smooth. Much of this remodelling is determined by the normal external forces to which it is submitted.

Conclusion

Wound healing involves the integrated action of a number of cell types, the ECM and soluble mediators. Clinically, our aim is to restore the integrity and function of the tissue as rapidly as possible after injury. The three overlapping phases of wound healing have been detailed. The inflammatory phase is marked by platelet accumulation, coagulation and leukocyte migration into the wound bed. The proliferative phase is characterized by (1) re-epithelialization restoring the cutaneous barrier; (2) angiogenesis, the neovasculature supplying much of the nutrition required for healing during this phase; (3) fibroplasia, forming the collagenous and noncollagenous matrix for the dermal component of the wound; and (4) wound contraction, reducing wound size and thus the need for scar tissue. Finally, the remodelling phase takes place over a period of months, during which the dermis responds to injury with a dynamic continuation of collagen synthesis and degradation, and the once highly vascular

granulation tissue undergoes a process of devascularization as it matures into less vascular scar tissue.

HOW DO WE NOW LINK THIS BASIC KNOWLEDGE TO PRACTICE?

Diagnosis, diagnosis, diagnosis – this is the key to successful wound healing. A wrong diagnosis can result, at best, in delayed healing, at worst, amputation or death of the patient.

When a patient with a wound first presents, a number of questions should be addressed which will aid the diagnosis:

1. What is the patient's age?
2. What is the patient's nutritional status?
3. Are there any underlying chronic conditions, such as diabetes, peripheral vascular insufficiency, etc.?
4. Is the patient on any drug regime?
5. Is there any infection present?

What is the patient's age?

Ageing affects all stages of wound healing. The onset of the inflammatory phase of repair is delayed and lasts longer. Cell proliferation and metabolism decreases. The rate of capillary growth into the wound bed and mast cell numbers decrease with age. The diminished blood flow causes decreased clearance of metabolites and foreign materials, and increased tissue hypoxia which delays healing.

Wound remodelling is also affected by age due to decreased fibroblast activity. There is also a reduction in the amount of collagen organization and cross-linkage which results in decreased tensile strength.[115]

What is the patient's nutritional status?

An adequate supply of nutrients is essential for wound healing. Malnutrition or any deficiencies of nutrients, e.g. zinc, vitamin C or iron, may delay wound healing and will lead to impaired immune resistance increasing the risk of infection. Lennard-Jones[116] highlighted the problems associated with malnutrition including loss of muscle tissue, impaired immune resistance to infection, increased risk of complications, prolonged recovery and increased length of hospital stay. These lead to not only the economical expense of prolonged hospital stay, but also the physical and emotional cost to the patient.

NUTRITIONAL ASSESSMENT

It is important for malnourished patients and those at risk of malnutrition to be identified early and referred to the dietitian for assessment.

By asking a few simple questions, nutritional problems can be highlighted and addressed on a patients' admission to hospital.

A simple tool including four questions is worth remembering:[117]

1. What is you normal weight?
2. How tall are you?
3. Have you unintentionally lost weight?
4. Have you been eating less than usual?

You may also wish to find out about activity levels; is this normal or reduced? Have there been any unusual losses such as chronic diarrhoea or vomiting?[116]

Other measurements of nutritional status include:

- serum albumin: (30–35 g/L is a possible indicator of moderate malnutrition; <30 g/L is a possible indicator of severe malnutrition);
- serum transferrin: (1.0–1.5 g/L is an indicator of moderate malnutrition; <1.0 g/L is an indicator of severe malnutrition);
- triceps skinfold thickness: (10 mm in males and <13 mm in females is an indicator of malnutrition.[118, 119, 120, 121]

Are there any underlying chronic conditions such as diabetes, peripheral vascular insufficiency, etc.?

Diseases that cause tissue hypoxia, such as diabetes, arteriosclerosis and chronic venous insufficiency, all retard wound healing.

Figure 8.7 shows a typical example of a diabetic wound and it occurs for a multitude of reasons, e.g. impaired vascular supply leading to reduced oxygen levels, elevated glucose levels leading to reduced vitamin C transport, reduced collagen synthesis, impairment of leukocyte function, etc. The primary aim should always

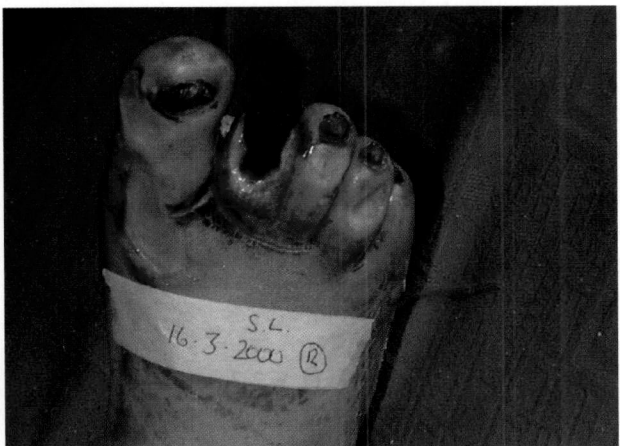

Figure 8.7 A diabetic wound. Image provided by TVU.

be to address the underlying diabetes first. This will make the problem of wound healing easier.

Is the patient on any drug regime?

Drugs that the patient may be taking include:

- antiinflammatory drugs;
- glucocorticosteroids depress the inflammatory phase of repair by inhibiting neutrophil and monocyte recruitment and by suppressing macrophage phagocytosis;
- cytotoxics;
- anticoagulants;
- immunosuppressives;
- penicillamine;
- HRT.[122]

Is there any infection present?

Bacterial contamination of a wound delays healing. Infection can prolong the inflammatory response, which causes further tissue damage. The susceptibility of a wound to infection is increased by a number of factors: the presence of necrotic tissue, foreign particles and haematoma in the wound. Apart from causing wound complications, bacteria may spread into the bloodstream causing bacteraemia and septicaemia.

Once these questions have been answered, the wound then needs to be fully classified and assessed. Classification falls under three main headings:

1. wound closure;
2. cause of the wound;
3. stage of healing.

It is important to be as accurate as possible with this classification because the subsequent treatment of the wound varies tremendously depending upon the answers obtained.

Categorization by wound closure

One of the most common ways to assess a wound is based on the degree of tissue loss, which in turn dictates the method of closure. The two basic types of wound closure are termed 'primary intention' and 'secondary intention', described under Healing by first intention and Healing by second intention.

In primary intention wounds where tissue loss has been minimal (see under Healing by first intention), it is possible to have the edges opposed and secured (usually with sutures, but possibly with clips, glue or adhesive strips).

In secondary intention wounds where tissue loss has been so great (see under Healing by second intention), it is not possible to bring the edges of the wound together and sutured in the same way as in the primary intention wounds. They have to heal by contraction and by filling up with granulation tissue. Examples of these are leg ulcers and pressure sores. The resulting scar from this type of healing is generally more pronounced than that produced by primary intention healing.

Categorization by the cause of the wound

ACUTE OR CHRONIC?

By categorizing wounds according to the way in which they occurred, they fit into a number of different groups. The two basic groups are termed 'acute' and 'chronic' wounds. Acute wounds are a result of trauma, e.g. thermal, mechanical, chemical, radiation, etc. In most acute wounds, when the cause of the injury is removed the wound tends to heal. In chronic wounds there tends to be an underlying pathology in the individual, e.g. diabetes, venous insufficiency, malignancy, which causes the wound to persist even when the original cause is removed. This is because the factors which are necessary for successful healing may be absent in the physiology of these individuals, e.g. cytokines, patent blood supply, etc.

ACUTE WOUNDS

There are a number of general categories of acute wounds:

- thermal wounds;
- postoperative wounds;
- mechanical injuries.

THERMAL WOUNDS

These wounds are caused by extremes of heat and cold and also radiation. Irradiation, which is frequently used to treat head and neck cancer, causes irreparable damage to the skin's microvasculature. As a consequence of reduced blood supply, resulting from irradiation, wounds heal poorly and are much more susceptible to infection than are nonirradiated tissue beds (**Figure 8.8**).

The major problem associated with this type of wound is in the assessment of the true extent of the injury. Burns are the most common type of this injury. Burns can be divided into three groups according to their severity.

1. **First degree:** This type of wound affects the upper layer of the epidermis and no intervention is generally needed. An example of this is sunburn.
2. **Second degree:** This type of burn generally results in blistering. It is advised that to reduce the chances of infection the blister should remain

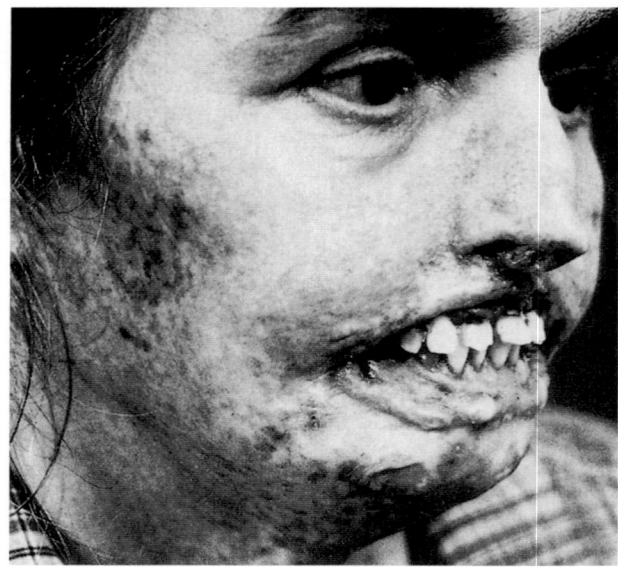

Figure 8.8 Patient had radiation treatment for acne 25 years previous to this photograph. Her lips are now infiltrated with invasive cancer. Note the extensive scarring resulting from the previous radiation. Courtesy William Panje.

intact. As with first-degree burns, minimal intervention is needed.

3. **Third degree:** This type of burn is the most serious and results in large areas of tissue necrosis. To allow new tissue to develop the necrotic tissue must be debrided, otherwise any intervention, such as grafting, will fail.

There have been many attempts to develop a tool to accurately measure the depth of second-degree burns. This measurement is critical in determining whether to treat the burn surgically or conservatively. Once debridement has been carried out, a range of grafting techniques are available depending upon individual circumstances:

- **autologous:** graft from one part of the body to another and also grafts which are grown in tissue culture from the patients own cells;
- **homologous:** graft from a donor to recipient of the same species, e.g. human to human;
- **heterologous:** donor and recipient are from different species, e.g. pig to human;
- **alloplastic:** temporary graft made from a foreign material such as plastic.

POSTOPERATIVE WOUNDS

There are numerous types of postoperative wounds, the most common are:

- incisions;
- skin biopsy;
- split thickness skin flaps;
- amputation.

Incisions

These wounds are typically made by a scalpel and will extend through the full thickness of the skin into the underlying tissues (see under Healing by first intention). Healing will be by primary intention.

Skin biopsy

This wound generally involves the surgical removal of a small area of full thickness skin for the purpose of histological examination of suspect tissue. Healing will normally be by primary intention.

Split thickness skin graft

This type of wound extends through the epidermis into the superficial layers of the dermis (papillary layer). This is not a full thickness wound and is equivalent to an abrasion resulting in minimal scarring.

Amputation

These wounds are caused by the surgical removal of a limb in order to save the individual. The wounds will generally heal by a mixture of primary and secondary intention depending upon the degree of tissue loss and the ability to graft a tissue flap to the injury site.

MECHANICAL INJURIES

These wounds are the most common and we have all experienced some form of mechanical injury at some point in our lives. Fortunately for most of us they are minor wounds and are not life threatening. However, some people face more serious mechanical injuries, which can at best disable and at worst kill. In addition to the initial mechanical injury there is also the possibility of infection, which can sometimes make a nonlife-threatening trauma become life threatening. Common examples of trauma wounds are:

- abrasions;
- blisters;
- bites;
- bruises;
- cuts;
- stabs;
- gunshots.

CHRONIC WOUNDS

The three most common types of chronic wound are:

1. diabetic wounds;
2. pressure ulcers;
3. leg ulcers.

Diabetic wounds

Diabetic wounds occur for a multitude of reasons, which have been previously discussed under Are there any underlying chronic conditions such as diabetes,

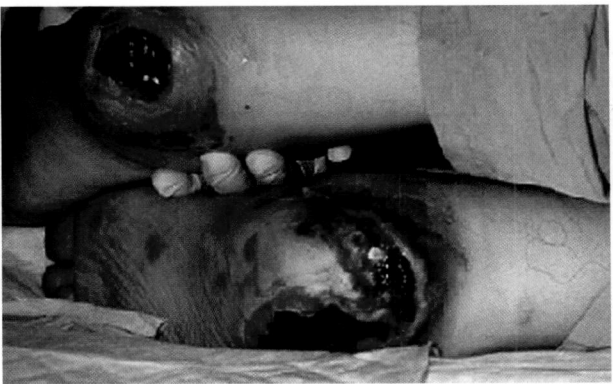

Figure 8.9   Typical pressure ulcers of the heels. Image provided by TVU.

peripheral vascular insufficiency, etc.? The primary aim should always be to address the underlying diabetes first, otherwise healing will be delayed.

Pressure ulcers

These wounds are typically caused by the action of pressure and shear forces on an already compromised tissue, which is overlying a bony prominence (**Figure 8.9**). Pressure ulcers tend to be divided into four groups depending upon the depth of the wound (**Figure 8.10**).

1. **Stage I**: This is a nonblanchable erythema of intact skin.
2. **Stage II**: This is defined as partial thickness skin loss involving the epidermis and the upper layer of the dermis (papillary zone).
3. **Stage III**: This is defined as a full thickness skin loss and extends into the underlying subcutaneous fat.
4. **Stage IV**: This is defined as a full thickness skin loss with extensive damage through the subcutaneous fat into the underlying muscle, bone and supporting tissue.

Leg ulcers

Legs ulcers are usually caused by deterioration in the arterial and/or the venous supply in the lower limb.

Venous leg ulcers

This type of ulcer accounts for approximately 70 percent of all leg ulcers. These wounds result because of a severe venous insufficiency in the lower limb. This results in reduced blood supply to and drainage from the tissues of this region. Once compromised in this way the tissues are easily damaged by the slightest injury, leading to ulceration.

Arterial leg ulcers

Approximately 10 percent of leg ulcers are arterial. The cause is due to blockage of an artery, which leads to a

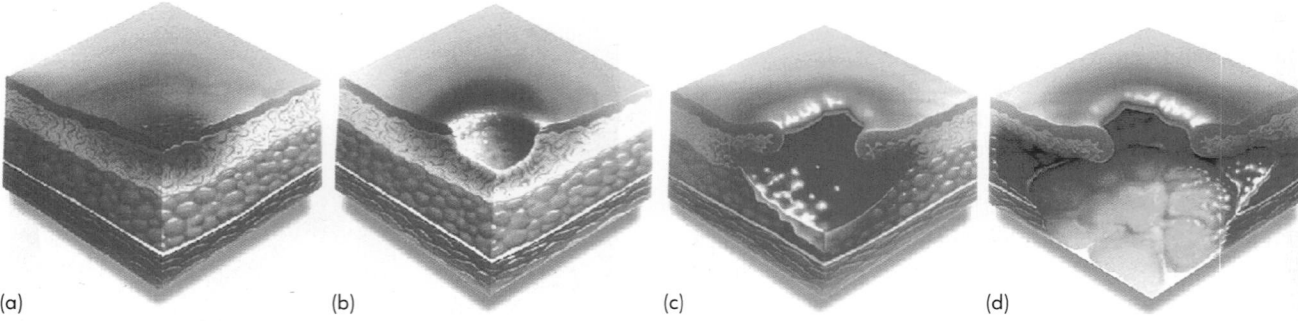

Figure 8.10 Pressure ulcer: (a) stage I; (b) stage II; (c) stage III; (d) stage IV. Artwork supplied courtesy of Hill-Rom®.

decrease in the blood flow to the tissues. This leads to a decrease in oxygen and nutrients to the area and so an ulcer is formed. The main cause of arterial blockage is smoking.

Categorization by stage of healing

A third way to categorize a wound is according to the type of tissue present within it. The type of tissue present will be directly related to the stage the wound is at in the healing process.

As discussed at the start of this chapter, there are three basic stages or phases of healing.

INFLAMMATION

Inflammation is characterized clinically by the common signs of heat, pain, swelling and redness and, microscopically, by the degranulation of mast cells and the presence of phagocytes, such as macrophages, in the wound (see under Inflammation above).

PROLIFERATION

Proliferation is the stage of new vessel and tissue growth (see under New tissue formation (proliferation)). It is characterized, clinically, by granulation and epithelial tissue and, microscopically, by the presence of fibroblasts (from approximately day 2 onwards), the synthesis of collagen, angiogenesis (the formation of new vessels) and the presence of epithelial cells.

REMODELLING

Remodelling is the stage where the collagen fibres that have been randomly laid down are reorganized (see under Matrix formation and remodelling). This may take several years to complete.

From these stages of healing, five different tissue types can emerge:

1. granulation;
2. epithelial;
3. slough;
4. necrotic;
5. infected.

Granulation tissue

This tissue can be recognized by its red, moist, shiny and granular appearance as shown in **Figure 8.3**. A biopsy of this tissue would reveal an abundance of blood capillaries, macrophages and fibroblasts.

Epithelial tissue

As the wound heals and fills with granulation tissue, the new epidermis will grow across it from the edges of the wound moving towards the centre of it. The appearance of the epithelial tissue is pinky/white (see **Figure 8.5**). Growth of epithelial tissue can also occur from hair follicles, sebaceous and sweat glands in the wound tissue itself. This means that source of growth of the new epidermis is not just restricted to the periphery of the wound, but can occur throughout the entire wound. This can give rise to islands of epithelial tissue often seen in the middle of expanses of granulation tissue.

Slough

This is seen as a yellow or white deposit in the wound (**Figure 8.11**). This deposit may be runny or fibrous in nature and is common in chronic and infected wounds. Epithelial tissue and tendons are often mistaken for slough, so care is needed when deciding whether to debride the tissue or not.

Necrotic tissue

This tissue is black or black/brown in colour with a leathery texture. This is dead tissue and has to be debrided before healing can commence.

Infected tissue

This tissue can be identified by a number of classical signs:

- erythema;
- presence of pus;
- excess exudate;
- odour;

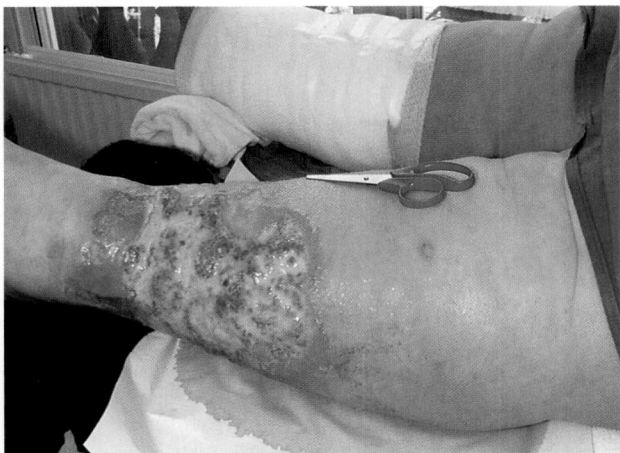

Figure 8.11 Wound covered with slough. Image provided by TVU.

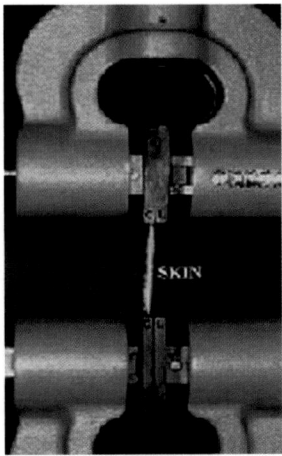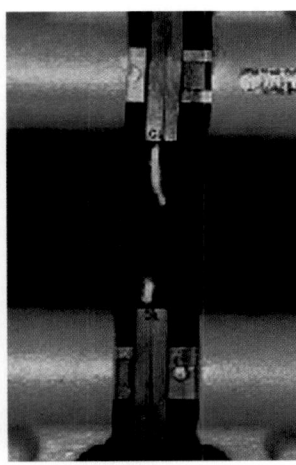

Figure 8.12 A tissue sample being tested for tensile strength using an Instron machine. Picture courtesy of M. Calvin.

- change in pain;
- pyrexia;
- delayed healing;
- friable granulation tissue;
- pocketing at base of wound;
- bridging of soft tissue and epithelium;
- wound breakdown.

IDENTIFYING INFECTION

Traditionally a swab is taken of the wound surface and sent to the laboratory for identification. 10^5 bacteria per gram has been the recognized point at which the bacteria are at a level which will inhibit wound healing. Therefore, this has been the level at which a wound is officially classified as being infected.

It must be understood that this level of bacteria in a wound may not necessarily be detrimental to all individuals. Some people can have this level of bacteria in their wound and will still heal successfully without delay or adverse reaction. Other individuals may suffer adverse reactions to this level of bacteria.

So interpreting what exactly your swab results mean can be very much an individual decision. Swabs provide some information about the type of bacteria present, but the important point is to identify whether the bacteria is causing delayed healing.

WOUND ASSESSMENT

Numerous techniques exist for the assessment of wounds. They can be divided into two basic categories: invasive or noninvasive.

Invasive

These techniques yield quantitative results and involve biopsy of the wound.

- **Histology** gives an indication of the number and type of cells present and therefore a good estimate on the stage of healing (see **Figure 8.4**).[123]
- **Biochemical analysis** gives an indication of what matrix materials are present, e.g. collagen type.[124]
- **Tensile strength** gives an indication of wound strength (**Figure 8.12**).[125]
- **Angiography** gives an indication of wound vascularity.[126]

Noninvasive

Whilst less quantitative than the invasive methods, these techniques are more acceptable to patients as they do not involve biopsy.

Wound area

Acetate or polythene film is placed over the wound and the outline traced using a permanent marker pen. The wound surface area is measured by computer or by placing tracing on to graph paper and counting the squares. Inaccuracies can be found when trying to define the wound edges. An alternative to tracing is photography, where the wound is photographed and measurements made from the image. A reference scale must always be included in the photograph (**Figure 8.13**).

Wound depth

A device known as the Kundin gauge[127] can be used to measure length, width and depth of a wound from which area and volume are calculated. Be aware that the method often underestimates area and volume; however, it is easy to use and is, disposable, objective and inexpensive.

Wound volume

By making moulds of the wound (silicone rubber, silastic foam, alginates, hydrocolloid gel), the wound volume can be estimated by placing the acquired mould into a beaker

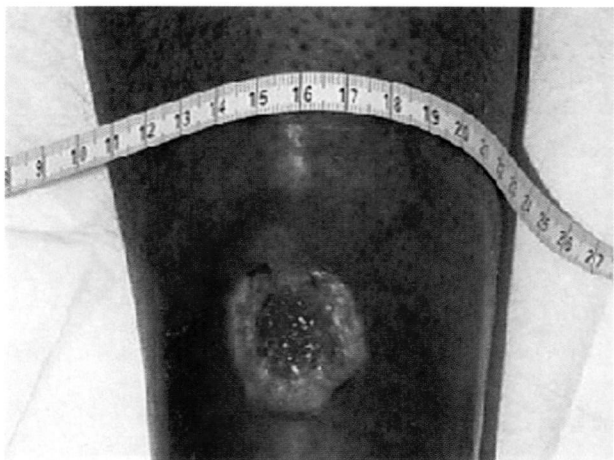

Figure 8.13 A wound with calibration reference present. Picture courtesy TVU.

of water and measuring the displaced water volume.[128] Other methods include covering the wound with a film and injecting saline into the wound. The amount of saline it takes to fill the cavity up to the film can then be measured; however, this is not satisfactory for superficial wounds.[129]

Stereoscopic photography can also be used to estimate volume.[130]

Thermal imaging

Infrared radiation (heat) emitted from the skin and wound is visualized using this technique. The more vascularized an area is the more heat is emitted. Interpretation of results can be difficult as the wound temperature can be subject to variations in factors other than vascularization, e.g. room temperature, underlying infection.

High-frequency diagnostic ultrasound

This relatively new noninvasive method allows the clinician a high resolution view deep into the skin and wound bed to assess the quality of the tissue.[131, 132, 133, 134, 135, 136]

This is a simple procedure and can even be carried out without the need to remove certain wound dressings. Because you can view under the surface of the skin, it is possible in certain cases to monitor changes in a wound even before they become clinically evident and therefore recognize whether the wound is deteriorating or improving. This ability can lead to considerable savings in treatment times. Wound depth can also be calculated using this technique, e.g. in burn injuries. This is a rapid, sensitive and repeatable method of quantifying wound healing.

Assessment of blood flow using Doppler ultrasonography

Combined with a full physical examination and clinical history, this assessment gives an indication of arterial blood flow to the lower limb.

Rationale for wound dressing choice

Once the wound has been correctly identified and assessed according to the above criteria, a choice has to be made as to which treatment or dressing will be applied to produce the best healing possible. The following is a guideline to aid the clinician in his/her choice:

DISCOLOURED, UNBROKEN SKIN

Dry skin

Simple, bland ointments, e.g. yellow/white soft paraffin. Avoid perfume/scented emollients. Nonsting barrier preparations, e.g. Cavilon and Supraskin – also for prevention and treatment of maceration or excoriation to the periwound area.

Skin conditions associated with wounds

Paste bandages, prescribed steroids may be necessary for eczema.

Skin subject to pressure or trauma

Primarily appropriate pressure relief, but foam dressings, low adherent dressings and vapour permeable films may occasionally be appropriate.

EPITHELIAZING WOUNDS

Dressing choice depends on the level of exudate: vapour permeable films, silicone membranes, low/nonadherent dressings, paraffin tulle, hydrocolloids, hydrogels, alginates, foams.

FLAT DRY WOUNDS

Choice of dressing for flat, dry wounds include low adherent dressings, vapour permeable films, membrane dressings and thin hydrocolloids.

FLAT MOIST WOUNDS

Choice of dressing for flat, moist wounds include low adherent dressings, nonmedicated tulles, vapour permeable films, membranes, hydrocolloids, hydrogels, foams, alginates and hydrofibre.

GRANULATING WOUNDS

Dressing choice depends on the level of exudate and depth of wound. Deep wounds that extend into the dermis will need to be packed gently with a suitable dressing. Dressings include hydrocolloids, alginates, foams, hydrogels and hydrofibre.

- **Exuding wounds**
  - Light–medium exudate:
    - foams;
    - alginates;
    - hydrocolloids, transparent or thin dressings;
    - hydrogel, sheets or gels;
    - hydroactives, transparent or thin dressings;
    - hydrofibre.
  - Medium–heavy exudate:
    - alginates;
    - hydrocolloids;
    - hydrofibre;
    - foams, extra or plus foams, i.e. those with greater absorbency;
    - hydroactives;
    - vacuum-assisted closure therapy (VAC).
  - Heavy exudate:
    - alginates;
    - hydrofibre;
    - foams, extra or plus foams, i.e. those with greater absorbency;
    - VAC therapy.
- **Cavity wounds**
  - Hydrofibre (Aquacel);
  - foams, cavity wound dressings, Cavicare;
  - alginate, rope, ribbon, cavity dressing;
  - hydroactives, cavity dressing;
  - hydrogels;
  - hydrocolloid paste;
  - sugar pastes, thick and thin;
  - Cadexemer iodine, infected or critically colonized cavities;
  - iodine ointment, infected or critically colonized cavities;
  - VAC therapy.
- **Sloughy wounds:** Modern products will remove slough and absorb exudate.
  - Hydrofibre;
  - hydrogels;
  - hydrocolloids;
  - alginates;
  - sugar pastes;
  - mechanical debridement;
  - scalpel (with or without local/general anaesthetic);
  - biosurgical debridement using larvae, e.g. Larv E;
  - enzymatic debridement, e.g. Varidase;
  - miscellaneous: whirlpool, hydrotherapy, high-pressure irrigation.
- **Infected wounds**
  - General infection control measures, e.g. hand washing;
  - systemic antibiotics, depending on local/systemic signs of infection;
  - topical antimicrobials.

- **Necrotic wounds**
  - Hydrocolloids;
  - hydrogels (ensure they do not macerate surrounding skin);
  - mechanical/surgical debridement;
  - biosurgical debridement using larvae, e.g. Larv E;
  - enzymatic debridement, e.g. Varidase.
- **Malodourous wounds**
  - Reduce levels of bacterial colonization;
  - activated charcoal dressings;
  - sugar paste (thick and thin);
  - metronidazole gels: use judiciously, e.g. for fungating, malodorous tumours.
- **Malignant/fungating wounds**
  - Control bleeding (topical Adrenalin or Leutral, Surgicel);
  - assess pain and analgesia requirements;
  - treat or mask odour;
  - debride wounds;
  - reduce volume of exudate;
  - reduce inflammation, e.g. by removing sensitizing agents;
  - care for surrounding skin;
  - improve cosmetic appearance, e.g. reduce tumour bulk, avoid bulk dressings;
  - enable patient to cope with altered body image.
- **Oedematous wounds**
  - Compression bandages;
  - exercise;
  - elevation of limb.

Over/hypergranulation tissue

Over/hypergranulation tissue occurs in many types of wounds when the inflammatory phase of healing is prolonged unnecessarily. Ideally any treatment should not further exacerbate the inflammatory reaction and should be nontraumatic.

There is no consensus as to the correct treatment, but the most frequently used methods are:

- change from an occlusive to a nonocclusive dressing, such as Lyofoam;
- application of light pressure to the wound bed by the addition of supplementary padding or bandages;
- short-term topical application of corticosteroid, e.g. Terracortril (tetracycline and hydrocortisone ointment) or Daktacort (miconazole and hydrocortisone cream);
- allowing the overgranulation to resolve itself without treatment.

CARE OF THE SURROUNDING SKIN

- Paste bandages;
- 50 percent white soft paraffin and 50 percent liquid paraffin for hydration of dry skin conditions;

- oily cream or 50:50 plus 2 percent salicylic acid for extremely dry scaly patches;
- diprobase for hydration.

SPECIFIC WOUNDS

A precise diagnosis and assessment of circulation is required.

- **Venous ulcers**
  - Treat tissue type in ulcer bed;
  - compression bandages, elevation, exercise;
  - paste bandages to treat skin conditions;
  - judicious use of Elocon topical steroid for eczema.
- **Arterial ulcers**
  - Treat tissue type in ulcer bed;
  - paste bandages to treat skin conditions, exercise;
  - compression bandages are contraindicated.
- **Mixed venous and arterial ulcers**
  - Treat as with arterial ulcers except that light compression may also be indicated.
- **Pressure ulcers**
  - Relief of pressure;
  - appropriate dressings for tissue type.
- **Burns and scalds**
  - Cold running water (10–15 minutes);
  - cling film prior to assessment of depth; flamazine often applied as an antimicrobial, but only after assessment;
  - emollient for hydration once healed.
  - **Superficial burns**
    - Semipermeable films;
    - hydrocolloids;
    - Aquacel®;
    - Mepitel™;
    - foams.
  - **Dermal burns**
    - Flamazine®;
    - Mepitel;
    - alginates;
    - Aquacel;
    - TransCyte®.
  - **Full thickness burns**
    - Assess at specialist centre;
    - Flamazine®;
    - Mepitel™;
    - hydrogels.

Diabetic ulcers

Diabetic ulcers require specialist care. There is evidence of effectiveness for the following prevention:

- identification of those at high risk, referral to foot care clinics, which offer education, podiatry and footwear;
- therapeutic shoes with custom-moulded insoles.

Dermatitis artefacta

Consider this in the differential diagnosis of a wound that fails to heal.

Care of haematoma

Skilled surgical techniques can prevent haematoma formation, but excess bleeding may arise from a tense haematoma beneath a suture line. The resulting dead space can act as a focus for infection, as well as weakening the suture line and delaying normal healing.

In severe cases, the suture line may have to be reopened and the haematoma surgically evacuated. Often one or two sutures or clips can be removed to allow the haematoma to drain, but occasionally complete dehiscence of the skin layers occurs.

An open wound with a visible haematoma can be cleaned out quickly and atraumatically with either hydrogen peroxide (3 percent) solution diluted with normal saline or an enzymatic debriding agent such as Varidase, which contains streptokinase and streptodornase. Once clean, the edges can be reapposed or more commonly, left to heal by secondary intention.

Care of suture lines

The tissue bonds together after 48 hours and forms a barrier against bacteria. Wound edges are held together with sutures, staples, clips or glue and these remain in place while the scar line epithializes and regains tensile strength.

Dressings applied after suturing do not need to be removed unless they are stained by discharge or there are clinical signs of infection.

Although technically the sutured wound has closed after 48 hours, a dressing is no longer needed over the suture line; however, a dressing prevents sutures catching on clothing and provides a cosmetic covering.

In order to prevent blister formation under adhesive-bordered, low adherent dressings, avoid application of dressings under tension and allow for swelling oedema of the surrounding tissue.

SUMMARY

The most important step in healing a wound is to diagnose the wound type accurately. This is particularly important in chronic wounds where the underlying pathology has to be addressed before prescribing a wound healing therapy. It should also be remembered that you are not merely treating a wound but the whole person. It is important to establish whether a patient is able to comply with treatment regimes once they are out of your care or will they need assistance. If assistance is needed, does the patient have relatives or friends at home willing and able to provide the necessary support or do they need this to be provided?

With the correct diagnosis and treatment regime, most wounds will heal in a straightforward manner.

KEY POINTS

- Wound healing subdivided into healing by primary and by secondary intention.
- Healing by first intention occurs in clean well-perfused wounds with minimal tissue destruction.
- Healing involves:
  - rapid epithelial proliferation within 24 hours;
  - minimal granulation tissue;
  - small scar.
- Healing by second intention occurs in:
  - gaping wounds with lacerated edges;
  - large defects that cannot be covered by grafting;
  - extensive trophic disturbances, such as leg ulcers;
  - highly suppurative wounds;
  - wounds interspersed with foreign bodies;
  - infected wounds that have undergone; primary closure;
  - wounds that heal better cosmetically as a result of contraction, e.g. fingertip injuries.
- Healing by second intention involves:
  - slow epithelial migration due to increased distance cells must travel;
  - more granulation tissue formation to fill the wound from the base;
  - wound contraction resulting in tissue distortion and extensive unsatisfactory scars often with impairment of function (repair).
- Wound repair can arbitrarily be divided into three phases:
  1. inflammation including early and late phases;
  2. new tissue formation (proliferation);
  3. matrix formation and remodelling.
- Inflammation can be defined as an essential localized protective tissue response elicited by injury or destruction of tissues which serves to destroy wall off both the injurious agent and the injured tissues.
- Early acute inflammation has two important components.
  1. Clot formation results in the cessation of haemorrhage and provides a provisional fibrin matrix for cell migration. Platelet induced mediators (PDGF, PF4, TGFα, TGFβ) vital to this process, modulate vascular tone and permeability and stimulate synthesis of extracellular matrix components. Blood clotting also activates complement cascades via Hagemann factor producing complement-derived anaphyllotoxins which together with bradikinin increase vascular permeability to produce extravascular clot. Anaphylotoxins stimulate release of vasoactive mediators from mast cells and attract neutrophils and monocytes into the wound.
  2. Neutrophils in the early neutrophil-rich phase of inflammation are attracted by a variety of chemotactic mediators including both general leukocyte and neutrophil-specific chemotactic factors. Their main function is the phagocytosis of bacteria and debris, although their role is not critical. In clean wounds, neutrophil infiltration ceases within a few days but persists in the presence of bacterial infection. Eventually, they are phagocytosed by macrophages or fibroblasts.
- Late inflammation is characterized by the accumulation of monocytes which rapidly differentiate into macrophages. Wound macrophages:
  - eliminate deleterious materials, e.g. microorganisms and wound debris by phagocytosis;
  - generate chemotactic factors responsible for the recruitment of additional inflammatory cells;
  - release collagenases that lyse necrotic material;
  - synthesize and release growth and regulatory factors critical to the coordination of granulation tissue formation.
- New tissue formation (proliferation day 5–14). This phase is characterized by granulation tissue consisting of macrophages, fibroblasts and endothelial cells embedded in a loose matrix of collagen, fibrin, fibronectin and proteoglycans rich in hyaluronic acid.
- Re-epithelialization is the reconstitution of the cells of the epidermis into an organized stratified squamous epithelium which covers the wound defect and restores the barrier properties of skin. In partial thickness wounds, hair follicles and ducts of sweat glands act as a source of epidermal skin cells, whereas in full thickness wounds the only source is the wound margin.
- Formation of granulation tissue consists of three phases.
  1. Fibroplasia defined as the process of fibroblast recruitment into the wound site and the ensuing synthesis and secretion of collagenous and noncollagenous matrix.

Fibroblast migration and proliferation necessary for granulation tissue formation and this occurs best in a mildly acidic medium provided by the accumulation of lactate from anaerobic metabolism;

2. Wound contraction (day 7–14) is the reduction of part or all of the skin defect by centripetal movement of the surrounding undamaged skin. There are two main theories of how fibroblasts generate the force necessary to facilitate wound contraction: (1) myofibroblast theory suggest that fibroblasts have some smooth muscle fibres; (2) cell to cell and cell to matrix contacts act as anchorage points. Together these allow wound contraction to take place. Fibroblast theory suggests that they exert traction forces;

3. Angiogenesis: the process of new blood vessel formation occurs simultaneously with fibroplasia. Capillaries bud from preexisting small venules close to the wound and extend into it. Angiogenic stimulants are released from macrophages, but their control is as yet poorly understood.

● Matrix formation and remodelling: During this phase the highly cellular and vascular granulation tissue is replaced by much less cellular and vascular scar tissue. This starts simultaneously with granulation tissue formation and can go on for months or years. Scar tissue is functionally inferior to the original, acting as a diffusional barrier to nutrients and oxygen and only ever reaches 75 percent of their tensile strength of normal skin. As a wound matrix matures:
  – hyaluronic acid and fibronectin associated with cellular ingrowth reduce;
  – accumulation type 1 collagen bundles, alteration in intermolecular cross-links providing an increase in tensile strength;
  – proteoglycan deposition increases the wound's resilience to deformation;
  – collagen remodelling and realignment into larger fibrillar bundles which become less randomly orientated.

Best clinical practice

✓ Take relevant points in patient history:
  – age: advancing age slows all aspects of wound healing;
  – nutritional status: malnutrition (albumin <30, transferring <1 = severe malnutrition) or

deficiencies in zinc, vitamin C and iron all impair wound healing;
  – underlying chronic disease, such as diabetes, arteriosclerosis and chronic venous insufficiency, all retard wound healing;
  – drugs which impair wound healing include antiinflammatory drugs especially steroids, cytotoxics, anticoagulants, immunosuppressives, penicillamine and HRT;
  – infection always delays wound healing.
✓ Classification and assessment:
  – wound closure: primary intention or secondary intention;
  – cause: acute or chronic: (1) acute: thermal wounds, postoperative wounds, mechanical injuries; (2) chronic: diabetic ulcers, pressure ulcers and leg ulcers;
  – categorization by stage of healing, i.e. by presence of inflammation, proliferation and remodelling. From these stages, five different tissue types can emerge: granulation, epithelial, slough, necrotic and infected tissue;
  – indicators of wound infection are erythema, pus, exudates, odour, change in pain, delayed healing, friable granulation tissue, pocketing at base of wound, bridging of soft tissue and epithelium, wound breakdown and wound swab counts > 105.
✓ Investigations used in wound assessment:
  – invasive: histology, biochemical analysis, tensile strength and angiography all of limited use because of the need to biopsy;
  – noninvasive: (1) wound area by tracing or photography; (2) wound depth using Kundin gauge can be used to estimate volume; (3) wound volume using a suitable mould or stereoscopic photography; (4) thermal imaging can give an idea of vascularity; (5) high frequency diagnostic ultrasound – can detect changes under the skin and is useful for monitoring progress; (6) Doppler ultrasonography can be used to measure blood flow.

Deficiencies in current knowledge and areas for future research

One of the biggest challenges in wound care is to give the right treatment at the right time. Wounds present an ever-changing environment; one day they may be dry and necrotic, the next, heavily exudating and infected. These different environments present different challenges to wound dressing, the former requiring a dressing that preserves or even donates moisture, the latter requiring enhanced absorptive properties. Research is needed to develop the 'ideal' wound dressing which can handle all environments that occur during the history of a wound. Also having a dressing, which can be left *in situ* for extended periods of time, would be of enormous benefit to both patient and carer.

Our knowledge of how wounds heal and how we can enhance this healing process continues to increase each year; however, the dissemination of this knowledge from researcher to practitioner often fails. For example, there are numerous high-tech wound dressings and highly specific care protocols available, yet how often do we see inappropriate care given. In addition to this, many wounds are preventable in the first instance if only the patient had been fully assessed using the correct assessment tools. There is a definite need for systems to be developed and put into practice so that as new techniques are developed they are delivered to the practitioner.

REFERENCES

1. Asmussen PD, Sollner B. *Wound care; principles of wound healing*. Germany: Beiersdorf Medical Bibliothek, 1993.
2. Goepel JR. Responses to cellular injury. In: Underwood JCE (ed.). *General and systemic pathology*, 2nd edn. London: Churchill Livingstone, 1996: 121–2.
3. Forrester JC. Mechanical, biochemical and architectural features of surgical repair. *Advances in Biological and Medical Physics*. 1973; **14**: 1–3.
4. Walter JB, Talbot IC. Wound healing. In: Walter JB and Israel MS (eds). *General pathology*, 7th edn. London: Churchill Livingstone, 1996: 165–80.
* 5. Clark RAF. Wound repair; overview and general considerations. In: Clark RAF (ed.). *The molecular and cellular biology of wound repair*, 2nd edn. London: Plenum Press, 1996: 3–50.
6. Gailit J, Clark RAF. Wound repair in the context of extracellular matrix. *Current Opinion in Cell Biology*. 1994; **6**: 717–25.
7. Thomas DW, O'Neill ID, Harding KG, Shepherd JP. Cutaneous wound healing: a current perspective. *Journal of Oral and Maxillofacial Surgery*. 1995; **53**: 442–7.
8. Yamada KM, Clark RAF. Provisional Matrix. In: Clark RAF (ed.). *The molecular and cellular biology of wound repair*, 2nd edn. London: Plenum Press, 1996: 51–94.
9. Lanir N, Ciano PS, van de Water L, McDonagh J, Dvorak AM, Dvorak HF. Macrophage migration in fibrin gel matrices II. Effects of clotting factor XIII, fibronectin and glycosaminoglycan content on cell migration. *Journal of Immunology*. 1988; **140**: 2340–9.
10. Koopmann Jr. CF. Cutaneous wound healing; an overview. *Otolaryngologic Clinics of North America*. 1995; **28**: 835–45.
11. Rudolph R, Shannon ML. The normal healing process. In: Eaglstein WH (ed.). *Wound care manual: New directions in wound healing*. New Jersey: Convatec, Princetown, 1990: 9–24.
12. Ginsberg M. Role of platelets in inflammation and rheumatic disease. *Advances in Inflammation Research*. 1981; **2**: 53–5.
13. Katz MH, Alvarez AV, Kirsner RS, Eaglstein WH, Falanga V. Human wound fluid from acute wounds stimulates fibroblast and endothelial cell growth. *Journal of the American Academy of Dermatology*. 1991; **25**: 1054–8.
14. Heldin C, Westermark B. Role of platelet-derived growth factor in vivo. In: Clark RAF (ed.). *The molecular and cellular biology of wound repair*, 2nd edn. London: Plenum Press, 1996: 249–74.
15. Deuel TF, Senior RM, Chang D, Griffin GL, Heinrikson RL, Kaiser ET. Platelet factor 4 is a chemotactic factor for neutrophils and monocytes. *Proceedings of the National Academy of Sciences of the United States of America*. 1981; **78**: 4584–7.
16. Schultz G, Rotari DS, Clark W. EGF and TGFα in wound healing and repair. *Journal of Cellular Biochemistry*. 1991; **45**: 346–52.
17. Sporn MB, Roberts AM. Transforming growth factor beta: recent progress and new challenges. *Journal of Cell Biology*. 1992; **119**: 1017–21.
18. Proud D, Kaplan AP. Kinin formation: mechanisms and role in inflammatory disorders. *Annual Review of Immunology*. 1988; **6**: 49–83.
19. Ghebrehiwet B, Silverberg M, Kaplan AP. Activation of classic pathway of complement, by hageman factor fragment. *Journal of Experimental Medicine*. 1981; **153**: 665–76.
20. Craddock P, Fehr J, Dalmasso A, Brighan KL, Jacob HS. Haemodialysis leukopenia: pulmonary vascular leukostasis resulting from complement activation by dialyzer cellophane membrane. *Journal of Clinical Investigation*. 1977; **59**: 879–88.
21. Williams TJ, Jose PL. Medication of increased vascular permeability after complement activation: histamine independent activation of C5a. *Journal of Experimental Medicine*. 1981; **153**: 136–53.
22. Terragno NA, Lonigro AJ, Malik KW, McGiff JC. The relationship of the renal vasodilator action of bradykinin to the release of PGE-like substances. *Experientia*. 1972; **28**: 437–9.
23. Williams TJ. Factors that affect vessel reactivity and leukocyte emigration. In: Clark RAF, Henson PM (eds). *The molecular and cellular biology of wound repair*. London: Plenum Press, 1988: 115–83.
24. Wedmore CV, Williams TJ. Control of vascular permeability by polymorphonuclear leukocytes, in inflammation. *Nature*. 1981; **289**: 646–50.
25. Marder SR, Chenoweth DE, Goldstein IM, Perez HD. Chemotactic responses of human peripheral blood monocytes to the complement-derived peptides C5a and C5a des Arg. *Journal of Immunology*. 1985; **134**: 3325–31.
26. Turk JL, Heather CJ, Diengdoh JV. A histochemical analysis of mononuclear cell infiltrates of the skin, with particular

reference to delayed hypersensitivity in the guinea pig. *International Archives of Allergy and Applied Immunology.* 1976; **29**: 278–89.

27. Senior RM, Skogen WF, Griffin GI. Effects of fibrinogen derivatives upon the inflammatory response. *Journal of Clinical Investigation.* 1986; **77**: 1014–9.

28. McKenzie R, Pepper DS, Kay AB. The generation of chemotactic activity for human leukocytes by the action of plasmin on human fibrinogen. *Thrombosis Research.* 1975; **6**: 1–8.

29. McKenzie R, Pepper DS, Kay AB. The generation of chemotactic activity for human leukocytes by the action of plasmin on human fibrinogen. *Thrombosis Research.* 1975; **6**: 1–8.

30. Ford-Hutchinson AW, Bray MA, Doig MV, Shipley ME, Smith MJ. Leukotriene B, a potent chemokinetic and aggregating substance, released from polymorphonuclear leukocytes. *Nature.* 1980; **286**: 264–5.

31. Freer RJ, Day AR, Radding JA, Schiffman E, Aswanikumar S, Showell HJ et al. Further studies on the structural requirement for synthetic peptide chemoattractants. *Biochemistry.* 1980; **19**: 2404–10.

32. Hanahan DJ. Platelet activating factor: a biologically active phosphoglyceride. *Annual Review of Biochemistry.* 1986; **55**: 483–509.

33. Ming WJ, Bersani L, Mantovani A. Tumour necrosis factor is chemotactic for moncytes and polymorhonuclear leukocytes. *Journal of Immunology.* 1987; **138**: 469–74.

34. Pierce GF, Mustoe TA, Lingelbach J, Masakowski VW, Griffin GL, Senior RM et al. Platelet derived growth factor and transforming growth factor-beta enhance tissue repair activities by unique mechanisms. *Journal of Cell Biology.* 1989; **109**: 429–40.

35. Riches DWH. Macrophage involvement in wound repair, remodelling and fibrosis. In: Clark RAF (ed.). *The molecular and cellular biology of wound repair,* 2nd edn. London: Plenum Press, 1996: 95–141.

36. Baggiolini M, Dewald B, Moser B. Interleukin-8 and related chemotactic cytokines-CXC and CC chemokines. *Advances in Immunology.* 1994; **55**: 97–179.

37. Kunkel SL, Standiford T, Kasahara K, Strieter RM. Stimulus specific induction of monocyte chemotactic protein-1 (MCP-1) gene expression. *Advances in Experimental Medicine and Biology.* 1991; **305**: 65–71.

38. Sherry B, Tekamp O, Gallegos C, Bauer D, Davatelis G, Wolpe SD et al. Resolution of the two components of macrophage inflammatory protein 1, and cloning and characterisation of one of those components, macrophage inflammatory protein 1 beta. *Journal of Experimental Medicine.* 1988; **168**: 2251–9.

39. Pierce GF, Yanagihara D, Costigan V et al. Platelet-derived endothelial cell growth factor (PD-ECGF) in angiogenesis and wound healing. First European Tissue Repair Society Meeting, Oxford, UK, 1991 (cited from abstract).

40. Bar-Shavit R, Kahn A, Fenton JW, Wilner GD. Chemotactic response of monocytes to thrombin. *Journal of Cell Biology.* 1983; **96**: 282–5.

41. Postlethwaite AE, Kang AH. Collagen and collagen peptide-induced chemotaxis of human blood monocytes. *Journal of Experimental Medicine.* 1976; **143**: 1299–307.

42. Senior RM, Griffin GL, Mecham RP. Chemotactic activity of elastin-derived peptides. *Journal of Clinical Investigation.* 1980; **66**: 859–62.

43. Senior RM, Griffin GL, Mecham RP, Wrenn DS, Prasad KU, Urry DW. Val-Gly-Val-Ala-Pro-Gly, a repeating peptide in elastin, is chemotactic for fibroblasts and monocytes. *Journal of Cell Biology.* 1984; **99**: 870–4.

44. Clark RAF. Cutaneous Wound Repair. In: Goldsmith LE (ed.). *Biochemistry and physiology of the skin.* Oxford: Oxford University Press, 1990: 576–601.

45. Williams PL, Warwick R, Dyson M, Bannister LH. *Gray's anatomy,* 38th edn. UK: Churchill Livingstone, 1995.

46. Wahl SM. Acute and chronic inflammation. In: Zembala M, Asherson GL (eds). *Human monocytes.* London: Academic Press, 1989: 361–71.

47. Halliwell B. Oxidants and human disease: some new concepts. *FASEB Journal.* 1987; **1**: 358–65.

48. Simpson DM, Ross R. The neutrophilic leukocyte in wound repair. A study with antineutrophil serum. *Journal of Clinical Investigation.* 1972; **51**: 2009–23.

49. Guirao X, Lowry SF. Biologic control of injury and inflammation: much more than too little or too late. *World Journal of Surgery.* 1996; **20**: 437–46.

50. Haslett C, Henson P. Resolution of inflammation. In: Clark RAF (ed.). *The molecular and cellular biology of wound repair,* 2nd edn. London: Plenum Press, 1996: 143–70.

51. Hosein B, Mosessens MW, Bianco C. Monocyte receptors for fibronectin. In: van Furth R (ed.). *Mononuclear phagocytes: Characteristics, physiology and function.* Holland: Martuus Nijhoff, Dordrecht, 1985.

* 52. Hunt TK. Prospective: a retrospective perspective on the nature of wounds. In: Barbul A, Pines E, Caldwell M et al. (eds). *Growth factors and other aspects of wound healing.* New York: Liss, 1987.

53. Ho YS, Lee WMF, Synderman R. Chemoattractant induced activation of c-fos gene expression in human monocytes. *Journal of Experimental Medicine.* 1987; **165**: 1524–38.

54. Newman SL, Henson JE, Henson PM. Phagocytosis of senescent neutrophils by human monocyte derived macrophages and rabbit inflammatory macrophages. *Journal of Experimental Medicine.* 1982; **156**: 430–42.

55. Tsukamoto Y, Helsel WE, Wahl SM. Macrophage production of fibronectin, a chemoattractant for fibroblasts. *Journal of Immunology.* 1981; **127**: 673–8.

56. Campbell EJ, Cury JD, Lazarus CJ, Welgus HG. Monocyte procollagenase and tissue inhibitor of metalloproteinases. Identification, characterisation and regulation of secretion. *Journal of Biological Chemistry.* 1987; **262**: 15862–8.

57. Moulin V. Growth factors in skin wound healing. *European Journal of Cell Biology.* 1995; **68**: 1–7.

58. Greenhalgh DG. The role of growth factors in wound healing. *Journal of Trauma.* 1996; **41**: 159–67.

59. Shimokado K, Raines EW, Madtes DK, Barrett TB, Benditt EP, Ross R. A significant part of macrophage derived growth factor consists of 2 forms of PDGF. *Cell.* 1985; **43**: 277–86.

60. Assoian RK, Fleurdelys BE, Stevenson HC, Miller PJ, Madtes PK, Raines EW *et al.* Expression and secretion of type beta TGF, by activated human macrophages. *Proceedings of the National Academy of Sciences of the United States of America.* 1987; **84**: 6020–4.

61. Madtes DK, Raines EW, Sakariassen KS, Assoian RK, Sporn MB, Bell GI *et al.* Induction of transforming growth factor alpha in activated human alveolar macrophages. *Cell.* 1988; **53**: 285–93.

62. Baird A, Mormede P, Bohlen P. Immunoreactive fibroblast growth factor in cells of peritoneal exudate suggest its identity with macrophage growth factor. *Biochemical and Biophysical Research Communications.* 1985; **126**: 358–64.

63. Eierman DF, Johnson CE, Haskill JS. Human monocyte inflammatory mediator gene expression is selectively regulated by adherence substrates. *Journal of Immunology.* 1989; **142**: 1970–6.

64. Leibovich SJ, Ross R. The role of macrophages in wound repair. A study of hydrocortisone and anti-macrophage serum. *American Journal of Pathology.* 1975; **78**: 71–100.

65. DiPietro LA. Wound healing: the role of the macrophage and other immune cells. *Shock.* 1995; **4**: 233–40.

66. Clark RAF. Basics of cutaneous wound repair. *Journal of Dermatologic Surgery and Oncology.* 1993a; **19**: 693–706.

67. Kanzler MH, Gorsulowsky DC, Swanson NA. Basic mechanisms in the healing cutaneous wound. *Journal of Dermatologic Surgery and Oncology.* 1986; **12**: 1156–64.

68. Hunt TK, van Winkle W. The fibroblast in normal repair. In: Hunt TK, Dunphy JE (eds). *Fundamentals of wound management.* New York: Appleton-Century-Crofts, 1979.

69. Ciano PS, Colvin RB, Dvorak AM, McDonagh J, Dvorak HF. Macrophage migration in fibrin gel matrices. *Laboratory Investigation.* 1986; **54**: 62–79.

70. Madri JA, Sankar SE, Romanic AM. Angiogenesis. In: Clark RAF (ed.). *The molecular and cellular biology of wound repair,* 2nd edn. London: Plenum Press, 1996: 355–72.

71. McCarthy JB, Iida J, Furcht LT. Mechanisms of parenchymal cell migration into wounds. In: Clark RAF (ed.). *The molecular and cellular biology of wound repair,* 2nd edn. London: Plenum Press, 1996: 373–90.

72. Woodley DT. Reepithelialisation. In: Clark RAF (ed.). *The molecular and cellular biology of wound repair,* 2nd edn. London: Plenum Press, 1996: 339–54.

* 73. Winter GD. Formation of the scab and the rate of epithelialization of superficial wounds in the skin of the young domestic pig. *Nature.* 1962; **193**: 293–4.

74. Kirsner RS, Eaglstein WH. The wound healing process. *Dermatologic Clinics.* 1993; **11**: 629–40.

75. Odland G, Ross R. Human wound repair I. Epidermal regeneration. *Journal of Cell Biology.* 1968; **39**: 135–51.

76. Grondahl-Hansen J, Lund LR, Ralfkiaer E, Ottevanger V, Dano K. Urokinase- and tissue-type plasminogen activators in keratinocytes during wound reepithelialisation *in vivo. Journal of Investigative Dermatology.* 1988; **90**: 790–5.

77. Stephens P, Davies KJ, al-Khateeb T, Shepherd JP, Thomas DW. A comparison of the ability of intra-oral and extra-oral fibroblasts to stimulate extracellular matrix reorganisation in a model of wound contraction. *Journal of Dental Research.* 1996; **75**: 1358–64.

78. Welch MP, Odland GF, Clark RAF. Temporal relationships of F-actin bundle formation, collagen and fibronectin matrix assembly, and fibronectin receptor expression in wound contraction. *Journal of Cell Biology.* 1990; **110**: 133–45.

79. Gabbiani G. The role of contractile proteins in wound healing, and fibrocontractive disease. *Methods and Achievements in Experimental Pathology.* 1979; **9**: 187–206.

80. Majno G. The story of myofibroblasts. *American Journal of Surgical Pathology.* 1979; **3**: 535–42.

81. Desmouliere A, Gabbiani G. The role of the myofibroblast in wound healing and fibrocontractive diseases. In: Clark RAF (ed.). *The molecular and cellular biology of wound repair,* 2nd edn. London: Plenum Press, 1996: 391–426.

82. Hom DB. Growth factors in wound healing. *Otolaryngologic Clinics of North America.* 1995; **28**: 933–53.

83. Clark RAF. Mechanisms of cutaneous wound repair. In: Fitzpatrick TB, Eisen AZ, Wolff K, Freedburg IM, Austin KF (eds). *Dermatology in general medicine,* 4th edn. New York: McGraw-Hill, 1993b: 473–86.

84. Kurkinen M, Vaheri A, Roberts PJ, Stenman S. Sequential appearance of fibronectin and collagen in experimental granulation tissue. *Laboratory Investigation.* 1980; **43**: 47–51.

85. Granstein RD, Murphy GF, Margolis RJ, Byrne MH, Amento EP. Gamma interferon inhibits collagen synthesis *in vivo* in the mouse. *Journal of Clinical Investigation.* 1987; **79**: 1254–8.

86. Clark RAF, Nielsen LD, Welch MP, McPherson JM. Collagen matrices attenuate the collagen synthetic response of cultured fibroblasts to TGFβ. *Journal of Cell Science.* 1995; **108**: 1251–61.

87. Peacock EE. Contraction. In: Peacock EE (ed.). *Wound repair,* 3rd edn. Philadelphia: WB Saunders, 1984: 39–55.

88. Gabbiani G, Ryan GB, Majno G. Presence of modified fibroblasts in granulation tissue, and their possible role in wound contraction. *Experientia.* 1971; **27**: 549–51.

89. Ehrlich HP, Rajaratnam JBM. Cell location forces versus cell contraction forces, for collagen lattice contraction. An *in vitro* model for wound contraction. *Tissue and Cell.* 1990; **22**: 407–11.

90. Rudolph R. Contraction and the control of contraction. *World Journal of Surgery.* 1980; **4**: 279–87.

91. Stopak D, Harris AK. Connective tissue morphogenesis by fibroblast traction I; tissue culture observations. *Developmental Biology.* 1982; **90**: 383–7.

92. Ehrlich HP. Wound closure: evidence of cooperation between fibroblasts and collagen matrix. *Eye.* 1988; **2**: 149–57.

93. Darby I, Skalli O, Gabbiani G. α-smooth muscle actin is transiently expressed by myofibroblasts during experimentla wound healing. *Laboratory Investigation.* 1990; **3**: 21–9.

94. Alison MR. Repair and regenerative responses. In: McGee J, Isaacson PG, Wright NA *et al.* (eds). *Oxford textbook of pathology; Volume 1 Principles of pathology.* Oxford: Oxford University Press, 1992: 365–88.

95. Findlay JK. Angiogenesis in reproductive tissues. *Journal of Endocrinology.* 1986; **111**: 357–66.

96. Folkman J, Shing T. Angiogenesis. *Journal of Biological Chemistry.* 1992; **267**: 10931–4.

97. Koch AE, Polverini PJ, Kunkel SL, Harlow LA, DiPietro LA, Elner VM *et al.* Interleukin 8 as a macrophage-derived mediator of angiogenesis. *Science.* 1992; **258**: 1798–801.

98. Imre G. Studies on the mechanism of retinal neovascularization. Role of lactic acid. *British Journal of Ophthalmology.* 1964; **48**: 75–82.

99. Zauberman H, Michaelson IC, Bergmann F, Maurice DM. Stimulation of neovascularization of the cornea by biogenic amines. *Experimental Eye Research.* 1969; **8**: 77–83.

100. Knighton DR, Hunt TK, Schevenstuhl H, Halliday BJ, Werb Z, Banda MJ. Oxygen tension regulates the expression of angiogenesis factor by macrophages. *Science.* 1983; **221**: 1283–5.

101. Ishikawa F, Miyazono K, Hellman U, Drexler H, Wernstedt C, Hagiwara K *et al.* Identification of angiogenic activity and the cloning and expression of PD-ECGF. *Nature.* 1989; **338**: 557–62.

102. Yang EY, Moses HL. Transforming growth factor-β1-induced changes in cell migration, proliferation and angiogenesis in the chicken chorioallantoic membrane. *Journal of Cell Biology.* 1990; **111**: 731–41.

103. Weisman DM, Polverini PJ, Kamp DW. Transforming growth factor beta is chemotactic for human monocytes and induces their expression of angiogenic activity. *Biochemical and Biophysical Research Communications.* 1988; **157**: 793–800.

104. Battegay EF, Rupp J, Iruela-Arispe L, Sage EM, Pech M. PDGF-BB modulates endothelial proliferation and angiogenesis *in vitro* via PDGF β receptors. *Journal of Cell Biology.* 1994; **125**: 917–28.

105. Azizkhan RG, Azizkhan JC, Zetter BR, Folkman J. Mast cell heparin stimulates migration of capillary endothelial cells *in vitro*. *Journal of Experimental Medicine.* 1980; **152**: 931–44.

106. Shepro D, Morel NM. Pericyte physiology. *FASEB J.* 1993; **7**: 1031–8.

107. Orlidge A, D'Amore PA. Inhibition of capillary endothelial cell growth by pericytes and smooth muscle cells. *Journal of Cell Biology.* 1987; **105**: 1455–62.

108. Chvapil M, Koopman CF. Scar formation: physiology and pathological states. *Otolaryngologic Clinics of North America.* 1984; **17**: 265–72.

109. Levenson SM, Geever EF, Crowley LV, Oates 3rd JF, Berard CW, Rosen H. The healing of rat skin wounds. *Annals of Surgery.* 1965; **161**: 293–308.

110. Pickett BP, Burgess LP, Livermore GH, Tzikas TL, Voussighi J. Wound healing. Tensile strength vs healing time for wounds closed under tension. *Archives of Otolaryngology-Head and Neck Surgery.* 1996; **122**: 565–8.

111. Compton CC, Gill JM, Bradford DA, Regauer S, Gallico GG, O'Connor NE. Skin regenerated from cultured epithelial autographs on full-thickness burn wounds from 6 days to 5 years after grafting. A light electron microscope and immunohistochemical study. *Laboratory Investigation.* 1989; **60**: 600–12.

112. Bailey AJ, Bazin S, Sims TJ, Le Lous M, Nicoletis C, Delaunay A. Characterization of the collagen of human hypertrophic and normal scars. *Biochimica et Biophysica Acta.* 1975; **405**: 412–21.

113. Kischer CW, Shetlar MR. Collagen and mucopolysaccharides in the hypertrophic scar. *Connective Tissue Research.* 1974; **2**: 205–13.

114. Stricklin GP, Li L, Jancic V, Wenczak BA, Nanney LB. Localisation of mRNAs representing collagenase and TIMP in sections of healing human burn wounds. *American Journal of Pathology.* 1993; **143**: 1657–66.

115. Lovell CR, Smolenski KA, Duance VC, Light ND, Young SR, Dyson M. A study of Type I and Type III collagen content and fibre distribution in normal human skin during ageing. *British Journal of Dermatology.* 1987; **117**: 419–28.

116. Lennard-Jones JE. *A positive approach to nutrition as treatment.* Kent: King's Fund Centre, 1992.

117. Lennard-Jones JE, Arrowsmith H, Davison C, Denham AF, Micklewright A. Screening by nurses and junior doctors to detect malnutrition when patients are first assessed in hospital. *Clinical Nutrition.* 1995; **14**: 336–40.

118. McLaren SMG. Nutrition and wound healing. *Journal of Wound Care.* 1992; **1**: 45–55.

119. Zador DA. Nutritional status on admission to a general surgical ward in a Sydney hospital. *Australia and New Zealand Journal of Medicine.* 1987; **17**: 234–40.

120. Anderson L, Dibble MV, Tukki PR. *Nutrition in health and diseases*, 17th edn. Philadelphia: Lippincott Company, 1982.

121. Thomas B. *Manual of dietetic practice*, 2nd edn. Cambridge: The University Press, 1994.

∗122. Calvin M, Young SR. Estrogens and wound healing. In: Brincat MP (ed.). *Hormone replacement therapy and the skin*, Lancaster: Parthenon Pub., 2001: 155–69.

123. Young SR. 'The effect of therapeutic ultrasound on the biological mechanisms involved in dermal repair'. PhD Thesis, University of London, 1988: 169–74.

124. Saperia D, Glassberg E, Lyons RF. Demonstration of elevated type I and II pro-collagen mRNA levels in cutaneous wounds treated with helium-neon laser. *Biochemical and Biophysical Research Communications.* 1986; **136**: 1123–8.

125. Charles D, Williams 3rd K, Perry LC, Fisher J, Rees RS. An improved method of in vivo wound disruption and

measurement. *Journal of Surgical Research*. 1992; **52**: 214–8.

126. Young SR, Dyson M. The effect of therapeutic ultrasound on angiogenesis. *Ultrasound in Medicine and Biology*. 1990; **16**: 261–9.

127. Kundin JI. A new way to size up a wound. *American Journal of Nursing*. 1989; **89**: 206–7.

128. Covington JS, Griffin JW, Mendius RK, Tooms RE, Clifft JK. Measurement of pressure ulcer volume using dental impression materials. *Physical Therapy*. 1989; **69**: 68–72.

129. Berg W, Tranroth C, Gunnarsson A, Lossing C. A method for measuring pressure sores. *Lancet*. 1990; **I**: 1445–6.

130. Bulstrode CJK, Goode JW, Scott PJ. Stereophotogrammetry for measuring rates of cutaneous healing: a conventional technique. *Clinical Science*. 1986; **71**: 440–3.

131. Young SR, Lynch JA, Leipins PJ, Dyson M. Non-invasive method of wound assessment using high-frequency ultrasound imaging. Paper presented at the Sixth Annual Symposium on Advanced Wound Care. Health Management Publications, 1993: 29–31.

132. Young SR, Erian A, Dyson M. High frequency diagnostic ultrasound: a noninvasive, quantitative aid for testing the efficacy of moisturizers. *International Journal of Aesthetic and Restorative Surgery*. 1996; **4**: 1–5.

133. Chen L, Dyson M, Rymer J, Bolton P, Young SR. The use of high frequency diagnostic ultrasound to investigate the effect of HRT on skin thickness. *Skin Research and Technology*. 2001; **7**: 95–7.

134. Mirpuri N, Young SR. The use of diagnostic ultrasound to assess the skin changes that occur during normal and hypertensive pregnancies. *Skin Research and Technology*. 2001; **7**: 63–9.

∗135. Young SR, Ballard K. Wound assessment: Diagnostic and assessment applications – Part 2. In: Electrotherapy-evidence based practice. London: Churchill-Livingstone, 2001: 308–312.

136. Chen L, Dyson M, Rymer J, Bolton P, Young SR. Evaluation of the effect of HRT on skin thickness using high frequency diagnostic ultrasound. *Menopause Digest*, **14**. 2002: 24.

9

Skin flap physiology

A GRAEME B PERKS

Definition	110	The compromised skin flap	112
History	110	Physical interventions	114
Skin flap design	111	Key points	115
Blood flow	111	Best clinical practice	115
Vessel wall tension	112	References	115
Sympathetic innervation	112		

SEARCH STRATEGY

The data in this chapter are supported by a Medline search using the key words vasculature, vessel, physiology, skin flap and tissue transfer.

DEFINITION

A skin flap is a piece of tissue transferred from the donor site and inserted into the recipient site while maintaining a continuous attachment to the body (the pedicle). The flap may consist of skin and subcutaneous fat but could also include fascia, muscle, bone, nerve or any combination of these tissues. Although alive when transferred, the flap may subsequently die due to vascular compromise.

Microvascular flap reconstruction adheres to the same principles, except that the pedicle is created in the recipient site by microanastomoses of donor artery and vein to recipient artery and vein.

HISTORY

The origin of the term 'flap' is alleged to originate from the Dutch *Flappe* meaning as something that hung broad and loose attached only at one side.[1]

Reconstructive skin flap surgery owes a great deal to the work of the Indian Ayurvedic medical practice of nasal reconstruction. The following description is from the classical text on this surgery, the *Sushruta Samhita*:

> Now I shall deal with the process of affixing an artificial nose, the leaf of a creeper, long and broad enough to fully cover the whole of the severed or clipped off part, should be gathered, and a patch of living flesh, equal in dimensions to the preceding leaf should be sliced off (from down upward) from the region of the cheek, and after scarifying it with a knife swiftly adhered to the severed nose.[2]

This heralds Sir Harold Gillies' third principle 'Make a plan and a pattern for this plan.'[3] The English surgeon Joseph Carpue (1764–1840) is given credit for introducing the Indian forehead rhinoplasty technique into the English language text based on a letter to the editor in 1794 relating the nasal reconstruction of one bullock driver called Cowasjee. An extremely well-referenced discussion of the history of this flap reconstructive technique is given by Nichter *et al.*[4]

Greater understanding of skin flaps has occurred in both the anatomical descriptions of the blood supply and through pharmacological manipulation of the circulation.

In 1889, Manchot published on many of the distinct cutaneous vascular territories served by identified named arteries. Spalteholz[5] described the fasciocutaneous vessels, as well as those passing through muscle, and provided the origin of the concept of the musculocutaneous blood supply to flaps. In France, Salmon[6] added to these ideas by performing radiographs on cadaver skin following intraarterial contrast injection.

In 1963, McGregor and Morgan[7] described how skin flaps could be considered as axial or random and therefore the length to width ratio was given an anatomical basis. Having studied intraarterial fluorescine injections in 14 patients, McGregor and Morgan deduced that an axial pattern flap could be safely raised beyond the standard dimensions of a random pattern flap of 1:1 length to width ratio. They went on to postulate that changes in pressure between one territory and an adjacent territory could create the effect of reverse flow in the adjacent axial vessels. This was further developed by Taylor and Palmer[8] who postulated that each of the composite blocks (angiosomes) were connected by true anastomoses or reduced calibre 'choke vessels'. These choke vessels are analogous with the description by Salmon of 'retiform anastomoses' and as such are the defining limits of the vascular territories. They name the accompanying veins 'oscillating veins' in which flow could occur in either direction. In 1970, Milton[9] reported that 'the surviving length of flaps made under similar conditions of blood supply is constant regardless of width. The only effect of decreasing width is to reduce the chance of the pedicle containing a large vessel.' As contemporary researchers have contributed increasing amounts to the anatomy of the skin circulation, larger flaps can now be raised on smaller but specifically identified vessels.

SKIN FLAP DESIGN

Skin flaps can be advanced, rotated or transposed, and initially all flaps were random pattern flaps meaning that it was a random chance whether the specific vessel was included within the pedicle and substance of the flap. The design of flaps relied on fixed length to width ratios which varies from 1:1 in the lower extremity to 4:1 in the head and neck where the blood supply was recognized to be more extensive and therefore robust. Conversely, a flap could be raised as an island based entirely on a subcutaneous pedicle.

BLOOD FLOW

Flap survival depends on blood flow through the pedicle of the flap.[10] Although the fluid mechanics of blood flow are complex, certain factors applicable to the small vessels supplying the flap are well established.

Vessel blood flow (Q) is determined by:

1. pressure difference (ΔP) between the two ends of the vessel;
2. the resistance to flow (R) produced in the vessel.

The mathematical expression of this blood flow is:

$$Q = \frac{\Delta P}{R}$$

where the letters are as defined above.

The flow of blood through a smooth, straight vessel behaves as if there are concentric laminae, with the fastest flow in the centre creating a paraboloid wave front. The smaller the vessel becomes, the closer the central lamina becomes to the vessel wall. While this formula and lamina flow holds true for a straight, smooth vessel, any deformity, such as vessel angulation, branching, obstruction or intraluminal irregularity, will interfere with lamina flow. Disturbance in lamina flow is known as turbulence. Because all the flow is no longer in the same concentric laminae, fluid flowing across the direction of flow down the vessel will increase resistance to flow. Resistance to lamina blood flow in a vessel is created by marginal adherence of molecules to the vessel wall.

The smaller the vessel diameter, the closer the fastest flowing central lamina becomes to the margin. Therefore, these molecules become closer to the slow moving marginal molecules which increases the resistance to flow. The effect of reducing the vessel diameter can be expressed as mean velocity of flow (v) and is described in the formula:

$$v = \frac{\Delta P\, r^2}{8\eta\, L}$$

where v is velocity in cm/s; ΔP is pressure gradient (dynes)/cm^2; r is the radius of the vessel in cm; η is the viscosity in poises; and L is the length of vessel in cm.

The rate of blood flow through a vessel (Q) is related to the velocity of flow (v) multiplied by the cross-sectional area:

$$Q = v\pi\, r^2.$$

From this and the previous formula can be derived Poiseuilles' law:

$$Q = \frac{\pi \Delta P\, r^4}{8\eta\, L}.$$

Thus it can be seen that if $Q = \Delta P/R$ and $Q = \pi\Delta P\, r^4/8\eta\, L$ such that the resistance of a blood vessel (R) is:

1. directly proportional to the viscosity of the fluid and the length of the vessel;
2. the resistance is inversely proportional to the fourth power of the radius. Therefore the smaller

the vessel (r), the greater the resistance of the flow. Thus, any interference with the resting tone in the blood vessel, which reduces the vessel radius, will have a detrimental effect on blood flow.

$$R = \frac{8\eta\,L}{\pi\,r^4}.$$

Viscosity varies with the speed of blood flow; the faster the flow, the lower the viscosity because Poiseuille's law does not apply fully *in vivo*. The Fahreus–Lindqvist affect appears with reducing vessel diameter below 1.5 mm. The viscosity of blood in vessels narrower than 1.5 mm is so much smaller that viscosity in the capillaries is half that of large vessels. In a 100-micron arteriole, red blood cells are randomly orientated whilst within a 15-micron vessel more regular orientation of red cells occurs. Bloch[11] postulated that the vessel flow has a marginal layer with few cells and red cells congregate in the centre of the stream which reduces the viscosity of the layer in contact with the vessel wall. In the 10-micron capillary, the red cells travel in single file paraboloids, rather than the usual biconcave disc shape.

VESSEL WALL TENSION

From Laplace's law, the tangential vessel wall tension (T) is proportional to the vessel diameter (D) and the pressure exerted across the vessel wall (P) such that:

$$T \propto DP.$$

This has critical importance in a small vessel in which vessel diameter reduces, as does the pressure within the vessel. The vessel will collapse at the point when elastic tension in the vessel wall exceeds the transmural pressure (P). This is known as the critical closing pressure. Any increase in the resting tone in the blood vessel (spasm in the clinical setting) which reduces the vessel radius, will thus have a deleterious effect on blood flow.

The control of blood supply to skin flaps occurs predominantly in the microcirculation. These vessels include arterioles which provide two-thirds of resting systemic peripheral vascular resistance, and venules, capillaries and arteriovenous anastomoses which provide the remainder of the peripheral resistance. Skin capillaries are 10–20 microns in diameter; arteriovenous anastomoses have a diameter of 10–30 microns, while the blood flow through them is approximately 325 mL/100 g/min at 20°C.

Regulating the distribution of blood flow occurs at the arteriolar level at which the muscle wall tone is under dual (systemic and local) control, and has been well discussed by Folkow and Neil[12] and Daniel and Kerrigan.[13] Skin is not considered a 'vital' organ and therefore has little autoregulation mechanism by which blood flow is

maintained to an organ at all costs (unlike the brain or cardiac muscle). The basal vascular tone in the skin is a neural regulation of both sympathetic vasoconstrictor fibres and cholinergic fibres passing to sweat glands with bradykinin-mediated vasodilatation.

Humoral factors acting on the vessel wall include prostaglandin, bradykinin, histamine, norepinephrine, epinephrine, serotonin and $PGF_2\alpha$.

The external temperature is the most obvious physical mechanism acting locally on the skin blood vessel. Hypothermia will produce vasoconstriction and reduce blood flow, while hyperthermia will have the opposite effect. Increasing blood viscosity will reduce blood flow, but usually only at extreme conditions of low temperature such as seen in the digits. The myogenic response induced by myogenically active 'pacemaker' cells within the muscle wall is less influential in skin blood vessels because the skin vascular bed is weakly autoregulated.

Local metabolic factors acting on the vessel wall act to promote vasodilatation in response to hypoxia and acidosis, hypercarbia or hypercalaemia.

SYMPATHETIC INNERVATION

The vasomotor response of the autonomic nervous system produces noradrenaline release from sympathetic vasoconstrictor fibres in the walls of arterials, veins and arteriovenous anastomoses. Noradrenaline release produces an alpha adrenergic vasoconstriction. There is no parasympathetic innervation to the skin.

THE COMPROMISED SKIN FLAP

'The after care is as important as the planning' is the fifteenth principle postulated by Sir Harold Gillies.[14] His principle reads, 'How futile it is to lose flap or graft for the lack of a little postoperative care. If in any doubt about the progress slip your hands out of your pockets and get down to that haematoma.' This advice holds as true today as it did when the book was published, the most common cause for flap failure being failure to recognize a compromised circulation. Factors affecting flap survival can be considered as either extrinsic or intrinsic.

Extrinsic factors

External compression of the circulation to the flap is either due to a tight dressing, tension in the skin wound closure which more commonly occurs if the flap is angulated over an underlying rigid bony surface or soft tissue swelling, and this can be due to oedema or a postoperative haematoma. The flap is usually blue and engorged, indicative of venous congestion. The prompt release of tight bandages, dressings and removal of wound sutures may salvage the situation. In very exceptional circumstances, the flap may be repositioned back on to the donor site if there is concern that the pedicle has been kinked, thus following the old adage 'It is better to have a live flap out of position than a dead flap in position'. [*]

Intrinsic factors

Vasospasm in the flap following raising of the flap is a normal physiological response to reduce blood loss. Under normal circumstances, this vasospasm resolves without intravascular thrombosis because the spasm empties the lumen of blood. In the presence of intact endothelium, the coagulation cascade is not activated. Endothelial cell integrity plays a vital role in the maintenance of blood flow. Where flow to the flap is not established (or is compromised for a prolonged period of time) it has been shown experimentally in rabbits that 'no reflow' occurs after a period of several hours of ischaemia. This has become known as the 'no reflow phenomenon' coined by Ames et al. in 1968[15] and studied first in flap reperfusion in 1978.[16] In the no reflow phenomenon, reperfusion of the ischaemic tissue results in the formation of oxygen-derived free radicals. Furthermore, it has been shown that the vasodilator effect of acetyl choline is mediated through endothelial production of nitric oxide.[17] The net effect of acetyl choline following reperfusion in the presence of damaged endothelial cells is vasoconstriction.

Nitric oxide is produced by nitric oxide synthase from the amino acid L-arginine. Elegant experimental research in mice with targeted disruption of the inducible nitric oxide synthase (iNOS) gene (iNOS knockout mice) has shown pharmacological and genetic evidence that iNOS activity promoted survival of ischaemic tissue. The administration of nitro-L-arginine methyl ester (a constitutive NOS, endothelial NOS and neuronal NOS inhibitor) significantly increased flap survival in these mice.

In a pig ischaemia-reperfusion injury flap model, there was a disruption of constitutive nitric oxide synthase expression and activity, which may have led to decreased nitric oxide production.

A great deal of laboratory research has been undertaken to reduce flap failure by pharmacological means. Much attention has been paid to drugs that could act as 'free radical scavengers.' Superoxide dismutase has been shown to improve flap survival in animals,[18, 19] but not in humans. Angel and coworkers[20, 21] have been at the forefront of superoxide radical scavenger therapy, publishing work on the beneficial effects of the iron chelator deferoxamine. These benefits, however, occur with significant toxicity which can be ameliorated (in pigs) by the conjugated form, deferoxamine-hespan (DFO-H). DFO-H has a longer half-life, but with reduced efficacy in augmenting flap survival. This was postulated to decrease its ability to reach the intracellular oxygen free radicals.[22]

It has also been shown that allopurinol can augment flap survival.[23, 24] Allopurinol is a xanthine oxidase inhibitor, although elevated levels of xanthine oxidase and malonyldialdehyde have been noted to be elevated in ischaemic flap tissue in animals.[25] A beneficial effect has yet to be shown in humans. Innumerable other animal experiments have been performed on such things as antiadrenergic drugs[26] and magnesium–ATP (a supply of high energy phosphometabolites),[27] both approaches being designed to increase the levels of ATP in the tissues.

Other researchers have looked at prostacycline (PGI_2) and prostaglandin-E1 (PGE_1). Both cause peripheral vasodilatation and inhibition of platelet aggregation.[28, 29, 30, 31]

Endothelin-1 (ET-1) is an endogenous vasoactive (vasoconstrictor) peptide, produced in ischaemic flap tissues. In human microvascular breast reconstruction flaps, a statistically significant increase in (skin biopsy) tissue levels of endothelin-1 after clamping of the flap pedicle has been demonstrated. The authors concluded that endothelin-1 levels were elevated in free flaps following reperfusion.[32]

Recent studies have shown that this detrimental effect can be blocked in experimental porcine transverse rectus abdominis myocutaneous (TRAM) flaps by tezosentan, a new endothelin receptor blocker. The authors suggest that 'tezosentan improves oxygenation and metabolism in the jeopardized contralateral flap tissue, probably as a result of a decrease in venous vascular resistance and fluid extravasation'.[33]

This beneficial effect on the venous outflow would fit with observations on the sensitivity of the human musculocutaneous perforator vessels to vasoconstrictors and vasodilators in vitro. The vasoconstrictor potency of norepinephrine, endothelin-1 and a thromboxane-A_2 mimetic were shown to be significantly higher in the vein than in the artery, hence the maximal venous effect of ET-1 blockade.[34] The severity of tissue necrosis correlated well with tissue levels of ET-1 in rat skin flaps, whilst topical nifedipine antagonized the vasoconstrictive effects of ET-1.

Topical nitroglycerin (GTN) has also been shown to exert a greater vasodilator effect on the venous circulation than on arterial vessels. Rohrich and colleagues[35] reported improved survival of axial flaps in pigs and rats treated with nitroglycerin ointment. Topical GTN paste is used in clinical practice but with variable success. [*]

Direct smooth muscle relaxants nifedipine and verapamil increased flap survival in rats.[36, 37, 38] These are calcium-channel blockers which act on the vascular smooth muscles to cause vasodilation but are restricted in clinical practice to topical application on to microvascular anastomoses, as there is no trial evidence to support their systemic use.

Surgically induced neutrophil recruitment in skin flaps has been shown to impair flap survival experimentally in the rat.[39] Myeloperoxidase (a marker for neutrophil recruitment) was significantly reduced by low-dose intraperitoneal calcitonin gene-related peptide (CGRP) without affecting the circulating neutrophil count, with improved random pattern flap survival.

One Japanese group[40] have studied sulphatide which binds to P- and L-selectin, important in the initiation of neutrophil-endothelial interactions. Pretreated experimental skin flaps showed little histological evidence of leukocyte invasion compared to that in the dermal layer of control flaps 48 hours after flap elevation. They went on to show augmented protection against ischaemia-reperfusion in rat skin flaps when combining sulphatide with anti-rat ICAM-1 and anti-rat LFA-1 antibodies.

The monoclonal antibody to the primary neutrophil adherence-mediating glycoprotein CD18 improves the survival length of the random pattern flap. Histological examination 24 hours after reperfusion in the treated group demonstrated only slight leukocyte invasion into the flap, and myeloperoxidase activity 24 hours after reperfusion was significantly reduced. This study indicated that sulphatide and monoclonal antibodies combined protect rat skin flaps from ischaemia-reperfusion injury.[41]

The platelet glycoprotein IIb/IIIa receptor antagonist Abciximab promoted experimental skin flap survival secondary to blocked platelet activation/aggregation and decreased activated-platelet deposition on the vascular endothelium in the rat.[42] Thus, administration may save the skin flap from reperfusion injury after a long period of ischaemia.

Dimethylsulfoxide (DMSO) is the only substance which has been shown experimentally to improve flap survival in animals and then been supported in a randomized control trial of mastectomy skin flap survival by Rand-Luby et al.[43] [***] This is one of only two controlled trials referenced by the Cochrane database. The authors concluded that the topical application of DMSO safely reduced human mastectomy skin flap ischaemia.

The other clinical trial on the Cochrane database reported a selective phosphodiesterase III inhibitor (Amrinone) which prevents breakdown of cyclic adenosine monophosphate.[44] Statistically proven to improve positively the microcirculatory blood flow of transferred flaps, the authors proposed that this occurred by relief of intraoperative vasospasm. [***]

More recent work in rats by Pang et al.[45] concluded that the administration of exogenous vascular endothelial growth factor (VEGF) 'could protect flaps from ischemia-reperfusion injury through the regulation of proinflammatory cytokines and the inhibition of cytotoxic nitric oxide production'.

Adenovirus-mediated gene therapy with vascular endothelial growth factor delivered into the subdermal space of compromised epigastric skin flaps in a rat model has improved skin flap survival.[46] Viral transfection with subdermal injections of adenovirus-encoding VEGF (Ad-VEGF) was performed two days before flap elevation.

Compared with controls, a significant reduction in the area of necrotic and hypoxic zones of the flap was demonstrated following both local and midline subdermal injections of Ad-VEGF.

Others have reported that the survival of flaps treated with VEGF A165 or B167 cDNA was significantly greater than that of controls.[47] However, neither study could produce evidence that the mechanism was due to angiogenesis using light microscopy, microvessel count or angiography on the treated flap. This is in contrast with histologically demonstrated angiogenesis at the skin paddle–recipient bed interface following the subcutaneous administration of VEGF into the recipient bed of a skin tube flap.[48]

Further support for VEGF therapy comes from Kryger et al.[49] who showed that all routes of administration (systemic, subdermal into the flap, subfascial into the recipient bed and topical on to the recipient bed) improved survival of a full thickness random pattern flap in the rat compared with controls.

By contrast, Rinsch et al.[50] demonstrated that FGF-2, was more efficacious than either VEGF(121) or VEGF(165) in treating acute skin ischaemia and improving skin flap survival when delivered from encapsulated cells positioned under the distal flap.

Thus, with improved delivery strategies, VEGF and FGF-2 may have a role in the management of surgical ischaemia. However, novel gene therapies to improve flap survival have not yet been translated into clinical flap surgery.

Dextran and heparin have been shown to improve flap survival in experimental studies of microvascular anastomoses, but not in improving survival of a failing flap.[51, 52] [*]

PHYSICAL INTERVENTIONS

Surgical delay

The only well-established technique to improve skin flap survival is by the 'delay procedure' with which all surgeons should be familiar. 'Delay' is a surgical procedure that renders a flap partially ischaemic several days prior to its transfer in order to increase its viability at transfer. Though much debate exists regarding the actual mechanism of vascular delay, most agree that changes in the microcirculation play a key role.

The latest work by Dhar and Taylor[53] showed that when a flap is delayed, there is dilation of existing vessels within the flap, not ingrowth of new vessels. The maximal anatomic effect on the arterial tree occurs at the level of the reduced-caliber 'choke' anastomotic vessels that link adjacent vascular territories.

They describe 'an active process associated with both an increase (hyperplasia) and an enlargement (hypertrophy) of the cells in all layers of the choke artery wall and a resultant increase in calibre of these vessels.'

Tissue expansion can be considered a form of skin flap delay, where expanded porcine flaps showed 150 percent greater length survival compared with acute nondelayed flaps.[54] The expanded flaps had 50 percent greater length survival compared with delayed flaps. Angiography showed increased axial vessel calibre in the tissue expanded flaps, subsequently confirmed by Taylor's work. A controlled clinical trial of TRAM flap breast reconstruction confirmed by colour flow Doppler showed an increase in the diameter of flap vessels in which surgical delay was performed one month prior to transfer.[55] A lower flap necrosis rate was found using a delayed TRAM (7.1 percent) compared with a standard standard TRAM (30 percent). [***]

Lasers

Low energy helium-neon (He-Ne) laser irradiation has been shown to improve the viability of skin flaps in rats[56] and in clinical flap repair after avulsion injury.[57] [***] In rat capillaries and fibroblasts, proliferation was demonstrated histologically while clinical improvement was attributed to improved superoxide dismutase activity.

Leeches

Hirudo medicinalis, the medicinal leech, exerts its effect by injecting hirudin, a naturally occuring anticoagulant, into the affected part. In addition, leeches secrete hyaluronidase into the tissues, as well as a vasodilator, which contributes to prolonged bleeding. The main use for leeches is in the congested microvascular flap when there is no other way of improving venous outflow.[58] [**] Useful in selected cases, there is nonetheless a serious risk of secondary infection with the leech enteric organism *Aeromonas hydrophila* which can kill the skin flap. Antibiotic cover should be provided when using leeches.

KEY POINTS

- Despite a great deal of research into the physiology and pharmacological manipulation of failing or compromised flaps there is no consensus about the clinical application of any of the research methods described.
- Dimethylsulphoxide, amrinone and low energy laser may have a role to play in the prevention of flap ischaemia.

Best clinical practice

- ✓ The only well-proven techniques for augmenting flap survival are preoperative surgical delay or tissue expansion (Recommendation B).
- ✓ 'Prevention is better than cure' is as true today as it was in times past. Meticulous flap planning to preserve a reliable vascular pedicle and avoidance of any extrinsic postoperative compression is vital.
- ✓ Relevant biennial updates beyond the scope of this review can be obtained through *Selected readings in plastic surgery.*[59]

REFERENCES

1. Cormack GC, Lamberty BGH. *The arterial anatomy of skin flaps*. London: Churchill Livingstone, 1986: 2–4.
2. Sushruta: Sushruta Samhita. In: Bhishagratna, K. An English translation of the Sushruta Samhita, based on original Sanskrit text. Calcutta: Bose, 1907. Quoted in Nichter LS, Morgan RF, Nichter MA (eds). The impact of indian methods for total nasal reconstruction (Historical perspectives of plastic surgery). *Clinics in Plastic Surgery* 1983; **10**: 637–8.
3. Gillies H, Millard DR. *The principles and art of plastic surgery*, Vol. 1. London: Butterworth and Co. (Publishers) Limited, 1957: 49–63.
4. Nichter LS, Morgan RF, Nichter MA. The impact of Indian methods for total nasal reconstruction. *Clinics in Plastic Surgery*. 1983; **10**: 635–47.
5. Spalteholz W. Die verteilung der blutgefasse in der haut. *Archives d'Anatomie Physiologie*. 1893; **1**: 1–4.
6. Salmon N. Arteres de la peau, Paris: Masson, 1936. Quoted Taylor GI, Razzaboni RM (eds). *Michel Salmon anatomic studies*. St Louis, MI: Quality Medical Press, 1994: 13–17.
7. McGregor IA, Morgan G. Axial and random pattern flaps. *British Journal of Plastic Surgery*. 1973; **26**: 202–13.
8. Taylor GI, Palmer JH. The vascular territories (angiosomes) of the body: Experimental date and clinical applications. *British Journal of Plastic Surgery*. 1987; **40**: 113–41.
9. Milton SH. Pedicle to skin flaps: the fallacy of the length: width ratio. *British Journal of Surgery*. 1970; **57**: 502–8.
10. Gumley GJ. Chapter 7. In: O'Brien B McC, Morrison WA (eds). *Reconstructive Microsurgery*. London: Churchill Livingstone, 1987: 65–73.
11. Bloch EH. A quantitative study of the haemodynamics in the living microvascular system. *American Journal of Anatomy*. 1962; **11**: 125–53.
12. Folkow B, Neil E. 1971 Circulation. Oxford University Press, Oxford Ch 25 Cutaneous Circulation 449–65.
13. Daniel RK, Kerrigan CL. Skin flaps: an anatomical and hemodynamic approach. *Clinics in Plastic Surgery*. 1979; **6**: 181–200.

14. Gillies H, Millard DR. *The principles and art of plastic surgery*, Vol. 1. London: Butterworths, 1957: 15–20.

15. Ames III A, Wright LR, Kowada M, Thurston JM, Majno G. Cerebral ischaemia II. The no reflow phenomenon. *American Journal of Pathology*. 1968; **52**: 437–45.

16. May Jr. JW, Chait LA, O'Brien BM, Hurley JV. The no-reflow phenomenon in experimental free flaps. *Plastic and Reconstructive Surgery*. 1978; **61**: 256–67.

17. Furchgott RF, Zawadzki JV. The obligatory role of endothelial cells in the relaxation of arterial smooth muscle by acetylcholine. *Nature*. 1980; **288**: 373–6.

18. Im MJ, Manson PN, Bulkley GB, Hoopes JE. Effects of superoxide dismutase and allopurinol on the survival of acute island skin flap. *Annals of Surgery*. 1985; **201**: 357–9.

19. Manson PN, Narayan KK, Im MJ, Bulkley GB, Hoopes JE. Improved survival in free skin flap transfers in rats. *Surgery*. 1986; **99**: 211–15.

20. Angel MF, Narayanan K, Swartz WM, Ramasastry SS, Kuhns DB, Basford RE *et al*. Deferoxamine increases skin flap survival: additional evidence of free radical involvement in ischaemic flap surgery. *British Journal of Plastic Surgery*. 1986; **39**: 469–72.

21. Angel MF, Mellow CG, Knight KR, Coe SA, O'Brien BMcC. A biochemical study of acute ischaemia in rodent skin free flaps with and without prior elevation. *Annals of Plastic Surgery*. 1991; **26**: 419–24.

22. Hom DB, Goding Jr. GS, Price JA, Pernell KJ, Maisel RH. The effects of conjugated deferoxamine in porcine skin flaps. *Head and Neck*. 2000; **22**: 579–84.

23. Im MJ, Shen WH, Pak CJ, Manson PN, Bulkley GB, Hoopes JE. Effect of allopurinol on the survival of hyperemic island skin flaps. *Plastic and Reconstructive Surgery*. 1984; **73**: 276–78.

24. Angel MF, Ramasastry SS, Swartz WM, Narayanan K, Basford RE, Futrell JW. Augmentation of skin flap survival with allopurinol. *Annals of Plastic Surgery*. 1987; **18**: 494–8.

25. Angel MF, Ramasastry SS, Swartz WM, Narayanan K, Kuhns DB, Basford RE *et al*. The critical relationship between free radicals and degrees of ischemia: evidence for tissue intolerance of marginal perfusion. *Plastic and Reconstructive Surgery*. 1988; **81**: 233–9.

26. Jurell G, Hjemdahl P, Fredholm BB. On the mechanism by which antiadrenergic drugs increase survival of critical skin flaps. *Plastic and Reconstructive Surgery*. 1983; **72**: 518–25.

27. Zimmerman TJ, Sasaki GH, Khattab S. Improved ischaemic island skin flap survival with continuous intra-arterial infusion of adenosine triphosphate – magnesium chloride and superoxide dismutase: A rat model. *Annals of Plastic Surgery*. 1987; **18**: 218–23.

28. Emerson DJM, Sykes PJ. The effect of prostacyclin on experimental random pattern flaps in the rat. *British Journal of Plastic Surgery*. 1981; **34**: 264–6.

29. Zachary LS. Effects of exogenous prostacyclin on flap survival. *Surgical Forum*. 1982; **33**: 588.

30. Suzuki S, Isshiki N, Ogawa Y, Nishimura R, Kurokawa M. Effect of intravenous prostaglandin E1 on experimental flaps. *Annals of Plastic Surgery*. 1987; **19**: 49–53.

31. Sasaki GH, Pang CY. Experimental evidence for involvement of prostaglandins in viability and acute skin flaps: effects on viability and mode of action. *Plastic and Reconstructive Surgery*. 1981; **67**: 335–40.

32. Lantieri LA, Carayon A, Maistre O, Evrin J, Hemery F, Torossian JM *et al*. Tissue and plasma levels of endothelin in free flaps. *Plastic and Reconstructive Surgery*. 2003; **111**: 85–91.

33. Erni D, Wessendorf R, Wettstein R, Schilling MK, Banic A. Endothelin receptor blockade improves oxygenation in contralateral TRAM flap tissue in pigs. *British Journal of Plastic Surgery*. 2001; **54**: 412–8.

34. Zhang J, Lipa JE, Black CE, Huang N, Nelligan PC, Ling FT *et al*. Pharmacological characterization of vasomotor activity of human musculocutaneous perforator artery and vein. *Journal of Applied Physiology*. 2000; **89**: 2268–75.

35. Rohrich R, Cherry GW, Spira M. Enhancement of skin-flap survival using nitroglycerin ointment. *Plastic and Reconstructive Surgery*. 1984; **73**: 943–8.

36. Hira M, Tajima S, Sano S. Increased survival length of experimental flap by calcium antagonist nifedipine. *Annals of Plastic Surgery*. 1990; **24**: 45–8.

37. Pal S, Khazanchi RK, Moudgil K. An experimental study on the effect of nifedipine on ischaemic skin flap survival in rats. *British Journal of Plastic Surgery*. 1991; **44**: 299–301.

38. Carpenter RJ, Angel MF, Amiss LR. Verapamil enhances the survival of primary ischemic venous obstructed rodent skin flaps. *Archives of Otolaryngology – Head and Neck Surgery*. 1993; **119**: 1015–7.

39. Jansen GB, Torkvist L, Lofgren O, Raud J, Lundeberg T. Effects of calcitonin gene-related peptide on tissue survival, blood flow and neutrophil recruitment in experimental skin flaps. *British Journal of Plastic Surgery*. 1999; **52**: 299–303.

40. Akamatsu J, Ueda K, Tajima S, Nozawa M. Sulfatide elongates dorsal skin flap survival in rats. *The Journal of Surgical Research*. 2000; **92**: 36–9.

41. Ueda K, Nozawa M, Nakao M, Miyasaka M, Byun SI, Tajima S. Sulfatide and monoclonal antibodies prevent reperfusion injury in skin flaps. *The Journal of Surgical Research*. 2000; **88**: 125–9.

42. Kuo YR, Jeng SF, Wang FS, Huang HC, Wei FC, Yang KD. Platelet glycoprotein IIb/IIIa receptor antagonist (abciximab) inhibited platelet activation and promoted skin flap survival after ischemia/reperfusion injury. *The Journal of Surgical Research*. 2002; **107**: 50–5.

43. Rand-Luby L, Pommier RF, Williams ST, Woltering EA, Small KA, Fletcher WS. Improved outcome of surgical flaps treated with topical dimethylsulfoxide. *Annals of Surgery*. 1996; **224**: 583–9.

44. Ichioka S, Nakatsuka T, Ohura N, Sato Y, Harii K. Clinical use of amrinone (a selective phosphodiesterase III inhibitor) in reconstructive surgery. *Plastic and Reconstructive Surgery*. 2001; **108**: 1931–7.

45. Pang Y, Lineaweaver WC, Lei MP, Oswald T, Shamburger S, Cai Z et al. Evaluation of the mechanism of vascular endothelial growth factor improvement of ischemic flap survival in rats. *Plastic and Reconstructive Surgery.* 2003; 112: 556–64.

46. Lubiatowski P, Goldman CK, Gurunluoglu R, Carnevale K, Siemionow M. Enhancement of epigastric skin flap survival by adenovirus-mediated VEGF gene therapy. *Plastic and Reconstructive Surgery.* 2002; 109: 1986–93.

47. O'Toole G, MacKenzie D, Lindeman R, Buckley MF, Marucci D, McCarthy N et al. Vascular endothelial growth factor gene therapy in ischaemic rat skin flaps. *British Journal of Plastic Surgery.* 2002; 55: 55–8.

48. Zhang F, Richards L, Angel MF, Zhang J, Liu H, Dorsett-Martin W et al. Accelerating flap maturation by vascular endothelium growth factor in a rat tube flap model. *British Journal of Plastic Surgery.* 2002; 55: 59–63.

49. Kryger Z, Zhang F, Dogan T, Cheng C, Lineaweaver WC, Buncke HJ. The effects of VEGF on survival of a random flap in the rat: examination of various routes of administration. *British Journal of Plastic Surgery.* 2000; 53: 234–9.

50. Rinsch C, Quinodoz P, Pittet B, Alizadeh N, Baetens D, Montandon D et al. Delivery of FGF-2 but not VEGF by encapsulated genetically engineered myoblasts improves survival and vascularization in a model of acute skin flap ischemia. *Gene Therapy.* 2001; 8: 523–33.

51. Salemark L, Knudsen F, Dougan P. The effect of dextran 40 on patency following severe trauma in small arteries and veins. *British Journal of Plastic Surgery.* 1995; 48: 121–6.

52. Cox GW, Runnels S, Hsu HSH, Das SK. A comparison of heparinised saline irrigation solutions in a model of microvascular thrombosis. *British Journal of Plastic Surgery.* 1992; 45: 345–8.

53. Dhar SC, Taylor GI. The delay phenomenon: the story unfolds. *Plastic and Reconstructive Surgery.* 1999; 104: 2079–91.

54. Saxby PJ. Survival of axial pattern flaps after tissue expansion: A pig model. *Plastic and Reconstructive Surgery.* 1988; 81: 30–4.

55. Ribuffo D, Muratori L, Antoniadou K, Fanini F, Martelli E, Marini M et al. A hemodynamic approach to clinical results in the TRAM flap after selective delay. *Plastic and Reconstructive Surgery.* 1997; 99: 1706–14.

56. Amir A, Solomon AS, Giler S, Cordoba M, Hauben DJ. The influence of helium-neon laser irradiation on the viability of skin flaps in the rat. *British Journal of Plastic Surgery.* 2000; 53: 58–62.

57. Luo Q, Xiong MG, Gu H. Effect of intravascular low level laser irradiation used in avulsion injury. *Chinese Journal of Reparative and Reconstructive Surgery.* 2000; 14: 7–9. *Plastic Surgery,* 53: 58–62.

58. Batchelor AGG, Davison P, Sully L. British Journal of Plastic Surgery. *The salvage of congested skin flaps by the application of leeches.* 1984; 37: 358–60.

59. *Selected Readings in Plastic Surgery,* ISSN 0739-5523, www.srps.org/index.html

10

Biomaterials, tissue engineering and their applications

COLIN A SCOTCHFORD, MATTHEW EVANS AND ARCHANA VATS

Introduction	118	Key points	127
Biocompatibility	119	Deficiencies in current knowledge and areas for future	
Tissue engineering	122	research	127
Conclusion	126	References	128

SEARCH STRATEGY

The data in this chapter are supported by a PubMed search using the key terms biomaterials, implants, tissue engineering, otology, rhinology, laryngology and otorhinolaryngology.

INTRODUCTION

Biomaterials have been defined as nonviable materials used in medical devices intended to interact with biological systems,[1] the aim being to replace or repair tissues. Many materials have been used in such roles, with the use of materials such as gold in dental applications being one of earliest described. Polymeric materials were used in dentistry and cardiovascular surgery around the middle of the twentieth century and this was paralleled by the use of metals and polymers in orthopaedics, leading to the Charnley total hip prosthesis in the early 1960s. The term 'biomaterials' was, however, not coined until the late 1960s and the Society for Biomaterials was formed in 1975, reflecting the growing field of biomaterial science.

In the field of otorhinolaryngology (ORL), the use of biomaterials has paralleled the development that has occurred with biomaterials in other fields such as dentistry, cardiovascular and orthopaedic surgery. Early applications were found in reconstructive middle ear surgery using materials such as vinyl-acrylic, polyethylene, polytetrafluoroethylene (PTFE) polyamide and stainless steel wire.[2, 3] Despite initial improvements in middle ear

reconstruction, early attempts were disappointing due to extrusion.[3, 4] It was not until the 1980s that biomaterial ossicular prostheses provided acceptable results with the introduction of hydroxyapatite devices.[3, 5] Hydroxyapatite, along with metals such as titanium, has also found applications in skeletal augmentation and reconstruction, whereas a range of polymers have been used in soft tissue augmentation and reconstruction. [***/**]

The field of biomaterials science is by necessity an interdisciplinary area. For the successful development and deployment of medical devices, a variety of critical areas need to be understood and optimized. These include toxicology, implant design, surgical technique, sterility, implant movement, biodegradation and the biological reaction to implant surfaces. Whilst it is true that there is tension between the surgical requirements and the properties that materials possess for many current applications, the majority of these areas have a good knowledge base. There remains, however, a poor understanding of the biological reaction to implant surfaces at the molecular level. Considerable research is currently being undertaken in this area, in parallel with efforts to tailor novel materials with specific properties, in an effort to engineer a third generation of biomaterials that better match their proposed function.[6] Whilst the previous generations of biomaterials were used primarily for tissue replacement, being selected for inertness or subsequently bioactivity, the emphasis is now on tissue repair, stimulating specific cellular responses at the molecular level, as highlighted by the developing field of tissue engineering.

BIOCOMPATIBILITY

Biomaterial and implant biocompatibility are essential requirements for the success of an implanted device. The concept of biocompatibility goes much further than merely assessing the cytotoxicity of a material, but takes into account the reaction of the body to the implant and, of equal importance, the reaction of the implant to the body. Indeed, biocompatibility has been defined as the ability of a material to perform with an appropriate host response in a specific application,[1] implying that materials may be defined in terms of their biocompatibility for specific applications rather than making a general designation.

A key factor in the success or failure of a biomaterial in a specific application is the interaction between the biological milieu and the material surface. Biomaterials have been classified according to the manner of interfacial reaction. A biomaterial may be termed 'bioinert' if the body does not react at all to the implant material. It is biotolerant if, after the initial reaction, the implant is well tolerated, although walled off by a fibrous capsule (almost all bionert materials show a minimal biotolerant-type response) or bioactive if the implant has a biologically active surface which results in an intimate interfacial bond at the implant site.

These responses are associated with wound repair and foreign body reactions.[7, 8] The type and severity of any response may vary according to the class of biomaterial. With biotolerant materials, the fibrous capsule may be more extensive and associated with the presence of inflammatory cells. A material that is considered bioactive would typically form an intimate chemical bond with the surrounding tissue without an intervening fibrous capsule. The thickness of a fibrous membrane has been used to assess metal reactivity. Titanium typically provokes a very slight fibrous response. Bioinert ceramics generate a minimal tissue reaction, whilst bioactive ceramics tend to form a direct interfacial bond, for example, with bone. Polymeric materials without additives tend to be relatively inert. However, the tissue response to reactive polymers differs from that of reactive metals in that membrane thickness does not correlate well with polymer reactivity, being better assessed by the degree of necrosis and inflammation produced by an implanted polymer in the surrounding tissue.

Biomaterials may be divided into three main groups: metals, polymers and ceramics. These may be further divided into composites, degradable materials, synthetic and natural polymers. Each of the main groups of materials will be considered in turn as they all have applications relevant to ORL.

Metals

Metals were the earliest class of material to be used as a biomaterial and are largely involved in skeletal and dental applications. The three main classes of metals and alloys currently used to construct surgical implants are:

1. 316L stainless steel;
2. cobalt-chromium (Vitallium being the trade name of the most popular formulation for surgical implants);
3. titanium and titanium alloys.

Metal plates are utilized for skeletal repair, based on their ability to match the supportive and protective functions of bone. However, other properties besides strength, such as corrosion resistance and biocompatibility, require consideration. Titanium is the preferred implant metal for craniomaxillofacial skeletal repair.

The effective use of stainless steel in the maxillofacial region is limited to wires, pins and plates.[9] Whilst possessing adequate physical properties for most maxillofacial applications, stainless steel loses its biocompatibility over time, has the potential for stress-shielding if it is not removed and has the greatest degree of corrosion of all the metals used for implantation. In contrast, titanium forms a stable titanium oxide layer on its surface upon exposure to oxygen. This is renewed even in biological fluids and allows titanium implants to remain chemically inert and stable to corrosion. Titanium has the additional advantage of osseointegration and when implanted in bone, the bone will grow in intimate proximity to the implant resulting in a permanent solid implant.[9] [***/**]

Both stainless steel and Vitallium are also known to leach nickel, chromium and molybdenum into surrounding tissues. Titanium plates release titanium dioxide, but no adverse reactions to this have been identified and titanium also possesses advantages in terms of imaging characteristics.[10] [***/**]

In ORL applications, titanium has been used for ossicular prostheses and virtually all long-term clinical studies have been favourable.[11] Migration or slippage of the ossicular prosthesis has replaced extrusion as the most common cause of failure that occurs with other prostheses, other than host factors.[12] A recent clinical study reported the extrusion rate to be less than 1 percent and these were associated with resorption of the interposed cartilage layer.[13] The main area of development has been in the design of the prosthesis, with the strength of titanium allowing for variety in the shapes and sizes of implant that can be machined. Both stainless steel and titanium are utilized in implantable hearing devices as coatings, wires, electrodes and casings. [***/**]

Ceramics

Ceramics can broadly be described as refractory poly-crystalline compounds, typically with high compressive strength. Ceramic biomaterials range from being relatively bioinert to bioactive. Attention will also be given to glass ceramics and ceramic-containing composite materials in this section. Bioactive ceramics, glasses and glass ceramics have long been known to interact and bond to living bone. Calcium phosphate-based bioceramics have been used for over 20 years as implants, in periodontal treatment, alveolar ridge augmentation, orthopaedics, maxillofacial surgery and ORL.

Hydroxyapatite (HA) is the most common calcium phosphate bioceramic used in ORL applications. It is similar in chemical composition to the inorganic constituents of living bone. Hydroxyapatite use in ORL was adapted from the field of dentistry and pioneered by Professor Jan Grote and others in the form of prosthetic ossicles for middle ear surgery. Development programmes with animal models indicated good integration without signs of extrusion.[14] These results have been shown to be consistent with studies in humans. For example, Goldenberg and colleagues reported that a HA/Plastipore hybrid implant for tympanoplasty can be placed in direct contact with the tympanic membrane without the requirement for an intervening tissue layer to prevent extrusion.[15] Evaluation of long-term clinical outcome using hydroxyapatite hybrid prostheses indicate stable hearing results with low extrusion (5 percent). Extrusion rates have been shown to rise when prostheses are placed in contact with the tympanic membrane, but this can be reduced (13.2–1.9 percent) by the interposition of autologous cartilage.[16, 17] Hydroxyapatite has also been used in a porous form as a canal wall prosthesis.[18] [***/**]

Composites containing hydroxyapatite have found ORL applications. Commercial examples of these include HAPEX, a high-density polyethylene (HDPE)/hydroxyapatite composite and Flex HA, a silicone rubber/hydroxyapatite combination. Applications for these include middle ear implants and skeletal augmentation (**Figure 10.1**).

For example, HAPEX has been used for an ossicular replacement prosthesis,[19] combining HA biocompatibility with mechanical advantages conferred by the composite form.[20] Hapex is a homogenous, osteoconductive biomaterial that is comprised of 40 percent hydroxyapatite and 60 percent polyethylene by volume. This results in a material that approximates the mechanical strength of cortical bone, yet is soft enough to cut with a knife. HAPEX also has good sound conduction properties because of its rigidity. [***]

Whilst hydroxyapatite remains the only ceramic that is widely used on a commercial basis for ORL applications, several other biomaterials require attention within this category. Two silicates (glass ceramics)

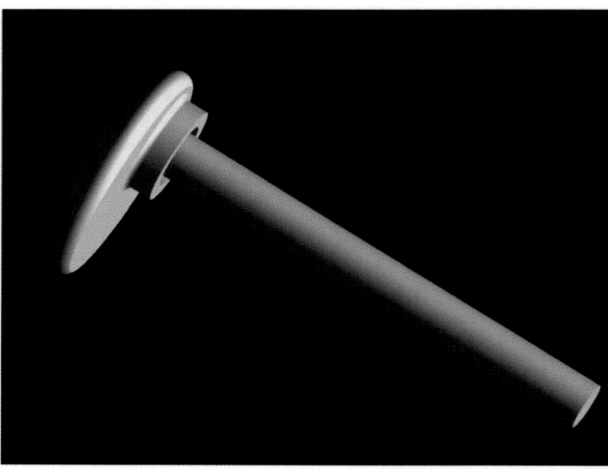

Figure 10.1 An example of a Richards OC HAPEX total ossicular replacement prosthesis. Courtesy of Gyrus ENT, Bartlett, TN, USA.

with middle ear applications are Bioglass and Ceravital®.[20, 21] Such materials demonstrate bioactive properties in that, on implantation, they develop an apatite-rich gel layer that results in deposition of collagen and bone mineral, producing a chemical bonding between implant and tissue. This interfacial response has been exploited in ossicular replacement and canal wall surgery. [****/***]

Ionomer cements are hybrid glass polymer composites formed by the neutralization reaction of a basic ion leachable inorganic glass and an organic polyelectrolyte (polyacrylic acid). Their properties include high compressive strength, the release of potentially osteoconductive ions such as calcium and fluoride, chemical adhesion to bone and metal and the ability to mould and shape to an implant site. Ionomer cements are established restorative dental materials and have been used as preformed implants and cements in ORL and cranial surgery.[22, 23] Possible complications include central nervous system (CNS) disturbances due to leakage of aluminum ions when the cement is in contact with cerebrospinal fluid (CSF), damage to structures (e.g. facial nerves, inner ear) by direct contact, foreign-body reaction and deficient wound healing of structures over implanted cement.[24] The successful clinical use of glass ionomer cement (GIC), both as bone cements and as preformed implants for hard tissue replacement, have been reported in cochlear implant fixation, the repair of the tympanic chain and eustachian tube obliteration. They have also been used for prosthetic implants such as ear ossicles, and as a bone substitute for oral and reconstructive surgery, for example Serenocem[TM25] (**Figure 10.2**).

The major application in otological surgery, where GICs have no near rival for clinical efficacy, is in the reconstruction of the ossicular chain, and where the cement can be used to repair the bony ossicles in their normal position and cement cochlear implants.[25] [***/**]

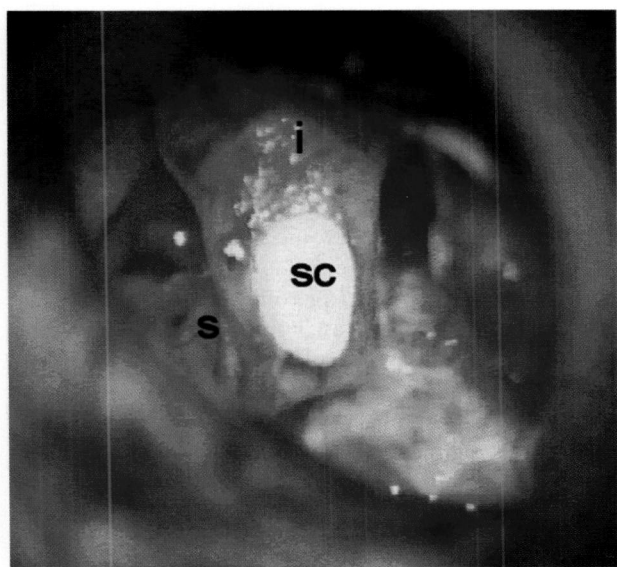

Figure 10.2 An example of ossicular chain repair using SerenoCem™ glass ionomer cement (sc). Incus (i) and crus anterior stapes (s) are indicated. Courtesy of Corinthian Medical Ltd, Nottingham, UK.

Polymers

There are many forms of polymer, both natural and synthetic, and a wide variety have been tested as some form of surgical implant. For a biomaterial implant, a polymer needs to be selected or developed, which has properties that are close to those required for a particular application.

Polymers possess certain advantages for use as biomaterials, including:

- variety of mechanical and physical properties;
- malleability;
- moderate inertness to host tissue;
- reasonable cost.

Their disadvantages include:

- general nonbiocompatibility (due to the leaching of toxic substances);
- a lack of resistance to the harsh tissue environment.[26]

Polymers have been extensively used in ORL for middle ear surgery, where they have been used as ossicular replacement prostheses, but their performance has varied. Synthetic polymers that have seen application in this regard include PTFE and polyethylene (PE).

Proplast is a PTFE-based material whose initial embodiment as an ossicular replacement was as a spongy graphite composite, but which evolved to include both alumina and hydroxyapatite. It was removed from the US market after released particulate debris led to many chronic inflammatory responses following implantation

in vivo.[26] A PTFE-based material used as a stapes prosthesis that is not reactive with the tissue, is Teflon. However, this feature can lead to slippage of the device if not placed properly.[27] [***/**]

Plastipore and Medpore are trade names for HDPE implants. They are noncompressive, chemically inert sponges that permit soft-tissue and bone ingrowth.[26] Two basic prosthesis types have been used in middle ear reconstructive surgery: total ossicular replacement prosthesis (TORP) and partial ossicular replacement prosthesis (PORP).

For all these synthetic polymer prostheses used in ossicular reconstruction, the major failing has been high extrusion rates in long-term clinical studies.[11] The insertion of a thin sheet of tissue (autograft cartilage) between the head of the prosthesis and the tympanic membrane can help reduce the extrusion of Plastipore implants.[28] Satisfactory long-term results with Plastipore using this procedure in large series have been reported by several sources (typical extrusion rates of 4 percent).[29, 30] [***/**]

PTFE has also been used in nasal dorsum surgery, both in injectable form and as a solid nasal dorsal implant.[31] A further application for PTFE been used in the form of Gore-Tex®, which has a long record of tissue compatibility by virtue of its use in vascular surgery. Gore-Tex sheets manufactured for facial surgery can be custom cut and layered to create a natural-appearing nasal dorsum.[32] Gore-Tex has also been used for facial reconstruction in areas including the frontal bone, orbital rim, malar complex and nasal tip. The mild foreign body reaction, minimal fibrous tissue ingrowth and its mouldable nature enables Gore-Tex to conform to surrounding profiles and lends itself to excellent visual tissue-filling capabilities with minimal palpability in subcutaneous augmented site.[33] However, Gore-Tex has been reported to have an infection rate of 2–3 percent.[34] [***/**]

Nasal reconstruction has also seen the application of polyethylene terephthalate (Mersilene) and HDPE (Medpore). Both implants allow tissue ingrowth, which reduces problems of implant mobility, but the stiffness of Medpore means it does not feel as natural over the nasal bridge.[32] Reported long-term clinical experience with Medpore used for nasal reconstruction and the correction of craniofacial deformity claim that 87 percent of patients remain free of complications.[35] [***/**]

Silicone is also of interest in ORL. A pure form of silicone rubber is marketed as Silastic. Clinical experience with Silastic as a solid silicone rubber implant in nonload-bearing areas (nasal dorsum, chin) is extensive. Complications of infection, migration, extrusion and changes in the overlying skin have been reported, occurring at widely varying incidence.[32, 36, 37] [***/**]

Silicone elastomer implantation has been used for medialization of a paralysed vocal cord. This proved more effective than Teflon injection, the shortcomings of which include its irreversibility and granuloma formation and acute reactions including erythema, fever, transient hoarseness and cervical lymphadenopathy.[38, 39] [***/**]

A further application for silicone elastomer is with the intracochlear electrode used in cochlear implants. The electronic unit is also covered by hard Silastic and sealed within a ceramic or titanium case, with further insulation of the electrode array by Teflon being necessary. Despite this range of biomaterials, there have been no documented cases of rejection of this type of cochlear implant.[40]

The advantages of silicone elastomer implants include shaping to precise dimensions at the time of surgery, the reversibility of the procedure and a more predictable result. However, concern is increasing regarding the safety and local and systemic effects of silicone implants.[38] [***/**]

TISSUE ENGINEERING

A large part of modern medical practice is aimed at the restoration of function by replacement of damaged or diseased tissues and organs. Replacement and repair is either by using artificial implants or by transplantation of tissues.[41] Such interventions are hindered by factors such as immune rejection, limited supply and donor site morbidity.

The fundamental premise of tissue engineering is the regeneration of tissues and restoration of function of organs through implantation of cells/tissues grown outside the body or stimulating cells to grow into an implanted matrix.[42] Tissue engineering has evolved from the use of biomaterials to repair or replace diseased or damaged tissue to using controlled 3D scaffolds in which cells can be seeded usually prior to implantation, as shown diagrammatically in **Figure 10.3**. This living tissue construct is functionally, structurally and mechanically equal (if not better) to the tissue it has been designed to replace.[42]

A major advantage with this approach is that tissues can be designed to grow in such a way that they precisely match the requirements of the individual in terms of size, shape and immunologic compatibility, minimizing the need for further treatment. The clinical success of the construct is largely dependent on the quality of the starting materials, i.e. scaffold composition, and of key importance is a suitable supply of cells. There are a number of different sources of cells that could be used for tissue repair and regeneration. These include mature (non-stem) cells from the patient, 'adult' stem cells from the patient such as bone marrow stromal (or mesenchymal) stem cells and embryonic stem (ES) cells/embryonic germ (EG) cells.[43] Scaffolds may be composed of polymers, metals, ceramics or composites. It is important to select a material that closely matches the properties of the tissue that it is to replace. Scaffolds intended to replace soft tissues such as skin, tendon, ligament, breast, eye, blood vessels and heart valves tend to be composed of natural and synthetic polymers. Replacement of hard tissues, such as bone and dentine, tend to use metals, ceramics, composites and polymers.

Characteristics of scaffolds

The primary function of a scaffold is to allow cell attachment, migration on to or within the scaffold, cell proliferation and cell differentiation. It must also provide an environment in which the cells can maintain their phenotype and synthesize required proteins and molecules. The characteristics required of scaffolds include high porosity, high surface area, structural strength, specific 3D shape and biodegradability if necessary. A porous structure provides an implant with two critical functions. Firstly, pore channels provide ports of entry for migrating cells or for capillary suction of blood. Secondly, a large area is available for specific and numerous cell interactions. An example of a porous scaffold, currently under investigation for bone repair,[44, 45] is shown in **Figure 10.4**.

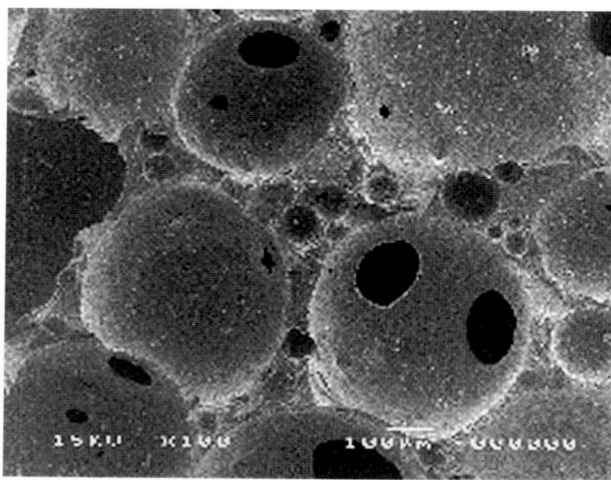

Figure 10.4   Scanning electron micrograph of a porous 58S bioactive glass produced using a foaming technique. Courtesy of Julian R Jones, Imperial College of Science, Technology and Medicine, London, UK.

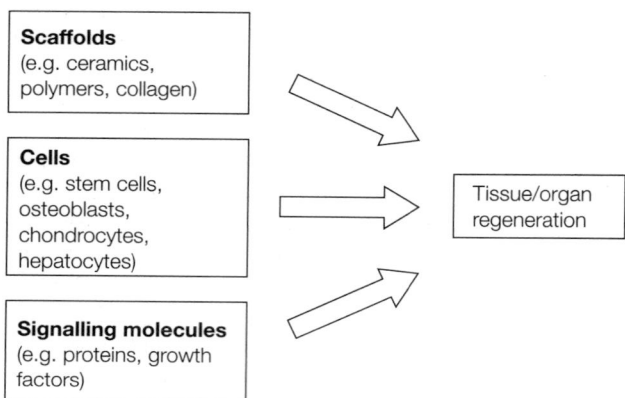

Figure 10.3   Key factors involved in tissue engineering.

Biodegradable materials are required for repair or remodelling and not necessarily long-term stability. Manufacturing feasibility, the ability to form final product design, and short-term mechanical properties with negligible toxicity from degradation products are prerequisites essential for these materials.

Types of scaffold materials

Materials can be subdivided into those derived from naturally occurring materials and those manufactured synthetically.

NATURAL MATERIALS

Examples of natural materials include collagen, glycosaminoglycans (GAG), chitosan and alginates. The advantages of natural materials are that they have low toxicity and a low chronic inflammatory response. They can be combined into a composite with other natural materials or synthetic materials (thereby having the mechanical strength of the synthetic material, as well as the biocompatibility of the natural material) and can be degraded by naturally occurring enzymes. The disadvantages, however, include poor mechanical strength, as well as a complex structure and hence manipulation becomes more difficult. They can be easily denatured and often require chemical modification, which can lead to toxicity.[46, 47, 48, 49] An example of a commonly used natural material is collagen. This is a major protein of the extracellular matrix, which is a component of connective tissues and can provide mechanical support. Collagen is a fibrous protein with a long, stiff, triple-stranded helical structure. The three predominant types are type I found in skin and bone, type II that is predominant in cartilage and type III which is predominant in the wall of blood vessels.[50]

As mentioned previously, natural materials often require chemical modification. Collagen can be modified to increase strength by a variety of methods including crosslinking by dehydrative methods or chemical methods, e.g. glutaraldehyde.[48, 51, 52] Collagen can also be made into a porous scaffold by freezing in a dilute suspension and then inducing sublimation of the ice crystals by exposure to a low temperature vacuum,[53] as shown in **Figure 10.5**. By adjusting the kinetics of ice crystal formation to the appropriate magnitude and direction, pores from the ice dendrites are eventually sublimed.[53]

Clinical applications of collagen scaffolds are highly relevant to otorhinolaryngological practice. These include the manufacture of sutures, haemostatic agents (powder, sponge, fleece), blood vessels (extruded collagen tubes), tendons and ligaments, dermal regeneration for burn treatment and peripheral nerve regeneration (e.g. porous collagen–GAG copolymer).[54]

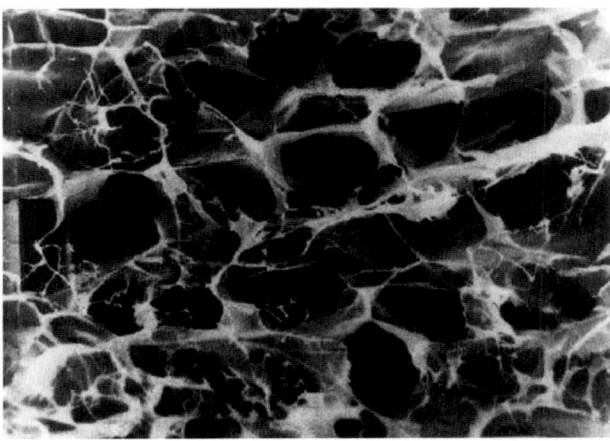

Figure 10.5   Collagen scaffold. Reproduced from Ratner *et al.*[53], © 1996, with permission from Elsevier Science.

SYNTHETIC SCAFFOLD MATERIALS

Polymers

Absorbable polymers include polyglycolide (PGA), polylactide (PLA) and polylactide-coglycolide (PLG) which are used for sutures and meshes, as well as polydioxanone which is also used for intramedullary pins. Nonabsorbable PTFE used in vascular grafts and periodontal inserts, nylon and polyethylene terephthalate (PET) used for sutures, meshes and vascular grafts (for a review of polymer applications see *Principles of tissue engineering*[55]).

Ceramics and glasses

Ceramics and glasses encompass a wide range of inorganic/nonmetallic compositions and are particularly used to repair or replace bone. **Table 10.1** shows examples of ceramics and bone tissue attachment to them.

Bioactive glasses

These are based on a silica (O–Si–O) network structure with ions such as calcium, sodium and phosphorus. Bioactive glasses have been investigated for applications in bone repair and engineering due to their ability to form a bond to living bone which has been attributed to the formation of a biologically active hydroxycarbonate apatite (HCA) layer.[56] This HCA layer is chemically equivalent to the inorganic part of bone.[57] Interestingly, they have been found to stimulate genes in osteoblasts[58] causing upregulation of various osteoblast-specific genes.

There are two categories of bioactive glass: melt derived and sol-gel derived. Melt-derived glasses are produced by the melting and mixing of oxide components in a furnace. They are mainly quaternary such as Bioglass® (46.1 percent SiO_2, 24.4 percent Na_2O, 26.9 percent CaO and 2.6 percent P_2O_5). Bioglass can be cast into any shape or powder size and is commercially available as Novabone® (US Biomaterials, Jacksonville Beach, FL, USA).

Sol-gel-derived glass is manufactured by the mixing of alkoxide components in solution in a fume hood (sol).

Table 10.1 Bone tissue attachment to bioceramics.

Bioceramic	Bone tissue attachment
Single crystal Al_2O_3	Dense nonporous nearly inert ceramics.
Polycrystalline Al_2O_3	Bone growth into surface irregularities by cementing the device into the tissues or by press fitting into a defect (morphological fixation).
Polycrystalline Al_2O_3 Hydroxyapatite (HA) coated porous metals	Porous inert implants – bone ingrowth occurs that mechanically attaches the bone to the material (biological fixation)
Bioactive glasses Bioactive glass ceramics HA	Dense porous/nonporous surface reactive ceramics, glasses and glass-ceramics attach directly by chemical bonding with bone (bioactive fixation)
Calcium sulphate Tricalcium phosphate (TCP) Calcium phosphate salts	Dense porous/nonporous resorbable ceramics slowly replaced by bone

Adapted from Ratner et al.[53], © 1996, with permission from Elsevier Science.

Polymer reactions then form a silica network (gel). They are mainly ternary, binary or pure silica materials, which have a mesoporous texture with enhanced bioactivity and resorbability.

Types of scaffolds

Scaffolds can be manufactured in many forms to give their required characteristics for specific applications. Fibre scaffolds have a large surface area to volume ratio with high porosity. They can be used in conjunction with other scaffolds to form a composite with added strength. They can be tubular, e.g. for nerve, blood vessel and intestine, or solid. Fibres and fibre scaffolds are commonly composed of PLA, PGA, PLG or glass. Textile fabrics are produced from woven, nonwoven and knitted fibres and are composed of a wide range of natural and synthetic, absorbable and nonabsorbable fibres. They can be used for wound repair in the form of sutures and reinforcing meshes, tendons and ligaments.

Clinical applications

Each tissue type has specific requirements, which are due to the cell types within the tissue, the function of the tissue, mechanical requirements such as load and flexibility and finally, the specific environment in which the tissue is located.

BONE

Bone is an example where mechanical strength is a predominant feature required of the scaffold. It needs to be strong enough for load-bearing sites, yet not too strong as stress shielding problems may occur.[59] For osteoblasts

to undergo an ideal process of new bone formation, the scaffold must have interconnective porosity. The ability of the scaffold to be produced as a 3D anatomical shape is also an essential feature.

Successful bone repair in a sheep model has been accomplished using a coral scaffold seeded with in vitro expanded marrow stromal cells/mesenchymal stem cells[60] as shown in **Figure 10.6**. Formation of new medullary bone with mature lamella cortical bone was achieved. Coral is a natural exoskeleton where inorganic calcium carbonate grows on to a charged organized organic template and has been used in various clinical applications.[61, 62, 63, 64, 65] This natural ceramic has the best mechanical properties of the porous calcium-based ceramics due to its interconnected porous architecture, similar to that of spongy bone.[66, 67]

CRANIOFACIAL BONE (RECONSTRUCTIVE AND COSMETIC)

This is a nonload-bearing site and patient-specific shapes are crucial. An example of such an area is repair of the orbital floor. Success of this procedure is crucial for binocular vision. Titanium is used most frequently but has many disadvantages, such as migration of the implant and hence occasionally necessitating further surgery for extrusion. Although there has been a move towards degradable materials in recent years, these also have the disadvantage of losing their mechanical strength, leading to sagging of the implant and potential loss of binocular vision. Recently, research has focussed on the development of new composite materials for improved craniofacial bone repair, comprising polycaprolactone reinforced with phosphate glass-long fibres.[68, 69, 70] Ideally, machining of a patient-specific implant controlled by computerized tomography (CT) scan data from the patient would be standard manufacturing protocol in the future (**Figure 10.7**).

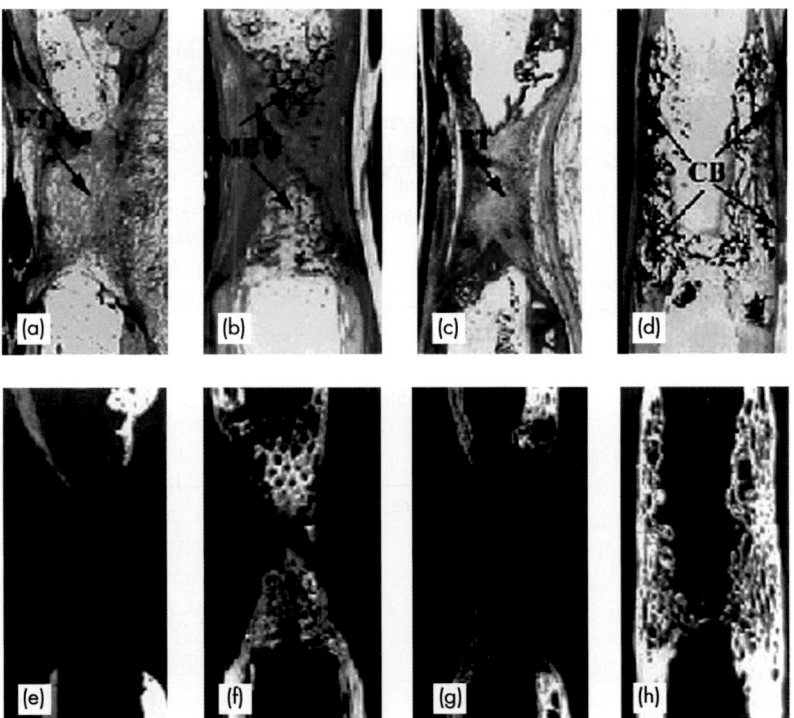

Figure 10.6   New bone formation using a cell–seeded coral scaffold. Microradiographs and photomicrographs after 16 weeks. Histological sections of defects (a) left empty or filled with (c) coral (e) coral-FBM (fresh bone marrow) and (g) coral-MSC. Fibrous tissue (FT) has invaded the defect in (a) and (e). In defects filled with coral alone (c), osteogenesis occurred within the medullary canal (MB). Defects filled with coral and MSC show cortical-like bone formation peripherally (CB). Cortical continuity was achieved between the edges of the defect. Microradiographs confirmed the histological observations. There was no bone formation in the defects left empty (b) or filled with coral-FBM (f). Bone formation occurred in the medullary area in defects filled with coral alone (d), but was insufficient for bone union. In contrast defects filled with coral-MSC (h) show osteogenesis chiefly at the periphery of the defect, leading to cortical bone union of the defect. Reproduced with kind permission from Petite *et al.*[60], © 2000, Nature.

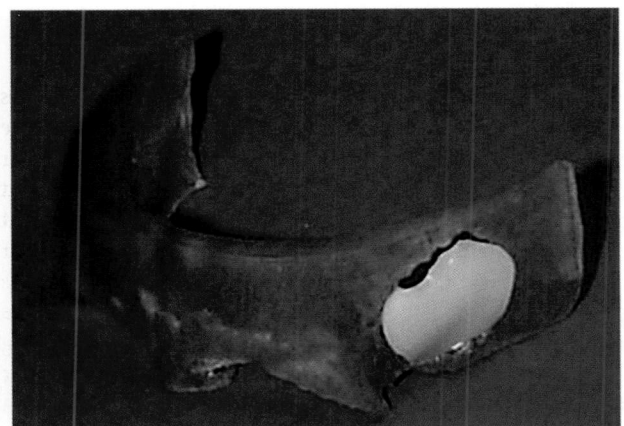

Figure 10.7   An example of the use of CT scan data in manufacture of a patient-specific implant (shown in white) for a skull defect. The image obtained from the CT scan data was manipulated via CAD and subsequently used to control machining of the implant. Courtesy of P. Christian, University of Nottingham, UK.

CARTILAGE

Cartilage is a nonvascular tissue and therefore has a limited capacity for self-repair. *In vivo* chondrocytes have a rounded morphology but often *in vitro*, become fibroblastic and lose their rounded phenotype and this may alter gene expression. Therefore, an ideal scaffold would retain the rounded morphology of chondrocytes. One such material that does possess this property is poly (ethylmethacrylate)/tetrahydrofurfuryl methacrylate (PEMA/THFMA),[71] which has been proposed as a material for cartilage repair.[72] Other materials that have been investigated for cartilage repair include hydrogels,[73] collagen matrices[74] and PGA/PLA.[75, 76]

The most widely held public perception of tissue engineering is research performed by Cao *et al.*[75] A scaffold was composed of PGA/PLA as a nonwoven mesh and produced in the shape of a human auricle. The mesh was then seeded with bovine articular cartilage chondrocytes and implanted into subcutaneous pockets on the back of athymic mice.

NERVE

Current surgical techniques employed to repair transected peripheral nerves, e.g. facial nerve, are based on suturing nonuniting ends. Improved nerve regeneration is facilitated by the use of conduits. Guided nerve regeneration would also be of benefit. This could be achieved by micropatterning polymer surfaces with extracellular matrix proteins or peptides or by a grooved topography, promoting cell adhesion and axonal outgrowth. Neuronal regeneration with conduit devices, including cellular components, e.g. Schwann cells, are currently being investigated.[77] For a review of this subject see Fine *et al.*[78]

VASCULAR

The replacement of small-diameter blood vessels by tissue-engineered vascular grafts is a further application that may be of benefit to the otolaryngologist-head and neck surgeon. For example, smooth muscle cells have been seeded into porous PGA tubes and then cultured under pulsing conditions of 165 times/minute.[79] The interior of the vessel is then coated with endothelial cells (**Figure 10.8**). Tissue-engineered arteries have lasted for more than three weeks without occluding in autologous pig models.

SKIN

A common application of tissue engineering is for the treatment of burn injuries. These cause loss of the skin's integrity, massive fluid loss and microbial invasion. Tissue engineering of skin would be applicable to ensuring adequate coverage in reconstructive surgery. Skin cells can regenerate and repair themselves in many instances, but deep second-degree (partial thickness) or third-degree (full thickness) burns have a decreased capacity for regeneration of tissue and can lose this capacity altogether.

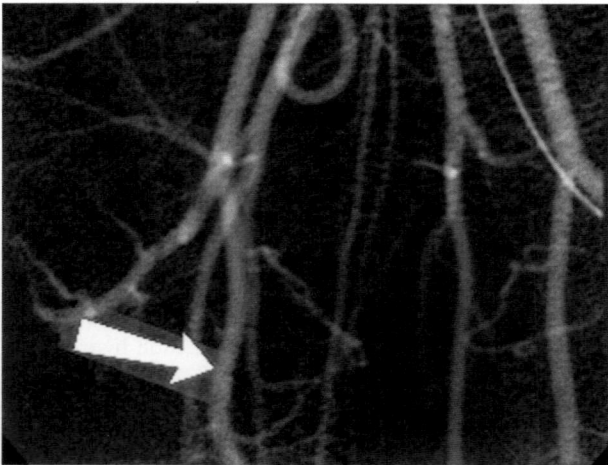

Figure 10.8 An example of a tissue-engineered blood vessel, which maintained successful function when implanted into a pig model. Reprinted with permission from Niklason *et al.*[79], © 1999, American Association for the Advancement of Science.

There are two well-known examples of skin regeneration scaffolds which are available commercially. They are Dermagraft® produced by Advanced BioHealing, Inc. (La Jolla, CA, USA)[80] and Apligraf® produced by Organogenesis (Canton, MA, USA).[81]

Dermagraft is produced by seeding stromal cells on to vicryl, a blend of PLA and PGA (produced by Johnson & Johnson, New Brunswick, NJ, USA). This scaffold is then kept under optimal conditions in a bioreactor where the cells multiply and produce collagen, ECM proteins and growth factors. Once it has served its purpose, the scaffold breaks down into glycolic and lactic acid, which is then transported away by the bloodstream and metabolized into CO_2, O_2 and H_2O. A 1-inch square sample yields cells sufficient for 250,000 square feet of final product, each 3×4 inch lot produces 1000 units of Dermagraft and is ready for use after 20 days of preparation.

This manufacturing process enables the skin cells to establish their natural organization and enables up to 200,000 units of Apligraf to be produced from a single piece of donated tissue (circumcized infant foreskin). Hence it is available to physicians upon demand, it is easy to use and does not require cryogenic storage.

CONCLUSION

Despite the relative successes in the use of biomaterials in ORL, there remain significant challenges where the desired parameters cannot be met using current materials. Other areas of the field can be said to be still in their infancy. For example, considering ossicular prostheses, whilst biocompatibility parameters are being established, little attention has been addressed to optimizing the acoustic properties of the material used. Similarly, in the field of tissue engineering, optimal materials and parameters are still to be established. Significant improvements in implant performance are associated with a corresponding development in materials, but for each new application of a biomaterial, testing to ensure safety and efficacy must be undertaken.[4] The most difficult and expensive development for a new medical implant involves materials that have no history as biomaterials, because of the costly and lengthy process of animal and human studies. The developments of new implants for use in ORL will be helped by people working in the area of biomaterials collaborating closely with clinicians. Areas which have posed a particular problem for biomaterials include repair of stenotic trachea, replacement of the larynx, total tympanic membrane replacement, accelerated mucosal healing after sinus surgery and reducing fibrous tissue formation after middle ear surgery. Biodegradable implants that promote tissue regeneration obviate the concern about long-term implant failure due to mechanical mismatch at the implant–tissue interface and show great promise for some of the above applications.

In tissue engineering, the search for a scaffold that will act as a template for tissue growth in three dimensions by having an interconnected macroporous network for tissue ingrowth, vascularization and nutrient delivery continues. The ideal scaffold would also bond to host tissue without formation of scar tissue, and influence the genes of the cells of the local tissue to enable efficient cell differentiation, proliferation and maintenance of the phenotype. Ideally, the scaffold would resorb at the same rate as tissue regeneration and be strong enough to withstand loading where necessary. An ideal scaffold would also be easily and cheaply manufactured and produced to ISO9001/FDA standards.

KEY POINTS

- Biocompatibility is defined as the ability of a material to perform with an appropriate host response in a specific application and is an essential requirement for the success of any implanted device.
- There are three main groups of materials that are used in ORL applications, i.e. metals, polymers and ceramics.
- Titanium is a widely used biomaterial in ORL applications. It has been used for ossicular prostheses with favourable clinical results, as the strength of titanium allows the implant to be manufactured into a variety of shapes and sizes.
- Hydroxyapatite, a calcium phosphate ceramic similar in chemical composition to the inorganic constituents of bone, is the most common bioceramic used in ORL applications, typically as a composite device with metals or polymers.
- Hydroxyapatite polymer composites have been used as implants for tympanoplasty in direct contact with the tympanic membrane, middle ear implants and skeletal augmentation.
- Polymer biomaterials have been extensively used in ORL applications for middle ear and facial reconstructive surgery, for example, total ossicular replacement prosthesis and nasal reconstruction.

Deficiencies in current knowledge and areas for future research

Biomaterials

The development of new materials is essential for progress in the field of implant technology. The majority of current commercial materials can be improved, whilst for certain conditions, for example laryngectomy, no candidate implant has been successful in restoring natural function. There is a general requirement for a greater understanding of the interfacial responses at the molecular level to improve the fabrication of the next generation of materials. Such materials are likely to include genetically engineered and immunologically prepared natural and synthetic substances, conjugates (probably bioresorbable)[26] or biomimetic materials.

It is anticipated that tissue repair will ultimately take over from tissue replacement, hence biomaterials will be utilized more as scaffolds or templates for tissue regeneration rather than using replacement materials. Such a shift will alter the properties sought from biomaterials.

Synthetic biodegradable polymers in the form of scaffolds are being increasingly used to engineer tissues to restore form and function. For example, a scaffold seeded with transplanted chondrocytes has potential for the regeneration of any cartilaginous structure possessing normal cartilage tissue. The scaffold must allow nutrient to pass to cells as well as maintain its 3D shape and have appropriate flexibility and strength. Polyglycolic acid (PGA) and polylactic acid (PLA) remain among the most widely used synthetic materials for such applications. PGA scaffolds, in preformed shapes, loaded with bovine chondrocytes have been implanted subcutaneously in athymic mice with the resulting tissue showing histological evidence of organized hyaline cartilage.[75, 82, 83] [**]

Natural polymers, such as alginates, have also been used to deliver chondrocytes for cartilage repair.[84] Natural materials may closely mimic the native cellular environment as they often comprise extracellular matrix components, whereas synthetic materials have the advantage of being able better to control material properties such as strength, degradation time, porosity and microstructure. Cellular attachment to these can be improved by modifying the polymer chemically or by coating it and growth factors to stimulate tissue formation can also be incorporated into such scaffolds.[85] [**]

Tissue engineering

Research is now focussing on 'third-generation biomaterials'[6] as materials for tissue-engineering scaffold production. When research into biomaterials began, materials were commonly inert. Research then began to focus on a second generation of bioactive materials that elicit action and reaction in the biological environment.[86] Now, however, there is a move to third-generation materials which stimulate specific cellular responses at the molecular level.[6] They are also bioresorbable and can be tailored to suit specific tissues.

REFERENCES

1. Williams DF. *Definitions in biomaterials. Proceedings of a Concensus Conference of the European Society for Biomaterials.* Amsterdam: Elsevier Science, 1987.
2. Emmett JR. Biocompatible implants in tympanoplasty. *American Journal of Otology.* 1989; **10**: 215–9.
3. Wehrs RE. Hydroxylapatite implants for otologic surgery. *Implants in Otolaryngology.* 1995; **28**: 273–86.
* 4. Portmann M. Management of ossicular chain defects. *Journal of Laryngology and Otology.* 1967; **81**: 1309–23.
5. Demane CQ. The development of implants and implantable materials. *Implants in Otolaryngology.* 1995; **28**: 225–34.
6. Hench LL, Polak JM. Third-generation biomedical materials. *Science.* 2002; **295**: 1014–7.
7. Clark RAF, Henson PM (eds). *The molecular and cellular biology of wound repair.* New York: Plenum Publishers, 1988.
8. Anderson JM. Inflammatory response to implants. *Journal of the American Society for Artificial Internal Organs.* 1988; **11**: 101–7.
9. Panje WR, Hetherington HE. Use of stainless steel implants in facial bone reconstruction. *Otolaryngologic Clinics of North America.* 1995; **28**: 341–9.
10. Ellerbe DM, Frodel JL. Comparison of implant materials used in maxillofacial rigid internal fixation. *Otolaryngologic Clinics of North America.* 1995; **28**: 325–40.
11. Yung MW, Brewis C. A comparison of the user-friendliness of hydroxyapatite and titanium ossicular prostheses. *Journal of Laryngology and Otology.* 2002; **116**: 97–102.
12. Goldenberg RA, Driver M. Long-term results with Hydroxylapatite middle ear implants. *Otolaryngology and Head and Neck Surgery.* 2000; **122**: 635–42.
13. Dalchow CV, Grun D, Stupp HF. Reconstruction of the ossicular chain with titanium implants. *Otolaryngology and Head and Neck Surgery.* 2001; **125**: 628–30.
14. Grote JJ. Reconstruction of the middle ear with hydroxyapatite implants. *Annals of Otology, Rhinology and Laryngology.* 1986; **95**: 1–12.
15. Goldenberg RA. Reconstruction of the middle ear using hydroxylapatite hybrid prosthesis. *Otolaryngology and Head and Neck Surgery.* 1992; **3**: 225–31.
16. Shinohara T, Gyo K, Saiki T, Yanagihara N. Ossiculoplasty using hydroxyapatite prostheses: long-term results. *Clinical Otolaryngology.* 2000; **25**: 287–92.
17. Kobayashi T, Gyo K, Shinohara T, Yanagihara N. Ossicular reconstruction using hydroxyapatite prostheses with interposed cartilage. *American Journal of Otolaryngology.* 2002; **23**: 222–7.
18. Weit RJ, Harvey SA, Pyle MG. Canal wall reconstruction: a newer implantation technique. *Laryngoscope.* 1993; **103**: 594–9.
19. Dornhoffer JL. Hearing results with the Dornhoffer ossicular replacement prosthesis. *Laryngoscope.* 1998; **108**: 531–7.
20. Merwin GE. Bioglass middle ear prosthesis: preliminary report. *Annals of Otology, Rhinology, and Laryngology.* 1986; **95**: 78–82.
21. Mangham CA, Lindeman RC. Ceravital versus plastipore in tympanoplasty: A randomised prospective trial. *Annals of Otology, Rhinology, and Laryngology.* 1990; **99**: 112–6.
22. Ramsden RT, Herdman RCD, Lye RH. Ionomeric bone cement in neuro-otological surgery. *Journal of Laryngology and Otology.* 1992; **160**: 949–53.
* 23. Babighian G. Use of glass ionomeric cement in otological surgery. *Journal of Laryngology and Otology.* 1992; **106**: 954–9.
24. Weber BP, Philipps B, Strauchmann B, Lenarz TH. Advances in the use of glass-ionomeric cement. *Journal for Otorhinolaryngology and its Related Species.* 1998; **60**: 111–5.
25. Brook IM, Hatton PV. Glass-ionomers: bioactive implant materials. *Biomaterials.* 1998; **19**: 565–71.
26. Dormer KJD, Bryce GE, Hough JVD. Selection of biomaterials for middle and inner ear implants. *Otolaryngologic Clinics of North America.* 1995; **28**: 17–27.
27. Slattery WH, House KW. Prostheses for stapes surgery. *Otolaryngologic Clinics of North America.* 1995; **28**: 253–64.
28. Emmett JR. Plasti-pore implants in middle ear surgery. *Otolaryngologic Clinics of North America – Implants in OTL.* 1995; **28**: 265–72.
29. Goldenberg RA, Emmett JR. Current use of implant in middle ear surgery. *Otology and Neurotology.* 2001; **22**: 145–52.
30. House JW, Teufert KB. Extrusion rates and ghearing results in ossicular reconstruction. *Otolaryngology and Head and Neck Surgery.* 2001; **125**: 135–41.
31. Schell JJ. Polytef injection for nasal deformity. *Archives of Otolaryngology.* 1970; **92**: 554–9.
32. Staffel GS, Shockley W. Nasal implants. *Otolaryngologic Clinics of North America – Implants in OTL.* 1995; **28**: 295–308.
33. Schoenrock LD, Chernoff WG. Subcutaneous implantation of Gore-Tex for facial reconstruction. *Otolaryngologic Clinics of North America – Implants in OTL.* 1995; **28**: 325–40.
34. Conrad K, Gillman G. A 6-year experience with the use of expanded polytetrafluoroethylene in rhinoplasty. *Plastic and Reconstructive Surgery.* 1998; **101**: 1675–83.
35. Wellisz T. Clinical experience with the Medpor porous polyethylene implant. *Aesthetic Plastic Surgery.* 1993; **17**: 339–44.
36. Porter JP. Grafts in rhinoplasty alloplastic vs autogenous. *Archives of Otolaryngology – Head and Neck Surgery.* 2000; **126**: 558–61.
37. Pak MW, Chan EY, van Hasselt CA. Late complications of nasal augmentation using silicone implants. *Journal of Laryngology and Otology.* 1998; **112**: 1074–7.
38. Righi PD, Wilson KM, Gluckman JL. Thyroplasty using a silicone elastomer implant. *Otolaryngologic Clinics of North America – Implants in OTL.* 1995; **28**: 309–16.

39. Kasperbauer JL. Injectable Teflon for vocal cord paralysis. *Otolaryngologic Clinics of North America.* 1995; **28**: 317–23.

40. Miyamoto RT. Cochlear implants. *Otolaryngologic Clinics of North America.* 1995; **28**: 287–94.

41. Vacanti JP, Langer R. Tissue engineering: the design and fabrication of living replacement devices for surgical reconstruction and transplantation. *The Lancet.* 1999; **354**: 32–4.

42. Stock UA, Vacanti JP. Tissue engineering: current state and prospects. *Annual Review of Medicine.* 2001; **52**: 443–51.

43. Vats A, Tolley NS, Polak JM, Buttery L. Stem Cells: sources and applications. *Clinical Otolaryngology and Allied Sciences.* **27**: 227–32.

44. Sepulveda P, Jones JR, Hench LL. Bioactive sol-gel foams for tissue repair. *Journal of Biomedical Materials Research.* 2002; **59**: 340–8.

45. Jones JR, Sepulveda P, Hench LL. The effect of temperature on the processing and properties of macroporous bioactive glass foams. *Key Engineering Materials.* 2002; **218–20**: 299–302.

46. Olde Damink LLH, Dijkstra PJ, van Luyn MJA, van Wachem PB, Nieuwenhuis P, Feijen J. Cross-linking of dermal sheep collagen using a water soluble carbodiimide. *Biomaterials.* 1996; **17**: 765–73.

47. Van Luyn MJA, van Wachem PB, Olde Damink L, Dijkstra PJ, Feijen J, Nieuwenhuis P. Relations between in vitro cytotoxicity and crosslinked dermal sheep collagen. *Journal of Biomedical Materials Research.* 1992; **26**: 1091–110.

* 48. Gough JE, Scotchford CA, Downes S. Cytotoxcity of glutaraldehyde crosslinked collagen/poly(vinyl alcohol) films is by the mechanism of apoptosis. *Journal of Biomedical Materials Research.* 2002; **61**: 121–30.

49. Eybl E, Grimm M, Grabenwoger M, Bock P, Muller MM, Wolner E. Endothelial cell lining of bioprosthetic heart valve materials. *Journal of Thoracic and Cardiovascular Surgery.* 1992; **104**: 763–9.

50. Alberts B, Bray D, Lewis J, Raff M, Roberts K, Watson JD (eds). *Molecular Biology of the Cell*, 2nd edn. New York: Garland Publishing Inc, 1994.

51. Scotchford CA, Cascone MG, Downes S, Giusti P. Osteoblast responses to collagen-PVA bioartificial polymers in vitro: the effects of cross-linking method and collagen content. *Biomaterials.* 1998; **19**: 1–11.

52. Jayakrishnan A, Jameela SR. Glutaraldehyde as fixative in bioprostheses and drug delivery matrices. *Biomaterials.* 1996; **17**: 471–84.

* 53. Ratner BD, Hoffman AS, Schoen FJ, Lemons JE (eds). *Biomaterials Science. An Introduction to Materials in Medicine.* London: Academic Press, 1996.

* 54. Gorham SD. Collagen as a biomaterial. In: Byron D (ed.). *Biomaterials, novel materials from biological sources.* Basingstoke: MacMillan, 1991: 57–121.

55. Lanza RP, Langer R, Vacanti J (eds). *Principles of Tissue Engineering,* 2nd edn. London: Academic Press, 2000.

56. Hench LL. Bioceramics. From concept to clinic. *Journal of the American Ceramic Society.* 1991; **74**: 1487–510.

57. Videau JJ, Dupuis V. Phosphates and biomaterials. *European Journal of Solid State Inorganic Chemistry.* 1991; **28**: 303–43.

58. Xynos ID, Edgar AJ, Buttery LDK, Hench LL, Polak JM. Gene expression profiling of human osteoblasts following treatment with the ionic products of Bioglass 45S5. *Journal of Biomedical Materials Research.* 2001; **55**: 151–7.

59. Simske SJ, Ayers RA, Bateman TA. Porous materials for bone engineering. *Materials Science Forum.* 1997; **250**: 151–82.

60. Petite H, Viateau V, Bensaid W, Meunier A, de Pollak C, Bourguignon M *et al.* Tissue engineered bone regeneration. *Nature Biotechnology.* 2000; **18**: 959–63.

61. Guillemin G, Patat JL, Fournie J, Chetail M. The use of coral as a bone graft substitute. *Journal of Biomedical Materials Research.* 1987; **21**: 557–67.

62. Yukna RA, Yukna CN. A 5-year follow up of 16 patients treated with coralline calcium carbonate (Biocoral) bone replacement grafts in infrabony defects. *Journal of Clincal Periodontology.* 1998; **25**: 1036–40.

63. Yukna RA. Clinical evaluation of coralline calcium carbonate as a bone replacement graft material in human periodontal osseous defects. *Journal of Periodontology.* 1994; **65**: 177–85.

64. Roux FX, Brasnu D, Loty B, Georges B, Guillemin G. Madreporic coral: a new bone graft substitute for cranial surgery. *Journal of the Neurological Sciences.* 1988; **69**: 510–3.

65. Pouliquen JC, Noat M, Guillemin G, Verneret C, Patal JL. Coral as a substitute for bone graft in posterior spine fusion in childhood. *French Journal Orthopaedic Surgery.* 1989; **3**: 272–80.

66. Guillemin G, Patat JL, Meunier A. Natural corals used as bone graft substitutes. *Bulletin de L'Institute oceanographique Monaco.* 1995; **14**: 67–77.

67. Piecuch JF, Goldberg AJ, Shastry CV, Chrzanowski RB. Compressive strength of implanted porous replamineform hydroxyapatite. *Journal of Biomedical Materials Research.* 1984; **18**: 39–45.

68. Corden T, Jones IA, Rudd CD, Christian P, Downes S, McDougall KE. Physical and biocompatibility properties of poly-epsilon-carpolactone produced using in situ polymerisation; a novel manufacturing technique for long fibre composite materials. *Biomaterials.* 2000; **21**: 713–24.

69. Christian P, Jones IA. Polymerisation and stabilisation of polycaprolactone using a borontrifluoride-glycerol catalyst system. *Polymer.* 2001; **42**: 3989–94.

70. Gough JE, Christian P, Scotchford CA, Rudd CD, Jones IA. Synthesis, degradation and in vitro cell responses of sodium phosphate glasses for craniofacial bone repair. *Journal of Biomedical Materials Research.* 2002; **59**: 481–9.

71. Sawtell RM, Kayser MV, Downes S. A morphological assessment of bovine chondrocytes cultured on poly(ethyl methacrylate)/tetrahydrofurfuryl methacrylate. *Cell Materials.* 1995; **5**: 63–71.

72. Downes S, Archer RS, Kayser MV, Patel MP, Braden M. The regeneration of articular cartilage using a new polymer system. *Journal of Materials Science: Materials in Medicine.* 1994; **5**: 88–95.

73. Risbud M, Ringe J, Bhonde R, Sittinger M. In vitro expression of cartilage specific markers by chondrocytes on a biocompatible hydrogel: Implications for engineering cartilage tissue. *Cell Transplantation.* 2001; **10**: 755–63.

74. Nehrer S, Breinan HA, Ramappa A, Hsu H-P, Shortkroff S, Minas T *et al.* Chondrocyte seeded collagen matrices implanted in a chondral defect in a canine model. *Biomaterials.* 1998; **19**: 2313–28.

* 75. Cao YC, Vacanti JP, Paige KT, Upton J, Vacanti CA. Transplantation of chondrocytes utilising a polymer-cell construct to produce tissue-engineered cartilage in the shape of a human ear. *Plastic and Reconstructive Surgery.* 1997; **100**: 297–302.

76. Freed LE, Vunjak-Novakovic G, Biron R, Eagles D, Lesnoy D, Barlow S *et al.* Biodegradable polymer scaffolds for tissue engineering. *BioTechnology.* 1994; **12**: 698–3.

77. Mosahebi A, Fuller P, Wiberg M, Terenghi G. Effect of allogenic schwann cell transplantation on peripheral nerve regeneration. *Experimental Neurology.* 2002; **173**: 213–23.

78. Fine EG, Valentini RF, Aebischer P. Nerve regeneration. In: Lanza RP, Langer R, Vacanti J (eds). *Principles of tissue engineering*, 2nd edn. London: Academic Press, 2000: 785–98.

79. Niklason LE, Gao J, Abbot WM, Hirschi KK, Houser S, Marini R *et al.* Functional arteries grown in vitro. *Science.* 1999; **284**: 489–93.

80. Dermagraft website. La Jolla, CA, USA: Advanced BioHealing, Inc. Cited March 2007. Available from: www.dermagraft.com/

81. Apligraf website. Canton, MA, USA: Organogenesis Inc. Cited March 2007. Available from: www.apligraf.com/

82. Puelacher WC, Mooney D, Langer R, Upton J, Vacanti JP, Vacanti CA. Design of nasospetal cartilage replacements synthesised from biodegradable polymers and chondrocytes. *Biomaterials.* 1994; **15**: 774–8.

83. Sakata J, Vacanti CA, Schloo B, Healy GB, Langer R, Vacanti JP. Tracheal composites tissue engineered from chondrocytes, tracheal epithelial cells, and synthetic degradable scaffolding. *Transplantation Proceedings.* 1994; **26**: 3309–10.

84. Chang SC, Rowley JA, Tobias G, Genes NG, Roy AK, Mooney DJ *et al.* Injection molding of chondrocyte/ alginate constructs in the shape of facial implants. *Journal of Biomedical Materials Research.* 2001; **55**: 503–11.

85. Fuchs JR, Nasseri BA, Vacanti JP. Tissue engineering: a 21st century solution to surgical reconstruction. *Annals of Thoracic Surgery.* 2001; **72**: 557–91.

86. Hench LL, Wilson J. Surface active biomaterials. *Science.* 1984; **226**: 630–6.

PART 3

IMMUNOLOGY

EDITED BY NICHOLAS S JONES

11 Defence mechanisms   133
   Ian Todd and Richard J Powell

12 Allergy: basic mechanisms and tests   144
   Stephen R Durham and Graham Banfield

13 Evaluation of the immune system   167
   Elizabeth Drewe and Richard J Powell

14 Primary immunodeficiencies   174
   Elizabeth Drewe and Richard J Powell

15 Rheumatological diseases   183
   Adrian Drake-Lee

11

Defence mechanisms

IAN TODD AND RICHARD J POWELL

Innate and adaptive immunity	133	Immunity to cytosolic infectious agents	140
Antigen recognition	134	Inflammation and hypersensitivity	140
Immunity to extracellular and vesicular infectious agents	137	Further reading	143

INNATE AND ADAPTIVE IMMUNITY

The immune system has evolved for protection against infective agents that invade the body. In order to achieve this, the immune system has recognition properties to locate and identify the invader, and to activate defence processes that repel or destroy the invader. There are an enormous number and variety of infectious agents within the main categories of viruses, bacteria, fungi, protozoa and parasitic worms. In order to provide effective immunity against each of these agents, the immune system has to be able to meet the challenges that they pose: this is achieved by a diverse range of molecular and cellular components of the body that cooperate with each other in order to maximize their defensive activities. Some of these components generate innate immunity, whereas others provide adaptive (or acquired) immunity. The main cell types of the immune system are the leukocytes that develop from stem cells in the bone marrow.

The innate immune system is evolutionarily older than the adaptive system and provides generic defence against categories of microbes. It is composed of a range of cells and proteins found in the circulation and in tissues: these include macrophages (and their monocyte precursors), granulocytes (i.e. neutrophils, eosinophils, basophils) and mast cells, natural killer cells, complement proteins and regulatory proteins called cytokines. The innate system employs an inherited repertoire of receptor proteins (known as pattern-recognition molecules) that recognize characteristic structures that are commonly expressed by microbes, and changes to cells brought about by infection. The advantage of this system is that it is rapidly activated by infective agents that penetrate tissues. However, it is only moderately efficient, which means that adaptive immunity is also required for the complete elimination of many pathogens.

Adaptive immunity is mediated by T lymphocytes and B lymphocytes (also known as T cells and B cells). Like the leukocytes of the innate system, lymphocytes develop from bone marrow stem cells, but the precursors of T cells migrate from the bone marrow to complete their maturation in the thymus. Each T or B cell expresses receptors that specifically recognize one particular chemical structure of a microbial molecule (known, in this context, as an antigen). Activated B cells also secrete a soluble form of their antigen receptors, known as antibodies or immunoglobulins (Ig). An enormously diverse repertoire of antigen receptors is somatically generated by recombination events involving the receptor genes during the development of lymphocytes, so that potentially millions of different antigens can be recognized. The recruitment, activation and proliferation of resting lymphocytes specific for the antigens of an invading microbe take some time (possibly several days), but the lymphocytes generate highly efficient defence. In addition, some of the lymphocytes activated by specific antigens are maintained in the body as resting cells after the elimination of the infection and constitute a memory population of cells that are able to generate a bigger and faster response upon subsequent exposure to the same antigens: this demonstrates the adaptive properties of lymphocytes.

The innate and adaptive systems are not independent, but interact with each other and synergize to generate optimal immunity. First, lymphocyte activation is dependent not only on antigen recognition, but also on costimulatory signals provided by cells and molecules of the innate system. Second, the antibodies produced by B cells and the cytokines secreted primarily by T cells enhance the defensive activities of the innate system.

Stages of an immune response

The immediate response to an invading pathogen is mounted by innate components resident within the infected tissues (**Figure 11.1a**). In particular, tissue macrophages express a range of receptors for microbial structures, including mannose receptor, scavenger receptors and Toll-like receptors, whose ligands include various microbial polysaccharides and lipids. Complement proteins are also directly activated by microbes via what is termed the alternative pathway (see under The complement system). Inflammatory products of macrophages and complement, together with those released by tissue mast cells activated by the complement peptides C3a and C5a (known as anaphylatoxins), induce the migration of granulocytes, natural killer cells and more complement proteins from the bloodstream into the infected tissues (**Figure 11.1b**).

Whilst these innate processes are providing early defence to limit growth and spread of the infection within the body, other processes are set in train to generate the antigen-specific adaptive response (**Figure 11.1c**). The activation of lymphocytes does not initially take place within the infected tissues themselves, but in specialized lymphoid tissues such as lymph nodes, the spleen and mucosa-associated lymphoid tissues (MALT) that include Waldeyer's ring. Antigens therefore have to be transported from the infected tissues to local lymphoid tissues. Some antigens may be passively carried in the tissue fluid forming the lymph that drains into regional lymph nodes. However, a major part is played by cells found in most tissues called dendritic cells. These, like the macrophages described above, express pattern-recognition receptors for microbial structures, and actively engulf microbial material. This induces the maturation of the dendritic cells, which migrate from the site of infection and carry the microbial antigens to the local lymphoid tissues where T and B lymphocytes have the opportunity to interact with the antigens and be activated by them. Only a very small proportion of the millions of lymphocytes in a particular lymphoid organ will have receptors that specifically recognize the antigens of a particular microbe. It is these specific lymphocytes that are activated by the antigens and proliferate and mature into effector cells that contribute to defence against the pathogen. These effector lymphocytes leave the lymphoid tissues and recirculate via the bloodstream to the site of infection in order to enhance the destruction and elimination of the pathogen in cooperation with the innate components described above.

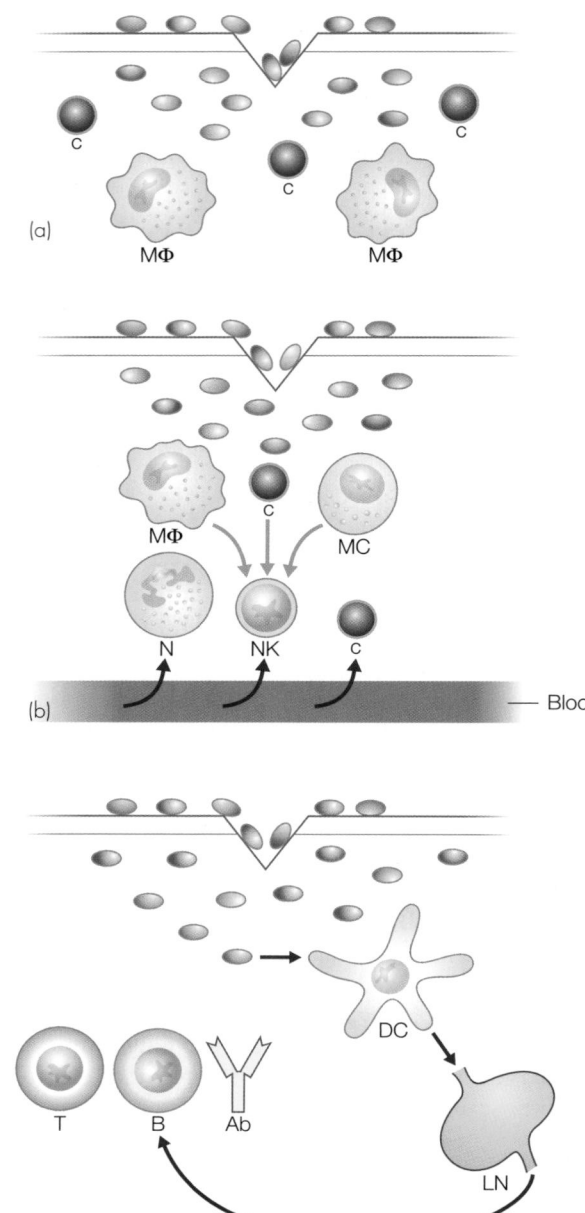

Figure 11.1 Stages of an immune response: see text for details. **(a)** Immediate local innate response; **(b)** early induced response (innate/inflammatory); **(c)** later adaptive response. Ab, antibody; B, B lymphocyte; C, complement; DC, dendritic cell; LN, lymph node; MΦ, macrophage; N, neutrophil; NK, natural killer cell; T, T lymphocyte.

ANTIGEN RECOGNITION

Antigen recognition involves a high affinity interaction between an antigen and the specialized antigen combining site of a lymphocyte's antigen receptor protein (or of an antibody molecule). The binding involves noncovalent intermolecular attractive forces that require a very close approach between the surfaces of the antigen and the combining site. In other words, the interacting surfaces must have complementary shapes that fit snugly together (rather like a lock and a key) so that significant attractive interactions occur between complementary chemical groups of the antigen and the combining site. Each lymphocyte clone (i.e. group of cells derived from a single parent lymphocyte) expresses antigen receptors with a single type of combining site that is essentially unique in shape and amino acid composition to that clone compared with the millions of other lymphocyte clones in the body: this is why millions of different antigens can be recognized by the adaptive immune system. Furthermore, the specificity of the adaptive response arises because those lymphocytes whose receptors have the highest affinity for an antigen that enters the body are the ones most likely to bind it and, therefore, to be activated by it: this is termed clonal selection.

B cells and antibodies (immunoglobulins)

The B cell's receptor is essentially a membrane bound form of the antibodies that the B cell secretes, and is called surface immunoglobulin (sIg) (**Figure 11.2**). It is made up of two identical large polypeptides (heavy chains) and two identical smaller light chains (which can be one of two types called kappa and lambda light chains). Each chain is composed of a series of homologous globular regions called Ig domains: two in the light chains and four or five in the heavy chains.

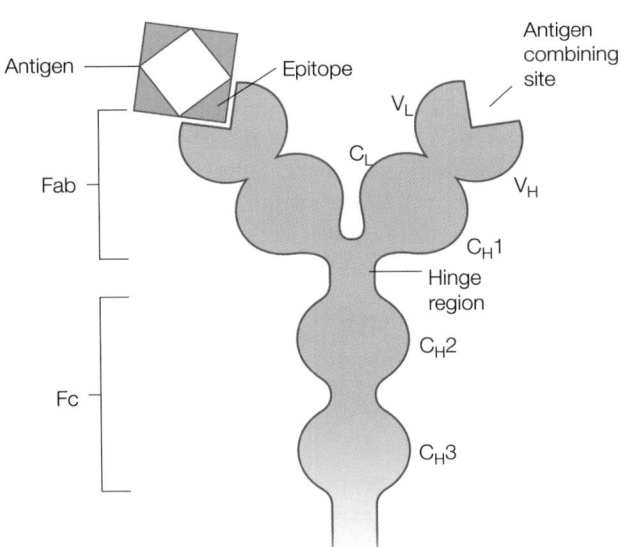

Figure 11.2 A schematic structure of a generic immunoglobulin (surface or secreted), see text for details. The variable domains of the heavy and light chains are labelled V_H and V_L, respectively. Similarly, the constant domains are labelled C_H1–3 and C_L. The region below C_H3 represents the transmembrane region and cytoplasmic tail present in sIg, but not in secreted antibodies.

The receptor has two identical antigen combining sites, each of which is composed of the amino terminal domains of a heavy and a light chain: these are called variable domains because they vary in structure between different B cell clones, thereby conferring the differences in antigenic specificity between B cells. Different types of chemicals can serve as antigens for direct interaction with different B cell receptors and antibodies, including proteins, carbohydrates, lipids and even nucleic acids. The combining site constitutes only a small part of a whole Ig molecule and, for example, can accommodate approximately four to six amino acids of a protein antigen: the precise region of an antigen molecule that interacts with a combining site is termed the antigenic determinant or epitope. Each variable domain contains three hypervariable loops, so called because they differ most in amino acid sequence between different clones of B cells; they are also known as complementarity determining regions because they are complementary to the epitope and form the main interactions with it. Following B cell activation, modifications can occur to the variable domains by somatic mutation. This involves nucleotide changes to the variable domain genes during B cell replication that affect the amino acid sequence (particularly of the complementarity determining regions), and therefore affect the antigenic specificity of the antigen combining sites. This can generate combining sites that fit even better with the epitope and therefore have improved affinity for the antigen.

The other domains are called constant domains because they have the same structure in the sIg of different B cells. Human B cells can express one of nine different forms or isotypes of Ig (both surface and secreted) that differ in the structure and number of their heavy chain constant region domains, and constitute five immunoglobulin classes. These are called IgM, IgG (with subclasses IgG1, IgG2, IgG3 and IgG4), IgA (with subclasses IgA1 and IgA2), IgE and IgD. All B cells are initially programmed to express IgM (plus IgD), but can undergo Ig class switching to produce one of the other isotypes following stimulation by antigen, without changing their antigenic specificity. They do this by changing the heavy chain constant region domains that they express, but maintain expression of the same heavy chain variable domain and the same light chain variable and constant domains.

The sIg is anchored in the surface membrane of a B cell by a transmembrane amino acid sequence at the carboxy terminus of the heavy chains. When a resting B cell is activated by antigen, it can differentiate into a plasma cell that produces large numbers of Ig molecules that lack the transmembrane sequence, and so are secreted from the cell as antibodies with the same antigenic specificity and isotype as the B cell's sIg. Because B cells initially express sIgM, the first antibodies produced during an immune response (i.e. on first exposure to a particular antigen) are also IgM (there is little, if any, secretion of IgD), but IgG, IgA and IgE antibodies appear later in the response as activated B cells undergo class switching. Furthermore, the memory population is derived from B cells that have undergone class switching, so that IgG, IgA and IgE are produced at the start of a secondary response on repeated exposure to the same antigen. The advantages of producing a range of antibody isotypes are because they have different physiological and defensive activities.

T cells and antigen presentation

The T cell receptor (TCR) for antigen shows both similarities and differences to B cell sIg (**Figure 11.3**). The TCR is a much smaller molecule, being made up of two polypeptide chains each of which is approximately the same size as an Ig light chain, with both expressing a transmembrane sequence: indeed, T cells do not produce a secreted form of the TCR, i.e. they do not release anything equivalent to antibodies. The TCR polypeptides expressed by the majority of T cells are called alpha and beta chains, whereas a minority express gamma and delta chains. Each chain is composed of two domains that show strong structural homologies with those of the immunoglobulins. Similar Ig-like domains are found in many other surface molecules of lymphocytes and other cells: this indicates evolutionary genetic relationships between these molecules, and they constitute the immunoglobulin superfamily. The two amino terminal, membrane-distal domains of the TCR chains are variable between T cells and constitute a single antigen combining site. The membrane-proximal domains are constant in structure.

Unlike B cell immunoglobulins, conventional TCR cannot interact directly with antigenic epitopes of proteins, but bind only to short peptides that are derived from protein antigens, and are expressed on the surface of other cells of the body that are known, in this context, as antigen presenting cells (APC). This is because the main function of T cells is to interact with other cells within the context of an immune response: binding to antigenic peptides held on the surface of a cell thereby directs a T cell to exert effects on that particular APC. There are two main functional types of T cells: T helper (Th) cells regulate the activity of other cells of the immune system, whereas T cytotoxic (Tc) cells kill cells that are infected. In order for this to happen, protein antigens that enter the cytoplasm of an APC are processed (i.e. degraded) into peptides, some of which associate with proteins of the major histocompatibility complex (MHC), known in humans as human leukocyte antigens (HLA). The MHC molecule/peptide complexes are then expressed on the surface of the APC where they can interact with T cells whose TCR have combining sites specific for the particular antigenic peptides presented, much in the same way as an Ig combining site interacts with an antigen epitope. This interaction binds the T cell to the surface of the APC thereby enabling these cells to exert effects on each other.

There are two types of MHC molecules called MHC class I and MHC class II (**Figure 11.3**). They have similar three-dimensional structures, but are made up of different types of polypeptide chains. The MHC class I protein is composed of a large alpha-chain noncovalently associated with the smaller $beta_2$-microglobulin, whereas MHC class II is composed of similarly sized alpha and beta chains. Both class I and class II have two Ig-like domains adjacent to the cell membrane (i.e. they are members of the Ig superfamily), whereas distal to the membrane is the antigen peptide binding cleft. Two alpha-helices form the walls of the cleft and sit on a platform of beta-pleated sheet; antigen peptide is held within the cleft in a linear conformation (rather like a hotdog sausage in a bun!) with its exposed surface available for interaction with a TCR. Peptides of eight or nine amino acids in length can be accommodated within the cleft of MHC class I molecules, whereas the peptides that associate with MHC class II molecules can be between 12 and 20 amino acids in length because they can extend beyond the ends of the peptide binding cleft.

MHC class I molecules present antigens primarily to Tc cells because these cells express a protein called CD8 that binds to the side of the class I alpha-chain when the TCR interacts with the peptide and binding cleft (**Figure 11.3a**). Most tissue cells of the body express MHC class I molecules on their surfaces and thus have the potential to be targets for Tc cells if they become infected by microbes that enter the cytosol, such as viruses. The processing pathway for cytosolic proteins delivers the peptides to MHC class I molecules for binding and presentation. Tc cell clones that specifically bind to these peptides have various ways of

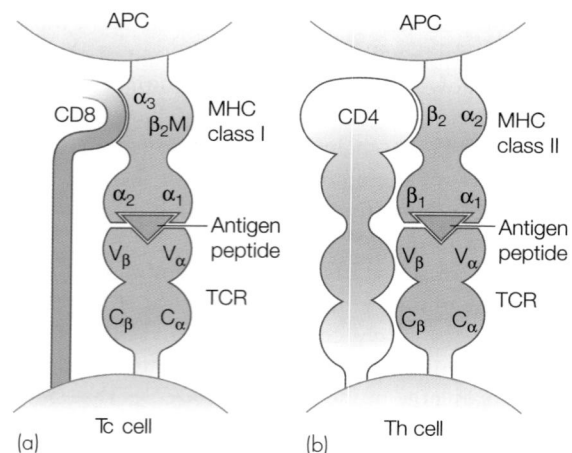

Figure 11.3 Antigen recognition by T cells, see text for details. APC, antigen presenting cell; $beta_2M$, $beta_2$-microglobulin; C, constant domain; MHC, major histocompatibility complex; Tc, cytotoxic T cell; TCR, T cell receptor; Th, helper T cell; V, variable domain.

killing infected cells by inducing them to undergo apoptosis (programmed cell death):

- the Tc cells secrete two types of proteins stored in cytoplasmic granules: these are perforins that polymerize to form pores through the plasma membranes of the target cells, and granzymes that enter the target cells through the perforin pores and induce apoptosis;
- Fas-ligand expressed on the surface of Tc cells, or tumour necrosis factor (TNF) secreted by Tc cells can induce apoptosis when they bind to their receptors on infected target cells (Fas and TNFR1, respectively).

MHC class II molecules present peptides mainly to Th cells because these cells express the CD4 protein that binds to the side of the class II beta-chain (**Figure 11.3b**). The expression of MHC class II molecules is mainly restricted to cells of the immune system whose functions are to activate, and be activated by, Th cells: these are dendritic cells, macrophages and B cells. These cells deliberately engulf exogenous antigens that, for example, bind to pattern recognition receptors expressed on macrophages and dendritic cells, or specifically bind to the sIg of selected B cell clones. In either case, the surface-bound antigens are endocytosed into membrane-bound vesicles within the cytoplasm. The processing pathway for these vesicular proteins delivers peptides to MHC class II molecules for binding and presentation. Th cell clones that specifically bind to these peptides can then be triggered by the APC to exert their regulatory activities. A range of cell surface and secreted molecules mediate the mutual effects of Th cells and APC on one another. First, there are the interactions of TCR and CD4 with the peptide/MHC class II complex, with the signal resulting from TCR binding being delivered to the interior of T cells by the CD3 protein. Second, a number of other membrane proteins interact between the surfaces of the T cells and

APC to deliver co-stimulatory signals: particularly important are interactions of CD28 with B7, and CD40-ligand with CD40, but others include the interactions of CD2 with LFA-3, and LFA-1 with ICAM (in each case on the T cells and APC, respectively). Third, both the APC and the T cells secrete cytokines as soluble regulatory proteins that bind to specific cell surface receptors. For example, interleukin (IL-1) and IL-12 are important T cell activators secreted by dendritic cells.

When activated, different Th cells preferentially secrete different combinations of cytokines (**Figure 11.4**). Th1 cells produce interferon-gamma (IFN-gamma) that is an important macrophage activator, and IL-2 that stimulates T cells (including Tc cells): thus, Th1 cells induce primarily cell-mediated immunity, although they do also stimulate some antibody production by B cells. Th2 cells produce IL-4, IL-10 and IL-13 that stimulate B cells to produce antibodies, and particularly induce Ig class switching to production of IgE; they also secrete IL-5 that stimulates eosinophils. In addition, Th1 and Th2 cells inhibit each other's activities via the cytokines they secrete. These patterns of type 1 and type 2 cytokine secretion are observed with other cell types, including Tc cells and B cells.

IMMUNITY TO EXTRACELLULAR AND VESICULAR INFECTIOUS AGENTS

Different defence mechanisms are required to deal with infective agents that occupy different compartments within the body. A major distinction is whether an infective agent is in an extracellular environment, or has entered the cytoplasm of cells and so is in an intracellular environment (**Figure 11.5**). This distinction is important because extracellular agents are directly accessible to defensive molecules secreted by cells of the immune

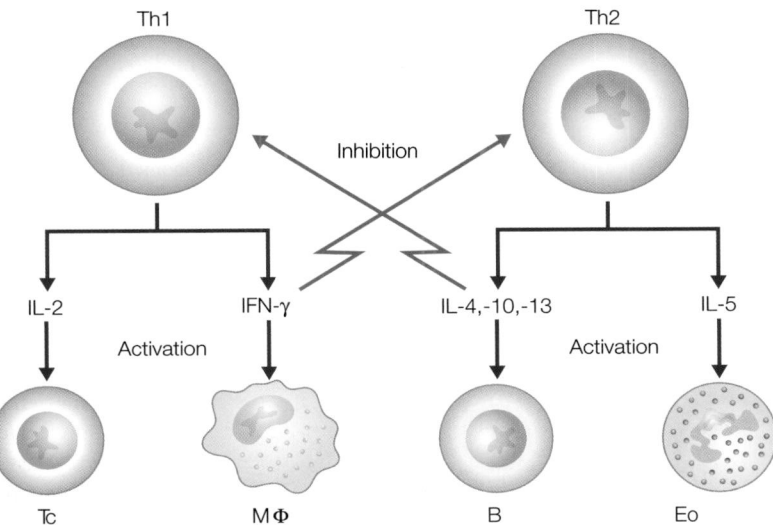

Figure 11.4 Cytokine-mediated regulation by Th1 and Th2 cells. B, B lymphocyte; Eo, eosinophil; IFN-γ, interferon-γ; IL, interleukin; MΦ, macrophage; Tc, cytotoxic T cell; Th1, T helper 1 cell; Th2, T helper 2 cell.

system, whereas intracellular ones are not. Antibodies therefore play a major role in the adaptive immune response to extracellular pathogens (**Figure 11.5a**).

Antibody effector functions

Antibodies are bifunctional molecules with one end having antigen binding properties while the other end triggers defensive activities. These functional regions are separated by a relatively flexible amino acid sequence between the first and second heavy chain constant domains called the hinge region (**Figure 11.2**). The two arms containing the antigen combining sites are called the Fragment antigen binding (Fab) regions: each is

composed of a light chain and the variable and first constant domain of a heavy chain. The other constant domains of the two heavy chains constitute the Fragment crystallizable (Fc) region (because it can form crystals when isolated experimentally).

As described under Antigen recognition above, there are five classes of Ig molecules expressed as B cell sIg, four of which are also secreted as antibodies (i.e. IgM, IgG, IgA, IgE, but not IgD). The classes have different heavy chain constant domains, and thus differ primarily in their Fc regions (**Table 11.1**). The heavy chains of IgG and IgA (and also IgD) each have two constant domains in the Fc region, whereas IgM and IgE have three. In addition, IgM forms pentamers of five Ig monomers held together by a J (joining) chain polypeptide, whereas IgA can similarly form dimers. The large size of IgM means that it is mainly restricted to the bloodstream (except at sites of inflammation), whereas the other classes more readily diffuse into tissues. IgG is the most abundant antibody class and also is transported across the placenta from the maternal to the foetal circulation during gestation. This maternal IgG provides initial protection against infection to newborn babies until their own immune system produces significant levels of antibodies, but is lacking in babies born very prematurely. In its dimeric form, IgA is transported across mucosal epithelia and thus constitutes the main antibody class conferring protection in secretions and at mucosal surfaces. Part of the mucosal receptor that binds and transports IgA across the epithelium remains associated with it as the secretory piece. IgA is also secreted into milk and thus confers protection to the gastrointestinal tract of suckling babies.

Antibodies can neutralize microbes and their toxins simply by binding to them, thereby inhibiting their functions and infectivity. However, antibodies can also contribute to the destruction of infectious agents by interacting with other defensive components, as described below.

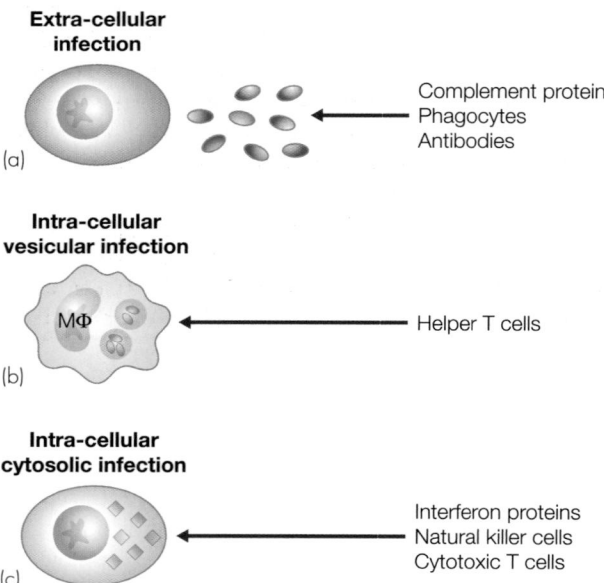

Figure 11.5 Immune responses to different types of infections.

Table 11.1 Properties of functional antibody classes and subclasses.

	IgM	IgG1	IgG2	IgG3	IgG4	IgA1	IgE
Molecular weight	970 (pentamer)	146	146	165	146	160 (monomer)	188
Adult serum level (mg/mL)	1.5	9	3	1	0.5	3	5×10^{-5}
Serum half-life (days)	10	21	20	7	21	6	2
Extravascular diffusion	±	+ + +	+ + +	+ + +	+ + +	+ + (monomer)	+
Transport across epithelium	+	−	−	−	−	+ + + (dimer)	−
Transport across placenta	−	+ + +	+	+ +	±	−	−
Neutralization	+	+ +	+ +	+ +	+ +	+ +	−
Binding to phagocytes	−	+ + +	±	+ +	+	+	−
Binding to NK cells	−	+ +	−	+ +	−	−	−
High affinity mast cell binding	−	−	−	−	−	−	+ + +
Classical complement pathway activation	+ + +	+ +	+	+ + +	−	−	−
Alternative complement pathway activation	−	−	−	−	−	+	−

The complement system

The complement proteins found in the circulation and tissue fluids constitute an important defensive system that can be activated by the Fc regions of IgM and IgG antibodies in what is termed the classical pathway of complement activation (**Figure 11.6**). This is triggered when IgM or several IgG antibodies that are bound to antigen interact with the complement C1 protein complex, resulting in the formation of a C3 convertase enzyme from C4 and C2 (C4b2a). This same C3 convertase can be generated when the pattern recognition molecule mannan-binding lectin (MBL) interacts with mannose residues of microbial surfaces. (MBL is a member of a family of secreted carbohydrate-binding collagenous defensive proteins called collectins.) A different C3 convertase is produced when certain complement proteins directly form a stable complex (C3bBbP) on microbial surfaces in what is termed the alternative pathway of complement activation. IgA can also activate the alternative pathway.

The conversion, or splitting, of complement protein C3 by the C3 convertase enzymes into fragments C3a and C3b is the central event of complement activation and generates a range of biological effects. Some of the C3b can be used to generate more of the alternative pathway C3 convertase; it also modifies the activity of the C3 convertase enzymes to split C5 into C5a and C5b. As mentioned under Innate and adaptive immunity above,

C3a and C5a activate mast cells and thus promote inflammation: they also attract and activate neutrophils (particularly C5a). The C5b fragment forms the membrane attack complex (MAC) with C6, C7, C8 and several molecules of C9: this last complement protein has structural and functional similarities to perforin (see under T cells and antigen presentation above) and forms pores through lipid bilayers. Thus, the MAC has direct antimicrobial effects by disrupting microbial membranes. Finally, in addition to its other activities, C3b opsonizes (i.e. coats) infectious agents, which facilitates their interaction with leukocytes, as described below.

Digestive and inflammatory leukocytes

Some leukocytes have surface receptor proteins that bind to the Fc regions of antibodies (FcR), and others that bind to complement C3b (CR). As described under Innate and adaptive immunity above, the phagocytes (macrophages and neutrophils) express pattern-recognition molecules that enable them to bind microbes directly. However, they also possess FcR specific for IgG or IgA and CR that have particularly high affinities for their respective ligands. Thus, microbes such as bacteria can be firmly bound to the surface of phagocytes when opsonized by antibodies and C3b. This facilitates and activates phagocytosis (i.e. engulfing) of the microbes into

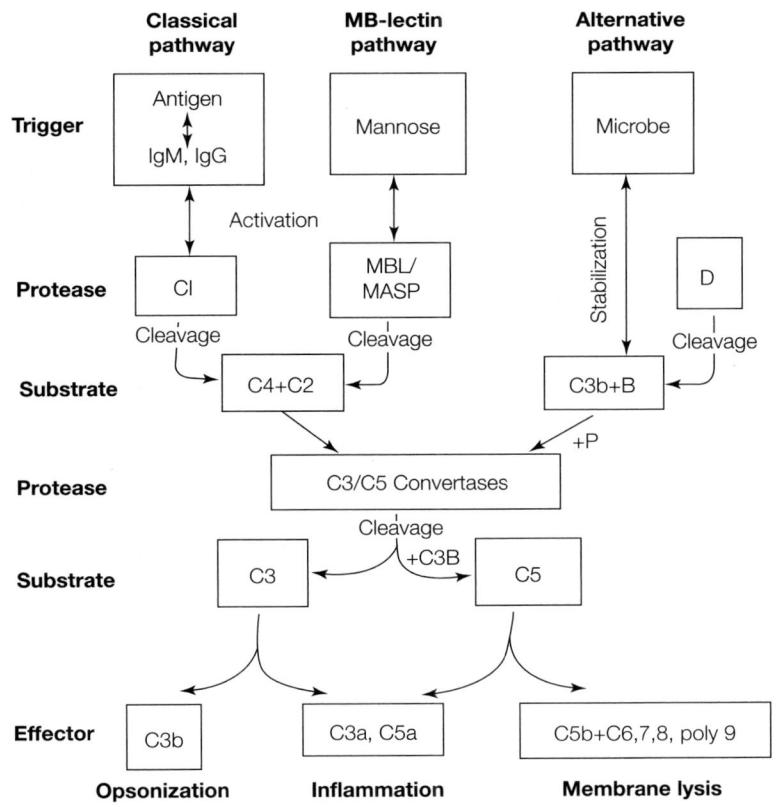

Figure 11.6 Complement activation pathways and effector functions. MBL is mannan-binding lectin; MASP is MBL-associated serine protease. Ig, immunoglobulin; MASP, MBL-associated serine protease; MBL, mannan-binding lectin.

membrane-bound cytoplasmic vesicles. The microbes can then be destroyed by lysosomal enzymes and reactive oxygen molecules.

Some microbes, such as the mycobacteria that cause tuberculosis and leprosy, are relatively resistant to the digestive activities of phagocytes and are able to survive and multiply within the cytoplasmic vesicles of macrophages. In this environment the microbes are protected from the activities of extracellular antibodies and complement proteins. The effective control of such infections is then dependent on the activity of Th1 cells that, as described under T cells and antigen presentation above, produce the potent macrophage activating cytokine IFN-gamma: this promotes macrophage digestive activity against microbes in intracellular vesicles (**Figure 11.5b**).

Other infective agents, particularly parasitic worms, such as schistosomes and helminths, are much too large to be engulfed for intracellular digestion by phagocytes. In such circumstances, eosinophils are recruited to undertake extracellular digestion by releasing their digestive proteins (e.g. major basic protein) onto the surface of the parasites. Eosinophils possess FcR (specific for IgG or IgE) and CR, and so again will bind most avidly to opsonized targets.

The other main cells that express FcR for IgE are the tissue mast cells and blood basophils, whose functions are inflammatory rather than directly defensive. These cells are activated when an antigen binds and cross-links several FcR-bound surface IgE molecules. This induces the immediate release of preformed inflammatory mediators, particularly histamine, that are stored in cytoplasmic granules. It also induces the *de novo* synthesis and later release of leukotrienes. (As mentioned above, mast cells are also activated by the complement peptides C3a and C5a.)

IMMUNITY TO CYTOSOLIC INFECTIOUS AGENTS

Some infectious agents actively infect cells by entering the fluid cytosol (**Figure 11.5c**). Viruses are prime examples of such pathogens because they are obliged to infect cells in order to use the machinery of the cells they parasitize in order to replicate themselves. Although antibodies and complement can neutralize viruses while they are outside cells, other immune mechanisms are necessary to deal with intracellular viruses.

An innate mechanism of antiviral defence is the production and secretion of interferon-alpha (IFN-alpha) and/or inteferon-beta (IFN-beta) by the infected cells. These type 1 interferons are structurally unrelated to the IFN-gamma (type 2 interferon) that is produced by activated T cells and natural killer (NK) cells: however, both types derive their name from their ability to *interfere* with viral replication. Type 1 interferons secreted by

virally infected cells induce an antiviral state in neighbouring noninfected cells by stimulating these cells to produce enzymes that block viral replication. In addition, type 1 interferons enhance MHC class I expression, which is necessary for Tc cell recognition of target cells, and type I interferons activate NK cells. Both these types of killer cells are important in the immune response to intracellular viruses because killing the infected cells inhibits the replication and spread of the virus within the body. NK cells are the first killer cells to be activated and they employ the perforin/granzyme mechanism of cytotoxicity described for Tc cells under T cells and antigen presentation above. However, unlike Tc, NK cells do not possess antigen-specific receptors, but detect abnormalities in the expression of a cell's own surface molecules that may be indicative of the cell being virally infected. NK cells possess two types of receptors that interact with potential target cells – killer activating receptors (KAR) and killer inhibitory receptors (KIR), with the latter providing a dominant inhibitory signal that prevents NK cells from killing normal, uninfected cells. The ligands for KIR are often MHC class I molecules, whose expression may be reduced by viral infection of a cell: this makes the cell susceptible to the activity of NK cells because they then bind predominantly via their KAR.

NK cells also express FcR specific for IgG and so can interact with, and kill, target cells via antibodies that have bound to antigens expressed in the surface membranes of the target cells, as may happen during the formation of budding viruses. This is termed antibody-dependent cellular cytotoxicity (ADCC).

Interferons and NK cells are very important in limiting the replication and spread of a virus during the early stages of an infection, but may not be able to eliminate the infection. The adaptive Tc cells will take longer to be activated, as described under Stages of an immune response above, but can then specifically and efficiently target the infected cells, as described under T cells and antigen presentation above.

INFLAMMATION AND HYPERSENSITIVITY

Inflammatory processes are necessary to recruit components of the immune system to sites of infection. The importance of tissue mast cells as a source of inflammatory mediators has been discussed in previous sections, but many cell types can produce a range of inflammatory mediators, including cytokines and other proteins as well as other types of chemicals (e.g. prostaglandins and leukotrienes). A number of these have particular effects on the vessels that supply blood to infected tissues, promoting vasodilatation, increased vascular permeability, and enhancing endothelial expression of adhesion molecules (particularly selectins and ligands for integrins). The interaction of circulating leukocytes with the adhesion molecules facilitates their migration across the blood vessel walls and into the infected tissues in response to chemotactic factors.

In addition to localized inflammatory events within infected tissues, systemic effects are induced by cytokines that enter the bloodstream: particularly IL-1, IL-6 and TNF. These have effects on the hypothalamus to induce fever, they promote leukocyte release from the bone marrow, and the release of acute phase proteins from the liver; in particular, the liver-derived pentraxins called C-reactive protein and serum amyloid P possess innate antimicrobial activities.

The enormous destructive potential of the immune system that is unleashed against invading microbes can be equally damaging to the body's own tissues. Thus, during every immune and inflammatory response, a balance must be struck between beneficial and tissue damaging effects. The immune system has evolved regulatory processes to limit the latter but, in some instances, immunological tissue damage becomes the main clinical feature, generating the problems of hypersensitivity.

Allergy and autoimmunity

Tissue damaging adaptive immune mechanisms can be triggered by foreign antigens or the body's own components. The former can be microbes, inducing the immune-mediated tissue damage associated with infective diseases, or can be inert (noninfective) materials that cause allergies. Up to 30 percent of the population is affected by allergies in developed countries, with a host of different allergens affecting different individuals, e.g. pollen, house dust mite, insect venom, food components, latex. On the other hand, reactivity to self-components can lead to autoimmune diseases. Collectively, these affect over 3 percent of the population, with a much higher incidence of subclinical autoimmunity. In organ-specific autoimmunity, the stimulating autoantigens are restricted to particular tissues or organs, e.g. thyroid peroxidase and thyroglobulin in autoimmune thyroiditis, insulin and glutamate decarboxylase in type 1 diabetes mellitus. By contrast, systemic autoimmunity involves reactivity against widely spread tissue components, e.g. DNA, histones and ribonucleoproteins in systemic lupus erythematosus, IgG in rheumatoid arthritis.

Mechanisms of hypersensitivity

Although allergic and autoimmune disorders differ in the nature of the stimulating antigens, they can involve similar mechanisms of tissue damage, referred to as the four mechanisms of hypersensitivity (**Figure 11.7**).

Type I (immediate or reaginic) hypersensitivity occurs in a variety of atopic allergies (**Figure 11.7a**). It involves activation of tissue mast cells when an inducing allergen specifically binds to several IgE antibodies on the surface of mast cells. The IgE cross-linking induces the release of inflammatory mediators, as described under Digestive and inflammatory leukocytes above, which induce vasodilatation, increased vascular permeability and smooth muscle contraction. For example, inhaled allergens that induce immediate mast cell activation commonly cause allergic rhinitis and extrinsic asthma. These conditions may be seasonal (e.g. hay fever) or perennial in allergies to house dust mite or animal danders, for example. Severe systemic acute forms of type 1 hypersensitivity are seen in anaphylaxis (e.g. to nuts, insect stings, latex).

Type II (cell or membrane reactive) hypersensitivity involves antibodies of the IgG, IgA or IgM classes that bind to antigens associated with cell surface membranes or basement membranes (**Figure 11.7b**). The antigen-bound antibodies then activate complement, which may damage the membranes directly via the membrane attack complex, but also attract and activate neutrophils via the actions of C5a and C3a. The release of digestive enzymes and reactive oxygen species by the neutrophils can then exacerbate the membrane damage. Bullous pemphigoid is an example of a disease involving antibodies to basement membrane antigens. Some of the autoantibodies of pemphigoid bind to hemidesmosomes associated with epidermal basement membranes (although these antibodies have not conclusively been proven to be pathogenic). In pemphigus, by contrast, autoantibodies bind to desmoglein in the epidermal intracellular cement, and clearly correlate with tissue damage. Goodpasture's syndrome is another example of a disease involving autoantibodies to basement membranes; in this case the autoantigen is type IV collagen in alveolar and glomerular basement membranes. The muscle weakness of myasthenia gravis is induced by autoantibodies to the acetylcholine receptors in the post-synaptic membranes of muscles: these antibodies induce complement-mediated damage, receptor internalization and blockade that inhibit neurotransmission by acetylcholine.

Type III (immune complex mediated) hypersensitivity, like type II hypersensitivity, involves IgG, IgA and IgM antibodies, but in this case reacts with soluble antigens to form cross-linked molecular lattices containing multiple antibody and antigen molecules known as immune complexes (**Figure 11.7c**). These complexes can become too large to remain soluble and so precipitate within tissues where they can activate complement and neutrophils, leading to tissue damage. Allergic immune complex disease is exemplified by extrinsic allergic alveolitis that is triggered by inhalation of allergens that form immune complexes in the alveolar walls leading to tissue damage and fibrosis. Common allergens are fungal spores (e.g. in farmers' lung) and animal proteins (e.g. in bird fanciers' lung). In systemic lupus erythematosus, immune complex deposition can occur in various tissues including the skin, joints, lungs, brain and kidneys: these complexes are frequently composed of DNA and

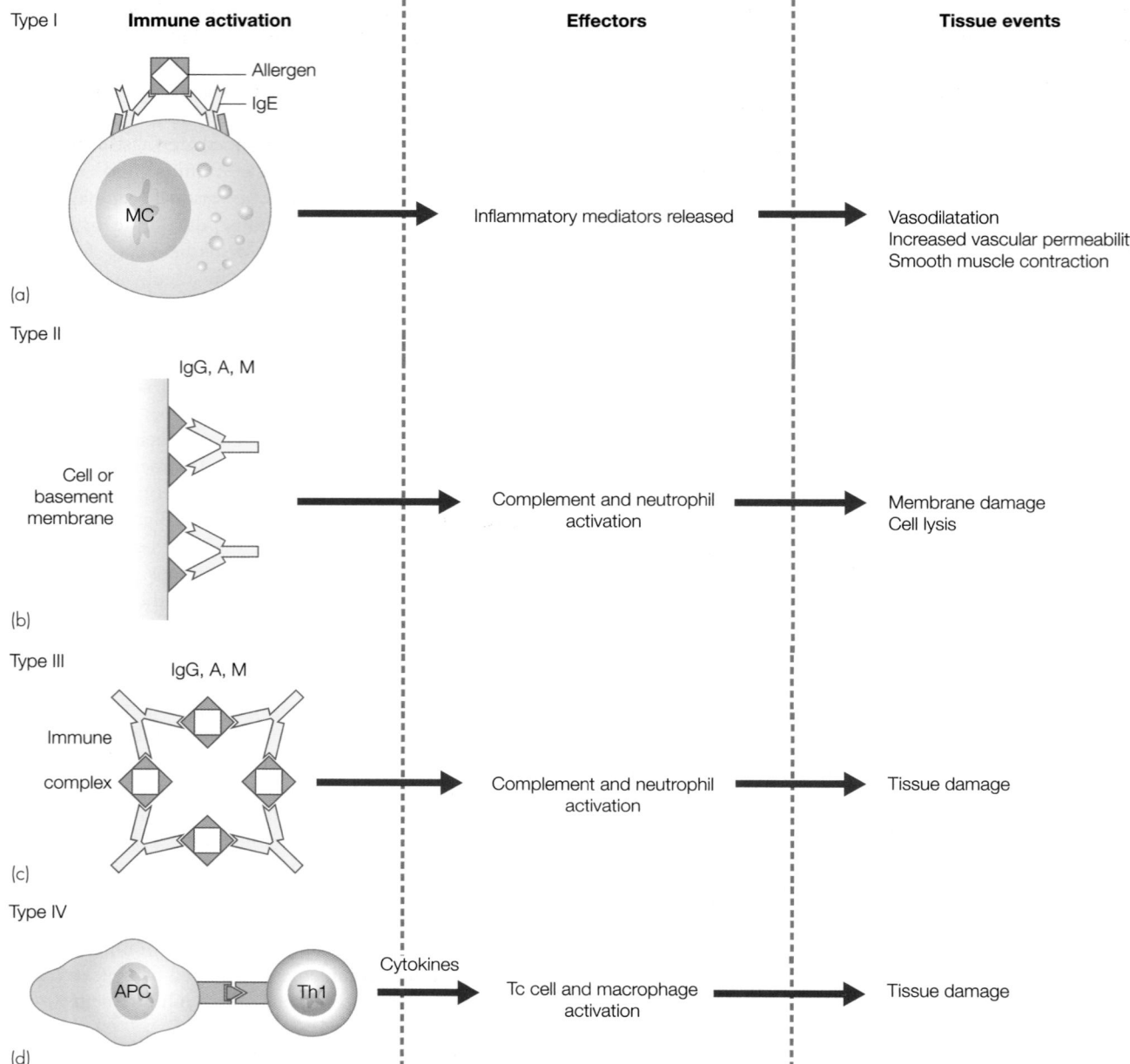

Figure 11.7 Mechanisms of hypersensitivity, see text for details. APC, antigen presenting cell; Ig, immunoglobulin; MC, mast cell; Th1, T helper 1 cell.

anti-DNA antibodies, with contributions from other nuclear and cytoplasmic autoantigens.

Type IV (cell mediated) hypersensitivity is distinguished from the other three types by not involving antibodies. It is principally dependent on the activities of T cell and macrophages with Th1 cells producing cytokines like IL-2 and IFN-gamma that activate cytotoxic T cells and macrophages, respectively (**Figure 11.7d**). Much of the tissue damage in a number of auto-immune diseases is brought about by cell-mediated mechanisms, although autoantibodies are also present, e.g. thyroiditis in the autoimmune thyroid diseases, insulitis in type 1 diabetes and synovitis in rheumatoid

arthritis. Sjogren's syndrome is characterized by lymphocytic destruction of exocrine tissues, particularly the lacrimal and salivary glands causing dry eyes and mouth. Tuberculosis is an example of an infectious disease in which much of the tissue damage is immune-mediated. Infection of lung macrophages by *Mycobacterium tuberculosis* that is resistant to intracellular digestion leads to chronic T cell activation and cytokine production.

Despite the clinical problems of hypersensitivity diseases, the severe, persistent, unusual and recurrent infection problems associated with the immuno-deficiency disorders, described in Chapter 14 Primary immunodeficiencies, highlight the vital defensive role of the immune system.

FURTHER READING

Chapel H, Haeney M, Misbah S, Snowden N. *Essentials of clinical immunology*, 5th edn. Oxford: Blackwell Publishers, 2006.

Janeway CA, Travers P, Walport M, Schlomchik M. *Immunobiology*, 6th edn. New York: Garland/Churchill Livingstone, 2005.

Male D, Brostoff J, Roth DB, Roitt I. *Immunology*, 7th edn. Edinburgh: Mosby, 2006.

Todd I, Spickett G. *Lecture notes on immunology*, 5th edn. Oxford: Blackwell Publishers, 2005.

12

Allergy: basic mechanisms and tests

STEPHEN R DURHAM AND GRAHAM BANFIELD

Introduction	144	Rhinitis/asthma link	158
Aetiology	144	Tests	158
Pathogenesis	146	Key points	161
Influence of treatment	152	Best clinical practice	161
Implications for therapy	155	References	163

SEARCH STRATEGY

The authors searched Pubmed using the key words allergy basic mechanisms, allergic rhinitis mechanisms, allergic rhinitis cytokines, allergic rhinitis chemokines, allergic rhinitis adhesion molecules. Major international allergy journals were also scanned.

INTRODUCTION

Atopy refers to a predisposition to develop exaggerated immunoglobulin E (IgE)-antibody responses against common inhaled aeroallergens. Atopy is defined clinically as a positive skin prick test and/or elevated serum allergen-specific IgE concentration to one or more common inhaled allergens, such as grass pollen, cat hair or house dust mite (HDM). Whereas a high proportion of atopic individuals develop allergic manifestations at some time during their lifetime, a substantial minority remain asymptomatic. In contrast to atopy, the term 'allergy' refers to the clinical expression of atopic allergic disease, such as allergic rhinitis, allergic bronchial asthma, atopic eczema and IgE-mediated food allergy.

In this chapter, the aetiology of allergic disease is briefly considered in relation to genetics and to environmental influences. Pathogenesis is considered, particularly in relation to allergic rhinitis, and considers mediators, IgE antibody, effector cells, mechanisms of cell recruitment, the role of T cells and T–B cell interactions, including local IgE regulation at allergic tissue sites and the role of IgE in facilitating allergen presentation to T cells. The influence of topical nasal corticosteroids and

allergen injection immunotherapy on these events are compared and contrasted.

A better understanding of basic mechanisms of allergy and the influence of current treatments has given rise to a number of novel, more targeted therapies for allergic rhinitis and asthma. New strategies for allergen immunotherapy are also briefly considered. Currently available tests for allergy diagnosis, including skin prick tests, allergen specific IgE concentrations and the role of serum tryptase measurements, are presented.

AETIOLOGY

Genetics

Allergic diseases result from a complex interaction between genetic and environmental influences. The contribution of genetics was illustrated by twin studies in which a higher concordance rate for atopy and allergic diseases was found in monozygotic compared with dizygotic twins.[1, 2] Over the past 15 years, two approaches have been used to identify disease-causing genes.[3] One

Table 12.1 Genetic associations with atopy, allergy and asthma.

Chromosome	Genetic association
1p	IL-12R
2q	IL-1, CTLA-4, CD28
5q	IL-3,4,5,9,13, GM-CSF, LTC4-S, β-R, GCS-R
6p	MHC
7q	TCR γ, IL-6
11q	Fcε R1 β chain
12q	IFN-γ, SCF, NO synthase, STAT-6
14q	TCR α δ NFκB inhibitor
16p	IL-4 R
17p	CC chemokines
19q	TGF-β1, CD22 (MDC)
20p	ADAM-33

Table 12.2 Inhaled allergens.

Seasonal	Perennial	Occupational
Grasses	Housedust mite	HMW: laboratory animals, flour, latex
Trees	Cats	LMW: colophony, isocyanates, acid anhydrides
Weeds	Dogs	
Moulds	Horses	

approach, entitled positional cloning, is based on the presence of highly polymorphic genetic markers with positions on a chromosome that are known. When multiple families are analysed, markers close to the disease gene will statistically be coinherited with the disease. Candidate gene approaches consist of directly studying a narrow region of the genome around the suspected gene with highly polymorphic markers. Interpretation of these studies has been complicated by variability in the strict definition of the clinical phenotypes within atopy, allergy and asthma. Nonetheless, multiple genetic loci have been identified. Examples,[3] classified according to their chromosomal localization, are given in **Table 12.1**. All of these genes have biologic functions consistent with a role in the pathogenesis of allergic disorders. Chromosome 5q is of particular interest, representing the loci of the major T helper (Th) lymphocyte 2 cytokine genes,[4] leukotriene C4 synthase (LTC4-S), the β-adrenergic receptor and the glucocorticosteroid receptor. A recent study which combined positional cloning techniques with candidate gene analysis identified strong linkage between asthma and bronchial hyperresponsiveness with the gene for A disintegrin and metalloprotease 33κ (ADAM-33), a cell surface protease which is part of the matrix metalloproteinase family, considered important in remodelling responses in the basement membrane to damaged epithelium and airway smooth muscle.[5]

Environment

ALLERGENS

The major allergens giving rise to allergic rhinitis and asthma are listed in **Table 12.2**. Within the UK, seasonal exposure to grass pollens is a major cause. In recent years, tree pollens that give rise to springtime hay fever have

become more prominent. Birch pollen allergy is commonly associated with oral allergy syndrome. Allergenic cross reactivity exists between birch pollen and apple, stone fruits and hazelnut, all of which may give rise to itching and swelling in the lips, mouth and pharynx. The common perennial allergens are house dust mite and animal danders. An occupational cause should be suspected in all patients whose symptoms are worse within the workplace or during the evening following work, with improvement at weekends and/or during holiday periods. Allergy to high molecular weight (HMW) allergens, including laboratory animals and latex, is commonly associated with rhinitis. In contrast, associations of rhinitis with exposure to low molecular weight (LMW) agents, such as isocyanates and acid anhydrides that are used as catalysts in paint and resin systems, are less well characterized. Further studies are needed.

HYGIENE HYPOTHESIS

There has been a marked increase in allergic disorders over the last 20 years in developed countries, including Western Europe, Australia, and New Zealand, where approximately 20 percent of the population have allergic rhinitis. Increases over such a short time period cannot be explained by genetic influences. Suggestions have included increases in allergen exposure due to changes in modern housing, such as fitted carpets, central heating and double glazing, which may have increased exposure to mite allergens. Other possible influences are increases in environmental pollution, and changes in the diet and the gut flora. Strachan coined the term 'hygiene hypothesis' which suggested that improved hygiene in industrialized societies, together with improved public health measures and use of vaccines and antibiotics, have reduced the incidence of infections.[6] Epidemiologic studies have shown that large family size, and presumed high exposure to infectious agents, protects against the development of allergic diseases. Similarly, exposure to farm animals early in life reduces atopic sensitization and asthma, possibly due to higher bacterial endotoxin levels.[7] The hypothesis is that lack of infections leads to less frequent stimulation of Th1-biased responses, thereby facilitating development of Th2-biased immune responses to environmental allergens.[8] However, the observed parallel increases in Th1-mediated autoimmune disorders, such as type-1 diabetes and multiple sclerosis, argue against this theory.[9] An alternative explanation that may possibly account for the observed increase in both Th1 and Th2 disorders in recent years is a failure of regulation of the immune response by so-called T regulatory cells that secrete the inhibitory cytokines interleukin (IL)-10 and transforming growth factor (TGF)-β. Since regulatory T cells control immune responses to bacteria, a reduced microbial pressure could suppress the development or function of T regulatory cells, which would have an impact on both allergic and autoimmune diseases.[10] Similar hypotheses underpin the mechanism of allergen specific immunotherapy, the only treatment which has been shown to modify the natural history of allergic disorders (see Allergen injection immunotherapy).

POLLUTION

It has been suggested that urban pollution, particularly from motor exhaust fumes, may be one factor responsible for the increasing prevalence of allergic disorders. For example, the increase in hay fever due to Japanese cedar pollen over the last 30 years has coincided with a dramatic increase in motor vehicle exhaust pollution. The increase in cedar pollen allergy in Japan is largely confined to urban, rather than rural, areas.[11] Diesel particulates have been shown to be adjuvant for IgE antibody production, whereas exposure to the combination of nitrogen dioxide and ozone may amplify subsequent pollen-induced immediate symptoms of rhinitis. However, studies comparing the prevalence of hay fever in heavily polluted districts in Leipzig compared with relative pollution-free areas of Munich[12] have shown that hay fever is more common in Munich. For these reasons, the role of pollution in hay fever and asthma remains controversial. Undoubtedly, pollutants may irritate or exacerbate symptoms, although the role of specific

pollutants in the development of pollen sensitivity and the persistence of hay fever symptoms remains in doubt.

PATHOGENESIS

Early and late allergic responses

The classic features of allergic inflammation include IgE-dependent activation of mast cells and tissue eosinophilia (**Figure 12.1**).[13] Following allergen provocation in sensitive subjects, there occurs an early allergic response that is maximal at 10–30 minutes and resolves within one to two hours. In the skin, this is manifest as a weal and flare response, in the nose as itching that occurs within seconds and watery nasal discharge and nasal congestion within minutes, whereas allergen inhalation results in immediate bronchospasm with associated wheezing, cough and chest tightness. In a proportion of subjects, approximately 50 percent of adults and 70 percent of children, there occurs a late phase response that begins at three to four hours, is maximal at 6–12 hours and resolves within 24–48 hours. The magnitude of early and late phase responses is dependent upon the sensitivity of the subject and the allergen dose used for provocation. In the nose, late responses are manifest largely as nasal obstruction and are far less pronounced than the airways hyperinflation, chest tightness and dyspnoea that accompany late asthmatic responses. Late asthmatic responses are accompanied by an increase in nonspecific bronchial hyperresponsiveness that may last for several days, or occasionally weeks, following a single allergen provocation. During this time, there is a heightened sensitivity to nonspecific triggers such as exercise, cold air and viral infections, and a reduced threshold for development of immediate allergic responses following allergen re-exposure.[14]

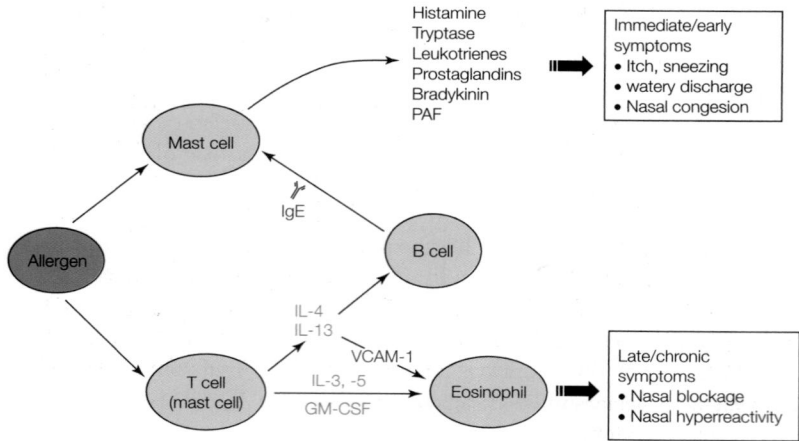

Figure 12.1 Basic mechanisms of human early and late allergic responses.

Mediators of hypersensitivity

The early allergic response is largely mast cell-dependent. Cross linking of adjacent IgE molecules on the mast cell surface by allergen results in mast cell degranulation and the release of mediators of hypersensitivity with known biological properties responsible for the early allergic response. Mediators released by the mast cell include histamine, leukotriene C4, D4 and E4 and tryptase.[15, 16]

Histamine stimulates H1 receptors on sensory nerves giving rise to immediate itching and sneezing within seconds of allergen exposure. In addition, histamine causes vascular dilatation and increased permeability with plasma exudation, contributing to the sensation of nasal congestion. Histamine may also provoke immediate bronchospasm and is responsible for most, but not all, the immediate skin weal and flare.

Leukotrienes increase vascular permeability, induce mucus secretion from nasal and bronchial glands and induce bronchoconstriction involving, in particular, the small airways. Whereas histamine and tryptase are preformed in mast cell granules, leukotrienes and the mast cell derived prostaglandin D2 are newly formed, membrane-derived mediators generated from membrane arachidonic acid under the influence of 5-lipoxygenase. The role of tryptase is unclear, although tryptase has potent enzymatic activity and breaks down kininogen from the blood, leading to the formation of potent inflammatory kinins, including bradykinin, an extremely potent mediator that promotes acute plasma extravasation and is likely to be a major factor in the formation of angio-oedema. In addition, mast cells and basophils produce IL-4 and other inflammatory cytokines that may contribute to the induction of late responses.

In contrast to the immediate response, the late phase response is characterized by T cell recruitment and activation and tissue eosinophilia (**Figure 12.1**).[16] Whereas mast cells and basophils are recognized sources of IL-4 and IL-13, T lymphocytes represent the principle source of Th2 cytokines during late responses.[17] Examples of mast cells, activated (EG2[+]) eosinophils, cluster of differentiation (CD)4[+] T cells and IL-5 messenger ribonucleic acid (mRNA)[+] cells present within the nasal epithelium and submucosa are shown in **Figure 12.2**.

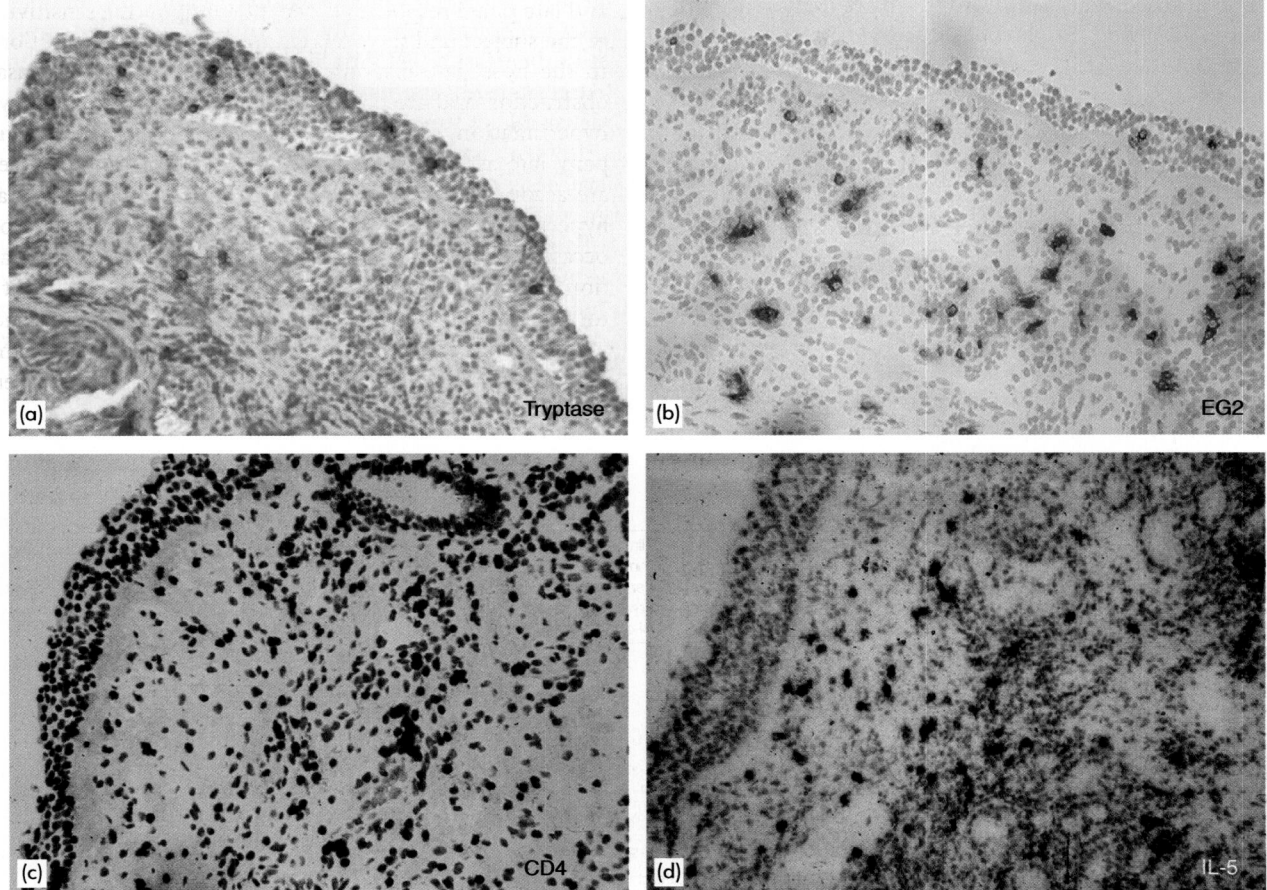

Figure 12.2   Immunohistochemistry and *in situ* hybridization studies demonstrating labelling of (a) mast cells, (b) activated eosinophils, (c) Th lymphocytes and (d) cells expressing mRNA for the cytokine IL-5.

Sensory nerves

Activation of sensory nerves is a pivotal event in the generation of acute symptoms of rhinitis.[18] Also, sensory innovation is, in large part, responsible for increased nasal hyperreactivity to nonspecific triggers in allergic individuals. For example, capsaicin is a potent stimulus for nerve C-fibres and provokes a 100-fold stronger secretory response in patients with allergic rhinitis compared to healthy control subjects following allergen challenge. Sensory nerves themselves may produce inflammation by an antidromic axon reflex which causes sensory nerves to release neuropeptides such as substance P and neurokinin A. This 'neurogenic inflammation' is self-perpetuating and represents an important component of the allergen–IgE interaction. Nerve growth factor, responsible for maturation and development of sensory nerves, is present in nasal fluids of patients with chronic allergic rhinitis and is increased after allergen challenge.[18] Thus, the immediate response represents a complex interaction between mediators of hypersensitivity released following mast cell activation and their interaction with sensory nerves, the vasculature and mucus-secreting glands. Increased allergen-induced target organ hyperresponsiveness that is associated with late responses and ongoing day-to-day allergic disease is likely to relate to a combination of both inflammation and heightened sensory nerve activation, the contribution of these components varying in different individuals.

Immunoglobulin E

The concentration of IgE in serum is the lowest of the five immunoglobulin classes, being around 100–400 ng/mL. The majority of IgE is tissue-bound with a half-life of approximately 11–14 days. IgE is bound to high affinity receptors (Fcε R1) on mast cells and basophils.[19] Recent studies have demonstrated that, in contrast to other immunoglobulins, Fcε R1 is present on dendritic cells in atopic individuals and in low numbers on monocytes/macrophages and eosinophils, although on these cell types, Fcε R1 lacks the β-chain subunit and is of doubtful functional significance, at least in terms of IgE-dependent activation.[20] IgE is also bound to low-affinity IgE receptors Fcε R2 (CD23) present on monocytes/macrophages and, in particular, on B cells.

B lymphocytes initially produce IgM antibodies. Heavy chain class switching in favour of IgE antibody production occurs in two steps.[21] Step one involves generation of a sterile ε-germline gene transcript under the influence of IL-4 and/or IL-13. Step two, heavy chain gene rearrangement, will only proceed following cross-linking of CD40 on the B cell surface by CD40 ligand. Th2 T-lymphocytes express IL-4, IL-13 and CD40 ligand and are essential for allergen-specific class switching in to IgE synthesis.

Additionally, mast cells and basophils express IL-4, IL-13 and CD40 ligand and therefore have the potential to augment/amplify IgE synthesis in a nonspecific manner.

The traditional view has been that IgE class switching occurs in the bone marrow and draining regional lymph nodes. However, the presence of Th2 cells and B cells and the expression locally of IL-4 and IL-13 in the nasal and bronchial mucosa raised the possibility that IgE synthesis might occur locally at these allergic tissue sites. In support of this concept, CD20[+] B cells that express ε germline transcripts and Cε heavy chain RNA are detectable in the nasal mucosa in allergic rhinitis[22] and in the bronchial mucosa of patients with both and atopic and nonatopic asthma.[23] Local increases in allergen-specific isotype-specific IgE are detectable in bronchoalveolar lavage fluid following allergen challenge in atopic asthma.[24] Coker and colleagues identified and sequenced IgE variable region heavy chain genes from B cells within the nasal mucosa.[24] In contrast to findings in peripheral blood, the detection of highly homologous variable segment genes within the nasal mucosa confirmed the clonality of local B cells, consistent with heavy chain class switching occurring within the nasal mucosa. By use of in situ hybridization of sections of cultured nasal mucosal biopsies, upregulation of IL-4 and ε germline gene transcripts were detectable within 24 hours of allergen stimulation.[25] By use of enzyme-linked immunosorbent assay (ELISA) of supernatants from cultured nasal biopsies, spontaneous synthesis of IgE protein was detectable at three to seven days.[26]

Taken together, these observations confirm local synthesis of IgE within the respiratory mucosa, thereby providing a long-lived source of IgE for local sensitization of mast cells and basophils in target organs. This may explain why some atopic individuals with elevated serum IgE concentrations develop rhinitis, whereas others develop bronchial asthma or atopic eczema, whereas others may exhibit positive skin prick tests without any clinical manifestations. The presence of IgE in the bronchial mucosa of nonatopic asthmatics and, as recently shown in the nasal mucosa of patients with so-called intrinsic rhinitis,[27] implies the potential importance of IgE in these subjects in the absence of positive skin prick tests or raised serum allergen-specific IgE concentrations. The findings raise the testable hypothesis that strategies directed against IgE may also be of value in patients with late onset 'intrinsic' rhinitis and asthma.

Effector cells

MAST CELLS

Mast cells are tissue-based inflammatory cells derived from cKIT[+] CD34[+] pluripotent bone marrow stem cells. Mast cell precursors circulate via the blood and lymphatic tissues where they mature under the influence of cKIT-ligand (stem cell factor (SCF)), produced from local structural cells.[19] Other cytokines involved in mast cell maturation and survival include IL-4, IL-5, IL-6, IL-9 and interferon gamma (IFN-γ). Mast cells have been classified traditionally as mucosal and connective tissue types. By use of specific immunostaining, mucosal mast cells are predominantly tryptase-only positive, whereas connective tissue mast cells are tryptase positive chymase positive. Although this classification has been questioned, there is clear evidence for a predominance of tryptase only-positive mast cells in the bronchial mucosa, and in patients with hayfever, natural allergen exposure results in transepithelial migration of tryptase-only positive mast cells to the epithelial surface.

BASOPHILS

Basophils are granulocytes that share many common features with mast cells, including expression of Fcε R1, metachromatic staining and the synthesis and release of histamine, and IL-4.[19] Basophils develop from CD34+ pluripotent bone marrow stem cells which circulate to the periphery where IL-3 is the dominant cytokine involved in differentiation of basophils from IL-3-receptor positive precursors. The role of basophils in allergic disease has recently been highlighted following the availability of two basophil granule-specific monoclonal antibody markers, namely BB-1 and 2D7. Basophils are increased in the nasal epithelium during seasonal grass pollen exposure and eliminated following successful immunotherapy. Basophils are detectable in the bronchial mucosa in asthma, and they increase in numbers and express IL-4 during allergen-induced late responses.[28]

EOSINOPHILS

Blood and tissue eosinophilia are hallmarks of allergy.[19] Eosinophils have a bilobed nucleus and multiple intracellular granules that contain highly basic proteins that include major basic protein (MBP) and eosinophil cationic protein (ECP). Eosinophils are derived from progenitors in the bone marrow under the influence of IL-3, IL-5 and granulocyte–macrophage colony stimulating factor. Eosinophils are present at allergic tissue sites and increase in numbers following allergen provocation[16] and during natural seasonal exposure. Eosinophil proteins have been localized to sites of epithelial damage in asthma and have been shown to be highly toxic *in vitro* to human bronchial epithelium. Eosinophils produce lipid mediators, including leukotriene C4 and platelet activating factor (PAF). They also produce a range of cytokines, including IL-4, IL-5 and granulocyte–macrophage colony stimulating factor (GM-CSF). Eosinophils have many surface receptors, including IL-3R, IL-5R and GM-CSFR. Characteristic chemokine receptors (CCR) include CCR3. They possess immunoglobulin receptors including Fc γR2 (CD32), Fc αR1 (secretory IgA), complement receptors (C3aR, C5aR) and adhesion molecules, particularly very late antigen (VLA)-4, the ligand for the eosinophil-selective vascular cell adhesion molecule-1 (VCAM-1).

CELLULAR RECRUITMENT

The presence of effector cells in allergic inflammation depends upon a balance between their recruitment, persistence and survival in tissues. Local mechanisms responsible for recruitment and activation of eosinophils are shown in **Figure 12.3**. Eosinophil recruitment is an active process involving four steps. Mast cell activation by allergen results in the release of inflammatory cytokines including IL-1 and tumour necrosis factor (TNF)-alpha that upregulate adhesion molecules present on the vascular endothelium. The transit of eosinophils is initially slowed by the early expression of E-selectin which binds to its ligand present on the eosinophil surface.[29] This results in the rolling of the eosinophil along the vascular endothelium. Cell activation with an increase in eosinophil surface expression of receptors such as CCR3 and VLA-4 occurs in response to chemokines, particularly eotaxin and RANTES (released from activated normal T cells expressed and secreted).[30] The adhesion of eosinophils to the vascular endothelium is dependent upon binding of VCAM-1 produced from the vascular endothelium to its ligand VLA-4 on the eosinophil surface.

Following adhesion, there follows the active migration of eosinophils through the vascular endothelium, followed by directional migration along a chemotactic gradient involving interaction between eotaxin and RANTES with CCR3. Other chemotactic factors, which may be involved in eosinophil recruitment, include the monocyte chemotactic proteins (MCP)-2, and 3. CCR3 is a common receptor for eotaxin, RANTES, and the monocyte chemokine proteins and is highly expressed on the surface of eosinophils, basophils, mast cells and Th2 T-lymphocytes, all of which are characteristic of allergic inflammation. Nasal administration of both RANTES[31] and eotaxin[32] has been shown to provoke nasal symptoms and increase local eosinophils. Both eotaxin[33] and RANTES are detectable in nasal lavage fluid and/or the nasal mucosa during natural disease and increase following allergen provocation.[34]

T–LYMPHOCYTES

T-lymphocytes are central to the pathogenesis of allergic diseases, since they are the only cells capable of recognizing antigenic material after processing by antigen pre;senting cells. T-cell responses are classified into two subtypes, depending on their cytokine profile in response to antigenic stimulation. Th1 cells express predominantly IFN-γ and IL-2, whereas Th2 cells express preferentially IL-4, IL-5 and IL-13.[35] Present evidence points to the

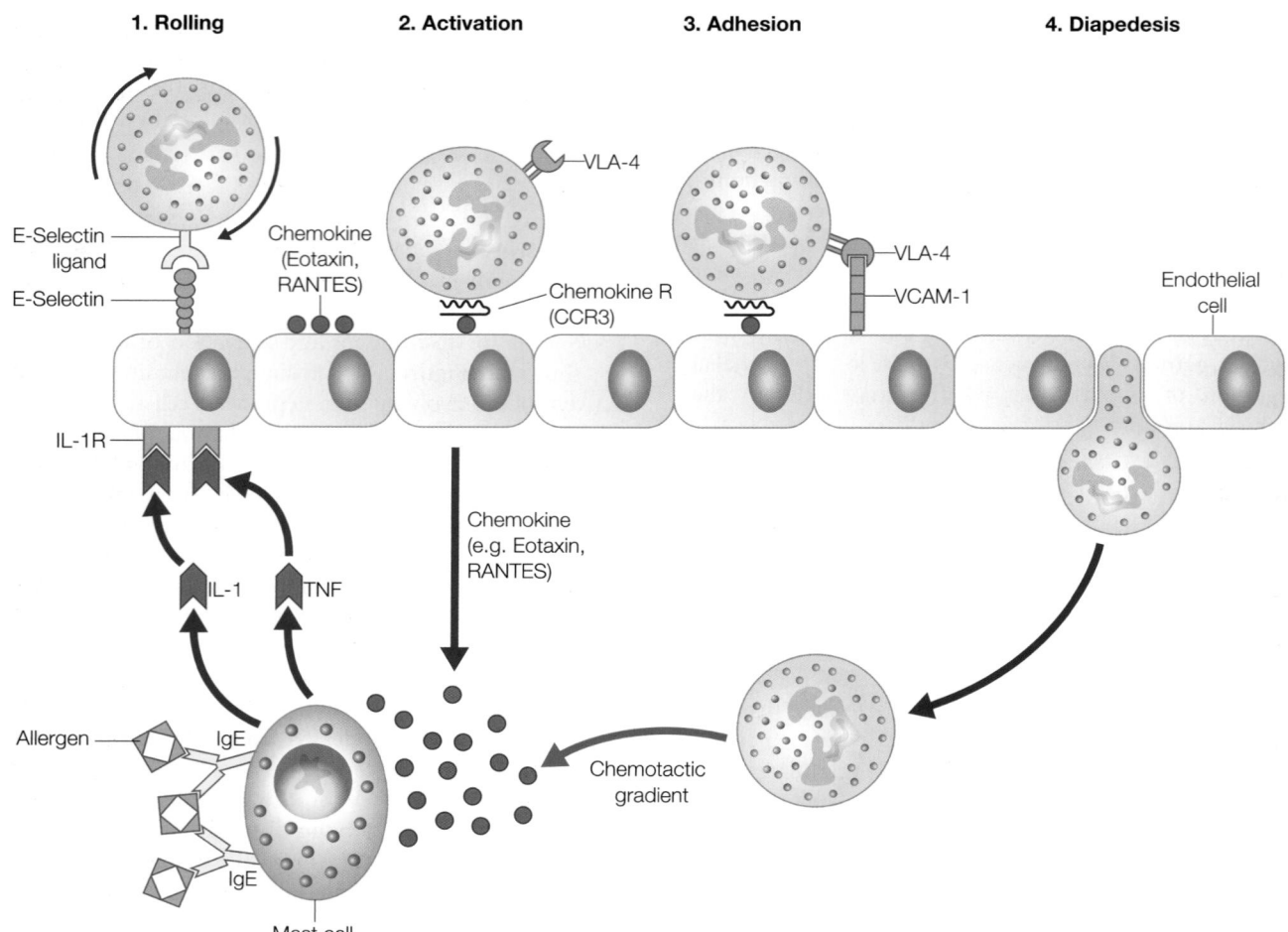

Figure 12.3 Schematic showing eosinophil recruitment from the vascular compartment to the tissues demonstrating the complex interplay between vascular adhesion molecules and chemokines.

recruitment of Th2 cells, their activation in tissues and generation of Th2 cytokines as cardinal features of both allergic rhinitis and asthma.[36] Allergenic peptides are presented to T-cell receptors as a high-affinity complex of peptide and major histocompatability complex (MHC) class II molecules. The binding of peptide alone to the T cell receptor (TCR) is insufficient to cause activation of T cells in the absence of costimulation. Costimulatory molecules involved include CD4, CD8, lymphocyte-function associated (LFA)-1, CD28 and cytotoxic T-lymphocyte-associated molecule (CTLA)-4 on the T-cell and MHC class II, intercellular adhesion molecule (ICAM)-1 and -2, and the B7 homologues, CD80/CD86 on the antigen presenting cell surface. In particular, CD28 ligation by B7-1 (CD80) and B7-2 (CD86) is a necessary requirement for the synthesis and secretion of the T-cell growth factor IL-2. In the absence of co-stimulation, signalling through the TCR results in a nonresponsive state known as 'anergy', which may last for several days or weeks.[37]

T cells may differentiate preferentially into Th1- or Th2-cells, depending on their location, the level (or dose)

of allergen stimulation, the nature of the antigen presenting cell, the level of co-stimulation and the local cytokine environment.[36] In general, low doses of soluble allergen presented at mucosal surfaces by B cells or dendritic cells, preferentially favour Th2 T cell development. These circumstances are typical of those occurring during natural seasonal pollen exposure and in the presence of low doses of perennial environmental allergens, such as cat fur and house dust mite. In contrast, high concentrations of allergen via injection as, for example, during allergen immunotherapy, and preferential presentation by monocyte/macrophages favour Th1 T lymphocyte development. The local cytokine milieu is a critical factor in T lymphocyte differentiation and activation. For example, IL-4 produced by mast cells and basophils, as well as T-lymphocytes[38] may induce Th2 T lymphocyte development at mucosal surfaces, whereas local IL-12 may induce preferential Th1 responses. An additional level of control of T-cell activation during IgE-dependent responses occurs at the level of the antigen presenting cell (APC). Allergen-specific IgE bound to inhaled allergens can be taken up and presented to T cells via low affinity IgE receptors (CD23 Fcε R2) expressed on B cells and other APCs or via high affinity IgE receptors (Fcε R1) expressed on monocytes or dendritic cells.[39] Formation of allergen–IgE complexes, with preferential uptake at low allergen concentration, as occurs at mucosal surfaces, results in a marked (10–100-fold) reduction in threshold levels of aeroallergen necessary to trigger T cell activation *in vivo*. Thus *in vivo* T cell-dependent late responses may be augmented by IgE-dependent mechanisms, including IL-4 and formation of allergen–IgE complexes. Conversely, interference with these IgE-dependent mechanisms by 'functional' immunoglobulin G (IgG) antibodies (see Allergen injection immunotherapy) may down-regulate antigen-specific T-cell responses, manifest as inhibition of late responses *in vivo*.[40]

Preferential Th1 or Th2 T-lymphocyte activation and cytokine synthesis is dependent on interactions between sequence-specific transcription factors, present within the cytoplasm of T cells that may translocate to the nucleus and interact with promotor and enhancer regions of RNA polymerase II-dependent genes.[41] For example, IL-4 signalling in favour of Th2 T lymphocyte development requires activation of the signal transducer and activator of transcription (STAT)-6. Th2 cytokine synthesis is dependent upon the transcription factors c-MAF (critical for the expression of IL-4) and GATA-3 (involved in the regulation of both IL-4 and IL-5). Conversely, IL-12-induced Th1 T lymphocyte development requires activation of STAT-4 and synthesis of the Th1 cytokine INF-γ is critically dependent upon the transcription factor T-bet.

Recent evidence from murine models points to an additional distinct subset of so-called T-regulatory cells which are capable of inhibiting the activation of T cells at peripheral sites.[42] These T cells are CD4+ CD25+, and their immunosuppressive properties have been linked to the production of the cytokines IL-10, TGF-β or both. Regulatory T cells might also down-regulate T-cell responses through cell–cell contact, as well as through the direct effect of these cytokines.[43] In man, IL-10 producing CD4+ CD25+ T regulatory cells have recently been recognized in peripheral blood[44] and have been shown to play a role in natural tolerance induction in bee keepers during high allergen exposure to bee venom.[45] T-regulatory cells have been associated with the co-expression of certain cell surface markers such as GITR and CTLA-4. The novel transcription factor Fox P3 has been shown to be important in gene regulation of IL-10 synthesis in these cells.

Over the last decade, studies in peripheral blood, the nose and the lung have confirmed the central role of Th2 T lymphocytes in allergic diseases. Th2 cytokines are detectable in the nasal mucosa during seasonal and perennial rhinitis. Following local allergen provocation, preferential T lymphocyte expression of IL-4 and IL-5, but not INF-γ, is detectable in bronchoalveolar lavage, the bronchial mucosa and in the nose (**Figures 12.4** and

12.5).[17] The combination of immunocytochemistry and *in situ* hybridization has co-localized the majority of Th2 cytokines detectable at 24 hours after allergen to T-lymphocytes, whereas at earlier time points, mast cells (IL-4) and eosinophils (IL-4 and IL-5) are more prominent sources of Th2 cytokines.[46] Th2-lymphocytes preferentially express the chemokine receptors CCR3, CCR4 and CCR8, all of which may be involved in their recruitment and activation in allergic rhinitis and asthma.[30]

DENDRITIC CELLS

Dendritic cells are professional antigen presenting cells which are abundant within the epithelium and submucosa of the upper and lower respiratory mucosa in patients with allergic diseases.[47] Expression of CD1a on the cell surface is a marker of a subclass of dendritic cells, Langerhans cells. Traditionally, dendritic cells have been classified as myeloid derived DC1 cells derived from human blood monocytes or DC2, plasmacytoid cells derived from lymphoid cells. Dendritic cells are highly efficient at capturing, processing and presenting antigen to T cells. It has been suggested that DC1 cells produce high levels of IL-12 and favour Th1 T-cell development, whereas DC2 cells are low-IL-12 producers and support preferential Th2 T-lymphocyte differentiation. However, it is likely that rather than distinct dendritic cell subpopulations, differential function may depend on their location, their degree of maturation and the local cytokine milieu. Immature cells express high levels of immunoglobulin receptors and are highly endocytic, in keeping with efficient allergen capture. In contrast, mature cells express high levels of MHC class II and have upregulated CD86 expression and produce abundant cytokines, features consistent with their role in allergen presentation and immune modulation. A recent study in rodents suggested that local allergen provocation in the bronchial mucosa resulted in the rapid maturation from immature to mature phenotype of dendritic cells within two hours of allergen exposure, with rapid upregulation of MHC class II and upregulated CD86 expression.[48] Interestingly, this rapid maturation was only observed in dendritic cells within the bronchial mucosa and not peripheral lung. Rapid dendritic cell recruitment to the bronchial mucosa in atopic asthmatic patients has also been observed within the time frame of late asthmatic responses following local segmental allergen challenge. Recruitment of so-called plasmacytoid (CD123) IL-3R α-chain positive, CD45 RA positive cells increase dramatically in numbers, as detected in nasal biopsies, following local allergen challenge repeated daily for seven days.[49] This is of particular interest since plasmacytoid dendritic cells matured *in vitro* can induce preferential Th2 T-cell development. Recently, Novak examined IgE receptor expression on dendritic cells

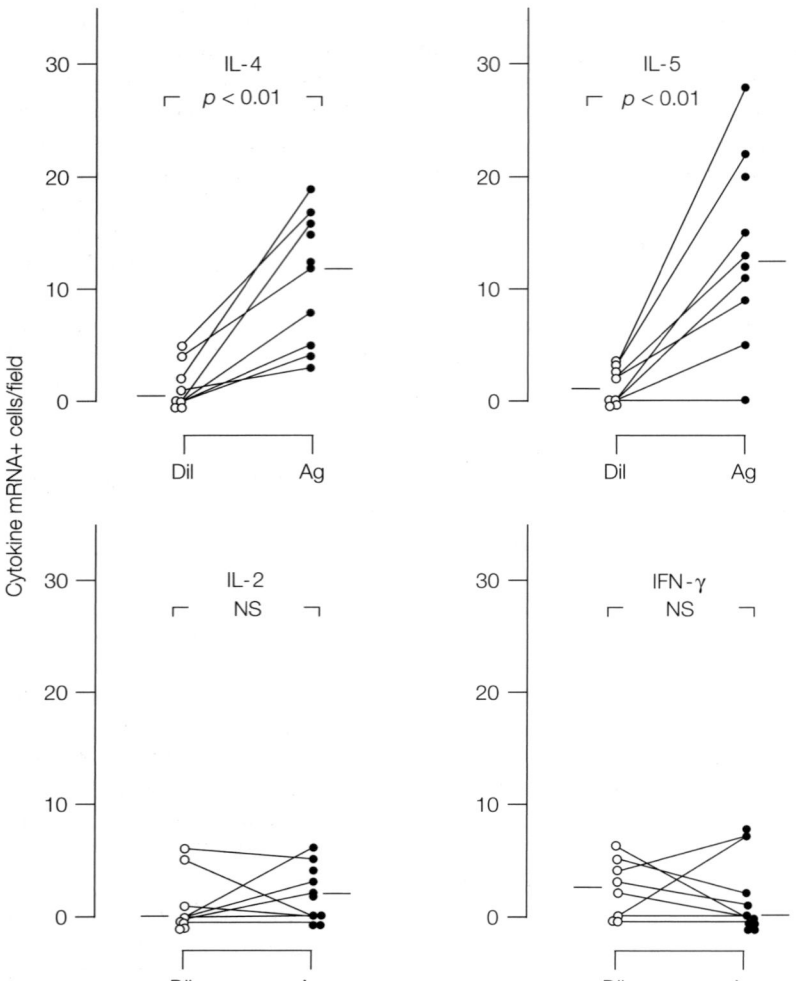

Figure 12.4 Preferential production of Th2 type cytokines, detected by *in situ* hybridization during allergen induced late responses in the nasal mucosa.

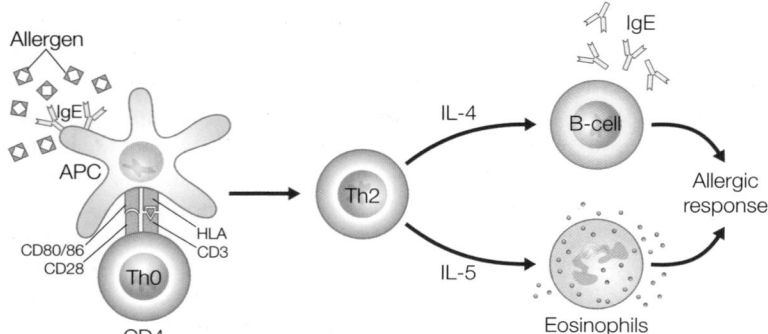

Figure 12.5 The pivotal role of Th2 lymphocytes and the cytokines IL-4 and IL-5 in the pathogenesis of the allergic response.

from atopic and nonatopic individuals. FCε R1α is expressed on dendritic cells from both groups, but differential expression of the gamma chain on dendritic cells from atopics is associated with sustained surface expression of Fcε R1, consistent with a more efficient antigen-presenting cell in the context of IgE-associated Th2 T-lymphocyte development.[50]

INFLUENCE OF TREATMENT

Antihistamines

Antihistamines are effective in the partial suppression of immediate allergen-induced responses in the skin, nose and lung. The particular importance of histamine as an inflammatory mediator in the upper airway is confirmed by the effectiveness of antihistamines in allergic rhinitis, whereas antihistamines have little or no effect on allergen-induced late asthmatic responses and are much less effective in bronchial asthma. In contrast, topical corticosteroids, the most effective agents in the treatment of chronic perennial allergic rhinitis and asthma, when given immediately before allergen provocation, have virtually no effect on allergen-induced early responses. In contrast, topical corticosteroids, when given immediately before challenge, are highly effective in inhibiting allergen-induced late responses in the skin, nose and lung. For example, in a controlled trial in patients with allergic asthma, inhaled beclomethasone, but not oral cetirizine, was effective in suppressing allergen-induced late asthmatic responses and associated increases in airway methacholine responsiveness.[51] [****] Similarly, in a controlled trial in patients with allergic rhinitis, six weeks treatment with intranasal aqueous fluticasone proprionate resulted in only a 50 percent inhibition of early nasal symptoms whereas complete inhibition of nasal symptoms at 1–24 hours after challenge was observed.[52] [****] These effects of corticosteroids *in vivo*, are consistent with their observed effects *in vitro*. Corticosteroids have no effect on IgE-dependent activation of mast cells and mediator release *in vitro*, whereas allergen-induced Th2 T-lymphocyte proliferation and cytokine secretion are exquisitely sensitive to corticosteroids in low 10^{-10} to 10^{-8} molar concentrations.[53] [****]

Topical corticosteroids

Topical corticosteroids and their effects on inflammatory cells, antigen presenting cells, cytokine synthesis and the expression of chemokines and adhesion molecules have been extensively studied in allergic rhinitis following allergen provocation and during natural seasonal exposure. For example, six weeks treatment with topical fluticasone proprionate resulted in a marked reduction in T lymphocytes, eosinophils and mast cells within the nasal mucosa.[52] [****] Effects were more pronounced on cell numbers in the epithelium compared to the lamina propria and submucosa. Neutrophil numbers were either unaffected or tended to increase following topical steroid therapy. Topical corticosteroids inhibited cytokine mRNA expression for IL-4 and resulted in a reduction in local Th2 cytokine protein levels.[54] [****] Corticosteroids inhibited adhesion molecule expression and RANTES secretion.[55] Local synthesis of IgE is also inhibited, as illustrated by a marked reduction in ε-germline gene transcripts and Cε mRNA for the IgE heavy chain.[22] [****] These effects of topical corticosteroids on the nasal mucosa during late responses have also been confirmed during natural seasonal grass pollen exposure. For example, topical corticosteroid resulted in a marked reduction in nasal mucosal eosinophils and a parallel reduction in IL-5 mRNA-expressing cells, principally T lymphocytes, within the nasal mucosa (**Figure 12.6**).[54] [****] Similarly, local upregulation of IL-4 and local IgE synthesis in the nasal during the pollen season was inhibited by topical corticosteroids.[56] [****] A characteristic feature of seasonal allergic rhinitis is the transepithelial migration of CD1a positive Langerhans cells. Following topical corticosteroids, nasal mucosal Langerhans cells were reduced in the submucosa and absent from the nasal epithelium.[57] [****]

In summary, topical corticosteroids are highly effective and have profound effects on cell recruitment and activation in allergic rhinitis. It seems likely that these effects are largely mediated either directly on Th2 cells, by downregulating their recruitment, activation and cytokine synthesis, or indirectly via suppression of antigen presenting cells, such as nasal mucosal Langerhans cells (**Figure 12.7**).

Allergen injection immunotherapy

Immunotherapy involves the step-wise incremental injection of increasing subcutaneous doses of allergen, in order to suppress symptoms on subsequent re-exposure to that allergen. Immunotherapy is highly effective in selected patients with a limited spectrum of IgE-dependent allergies.[58] [****] Immunotherapy is particularly effective in seasonal pollinosis, although less effective in polysensitized patients with perennial disease. Risks are increased in patients with bronchial asthma, in whom immunotherapy is not currently recommended within the UK. In contrast to topical corticosteroids, immunotherapy, when given monthly for three to four years, has been shown to induce long-term remission for at least three years following discontinuation of treatment.[59] [****] In children, immunotherapy has been shown to reduce the risk of physician-diagnosed asthma at three to five years after commencing treatment[60] [****] and to prevent the onset of new allergen sensitivities in children.[61] [***] These studies strongly suggest that immunotherapy is the only treatment that has the potential to modify the course of allergic disease.

Immunotherapy has been associated with a decrease in the mucosal recruitment and activation of inflammatory cells, a reduction in the release of inflammatory mediators in target organs and increases in 'protective' serum IgG antibodies.[62] Immunotherapy suppresses both early and late nasal responses after allergen challenge. Suppression of late responses in the skin and nose has been associated with immune deviation with a reduction in the local expression of Th2 cytokines and an increase in the Th1 cytokine INF-γ. Recently, pollen immunotherapy was shown to reduce nasal mucosal eosinophil and basophil numbers during the pollen season.[63] There were also seasonal increases in the ratio of local INF-γ to IL-5-producing cells in the nasal mucosa after immunotherapy,

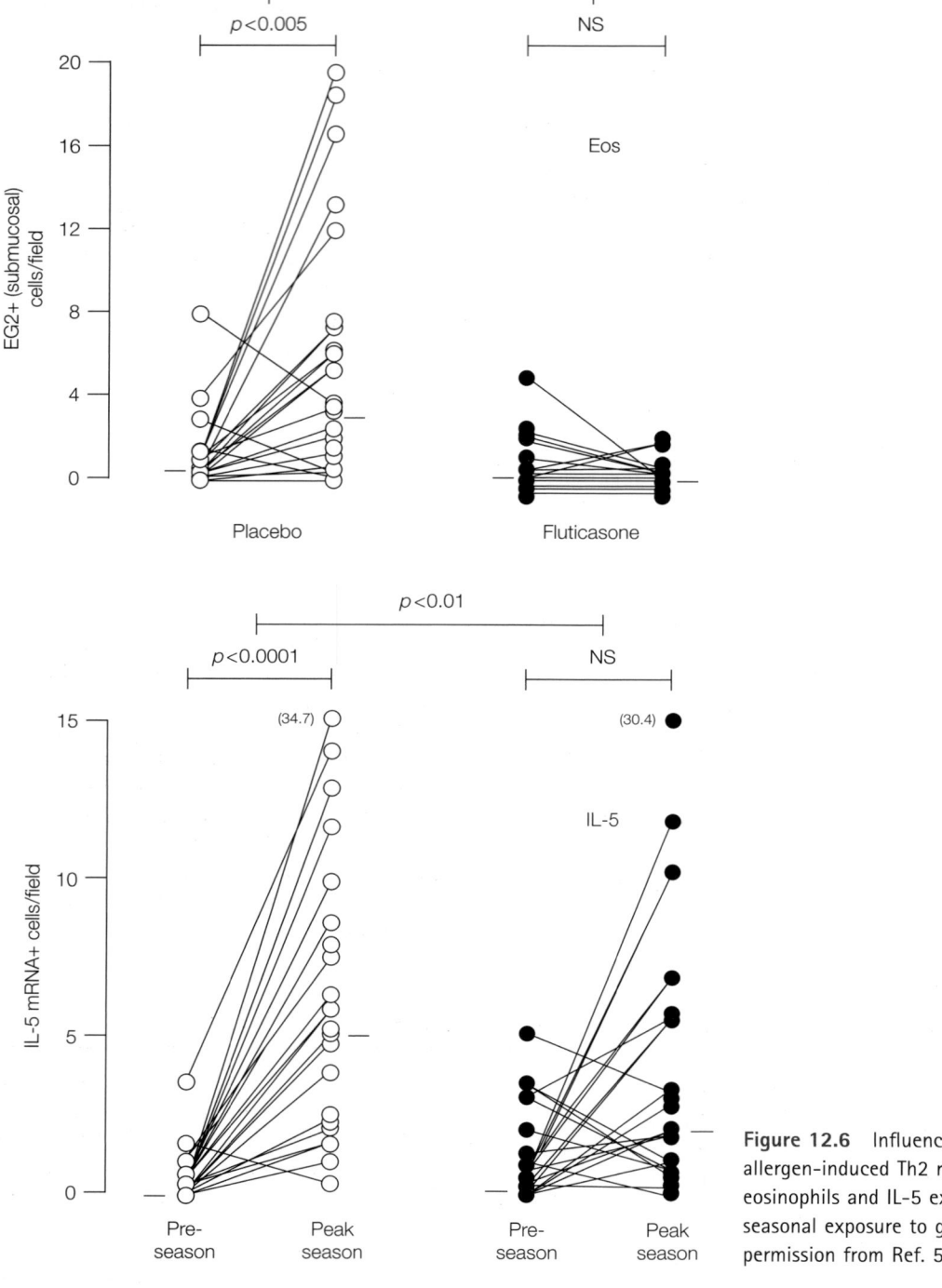

Figure 12.6 Influence of corticosteroids on allergen-induced Th2 responses (nasal mucosal eosinophils and IL-5 expression) during natural seasonal exposure to grass pollen. Reproduced with permission from Ref. 53.

consistent with immune deviation of local T cell responses in favour of Th1 responses (**Figure 12.8**).[64] In the same nasal biopsies, we identified increases in the number of IL-10 and TGF-β producing cells, detectable at both messenger RNA and protein levels.[65] Co-localization confirmed that 15–20 percent of these IL-10 and TGF-β producing cells were T cells, results consistent with an immunotherapy induced local mucosal T-regulatory response during natural seasonal exposure. These local increases in IL-10 (and INF-γ) were accompanied by

30–100 fold increases in serum allergen-specific IgG and IgG4 antibody concentrations (**Figure 12.9**). [****] Whereas crude serum IgG antibody levels, in general, have failed to correlate with clinical improvement following immunotherapy, we detected a serum 'blocking' activity present within the IgG4 fraction of serum capable of inhibiting IgE-facilitated allergen presentation to T cells.[40] We have developed a simple flow cytometry assay that measures the binding of allergen-IgE complexes to B cells and its inhibition by the IgG4 fraction contained

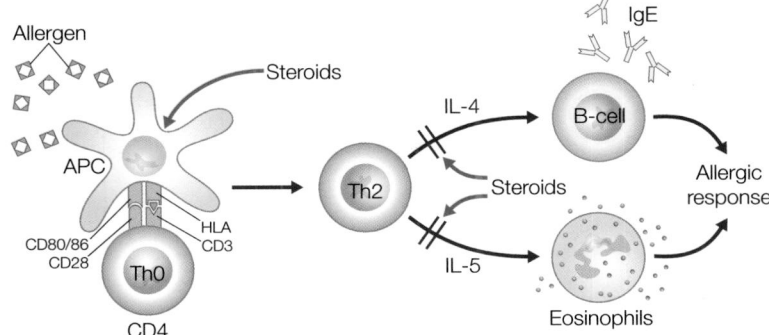

Figure 12.7 The mechanisms of steroid suppression of the late phase allergic response.

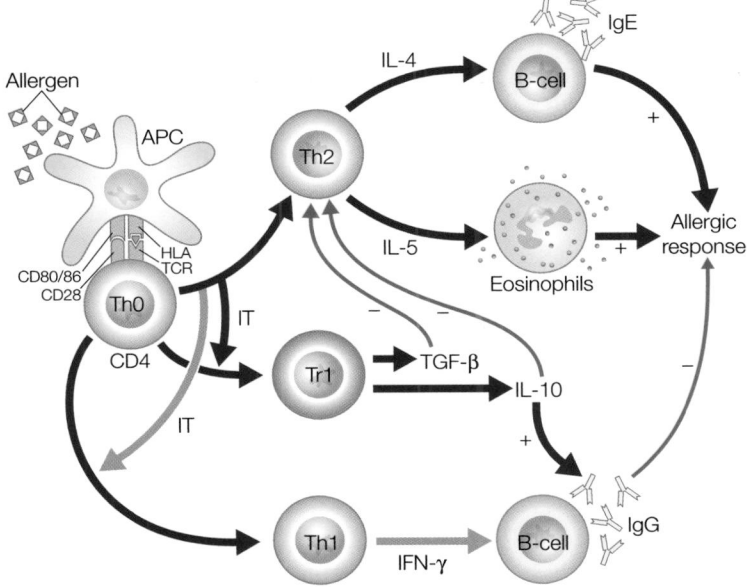

Figure 12.8 Influence of allergen injection immunotherapy on allergen induced Th2 allergic responses. Immunotherapy induces immune deviation in favour of Th1 responses, as well as Th2 T-cell unresponsiveness, under the influence of the inhibitory cytokines IL-10 and TGF-β, derived, at least in part, from $CD4^+$ $CD25^+$ T cells. These events result in the emergence of 'protective' IgG, particularly IgG4, antibody responses and downregulation of IgE and tissue eosinophilia.

within post-immunotherapy serum. It seems likely that IgE-facilitated allergen presentation may represent a rate-limiting step in allergen-driven Th2 T-cell responses. Whether or not detection of this 'functional' IgG blocking activity is surrogate and/or predictive of the clinical response to immunotherapy remains to be determined.

In summary, both topical nasal corticosteroids and allergen immunotherapy are highly effective treatments for allergic rhinitis. In contrast to topical steroids, allergen immunotherapy has the potential to induce long-term disease remission. Whereas topical steroids act by downregulation of Th2 T-lymphocyte function (**Figure 12.7**), immunotherapy appears to act either by immune deviation of Th2 in favour of Th1 responses and/or induction of a population of IL-10 producing T-regulatory cells (**Figure 12.8**) which may downregulate Th2 responses directly or via induction of IgG blocking activity which inhibits IgE-facilitated allergen presentation.

IMPLICATIONS FOR THERAPY

New knowledge concerning the mechanisms of allergic rhinitis and the influence of treatment has identified a number of novel, more targeted strategies (**Figure 12.10**). Obvious candidates are the Th2 cytokines IL-4 and IL-5. IL-4 induces B cell switching, upregulates IgE receptors on mast cells, increases VCAM-1 expression on vascular endothelium, induces mucus secretion and promotes Th2 T-lymphocyte polarization. One study examined the effects of inhaled soluble IL-4-receptor during withdrawal of inhaled corticosteroids in patients with moderately severe atopic asthma. In this small pilot study of two weeks treatment, soluble IL-4 receptor 1500 μg was effective in preventing relapse, as reflected by increases in asthma symptom scores, increase in beta agonist use, and a reduction in FEV_1 in patients on placebo therapy.[66] Further trials are needed.

Interleukin-5 is a major factor responsible for terminal differentiation of eosinophils from bone marrow

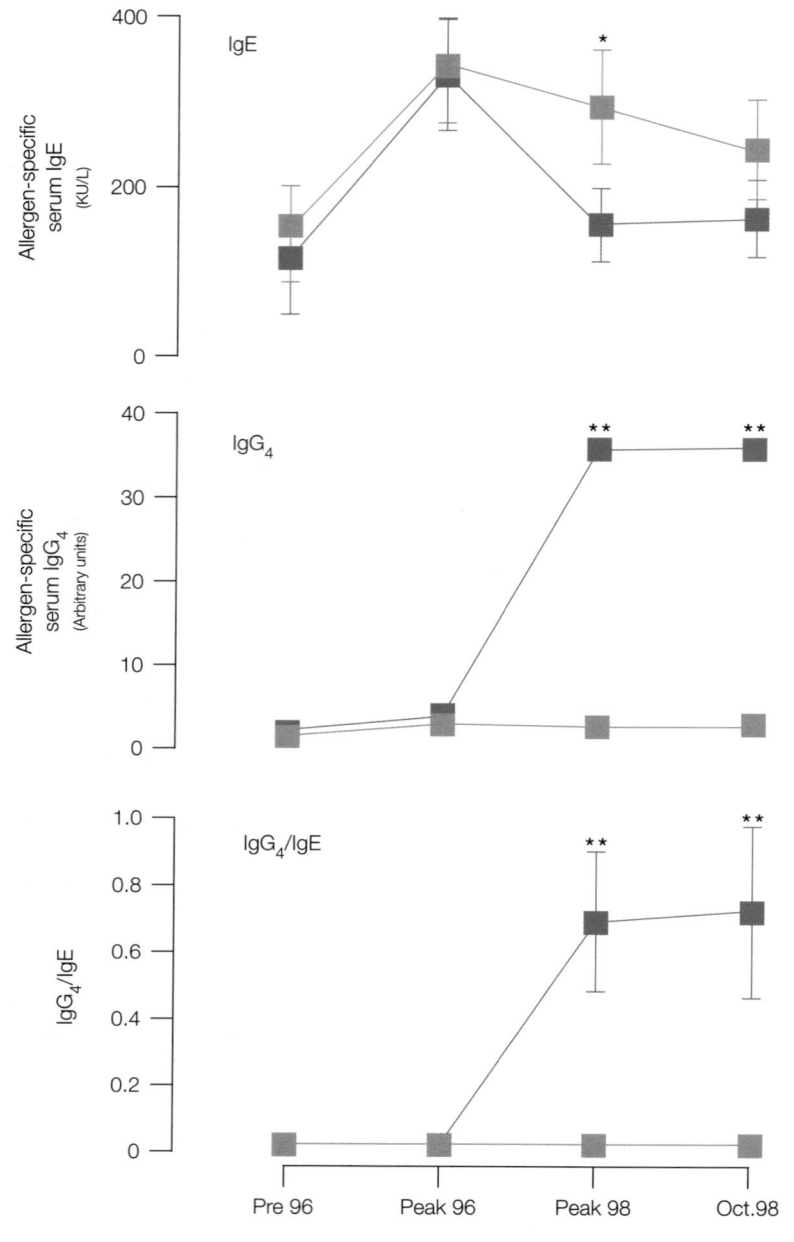

Figure 12.9 Changes in allergen specific IgE, IgG4 and IgE/IgG4 ratio (mean ± standard error) during two years allergen injection immunotherapy. Data shown are for baseline, peak season before treatment, and peak season and out of season following two years immunotherapy. *P*-values refer to comparisons between immunotherapy and placebo groups (Mann–Whitney *U* test).

*p = 0.09   **p < 0.001   ∎ IT   ∎ Placebo

precursors. Inhaled IL-5 induces airway hyperresponsiveness and sputum eosinophilia. In patients with atopic asthma, an anti-IL-5 blocking monoclonal antibody was effective in reducing allergen-induced blood eosinophilia, whereas no detectable effect on allergen-induced late asthmatic responses or the associated increases in airway hyperresponsiveness was observed.[67] Recently, anti-IL-5 has been shown to reduce deposition of extracellular matrix proteins in the bronchial subepithelial basement membrane zone in patients with mild asthma,[68] raising the possibility that long-term anti-IL-5 monoclonal antibody therapy may have a role in preventing airway remodelling in asthma. Recombinant IL-12 in atopic asthmatics, like anti-IL-5 therapy, was effective in reducing blood eosinophils during four weeks treatment, although had no effect on allergen-induced late asthmatic responses.[69]

In a pilot study in patients with severe bronchial asthma, a more global strategy against T cells was adopted by use of an anti-CD4 monoclonal antibody.[70] Although there was a modest improvement in peak expiratory flow and symptoms in the high-dose group, further studies have not been performed, presumably in view of concerns of the safety of a general suppression of CD4+ helper T-lymphocyte function.

The most successful targeted approach has been with strategies directed against IgE antibody. [****] Subcutaneous anti-IgE antibody given at two to three weekly

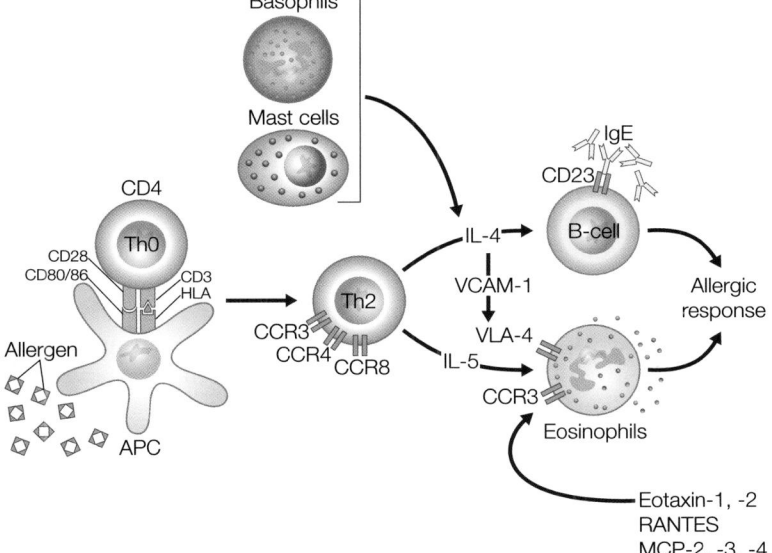

Figure 12.10 New knowledge about mechanisms of allergy has resulted in a number of individual more targeted therapeutic strategies. Both anti-IL-5 and IL-12 therapy inhibited eosinophilia but had no effect on allergen-induced late responses. To date, only anti-IgE therapy has proved successful in phase 3 clinical trials of allergic asthma and rhinitis.

intervals has been shown to be moderately effective in seasonal allergic rhinitis.[71] In the first trial of anti-IgE therapy in moderate to severe perennial allergic asthma, a modest reduction in symptoms was noted, and a more convincing reduction in steroid requirements.[72] In subsequent trials in both adults and children, anti-IgE treatment resulted in clinical improvement, a reduction in corticosteroid use and, importantly, a decrease in the frequency of asthma exacerbations. Anti-IgE therapy is now registered in some countries, although more studies are required to define patients most likely to benefit. A recent study targeted the low-affinity IgE receptor CD23. An anti-CD23 monoclonal antibody (IDEC-152) was well tolerated in man,[73] although further studies are required to evaluate clinical activity in allergic asthma.

Of particular current interest are strategies directed against adhesion molecules and chemokine receptors. CCR3 is particularly attractive as a target since it is the dominant receptor expressed by mast cells, eosinophils, basophils and Th2 T-lymphocytes. Also, CCR3 is the common receptor for Eotaxin, RANTES and MCP2, 3 and 4. It is possible that the combination of anti-IL-5 and CCR4 antagonism may more effectively suppress tissue eosinophilia where targeting either alone may be less effective. Alternatively, CCR4 and CCR8 have been identified as putative phenotype-specific receptors for Th2-type T-lymphocytes.[30] Increases in CCR4 expression on T-cells in the bronchial mucosa and, more recently, increases in the CCR4-specific ligands macrophage derived chemokine (MDC) and thymus and activation-regulated chemokine (TARC) in bronchoalveolar lavage fluid have been detected during allergen-induced late asthmatic responses. However, to date, no clinical trials of chemokine receptor antagonism in humans have been reported.

Conventional high-dose allergen injection immunotherapy is highly effective in allergic asthma and rhinitis,

although, at present, its use is confined to specialist centres on the grounds of safety. Novel approaches are aimed at retaining or improving efficacy whilst reducing side effects. In general, this involves strategies that increase the immunogenicity (potential to modify T cell responses) whilst reducing the allergenicity (the potential to crosslink IgE on mast cells) of allergen extracts. This may be achieved by the use of alternative routes, the use of adjuvants and the development of modified recombinant major allergens. Sublingual immunotherapy is the most promising alternative route. A recent meta-analysis of 22 randomized controlled trials of sublingual immunotherapy in adults with seasonal and perennial allergic rhinitis confirmed efficacy with minimal side effects.[74] [****] However, overall, clinical efficacy was modest and further studies are needed to establish the optimal dose and duration of therapy. Alum is a longstanding effective depot adjuvant. Monophosphoryl lipid A (MPL) is a novel derivative of a lipopolysaccharide from salmonella.[75] MPL may act by inducing IL-12-dependent immune deviation in favour of Th1 responses and has been shown to be effective in seasonal allergic rhinitis. Similarly, the use of short oligonucleotide sequences of bacterial DNA containing an excess of unmethylated CG sequences (immunostimulatory DNA sequences (ISS)) has been explored.[76] ISS are recognized by Toll-like receptor 9 present on antigen-presenting cells and induce immune deviation of T-lymphocyte responses in favour of Th1 responses. The presence of conjugated ISS sequences also appears to inhibit IgE-crosslinking on mast cells. Preliminary studies in ragweed hay fever have demonstrated modest reductions in seasonal symptoms, accompanied by increases in allergen specific IgG antibody. Another novel approach that has been employed in cat-sensitive patients is the use of small T cell peptide epitopes by intradermal injection.[77] These peptides are highly immunogenic and repeated administration in man has demonstrated marked suppression of allergen-induced late cutaneous responses, although further studies are required to assess clinical efficacy.

Alternative approaches involve the combination of conventional immunotherapy with more targeted therapies. For example, the combination of anti-IgE with allergen immunotherapy,[78] particularly during the updosing phase, is likely to reduce IgE-dependent side effects, whilst allowing administration of optimal doses of allergen to achieve allergen-specific tolerance.

RHINITIS/ASTHMA LINK

The link between rhinitis and asthma has recently been highlighted in a World Health Organization report: Allergic rhinitis and its impact on asthma (ARIA).[79] Approximately 30 percent of patients with rhinitis develop asthma and up to 80 percent of patients with perennial asthma have rhinitis. The upper and lower airway share the same respiratory pseudostratified respiratory epithelium. Both allergic rhinitis and asthma are characterized by IgE-dependent mast cell activation, tissue eosinophila and upregulation of Th2-type cytokines.[80] Both diseases are characterized by epithelial migration of mast cells, eosinophils and basophils and the presence of Langerhans cells within the respiratory epithelium. Both diseases are corticosteroid responsive. Anticholinergics are effective in suppressing mucus rhinorrhoea and bronchospasm and anti-leukotriene drugs have been shown to be at least partially effective in both upper and lower airway allergic disease. [****]

Despite these similarities, important differences between rhinitis and asthma also exist. Whereas in the nose, there are prominent erectile venous sinusoids, there are no venous sinusoids in the bronchial mucosa. Submucosal glands are far more prominent in the upper airway compared to the bronchial mucosa. Airway smooth muscle is a prominent feature in the bronchi and increased in asthma, whereas no airway smooth muscle exists in the upper airway. A prominent feature of even mild allergic asthma is disruption of the bronchial epithelium, whereas in rhinitis, even in longstanding persistent rhinitis, the epithelium remains intact. In asthma, there is a thickening of the sub-basement membrane zone with an increase in collagen deposition, whereas in rhinitis, the basement membrane zone appears normal. Therapeutic differences include the selective effectiveness of β_2-agonists in asthma and antihistamines in rhinitis. It seems likely that, in general, allergic rhinitis and asthma share a common Th2-driven pathogenesis and that the above differences may largely be explained by the presence of different effector organs (smooth muscle in the lower airway, mucus glands in the upper airway). However, chronic perennial asthma is a more heterogeneous, less Th2-polarized disease and

the relative lack of evidence for airway remodelling in rhinitis compared to asthma remains unexplained.

Although rhinitis and asthma frequently co-exist, it is not clear whether this simply reflects a common mucosal susceptibility to disease in the upper and lower airway or alternatively whether there exists a causal link. Early studies suggested that topical intranasal corticosteroid treatment may improve bronchial asthma symptoms and reduce bronchial hyperresponsiveness. However, these studies were small scale and may possibly reflect a 'positive publication' bias. A recent study examined symptoms and inflammatory changes in the upper and lower airway following nasal allergen provocation.[81] Biopsies from the nasal and bronchial mucosa were taken before and at 24 hours after nasal provocation. Patients developed both nasal and bronchial symptoms and changes in both nasal peak inspiratory and bronchial peak expiratory flow rates. Immunocytochemistry revealed marked increases in the local expression of the adhesion molecules ICAM-1 and VCAM-1, that correlated with eosinophil numbers in both the nasal and bronchial mucosa. Whether there exists a true causal link between allergic rhinitis could be resolved by a large definitive trial comparing the effects of topical nasal versus inhaled corticosteroid treatment on symptoms and inflammatory markers in both the upper and lower airways. As emphasized in ARIA,[79] whether or not the link is causal, it is clearly important to recognize and treat asthma in patients presenting with allergic rhinitis. All patients should be asked whether they have chest symptoms, including cough, chest tightness, wheeze and shortness of breath. Asthma symptoms tend to be episodic, worse at night and respond to inhaled bronchodilators. Particular triggers include exercise, viral colds and common aeroallergens. A peak expiratory flow (best of three recordings), with reference to predicted normal values, is the minimum requirement for an objective test of airflow limitation in the ENT clinic. Where doubt remains, consideration should be given to the performance of spirometry, reversibility testing in response to an inhaled bronchodilator and the request of serial peak flow measurements at home/in the work place. Alternatively, if such tests are unavailable, early referral to a chest physician would be appropriate.

TESTS

A skin prick test (SPT) provides objective confirmation of IgE sensitivity although must always be interpreted in the light of the clinical history. SPTs (or radioallergosorbent assay tests (RAST)) using a limited number of allergens (grass, house dust mite, cat) may confirm or exclude the diagnosis of atopy. SPTs identify sensitization although cannot predict clinical relevance independent of the history. In general, SPTs are more sensitive, whereas serum allergen-specific IgE measurements may be more specific. The reliability of SPTs depends upon the competence of the operator, the content of major allergenic determinants in the extract, its shelf-life, and the need for storage of extracts at +4°C.

Skin prick testing requires training in performance and interpretation of results. Antihistamines should be avoided for two to three days before skin testing, whereas oral corticosteroids do not significantly inhibit SPT results. They should be performed on the flexor aspect of the forearm using sterile lancets. The procedure should be painless and not draw blood. An unequivocal positive test is one 3 mm greater than the negative control test with allergen diluent. Skin tests should not be performed in the presence of severe eczema. The presence of dermographism may confound results. However, dermographism will be identified by the presence of a positive prick test with the negative control solution, due to the minor trauma of the procedure. For routine clinical use, the skin test result is recorded as the mean diameter of the skin weal, excluding pseudopodia, expressed in millimetres and compared with the negative control (allergen diluent). Examples of skin tests are shown in **Figure 12.11**. The value of SPTs is summarized below:

- diagnosis of atopy;
- supportive evidence (positive or negative) for clinical history;
- essential if avoidance measures are being considered;
- educational value: visual reinforcement of verbal advice.

In hospital practice, a routine panel of SPTs might include house dust mite, animal danders (cat fur, dog hair and horse hair), moulds (aspergillus, cladosporium and alternaria), and pollens (birch, mixed trees, timothy or mixed grasses and weeds), and a positive (histamine 10 mg/mL) and negative (allergen diluent) control. Skin testing with fresh food may be more sensitive and specific than the use of allergen extracts, particularly for fresh fruit and egg that are unstable, heat-labile allergens. Skin testing may also be useful for certain drug allergies including penicillin, general anaesthetics and neuromuscular blocking drugs in addition to latex allergy. It is debatable whether SPTs should routinely be performed in general practice. A pilot study of patients with newly diagnosed asthma, performed by nurses in the context of primary care, suggested that the procedure raised nurses' awareness of the role of allergy in asthma and rhinitis.[82] In particular, the study highlighted the value of negative skin prick tests for excluding atopic allergy in these subjects. [***] However, the downside was that, despite training in performance and interpretation, nurses tended to place more reliance on the skin test rather than the clinical history of allergic sensitivities.

Total IgE

Total IgE levels are usually below 200 ng/mL in non-allergic adults. In atopic adults, results may vary from within the normal range up to 600 ng/mL, or higher levels. Cord blood levels are around 1 ng/mL and it is debatable whether cord blood IgE has any prognostic value. Approximately half of IgE-allergic adults will have a total IgE within the normal range, such that the predictive value of total IgE is poor. However, the presence of very high total IgE levels in serum, such as may occur in disorders such as atopic eczema, may give rise to false positive marginally raised allergen-specific IgE tests. It is therefore valuable to know the total IgE level when interpreting the results of borderline allergen-specific IgE tests.

Allergen-specific IgE

Allergen-specific IgE in serum is measured in specialist immunology or clinical chemistry laboratories by radio-immuno assay (RIA), enzyme-linked immunosorbent assays (ELISA) or chemiluminescence methods. The best-known test for allergen-specific IgE is the radio-allergosorbent test (**Figure 12.12**). In this test, allergen extract is covalently bound to a paper disc. A small amount of patient serum is added and any immunoglobulin specific for that particular allergen binds to the allergen. After vigorous washing, radiolabelled anti-IgE is incubated for a defined period. After further washing, the level of radioactivity is counted. In an ELISA, the anti-IgE is linked to an enzyme. When the relevant substrate is added the enzyme yields a coloured product that is measured in a colorimeter. In chemiluminescence assays, anti-IgE is linked to luciferase that emits photons which can be measured. The sensitivity of the tests varies, depending on the quality of the allergen extract used, the need to optimize the detection system and the proficiency of the operator. For inhalant allergies, the sensitivity of

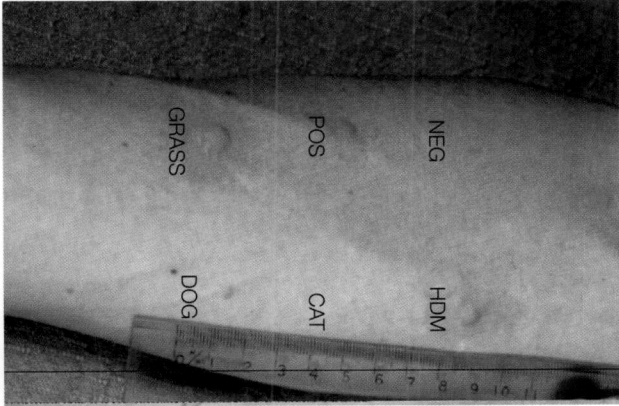

Figure 12.11 Skin prick tests in allergy diagnosis. The weal size is recorded as mean diameter in millimetres. A positive test is 3 mm greater than the negative control test using allergen diluent.

In vitro allergy diagnosis

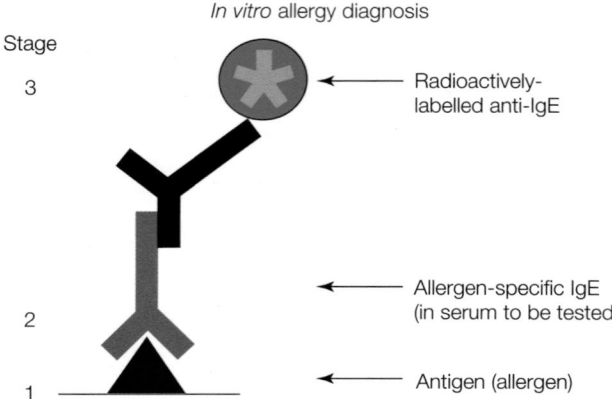

Stage 3

Radioactively-labelled anti-IgE

Stage 2

Allergen-specific IgE (in serum to be tested)

Stage 1

Antigen (allergen)

Figure 12.12 Allergen-specific IgE measurements: RAST. The detection system measures binding of radiolabelled anti-IgE. ELISA employs an enzyme label that is detected by addition of enzyme substrate. Enzyme–substrate interaction results in a coloured product that is detected by spectrophotometry.

the RAST test is around 80 percent and specificity is higher than for skin tests, often greater than 90 percent. The test will therefore occasionally 'miss' IgE-sensitive patients, but if the RAST is positive, most patients will be IgE-sensitive. RAST tests have the advantage of complete safety, and testing is possible with a wider range of allergens than for skin tests. Also, drugs such as antihistamines or the presence of skin disease do not influence RAST tests.

Basophil histamine release

This test relies on assessing histamine release from blood basophils added to allergen extract. Whole blood is added to an ELISA plate precoated with the relevant allergen. After incubation at 37°C for one hour, histamine release is measured by fluorescence assay or by RIA. This test requires fresh blood and needs to be performed in specialist laboratories, although it only takes a few hours to obtain a result. One disadvantage is that 5 percent of the population have basophils which do not release histamine. For this reason, a positive control such as anti-IgE should be included with all tests, in order to validate a negative test.

Provocation tests

Provocation testing with allergen in target organs is only very rarely used in routine allergy diagnosis. They may be employed in tertiary centres where there is discordance between the results of SPTs and the clinical history. However, there are problems with interpretation since accurate threshold levels for a positive or negative response have not been determined in relation to their clinical relevance. However, in view of new knowledge concerning local IgE synthesis, such tests may be of value,

for example in a patient with a clear cut history of allergic symptoms on exposure to an allergen, but with negative skin test/RAST test results to that allergen.

In contrast, measurement of nonspecific hyperresponsiveness, for example by histamine or methacholine inhalation testing, is helpful in assessing the presence and severity of asthma, particularly in patients with a clear history of bronchial asthma, when baseline lung function is normal and there is no detectable immediate response to a bronchodilator. In such cases, detection of increased methacholine or histamine airway responsiveness indicates the need for a therapeutic trial of a bronchodilator and further monitoring.

Serum tryptase

Tryptase is a serine protease, molecular weight 130,000. There are two distinct forms with 90 percent sequence homology, α-tryptase and β-tryptase, of which only β-tryptase is enzymatically active. β-tryptase predominates in allergic reactions, whereas both α- and β-tryptase are detectable in systemic mastocytosis. An elevated serum tryptase level indicates mast cell activation and mediator release. Tryptase assays may be valuable in the differential diagnosis of anaphylaxis from other problems such as vasovagal syndrome, angio-oedema, and carcinoid syndrome.[83] Blood should be taken approximately one hour after the reaction (tryptase levels peak at around 45–60 minutes and then gradually fall over four to six hours). Advantages of the test are that, unlike histamine, blood may be stored, if necessary overnight, and serum separated the following day.

Diagnostic approach

The diagnostic approach to allergy is summarized in **Figure 12.13**. The following questions should be asked:

- Is the patient atopic?
- Does allergy contribute to the patient's symptoms?
- Which are the clinically relevant allergens?

All patients presenting with asthma, rhinitis, eczema or gastrointestinal symptoms should be questioned about potential allergic causes. Also, whether or not allergy is suspected, in the authors' view, SPT to house dust mite, cat and grass pollen should be performed in order to confirm or exclude the presence of atopy. Additional tests should only be based on possible relevance determined by the clinical history. In the majority of patients, there will be concordance between the history and skin test or RAST test results. A negative history and negative tests excludes allergy and indicates that no allergy-specific treatment is required. In patients with a positive history confirmed with objective confirmation by skin or RAST testing, allergen specific measures such as allergen avoidance or, in selected

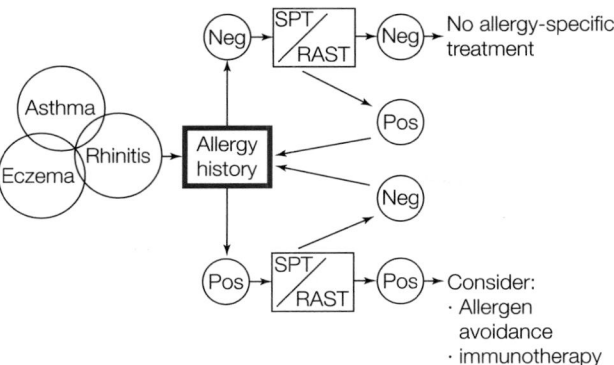

Figure 12.13 An approach to allergy diagnosis.

patients, immunotherapy should be considered. Where there is discordance, then initially, the history should be retaken and, if necessary, tests repeated. If doubt remains, specialist referral for re-evaluation and, if necessary, specific provocation testing can be performed. Ultimately, a therapeutic trial of intervention may be necessary. For example, in patients suspected of IgE-mediated food allergy, a period of dietary exclusion and/or double-blind placebo-controlled food challenge may be indicated. A skilled specialist allergy nurse and the availability of a dietitian with expertise in food allergy are essential for an effective specialist allergy diagnostic service.

KEY POINTS

- Genetic and environmental factors interact as causes of allergic disease.
- Allergic inflammation is characterized by IgE-dependent activation of mast cells and tissue eosinophilia.
- These events are under the regulation of Th2 T lymphocytes.
- Corticosteroids suppress Th2 T lymphocyte responses.
- Immunotherapy induces allergen-specific immune deviation in favour of Th1 responses and/or allergen specific T cell tolerance, probably under the influence of T regulatory cells.
- A number of novel targeted immunotherapeutic approaches have been tested in clinical trials. So far, only anti-IgE has been successful.
- Allergic rhinitis and asthma are commonly associated. Always check for asthma in patients presenting with rhinitis.
- Skin tests and RAST tests indicate IgE sensitivity only and must always be interpreted in the context of the clinical history.

Best clinical practice

✓ The diagnosis of allergic disease is based principally upon a careful clinical history. Allergic rhinitis is characterized by nasal itch, sneeze and watery discharge and the seasonal or perennial nature of these symptoms should be noted. Summer hay fever is recognized to cause significant morbidity and the impact of the disease upon the patient's work and leisure activities should be considered.[84] Chest symptoms, in particular shortness of breath and wheeze, may indicate the presence of associated allergic asthma.

✓ The examination of patients with allergic rhinitis is often unremarkable, but the nasal mucosa should be inspected with either a flexible or rigid nasendoscope to rule out other conditions or exacerbating factors, in particular septal deflection, nasal polyps or chronic rhinosinusitis.

✓ Atopic individuals produce allergen-specific IgE to one or more of the common aeroallergens and may be quickly and reliably identified by skin prick testing in the clinic. In hospital practice, a routine panel of skin prick tests includes house dust mite, animal danders (cat fur, dog hair and horse hair), moulds (*Aspergillus*, *Cladosporium* and *Alternaria*) and pollens (birch, mixed trees, Timothy or mixed grasses, and weeds), and positive (histamine 10 mg/mL) and negative (allergen diluent) controls. Responses are recorded as the weal diameter, excluding pseudopodia, at 15 minutes. A positive prick test is defined as a weal diameter 3 mm or greater than that of the negative control test. The results should only be interpreted in conjunction with the clinical history and tests should not be performed when the patient is taking antihistamines as these will reduce the clinical response.

✓ In the presence of dermographism or eczema, serum IgE antibodies to specific antigen may be measured by RAST. In general, skin prick tests are a more sensitive test of atopy, whereas serum allergen specific IgE measurements are available for a wider panel of allergens than skin test reagents. A raised total IgE level is usually found in atopic individuals, but may also be found in other conditions such as helminth disease.

✓ Pharmacotherapy is the mainstay of treatment for allergic rhinitis and most medications are designed to target inflammatory mediators.

✓ Antihistamines are H1 receptor antagonists that have been used as first-line treatment for seasonal allergic rhinitis for many years.[85, 86] They are effective at relieving the early symptoms of hay fever in particular sneeze, itch and nasal discharge, but considered less effective at reducing nasal congestion.[87] The first generation antihistamines

(Chlorpheniramine, Bropheniramine) were recognized to cause drowsiness in a proportion of patients and indeed have been associated with impaired performance at home and at work.[88] The second generation antihistamines such as Loratidine, Fexofenadine and Desloratadine are nonsedating.

✓ Intranasal corticosteroids are considered first-line treatment for more severe symptoms of allergic rhinitis and are highly effective in suppressing all symptoms of allergic rhinitis, including nasal obstruction. Preparations include Beclometasone, Budesonide, Fluticasone, Triamcinolone and Mometasone. Topical corticosteroids are effective at improving nasal airflow,[89] in addition to relieving the symptoms of itch, sneeze and nasal discharge.[90] Traditionally, topical corticosteroids have been administered on a regular basis, but more recently as needed use of Fluticasone propionate has been found to be effective in the treatment of seasonal allergic rhinitis.[91]

✓ Weiner et al.[92] reported in a meta-analysis of 16 randomized controlled trials that intranasal steroids were more effective than oral antihistamines at relieving the symptoms of allergic rhinitis. Others have reported that both medications may be required to provide optimum treatment in more severe cases.[93]

✓ However, in a large postal survey in the UK, of those patients who were regularly using a nonsedating antihistamine and nasal steroid spray, 62 percent still experienced troublesome residual symptoms and described symptom control as partial or poor.[94]

✓ In a small proportion of patients whose symptoms are not otherwise controlled, a short course of prednisolone (20 mg daily for five days) may be prescribed and is highly effective at relieving all nasal symptoms, including nasal obstruction in the majority of patients.[95]

✓ Sodium cromoglycate is a membrane stabilizer that inhibits mast cell degranulation and the release of mediators. It reduces nasal discharge and congestion, but is less effective than topical corticosteroids and must be administered to the nasal mucosa four times daily.[90] Topical Cromoglycate eye drops are useful for allergic eye symptoms in many, but must also be administered three to four times daily. Intranasal anticholinergics relieve rhinorrhoea but do not greatly improve the other symptoms of allergic rhinitis.

✓ Leukotriene receptor antagonists, such as Monteleukast, have been shown to have antiinflammatory properties and to have beneficial effects on asthma disease control.[96] However, a metaanalysis of 11 studies involving over 4000 patients reported that leukotriene receptor antagonists are minimally better than placebo, but less effective than nasal corticosteroids at improving symptoms and quality of life in patients with seasonal allergic rhinitis.[97]

✓ Allergen avoidance is possible for some allergens, such as latex and certain foods, but is less effective for hay fever owing to the ubiquitous nature of pollen. Avoidance of wide open and grassy spaces may be helpful, particularly in the late afternoon and evening when pollen counts are highest. Cars may be fitted with pollen filters and windows in cars and buildings may be kept tight shut.

✓ Measures to reduce house dust mite exposure are often recommended and include the removal of soft furnishings, such as carpets and curtains, and the provision of mite proof covers for the pillows, duvets and mattresses. However, trials to date have been small and of poor methodological quality. This has made it difficult to offer any definitive recommendations on the role, if any, of house dust mite avoidance measures in the management of house dust mite-sensitive perennial allergic rhinitis.[98] Allergen-impermeable covers, as a single intervention for the avoidance of exposure to dust-mite allergen, are clinically ineffective in adults with asthma.[99]

✓ Allergen-specific immunotherapy is an effective intervention that involves the incremental administration of subcutaneous allergen extract for 8–16 weeks followed by monthly injections for up to three to five years. It is the only currently available intervention that can modify the disease process and long-lasting benefit has been reported.[59] A recent review of 51 randomized, placebo-controlled clinical trials confirmed that specific allergen injection immunotherapy in suitably selected patients with seasonal allergic rhinitis results in a significant reduction in symptom scores and medication use.[100]

✓ The treatment, however, requires injections for a number of years and carries the risk of local skin reactions and rare, but potentially fatal, anaphylaxis. The risks of systemic reactions are significantly increased in those patients with concomitant asthma. Efficacy is limited in those with multiple sensitivities. In the UK allergen-specific immunotherapy is restricted to tertiary referral centres thereby limiting patient access to this form of treatment.

✓ More recently sublingual immunotherapy has become available as a mainstream treatment for seasonal allergic rhinitis. A review and metaanalysis of 22 trials involving 979 patients concluded that overall there was a significant reduction in both symptoms (SMD-0.42, 95 percent confidence interval -0.69 to -0.15; $p = 0.002$) and medication requirements (SMD-0.43 (-0.63, -0.23); $p = 0.00003$) following immunotherapy.[101]

REFERENCES

1. Hopp RJ, Bewtra AK, Watt GD, Nair NM, Townley RG. Genetic analysis of allergic disease in twins. *Journal of Allergy and Clinical Immunology.* 1984; **73**: 265–70.
2. Koppelman GH, Los H, Postma DS. Genetic and environment in asthma: the answer of twin studies. *European Respiratory Journal.* 1999; **13**: 2–4.
3. Steinke JW, Borish L, Rosenwasser LJ. 5. Genetics of hypersensitivity. *Journal of Allergy and Clinical Immunology.* 2003; **111**: S495–501.
4. Marsh DG, Neely JD, Breazeale DR, Ghosh B, Freidhoff LR, Ehrlich-Kautzky E et al. Linkage analysis of IL4 and other chromosome 5q31.1 markers and total serum immunoglobulin E concentrations. *Science.* 1994; **264**: 1152–6.
5. Van Eerdewegh P, Little RD, Dupuis J, Del Mastro RG, Falls K, Simon J et al. Association of the ADAM33 gene with asthma and bronchial hyperresponsiveness. *Nature.* 2002; **418**: 426–30.
* 6. Strachan DP. Hay fever, hygiene, and household size. *British Medical Journal.* 1989; **299**: 1259–60.
* 7. Braun-Fahrlander C, Riedler J, Herz U, Eder W, Waser M, Grize L et al. Environmental exposure to endotoxin and its relation to asthma in school-age children. *New England Journal of Medicine.* 2002; **347**: 869–77.
8. Umetsu DT, McIntire JJ, Akbari O, Macaubas C, DeKruyff RH. Asthma: an epidemic of dysregulated immunity. *Nature Immunology.* 2002; **3**: 715–20.
9. Black P. Why is the prevalence of allergy and autoimmunity increasing? *Trends in Immunology.* 2001; **22**: 354–5.
10. Caramalho I, Lopes-Carvalho T, Ostler D, Zelenay S, Haury M, Demengeot J. Regulatory T cells selectively express toll-like receptors and are activated by lipopolysaccharide. *Journal of Experimental Medicine.* 2003; **197**: 403–11.
11. Muranaka M, Suzuki S, Koizumi K, Takafuji S, Miyamoto T, Ikemori R et al. Adjuvant activity of diesel-exhaust particulates for the production of IgE antibody in mice. *Journal of Allergy and Clinical Immunology.* 1986; **77**: 616–23.
12. von Mutius E, Fritzsch C, Weiland SK, Roll G, Magnussen H. Prevalence of asthma and allergic disorders among children in united Germany: a descriptive comparison. *British Medical Journal.* 1992; **305**: 1395–9.
* 13. Durham SR. Allergic inflammation: cellular aspects. *Allergy.* 1999; **54**: 18–20.
14. Cockcroft DW. Mechanism of perennial allergic asthma. *Lancet.* 1983; **2**: 253–6.
15. Lund VJ. Seasonal allergic rhinitis – a review of current therapy. *Allergy.* 1996; **51**: 5–7.
16. Varney VA, Jacobson MR, Sudderick RM, Robinson DS, Irani AM, Schwartz LB et al. Immunohistology of the nasal mucosa following allergen-induced rhinitis. Identification of activated T lymphocytes, eosinophils, and neutrophils. *American Review of Respiratory Disease.* 1992; **146**: 170–6.

17. Durham SR, Ying S, Varney VA, Jacobson MR, Sudderick RM, Mackay IS et al. Cytokine messenger RNA expression for IL-3, IL-4, IL-5, and granulocyte/macrophage-colony-stimulating factor in the nasal mucosa after local allergen provocation: relationship to tissue eosinophilia. *Journal of Immunology.* 1992; **148**: 2390–4.
18. Togias A. Unique mechanistic features of allergic rhinitis. *Journal of Allergy and Clinical Immunology.* 2000; **105**: S599–604.
19. Prussin C, Metcalfe DD. 4. IgE, mast cells, basophils, and eosinophils. *Journal of Allergy and Clinical Immunology.* 2003; **111**: S486–94.
20. Kita H, Kaneko M, Bartemes KR, Weiler DA, Schimming AW, Reed CE et al. Does IgE bind to and activate eosinophils from patients with allergy. *Journal of Immunology.* 1999; **162**: 6901–11.
21. Vercelli D, Geha RS. Regulation of IgE synthesis in humans: a tale of two signals? *Journal of Allergy and Clinical Immunology.* 1991; **88**: 285–95.
22. Durham SR, Gould HJ, Thienes CP, Jacobson MR, Masuyama K, Rak S et al. Expression of epsilon germ-line gene transcripts and mRNA for the epsilon heavy chain of IgE in nasal B cells and the effects of topical corticosteroid. *European Journal of Immunology.* 1997; **27**: 2899–906.
23. Ying S, Humbert M, Meng Q, Pfister R, Menz G, Gould HJ et al. Local expression of epsilon germline gene transcripts and RNA for the epsilon heavy chain of IgE in the bronchial mucosa in atopic and nonatopic asthma. *Journal of Allergy and Clinical Immunology.* 2001; **107**: 686–92.
24. Coker HA, Durham SR, Gould HJ. Local somatic hypermutation and class switch recombination in the nasal mucosa of allergic rhinitis patients. *Journal of Immunology.* 2003; **171**: 5602–10.
25. Cameron L, Hamid Q, Wright E, Nakamura Y, Christodoulopoulos P, Muro S et al. Local synthesis of epsilon germline gene transcripts, IL-4, and IL-13 in allergic nasal mucosa after ex vivo allergen exposure. *Journal of Allergy and Clinical Immunology.* 2000; **106**: 46–52.
* 26. Smurthwaite L, Walker SN, Wilson DR, Birch DS, Merrett TG, Durham SR et al. Persistent IgE synthesis in the nasal mucosa of hay fever patients. *European Journal of Immunology.* 2001; **31**: 3422–31.
* 27. Powe DG, Jagger C, KleinJan A, Carney AS, Jenkins D, Jones NS. 'Entopy': localized mucosal allergic disease in the absence of systemic responses for atopy. *Clinical and Experimental Allergy.* 2003; **33**: 1374–9.
28. Nouri-Aria KT, Irani AM, Jacobson MR, O'Brien F, Varga EM, Till SJ et al. Basophil recruitment and IL-4 production during human allergen-induced late asthma. *Journal of Allergy and Clinical Immunology.* 2001; **108**: 205–11.
29. Gangur V, Oppenheim JJ. Are chemokines essential or secondary participants in allergic responses? *Annals of Allergy, Asthma and Immunology.* 2000; **84**: 569–79.
30. Ono SJ, Nakamura T, Miyazaki D, Ohbayashi M, Dawson M, Toda M. Chemokines: roles in leukocyte development,

trafficking, and effector function. *Journal of Allergy and Clinical Immunology*. 2003; **111**: 1185–99.

31. Kuna P, Alam R, Ruta U, Gorski P. RANTES induces nasal mucosal inflammation rich in eosinophils, basophils, and lymphocytes in vivo. *American Journal of Respiratory and Critical Care Medicine*. 1998; **157**: 873–9.

32. Hanazawa T, Antuni JD, Kharitonov SA, Barnes PJ. Intranasal administration of eotaxin increases nasal eosinophils and nitric oxide in patients with allergic rhinitis. *Journal of Allergy and Clinical Immunology*. 2000; **105**: 58–64.

33. Terada N, Hamano N, Kim WJ, Hirai K, Nakajima T, Yamada H *et al*. The kinetics of allergen-induced eotaxin level in nasal lavage fluid: its key role in eosinophil recruitment in nasal mucosa. *American Journal of Respiratory and Critical Care Medicine*. 2001; **164**: 575–9.

34. Rajakulasingam K, Hamid Q, O'Brien F, Shotman E, Jose PJ, Williams TJ *et al*. RANTES in human allergen-induced rhinitis: cellular source and relation to tissue eosinophilia. *American Journal of Respiratory and Critical Care Medicine*. 1997; **155**: 696–703.

* 35. Mosmann TR, Cherwinski H, Bond MW, Giedlin MA, Coffman RL. Two types of murine helper T cell clone. I. Definition according to profiles of lymphokine activities and secreted proteins. *Journal of Immunology*. 1986; **136**: 2348–57.

36. Durham SR, Till SJ, Corrigan CJ. T lymphocytes in asthma: bronchial versus peripheral responses. *Journal of Allergy and Clinical Immunology*. 2000; **106**: S221–6.

37. Alam R, Gorska M. 3. Lymphocytes. *Journal of Allergy and Clinical Immunology*. 2003; **111**: S476–85.

38. Wierenga EA, Snoek M, de Groot C, Chretien I, Bos JD, Jansen HM *et al*. Evidence for compartmentalization of functional subsets of CD2+ T lymphocytes in atopic patients. *Journal of Immunology*. 1990; **144**: 4651–6.

39. van der Heijden FL, van Neerven RJ, van Katwijk M, Bos JD, Kapsenberg ML. Serum-IgE-facilitated allergen presentation in atopic disease. *Journal of Immunology*. 1993; **150**: 3643–50.

40. Wachholz PA, Soni NK, Till SJ, Durham SR. Inhibition of allergen-IgE binding to B cells by IgG antibodies after grass pollen immunotherapy. *Journal of Allergy and Clinical Immunology*. 2003; **112**: 915–22.

41. Escoubet-Lozach L, Glass CK, Wasserman SI. The role of transcription factors in allergic inflammation. *Journal of Allergy and Clinical Immunology*. 2002; **110**: 553–64.

* 42. Nakamura K, Kitani A, Strober W. Cell contact-dependent immunosuppression by CD4(+) CD25(+) regulatory T cells is mediated by cell surface-bound transforming growth factor beta. *Journal of Experimental Medicine*. 2001; **194**: 629–44.

43. Zhang X, Izikson L, Liu L, Weiner HL. Activation of CD25(+) CD4(+) regulatory T cells by oral antigen administration. *Journal of Immunology*. 2001; **167**: 4245–53.

44. Dieckmann D, Plottner H, Berchtold S, Berger T, Schuler G. Ex vivo isolation and characterization of CD4(+)CD25(+) T cells with regulatory properties from human blood. *Journal of Experimental Medicine*. 2001; **193**: 1303–10.

45. Akdis CA, Blesken T, Akdis M, Wuthrich B, Blaser K. Role of interleukin 10 in specific immunotherapy. *Journal of Clinical Investigation*. 1998; **102**: 98–106.

46. Nouri-Aria KT, O'Brien F, Noble W, Jabcobson MR, Rajakulasingam K, Durham SR. Cytokine expression during allergen-induced late nasal responses: IL-4 and IL-5 mRNA is expressed early (at 6 h) predominantly by eosinophils. *Clinical and Experimental Allergy*. 2000; **30**: 1709–16.

47. Holt PG, Upham JW. The role of dendritic cells in asthma. *Current Opinion in Allergy and Clinical Immunology*. 2004; **4**: 39–44.

48. Huh JC, Strickland DH, Jahnsen FL, Turner DJ, Thomas JA, Napoli S *et al*. Bidirectional interactions between antigen-bearing respiratory tract dendritic cells (DCs) and T cells precede the late phase reaction in experimental asthma: DC activation occurs in the airway mucosa but not in the lung parenchyma. *Journal of Experimental Medicine*. 2003; **198**: 19–30.

49. Jahnsen FL, Lund-Johansen F, Dunne JF, Farkas L, Haye R, Brandtzaeg P. Experimentally induced recruitment of plasmacytoid (CD123high) dendritic cells in human nasal allergy. *Journal of Immunology*. 2000; **165**: 4062–8.

50. Novak N, Tepel C, Koch S, Brix K, Bieber T, Kraft S. Evidence for a differential expression of the Fcε RIγ chain in dendritic cells of atopic and nonatopic donors. *Journal of Clinical Investigation*. 2003; **111**: 1047–56.

51. Bentley AM, Walker S, Hanotte F, De Vos C, Durham SR. A comparison of the effects of oral cetirizine and inhaled beclomethasone on early and late asthmatic responses to allergen and the associated increase in airways hyperresponsiveness. *Clinical and Experimental Allergy*. 1996; **26**: 909–17.

52. Rak S, Jacobson MR, Sudderick RM, Masuyama K, Juliusson S, Kay AB *et al*. Influence of prolonged treatment with topical corticosteroid (fluticasone propionate) on early and late phase nasal responses and cellular infiltration in the nasal mucosa after allergen challenge. *Clinical and Experimental Allergy*. 1994; **24**: 930–9.

53. Masuyama K, Till SJ, Jacobson MR, Kamil A, Cameron L, Juliusson S *et al*. Nasal eosinophilia and IL-5 mRNA expression in seasonal allergic rhinitis induced by natural allergen exposure: effect of topical corticosteroids. *Journal of Allergy and Clinical Immunology*. 1998; **102**: 610–7.

54. Masuyama K, Jacobson MR, Rak S, Meng Q, Sudderick RM, Kay AB *et al*. Topical glucocorticosteroid (fluticasone propionate) inhibits cells expressing cytokine mRNA for interleukin-4 in the nasal mucosa in allergen-induced rhinitis. *Immunology*. 1994; **82**: 192–9.

55. Stellato C, Beck LA, Gorgone GA, Proud D, Schall TJ, Ono SJ *et al*. Expression of the chemokine RANTES by a human bronchial epithelial cell line. Modulation by cytokines and glucocorticoids. *Journal of Immunology*. 1995; **155**: 410–8.

56. Cameron LA, Durham SR, Jacobson MR, Masuyama K, Juliusson S, Gould HJ *et al.* Expression of IL-4, Cepsilon RNA, and Iepsilon RNA in the nasal mucosa of patients with seasonal rhinitis: effect of topical corticosteroids. *Journal of Allergy and Clinical Immunology.* 1998; **101**: 330–6.

57. Till SJ, Jacobson MR, O'Brien F, Durham SR, KleinJan A, Fokkens WJ *et al.* Recruitment of CD1a+ Langerhans cells to the nasal mucosa in seasonal allergic rhinitis and effects of topical corticosteroid therapy. *Allergy.* 2001; **56**: 126–31.

58. Bousquet J, Lockey R, Malling HJ, Alvarez-Cuesta E, Canonica GW, Chapman MD *et al.* Allergen immunotherapy: therapeutic vaccines for allergic diseases. World Health Organization. American Academy of Allergy, Asthma and Immunology. *Annals of Allergy, Asthma and Immunology.* 1998; **81**: 401–5.

∗ 59. Durham SR, Walker SM, Varga EM, Jacobson MR, O'Brien F, Noble W *et al.* Long-term clinical efficacy of grass-pollen immunotherapy. *New England Journal of Medicine.* 1999; **341**: 468–75.

60. Moller C, Dreborg S, Ferdousi HA, Halken S, Host A, Jacobsen L *et al.* Pollen immunotherapy reduces the development of asthma in children with seasonal rhinoconjunctivitis (the PAT-study). *Journal of Allergy and Clinical Immunology.* 2002; **109**: 251–6.

61. Des RA, Paradis L, Menardo JL, Bouges S, Daures JP, Bousquet J. Immunotherapy with a standardized Dermatophagoides pteronyssinus extract. VI. Specific immunotherapy prevents the onset of new sensitizations in children. *Journal of Allergy and Clinical Immunology.* 1997; **99**: 450–3.

∗ 62. Durham SR, Till SJ. Immunologic changes associated with allergen immunotherapy. *Journal of Allergy and Clinical Immunology.* 1998; **102**: 157–64.

63. Wilson DR, Irani AM, Walker SM, Jacobson MR, Mackay IS, Schwartz LB *et al.* Grass pollen immunotherapy inhibits seasonal increases in basophils and eosinophils in the nasal epithelium. *Clinical and Experimental Allergy.* 2001; **31**: 1705–13.

64. Wachholz PA, Nouri-Aria KT, Wilson DR, Walker SM, Verhoef A, Till SJ *et al.* Grass pollen immunotherapy for hayfever is associated with increases in local nasal but not peripheral Th1:Th2 cytokine ratios. *Immunology.* 2002; **105**: 56–62.

65. Nouri-Aria KT, Wachholz PA, Francis JN, Jacobson MR, Walker SM, Wilcock LK *et al.* Grass pollen immunotherapy induces mucosal and peripheral IL-10 responses and blocking IgG activity. *Journal of Immunology.* 2004; **172**: 3252–9.

66. Borish LC, Nelson HS, Lanz MJ, Claussen L, Whitmore JB, Agosti JM *et al.* Interleukin-4 receptor in moderate atopic asthma. A phase I/II randomized, placebo-controlled trial. *American Journal of Respiratory and Critical Care Medicine.* 1999; **160**: 1816–23.

67. Leckie MJ, ten Brinke A, Khan J, Diamant Z, O'Connor BJ, Walls CM *et al.* Effects of an interleukin-5 blocking monoclonal antibody on eosinophils, airway hyper-responsiveness, and the late asthmatic response. *Lancet.* 2000; **356**: 2144–8.

68. Flood-Page P, Menzies-Gow A, Phipps S, Ying S, Wangoo A, Ludwig MS *et al.* Anti-IL-5 treatment reduces deposition of ECM proteins in the bronchial subepithelial basement membrane of mild atopic asthmatics. *Journal of Clinical Investigation.* 2003; **112**: 1029–36.

69. Bryan SA, O'Connor BJ, Matti S, Leckie MJ, Kanabar V, Khan J *et al.* Effects of recombinant human interleukin-12 on eosinophils, airway hyper-responsiveness, and the late asthmatic response. *Lancet.* 2000; **356**: 2149–53.

70. Kon OM, Sihra BS, Compton CH, Leonard TB, Kay AB, Barnes NC. Randomised, dose-ranging, placebo-controlled study of chimeric antibody to CD4 (keliximab) in chronic severe asthma. *Lancet.* 1998; **352**: 1109–13.

71. Casale TB, Condemi J, LaForce C, Nayak A, Rowe M, Watrous M *et al.* Effect of omalizumab on symptoms of seasonal allergic rhinitis: a randomized controlled trial. *Journal of the American Medical Association.* 2001; **286**: 2956–67.

∗ 72. Frew AJ. Anti-IgE and asthma. *Annals of Allergy, Asthma and Immunology.* 2003; **91**: 117–8.

73. Rosenwasser LJ, Busse WW, Lizambri RG, Olejnik TA, Totoritis MC. Allergic asthma and an anti-CD23 mAb (IDEC-152): results of a phase I, single-dose, dose-escalating clinical trial. *Journal of Allergy and Clinical Immunology.* 2003; **112**: 563–70.

∗ 74. Wilson DR, Torres LI, Durham SR. Sublingual immunotherapy for allergic rhinitis. *Cochrane Database of Systematic Reviews.* 2003: CD002893.

75. Drachenberg KJ, Wheeler AW, Stuebner P, Horak F. A well-tolerated grass pollen-specific allergy vaccine containing a novel adjuvant, monophosphoryl lipid A, reduces allergic symptoms after only four preseasonal injections. *Allergy.* 2001; **56**: 498–505.

76. Marshall JD, Abtahi S, Eiden JJ, Tuck S, Milley R, Haycock F *et al.* Immunostimulatory sequence DNA linked to the Amb a 1 allergen promotes T(H)1 cytokine expression while downregulating T(H)2 cytokine expression in PBMCs from human patients with ragweed allergy. *Journal of Allergy and Clinical Immunology.* 2001; **108**: 191–7.

77. Oldfield WL, Larche M, Kay AB. Effect of T-cell peptides derived from Fel d 1 on allergic reactions and cytokine production in patients sensitive to cats: a randomised controlled trial. *Lancet.* 2002; **360**: 47–53.

78. Kuehr J, Brauburger J, Zielen S, Schauer U, Kamin W, Von Berg A *et al.* Efficacy of combination treatment with anti-IgE plus specific immunotherapy in polysensitized children and adolescents with seasonal allergic rhinitis. *Journal of Allergy and Clinical Immunology.* 2002; **109**: 274–80.

79. Bousquet J, van Cauwenberge P, Khaltaev N. Allergic rhinitis and its impact on asthma. *Journal of Allergy and Clinical Immunology.* 2001; **108**: S147–334.

80. Durham SR. The inflammatory nature of allergic disease. *Clinical and Experimental Allergy.* 1998; **28**: 20–4.

∗ 81. Braunstahl GJ, Fokkens W. Nasal involvement in allergic asthma. *Allergy*. 2003; **58**: 1235–43.

82. Sibbald B, Barnes G, Durham SR. Skin prick testing in general practice: a pilot study. *Journal of Advanced Nursing*. 1997; **26**: 537–42.

83. Lin RY, Schwartz LB, Curry A, Pesola GR, Knight RJ, Lee HS et al. Histamine and tryptase levels in patients with acute allergic reactions: An emergency department-based study. *Journal of Allergy and Clinical Immunology*. 2000; **106**: 65–71.

84. Turvey SE. Atopic diseases of childhood. *Current Opinion in Pediatrics*. 2001; **13**: 487–95.

85. Druce HM, Kaliner MA. Allergic rhinitis. *Journal of the American Medical Association*. 1988; **259**: 260–3.

86. Tarnasky PR, Van Arsdel Jr. PP. Antihistamine therapy in allergic rhinitis. *Journal of Family Practice*. 1990; **30**: 71–80.

87. Casale TB, Andrade C, Qu R. Safety and efficacy of once-daily fexofenadine HCl in the treatment of autumn seasonal allergic rhinitis. *Allergy and Asthma Proceedings*. 1999; **20**: 193–8.

88. Kay GG. The effects of antihistamines on cognition and performance. *Journal of Allergy and Clinical Immunology*. 2000; **105**: S622–7.

89. Meltzer EO, Gallet CL, Jalowayski AA, Garcia J, Diener P, Liao Y et al. Triamcinolone acetonide and fluticasone propionate aqueous nasal sprays significantly improve nasal airflow in patients with seasonal allergic rhinitis. *Allergy and Asthma Proceedings*. 2004; **25**: 53–8.

90. Dykewicz MS, Fineman S, Skoner DP. Joint Task Force summary statements on diagnosis and management of rhinitis. *Annals of Allergy, Asthma and Immunology*. 1998; **81**: 474–7.

91. Jen A, Baroody F, de Tineo M, Haney L, Blair C, Naclerio R. As-needed use of fluticasone propionate nasal spray reduces symptoms of seasonal allergic rhinitis. *Journal of Allergy and Clinical Immunology*. 2000; **105**: 732–8.

92. Weiner JM, Abramson MJ, Puy RM. Intranasal corticosteroids versus oral H1 receptor antagonists in allergic rhinitis: systematic review of randomised controlled trials. *British Medical Journal*. 1998; **317**: 1624–9.

93. Juniper EF, Guyatt GH, Ferrie PJ, Griffith LE. First-line treatment of seasonal (ragweed) rhinoconjunctivitis. A randomized management trial comparing a nasal steroid spray and a nonsedating antihistamine. *Canadian Medical Association Journal*. 1997; **156**: 1123–31.

94. White P, Smith H, Baker N, Davis W, Frew A. Symptom control in patients with hay fever in UK general practice: how well are we doing and is there a need for allergen immunotherapy? *Clinical and Experimental Allergy*. 1998; **28**: 266–70.

95. Mygind N, Laursen LC, Dahl M. Systemic corticosteroid treatment for seasonal allergic rhinitis: a common but poorly documented therapy. *Allergy*. 2000; **55**: 11–5.

96. Lipworth BJ. The emerging role of leukotriene antagonists in asthma therapy. *Chest*. 1999; **115**: 313–6.

97. Wilson AM, O'Byrne PM, Parameswaran K. Leukotriene receptor antagonists for allergic rhinitis: a systematic review and meta-analysis. *American Journal of Medicine*. 2004; **116**: 338–44.

98. Sheikh A, Hurwitz B. House dust mite avoidance measures for perennial allergic rhinitis. Cochrane Database of Systematic Reviews. 2001: CD001563.

99. Woodcock A, Forster L, Matthews E, Martin J, Letley T, Vickers M et al. Medical Research Council General Practice Research Framework. Control of exposure to mite allergen and allergen-impermeable bed covers for adults with asthma. *New England Journal of Medicine*. 2003; **349**: 225–36.

100. Calderon M, Alves B, Jacobson M, Hurwitz B, Sheikh A, Durham S et al. Allergen injection immunotherapy for seasonal allergic rhinitis. *Cochrane Database of Systematic Reviews*. 2007; **24**.

∗101. Wilson DR, Lima MT, Durham S. Sublingual immunotherapy for allergic rhinitis: systematic review and meta-analysis. *Allergy*. 2005; **60**: 4–12.

13

Evaluation of the immune system

ELIZABETH DREWE AND RICHARD J POWELL

Introduction to evaluation of the immune system	167	Deficiencies in current knowledge and areas for future research	172
Immunological tests	167	References	173
Key points	172		
Best clinical practice	172		

SEARCH STRATEGY AND EVIDENCE-BASE

The information in this chapter is taken from standard UK immunology laboratory practice. It reflects expert opinion (level 4 evidence) with regards to immunology tests currently performed in the UK.

INTRODUCTION TO EVALUATION OF THE IMMUNE SYSTEM

Evaluation of the immune system broadly encompasses the investigation of immunodeficiency, autoimmune disease including vasculitis, allergy and lymphoproliferative disease. Diagnosis results from studying the combination of clinical presentation and investigations including immunological, haematological, microbiological and histopathological, with increasing recognition of the place of genetic and molecular biological approaches. However, tests in isolation are rarely diagnostic. Some understanding of the sensitivity (proportion of true positives correctly identified), specificity (proportion of true negatives correctly identified) and the positive predictive value (likelihood an individual has a disease given a positive result) for each test is required.

Interpretation of results reflects the age and sex of the patient. This is particularly evident for the investigation of childhood immunodeficiency when a lymphocyte count that would be normal for an adult, may signify an underlying immunodeficiency in an infant. Similarly, a low positive anti-nuclear antibody (ANA) titre may be a normal finding in a middle-aged female, but be highly suggestive of an autoimmune process in female teenagers or in males of any age.

The investigations will ultimately depend on the clinical presentation and may be guided through discussion with a clinical immunologist. Whilst rare immunological diseases will only be recognized by the appropriate investigation, consideration must also be given to commoner diseases with a similar presentation, for example, cystic fibrosis.

IMMUNOLOGICAL TESTS

Immunodeficiency

Investigation for immunodeficiency should be targeted at patients with persistent or recurrent infections not responding to antibiotics, or patients with unusual or opportunistic infections.[1] Recurrent sinopulmonary infections are a common presentation of primary immunodeficiency and ENT workers should look out for these individuals and initiate the appropriate investigations. It is estimated that half of the patients with primary antibody deficiency in the UK remain undiagnosed.[2] Remember that early diagnosis of primary immunodeficiency does lead to an improved outcome, emphasizing the need to consider this diagnosis.

Table 13.1 Outline of associations between pathogens and specific immunodeficiencies.

Pathology	Immunodeficiency
Bacterial infections	Antibody deficiency
	T cell deficiency
	Complement
	Neutrophil disorders
Viral infections	T cells
	Antibody deficiency
Fungal infections	Neutrophil disorders
	T cells
Neisserial infections	Complement
Abscess formation	Neutrophil disorders
Mycobacterial infection	T cells
	Macrophage/cytokines

Table 13.2 Outline of immunological tests for primary immunodeficiency.

Deficiency	Tests
T lymphocytes	Number
	Surface marker analysis
	Lymphocyte proliferation studies
Antibody deficiency	Total immunoglobulins
	Vaccine specific immunoglobulins
	IgG subclasses
	B cell number
Phagocyte disorders	Neutrophil number
	NBT test
	Phagocytosis and killing studies
Complement disorders	Functional complement assays
	Assay individual complement components

When considering immunodeficiency, the type of pathogen may provide a clue to the underlying disease and appropriate tests required (**Tables 13.1** and **13.2**). Certain tests require laboratory preparation, hence require prior arrangements.

C-REACTIVE PROTEIN

C-reactive protein (CRP) levels reflect the acute phase response and are particularly elevated in bacterial infections, malignancy and active vasculitis. An elevated CRP may be helpful in diagnosing intercurrent infection in immunodeficiency and in individuals on high dose steroids.

IMMUNOGLOBULINS

Serum levels of immunoglobulin classes IgG, IgA and IgM are a first line test for investigation of immunodeficiency.

IgG and IgA levels are typically low in common variable immunodeficiency, although a raised IgM with low IgG and IgA is characteristic of hyper IgM syndrome. An elevated IgG is often seen in chronic granulomatous disease. Other indications for immunoglobulin testing include infective and inflammatory diseases and the evaluation of lymphoproliferative disease.

IMMUNOGLOBULIN SUBCLASSES

Testing of IgG subclasses may be an adjunct to the diagnosis of immunodeficiency. Isolated low IgG2 levels may be normal in childhood, but may amount to significant immunodeficiency in combination with IgA deficiency or failure to respond to pathogens, e.g. pneumococcus. Specific vaccine responses appear more informative in the evaluation of humoral immunodeficiency than IgG subclass quantification.

SPECIFIC ANTIBODIES

Assessing if a patient has produced IgG antibodies to a previously encountered pathogen or vaccination plays an important part in diagnosing antibody deficiency, especially in patients who have borderline or normal immunoglobulin levels. Additional immunization, for example tetanus, pneumococcus and haemophilus b, may be given followed by repeat measurements of specific antibody levels after four to six weeks. Failure to mount an adequate response is a pointer to an underlying immunodeficiency. Live vaccines must not be given to patients with a suspected immunodeficiency.

LYMPHOCYTE PHENOTYPING

A reduced lymphocyte count may require evaluation of lymphocyte subsets. Lymphocyte phenotyping by flow cytometry allows accurate quantitative measurements of cell subsets by detection of cell surface markers. The two main T cell subsets are evaluated by assessing $CD3^+$ $CD4^+$ and $CD3^+$ $CD8^+$ numbers whilst $CD19^+$ cells identify B cells. Low T and/or B cells may occur with severe combined immunodeficiency whereas absence of B cells is a feature of X-linked agammaglobulinaemia. However, these findings are not diagnostic and may be affected by drugs or an intercurrent infection. Low $CD3^+$ $CD4^+$ cell numbers are characteristic of human immunodeficiency virus (HIV) infection. However, a normal CD4 count does not exclude HIV nor should it be used as a covert screening test. Phenotypic markers can be valuable in the diagnosis of lymphoproliferative disease.

LYMPHOCYTE PROLIFERATION

This specialized test is reserved for the investigation of suspected cellular immunodeficiency following liasion with an immunologist. The proliferation of lymphocytes can be measured following *in vitro* stimulation by mitogens such as phytohaemagglutinin, or antigens such as tetanus, to which the patient has previously been exposed.

COMPLEMENT PATHWAY LEVELS (C3, C4, C1 INHIBITOR)

Specific components of the complement pathway can be measured, and C3 and C4 levels in particular. Raised levels may suggest an acute phase response where low levels may occur with inflammatory diseases and rare hereditary immunodeficiencies. A low C4 may also occur with C1 inhibitor deficiency (hereditary angioedema (HAE)) and a normal level during an attack excludes this diagnosis. C1 inhibitor levels can also be measured, with functional tests being reserved for those few individuals with a high clinical index of suspicion when normal C1 inhibitor levels are found. Defects in functional assays of complement activity (discussed below) may suggest a rare hereditary complement deficiency that requires individual components of the complement pathway to be assayed at a specialist laboratory.

COMPLEMENT ACTIVITY (CH50 AND AP50)

These tests are reserved for atypical cases of lupus (classical pathway deficiencies), recurrent bacterial infections (alternative pathway defects) and recurrent neisserial infections (terminal pathway deficiencies). Low activity during a period of health suggests an underlying hereditary defect requiring identification.

NITRO BLUE TETRAZOLIUM TEST

The traditional test for the diagnosis of chronic granulomatous disease (CGD) is the nitro blue tetrazolium (NBT) test, where the absence of a neutrophil oxidative burst results in patients' leukocytes failing to reduce NBT dye to a blue precipitate during phagocytosis. Carriers may also be detected by this method.

PHAGOCYTOSIS AND KILLING

This test is technically difficult but remains helpful for the evaluation of neutrophil disorders. Patients' cells are mixed *in vitro* with bacteria or fungi. The presence of viable microorganisms outside the cells is compatible with phagocytic defects whereas intracellular killing defects, for example CGD, are characterized by a reduction in killed intracellular microorganisms.

MOLECULAR AND GENETIC STUDIES

Over the last decade, the molecular defects underlying many primary immunodeficiencies have been recognized, allowing confirmation of disease by detection of genetic mutations. Examples include some forms of severe combined immunodeficiency, X-linked agammaglobulinaemia, X-linked hyper-IgM syndrome, CGD and X-linked lymphoproliferative disease.

Allergy

A brief discussion of allergy tests follows, although this subject will be discussed further in Chapter 12, Allergy: basic mechanisms and tests. When diagnosing allergy, a clear and detailed history is paramount. Detection of allergen specific IgE can be used to test for a wide range of inhaled and food allergens.[3] This can be performed *in vivo* by skin prick tests or *in vitro* on serum using the outdated term radioallergosorbent assay test (RAST). Modern enzyme-linked immunosorbent assay (ELISA) tests have replaced RASTs. The presence of specific IgE *in vivo* or *in vitro* does not necessarily indicate clinical allergy, emphasizing the importance of the patient's history. Results in both circumstances are also dependent on the sensitivity or specificity of the allergen in the solution or assay.

SKIN PRICK TESTS

Drops of aqueous solutions of relevant allergens, negative (allergen buffer) and positive controls (histamine) are applied to the skin. A pinprick is made through the drop placed on the epidermis and excess solution removed with tissue. The size of any localized skin reaction is measured at 15 minutes, and results >2–3 mm diameter larger than the negative control are considered positive. Antihistamines should be stopped several days before testing, to prevent false negative results.

IgE

IgE levels may be raised in allergic diseases, particularly eczema, and also with certain parasitic infections, immunodeficiencies and lymphomas. A total serum IgE is useful when interpreting *in vitro* allergen specific IgE levels as patients with very high serum IgE levels may give false positive results.

SPECIFIC IgE

Measuring serum IgE antibodies specific to relevant antigens is an *in vitro* method for diagnosing allergy. It is especially useful if patients have widespread skin disease which would make skin prick testing difficult. However, this test has poor specificity when compared with the skin prick test.

ANAESTHETIC REACTION TESTING

Hypersensitivity reactions occurring during surgery may be difficult to differentiate from other simultaneous

Table 13.3 Interpretation of autoantibodies in typical autoimmune screen.

Autoantibodies	Disease	Further tests
Thyroid microsomal	Autoimmune hypo and hyperthyroidism	Thyroid function tests
Gastric parietal cell	Pernicious anaemia	B12 levels
		Intrinsic factor antibodies
Mitochondrial	Primary biliary cirrhosis	Immunoglobulins
		Liver function tests
Smooth muscle	Autoimmune liver disease	Liver function tests
	Viral infections, e.g. EBV	
Anti-nuclear antibodies	Connective tissue disease, e.g. lupus	dsDNA, ENA antibodies
		Complement levels
		BP and urinalysis

haemodynamic events. Serial evaluation of serum tryptase may be helpful in this situation. A clear history detailing all drugs and fluids given and possible peri-operative sources of latex exposure is essential if the precipitating cause is to be identified. Subsequent skin testing to general anaesthetic agents and latex, may be appropriate in some cases.

Autoimmune disease including vasculitis

The presence of serum autoantibodies is a helpful aid in the management of a variety of autoimmune diseases and vasculitis and should be considered in the light of the clinical history and the outcome of appropriate tissue biopsies.[4] Some autoantibodies are considered to contribute to disease pathogenesis whilst others are secondary to tissue damage but are nevertheless useful disease markers. High levels of IgG class autoantibodies, are more likely to reflect autoimmunity and disease compared to those of the IgM class. The major use of autoantibody testing is for diagnosing disease. Certain tests are helpful for monitoring disease, for example anti-glomerular basement membrane antibodies, whilst some provide information on disease prognosis, for example cytoplasmic anti-neutrophil cytoplasmic antibodies (ANCA) and anti-proteinase-3 antibodies in Wegener's granulomatosis. In some circumstances, for example thyroid disease, autoantibodies may predate clinical disease identifying patients who require observation. False positive autoantibodies may occur with a range of infections, drugs and malignancy and some may also occur in healthy individuals. The most frequently performed autoantibody tests will be discussed, other tests not mentioned may require liaison with the immunologist.

AUTOIMMUNE SCREEN

An autoimmune screen evaluates autoantibodies associated with some of the commoner autoimmune diseases.

There is, however, some variation between laboratories in which autoantibodies are evaluated. Autoimmune thyroid and liver disease, pernicious anaemia and lupus are typically sought. The corresponding autoantibodies are outlined in **Table 13.3**.

RHEUMATOID FACTOR AND RHEUMATOID ARTHRITIS

A positive rheumatoid factor (an autoantibody against IgG) occurs in approximately 75 percent of cases of rheumatoid arthritis although its absence does not exclude this diagnosis. It also occurs in Sjogren's disease, SLE, cryoglobulinaemia and certain infections.

dsDNA ANTIBODIES AND LUPUS

The presence of high titre IgG anti-dsDNA (double stranded DNA) antibodies in a patient with positive ANA antibodies is highly suggestive of lupus. However, only 50 percent of patients with lupus will have positive dsDNA antibodies at some time in their illness; some of the remainder have positive extra nuclear antigen (ENA) antibodies, as described below.

ENA ANTIBODIES AND CONNECTIVE TISSUE DISEASE

The detection of positive ENA autoantibodies in a patient with a positive ANA is suggestive of connective tissue disease and may help categorize the illness. For example, Ro, and sometimes La, antibodies occur with Sjogren's disease, Sm antibodies are associated with lupus and are predictive of increased risk of renal lupus and anti-ribonucleoprotein (RNP) antibodies occur with lupus and its overlap syndromes.

CENTROMERE, SCL-70 ANTIBODIES AND SCLERODERMA

Scleroderma (progressive systemic sclerosis) is a connective tissue disease characterized by skin sclerosis and internal organ fibrosis involving lungs, oesophagus and kidney. It can present with dysphagia, and the presence of telengiectasia or a history of Raynaud's phenomenon are clues to the diagnosis. A positive ANA with Scl-70 antibodies occurs in widespread disease whereas anti-centromere antibodies are typically associated with calcinosis, Raynauds, esophageal dysmotility, sclerodactyl and telangiectasia (CREST) syndrome.

ANCA AND VASCULITIS

The diagnosis of vasculitis, wherever possible, relies on tissue biopsy. However, autoantibody evaluation has a role in reaching a definitive diagnosis, identifying patients who need urgent assessment and, in some cases, monitoring disease. Great care is needed in interpreting these autoantibodies. Infective endocarditis and HIV infection clinically mimic vasculitis and may give rise to false positive test results. A positive c-ANCA is typically associated with Wegener's granulomatosis whereas a p-ANCA (perinuclear ANCA) is compatible with microscopic polyangiitis (MPA) or Churg–Strauss syndrome. The presence of anti-proteinase-3 (PR3) and anti-myeloperoxidase (MPO) antibodies respectively, add specificity to these diagnoses. A negative ANCA will occur in 15–20 percent of patients with these vasculitides (**Table 13.4**).

CARDIOLIPIN ANTIBODIES AND ANTIPHOSPHOLIPID SYNDROME

The anti-phospholipid syndrome has great clinical diversity and features include recurrent venous and arterial thrombosis, recurrent pregnancy loss and thrombocytopaenia, and neurological disease due to both small and large vessel occlusion. Presentation to an ENT surgeon might include vertigo or a nasal perforation. Anti-cardiolipin antibodies (and also anti β-2 glycoprotein 1 antibodies) may suggest a diagnosis of anti-phospholipid (APL) syndrome. Anti-cardiolipin antibodies may also occur in association with connective tissue diseases, for example lupus, but also occur with infections (including HIV), lymphoproliferative disease and drugs, for example anti-epileptics and anti-psychotics. Repeat testing may be indicated to exclude transient autoantibody production secondary to infection. The lupus anti-coagulant assay (usually performed in haematology) is a functional test assessing blood coagulation, and should be performed concurrently.

CRYOGLOBULINAEMIA

Cryoglobulins are immunoglobulins that form gels or precipitates on cooling. Clinical features include purpura, Raynauds syndrome, thrombosis, neuropathy and vasculitis. They are associated with infections, connective tissue disease and lymphoproliferative disease. Detection relies on the appropriate collection into a prewarmed blood tube in a waterbath/vacuum flask. Cold agglutinins are autoantibodies that reversibly agglutinate erythrocytes in the cold and should not be confused with cryoglobulins.

COELIAC DISEASE

Coeliac disease is characterized by malabsorbtion and weight loss but can present with oral ulceration, anaemia and malaise. The presence of villous atrophy on duodenal biopsy remains the gold standard for diagnosis but serological tests are an invaluable screen. IgA endomysial antibodies occur in over 95 percent of Coeliac disease patients although they may be negative in individuals with IgA deficiency or in patients established on a gluten free diet. IgA anti-transglutaminase antibodies are emerging as an alternative test. Anti-gliadin antibodies may be helpful for diagnosing Coeliac disease in children and IgA deficiency but they are less specific, occurring with gastrointestinal infection and inflammation.

BULLOUS PEMPHIGOID AND PEMPHIGUS

Bullous pemphigoid is associated with autoantibodies to the dermo-epidermal junction or mucosal basement membrane zone leading to cutaneous and mucosal blisters, particularly in the elderly. Circulating autoantibodies are positive in approximately 75 percent of cases. Direct immunofluorescence examination of perilesional biopsy material, however, reveals linear deposits of C3 and IgG at the basement membrane in nearly all cases. Pemphigus is a blistering disease associated with serum intercellular autoantibodies in nearly all cases. These antibodies, usually at low titre, may also occur with burns and infections. Direct immunofluorescence examination is helpful for the diagnosis of pemphigus revealing linear intraepithelial IgG. The intraepithelial pathology in pemphigus predisposes to increased mortality.

Table 13.4 Guide to interpretation of ANCA.

Result	Guide to interpretation
Positive C-ANCA with PR3 antibodies	Wegeners granulomatosis
Positive P-ANCA with MPO antibodies	Microscopic polyangiitis Churg–Strauss syndrome
Positive C-ANCA without PR3 antibodies	Inflammatory bowel disease Infection, malignancy
Positive P-ANCA without MPO antibodies	Vasculitis, connective tissue disease Infection, malignancy

ACETYL CHOLINE RECEPTOR ANTIBODIES, MYASTHAENIA GRAVIS AND THYMOMA

Myasthaenia gravis is characterized by increased skeletal muscle fatiguability. Facial and bulbar muscle involvement may cause nasal speech and difficulty in swallowing. Generalized weakness occurs in approximately 85 percent of patients. Autoantibodies to the acetyl choline receptor (AchR) at the neuromuscular junction are detectable in 90 percent of patients. Myasthenia gravis is associated with thymoma (when anti-striated muscle antibodies may also be present) and other autoimmune diseases.

IMMUNOFLUORESCENCE STUDIES/BIOPSY

Detecting immunoglobulin and complement deposits in biopsies by means of fluorescent antibodies to these components may be helpful in the diagnosis of bullous skin disease, as mentioned above. Other indications include a variety of dermatological and renal diseases.

Lymphoproliferative disease

Many of the immunological tests required to investigate lymphoproliferative disease have already been mentioned and are used in combination with bone marrow and lymph node biopsies. A diagnosis of multiple myeloma is derived from the presence of two from three of the following: urinary or serum paraprotein (immunoglobulins detectable as a discrete band on electrophoresis and produced from a single clone of plasma cells); 10 percent plasma cells on bone marrow examination; and bone involvement on skeletal survey or bone scan.

IMMUNOGLOBULINS AND SERUM AND URINE PARAPROTEIN

A paraprotein should be sought when analysing total immunoglobulin levels. They may be detectable in both serum and/or urine, the presence of free light chains in the urine (Bence–Jones proteins) being particularly suggestive of a lymphoproliferative disease. High levels of serum paraproteins associated with reduced serum immunoglobulins (immunoparesis) is also suggestive of malignant disease. Low paraprotein concentrations, e.g. $<10\,g/L$ may occur in infections, inflammatory diseases and with monoclonal gammopathy of uncertain significance (MGUS). MGUS may progress to lymphoproliferative disease.

PHENOTYPING

Cellular phenotyping may contribute to the diagnosis of lymphoproliferative disease, for example chronic lymphatic leukaemia (CLL). Similar techniques can also be applied to peripheral blood and bone marrow aspirates for the evaluation of myeloid disease.

KEY POINTS

- Immunodeficiency is uncommon but patients will present or be undiagnosed in ENT clinics. Targeting investigations to the relevant group, for example refractory sinusitis, will avoid missing cases of immunodeficiency.
- Immunological tests may help in diagnosis and monitoring of disease but must always be considered in association with clinical presentation and biopsy findings.
- Liaise with your clinical immunologist/ immunology laboratory to ensure the appropriate tests are being requested. If clinical history is particularly suggestive of a disease, further tests may be required even in the presence of initial negative investigations.

Best clinical practice

✓ Immunological tests always need to be interpreted in the context of the clinical case.

Deficiencies in current knowledge and areas for future research

➤ The majority of current tests are performed on peripheral blood due to its accessibility. Tests that reflect activity at local surfaces, for example defensins, and tests that are more reflective of *in vivo* pathology, such as intracellular cytokine analysis, may enter clinical practice.

➤ Many patients that have severe, persistent, unusual and recurrent infections yet no immunological cause is identified. Advancing knowledge, particularly regarding the innate immune system, e.g. toll receptors, may account for such disease and diagnostic tests will subsequently follow.

➤ Increasing use of molecular diagnosis and development of tests looking at functional pathways will occur. It is becoming increasingly apparent that individuals with the same genetic mutation may have diverse disease phenotypes, e.g. btk mutation associated with complete absence of B cells or IgG subclass defect. Identification of genetic polymorphisms may predict patients at risk of severe disease requiring a more aggressive management strategy.

➤ Tests are being developed that reflect patient response to treatment, e.g. antiviral drugs in HIV, or side effects to azathioprine, for example. This will help optimize treatments whilst minimizing harm.

REFERENCES

1. Report of an IUIS Scientific Committee. Primary Immunodeficiency Diseases. *Clinical and Experimental Immunology.* 1999; **118**: 1–28.
2. Spickett GP, Misbah SA, Chapel HM. Primary antibody deficiency in adults. *Lancet.* **337**: 281–4.
3. Rusznak C, Davis RJ. ABC of allergies. *British Medical Journal.* 1998; **316**: 686–9.
4. Jury EC, D'Cruz D, Morrow WJW. Autoantibodies and overlap syndromes in autoimmune rheumatic disease. *Journal of Clinical Pathology.* 2002; **54**: 340–7.

14

Primary immunodeficiencies

ELIZABETH DREWE AND RICHARD J POWELL

Introduction: primary and secondary immunodeficiency	174	Deficiencies in current knowledge and areas for future research	181
Primary immunodeficiency diseases	174	References	182
Key points	181		
Best clinical practice	181		

SEARCH STRATEGY

The data for this chapter are supported by a Medline search using the key words immunodeficiency and ear/nose/throat. The classification of primary immunodeficiency is based on the report of the IUIS Scientific Committee.[1]

INTRODUCTION: PRIMARY AND SECONDARY IMMUNODEFICIENCY

Primary and secondary immunodeficiency may both present with severe, recurrent, unusual or persistent infections with the specific defect influencing the type of presentation or organism involved. Primary immunodeficiency refers to rare deficiencies of the innate or adaptive immune system. Secondary immunodeficiency is commoner and reflects immunological defects secondary to other pathology including cancer and infections such as human immunodeficiency virus (HIV). It is, however, important to differentiate these two groups of conditions to allow initiation of the correct treatment which may, for both conditions, reduce morbidity and mortality. Features that may point to primary immunodeficiency include failure to thrive, a positive family history and associated autoimmune features, for example, idiopathic thrombocytopaenic purpura (ITP). Lymphoproliferative disease may also be a complication.

Patients with immunodeficiency present to a variety of specialties, but particularly ENT and respiratory departments. A multidisciplinary approach is essential for both diagnosis and treatment. Deficiencies affecting most parts of the immune system are documented and those affecting T and B cells, phagocytes and complement will be described along with certain specific diseases characterized by major immunological deficits. When managing immunodeficiency, liaison with a clinical immunologist is required at an early stage in each individual case. Infections in immunodeficient patients must also be treated with higher doses of antibiotics and for longer periods, compared to immunocompetent individuals.

PRIMARY IMMUNODEFICIENCY DISEASES

Combined immunodeficiency

SEVERE COMBINED IMMUNODEFICIENCY

Severe combined immunodeficiency (SCID) describes the most severe forms of primary immunodeficiency affecting both T and B lymphocytes. It has an incidence of 1/30–70,000 live births.[2] A variety of genetic defects, e.g. cytokine (interleukin (IL)-2, 4, 7, 9 and 15) receptor gamma chain, janus kinase 3 and recombinase activation gene mutations, prevent T cell and also sometimes B cell and NK cell development and function. Untreated SCID leads to early death from overwhelming infection, typically within the first year of life.[2] Respiratory infections are common and include *Pneumocystis carinii*,

Cytomegalovirus pneumonitis and viral bronchiolitis. *Candida* frequently colonizes the skin, oropharynx and nappy area, and skin sepsis, e.g. *Staphylococcus*, may also be problematic. Other features compatible with SCID are failure to thrive and disseminated BCG infection. Once the diagnosis is suspected, antibiotics, anti-fungal and immunoglobulin therapy should be commenced. Live vaccines must be avoided and if blood transfusion is required it must be cytomegalovirus negative. Blood must also be irradiated to kill any donor lymphocytes that could cause graft versus host disease. Early bone marrow transplantation, prior to infection becoming established, is curative for some forms of SCID. Early experiences with gene therapy for cytokine receptor gamma chain SCID are also impressive.

Reticular dysgenesis is a form of SCID characterized by severe neutropenia as well as lymphopaenia. It reflects aberrant stem cell development and follows autosomal recessive inheritance. Some defects, for example adenosine deaminase (ADA) deficiency and purine nucleoside phosphorylase deficiency, may present as a SCID but may also present later in life with recurrent infections accompanied by neurological disturbance in combination with bony defects (for ADA deficiency) or autoimmune manifestations (for purine nucleoside phosphorylase (PNP) deficiency) (**Table 14.1**).

X-LINKED HYPER IgM SYNDROME

X-linked hyper IgM (XHIM) syndrome results from defects in the gene for CD40 ligand (see Chapter 11, Defence mechanisms) which is expressed on T cells and whose interaction with B cells induces B cells to switch from producing IgM antibodies to IgG and IgA

Table 14.1 Disorders of T and B lymphocytes and antibodies.

Disease	Defect	Clinical	Laboratory	Treatment
SCID	Mutations affecting T and B cell development and function	Respiratory Candida Failure to thrive	Low lymphocyte count Low T/B cell number Reduced T cell proliferation Specific defects	Antibiotics Anti-fungals Immunoglobulin BMT Gene therapy
Hyper IgM syndrome	Mutations CD40 ligand on T cells needed for immunoglobulin class switching and T cell priming	Respiratory infections Diarrhoea Oral ulcers Tumours	Normal or high IgM Low IgG and IgA Neutropenia +/− Lack of CD40 ligand expression Mutations CD40 ligand	Cotrimaoxazole Immunoglobulin BMT
X linked agammaglobulinaemia	Mutations in btk gene needed for B cell development	Sinusitis Otitis media Pneumonia Arthritis Meningoencephalitis	Absent/low B cells Low immunoglobulins Neutropenia +/− Btk mutations	Immunoglobulins Antibiotics
CVI	Most unknown	Sinusitis Otitis media Pneumonia Gastrointestinal infection Autoimmunity Granuloma Tumours	Low immunoglobulins B cells present	Immunoglobulin Antibiotics
Selective antibody deficiency	Unknown	Well Sinusitis Pneumonia	Low IgA Low IgG subclass Lack of response to immunizations	None Antibiotics Immunoglobulin
Transient hypo-gammaglobulinaemia newborn	Disparity resolution maternal IgG and IgG production	Well Bacterial infections	IgM low/normal IgG and IgA low	None Antibiotics Immunoglobulin

antibodies. This condition usually presents in infancy with upper and lower respiratory tract infections.[3] CD40 ligand defects also result in poor T cell priming leading to infection with *Pneumocystis jerovici* and *Cryptosporidium*. Recurrent oral ulcers are also common and may be associated with neutropenia. Regular immunoglobulin replacement and prophylactic co-trimoxazole are the cornerstone to management. Life expectancy is poor with <30 percent of patients alive at 25 years of age and major causes of death including *Pneumocystis jerovici* pneumonia, liver failure and tumours. Bone marrow transplantation performed early in life offers the potential for a cure.

Predominantly antibody deficiency

Defects in B lymphocyte development and antibody production commonly produce recurrent bacterial infections presenting at any age. Antibody deficiencies are a spectrum ranging from the absence of a single antibody class of antibody, namely IgA, through to essentially no antibody (panhypogammaglobulinaemia). There are even certain individuals that have normal antibody levels but are unable to respond to specific microorganisms. Treatment, if required, is centred on intravenous immunoglobulin (IVIg) therapy, although concerns about supply and potential transmission of infections require the use of IVIg to be justified on an individual basis. Immunoglobulin therapy (0.6 g/kg/month) has been shown to significantly reduce the frequency of acute infections and improve lung function tests.[4] [****] Intravenous and subcutaneous immunoglobulin administration appear to be equally beneficial whilst intramuscular replacement is less effective.[5, 6] [****] Home therapy programmes which involve self-administration, intravenous and subcutaneous, may enhance quality of life and allow patients optimal control of their disease.

X-LINKED AGAMMAGLOBULINAEMIA

X-linked agammaglobulinaemia (XLA) is characterized by a profound deficiency of B cells due to a mutation in the btk gene producing arrest of B cell development. Lymphoid hypoplasia with a lack of tonsils may be a diagnostic clue.[7] Susceptibility to infection manifests as transplacentally transferred maternal IgG levels wane at four to six months, although some patients may not present until five years of age or older. Sinusitis, otitis media and lower respiratory infections are the most common infected sites with *Haemophilus influenzae*, *Staphylococcus aureus*, *Streptococcus pneumonia* and *Pseudomonas*, the most frequent pathogens.[8] Mycoplasma arthritis and enteroviral meningoencephalitis contribute both to morbidity and mortality. Treatment is based on immunoglobulin replacement and whilst low dose regimes may prevent severe acute bacterial infections, higher doses

may be required to prevent the development of bronchiectasis, chronic sinusitis and enteroviral infections.[9]

COMMON VARIABLE IMMUNODEFICIENCY

Common variable immunodeficiency (CVI) probably encompasses a variety of antibody deficiencies and a handful of genetic causes have been found to account for a small percentage of cases. It is characterized by recurrent bacterial infections. Patients have circulating B cells but are unable to secrete immunoglobulin resulting in hypogammaglobulinaemia. A family history occurs in approximately 20 percent of cases of CVI and IgA deficiency. Mean age at diagnosis is 30 years but, regrettably, symptoms are often present up to six years prior to diagnosis.[10] Recurrent pneumonia and maxillary sinusitis are the commonest prediagnostic finding and chronic pulmonary complications may have already developed prior to diagnosis.[11] Recurrent bronchitis, sinusitis and otitis media, most frequently due to *Haemophilus influenzae* and *Streptococcus pneumoniae*, occur in 98 percent of patients. Seventy-five percent of patients also have pneumonia. Gastrointestinal infection, for example *Salmonella* and *Giardiasis*, is also common whilst septic arthritis and meningitis are recognized, but less frequent, complications. Over 20 percent of patients have associated autoimmunity, e.g. haemolytic anaemia and idiopathic thrombocytopaenia. Granuloma and inflammatory bowel disease are also common. Non-Hodgkin's lymphoma occurs in <8 percent of patients and the risk of other malignancies, including squamous cell tumours and adenocarcinomas, is also increased. Life expectancy is reduced with 20-year survival rates of approximately 65 percent. Treatment is based on regular immunoglobulin therapy with aggressive and appropriate treatment of intercurrent infections.

SELECTIVE IMMUNOGLOBULIN IMMUNODEFICIENCY

This broad term includes isolated IgA deficiency, selective IgG subclass deficiency (normally IgG2) and specific antibody deficiency, or any combination of these. Diverse clinical presentations require management decisions to be made on an individual basis with the clinical phenotype ranging from normal health to recurrent otitis media and sinopulmonary infections.

IgA deficiency occurs in 1/600 Caucasians and it is important to screen those individuals who in addition have recurrent infections, for a functional antibody defect. Complete IgA deficient patients may also develop anti-IgA antibodies posing a risk of anaphylaxis on exposure to IgA via blood products.

A primary diagnosis of IgG subclass deficiency is based on a normal total IgG with low levels of one or more IgG subclasses. IgG subclasses are, however, reduced as part of other immunodeficiencies. In early childhood, normal

IgG subclass ranges may be difficult to define and IgG2 levels are frequently reduced. IgG2 deficiency may be associated with an inability to respond to polysaccharide antigens, for example pneumococcus, and one clue is that it is often associated with IgA deficiency.

Specific or functional antibody deficiencies refers to individuals who cannot mount an antibody response to a pathogen or immunization and can be present in individuals with normal or low levels of IgG. This most commonly occurs with pneumococcal antigens but the diagnosis can also be applied to patients who fail to respond to hepatitis vaccine.

TRANSIENT HYPOGAMMAGLOBULINAEMIA OF INFANCY

This condition reflects an imbalance between neonatal catabolism of maternal IgG that was transported across the placenta during the last trimester of pregnancy, and initiation of immunoglobulin synthesis by the maturing infant. A period may occur where infants have immunoglobulin levels in the immunodeficiency range and hence may be susceptible to infections. This condition is exacerbated by prematurity where the opportunity for maternal transfer of IgG is reduced. Infants require monitoring which should demonstrate initial production of IgM, followed by responses to vaccinations and rising levels of IgG. In cases of severe infection, immunoglobulin therapy may be required during the period of immunodeficiency and a definitive diagnosis may only be made retrospectively.

Defects in phagocyte number and function

Phagocyte defects are characterized by early age of onset of recurrent infections with opportunistic bacterial and fungal infections. Neutrophil disorders may be divided into neutropenia reflecting decreased production (e.g. secondary to cytotoxics) or increased consumption of neutrophils (e.g. systemic lupus erythematosus (SLE)), and disorders of neutrophil function.[12] Neutrophil dysfunction may reflect defects of intracellular killing, for example chronic granulomatous disease (CGD), defects in the formation and function of neutrophil granules, for example Chediak–Higashi syndrome, or defective neutrophil adhesion, for example leukocyte adhesion deficiency (LAD). Defective cytokine signalling involving macrophages may also account for susceptibility to mycobacterial infections. Early diagnosis resulting in initiation of appropriate treatment, for example prophylactic antibiotics and antifungals, granulocyte colony stimulating factors (G-CSF) or bone marrow transplantation may improve survival. Several specific immunodeficiency diseases are detailed below (**Table 14.2**).

Table 14.2 Disorders of phagocyte number and function.

Disease	Defect	Clinical	Laboratory	Treatment
Severe congenital neutropenia	Mutations in G-SCF receptor in some cases	Septicaemia Meningitis Peritonitis	Absolute neutropenia Bone marrow myeloid hyperplasia with maturation arrest	G-CSF Antibiotics
Cyclical neutropenia	Neutrophil elastase 2 mutations	Oral ulceration Stomatitis Cellulitis	Neutropenia for 3–10 days every 15–35 days	Antibiotics
LAD	Mutations in CD18	Delay umbilical cord separation Stomatitis Otitis media Peridontitis Intestinal fistulas	Neutrophilia with infection Reduced CD18 expression	BMT (severe) Antibiotics
CGD	Defects in NADPH complex for reactive oxygen metabolites	Pneumonia Abscess Osteomyelitis Granuloma	Abnormal NBT test Abnormal phagocytosis and killing	Antibiotics Antifungals Bone marrow transplant
Leukocyte mycobacterial deficiency	IL-12, IL-12 R IFN-γR	Disseminated Mycobacterial infection		IFN-γ in some cases BMT (severe)

SEVERE CONGENITAL NEUTROPENIA

Severe congenital neutropenia (SCN) is related to maturation arrest at the myelocyte to promyelocyte stage and both autosomal dominant and recessive forms as well as sporadic cases are recognized. Some patients have mutations in the G-CSF receptor gene resulting in hyporesponsiveness to G-CSF. SCN usually manifests in the first few months of life with overwhelming infections, for example septicaemia, meningitis, peritonitis and pneumonia. Other presentations include lymphadenitis, stomatitis, cellulitis and omphalitis with *Staphylococcal aureus* and *Pseudomonas* representing common pathogens. Life expectancy is increased with G-CSF therapy but transformation into acute myelogenous leukaemia or myelodysplasia occurs in 10 percent of cases.

CYCLICAL NEUTROPENIA

This condition reflects cyclical disturbances in bone marrow myelocyte production translating into recurrent neutropenia, often with a 21-day cycle. An autosomal dominant pattern of inheritance is recognized and mutations in the neutrophil elastase gene (ELA2) are described, although how this leads to pathology is currently unknown. Cyclical neutropenia typically presents in the first decade of life with episodic oral ulceration, stomatitis, fevers and cellulitis. Whilst this condition may improve with age, 10 percent of patients have fatal infections including pneumonia and peritonitis, or gangrene.

LEUKOCYTE ADHESION DEFECTS

Defects in adhesion molecules (see Chapter 11, Defence mechanisms), for example intergrins (CD18 deficiency) and selectins, may disrupt neutrophil adherence to activated endothelium and migration to inflammatory sites. When an individual with leukocyte adhesion defects (LAD) encounters a pathogen, the bone marrow responds appropriately upregulating neutrophil production and release. However, these cells will not reach their destination, making individuals susceptible to overwhelming infection whilst exhibiting a profound neutrophilia.

CHRONIC GRANULOMATOUS DISEASE

Chronic granulomatous disease (CGD) is caused by mutations in the components of the nicotinamide adenine dinucleotide phosphate (NADPH) oxidase complex in phagocytes that produce reactive oxygen metabolites necessary to kill bacteria and fungi. CGD occurs in 1/200,000 live births with an X-linked recessive inheritance accounting for 70 percent of cases whilst the remainder are autosomal recessive.[13] Seventy-five percent of individuals are diagnosed at less than five years of age,

in 4 percent the diagnosis is delayed to the third decade or later; the oldest patient was 69 years at diagnosis. The clinical picture is dominated by pneumonia, abscesses, suppurative rhinosinusitis and osteomyelitis. *Aspergillus, Staphylococcus, Burkholderia* and *Serratia* are the common pathogens. Prophylactic anti-bacterials (Cotrimoxazole) and anti-fungals (Itraconazole) appear to reduce the incidence of infection. *Aspergillus* infection is the most frequent cause of death and established infection requires aggressive treatment. Granulomatous complications may lead to gastric outlet or urinary obstruction and may be helped by corticosteroids. The role of interferon (IFN)-γ therapy in CGD remains controversial but is helpful in some cases. Bone marrow transplantation may be curative but carries a 10 percent mortality rate.

LEUKOCYTE MYCOBACTERIAL DEFECTS

This covers mutations in IFN-γ receptor, IL-12 and IL-12 receptor, which are all required for defence against intracellular microbes by macrophages, and effective granuloma formation. Patients are susceptible to disseminated non-tuberculous *mycobacteria*, BCG, *Salmonella* and *Listeria monocytogenes*.

Complement deficiencies

Genetic deficiencies have been documented in most components in the classical, alternative and terminal complement pathways. Each defect is associated with a specific immunological presentation, for example recurrent infections, systemic lupus erythematous (SLE) or angioedema. Mannan binding lectin (MBL) interacts with the complement system and deficiencies of MBL also predispose to recurrent bacterial infections, for example otitis media. MBL polymorphisms also influence the clinical expression of other immunodeficiencies, for example CGD, and affect the susceptibility to certain pathogens such as meningococcus and aspergillus (**Table 14.3**).

CLASSICAL PATHWAY

C1q, C1r, C2 and C4 deficiency

Defects of the classical pathway, for example C1q, C1r, C2 and C4 deficiency, have an autosomal recessive mode of inheritance. They are associated with an SLE-like syndrome, rheumatoid disease and recurrent infections. Treatment is centred on management of the connective tissue disease with antibiotics for infection.

C1 esterase inhibitor deficiency

C1 inhibitor is part of the classical pathway but in contrast to the above, its deficiency (hereditary

Table 14.3 Disorders of complement pathway.

Disease	Defect	Clinical	Laboratory	Treatment
C1q, C1r, C2 and C4 deficiency	Genetic defects (AR)	Pyogenic infections	Reduced CH50 Low level component	Antibiotics
C1 esterase inhibitor deficiency	Absence or dysfunction C1 esterase (AD)	Angioedema	Reduced C1 esterase inhibitor levels (85%) Low C3 and C4 in attack	C1 esterase concentrate Danazol Tranexamic acid
C3, factor H and I deficiency	Genetic defect (AR)	Pyogenic infection	Reduced AP 50 Low level component	Antibiotics
Factor D and properidin deficiency	Genetic defects (AR/XL)	Meningitis	Reduced AP 50 Low level component	Antibiotics
Terminal complement	Defects in C5-9	Meningitis Gonorrhoea	Reduced CH50 and AP50 Low level component	Antibiotics
MBL	Point mutations in MBL, low levels MBL	Otitis media	Low levels MBL	Antibiotics

angioedema (HAE)) is characterized by autosomal dominant inheritance and recurrent attacks of angioedema either externally or internally. This can result in potentially fatal epiglottic and laryngeal oedema or oedema of the gut causing recurrent abdominal pain. Attacks often start in adolescence and may be precipitated by physical pressure, for example dental work and oral contraception. Patients have an absent or dysfunctional C1 inhibitor. Acute attacks resolve quickly with C1 inhibitor concentrate. Prophylactic measures for HAE include danazol, tranexamic acid and preoperative C1 esterase concentrate to cover surgery. In contrast to the oedema of immediate allergic reactions (Type 1 hypersensitivity), the oedema of HAE evolves less quickly, is never associated with urticaria and does not respond to adrenaline but is associated with a low plasma C4.

ALTERNATIVE PATHWAY

Alternative pathway defects, for example C3, Factor H and I deficiency, follow autosomal recessive inheritance and predispose to recurrent pyogenic infections. Factor D (autosomal recessive) and Properidin (X-linked) deficiency, however, predispose to neisserial infections in a manner similar to terminal pathway defects.

TERMINAL PATHWAY

Terminal pathway defects (C5–C9) pose an increased susceptibility to neisserial infections with both meningococcus and gonococcus. Meningitis may actually take a less fulminant form than in immunocompetent individuals. However, optimum immunization should be achieved whilst prophylactic antibiotics are usually recommended although evidence is lacking.

Other well-defined immunodeficiency syndromes

WISKOTT ALDRICH SYNDROME

Wiskott Aldrich syndrome (WAS) results from defects in the WAS protein which appears to be involved in cytoskeletal reorganization resulting in defective signal transduction, cell motility and phagocytosis. This X-linked disease is characterized by recurrent infections (particularly otitis media), eczema, thrombocytopaenia, autoimmune phenomena and increased risk of lymphoproliferative disease.[14] IgG levels may fall with increasing age, particularly impaired pneumococcal antibody responses. Treatment is based on prophylactic antibiotics, immunoglobulin replacement therapy, splenectomy for thrombocytopaenia and platelet transfusions for life threatening haemorrhage.[15] Median survival is around 15 years of age. Bone marrow transplantation remains a realistic option for children under five years with survival rates becoming poor in later life (**Table 14.4**).

ATAXIA TELANGIECTASIA

Ataxia telangiectasia (AT) is an autosomal recessive disorder caused by mutations in the ATM gene which encodes a large protein kinase that detects DNA breaks, facilitating DNA repair. Patients exhibit a particular sensitivity to radiation such that immunoglobulin and T cell receptor genes are subject to frequent chromosomal breakages, inversions and translocations. It is clinically characterized by immunodeficiency, oculocutaneous telangiectasia, progressive cerebellar disease and a susceptibility to cancer. Immunodeficiency may be progressive and is associated with reduced IgA and IgG2 levels with

Table 14.4 Other well-defined syndromes.

Disease	Defect	Clinical	Laboratory	Treatment
WAS	Mutations in WASP	Bacterial infections Eczema Thrombocytopaenia Autoimmunity Lymphoma	Low IgM Falling IgG Low pneumococcal response Lymphopaenia Low mean platelet volume	Antibiotics Immunoglobulins Splenectomy BMT
AT	Mutations in ATM gene which detects DNA breaks in T and B cells	Sinopulmonary infections Telangiectasia Cerebellar ataxia Cancer	Low IgA and IgG2 Poor response polysacharride	Antibiotics Immunoglobulins
Chromosome 22q11.2 deletions	Defect unclear Abnormal differentiation of branchial arches	Viral infections Hypocalcaemia Dysphagia	T lymphopaenia Reduced T cell proliferation	Antibiotics
XLP	SAP and SLAM gene mutations causing lymphocyte proliferation post EBV	Bacterial infections Fulminant EBV Aplastic anaemia Lymphoma	Agammaglobulinaemia to hypergammaglobulinaemia	BMT
Hyper IgE syndrome	Unknown	Pneumonia Pneumatocele Abscess Eczema Abnormal facies Bony abnormalities	Raised IgE	Antibiotics Anti-fungals
Autoimmune lymphoproliferative syndrome	Defects in apoptosis, e.g. Fas, Fas ligand	Lymphadenopathy Organomegaly	Defective apoptosis	Cytotoxics BMT
Chronic mucocutaneous candidiasis	Mutations in AIRE	Mucosal candida Endocrinopathy Autoimmunity	Reduced T cell proliferation to candida	Fluconazole

failure to respond to polysaccharide antigens. Recurrent bacterial sinus and pulmonary infections are common and may be exacerbated by aspiration and malnutrition. Twelve to fifteen percent of patients develop lymphoproliferative disease with other malignancies, for example adenocarcinoma also increased.

DI GEORGE SYNDROME/CHROMOSOME 22 DELETIONS

Di George syndrome (cardiac anomalies and parathyroid and thymic hypoplasia with immunodeficiency), Velocardiofacial syndrome (cardiac anomalies, hypotonia, palatal anomalies and mild developmental delay) and cardiac defects, abnormal facies, thymic hypoplasia, cleft palate and hypocalcaemia-22 (CATCH-22) are all associated with 22q11.2 deletions. These specific gene defects disrupt differentiation of the branchial arches and the clinical phenotype of these conditions may blend. Immunodeficiency does not correlate with a specific clinical presentation and needs to be assessed on an individual basis.[16] T cell lymphopaenia is common and can be associated with both impaired T cell and antibody function. Recurrent infections are common and viral infections, such as *Varicella*, *Parainfluenza* and *Rotavirus*, may be particularly severe. Conductive hearing impairment occurs in 45 percent of cases and may be associated with otitis media and speech delay.[17] Sensorineural hearing loss is also reported but may partly reflect peri-natal ischaemia. Persisting feeding difficulties related to cleft palate, increased depth of nasopharynx and pharyngo-esophageal dysmotility are common.

X-LINKED LYMPHOPROLIFERATIVE SYNDROME

X-linked lymphoproliferative syndrome (XLP) is caused by mutations either in the SLAM associated protein (SAP) gene whose protein is expressed on T cells, or its counterpart the SLAM gene, which encodes a costimulatory receptor on T and B cells.[18] In XLP, Epstein Barr virus (EBV) infected B cells may trigger uncontrolled polyclonal T and B cell proliferation and immune dysregulation. Patients may present with a clinical picture resembling common variable immunodeficiency (CVI). Hypogammaglobulinaemia may actually predate EBV infection in one-third of cases. Other presentations include fulminant EBV infection with diffuse lymphadenopathy, hepatitis and bone marrow failure, aplastic anaemia and B cell lymphoma. Prognosis is generally poor although immunoglobulin therapy containing antibodies to EBV may potentially help those patients diagnosed prior to primary EBV infection. Bone marrow transplantation has been curative in some cases.

HYPER IgE SYNDROME

The genetic basis of this autosomal dominant inherited multisystem disorder is unclear.[19] Hyper IgE syndrome is characterized by recurrent skin and pulmonary abscesses, eczema and extremely high IgE levels. *Staphylococcus aureus* and *Haemophilus influenzae* pneumonia are common and may lead to pneumatocele formation with susbsequent superinfection with *Pseudomonas aeruginosa* and *Aspergillus fumigatus*. Opportunistic infection including *Pneumocystis jerovici* pneumonia and chronic candidiasis may also occur. Associated nonimmunological conditions include delay of shedding of primary teeth due to lack of root resorption, abnormal facies with facial hemihypertrophy, prominent forehead, deep-set eyes, broad nasal bridge, wide fleshy nasal tip, mild prognathism and high arched palate. Bone fractures, hyperextensibility and scoliosis can also be features.

AUTOIMMUNE LYMPHOPROLIFERATIVE SYNDROME

Autoimmune lymphoproliferative syndrome (ALPS) is due to defects in genes encoding proteins that regulate apoptosis (see Chapter 11, Defence mechanisms), for example Fas, Fas ligand and caspases. The resultant failure of control of programmed cell death manifests as lymphoid proliferation with enlarged lymph nodes and spleen, B and T cell lymphomas and autoimmune phenomena. A characteristic immunological finding is the presence of double negative T cells (CD3$^+$CD4$^-$CD8$^-$).

CHRONIC MUCOCUTANEOUS CANDIDIASIS

This condition is characterized by persistent candidiasis affecting the skin, nails and mucosa. It contributes to a spectrum of disease associated with multiple endocrinopathies involving the parathyroid, adrenal glands, thyroid, pituitary and ovaries and autoimmune phenomena, for example vitiligo and haemolytic anaemia. The disease may be known as autoimmune polyendocrinopathy–candidiasis–ectodermal dystrophy (APECED) and be due to mutations in autoimmune regulator gene (AIRE) which effects immune tolerance.[20] The immunological defects are poorly defined but include reduced T cell proliferative responses.[21] Fluconazole treatment may be effective for Candidiasis.

KEY POINTS

- Primary immunodeficiency is a rare disease but early diagnosis and treatment improves outcome.
- Primary immunodeficiency can target most parts of the immune system and specific defects are associated with clinical presentation.
- Always consult your local immunologist as he/she should be aware of new developments.

Best clinical practice

✓ Consider immunodeficiency if history of recurrent or unusual infections.
✓ Early liaison with a clinical immunologist can reduce long-term complications of immunodeficiency.

Deficiencies in current knowledge and areas for future research

➤ The definition of primary immunodeficiency may be challenged with advancing knowledge of disease pathogenesis. Disease could be classified according to innate immunological molecular defect or clinical presentation dominated by infection. This is illustrated by the finding of an immunological cause (defective TAP genes resulting in low expression of surface HLA class 1 molecules) causing a condition resembling Wegeners granulomatosis, a disease that would traditionally not be considered to be an immunodeficiency.[22]

➤ New immunodeficiencies will be characterized. A new form of X-linked dominant hereditary angioedema with normal C1 inhibitor levels has already been described although the cause is yet undefined.[23] Knowledge of such diseases will provide insights into the immunopathogenesis of disease.

➤ Whilst major advances in understanding the genetic cause of disease have occurred in the last decade, new treatments are still required. Advances in the current practices of transplantation and gene therapy will occur, along with the use of biological agents and drugs targeting intracellular signalling. Experimental animal models suggest injection of B-lys (a TNF-receptor superfamily ligand) may actually increase total immunoglobulin levels and specific antibody responses in immunodeficient mice.

➤ Increasing understanding of the psychological impact of a diagnosis of immunodeficiency and its interaction with disease will occur which may translate into better quality of life.

REFERENCES

* 1. Report of an IUIS Scientific Committee. Primary Immunodeficiency Diseases. *Clinical and Experimental Immunology.* 1999; **118**: 1–28.

2. Gennery AR, Cant AJ. Diagnosis of severe combined immunodeficiency. *Journal of Clinical Pathology.* 2002; **54**: 191–5.

3. Notarangelo LD, Hayward AR. X-linked immunodeficiency with hyper-IgM. *Clinical and Experimental Immunology.* 2000; **120**: 399–405.

4. Roifman CM, Levison H, Gelfand EW. High-dose versus low-dose intravenous immunoglobulin in hypogammaglobulinaemia and chronic lung disease. *Lancet.* 1987; **8541**: 1075–7.

5. Chapel HM, Spickett GP, Ericson D, Engl W, Eibl MM, Bjorkander J. The comparison of the efficacy and safety of intravenous versus subcutaneous immunoglobulin replacement. *Journal of Clinical Immunology.* 2000; **20**: 94–100.

6. Nolte MT, Pirofsky B, Geeritz GA, Golding B. Intravenous immunoglobulin therapy for antibody deficiency. *Clinical and Experimental Immunology.* 1979; **36**: 237–43.

7. Ochs HD, Smith CI. X-linked aggamaglobulinaemia. A clinical and molecular analysis. *Medicine (Baltimore).* 1996; **75**: 287–99.

8. Lederman HM, Winkelstein JA. X-linked agammaglobulinaemia: An analysis of 96 patients. *Medicine (Baltimore).* 1985; **64**: 145–56.

9. Quartier P, Debre M, De Bilc J, de Sauverzac R, Sayegh N, Jabado N et al. Early and prolonged use of intravenous immunoglobulin replacement therapy in childhood agammaglobulinaemia. *Journal of Pediatrics.* 1999; **134**: 589–96.

10. Cunningham-Rundles C, Bodian C. CVID: Clinical and immunological features of 248 patients. *Clinical Immunology.* 1999; **92**: 34–8.

11. Kainulainen L, Nikoskelainen J, Ruuskanen O. Diagnostic findings in 95 Finnish patients with CVID. *Journal of Clinical Immunology.* 2001; **21**: 145–9.

12. Lakshman R, Finn A. Neutrophil disorders and their management. *Journal of Clinical Pathology.* 2001; **54**: 7–19.

13. Winkelstein JA, Marino MC, Johnston Jr. RB, Boyle J, Curnette J, Gallin JI et al. Chronic granulomatous disease. *Medicine.* 2000; **79**: 155–69.

14. Sullivan KE, Mullen CA, Blaese RM, Winkelstein JA. A multi-institutional survey of the Wiskott–Aldrich syndrome. *Journal of Pediatrics.* 1994; **125**: 876–85.

15. Thrasher AJ, Kinnon C. The Wiskott–Aldrich syndrome. *Clinical and Experimental Immunology.* 2000; **120**: 2–9.

16. Sullivan KE, Jawad AF, Randall P, Driscoll DA, Emanuel BS, McDonald-McGinn DM et al. Lack of correlation between impaired T cell production, immunodeficiency, and other phenotypic features in chromosome 22q11.2 deletion syndromes. *Clinical Immunology and Immunopathology.* 1998; **86**: 141–6.

17. Digilio MC, Pacifico C, Tieri L, Marino B, Giannotti A, Dallapiccola B. Audiological findings in patients with microdeletion 22q11. *British Journal of Audiology.* 1999; **33**: 329–33.

18. Nelson DL, Terhorst C. X-linked lymphoproliferative syndrome. *Clinical and Experimental Immunology.* 2000; **122**: 291–5.

19. Grimbacher B, Holland SM, Gallin JI, Greenberg F, Hill SM, Malech HL et al. Hyper-IgE syndrome with recurrent infections – an autosomal dominant multisystem disorder. *New England Journal of Medicine.* 1999; **340**: 692–702.

20. The Finnish–German APECED Consortium. An autoimmune disease, APECED, caused by a mutation in a novel gene featuring two PHD-type zinc-finger domains. *Nature Genetics.* 1997; **17**: 399–403.

21. De Moraes-Vasconcelos D, Orii NM, Romano CC, Iqueoka RY, Duarte AJ. Characterization of the cellular immune function of patients with chronic mucocutaneous disease. *Clinical and Experimental Immunology.* 2001; **123**: 247–53.

22. Moins-Teisserenc HT, Gadola SD, Cella M, Dunbar PR, Exley A, Blake N et al. Association of a syndrome resembling Wegener's granulomatosis with low surface expression of HLA class-I molecules. *Lancet.* 1999; **354**: 1598–603.

23. Bork K, Barnstedt SE, Koch P, Traupe H. Herediary angioedema with normal C1 inhibitor activity in women. *Lancet.* 2000; **356**: 213–7.

15

Rheumatological diseases

ADRIAN DRAKE-LEE

Introduction	183	Behçet's syndrome	189
Symptoms and signs	184	Churg–Strauss syndrome	189
Rheumatoid arthritis	185	Overlap syndromes	189
Osteoarthritis	186	Sarcoidosis	189
Spondylarthropthy	186	Relapsing polychondritis	190
SLE	186	Amyloidosis	190
Sjögren's syndrome	186	Drugs	190
Scleroderma	186	Conclusions	190
Polymyositis and dermatitis	186	Key points	190
Vasculitides	187	Best clinical practice	190
Crystal arthropathies	188	Deficiencies in current knowledge and areas for future	
SLE	188	research	190
Paget's disease (osteitis deformans)	188	References	190
Inflammatory diseases including infections	189		

SEARCH STRATEGY AND EVIDENCE-BASE

The data in this chapter are supported by a Medline search using the key words: rheumatology, rheumatoid arthritis, osteoarthritis, spondylarthropthy, SLE, Sjögren's syndrome, scleroderma, polymyositis, vasculitides, systemic lupus erythematosus, Paget's disease, Behçet's syndrome, Churg–Strauss syndrome, sarcoidosis, relapsing polychondritis, amyloidosis. Evidence throughout is level 4.

INTRODUCTION

The ENT manifestations of rheumatological diseases in the ear, nose and throat are diverse and although they are relatively uncommon, it is important that they are considered in the differential diagnosis of many conditions and are not overlooked (see **Table 15.1**). This chapter will not discuss the treatment, except where it may cause symptoms, for these are many and varied and are usually monitored by the physician. They are covered in a standard textbook on the subject, such as the *Oxford handbook of rheumatology*.[1] This chapter will look at the possible relationship between the diverse range of rheumatological conditions along with various ENT diseases and examine the validity of many of the proposed links that have been advocated between them and examine whether they are coincidental or not.

The word *rheum* comes from the Greek meaning to flow down as of mucus. It was applied to the musculoskeletal system following its usage in rheumatic fever, which presented with upper respiratory tract symptoms. Many diseases give rise to both ENT manifestations and musculoskeletal problems, and they range from the common cold to severe necrotizing granulomata. This presents a problem to the ENT surgeon in the differential diagnosis of ear, nose and throat symptoms in patients who come with nonspecific musculoskeletal complaints. Examination of the ear, nose and throat may show nonspecific

Table 15.1 Manifestations of rheumatological diseases in the ear, nose and throat.

Condition	Nose	Ear	TMJ	Mouth	Larynx	Salivary
Rheumatoid arthritis	+	+	+	+	+	+
Osteoarthritis			+			
Spondylarthropthy			+			
SLE	+	+ +	+	+	+	+
Sjögren's syndrome	+	+ +	+	+	+	+ + +
Scleroderma	+			+		
Polymyositis etc.						
Vasculitides	+ + +	+ +			+	
Crystal arthropathies		+				
Paget's disease		+ +	+			
Inflammatory diseases	+ +	+ +		+ +	+	
Behçet's syndrome	+			+ + +		
Sarcoidosis	+ +				+	+
Relapsing polychondritis		+				
Amyloidosis				+	+ +	+ / −

Key: +, <20%; + +, 20–50%; + + +, >50%.

changes prior to the development of florid signs. The skin may also be involved in some of these conditions. An ENT surgeon may be asked to see a patient with an established rheumatological condition, and be asked if there is any connection between it and, say, sensorineural deafness. As both sets of conditions may be common, particularly in the elderly, it may be easy to falsely link the two conditions.

There are essentially four relationships between the two sets of conditions; a chance finding, the natural occurrence, an association and a direct causal relationship. It is easy to confuse the first two relationships with the last two. This happens in many areas and is particularly true for Ménière's syndrome where a large number of tests have been advocated on poor epidemiological evidence.

SYMPTOMS AND SIGNS

Ear

Symptoms may be unilateral or bilateral and depend on whether the middle ear, inner ear or both are involved. Hearing loss is the commonest complaint but all symptoms, including Ménière's-like phenomenon, have been described. If the ear is abnormal, the commonest abnormality is a middle ear effusion. When the mucosa is ulcerated and scarred, adhesive otitis media results in a fixed middle ear mass. This is virtually impossible to correct surgically. Sensorineural hearing loss can either be fluctuant as in Wegener's granulomatosis, particularly prior to or as a response to treatment, or progressive as in some cases with rheumatoid diseases, particularly systemic lupus erythematosus (SLE). It may be due to either a vasculitis or deposition of immune complexes.

Oral cavity and temporomandibular joint

Aphthous ulceration in the oral cavity and pharynx frequently results in extremely painful, small, punched-out white lesions. If the ulcers are deep and large, cercarial scaring results. When this extends into the oesophagus, stenosis and dysphagia may be extreme. If the salivary glands are involved, the mouth may be dry and dental caries result from this. Patients complain of a foul taste. Burning may be a problem but is frequently a nonspecific complaint of patients, particularly affecting women in the sixth decade. The major salivary glands may be palpable. Pain and reduction of movement can occur in the temporomandibular joint (TMJ). This fluctuates with the severity of the disease and rarely results in ankylosis.

Larynx and pharynx

Patients can have hoarseness due to involvement of the synovial joints in the larynx. Salivary gland involvement gives rise to lowering the production of saliva and this can produce a feeling of a lump in the throat or dysphagia. If there is ulceration in the subglottis, hemoptysis and crusting may occur. This heals by fibrosis and stenosis. Poor movement of the vocal cords occurs particularly when there is involvement of the synovial joints of the arytenoids cartilages. Rarely, plaques may be seen in amyloidosis.

Nose

The symptoms range from blockage alone to a serosanguinous discharge and crusting. Facial pain is usually a symptom of active disease but may occur with an intercurrent infection. The nose may be affected by ulceration and granulomata with and without haemorrhage. Mucus will crust on denuded areas, or on fibrotic atrophic sites. Septal perforation and nasal collapse may also develop. Nasal bone cysts are very uncommon and have been described in sarcoidosis.

Lymphadenopathy

Nonspecific lymphadenopathy can accompany connective tissue diseases. Sarcoid produces a granulomatous lymphadenopathy as part of the condition, whereas the generalized inflammation in SLE and Sjögren's syndrome, for example, results in a higher rate of lymphoma. Any unexplained and persistent lymphadenopathy must be taken seriously and investigated appropriately.

Investigations

Most patients will have been investigated already, but some patients will present to the ENT surgeon or may no longer be under the care of the physician. As up to one-third of the patients may have anaemia, it will be worth performing a full blood count if the patients are lethargic. The erythrocyte sedimentation rate (ESR) or equivalent will often be raised in suspected vasculitis or in chronic diseases. Acute phase proteins are often raised in inflammatory conditions. The raised ESR may relate to the presence of autoantibodies.

Serological tests are the most useful and may be diagnostic for rheumatoid arthritis. Most laboratories run a batch of screening tests using histofluorescence and measure antibodies directed at different parts of the cell. Two cells are used, immortalized epithelial cells and polymorph leukocytes. Perhaps the most surprising connection between the connective tissue diseases and ENT is the use of the immortalized HEp-2 (human epithelial type 2 cells) cells as the substrate. These cells were derived from a human laryngeal carcinoma removed from a patient in the USA. The staining patterns help determine the enzyme-linked immunosorbent assay (ELISA) tests undertaken subsequently and these give a quantitative result.

Polymorph leukocytes are used for the presence of anti-neutrophil cytoplasmic antibody, and this test is probably the most useful one. It has two patterns, the perinuclear and the cytoplasmic patterns. The cytoplasmic pattern is found in Wegener's granulomatosis but may be raised in other vasculitides.[2] This study examined 871 sera that were positive in 10/11 (90 percent) of the active cases of Wegener's granulomatosis and there was a perinuclear positive pattern in 9/22 (40 percent) of patients with Sjögren's syndrome. It was occasionally raised in other conditions. Antibodies to proteinase 3 (PR3) from the polymorph leukocyte may be raised. The antibodies can disappear during treatment, and so levels

may be used as an indicator to monitor the disease but it should not be used in isolation as it is not accurate on its own. None of the tests is diagnostic but positive tests confirm connective tissue diseases.

A serum angiotensin converting enzyme level may be raised in sarcoidosis. Protein electrophoresis may help in excluding the 15 percent of patients with amyloid who have an underlying myeloma.

Biopsies of lesions and minor salivary glands may help in the diagnosis of these conditions. Some studies have looked at physical findings, such as nasal septal ulcers and perforations.[3] Biopsy did not help in the diagnosis of 71 patients, six had Wegener's granulomatosis and one had sarcoid on further testing. If granulomata are found, the diagnostic yield is higher and may help in the diagnosis.[4] The author undertakes biopsies in the operating theatre using an endoscope and samples any granulomata in preference to ulcers and perforations.

Imaging

CT and MRI have a role in evaluating the extent of disease in the organ affected but are usually unable to tell the current activity. An MR scan is best for determining inflammatory activity in joints but may show nonspecific changes in the nose and sinuses. CT is best for demonstrating bony erosion and new bone formation. Similar, but far more pronounced, changes are found when patients have a T-cell lymphoma. Patients with Wegener's granulomatosis have residual changes after the acute phase has been treated and this can confuse the clinician. Bony erosion may also occur in sarcoidosis and bone cysts can develop in the nasal bones very rarely. Imaging is helpful but is not diagnostic except in scleroderma when the contrast study demonstrates the oesophageal lesion.

RHEUMATOID ARTHRITIS

Rheumatoid arthritis is a persistent, fluctuating, destructive and chronic inflammatory condition, which produces synovitis and joint destruction. Women are more frequently affected than are men, and pregnancy improves the condition. There is a familial predisposition and HLA-DR1 and 4 are found more frequently than expected. It is a symmetrical disease affecting the small synovial joints. It may affect the cervical spine and great care must be taken when such patients have general anaesthesia as damage to the spinal cord is possible. Morrell MacKenzie first described this condition affecting the joints of the adult larynx. Similar but less pronounced changes occur in juvenile cases. A post-mortem study of five patients showed that it affected the synovial joints of the larynx and other surrounding structures.[5] Symptomatic involvement may occur in 25 percent of patients and up to 80 percent have asymptomatic involvement.[6] The pathology ranges from synovial involvement of the small joints through to ankylosis. Rheumatoid nodules may occur in the larynx and necrosis and involvement of the recurrent laryngeal nerves have been described. The TMJ may also be involved by the disease and is usually dealt with by the maxillofacial surgeons.[7]

Both conductive and sensorineural hearing loss may occur but the commonest finding is a hypermobile tympanic membrane and is contrary to expectation. This occurred in 25 percent of patients and 8 percent of controls.[8]

Lymphocytes are not antigen specific. Attention has moved away from the T cell being the most important cell to the increasing importance of macrophages and fibroblasts in the pathogenesis. They induce lymphoid aggregations that are micro-anatomical structures similar to lymph nodes. They produce cytokines such as interferon (IFN)-γ, which delay apoptosis and perpetuate the inflammation.[9]

OSTEOARTHRITIS

This degenerative condition may give rise to problems in any synovial joint but rarely affects the jaw joint. Cervical spine disease may present with neck pain that can be referred to the cranium. Patients confuse the pain with sinusitis but the symmetrical distribution and lack of any nasal symptoms rule this out. Patients with facial pain should have their neck examined carefully. Radiology and an MR scan of the affected areas, particularly the neck, may be helpful.

SPONDYLARTHROPHY

Ankylosing spondylitis is the most common condition. It is associated with nonspecific complaints in the head and neck but the literature does not reveal any obvious associations.

SLE

SLE is a multifactorial condition with a large number of different autoantibodies. Clinical classification includes a group with oral ulceration. Aphthous ulceration occurs in one-third of patients and so undiagnosed patients may present to the dental, maxillofacial and ENT surgeons. The diagnosis should be considered in all cases of multiple oral ulcers that fail to heal. A polyarteritis may cause a vasculitis that causes ulceration or an atrophic nasal mucous membrane and may result in a septal perforation. The symptoms of crusting and blockage are similar to Wegener's granulomatosis and there is overlap between the two conditions pathologically. Laryngeal involvement may also occur is a similar manner to rheumatoid arthritis.[6] A recent study of ear involvement compared 43 patients with 50 age-matched controls.[10] It showed that one-quarter of patients have a greater hearing loss in higher frequencies compared with controls. Overall, approximately three-quarters of the patients have some manifestations in the head and neck. Non-Hodgkin's lymphoma is more common in these patients than in the normal population and so unexplained and persistent cervical lymphadenopathy should be investigated promptly.

SJÖGREN'S SYNDROME

This is either a primary condition or it can be part of a generalized rheumatological condition. While a dry mouth and eyes are common, it may also result in hoarseness because of dryness and frequent throat clearing. Nasal symptoms are described with dryness, blockage and crusting. The condition is an immune-mediated chronic inflammatory disease of the salivary and lacrimal glands. The lymphocytic infiltration and inflammation lead to acinar destruction. Various autoantigens are found and include salivary duct antibodies. Nonspecific autoantibodies are present when it complicates autoimmune deficiency syndrome (AIDS) (e.g. antinuclear antibodies to antigens Ro and La). Loss of regulatory T cell function results in a polyclonal B cell proliferation and production of autoantibodies. The ENT surgeon may be asked to diagnose the condition with an intra-oral salivary gland biopsy, which can be undertaken under local anaesthesia infiltrated into the lower lip. The condition must be differentiated from other causes of diffuse parotid gland enlargement. Sjögren's syndrome is associated with a 40-fold increase in the development of lymphoma. The architecture of the lymphatic aggregations in the glands is similar to the germinal centres in lymph nodes.[11] Any lymphadenopathy must be investigated with fine needle aspiration cytology (FNAC).

SCLERODERMA

This heterogeneous disease affects women more commonly than men. The primary lesion is the formation of extra collagen. While there are many variations, both localized and diffuse, localized skin disease accounts for 60 percent of the cases. Raynaud's phenomenon is often the earliest presentation. The oesophagus is involved later, which may present as dysphagia to an ENT surgeon. The barium swallow has characteristic diffuse changes with cicatrization, often along a long segment.

POLYMYOSITIS AND DERMATITIS

There are many nonspecific symptoms other than the neck symptoms, the most common complaint is arthralgia in the larynx. The examination rarely adds anything further.

VASCULITIDES

While the rheumatologists and renal physicians categorize conditions by the size of the vessels involved, ENT surgeons group conditions by the extent of the inflammatory response – granulomata formation (**Figure 15.1**, **Table 15.2**). We have recently reviewed the classification of the specific and nonspecific nasal granulomata.[12] Wegener's granulomatosis is the most common multisystem disease and is seen at some time by every ENT surgeon (**Table 15.3**). The clinical division is split into limited disease and generalized disease when the kidney is involved. The lymphocyte response may initiate the vasculitis secondarily through the inflammatory chemokines. The lymphocyte response is commonly divided into a Th1 or a Th2 response by the cytokine profiles. Allergic diseases are driven by Th2 helper lymphocytes and the granulomatous diseases by a Th1 response. This is an over-simplification for there is evidence of a Th2 response in the nose in Wegener's syndrome while a Th1 response occurs in the blood and the kidney.[13] This suggests that the end organ is important in the type of inflammatory response.

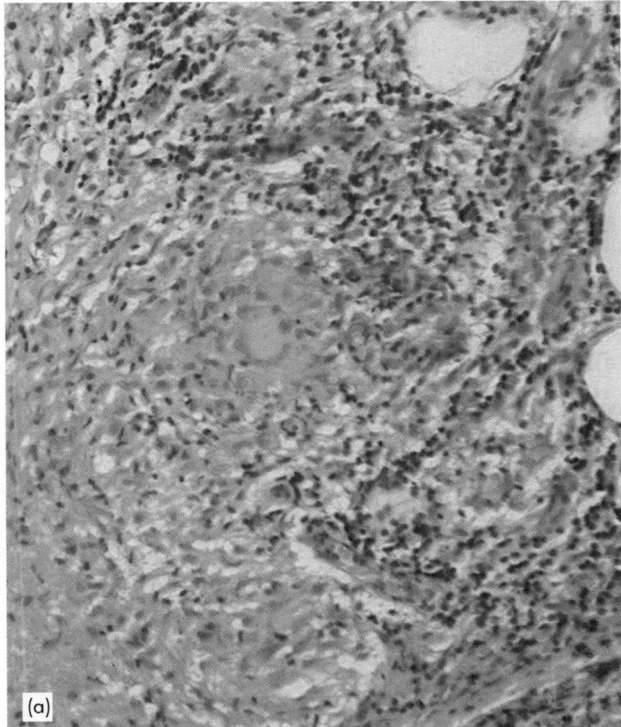

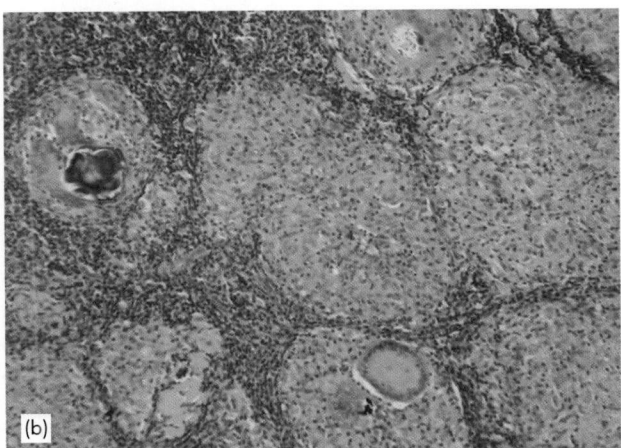

Figure 15.1 (a) and (b) The characteristic granulomata from a nasal biopsy removed from a patient with sarcoidosis. Histologically these are nonspecific but there is no caseation here and (b) shows giant cells and calcification. The latter is called a Schaumann body (Courtesy of Dr A Warfield).

Table 15.2 Diagnostic paradigms – ENT surgeons compared with rheumatologist and renal physicians or granulomata versus vasculitides.

ENT surgeons	Physicians
Granulomata	Vasculitis
Specific or infectious	Large vessel
Tuberculosis	Giant-cell arteritis (temporal)
Syphilis	Takayasu
Leprosy	Medium
Rhinoscleroma	Classical polyarteritis nodosa
Leishmaniasis	Kawasaki's
Nonspecific or noninfective	Small
Wegener's	+ immune deposits
Sarcoid	Henoch–Schönlein purpura
Pyogenic granuloma	Cryoglobulinemia
Malignant	Goodpasture's disease
T cell lymphoma (lethal	SLE
midline)	– immune deposits
	Microscopic polyangiitis
	Wegener's
	Churg–Strauss syndrome

Table 15.3 System involvement in Wegener's granulomatosis.

	%
Nose	
Intranasal	80–95
External	25–40
Ear	
Middle	25–40
Inner	5–15
Larynx	25–40
Lung	80–90
Kidney	40–65
Eye	25–40
Musculoskeletal	25–50
Gastrointestinal	5–15

This table is taken from published studies. The variations reflect the different specialties that report patients.

Wegener's granulomatosis typifies all that may go wrong in rheumatological diseases, together with the variability of the severity of the condition. It is the condition with which ENT surgeons have the greatest familiarity as over 50 percent of patients have nasal symptoms on presentation[14] and primarily complain of crusting, nasal obstruction, epistaxis and whistling from a septal perforation (**Figure 15.2**). The condition is considered in Chapter 130, Granulomatous conditions of the nose. Series range from a few cases to over a hundred. The author has between 30 and 40 under review at any one time. The vast majority of patients have nasal involvement. Those with middle ear involvement usually also have the nasal manifestations. Patients may present with a fluctuating sensorineural hearing loss and this often recovers on treatment.[15] Nasal surgery, other than a biopsy, should be avoided in active Wegener's granulomatosis as it will induce adhesions. Biopsying normal looking nasal mucosa is of no value.[3, 14] Reconstruction of the nose should be undertaken at least one year after the disease is inactive and no medication is required. Airway support with a tracheostomy is required if the subglottic stenosis is severe.

CRYSTAL ARTHROPATHIES

Gout is the most common condition and has a number of causes, including familial, and it is more common in men. The pinna may have tophi in patients who have a very high and untreated uric acid. This is rare now that the condition is better managed. The condition may affect the TMJ very rarely. Tophi have been described in the larynx, and may cause hoarseness. If these ulcerate, uric acid may be demonstrated in the sputum.[6]

SLE

The skin of the nose and nasal vestibule can be involved but this is usually long after the diagnosis has become apparent through its other manifestations. The manifestations are similar to Wegener's granulomatosis but are milder and less common.

PAGET'S DISEASE (OSTEITIS DEFORMANS)

Paget's disease is a common condition which occurs in 5 percent of the population over 60. It varies in severity and it involves the pelvis, long bones and the skull and is associated with various medical problems due to excessive new bone, which is vascular. When it involves the base of the skull, it gives rise to tinnitus, deafness and dysequilibrium in addition to headache. The deafness is sensorineural or may be mixed.[16, 17] The middle ear may be reduced in volume by new bone, the bony changes may affect the ossicles including stapedial fixation, and fibrosis

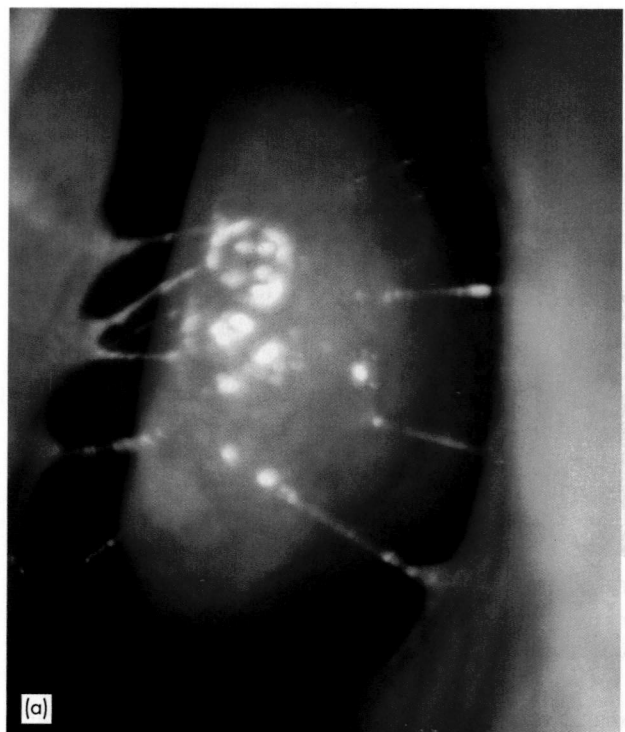

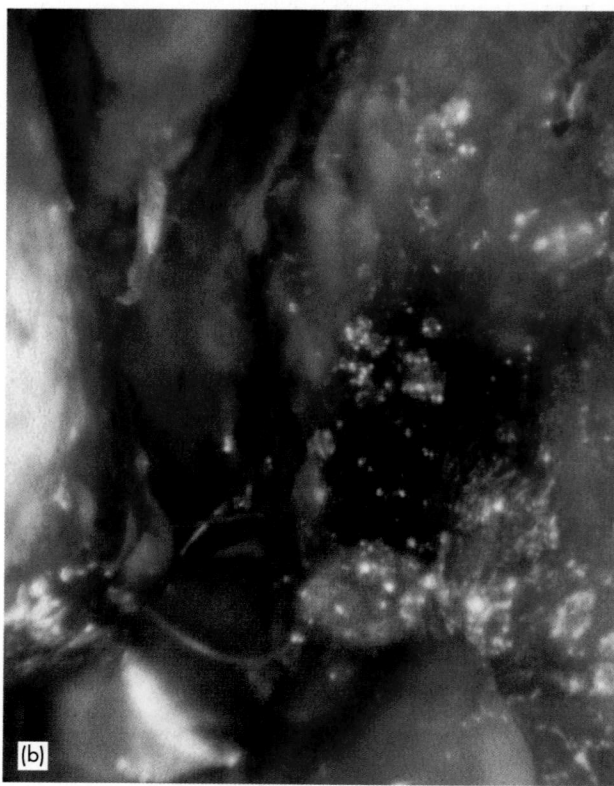

Figure 15.2 The changes in crusting found inside the nose from a patient with active Wegener's granulomatosis: **(a)** shows early changes with an angry mucosa and mucous hypersecretion; **(b)** demonstrates the end result of gross activity.

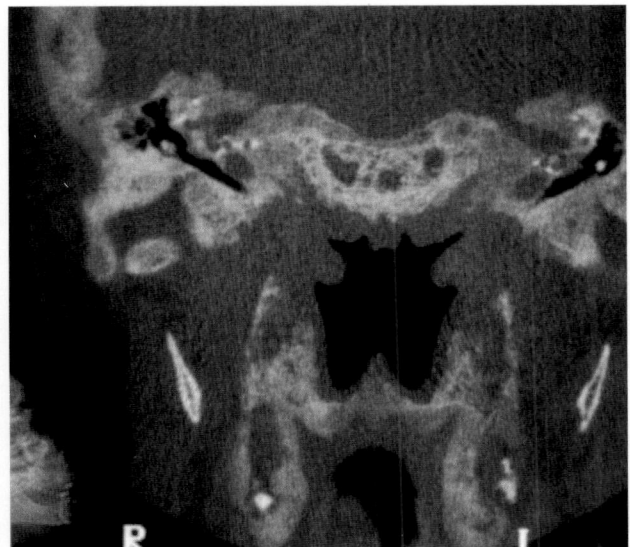

Figure 15.3 A CT scan taken of a patient with Paget's disease of the base of the skull, the patchy new bone can be seen throughout. Courtesy of Mr D Proops.

may occur. Presbyacusis is common in this age group and is exacerbated by the condition and the damage is probably multifactorial. The findings on a skull radiograph are characteristic (**Figure 15.3**) and MRI findings have been described.[18]

INFLAMMATORY DISEASES INCLUDING INFECTIONS

Acute sore throat and tonsillitis are the prodromal symptoms of rheumatic fever, which is fortunately rare now. Many acute infections have a generalized arthralgia as part of their picture. Most do not present to the ENT surgeon. Other chronic infections may present with laryngeal involvement such as tuberculosis.

BEHÇET'S SYNDROME

Although the eye manifestations are more commonly encountered, a Sjögren's syndrome-like picture is present in 10 percent of patients. The oral ulceration is often overshadowed by severe genital ulceration.

CHURG–STRAUSS SYNDROME

This is rare and typically presents with marked nasal polyposis, asthma and eosinophilia and patients are systemically unwell and may have a pyrexia of unknown origin. The management is similar to patients with severe polyposis.

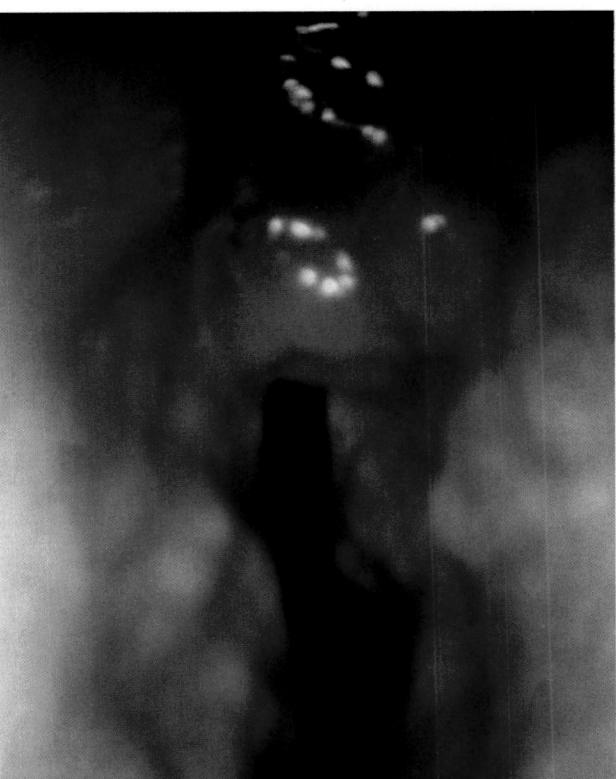

Figure 15.4 Examination of the nasal mucosa from a patient with sarcoidosis reveals apple jelly nodules.

OVERLAP SYNDROMES

These have a variety of features consistent with different aspects of connective tissue diseases but they are disparate enough that each patient with one or two of their features escapes categorization.

SARCOIDOSIS

The ear nose and throat may be involved in 5 percent of patients with sarcoidosis. They have the more severe manifestations of the disease and it tends to be more chronic than those presenting with erythema nodosum and hilar lymphadenopathy. The nasal mucosa has yellow submucosal nodules with a cobblestone appearance.[19] If there is more advanced nasal disease it can have a similar appearance to Wegener's granulomatosis with crusts and mucus stagnation. A notable difference compared with Wegener's granulomatosis is that patients often feel well. Intracranial involvement is the most worrying complication as mortality is high and similar to cardiac involvement. The local cervical lymph nodes may be enlarged either alone or in combination with the intranasal involvement. The nose is most commonly involved and around 5 percent of patients have intranasal granulomata (**Figure 15.4**). The surrounding skin may be involved and produce a violaceous discolouration with small nodules to large plaques known as lupus pernio. Bony involvement is rare, but lytic lesions may occur in the nasal bones. A chest radiograph shows hilar lymphadenopathy in approximately 80 percent of patients. Other ENT manifestations include lacrimal and salivary gland enlargement and facial palsy.

RELAPSING POLYCHONDRITIS

Tietze's syndrome is a relapsing polychondritis that affects the ribs and the cartilage of the external ear. The ear is very painful and the condition is distinguished from cellulitis by the distribution of the erythema, which spares the lobule. Deformity may result after resolution of the condition. For the diagnosis to be made, there have to be at least three of the following: chondritis of the pinna, the nose, the larynx or trachea, ocular involvement, a seronegative arthritis or a sensorineural hearing loss with or without vertigo.[20]

AMYLOIDOSIS

Amyloidosis complicates patients with rheumatoid arthritis, juvenile arthritis and ankylosing spondylitis. The condition affects the larynx and tongue, but it has been described throughout the head and neck.[21] Although the larynx is the most frequently affected area in the head and neck, it is usually involved in isolation.[22] Patients have hoarseness. Deposits are found in the glottis and are firm red lesions lying under the mucosa. The tongue is usually involved in the generalized condition and sampling of abdominal fat by FNAC may confirm generalized amyloidosis. Macroglossia is rare and the tongue is firm and dry and some areas are raised and red. The biopsies of suspected areas are examined under polarized light, following staining with Congo red. The patients are grouped clinically into eight main types, primary, secondary, myeloma associated, isolated laryngeal, familiar Mediterranean fever, familial, senile and dialysis-associated amyloidosis. The chemical composition groups the conditions into four. The vast majority of patients with ENT manifestations have IgG light chains in the deposit. Serum and urine analysis will exclude multiple myeloma.

DRUGS

Cyclophosphamide and azathioprine depress the marrow, which may result in oral infection and occasionally ulceration. The full blood count needs monitoring when patients are being treated with these. Aspirin may cause a self-limiting and dose-dependent tinnitus.

CONCLUSIONS

The rheumatological conditions are a heterogenous group of diseases that may present to the ENT surgeon. The manifestations depend on the nature of the condition but every area in the head and neck may be involved. The role of the otorhinolaryngologist is to collaborate with clinicians who have an interest in this area. If there is evidence of abnormal mucosa, a biopsy can help to arrive at a diagnosis although this is not a very sensitive test, a positive result has a high predictive value. A negative biopsy does not exclude a vasculitis. In a patient with suspected Wegener's granulomatosis in whom the antineutrophil cytoplasmic antibodies (ANCA) test and biopsy are negative, the ANCA test should be repeated as it can take up to four years to become positive.[14] It is sensible to transfer the care of the patient with the more active manifestations of these diseases to a subspecialist.

KEY POINTS

- Connective tissue diseases present to ENT surgeons.
- Wegener's granulomatosis has nasal manifestations in 90 percent of cases.
- Clinical management is best carried out by the appropriate physician.

Best clinical practice

✓ The role of the ENT specialist is in the diagnosis and monitoring of the condition.

Deficiencies in current knowledge and areas for future research

➤ Improved understanding of the pathophysiology is required, so that treatment can be improved.

REFERENCES

1. Hakim A, Clunie G. *Oxford handbook of rheumatology*, 1st edn. Oxford Handbooks. Oxford: Oxford University Press, 2002: 561.
2. Fukase S, Ohta N, Inamura K, Kimura Y, Aoyagi M, Koike Y. Diagnostic specificity of anti-neutrophil cytoplasmic

antibodies (ANCA) in otorhinolaryngological diseases. *Acta Oto-Laryngologica - Supplement.* 1994; **511**: 204–7.

3. Diamantopoulos II, Jones NS. The investigation of nasal septal perforations and ulcers. *Journal of Laryngology and Otology.* 2001; **115**: 541–4.

4. Coup AJ, Hopper IP. Granulomatous lesions in nasal biopsies. *Histopathology.* 1980; **4**: 293–308.

5. Bridger M, Jahn A, Van Norstrand A. Laryngeal rheumatoid arthritis. *Laryngoscope.* 1980; **90**: 296–303.

6. Kovarsky J. Otorhinolaryngologic complications of rheumatic diseases. *Seminars in Arthritis and Rheumatism.* 1984; **14**: 141–50.

7. Chalmers I, Blair G. Rheumatoid arthritis of the temporomandibular joint. *Quarterly Journal of Medicine.* 1973; **42**: 369–86.

8. Moffatt D, Ramsden R, Resenberg J. Otoadmittance measurements in patients with rheumatoid arthritis. *Journal of Laryngology and Otology.* 1977; **91**: 917–27.

9. Buckley C, Salmon M. Why do leukocytes accumulate in the inflamed rheumatoid synovium? *Rheumatology Highlights.* 2001-2: 15–21.

10. Kastanioudakis I, Ziavra N, Voulgari PV, Exarchakos G, Skevas A, Drosos AA. Ear involvement in systemic lupus erythematosus patients: a comparative study. *Journal of Laryngology and Otology.* 2002; **116**: 103–7.

11. Amft N, Curnow SJ, Scheel-Toellner D, Devadas A, Oates J, Crocker J *et al.* Ectopic expression of the B cell-attracting chemokine BCA-1 (CXCL13) on endothelial cells and within the lymphoid follicules contributes to the establishment of germinal center-like structures in Sjogren's syndrome. *Arthritis and Rheumatism.* 2001; **22**: 2633–41.

12. Hughes RG, Drake-Lee A. Nasal manifestations of granulomatous disease. *Hospital Medicine (London).* 2001; **62**: 417–21.

13. Balding C, Howie AJ, Drake-Lee A, Savage CO. Th2 dominance in nasal mucosa in patients with Wegener's granulomatosis. *Clinical and Experimental Immunology.* 2001; **125**: 332–9.

14. Jennings CR, Jones NS, Dugar J, Powell R, Lowe J. Wegeners granulomatosis – a review of diagnosis and treatment in 53 subjects. *Rhinology.* 1998; **36**: 188–91.

15. McDonald TJ, DeRemee RA. Head neck involvement in Wegener's granulomatosis (WG). *Advances in Experimental Medicine and Biology.* 1993; **336**: 309–13.

16. Proops D, Bayley D, Hawke M. Paget's disease and the temporal bone – a clinical and histopathological review of six temporal bones. *Journal of Otolaryngology.* 1985; **14**: 20–9.

17. Ramsay HA, Linthicum Jr. FH. Cochlear histopathology in Paget's disease. *American Journal of Otolaryngology.* 1993; **14**: 60–1.

18. Ginsberg LE, Elster AD, Moody DM. MRI of Paget disease with temporal bone involvement presenting with sensorineural hearing loss. *Journal of Computer Assisted Tomography.* 1992; **16**: 314–6.

19. Fergie N, Jones NS, Halvat MF. Nasal sarcoidosis. *The Journal of Laryngology and Otology.* 1999; **113**: 893–8.

20. McAdam LP, O'Hanion MA, Bluestone R, Pearson CM. Relapsing polychondritis: prospective study of 23 patients and a review of the literature. *Medicine.* 1976; **55**: 193–215.

21. Barnes L. Miscellaneous disorders of the head and neck. In: Barnes L (ed.). *Surgical pathology of the head and neck,* Vol. 3. New York: Marcel Dekker, 2001: 2191–206.

22. Zundel R, Pyle G, Vovtovitch M. Head and neck manifestations of amylodosis. *Otolaryngology – Head and Neck Surgery.* 1999; **120**: 553–8.

PART 4

MICROBIOLOGY

EDITED BY NICHOLAS S. JONES

16 Microorganisms   195
Vivienne Weston

17 Viruses and antiviral agents   204
Paul Simons and Karl G Nicholson

18 Fungi   213
Juliette Morgan and David W Warnock

19 Antimicrobial therapy   228
Vivienne Weston

20 HIV and otolaryngology   238
Thomas A Tami and Jahmal A Hairston

Microorganisms

VIVIENNE WESTON

Introduction	195	Anaerobes and microaerophilic bacteria	200
Normal microflora	195	Other bacteria	201
Gram-positive bacteria	196	Key points	202
Gram-negative bacteria	199	References	202

SEARCH STRATEGY

The information in this chapter is supported by a Medline search of review articles using the key words of each of the organisms, upper respiratory tract infections focusing on bacterial causes, respiratory and nasopharyngeal microflora.

INTRODUCTION

With the rise in incidence of bacteria resistant to antimicrobial agents, the emergence of new and resurgence of old pathogens, the ability to recognize, investigate and treat infection appropriately is important for clinicians of all specialties.

The aim of this chapter is to summarize our current understanding of bacterial microorganisms of human importance, with specific emphasis on bacteria which are found as part of the normal microflora of and those responsible for, infections of the ear, nose and throat. Viruses and fungi will be covered in Chapter 17, Viruses and antiviral agents; and Chapter 18, Fungi.

Bacteria are single-cell organisms, seen by light microscopy, which unlike viruses are able to multiply by binary fission as well as survive outside other cells. Bacteria traditionally are separated on the basis of a combination of their cell wall structure using Gram stain, shape, results of simple biochemical reactions, for example catalase reaction, and more recently, ribosomal RNA analysis.

NORMAL MICROFLORA

After birth the nasopharynx of a newborn does not remain a sterile site for more than 48 hours, with rapid acquisition of colonizing bacteria initially from the mother's genital tract, later followed by organisms which are ingested or from a carer's skin.

The normal indigenous flora consists of Gram-positive and -negative aerobic and anaerobic bacteria, including the oral streptococci, *Bacteroides* sp., *Corynebacteria* sp. and *Neisseria* sp. In addition, the nasopharynx can be colonized with potentially pathogenic bacteria such as *Streptococcus pneumoniae* (see **Table 16.1**). Carriage rates of these potential respiratory pathogens have been found to be higher in children during episodes of otitis media compared with healthy children.[1] [**] Both *Staphylococcus aureus* and *Streptococcus pyogenes* can be found in significant numbers in the nasopharynx of healthy adults (25 and 5 percent, respectively). Why these potential pathogenic bacteria can be carried without ill effect in the vast majority of people is not entirely clear. There seems to be a fine balance between underlying host risk factors which affect susceptibility to disease, the natural mucosal barrier to infection, the pathogenicity of the organism, and the presence of infection with other organisms, such as influenza A and respiratory syncitial virus.[2] [**] Also, some of the oral streptococci have been shown to inhibit the adherence of pathogenic bacteria, a phenomenon known as bacterial interference, and it is well recognized that the use of broad-spectrum antimicrobial chemotherapy can result in the reduction of these commensal

Table 16.1 Bacterial microflora of the nasopharynx.

Bacteria carried in the majority of people	'Respiratory bacterial pathogens' that may be carried asymptomatically	Organisms associated with transient carriage (e.g. sick patients, antibiotic therapy)
Oral streptococci	*S. pyogenes*	Enterobacteriaceae, e.g. *Klebsiella* sp., *E. coli*
Neisseria sp.	*M. catarrhalis*	*P. aeruginosa*
Haemophilus sp.	*S. pneumoniae*	
Candida albicans	*H. influenzae*	
Corynebacteria sp. (diphtheroids)	*N. meningitidis*	
Anaerobes		

organisms. Studies have shown that in otitis-prone children the numbers of oral streptococci are reduced and the numbers of *S. pneumoniae* and nontypable *Haemophilus influenzae* are increased.[3] [**] A recent approach which warrants further investigation is to try and restore the bacterial flora back to normal using bacteriotherapy, for example the administration of nasal oral streptococci to prevent or reduce recurrent bouts of otitis media.[4, 5] [****/*]

The nasopharyngeal flora can change with antibiotic therapy, underlying severe disease in the patient and hospitalization, with the replacement of the normal flora with aerobic Gram-negative bacilli (enterobacteriaceae) and the yeast *Candida albicans*.

GRAM–POSITIVE BACTERIA

Staphylococci

Staphylococci are Gram-positive, catalase-positive cocci that divide in two planes producing characteristic grape-like clusters on Gram stain. They grow well on most media at 18–40°C and will grow in the presence of sodium chloride and therefore are found on the skin and mucous membranes of warm-blooded animals. The genus contains 24 different species, only a few of which produce human disease. The coagulase test, which tests for the ability to coagulate plasma, separates the genus into two groups. *Staphylococcus aureus* is coagulase positive and is the main pathogenic species of the genus. There are 23 different coagulase-negative staphylococci. Other related genera are the micrococci and stomatococci, which rarely produce disease.

Staphylococcus aureus

Staphylococcus aureus is a coagulase-positive staphylococcus that has characteristically golden colonies when cultured on blood agar. At any one time 10–40 percent of the population carry *S. aureus* in their anterior nares and other skin sites, such as the perineum, with higher carriage rates in hospital inpatients.

Staphylococcus aureus has a number of virulence factors which enable it to invade human tissue, avoid the immune system and produce disease. They include capsular polysaccharide, collagen receptors and fibronectin-binding protein (promotes adhesion to host-cell surfaces), protein A (inhibits phagocytosis), coagulase, haemolytic toxins, staphylokinase (causes cellular damage) and a range of toxins.[6, 7] [**]

Staphylococcus aureus is the most common cause for wound and skin sepsis, is responsible for invasive infections by haematogenous spread or direct invasion, producing focal infections, for example osteomyelitis, lung abscesses, and is the commonest organism recovered from blood cultures of patients presenting with bacteraemia/septicaemia in England and Wales. The isolation of epidemic methicillin-resistant *S. aureus* strains which are resistant to the β-lactam antibiotics and varying classes of other antibiotics has been increasing in clinical isolates in the UK over the last decade.

Staphylococcus aureus can also produce nonsuppurative disease either by the production of toxins outside the body which are then ingested, for example staphylococcal food poisoning due to enterotoxin production, or the production of the toxin at a site of colonization or minor infection, for example toxic shock syndrome due to staphylococcal toxic shock syndrome toxin which acts as a superantigen.

COAGULASE–NEGATIVE STAPHYLOCOCCI

The coagulase-negative staphylococci make up a large part of the normal skin and mucous membrane microflora, and there are 23 species of which *Staphylococcus epidermidis* is the commonest human isolate.

Most of the coagulase-negative staphylococci do not produce as many of the virulence factors as *S. aureus* and therefore are relatively nonpathogenic. They have been shown to be able to survive on inanimate objects, such as implants, by the production of a extracellular polysaccharide adhesin or biofilm in which they are protected from the immune system and multiply slowly.[8] [**]

The coagulase-negative staphylococci were therefore generally thought to be nonpathogenic. Over the last two decades the importance of these organisms has been recognized as the number of patients with prosthetic orthopaedic implants, intravascular lines and prosthetic valves has increased. They are a major cause for orthopaedic prosthesis failure, which usually results in implant removal and revision.

Streptococci (including enterococci)

Streptococci are Gram-positive catalase-negative cocci, which divide in one plane producing chains in broth culture. Streptococci are separated using a combination of haemolysis when cultured on blood agar and cell wall polysaccharide antigen detection using the Lancefield grouping antisera, biochemical tests and growth characteristics. Analysis of the ribosomal RNA has lead to the separation of the faecal streptococci into the genus enterococci, producing the following groups:

- pyogenic streptococci (β-haemolytic streptococci);
- oral streptococci (viridans streptococci);
- anginosus-milleri group of streptococci;
- *Streptococcus pneumoniae*;
- enterococci (faecal or group D streptococci).

Apart from enterococci they are generally sensitive to all the β-lactam antimicrobial agents and the macrolide antibiotics.

Other closely related genera, which rarely produce human infections, are *Leuconostoc* sp., *Lactococcus* sp., *Pediococcus* sp., *Aerococcus* sp. and *Gemella* sp.

PYOGENIC STREPTOCOCCI (β-HAEMOLYTIC STREPTOCOCCI)

Streptococci which produce complete haemolysis of blood when isolated on blood agar (**Figure 16.1**) are separated using the Lancefield group antisera. The main human isolates group with A, B, C, D (enterococci see below) and G antisera.

Group A (*Streptococcus pyogenes*), C and G streptococci

Streptococcus pyogenes (group A streptococcus) is the most important of the β-haemolytic streptococci, producing the suppurative diseases of tonsillitis, skin sepsis, for example cellulitis and, rarely, severe necrotizing fasciitis, invasive disease, for example septicaemia, septic arthritis and streptococcal toxic shock syndrome.[9, 10] [**/*] Groups C and G streptococci can occasionally produce similar disease.[11, 12] [**]

They all produce two haemolysins, streptolysin O and S, streptokinase and hyaluronidase; in addition, *S. pyogenes* can produce erythrogenic toxins, proteinase and nucleases.

Groups A, C and G streptococci can be found colonizing the nasopharynx in apparently healthy

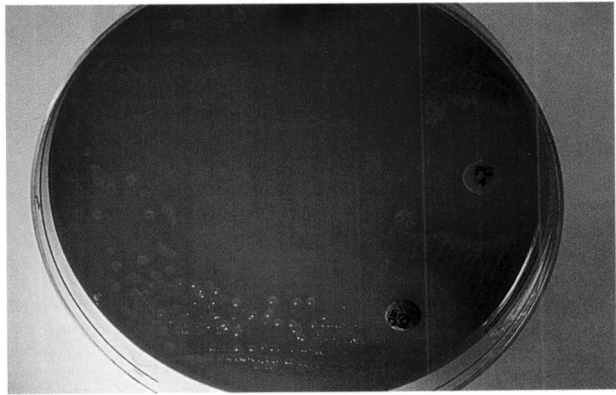

Figure 16.1   Group A streptococcus (*S. pyogenes*) on blood agar demonstrating β-haemolysis and sensitivity to penicillin (PG 4).

subjects, in up to 11 and 1.4 percent for groups A and C, respectively.[11, 13] [**]

Nonsuppurative diseases also occur with group A streptococcal infection, such as glomerulonephritis, and rheumatic fever. Group A streptococci can be further separated by antisera raised to the M protein epitopes, M1, M18 and M3 serotypes are associated with more invasive disease and M3 and M18 with cases of rheumatic fever.[14] [**] Several studies have shown that the epidemiology of group A serotypes is dynamic, with the replacement of one serotype with another in populations over time.[15] [**] At the present time, rheumatic fever is rarely seen in the UK, but in the USA there have been outbreaks associated with the carriage of serotypes M3 and 18.[16] [**]

Streptococcus agalactiae (group B streptococcus)

Group B streptococci rarely produce disease as they are not found in the nasopharynx but are the commonest cause of neonatal sepsis, and produce invasive disease in diabetics, alcoholic and immunocompromised patients.

STREPTOCOCCUS PNEUMONIAE (PNEUMOCOCCUS)

Pneumococci produce incomplete or alpha haemolysis on blood agar with draughtsman-like colonies, which are bile soluble and sensitive to the chemical agent optochin (**Figure 16.2**). In the diagnostic laboratory this characteristic is used to separate them from the oral streptococci which can be found in clinical samples. They are characteristically seen as capsulated diplococci in Gram stains of infected samples (**Figure 16.3**). The capsular polysaccharide is the main virulence factor and 90 different capsular polysaccharide serotypes have been described. They can be found as part of the normal nasopharyngeal flora particularly in the first two years of life, and are the commonest bacterial cause in all age groups for otitis media, sinusitis and pneumonia. Pneumococcal meningitis is more common in the very

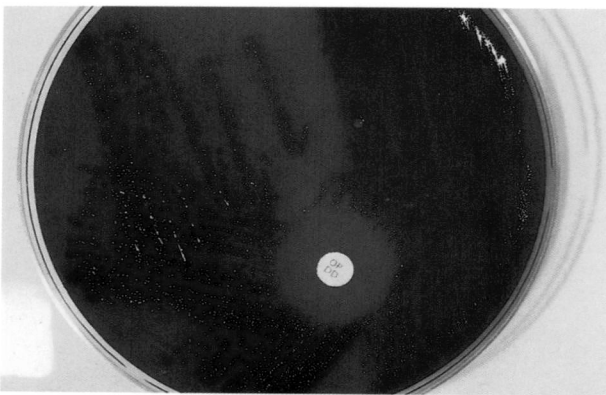

Figure 16.2   *Streptococcus pneumoniae* on blood agar demonstrating α-haemolysis.

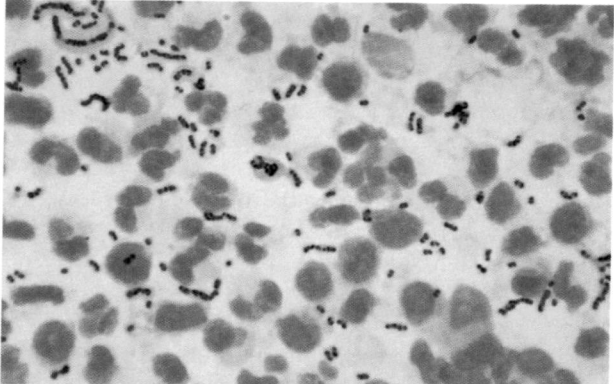

Figure 16.3   *Streptococcus pneumoniae* in Gram stain of sputum demonstrating characteristic Gram-positive diplococci.

young and elderly, where pneumococci gain entry to the meninges via haematogenous spread from respiratory infection. Pneumococci have been traditionally very sensitive to penicillins, but a rising incidence of penicillin resistance has been seen in the last decade, particularly in isolates from Eastern Europe, Spain and some parts of the USA, resulting in failures of penicillin therapy for meningitis. In view of the severity of disease produced by pneumococci and the emergence of antibiotic resistance, prevention of disease by vaccination has been widely studied. Until recently, polysaccharide vaccines which contained 23 of the commonest invasive serotypes were available but protection was short-lived with no protection for young children. Conjugate pneumococcal vaccines are now available (7, 9 and 11 valent) and have been introduced as part of the childhood vaccine schedule in the USA, and more recently in the UK, as they have been shown to reduce invasive disease, lobar pneumonia and 6–7 percent of cases of acute otitis media.[17] [**/*] Further studies are required to determine the effect of these vaccines on the epidemiology of carriage strains.

ORAL STREPTOCOCCI (VIRIDANS STREPTOCOCCI)

The oral streptococci produce incomplete α-haemolysis when grown on blood agar, but are resistant to the agent optochin and are found as part of the normal oral and nasopharyngeal flora. They occasionally cause local disease, such as tooth decay and dental abscesses, but more importantly, they are the commonest cause for native valve endocarditis, against which antibiotic prophylaxis is given for high-risk dental and surgical procedures. Some species of oral streptococci have been shown to inhibit the colonization of the nasopharynx by other bacteria, and some preliminary studies suggest that the use of these bacteria as bacteriotherapy may reduce the incidence of recurrent otitis media in otitis-prone children.[4, 5] [****/*]

ANGINOSUS–MILLERI GROUP

Previously *Streptococcus intermedius*, *Streptococcus anginosus* and *Streptococcus constellatus* were separate species, but they are now all included under the genus name *S. anginosus* but are still often referred to as *Streptococcus milleri* in clinical diagnostic laboratories because of their specific disease associations. They are part of the normal nasopharyngeal flora, but can produce invasive disease and are one of the commonest causative isolates found in deep pyogenic lesions, liver, lung and brain abscesses.[18] [**]

ENTEROCOCCI

The enterococci look like streptococci on microscopy but group with group D antisera, are bile tolerant and inherently resistant to a number of antibiotics including the cephalosporins and fluoroquinolones. Outbreaks due to vancomycin-resistant enterococci are increasing in incidence in high-risk areas, such as haematology and renal units. They are part of the normal faecal flora and owing to the antibiotic resistance will often colonize open wounds and the nasopharyngeal flora when a patient is on antibiotics. They are a cause of urinary tract infections, line and implant infections and intraabdominal sepsis.

Corynebacteria species including *Corynebacterium diphtheriae*

Corynebacteria are Gram-positive pleomorphic bacilli with a Chinese lettering-like appearance on Gram stain. Generally, *Corynebacteria* sp. do not produce disease but constitute a major component of the bacterial flora of the human skin and mucous membranes. Only a few species produce human disease in addition to the notable pathogen of this genus *Corynebacterium diphtheriae*, which produces disease by production of the exotoxin diphtheria toxin that is only produced by strains which have become infected with a lysogenic bacteriophage carrying a specific 'tox gene'. Nontoxigenic strains rarely cause more than local self-limiting disease but lysogenic conversion can occur at a site of colonization, and this has been suspected to have happened in several outbreaks; treatment with a macrolide to eradicate the organism is therefore advised.[19, 20] [**] The diphtheria toxin exerts a lethal effect on all human cells by inhibition of protein synthesis with resulting pharyngeal damage and with absorption into the bloodstream, subsequent myocardial and neurological toxicity. Three biotypes of *C. diphtheriae* exist: gravis, mitis and intermedius types; the gravis and intermedius types are associated with a higher rate of mortality which is probably related to the amount of toxin production (**Figure 16.4**). Less commonly *Corynebacterium ulcerans* can also be infected by this bacteriophage and produce a diphtheria-like presentation.[21] [**]

GRAM–NEGATIVE BACTERIA

Neisseria species

There are ten different members of this genus, of which *Neisseria meningitidis* and *Neisseria gonorrhoeae* are the important pathogens of man. The other species, which include *Neisseria lactamica* and *Neisseria sicca*, are part of the normal upper respiratory tract microflora. These are Gram-negative cocci, which appear in pairs or diplococci in clinical specimens. Gonococci and meningococci have become adapted to survival in man; they therefore require CO_2, 37°C and enriched media for isolation within the laboratory. They are identified on the basis of their biochemical reactions and using monoclonal antisera.

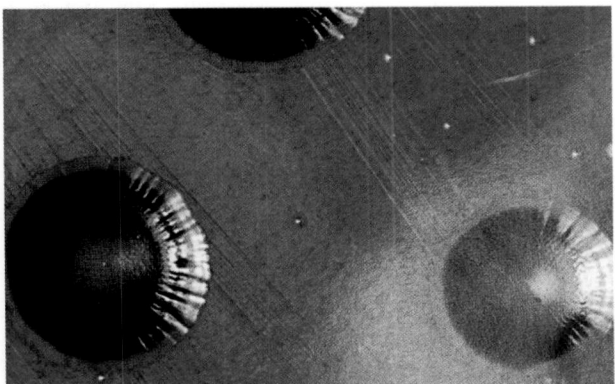

Figure 16.4 *Corynebacterium diphtheriae* var gravis on tellurite-containing media showing a typical 'daisy head'-like appearance.

NEISSERIA GONORRHOEAE (GONOCOCCUS)

Gonococci classically produce disease of the genital tract with cervicitis, urethritis and pelvic inflammatory disease. They are also occasionally responsible for sexually acquired pharyngitis and can be carried in the nasopharynx asymptomatically.

NEISSERIA MENINGITIDIS (MENINGOCOCCUS)

Meningococci are further separated with antisera into serogroups A, B, C, W135 and Y. Meningococci can be found as part of the commensal nasopharyngeal microflora in up to 10 percent of the population with higher carriage rates found in institutions and during outbreaks. Investigations of the carriage of meningococci in university students have identified that carriage is a dynamic process with acquisition of loss of strains over time.[22] [***] Invasive disease occurs in only a small percentage of carriers with severe disease such as meningitis, meningococcal septicaemia, and rarely, septic arthritis. Currently, in the UK, the main serogroups responsible for invasive disease are B and C. Since 1999 a conjugate serogroup C meningococcal vaccine has been introduced for young teenagers and children, with a dramatic reduction in invasive serogroup C disease.

Moraxella catarrhalis

This organism is morphologically similar to *Neisseria* and thought to be a harmless commensal of the upper respiratory tract. It is now recognized as a cause of infective exacerbations of chronic obstructive pulmonary disease, the third commonest cause of otitis media and a cause of acute sinusitis.[23] [**] They are inherently resistant to penicillins including ampicillin by the production of β-lactamase.

Haemophilus species

Haemophili are Gram-negative pleomorphic coccobacilli and form a major part of the normal respiratory microflora. They have varying requirements for specific growth factors (X) haemin and (V) nicotinamide adenine dinucleotide and will not grow on laboratory media without these nutrients. *Haemophilus influenzae* is the important pathogen of this genus; the other species rarely cause disease and are commonly found as part of the normal nasopharyngeal flora, for example *Haemophilus parainfluenzae*.

HAEMOPHILUS INFLUENZAE

Haemophilus influenzae is identified by its poor growth on blood agar owing to its need for X and V factors, and contributes about 10 percent of the nasopharyngeal microflora, the majority of which are noncapsulated strains that are one of the commonest causes of otitis media and sinusitis.[23, 24, 25] [**/*] Both capsulated and noncapsulated strains exist, capsulated being associated with pathogenicity. Capsulated strains can be separated further using antisera against capsular types a–f; the presence of capsular type b is associated with severe invasive disease, most notably meningitis, septic arthritis and epiglottitis. The introduction of the conjugated *H. influenzae* type b (Hib) capsular polysaccharide vaccine in the autumn of 1992 in the UK has been associated with a dramatic reduction in the incidence of Hib invasive disease, both in vaccinated children and nonvaccinated individuals, with the almost disappearance of epiglottitis in children. A slight rise in the incidence of invasive disease has been noted since 1999; clinical recognition and microbiological investigation of this disease is therefore still important.[26] [**]

Bordetella pertussis

Bordetella pertussis is the causative organism of pertussis (whooping cough), a small Gram-negative coccobacillus which is fastidious in its growth requirements, requiring up to five days incubation on charcoal-containing media. Virulence factors that contribute to disease include filamentous haemagglutinin, a cell-surface associated adherence protein that mediates bacterial host–cell interaction and pertussis toxin, which mediates the paroxysmal cough and induces lymphocytes producing the characteristic lymphocytosis. Disease is most commonly seen in infants too young to have been vaccinated and in families who have declined immunization. The reservoir of infection is adult carriers and subclinical cases, as immunity from the vaccine wanes after childhood.

Enterobacteriaceae (aerobic Gram–negative bacilli)

There are over 100 different species in this family, which are normally found as part of the bowel microflora and are able to grow under aerobic and anaerobic conditions and in the presence of bile salts. They are not normally found in the nasopharynx of fit individuals in the community, but become part of the nasopharyngeal flora in sick, hospitalized patients, such as ventilated patients on intensive care units, from where they can produce lower respiratory tract infection. They are separated in the clinical laboratory on the basis of simple biochemical reactions such as fermentation of sugars. Only a few of the genera and species commonly produce disease, for example *Escherichia coli*, *Klebsiella* sp. They are the isolates commonly found from cases of urinary and abdominal sepsis, but rarely produce infection in the upper respiratory tract in the UK. *Klebsiella rhinoscleromatis* is a Gram-negative organism that can produce chronic granulomatosis infection of the upper respiratory tract, rarely found in the UK but is endemic in some parts of South America, Asia and Eastern Europe.

Pseudomonas species

These are environmental unreactive thin Gram-negative bacilli, which are inherently resistant to most antimicrobials and disinfectants, and survive well in moist warm environments. They cause opportunistic infection, when the host normal barrier to infection is compromised by disease, for example skin damage by burns.

Pseudomonas aeruginosa is the commonest pseudomonad to produce opportunistic infections. It is recognized in culture and sometimes in clinical samples by its ability to produce pigments or pyocyanins. It is commonly found colonizing breaks in the skin, such as leg ulcers and surgical wounds, particularly when the patient has been on antibiotics. In chronic otitis externa *P. aeruginosa* is often found to colonize the damaged ear canal. Invasive disease and infection is rare but is occasionally seen in immunosuppressed and poorly controlled diabetic patients.[27, 28]

ANAEROBES AND MICROAEROPHILIC BACTERIA

Anaerobes

There are a number of both Gram-positive and -negative organisms which only survive in strict anaerobic conditions, i.e. in the complete absence of oxygen. They make up a large part of the normal oral and large bowel microflora, and only a few of the anaerobic genera found in man commonly produce infection. The restricted activity of metronidazole against anaerobes is used in the diagnostic laboratory to help detect the presence in polymicrobial mixtures of the relatively slower growing anaerobes. Anaerobes are more likely to be isolated from clinical samples if a large volume of the pus rather than a swab is sent quickly to the laboratory and strict anaerobic conditions with prolonged incubation are maintained in the laboratory.

Bacteroides fragilis is a Gram-negative bacillus found in small numbers in the oral and large bowel microflora but is the commonest anaerobe found in infections, which are usually polymicrobial with a synergistic mixture of aerobic and anaerobic bacteria. The characteristically fusiform Gram-negative bacillus *Fusobacterium necrophorum*, which is part of the normal oral flora, occasionally produces the rapidly progressive invasive disease 'necrobacillosis' without the need for the presence of other bacteria.[29] [**]

Microaerophilic bacteria, for example *Actinomycetes*

Unlike anaerobic bacteria, some organisms are able to tolerate microaerophilic conditions with very low concentrations of oxygen, for example *Actinomyces* sp. *Actinomyces* are usually found as part of the normal oral and large bowel microflora. If there is trauma or injury they can penetrate deep tissues and produce disease, which is often polymicrobial in nature and known as actinomycosis. Characteristically clumps of Gram-positive bacilli can be seen on histology or Gram staining but also sometimes in the sample of pus, producing sulphur-like granules. *Actinomyces israelii*, *Actinomyces meyeri* and *Actinomyces odontolyticus* are the species which are usually isolated from clinical samples. They are difficult to isolate as they are slow growing, often mixed with other organisms and require microaerophilic conditions; they are generally sensitive to penicillin.

OTHER BACTERIA

Mycobacteria

Mycobacteria are acid- and alcohol-fast bacilli that usually grow slowly in aerobic conditions and are not isolated on routine agar media. There are 25 *Mycobacterium* sp., which are usually split into *Mycobacterium tuberculosis* and the 'atypical' mycobacteria.

MYCOBACTERIUM TUBERCULOSIS (INCLUDES MYCOBACTERIUM BOVIS)

It characteristically grows slowly on agar containing fatty acids, such as the egg-containing Löwenstein-Jensen media, taking four to six weeks for visible colonies to appear, so it cannot be isolated by conventional culture (**Figure 16.5**). It is looked for in clinical samples using the Ziehl-Nielsen stain or a modification of this using auramine, exploiting the acid- and alcohol-fast characteristics of the mycobacterial cell wall. In the laboratory, samples and cultures for tuberculosis have to be handled in a category 3 laboratory using a safety cabinet to minimize the risk of laboratory-acquired infections. On being sent to the clinical laboratory, specimens that may contain *M. tuberculosis* must therefore be labelled as such, so that they can be handled safely, but also so that specific stains and cultures are performed which will not be routinely carried out. The use of liquid culture media with automated detection of growth and DNA probes to identify any acid-fast bacilli isolated can decrease the isolation time of these organisms.

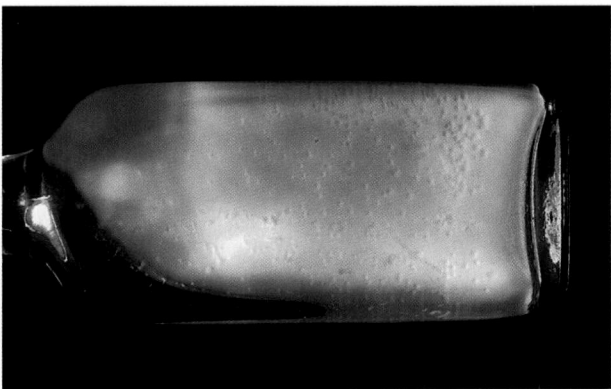

Figure 16.5 *Mycobacterium tuberculosis* on Löwenstein-Jensen media demonstrating the characteristic buff-coloured breadcrumb-like appearance.

'ATYPICAL' MYCOBACTERIA

This includes *Mycobacterium avium intracellulare*, *Mycobacterium kansasii*, *Mycobacterium scrofulaceum* and *Mycobacterium malmoense* which are responsible for cervical adenitis in children under 12 years of age.[30, 31] [**] They vary in their colonial appearance and time to positive culture and sensitivity to antimicrobials from *M. tuberculosis*. Disseminated *M. avium intracellulare* infection can be a late opportunistic infection in HIV patients.

Mycoplasmas

Mycoplasmas do not have a cell wall and are therefore difficult to isolate on routine culture media, thus diagnosis is therefore based on serological tests. *Mycoplasma orale* and *Mycoplasma salivarum* are part of the normal nasopharyngeal flora but do not produce disease. *Mycoplasma pneumoniae* is the important pathogen of this group, as it is a common cause of pneumonia in children and young adults with epidemics every four years, but it is probably a rare cause of otitis media. Owing to the lack of a cell wall, antibiotics which target cell wall synthesis are inactive against mycoplasmas; the macrolides, tetracyclines and fluoroquinolones are effective.

Chlamydiae

These are tiny Gram-negative intracellular bacteria, which form inclusion bodies in the cytoplasm of infected cells. They lack some of the enzymes required for independent existence and must replicate intracellularly. There are three main species which produce disease in humans:

1. *Chlamydophila psittaci*: severe lower respiratory tract infection, infections in birds;
2. *Chlamydophila trachomatis*: ocular, genital and occasionally respiratory tract infection;

3. *Chlamydophila pneumoniae*: upper and lower respiratory tract infection.

In the mid-1980s it was recognized that *C. psittaci* actually contained two differing species: *C. pneumoniae* which generally produces less severe disease only in humans and *C. psittaci* which produces more severe systemic disease and pneumonia.[32] [**/*]

Laboratory diagnosis of chlamydial infections is difficult as they require cell culture to be isolated, so it is usually based on finding rising titres of complement-fixing antibodies to whole cell antigen preparations (except genital *C. trachomatis* infections). There is cross reaction between the antibodies to the different species. Species-specific antibodies can be detected by microimmunofluorescence techniques. Detection of species-specific DNA using polymerase chain reaction has been used in studies of upper respiratory tract infections but not routinely.

Cell wall active antimicrobials are inactive and treatment is usually with macrolides, tetracyclines and the newer fluoroquinolone antibiotics.

Spirochaetes

These are irregular curved motile bacteria which have a characteristic appearance on microscopy but are not isolated on routine culture.

Borrelia species

Borrelia vincentii is the organism found in acute necrotizing gingivitis and Vincent's angina, accompanied by anaerobic fusobacteria organisms. *Borrelia burgdorferi* is the causative organism of Lyme disease.

Treponema pallidum

This is the causative organism of syphilis in the primary or secondary stages and can be seen in dark ground microscopy of lesions, but it cannot be isolated on artificial media. Diagnosis is based on a combination of serological tests. The syphilis enzyme immunoassay has replaced the traditional cardiolipin antibody tests (e.g. Venereal Disease Research Laboratory (VDRL)) as a screening test, as the VDRL was troubled by biological false positives. Specific treponemal tests, for example TPHA and TPPA are positive later in the course of an infection but remain positive for life and are positive after other treponemal infections, for example yaws. Syphilis has recently re-emerged as a public health problem in the UK with outbreaks of primary and secondary infections occurring in individuals with high-risk sexual behaviour. This disease therefore needs to be considered as a cause of painless mucosal or cutaneous lesions.

KEY POINTS

- The nasopharynx has resident commensal bacteria which can include pathogens.
- There is some evidence to suggest that the commensal bacterial flora protects against invasive disease.
- Nearly all bacteria are separated on the basis of the Gram stain, growth characteristics and biochemical reactions.
- New pathogens have recently been identified, e.g. *C. pneumoniae*, while others await identification and old diseases and pathogens are re-emerging, e.g. syphilis.

REFERENCES

1. Faden H, Stanievich J, Brodsky L, Bernstein J, Ogra PL. Changes in nasopharyngeal flora during otitis media of childhood. *Pediatric Infectious Disease Journal.* 1990; **9**: 623–6.
 * 2. Ruuskanen O, Heikkinen T. Viral–bacterial interaction in acute otitis media. *Pediatric Infectious Disease Journal.* 1994; **13**: 1047–9.
3. Bernstein LM, Faden HF, Dryia DM, Wactawski-Wende J. Micro-ecology of the naso-pharyngeal bacterial flora in otitis-prone and non-otitis-prone children. *Acta Otolaryngology.* 1993; **113**: 88–92.
4. Huovinen P. Bacteriotherapy: the time has come. *British Medical Journal.* 2001; **323**: 353–4.
 * 5. Roos K, Håkansson EG, Holm S. Effect of recolonisation with 'interfering' α streptococci on recurrences of acute and secretory otitis media in children; randomised placebo controlled trial. *British Medical Journal.* 2001; **322**: 210–2.
6. Cunningham R, Cockayne A, Humphreys H. Clinical and molecular aspects of the pathogenesis of *Staphylococcus aureus* bone and joint infections. *Journal of Medical Microbiology.* 1996; **44**: 157–64.
7. Humphreys H, Keane CT, Hone R, Pomeroy H, Russell RJ, Arbuthnott JP, Coleman DC. Enterotoxin production by *Staphylococcus aureus* isolates from cases of septicaemia and from healthy carriers. *Journal of Medical Microbiology.* 1989; **28**: 163–72.
8. O'Gara JP, Humphreys H. *Staphylococcus epidermidis* biofilms: importance and implications. *Journal of Medical Microbiology.* 2001; **50**: 582–7.
9. Stevens DL, Tanner MH, Winship J, Swarts R, Ries KM, Schlievert PM, Kaplan EL. Severe group A streptococcal infections associated with a toxic shock-like syndrome and scarlet fever toxin A. *New England Journal of Medicine.* 1989; **321**: 1–17.

* 10. Stevens DL. Invasive group A streptococcal infections: the past, present and future. *Pediatric Infectious Disease Journal.* 1994; **13**: 561–6.

11. Cimolai N, Elford RW, Bryan L, Anand C. Do the β-haemolytic non-group A streptococci cause pharyngitis? *Reviews of Infectious Diseases.* 1988; **10**: 587–601.

12. Meier FA, Centor RM, Graham L, Dalton HP. Clinical and microbiological evidence for endemic pharyngitis among adults due to group C streptococci. *Archives of Internal Medicine.* 1990; **150**: 825–9.

13. McMillan JA, Sandstrom C, Weiner LB, Forbes B, Woods M, Howard T *et al.* Viral and bacterial organisms associated with acute pharyngitis in a school-aged population. *Journal of Pediatrics.* 1986; **109**: 747–52.

14. Johnson DR, Stevens DI, Kaplan EL. Epidemiologic analysis of group A streptococcal serotypes associated with severe systemic infections, rheumatic fever, or uncomplicated pharyngitis. *Journal of Infectious Diseases.* 1992; **166**: 374–82.

15. Kaplan EL, Wotton JT, Johnson DR. Dynamic epidemiology of group A streptococcal serotypes associated with pharyngitis. *Lancet.* 2001; **358**: 1334–7.

16. Veasy LG, Wiedmeier SE, Orsmond GS, Ruttenberg HD, Boucek MM, Roth SJ *et al.* Resurgence of acute rheumatic fever in the intermountain area of the United States. *New England Journal of Medicine.* 1987; **316**: 421–7.

* 17. Choo S, Finn A. New pneumococcal vaccines for children. *Archives of Childhood Diseases.* 2001; **84**: 289–94.

18. DeLouvois J, Gortval P, Hurley R. Bacteriology of abscesses of the central nervous system: a multicentre study. *British Medical Journal.* 1977; **2**: 981–4.

19. Pappenheimer Jr AM, Murphy JR. Studies on the molecular epidemiology of diphtheria. *Lancet.* 1983; **2**: 923–6.

20. Wilson AP. Treatment of infection caused by toxigenic and non-toxigenic strains of *Corynebacterium diphtheriae.* *Journal of Antimicrobial Chemotherapy.* 1995; **35**: 712–20.

21. Lipsky BA, Goldberger AC, Tompkins LS, Plorde JJ. Infections caused by nondiphtheria corynebacteria. *Review of Infectious Diseases.* 1982; **4**: 1220–35.

22. Neal KR, Nguyen-Van-Tam JS, Jeffrey N, Slack RC, Madeley RJ, Ait-tahar K *et al.* Changing carriage rate of *Neisseria meningitidis* among university students during the first week of term: cross sectional study. *British Medical Journal.* 2000; **320**: 846–9.

23. Bluestone CD, Stephenson JS, Martin LM. Ten-year review of otitis media pathogens. *Pediatric Infectious Diseases Journal.* 1992; **11**: S7–11.

24. Klossek J, Dubreuil L, Richet H, Richet B, Beutter P. Bacteriology of chronic purulent secretions in chronic rhinosinusitis. *Journal of Laryngology and Otology.* 1998; **112**: 1162–5.

25. Musher D, Dagan R. Is the pneumococcus the one and only in acute otitis media? *Pediatric Infectious Disease Journal.* 2000; **19**: 399–400.

26. Anon. Surveillance of invasive *Haemophilus influenzae* infections in children. *Communicable Disease Report. CDR Weekly.* 2001; **11**: 3–4.

27. Rubin J, Yu VL. Malignant external otitis: insights into pathogenesis, clinical manifestations, diagnosis and therapy. *American Journal of Medicine.* 1988; **85**: 391–8.

28. Brook I, Frazier EH, Thompson DH. Aerobic and anaerobic microbiology of external otitis media. *Clinical Infectious Diseases.* 1992; **15**: 955–8.

29. Brazier JS, Hall V, Yusuf E, Duerden BI. *Fusobacterium necrophorum* infections in England and Wales 1990-2000. *Journal of Medical Microbiology.* 2002; **51**: 269–72.

30. Zaugg, Salfinger M, Opravil M, Luthy R. Extrapulmonary and disseminated infections due to *Mycobacterium malmoense*: case report and review. *Clinical Infectious Diseases.* 1993; **16**: 540–9.

31. Hazra R, Robson CD, Perez-Atayde AR, Husson RN. Lymphadenitis due to nontuberculous Mycobacteria in children: presentation and response to therapy. *Clinical Infectious Diseases.* 1999; **28**: 123–9.

32. Grayston JT. Infections caused by *Chlamydia pneumoniae* strain TWAR. *Clinical Infectious Diseases.* 1992; **15**: 757–63.

17

Viruses and antiviral agents

PAUL SIMONS AND KARL G NICHOLSON

Introduction	204	Key points	211
Respiratory tract viral infections	204	Best clinical practice	211
Herpes viruses	207	Deficiencies in current knowledge and areas for future	
Viruses and malignancy	208	research	211
Antivirals	209	References	211
Conditions with a viral aetiology	210		

SEARCH STRATEGY

Medline searches were undertaken for conditions with viral aetiology. For example, for the viral aetiology of sensorineural hearing loss, the key words used were sensorineural hearing loss and virus. Searches were also undertaken using specific viruses as key words, for example influenza and mumps, in conjunction with serology.

INTRODUCTION

Viruses frequently infect the ear, nose and throat. As well as causing local symptoms and complications they can also be involved in the pathogenesis of malignancy. This chapter covers viruses that primarily infect the respiratory tract; others, such as hepatitis B and C, are not dealt with here but are of relevance to all surgical specialties. Human immunodeficiency virus (HIV) is covered in a dedicated chapter (Chapter 20, HIV and otolaryngology) and not discussed here.

RESPIRATORY TRACT VIRAL INFECTIONS

Respiratory tract viral infections are the commonest diseases affecting humans worldwide, and account for 30 percent of all childhood deaths in the developing world.[1] Most preschool children experience six to eight viral respiratory infections per year; episodes in adults are responsible for a significant number of lost working days. The respiratory tract is one of the commonest sites for viral infection, partly due to its accessibility and large surface area.

Annual illness rates are almost 85 percent with one-third requiring medical attention. Many viruses have characteristic seasonal activity. For example, parainfluenza types 1 and 2 outbreaks happen predominantly in autumn, type 3 in spring and respiratory syncytial virus (RSV) outbreaks during winter.

Pathogenesis

Respiratory viruses infect cells by binding host-cell receptors. Most rhinoviruses, for example, bind the intercellular adhesion molecule receptor (ICAM-1). In influenza the resulting interferon response is likely to account for the majority of systemic symptoms, and mediators such as bradykinins are largely responsible for local symptoms.

Diagnosis

Viral pathogens are diagnosed by a variety of techniques. Inoculation of respiratory secretions on to tissue culture has traditionally been the mainstay of diagnosis. Enzyme

Table 17.1 Viruses causing respiratory illness.

Illness	Virus
Pharyngitis	PIV/CMV/adenovirus/influenza A and B/HSV/Coxsackie/enterovirus
Pneumonia/pneumonitis	RSV/parainfluenza type 3/rhinovirus/coronavirus
Common cold	Rhinovirus/coronavirus/parainfluenza type 4
Croup	Parainfluenza types 1, 2 and 3/RSV/influenza
Bronchioloitis	RSV/parainfluenza type 3/influenza
Flu'	Influenza A and B
Bronchitis	PIV/RSV

immunoassay and immunofluorescent-labelled antibody against viral antigens allow more rapid detection. Viral nucleic acid can be detected by polymerase chain reaction (PCR) giving greater sensitivity and not necessitating live virus to be present. Nasopharyngeal aspirates are the preferred specimen as nose and throat swabs produce a lower yield. Serology is widely used, and although some viruses are detected by specific immunoglobulin (Ig)M antibody tests, diagnosis based on convalescent IgG rise is retrospective and entails delay. Viruses causing respiratory illness are shown in **Table 17.1**.

Coronavirus

Coronavirus is the largest human RNA virus and is transmitted predominantly by aerosol spread. There are two human strains (229E and OC4) that infect epithelium of the trachea, nasal mucosa and alveolar cells of the lung. Coronavirus causes up to 10 percent of cases of 'common cold', particularly in the winter. Infection causes nasal discharge, malaise and exacerbations of airways disease; cervical lymphadenititis, cough and fever are less common.

Adenovirus

Adenovirus is a double-stranded DNA virus originally isolated from human adenoid tissue; over 45 serotypes exist. Most children are asymptomatically infected with types 1 and 2 in early childhood and types 3 and 5 predominate in later life. Transmission is by aerosol and probably faecal and oral spread.

Adenovirus causes outbreaks of upper and lower tract illness in institutions and small communities, particularly in winter. Certain types present with specific features, for example type 2 causes mild illness compared with types 3 and 7, which are associated with pneumonia in young children. Pharyngoconjunctival fever often occurs in swimming pool outbreaks involving children and young adults, and epidemics of keratoconjunctivitis are associated with inadequately sterilized instruments. Adenovirus causes a variety of respiratory tract syndromes including exudative tonsillitis with a high fever, pharyngitis and pneumonia, and type 7 may cause disseminated disease.

Animal models suggest that the virus directly infects bronchiolar epithelium with most local damage being due to the immune responses rather than the virus itself. There are case reports of success using ribavirin in treating childhood adenoviral pneumonia.[2] [**]

Rhinovirus

Rhinovirus is a small, nonenveloped RNA virus with well over a hundred serotypes. Replication is restricted to cells of the upper respiratory tract with optimal growth at lower temperatures of about 33°C. Transmission is by aerosol and contact with contaminated surfaces, such as hands and utensils. Symptoms are partly due to bradykinin release and include nasal congestion, sneezing, sore throat, headache and cough. Infection occurs throughout the year with several serotypes in circulation which results in people succumbing to repeated infection. Although symptoms are usually minor they can cause a significant amount of time off work, and important complications, such as exacerbation of airways disease. Infection with one serotype does not result in immunity to another and vaccination is not practical owing to the large number of serotypes. Antiviral agents such as enviroxime and dichloroflavan have shown no therapeutic benefit in randomized double-blind controlled trials.[3, 4] Controlled trials of vitamin C have also shown no definite benefit.[5] [****]

Influenza

Influenza is an RNA orthomyxovirus with subtypes A, B and C (**Figures 17.1**, **17.2** and **17.3**). Transmission occurs by droplet spread and the incubation period is one to three days. Outbreaks often begin suddenly, peaking within four weeks and usually last between eight and ten weeks. In the UK there are up to 25,000 deaths per year, mainly in older people and those with chronic illness. Pandemics of influenza are unpredictable and during the last century occurred at intervals of 11–39 years; the pandemic of 1918 killed 20–40 million people.

Typical symptoms include fever, chills, headache, myalgia, anorexia and malaise. Although a primary viral

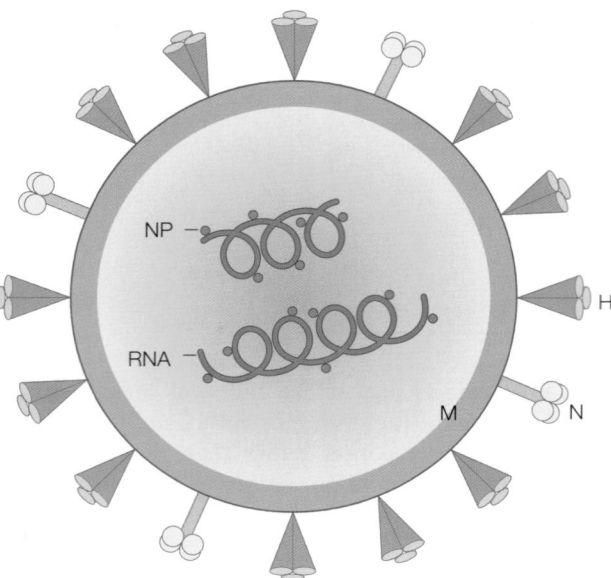

Figure 17.1 Diagram of influenza virus. H, haemagglutinin; M, matrix protein; N, neuraminidase; NP, nucleoprotein; RNA, ribonucleic acid.

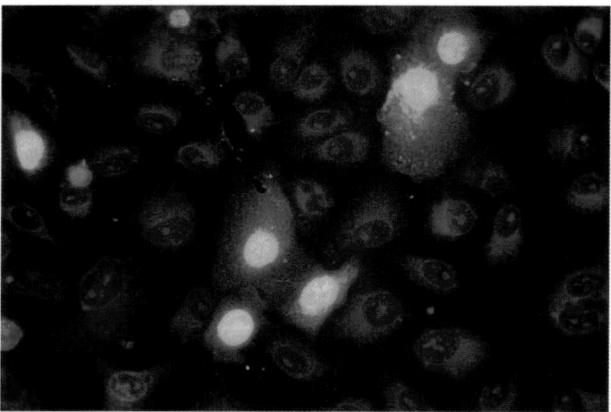

Figure 17.2 Influenza virus detected by immunofluorescence. Courtesy of Dr Zambon, HPA.

pneumonia may occur, pneumonia is often due to secondary *Staphylococcus aureus* superinfection. Other less common complications include myocarditis and pericarditis. In susceptible people infections may cause exacerbations of chronic obstructive pulmonary disease (COPD), asthma and heart failure. In children, complications include otitis media, croup, bronchiolitis and febrile convulsions. Ciliated columnar cells are primarily infected with necrosis and impairment of the mucociliary escalator which predisposes to bacterial infection. Annual immunization is recommended each autumn for those considered at greatest risk of serious complications including the elderly, diabetics, patients with chronic liver, cardiac, respiratory and renal disease, the immuno-suppressed and those in long-stay care. Comparatively

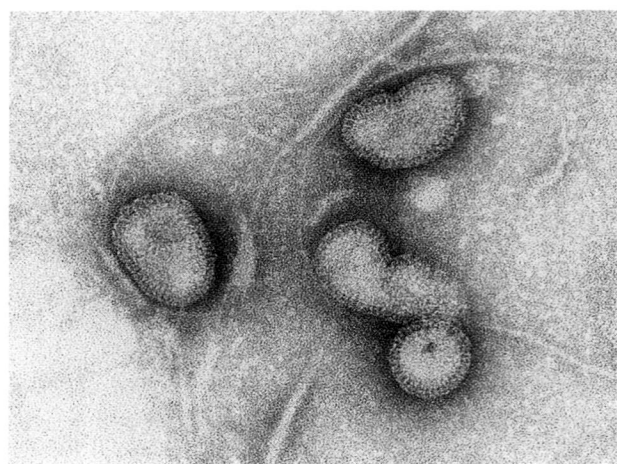

Figure 17.3 Electron micrograph of influenza virus. Courtesy of Dr Appleton, HPA.

little is known about the epidemiology and burden of influenza C which typically causes sporadic infections with common cold symptoms or is subclinical. Sporadic infections are the rule. Avian H5N1 influenza is particularly virulent and has the capacity to infect humans resulting in significant mortality. It originates from wild and domestic birds in South East Asia and has recently spread into Europe.

Mumps

Mumps is a highly infectious RNA virus with an incubation period of two to three weeks. Infection is transmitted to the respiratory tract by droplet transmission and close contact.

Fever and malaise occur at the onset and parotid enlargement develops within one to two days. Swelling usually subsides over a few days but may cause transient facial nerve palsy. One in five men develops orchitis (usually if mumps is contracted after puberty) and atrophy occurs in one-third, although sterility is uncommon. Other complications include encephalitis and aseptic meningitis with residual deafness. Serum amylase may be elevated for several weeks after parotitis and pancreatitis. Vaccination with live attenuated vaccine (trivalent mumps–measles–rubella) (MMR) has dramatically reduced cases of infection.

Measles

Measles has an incubation period of 14 days and causes infection in children between three and six years of age, particularly in winter and spring. The virus replicates in the respiratory and conjunctival epithelium, several days later it is found in reticuloendothelial organs. Typical symptoms are rhinorrhoea, cough, fever and 'Koplik's spots' on mucous membranes of the cheeks. A few days later a maculopapular rash appears, starting on the face, then affecting the trunk and limbs. There may be high fever and other features of the illness include bronchitis, pneumonitis and diarrhoea. Complications include croup, otitis media, conjunctivitis, enteritis, febrile convulsions (and rarely post-exposure encephalitis and subacute sclerosing panencephalitis). Live-attenuated vaccine is given in combination with mumps and rubella. In developing countries over one million children die every year due to insufficient vaccine coverage, younger age of infection and concurrent malnutrition.

Respiratory syncytial virus

Respiratory syncytial virus is an RNA virus with two serotypes A and B. The virus is particularly contagious and causes winter outbreaks in infants and epidemics that last for months. It is sometimes misdiagnosed as influenza in older people and is responsible for approximately one million childhood deaths annually in developing countries. Transmission is through contact with respiratory secretions rather than by aerosol. The incubation period is between two and eight days. Infants from six weeks to six months are predominantly infected and most children have been exposed to the virus by two years of age. Coryzal symptoms occur initially but the illness may progress rapidly to cause respiratory distress within 24 hours, particularly in those with underlying cardiac or pulmonary disease. Significant morbidity and mortality is seen at the extremes of age.

Respiratory syncytial virus causes necrosis of bronchiolar epithelium and lung parenchyma causing bronchiolitis and, less commonly, pneumonitis. Infection is associated with recurrent wheezing but does not necessarily cause asthma in older children. The interferon response is greater than with other paramyxovirus infections resulting in more severe systemic symptoms. Reinfection is frequent and likely to be due to antigenic variation.

As vaccine development has not been successful, preventative measures, such as limiting aerosol spread, cohorting and hand washing, are important.

It is unclear whether the use of ribavirin or steroids reduces morbidity or mortality and their use remains controversial. Ribavirin as a prophylaxis is generally reserved for high-risk infants.[6]

Parainfluenza virus

Parainfluenza virus (PIV) causes nearly a third of all respiratory tract infections. PIV 1 and 2 cause autumn croup outbreaks every one to two years. PIV 3 is endemic and usually causes infantile bronchiolitis and pneumonia. Type 4 is less common and can cause both upper and lower tract infection. Parainfluenza virus infection causes exacerbations of COPD, asthma and cystic fibrosis. Person to person spread is the main mode of transmission. Detection is by indirect immunofluorescence of antigen and PCR of nasopharyngeal aspirates. Nebulized ribavirin has been used in PIV infection in children with immunodeficiency. Vaccines are currently being evaluated clinically.

HERPES VIRUSES

Herpes simplex virus

Herpes simplex viruses (HSV) are double-stranded DNA viruses. Types 1 and 2 both cause primary infection and reactivation. After entry into the skin, the virus replicates locally forming vesicles of degenerating cells and fluid. HSV then tracks along sensory nerves and remains dormant in sensory ganglia. Reactivation is precipitated by several factors including trauma, stress, menstruation, fever, extremes in temperature and ultraviolet light.[7, 8] Humans are the only known host and transmission is by direct contact with infected mucosal secretions from active lesions or asymptomatic secretors. HSV-1 is mostly contracted from oral and HSV-2 from genitourinary secretions.

During primary oral disease, an incubation period of between two days and two weeks is followed by sore throat, pharyngitis and febrile illness. Painful vesicles may develop on the oropharynx with progression resulting in extensive gingivostomatitis and lesions extending onto the cheeks and lips, persisting for several days (**Figure 17.4**). Other complications include HSV encephalitis, meningitis, erythema multiforme and eczema herpeticum. HSV is implicated in the aetiology of Bell's palsy.

Recurrent infections

Recurrent labial herpes begins with symptoms of itching, burning, tingling and pain lasting between six hours and

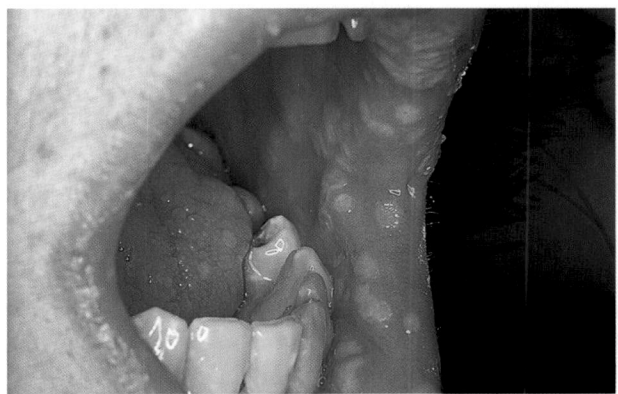

Figure 17.4 Herpetic gingivostomatitis.

two days. Lesions often occur on the lips and perioral skin and may extend into the nostrils. Multiple recurrences are usually at the same site, some become secondarily infected with *Staphylococcus aureus*. Complete healing may take up to two weeks. Of those infected with latent virus, less that 10 percent have one attack per month and 50 percent have approximately two attacks per year.[9]

Although the diagnosis is usually clinical, the virus can be isolated and detected by electron microscopy, antibody tests and tissue culture.

Treatment

Although topical preparations are used for labial herpes, systemic treatment is required for severe or recurrent episodes. Famciclovir and valacyclovir are generally used in preference to acyclovir as they have better oral absorption. Although drugs reduce the severity and duration of symptoms, they do not eradicate the virus. Antivirals should be used immediately symptoms arise and preferably before any vesicles develop. Other approaches include preventative intermittent therapy where treatment is taken before exposure to the trigger factor. Using this approach, recurrence has been reduced by 80 percent using famcyclovir[10] and by 50–78 percent with acyclovir.[11] Patients who experience more than 6–12 episodes per year should be considered for long-term prophylaxis with the minimum dose to prevent recurrence.[12] It should be noted that data are extrapolated from the outcome of genitourinary tract lesions. [****]

Treatment of recurrent infection in the immunocompetent host is often unnecessary unless symptoms include neuralgia and systemic upset. In immunocompromised patients, however, recurrences may be prolonged and severe. Long-term therapy may be required and carries the risk of drug resistance. Prevention is difficult as many carriers are asymptomatic; gloves should be used if contact is likely.

A number of HSV vaccines are under investigation. It is hoped that as well as preventing primary HSV infection, increased immunity will reduce the severity and frequency of recurrent episodes.[9]

Epstein–Barr virus

Epstein-Barr virus (EBV) is a DNA virus that infects B lymphocytes and epithelial cells of both oral and genital tracts. Primary infection is often subclinical resulting in asymptomatic lifelong carriage. Infectious mononucleosis arises in approximately half of young adults who are not infected during childhood. Symptoms include sore throat, fever and disproportionate fatigue. There may be transient periorbital oedema and a characteristic maculopapular rash is typical in those taking ampicillin. Dysphagia occurs with tonsillar and pharyngeal oedema

in 50 percent, sometimes with greyish exudates. Generalized lymphadenopathy and hepatosplenomegally usually resolve within one to two weeks. A minority of patients have protracted lethargy and lymphadenopathy. The infection appears to initiate the onset of recurrent bacterial tonsillitis in a proportion of patients. These patients often fail to resolve with time and some require tonsillectomy. Rarely, the degree of tonsillar hypertrophy is so marked that the upper airway can become obstructed. The use of parenteral steroids helps tonsillar swelling to resolve, avoiding the need for tracheostomy. Complications include airway obstruction, splenic rupture, secondary bacterial pharyngitis, haematological problems and Guillain-Barré syndrome. Malignant disease associated with EBV is discussed below.

VIRUSES AND MALIGNANCY

Several human viruses are associated with malignancy by interfering with cell proliferation and growth. Insertion of viral oncogenes or integration of viral DNA into a region which disrupts a tumour suppressor gene can confer malignant properties to the host cell. Human papilloma virus (HPV) may cause carcinoma of the skin, genitalia and larynx. 'High-risk' genotypes 16 and 18 cause malignancy owing to the ability of E6 and E7 protein to bind to cell-suppressor proteins Rb and p53.[13]

Epstein–Barr virus

Epstein–Barr virus causes a number of malignant diseases including nasopharyngeal carcinoma, Burkitt's lymphoma (BL) and B-cell lymphoma. BL is a B-cell tumour typically involving the mandibular area and occurs in children aged 4–12 years. Malaria is considered a cofactor as BL is endemic in certain areas of Africa where malaria is hyperendemic. EBV can be detected in 95 percent of tumours, the malignancy is thought to be due to translocation of immunoglobulin genes to the region of the c-myc oncogene which then becomes deregulated.[13] Cyclophosphamide is the treatment of choice, often giving good results.

Nasopharyngeal carcinoma has a high incidence in south China, Indonesia, Vietnam and those with an A2BW36 haplotype. It arises primarily in the post-nasal space from squamous epithelial cells. EBV is widely accepted as a cofactor along with racial predisposition.

Epstein–Barr virus is present in malignant cells and serum antibody titres correlate with tumour burden, although the mechanism of oncogenesis is unclear.

Hairy oral leukoplakia is considered a premalignant condition consisting of painless, white, raised lesions on the lateral aspect of the tongue. The condition occurs in HIV infection and other causes of immunosuppression. Squamous epithelial cells have been demonstrated to

Table 17.2 Associations of pathology and HPV type.

Condition	HPV type	Less common
Oral papilloma	Various	
Heck's tumour	13, 32	
Multiple papillomatosis	6, 11	67
Laryngeal papillomatosis	16, 11	6
Laryngeal carcinoma	16, 18	6, 11, 30
Inverted papilloma	6, 11	18

contain large amounts of actively replicating EBV. Acyclovir inhibits EBV replication but only to an extent to allow transient lesion regression.

Lymphomas occur more commonly in immunocompromised and HIV-infected individuals. In Hodgkin's and oral T-cell lymphoma, EBV DNA is expressed by tumour cells. Persistent EBV infection becomes uncontrolled in the immunosuppressed and there is an increase in viral replication and the numbers of virus-carrying B lymphocytes. Although this condition can remain 'silent', loss of immune control can lead to EBV-associated lymphomas.[14]

Human papilloma virus

Human papilloma virus is a double-stranded DNA papovavirus with a predilection for human epithelial cells. Of the 60 types that exist, perinatal acquisition of types 6 and 11 from an infected maternal genital tract may result in juvenile-onset recurrent respiratory papillomatosis. Respiratory papillomas are the most common laryngeal tumour and occur in young adults and the under 5 age group. They are usually single and pedunculated and rarely recur after excision. Although rare, the condition may be life-threatening if airway obstruction develops. The vocal cords are most commonly affected, resulting in hoarseness and dysphonia. Infection with types 13 and 32 appear to be confined to the mouth, types 6 and 11 may rarely progress to cause invasive cancer. Although Caesarean section is effective in reducing transmission, it is not routinely practised owing to the large number needed to avoid one case of infection. Trials of HPV vaccination are currently being evaluated.

ASSOCIATIONS OF PATHOLOGY AND HUMAN PAPILLOMA VIRUS TYPE

Associations of pathology and HPV type are presented in **Table 17.2**.

ANTIVIRALS

Vaccination has been highly effective in controlling certain viral diseases such as measles but is ineffective against others, such as those with multiple serotypes, for example rhinovirus. Of the antiviral agents that have been developed some theoretically have a broad range of activity, such as interferon, other drugs, such as aciclovir, are more virus specific.

Antiviral agents **target specific points** of the virus replication cycle. Virus **uncoating** is inhibited by amantadine with activity against influenza A. Herpes DNA **polymerase** is inhibited by acyclovir and foscarnet; inosine-5-monophosphate dehydrogenase is inhibited by ribavirin. **Virus release** is blocked by the influenza neuraminidase inhibitors, zanimivir and oseltamivir.

Interferon

Interferons (IFN) are naturally occurring substances with antiviral properties. Virus-infected cells release soluble factors in response to viral infection. Surrounding cells release ribonuclease, 2–5A synthetase and protein kinase which together degrade RNA and inhibit viral protein synthesis. Interferon as a therapeutic agent is less effective *in vivo* than hoped. Unpleasant adverse effects such as 'flu-like' symptoms and haematological complications limit its use. Alpha interferon is used with success, however, in chronic hepatitis B and C infection, often in conjunction with lamivudine and ribavirin, respectively.

Acyclovir

Acyclovir, a pro-drug, is phosphorylated by the thymidine kinase of the herpes virus. The active monophosphate inhibits herpes DNA replication. Acyclovir is used in the treatment of HSV and herpes zoster (HZV) infections and given as prolonged courses in those with recurrent HSV-1 and -2 infections. It is used as prophylaxis in bone marrow and organ transplant patients. High doses are given for varicella zoster virus (VZV) or HSV in the immunocompromised and HSV encephalitis.

Ganciclovir is a related compound with more activity against cytomegalovirus (CMV) than acyclovir. It is also more toxic and usually reserved to treat conditions such as CMV oesophagitis and retinitis in the immunocompromised.

Influenza neuraminidase inhibitors

Zanamivir is an influenza A and B neuraminidase inhibitor administered by powder inhalation. Administration is recommended within 48 hours of symptoms. Although it does not appear to reduce serious complications or mortality, it shortens illness duration by approximately one day. There is insufficient evidence as to whether it affects hospitalization rates and is intended currently for 'at risk adults' only.[15] Oseltamivir is similarly effective and is safe and well tolerated.

Other antivirals used against influenza include amantidine and rimantidine. These block membrane ion channels and inhibit induction of RNA synthesis. Although rimantidine is used in the USA and Canada, it is not available in the UK and most other European countries. Amantadine is effective against influenza A only, it is poorly tolerated and is associated with a high incidence of drug resistance.

Ribavirin

Ribavirin is a synthetic analogue of guanosine. *In vitro* it has good activity against a range of viruses including RSV, measles, influenza A and B, hepatitis A, B and C as well as HIV. However, *in vivo* it has dose-limiting toxic effects and few clinical indications. It is used in hepatitis C infection and is administered by aerosol inhalation in pediatric cases of severe RSV infection. Its efficacy is controversial with many studies failing to show significant benefit.[16] Ribavirin has activity against influenza A and B *in vitro*, but is not licensed or used clinically as no real efficacy has been demonstrated in humans.

CONDITIONS WITH A VIRAL AETIOLOGY

Bell's palsy

Bell's palsy is an acute, idiopathic, lower motor neurone unilateral facial paralysis. The incidence is approximately 20 per 100,000 per year and increases with age. There is equal sex predominance. The lifetime incidence is 1 in 60–70 with a peak between ages 10 and 40.[17] The course is usually benign but significant sequelae are seen in 16 percent of those affected.[18] Although the cause is unclear a number of aetiologies has been suspected, including viral infection, vascular ischaemia and autoimmune dysfunction. The viral reactivation theory became popular after detection of the HSV-1 genome in endoneurial fluid in patients with Bell's palsy. The viral theory is widely[19] but not universally accepted.[17]

Treatment

There have been studies comparing the efficacy of steroids, acyclovir and facial nerve decompression. In a review of studies there were no adequately powered class 1 studies, and no significant difference in outcome using steroids. One randomized control trial with limitations demonstrated decreased frequency of motor synkinesis with steroids.[20] Two randomized control trials showed an increased proportion of those with good recovery of motor function in the group who received acyclovir and prednisolone compared with using prednisolone alone. There was no difference in incidence of longer-term sequelae, and authors have encouraged results to be interpreted with caution.[21] [****]

Santos-Lasaosa *et al.* have stated that 'in spite of recent trials' the generally accepted treatment is prednisolone (1 mg/kg per day).[18] Further well-designed studies of treatment efficacy are still needed.[20]

In view of the above it should be noted that HSV and VZV viruses are ubiquitous in the population and often found in cranial nerve ganglia of unaffected as well as affected individuals. A significant difference has yet to be demonstrated before an aetiological role can be attributed to the virus.[22]

Other conditions, such as postoperative trigeminal sensory deficit, have been attributed to viral reactivation and prompted interest in prophylactic acyclovir.[23]

Inverted nasal papilloma

Human papilloma virus has been implicated in the aetiology of inverted sinonasal papilloma using PCR techniques.[24, 25] It may also cause malignant transformation and is possibly associated with disease recurrence.[26] The prevalence of HPV in samples using PCR varies from between 11 percent[27] and almost 80 percent;[25] type 11 is most commonly detected.[24, 26, 27]

Opinion is divided whether histopathological dysplasia predicts the prognosis of lesions and there is considerable interest as those with a benign or malignant clinical course have been shown to be separable on the basis of HPV type.[24] HPV types 6 and 11 are associated with benign lesions and HPV-18 with malignant lesions. Other studies (with lower HPV detection) dispute whether screening for HPV is a useful prognostic parameter.[27] [****/***]

Sensorineural hearing loss

Many viruses, even the common cold, are capable of producing sensory neural hearing loss (SNHL).[28] Specific viruses implicated in acute hearing loss include, rubella, mumps, measles, herpes zoster, CMV and influenza.

In a study of 77 cases of idiopathic sensory hearing loss, 65 percent of cases had serological evidence of viral infection as follows: influenza A in 8, influenza B 18, rubella 16, HSV 8, mumps 8 and rubella 7 percent. Almost 50 percent of samples showed evidence of multiple infectious agents.[29]

Mumps and 'silent mumps' are considered causative factors of 'idiopathic sudden sensory neural hearing loss' with serological evidence of infection of approximately 7 percent.[30]

A number of respiratory viruses have been linked to the postviral olfactory disorder. Although RSV, herpes and influenza have been implicated, parainfluenza 3 is the most likely causative virus based on serology.[31]

Live attenuated virus vaccines have also been implicated in SNHL. Cases of otherwise unexplained SNHL have been reported following MMR vaccination.[32] [****/**]

Viral acute otitis media

Viruses causing upper respiratory tract infection are important in the aetiology of acute otitis media (AOM). Rhinovirus and RSV are most commonly detected; adenovirus, coronavirus and PIV are found less frequently.[33] Recent data indicate that some viruses actively invade the middle ear. There is optimism that vaccination may be effective in preventing virally mediated AOM.[34] It has been shown that influenza vaccination is 30–36 percent effective against the development of AOM.[35] As viral and bacterial infection often coexist antimicrobials are still advised,[33] although a poor clinical response is often seen in children.[34]

KEY POINTS

- Respiratory viruses are very common and cause significant morbidity and mortality.
- A variety of viruses cause respiratory illness; RSV can cause a rapid deterioration in children.
- EBV and HPV are associated with a variety of malignant and premalignant conditions in the head and neck.
- Vaccination is highly effective in certain viral diseases. In others the characteristics of the virus have prevented effective vaccine development.
- Some antivirals, such as acyclovir, are highly effective while others have a limited role in controlling illness.
- In recurrent herpes infection, acyclovir and famciclovir are effective in reducing episodes by up to 80 percent.

Best clinical practice

✓ Influenza immunization is recommended for at risk groups including those over 65, patients with chronic liver, cardiac, respiratory and renal disease, diabetes, immunosupression and those in institutions.

✓ Although acyclovir is not always necessary in the immunocompetent patient it is recommended in the immunocompromised, and at high dose in serious infection.

✓ In recurrent herpes simplex famciclovir or valacyclovir should be taken immediately symptoms begin.

Deficiencies in current knowledge and areas for future research

➤ Further quality studies of steroids and antivirals are needed in the management of Bell's palsy.
➤ Vaccine development for respiratory viruses, including RSV and PIV.
➤ Development of further effective antivirals against influenza and other respiratory viruses.

REFERENCES

1. Hinman AR. Global progress in infectious disease control. *Vaccine*. 1998; **16**: 1116–21.
2. Shetty AK, Gans HA, So S, Millan MT, Arvin AM, Gutierrez KM. Intravenous ribavirin therapy for adenovirus pneumonia. *Pediatric Pulmonology*. 2000; **29**: 69–73.
3. Miller FD, Monto AS, DeLong DC, Exelby A, Bryan ER, Srivastava S. Controlled trial of enviroxime against natural rhinovirus infections in a community. *Antimicrobial Agents and Chemotherapy*. 1985; **27**: 102–6.
4. Phillpotts RJ, Wallace J, Tyrrell DA, Freestone DS, Sheperherd WM. Failure of oral 4', 6-dichloroflavan to protect against rhinovirus infection in man. *Archives of Virology*. 1983; **75**: 115–21.
5. Karlowski TR, Chalmers TC, Frenkel LD, Kapikian AZ, Lewis TL, Lynch JM. Ascorbic acid for the common cold. A prophylactic and therapeutic trial. *Journal of the American Medical Association*. 1975; **231**: 1038–42.
6. Greenough A. Respiratory syncytial virus infection: clinical features, management, and prophylaxis. *Current Opinion in Pulmonary Medicine*. 2000; **8**: 214–7.
7. Pereira FA. Herpes simplex: evolving concepts. *Journal of the American Academy of Dermatology*. 1996; **35**: 503–20.
8. Spruance SL, Freeman DJ, Stewart JC, McKeough MB, Wenerstrom LG, Krueger GG *et al*. The natural history of ultraviolet radiation-induced herpes simplex labialis and response to therapy with peroral and topical formulations of acyclovir. *Journal of Infectious Diseases*. 1991; **163**: 728–34.
* 9. Kurtz JB. Herpes simplex virus infections. In: Ledingham JGG, Warrell DA (eds). *Concise Oxford textbook of*

medicine. Oxford: Oxford University Press, 2000: 1497–501. *Detailed coverage of HSV.*

10. Diaz-Mitoma F, Sibbald RG, Shafran SD, Boon R, Saltzman RL. Oral famciclovir for the suppression of recurrent genital herpes: a randomised control trial. *Journal of the American Medical Association*. 1998; **280**: 887–92.

11. Spruance SL. Prophylactic chemotherapy with acyclovir for recurrent herpes simplex labialis. *Journal of Medical Virology*. 1993: 27–32.

12. Tyring SK, Douglas JM, Corey L, Spruance SL, Esman J. A randomised, placebo-controlled comparison of oral valacyclovir and acyclovir in immunocompetent patients with recurrent genital herpes. *Archives of Dermatology*. 1998; **134**: 185–91.

* 13. Collier L, Oxford J. Viruses and cancer. In: Collier L, Oxford J (eds). *Human virology*. Oxford: Oxford University Press, 2000: 49–56.

14. Epstein MA, Crawford DH. The Epstein-Barr virus. In: Ledingham JGG, Warrell DA (eds). *Concise Oxford textbook of medicine*. Oxford: Oxford University Press, 2000: 1505–8.

15. National Institute for Clinical Excellence. Guidance on the use of zanamivir (Relenza) in the treatment of influenza. Technology appraisal Guidance – No. 15 [21 November 2000].

16. DeVincenzo J. Prevention and treatment of respiratory syncytial virus infections (for advances in paediatric infectious diseases). *Advances in Paediatric Infectious Diseases*. 1997; **13**: 1–47.

17. Rowlands S, Hooper R, Hughes R, Burney P. The epidemiology and treatment of Bell's palsy in the UK. *European Journal of Neurology*. 2002; **9**: 63–7.

18. Santos-Lasaosa SR, Pascual-Millan LF, Tejero-Juste C. Morales-Asin. Peripheral facial paralysis: etiology, diagnosis and treatment. *Revista de Neurologia*. 2000; **30**: 1048–53.

19. De Diego JI, Ptim MP, Gavilan J. Aetiopathogenesis of Bell's idiopathic peripheral facial palsy. *Revista de Neurologia*. 2001; **32**: 1055–59.

20. Grogan PM, Gronseth GS. Practice parameter: Steroids, acyclovir, and surgery for Bell's palsy (an evidence-based review): report of the Quality Standards Subcommittee of the American Academy of Neurology. *Neurology*. 2001; **56**: 830–6.

* 21. Salinas R. Bell's palsy. *Clinical Evidence*. 2000; **4**: 706–9. *Good review of recent studies.*

22. Vrabec JT, Payne DA. Prevalence of herpesviruses in cranial nerve ganglia. *Acta Otolaryngologica*. 2001; **121**: 8831–35.

23. Gianoli GJ, Kartush JM. Delayed facial palsy after acoustic neuroma resection: the role of viral reactivation. *American Journal of Otology*. 1996; **17**: 625–9.

24. Kashima HK, Keissis T, Hruban RH, Wu TC, Zinreich SJ, Shah KV. Human papillomavirus in sinonasal papillomas and squamous cell carcinoma. *Laryngoscope*. 1992; **102**: 973–6.

25. Zhou Y, Hu M, Li Z. Human papillomavirus (HPV) and DNA test in inverted nasal papilloma of the nasal cavities and paranasal sinuses. *Zhonghua Er Bi Yan Hou Ke Za Zhi*. 1997; **32**: 345–7.

26. Hwang CS, Yang HS, Hong MK. Detection of human papilloma virus (HPV) in sinonasal inverted papillomas using polymerase chain reaction (PCR). *American Journal of Rhinology*. 1998; **12**: 363–6.

27. Kraft M, Simmen D, Casas R, Pfaltz M. Significance of human papillomavirus in sinonasal papilloma. *Journal of Laryngology and Otology*. 2001; **115**: 7-9–14.

28. Linthicum Jr. FH. Viral causes of sensoryneural hearing loss. *Otolaryngolic Clinics of North America*. 1978; **11**: 29–33.

29. Veltri RW, Wilson WR, Sprinkle PM, Rodman SM, Kavesh DA. The implication of viruses in idiopathic sudden hearing loss infection or reactivation of latent viruses. *Otolaryngology and Head and Neck Surgery*. 1981; **89**: 137–41.

30. Fukuda S, Chida E, Kuroda T, Kashiwamura M, Inuyama Y. An anti-mumps IgM antibody level in the serum of idiopathic sensoryneural hearing loss. *Auris Nasus Larynx*. 2001; **28**: S3–5.

31. Sugiura M, Aiba T, Mori J, Nakai Y. An epidemiological study of postviral olfactory disorder. *Acta Otolaryngologica Supplementum*. 1998; **538**: 191–6.

32. Stewart BJ, Prabhu PU. Reports of sensorineural deafness after measles, mumps, and rubella immunisation. *Archives of Disease in Childhood*. 1993; **69**: 153–4.

33. Arola M, Ruuskanen O, Ziegler T, Mertsola J, Nanto-Salonen K, Putto-Laurila A *et al*. Clinical role of respiratory virus infection in acute otitis media. *Pediatrics*. 1990; **86**: 848–55.

34. Heikkinen T, Thint M, Chonmaaitree T. Prevalence of various respiratory viruses in the middle ear during acute otitis media. *New England Journal of Medicine*. 1999; **34**: 312–4.

35. Greenberg DP. Update on the development and use of viral and bacterial vaccines for the prevention of acute otitis media. *Allergy and Asthma Proceedings*. 2001; **22**: 353–7.

18

Fungi

JULIETTE MORGAN AND DAVID W WARNOCK

Introduction	213	Best clinical practice	222
Mycotic diseases of the ear	213	Mycotic diseases of the throat	223
Key points	214	Key points	225
Mycotic diseases of the nose and nasal passages	215	Best clinical practice	225
Key points	216	Deficiencies in current knowledge and areas for future	
Mycotic diseases of the paranasal sinuses	216	research	226
Key points	222	References	226

SEARCH STRATEGY

The data in this chapter are supported by a Medline search using the following key words: ear, nose, sinus, larynx, throat, *Aspergillus, Blastomyces, Candida, Coccidioides, Conidiobolus, Cryptococcus, Histoplasma, Rhinosporidium, Zygomycetes,* fungi, aspergillosis, blastomycosis, candidiasis, coccidioidomycosis, cryptococcosis, entomophthoramycosis, histoplasmosis, mucormycosis, otomycosis, rhinosporidiosis, sinusitis and zygomycosis.

INTRODUCTION

With the exception of two conditions, otomycosis and oropharyngeal candidiasis, fungal infections are uncommon in ear, nose and throat practice. There are, however, a number of different mycotic diseases that the otorhinolaryngologist should be aware of as they can mimic other conditions and occasionally have serious consequences if they are not recognized.

MYCOTIC DISEASES OF THE EAR

Otomycosis

DEFINITION

The term otomycosis is used to describe a superficial, diffuse, fungal infection of the ear canal. Otomycosis generally occurs unilaterally among healthy individuals; however, a predisposing condition is usually present.

AETIOLOGICAL AGENTS

Otomycosis is most commonly caused by *Aspergillus* species, particularly *A. niger, A. flavus,* and *A. fumigatus,* and *Candida* species, particularly *C. albicans, C. parapsilosis* and *C. tropicalis.*[1, 2, 3, 4] Studies conducted in temperate regions showed a slight preponderance of *Candida* species while those conducted in tropical and subtropical regions found *A. niger* to be the commonest cause of infection.[1, 2, 3, 4] Other moulds that have been implicated include *Penicillium* species and *Rhizopus* species. Mixed bacterial and fungal cultures are common and account for more than 50 percent of all cultures in otomycosis.[1] [**]

EPIDEMIOLOGY

The aetiological agents of otomycosis are commonly found in indoor and outdoor air, in the soil and dust, and on decomposing plant matter. Their prevalence varies with climatic conditions, but warm humid environments support their growth and the human ear canal is ideal for their proliferation. In tropical countries, otomycosis has been reported to account for 6 percent of patients with symptoms of ear disease,[2] but the disease is less common in temperate climates. Otomycosis occurs in adults of all ages and of both sexes, but children are less commonly affected.[1, 2, 3] It is not contagious. Otomycosis often develops in individuals with pre-existing dermatological conditions of the ear, such as seborrhoeic dermatitis or psoriasis. Bacterial infection is common in such cases, and prolonged use of topical antibiotics and corticosteroids will often result in fungal superinfection. [**/*]

CLINICAL MANIFESTATIONS

The initial symptoms of fungal and bacterial otitis externa are often indistinguishable. However, while pain is the dominant symptom in bacterial infection, the most common complaint in otomycosis is aural fullness and pruritis deep inside the canal.[2] Sometimes, discharge is present but it is not mucoid that would suggest that there is a tympanic perforation. Obstruction of the meatus can lead to partial hearing loss and tinnitus. Otoscopic examination often reveals the presence of debris and an oedematous and erythematous canal. If *A. niger* is the causative agent, a mat of fungus, often covered with black sporing heads, can be seen (**Figure 18.1**). This mass lining the meatus, which it can obstruct, is often described as resembling blotting paper. In chronic infections, eczematoid changes and lichenification of the canal can become marked. [**/*]

DIAGNOSIS

Fungal infection should be suspected when a patient with otitis externa fails to respond to topical antibiotics and

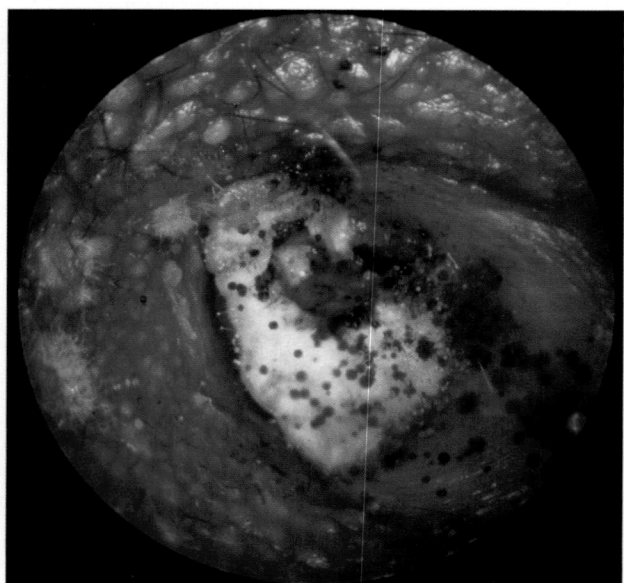

Figure 18.1 Otitis externa due to *Aspergillus niger.*

corticosteroids. Material taken for microscopic examination using a potassium hydroxide preparation will reveal branching hyphae, budding cells or both. In cases of *Aspergillus* infection, the typical sporing heads can sometimes be seen. Isolation of the aetiological agent in culture will enable the species of the fungus involved to be identified. [**/*]

MANAGEMENT OPTIONS

Treatment primarily consists of the removal of debris from the ear canal and thorough cleaning, together with the local application of an antifungal agent. Topical nystatin can be applied three times a day for two to three weeks. The local application of an imidazole cream, such as clotrimazole or econazole nitrate also gives good results. Another method is to insert gauze packs, soaked in amphotericin B or an imidazole preparation for one week and these should be replaced at frequent intervals. [Grade D] In developing countries, or when these agents are not readily available, mercurochrome solution and boric acid have been used with success. [Grade D]

OUTCOMES AND COMPLICATIONS

The majority of patients with otomycosis respond to treatment. Complications are rare, but include recurrence, or perforation of the tympanic membrane. Most perforations heal spontaneously, usually within a month.[5] In immunosuppressed individuals (with haematological malignancies or end-stage acquired immune deficiency syndrome (AIDS)), the infection may progress to a necrotizing (malignant) otitis externa. This is most commonly caused by *A. fumigatus*, but *Scedosporium apiospermum* has also been implicated.[6] [**/*]

Disease of the external ear

The external ear is sometimes the site of fungal infection. The commonest cause is dermatophytosis, with infection caused by *Trichophyton rubrum* being the most frequent. However, mycotic diseases of implantation, such as chromoblastomycosis and sporotrichosis, may also affect this site. The clinical manifestations are similar to those seen with cutaneous or subcutaneous infections caused by these organisms. [*]

KEY POINTS

- Otomycosis is more commonly seen in adults and in tropical climates.
- The symptoms of otomycosis are often indistinguishable from bacterial otitis externa.

- Prolonged use of topical antibiotics and corticosteroids often leads to otomycosis.
- Laboratory tests are often required to confirm the diagnosis of otomycosis.
- Topical antifungal treatment is usually effective.

MYCOTIC DISEASES OF THE NOSE AND NASAL PASSAGES

Nasal involvement can occur when invasive aspergillosis or mucormycosis extends outside the paranasal sinuses. However, two diseases are specifically associated with nasal invasion: entomophthoramycosis and rhinosporidiosis.

Entomophthoramycosis

DEFINITION

This is a chronic localized subcutaneous fungal infection that originates in the nasal mucosa and spreads painlessly to the adjacent subcutaneous tissue of the face. This rare infection is seen in healthy individuals, but its progressive nature can lead to severe facial disfigurement.

AETIOLOGICAL AGENT

Conidiobolus coronatus is found in the soil and on decomposing vegetation in tropical rain forests. It is also an insect pathogen.

EPIDEMIOLOGY

The disease is most common in West Africa, in particular, Nigeria, but cases have also been reported from India, and from South and Central America.[7, 8] The disease can occur at any age, but is uncommon in children. Most cases affect men living or working in tropical rain forests. In most cases the organism is introduced on the soiled hands of the patient. In some instances, the infection follows spore inhalation. [**/*]

CLINICAL MANIFESTATIONS

The clinical appearances are typical. The spread of the infection from the nose to the facial tissues is slow but relentless leading to severe facial disfigurement. The commonest symptom is nasal obstruction, due to tissue expansion. Pain and ulceration are uncommon, but nasal discharge is frequent. The lesions have a distinct margin, but the mass is not movable over the underlying tissue. The swelling is hard but not tender. The skin remains intact. [**/*]

DIAGNOSIS

Even if, in advanced cases, the diagnosis is obvious from the typical clinical appearance, laboratory investigation is essential for its confirmation. The diagnosis is best established by microscopic examination of smears or tissue from the nasal mucosa. In haematoxylin-eosin stained tissue sections, the organisms appear as broad, nonseptate, thin-walled, irregularly branching hyphae and in some cases are surrounded by Splendore-Hoeppli material. Culture is difficult. [**/*]

MANAGEMENT OPTIONS

Patients often respond to oral treatment with fluconazole (200 mg/day), itraconazole (200–400 mg/day) or ketoconazole (200–400 mg/day). [Grade D] Treatment should be continued for at least one month after the lesions have cleared. Saturated potassium iodide solution can be useful. The starting dose is 1 mL three times daily, and this is increased up to 4–6 mL three times daily as tolerated. [Grade D] Treatment must be continued for at least one month after the lesions have disappeared. Surgical resection of infected tissue is seldom successful; it may hasten the spread of infection.

OUTCOMES AND COMPLICATIONS

Relapse is common and can happen long after apparently successful treatment. [**/*]

Rhinosporidiosis

DEFINITION

This is an uncommon chronic granulomatous infection that affects the nasal mucosa, ocular conjunctiva and other mucosa.

AETIOLOGICAL AGENT

The causal agent of rhinosporidiosis is *Rhinosporidium seeberi*. In tissue, this organism forms characteristic abundant, large, thick-walled sporangium-like structures containing large numbers of endospores. It has long been unclear whether this organism is a fungus, but sequencing of the 18S small subunit ribosomal DNA sequence from *R. seeberi* has led to its recent reclassification as a member of the protoctistan Mesomycetozoa.[9] Attempts to isolate *R. seeberi* in culture have failed and thus far it has not been recovered from an environmental source.

EPIDEMIOLOGY

The disease is most common in southern India and Sri Lanka, but sporadic cases have been reported from

East Africa, Central and South America, South East Asia and other parts of the world.[10] The natural habitat of the organism is unknown, but it is believed, based on the epidemiologic data, that stagnant pools of fresh water are an important source. The disease is most prevalent in rural districts, among persons bathing in public ponds or working in stagnant water, such as rice fields. Rhinosporidiosis is most common in persons in the age range of 15–40; males are more commonly affected than females. [**/*]

CLINICAL MANIFESTATIONS

The nose is the commonest site of rhinosporidiosis, being affected in more than 70 percent of cases. The fungus causes the production of large sessile or pedunculated lesions that affect one or both nostrils. The infection is insidious in onset and the patient remains unaware of its existence until obstruction develops. Rhinoscopic examination will reveal papular or nodular, smooth-surfaced lesions that become pedunculated and acquire a papillomatous or proliferative appearance. The lesions are pink, red or purple in colour. In most cases the general health of the patient is unimpaired. Spontaneous remission is unusual and, left untreated, the polyps will continue to enlarge. [**/*]

DIAGNOSIS

The diagnosis is established by histopathologic examination of tissue sections. These contain large, round or oval sporangia up to 350 μm in diameter, with a thick wall and an operculum. The largest sporangia are filled with spores.

MANAGEMENT OPTIONS

The treatment of choice is surgical excision of lesions, with or without cauterization. No drug treatment has proved effective. [Grade D]

OUTCOMES AND COMPLICATIONS

Recurrence is common and patients should be followed up where possible. [**/*]

KEY POINTS

Entomophthoramycosis

- Entomophthoramycosis is a rare infection, but can lead to severe facial disfigurement.
- Laboratory tests are essential to confirm the diagnosis.
- Surgical resection is seldom successful and can hasten the spread of infection.
- Relapse is common after medical treatment.

Rhinosporidiosis

- Bathing or working in stagnant water is an important risk factor for rhinosporidiosis.
- Histopathological examination is important to confirm the clinical diagnosis.
- Medical treatment is ineffective.
- Patients often relapse following surgical removal of lesions.

MYCOTIC DISEASES OF THE PARANASAL SINUSES

Mycotic diseases of the paranasal sinuses range from an indolent infection in an otherwise normal person, to a lethal fulminant infection in an immunocompromised individual, reflecting the interaction between host and aetiological agent. Until the 1990s, no criteria for diagnosis or consensus on the classification of fungal sinusitis existed. Several recent investigations have addressed these problems and have led to the development of both diagnostic criteria and a new system of classification.[11, 12, 13] Based on histopathologic findings and clinical presentation, fungal sinusitis is now classified into three categories: invasive sinusitis, noninvasive sinusitis and allergic fungal sinusitis.

Invasive fungal sinusitis

DEFINITION

Invasive fungal sinus disease can be subdivided into the following three syndromes: acute fulminant invasive sinusitis, chronic invasive sinusitis and chronic granulomatous invasive sinusitis or paranasal granuloma.[11, 12, 13] The diagnosis of these disorders requires radiographic or nasal endoscopic evidence of sinusitis, together with histopathological evidence of the presence of fungal hyphae in the sinus mucosa, submucosa or bone.

Active invasive sinusitis

Acute fulminant (invasive) fungal sinusitis is a rapidly progressive disease that is most commonly seen in immunocompromised individuals or diabetics with uncontrolled ketoacidosis. Immunocompetent individuals are seldom affected. The infection can spread from the nasal mucosa and sinus into the orbit and brain. The aetiological agents have a predilection for vascular invasion, causing thrombosis, infarction and ischaemic necrosis of tissues.

Chronic invasive sinusitis

Chronic (invasive) fungal sinusitis is a slowly progressive disease that is seen in both immunocompromised and immunocompetent individuals. This condition may begin as a paranasal sinus fungus ball (see under Noninvasive fungal sinusitis) and then become invasive, perhaps as a result of the immunosuppression associated with diabetes mellitus or corticosteroid treatment. If left untreated, the infection can spread to invade adjacent structures, including the orbit and brain.

Chronic granulomatous invasive sinusitis

Granulomatous invasive fungal sinusitis (paranasal granuloma) is a slowly progressive disease that occurs in immunocompetent persons who often have had chronic sinusitis. There is profuse fungal growth with localized tissue invasion, and noncaseating granulomas with giant cells. The granulomatous response is often intense enough to cause pressure necrosis of bone and can cause proptosis. Unless removed, the fungal mass can spread into the orbit and brain.

AETIOLOGICAL AGENTS

Many different organisms have been implicated as aetiological agents of invasive fungal sinusitis. However, the commonest causes of acute fulminant sinusitis are moulds belonging to the order Mucorales, including *Rhizopus* species, particularly *R. arrhizus*, *Absidia* species and *Rhizomucor* species. Other less frequent causes of fulminant sinusitis include *Aspergillus* species, particularly *A. flavus* and *A. fumigatus*, *Fusarium* species and *S. apiospermum*. Among the more important aetiological agents of chronic invasive sinusitis are *Alternaria* species, *Aspergillus* species, *Bipolaris* species, *Curvularia* species and *Exserohilum* species. Many of these organisms are ubiquitous in the environment, being found in the air, in soil and on decomposing organic matter; others are plant pathogens. [**]

Most cases of granulomatous invasive fungal sinusitis have been caused by *A. flavus* infection. [**/*]

EPIDEMIOLOGY

Acute invasive fungal sinusitis has a worldwide distribution. Most cases have been reported in adults, but immunocompromised children are also at risk; men and women are equally affected.[14, 15, 16] The aetiological agents are ubiquitous in the environment, and the likelihood that infection will occur following inhalation of fungal spores largely depends on host factors. Prolonged neutropenia and metabolic acidosis are well recognized as important risk factors for rhinocerebral mucormycosis and fulminant aspergillus sinusitis among patients with haematological malignancies, haematopoietic stem cell transplant recipients and individuals with diabetes mellitus.[14, 15, 16] Other contributing factors include the use of corticosteroids, deferoxamine treatment and human immunodeficiency virus (HIV) infection.[14, 15, 16] [**]

Chronic invasive fungal sinusitis also has a worldwide distribution, but the largest number of cases has been reported from North America. The more indolent invasive presentations are seen in both immunocompromised and immunocompetent individuals, including patients with well-controlled diabetes mellitus and those receiving corticosteroid treatment. Affected individuals often complain of long-standing allergic rhinitis, or chronic bacterial sinusitis. [**]

Most cases of granulomatous invasive fungal sinusitis occur in immunocompetent individuals and have been reported from North Africa. However, reports of this condition have also come from India, Pakistan and the United States. [**]

CLINICAL MANIFESTATIONS

In immunocompromised persons, acute invasive fungal sinusitis presents with fever, unilateral facial swelling, unilateral headache, nasal obstruction or pain and a serosanguinous nasal discharge.[14, 15, 16] Necrotic black lesions on the hard palate or nasal turbinate are a characteristic diagnostic sign.[14, 15, 16] As the infection spreads into the orbit, periorbital or perinasal swelling occurs and progresses to disfiguring destruction of facial tissue. Ptosis, proptosis, ophthalmoplegia and loss of vision can occur (**Figure 18.2**).[14, 15, 16] [**]

Chronic invasive fungal sinusitis has been reported in nonimmunocompromised persons as well as in individuals who had received corticosteroids or had diabetes mellitus. Patients with AIDS can also present with this form of fungal sinusitis, although the classification in this population is not always clear.[17] Many patients present with a history of nasal obstruction and chronic sinusitis.

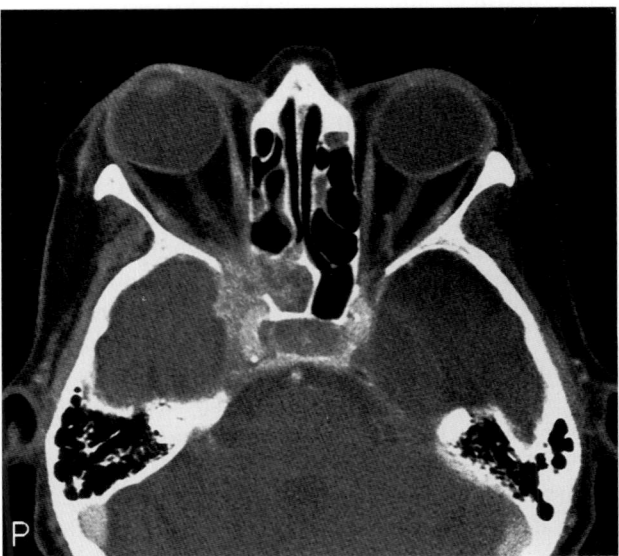

Figure 18.2 An axial CT scan of chronic invasive aspergillosis in an elderly woman treated with steroids for polymyalgia rheumatica. She presented with blindness. Note the disease invading the cavernous sinus. She remains well 18 months later after 12 months of itraconazole.

Thick nasal polyposis and thick purulent mucus are common. If the infection spreads from the ethmoid sinuses into the orbit, the orbital apex syndrome is a common clinical presentation.[11, 12, 13] This condition results from erosion of the fungal mass into the orbital apex causing impaired vision and restricted ocular movement. Proptosis can also occur. Chronic invasive sinusitis is often advanced by the time of diagnosis, with posterior erosion out of the ethmoid sinus, resulting in cavernous venous thrombosis. [**]

Granulomatous invasive fungal sinusitis (paranasal granuloma) occurs in immunocompetent persons who often present with long-standing symptoms of nasal obstruction, unilateral facial discomfort and/or enlarging mass, or with a silent proptosis.[11, 12, 13] [**]

DIAGNOSIS

Imaging studies can assist in determining the presence and the anatomic extent of sinus disease, however, plain radiographs are insensitive and do not allow distinction between bacterial and fungal infections. Computed tomography (CT) scanning is more discriminating and can be used to assess the extent of bone destruction and pattern of sinus and orbital involvement. The commonest findings in patients with acute invasive fungal sinusitis include involvement of several sinuses (in particular ethmoid and sphenoid) but with a clear unilateral predilection, no air-fluid levels, thickening of sinus linings and destruction of surrounding bone.[18, 19] Magnetic resonance imaging (MRI) is not clearly superior to CT, but it is deemed more accurate in providing information about cavernous sinus and cerebral involvement.[19] [**]

In patients with chronic invasive sinusitis, noncontrast CT scans reveal a hyperdense mass (owing to a dense accumulation of fungal hyphae) within the involved sinus with associated erosion of the sinus walls.[11, 13] The most common radiographic findings in patients with granulomatous invasive fungal sinusitis (paranasal granuloma) are opacification of ethmoid, maxillary or all sinuses (pansinusitis), together with erosion of bone. [**/*]

Local biopsy with histopathological examination and culture of tissue or sinus contents confirms the clinical and radiological diagnosis of invasive fungal sinusitis. In cases of acute invasive infection, where delay may have a serious impact on the outcome, the diagnosis is often best made by direct microscopic examination of a potassium hydroxide preparation of material taken from necrotic lesions. The Mucorales can be distinguished from other moulds, such as *Aspergillus* species, by their characteristic broad nonseptate hyphae with right-angled branching. It is not possible, however, to differentiate *Aspergillus* species from *Fusarium* species, *S. apiospermum* or other nonpigmented moulds by their microscopic appearance in tissue. All produce branching septate nonpigmented hyphae. Isolation of the aetiological agent in culture is essential for the species of fungus involved to be identified. [**/*]

MANAGEMENT OPTIONS

If treatment of acute invasive fungal sinusitis is to be successful, a prompt diagnosis is essential. Underlying host disorders must be controlled: correction of acidosis is essential and immunosuppressive drugs should be reduced in dose if possible. Infected and necrotic tissue must be removed immediately and an effective antifungal agent must be administered. [Grade B]

In acute fulminant fungal sinusitis with invasion of blood vessels, amphotericin B has been considered the drug of choice (at a dose of 1–1.5 mg/kg per day). However, there is a growing consensus, based on animal models and retrospective clinical data, that the newer lipid-based formulations of the drug, in particular high doses of liposomal amphotericin B (10–15 mg/kg per day), should be considered the first line of treatment.[20] This should be continued until the patient recovers. [Grade B]

The optimum duration and total dose of amphotericin B that should be given in acute invasive sinusitis has not been determined. Treatment must be individualized according to the patient's clinical response and the rate of clearing of the infection. Treatment should be continued at least until progression of disease ceases and the underlying disorder is well controlled.

Itraconazole should not be regarded as a first-line agent against mucormycosis,[20] but its use may be considered for infections with susceptible organisms, such as *S. apiospermum*, that are resistant to amphotericin B. However, the optimum dosage and duration of treatment have not been defined. [Grade D] The role of voriconazole in acute invasive sinusitis is unclear. This drug is effective against *Aspergillus* species, but inactive against the Mucorales.[20] Posaconazole, a new broad-spectrum triazole, is active against *Aspergillus* species and the Mucorales. There are anecdotal reports of successful salvage treatment of acute rhinocerebral mucormycosis with this drug.[21, 22] [Grade D]

Other treatment options of unclear effectiveness are administration of hyperbaric oxygen, iron chelators and cytokines.[20] The usefulness of these approaches cannot be evaluated on the basis of published uncontrolled reports.

In chronic invasive sinusitis, a histological diagnosis is needed to exclude blood vessel invasion found in acute fulminant fungal sinusitis. Invasion of adjacent structures is a common complication of chronic invasive fungal sinusitis. Extensive surgical debridement with removal of all necrotic material, combined with antifungal treatment, has been recommended. [Grade B] The optimum duration of itraconazole (100 mg bd) has not been defined. The role of the newer triazole antifungal agents, such as itraconazole, voriconazole and posaconazole, is unclear but promising. [Grade D] There is evidence that long-term treatment with itraconazole can reduce the rate of recurrence following surgical resection or cure the condition on its own. [Grade D]

In patients with granulomatous invasive sinusitis, surgical removal of the paranasal granuloma has been recommended. Complete removal is often difficult and the condition can recur. However, there is some evidence that long-term oral treatment with itraconazole reduces the rate of recurrence [Grade C], or can cure the disease on its own.[23] [Grade D]

OUTCOMES AND COMPLICATIONS

More than 70 percent of diabetic patients with acute invasive fungal sinusitis will recover following prompt correction of acidosis, amphotericin B and aggressive surgical treatment.[14, 15] In contrast, the outcome in individuals with other underlying disorders is less favourable. Factors associated with a lower survival rate include delayed diagnosis and treatment, hemiparesis or hemiplegia, bilateral sinus involvement, leukaemia, renal disease and treatment with desferroxamine mesilate.[14, 15] Survival is unusual in neutropenic patients with leukaemia in relapse.[15] [**]

Although the combination of aggressive surgical debridement and amphotericin B treatment is recommended for the management of acute invasive sinusitis, it is not without complications. Surgical debridement is often mutilating and the conventional formulation of amphotericin B is nephrotoxic. Debridement carries the risk of bleeding in thrombocytopenic patients, as well as the risk of inadvertent damage to the orbit and brain. Patients who receive amphotericin B must be monitored for signs of renal damage. [**]

In patients with chronic invasive sinusitis, prolonged duration of symptoms prior to diagnosis and intracranial extension of the infection have been identified as factors associated with a lower survival rate.[24] According to a recent review of published cases of aspergillus sinusitis in immunocompetent individuals, the mortality rate for patients with intracranial extension was 44 percent, compared with 15 percent for those without intracranial infection. Furthermore, only 6 percent of patients with intracranial extension were cured by antifungal and surgical treatment, compared with 46 percent of those without intracranial infection.[24] [**]

No long-term follow up of patients with granulomatous invasive sinusitis has been published.

Noninvasive fungal sinusitis

DEFINITION

A paranasal sinus fungus ball (or sinus mycetoma) is a chronic noninvasive fungal infection that is seen in immunocompetent persons. However, if immunocompromise should occur, then the condition may become invasive and life-threatening.[25, 26] Fungus balls consist of a dense mass of fungal hyphae. They are sometimes found in the sinus cavities of patients undergoing investigation for chronic sinusitis, nasal obstruction, facial pain or other conditions.

AETIOLOGICAL AGENTS

Aspergillus fumigatus is the most frequently isolated organism.[25] Less commonly, other *Aspergillus* species (including *A. flavus*), *S. apiospermum* and *Alternaria* species have been incriminated.[26] These moulds are ubiquitous in the environment. In many cases, however, the content of sinus fungus balls has failed to grow on culture. [**]

EPIDEMIOLOGY

Older individuals appear to be more susceptible. The average age reported in one review of 29 cases was 64 years.[25] No cases have been reported in children, but women account for around 64 percent of published cases.[26] Associated medical conditions are uncommon. The incidence of allergic rhinitis is no higher than in the general population. [**/*]

CLINICAL MANIFESTATIONS

The symptoms are often similar to those of chronic bacterial rhinosinusitis, but sometimes patients are asymptomatic. Affected persons often present with long-standing symptoms of nasal obstruction, purulent nasal discharge, cacosmia (fetid smell) or facial pain.[25, 26] The symptoms are often unilateral. Unusual symptoms include fever, cough, proptosis, epistaxis, and diplopia. Nasal polyps are found in 10 percent of patients.[26] [**]

The maxillary sinus is most commonly involved, with partial or complete opacification, bone thickening and sclerosis; occasionally bone destruction can occur. The sphenoid sinus is the second most common site of involvement (**Figure 18.3**). Frontal sinus involvement is uncommon. Air–fluid levels, which are characteristic of acute bacterial sinusitis, are uncommon in fungus balls of the paranasal sinuses. [**]

DIAGNOSIS

Various features are required to confirm the diagnosis of fungus ball of the sinuses.[25] First, CT scans should reveal partial or total opacification of the involved sinus, often associated with flocculent calcifications. Mucopurulent sinus material should be found at the time of surgical intervention. Histopathological investigation should reveal that this material is composed of a dense matted

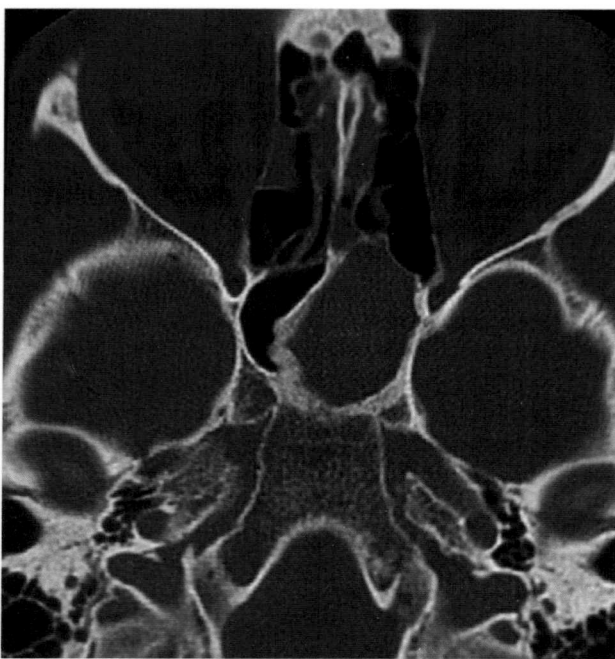

Figure 18.3 An axial CT scan showing a mycetoma caused by aspergillosis of the sphenoid sinus. Note the reactive hyperostosis.

conglomeration of fungal hyphae, separate from but adjacent to the mucosa of the sinus. Histopathological investigation should also demonstrate no evidence of allergic mucin in the sinus or granulomatous reaction in the mucosa. There should be no fungal invasion of the mucosa, associated blood vessels or bone. [**]

MANAGEMENT OPTIONS

Surgical removal of the fungus ball is the treatment of choice.[25, 26] No local or systemic antifungal medication is needed. [Grade B]

OUTCOME AND COMPLICATIONS

Recurrence is rare, but has been described as late as two years following the endoscopic removal of a paranasal fungus ball. Patients with sphenoid sinus balls are at risk of an intracerebral bleed or infarct as a complication of their surgical treatment. Patients who become immuno-suppressed are at risk of developing an invasive fungal sinusitis. [**]

Allergic fungal sinusitis

DEFINITION

Allergic fungal sinusitis is a noninvasive disorder, seen in immunocompetent individuals, which is increasingly

being recognized as a cause of chronic rhinosinusitis. The reported incidence of this disorder ranges from 5 to 10 percent of patients with chronic rhinosinusitis in some studies,[27, 28] to a much higher percentage in others.[29] The criteria for diagnosis of this condition have undergone numerous revisions, however, most authors agree on the following: the presence in patients with chronic rhinosinusitis (confirmed by CT scan) of characteristic 'allergic' mucin containing clusters of eosinophils and their byproducts; and the presence of noninvasive fungal elements within that mucin detectable on staining or culture.[27, 28, 29, 30] Most experts also require the presence of documented type 1 (immunoglobulin (Ig)E-mediated) hypersensitivity to cultured fungi, and nasal polyposis.[27, 28, 30] The diagnosis of allergic fungal sinusitis should not, however, be established, or eliminated, on the basis of the results of the fungal cultures because of the variable yield of these cultures.[30]

In 1999, Ponikau *et al.*,[29] using ultrasensitive mucus collection and staining methods, reported finding fungus in nasal mucus from 202 (96 percent) of 210 consecutive patients with chronic rhinosinusitis at the Mayo Clinic, as well as 14 of 14 control patients. Allergic mucin, containing degenerating eosinophils and their byproducts, was found in 97 (96 percent) of a subset of 101 consecutive patients who underwent surgical treatment; in the four cases in which allergic mucin was absent, eosinophils were also absent. Fungal elements were detected in histopathological specimens from 82 (81 percent) of these 101 cases. Conventional IgE-mediated hypersensitivity to fungi was not a consistent finding in the patients with chronic rhinosinusitis. These observations led Ponikau *et al.*[29] to conclude that allergic fungal sinusitis is an under-diagnosed disorder that is, in fact, present in most patients with chronic rhinosinusitis. More recently, an Austrian group[31] used the Mayo Clinic procedure and detected fungus in cultures of nasal mucus from 87 percent of patients with chronic rhinosinusitis, as well as from 91.3 percent of a control group. Ponikau *et al.*[29] speculated that IgE-mediated type 1 hypersensitivity to fungi is not the dominant pathophysiological mechanism, rather this role is played by eosinophils. They suggested that the disorder be renamed 'eosinophilic fungal sinusitis'. These conclusions have proved controversial and have been criticized on the grounds that the 'causative agents' (i.e. fungi) were detected in all the control subjects, and because of the small number of cases studied in which eosinophils were not found in tissue specimens. The current consensus is that the term 'allergic fungal rhinosinusitis' should be retained for the subgroup of patients with classical distinct immunologic, allergic, clinical and histologic features.[30]

The term 'eosinophilic mucin rhinosinusitis' has been proposed to describe those patients with chronic rhinosinusitis and allergic mucin in whom no fungal elements can be detected.[32] It has been suggested that allergic fungal sinusitis is an allergic response to fungi in predisposed individuals, while eosinophilic mucin rhino-sinusitis represents a heterogenous group of pathophy-siological mechanisms all associated with eosinophilia, but in which the predominant mechanism is a systemic dysregulation of immunological controls.

AETIOLOGICAL AGENTS

In earlier reports, *Aspergillus* species were believed to be the predominant cause of allergic fungal sinusitis. More recent series suggest that it is predominantly due to various dematiaceous (brown-pigmented) environmental moulds, including *Alternaria*, *Bipolaris*, *Cladosporium*, *Curvularia* and *Drechslera* species.[28] [**]

EPIDEMIOLOGY

This condition occurs in young immunocompetent adults with chronic relapsing rhinosinusitis, unresponsive to antibiotics, antihistamines or corticosteroids. Although patients do not have underlying immunodeficiencies, 50–70 percent are atopic.[28] There is no male or female predominance. Cases of allergic fungal sinusitis have been described from different parts of the world, but the largest number of reports have come from the warm humid areas of the southern United States where the disorder accounts for about 7 percent of all sinus surgeries. [**]

CLINICAL MANIFESTATIONS

Many patients with allergic fungal sinusitis have a history of chronic rhinosinusitis and have undergone multiple operations prior to diagnosis.[27, 28] Although there are no unique pathognomonic symptoms, patients often present with unilateral nasal polyposis and thick yellow-green nasal or sinus mucus. The nasal polyposis may form an expansive mass that causes bone necrosis of the thin walls of the sinuses. Should the lamina papyracea of the ethmoid bone be traversed it may cause proptosis. Polypoid material can also push the nasal septum into the contralateral airway. CT scans often reveal a characteristic serpiginous sinus opacification of more than one sinus, mucosal thickening and erosion of bone, but this does not represent tissue invasion (**Figure 18.4**). In addition, allergic fungal sinusitis may be suspected when a patient with nasal polyposis, having no other known disease, responds only to oral corticosteroids. [**]

DIAGNOSIS

The diagnosis of allergic fungal sinusitis requires the presence of chronic rhinosinusitis in an otherwise immunocompetent individual; the microscopic examina-tion of the characteristic allergic mucin (either at the time of surgical debridement for chronic sinusitis or

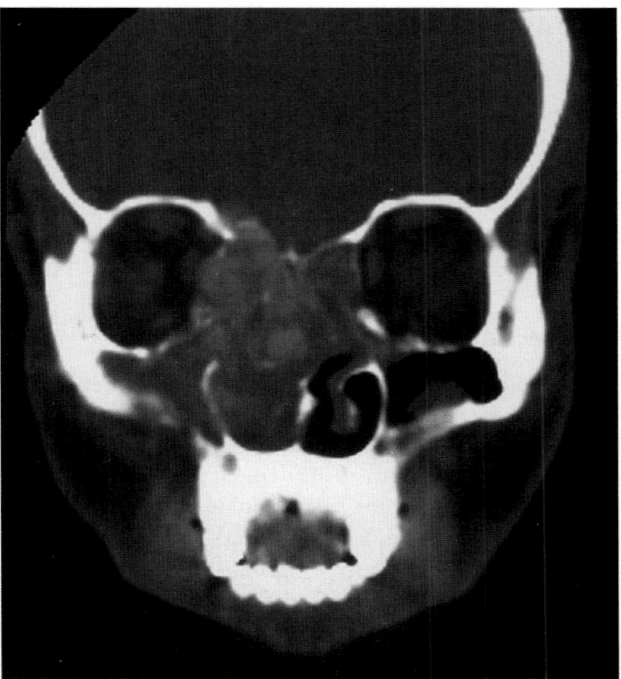

Figure 18.4 A coronal CT scan showing allergic polyposis due to aspergillosis of the paranasal sinuses with expansion into the orbit and anterior cranial fossa simulating invasive disease. The patient had raised IgE levels to Aspergillus. At surgery the dura and periosteum were intact, histologically Aspergillus was present with Charcot Leyden crystals and there was no invasion. The patient remains well five years after surgery and topical nasal steroids.

endoscopic examination for drainage) to determine the presence of eosinophils and fungal elements; histologic examination of sinus tissue to rule out invasion; radio-graphic studies to assess the extent of disease; and laboratory testing for eosinophilia, total serum IgE, specific IgE against fungal antigens, and a positive skin prick test to fungal antigens. Fungal cultures are used to identify the responsible fungus. [**]

MANAGEMENT OPTIONS

The treatment of allergic fungal sinusitis includes surgical debridement to remove polyps and the allergic mucin containing fungal debris which is thought to be the cause of the immune reaction in the sinus mucosa. [Grade B] More than one surgical procedure may be required to accomplish this goal. Adjunctive medical management is also required because it is unlikely that all fungal elements can be removed. In small studies, use of postoperative oral corticosteroids reduced recurrence of disease.[33, 34] [Grade D] Other commonly used adjunctive medical treatments for allergic fungal sinusitis include specific allergen immunotherapy, nasal corticosteroids, antihistamines, antileukotrienes and sinonasal saline lavage.[32] However, there have been no controlled studies. [Grade D]

Systemic antifungal drug treatment has not proved effective for the management of allergic fungal sinusitis other than preoperatively to reduce swelling and pre-operative bleeding. In most cases, even patients whose symptoms, endoscopic signs and CT scans cleared with systemic antifungal treatment relapsed soon after this was discontinued.[35] [Grade D] There is poor evidence that topical antifungal treatment might be of benefit in allergic fungal sinusitis.

OUTCOMES AND COMPLICATIONS

Postoperative endoscopic follow up is recommended because there is a poor correlation between subjective improvement and the presence of objective regression of disease. Despite surgical debridement and corticosteroid treatment, the condition recurs in up to two-thirds of patients. In addition, corticosteroid use is sometimes associated with limiting side effects. [**]

KEY POINTS

Fulminant acute invasive sinusitis

- The infection often spreads into the orbit and brain.
- Prolonged neutropenia and metabolic acidosis are important risk factors.
- The commonest aetiological agents are moulds belonging to the order Mucorales.
- For treatment to be successful, prompt diagnosis is essential.
- Aggressive medical and surgical treatment are both required.
- Blood vessel invasion is seen histologically.

Chronic invasive sinusitis

- The most common aetiological agents include *Aspergillus*, *Bipolaris* and *Curvularia* species.
- Invasion of adjacent structures is a common complication.
- MRI is useful for assessing cavernous sinus and cerebral involvement.
- Medical treatment is sufficient in most cases.
- Itraconazole (100 mg bd) results in remineralization of the eroded skull base.

Chronic granulomatous invasive sinusitis

- Most cases have been reported from North Africa.
- *A. flavus* is the most common aetiological agent.
- Medical treatment is itraconazole 100 mg bd.
- Complete surgical removal of the granuloma is difficult.

Noninvasive fungal sinusitis

- Paranasal sinus fungus balls are most often seen in older persons.
- *A. fumigatus* is the commonest aetiological agent.
- The symptoms are often unilateral and include nasal obstruction, purulent discharge and cacosmia.
- CT scans should reveal partial or total opacification of the involved sinus.
- Surgical removal of the fungus ball is the recommended treatment.

Allergic fungal sinusitis

- Allergic fungal sinusitis is an important cause of chronic rhinosinusitis.
- The criteria for diagnosis of this condition are:
  - characteristic allergic mucin
  - clusters of eosinophils
  - Charcot Leyden
  - the presence of fungal organisms detectable on staining and culture
  - the presence of type I hypersensitivity.
- The predominant causes of this condition are dematiaceous (brown-pigmented) moulds.
- Management includes surgical debridement with adjunctive medical treatment.
- Systemic antifungal treatment is ineffective on its own, but may reduce inflammation and peroperative bleeding and if given postoperatively may reduce the recurrence rate.

Best clinical practice

Acute invasive sinusitis

✓ Underlying host disorders must be controlled: correction of acidosis is essential and immunosuppressive drugs should be reduced in dose if possible.

✓ Aggressive surgical debridement of infected and necrotic tissue is essential.

✓ Lipid-based formulations of amphotericin B, in particular high doses of the liposomal formulation (10–15 mg/kg per day), are considered the first choice treatment.

✓ Patients who receive amphotericin B should be monitored for signs of renal damage.

✓ Treatment should be continued at least until progression of disease ceases and the underlying disorder is well controlled.

Chronic invasive sinusitis

- ✓ Itraconazole (200 mg bd) has made surgery unnecessary in most cases.
- ✓ It is important to exclude fulminant acute sinusitis by histology.

MYCOTIC DISEASES OF THE THROAT

With the exception of pharyngeal candidiasis (which occurs as an extension of oral disease), mycotic infections of the pharynx and larynx are uncommon in ear, nose and throat practice.

Candidiasis

DEFINITION

The term candidiasis is used to refer to infections caused by organisms belonging to the genus *Candida*. These opportunistic pathogens can cause acute or chronic deep-seated infection, but are more often seen causing mucosal, cutaneous or nail infection. Oropharyngeal candidiasis is a common problem in debilitated or immunocompromised persons. Isolated laryngeal candidiasis can also occur in these individuals, but is much less common.

AETIOLOGICAL AGENTS

Oropharyngeal and laryngeal candidiasis is most commonly caused by *C. albicans*. However, several other members of the genus, including *C. glabrata*, *C. krusei*, *C. tropicalis* and *C. parapsilosis*, have sometimes been associated with oropharyngeal disease. [***/**]

EPIDEMIOLOGY

In most cases, infection is derived from an individual's own endogenous reservoir in the mouth and upper respiratory tract. *Candida albicans* is present as a commensal in the mouth of up to 40 percent of the normal adult population. The number of organisms in the saliva of carriers increases with tobacco smoking and when dentures are worn. [***/**]

Both general and local predisposing factors are important in the development of oropharyngeal and laryngeal candidiasis. Debilitated patients, such as those receiving broad-spectrum antibiotics or corticosteroids, patients with diabetes mellitus, individuals with severe nutritional deficiencies and immunosuppressive diseases, such as AIDS, are more susceptible to oropharyngeal candidiasis. Local factors, such as trauma from unhygienic or ill-fitting dentures and tobacco smoking, are also important. Isolated laryngeal candidiasis has usually been

described in immunocompromised patients, but it may also occur in immunocompetent individuals. Most patients have some associated disease and/or predisposing factors. These include previous radiation therapy, broad-spectrum antibiotics and corticosteroid use. [***/**]

Prior to the introduction of combination antiretroviral treatment, oropharyngeal candidiasis was the most common opportunistic infection seen in persons with HIV infection. Up to 90 percent of untreated HIV-positive individuals developed candidiasis at some time during the course of HIV disease.[36] Furthermore, oropharyngeal candidiasis occurred in about 60 percent of those with a CD4 cell count of less than 100–200 cells/mm^3, more than half of whom experienced recurrent infection.[36] Recent epidemiological data indicate that the incidence of oropharyngeal and oesophageal candidiasis has fallen since the widespread introduction of new antiretroviral therapies, including protease inhibitors, perhaps by as much as 50–60 percent.[37] The development of oropharyngeal candidiasis is often one of the earliest clinical manifestations of HIV infection in asymptomatic individuals and is a reliable marker of disease progression. Although it is not life-threatening, it can be most uncomfortable for the patient, contributing to inadequate oral nutrition and weight loss. Of greater concern, it can predispose patients to develop a more invasive disease, such as oesophageal candidiasis. [***/**]

CLINICAL MANIFESTATIONS

Oral candidiasis can be classified into a number of distinct clinical forms: pseudomembranous, erythematous (or atrophic) and hyperplastic (or hypertrophic) candidiasis.

Pseudomembranous candidiasis is an acute infection, but it can recur in patients using steroid inhalers and in immunocompromised individuals. It is also seen in neonates and among terminally ill patients, particularly in association with serious underlying disorders, such as leukaemia and other malignancies. It is the most common form of candidiasis in HIV disease. Pseudomembranous candidiasis presents as white raised lesions on the surfaces of the tongue, hard and soft palate, buccal mucosa and tonsils. If left untreated, these can develop to form confluent plaques. The lesions are often painless, although mucosal erosion and ulceration may occur. The infection may spread to involve the throat, giving rise to severe dysphagia. It is important to distinguish this condition from hyperplastic candidiasis (oral leukoplakia). The simplest test is to determine whether the white pseudomembrane can be dislodged. If it can be wiped off to reveal an eroded, erythematous, and sometimes bleeding base, then this is diagnostic for pseudomembranous candidiasis. [**]

Erythematous candidiasis is often associated with broad-spectrum antibiotic treatment, chronic corticosteroid use and with HIV disease. It can arise as a consequence of persistent pseudomembranous candidiasis, when pseudomembranes are shed, or, in HIV infection, may precede pseudomembranous candidiasis. It can affect any part of the oral mucosa and manifests as a flat, red lesion, usually on the palate or dorsum of the tongue. Lesions on the tongue present as depapillated areas. [**]

Hyperplastic candidiasis (candida leukoplakia) is an important condition because the lesions can undergo malignant transformation. The lesions range from small, palpable, translucent white areas to large, dense opaque plaques, hard and rough on palpation. In contrast to the pseudomembranous form of oral candidiasis, the lesions cannot be removed. The lesions usually occur on the inside surface of one or both cheeks and, less commonly, on the tongue. They are usually asymptomatic. Lesions that contain both red erythroplakic and white leukoplakic areas must be regarded with great suspicion as malignant change is often present. [**]

In addition to the foregoing three major forms of oropharyngeal candidiasis, there are several other lesions associated with candida infection. Chronic atrophic candidiasis (or denture stomatitis) is usually associated with oral prostheses, occurring in up to 60 percent of denture wearers. Apart from soreness, the condition is usually asymptomatic. The only presenting complaint may be associated angular stomatitis (or cheilitis). Lower dentures are seldom involved. The characteristic presenting signs are chronic mucosal erythema and oedema of the portion of the hard palate that comes into contact with the fitting surface of the upper denture. The condition is mainly due to the overgrowth of *C. albicans* beneath the dentures. The mucosa beneath the dentures is rarely involved. [**]

Hoarseness and dysphagia are the most common symptoms of laryngeal candidiasis. Some patients present with stridor. The characteristic signs of the infection are white plaques on the laryngeal mucosa. If left untreated, the infection can progress to airway obstruction. [**]

DIAGNOSIS

The clinical manifestations of oropharyngeal candidiasis are often characteristic, but can be confused with other disorders. For this reason, the diagnosis should be confirmed by demonstration of the various morphological forms of the fungus in smears prepared from swabs or scrapings of lesions and its isolation in culture. As *C. albicans* is a normal commensal in the mouth, its isolation alone cannot be considered diagnostic of infection. [**]

The diagnosis of laryngeal candidiasis should be considered in any immunodeficient patient presenting with symptoms of laryngeal disease. The most effective diagnostic procedure is fibreoptic or indirect laryngoscopy.[38] Mucosal biopsy specimens should be submitted for histopathological examination and culture. [**]

MANAGEMENT OPTIONS

In infants, pseudomembranous candidiasis can be treated with nystatin oral suspension (100,000 units/mL) or amphotericin B oral suspension (100 mg/mL). This should be dropped into the mouth after each feed or at four to six hour intervals. In most cases the lesions will clear within two weeks. [Grade D] Older children and adults with pseudomembranous candidiasis can be treated with clotrimazole troches (one 10-mg troche five times daily) nystatin or amphotericin B oral suspension (1 mL at six hour intervals for about two to three weeks) or miconazole oral gel (250 mg at six hour intervals). Treatment should be continued for at least 48 hours after all lesions have cleared and symptoms have disappeared. [Grade C/D]

Oral fluconazole (100–200 mg/day for 7–14 days) has been found to be more effective than ketoconazole in controlling oropharyngeal candidiasis in AIDS patients.[39, 40] [Grade B] Itraconazole capsules (200–400 mg/day for 14 days) are as effective as ketoconazole.[39, 40] [Grade B] Itraconazole oral solution (200–400 mg/day for 7–14 days) is better absorbed than the capsules, and it is as effective as fluconazole.[39, 40] [Grade B] This may reflect the improved absorption of the solution or an additional topical effect.

Chronic suppressive treatment with fluconazole is effective in the prevention of oropharyngeal candidiasis in both AIDS and cancer patients.[40] To reduce the likelihood of development of antifungal resistance, it should only be used if recurrence is frequent or disabling. [Grade C] Up to two-thirds of AIDS patients with fluconazole-resistant oropharyngeal candidiasis will respond to itraconazole oral solution.[39, 40] [Grade B] Amphotericin B oral suspension (1 mL at six hour intervals) is sometimes effective in patients who do not respond to itraconazole. [Grade C] Refractory candidiasis can be managed with parenteral amphotericin B (0.3–0.5 mg/kg per day for one week) or caspofungin (50 mg/day).[40] [Grade B]

The treatment of choice for laryngeal candidiasis is parenteral amphotericin B (0.7–1.0 mg/kg per day).[40] [Grade D] Oral fluconazole may be appropriate for treatment once symptoms and signs are improving.[40] [Grade D] Airway obstruction is managed by endotracheal intubation. [Grade D]

OUTCOMES AND COMPLICATIONS

Most individuals with oropharyngeal candidiasis will respond initially to topical or oral antifungal treatment. Prior to the introduction of the new highly active antiretroviral drug regimens, up to 60 percent of patients with HIV disease relapsed within three months of the successful completion of azole treatment for oropharyngeal candidiasis. However, recent data indicate that the incidence of relapse has decreased.[37] In HIV-positive individuals, symptomatic relapses are apt to occur sooner with topical than with oral azole treatment. Resistance can develop with either regimen, but it is important to recognize that recurrence does not necessarily denote the development of resistant *C. albicans* strains, nor does it imply that the recurrent episode will be unresponsive to standard treatment.[39, 40] [****/***]

Most patients with laryngeal candidiasis will respond to amphotericin B treatment. If not diagnosed and treated promptly, airway obstruction and, potentially, respiratory arrest can ensue. [**]

Other mycotic infections of the pharynx and larynx

A number of fungi can cause pharyngeal and laryngeal lesions as part of a disseminated mycosis. The most frequently seen of the systemic infections to affect this site are histoplasmosis and paracoccidioidomycosis. Occasional cases of blastomycosis, coccidioidomycosis and cryptococcosis have also been reported. [**]

Histoplasmosis and paracoccidioidomycosis both present in a similar way, usually with hoarseness or altered vocalization. Patients sometimes complain of sore throat, dysphagia, dyspnoea and cough.[41, 42] Laryngoscopy will reveal an ulcer or granuloma on the vocal chords or on the laryngeal epithelium. The lesions are similar to those of laryngeal cancer, and biopsy with histopathological examination and culture is essential to establish the diagnosis.[41, 42] [**/*]

Treatment of these infections is similar and, for paracoccidioidomycosis and histoplasmosis, itraconazole (200–400 mg/day for 6–18 months) is the drug of choice. [Grade D] Ketoconazole (200–400 mg/day) is also effective, but is less well tolerated than itraconazole. [Grade D] Lesions in the pharynx and larynx are usually part of a chronic disseminated infection and it is important to investigate the patient for other sites of involvement, including the oral mucosa, adrenals, lymph nodes, heart, liver and lungs.

Delay in the diagnosis may worsen the prognosis. In the case of paracoccidioidomycosis, the onset of fibrosis may cause laryngeal stenosis with permanent problems in both breathing and speech. Once it has been established it is not possible to stop fibrotic scarring. Other deep fungal infections in this site seldom cause such severe fibrosis. [**]

Mycotic colonization of tracheo–oesophageal voice prostheses

Silastic tracheo-oesophageal voice prostheses, which are used for speech rehabilitation in laryngectomized cancer patients, often deteriorate and require replacement. This deterioration is usually associated with biofilm formation

and invasion of the structure of the silastic by *Candida* species, including *C. albicans*, *C. glabrata*, *C. krusei* and *C. tropicalis*. This can occur within two to four months of implantation. In one report, 257 prosthesis replacements were required in a group of 31 patients over a 40-month period.[43] Radiation therapy-induced xerostomia was an important factor in shortening the lifetime of the prostheses that required replacement. [**]

Fungal damage to silastic tracheo-oesophageal prostheses results in valve failure and necessitates the replacement of the device. Local antifungal treatment is inadequate to eliminate deep infiltration of *Candida* species into the silastic material. However, a double-blind randomized trial has shown that the use of a buccal bioadhesive slow-release tablet containing miconazole nitrate might be an adequate method of preventing fungal colonization and deterioration.[44] [Grade C] Another potential new approach is metal coating of prostheses to prevent the adhesion of microorganisms.[45]

KEY POINTS

- Oropharyngeal candidiasis is common in debilitated or immunocompromised persons.
- It is one of the earliest clinical manifestations of HIV infection, but has fallen in incidence since the introduction of combination antiretroviral therapies.
- Topical or oral antifungal treatment is usually highly effective.
- Azole drug resistance can develop in HIV-positive individuals receiving long-term treatment for recurrent infection.

Best clinical practice

✓ Because the clinical manifestations of oropharyngeal candidiasis can be confused with other disorders, the diagnosis should be confirmed by microscopic examination and culture.
✓ Patients can often be managed with topical clotrimazole, miconazole or nystatin.
✓ In persons with AIDS, oral fluconazole is more palatable than itraconazole oral solution, and more effective than ketoconazole.
✓ To reduce the likelihood of resistance developing, long-term azole treatment should be avoided unless relapse is frequent or disabling.
✓ Patients unresponsive to azole treatment can be managed with amphotericin B or caspofungin.

Deficiencies in current knowledge and areas for future research

➤ The role of azole antifungals, in particular voriconazole and posaconazole, in the treatment of acute invasive sinusitis is unclear and needs to be evaluated.
➤ The role of fungi in the pathogenesis of chronic sinusitis needs to be determined, as does the role of antifungal and other adjunctive medical treatments in the management of this disorder.

REFERENCES

1. Mugliston T, O'Donoghue G. Otomycosis: a continuing problem. *Journal of Laryngology and Otology.* 1985; **99**: 327–33.
2. Paulose KO, Al Khalifa S, Shenoy P, Sharma RK. Mycotic infection of the ear (otomycosis): a prospective study. *Journal of Laryngology and Otology.* 1989; **103**: 30–5.
3. Kaur R, Mittal N, Kakkar M, Aggarwal AK, Mathur MD. Otomycosis: a clinicomycologic study. *Ear, Nose, and Throat Journal.* 2000; **79**: 606–9.
4. Kurnatowski P, Filipiak A. Otomycosis: prevalence, clinical symptoms, therapeutic procedures. *Mycoses.* 2001; **44**: 472–9.
5. Hurst WB. Outcome of 22 cases of perforated tympanic membrane caused by otomycosis. *Journal of Laryngology and Otology.* 2001; **115**: 879–80.
6. Yao M, Messner AH. Fungal malignant otitis externa due to Scedosporium apiospermum. *Annals of Otology, Rhinology, and Laryngology.* 2001; **110**: 377–80.
7. Martinson FD. Chronic phycomycosis of the upper respiratory tract: rhinophycomycosis entomophthorae. *American Journal of Tropical Medicine and Hygiene.* 1971; **20**: 449–55.
8. Drouhet E, Ravisse P. Entomophthoromycosis. *Current Topics in Medical Mycology.* 1993; **5**: 215–45.
9. Herr RA, Ajello L, Taylor JW, Arseculeratne SN, Mendoza L. Phylogenetic analysis of Rhinosporidium seeberi's 18S small-subunit ribosomal DNA groups this pathogen among members of the protoctistan Mesomycetozoa clade. *Journal of Clinical Microbiology.* 1999; **37**: 2750–4.
10. Arsecularatne SN, Ajello L. Rhinosporidium seeberi. In: Ajello L, Hay RJ (eds). *Microbiology and Microbial Infections,* vol. 4. London: Arnold, 1998: 67–73.
* 11. deShazo RD, Chapin K, Swain RE. Fungal sinusitis. *New England Journal of Medicine.* 1997; **337**: 254–9.
12. deShazo RD, O'Brien M, Chapin K, Soto-Aguilar M, Gardner L, Swain R. A new classification and diagnostic criteria for invasive fungal sinusitis. *Archieves of Laryngology – Head and Neck Surgery.* 1997; **123**: 1181–8.
* 13. Fatterpekar G, Mukherji S, Arbealez A, Maheshwari S, Castillo M. Fungal diseases of the paranasal sinuses. *Seminars in Ultrasound, CT, and MR.* 1999; **20**: 391–401.

14. Blitzer A, Lawson W, Meyers BR, Biller HF. Patient survival factors in paranasal sinus mucormycosis. *Laryngoscope.* 1980; **90**: 635–48.
15. Yohai RA, Bullock JD, Aziz AA, Markert RJ. Survival factors in rhino-orbital-cerebral mucormycosis. *Survey of Ophthalmology.* 1994; **39**: 3–22.
16. Iwen PC, Rupp ME, Hinrichs SH. Invasive mold sinusitis: 17 cases in immunocompromised patients and review of the literature. *Clinical Infectious Diseases.* 1997; **24**: 1178–84.
17. Hunt SM, Miyamoto C, Cornelius RS, Tami TA. Invasive fungal sinusitis in the acquired immunodeficiency syndrome. *Otolaryngologic Clinics of North America.* 2000; **33**: 335–47.
18. Centeno RS, Bentson JR, Mancuso AA. CT scanning in rhinocerebral mucormycosis and aspergillosis. *Radiology.* 1981; **140**: 383–9.
19. de Carpentier JP, Ramamurthy L, Denning DW, Taylor PH. An algorithmic approach to aspergillus sinusitis. *Journal of Laryngology and Otology.* 1994; **108**: 314–8.
* 20. Spellberg B, Edwards J, Ibrahim A. Novel perspectives on mucormycosis: pathophysiology, presentation and management. *Clinical Microbiology Reviews.* 2005; **18**: 556–69.
21. Tobon AM, Arango M, Fernandez D, Restrepo A. Mucormycosis (zygomycosis) in a heart-kidney transplant recipient: recovery after posaconazole therapy. *Clinical Infectious Diseases.* 2003; **36**: 1488–91.
22. Greenberg RN, Scott LJ, Vaughn HH, Ribes JA. Zygomycosis (mucormycosis): emerging clinical importance and new treatments. *Current Opinion in Infectious Diseases.* 2004; **17**: 517–25.
23. Browning AC, Sim KT, Timms JM, Vernon SA, McConachie NS, Allibone R et al. Successful treatment of invasive cavernous sinus aspergillosis with oral itraconazole monotherapy. *Journal of Neuroophthalmology.* 2006; **26**: 103–6.
24. Clancy CJ, Nguyen MH. Invasive sinus aspergillosis in apparently immunocompetent hosts. *Journal of Infection.* 1998; **37**: 229–40.
25. DeShazo RD, O'Brien M, Chapin K, Soto-Aquilar M, Swain R, Lyous M et al. Criteria for diagnosis of sinus mycetoma. *Journal of Allergy and Clinical Immunology.* 1997; **99**: 475–85.
26. Ferguson BJ. Fungus balls of the paranasal sinuses. *Otolaryngologic Clinics of North America.* 2000; **33**: 389–98.
27. Bent JP, Kuhn FA. The diagnosis of allergic fungal sinusitis. *Otolaryngology and Head and Neck Surgery.* 1994; **111**: 580–8.
28. DeShazo RD, Swain RE. Diagnostic criteria for allergic fungal sinusitis. *Journal of Allergy and Clinical Immunology.* 1995; **96**: 24–35.
29. Ponikau JU, Sherris DA, Kern EB, Homberger HA, Frigas E, Gaffey TA et al. The diagnosis and incidence of allergic fungal sinusitis. *Mayo Clinic Proceedings. Mayo Clinic.* 1999; **74**: 877–84.

30. Meltzer EO, Hamilos DK, Hadley JA, Lanza DC, Marple BF, Nicklas RA *et al.* Rhinosinusitis: establishing definitions for clinical research and patient care. *Journal of Allergy and Clinical Immunology.* 2004; **114**: 155–212.

31. Braun H, Stammberger H, Buzina W, Freudenschuss K, Lackner A, Beham A. Haufigkeit und nachweis von pilzen und eosinophilen granulozyten bei chronischer rhinosinusitis. *Laryngo-Rhino-Otologie.* 2003; **82**: 330–40.

32. Ferguson BJ. Eosinophilic mucin rhinosinusitis: a distinct clinicopathological entity. *Laryngoscope.* 2000; **110**: 799–813.

33. Schubert MS, Goetz DW. Evaluation and treatment of allergic fungal sinusitis. II: treatment and follow-up. *Journal of Allergy and Clinical Immunology.* 1998; **102**: 395–402.

34. Schubert MS. Allergic fungal sinusitis: pathogenesis and management strategies. *Drugs.* 2004; **64**: 363–74.

35. Kuhn FA, Javer AR. Allergic fungal rhinosinusitis. Perioperative management, prevention of recurrence, and role of steroids and antifungal agents. *Otolaryngologic Clinics of North America.* 2000; **33**: 419–32.

36. Powderly WG, Mayer KH, Perfect JR. Diagnosis and treatment of oropharyngeal candidiasis in patients infected with HIV: a critical reassessment. *AIDS Research and Human Retroviruses.* 1999; **15**: 1405–12.

37. Martins MD, Lozano-Chiu M, Rex JH. Declining rates of oropharyngeal candidiasis and carriage of Candida albicans associated with trends towards reduced rates of carriage of fluconazole-resistant C. albicans in human immunodeficiency virus-infected patients. *Clinical Infectious Diseases.* 1998; **27**: 1291–4.

38. Alba D, Perna C, Molina F, Ortega L, Varquez JJ. Isolated laryngeal candidiasis. Description of 2 cases and review of the literature. *Archivos de Bronchoneumologia.* 1996; **32**: 205–8.

39. Darouiche RO. Oropharyngeal and esophageal candidiasis in immunocompromised patients. *Clinical Infectious Diseases.* 1998; **26**: 259–74.

∗ 40. Pappas PG, Rex JH, Sobel JD *et al.* Guidelines for treatment of candidiasis. *Clinical Infectious Diseases.* 2004; **38**: 161–89.

41. Sant'Anna GD, Mauri M, Arrarte JL, Camargo H. Laryngeal manifestations of paracoccidioidomycosis (South American blastomycosis). *Archives of Otolaryngology – Head and Neck Surgery.* 1999; **125**: 1375–8.

42. Gerber ME, Rosdeutscher JD, Seiden AM, Tami TA. Histoplasmosis: the otolaryngologist's perspective. *Laryngoscope.* 1995; **105**: 919–23.

43. Eerenstein SE, Grollman W, Schouwenburg PF. Microbial colonization of silicone voice prostheses used in laryngectomized patients. *Clinical Otolaryngology.* 1999; **24**: 398–403.

44. Van Weissenbruch R, Bouckaert S, Remon JP, Nelis HJ, Aerts R, Albers FW. Chemoprophylaxis of fungal deterioration of the Provox silicone tracheoesophageal prosthesis in postlaryngectomy patients. *Annals of Otology, Rhinology, and Laryngology.* 1997; **106**: 329–37.

45. Arweiler-Harbeck D, Sanders A, Held M, Jerman M, Ehrlich H, Jahnke K. Does metal coating improve the durability of silicone voice prostheses? *Acta Otolaryngologica.* 2001; **121**: 643–6.

19

Antimicrobial therapy

VIVIENNE WESTON

Introduction	228	Adverse effects of antimicrobial agents	235
Principles of antimicrobial therapy	228	Key points	236
Antimicrobial activity and pharmokinetics	229	Best clinical practice	236
Antimicrobial resistance	234	References	237

SEARCH STRATEGY

The information in this chapter is supported by a Medline search of review articles using the key words antibiotic, antifungal and antimicrobial resistance.

INTRODUCTION

The discovery of potent nontoxic chemotherapeutic agents selectively active against bacteria in the late 1930s revolutionized the treatment of infections. Unfortunately, microbes have demonstrated their ability to avoid, withstand or repel the antimicrobial onslaught. In addition, the pattern of infection has altered considerably, due to the impact of new operative and invasive procedures, and treatment regimens that severely compromise the patient's own capacity to withstand infection. No antimicrobial drug is entirely free from toxic side effects, and the use of antibiotics can disturb the delicate bacterial ecology of the body allowing the proliferation of resistant organisms. In the last two decades the pace of the development of antibiotic resistance has been faster than the development of new antibacterial agents, resulting in antibiotic resistance becoming a major threat to the effective treatment of infections, both in the community and in hospital. Thus, penicillin therapy can no longer be relied upon for the empirical treatment of pneumococcal meningitis and with the continuing rise of meticillin-resistant *Staphylococcus aureus* (MRSA) isolation rates, flucloxacillin therapy is under threat.[1] [**] Both national (UK) and international concern has risen since the late 1990s, with the formation of working parties to try and

stem the rising tide of antimicrobial resistance. These have identified the association of antimicrobial resistance with the use and abuse of antibiotics, and have emphasized the importance of the appropriate use of antibiotics, education on antimicrobial therapy and the proper selection of patients for treatment.[2, 3] [*]

The aim of this chapter is to explore the principles of antimicrobial therapy, provide brief details on the mechanism of action, spectrum of antimicrobial activity and pharmokinetic features of each of the main classes of antimicrobials, and give a brief description of resistance mechanisms and adverse effects of antimicrobial agents.

PRINCIPLES OF ANTIMICROBIAL THERAPY

Effective treatment of an infection is based on the knowledge of the likely infecting organisms and antimicrobial susceptibility, the natural history of the disease, the site of the infection, the spectrum of action of antimicrobial agents and the risk of the treatment. Knowledge of the pharmacokinetics of an antimicrobial agent is important in ensuring that the agent reaches the site of the infection. Infection in difficult sites, such as cerebrospinal fluid (CSF), cannot be treated by an antimicrobial agent which does not cross the blood–brain barrier in sufficient amounts at nontoxic doses. The pharmacological principles which apply to other drugs apply to antimicrobial agents, so that lipid-soluble agents such as chloramphenicol are well absorbed orally and cross the blood–brain barrier. Conditions at the site of infection can affect the activity of the antimicrobial agent, for example the lower pH found in an abscess reduces the efficacy of aminoglycosides and macrolides. The route of excretion can also affect the efficacy of an antimicrobial agent, for example those which are excreted in the urine are more likely to be effective in urinary tract infections.

Where antimicrobials are being used for surgical prophylaxis they should be administered immediately before or during a procedure and there is no published benefit from extending the duration of prophylaxis beyond wound closure. By giving extended prophylaxis the risks of treatment outweigh the benefit, due to the potential for further disturbance to the patient's natural flora and hence selecting for resistant organisms or infection with *Clostridium difficile*.

The antimicrobial activity of antibiotics depends on the bacterial target site, the ability of the antibiotic to get to that target site and whether the bacteria can break down the antibiotic before it is able to act. The cellular target sites for the main antibiotics are summarized in **Figure 19.1**. Similar principles apply to antifungal and antiviral agents.

ANTIMICROBIAL ACTIVITY AND PHARMOKINETICS

Antibiotics

INHIBITORS OF BACTERIAL CELL WALL SYNTHESIS

The bacterial cell wall is a common target as it differs from that of human cells. The structure is different in Gram-negative and -positive organisms and, in addition, some bacteria, such as chlamydiae, do not possess a bacterial cell wall.

β-LACTAM ANTIBIOTICS

Penicillins, cephalosporins, monobactams and carbapenems are similar compounds, containing a β-lactam ring, which mimics the cross-link of the peptidoglycan 'backbone' of the cell wall. Inhibition of this cross-linking occurs, weakening the cell wall and resulting in cell death by lysis.

PENICILLINS

Penicillins vary markedly in their oral absorption, penicillin V and aminopenicillins are absorbed orally but the remainder have to be given parenterally. They are divided on the basis of bacterial activity.

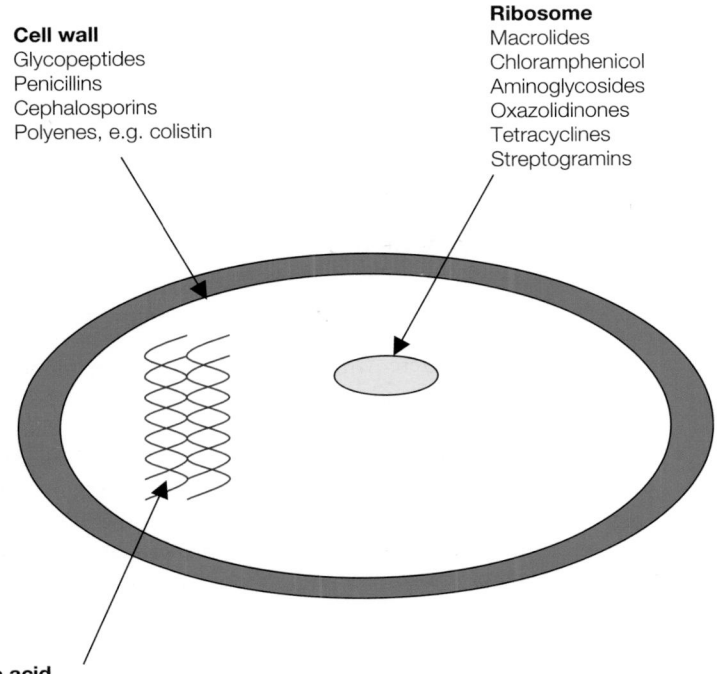

Cell wall
Glycopeptides
Penicillins
Cephalosporins
Polyenes, e.g. colistin

Ribosome
Macrolides
Chloramphenicol
Aminoglycosides
Oxazolidinones
Tetracyclines
Streptogramins

Nucleic acid
Quinolones
Nitroimidazoles, e.g. metronidazole
Rifamycins
Sulphonamides
Diaminopyrimidines e.g. trimethoprim

Figure 19.1 Bacterial sites of activity of the main classes of antibiotics.

- Natural penicillins, e.g. penicillin V: Gram-positive bacteria including streptococci, clostridia and corynebacteria (excluding most staphylococci), and some Gram-negative cocci including meningococci and most anaerobes (excluding *Bacteroides fragilis*).
- Penicillinase-resistant penicillins, e.g. flucloxacillin: As above with additional activity against penicillin-resistant *Staphylococcus aureus*.
- Aminopenicillins, e.g. ampicillin, and expanded-spectrum penicillins, e.g. piperacillin: Additional activity against Gram-negative bacilli including haemophili and many of the enterobacteriaceae. The expanded-spectrum penicillins have increased activity against enterobacteriaceae and pseudomonads, but resistance is increasing.
- Carbapenems, e.g. imipenem: Broad spectrum against Gram-positive and negative bacteria, including the β-lactamase producing Gram-negative organisms and anaerobic activity including *B. fragilis*.
- Monobactams, e.g. aztreonam: No Gram-positive but good Gram-negative activity including pseudomonads.
- β-lactamase inhibitors, e.g. clavulanic acid: In combination with a β-lactam with similar pharmokinetic properties they have increased activity against anaerobes and enterobacteriaceae.

The most serious but uncommon side effect is acute anaphylaxis. Other allergic manifestations include angio-neurotic oedema, urticaria, Stevens-Johnson syndrome, dermatitis, morbilliform eruptions and allergic vasculitis. Reversible neutropenia sometimes occurs with prolonged high-dose penicillin therapy. High-dose therapy in renal failure can precipitate epilepsy if dose adjustments are not made. Diarrhoea including *C. difficile* infection is more commonly associated with ampicillin and amoxicillin.

Penicillins are used to treat streptococcal infections (including pneumococcal meningitis once penicillin sensitivity is confirmed), meningococcal and penicillin-sensitive gonococcal infections. Aminopenicillins are used to treat upper and lower respiratory tract infections, as they are also active against *Haemophilus influenzae*, whereas the penicillinase-resistant penicillins are used to treat meticillin-sensitive staphylococcal infections, as the majority of *S. aureus* isolates are resistant to penicillin due to the production of penicillinase.

CEPHALOSPORINS

These compounds are closely related to the penicillins and classified into four main generations.

The first-generation cephalosporins, such as cefradine are absorbed well orally; the second-generation cephalosporins are usually given intravenously but are available in oral formulations. The third-generation cephalosporins are injectable agents, cefotaxime and ceftriaxone are able to cross the blood–brain barrier in sufficient amounts to be used to treat meningitis.

As Gram-negative activity increases Gram-positive activity decreases. The first-generation cephalosporins are more active against meticillin-sensitive *S. aureus* and streptococci, while the third- and fourth-generation cephalosporins have increased Gram-negative activity and some pseudomonal activity, for example ceftazidime. They are not active against enterococci and, except for some of the fourth-generation compounds, are not active against *B. fragilis*.

There is a low incidence of anaphylaxis, but cross-reactivity in approximately 10 percent of penicillin-allergic patients, and rashes can occur. The third-generation cephalosporins are associated with a higher risk of *C. difficile* diarrhoea.

GLYCOPEPTIDES, FOR EXAMPLE VANCOMYCIN AND TEICOPLANIN

They affect bacterial cell wall synthesis by binding to the D-alanine of the peptide chain of Gram-positive cell walls inhibiting the cross-linking process. They only have Gram-positive activity as they are unable to penetrate Gram-negative cell walls. Resistance is uncommon but increasing, particularly in enterococci. As they are large molecules they are not absorbed orally and do not penetrate the blood–brain barrier and 80 percent of the drug is excreted in the urine. 'Red-man' syndrome can occur with rapid infusions of vancomycin due to the release of histamine and renal toxicity with high serum levels, which is more likely with the concomitant use of aminoglycosides. These toxic effects are minimized by dosage schedules and monitoring of serum levels. They are used for treatment of sepsis due to resistant Gram-positive infections, such as MRSA, or if the patient is penicillin allergic. Orally, vancomycin is a second-line therapy for *C. difficile* diarrhoea.

Inhibitors of nucleic acid synthesis

QUINOLONE ANTIBIOTICS, FOR EXAMPLE CIPROFLOXACIN

They interfere with the bacterial enzyme DNA gyrase which is required for supercoiling of DNA during transcription and replication. Nalidixic acid had limited Gram-negative activity, and the fluoroquinolones have replaced it with increased Gram-negative, pseudomonal and Gram-positive activity due to the addition of a fluorine atom. The newer quinolones are active against anaerobic bacteria and streptococci. There is good oral absorption and wide tissue distribution except for the CSF. Adverse effects include central nervous system effects which include epileptic seizures, and interaction with other drugs, such as increasing theophylline levels. Photosensitivity has been a problem with some of the newer quinolones and also limited use. Invasive Gram-negative infections, particularly where pseudomonal infection is a possibility, and more difficult infections, such as typhoid, are typical clinical uses. The rise in resistance, particularly in *Salmonella typhi* and *Neisseria gonorrhoeae*, is beginning to limit their use.

SULPHONAMIDES AND TRIMETHOPRIM

These interfere with bacterial folic acid synthesis, and as they act at different stages producing synergistic activity in combination, for example co-trimoxazole, and display good oral absorption and tissue penetration. They have Gram-positive and -negative activity, and activity against *Pneumocystis carinii* and *Nocardia* sp., but resistance in enterobacteriaceae has increased. Sulphonamides are associated with severe allergic skin rashes including Stevens-Johnson syndrome. Combination agents are only licensed for severe infections in the UK. Trimethoprim is used in isolation for simple urinary and respiratory tract infections.

RIFAMYCINS

Rifamycins inhibit DNA-dependent RNA polymerase with inhibition of transcription to mRNA. Although good Gram-positive and mycobacterial activity, with some Gram-negative activity, for example meningococci, is shown, resistance develops rapidly if used as a single agent. They are well absorbed orally with good tissue, CSF and intracellular penetration. Hepatitis and occasionally haemolytic anaemia are important adverse effects used for prophylaxis against meningococcal and *H. influenzae* type b disease, in combination for mycobacterial disease and severe staphylococcal infections.

METRONIDAZOLE

It is active at low redox potentials producing toxic metabolites which damage DNA. The spectrum of activity is against anaerobic bacteria and protozoal organisms such as *Giardia* sp. Metronidazole is well absorbed orally and penetrates tissues and crosses the blood–brain barrier. Dizziness and a metallic taste can be present and peripheral neuropathy and encephalopathy can occur with long-term treatment. It is used for the treatment of and prophylaxis against infections that may include anaerobic bacteria, such as abdominal sepsis, and some protozoal infections, for example giardiasis.

Inhibitors of bacterial protein synthesis

TETRACYCLINES

They bind to the 30s ribosomal subunit and inhibit binding of the transfer RNA to the 30s ribosome. Activity is in Gram-positive bacteria including *S. aureus* and pneumococci, and some of the Gram-negative organisms

such as *H. influenzae* and gonococci. They have some anaerobic activity and are effective against the atypical bacteria, such as chlamydiae, mycoplasmas, rickettsiae and spirochaetes, and have limited protozoal activity. Tetracyclines are absorbed well orally but the different formulations vary in their half-life, so that doxycycline can be given once daily. They are well distributed in tissues but do not penetrate the CSF and should be used with caution in renal and liver failure. The commonest side effect is gastrointestinal intolerance, but photosensitivity reactions can be troublesome. Tetracyclines cannot be used in childhood or pregnancy because they are concentrated in developing bones and teeth. Owing to these side effects they are not used as first-line treatment of infections apart from rickettsial infections.

CHLORAMPHENICOL

It inhibits protein synthesis by binding to the 50s ribosome, is absorbed well orally, widely distributed in tissues and crosses the blood–brain barrier. Active in Gram-positive and -negative aerobic bacteria and many anaerobic bacteria, mycoplasmas, spirochaetes and rickettsiae. It is bacteriostatic against most microorganisms which limits its use but bactericidal against *H. influenzae* and *Neisseria* sp. The main adverse effect is 'grey-baby' syndrome in neonates due to a lack of hepatic enzyme activity with build-up of unconjugated chloramphenicol, resulting in circulatory collapse. In adults there is reversible dose-dependent bone marrow suppression, but 1 in 40,000 patients develop an irreversible aplastic anaemia. Potential toxic effects have limited its use, so that in the UK it is mainly used topically for ophthalmic infections.

MACROLIDES, FOR EXAMPLE ERYTHROMYCIN AND CLARITHROMYCIN

They inhibit the binding of tRNA to the 50s ribosome. The spectrum of activity is in Gram-positive organisms, *Neisseria* sp., *Haemophilus* sp., *Bordetella* sp. and some Gram-negative anaerobes. They are also active against *Mycoplasmas*, *Rickettsiae* and *Legionella* sp. Absorbed well orally, the newer macrolides such as clarithromycin have better pharmokinetics with a longer half-life and azithromycin is concentrated intracellularly. Important adverse effects include nausea and vomiting as they increase gastric motility, and the intravenous preparations are associated with thrombophlebitis. Macrolides are an alternative therapy for respiratory infections if atypical organism or penicillin allergy is likely and an alternative treatment for chlamydial and campylobacter infections.

FUSIDIC ACID

Fusidic acid inhibits the translocation step of protein synthesis, and is mainly active against *S. aureus*.

Resistance emerges rapidly during treatment unless a second agent is given. It is absorbed well orally with good tissue penetration including brain abscesses, but does not reach the CSF. Generally it is well tolerated but cholestasis and jaundice can develop during therapy but this is much more common if the intravenous formulation is used. Clinical use is in severe staphylococcal infections, particularly bone and joint infections in combination with another anti-staphylococcal agent, and some superficial staphylococcal infections, such as impetigo, but resistance is increasing.

AMINOGLYCOSIDES

Aminoglycosides inhibit bacterial protein synthesis by binding to both subunits of the ribosome, resulting in misreading of the genetic code. They are active in Gram-negative bacilli, *S. aureus*, mycobacteria and *Brucella*, but there is no anaerobic activity and only synergistic activity against streptococci in combination with β-lactam agents. They are not absorbed orally, and therefore have to be given parenterally, and have reduced activity at a low pH. Ototoxicity, nephrotoxicity and neuromuscular paralysis are important side effects, with variations in the degree of toxicity between the different agents with neomycin being the most toxic. Therapeutic monitoring is mandatory because of their narrow therapeutic window and dose is adjusted according to age, renal function and weight. They are used to treat severe Gram-negative and staphylococcal sepsis, in combination with β-lactam agents in endocarditis and streptomycin is used as a second-line treatment for mycobacterial infections and brucellosis.

STREPTOGRAMINS

A combination of compounds binds to the 50s ribosome and cooperate to inhibit protein synthesis. Gram-positive activity includes some multiresistant enterococci, with additional activity against *Mycoplasma* sp., *Chlamydia* sp. and *Legionella* sp. Thrombophlebitis is an important adverse effect and usage is mainly limited to the treatment of resistant Gram-positive infections.

OXAZOLIDINONES, FOR EXAMPLE LINEZOLID

These are a new class of agents, which act on the bacterial ribosome, and display bacteriostatic Gram-positive activity, particularly against resistant staphylococci such as MRSA and vancomycin-resistant enterococci (VRE). Resistance has already been described. They are well absorbed orally. Thrombocytopenia is an adverse effect with prolonged therapy. They may be used as an alternative therapy for resistant Gram-positive infections such as VRE.

Antiviral agents

The scope of antiviral therapy is rapidly expanding as we understand the mechanism of antiviral replication. The need for antiviral agents has increased with the use of immunosuppressive therapies and the emergence of human immunodeficiency virus (HIV) infection. As RNA viruses, for example HIV, have a highly variable genome, drug-resistant mutants are readily produced, which is a particular problem when resistance is encoded by a single mutation event. Thus, combination therapy as with the treatment of tuberculosis (TB) is warranted for some viral infections.

AMANTADINE

Cell penetration of the virus and viral uncoating is inhibited. The spectrum of activity is in influenza A, but resistance can occur when it is used prophylactically. It is well absorbed orally, but central nervous system side effects reduce its use in the elderly. Clinically it is used for both the prophylaxis and treatment of influenza A. With the introduction of the newer agents active against the influenza viruses, usage is likely to be limited in the future.

NUCLEOSIDE ANALOGUES, FOR EXAMPLE ACICLOVIR, VALCICLOVIR, FAMCICLOVIR AND GANCICLOVIR

Chemical analogues of the natural purine or pyrimidine nucleosides, they are only active once they have phosphorylated within the host cell and then interact with the viral DNA or RNA polymerase, becoming incorporated in the nucleotide chain and distorting it or terminating further elongation. Aciclovir, valciclovir and famciclovir are active against herpes simplex virus types 1 and 2 and herpes zoster virus. Resistant mutants can be produced but as they are of low pathogenicity they rarely produce a clinical problem. Ganciclovir is more active against cytomegalovirus (CMV), which has a different thymidine kinase. Aciclovir can be given orally with 15–20 percent bioavailablity and is widely distributed including the CSF, and is excreted renally so doses must be reduced in renal impairment. Valciclovir is an ester of aciclovir and famciclovir an ester of penciclovir with increased bioavailablity, both of which can be used orally. Ganciclovir is poorly absorbed orally and only given intravenously. Among adverse effects are neurotoxicity with toxic levels of aciclovir and bone marrow toxicity with ganciclovir. Aciclovir is used to treat severe herpes simplex and zoster infections, i.e. encephalitis and ganciclovir for severe life-threatening CMV infections.

OTHER ANTIVIRAL DRUGS

Zanamivir and ostelamivir

They inhibit neuraminidase of influenza A and B viruses, thereby inhibiting their release from cells and reducing disease and infectivity. Studies of the inhaled formulation have demonstrated a reduction in the duration of symptoms if used within 48 hours of onset. They are active in influenza A and B viruses. Zanamivir is given locally by inhalation which can precipitate bronchospasm. In the UK both are licensed for the treatment of influenza-like disease in at-risk adults who present within 48 hours of onset, and oseltamivir is also licensed for the treatment of at-risk children and for post-exposure prophylaxis in at-risk adults and adolescents over 13 years of age, when influenza is circulating in the community. Further studies of this and similar agents are awaited.

ANTIRETROVIRAL THERAPY

The introduction of highly active antiretroviral therapy has transformed the treatment of HIV infection, with dramatic sustained reductions in viral load and opportunistic infections. They fall into three main classes.

Nucleoside reverse transcriptase inhibitors, for example zidovudine and lamuvidine

They are nucleoside analogues that inhibit reverse transcriptase thereby inhibiting the conversion from RNA to a DNA copy, and are active in HIV and lamuvidine is also active against hepatitis B virus. Zidovudine is well absorbed orally and crosses the placenta and blood–brain barrier, and the main side effects are anaemia and neutropenia in the first six weeks of therapy. They are the mainstay of antiretroviral therapy and are used in combination to inhibit emergence of resistant strains.

Non–nucleoside reverse transcriptase inhibitors

These agents also inhibit the reverse trancriptase enzyme, but resistance emerges quickly on monotherapy, so that they can only be used in combination.

Protease inhibitors

Protease inhibitors include the antiretroviral agents indinavir, ritonavir and saquinavir which have activity against HIV. Some also have activity against enteroviruses, hepatitis C and rhinoviruses and are under investigation. They produce the greatest fall in HIV viral load but can cause significant toxicity, for example renal stones and lipodystrophy.

Antifungal therapy

Systemic fungal infections are an increasing problem with the emergence of resistant *Candida* sp. and the increased incidence of infections due to invasive moulds. Many antifungal therapies exist but a large number are toxic and therefore can only be used topically. Development of newer antifungal agents, such as the echinocandins, which

target the fungal cell wall more specifically, are promising. Antifungal resistance can be either primary, i.e. the organism is resistant prior to treatment, secondary, i.e. develops after exposure to antifungals, or clinical resistance, i.e. progression of the fungal infection despite treatment to which the organism is sensitive. Clinical resistance is particularly seen in profoundly immunosuppressed patients or where there is infected prosthetic material. Sensitivity testing of fungi is difficult to carry out and reproduce and does not always correlate with the clinical response. The main classes of systemic and topical antifungals are discussed below.

POLYENES

Polyenes, for example amphotericin and nystatin, bind to the sterols of eukaryotic cell membranes, causing leakage of cell contents, most can only be used topically as they can act on mammalian cell walls. Amphotericin B is active against nearly all fungi which produce human disease, and in addition, is active against *Leishmania* sp. Development of resistance has only rarely been described. Amphotericin is given parenterally for systemic infection as it is not absorbed orally and, as it is highly protein bound, and therefore enters the CSF poorly. Adverse effects include the infusion-related side effects of fever, rigors and headaches which can be reduced with the co-administration of steroids, also renal toxicity and hyperkalaemia. The incidence of serious side effects has been reduced by the incorporation of the amphotericin B into liposomes or other lipid carriers. This allows higher doses to be given with fewer toxic reactions. Nystatin is only used topically for yeast infections, whereas amphotericin is mainly used parenterally for severe invasive yeast infections, aspergillosis and other mould infections.

AZOLES

The azoles are the largest group of antifungal agents, inhibiting cytochrome P450 14α-demethylase that is required for fungal cell wall synthesis. They are active in *Candida* sp., dermatophytes, with some activity against *Aspergillus* sp.

Imidazoles

The topical imidazoles, such as clotrimazole are powerful agents against oral, vaginal and skin candidiasis and dermatophytes infections. The oral formulation of the imidazole ketoconazole is generally more toxic than the triazoles, as 1 in 15,000 patients develop hepatitis.

Triazoles

Fluconazole has activity against most *Candida* sp. and *Cryptococcus* sp., but no activity against invasive moulds. Primary resistance is common with some non-albicans *Candida* sp., particularly *Candida krusei* and *Candida glabrata.*[4] Itraconazole and variconazole have improved activity over invasive moulds including *Aspergillus* sp. and *Fusarium* sp., but not the zygomycetes.

ECHINOCANDINS, FOR EXAMPLE CAPSOFUNGIN

Echinocandins are a new class of antifungals, which inhibit cell-wall glucan synthesis, leading to fungal cell lysis. Rapidly fungicidal against *Candida* sp., including azole-resistant species, they are active against *Aspergillus* sp., but not other moulds or *Cryptococcus* sp.

ALLYLAMINES, FOR EXAMPLE TERBINAFINE

Allylamines reduce ergosterol synthesis. The spectrum of activity is in dermatophytes, with poor intrinsic activity against yeasts and moulds, and are used in extensive skin and nail dermatophyte infections.

Other antifungal agents

FLUCYTOSINE

Flucytosine incorporates into fungal mRNA in the place of uracil, causing disruption to protein synthesis and DNA synthesis. Activity is in *Candida* sp. and *Cryptococcus* sp. only. Resistance is a common problem arising during treatment. Levels should be monitored and the dose reduced in renal failure. Important adverse effects are bone marrow toxicity and hepatotoxicity. It is used in combination therapy for severe candidal and cryptococcal infections such as meningitis.

GRISEOFULVIN

Griseofluvin is used to treat nail infections as it has restricted activity against dermatophytes but the mechanism of action is unclear.

ANTIMICROBIAL RESISTANCE

In the UK, the prevalence of resistant Gram-positive isolates is increasing, with 1.5 percent in 1990 and 3.9 percent in 1995 of pneumococcal isolates demonstrating low-level penicillin resistance, and 2.8 percent in 1990 and 8.6 percent in 1995 macrolide resistance.[5] [**] In Eastern Europe, Spain and the USA the rates of penicillin and macrolides resistance in pneumococci are even higher.[6] [**] There has also been an increase in glycopeptide-resistant enterococci. Although new agents with Gram-positive activity are being developed there is no reason to believe that resistance to these agents will not emerge.[7] [**]

In addition, the number of multiresistant Gram-negative organisms, resistant to all the main Gram-negative antimicrobials are becoming an increasing problem in hospitals, and multidrug-resistant TB isolates have resulted in failures of TB treatment.

Antimicrobial resistance is not new, as some organisms are inherently resistant to antimicrobial agents either due to differences in the cellular target of the antimicrobial agent or inactivation of the antimicrobial. These mechanisms can be acquired by other organisms either by genetic mutation and selection of the resistant clone or acquisition of the genetic material required to produce the resistance in the form of plasmids, transposons or naked DNA. In the presence of antimicrobial selection pressure, organisms able to produce resistance determinants will be favoured. Unfortunately, some strains possess multiple resistance determinants which are more difficult to control as any of the antimicrobials can exert a positive selective pressure, for example MRSA strains currently circulating are resistant to all the β-lactam agents, quinolones and can be resistant to the macrolide antibiotics.

Antimicrobial sensitivity testing

An organism is defined as sensitive to an antimicrobial if the antimicrobial is active at concentrations that can be achieved therapeutically. The minimum inhibitory concentration (MIC) is the lowest concentration of the antimicrobial agent at which growth of the test organism is completely inhibited, whereas the minimal bactericidal concentration is the lowest concentration of the antimicrobial agent which achieves 99.9 percent killing of the test organism. Bactericidal activity is particularly important if infection is in a difficult site, such as a vegetation in endocarditis or in immunocompromised patients, where the additional effects of phagocytosis and antibody-dependent killing cannot be achieved. Agents that only achieve bacterial inhibition of replication are known as bacteriostatic agents.

Sensitivity testing can be performed by a number of methods. In a routine diagnostic laboratory determination of the MIC is time-consuming and too cumbersome to be carried out routinely. More rapid indirect methods are used which allow a number of organisms to be tested against a range of antimicrobials. A common method is the Stokes method, in which known concentrations of the antibiotic are impregnated into a disc that is released into the agar onto which the test organism and a control organism have been inoculated (**Figure 19.2**). The zone of inhibition of growth is compared with the known test organism after overnight incubation. The breakpoint method is used to test multiple organisms that are inoculated onto different agar plates containing high and low concentrations of a range of antimicrobials (**Figure 19.3**).

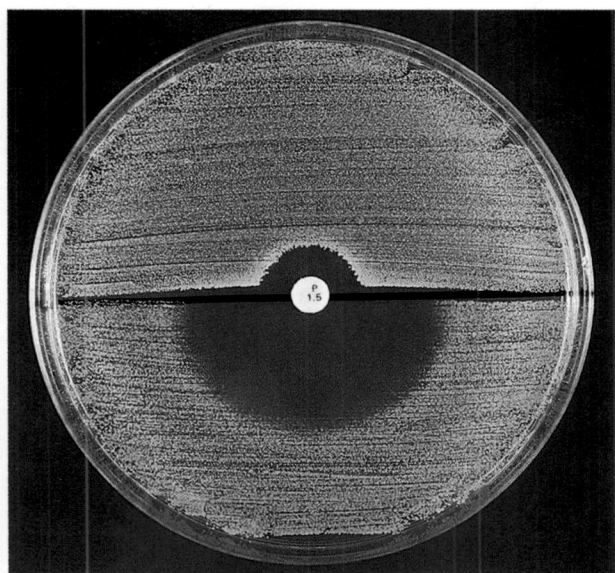

Figure 19.2 Antimicrobial sensitivity testing of *S. aureus* against penicillin (P 1.5) using the modified Stokes method, demonstrating penicillin resistance in the test organism (top) and penicillin sensitivity in the control organism (bottom).

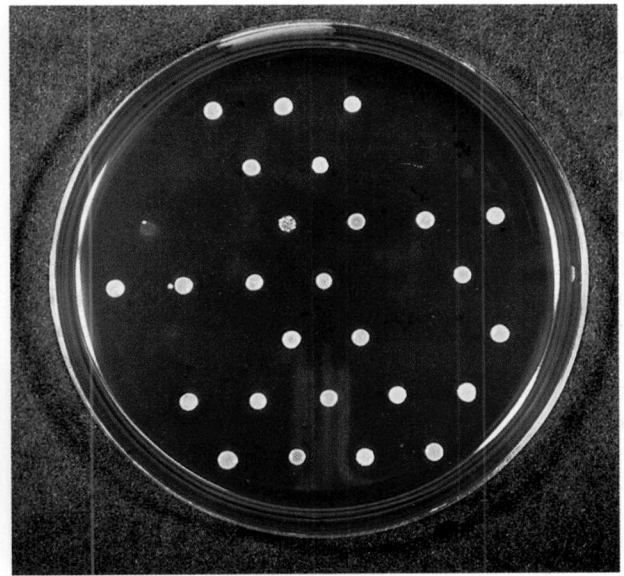

Figure 19.3 Breakpoint sensitivity testing of multiple staphylococcal isolates against penicillin at a concentration of 0.1 mg/L. Growth of organisms at that concentration demonstrates penicillin resistance and where there is no growth there is penicillin sensitivity.

For more slow-growing organisms antimicrobial sensitivity testing can be slow, difficult to reproduce and technically difficult. Newer molecular methods have been developed for some of the slow-growing organisms where the genetic basis for the resistance is known, such as polymerase chain reaction to detect the rifampicin resistance gene in *Mycobacterium tuberculosis* isolates.

Laboratory sensitivity testing measures the activity of a known concentration of the pure drug against an organism growing exponentially in an artificial culture, which does not reflect the situation at the site of an active infection. Results should therefore be used as a guide to likely active antimicrobial therapy.

The main mechanisms of antimicrobial resistance are described below.

Antimicrobial-inactivating enzymes

Some organisms naturally produce enzymes that will inactivate antimicrobial agents, for example the β-lactamases, with over 95 percent of *S. aureus* isolates resistant due to the production of this enzyme. Other β-lactamases are able to break down the β-lactam bond of the cephalosporins and have been acquired by Gram-negative organisms. Enzymes can also inactivate the aminoglycosides.

Altered antimicrobial binding site

The action of an antimicrobial can be reduced or inhibited by alterations in the cellular target. Penicillin resistance in pneumococci results from an alteration in the affinity of the penicillin-binding protein, with production of a cell wall that will not bind penicillin, the genetic mechanism for which has been acquired from commensal oral streptococci. Resistance to the sulphonamides and trimethoprim can occur due to alterations in the target enzymes in the folate synthesis pathway. Many viruses develop resistance to antiviral agents by point mutations in the genes which encode the antiviral target protein, for example HIV resistance to lamivudine.

Altered antimicrobial penetration

Alteration of the bacterial outer cell membrane may prevent penetration of a particular class of antimicrobials into the cell, for example in *Pseudomonas aeruginosa*. Bacteria may also become resistant by rapid removal of the antimicrobial from the cell before it is able to act, as seen with the tetracyclines.

ADVERSE EFFECTS OF ANTIMICROBIAL AGENTS

The basic principle of antimicrobial chemotherapy is selective toxicity, i.e. killing of the microorganism with no toxic effects to the patient. Most antimicrobial agents have a wide therapeutic window. Adverse events are either dose dependent, such as renal toxicity of aminoglycosides, or idiosyncratic reactions, such as anaphylaxis with penicillins.

Cutaneous adverse effects

These vary from fixed drug eruptions, photosensitivity rashes through to life-threatening Stevens-Johnson syndrome. The sulphonamides are well known to be a common cause of these cutaneous reactions. Mild itchy rashes are common with penicillins and cephalosporins. Anaphylaxis occurs if the antimicrobial agent initiates a type I hypersensitivy reaction; this is an uncommon event that occurs in about 1 in 100,000 treatments.

Haematological effects

Bone marrow toxicity can result from the normal action of the drug, an idiosyncratic reaction or immune mechanisms. Irreversible aplastic anaemia is an uncommon but serious idiosyncratic side effect of chloramphenicol therapy. Metabolic bone marrow suppression can occur in agents which affect nucleic acid synthesis, such as the antivirals zidovudine and ganciclovir, or those which reduce folate synthesis, such as the sulphonamides. Reversible granulocytopenia alone can also occur with the sulphonamides and with prolonged high doses of the penicillins and cephalosporins usually after two to three weeks of high-dose therapy. Occasionally, antibiotics can induce the production of antibodies to red cells or platelets, producing Coombs' positive haemolytic anaemia, such as with rifampicin or immune thrombocytopenia.

Liver toxicity

Damage to the liver can be acute or chronic hepatitis, cholestasis, fatty degeneration or granulomatous hepatitis. Hepatocellular damage is the commonest form of damage to the liver, most often seen with the antituberculous agents rifampicin and isoniazid, which in combination cause hepatitis in about 5 percent of cases. Granulomatous hepatitis is a rare side effect of high-dose ampicillin and flucloxacillin therapy and after prolonged quinine therapy. Cholestatic jaundice is most commonly seen with fusidic acid therapy particularly with doses above 2 g/day and with the intravenous preparation.

Gastrointestinal side effects

Antimicrobials similar to other drugs can produce nausea, vomiting and diarrhoea, but with antimicrobial agents, diarrhoea can be caused by the alteration of the colonic microflora and the overgrowth of toxin producing

C. difficile. Clostridium difficile infection can result in a spectrum of disease from asymptomatic carriage or mild diarrhoea through to severe diarrhoea with pseudomembranous colitis. Although most antibiotics have been associated with a predisposition to *C. difficile* infection, the most commonly implicated agents have been clindamycin, cephalosporins and ampicillin.[8] [**] More recently, the quinolone antibiotics have also been implicated.

Renal toxicity

Renal damage can happen for a number of reasons during therapy. Direct renal cell damage or nephrotoxicity can occur with a number of antimicrobials, particularly the aminoglycosides and amphotericin. The aminoglycosides are toxic to the cells of the proximal renal tubules at serum levels close to the levels required to produce an antimicrobial affect, i.e. there is a narrow therapeutic index. This toxicity is more likely to arise in the elderly and those with pre-existing renal impairment and treatment with other potentially nephrotoxic agents. They can also be ototoxic leading to impaired hearing and vestibular damage. To prevent this happening therapy must be closely monitored and doses adjusted according to age, weight and renal function. Renal toxicity is commonly seen with amphotericin therapy, which has led to the production of liposonal formulations that are less nephrotoxic.

KEY POINTS

- The pace of development of antibiotic resistance has become faster than the development of new antibacterial agents.
- Antibiotic resistance is threatening the effective treatment of infections both in the community and hospital.
- Novel new antifungal and antiviral therapies are under development.

Best clinical practice

✓ The decision to use antimicrobials should be with knowledge of the likely causative organism(s), antimicrobial sensitivity, site of infection, spectrum of activity of the antimicrobial and the risks of treatment and of untreated infection.
✓ Use antibiotics for surgical prophylaxis where there is proven benefit.
✓ Do not give repeated or prolonged courses of antimicrobials without evidence of benefit.

✓ Try and use narrow-spectrum agents where adequate cover for the likely organism(s) is achieved.
✓ Follow your local antimicrobial guidelines and liaise with your local microbiologist for difficult infections, as rates of resistant organisms vary from area to area.

REFERENCES

1. Reacher MH, Shah A, Livermore DM, Wale MC, Graham C, Johanson AP et al. Bacteraemia and antibiotic resistance of its pathogens reported in England and Wales between 1990 and 1998: trend analysis. *British Medical Journal.* 2000; **320**: 213–6.

∗ 2. House of Lords Select Committee on Science and Technology. *Resistance to antibiotics and other antimicrobial agents.* London: HMSO, 1998.

∗ 3. Standing Medical Advisory Committee Subgroup on Antimicrobial Resistance. *The path of least resistance.* London: Department of Health, 1998.

4. Kontoyiannis DP, Lewis R. Antifungal resistance of pathogenic fungi. *Lancet.* 2002; **359**: 1135–44.

∗ 5. Johnson AP. Antibiotic resistance among clinically important Gram-positive bacteria in the UK. *Journal of Hospital Infection.* 1998; **40**: 17–26.

6. Appelbaum PC. Antimicrobial resistance in *Streptococcus pneumoniae*: An overview. *Clinical Infectious Diseases.* 1992; **15**: 77–83.

7. Andrews J, Ashby J, Jevons G, Marshall T, Lines N, Wise R. A comparison of antimicrobial resistance rates in Gram-positive pathogens isolated in the UK from October 1996 to January 1997 and October 1997 to January 1998. *Journal of Antimicrobial Chemotherapy.* 2000; **45**: 285–93.

8. Spencer RC. The role of antimicrobial agents in the aetiology of Clostridium difficile-associated disease. *Journal of Antimicrobial Chemotherapy.* 1998; **41**: 21–7.

20

HIV and otolaryngology

THOMAS A TAMI AND JAHMAL A HAIRSTON

Introduction	238	Pharynx and larynx	243
Human immunodeficiency virus	238	Oesophagus	244
Therapy	239	Salivary glands	245
Occupational exposure	239	Neck	246
Head and neck manifestations	240	Dermatologic	247
Nose and paranasal sinus	241	Key points	248
Oral cavity	242	References	248

SEARCH STRATEGY

The information and data in this chapter were produced from a Medline search using the key words otolaryngology, HIV, AIDS, otology, occupational exposure and lymphoma.

INTRODUCTION

Human immunodeficiency virus (HIV) and the acquired immunodeficiency syndrome (AIDS) has had a profound effect on the practice of medicine in the 20 years since its discovery. Initially a disease of homosexual men and haemophiliacs, it is now a disease that affects individuals of every age, sex and socioeconomic group, becoming a worldwide epidemic and spreading into regions of the globe such as Southeast Asia. There are over one million HIV-positive people in China alone, and the number is steadily growing. Women form an increasing subset of patients and with this comes vertical transmission of the virus from mother to child. Head and neck manifestations of the disease are prevalent, and up to 100 percent of HIV patients will have some head and neck presentation of the disease during the course of their illness.

HUMAN IMMUNODEFICIENCY VIRUS

HIV is an example of a retrovirus, a virus whose genetic material is present in the form of ribonucleic acid (RNA) instead of DNA. Its genetic material is a diploid, single-stranded RNA that uses the enzyme reverse transcriptase to convert its ssRNA into double-stranded DNA. The HIV has a lipid bilayer membrane for an outer cell envelope that is acquired from the host cell from which it was produced. This envelope contains two glycoproteins, (gp)41 and gp120, which form a complex essential for cell proliferation. The gp120 glycoprotein binds to the CD4 receptor on the host-cell membrane. CD4 receptor is found in highest concentrations in T helper lymphocytes, and it is through these cells that HIV primarily proliferates. CD4 receptors are also found in lesser numbers in monocytes/macrophages. Once gp120 and the CD4 receptor are bound, the viral and host-cell membranes fuse. This allows the viral contents to be injected into the host cell. Reverse transcriptase then catalyzes the synthesis of viral DNA from RNA. The viral DNA then migrates into the host-cell nucleus and integrates itself into the host DNA. Once incorporated, the viral DNA is replicated along with the host cell DNA and passed onto progeny cells. The provirus, once activated, begins to synthesize new virus particles (RNA, reverse transcriptase and other enzymes) using host cell transcription machinery. These particles assemble beneath the host-cell membrane and then bud through, thus acquiring their own membrane from the host. The host cell is subsequently destroyed during this process and the viral particles infect new CD4-positive cells. As helper T lymphocytes are the primary cells infected, their destruction is what primarily causes immunodeficiency in the host. Cells of the monocyte/macrophage lineage have also been shown to express CD4 and thus can be infected by HIV and act as reservoirs.[1, 2]

Once initial infection occurs there is often a clinical latency period of approximately six to ten years, during which time there may be no symptoms. During this latency period, viral replication and $CD4^+$ lymphocyte destruction continues. As the $CD4^+$ count decreases, the patient's clinical course worsens. In 1986, the Centers for Disease Control (CDC), together with the World Health Organization, attempted to establish a staging system for AIDS which used clinical criteria to stage disease progression. A second staging system by the CDC followed which classified the different stages of HIV infection from asymptomatic to full-blown disease.[3] The Walter Reed Staging Classification was developed in 1986, dividing HIV infection into six stages and including analysis of CD4 counts. The absolute T helper lymphocyte count is still currently used to measure disease progression.

Upon initial infection with HIV, the patient may be asymptomatic. However, 50–70 percent of people will have an acute illness within two to six weeks of infection consisting of acute onset of fever, mucocutaneous ulceration, maculopapular rash and pharyngitis. This syndrome lasts about two weeks. These patients may be seronegative, but have high titres of virus in the bloodstream and are highly infectious. Viral loads decrease as serum antibody to HIV increases, and by six months most patients are seropositive. Patients at this stage are generally asymptomatic. Circulating CD4 counts are generally high during this period, which may last for years. Once the CD4 counts start to decrease, symptomatology may resume beginning with fatigue and generalized lymphadenopathy. Further decreases in CD4 count produce more constitutional symptoms including fever, sweats, chills, weight loss, night sweats and diarrhoea. With further declines, the patient becomes susceptible to more opportunistic infections and neoplasms, some of which (e.g. *Pneumocystis carinii* pneumonia) are essentially diagnostic for AIDS.

THERAPY

Currently, there is no vaccine or cure for infection with HIV, which is universally fatal. However, with further elucidation not only of the life cycle of the virus but the progression of infection, various agents have been created which have helped to extend the life of HIV-infected individuals. Secondary treatment for HIV includes symptomatic treatment of opportunistic infections. Primary treatment consists of a variety of drugs that inhibit viral progression at different stages of its life cycle.

One of the earliest classes of drugs created was the nucleoside analogues, one of the first being 3′azido3′deoxythymidone zidovudine (AZT). This class of drugs acts as an antimetabolite by becoming phosphorylated and binding to and inhibiting reverse transcriptase. The benefits of this class of drugs are limited by the emergence of viral resistance. Toxicity of this class of drugs includes fatigue, nausea, headache, macrocytic anaemia and neutropenia.

Another class of antiretroviral drugs is the non-nucleoside analogues. Nevirapine and delavirdine are two agents in this class.[2, 4] The major side effect of these drugs is a rash.

The protease inhibitors are a class of drugs that act by inhibiting the protease used to cleave polypeptides in the budding virion into their functional form, thus halting viral maturation. Drugs in this class include saquinavir, ritonavir, indinavir and nelfinavir. Toxicities are variable among the different drugs. Saquinavir has the least side effects (diarrhoea, nausea, abdominal discomfort), but also has the least efficacy and bioavailability. Ritonavir is on the opposite side of the spectrum with high efficacy but also more side effects including more severe gastrointestinal side effects and elevations in liver function tests and triglycerides.

OCCUPATIONAL EXPOSURE

Physician exposure to HIV-infected individuals will continue to rise as the prevalence of HIV infection increases. Many of these encounters will occur without the physician or the patient having any knowledge of infection. Of HIV-infected patients 70–80 percent will have some manifestation necessitating evaluation by an otolaryngologist. Very few seroconversions have occurred despite numerous job-related exposures to body fluid contaminated with HIV. The risk of contracting HIV after a single hollow needlestick injury is 0.36–0.5 percent if the incident involves blood known to have the HIV virus.[5] Sticks involving solid needles, metal wires and scalpels have a lower risk. Universal Blood and Body Precautions was issued by the CDC in 1987, and was an attempt to set out standards that can be used by all healthcare providers to decrease the risk of HIV exposure. The basis of these precautions is that every patient should be seen as potentially HIV positive, and protective measures instituted. The use of latex gloves and double gloving, to decrease risk of exposure from puncture injury, has been advocated. There were specific recommendations for handling sharp instruments as they are involved in most accidental stick injuries. Needle stick injuries are a common source of injury, and therefore needles should never be recapped. In the operating theatre or the office, avoidance of direct hand-to-hand passage can be avoided by using a magnetic pad, kidney basin or Mayo stand. Using staples during wound closure instead of sutures also decreases the risk of inadvertent stick injury. Protective eye wear and gowns should always be worn in the operating theatre and are even recommended in some office encounters where the risk of encountering contaminated secretions is high.

In cases where the physician or healthcare worker is exposed to blood or bodily secretions, the area of skin or wound that was exposed should be immediately washed with soap and water. If the patient's HIV status is unknown, informed consent should be obtained for testing of the patient for HIV as well as hepatitis B and C. The involved healthcare worker should have a baseline HIV test performed, with subsequent tests at six weeks and three months.[6] Chemoprophylaxis is recommended for workers sustaining puncture injuries or high-risk contact with contaminated body fluids and should be instituted within two hours after exposure. AZT is recommended for all prophylaxis regimens with the addition of a protease inhibitor for higher-risk exposures.

HEAD AND NECK MANIFESTATIONS

Otologic

EXTERNAL EAR

Seborrhoeic dermatitis and Kaposi's sarcoma (KS) are dermatologic lesions that can occur on the pinna and the external auditory canal (EAC). Seborrhoeic dermatitis can occur in the periauricular region and the EAC as well as the face and scalp. Applying a zinc pyrithone-containing shampoo over the affected area typically treats it. Other treatments include washing with coal tar, selenium sulphide or ketoconazole. A 1-percent hydrocortisone lotion may be used as adjunctive treatment in refractory cases. Seborrhoeic dermatitis often recurs and this fact should be included in patient education. Karposi's sarcoma has an incidence higher in the AIDS population than the general population. When the pinna or external auditory canal is involved, a conductive hearing loss may manifest secondary to obstruction. Treatment of KS will be further detailed under dermatologic manifestations.

Staphylococcus aureus is the usual bacteria involved when there is a cellulitis of the pinna, and usually resolves with either oral antibiotics or i.v. antibiotics in more severe cases. Otitis externa is a severe infection of the external auditory canal most frequently caused by Pseudomonas aeruginosa. Symptoms include severe otalgia, otorrhoea and fever. Treatment involves topical antibiotics and/or 2-percent acetic acid and steroid drops in addition to canal debridement as often as is necessary. If severe swelling occurs, a wick should be placed in the EAC to maintain patency and further direct topical drops.

In HIV and/or diabetic patients in whom the above measures do not result in improvement, osteomyelitis of the skull base should be suspected. Other warning symptoms include facial nerve or cranial nerve dysfunction. Diagnosis can be confirmed using a computed tomography (CT) scan of the temporal bone or technetium 99m-bone scan. Treatment is six weeks of antibiotics. Coverage should be broad spectrum and include coverage against P. aeruginosa.[7] [**] Surgical debridement may be necessary in more severe cases. Aspergillus fumigata can also present as a chronic otitis externa. In severely immunocompromised individuals, Aspergillus infection can become invasive with subsequent skull base and intracranial extension.

Any subcutaneous cyst or polyp in the EAC should be biopsied. Pneumocystis carinii may present as either a cyst or polyp, and the cyst if allowed to grow can occlude the EAC.[2] The diagnosis is made by biopsy and staining with Gomori's methenamine silver stain, and treatment with trimethoprim/sulphamethoxazole usually results in resolution of infection. Mycobacterium tuberculosis can also present as a polyp in the external auditory canal.

MIDDLE EAR

The most common otologic entities seen in HIV-positive individuals are serous and recurrent otitis media. Pathogenic organisms involved include Streptococcus pneumonia, Haemophilus influenzae and Moraxcella catarrhalis. Pseudomonas and Staphylococcus organisms have been isolated more commonly from the AIDS population than the general population. There is a variety of aetiologies that includes Eustachian tube dysfunction, nasopharyngeal neoplasms, adenoid hypertrophy and sinusitis/allergies. Nasopharyngeal neoplasms should be ruled out in HIV-infected individuals, particularly with unilateral otitis media. Myringotomy and tympanostomy tube placement can offer symptomatic relief easily and quickly. Treatment of associated sinusitis or allergies should also be instituted. Adenoidectomy is indicated when more conservative measures fail.

Mastoiditis in the AIDS population is usually caused by S. pneumonia. Its incidence does not appear to be increased in the AIDS population versus the general population. Antibiotic therapy directed towards the pathogens most commonly responsible for otitis media is usually sufficient treatment, although there have been reported cases of atypical organisms causing mastoiditis such as A. fumigata.[8] Intravenous antibiotics and surgical drainage is indicated for coalescing suppurative mastoiditis.

INNER EAR

Individuals with HIV and AIDS can have a high rate of otologic symptoms referable to the inner ear. They can present with aural fullness, vertigo, tinnitus and sensorineural hearing loss. These symptoms can be caused by the virus itself which can affect the central nervous system or CN VIII; or can be a side effect of the many medications that these patients often take. Many of the opportunistic infections that this population is prone to can cause sensorineural hearing loss, infections such as cytomegalovirus (CMV), herpes simplex virus (HSV) and herpes zoster virus. Cytomegalovirus, although well documented as a cause of congenital deafness, has not been directly implicated in adult onset hearing loss. It has been shown in temporal bone autopsy studies to have infected the inner ear in approximately 20 percent of those bones studied. Some of the ototoxic medications that these patients take include acyclovir, gancyclovir, AZT and isoniazid. Otosyphilis can present at any stage of HIV infection, and HIV infection can hasten development of otosyphilis in the latent stage of the disease. Diagnosis is primarily by clinical history with confirmatory serologic studies (fluorescent treponemal antibody absorption test. Symptoms primarily consist of low frequency hearing loss, labyrinthine symptoms and aural fullness may or may not be present.[9] Treatment is with high-dose penicillin and steroids. In AIDS patients, long-term steroid use should be avoided and it is suggested that any patient in a high-risk population who presents with sudden onset unilateral or bilateral hearing loss be tested for HIV prior to institution of steroid therapy. Steroid use may be contraindicated if there is concomitant opportunistic infection.

The work-up for hearing loss by the otolaryngologist in an HIV-infected individual with hearing loss should include an audiogram, auditory brain stem response and serologic treponemal testing. Imaging with CT is appropriate when neurologic findings are found on neurologic examination.

Facial nerve palsy can occur in up to 7.2 percent of HIV patients and is referable to direct infection by the HIV, neoplasms, opportunistic infections, AIDS encephalopathy and toxoplasmosis. Bell's palsy is the most frequent diagnosis given for CN VII paralysis. It is postulated to be caused by HSV and is a diagnosis of exclusion. Complete recovery usually occurs within three weeks to three months.[2, 10] Ramsay Hunt syndrome (herpes zoster oticus) usually occurs later in HIV infection and is more prevalent in AIDS patients. Symptoms include peripheral facial nerve palsy, herpetic vesicles along the seventh nerve dermatome and in the conchal bowl, and severe herpetic pain. The aetiology of this syndrome is varicella zoster virus infection of the geniculate ganglion. The diagnosis is clinical, and evaluation should include an audiogram and electrophysiological tests. Treatment is with high-dose acyclovir and high-dose steroids when not contraindicated.

NOSE AND PARANASAL SINUS

Thirty to sixty-eight percent of HIV-positive patients will manifest some form of nasal and/or sinus symptom.[11]

Nasal obstruction secondary to a variety of aetiologies is a complaint that commonly causes these patients to see an otolaryngologist. Adenoidal hypertrophy can present as nasal obstruction, as can hypertrophy of any of the tissues in Waldeyer's ring. Any nonpediatric patient with adenoid hypertrophy should be tested for HIV. The obstruction caused by lymphoid hyperplasia can lead to a variety of other aetiologies including otitis media with effusion and upper airway obstruction. As with any nonimmunocompromised adult, unilateral otitis media with effusion warrants a thorough nasopharyngeal examination. Treatment should start with medical therapy that consists of topical steroid sprays and antibiotics. Surgical measures include adenoidectomy and a pressure equalization tube placement in refractory cases.

Neoplasms such as KS or non-Hodgkin's lymphoma (NHL) can also cause nasal obstruction.[12] Both lesions can arise from the nasal cavity or nasopharynx. Kaposi's sarcoma can also arise from the nasal septum. Non-Hodgkin's lymphoma can also arise from the sinuses.

Sinusitis in HIV-positive individuals is similar in symptomotology to that in noninfected persons. Symptoms include purulent nasal discharge, facial pain, headache and congestion. In HIV-positive persons with fever of unknown origin, the sinuses should always be investigated for possible infection. The bacteria involved in sinusitis include *S. pneumonia*, *M. catarrhalis* and *H. influenzae* and are similar to that of nonimmunocompromised patients. In chronic sinusitis, *S. aureus* and anaerobic bacteria become more common. As the CD4 count decreases below 50/μL, fungal infection of the sinuses can occur (**Figure 20.1**), with the majority of fungal infections the result of *Aspergillus*.[13] Other pathogens reported in the literature include CMV,[14]

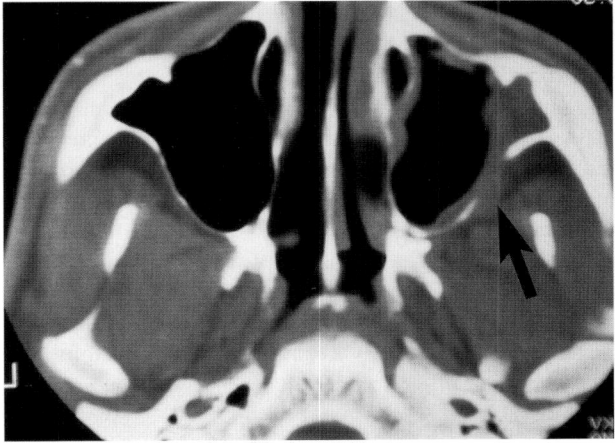

Figure 20.1 In advanced HIV disease, invasive fungal infection of the paranasal sinuses must be considered. As seen in this axial CT scan, subtle bony erosion with extension into the infratemporal fossa (arrow) indicates an invasive fungal process.

Microsporidia,[15] *Acanthamoeba castellani*[16] and *Legionella pneumophila*.

Evaluation of sinusitis in HIV-positive patients is similar to that of HIV-negative patients. Nasal endoscopy can be performed in the office, and the physician should not only look for signs of sinusitis (purulent discharge), but also evaluate the nose and posterior choanae for adenoid hypertrophy, nasal masses/neoplasms, destructive lesions, etc. In addition, endoscopy is simple to perform and can be used to follow the patient's response to management. Imaging should be performed by CT scan, which gives superior visualization of all the sinuses, particularly the sphenoid sinuses and posterior ethmoids.

The hallmarks of medical management of sinusitis are antibiotics and decongestants. Oral antibiotics should be instituted for three to four weeks. First-line antibiotics include amoxicillin, Augmentin (amoxicillin/clavulanate), cephalosporins and Bactrim (sulphamethoxazole/trimethoprim). Augmentin and the cephalosporins offer more broad-spectrum coverage. During the three to four week period of antibiotics, decongestants should also be part of the medical therapy. Systemic decongestants, such as pseudoephedrine, are recommended but their use may be limited in patients with underlying hypertension or cardiac problems. Topical decongestants such as oxymetazoline may be used, but their use should be limited to three to five days secondary to possible rebound congestion upon cessation of use. Topical nasal steroids may also be considered as an adjunctive therapy. There is also evidence suggesting a role for quaifensin therapy for these patients.[17]

The bacteriology of chronic sinusitis differs from that of acute sinusitis. In patients with CD4 counts $< 200/\mu$L, *S. aureus*, *P. aeruginosa* and anaerobes become more prominent, and antibiotic therapy should be broadened to include these organisms. Cultures should be obtained to confirm the bacteriology and further direct treatment. Antibiotics should be instituted for up to six weeks.[18]

Surgery is advocated in patients with persistent symptoms despite medical therapy, or in any patient at any time with extra-sinus symptoms (mental status changes, cranial nerve dysfunction, intracranial extension, abscess, etc.). Endoscopic sinus surgery is particularly effective. It can be performed as an outpatient procedure, and has low morbidity. The goal of surgery should be symptomatic relief, as well as optimizing nasal anatomy to facilitate drainage of the sinuses. However, as HIV disease progression continues and CD4 counts decrease, the physician can expect recurrent sinus infections that become more difficult to treat.

ORAL CAVITY

Oral cavity manifestations of AIDS are extremely common and can occur in up to 100 percent of AIDS patients. Recurrent apthous ulcers are common in immunocompromised patients, are generally larger than those in nonimmunocompromised patients and can vary in size from 1 mm to 4 cm. On physical examination, the lesions are solitary or multiple appearing, have an erythematous halo that is well circumscribed, and may have an exudate or pseudomembrane. The lesions are tender to palpation, and in giant apthous ulcers can cause severe odynophagia and pain. In severe cases, the pain may accentuate the anorexia and dehydration that can be seen in AIDS patients. Treatment is primarily to provide symptomatic relief. Topical anesthetics or steroids are often effective in less severe cases. Miles' mixture (liquid tetracycline, hydrocortisone and viscous lidocaine in Orabase with nystatin) is a combination of various topical agents that is often effective. Topical tetracycline has also been shown to be an effective analgesic agent. Topical tetracycline or systemic clindamycin are effective agents when superimposed infection is present.

An intralesional steroid injection with triamcinolone acetonide has been shown to have analgesic effects within 24–48 hours after injection, and has very few side effects.[19] [**] Oral thalidomide has been shown in some studies to heal ulcers completely in 55 percent of patients and partially in 90 percent of patients, but is only recommended to be used for two to four weeks at a time secondary to increased production of HIV and tumour necrosis factor-alpha.[20] [**] Thalidomide also has teratogenic effects limiting its use in women, who comprise an increasing number of AIDS patients.

Oral candidiasis is an infection that presents as a tender white plaque atop an erythematous and erosive mucosal surface. In some forms, the lesions can be removed with scraping, leaving a friable, bleeding base. In the chronic hypertrophic form, the plaques are heaped up and not easily removed with scraping. As with recurrent apthous ulcers, the lesions can be extremely painful, leading to malnutrition, dehydration and wasting if not effectively treated. Treatment in patients who are not severely immunocompromised consists of Nystatin solution that is swished around the mouth and swallowed. Clotrimazole troches are also effective. Systemic therapy is indicated in patients with worsening immunocompromise or thrush unresponsive to topical agents. Ketoconazole or fluconazole are two agents frequently used. Severe cases require amphotericin administered intravenously.

Hairy leukoplakia is unique to HIV-positive individuals and typically arises on the lateral border of the tongue as a white, raised, corrugated or filiform lesion. It can also arise on the dorsal tongue, buccal and labial mucosa, floor of mouth or soft palate. It requires no treatment and is usually asymptomatic.

Oral herpes simplex commonly presents as herpes labialis (fever blisters, cold sores), the most common manifestation of infection in HIV patients. The lesions frequently present as small bullae that form ulcerations after they rupture. These lesions are painful and in HIV patients, generally larger than in immunocompetent individuals. Treatment consists of oral acyclovir.

Gingivitis in HIV patients tends to be more severe than in noninfected patients. It can easily progress to a necrotizing gingivitis or severe periodontal disease. Gingivitis presents as erythema of the gum line with inflammation and interdental soft tissue papillae edema. Bleeding from the gums can occur with seemingly light or no trauma. Periodontitis presents as loosening of periodontal attachments. It can progress to acute necrotizing ulcerative gingivitis which is an ulcerative process along the gingival margin leading to destruction of the periodontal soft tissues. Treatment consists of antibiotics aimed at anaerobic organisms and topical irrigations with chlorhexidine gluconate. If available, a referral to a dentist or oral surgeon should be made early in the process.[21]

Human papilloma virus can present as a verrucous, flat or spiky lesion in the oral cavity. It appears similar to venereal warts and usually appears in synchrony with anal or genital lesions. While often solitary lesions, these can occur as widespread involvement of the entire oral cavity and oropharyngeal mucosa (**Figure 20.2**). Treatment consists of surgical excision, but recurrence is likely.

Xerostomia secondary to chronic inflammation of the major and minor salivary glands is frequently seen in HIV patients. As with xerostomia from other causes, the development of dental caries and periodontal disease is a major concern. Also, nutritional deficiencies secondary to impaired deglutition can occur. The treatment is for symptomatic relief and consists of oral irrigations, saline rinses, salivary substitutes and sialogogues.[22]

Kaposi's sarcoma is the most common HIV-related oral malignancy, with the majority arising on the palate. This tumour can also appear on the gingival (**Figure 20.3**) or oropharynx. Diagnosis is by either excisional or punch biopsy. Treatment is necessary only for lesions that cause functional impairment or for cosmesis with enlarging lesions. There is a variety of therapeutic options. Intralesional vinblastine injection has been shown to be effective in bringing about regression by inducing local fibrosis.[23] [**] Sodium tetradecyl sulphate works in a similar manner and has also been shown to be effective. Kaposi's sarcoma has been shown to respond well to radiation, however its side effects include mucositis and can exacerbate existing xerostomia.[24] Surgical excision using a laser is helpful in debulking larger lesions.

Non-Hodgkin's lymphoma may also arise in the oral cavity. In AIDS patients, NHL is usually a poor prognostic indicator of disease progression. Recurrences are common despite chemotherapy and radiation. The lesions may present as an ulcerative lesions, but typically appear red and exophytic. They usually involve the gingiva and alveolar ridges and may arise from Waldeyer's ring.[25]

Table 20.1 reviews the characteristics and treatment of many of the most common oral manifestations of HIV disease.

PHARYNX AND LARYNX

Many of the same processes that affect the oral cavity can also affect the larynx and pharynx. Many of these processes present with similar symptoms: odynophagia, dysphagia and in some cases, chest pain. Correctly identifying and treating these processes can not only provide symptomatic relief, but in many cases, also help in dealing with the wasting and malnutrition that can occur.

Barium swallow and oesophagoscopy should be performed if the diagnosis of oesophageal candidiasis is

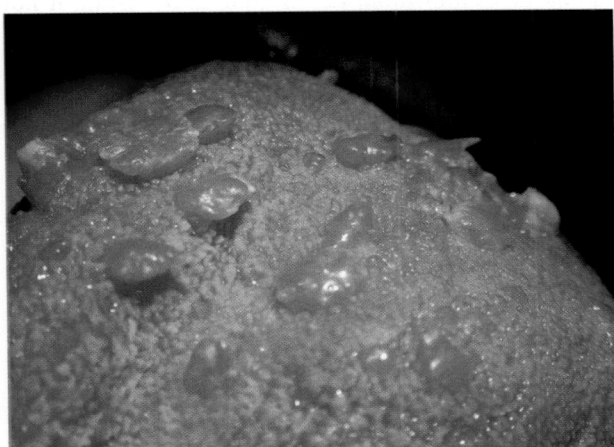

Figure 20.2 While often presenting as solitary lesions, oral papillomas can be widespread covering much of the oral and oropharyngeal mucosa. This patient has multiple papillomas of the dorsal tongue, which predictably recurred following surgical management.

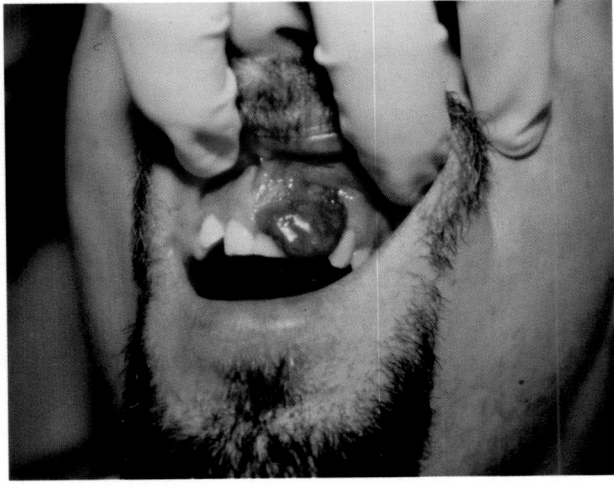

Figure 20.3 The gingival is a common site for presentation of Kaposi's sarcoma.

Table 20.1 Characteristics and treatment of the most common oral manifestations of HIV.

Disease		Management	Comment
Gingival disease	Can develop gingival tissue loss, tooth loosening/loss, bone exposure	Best treatment is frequent dental cleanings, flossing, etc. Aggressive antibiotics and/or surgical management when advanced	Common in HIV Requires close dental evaluations and frequent management
Oral thrush	Pseudomembranous candidiasis: Typical plaque-like lesions Atrophic form with erythematous lesions on palate, buccal mucosa, tongue Angular cheilitis	Topical agents such as clotrimazole Systemic agents (e.g. fluconazole) for refractory cases in patients with advanced disease	Prolonged or frequent use of fluconazole increases risk of azole-resistance candidiasis
Oral aphthous ulcers	Lesions may be large Biopsy confirms non-neoplastic, nonviral aetiology	Topical steroid therapy Intralesional or systemic steroids Thalidomide Antiretroviral therapy	Are usually difficult to treat Produce severe pain, odynophagia Often cause substantial morbidity
Kaposi's sarcoma	Typically on hard, soft palate Occasionally on gingival, buccal mucosa	Symptomatic relief When functionally problematic, low-dose radiotherapy or intralesional vinblastine or systemic chemotherapy	
Radiation mucositis	Side effect of treatment for other oral lesions	Topical therapy (steroids, antifungals, etc.) Supportive care – nutrition, pain management, hydration	Can result even from low doses of radiation
Hairy leukoplakia	Usually occurs on side of tongue Probably Epstein–Barr virus related	No treatment necessary if asymptomatic	Must be differentiated from other more serious oral disorders

suspected. Symptoms include retrosternal pain, odynophagia and/or dysphagia. Barium swallow will show an irregular surface to the mucosa secondary to ulcerations and candidal lesions. Direct visualization and biopsy can be obtained with oesophagoscopy. Treatment is with systemic amphotericin B or fluconazole. Laryngeal candidiasis presents as hoarseness and, in severe cases, stridor or shortness of breath. Fibreoptic laryngoscopy confirms the diagnosis along with biopsy. Again, treatment is with systemic antifungal agents.

Herpes simplex viral infection in the pharynx or larynx can present with similar symptoms as oesophageal and laryngeal candidiasis. Examination reveals discrete vesicles with mucosal ulceration. Biopsy and viral culture of lesions confirm diagnosis.

Kaposi's sarcoma can present primarily in the pharynx and/or larynx or extend to adjacent areas including the oral cavity. Ophageal KS may present with dysphagia secondary to obstruction or haematemesis secondary bleeding from the lesion. Laryngeal lesions may present as shortness of breath, hoarseness or severe airway compromise. Such lesions are treated aggressively. First, the airway should be secured. In acute settings of airway compromise, intubation and/or tracheostomy should be considered. Treatment, unlike with oral cavity lesions, is

typically radiation. Intralesional vinblastine has been shown to yield a complete response in certain lesions of the upper aerodigestive tract.[26]

OESOPHAGUS

Oesophageal inflammatory diseases are commonly seen in advanced HIV disease. The most common causes of this conditions are oesophageal candidiasis, herpetic oesophagitis, CMV infection and aphthous ulceration.

Oesophageal candidiasis is the most common, accounting for over 50 percent of the cases of oesophagitis in this population.[27] Although it can occur as an isolated infection, it is usually associated with oropharyngeal thrush. This association is so common that patients with oesophageal symptoms, also presenting with oral thrush, can be treated empirically for candida oesophagitis.[28] The symptoms of candidiasis consist of dysphagia (a feeling of difficulty in swallowing), odynophagia (pain when swallowing) and occasionally substernal chest pain. While the diagnosis occasionally requires endoscopy, empiric treatment can usually be instituted using a systemic antifungal agent, such as fluconazole for up to two weeks, especially in the setting of significant oropharyngeal thrush. If a clinical response is not noted early in the treatment regimen, then an alternative diagnosis should be considered, and also endoscopy.[29] [**]

Cytomegalovirus is the second most common infectious ulcerative condition of the oesophagus. Of patients who fail empirical antifungal therapy, approximately one-third will have CMV ulcerations.[30, 31] These ulcers tend to occur more commonly in the distal oesophagus with a raised indurated border and necrotic base. While occasionally occurring as solitary ulcers, CMV can also form multiple or diffuse ulcerations and lacking any defined pathognomonic appearance.[31] Unfortunately, other than biopsy and culture, there are also no disease-specific clinical characteristics that differentiate this from other forms of ulcerative oesophagitis. Once the diagnosis has been established, treatment can be instituted using intravenous gancyclovir or foscarnet.

Herpes simplex virus is a much less common cause of HIV-related oesophagitis (5 percent in some studies).[31] The symptoms are similar to those of other oesophageal diseases; however, on gastrointestinal endoscopy the ulcerative lesions tend to be smaller and sometimes confluent. The occurrence of HSV is usually associated with significant immune dysfunction, usually occurring only when the CD4 level is well below $100/mm^3$.[32] Treatment usually starts with intravenous acyclovir followed by oral agents.

Idiopathic oesophageal ulcer arises with the same frequency as CMV oesophagitis, and although its aetiology is unclear, there is usually no associated specific infectious aetiology. These lesions also usually occur with severe immunocompromise. The endoscopic appearance is similar to CMV lesions, often with solitary, large ulcerations with raised indurated margins. Treatment has been effective using systemic steroids.[33] Recent success has also been described with thalidomide, although this agent is currently not widely available.[34] [**]

SALIVARY GLANDS

Both major and minor salivary glands can be involved in disease processes in the HIV-infected individual. The most common complaint is xerostomia. The parotid gland, in particular, may be involved in some disease processes secondary to intraglandular lymph node involvement. The differential diagnosis for a person with parotid gland enlargement must include infection and salivary gland neoplasm (HIV-associated as well as the standard salivary gland neoplasms).

Included in the differential is the lymphoepithelial cyst, a disease process that is almost diagnostic of HIV infection as it was extremely rare prior to the AIDS era.[35] Lymphoepithelial cysts present as a parotid swelling, unilateral or bilateral, which progresses over months and is generally nontender (**Figures 20.4** and **20.5**). Facial nerve dysfunction should lead the physician to suspect a

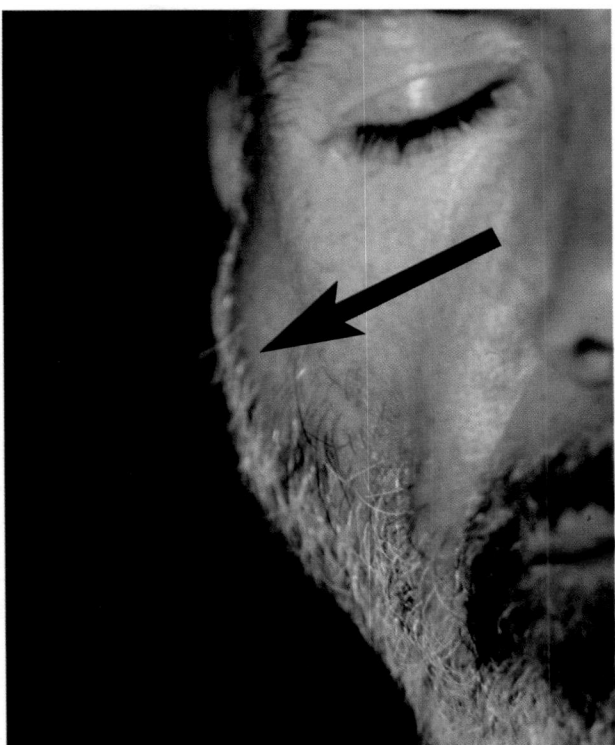

Figure 20.4 The most common etiology of an asymptomatic parotid mass in the HIV-infected patient is the lymphoepithelial cyst (arrow).

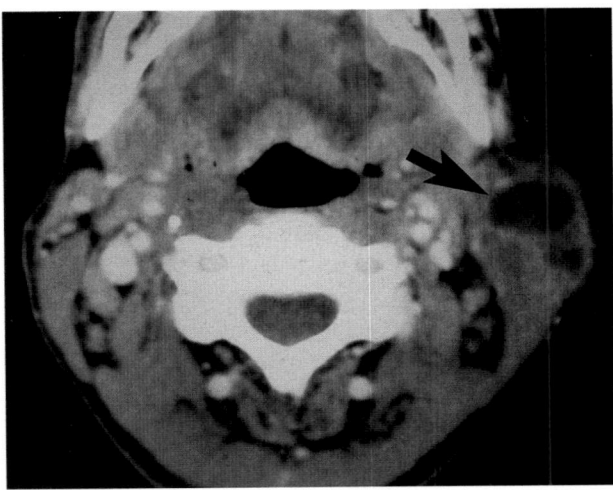

Figure 20.5 This axial CT scan demonstrates the typical findings (arrow) of a benign parotid lymphoepithelial cyst.

malignant neoplasm. Fine-needle aspiration reveals fluid with lymphocytes and squamous epithelial cells. Computed tomography imaging will show multiple thin-walled cysts in the parotid gland. With fine-needle aspiration biopsy (FNAB) and imaging, open biopsies or surgical excision for diagnosis is rarely indicated. Lymphoepithelial cysts are usually benign, and surgery is only necessary for enlarged lesions that are a cosmetic challenge or where the diagnosis is equivocal. Needle aspiration of cyst contents is ineffective for long-term cure as recurrence almost always happens.[36] [**] However, it is effective as a temporary treatment and for diagnostic purposes. Radiation therapy has shown some efficacy although, as when used to treat KS, it can cause severe mucositis locally. Superficial parotidectomy is the only permanent treatment and carries its own share of potential morbidities including damage to the facial nerve.

NECK

The majority of HIV patients may present with a neck mass at some point during their illness. In this population, the differential diagnosis includes four categories of disease process: neoplasm, infectious, HIV lymphadenopathy and parotid disease.

Neoplasms that can present as neck mass include KS, NHL and squamous cell carcinoma. Kaposi's sarcoma is one of the disease processes that define AIDS. Prior to the AIDS epidemic, it was mostly encountered on the lower extremities of people of Mediterranean or Ashkenazi Jewish descent. During the AIDS epidemic, its incidence increased in the male homosexual and bisexual population. With increasing spread via intravenous drug use and the increasing incidence in women worldwide, this distribution may change. The risk of KS increases with CD4 counts $<100/\mu L$ and tends to be more aggressive. Lesions can occur as cervical lymphadenopathy in the neck, skin, oral cavity and lungs. In the neck, diagnosis can be made by FNAB or open biopsy.

Non-Hodgkin's lymphoma is more aggressive in immunocompromised patients and is the second most common neoplasm in HIV patients. It can present as a neck mass that is rapidly enlarging and usually nontender. Although it can present as nodal mass, NHL localized to the neck is uncommon in HIV-infected patients and systemic disease is the norm. Extranodal presentations are also more common in HIV-infected patients (**Figure 20.6**). Constitutional symptoms (fever, night sweats and weight loss) usually occur with disease. Diagnosis is normally made by open biopsy with subsequent immunohistochemical staining and evaluation of cell architecture.

Hodgkin's disease can also present as a painless, enlarging neck mass in HIV patients. At the time of presentation, most patients have disseminated disease. As with NHL, Hodgkin's disease can be difficult to manage in HIV patients.

There have been reported cases of squamous cell carcinoma presenting as a cervical mass in AIDS patients. Evaluation is similar to that of cancer of unknown primary in non-HIV patients. Treatment is usually surgical.

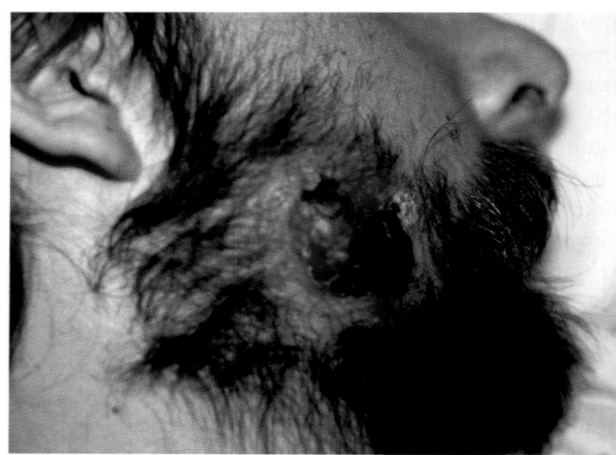

Figure 20.6 This patient presented with a non-Hodgkin's lymphoma of the right cheek. Extranodal presentations are common in patients with HIV disease.

Infectious processes that can cause neck masses in HIV-positive patients are numerous. There are a few that deserve special mention, as misdiagnosis of them can ultimately prove fatal in immunocompromised patients. Toxoplasmosis is a condition caused by the organism *Toxoplasma gondii*, a protozoan which infects humans who ingest tissue cysts contained in the meat of certain animals. In immunocompetent patients, symptoms include a self-limiting course of constitutional symptoms and cervical lymphadenopathy. In immunocompromised patients, toxoplasmic encephalitis can result in a central nervous system space-occupying lesion that is usually bilateral. Computed tomography scans of the head are useful for identifying these lesions. Definitive diagnosis is by biopsy and tissue culture; however, tissue culture ultimately takes anywhere from six days to several months. Therapy should be started presumptively based on history and CT scan. Treatment consists of pyrimethamine and sulphadiazine for six weeks.

Pneumocystis carinii is the most common opportunistic pathogen in AIDS patients. It is an opportunistic organism that only becomes pathogenic in immunocompromised individuals. Primarily it causes a pneumonia that presents as a progressive consolidation of the lungs. *Pneumocystis* prophylaxis is widely instituted in HIV patients, leading to more extrapulmonary manifestations. Since it is primarily a pulmonary process, any person with an extrapulmonary manifestation of *P. carinii* should have a pulmonary work-up. Head and neck manifestations include a lymphadenitis or a thyroiditis. Fine-needle aspiration biopsy specimens should be examined using the Gomori methenamine-silver stain that stains the cyst form of the organism, and histopathologic examination. Cervical infections respond to dapsone, trimethoprim/sulphamethoxazole or pentamidine.

Extrapulmonary *M. tuberculosis* infection in an HIV patient can present as an enlarging neck mass. It is usually firm, nontender, has a rubbery consistency, and may present with a draining sinus tract. Cervical lymphadenopathy may be the only symptom of tuberculous infection, therefore tuberculosis should always be on the differential diagnosis for neck masses. HIV-positive patients have a higher rate of reactivation of latent disease than their immunocompetent counterparts. Diagnosis is via administration of the purified protein derivative skin test. In immunocompetent individuals, a 10-mm reaction is considered positive. This criterion is lowered to 5 mm in immunocompromised individuals. Controls to test for anergy should also be placed. Positive results may also be seen with nontuberculous mycobacterial infections.

Nontuberculous mycobacterial infections, particularly *Mycobacterium avium* complex (MAC), are the most common mycobacterial infections seen in HIV patients, whereas in their immunocompetent counterparts, *M. tuberculosis* is more common. MAC infection, in the later stages of AIDS, presents as disseminated infection. Therefore, MAC infection of cervical lymph nodes should lead to a thorough investigation for disseminated infection. Treatment is with ciprofloxacin and clofazimine, as MAC is resistant to standard antimycobacterial medications.

Fungal infections may also manifest as a cervical mass. Rarely do they present as isolated cervical lymphadenopathy. Disseminated infection should be suspected in patients with fungal lymphadenopathy. Treatment is usually with amphotericin B, and lifelong suppressive therapy is necessary following successful treatment. In HIV-infected patients, *Cryptococcus neoformans* is the most prevalent form of infection. Cryptococcal meningitis is the most frequent presentation of cryptococcosis in HIV patients. Cultures for fungus should be obtained with all neck node biopsies.

Human immunodeficiency virus lympadenopathy (also called persistent generalized lymphadenopathy) can arise early in HIV infection, often within months of initial seroconversion. The syndrome is defined as two or more extrainguinal sites of lymphadenopathy which last for more than three months and have no obvious source. Lymphadenopathy in the head and neck region can occur anywhere, but particularly in the posterior triangle, periauricular areas and submental and submandibular lymph nodes. Routine biopsy (fine-needle or excisional) is not recommended.

The work-up for a neck mass in an HIV-positive patient begins with a thorough history and physical including questions about time of onset, duration and possible precipitating events. Any constitutional symptoms, or lack thereof, should be well documented. A thorough review of systems, focusing particularly on pulmonary and central nervous system symptoms, should be obtained. The patient's recent travel history should be ascertained. There should be a thorough physical examination, detailing not only the cervical lesion in question, but also any other oral cavity or nasal lesions.

Computed tomography or magnetic resonance imaging should be obtained to evaluate the size of the lesion, location and composition. Fine-needle aspiration biopsy can be used to obtain a tissue sample and perhaps guide therapy. Criteria exist for determining whether to perform open biopsy of a suspicious lymph node. Biopsy is indicated in individuals with a single lymph node >3 cm in patients with HIV lymphadenopathy, localized/enlarging/unilateral lymphadenopathy, constitutional symptoms, cytopenia/elevated erythrocyte sedimentation rate, or substantial mediastinal or abdominal lymphadenopathy.[37] Using these criteria, the physician can decrease the likelihood of biopsy morbidity in the patient, decrease the risk to the surgeon and medical personnel, and decrease the likelihood of the results returning as simple HIV lymphadenopathy.

DERMATOLOGIC

Seborrhoeic dermatitis is a common inflammatory disorder seen in HIV patients. It may present as scaly patches over the scalp. Treatment is with steroid creams and shampoos (see under Otologic above).

Herpes simplex virus can present as large ulcers on the face that are extremely tender. Ulcerative lesions in AIDS patients are presumed to be HSV until proven otherwise. Herpes simplex virus infection lasting more than one month is an indicator of AIDS. Diagnosis is made by Tzanck smear, viral cultures, skin biopsy or fluorescent antibody staining of scrapings from lesions.

Herpes zoster may present in immunocompromised patients secondary to reactivation of latent virus. It presents as vesicular lesions that appear over a particular dermatome. There can be severe pain during and after acute episodes. Ramsay Hunt syndrome can occur with facial nerve involvement and there may be ocular complications with involvement of the trigeminal nerve. The diagnosis is clinical, however Tzanck smear can be used for confirmation. Episodes are usually self-limited. Treatment of simple cases consists of oral acyclovir, which helps to shorten the course. Disseminated cases, Ramsay Hunt syndrome or ophthalmic involvement should be treated with intravenous acyclovir.

Molloscum contagiosum is a skin lesion caused by a poxvirus, which presents as a pearly, umbilicated papule, in approximately 10–20 percent of AIDS patients. Treatment is with curettage. Retinoic acid applied topically may assist in decreasing the size and rate of appearance of new lesions.

Bacillary angiomatosis is a caused by infection with Gram-negative bacteria related to the organism that causes trench fever, and occurs with immunosuppression. It can present in a variety of different ways, most frequently as a bright red, papular lesion that is friable. It may also present as a cellulitic plaque or a subcutaneous nodule. It can occur in skin or viscera. Diagnosis is by biopsy and is identified with the Warthin-Starry stain. Since visceral lesions can also arise, investigation of suspicous skin lesions is imperative. Treatment is with erythromycin for skin manifestations.

Staphylococcus aureus infection can present on the skin as a folliculitis, furuncle, carbuncle or abscess. The nares is the most common site of colonization. In HIV-positive homosexual men, the carriage rate is double that of noninfected homosexual men.[38] It is the most common cause of cutaneous bacterial infection in HIV infection. Infection typically occurs through breaks in skin secondary to needle sticks and indwelling venous catheters. Infection is precipitated in general by neutropenia secondary to bone marrow suppression from medications, and defective chemotaxis of neutrophils secondary to HIV infection. Treatment is with oral antistaphylococcal antibiotics and incision and drainage of abscesses.

Kaposi's sarcoma is a malignant tumour of endothelial cell origin and is the most common AIDS-associated neoplasm. In the head and neck region, it can affect any cutaneous surface as well as upper aerodigestive tract mucosa. Skin lesions are painful and appear as purple or brown skin nodules varying in diameter size from 1 mm to 2 cm. Smaller lesions may coalesce to form large lesions. The diagnosis is made by appearance and biopsy. Histologic appearance is variable and may resemble a simple haemangioma with haemosiderin-laden macrophages and tightly packed capillaries. Although vascular in appearance, bleeding is not considered a risk of biopsy. Treatment options include intralesional vinblastine, carbon dioxide laser excision, cryotherapy and low-dose radiation.

KEY POINTS

- One hundred percent of HIV patients will present head and neck manifestations at some point during the course of their illness.
- Lymphoepithelial cyst in the parotid is virtually diagnostic of AIDS.
- Oral hair leukoplakia is a benign process which must be distinguished from other more serious oral conditions.
- Candida oesophagitis is the most common aetiology of serious oesophageal inflammatory conditions; however, when empiric therapy is ineffective, oesophagoscopy with biopsy may be necessary to direct therapy.
- Sensorineural hearing loss in AIDS patients can be multifactorial and include the neurotropic effects of the HIV virus, ototoxic medications used to treat HIV and opportunistic infections.

- Otitis media with effusion in HIV patients warrants an evaluation of the nasopharynx to rule out a nasopharyngeal mass.
- Any nonpediatric patient with adenoid hypertrophy should be tested for HIV.
- Kaposi's sarcoma is a malignant tumour with increased incidence in HIV-positive individuals versus the general population. It can present at a variety of sites including the ear, nose, face and oral cavity.
- The differential diagnosis for a neck mass in HIV patients is vast and includes HIV lymphadenopathy, infectious, neoplastic and parotid disease. Specific recommendations exist for when biopsy of a neck node should be performed.

REFERENCES

1. McElrath MJ, Pruett JE, Cohn ZA. Mononuclear phagocytes of blood and bone marrow: comparative roles as viral reservoirs in human immunodeficiency virus type 1 infections. *Proceedings of the National Academy of Sciences of the United States of America.* 1989; **86**: 675–9.
2. Witiak DG, Tami TA. AIDS and otolaryngology. In: English GM (ed.). *Otolaryngology.* Philadelphia: Lippincott, Williams and Wilkins. Chapter 63.
3. Burke DS, Redfield RR. Classification of infections with human immunodeficiency virus. *Annals of Internal Medicine.* 1986; **105**: 968.
4. Friemuth WW, Wathen LK, Cox SR, *et al.* Delavirdine in combination with zidovudine causes sustained antiviral and immunological effects in HIV-1 infected individuals. Washington, DC: Third Conference on Retroviruses and Opportunistic Infections, 1996: 40 (abstract).
5. Murr AH, Lee KC. Universal precautions for the otolaryngologist: techniques and equipment for minimizing exposure risk. *Ear, Nose, and Throat Journal.* 1995; **338**: 341–36.
6. Centers for Disease Control: Public health service statement on management of occupational exposure to human immunodeficiency virus, including considerations regarding zidovudine postexposure use. *MMWR. Morbidity and Mortality Weekly Report* 1990; **39**: 1.
7. Hern JD, Almeyda J, Thomas DM, Main J, Patel KS. Malignant otitis externa in HIV and AIDS. *Journal of Laryngology and Otology.* 1996; **110**: 770–5.
8. Yates PD, Upile T, Axon PR, de Carpentier J. Aspergillus mastoiditis in a patient with acquired immunodeficiency syndrome. *Journal of Laryngology and Otology.* 1997; **111**: 560–1.

9. Smith ME, Canalis RF. Otologic manifestations of AIDS: the otosyphilis connection. *Laryngoscope*. 1989; **99**: 365–72.

10. Tami TA, Lee KC. Otolaryngologic manifestations of HIV disease. In: Cohen PT, Sande MA, Volberding PA (eds). The AIDS knowledge base, 2nd edn. London: Little, Brown, 1994, Chapter 5.29.

11. Tami TA, Wawrose S. Diseases of the nose and paranasal sinus in the human immunodeficiency virus-infected population. *Otolaryngologic Clinics of North America*. 1992; **25**: 1199–210.

12. Del Forno A, Del Borgo C, Turriziani A, Ottaviani F, Antinori A, Fantoni M. Non-Hodgkin's lymphoma of the maxillary sinus in a patient with acquired immunodeficiency syndrome. *Journal of Laryngology and Otology*. 1998; **112**: 982–5.

13. Hunt SM, Miyamoto C, Cornelius RS, Tami TA. Invasive fungal sinusitis in the acquired immunodeficiency syndrome. *Otolaryngologic Clinics of North America*. 2000; **33**: 335–47.

14. Brillhart T, Gath J, Pio D *et al.* Symptomatic cytomegaloviral rhinosinusitis in patients with AIDS. Florence: VII International Conference on AIDS, M.B.2182, 1991.

15. Rossi RM, Wanke C, Federman M. Microsporidian sinusitis in patients with the acquired immunodeficiency syndrome. *Laryngoscope*. 1996; **106**: 966–71.

16. Gonzalez MM, Gould E, Dickinson G, Martinez AJ, Visvesvara G, Cleary TJ *et al.* Acquired immunodeficiency syndrome associated with Acanthamoeba infection and other opportunistic organisms. *Archives of Pathology and Laboratory Medicine*. 1986; **110**: 749–51.

17. Wawrose SF, Tami TA, Amoils CP. The role of guaifenesin in the treatment of sinonasal disease in patients infected with the human immunodeficiency virus (HIV). *Laryngoscope*. 1992; **102**: 1225–8.

18. Tami TA. The management of sinusitis in patients infected with the human immunodeficiency virus (HIV). *Ear, Nose, and Throat Journal*. 1995; **74**: 360–3.

19. Friedman M, Brenski A, Taylor L. Treatment of aphthous ulcers in AIDS patients. *Laryngoscope*. 1994; **104**: 566–70.

20. Jacobson JM, Greenspan JS, Spritzler J, Ketter N, Fahey JL, Jackson JB *et al.* Thalidomide for the treatment of oral aphthous ulcers in patients with human immunodeficiency virus infection. National Institute of Allergy and Infectious Diseases AIDS Clinical Trials Group. *New England Journal of Medicine*. 1997; **336**: 1487–93.

21. Dichtel WJ. Oral manifestations of human immunodeficiency virus infection. *Otolaryngologic Clinics of North America*. 1992; **25**: 1211–24.

22. Schiodt M, Dodd CL, Greenspan D, Daniels TE, Chernoff D, Hollander H *et al.* Natural history of HIV-associated salivary gland disease. *Oral Surgery, Oral Medicine, and Oral Pathology*. 1992; **74**: 326–31.

23. McCormick SU. Intralesional vinblastine injections for the treatment of oral Kaposi's sarcoma: report of 10 patients with 2-year follow-up. *Journal of Oral Maxillofacial Surgery*. 1996; **54**: 583–7; discussion 588–9.

24. Cooper JS, Fried PR. Toxicity of oral radiotherapy in patients with acquired immunodeficiency syndrome. *Archives of Otolaryngology – Head and Neck Surgery*. 1987; **113**: 327–8.

25. Finn DG. Lymphoma of the head and neck and acquired immunodeficiency syndrome: clinical investigation and immunohistological study. *Laryngoscope*. 1995; **105**: 1–18.

26. Tami TA, Ferlito A, Rinaldo A, Lee KC, Singh B. Laryngeal pathology in the acquired immunodeficiency syndrome: diagnostic and therapeutic dilemmas. *Annals of Otology, Rhinology, and Laryngology*. 1999; **108**: 214–20.

27. Wilcox CM, Monkemuller KE. Diagnosis and management of esophageal disease in the acquired immunodeficiency syndrome. *Southern Medical Journal*. 1998; **91**: 1002–8.

28. Dieterich DT, Wilcox CM. Diagnosis and treatment of esophageal diseases associated with HIV infection. Practice Parameters Committee of the American College of Gastroenterology. *American Journal of Gastroenterology*. 1996; **91**: 2265–9.

29. Wilcox CM, Alexander LN, Clark WS, Thompson SE 3rd. Fluconazole compared with endoscopy for human immunodeficiency virus-infected patients with esophageal symptoms. *Gastroenterology*. 1996; **110**: 1803–9.

30. Parente F, Cernuschi M, Rizzardini G, Lazzarin A, Valsecchi L, Bianchi Porro G. Opportunistic infections of the esophagus not responding to oral systemic antifungals in patients with AIDS: their frequency and treatment. *American Journal of Gastroenterology*. 1991; **86**: 1729–34.

31. Wilcox CM, Straub RF, Schwartz DA. Prospective endoscopic characterization of cytomegalovirus esophagitis in AIDS. *Gastrointestinal Endoscopy*. 1994; **40**: 481–4.

32. Genereau T, Lortholary O, Bouchaud O, Lacassin F, Vinceneux P, De Truchis P *et al.* Herpes simplex eso-phagitis in patients with AIDS: report of 34 cases. The Cooperative Study Group on Herpetic Esophagitis in HIV Infection. *Clinical Infectious Diseases*. 1996; **22**: 926–31.

33. Kotler DP, Reka S, Orenstein JM, Fox CH. Chronic idiopathic esophageal ulceration in the acquired immunodeficiency syndrome. Characterization and treatment with corticosteroids. *Journal of Clinical Gastroenterology*. 1992; **15**: 284–90.

34. Jacobson JM, Spritzler J, Fox L, Fahey JL, Jackson JB, Chernoff M *et al.* Thalidomide for the treatment of esophageal aphthous ulcers in patients with human immunodeficiency virus infection. National Institute of Allergy and Infectious Disease AIDS Clinical Trials Group. *Journal of Infectious Diseases*. 1999; **180**: 61–7.

35. Huang RD, Pearlman S, Friedman WH, Loree T. Benign cystic vs. solid lesions of the parotid gland in HIV patients. *Head and Neck*. 1991; **13**: 522–7.

36. Echavez MI, Lee KC, Sooy CD. Tetracycline sclerosis for treatment of benign lymphoepithelial cysts of the parotid gland in patients infected with human immunodeficiency virus. *Laryngoscope.* 1994; **104**: 1499–502.

37. Lee KC, Cheung SW. Evaluation of the neck mass in human immunodeficiency virus-infected patients. *Otolaryngologic Clinics of North America.* 1992; **25**: 1287–305.

38. Berger TG. Dermatologic findings in the head and neck in human immunodeficiency virus-infected persons. *Otolaryngologic Clinics of North America.* 1992; **25**: 1227–43.

HAEMATOLOGY

EDITED BY NICHOLAS S JONES

21 Blood groups, blood components and alternatives to transfusion   253
     Fiona Regan and Ian Gabriel

22 Haemato-oncology   265
     Clare Wykes and Fiona Regan

23 Haemostasis: normal physiology, disorders of haemostasis and thrombosis and their management   278
     Fiona Regan

HAEMATOLOGY

Blood groups, blood components and alternatives to transfusion

FIONA REGAN AND IAN GABRIEL

Introduction	253	Key points	263
Human blood groups and their clinical significance	253	Best clinical practice	263
Blood components	255	Deficiencies in current knowledge and areas for future	
Adverse reactions	260	research	264
Alternatives to transfusion	262	References	264

SEARCH STRATEGY

The data in this chapter are supported by a Medline search using the key words transfusion, components, blood sparing agents, alternative, adverse events.

INTRODUCTION

Widely available and practised worldwide, the transfusion of blood and its constituent components has played a major role in allowing significant advances through greater medical and surgical intervention. However, the scientific basis of transfusion and the complications which can follow transfusion are not always used to make an informed decision to transfuse patients. This chapter reviews the biology of the major blood groups, the constituents of blood and their indications, the problems encountered when transfusion causes adverse effects and potential alternatives to blood transfusion.

HUMAN BLOOD GROUPS AND THEIR CLINICAL SIGNIFICANCE

There are 23 human blood group systems, leading to a huge variety of red cell phenotypes. The most important of these is the ABO system.

ABO blood groups

Patients are grouped by serological testing into either group O, A, B or AB. Patients of all groups have a common H antigen on the red cell membrane surface, which is coded for by the H gene on chromosome 19. This H antigen may then be acted upon by further enzymes, depending on the presence of ABO genes on chromosome 9. Each person inherits two ABO genes. The O gene is nonfunctional so that if an individual has not inherited either the A or B gene, then the H antigen alone is detected on the red cell surface. Such individuals are Group O. However, if an individual has inherited an A or B gene then each codes for a specific enzyme which adds a specific sugar to the H gene product producing either the A, B or AB phenotype (**Table 21.1**). People form antibodies to any of the ABO antigens that they lack. These antibodies appear during the first few months of life due to the exposure to ABH-like antigens in the environment. The ABO system is significant because these antibodies are of the immunoglobulin (Ig)M type and thus are capable of

Table 21.1 ABO blood groups.

Blood group	Frequency in UK population (%)	Genotype	Red cell antigens	Antibodies in plasma
O	47	OO	Nil	Anti-A, anti-B
A	42	AO	A	Anti-B
		AA		
B	8	BO	B	Anti-A
		BB		
AB	3	AB	A and B	Nil

Table 21.2 Rh D blood group.

Blood group	Frequency in UK population (%)	Genotype	Antigens	Antibody
Rh D-positive	85	DD or Dd	D	–
Rh D-negative	15	dd	Nil	Anti-D after first exposure

D gene is dominant, codes for D antigen; d gene is recessive, codes for no antigen.

complete activation of complement through to red cell lysis. Therefore, if the wrong (mismatched) blood is transfused into a patient, a potentially fatal reaction may ensue.

The Rh blood group system

The Rh system (originally termed 'Rhesus' system, when discovered in Rhesus monkeys) is a complex system of 45 antigens encoded on chromosome 1. The most important is the Rh D antigen, which is highly immunogenic and 90 percent of individuals exposed to Rh D-positive blood by transfusion will produce anti-D antibodies, which are of IgG type (**Table 21.2**).

Rh D-negative women may also become sensitized and form anti-D by an Rh D-positive foetus at times when fetomaternal haemorrhage occurs, e.g. at delivery. Anti-D is important as it can not only cause a delayed haemolytic transfusion reaction if Rh D-positive blood is transfused, but anti-D antibodies can also cross the placenta. Therefore, if a Rh D-negative woman has anti-D and she carries a Rh D-positive baby, anti-D may attach to the foetal red cells and cause haemolysis. This may cause either haemolytic disease of the newborn or even death of the foetus due to hydrops fetalis.

Therefore, a Rh D-negative woman of childbearing age must always receive Rh D-negative blood.

Other blood group systems

It is impossible to provide 'identical' or fully matched red cells for transfusion. In practice, ABO and Rh D identical blood is provided and in addition, all patients are tested to determine if they have any antibodies to other clinically significant red cell antigens – if so, antigen negative blood must be provided to prevent a delayed haemolytic transfusion reaction from occurring. Red cell antibodies occur in 3.8 percent of patients. For some antibodies, antigen negative blood may need to be obtained from a regional blood centre. Therefore, a patient is tested before each transfusion episode to screen for the presence of antibodies, i.e. a group and screen (G&S) test, by incubating the patient's plasma with two different fully antigen typed 'screening' red cells which are known to possess all the blood group antigens which matter clinically. If the antibody screen is negative, any blood which is ABO- and Rh D-compatible could be given. If the antibody screen is positive, the antibody(ies) must be identified using a large panel of red cells of known antigen types. As antibodies can develop 2 days to 20 weeks after a transfusion episode, a new blood sample is required for antibody screening if the patient has been transfused recently. [***] [Grade C/D].

Crossmatch

The patient's plasma is incubated with the donor red cells from units of blood selected for transfusion to double check that the patient has no antibodies present which could react with antigens on the donor's red cells to cause a delayed haemolytic transfusion reaction. Blood is normally reserved for a particular patient for 48 hours.

Maximum surgical blood ordering schedule

For some elective surgical procedures, blood may only rarely be used so to crossmatch blood for all patients undergoing such a procedure would be a waste of staff time, reagents and blood may be reserved for sequential patients and expire without being used. Therefore, for operations where blood is used in less than a third of procedures, if a patient's group and screen test shows no antibodies are present, a crossmatch is not performed. This is safe as in the event of an unexpected bleeding emergency, as no antibodies are present, ABO- and Rh D-compatible blood can be provided within 10 minutes. However, the corollary is that if a patient's group and screen does show an antibody, a full crossmatch must be done before surgery. A maximum surgical blood ordering schedule (MSBOS) is normally compiled by agreement between surgeons, anaesthetists and haematologists and is individually tailored to each hospital, taking into account the procedures performed, operators, logistical arrangements of the blood bank, etc. **Table 21.3** shows an example. This only applies to elective and not emergency surgery and the blood provided can be altered on discussion, if there are clinical factors which make significant bleeding more likely, for example, if a patient has a coagulopathy. [Grade D]

TIMING OF GROUP AND SCREEN OR CROSSMATCH SAMPLES BEFORE ELECTIVE SURGERY

Routine samples are tested in batches, so normally, a G&S requires approximately half a working day to complete, but if the antibody screen is positive, an additional half a working day or more is required. Therefore a G&S or crossmatch sample should be sent 24 hours before surgery to ensure that blood can be provided if the patient has an antibody. It is usual for anaesthetists to check that any crossmatched blood requested is available before surgery is started, but the equally important check that results of a G&S are available so that blood could be provided during surgery if needed, is not commonplace. With ever-reducing time between patient admission and elective surgery, patients may have G&S or crossmatch samples taken instead at pre-assessment clinics several days or weeks before surgery. It is safe practice to perform a G&S test on these samples and freeze the plasma until a few days before surgery, then crossmatch blood if required

Table 21.3 Example of a surgical blood ordering schedule.

Procedure	Blood order
Tumour of palate	G&S
Laryngectomy	2 units
Radical neck dissection	2 units
Commando	4 units

using this sample, provided that the patient's doctor, has ensured that the patient had not been transfused in the six months prior to the sample being taken so that new red cell antibodies cannot develop between obtaining the sample and transfusing the patient. If a patient has been transfused, a new sample is required before transfusion can be given. [Grade C/D]

EMERGENCY SURGERY

In an emergency, a patient's blood group and antibody screening can be tested manually. A test for the patient's ABO and Rh D group takes approximately 10 minutes and an antibody screen takes approximately 30 minutes: the times taken for samples to be sent to the laboratory and for blood to be taken to the patient are not included. **Figure 21.1** shows a typical example of what blood can be provided in an emergency. To avoid misunderstandings, communication between clinicians and laboratory staff to establish 'how long from now until blood is needed at the bedside' is crucial.

BLOOD COMPONENTS

Whole blood may be split into various components, to allow for efficient use of donated blood, as illustrated in **Figure 21.2**.

Red cell transfusions

Whole blood is rarely used in modern clinical practice: red cell concentrates, which have had plasma removed for other products, are used in preference. Each unit is estimated to raise the Hb concentration in an adult by 1 g/dL. Donated blood is collected into a pack containing the anticoagulant citrate phosphate dextrose (CPD) and then after centrifugation, transferred to a pack containing saline-adenine-glucose-mannitol (SAGM) medium suitable for optimal red cell storage. Red cells are then stored at 4°C for up to 35 days to minimize proliferation of any contaminant bacteria.

PREOPERATIVE PREPARATION

To avoid unnecessary transfusion, patients should be assessed well in advance of surgery so that simple measures can be taken, e.g. correction of iron deficiency anaemia and arrangements made for stopping nonsteroidal antiinflammatory drugs or anticoagulants, where appropriate.

INDICATIONS FOR TRANSFUSION

It is difficult to answer the question 'when should red cells be transfused'. Broadly, blood should be given when the

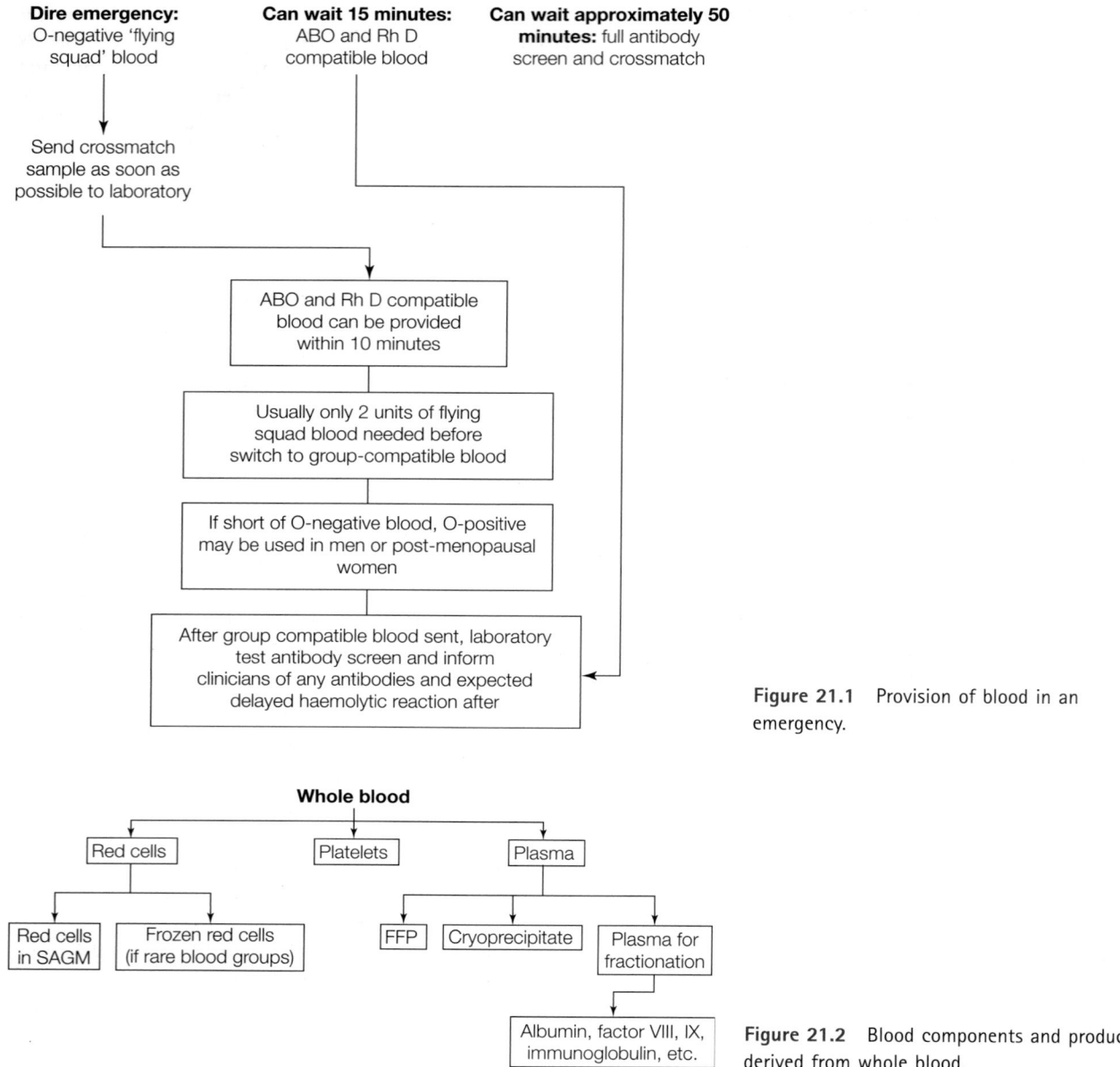

Figure 21.1 Provision of blood in an emergency.

Figure 21.2 Blood components and products derived from whole blood.

potential benefits outweigh the risks. Most hospitals have policies addressing the use of blood and components, as agreed among surgeons and haematologists and based on national guidelines. The British Committee for Safety in Haematology guidelines, *The clinical use of red cell transfusion*, published in 2001, provides useful guidance on when to transfuse patients, as summarized below.[1] [Grade C/D]

British Committee for Safety in Haematology guidelines 2001

ACUTE BLOOD LOSS

Patients with acute massive loss should ideally be managed by experienced clinicians in a suitable setting.

A blood sample should be sent for the urgent provision of blood according to hospital policy.

As it is often difficult in such circumstances to estimate blood loss, the classification given in **Table 21.4** is a useful guide to measuring hypovolaemic shock. According to the British Committee for Safety in Haematology (BCSH) guidelines:[1]

Requirement for transfusion based on an estimation of blood loss

- 15 percent loss of volume (750 mL in an adult or estimate the circulating blood volume by 75× weight in kg): No need for blood transfusion unless blood loss is superimposed on pre-existing anaemia or when the patient is unable to compensate for this

Table 21.4 Clarification of hypovolaemic shock according to blood loss.[2]

	Class I	Class II	Class III	Class IV
Blood loss				
Percentage	<15	15–30	30–40	>40
Volume (mL)	750	800–1500	1500–2000	>2000
Blood pressure				
Systolic	Unchanged	Normal	Reduced	Very low
Diastolic	Unchanged	Raised	Reduced	Very low unrecordable
Pulse (beats/min)	Slight tachycardia	100–120	120 (thready)	>120 (very thready)
Capillary refill	Normal	Slow (>2 s)	Slow (>2 s)	Undetectable
Respiratory rate	Normal	Normal	Tachypnoea (>20/min)	Tachypnoea (>20/min)
Urinary flow rate (mL/h)	>30	20–30	10–20	0–10
Extremities	Colour normal	Pale	Pale	Pale and cold
Complexion	Normal	Pale	Pale	Ashen
Mental state	Alert	Anxious or aggressive	Anxious, aggressive, or drowsy	Drowsy, confused, or unconscious

Reproduced with permission from the BMJ Publishing Group.

loss due to pre-existing cardiac or respiratory disease.
- 15–30 percent loss of volume (800–1500 mL in an adult): Need to transfuse crystalloids or colloids. The need for red cells is unlikely unless the patient has pre-existing anaemia, reduced cardiorespiratory reserve or if blood loss continues.
- 30–40 percent loss of blood volume (1500–2000 mL): Rapid volume replacement is required with crystalloid or synthetic colloids, and red cell transfusion will probably be required.
- 40 percent loss of blood volume (>2000 mL) rapid volume replacement including red cells is required. [Grade D]

Requirements for red cell transfusion based on haemoglobin concentration

- Red cell transfusion is not indicated when estimates of actual and anticipated haemoglobin concentrations are >10 g/dL.
- Red cell transfusion is indicated when the rate of concentration is <7 g/dL. Red cells should be given in relation to ongoing red cell loss. If the patient is otherwise stable, two units of red cells should be transfused in adults (or the equivalent in children according to size) and then the clinical situation and haemoglobin concentration should be reassessed.
- The correct strategy for transfusion of patients with haemoglobin concentrations between 7 and 10 g/dL is less clear. Clinicians often transfuse red cells, although the available evidence suggests this is not often justified.
- In patients who may tolerate anaemia poorly, e.g. patients over the age of 65 and patients with cardiovascular disease, consider adopting a higher haemoglobin level at which transfusions are indicated.

These guidelines provide a framework for clinical transfusion, but the decision to transfuse should be based on the individual patient's circumstances. [Grade D]

A retrospective review of transfusion in sinus surgery in Germany found that 0.46 percent of patients needed a transfusion, but that blood loss and therefore the need for transfusion decreased when a combination of endonasal surgery and controlled intraoperative hypotension were used.[3] Risk factors for requiring a transfusion were extensive polyposis and purulent exacerbation of sinus disease. A study in the United States concluded that transfusion is no longer necessary during routine bimaxillary orthognathic surgery[4] and another study found that using hypotensive anaesthesia and consistent surgical techniques, 0.8 percent of patients required transfusion.[5] Small patients requiring double-jaw procedures were the ones most likely to need blood. [Grade C/D]

Fresh frozen plasma

The use of fresh frozen plasma (FFP) in the UK has increased over many years, but there is evidence that it is often given unnecessarily.[6] It is usual practice for requests for FFP, platelets and cryoprecipitate to be discussed with a haematologist.

CHARACTERISTICS OF FRESH FROZEN PLASMA

Plasma is separated from whole blood by centrifugation and frozen to $-30°C$ within six hours of its collection (**Table 21.5**). Thawing of FFP takes about 30 minutes from the time of request and should be used within two hours for it to maintain its optimal clinical effectiveness. It cannot be refrozen for further storage.

FFP should be ABO-compatible to avoid a mild haemolytic reaction due to anti-A or anti-B in the FFP.

Table 21.5 Blood components.

	Storage (°C)	Shelf–life	Dose	Outcome measures
Red cells	4°C ±2	35 days	1 unit	Rise Hb 1 g/dL in adult
Platelets	Room temp – keep agitated	5 days	1 pool	Rise in platelet count of approximately 40 and monitor bleeding
FFP	Frozen	1 year	12–15 mL/kg	Monitor APTT and PT and bleeding
Cryoprecipitate	Frozen	1 year	10 donor units (may be pooled)	Monitor fibrinogen level

FFP is not crossmatched, but the patient needs to have had a G&S test. A small amount of red cell contamination may be present in FFP so women of childbearing age should therefore receive Rh D-compatible FFP to prevent possible sensitization. In an emergency situation if Rh-positive FFP has to be issued to Rh D-negative women, i.m. anti-D can be administered to prevent immunization.

INDICATIONS FOR FRESH FROZEN PLASMA

National BCSH guidelines give recommendations for the use of FFP.[7] [Grade C/D]

Definite

- thrombotic thrombocytopenic purpura (TTP);
- acute disseminated intravascular coagulation (DIC);
- immediate reversal of warfarin effect;
- replacement of single coagulation deficiencies where a specific or combined concentrate is unavailable;
- vitamin K deficiency;
- C1 esterase inhibitor deficiency.

Disseminated intravascular coagulation

Disseminated intravascular coagulation leads to deficiencies in coagulation factors particularly V, VIII and fibrinogen, and platelets. In patients who are actively bleeding and in whom laboratory tests indicate DIC, FFP, platelets and cryoprecipitate are often required. Subsequent therapy should be based on repeat coagulation tests and with the guidance of haematological colleagues. In chronic DIC or DIC without haemorrhage, there is no indication for FFP just to normalize laboratory results.

Vitamin K deficiency

Patients who present to surgical teams with biliary obstruction may have impaired absorption of the fat soluble vitamin K and therefore have a deficiency of vitamin K-dependent coagulation factors. If immediate correction is required, e.g. for haemorrhage or imminent surgery, FFP is indicated.

Reversal of warfarin effect

In an emergency, FFP (or prothrombin complex concentrate) can be used to reverse warfarin effects. In elective surgery, the risks of potential adverse effects of FFP must be balanced against the urgency of the surgery, and should be discussed with the patient, before deciding whether to reverse the effect of warfarin or postpone the elective surgery to allow the warfarin to be stopped ahead of surgery. Recommendations from the BCSH guidelines are summarized in **Table 21.6**.

Conditional use of fresh frozen plasma

In cases of massive transfusion (>5 L in 24 hours), dilution of clotting factors may occur. In patients who are hypotensive or septic, DIC may also complicate cases of massive transfusion. In most hospitals, the first dose of FFP (12–15 mL/kg) is given empirically, as laboratory coagulation results take at least 25 minutes to obtain, but subsequent use of FFP should be based on the results of repeated coagulation screens and guidance should be taken from a haematologist. Platelet and fibrinogen levels may also be required. The platelet count should be kept above 50×10^9/L. If the fibrinogen level is <0.8 g/L, cryoprecipitate should be given. 'Formula replacement', e.g. after a certain number of units of red cells is not proven to be of benefit, so is not indicated. [Grade B/C/D]

Liver disease

Patients who have liver disease may need FFP if they have bleeding associated with a coagulopathy. They may have significantly expanded plasma volumes (due to ascites and/or oedema) and the coagulopathy may be difficult to correct with FFP alone. If six to eight units of FFP fail to correct the coagulation tests in a bleeding patient prothrombin complex concentrate may be indicated, in spite of the associated increased risk of thrombosis. Such cases should be discussed with a haematologist. [Grade D]

No indication for fresh frozen plasma

Fresh frozen plasma is not indicated in the following:

- hypovolaemia;
- immunodeficiency;

Table 21.6 Reversal of warfarin anticoagulant effect.

Condition	Treatment
Life-threatening haemorrhage	Immediately give 5 mg vitamin K by slow intravenous infusion and a concentrate of factor II, IX, X (PCC) with factor VII concentrate if available
	The dose of concentrate should be calculated based on 50 IU factor IX/kg body weight. If no concentrate is available, FFP should be infused (15 mL/kg), but this may not be as effective
Less severe haemorrhage such as haematuria or epistaxis	Withhold warfarin for one or more days and consider giving vitamin K 0.5–2.0 mg i.v.
INR of > 4.5 without haemorrhage	Withdraw warfarin for 1 or 2 days then review
Unexpected bleeding at therapeutic levels	Investigate possibility of underlying cause such as unsuspected renal or alimentary tract disease

- nutritional support/protein loss states;
- plasma exchange procedures, unless there is an underlying coagulopathy.

CRYOPRECIPITATE

This is a product rich in factor VIII and fibrinogen and is made by thawing fresh frozen plasma overnight at 4–8°C. Indications for cryoprecipitate include treatment of DIC, where the fibrinogen is <1 g/L and in rare cases of fibrinogen deficiency.

PLATELETS

Platelet concentrates have made a major contribution to modern clinical practice, in particular in allowing the development of intensive treatment regimes for haematological and other malignancies.

Platelet collection and storage

Platelet concentrates are produced either by pooling platelets derived from four separate donations of whole blood or as single donor platelets which are obtained by apheresis.

For optimal platelet function, platelets, unlike red cells, are stored under conditions of gentle agitation (to prevent clumping) at a temperature of $22 \pm 2°C$. However, the shelf-life is limited to five days because of the risk of bacterial proliferation at this storage temperature. Sepsis secondary to platelet transfusion is more common than red cell infusion and therefore platelets should only be used when necessary. In the ENT setting, if patients have mild oral haemorrhage, the antifibrinolytic agent tranexamic acid (see Chapter 23, Haemostasis: Normal physiology, disorders of haemostasis and thrombosis and their management) may be a valuable alternative either as tablets or as an effective mouthwash suspension.

Indications for platelet transfusion

The cause of thrombocytopenia should be established as soon as possible so that the most appropriate treatment can be given and so that platelets are not given in conditions where they could cause harm. Serious spontaneous haemorrhage due to a low platelet count alone is unlikely to occur at platelet counts $>10 \times 10^9$/L.[8] BCSH guidelines suggest in stable thrombocytopenia, a threshold of 10×10^9/L for platelet transfusion, in the absence of any additional risk factors, e.g. sepsis antibiotic use or other abnormalities of haemostasis.[9]

Recommendations for platelets as surgical prophylaxis

Recommendations for various surgical procedures are as follows: [Grade D]

The platelet count should be kept above $>50 \times 10^9$/L for:

- lumbar puncture;
- epidural anaesthesia;
- gastroscopy and biopsy;
- insertion of indwelling lines;
- transbronchial biopsy;
- liver biopsy;
- laparotomy or similar procedures.

For operations at critical sites such as the eye and brain, the platelet count should be kept $>100 \times 10^9$/L.

Prior to a procedure, it is essential to repeat the platelet count after platelets have been transfused to ensure an adequate increment has been achieved.

Platelets may be required in massive transfusion or in acute DIC and in each the platelets should be kept $>50 \times 10^9$/L. Again repeated platelet counts are invaluable in acting as a guide to therapy. In chronic DIC, platelet transfusion is not routinely given to correct the thrombocytopenia. [Grade D]

Contraindications to platelet transfusion

- Heparin-induced thrombocytopenia (HIT) (see Chapter 23, Haemostasis: Normal physiology, disorders of haemostasis and thrombosis and their management). In such cases, platelet transfusion has been associated with acute arterial thrombosis. [Grade D]
- Thrombotic thrombocytopenia purpura (TTP) (see Chapter 23, Haemostasis: Normal physiology, disorders of haemostasis and thrombosis and their

management). Platelet infusions are contraindicated as they have been associated with TTP exacerbation: FFP (preferably by exchange transfusion) is the treatment of choice. [Grade B]

MEASURES TO AVOID TRANSMISSION OF BACTERIAL INFECTION VIA BLOOD COMPONENTS

In spite of stringent measures to minimize bacterial contamination of donated blood, bacterial contamination still rarely occurs. Therefore, all platelets in particular, should be checked at all stages, including at the bedside, for any possible leak or damage to the bag. Any change of colour or turbidity must be regarded as suspicious of contamination and discussed with the transfusion laboratory.

BLOOD DONATION

Strict eligibility criteria are applied to prevent harm to either the patient or the donor as a result of blood donation. Blood is taken from healthy adult donors aged between 17 and 70 years. Blood donation is voluntary so that there are no incentives for donors to withhold information about their health and put patients or themselves at risk. The avoidance of the transmission of infection to the recipient of blood products is of paramount importance in transfusion medicine. Donors at high risk of infections are excluded. Donors are therefore questioned extensively before donation proceeds.

Collection of 450 mL of blood is by strict aseptic technique. Blood in the UK is currently tested for a number of markers of infection (Table 21.7), but there is a 'window period' for each, when the donor may have recently acquired an infection but the marker will not yet be detected. *Cytomegalovirus* (CMV) negative components are only provided for patients at risk of developing severe manifestations of CMV, e.g. neonates, pregnant women, bone marrow transplant patients. Testing for malaria and *Trypanosoma cruzi* is also undertaken where appropriate.

There is no evidence at present to suggest that Creutzfeldt–Jakob disease (CJD) or variant CJD (vCJD) is transmissible to humans via blood products. However,

one study shows transfusion transmitted prion disease in sheep. Additionally, prion proteins have been located on the membranes of lymphocytes and platelets and in lymphoreticular tissue. For this reason and as our knowledge of prion disease is limited, the following precautions have been adopted in the UK: Firstly fractionated plasma products, e.g. albumin and IVIg, made from pooled plasma from thousands of donors, are now made using plasma from US donors, not UK donors. Secondly, all blood components are leukodepleted, as white cells were thought to play a key role in the pathogenesis of vCJD.

BLOOD GROUPING

Blood donations are tested for ABO and Rh D groups. Most UK donations are also labelled with their c, C, e, E and Kell antigen groups so that for 80 percent of antibodies that patients have, hospitals can provide antigen-negative blood from blood kept on site.

ADVERSE REACTIONS

The complications of transfusion can be for convenience divided into immediate and delayed and those caused by immune mechanisms and nonimmune complications (Table 21.8).

Immediate transfusion reactions

ABO INCOMPATIBILITY

This is the most dangerous of transfusion reactions and can prove fatal. The reaction often starts within the first hour of the transfusion and monitoring the patient's observations is important in detecting a reaction early.

ABO mismatch is totally preventable and most are due to human error in checking the patient's identity at the bedside before transfusion begins.[10] In addition, errors in labelling of crossmatch or G&S samples can be prevented by labelling the sample at the bedside, from the patient's wristband only. Mortality in cases of intravascular lysis

Table 21.7 Tests for infection in blood products in the UK.

Infection	Test	Window period	Residual risk per unit transfusion
HIV	Anti-HIV 1 and 2	22 days	1 in 4 million
Hepatitis B	HBsAg	3 weeks	1 in 100,000 to 400,000
Hepatitis C	Anti-HCV, HCV NAT	13 days	1 in 3 million
Syphilis	TPHA		Less well defined
HTLV	Anti-HTLV I and II		Less well defined
CMV	Anti-CMV		

Table 21.8 Complications of transfusion.

	Immune	Nonimmune
Immediate	ABO incompatibility	Bacterial sepsis ± endotoxic shock
	Febrile, nonhaemolytic reaction	Cardiac failure (overload)
	Urticarial rash	In large volume transfusions: hypothermia, hyperkalaemia, hypocalcaemia
	Anaphylactic reaction	Air embolism (rare)
	Transfusion-related acute lung injury (TRALI)	
Delayed	Delayed haemolytic transfusion reaction (DHTR) (red cell antibodies)	Viral: hepatitis B, C, HIV, HTLV, CMV, parvovirus
	Post-transfusion purpura (PTP)	
	Transfusion-associated graft-versus-host disease (TAGVHD)	Other infections: malaria, trypanosomiasis, etc.
	Immunomodulatory effects	Iron overload (long term)

secondary to ABO incompatibility is significant and of the order of 10 percent. From the annual Serious Hazards of Transfusion (SHOT) reporting scheme in the UK, two to four patients die each year and a further five to ten have serious morbidity (e.g. require renal dialysis or admission to the intensive therapy unit (ITU)) as a result of 'wrong blood' errors. A further 25–30 have the wrong blood given, but with no adverse effect, e.g. because they receive group O in error.

Clinically, the patient experiences headache, lumbar back pain, chest tightness, nausea or facial flushing. Examination of the patient may reveal tachycardia and hypotension. Fever and rigors typically follow. Microscopic or in severe cases macroscopic haematuria may be seen. Treatment consists of stopping the transfusion, giving i.v. fluids, resuscitation and management of renal failure. The blood unit and further samples for G&S, DAT, full blood count, coagulation screen, biochemistry and a urine for haemoglobinuria should be sent to the laboratory and discussed with a haematologist. [Grade D]

BACTERIAL INFECTION

Very similar symptoms of fever, tachycardia and hypotension also occur with infected blood components being transfused. Antibiotics need to be given before a definitive diagnosis is made. This should be done in accordance with the hospital's current antibiotic protocol. Management of the patient is again by resuscitation and plain fluids and treatment of any renal failure. [Grade D]

FEBRILE, NONHAEMOLYTIC TRANSFUSION REACTIONS

Patients may develop a fever and sometimes rigors during transfusions. This is thought to be due to release of cytokines during storage, but has not been prevented totally by leukodepletion. These reactions are harmless but clinicians must make sure that severe reactions, e.g. bacterial sepsis or wrong blood reactions are not mistaken for these.

ALLERGIC REACTIONS

These may occur when a blood component contains a plasma protein to which the patient is allergic and has IgE antibodies and occur in about 1 percent of transfusions. They often result in mild urticarial reactions and are usually treated with an antihistamine with or without hydrocortisone. However, severe reactions may rarely occur leading to anaphylaxis. These may be seen in patients who are deficient in IgA, who may make anti-IgA antibodies, which can react with IgA normally present in blood components, causing anaphylaxis. In known IgA-deficient patients undergoing surgery, it is important that the haematology department is told well in advance of any elective procedure as it requires planning in order to have an IgA-deficient donor or washed products on standby.

TRANSFUSION-RELATED ACUTE LUNG INJURY

This is a rare but often severe complication. During, or soon after transfusion, particularly of FFP or platelets, patients became markedly hypoxic, dyspnoeic and may require ventilation and it is sometimes fatal. Transfusion-related acute lung injury (TRALI) is caused by anti-leukocyte (or neutrophil) antibodies in the donor's plasma, which match the specificity of the patient's white blood cells (WBC), causing aggregation of WBC in the patient's lung vasculative, causing tissue destruction.

FLUID OVERLOAD

This can be avoided by giving a diuretic with alternate units of blood if necessary.

LARGE VOLUME TRANSFUSION

Hypothermia may occur and can be minimized by infusing blood via a blood warmer. Hyperkalaemia, due to a large volume of stored blood, in which red cells have leaked some potassium, does not usually require treatment but electrocardiogram (ECG) monitoring is advisable. Hypocalcaemia, due to citrate anti-coagulant in stored blood, does not usually require treatment.

Delayed haemolytic transfusion reactions

PREMATURE DESTRUCTION OF TRANSFUSED RED CELLS

Transfused red cells are destroyed prematurely (normal red cell lifespan 120 days) due to the presence of antibodies in the patient's plasma which are directed at antigens on the donor's red cells.

Such reactions usually occur between seven and ten days post-transfusion and may manifest as a mild anaemia, a rise in serum bilirubin level and often an accompanying fever. The drop in haemoglobin is proportional to the quantity of red cells transfused, i.e. larger volume transfusions manifest with a greater drop in haemoglobin. Occasionally, transfusion reactions occur within 24 hours of the transfusion.

POST-TRANSFUSION PURPURA

Profound thrombocytopenia (<10) associated with purpura and occasionally severe bleeding, may occur about seven and ten days post-transfusion and is caused by the presence of antiplatelet antibodies, usually anti-HPA 1a in the recipient. The resulting platelet destruction occurs in both autologous and transfused platelets due to cross-reaction or by the formation of immune complexes. Intravenous immunoglobulin is the treatment of choice. Platelet transfusion is unhelpful and not warranted unless life-threatening bleeding occurs. The differential diagnosis postoperatively often includes heparin-induced thrombocytopenia.

TRANSFUSION-ASSOCIATED GRAFT-VERSUS-HOST DISEASE

Transfusion-associated graft-versus-host disease (TAG-VHD) occurs in severely immunosuppressed patients or could occur in those receiving blood from first-degree relatives. It is caused by viable T lymphocytes in the donor's blood which attack the patient's tissues causing a skin rash, liver failure, severe diarrhoea and bone marrow failure and is uniformly fatal. It is preventable by irradiating blood components for susceptible patients.

IMMUNOMODULATORY EFFECTS

Transfusion may be associated with an increase in post-operative sepsis (away from the wound site) and increased tumour recurrence rates (e.g. in cancer of the colon), but there are conflicting results and the same results are apparent whenever allogeneic (donor) blood or autologous blood is used. Further studies are needed to clarify this.

IRON OVERLOAD

Repeated transfusions in some patients, such as those with thalassaemia or sickle cell disease, may result in the gradual accumulation of iron with subsequent organ deposition (heart, pancreas, etc.). Such patients are managed with iron-chelating agents. Any patient with a haemoglobinopathy, who is due to undergo surgery, should be discussed jointly with both the haematologist and anaesthetist well in advance of any procedure.

ALTERNATIVES TO TRANSFUSION

The fact that blood transfusion is not a zero risk intervention has led to attempts to introduce alternative therapies which reduce the need for allogeneic blood components. Such technologies may be useful for individual patients who decline transfusion on the grounds of religious teachings and beliefs. This section will concentrate primarily on alternatives to allogeneic red cell transfusion.

Autologous transfusion

PREOPERATIVE AUTOLOGOUS DEPOSIT

Preoperative autologous deposit (PAD) is of use only in those patients who have planned elective surgical procedures. Patients who are fit enough to donate blood, can take oral iron supplements and donate one unit (450 mL) of blood at weekly intervals in the four weeks leading up to surgery, provided their haemoglobin recovers adequately between weekly donations. In practice, patients donate two or three units at most. These donations are then subject to the same storage and handling procedures as for other donated units but kept solely for the use of the donor at a subsequent time. Such a procedure requires considerable planning and liaison between surgical firms and the local blood service. The other pitfall of autologous donation in clinical practice, is that as the amount of blood that can be used from autologous donation is limited, complications at the time of the planned procedure may mean that allogeneic transfusion may be needed in addition. Although regarded as safer than allogeneic transfusion from the point of view of viral transmission, it does not eliminate the risk of bacterial contamination or receiving the 'wrong blood'. Autologous transfusion in clinical practice is also limited by the five-week shelf-life of red cells so that if surgery is postponed, the blood expires. In recent years, PAD has became less poplar, as in practice, may patients do not make up their haemoglobin between donations and often undergo surgery with a haemoglobin level lower than it was before predeposit was started.[11] Many clinicians now prefer to ensure that patients are not anaemic before surgery, allow patients to run a lower haemoglobin postoperatively before requiring transfusion and give patients iron supplements.

ACUTE NORMOVOLAEMIC HAEMODILUTION

Just before induction of anaesthesia at operation, 0.5–1 L (one to two units) of a patient's blood can be removed, using a blood collection pack containing anticoagulant, and replaced with crystalloid fluid to maintain normovolaemia. Following blood loss during surgery, the patient's own blood can be returned. This technique has very limited use as the amount of blood that can be removed is limited, the patient must be fit enough to withstand this and often, allogeneic blood is still needed in addition to the patient's own.

CELL SALVAGE

Blood lost can be salvaged either (1) during surgery: intraoperative cell salvage, which requires expensive equipment to suction, anticoagulate, wash, centrifuge and filter the blood or (2) after surgery: postoperative cell salvage, which requires just a modified drain, in which blood is collected for six hours then simply filtered and reinfused. These techniques can be used in a variety of surgical operations, but generally, intraoperative cell salvage is used only where >1 L blood loss is likely and neither is appropriate where the surgical field is bacterially contaminated.

Other methods to reduce red blood cell transfusion

RECOMBINANT ERYTHROPOIETIN

Recombinant erythropoietin (rEpo) (see Chapter 22, Haemato-oncology) is currently widely used in a number of chronic and malignant conditions, such as chronic renal failure and multiple myeloma, to avoid repeated transfusions and the complications that accompany them. It can be used in the weeks prior to surgery in patients in whom transfusion with allogeneic blood would be a problem (e.g. Jehovah's witnesses).

Other alternative treatments to avoid the use of allogeneic blood are directed at reducing blood loss.

FIBRIN GLUE

One syringe containing calcium and human thrombin and another containing human fibrinogen are mixed directly when injected simultaneously at the point of bleeding. Subsequent reaction leads to the formation of fibrin clot achieving haemostasis. This 'glue' is now widely used in accident and emergency departments and at minor injury clinics for the treatment of minor cutaneous bleeds.

TRANEXAMIC ACID

Tranexamic acid is an antifibrinolytic agent and can be used for the treatment of minor bleeds, such as bleeds in the oral cavity, and is available both as tablets and in a mouthwash form and is available in most hospital pharmacies.

HAEMOGLOBIN SUBSTITUTES

There are available acellular preparations of human haemoglobin. Such products are interesting prospects in that they would remove the risk of bacterial, viral and prion transfusion. Unfortunately, at the present time, such preparations are of limited clinical use in areas of acute trauma resuscitation mainly became of their relatively short half-life of around 24 hours. Such preparations are only currently on limited licences in the United States and South Africa.

SYNTHETIC OXYGEN CARRIERS

O_2-carrying synthetic compounds such as perfluorocarbons (PFC) require high flow oxygen available to the patient for them to be of any significant value to the patient. Therefore, their application in the clinical arena is limited to situations such as intensive therapy where patients can be highly monitored. Again, their half-life is very short.

Overall, there is a range of measures that can be taken to avoid the use of allogeneic blood where required, but many require planning ahead and liaison in advance with haematologists is advisable.

KEY POINTS

- For elective surgery, a group and screen or crossmatch sample is needed 24 hours in advance, to ensure that compatible blood is available.
- In an emergency, indicate how long until blood is needed at the bedside, so that the laboratory staff can curtail testing if the clinical balance of risks warrants it
- Preoperative assessment and correction of anaemia can reduce perioperative transfusion.

Best clinical practice

✓ In an emergency, prothrombin complex concentrate (or FFP) can be used to reverse warfarin, but in elective surgery, the potential adverse effects of FFP should be balanced against the urgency of surgery and options discussed with the patient.

✓ If a patient has a marked reaction during a blood
transfusion, stop the transfusion and discuss urgently
with the transfusion laboratory and a haematology
doctor. 'Wrong blood' (ABO incompatible) or bacterial
infection of blood should be considered and treated
promptly. Other possibilities include TRALI and
anaphylaxis due to IgA deficiency.

Deficiencies in current knowledge and areas for future research

For a decade, considerable sums of money have been
spent on reducing infectious risks of transfusion in the
UK, yet it is often used unnecessarily. There is a lack of,
and a need for, good clinical trials to understand when
transfusion will be effective. These could then facilitate a
balanced approach to risk reduction which could be
understood and accepted by a well-informed public.

REFERENCES

1. Murphy MF, Wallington TB, Kelsey P, Boulton F, Bruce M, Cohen H et al. Guidelines for the Clinical Use of Red Cell Transfusions. BCSH Blood Transfusion Task Force. British Journal of Haematology. 2001; 113: 24–31.
2. Baskett PJF. Management of hypovolaemic shock. British Medical Journal. 1990; 300: 1453–7.
3. Maunes, Jeckstrom W, Thomsen H, Rudert H. Indication, incidence and management of blood transfusion during sinus surgery: a review over 12 years. Rhinology. 1997; 35: 2–5.
4. Gong SG, Krishnan V, Waack D. Blood transfusions in bimaxillary or orthognathic surgery: are they necessary? International Journal of Adult Orthodontics and Orthognathic Surgery. 2002; 17: 314–7.
5. Moenning JE, Bussard DA, Lapp TH, Garrison BT. Average blood loss and the risk of requiring perioperative blood transfusion in 506 orthognathic surgical procedures. Journal of Oral and Maxillofacial Surgery. 1995; 53: 880–3.
6. The Sanguis Study Group. Use of blood products for Electives Surgery in 43 European hospitals. Transfusion Medicine. 1994; 4: 251–68.
7. Contreras M, Ala FA, Greaves M, Jones J, Levin M, Machin SJ et al. Guidelines for the use of Fresh Frozen Plasma. BCSH Transfusion Task Force. Transfusion Medicine. 1992; 2: 57–63.
8. Schlicter SJ. Controversies in platelet transfusion therapy. Annual Reviews of Medicine. 1980; 31: 509–40.
9. Guidelines for the use of Platelet Transfusions. BCSH Transfusion Task Force. British Journal of Haematology. 2003; 122: 10–23.
10. The Serious Hazards of Transfusion Steering Group. Serious hazards of transfusion: Annual report 2001–2002. Published July 17, 2003; last accessed Spring 2004. Available from http://www.shotuk.org.
11. Brecher ME, Goodenough LT. The rise and fall of pre-operative autologous blood donation. Transfusion. 2001; 41: 1459–62.

22

Haemato-oncology

CLARE WYKES AND FIONA REGAN

Introduction	265	Key points	276
Normal haemopoiesis	265	Best clinical practice	276
Red cells	266	Deficiencies in current knowledge and areas for future	
White cells	272	research	276
Platelets	275	References	277
Splenectomy	276		

SEARCH STRATEGY

The data in this chapter are supported by a Medline search using the key words erythropoiesis, blood dyscrasias, leukaemia, lymphoma and plasma cell.

PERIOPERATIVE MANAGEMENT OF SICKLE CELL DISEASE

The data in this section are supported by a Medline search using the key words sickle cell disease, operative management, tonsillectomy, adenoidectomy and myringotomy.

INTRODUCTION

Patients with underlying haematological disease may present initially to the otorhinolaryngology surgeon, for example with epistaxis or lymphadenopathy. Many diseases affecting the ear, nose and throat or their treatments may have significant haematological effects. This chapter seeks to provide an understanding of the oncological aspects of the haematological system and haemato-oncology as a means of assisting prompt diagnosis.

NORMAL HAEMOPOIESIS

Physiology of blood

Blood consists of:

- red cells;
- white cells:
  - granulocytes: neutrophils, eosinophils, basophils;
  - mononuclear cells: lymphocytes, monocytes/macrophages.
- platelets;
- plasma, which contains soluble fibrinogen (serum is what remains after fibrin clot has formed).

Haemopoiesis (blood cell formation)

SITE OF HAEMOPOIESIS

Foetal haemopoiesis occurs in the yolk sac for the first few weeks of gestation and then in the liver and spleen. From about six months' gestation, haemopoietic stem cells migrate to the bone marrow and this becomes the principal site of haemopoiesis. In infancy, the majority of bone marrow is haemopoietic but during childhood there is progressive replacement by fatty tissue. By adulthood only the proximal ends of long bones and the central skeleton are haemopoietic.

Extramedullary haemopoiesis, i.e. resumption of blood cell formation in the liver or spleen, occurs in pathological states such as thalassaemias and myelofibrosis as a means of increasing production of haemopoietic cells.

HAEMOPOIETIC STEM CELLS

All blood cells are derived from pluripotential stem cells within the bone marrow, which differentiate into progenitor cells that are committed to a specific lineage, e.g. the erythroid progenitor (burst-forming unit erythroid (BFU-E)), the granulocyte/macrophage progenitor (colony-forming unit, granulocyte-macrophage (CFU-GM)) and the megakaryocyte progenitor (colony-forming unit, megakaryocyte (CFU-Mk)) (**Figure 22.1**). Pluripotential stem cells also have the capability of self-renewal which ensures a constant cellularity and ability to respond with increased production of a particular cell line when needed. Stromal cells within the bone marrow microenvironment produce growth factors which coordinate the production of lineage-specific progenitors. These include glycoproteins such as stem cell factor, interleukin-3 and granulocyte colony-stimulating factor (G-CSF). Erythropoietin (EPO) is produced by renal interstitial cells in response to low oxygen tissue tensions. It acts on committed erythroid precursors to induce proliferation and inhibit apoptosis. Recombinant G-CSF and EPO are available for therapeutic use.

RED CELLS

Erythropoiesis

For effective erythropoiesis, the marrow requires:

- metals – iron, cobalt;
- vitamins – B_{12}, folate, C, E, thiamine, B_6 and riboflavin;
- hormones – thyroxine and androgens.

As red cell precursors mature in the bone marrow, the haemoglobin (Hb) content in the cytoplasm increases, the nuclear material condenses and the nucleus is eventually lost before the red cell is released from the marrow as a reticulocyte, which still contains RNA for globin chain synthesis. These cells circulate for one to two days and lose their RNA whilst passing through the spleen, leaving a mature erythrocyte, which is a non-nucleated biconcave disc. If nucleated red blood cells (RBC) are seen in a blood film, this is abnormal and indicates extramedullary haemopoiesis, bone marrow infiltration or severe sepsis. Red cells normally survive for 120 days before destruction in the reticuloendothelial system. Reticulocytes normally comprise 1–2 percent of the red cell population.

Haemoglobin

Adult haemoglobin (HbA) is a tetramer of two α and two β globin chains (α2β2). The minor haemoglobin, HbA2 (α2δ2), is present in adults and is less than 3 percent of

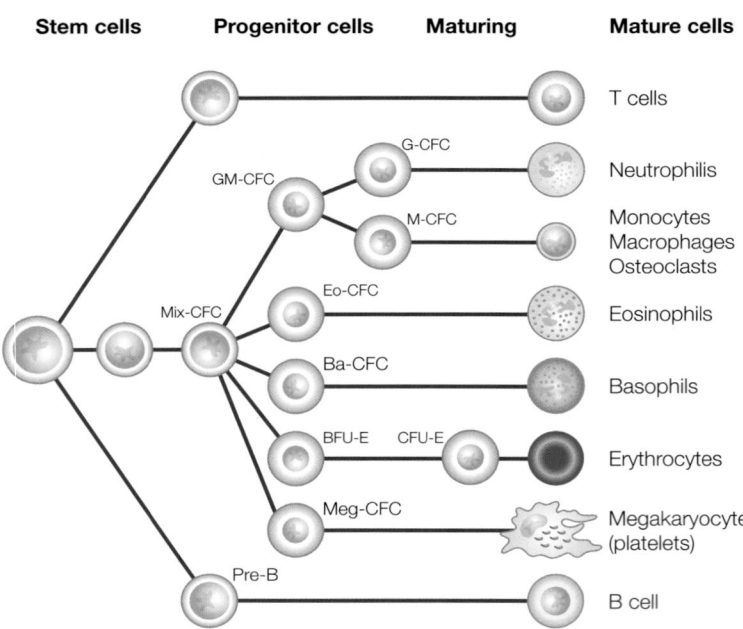

Figure 22.1 Schematic representation of haemopoiesis.

total haemoglobin. Foetal haemoglobin ($\alpha2\gamma2$) is normally replaced by HbA during the first six months of life.

Haem synthesis occurs in the mitochondria and requires vitamin B6. Each haem molecule combines with a globin chain and when a tetramer is formed, the four haem groups reside in 'haem pockets' in which the amino acids in the globin chains are positioned to keep the iron in a ferrous state such that it can associate reversibly with oxygen. The main function of erythrocytes is to carry Hb in adequate concentration to enable oxygen delivery to the tissues. When oxygen combines with the haem group, conformational change occurs so that the molecule has a greater affinity for oxygen. Other molecules, such as hydrogen ions and 2,3-diphosphoglycerate (2,3DPG), maintain the haem in its low affinity form and thus permit unloading of oxygen at the low pH of tissues. This property of the haem molecule explains the sigmoid form of the oxygen dissociation curve. For example, in anaemia 2,3DPG levels are increased and thus unload oxygen more readily.

Haematological blood investigations

THE FULL BLOOD COUNT

Automated cell counters are used to measure Hb and the number and size of red cells, white cells and platelets. Other indices such as the mean corpuscular volume (MCV) are derived from these results (**Table 22.1**). Blood for a full blood count (FBC) is taken in a tube anticoagulated with ethylenediaminetetraacetic acid (EDTA) and analysed as soon as possible to prevent storage artefacts. Increasingly, near-patient testing facilities such as the 'HemoCue' are available in the operating theatre or recovery room to provide more rapid results,

albeit for the Hb concentration. In anaemia or acute blood loss, the absolute reticulocyte count should rise because of erythropoietin increase.

Erythrocyte sedimentation rate

Erythrocyte sedimentation rate (ESR) is the rate of fall of red cells in a column of blood and is a measure of the acute phase response. A raised ESR reflects an increase in the number of large plasma proteins such as immunoglobulins and fibrinogen, which cause the red cells to clump together and fall more rapidly. Causes of a markedly raised ESR (e.g. > 100 mm/hour) include malignancy, tuberculosis, temporal arteritis and myeloma. Causes of a mildly raised ESR include anaemia, female sex and increasing age. The ESR may be a useful pointer if one of the above diseases is suspected, but is not specific and further definitive tests would be needed.

Plasma viscosity

Viscosity provides similar information to the ESR but is not affected by sex or Hb.

Anaemias

Anaemia is a reduction in the Hb concentration of blood below normal values. This may be caused by an increased plasma volume, for example haemodilution, as well as a reduced circulating red cell mass.

CLINICAL ASSESSMENT

Anaemia is not a specific condition and the underlying cause must be sought. If anaemia is detected preoperatively the clinical history and simple investigations will

Table 22.1 Normal adult ranges.

	Males	Females	Males and females
Haemoglobin	13.5–17.5 g/dL	11.5–15.5 g/dL	
Red cells	$4.5–6.5 \times 10^{12}$/L	$3.9–5.6 \times 10^{12}$/L	
Haematocrit	0.40–0.52	0.36–0.48	
MCV			80–95 fL
MCH			27–34 pg
MCHC			20–35 g/dL
White cells			
Total			$4.0–11 \times 10^9$/L
Neutrophils			$2.5–7.5 \times 10^9$/L
Lymphocytes			$1.5–3.5 \times 10^9$/L
Monocytes			$0.2–0.8 \times 10^9$/L
Eosinophils			$0.04–0.44 \times 10^9$/L
Basophils			$0.01–0.1 \times 10^9$/L
Platelets			$150–400 \times 10^9$/L
Reticulocytes			$20–130 \times 10^9$/L

MCH, mean corpuscular haemoglobin; MCHC, mean corpuscular haemoglobin concentration.

usually reveal the diagnosis, allow correction of anaemia and prevent unnecessary blood transfusions.

The history should focus on:

- duration of symptoms such as shortness of breath, fatigue, lethargy;
- bleeding especially from the gastrointestinal (GI) tract;
- family history;
- past history including gastrectomy;
- dietary history;
- drug history, including non-prescribed medication.

The examination may be unhelpful, but general signs of anaemia such as tachycardia, flow murmurs and congestive cardiac failure and more specific signs such as koilonychia ('spooning' of the nails seen in iron deficiency anaemia), jaundice and stomatitis should be sought.

Investigations

The most useful guide to further investigating anaemia is the MCV. This divides anaemia into microcytic, normocytic and macrocytic (**Table 22.2**).

Clues can also be gained from the WBC and platelet count: pancytopenia is suggestive of a more generalized marrow defect and during bleeding the anaemia is often accompanied by a reactive thrombocytosis.

MICROCYTIC ANAEMIAS

Iron deficiency is the most common cause of a microcytic, hypochromic anaemia worldwide. The major differential diagnoses are anaemia of chronic disease and thalassaemia, which is discussed below under Thalassaemias. The investigation of a microcytic anaemia (MCV <80) should therefore include serum iron, transferrin saturation, serum transferrin receptor, total iron binding capacity (TIBC), ferritin and haemoglobin electrophoresis (if indicated by the patient's ethnic origin) (**Table 22.3**).

Iron-deficiency anaemia

In men the daily iron requirement is 1 mg/day and in menstruating women it is 2–3 mg/day. Circulating Hb accounts for about 75 percent of total body iron (3–4 g) and the remainder is stored as ferritin and haemosiderin. There is no physiological route for iron excretion and homeostasis is achieved by regulation of the absorption of ferrous iron across the duodenal enterocytes. Hepcidin has been putatively proposed as the mediator of iron homeostasis.

The blood film characteristically shows hypochromic microcytic red cells and pencil cells. The underlying cause should be presumed to be blood loss until proven otherwise. Patients should be asked about diet, menstrual losses, GI symptoms and bleeding. Oral iron supplementation (i.e. ferrous sulphate 200 mg three times a day) can be started whilst the cause is being elucidated and a rise in Hb of 1 g per week and a reticulocytosis within a few days of starting iron should be expected.

Anaemia of chronic disease

This is common in chronic infection, inflammation, connective tissue diseases and malignancy. The mechanisms

Table 22.3   Identification of causes of anaemia from iron studies.

	IDA	AoCD	Thalassaemia
MCV/MCH	↓	↓↑	↓↓
Serum iron	↓	↓	↔
TIBC	↑	↓	↔
Transferrin saturation	↓	↓	↔
Serum transferrin receptor	↑	↔↓	Variable
Ferritin	↓	↑	↔
Hb electrophoresis	Normal	Normal	Raised HbA₂

AoCD, anaemia of chronic disease; IDA, iron deficiency anaemia; TIBC, total iron binding capacity.

Table 22.2   Identification of causes of anaemia by mean corpuscular volume result.

Microcytic	Normocytic	Macrocytic
MCV <80 fL	MCV 80–100 fL	MCV >80 fL If MCV >100
Iron deficiency	With reticulocytosis: haemolysis or acute blood loss	Megaloblastic: vitamin B_{12} or folate deficiency
Thalassaemia	With normal or low reticulocyte count: Anaemia of chronic disease (some cases), renal disease, bone marrow failure, mixed deficiencies	Nonmegaloblastic: alcohol, liver disease, myelodysplasia
Anaemia of chronic disease (some cases)		
Lead poisoning		
Sideroblastic anaemia (some cases)		

responsible include an increase in iron retention in the reticuloendothelial system, cytokine-mediated inhibition of erythroid progenitor proliferation and a blunted erythropoietin response.

The blood film shows hypochromic microcytic red cells as seen in iron deficiency anaemia (IDA). If the markers in **Table 22.3** cannot differentiate between IDA and anaemia of chronic disease (AoCD), a bone marrow aspirate may be required to determine if iron stores are absent, indicating iron deficiency.

Thalassaemias

This group of disorders is discussed below under Thalassaemias.

Congenital sideroblastic anaemia

This group of disorders is characterized by a defect in protoporphyrin incorporation into the haem molecule. It is diagnosed by finding sideroblasts in the bone marrow which are abnormal erythroblasts with rings of iron granules.

Lead poisoning

A blood film shows hypochromic microcytic red cells and many red cells with basophilic stippling (of which there are many causes). Lead levels would be required.

MACROCYTIC ANAEMIAS

The causes of a macrocytic anaemia (MCV > 100) are broadly divided into megaloblastic and nonmegaloblastic causes (see **Table 22.2**). Megaloblasts are premature erythrocytes with delayed nuclear maturation relative to that of the cytoplasm due to defective DNA synthesis. Initial investigations should include B_{12} and red cell folate levels.

Megaloblastic

In B_{12} or folate deficiency, there are oval macrocytes and hypersegmented neutrophils. Once B_{12} and red cell folate levels have been requested, then both B_{12} and folate replacement may be started until results are available. A rise in reticulocyte count and a rise in Hb of 1 g per week would be expected.

Vitamin B_{12} deficiency

Vitamin B_{12} is synthesized solely by microorganisms and is present only in food of animal origin. Absorption is dependent on intrinsic factor (IF), which is secreted by gastric parietal cells. The B_{12} complex is absorbed at the terminal ileum and is transported into the blood by transcobalamin II. Body stores, of which over half is in the liver, equate to approximately 3 mg, which is sufficient for three years.

Cause of vitamin B_{12} deficiency include inadequate intake, IF deficiency (e.g. pernicious anaemia (PA)),

post-gastrectomy or small intestinal disease. Particular attention should be paid to dietary history, family history of autoimmune disease and signs and symptoms of small bowel disease. Patients should be examined for evidence of a peripheral neuropathy. Intrinsic factor and parietal cell antibodies should be checked if PA is suspected. This is an autoimmune disease in which the gastric mucosa becomes atrophied. Intestinal metaplasia may occur and there is an increased risk of gastric carcinoma (2–3 percent of all cases of PA). Endoscopy should therefore be performed if there are symptoms of dyspepsia.

It is important to ascertain whether B_{12}-deficient patients have the capacity to absorb the vitamin normally. In the UK this is done by the Schilling test, which measures urinary excretion of B_{12}. The patient is given an oral dose of radioactively labelled B_{12} and a large dose of nonlabelled B_{12}. This serves to 'flush' the labelled B_{12} into the urine. In patients with dietary deficiency, absorption and excretion will be normal. In patients with PA, previous gastrectomy or intestinal malabsorption, the excretion is reduced. Such patients are then given a second dose of labelled B_{12} with IF. Patients with PA or gastrectomy will then show normal excretion whereas those with intestinal malabsorption will still fail to absorb B_{12}. If B_{12} and iron deficiency are found, coeliac disease needs to be considered and an endoscopy is required.

Folic acid deficiency

Folic acid is present in most foodstuffs, the highest concentrations in liver and green vegetables. Body stores are sufficient for only four months.

Causes of folic acid deficiency include poor diet, malabsorption (for example, with coeliac disease), excess utilization (for example, pregnancy, haemolysis, malignancy, inflammatory disease), drugs (for example, anticonvulsants), alcoholism and liver disease.

Nonmegaloblastic (MCV < 100)

In myelodysplastic syndrome (MDS), the blood film may reveal dysplastic red cells, neutrophils and abnormal platelets. There may be a pancytopenia. A bone marrow including cytogenetic analysis is needed to confirm the diagnosis. The blood film in liver disease may show target cells and thrombocytopenia.

NORMOCYTIC ANAEMIA

A normochromic, normocytic anaemia is seen in a wide variety of disorders. Depending on findings of the clinical history, initial investigations may include a reticulocyte count, blood film, renal function, liver and thyroid function tests, acute phase reactants and clotting screen. If these are not diagnostic, a bone marrow aspirate may be required.

Causes of this type of anaemia are outlined in **Table 22.2**.

Preoperative management of normochromic/normocytic anaemias

If the underlying cause of anaemia cannot be treated before surgery, blood transfusion should only be given when necessary, because of the residual risks of bacterial infection or receiving the incorrect transfusion (see Chapter 21, Blood groups, blood components and alternatives to transfusion). There has been one prospective series of ten patients awaiting major head and neck oncology surgery who received erythropoietin preoperatively. Eight patients experienced a significant increase in Hb.[1] There are no randomized controlled trials using erythropoietin peri-operatively, but it may be useful in patients with cultural or religious objections to allogeneic transfusion.[2] [Grade D]

HAEMOLYTIC ANAEMIA

The rate of red cell destruction is increased, but as the normal adult marrow is capable of producing red cells at six times the normal rate, anaemia may not be seen clinically until red cell survival is less than 30 days.

Patients should be questioned regarding family history, racial origin, drug and toxin exposure, recent blood transfusions and infective symptoms. Clinically the patient may show fluctuating jaundice, splenomegaly, acrocyanosis (including of the ears) and urine that darkens on standing due to the presence of excess urobilinogen. Intravascular haemolysis can cause haemoglobinuria.

Causes of a haemolytic anaemia include:

- intrinsic RBC abnormality:
  - membrane defects, e.g. hereditary spherocytosis;
  - metabolic defects, e.g. glucose-6-phosphate deficiency (G6PD);
  - Hb defect, e.g. sickle cell, thalassaemia.
- extrinsic RBC abnormality:
  - antibody-mediated, e.g. haemolytic transfusion reactions, autoimmune;
  - RBC fragmentation.
    - prosthetic heart valves;
    - microangiopathic haemolytic anaemia;
    - disseminated intravascular coagulation.
  - infections:
    - EBV;
    - Mycoplasma;
    - *Plasmodium falciparum* malaria;
  - chemicals and drug damage;
  - paroxysmal nocturnal haemoglobinuria.

Table 22.4 shows the investigations that confirm a haemolytic anaemia and further investigations should be directed by the history. In a postoperative setting, drugs and transfusion history should be elucidated. Depending on the blood film, haemoglobin electrophoresis (if not done preoperatively), G6PD and a direct antiglobulin test should be considered. The management of these conditions is tailored to the underlying condition, but all

Table 22.4 Laboratory investigations for haemolytic anaemia.

Presence of haemolysis	Compensatory increase in erythropoiesis
Increased unconjugated bilirubin	Reticulocytosis (a bone marrow test, if required, would show erythroid hyperplasia)
Increased LDH	
Absent haptoglobin (circulating protein which binds Hb)	
Increased urinary urobilinogen	

LDH, lactate dehydrogenase.

benefit from folic acid 5 mg daily. Iron deficiency does not occur unless there is intravascular haemolysis and iron is lost through the urine. Autoimmune cases are often managed with immunosuppression and if longstanding, this should not be stopped perioperatively. Patients with known haemolytic anaemias should be discussed with a haematologist preoperatively.

HAEMOGLOBINOPATHIES

The haemoglobinopathies are inherited disorders of haemoglobin structure or its production.

SICKLING DISORDERS

This group of disorders includes the homozygous state (HbSS), and co-inheritance of the sickle cell gene with β thalassaemia or with other Hb variants, e.g. HbSC disease. HbSS is found most commonly in Afro-Caribbeans but also seen in Mediterranean populations, the Middle East and India. HbS differs from HbA by the substitution of valine for glutamic acid at position 6 of the β chain. During deoxygenation, the abnormal Hb molecules form linear stacks causing the RBC to deform into a rigid sickle shape. These cells have difficulty passing through the microcirculation resulting in obstruction of small vessels and tissue infarction. Sickle cells also have a shortened survival.

The clinical course is highly variable but usually presents from three months onwards with anaemia and mild jaundice. In older patients vaso-occlusive problems occur as a result of sickling in the small vessels of any organ. Patients may present with:

- painful crises;
- aplastic crises;
- sequestration crises when sickled RBC pool in the liver or spleen;
- chest syndrome which is characterized by tachycardia, fever, profound hypoxaemia, falling Hb and bilateral chest signs;
- cerebrovascular accident.

Investigations reveal a steady state Hb between 5 and 11 g/dL, mildly raised WBC and platelets. There is a reticulocytosis and mildly elevated lactate dehydrogenase (LDH) and bilirubin. A sickle solubility test detects the presence of HbS, but cannot distinguish sickle trait from HbSS or HbSC. Hb electrophoresis is required to confirm the diagnosis. All patients from at-risk populations should have Hb electrophoresis (or at least a sickle solubility test) done prior to a general anaesthetic.[3] [Grade D] In patients with recurrent crises, hydroxyurea has been shown to improve the clinical course which is, in part, explained by its ability to increase HbF levels.[4] [Grade C]

Perioperative management of sickle cell disease

Surgery of the ear, nose and throat accounts for about 20 percent of all surgical procedures in this group. Surgical procedures may be complicated by hypoxia, acidosis or hypothermia leading to an increased risk of sickle cell-related complications. The observed complication rate of 32 percent for tonsillectomy and/or adenoidectomy (T/A) was twice the frequency that has been reported among patients without sickle cell disease.[5] The Cooperative Study of Sickle Cell Disease retrospectively analysed 1079 operations in patients with sickling disorders.[6] The sickle-related complication rate (painful crisis, acute chest syndrome, cerebrovascular accident) varied with the type of procedure; in patients undergoing T/A there were no sickle cell disease-related complications in HbSS patients. In patients undergoing myringotomy, there was one sickle-related complication. In both types of operation there was no significant difference between the overall postoperative complication rate and transfusion status. Blood transfusion regimes can be used preoperatively to dilute the percentage of sickle cells, thus potentially reducing the risk of vaso-occlusive crises. The multi-institutional Preoperative Transfusion Study[6] directly compared an aggressive transfusion approach in which the percentage of HbS was reduced to less than 30 percent (achieved by exchange transfusion), to a conservative approach in which the target Hb was 10 g/dL (achieved by top-up transfusion). This included 165 patients who underwent T/A or myringotomy. There was no difference in complication rates between the two groups. A previous history of pulmonary disease identified patients as at risk for sickle cell-related events undergoing T/A. This was the only trial that met the criteria for the Cochrane Database Review assessing preoperative blood transfusions for sickle cell disease (SCD).[7] There are no available data comparing exchange transfusion with no transfusion at all. [****/***]

In the absence of a study comparing transfusion versus no transfusion it seems reasonable to consider top-up transfusion in HbSS to a Hb of 10 g/dL, unless there is a history of pulmonary complications or other markers of severe disease. [Grade C] In such cases it would seem more appropriate to exchange transfuse preoperatively

aiming for ≤30 percent Hbs. [Grade D] Other cases are considered on an individual basis. Factors such as length of operation and presence of alloantibodies should be taken into account. [Grade D] Adenotonsillar hypertrophy is linked with obstructive sleep apnoea which in turn is a risk factor for cerebrovascular disease in SCD.[8] Careful preoperative assessment is therefore needed as a more aggressive transfusion approach may be indicated in such patients. [Grade D]

All patients with sickling disorders should be:

- discussed with an anaesthetist and haematologist;
- kept warm, well hydrated and oxygenated; [Grade C]
- monitored closely from a respiratory viewpoint postoperatively and measures such as spirometry and physiotherapy instituted to reduce the risk of chest syndrome;[9] [Grade C]
- given thromboprophylaxis. [Grade D]

Postoperative blood transfusion should be discussed with a haematologist. Most patients with sickle cell trait do not require transfusion and simple precautions, such as avoiding dehydration and hypoxia, should be followed.

THALASSAEMIAS

These disorders are caused by an inherited defect in the rate of globin chain synthesis, causing underproduction of haemoglobin and imbalanced globin chain synthesis. The chains that are in excess precipitate and cause premature red cell destruction. β thalassaemias, i.e. deficiency of β chains, predominantly occur in people from the Mediterranean region, whereas α thalassaemias, i.e. a reduction of α chains, occur predominantly in people of Middle and Far Eastern origin.

α and β thalassaemia traits, where only one α and β gene has been deleted or altered, are not usually associated with anaemia but have a markedly reduced MCV. The ethnic origin, clinical history and blood film are helpful in distinguishing these conditions from IDA.

α Thalassaemias

If more than two copies of the α gene have been deleted then HbH disease results with a marked hypochromic microcytic anaemia. Complete deletion of all four α genes is not compatible with life (HbBarts).

β Thalassaemias

Patients who have mutations causing failure to produce any β chains have a serious course. Such patients usually present from three months of age with failure to thrive, anaemia and marked hepatosplenomegaly. The blood picture is grossly abnormal with marked anaemia, hypochromia, nucleated red cells, target cells and stippled cells. Most patients require lifelong regular blood transfusion. By maintaining a near normal Hb, the erythropoietic drive is suppressed and the skeleton-deforming extramedullary haemopoiesis is curtailed. The downside for this is that patients require iron chelation to prevent organ damage from iron overload, using subcutaneous desferrioxamine infusions with or without oral deferriprone. Most patients with thalassaemia require no major preparation perioperatively. Those patients with iron overload, however, should have their cardiac function assessed prior to a general anaesthetic.[10] [Grade D] During any episode of infection, chelation therapy should be ceased until the source of the fever has been identified, as some bacteria, for example *Yersinia enterocolitica* proliferate rapidly in high blood concentrations of iron. Desferrioxamine is known to cause high frequency sensorineural hearing loss and patients should be monitored annually.

Polycythaemia

This is defined as an increase in Hb, haematocrit and red cell count. Haematocrit is a more reliable indicator of polycythaemia as Hb may be low in associated iron deficiency. Polycythaemia can be divided into:

- **Absolute** in which there is a true increase in red cell mass, or
- **Relative** in which the red cell volume is normal, but the circulating plasma volume is reduced.
  Table 22.5 shows the underlying causes.

INVESTIGATIONS

Red cell isotope studies to distinguish absolute from relative polycythaemia are indicated after overt dehydration has been excluded as a cause. Secondary causes need to be considered and pulse oximetry, erythropoietin levels and carboxyHb may be required, depending on clinical findings. A bone marrow aspirate and trephine may be required to diagnose polycythaemia rubra vera (PRV).

Polycythaemia rubra vera

PRV is a clonal stem cell disorder in which there is excessive proliferation of erythroid, myeloid and megakaryocytic progenitors. It usually presents in patients over 60 years with tiredness, visual disturbance, vertigo and tinnitus. Gout, pruritis, injected conjunctivae and splenomegaly may also be features. Increased viscosity caused by raised haematocrit and thrombocytosis (often with abnormal function) contribute to the vascular occlusive tendency. There is a paradoxical increased risk of haemorrhage and patients can present with epistaxis.

Without treatment, the median survival is 18 months; most die from cerebral thromboses. Survival is improved by repeated venesections to maintain haematocrit (Hct) below 0.45.[11] Hydroxyurea is also used and patients with previous vaso-occlusive events should be prescribed low-dose aspirin. [Grade C/D]

Surgery in these patients should be planned and the Hct should be less than 0.45. Abnormal platelet function should be expected and aspirin stopped. Platelet transfusions may sometimes be required: this should be discussed with a haematologist. Antithrombotic measures should be in place. Associated thrombocytosis cannot be quickly corrected – venesection may actually worsen this. [Grade C/D]

There is no evidence available to guide the management of patients who have secondary and relative polycythaemia. Perioperative management of such patients is therefore guided by the individual patient and operative risk and should be discussed with a haematologist.

WHITE CELLS

Granulopoiesis

White blood cells (WBC) can be broadly divided into granulocytes (neutrophils, eosinophils and basophils), monocytes and the immunocytes (lymphocytes and plasma cells). The major role of human WBC is host defence against microbial invaders. This is discussed in more detail in Chapter 11, Defence mechanisms.

Table 22.5 Causes of polycythaemia.

Absolute		Relative
Primary	Secondary	
Polycythaemia rubra vera (PRV)	Compensatory increase in erythropoietin	Pseudopolycythaemia, ie: no underlying cause found
	High altitudes	Cigarette smoking
	Pulmonary disease	Dehydration: diuretics, alcohol
	Cardiovascular disease	Plasma loss: burns, enteropathy
	Familial polycythaemia	
	Heavy cigarette smoking	
	Inappropriate increase in erythropoietin	
	Renal disease: cysts, renal cell carcinoma	

Granulocytes mature in the bone marrow until they become segmented neutrophils, eosinophils and basophils. Their lifespan is six to ten hours following their release into the peripheral circulation. The monocyte precursors spend only a short time in the marrow and mature in the peripheral tissues to macrophages.

Benign white cell disorders

The normal adult ranges are shown in **Table 22.1**.

NEUTROPHILIA

The primary role of the neutrophil is to engulf and kill any microbe it encounters in the extravascular tissues. The causes of neutrophilia are as follows:

- bacterial infections;
- inflammation/tissue necrosis: myocardial infarction (MI), trauma;
- metabolic disorders: uraemia, acidosis;
- neoplasia;
- acute haemorrhage and haemolysis;
- steroids;
- myeloproliferative disorders;
- treatment with myeloid growth factors.

The blood film may show a 'left shift' in which there is an increase in the number of neutrophil precursors. Neutrophilia and a 'left shift' together are called a 'leukaemoid reaction', which is seen in severe sepsis, with G-CSF administration and in chronic myeloid leukaemia (CML). A 'leukoerythroblastic blood film' refers to the presence of immature granulocytes and nucleated red cells and if it is not explained by severe sepsis or hypoxia indicates bone marrow infiltration by tumour or fibrosis and is an indication for a bone marrow biopsy.

NEUTROPENIA

This is defined as a neutrophil count of $< 2.0 \times 10^9$. In Blacks, the lower range is 1.5. The causes are outlined in **Table 22.6**. The risk of infection is more severe when the count is < 1.0 and when the cause reflects bone marrow failure or chemotherapy. Isolated neutropenia can simply be observed but if any other counts are affected then a bone marrow biopsy should be performed.

Any patient with neutropenia undergoing instrumentation should have antibiotic prophylaxis.[12] [Grade D]

PANCYTOPENIA

Neutropenia may be one manifestation of pancytopenia which is defined as a reduction in the blood count of all the major cell lines – red cells, white cells and platelets. It reflects either reduced bone marrow production or increased peripheral destruction. The causes of pancytopenia are outlined in **Table 22.7**. Bone marrow examination should be performed in all patients with pancytopenia.

Table 22.7   Causes of pancytopenia.

Decreased bone marrow function	Increased peripheral destruction
Aplasia	Splenomegaly
Acute leukaemia, myelodysplasia, myeloma	
Infiltration with lymphoma, solid tumours, tuberculosis	
Megaloblastic anaemia	
Paroxysmal nocturnal haemoglobinuria	
Myelofibrosis	
Haemophagocytic syndrome	

Table 22.6   Causes of neutropenia.

Congenital	Acquired	
Kostmanns syndrome	Drug induced:	Antibacterials (co-trimoxazole, chloramphenicol, imipenem)
		Anticonvulsants (phenytoin, carbamazepine)
		Antithyroids (carbimazole)
		Immunosuppressive agents (azathioprine, chemotherapy)
	Infections:	Viral (HIV, hepatitis, influenza)
		Fulminant bacterial infection
	Racial	
	Familial	
	Cyclical	
	Immune:	Autoimmune
		Systemic lupus erythematosus
		Felty's syndrome
		Anaphylaxis
	Part of pancytopenia	

EOSINOPHILS

Eosinophils have important antiparasitic activity and play a role in allergic responses. The causes of eosinphilia (>0.4) are outlined in **Table 22.8**.

LYMPHOCYTOSIS

Lymphocytes are responsible for adaptive immunity; T lymphocytes are responsible for cell-mediated immunity and B lymphocytes for humoral immunity. This is further explored in Chapter 11, Defence mechanisms. The causes of a lymphocytosis are outlined in **Table 22.9**. In children, lymphocytosis occurs as a response to acute infections; in adults a neutrophilia is more often seen in glandular fever. Large numbers of atypical lymphocytes are seen in the peripheral blood. A monospot test is usually positive by the second week if this is the underlying diagnosis.

Table 22.8 Causes of eosinophilia.

Cause	Example
Allergic diseases	Asthma, hayfever, urticaria, Churg–Strauss syndrome
Parasitic diseases	Amoebiasis, hookworm, ascariasis, tapeworm
Recovery from acute infection	
Skin disorders	Psoriasis, pemphigus, dermatitis herpetiformis
Pulmonary eosinophilia and the hypereosinophilic syndrome	
Drug sensitivity	
Polyarteritis nodosum	
Hodgkin's disease	
Metastatic malignancy	
Eosinophilic leukaemia	
Treatment with G-CSF	

Table 22.9 Causes of lymphocytosis.

Cause	Example
Infections	Acute: infectious mononucleosis, rubella, pertussis, mumps, hepatitis, cytomegalovirus, HIV, herpes simplex or zoster
Chronic: tuberculosis, toxoplasmosis, brucellosis, syphilis
Chronic lymphocytic leukaemias	
Acute lymphoblastic leukaemia	
Non-Hodgkin's lymphoma	
Thyrotoxicosis	

LYMPHOPENIA

Lymphopenia (peripheral blood lymphocytes <1.0) may occur in severe bone marrow failure, in autoimmune disorders, with immunosuppressive therapy, post-viral infection and in immune deficiency syndromes, such as human immunodeficiency virus (HIV).

MALIGNANT WHITE CELL DISORDERS

The haemopoietic malignancies are clonal disorders that derive from a single cell in the bone marrow or lymphoid tissue that has undergone genetic alteration. In the majority of cases neither a genetic susceptibility nor an environmental agent can be implicated. Increasingly, specific genetic abnormalities are used to tailor treatment protocols. For example, acute myeloid leukaemia associated with the t(15;17) translocation results in fusion of the PML gene to the retinoic acid receptor α gene, RARα. The resultant PML-RARα fusion protein acts as a transcription repressor instead of the wild type, which is an activator. Patients are therefore treated with high doses of all-trans retinoic acid (ATRA), which causes differentiation of the leukaemia cells and an improved prognosis.

ACUTE LEUKAEMIAS

This group of disorders is defined as a malignant proliferation of myeloid stem cells showing defective maturation. For the diagnosis to be confirmed, the bone marrow must contain greater than 20 percent blasts. Acute lymphoblastic leukaemia (ALL) is more common in children, whereas, acute myeloid leukaemia (AML) is more frequently seen in adults. Patients present acutely, often critically unwell with signs and symptoms related to bone marrow failure or leukostasis.

Both AML and ALL can present with:

- signs and symptoms related to anaemia;
- bleeding including DIC in AML with t(15;17);
- headaches, blurred vision, dizziness, shortness of breath secondary to leukostasis;
- infections secondary to neutropenia:

oral herpetic lesions;
oral candidiasis;
chest, perianal and skin infections.

AML with monocytoid blasts can also present with gum and skin infiltration. Patients with ALL can have lymphadenopathy, hepatosplenomegaly and CNS involvement. Any patient presenting with atypical oral infections should have a FBC and blood film at presentation. Abnormal leukaemic cells are often present in the blood film, but a bone marrow test is required to establish the exact diagnosis. These patients must be referred to the haematology team without delay. Treatment involves high-dose combination chemotherapy and sometimes a bone marrow or stem cell transplant.

Lymphomas, which involve the reticuloendothelial system, can also have a leukaemic component to them, i.e. overspill into the peripheral circulation. Although bone marrow biopsy is important in staging lymphoma, it is not often infiltrated, so is not a first-line test in establishing the diagnosis. A lymph node biopsy is usually required to make a diagnosis.

CHRONIC LEUKAEMIAS

The chronic leukaemias are distinguished from the acute leukaemias by their slower progression. They are also more difficult to cure.

CHRONIC MYELOID LEUKAEMIA

This is a clonal disorder of a pluripotent stem cell. The clinical features such as weight loss, lassitude and splenomegaly can be explained by the great increase in total body myeloid cell mass. The diagnosis is usually relatively straightforward due to the finding of the BCR-ABL gene in 95 percent of patients. This codes for a fusion protein with excess tyrosine kinase activity. Patients have a grossly elevated WCC, usually above 50, which are predominantly neutrophils and myelocytes. The term 'white blood cell' was originally coined due to the appearance of these patients' blood. Patients may also present with bruising and epistaxis due to impaired platelet function.

Since 2001, STI 571, a tyrosine kinase inhibitor, has been used to treat such patients with 30 percent achieving a molecular remission. Other chemotherapy or a bone marrow or stem cell transplant may be required.[13] [Grade C/D]

CHRONIC LYMPHOCYTIC LEUKAEMIA

Chronic lymphocytic leukaemia (CLL) is the most common adult leukaemia and is defined as a clonal proliferation of mature lymphocytes. Most cases occur in older patients and are found incidentally on a routine blood count with a mild lymphocytosis and characteristic smear cells on the blood film. Some patients, however, present with fatigue, recurrent infections (due to hypo-gammaglobulinaemia), hepatosplenomegaly, lymphadenopathy and autoimmune haemolytic anaemia. Diagnosis is by the immunophenotyping of peripheral blood. Treatment is reserved for those with symptoms, increasing lymphadenopathy or hepatosplenomegaly or doubling of lymphocytosis in <6 months.

PLASMA CELL DYSCRASIAS

These monoclonal proliferations of plasma cells are characterized by secretion of a single homogenous immunoglobulin product known as the M-component.

This group includes the following diseases:

- multiple myeloma;
- Waldenström's macroglobulinaemia;
- monoclonal gammopathy of uncertain significance (10 percent of patients with an isolated paraprotein eventually develop myeloma or Waldenström's macroglobulinaemia);
- AL amyloidosis;
- plasmacytomas (solitary or extramedullary).

These patients can present with:

- signs of bone marrow failure, especially infections;
- hyperviscosity, including haemorrhage, due to high levels of paraprotein (the M-component);
- bone pain or fractures;
- hypercalcaemia.

Over 80 percent of extramedullary plasmacytomas are localized to the oropharynx, nasopharynx, sinuses and larynx. Such patients should be investigated for the presence of multiple myeloma and treated with radiotherapy. Investigations should include plasma protein electrophoresis, urine for Bence–Jones protein, a skeletal survey plus a calcium level, renal function tests and a full blood count and blood film.

Bone marrow/stem cell transplantation

Bone marrow/stem cell transplantation (BMT/SCT) is used in the treatment of a wide range of haematological malignancies. Such patients, especially those receiving allogeneic transplants, are at risk of overwhelming infections. Sinus infections have been shown to occur in about one-fifth of patients undergoing allogeneic BMT[14] and invasive rhinocerebral aspergillosis in 2 percent.[15] Mucormycoses are also well recognized. Although there are no randomized trials to assess how such patients should be managed, the majority of such patients will be treated with systemic antifungal therapy and radical surgery. [Grade D]

PLATELETS

Thrombocytosis

Thrombocytosis is defined as a platelet count greater than 450×10^9/L. It is either primary, i.e due to a myeloproliferative disorder such as essential thrombocytosis (ET) or a secondary, reactive phenomenon. The secondary causes are outlined in **Table 22.10**.

About one half of patients with ET are asymptomatic and the thrombocytosis is an incidental finding. The most common symptoms at presentation relate to vascular occlusion, particularly of small vessels.

Patients with ET should receive an antiplatelet agent, usually aspirin. It is important to remember that such

Table 22.10 Causes of thrombocytosis.

Primary	Secondary
Essential thrombocythaemia	Following surgery
	Chronic infection
	Inflammatory states
	Malignancy
	Chronic blood loss and iron deficiency
	Severely ill patients, e.g. on ITU

patients, as well as being prothrombotic are also, paradoxically, at risk of haemorrhage. Surgery in these patients needs to be planned well in advance to ensure the platelet count is <600 to reduce the risk of cerebrovascular disease. The majority of patients are controlled with hydroxyurea.[16] [Grade C/D]

Secondary causes rarely cause a platelet count above 1000. Treatment is of the underlying condition. The use of antiplatelet agents in such circumstances is not clear.

Thrombocytopenias

See Chapter 23, Haemostasis: normal physiology, disorders of haemostasis and thrombosis and their management for the investigation and management of thrombocytopenias.

SPLENECTOMY

Patients who have had a splenectomy or who are functionally hyposplenic are at increased risk of overwhelming sepsis especially from encapsulated bacteria such as *Streptococcus pneumoniae*, *Haemophilus influenzae* type B and *Neisseria meningitides*. Functional hyposplenism occurs secondary to sickle cell anaemia, thalassaemia major, lymphoproliferative disease and coeliac disease.

The guidelines for the prevention and treatment of infection in patients with an absent or dysfunctional spleen produced by the British Committee for Standards in Haematology (BCSH) are summarized below:[17]

- All splenectomized patients and those with functional hyposplenism should receive pneumococcal immunization. Patients not previously immunized should receive haemophilus influenza type B vaccine. [Grade C/D] Patients not previously immunized should receive meningococcal group C conjugate vaccine. [Grade D] Influenza immunization should be given. [Grade D] Lifelong prophylactic antibiotics are still recommended (oral phenoxymethylpenicillin or erythromycin). [Grade C/D]
- Patients developing infection despite measures must be given systemic antibiotics and admitted urgently to hospital. [Grade C/D]

- Patients should be given written information and carry a card to alert health professionals to the risk of overwhelming infection. Patients may wish to invest in an alert bracelet or pendant. [Grade D]
- Patients should be educated about the potential risks of overseas travel, particularly with regard to malaria and unusual infections, for example those resulting from animal bites. [Grade C/D]
- Patient records should be clearly labelled to indicate the underlying risk of infection. Vaccination and revaccination status should be clearly and adequately documented. [Grade C/D]

KEY POINTS

- Many haematological disorders are complicated by ENT disorders.
- Anaemia should be investigated and treated preoperatively where possible – starting with FBC indices and a blood film.
- Abnormal FBC indices or symptoms suggestive of hyperviscosity should be referred to a haematologist for investigation.
- Patients without a functioning spleen are at greater risk of severe sepsis and need antibiotic cover for invasive procedures and urgent treatment for any overt sepsis.

Best clinical practice

- Preoperatively, discuss all patients with sickling disorders with an anaesthetist and haematologist – particularly any with adenotonsillar hypertrophy as associated obstructive sleep apnoea is a risk factor for cerebrovascular disease in sicklers.
- Neutropenic patients undergoing instrumental procedures should be discussed with a haematologist and have antibiotic prophylaxis.
- Patients without a spleen are at an increased risk of severe sepsis and need antibiotic cover for invasive procedures and urgent treatment of sepsis.

Deficiencies in current knowledge and areas for future research

- Further trials are needed for the optimal management of essential thrombocythaemia, polycythaemia rubra vera and chronic myeloid leukaemia.

- Further trials are needed to determine the optimal transfusion management of sickle cell disease patients perioperatively.

REFERENCES

1. Gall RM, Kerr PD. Use of preoperative erythropoietin in head and neck surgery. *Journal of Otolaryngology.* 2000; **29**: 131–4.

2. Prowse CV. Alternatives to blood transfusion: availability and promise [Review]. *Transfusion Medicine.* 1999; **9**: 287–99.

3. Working Party of the General Haematology Task Force of the British Committee for Standards in Haematology. Guideline: The Laboratory Diagnosis of Haemoglobinopathies. *British Journal Of Haematology.* 1998; **101**: 783–92.

4. Davies S, Olujohungbe A. Hydroxyurea for sickle cell disease. Cochrane Database of Systematic Reviews (Online) 2001; CD002202.

5. Waldron P, Pegelow C, Neumayr L, Haberkern C, Earles A, Wesman R et al. Tonsillectomy, adenoidectomy and myringotomy in sickle cell disease: perioperative morbidity. *Journal of Paediatric Hematology/Oncology.* 1999; **21**: 129–35.

6. Koshy M, Weiner S, Miller ST, Sleeper LA, Vichinsky E, Brown AK et al. The Cooperative Study of Sickle Cell Disease. *Surgery and Anesthesia in Sickle Cell Disease. Blood.* 1995; **86**: 3676–84.

7. Riddington C, Williamson L. Preoperative blood transfusions for sickle cell disease. Cochrane Database of Systematic Reviews 2001; CD003149. Review.

8. Kemp SJ. Obsructive sleep apnea and sickle cell disease. *Journal of Pediatric Hematology/Oncology.* 1996; **18**: 104–5.

9. Bellet PS, Kalinyak KA, Shukla R, Gelfand MJ, Rucknagel DL. Incentive spirometry to prevent acute pulmonary complications in sickle cell disease. *New England Journal of Medicine.* 1995; **333**: 699–703.

10. Anderson LJ, Holden S, Davis B, Prescott E, Charrier CC, Bunce NH et al. Cardiovascular T2-star (T2*) magnetic resonance for the early diagnosis of myocardial iron overload. *European Heart Journal.* 2001; **22**: 2171–9.

11. Tefferi A. Polycythemia vera: a comprehensive review and clinical recommendations. *Mayo Clinic Proceedings.* 2003; **78**: 174–94.

12. Walter TH, Donald A, Gerald PB, Eric JB, Arthur EB, Thierry C et al. Guidelines for the use of antimicrobial agents in neutropenic patients with cancer. *Clinical Infectious Diseases.* 2002; **34**: 730–51.

13. Goldman JM, Melo JV. Chronic myeloid leukaemia-advances in biology and new approaches to treatment. *New England Journal of Medicine.* 2003; **349**: 1451–64.

14. Shibuya TY, Momin F, Abella E, Jacobs JR, Karanes C, Ratanatharathorn V et al. Sinus disease in the bone marrow transplant population: incidence, risk factors, and complications. *Otolaryngology Head and Neck Surgery.* 1995; **113**: 705–11.

15. Saah D, Sichel JY, Schwartz A, Nagler A, Eliashar R. CT assessment of bone marrow transplant patients with rhinocerebral aspergillosis. *American Journal of Otolaryngology.* 2002; **23**: 328–31.

16. Cortelazzo S, Finazzi G, Ruggeri M, Vestri O, Galli M, Rodhieghero F et al. Hydroxyurea for patients with essential thrombocythaemia and a high risk of thrombosis. *New England Journal of Medicine.* 1995; **322**: 1132–6.

* 17. Davies JM, Barnes R, Milligan D. British Committee for Standards in Haematology. Working Party of the Haematology/Oncology Task Force. Update of guidelines for the prevention and treatment of infections in patients with an absent or dysfunctional spleen. *Clinical Medicine.* 2002; **2**: 440–3.

Haemostasis: normal physiology, disorders of haemostasis and thrombosis and their management

FIONA REGAN

Normal haemostasis	278	Best clinical practice	290
Bleeding disorders	280	Deficiencies in current knowledge and areas for future	
Thrombotic disorders	288	research	290
Key points	290	References	290

SEARCH STRATEGY

The data in this chapter are supported by a Medline search using the key words haemostasis, thrombosis, coagulation.

NORMAL HAEMOSTASIS

Bleeding or thrombotic problems in surgical patients are not uncommon and may occur for a variety of reasons. In order to understand the basis for these, it is important to understand the mechanisms for normal haemostasis. The haemostatic system comprises five major components: blood vessels, platelets, coagulation factors, coagulation inhibitors and fibrinolysis. These interact, using complex activating or inhibitory feedback mechanisms in order to ensure a powerful, quick, localized procoagulant response to minimize blood loss from sites of vascular injury, but without inappropriate and potentially harmful extension of the clot beyond the area of injury.[1]

Blood vessels

Normally, vessel endothelial cells inhibit haemostasis as they synthesize prostaglandin I_2 (PGI_2 or prostacyclin) and nitric oxide (NO), which cause vasodilation and inhibit platelet function. However, when a vessel is injured vasoconstriction occurs and platelets come into contact with vessel wall components which causes adhesion of platelets to the vessel wall. Von Willebrand factor (VWF), acts to further anchor platelets to vessel wall collagen.

Platelets

Platelets are fragments of cytoplasm derived from megakaryocytes in the bone marrow. About 20–30 percent of circulating platelets are normally sequestered in the spleen and the normal lifespan of platelets is 8–14 days. Following adhesion of platelets to the vessel wall, a variety of substances including ADP and thromboxane A_2 (TXA_2), induce platelet aggregation, resulting in the formation of a platelet plug at the site of vessel injury. In capillaries, platelet aggregation and vasoconstriction alone may be enough to sustain haemostasis, but in larger vessels, stabilization of the platelet plug by fibrin is required to prevent it breaking off. Coagulation factors interact with one another on the surface of activated platelets, promoting coagulation but thus localizing it to the site of injury.

Coagulation factors

FIBRIN FORMATION

In the last decade, a better understanding has been gained of the mechanisms resulting in formation of fibrin strands to stabilize the platelet plug (**Figure 23.1**).

The initiator of coagulation is the complex of tissue factor and factor VIIa (which is found in vascular endothelium and smooth muscle cells). A minute concentration of this complex can activate factor X, which has a central role in both the extrinsic and intrinsic pathways. Factor X forms a complex with calcium and factor V (the prothrombinase complex), which then cleaves prothrombin (II) to produce a minute amount of thrombin. This in turn feeds back to initiate massive activation of factors V and VIII, leading to rapid generation of vast amounts of thrombin. Thrombin in turn, as a proteolytic enzyme, cleaves fibrinogen to give polymerized insoluble fibrin strands. Factor XIII is also activated by thrombin and serves to cross-link fibrin and other proteins in the clot.

VWF is formed in endothelial cells and platelets and has two functions: it acts as a carrier for factor VIII in the circulation, stabilizing it to prevent metabolic breakdown, and it mediates platelet adhesion to collagen in the injured vessel wall.

COAGULATION INHIBITORS

Potentially, a small amount of plasma could generate enough thrombin to clot all the fibrinogen in the body in 30 seconds. Physiological anticoagulants exist to prevent this.

- Antithrombins (**Table 23.1**) inhibit a variety of the coagulation factors. Of note, heparin acts by both inducing a 2000-fold increase in the rate of inactivation of thrombin by antithrombin and also by enhancing the speed of neutralization of factor Xa.
- The components of the protein C system act to neutralize active coagulation factors once they have formed. The 'protein C pathway' which includes thrombomodulins, results in formation of activated protein C, which rapidly degrades the catalytic factors VIIIa and Va. Protein S, like protein C, is a vitamin K-dependent factor synthesized in the liver. It binds to the activated protein C complex and enhances its activity ten-fold.

FIBRINOLYSIS

Fibrinolysis prevents excessive deposition of fibrin which could impede blood circulation (**Figure 23.2**). Fibrin binds plasminogen, which is converted to the active form, plasmin by plasminogen activators, e.g. tPA, uPA. Plasmin then degrades fibrin. There are in turn a number of inhibitors of fibrinolysis to curb the potential for degradation of all the fibrinogen in the body quickly. α_2-antiplasmin inactivates free plasmin and plasminogen activator inhibitor type 1 (PAI-1) inactivates tPA.

Table 23.1 Antithrombins.

Inhibitor	Main substrates
Antithrombin[a]	IIa, Xa
Heparin cofactor II	IIa
α_1-antitrypsin	XIa, Xa
C_1 esterase inhibitor	Kallikrein, XIa
α_2-anti-plasmin	Plasmin
α_2-macroglobulin	Kallikrein
Tissues factor pathway inhibitor	Tissue factor VIIa

[a]Antithrombin was formerly known as antithrombin III (ATIII).

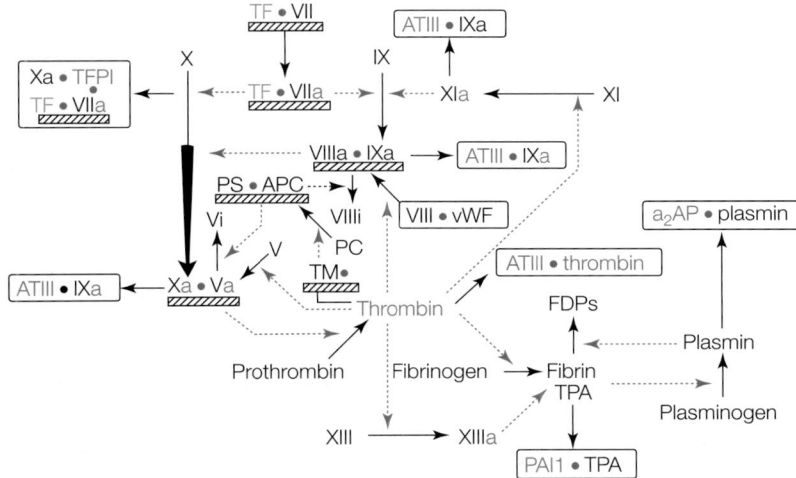

Figure 23.1 Mechanism of normal haemostasis.

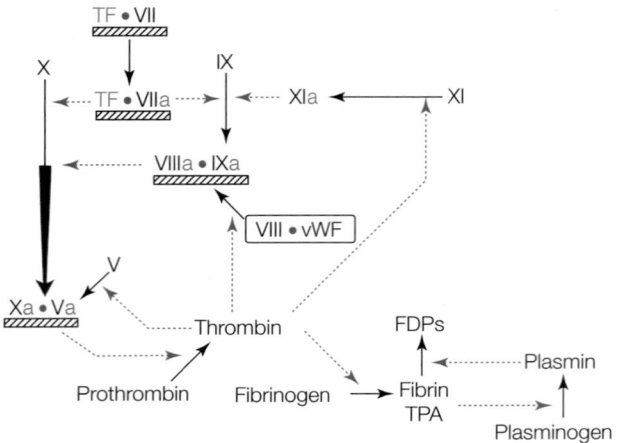

Figure 23.2 The fibrinolytic system.

Laboratory tests of haemostasis

COAGULATION TESTS

These are carried out on blood samples taken into tubes containing sodium citrate, which anticoagulates blood by depleting calcium. It is crucial that the correct volume of blood is taken for the amount of citrate present in the tube, otherwise test results are rendered meaningless. Similarly, spurious results can be caused by samples taken a long time previously or by contamination with heparin, e.g. from heparin-flushed cannulae. Laboratories vary slightly in the techniques and reagents used, so each defines its own normal ranges.

PROTHROMBIN TIME

Brain extract, as a source of tissue factor, and calcium are added to the test plasma and the time to clot formation is measured. The prothrombin time (PT) is sensitive to deficiencies in factors II, V, VII, X and fibrinogen (I). The prothrombin time can be expressed as a ratio of the result obtained using normal plasma (PTR). This ratio should normally be approximately 1.0 (often it is given as the international normalized ratio (INR)).

ACTIVATED PARTIAL THROMBOPLASTIM TIME

After adding phospholipid, calcium and an activator, e.g. kaolin to the test plasma, the time to clot formation is measured. The activated partial thromboplastim time (APTT) is sensitive to deficiencies in factors XII, XI, X, IX, VIII, V, II and fibrinogen. It should be noted that it is also prolonged if there is heparin contamination, either if samples are taken from heparized lines, or if the patient is on heparin.

THROMBIN TIME

Thrombin and calcium are added to patient plasma and the time to clot formation is measured. The thrombin time (TT) is prolonged when fibrinogen is reduced in level or dysfunctional or in the presence of thrombin inhibitors, e.g. heparin.

PLATELET COUNT

The normal range is $150–400 \times 10^9/L$. Significant bleeding would not normally be expected until the platelet count falls below $80 \times 10^9/L$.

BLEEDING DISORDERS

General assessment

Bleeding disorders may be due to abnormalities of coagulation, platelets (or rarely vascular origin) and may be inherited or acquired (**Table 23.2**). If a bleeding disorder is suspected, a careful clinical history and examination make important contributions in reaching a diagnosis.

TIMING

A congenital bleeding disorder may be suggested if there is a history of spontaneous bleeding (e.g. epistaxis, haemarthrosis, gastrointestinal bleeding) or bleeding after previous surgery (e.g. tonsillectomy, appendectomy, circumcision, dental extractions) or menorrhagia may be present. There may be a family history of bleeding, although not always, as for example, in haemophilia A, one-third of cases are due to new genetic mutations. Symptoms of congenital coagulation disorders usually appear early in life, but mild forms may only present after surgery or significant trauma. A history of operations including wisdom teeth extractions or childbirth without excessive bleeding makes a congenital bleeding disorder unlikely. Results of any previous platelet counts and coagulation screens are also useful.

PATTERNS OF INHERITANCE

Haemophilia A and B are X-linked disorders, so affect males, and females are carriers only (with very rare exceptions). Von Willebrand disease (VWD) and other coagulation factor and platelet disorders are not X-linked, so can affect males or females. Most forms of VWD are autosomal dominant; most other deficiencies are autosomal recessive and are much rarer than haemophilia A and B and VWD.

Table 23.2 Bleeding disorders.

	Coagulation	Platelets
Acquired	Vitamin K deficiency/liver disease	↑destruction
	Drugs (e.g. warfarin, heparin)	ITP
	DIC	TTP
	Massive transfusion	PTP
	Acquired inhibitors (rare)	Splenic pooling
		Splenomegaly
		Senile purpura
		Hereditary haemorrhagic telangiectasia
		Connective tissue disorders
		↓production
		Bone marrow failure, e.g. leukaemia
		Aplastic anaemia
		Chemotherapy
		Dysfunction
		NSAIDs
		Cardiac bypass/ECCs
		Renal failure
Inherited	Haemophilia A (VIII deficiency)	(rare)
	Haemophilia B (IX deficiency)	May–Hegglin thrombocytopenia
	vWD	TAR (thrombocytopenia with absent radii)
	Factor XI deficiency	Bernard Soulier syndrome
	Rarer deficiencies, e.g. V, I	Wiscott–Aldrich syndrome
		Glanzmann's disease
		Other rare abnormalities of platelet adhesion or aggregation

PATTERNS OF BLEEDING

Coagulation disorders, for example haemophilia A or B, usually present with bleeding into joints or muscles, whereas platelet disorders or vasculitic disorders cause more bleeding from mucosal surfaces, e.g. epistaxis, menorrhagia, skin purpura, haematuria. Von Willebrand disease, in which a lack of VWF results in decreased blood levels of factor VIII and failure of platelet aggregation, can present with joint bleeding or mucosal bleeding.

Factor XI deficiency is usually mild in terms of causing joint bleeds but results in post-surgical bleeding of variable severity and does not correlate well with factor XI levels. Often, in retrospect, a history of menorrhagia or mucosal bleeding was present. Factor XIII deficiency causes 'late' severe bleeding postoperatively because the initial clot formed is not properly stabilized, so it breaks down. It usually presents early in life, with prolonged bleeding from the umbilical cord. Whilst deficiencies of all other coagulation factors will be detected by abnormalities of the PT, APTT or TT, in factor XIII deficiency, the usual coagulation screen tests will be normal. However, a fibrin clot solubility test can be done, to show that the clot is more easily soluble than normal. Of note, factor XII deficiency does not cause bleeding. It is often picked up when the APTT is found to be prolonged and it simply needs to be identified to ascertain

that there is not a clinically significant factor deficiency present.

DRUG HISTORY

As part of the clinical history, a drug history should be taken and any drugs which interfere with haemostasis, e.g. nonsteroidal antiinflammatory drugs (NSAID), may need to be stopped.

Diagnostic tests

A full blood count (FBC), PT, APTT and TT will identify most inherited or acquired coagulation factor deficiencies and thrombocytopenias, apart from factor XIII deficiency as above. Further testing should be discussed with a haematologist. A typical algorithm is shown in **Figure 23.3**.

The lupus anticoagulant causes a prolonged APTT *in vitro*, but *in vivo* causes a thrombotic tendency.

If FBC, APTT, PT and fibrinogen results are all normal and a bleeding tendency is still suspected, a platelet dysfunction disorder or vasculitic problem may be present. A bleeding time test can be performed. It would be prolonged in both types of disorder. A

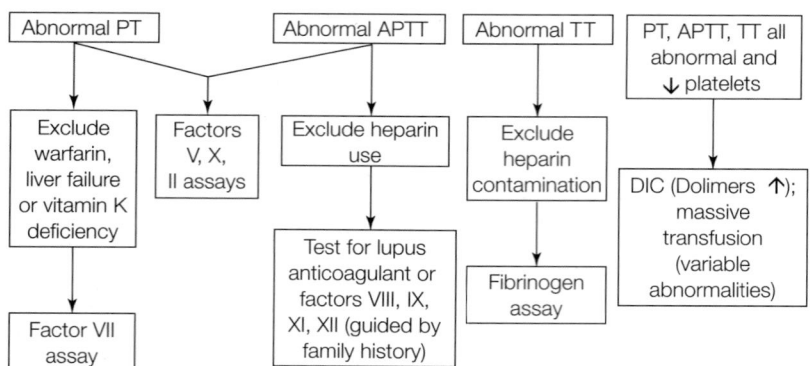

Figure 23.3 Algorithm for managing abnormal coagulation results.

sphygmanometer cuff is inflated to 40 mmHg around the upper arm and using an automated device a standardized 5-mm incision is made on the forearm avoiding superficial veins and warning the patient about scarring. The incision is blotted every 30 seconds, without disturbing the forming clot and the time taken for bleeding to stop is taken. A normal bleeding time is < 9 minutes. An abnormal bleeding time can indicate a platelet dysfunction problem (congenital or acquired) or a vasculitic problem. Platelet function tests can be performed. These are not routinely available and are done manually on approximately 20 mL of EDTA fresh samples.

Acquired coagulation disorders

LIVER DISEASE

Acute and chronic liver diseases often cause haemostatic abnormalities as the liver is the main site of synthesis of many coagulation and anticoagulant factors. Bleeding most commonly occurs in the upper gastrointestinal tract, from biopsy sites and following surgery. Bleeding into soft tissues is rare.

The PT and APTT are prolonged with a reduction in all coagulation factors, except factor VIII. Platelets may be reduced with alcohol excess.

Treatment

Vitamin K should be given if deficiency is likely. Blood component therapy should only be given when the coagulation screen is abnormal and there is bleeding or an invasive procedure is performed. The outcome should be monitored clinically and by coagulation tests. Fresh frozen plasma (FFP) 12–15 mL/kg contains all of the coagulation factors to replace those deficient in liver disease. Platelets should be given to keep the platelet count greater than 50×10^9/L: one pool is usually adequate. Inhibitors of fibrinolysis, e.g. tranexamic acid, may be useful. [Grade D]

VITAMIN K DEFICIENCY

Debilitated patients undergoing surgery are particularly vulnerable as broad spectrum antibiotics given in the context of a dietary deficiency may result in reduced absorption of vitamin K, which is necessary for the synthesis of factors II, VII, IX and X and protein C and S. The PT is prolonged and an injection of i.v. vitamin K is appropriate.

ANTICOAGULANTS

Warfarin inhibits formation of the vitamin K-dependent coagulation factors II, VII, IX and X (and protein C and S) and after stopping warfarin its effects diminish over several days. Heparin potentiates the natural anticoagulant antithrombin and its effects wear off in approximately six hours after stopping unfractionated heparin. Low molecular weight heparins (LMWH) act more specifically to inhibit factor X than as an antithrombin and have a longer half-life than unfractionated heparin. They are useful as they can be given subcutaneously twice a day rather than by continuous i.v. infusion. Protamine sulphate can be used to reverse heparin effects, but it is less effective against LMWH than unfractionated heparin. [*] [Grade C]

Skin necrosis and warfarin

If a patient develops skin necrosis when warfarin is started, protein C or protein S deficiency should be suspected as these are inhibited sooner than coagulation factors. If a patient is already known to have protein C or S deficiency, warfarin should be started under heparin cover and on stopping warfarin, the dose should be tailed off slowly. [*] [Grade C]

Managing patients already on anticoagulation perioperatively

This should be planned and discussed with a haematologist where appropriate at the stage of preassessment clinics or at least well before admission for surgery. National guidelines are available and recommendations are summarized below.[2]

- For minor surgical procedures, warfarin should be stopped or reduced to achieve a target INR of approximately 2.0 on the day of surgery[3, 4] [**] [Grade B] If the INR is less than 2.5 preoperatively, surgery can proceed. If the INR is greater than 2.5, the surgeon and haematologist should discuss options.

— Elective surgery could be postponed.
— Warfarin could be reversed using FFP or prothrombin complex concentrate (PCC), but the risks of deferring surgery would have to outweigh the risks associated with FFP or PCC (see Chapter 21, Blood groups, blood components and alternatives to transfusion) to justify using either.
— Surgical opinion may decide that the level of anticoagulation is safe for surgery to take place.

- For dental extraction, oral tranexamic acid mouthwash (4.8 percent) can secure homeostasis while continuing warfarin.[5] [***] [Grade A]
- For major surgery, oral anticoagulants should be stopped at least three days before surgery. Depending on the degree of thrombotic risk, heparin may be required instead, once the INR is below the theraputic range – this should be discussed with a haematologist beforehand. [Grade C] The risk of bleeding associated with heparin used in a particular operation should also be considered. When to restart warfarin also depends on the risk of bleeding, but in many instances, warfarin can be started once the patient manages oral intake.
- In all cases, subsequent monitoring of warfarin must be arranged before the patient is discharged.

Managing bleeding and excessive anticoagulation

The risk of bleeding while on warfarin increases significantly when the INR >5.0, but the decision to reverse warfarin depends on whether there is major or minor bleeding, whether surgery or invasive procedures are urgent. If the patient is warfarinized to prevent thrombi forming on prosthetic heart valves, vitamin K must be used with caution, as it may cause prolonged warfarin resistance and may result in thromboembolism. The degree of reversal must be decided on an individual basis. Recommendations according to national guidelines[3] are summarized in **Table 23.3**. Oral vitamin K (5 mg tablets) is quickly and efficiently absorbed so is as effective as i.v. vitamin K, except in patients who have any condition causing malabsorption of fats. In major bleeding, PCC is preferred where available, as reversal of warfarin is quicker and more effective than with FFP as it can be infused faster. FFP is a suitable alternative if PCC is not available. [Grade C]

Drug interactions

Many drugs interact with warfarin, as listed in the British National Formulary. If a patient is on warfarin any doctor starting, stopping or altering the dose of any other drug should check to see if it will change the anticoagulant effect. It is recommended that if the drug change lasts less than five days and could potentiate anticoagulation, then either no change or a minor reduction may be required. If the drug alteration lasts >5 days, the INR should be checked shortly after the changes and warfarin adjusted accordingly. [*] [Grade C] Most, but not all, potentiate the effect of warfarin. Correspondingly, warfarin can alter the efficacy of other drugs, e.g. anti-epileptics and oral contraceptives. Apart from drugs which directly affect warfarin metabolism, other drugs which affect haemostasis should be borne in mind, e.g. analgesics with anti-platelet effects, such as aspirin and other nonsteroidal antiinflammatory drugs.

Other anticoagulants

Occasionally, other anticoagulants are used. Thrombolytic drugs, e.g. streptokinase, given for myocardial infarct, within ten days of surgery or invasive procedure, can cause severe bleeding. It may be reversed using aprotinin.

DISSEMINATED INTRAVASCULAR COAGULATION

The coagulation cascade is activated to form clots far beyond the normal restrictions of clot formation local to the site of a vessel injury. There is resultant widespread clot formation and vascular occlusion causing limb and organ damage plus, paradoxically, a bleeding tendency due to depletion of coagulation factors, fibrinogen and platelets. The main underlying causes of disseminated intravascular coagulation (DIC) are as follows:

- severe infections (particularly Gram-negative cocci, e.g. menigococcal septicaemia);

Table 23.3 Recommendations for management of bleeding and excessive anticoagulation.

International normalized ratio	Recommendations	
3.0 < INR < 6.0 (target INR 2.5)	Reduce warfarin dose or stop	
4.0 < INR < 6.0 (target INR 3.5)	Restart warfarin when INR < 5.0	
6.0 < INR < 8.0, no bleeding or minor bleeding	Stop warfarin, restart when INR < 5.0	
INR > 8.0, no bleeding or minor bleeding	Stop warfarin, restart when INR < 5.0. If other risk factors for bleeding give 0.5–2.5 mg of vitamin K (oral)	[**] [Grade B]
Major bleeding	Stop warfarin. Give prothrombin complex concentrate 50 units/kg or FFP 15 mL/kg. Give 5 mg of vitamin (oral or i.v.)	[**] [Grade B]

- shock;
- obstetric disorders (eclampsia, antepartum haemorrhage, amniotic fluid embolism, retained dead foetus);
- severe burns;
- ABO-incompatible transfusion;
- intravascular haemolysis (for example, hypotonic saline, hypotonic fluids after prostatectomy, etc.);
- malignancy (for example, cancer of prostate, pancreas, lung, stomach, usually chronic DIC).

If severe, there is widespread bruising and oozing from venepuncture sites or surgical wounds and mucosal surfaces, for example, epistaxis. There may also be evidence of vascular occlusion in the limbs.

Laboratory tests

Platelets are low; the APTT, PT, TT are prolonged; the fibrinogen level is low and fibrinogen degradation products (e.g. D-dimers) are raised, indicating increased fibriolysis.

Treatment

In acute DIC, treatment of the underlying condition is crucial. Fresh frozen plasma at 15 mL/kg should be given, and if the fibrinogen is less than 1.0 g/L then one adult dose of cryoprecipitate (from ten donors) should be given. Platelets should be given to keep the platelet count above 50 – so initially one or sometimes two pools of platelets are needed. Subsequent component therapy should be given according to an FBC and coagulation tests repeated 15 minutes after the infusion of the relevant component. Transfusion of red cells may also be needed. There is no conclusive evidence to support the use of antithrombin concentrates, antifibriolytics or low-dose heparin. Aprotinin may be used where continued bleeding is life-threatening. In chronic DIC, e.g. associated with malignancies, unless there is active problematic bleeding, no treatment is indicated. [Grade C/D]

MASSIVE TRANSFUSION

Levels of coagulation factors and platelet function decline rapidly during storage of blood. The use of 'fresh blood' within 24 hours of collection to overcome this, is not justified, as testing for viral infections in the donor, for example, human immunodeficiency virus (HIV) and hepatitis B and C, could not be completed. Therefore, when large quantities of stored blood are given in a short time period (for example total blood volume replacement), bleeding may occur. Prolonged hypovolaemia worsens the coagulopathy. Where there are no underlying medical complications, replacement of one adult blood volume (8–10 units of blood) is not usually associated with significant haemostatic problems but these often occur once 1.5–2 times the blood volume has been replaced. There is considerable variation between patients. Therefore, an FBC and coagulation tests help to guide component therapy. Platelets should be kept above 50×10^9/L and the PT and APTT kept near to normal and the fibrinogen greater than 1.0 g/L. Microvascular bleeding is typical, e.g. bleeding from mucus membranes and oozing from surgical wounds or catheter sites. It should be noted that dextran can interfere with haemostasis.

ACQUIRED INHIBITORS

These are rare and usually present with unexplained severe and persistent mucosal bleeding (e.g. gastrointestinal tract, genitourinary tract), wound haematomas, massive skin bruises or muscle bleeding. Coagulation tests show a prolonged APTT or PT or TT depending on the coagulation factor affected. The most common is an inhibitor to factor VIII, which may occur secondary to drugs (e.g. penicillin, cephalosporin), rheumatoid arthritis and other connective tissue disorders or post-partum. Management should be discussed with a haematologist.

Inherited coagulation disorders

There may be a family history of haemophilia or VWD or other factor deficiency, or the patient may give a history of excessive bleeding after an operation, invasive procedure or childbirth. If there is an absence of excess bleeding during these procedures, then an inherited coagulation disorder is unlikely. The frequency of inherited bleeding disorders is given in **Table 23.4**.

Table 23.4 Inherited bleeding disorders.

Disorder	Deficiency	Inheritance	Approximate incidence
Haemophilia A	Factor VIII	X-linked	100 per 10^6
VWD	VWF	Autosomal dominant (rarely recessive)	100 per 10^6
Haemophilia B = Christmas disease	Factor IX	X-linked	20 per 10^6
Factor XI deficiency	Factor XI	Automsomal dominant or recessive	5 percent in Ashkenazi Jews, rare in others
Deficiencies of factors X, V, VII, II, I, XIII, V, plus VIII		Autosomal recessive	Each approximately 1 per 10^6

HAEMOPHILIA A AND B

Haemophilia A (due to factor VIII deficiency) is the most common and affects one in 10,000 males. Haemophilia B (due to factor IX deficiency) or Christmas disease is clinically identical, but less common. Both are X-linked disorders, but a third are due to new mutations. Female carriers rarely have a low enough factor level to cause problems, but occasionally, in cases of extreme lyonization, levels may be low enough to warrant treatment before major surgery. Patients with mild forms of haemophilia (factor levels >10 percent) rarely have spontaneous bleeding episodes, but may require treatment before surgery. Severely affected patients (levels less than two percent) may have spontaneous bleeding into joints (particularly weight-bearing joints, e.g. knees) or muscles (of limbs or internally, e.g. psoas muscle haematoma) with associated pain and some severely affected patients have proplylactic treatment with factor concentrate several times per week. Some patients develop inhibitor antibodies in response to treatment with either human or recombinant factor VIII. [**/*]

MANAGEMENT OF HAEMOPHILIA BEFORE SURGERY

Ideally, patients should be treated in a centre experienced in the management of haemophilia. Haemophiliac patients should carry a medical card stating their diagnosis including the level of deficiency and whether inhibitors are present.

ELECTIVE SURGERY

Patients with coagulation factor deficiencies and female carriers of haemophilia A or B, should be assessed well before surgery, ideally at a preassessment clinic. Their management should be discussed with a haematologist and adequate supplies of the relevant coagulation factor arranged. Recommended blood tests are shown in **Table 23.5**. Because the formation of inhibitors is unpredictable, it is important to test for these at preoperative clinic assessments. If present, treatment is far more difficult and needs careful planning. Do not give intramuscular injections to haemophiliacs and avoid using nonsteroidal antiinflammatory drugs. Prophylaxis with heparin or warfarin against thromboembolism is not necessary and can interfere with laboratory monitoring of treatment with the relevant factor.

In mild haemophilia A or VWD, provided there are no contraindications, some procedures can be carried out using an infusion of DDAVP, which raises the level of factor VIII by releasing stored factor VIII. For all other patients with coagulation factor deficiencies an infusion of the relevant factor is needed. The dose, timing and form of concentrate used (whether human or recombinant) should be discussed with a haematologist. Normally, a preinfusion coagulation sample is taken as a

Table 23.5 Blood tests before surgery in haemophiliac patients.

Test	Reason
Baseline factor level	To assess response to treatment
Inhibitor screen	To check if an inhibitor has developed since the last infusion of factor; a different treatment strategy would be required
Virological testing	As factor concentrates before the late 1980s could transmit viral infections
HBsAg and anti-HBs	To determine if a carrier of hepatitis B or if adequately immunized
Anti-HCV	
Anti-HIV	
Full blood count	
Blood group and antibody screen/crossmatch	As appropriate

baseline factor level measurement, then concentrate is infused an hour before surgery and a post-infusion sample is taken to confirm that the factor level has been boosted to well within the normal range (target 80–100 percent). Postoperatively, in severe haemophiliacs an infusion of factor concentrates is required for seven to ten days and patients cannot be discharged quickly after 'minor' surgery. Factor VIII infusions are needed twice a day, but factor IX has a longer half-life so is required once daily. Human derived factor VIII (or IX) concentrates are derived from pools of plasma from thousands of donors and are heat-treated for viral inactivation. Recombinant factor VIII is available and used to some extent, but is very expensive. In addition, tranexamic acid can be useful especially to treat mucosal bleeding, and can be given as a mouthwash (5 percent) for bleeding in the mouth. [Grade C/D]

EMERGENCY SURGERY

This should be discussed promptly with a haematologist. Depending on surgical and haematological considerations, the patient may be best managed by transferring to a hospital with a haemophilia centre, or it may be better to transport supplies of the relevant coagulation factor from a haemophilia centre as soon as possible. When assessing a patient, the exact diagnosis including the level of factor deficiency, needs confirmation either from a card carried by the patient or from the database at the haemophilia centre which cares for them. In a dire emergency where no coagulation factor is available quickly enough, FFP (or cryoprecipitate for factor VIII or fibrinogen deficiencies) may be needed as a holding measure, though it is difficult to raise the levels of factors quickly with FFP alone. The patient or their relatives may have a supply of the relevant coagulation factor if they are on 'home treatment', i.e. they manage joint bleeds, etc., at home by self-injecting the factor concentrate. Central nervous system bleeding is uncommon, but can occur even after a slight head injury and used to be the most common cause of death in haemophiliacs. Factor treatment must be continued for at least ten days, otherwise late recurrent bleeding can occur. Oropharyngeal bleeding is uncommon, but is clinically dangerous, as extension through soft tissues in the floor of the mouth can cause respiratory obstruction. Laceration of the tongue can be difficult as it cannot be immobilized.

Generally, it is preferable to time the change of wound dressings or physiotherapy after an infusion of factor concentrate, to minimize the risk of bleeding from wounds.

In an untreated haemophilac, bleeding is not so much profuse, as persistent. Clots may initially form, but are bulky and friable and tend to shear off with further bleeding, which may recur over days to weeks. However, this picture is now seen only in haemophiliacs resistant to treatment or in undiagnosed mild to moderate haemophiliacs after their first surgical or dental procedure. If the diagnosis is not known, a coagulation screen and a bleeding history will be required. [**/*]

Acquired platelet disorders

If thrombocytopenia is found without coagulation abnormalities, the patient's history, including a bleeding history, may indicate whether it is a chronic condition or whether the onset is recent. Results of previous platelet counts are useful. Unless surgery is urgent, the cause of the thrombocytopenia should be investigated first, as optimal treatment depends on the underlying cause and platelet transfusions may be contraindicated in some conditions.

INCREASED CONSUMPTION/DESTRUCTION OF PLATELETS

Idiopathic thrombocytopenic purpura (or autoimmune thrombocytopenia)

This is a common condition in which platelets are coated with an autoantibody (usually IgG) resulting in increased platelet destruction in the spleen and thrombocytopenia of variable severity. Idiopathic thrombocytopenic purpura (ITP) may be idiopathic or secondary to other auto-immune diseases, malignancies, drugs (e.g. trimethoprim, sulphonamides, quinidine) especially in children, HIV or viral infections. In adults, ITP may manifest as a single episode, may be recurrent or may cause chronic thrombocytopenia. Treatment is usually with predniso-lone or IVIg and a history of a previous good response to these indicates the patient is likely to respond again. Patients who fail to respond long term may require a

splenectomy (and long-term penicillin) or other immu-nosuppressive agents. Treatment prior to any surgical procedure depends on the starting platelet count and the nature of the surgery. For most major surgery, the platelets should be kept above 50; for central nervous system (CNS) and eye surgery platelets should be kept above 100. For minor surgery it is not necessary to keep platelets above 50. If treatment is required, steroids or IVIg can be given, but the response may take up to a week to achieve, so planning in advance is essential. In an emergency, giving platelet transfusions is not indicated except where there is life-threatening bleeding, e.g. CNS bleeding, as the platelets transfused are consumed very rapidly. In this setting, IVIg 1 mg/kg before platelet transfusion may be of benefit. [Grade D]

Thrombotic thrombocytopenia and haemolytic uraemic syndrome

The thrombotic microangiopathies are a spectrum of clinical syndromes characterized by microangiopathic haemolytic anaemia, thrombocytopenia, microvascular thrombosis and multiple organ failure. Thrombotic thrombocytopenia occurs in one per million of the population per year and presents with fever, intravascular haemolytic anaemia, thrombocytopenia, renal failure and neurological deficits. It may be acute, chronic or recurrent and may be associated with systemic lupus erythematosus (SLE), other connective tissue diseases, pregnancy or HIV. Haemolytic uraemic syndrome presents with haemolytic anaemia, thrombocytopenia and renal failure and may be associated with a viral or gastrointestinal infection (especially in children) or HIV. The mechanisms of these are not well understood, but are believed to involve vascular endothelial injury resulting in abnormal clump-ing of platelets and microvascular thrombosis. In thrombotic thrombocytopenia (TTP), it is proposed that there is a deficiency in the patient's plasma of a factor that normally inhibits platelet aggregation. This concurs with the finding that the most effective treatment is plasma infusion or exchange. It should be noted that these disorders cause thrombosis rather than bleeding, but are important to include in the differential diagnosis of thrombocytopenia.

Diagnosis

Once the possibility of haemolytic uraemic syndrome (HUS) or TTP has been considered, a blood film will show fragmented red cells and reduced numbers of platelets. A coagulation screen will be normal and urea and electrolytes are often abnormal.

Treatment

Platelet transfusions are normally contraindicated, as they may worsen the condition and result in death. Plasma exchange is optimal for TTP, giving an 80 percent response rate. It is less effective in HUS, but sometimes FFP infusions alone may be helpful. [Grade C/D]

Post-transfusion purpura

This is an uncommon condition in which the patient has a sudden dramatic fall in platelet count (less than 10×10^9/L) about five to ten days after a transfusion. They have purpura, mucosal bleeding and bleeding from surgical wounds. It is more common in women, as it is due to an antiplatelet antibody which formed after previous exposure to platelet antigens, usually from a foetus during pregnancy. In men, previous transfusion is the source of platelet antibody sensitization. The mechanism of post-transfusion purpura (PTP) is not well understood as the anti-HPA 1a antibody destroys any transfused platelets which are HPA 1a-positive, but also destroys the patient's own platelets which are HPA 1a-negative.

Diagnosis

A blood film is normal apart from low numbers of platelets, and the coagulation screen is normal. Anti-HPA 1a antibodies are found (results may take several days). Postoperatively, the differential diagnosis often includes heparin-induced thrombocytopenia (see below).

Treatment

Thrombocytopenia may resolve after a couple of weeks, but this is variable and the risk of significant bleeding during that time is high. Therefore, IVIg is given to minimize the duration of thrombocytopenia. Platelet transfusions are ineffective. Future transfusions should ideally be avoided, as even small amounts of platelets in red cell transfusions can precipitate an episode, but if needed, special components can be provided. [Grade D]

Heparin-induced thrombocytopenia with thrombosis

Type 1 heparin-induced thrombocytopenia is common and benign. The platelet count falls early after heparin is started and is not severe. Heparin-induced thrombocytopenia with thrombosis (HITT) type 2 is potentially lethal, and although it does not cause bleeding, it is crucial to consider in the differential diagnosis of thrombocytopenia after surgery, as heparin must be stopped. It is due to development of a platelet activating autoantibody against the heparin-platelet factor 4 complex. It presents five days or more after heparin is started and thrombocytopenia may be moderate to severe. Thrombosis causes occlusion of major vessels (sometimes while the platelet count is falling but still within normal range) and is fatal in 30 percent. Sometimes DIC and skin necrosis occur at the site of subcutaneous injections. HITT type 2 is much less common with low molecular weight heparin compared to unfractionated heparin.

Diagnosis

After starting heparin, the platelet count must be monitored beyond the fifth day and a high index of suspicion is needed. A PF4/heparin enzyme-linked immunosorbent assay (ELISA) test is available.

Treatment

Heparin must be stopped whenever HITT type 2 is suspected. Instead, the heparinoid 'orgaran' or warfarin can be used. Platelets are contraindicated. [Grade D]

Splenomegaly

Splenomegaly may result in thrombocytopenia due to pooling of platelets in the spleen.

REDUCED PRODUCTION OF PLATELETS

Conditions resulting in failure of production of megakaryocytes in the bone marrow are less common than conditions due to increased consumption. They include leukaemias, aplastic anaemia, myelodysplasia, systemic chemotherapy and metastatic infiltration by carcinomas. Severe thrombocytopenia may present with mucosal bleeding. A history of other symptoms and signs will aid diagnosis and a full blood count and blood film followed by a bone marrow examination if appropriate can elucidate the cause.

Treatment

Unless the patient is bleeding or requires an invasive procedure, platelet transfusions are only required when the platelet count is less than 10 (or <20 if the patient has sepsis or a coagulopathy). Platelets should be kept >50 for major surgery, lumbar punctures, liver biopsy or insertion of a central line, but >100 if eye or CNS surgery is performed.[6] [**] [Grade B] Tranexamic acid may also be useful.

PLATELET DYSFUNCTION

Drugs

NSAID act by inhibiting the cyclooxygenase pathway in platelets and therefore inhibit production of thromboxane A_2, which is required for platelet aggregation. To reverse the effects of aspirin, and other NSAID, they should be stopped five days before surgery. Specific antiplatelet drugs are also used in some patients, e.g. with ischaemic heart disease.

Extracorporeal circuits

Cardiopulmonary bypass and other extracorporeal circuits (ECC) result in platelet dysfunction through a number of mechanisms including a reversible depression of TXA_2 by hypothermia, fragmentation and loss of platelet surface receptors due to sheer stress, turbulent blood flow and adhesion to foreign surfaces. Heparinization of ECC should be adequately reversed when use of the circuit is stopped. Platelet function normally corrects itself by three hours after cardiac bypass. Platelets are not routinely indicated, unless antiplatelet drugs are also in use.

Renal failure

Uraemia may cause defective platelet–vessel wall interaction, but the most important factor in causing bleeding is the low haematocrit associated with chronic renal failure. Transfusion or administration of erythropoietin to raise the haematocrit (Hct) to greater than 0.30 usually corrects the bleeding tendency. DDAVP may also be useful in lessening bleeding, by increasing release of VWF to overcome a VWF inhibitor sometimes present in renal failure, with shortening of the bleeding time for about four hours afterwards. These measures may allow surgery to take place with a reduced risk of bleeding. [Grade D]

Inherited platelet disorders

These are rare and include a range of disorders of platelet function and thrombocytopenias. Bernard Soulier syndrome is due to a defect in platelet glycoprotein Ib which causes defective platelet adhesion to vessel subendothelium, with mucocutaneous bleeding, which is sometimes severe. The platelet count is mildly reduced and the platelets are large and abnormal. Glanzmann's disease is due to a defect in the platelet glycoprotein complex IIb/IIIa, so that platelet aggregation is impaired. The platelet count is normal. Skin and mucous membrane bleeding, especially in the nasopharynx, are common. In May–Hegglin thrombocytopenia, platelet numbers are often markedly reduced and the platelets are giant. The diagnosis of each is made based on a FBC, blood film and platelet aggregation followed by immunological tests to measure levels of glycoproteins studies where needed.

TREATMENT

Patients should avoid the risk of trauma where possible. There is no prophylactic treatment for spontaneous bleeding, but patients should avoid drugs which affect platelet function, e.g. NSAIDs. For bleeding episodes, local measures are often successful, so that platelet transfusions are not often needed. Arterial embolism has been used effectively for severe epistaxis. Ideally, platelet transfusions should be HLA-matched in order to prevent HLA antibody formation and platelet refractoriness in these patients. Specific blood donors would need to be called, once the patient's HLA type is known, so this should be arranged several weeks in advance. [Grade D]

THROMBOTIC DISORDERS

Management of a thrombotic episode

The pathogeneses of venous and arterial thrombosis are different and a patient's predisposition to either depends on a combination of environmental or acquired and inherited factors. Stasis is a prominent factor in venous thrombosis, whereas damage to the vascular endothelium is central to arterial thrombosis. Acquired and inherited risk factors for venous and arterial thrombosis are given in **Tables 23.6**, **23.7** and **23.8**.

TREATMENT OF A NEW DEEP VEIN THROMBOSIS OR PULMONARY EMBOLISM

According to local hospital practice, deep vein thrombosis (DVT) and pulmonary embolism (PE) may be treated with an i.v. infusion of unfractionated heparin, which requires monitoring, aiming for an APTR of 1.5–2.5; or using LMWH given subcutaneously once or twice daily (depending on the individual product) using a weight-based dose.

REFERRAL FOR INVESTIGATION OF THROMBOPHILIA

The majority of thrombotic episodes have no obvious underlying cause, but it is worth referring a patient for investigation if thromboses are recurrent, there is a family history, or there are unusual features, e.g. young age, unusual site, etc. They may have a 'thrombophilia', i.e. an inherited or acquired disorder which predisposes them to thrombosis. Interpretation of laboratory tests for these is difficult while the patient is on anticoagulants or in the acute phase of a thrombotic episode. Testing is best performed when anticoagulants have been stopped for at least one month.[7] [Grade D]

Table 23.6 Acquired risk factors for venous thromboembolism.

Risk factor
Immobility
Dehydration
Tissue trauma, including surgery
Myocardial infarction
Pregnancy and puerperium
Oestrogens
Obesity
Varicose veins
Previous deep venous thrombosis
Congestive cardiac failure
Malignancy
Nephrotic syndrome
Advancing age
Hyperviscosity states
Connective tissue diseases (especially lupus anticoagulant)
Behcet's syndrome
Paroxysmal nocturnal haemoglobinuria
Myeloproliferative disorders
Therapy with coagulation factor concentrates containing activated factors (II, IX, X concentrates)

Table 23.7 Genetic risk factors for venous thromboembolism.

Risk factor	
Deficiency of anticoagulant	Antithrombin
	Protein C
	Protein S
Abnormal protein	Factor V Leiden
	Dysfibrinogenaemia
Increased procoagulant	Prothrombin
	Factor VIII
Abnormal metabolism	Homocystinuria
Putative mechanisms	Thrombomodulin defects
	Fibrinolytic defects

Table 23.8 Acquired and genetic risk factors for arterial artherothrombosis.

Risk factor	
Increased procoagulant	Fibrinogen
	Factor VII
	Factor VIII
Abnormal metabolism	Hypercholesterolaemia
	Diabetes
	Hyperhomocysteinaemia
Autoimmune disease	Antiphospholipid antibodies
Environmental	Smoking
	Diet

PERIOPERATIVE MANAGEMENT

Whether to treat patients with thrombophilia any differently from other patients depends on a number of factors including their diagnosis, history of thrombosis and nature of surgery and should be discussed with a haematologist. National guidelines recommend that:[7]

- All patients with a previous DVT (with or without a thrombophilic defect) receive prophylactic anticoagulation to cover surgery, trauma or immobilization including plaster casts. Equally, so should patients who are known to have a thrombophilic disorder, have had no thrombotic episode themselves, but have a relative with the same disorder who has had a thrombosis. [Grade C]
- There is no evidence that the dose or duration of anticoagulation should be different in patients with a thrombophilia than other patients, except that patients with antithrombin deficiency may require larger doses of heparin.

Heparin is required for four to five days (with no monitoring required), but should be continued until the oral anticoagulant warfarin achieves a therapeutic level, as monitored by the INR. The recommended warfarin loading schedule for different conditions and target INRs are given in **Table 23.9** and in the Haemostasis and

Table 23.9 Warfarin loading schedule.

Day	INR	Warfarin dose (mg)
First	<1.4	10
Second	<1.8	10
	1.8	1
	>1.8	0.5
Third	<2.0	10
	2.0–2.1	5
	2.2–2.3	4.5
	2.4–2.5	4
	2.6–2.7	3.5
	2.8–2.9	3
	3.0–3.1	2.5
	3.2–3.3	2
	3.4	1.5
	3.5	1
	3.6–4.0	0.5
	>4.0	0
		(Predicted maintenance dose)
Fourth	<1.4	>8
	1.4	8
	1.5	7.5
	1.6–1.7	7
	1.8	6.5
	1.9	6
	2.0–2.1	5.5
	2.2–2.3	5
	2.4–2.6	4.5
	2.7–3.0	4
	3.1–3.5	3.5
	3.6–4.0	3
	4.1–4.5	Miss out next day's dose then give 2 mg
	>4.5	Miss out 2 days' doses then give 1 mg

Thrombosis Task Force for the British Committee for Standards in Haematology's Guidelines on Oral Anticoagulation.[2] Patients should have the dose and side effects of warfarin explained to them and be referred for subsequent monitoring of warfarin. [Grade B]

Perioperative heparin prophylaxis for high risk patients

For patients at high risk of venous thromboembolisms, unfractionated or LMWH heparin may be used according to local hospital practice, subcutaneously 5000 units twice or three times a day starting two hours preoperatively and continuing until the patient is mobile.

ORAL CONTRACEPTIVES

Because of the increased risk of venous thromboembolism associated with oestrogen-containing contraceptives around the time of surgery, these should be stopped (and adequate alternative arrangements made) at least four weeks before major elective surgery, including surgery to the legs or any surgery resulting in prolonged immobilization of the legs. It can be restarted at least two weeks after full mobilization, when the first period occurs. However, oral contraceptives need not be stopped for minor surgery involving a short anaesthetic, e.g. dental extractions. For major surgery, if stopping oestrogen-containing oral contraceptives in advance is not an option, heparin prophylaxis is indicated.

Inherited and acquired thrombophilias

ACQUIRED

The pathogenesis of thrombosis is often multifactorial. Tissue trauma, whether surgical or accidental, and malignant disease both predispose patients to venous thromboembolism, though the exact mechanisms are poorly understood. Myeloproliferative disorders (e.g. polycythaemia rubra vera and essential thrombocythaemia), hyperhomocysteinaemia and Behçet's syndrome predispose patients to both venous and arterial thromboembolism. The primary antiphospholipid syndrome also predisposes to both venous and arterial thromboembolism. The lupus anticoagulant is only one of the antiphospholipid antibodies which can predispose to thromboembolism, so for screening purposes, 'antiphospholipid antibodies' rather than the lupus anticoagulant should be requested.

INHERITED

Antithrombin, protein C and protein S deficiency are all usually autosomal dominant conditions: rare homozygous individuals are usually very severely affected almost from birth. All predispose to venous thromboembolism often at an early age (<45 years). However, the more recently discovered factor V Leiden variant, which is present in 4 percent of Caucasians, is the most common cause of early onset venous thrombosis. Raised factor VIII levels are also associated with increased venous thrombosis. [***/**]

If thrombophilia is suspected, referral for further investigation should be discussed with a haematologist.[7]

KEY POINTS

- Patients with abnormal PT, APTT, TT or platelet count should be investigated on the basis of their medical history.
- Elective surgery on patients taking warfarin needs advanced planning to minimize the risk of bleeding or thrombosis, with the minimum use of blood components.

- Surgery in haemophiliac patients needs planning in advance to ensure adequate factor therapy and an adequate response.
- Patients with thrombocytopenia should be discussed with a haematologist, to ensure the optimal treatment depending on the underlying cause and to avoid the use of platelets in conditions where this is contraindicated.

Best clinical practice

✓ Haemophiliacs: do not give intramuscular injections or nonsteroidal antiinflammatory drugs, or routine heparin prophylaxis.
✓ Haemophiliacs: in central nervous system bleeding, e.g. following head injury, factor replacement treatment must continue for at least ten days, or later bleeding recurs.

Deficiencies in current knowledge and areas for future research

➤ Further studies are needed towards optimal antiplatelet agents.
➤ Further work is needed to understand more fully the causes of thrombophilia.
➤ Further work towards an optimal anticoagulant agent, taken orally, with minimum side effects and with minimum monitoring required, is needed.

REFERENCES

1. Hutton RA, Laffan MA, Tuddenham EGH. Normal haemostasis. In: Hoffbrand AV, Lewis SM, Tuddenham EGD (eds). *Postgraduate haematology*. Oxford: Butterworth Heinemann, 1999: 550–80.
* 2. Haemostasis and Thrombosis Task Force for the British Committee for Standards in Haematology. Guidelines on Oral Anticoagulation, 3rd edn. *British Journal of Haematology*. 1998; **101**: 374–87.
3. Taberner D, Poller L, Burslem R, Jones J. Oral anticoagulants controlled by the British comparative thromboplastin versus low dose heparin prophylaxis of deep vein thrombosis. *British Medical Journal*. 1978; ii: 272–4.
4. Francis C, Marder V, Evarts C, Yaukoolbodi S. Two-step warfarin therapy: prevention of post operative venous

thrombosis without excessive bleeding. *Journal of the American Medical Association*. 1983; **249**: 374–8.

5. Ramstrom G, Sindet-Pederson S, Hall G, Blomback M, Alander U. Prevention of post surgical bleeding in oral surgery using tranexamic acid without dose modification of oral anticoagulants. *Journal of Oral and Maxillofacial Surgery*. 1993; **51**: 1211–6.

* 6. British Committee for Standards in Haematology. Guidelines for the Use of Platelet Transfusions. *British Journal of Haematology*. 2003; **122**: 10–23.

7. British Committee for Standards in Haematology. Guideline for the Investigation and Management of Heritable Thrombophilia. *British Journal of Haematology*. 2001; **114**: 512–28.

PART 6

ENDOCRINOLOGY

EDITED BY NICHOLAS S JONES

24 The pituitary gland: anatomy and physiology   295
John Hill

25 The pituitary: imaging and tests of function   303
Alan P Johnson, Swarupsinh Chavda and Paul Stewart

26 The thyroid gland: anatomy and physiology   314
Julian A McGlashan

27 The thyroid gland: function tests and imaging   327
Susan Clarke

28 The thyroid: nonmalignant disease   338
Lorraine M Albon and Jayne A Franklyn

29 The parathyroid glands: anatomy and physiology   367
Mateen H Arastu and William J Owen†

30 Parathyroid function tests and imaging   379
David Hosking

31 Parathyroid dysfunction: medical and surgical therapy   387
E Dinakara Babu, Bill Fleming and JA Lynn

32 Head and neck manifestations of endocrine disease   398
Jonathan M Morgan and Thomas McCaffrey

24

The pituitary gland: anatomy and physiology

JOHN HILL

Anatomy	295	Key points	302
Pituitary gland	295	References	302
The sella turcica	298	Further reading	302
Physiology of the hypothalamus and pituitary gland	300		

SEARCH STRATEGY AND EVIDENCE-BASE

This chapter was prepared from anatomy and physiology texts and supported by a Medline search using the key words anatomy, pituitary and cavernous sinus. The anatomical studies quoted constitute level 3 evidence.

ANATOMY

Embryology

The adenohypophysis is derived from the placodal ectoderm of the roof of the stomodeal. The neurohypophysis is derived from an evagination of the floor of the forebrain and the third ventricle.

There is a saccular depression in the roof of the stomodeum immediately in front of the oropharyngeal membrane. This saccular depression evaginates to form the pouch of Rathke. This area remains in close contact with the ventral surface of the forebrain. The pouch of Rathke develops into the adenohypophysis. The anterior part becomes the pars anterior and the posterior part, in contact with the forebrain, becomes the pars intermedia. The section of the forebrain in close contact with the pars intermedia becomes the neurohypophysis (see **Figure 24.1**).[1] In foetal life and childhood, the vestige of Rathke's pouch remains as the hypophyseal cleft separating the pars anterior and pars intermedia. The pars intermedia is rudimentary in humans and is of little functional significance. Remnants of Rathke's pouch may persist below the sphenoid in the roof of the nasopharynx forming a pharyngeal pituitary. The clivus and the dorsum sellae of the future sphenoid bone are formed from mesenchymal condensations surrounding the hypophysis. The cavernous sinus is derived from the primary head vein (see **Figure 24.1**).

PITUITARY GLAND

The pituitary gland or hypophysis cerebri is an ovoid body measuring approximately 8 mm in the anteroposterior diameter by 12 mm transversely by 4 mm high. By the age of puberty it weighs approximately 100–500 mg. It doubles in size during pregnancy and usually remains larger in females. The adenohypophysis constitutes two-thirds of its volume.

There are two major parts to the hypophysis:[2]

- adenohypophysis: includes the pars anterior, pars intermedia and pars tuberalis;
- neurohypophysis: includes the pars posterior, infundibular stem and median eminence.

Both these parts include parts of the infundibulum and are preferred to the old terms anterior and posterior lobes (see **Figure 24.2**).

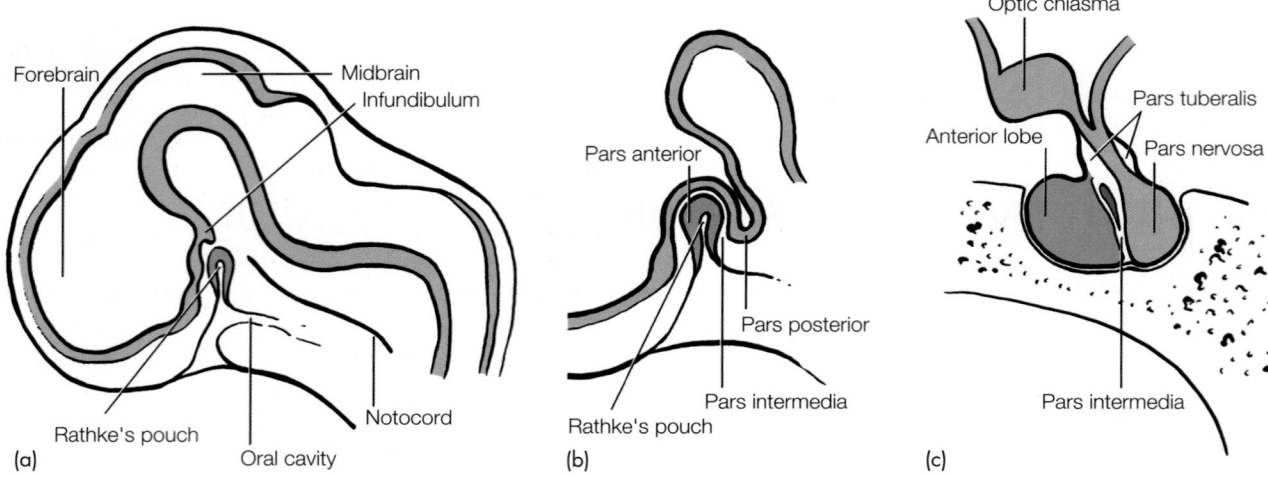

Figure 24.1 Embryological development of the hypophysis.

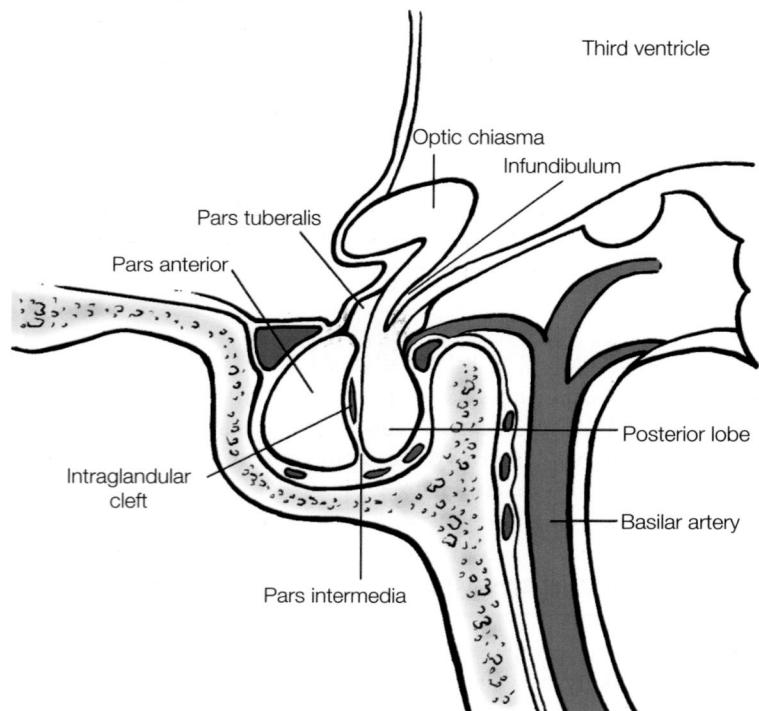

Figure 24.2 Lateral view of the hypophysis in the sella turcica with the intercavernous venous sinuses demonstrated (blue).

Adenohypophysis

This structure is highly vascular and consists of epithelial cells arranged in follicles and cords between thin walled vascular sinuses. This arrangement is supported by a delicate skeleton of reticular tissue.

Pars tuberalis contains a large number of blood vessels as well as the secreting cells listed above. In some species this area is rich in receptors for the pineal hormone melatonin.

Traditionally, cell types of the adenohypophysis have been divided up by their staining characteristics into chromphil (acidophilic, basophilic) and chromophobe cells. Modern immunohistochemical techniques allow us to identify cells by the hormones that they produce as follows:

- somatotrophs: (acidophilic) the largest and most abundant chromphil cells these secrete the protein somatotrophin or growth hormone (GH);

- mammotrophs: (acidophilic) secrete the polypeptide hormone prolactin (PRL) and become the dominant cell during pregnancy and lactation;
- mammosomatotrophs: (acidophilic) secrete growth hormone and prolactin simultaneously;
- corticotrophs: (basophilic) produce the precursor molecule pro-opiomelanocorticotropin, which is broken down into adrenocorticotropin (ACTH), beta-lipotropin and beta-endorphin;
- thyrotrophs: (basophilic) secrete thyroid-stimulating hormone (TSH);
- gonadotrophs: (basophilic) secrete follicle-stimulating hormone (FSH) and luteinizing hormone (LH);
- chromophobe cells: these small cells form the majority of the cells in the adenohypophysis. They include stem cells and degranulated secretory cells;
- folliculostellate cells (FS): these are the supporting cells of the adenohypophysis, with growth factor and cytokine activity. Their expression of cytokeratins supports the theory that the adenohypophysis is derived from Rathke's pouch.[3]

Neurohypophysis

Axons with their cell bodies in the supra optic and paraventricular nuclei of the hypothalamus run to the neurohypophysis. Some terminate in the median eminence from where they can influence the action of the adenohypophysis (see below), others run down through the stalk of the hypophysis to the main mass of the neurohypophysis where they terminate close to the sinusoids. The latter transport polypeptide hormones in conjunction with a glycoprotein (neurophysin) to the neurohypophysis where they are stored prior to release. The two hormones secreted in this way are:

1. antidiuretic hormone (ADH) or vasopressin;
2. oxytocin.

BLOOD SUPPLY OF THE HYPOPHYSIS

The arterial supply of the hypophysis is from single inferior hypophyseal arteries and several superior hypophyseal arteries on each side, all of which are branches from the internal carotid. The superior hypophyseal arteries supply the median eminence and the infundibulum. The inferior hypophyseal arteries anastamose to form an arterial ring around the infundibulum, which gives fine branches supplying the capillary bed of the neurohypophysis. The adenohypophysis does not have a direct arterial supply[4] but is supplied by long and short portal vessels, which run from the median eminence and the lower infundibulum, respectively, to the capillary bed of the adenohypophysis (**Figure 24.3**).

The hormones of the adenohypophysis are secreted by exocytosis into the nearby sinusoids. The major signal for this secretion involves the release of specific releasing factors from neurones in the median eminence, which are then transported to the adenohypophysis by the portal system.

The venous drainage of the hypophysis is less clear but has important implications in understanding the control of pituitary hormone secretion.[4] Possible drainage is via:

- long and short portal vessels to the infundibulum;
- large inferior hypophyseal veins into the dural venous sinuses;
- to the hypothalamus via the median eminence;
- reversible flow between the adenohypophysis and neurohypophysis.

Pituitary gland capsule

The gland has a capsule which is made up of very dense fibrous tissue, which is in continuity with the fibrous connective tissue of the gland. The gland appears to be loosely attached to the surrounding connective tissue, which forms a smooth nest for the hypophysis. Bridging veins, capsular arteries and fibrous bundles cross this space.[5]

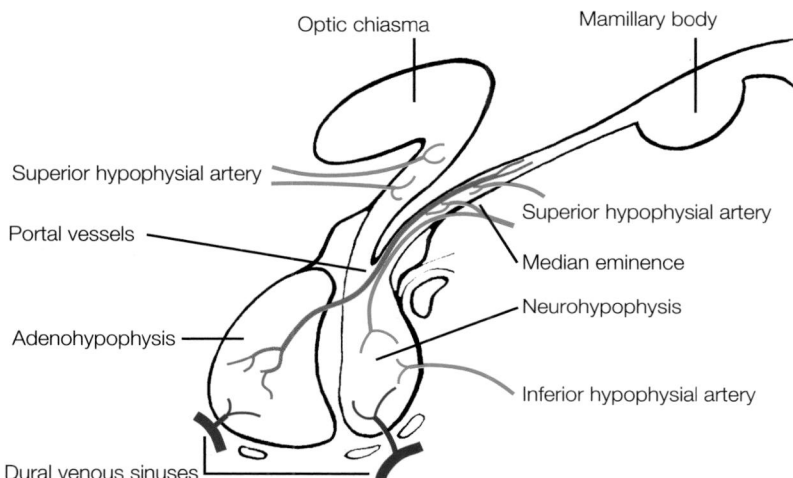

Figure 24.3 Vasculature of the hypophysis.

THE SELLA TURCICA

The sella turcica, or Turkish saddle, is the deep depression in the body of the sphenoid bone. It contains the hypophysis cerebri, dural layers and the inter-cavernous sinuses. The hypophysis fills 50 to 85 percent of the fossa.[6]

The bony landmarks around the fossa are as follows (see **Figure 24.4**).

- **Optic canal.** Between the roots of the lesser wing and the body of the sphenoid medially. Descends slightly anterolaterally, contains the optic nerve, ophthalmic artery and meninges.
- **Anterior clinoid process.** This is the posterior projection from the lesser wing of the sphenoid.
- **Tuberculum sellae** is a midline ridge in the anterior slope of the sella tunica.
- The **dorsum sellae** is the posterior wall of the sella turcica, the superiolateral projections of the dorsum form the posterior clinoid processes.
- The **groove** for the internal carotid artery is formed as the artery turns anteriorly from the foramen lacerum. The groove can be seen on the sphenoid lateral to the sella turcica.
- The **middle clinoid process** is a small elevation in the median edge of the groove. In approximately 10 percent of skulls the middle and anterior clinoid processes are joined to form a continuous ring called the carotico-clinoid foramen.[7]
- The **lingula** is a small projection arising on the posterolateral aspect of the carotid groove.
- The **clivus** is made up of the body of the sphenoid bone behind the dorsum sellae and the basioccipital bone. The upper part of the pons lies adjacent to the clivus.

In approximately 2 percent of skulls there is a bony bridge joining the anterior clinoid and posterior clinoid processes called the tinea interclinoidea. In approximately 1 percent of skulls there is a bony projection in the floor of the sella called the sella spine. It is a bony spicule that projects from the junction of the anterior and inferior walls of the sella towards the middle of the hypophyseal fossa. It is usually 1 mm in diameter and 2–5 mm in length. It probably represents an ossified remnant of the notochord.[6, 8]

Dural reflections

The diaphragmatica sella is a sheet of dura mater that forms the roof of the sella turcica. This small flat horizontal circular sheet covers over the fossa between the clinoid processes and is continuous with the roof of the cavernous sinus. There is a central defect in the diaphragm called the 'foramen diaphragmatis' which the pituitary stalk or infundibulum passes through. It is of variable diameter up to 5 mm.[9] In the region of the foramen of the dura, arachnoid and pia mater fuse with each other and with the capsule of the pituitary gland to form one fibrous layer that lines the hypophyseal fossa. In the fossa it is not possible to differentiate the fibrous layers and there are no subdural or subarachnoid spaces. Therefore, there is no cerebrospinal fluid (CSF) in the normal pituitary fossa. The diaphragmatica sella separates the contents of the pituitary fossa from the CSF. In the region of the foramen, the barrier may be very thin and consist of only arachnoid mater.[10]

The tentorium cerebelli is the main dural sheet that loops around the brainstem and separates the cerebral hemispheres from the cerebellum, forming the floor of

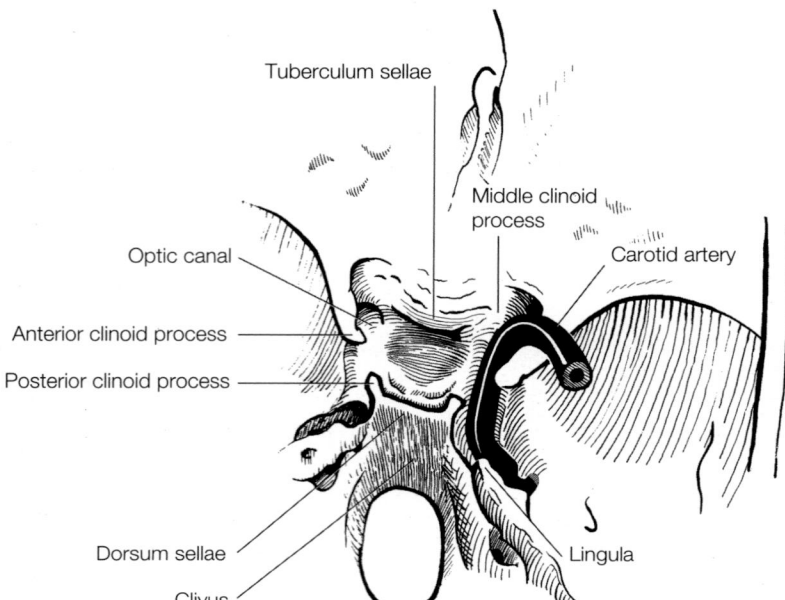

Figure 24.4 Posterio–superior view of the sella turcica of a skull. The position of the right internal carotid is demonstrated.

the middle cranial fossa. It arises from the anterior clinoid processes and has a 'U' shaped free border looping posteriorly. The peripheral attachments of the tentorium run from the anterior clinoid process backwards as a ridge of dura mater to the apex of the petrous temple bone. This ridge is at the junction of the roof and the lateral part of the cavernous sinus. From here, the attachment runs backwards to the posterior clinoid process forming the roof of the cavernous sinus and is continuous with the diaphragmatica sella. The remainder of the peripheral attachment of the tentorium is to the superior surface of the petrous temporal bone in the region of the superior petrosal sinus and to the occipital bone in the region of the transverse sinuses.

The cavernous sinus

These sinuses lie on the lateral aspect of the sphenoid body and are the lateral relations of the sella turcica. The term cavernous was adopted when it was thought that these sinuses were a single cavern with a few trabeculae. More recent work using corrosion casts has established that these sinuses are plexiform in nature, i.e. they are made up of an intertwined network of thin walled venous channels of varying sizes that divide and coalesce and incompletely surround the carotid arteries.[11]

The sinuses are approximately 1 cm wide and up to 2 cm long. They extend forwards from the apex of the petrous temporal bone to the superior orbital fissure. They are wider at the roof than at the base. The carotid arteries have a variable course in the sinuses. They enter postero–inferiorly, having passed through the carotid canal, and then turn anteriorly passing horizontally through the sinus before turning superiorly to enter the anterior cranial fossa medial to the anterior clinoid processes. The horizontal portion of the artery is usually the lateral relation of the hypophysis. There is significant individual variation and the artery may be up to 7 mm away from the gland with the intervening space filled with venous plexus, or it may be as close as 1 mm to intervening venous tissue.[12]

The oculomotor nerve, trochlear nerve and ophthalmic division of the trigeminal nerve are closely related to, but not in the lateral wall of the sinus as they pass anteriorly towards the superior orbital fissure.[12] The abducens nerve runs inferiolaterally to the carotid artery in its horizontal portion. The sympathetic plexus runs with the carotid artery.

The sinus receives tributaries from the superficial middle cerebral vein, inferior cerebral vein, spheno-parietal sinus, inferior ophthalmic vein and sometimes the central retinal vein and frontal tributaries of the middle meningeal vein. The sinus then drains into the internal jugular vein via the inferior petrosal sinus to the transverse sinus via the superior petrosal sinus, and small emissary veins drain through the foreman lacerum and ovale to the pterygoid plexus.[2]

Intercavernous venous sinuses

The two cavernous sinuses are connected across the floor of the pituitary fossa by the intercavernous venous sinuses. Some texts indicate that there is a single anterior and single posterior vein in the floor of the fossa, hence the old term 'inferior circular sinus of Winslow'. Cast studies have shown that the arrangement is much more variable with multiple interconnections across the floor possible. The superior and inferior connections may be found behind the anterior wall of the fossa and the connections may widen out laterally as they enter the cavernous sinuses (see **Figure 24.1**).[13]

Relations of the pituitary fossa

- **Superior:**
  - the diaphragmatica sella;
  - the pituitary stalk and infundibulum;
  - the optic chiasm anterior to the infundibulum 5–10 mm above the diaphragm;
  - anterior cerebral artery and anterior communicating artery anterior to the optic chiasm;
  - internal carotid artery/middle cerebral artery lateral to the infundibulum;
  - CSF surrounds the above structures above the diaphragmatica sella;
  - the third ventricle lies above the infundibulum.
- **Posterior:**
  - Lamellar bone of the dorsum sella behind which is the dura mater of the poster fossa behind which is the basilar artery;
  - CSF.
- **Lateral:**
  - upper part of the cavernous sinus containing
    - horizontal portion of the internal carotid artery
    - oculomotor, trochlear and abducens nerves.

The lateral wall of the cavernous sinus is a thick sheet of dura mater, the medial wall is much thinner. There is no thick dural sheet and the capsule of the pituitary is the only barrier against spread of adenoma from the pituitary fossa.[6]

- **Anterior and inferior:**
  - sphenoid sinus;
  - intrasphenoid sinus septum.

The anterior wall of pituitary fossa usually forms an angle of 90° with the roof of the sphenoid sinus or planum sphenoidale, although this angle may become more acute if fossa is expanded by a pituitary adenoma.[14]

The degree of pneumatization of the sphenoid is variable. In 88 percent pneumatization, aeration of the sinus extends posteriorly at least as far as the posterior limit of the pituitary fossa. In 10–12 percent, the sinus extends to the anterior wall of the pituitary fossa and in less than 1 percent the pituitary sinus is not pneumatized.[14]

The intrasphenoid sinus septae are thin, variable sheets of bone that have significant anatomical importance to the pituitary surgeon. If it is in contact with the anterior wall of the sphenoid, the septum is usually in the midline at this point, i.e. in a plane continuous with the nasal septum. The intrasphenoid sinus septum remains in the midline and attaches to the anterior wall of the pituitary fossa in 41.9 percent. In the remainder it deviates laterally where it may insert over the internal carotid artery. In addition, 20 percent of sphenoids have an additional intrasphenoid sinus septum running parasagittally. These septae are usually deficient anteriorly and, again, often insert posteriorly over the internal carotid artery.[14]

PHYSIOLOGY OF THE HYPOTHALAMUS AND PITUITARY GLAND

The hypothalamus and the pituitary act as a functional unit representing the main interface between the endocrine system and the nervous system. The hypothalamus controls the secretion of hormones from both the adenohypophysis and neurohypophysis. The secreted hormones, in turn, influence the hypothalamus by negative feedback loops.

Hypothalamic hormones

The following are secreted directly by the hypothalamus and the median eminence and influence the adenohypophysis via the portal system.[15]

- Growth hormone releasing hormone (GHRH). Causes release of growth hormone. Cell bodies in arcuate nuclei.
- Somatostatin. Inhibits secretion of GH and TSH. Cell bodies in periventricular region.
- Dopamine. Inhibits PRL secretion via portal system. PRL secretion is predominantly inhibitory; therefore disruption of the hypothalamus/pituitary connection results in hyperprolactinaemia. This is often seen in nonsecreting pituitary adenomas.
- Thyrotropin-releasing hormone (TRH). Stimulates release of TSH.
- Corticotropin-releasing hormone (CRH). Stimulates the release of ACTH and its precursor pro-opiomelanocorticotropin. Cell bodies in the paraventricular nuclei together with TRH releasing neurones.
- Gonadotropin-releasing hormone (GnRH). Cell bodies in the optic area. Stimulates release of both LH and FSH.

Neurohypophyseal hormones

These two hormones are both nonopeptides. They are transported down the axons from the cell bodies in the supraoptic and paraventricular nuclei bound to neurophysin.

ADH, or arginine vasopressin, regulates water balance and is a potent vasoconstrictor in hypovolaemic shock.

Oxytocin causes contraction of smooth muscle, particularly the myoepithelial cells lining the mammary gland ducts.

Adenohypophyseal hormones

ACTH

Circulating levels

ACTH has a half-life of only 7–12 minutes and is secreted episodically. Its plasma concentrations and those of cortisol therefore fluctuate greatly.

Tests for ACTH deficiency

The diurnal rhythm results in a wide variation in levels of ACTH and cortisol throughout the day. Single samples, even when taken at a fixed time (e.g. early morning cortisol) are therefore only an approximate guide. The hypothalamic-pituitary-adrenal axis can be tested by the following.

- ACTH stimulation. Plasma cortisol levels are measured in response to an injection of synthetic ACTH. This tests the adrenal glands ability to respond to ACTH.
- Insulin-induced hypoglycaemia. Hypoglycaemia stimulates the production of CRH, then ACTH and finally cortisol, which can be measured reliably.
- Metyrapone stimulation test. Metyrapone blocks the conversion of cortisol from its precursor 11-deoxy cortisol. In the presence of the normally functioning axis it leads to a drop in cortisol secretion, an increase in CRH, ACTH and 11-deoxycortisol levels, the last of which can be reliably measured in circulation.

Effects

Stimulates the adrenal cortex to secrete glucocorticoids, mineralocorticoids and androgenic steroids. The hyperpigmentation seen in excess ACTH secretion states (Addison's disease, Nelson's syndrome) is due to ACTH binding to MSH receptors.

Control of secretion

CRH stimulates secretion in a diurnal rhythm with the peak for waking and a gradual decline through the day. There is also an increase in ACTH secretion in response to stress, which can be emotional, physical or biochemical.

Cortisol acting on the hypothalamus and the pituitary levels provides negative feedback.

GROWTH HORMONE

Circulating levels

The half-life of growth hormone is 20–50 minutes. Normal early morning levels are 0–40 µg/L. Insulin-like growth factor (IGF)-1 levels are less variable and are age and sex related, but are better indications of growth hormone levels.[16]

Effects

Its main function is to promote growth. This action is mediated by the IGF-1, which increases protein synthesis and fat metabolism for energy production. It counteracts the effects of insulin, impairing glucose uptake into cells.

Control of secretion

This is mediated by GHRH (stimulation) and somatostatin (inhibition). Somatostatin analogues are being increasingly used in the treatment of acromegaly. Peak levels of growth hormone occur one to four hours after the onset of sleep and this is when the majority of growth hormone is produced. Less growth hormone is secreted with advancing age. Levels are increased by exercise, physical, metabolic and emotional stress. Decreased levels are seen in children with severe emotional deprivation.

Tests of growth hormone secretion

- Insulin-induced hypoglycaemia: in normal individuals hypoglycaemia will result in an increase in growth hormone levels and is easily measured. This response may be lacking in individuals with growth hormone deficiency.
- Glucose tolerance test: increased circulating glucose level lowers growth hormone levels in normal subjects but not in acromegalics and therefore this test is useful in the diagnosis of acromegaly.

PROLACTIN

Circulating levels

The half-life is 50 minutes. The normal range is less than 20 µg/L.[16]

Effects

Prolactin stimulates lactation. During pregnancy, oestrogen together with progesterone and cortisol help promote breast development. Prolactin levels increase during pregnancy but the high levels of oestrogen inhibit lactation. The oestrogen and progesterone levels fall at parturition and the high prolactin levels then stimulate lactation. Prolactin does not have a role in the development of normal breast tissue.

Prolactin does not affect gonadal function physiologically but in hyperprolactinanaemia gonadal function is affected. There is shortening of the luteal phase of the cycle in women with failure of ovulation, amenorrhoea and infertility. Men develop decreased testosterone production, decreased libido, impotence and infertility.

Control of secretion

Peak secretion is usually between 4 and 7 a.m. and is episodic.

Increased secretion is seen following physical stress, surgery, nipple stimulation, hypoglycaemia and myocardial infarction.

Prolactin secretion is predominantly controlled in an inhibitory fashion by dopamine. Drugs that interfere with dopamine receptors, such as phenothiazines, metoclopramide, reserpine and methyldopa, can increase prolactin release.

Dopamine agonists, such as bromocriptine and its derivatives, lower prolactin levels and are used in the treatment of hyperprolactinaemia.

THYROTROPIN

Circulating levels

The half-life of thyrotropin (TSH) is 50–60 minutes. Circulating TSH levels are readily measurable and used in the diagnosis of hypothyroidism and hyperthyroidism but are less use in diagnosing pituitary disorders. There is an early morning surge in TSH levels.

Effects

TSH, like LH, FSH and human chorionic gonadotrophin (HCG) are glycoproteins with an alpha and beta subunit. The alpha unit in all four hormones is identical. The beta subunit of TSH stimulates T4 and T3 release, and iodine uptake in the thyroid gland.

Control of secretion

TRH stimulates the release of the TSH and somatostatin inhibits it. T3 and T4 are also significant inhibitors of TSH release. They act at the pituitary level by reducing the amount of TSH that has released in response to TRH. Dopamine also inhibits TSH secretion. Bromocriptine will therefore decrease the TSH secretion and has been used to treat encountered TSH secreting pituitary adenomas that are uncommon.

GONADOTROPINS, LH AND FSH

Circulating levels

Levels of both hormones are low before the onset of puberty. In girls, the hormones are secreted cyclically at the onset of puberty and in boys there is a nocturnal rise in the secretion of LH at puberty.

In women, LH steadily increases and then peaks in the middle of the menstrual cycle stimulating ovulation. FSH is high early in the cycle, then steadily declines until mid-cycle when it surges. Both FSH and LH decrease in the second half of the cycle.

Both FSH and LH levels are high in postmenopausal women. In men, levels mirror those of the follicular phase in adult women.

Effects

These glycoprotein hormones differ only in their beta subunits and are secreted by the same cell. They regulate the noble function by stimulating sex steroid production and gametogenesis by the ovary and testis.

In women, LH stimulates oestrogen and progesterone production, stimulates ovulation and stimulates the corpus luteum to produce progesterone in the second half of the cycle. FSH controls the development of the ovarian follicle.

In men, FSH stimulates the Sertoli cells in their role in spermatogenesis and LH stimulates the Leydig to produce testosterone.

Control of secretion

GnRH stimulates the release of LH and FSH. It is released episodically and this pattern of release is necessary for controlling the onset of puberty and ovulation. In women, the circulating sex hormones influence GnRH secretion by both negative and positive feedback mechanisms at different parts of the menstrual cycle. Switching from negative to positive feedback results in the surges of FSH and LH seen in midcycle. In men, androgens stimulate the production of inhibin by the Sertoli cells and this hormone in turn inhibits GnRH secretion.

KEY POINTS

- A normal pituitary is approximately $8 \times 12 \times 4$ mm in size, weighing up to 500 mg.
- The lateral relation to the internal carotid artery and the rest of the contents of the cavernous sinus is variable.
- The sella turcica does not normally contain CSF.
- The anterior lobe hormones are ACTH; and growth hormones are TSH, LH, FSH and prolactin.
- The posterior lobe hormones are oxytocin and ADH.

REFERENCES

1. Langman J (ed.). *Medical embryology*, 4th edn. Baltimore and London: Williams and Wilkins, 1981.

2. Williams PL (ed.). *Gray's anatomy*, 38th edn. Edinburgh: Churchill Livingstone, 1995.

3. Tsuchida T, Hruban RH, Carson BS, Philips PC. Folliculo-stellate cells in the human anterior pituitary express cytokeratins. *Pathology, Research and Practice.* 1993; **189**: 184–8.

4. Page RB, Bergland RM. Pituitary vasculature. In: Allen MB, Makesh VB (eds). *The pituitary. A current review.* New York: Academic Press, 1977: 9–17.

5. Dieteman JL, Kehrli P, Maillot C, Diniz R, Reis M, Neugroschl C *et al.* Is there a dural wall between the cavernous sinus and the pituitary fossa? Anatomical and MRI findings. *Neuroradiology.* 1998; **40**: 627–30.

6. Di Chiro G, Nelson KB. The volume of the sella turcica. *American Journal of Roentgenology.* 1962; **87**: 989–1008.

7. Lang J. Structure and postnatal organisation of the heretofore uninvestigated and infrequent ossifications of the sella turcica region. *Acta Anatomica.* 1977; **99**: 121–30.

8. Dietemann JL, Lang J, Francke JP, Bonneville JF, Clarisse J, Wackenhiem A. Anatomy and radiology of the sella spine. *Neuroradiology.* 1981; **21**: 5–7.

9. Hempel KJ. Zur Pathologie der sellaregion. *Radiologe.* 1970; **10**: 425–9.

10. Sheahy CN, Jackson CCR, Pearson O, Kaufman B. Submucosal infranasal transphenoid hypophysectomy. *Bulletin of Los Angeles Neurological Society.* 1968; **33**: 564–73.

11. Parkinson D. Carotid cavernous fistula: direct repair with preservation of the carotid artery. Technical note. *Journal of Neurosurgery.* 1973; **38**: 99–106.

12. McGrath P. The cavernous sinus: anatomical survey. *Australian and New Zealand Journal of Surgery.* 1977; **47**: 601–13.

13. Kaplan HA, Browder J, Krieger AJ. Intercavernous connections of the cavernous sinuses. The superior and inferior circular sinuses. *Journal of Neurosurgery.* 1976; **45**: 166–8.

14. Kinman J. Surgical aspects of the anatomy of the sphenoidal sinuses and the sella turcica. *Journal of Anatomy.* 1977; **124**: 541–53.

15. Greenspan FS, Gardner DG. *Basic and clinical endocrinology.* New York: Lange Medical Books/McGraw-Hill, 2001.

16. Weatherall DJ, Ledingham JGC, Warrell DA. *Oxford textbook of medicine*, 3rd edn. Oxford: Oxford University Press, 1996.

FURTHER READING

Cappabianca P, Alfieri AR, De Divitis E, Tschabitscher M. *Atlas of endoscopic anatomy for endonasal intracranial surgery.* New York: Springer-Verlag, 2001. *Demonstrates the endoscopic views of sphenoid and pituitary fossa.*

Cushing HJB. *Pituitary body and its disorders.* Philadelphia: Lippincott Co, 1912. *Historical perspective on surgical anatomy.*

25

The pituitary: imaging and tests of function

ALAN P JOHNSON, SWARUPSINH CHAVDA AND PAUL STEWART

Pituitary anatomy as it relates to imaging	303	Visual field assessment	312
The use of imaging in pituitary disease	304	Pituitary function in the postoperative period	312
MRI	305	Key points	312
Pituitary physiology as it relates to tests for normal function	307	Best clinical practice	313
The biochemical investigation of functioning and nonfunctioning adenomas and lesions arising adjacent to the pituitary	308	Deficiencies in current knowledge and areas for future research	313
		References	313

SEARCH STRATEGY

All searches were carried out using Ovid Medline. Individual references used the terms and key words related to the relevant text as follows: pituitary, adenoma, imaging and diagnosis.

PITUITARY ANATOMY AS IT RELATES TO IMAGING

High quality imaging of the pituitary and adjacent structures is essential in the management of pituitary adenomas. The development of magnetic resonance imaging (MRI) has been the greatest advance in this field in recent decades. Computed tomography (CT) scanning has a role, particularly for bone detail. On occasions conventional digital subtraction angiography (DSA) may be of use. These techniques have rendered more invasive and less effective imaging methods, such as air and contrast encephalography, redundant.

The detail of pituitary anatomy is described in Chapter 24, The pituitary gland: anatomy and physiology. In brief, the pituitary fossa lies in the posterior superior corner of the sphenoid sinuses. Its boundaries are as follows.

- **Anterior and inferior** – in well-aerated sphenoid sinuses, the bony walls of the sinuses form the anterior wall and the floor of the pituitary fossa. If the body of the sphenoid bone is poorly aerated, the fossa is a recess in the posterior superior part of the body of the sphenoid bone itself.
- **Posterior** – the superior extension of the clivus, the dorsum sellae, forms the posterior wall of the fossa.

Together, these structures form a bony saddle in the skull floor, the sella turcica or Turk's saddle, in which the gland sits.

- **Lateral** – the cavernous sinuses are the soft tissue structures which form the lateral aspects of the pituitary fossa. They are venous lakes, which have dura mater and vein wall on their medial aspects separating them from the pituitary gland. Blood flows into them from the opthalmic veins and pterygoid plexuses and out of them into the superior and inferior petrosal sinuses. They communicate across the midline by means of intercavernous connecting veins, whose size and position are extremely variable. They contain a range of important structures – the internal carotid arteries, and the oculomotor (III), trochlear (IV), abducent (VI), ophthamlic (V^1) and maxillary (V^2) nerves.

- **Superior** – a thin structure called the diaphragma sellae forms the roof of the pituitary fossa. It is formed from the thin inner layer of the dura and the pia-arachnoid. This is perforated by the pituitary stalk and may actually be deficient at this point. Immediately above this is the suprasellar cistern, a space filled with cerebrospinal fluid (CSF).

THE USE OF IMAGING IN PITUITARY DISEASE

Imaging is used to identify the following.

- Normality (**Figure 25.1**). Imaging gives details of the size, shape, signal intensity (MRI) and signal density (CT) of the pituitary gland and adjacent structures.
- Intrinsic abnormality (**Figure 25.2**). MRI is the best technique to identify an intrinsic abnormality in a normal sized pituitary gland (tumour <10 mm in diameter – a microadenoma). However, in a patient with clinical features of a functioning adenoma, the presence of a localized abnormality within the pituitary can be misleading because:
  - there is a 10 percent incidence of asymptomatic pituitary adenomas in the general population and 10 percent of these are multiple;[1, 2] [***/**]
  - small functioning adenomas may not be visible on imaging – 25 percent in Cushing's disease;[3] [***]
  - in Cushing's disease, there may be hyperplasia rather than an adenoma.[4] [**]
- Extrinsic abnormality (**Figure 25.3**). If a tumour extends out of the fossa (tumour >10 mm diameter – a macroadenoma) imaging provides information on invasion or displacement of adjacent structures.
  - Superior extension (**Figures 25.3** and **25.4**). Pituitary adenomas most often extend superiorly into the suprasellar cistern where they may cause

symptoms by compression. Visual disturbance is the classical presentation, with superior temporal quadrantanopia as the presenting symptom due to compression of the inferomedial fibres in the optic nerves. The shape of the superior extension is

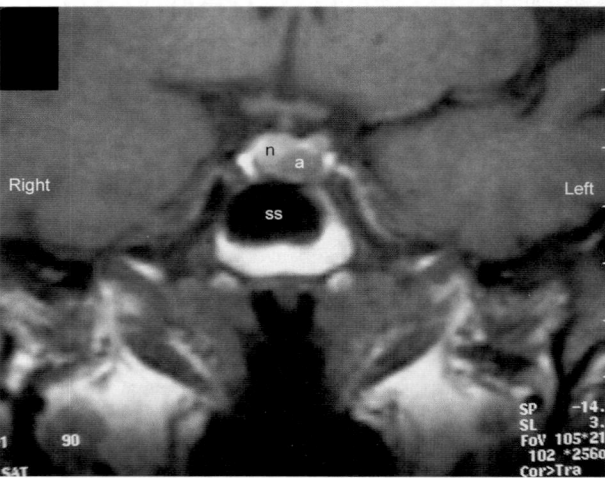

Figure 25.2 T1-weighted MR scan without contrast showing a left-sided microadenoma as a hypointense area. a, adenoma; n, normal pituitary; ss, sphenoid sinus.

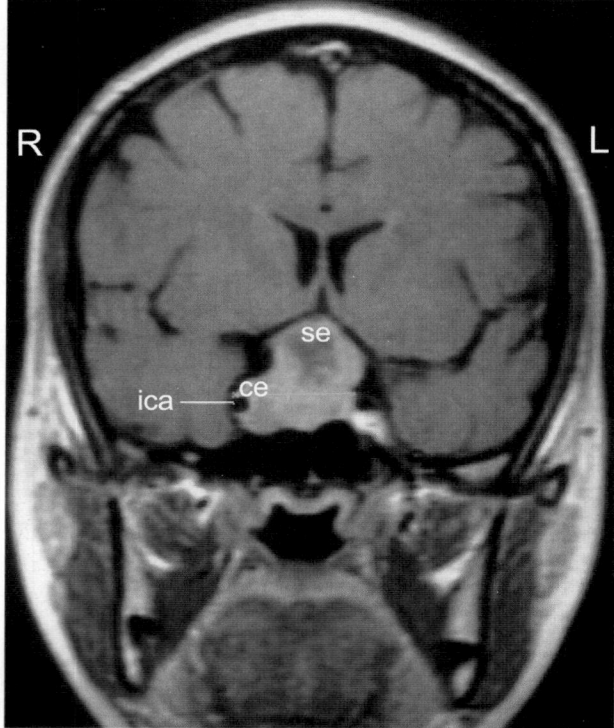

Figure 25.3 Macroadenoma of the pituitary with suprasellar extension and extension into the right cavernous sinus. ce, cavernous sinus extension; ica, internal carotid artery; se, suprasellar extension.

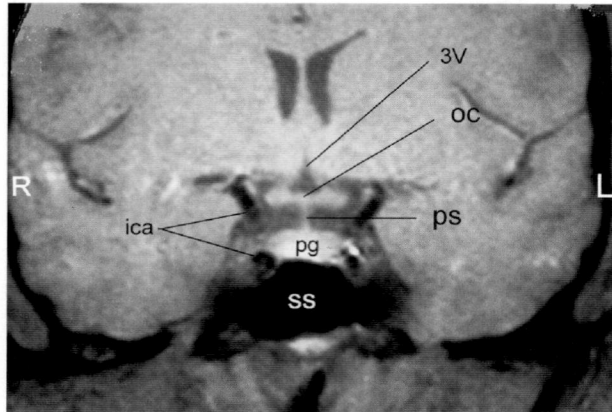

Figure 25.1 Normal pituitary gland. 3V, third ventricle; ica, internal carotid artery; oc, optic chiasm; pg, pituitary gland; ps, pituitary stalk; ss, sphenoid sinus.

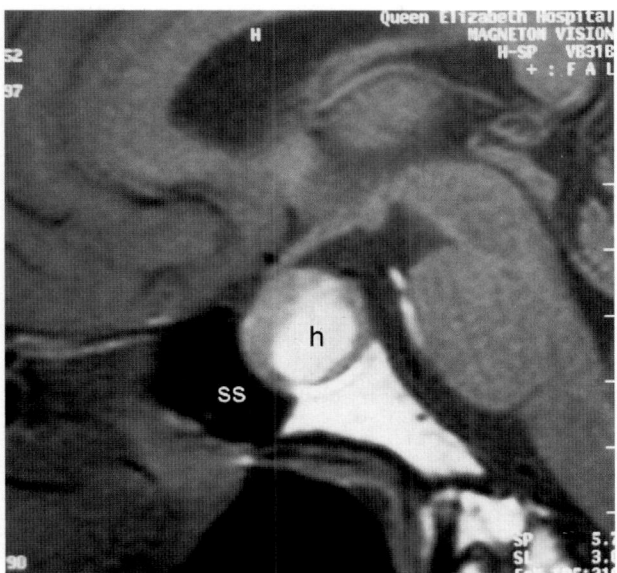

Figure 25.4 Saggital T1 weighted MRI showing haemorrage into a macroadenoma. h, area of haemorrhage; ss, sphenoid sinus.

important, because a concentric tumour will be more easily removed from below than a so-called 'cottage loaf' tumour, where there is a waist in the tumour at the level of the diaphragma sellae (see Chapter 258, Pituitary tumours: medical and surgical management).

- Lateral extension into the cavernous sinus is usually asymptomatic. If there is evidence of an oculomotor palsy, it is important to consider alternative pathology such as an invasive tumour or an aneurysm (**Figure 25.3**).
- Inferior extension into the sphenoid sinus. Once again, this is usually asymptomatic, but if a connection develops through the pituitary fossa between the CSF spaces and the nose, the patient can present with either a CSF rhinorrhoea or meningitis. This can occur if infarction or medical treatment of an extensive prolactinoma leads to marked tumour shrinkage of a locally invasive tumour. CT scanning is useful in this situation because it will define the extent of any bone defect.
- Features on imaging which suggest alternative pathology. There are a range of other conditions which can arise in this area and mimic nonfunctioning pituitary adenomas (see Chapter 258, Pituitary tumours: medical and surgical management).

MRI

MRI should include thin section T1-weighted images (T1WI) with and without contrast and T2-weighted images (T2WI), in the axial, coronal and sagittal planes. Fat suppressed T1WI with contrast and dynamic contrast imaging and magnetic resonance angiography (MRA) are useful additional techniques.

- T1WI without contrast (**Figures 25.1** and **25.2**).
  - Soft tissue detail within the gland.
    - The appearance of normal anterior pituitary is uniform and in normal adults the adenohypophysis is isointense to cerebral white matter on standard T1WI. The adenohypophysis makes up approximately 70–80 percent of the total gland volume. The neurohypophysis can appear hyperintense on T1WI. This is due to the effect of stored neurosecretory phospholipid granules on T1WI. This hyperintense region is seen in up to 90 percent of children but is a less consistent finding in adults. In adults, the gland ranges from 8–10 mm in height in the sagittal plane, but may exceed 12 mm in height in the postpartum period. The upper contour of the gland is normally flat or concave but it may have a convex upper border in menstruating or lactating females and during puberty.
    - Asymptomatic non-neoplastic cysts, found in approximately 20 percent of autopsy specimens, may be hypointense, isointense or hyperintense, depending on their content. If a cyst has a high cholesterol, fat or protein content, it will be hyperintense on T1WI.
    - Microadenomas may be either hypointense or isointense (**Figure 25.2**). They may be homogeneous or have areas of cystic change. Haemorrhage into an adenoma can cause sudden visual deterioration and the T1WI may help to confirm this with an area of hyperintensity within the adenoma (**Figure 25.4**).
  - Adjacent structures.
    - T1WI also shows fat within the clivus and body of the sphenoid as high intensity and demonstrates cortical bone as low intensity (**Figure 25.4**).
    - The pituitary stalk is well seen in the CSF in the suprasellar cistern (**Figures 25.1** and **25.2**). The infundibulum tapers from the floor of the third ventricle to the pituitary gland. The diameter of the stalk normally does not exceed that of the basilar artery or 3 mm in diameter. It enhances after the administration of intravenous contrast, because it lacks a blood–brain barrier. Stalk deviation is best seen on coronal views and although it usually has a midline position it may deviate slightly from the midline.

- The optic chiasm is well seen, although it is often difficult to define the optic nerves at the orbital apex on more anterior coronal cuts.
- The cavernous sinuses and the nerves within them are isointense. On coronal views, a clear line can often be seen between the anterior pituitary and the cavernous sinus. Invasion of the cavernous sinus by an adenoma may be clearly visible.
- The internal carotid arteries show well as flow voids.
- The air within the sphenoid sinuses and the cortical bone margins will appear black while the mucosa of the sphenoid sinus is easily seen to indicate the anatomy of the interior of the sinus. Extensive soft tissue encroaching from the pituitary into the sphenoid sinus indicates inferior extension of the tumour. Bone detail is best seen on CT (see below under CT scanning). Mucosal thickening or fluid levels seen within the sphenoids or other sinuses (on MRI or CT) raises the possibility of sinusitis.
- T1WI with contrast. The use of intravenous gadolinium as contrast is part of the routine imaging technique for investigating the pituitary.
  – Soft tissue detail within the gland.
    - Normal anterior pituitary enhances uniformly with contrast as it has no blood–brain barrier.
    - Cystic areas will have an impaired circulation, and will retain the intensity they had on the noncontrast image.
    - Microadenomas normally enhance less rapidly than normal pituitary tissue and hence appear hypointense on immediate contrast studies facilitating the diagnosis. They may appear hyperintense on delayed scans.
    - Macroadenomas may enhance to a variable degree and appear more heterogeneous than without contrast.
    - The cavernous sinuses will enhance with contrast. Depending on the imaging characteristics of any tissue extending into them, this can add information on the extent of a pituitary lesion. Other structures do not change significantly with contrast.
- T2WI is useful because of the high signal of CSF. This allows a clear definition of the upper surface of a small gland or a tumour extending out of the fossa into the suprasellar cistern. T2WI is also very useful to define an empty sella or an arachnoid cyst. The signal characteristics follow CSF on fluid attenuated inversion recovery (FLAIR) and diffusion weighted images (DWI).

CT scanning

This form of imaging can be used to enhance the information obtained from MRI. It is widely used in sinus surgery because of the precise information it gives with good demonstration of the air, soft tissue and bone details within the sinuses. Images can be acquired in the axial or coronal planes, and reformatted into any plane required. Good reformatting requires thin slice CT with contiguous images and the newer spiral/helical scans make this feasible. The use of CT scans does result in exposure of patients to moderate doses of radiation. It is indicated in pituitary tumours for the following reasons:

- to define bone detail in the sphenoid sinuses and the nasal anatomy;
- to demonstrate bone destruction of the pituitary fossa. This can be of the anterior wall, the floor or the dorsum sellae;
- to define the extent and severity of sinus infection;
- to assist in the diagnosis of other lesions such as meningioma or craniopharyngioma which may be partially calcified as calcification is best seen on CT.

Digital subtraction angiography

Digital subtraction angiography can be used if there are reasons to suspect a vascular lesion, such as an aneurysm or an arterio-venous malformation, although MRA may be used instead. In a pituitary lesion with an associated oculomotor palsy, an aneurysm should be part of the differential diagnosis because pituitary adenomas very seldom cause diplopia.

IMAGING OF THE PITUITARY AFTER SURGERY

Macroadenomas

Serial postoperative MR scanning is particularly valuable in large tumours. The 'base line' postoperative scan should be timed to allow the early effects of surgery, such as oedema and organization of tissue, to resolve. Subsequent scans then allow accurate monitoring of any change in the volume of residual tissue within the pituitary fossa and can be used to detect recurrence.

Microadenomas

Where the surgeon has performed an adenectomy or partial hypophysectomy for a microadenoma, interpretation is more difficult, because residual tissue within the fossa may be either the remaining normal tissue, or material which the surgeon inserted at the time of surgery, or recurrent adenoma. Serial scans can demonstrate growth of persistent tissue, which may indicate recurrent adenoma. In functioning adenomas, endocrine assessment is probably a more reliable indication of cure, persistence or recurrence of disease.

The future of imaging

Recent advances in imaging technology will considerably improve the assessment of the sella and the parasellar pathologies. These include:

- an increase in magnetic strength of MR scanners with research scanners available at 9.4T with the potential for MR imaging to display very fine anatomic detail within CNS;
- open bore MR scanners which can allow real time image guided surgery;[5] [*]
- image fusion for stereotactic surgery and radiotherapy planning;
- MR spectroscopy for correct diagnosis of lesions including post-radiotherapy necrosis;
- multislice CT scanners for quick scans which will prove excellent for noninvasive CT angiography;
- the development of positron emission tomography (PET) of pituitary tumours.

PITUITARY PHYSIOLOGY AS IT RELATES TO TESTS FOR NORMAL FUNCTION

The pituitary gland consists of an anterior part, the adenohypophysis, and a posterior part, the neurohypophysis, attached to the hypothalamus by the pituitary stalk. Both adenohypophysis and neurohypophysis are physically attached and physiologically intimately related to the hypothalamus, which lies immediately above the pituitary in the lateral walls of the third ventricle (see also Chapter 24, The pituitary gland: anatomy and physiology).[6]

The arterial blood supply of the whole gland is from the superior and inferior hypophyseal arteries, both of which are branches of the internal carotid artery. The superior hypophyseal arteries supply a plexus which is closely associated with the median eminence of the hypothalamus and the axons of the hypophysiotropic neurones within the hypothalamus. These vessels then form a pituitary portal circulation, which runs down the pituitary stalk into sinusoids in the anterior pituitary. The venous drainage of the gland is into the cavernous sinuses. These are venous lakes, which contain the last part of the internal carotid arteries, and the IIIrd, IVth, Vth and VIth cranial nerves. They are connected across the midline by a variable array of intercavernous connecting veins and they drain into the superior and inferior petrosal sinuses. The venous connections are of importance when considering inferior petrosal sinus sampling as a method of locating secreting adenomas.

The function of the hypothalamus and pituitary is highly complex and the pituitary is often described as the conductor of the endocrine orchestra. Neural and hormonal factors act on the hypothalamus to control the secretion from the pituitary. The hormones released from the pituitary either act on target organs (thyroid, adrenals and gonads), which then secrete the active hormones, or they act directly on target cells (prolactin, growth hormone/IGF1, vasopressin).

Hypothalamus

The hypothalamus exerts control over both the anterior and posterior pituitary. The control of the anterior part is via the portal circulation, and the hypothalamic axons extend directly into the posterior part.

In the case of the anterior gland, the hypophysiotropic cells within the hypothalamus are regulated by neural stimuli and feedback from the circulating levels of active hormones, whether secreted by the adenohypophysis itself (e.g. GH) or a target organ (e.g. thyroxine). Neurohormones are synthesized by the hypophysiotropic neurones, transported down their axons and released into the pituitary portal circulation, which carries them to target cells in the anterior pituitary. There is also a lesser direct feedback effect of circulating active hormones on the anterior pituitary cells themselves.

The neurohormones can have either a stimulatory or inhibitory effect on the cells of the anterior pituitary. The identified stimulatory neurohormones are gonadotrophin releasing hormone (GnRH), thyrotrophin releasing hormone (TRH), corticotrophin releasing factor (CRF) and growth hormone releasing hormone (GHRH). Examples of inhibitory neurohormones are somatostatin, inhibiting the release of growth hormone, and prolactin release inhibiting factor (PIF) hormone. Dopamine is either PIF or at least one PIF. When these neurohormones reach the target cells in the adenohypophysis they stimulate or inhibit the release of the specific hormone in question.

Adenohypophysis

The adenohypophysis is made up of three parts, the pars anterior which is 80 percent of the gland, the pars intermedia, which is small in adults but well developed in the foetus, and the pars tuberalis which is an upward extension of the anterior part wrapped around the lower end of the pituitary stalk.

The adenohypophysis secretes thyroid stimulating hormone (TSH), adrenocorticotrophic hormone (ACTH), growth hormone (GH), prolactin (PRL) and two gonadotrophins, follicle stimulating hormone (FSH) and luteinizing hormone (LH).

Hormone secretion by the adenohypophysis is subject to marked cyclical rhythms. The cycle of secretion can vary widely with particular hormones. Seasonal rhythms are well recognized in the breeding cycles of many animals, but are probably unimportant in humans. In women, gonadotrophin secretion has a 28-day cycle which is critical for ovulation and implantation. The circadian rhythmic nature of ACTH release is well recognized. Normal growth hormone secretion has a diurnal rhythm and is pulsatile, with more pulses secreted during sleep.

Fluctuations in hormone secretion are important when assessing the level of a particular hormone for two reasons. First, the loss of the diurnal rhythm may be an important indicator of disease, as in Cushing's disease. Second, if the hormone has a short half-life, an isolated measurement of the hormone level can be very misleading if the rhythmic or pulsatile nature of its secretion is not taken into account. This is particularly true of growth hormone assays.

Neurohypophysis

The neurohypophysis is in continuity with the supraoptic and paraventricular neurones in the hypothalamus. Axons from these cells run through the stalk to the posterior pituitary. These cells synthesize and contain granules which pass down the axons. The granules are stored in the distal ends of the axons in the posterior pituitary and release oxytocin and vasopressin (ADH or antidiuretic hormone) into the systemic circulation when stimulated to do so.

Vasopressin has a direct effect on the distal convoluted tubules and medullary collecting ducts of the kidney, which it stimulates to reabsorb water. It also has a direct vasoconstrictive effect on vascular smooth muscle. Diabetes insipidus arises when vasopressin secretion is deficient and can be seen following pituitary surgery. However, this is not the only cause of a postoperative diuresis in hypophysectomy, and the syndrome of inappropriate antidiuretic hormone (SIADH) can arise in the postoperative period. It is essential to confirm that a diuresis is due to diabetes insipidus, by confirming that the plasma sodium levels are normal in the presence of a high output of dilute urine, before treating it with a vasopressin analogue such as DDAVP. Treating a diuresis with DDAVP in the presence of SAIDH may cause a serious fall in sodium levels, which may cause severe complications.

Oxytocin secretion causes milk ejection during lactation and uterine contraction during labour. Oxytocin release is stimulated by mechanical stimulation of the nipple during lactation. During labour, stimulation of receptors in the pelvic wall leads to stimulation of the hypothalamic neurones which release oxytocin.

THE BIOCHEMICAL INVESTIGATION OF FUNCTIONING AND NONFUNCTIONING ADENOMAS AND LESIONS ARISING ADJACENT TO THE PITUITARY

Anterior pituitary

PROLACTIN AND PROLACTINOMA

Human prolactin is a protein consisting of 199 amino acids. It has similarities with growth hormone. Its predominant and most active form is a monomer, but it also circulates as a dimer and a polymer. The serum prolactin level is a reliable measure of this hormone. It is used to diagnose prolactinoma and to monitor the effect of treatment. The normal circulating level will depend on the laboratory, but the normal range in our centre is 60–620 mU/L. Circulating levels are higher in women than in men.

Prolactin regulation is via neural and feedback pathways to the hypothalamus and anterior pituitary. Inhibitory factors – PIF – and releasing factors are involved in the control of prolactin release. The main PIF is dopamine. Twelve to twenty-eight percent of cells in the normal anterior lobe produce prolactin. The control of secretion is complex and a wide range of factors and conditions influence prolactin secretion.

The main site of action of prolactin is the mammary gland where it acts to prepare for milk production and maintain it. Physiological and pathological hyperprolactinaemia also suppresses the hypothalamo-pituitary axis and suppresses the release of GnRH and therefore gonadotrophins. These effects can cause galactorrhoea and amenorrhoea in women. In men there may be little effect but low gonadotrophin levels may reduce the secretion of testosterone, causing loss of libido.

Physiologically high levels of prolactin are to be expected during pregnancy and lactation. Pathological causes of high prolactin levels are due to autonomous secretion of prolactin by the pituitary as in a prolactinoma, or because of loss of PIF from the hypothalamus. In prolactinomas the prolactin levels can be very high – over 10,000 mU/L. In nonfunctioning adenomas there may be a moderate rise in prolactin levels, up to approximately 2000 mU/L, probably because of a loss of PIF due to the effect of the adenoma and stalk compression. In other functioning adenomas, such as GH secreting adenomas, prolactin may be elevated because this hormone can be produced in excess along with growth hormone.

It is important to remember that when a pituitary macroadenoma is identified on imaging, a modest elevation of serum prolactin (up to 2000 mU/L) can be anticipated in a nonfunctioning tumour. Conversely, prolactinomas may cause little in the way of symptoms, particularly in men, and no pituitary macroadenoma should be assumed to be nonfunctioning unless the serum prolactin is less than 2000 mU/L.

Dopamine agonists, such as bromocriptine and cabergoline, are the first line treatment for prolactinomas. Serum prolactin levels can be used to monitor their effect, but imaging should also be used, particularly in the presence of a macroadenoma (>10 mm in diameter on imaging). On this treatment the levels of circulating prolactin should fall and the tumour shrink. However, a biochemical response is not invariable and if it occurs it does not guarantee tumour shrinkage. The indications for surgery and its results are discussed in Chapter 258, Pituitary tumours: medical and surgical management. Serum prolactin levels are also used to monitor the results of other forms of treatment, namely surgery or radiotherapy.

GROWTH HORMONE AND ACROMEGALY

Seventy to eighty percent of GH is a single chain 191 amino acid protein. Other forms of the hormone are also secreted. Approximately half the cells in the anterior pituitary secrete GH. GH acts either directly on cells when it binds to GH receptors, or indirectly when it triggers the production of insulin-like growth factors (IGFs) which are mainly synthesized in the liver. IGF1 is the most important of these. The serum concentration of IGF1 is a good indicator of the mean concentration of GH over time. Concentrations of GH and IGF1 can be measured in serum, but because normal secretion of GH is pulsatile and the hormone has a short half-life in circulation and IGF1 has a long half-life, IGF1 concentration is a very useful indicator of the mean GH output.

The regulation of GH output is highly complex, but it is both neural and by the feedback mechanism. Secretion is controlled by at least two antagonistic peptides from the hypothalamus, GHRH, which stimulates secretion and somatostatin, which inhibits it.

Because GH secretion is pulsatile, the quantity secreted can be varied by the frequency or the amplitude of the pulses. When considering the diurnal rhythm, output is highest during slow wave sleep. Over a lifetime, output is highest during adolescence and decreases with age. A random GH is normally less than 5.5 mU/L.

GH is anabolic and stimulates protein synthesis. It is essential for normal growth and protein metabolism. It also induces lipolysis. It is secreted during hypoglycaemia, releasing energy from body stores. Conversely, hyperglycaemia suppresses GH output. GH antagonises insulin and induces hyperglycaemia. This is why acromegaly may induce the onset of diabetes mellitus or make it worse.

Because of the way in which GH is secreted in normal individuals, it may be high at times and undetectable at others, making a random estimation of serum GH levels unreliable in the assessment of pituitary function. In order to confirm that GH levels are elevated, it is important to measure GH during an oral glucose tolerance test (OGTT). A high blood sugar should suppress GH output, but it will not do so if an adenoma is secreting GH autonomously. During such a test, as long as the blood glucose level rises above 6 mmol/L, GH should suppress to less than 2 mU/L. It is important to measure the blood glucose levels during the test.

Levels of GH during an OGTT and IGF1 are reliable in the diagnosis of acromegaly and to monitor the effects of all forms of treatment.

The diagnosis of GH deficiency in childhood is critical as treatment has to be instituted early for the patient to achieve normal growth. Post-surgical GH deficiency in adults is an area of increasing interest. Patients who have received treatment to the pituitary may become GH deficient. Symptoms are often nonspecific, diagnosis may be difficult but there is increasing evidence that some patients derive significant benefit from receiving replacement GH.

ACTH, CUSHING'S DISEASE, CUSHING'S SYNDROME AND NELSON'S SYNDROME

ACTH is a 39 amino acid peptide. It is derived from a large precursor protein which is found in the cortico-trophic cells of the anterior and intermediate lobes of the pituitary, in some neuronal cell groups, in peripheral chromaffin cells and some immune cells. In the anterior pituitary, 6–10 percent of cells are corticotrophs.

ACTH has a short circulating half-life and it is more usual to assay plasma cortisol levels and 24 hour urinary free cortisol production to screen patients for Cushing's syndrome. Both these can be reliably measured. In normal subjects, plasma cortisol levels are highest in the morning and lowest at night. This diurnal rhythm can be measured. In Cushing's syndrome, this rhythm is absent and plasma cortisol and urinary free cortisol levels are elevated.

Normal ACTH output is regulated by CRF and vasopressin. These two potentiate each other, but CRF output is suppressed by high circulating levels of glucocorticoids, whereas vasopressin is not. ACTH acts mainly on the adrenal cortex which secretes glucocorticoids, mineralocorticoids and androgens.[7]

Diagnosing Cushing's syndrome

- Circulating glucocorticoid levels and 24 hour urinary free cortisol can be measured by routine laboratory assays. Normal plasma cortisol levels are subject to large diurnal variation and the precise levels will depend on the laboratory used. In this institution the normal levels are 180–550 nmol/L at 9.00 a.m. and <130 nmol/L at 12 midnight. Loss of the diurnal rhythm is a feature of Cushing's syndrome. Measurement of 24 hour urinary free cortisol output is also a useful measure of glucocorticoid production and provides a screening test for Cushing's syndrome.

- The low-dose dexamethasone test (see Differentiating Cushing's disease from Cushing's syndrome) is also of value to diagnose Cushing's syndrome. In this test, plasma cortisol is effectively suppressed in normals, but not in those with autonomous ACTH secretion.
- Insulin tolerance test. Depressed patients may show some of the clinical features of Cushing's syndrome and lose the circadian rhythm of cortisol output. Insulin-induced hypoglycaemia can be used to distinguish depressed patients from those with Cushing's syndrome because it will induce a rise in ACTH in the former but not the latter. Adequate hypoglycaemia must be induced and in Cushing's syndrome, this may require quite large doses of insulin.

Differentiating Cushing's disease from Cushing's syndrome

In suspected Cushing's syndrome, once raised plasma cortisol and urinary free cortisol levels have been detected, it is important to establish the cause. This could be due to excess production from the adrenal glands themselves, as in an adrenal adenoma or carcinoma, or due to excessive stimulation of the adrenal cortex by overproduction of ACTH, secreted from the pituitary or from an ectopic source. The commonest cause of Cushing's syndrome is excess ACTH from the pituitary (70 percent) – Cushing's disease – but this must be defined if treatment is to be appropriate and effective. A number of tests exist to achieve this.

- If the source of glucocorticoids is adrenal, the plasma ACTH level is low.
- Hypokalaemic alkalosis is a feature of Cushing's syndrome due to ectopic ACTH, but not of Cushing's disease.
- The dexamethasone suppression test. The high-dose part of this test is used to differentiate between a pituitary source and an ectopic source of excess ACTH. There are several variations in the test, but they hinge on the fact that there is a differential sensitivity on the feedback mechanism with increasing doses of dexamethasone in the different causes of Cushing's syndrome. Dexamethasone is a powerful glucocorticoid, which acts centrally via the feedback mechanism to suppress ACTH output. At low dose (0.5 mg four times a day) it will suppress secretion of ACTH in normal subjects, but the effect is insufficient in those with autonomous ACTH

secretion. However, pituitary secretion of excess ACTH is not totally autonomous, and so high doses of dexamethasone (2 mg four times a day) will suppress ACTH output from the pituitary. Ectopic sources of ACTH are more autonomous and suppression does not occur on either low-or high-dose dexamethasone. There are a number of variations in this test, but the full test is run over four days, with the low dose being given for 48 hours, then the high dose being given for 48 hours. The plasma cortisol levels and the urinary free cortisol levels are measured during the test. Unfortunately, this test is not invariably accurate because 10–20 percent of ACTH secreting pituitary adenomas do not suppress on high dose whereas 50 percent of ACTH secreting bronchial carcinoid tumours show some suppression on high dose. It is therefore important to have additional evidence of a pituitary adenoma before concluding that the cause of Cushing's syndrome is a pituitary adenoma as opposed to an ectopic source of ACTH. The test is summarized in **Table 25.1**.

- CRF test. If CRF is administered, ACTH levels will rise in normals and this response is exaggerated in Cushing's disease, but it is typically absent if the source of ACTH is ectopic. In most cases, CRF has more effect on ACTH levels if the source is the pituitary rather than if it is an ectopic source, but once again this test is not foolproof. Up to 10 percent of pituitary adenomas do not respond to infused CRF as would be expected and a few ectopic ACTH producing tumours do respond by secreting more ACTH.
- Metyrapone test. This drug blocks glucocorticoid metabolism and if given to normal people it will cause a rise in ACTH. This response is usually exaggerated in Cushing's disease, but not if the source of ACTH is ectopic.
- Inferior petrosal sinus sampling (IPSS). This test is used as a further means of defining the source of excess ACTH. It also holds out the prospect of localizing the source of ACTH within the pituitary itself. Because some adenomas are so small that they cannot be demonstrated on scanning (see below), this is an attractive prospect, but localization is not as accurate as might be anticipated. This is an invasive technique, requiring selective cannulation of both inferior petrosal sinuses under radiographic control via the femoral vein. With the catheters in place, samples

Table 25.1   The dexamethasone suppression test.

	Normal	Pituitary Cushing's	Ectopic Cushing's
Low-dose dexamethasone	Suppression of plasma cortisol and UFC	No effect	No effect
High-dose dexamethasone	Suppression of plasma cortisol and UFC	Suppression of plasma cortisol and UFC	No effect

can be taken for hormonal assay. After baseline samples have been taken to assay the pituitary hormone levels from each side, CRF is administered intravenously and further samples are taken to measure the effect on pituitary hormone output. IPSS is most useful to confirm that the source of ACTH is the pituitary. It is therefore used when Cushing's disease is suspected but imaging does not confirm the presence of an adenoma and there is doubt as to whether the source of excess ACTH is the pituitary or ectopic. High levels of ACTH in blood obtained from IPSS are strongly indicative of a pituitary source of ACTH. A differential between the levels of ACTH in the IPS and a peripheral sample is further evidence of a pituitary source. If this is combined with a CRF test, a rise in the ACTH levels can be demonstrated with CRF. This raises the sensitivity of the test to 95 percent.[8] [***] Although there are large venous connections between the cavernous sinuses, the venous blood between the two may not mix very much.[9] [**] If there is a marked difference in the ACTH levels between the two sides, without a similar asymmetry in the levels of the other pituitary hormones (prolactin, GH, FSH and LH), tumours can be localized by this technique. Unfortunately, venous drainage is variable and IPSS only assists localization in 50–70 percent of cases.[8, 10] [***/**] In summary, this technique is quite invasive and is reserved for more difficult diagnostic cases. It is certainly useful to confirm high levels of ACTH output and so to confirm a pituitary source of Cushing's but, disappointingly, localization is less accurate.

Nelson's syndrome

This is a condition which arises when bilateral adrenalectomy is performed to relieve Cushing's disease and the pituitary lesion then expands more rapidly because of the loss of feedback from the high circulating steroid levels. The clinical features are those of an expanding pituitary mass with visual and ocular effects and hyperpigmentation due to the high circulating levels of ACTH.

Details of the biochemical tests used to diagnose and define Cushing's disease and syndrome are widely discussed in most textbooks of endocrinology. The conclusion is that biochemical testing does not yet provide 100 percent accuracy in distinguishing ACTH generated by a pituitary microadenoma from that produced by an ectopic tumour.

TSH AND TSHOMA

TSH secreting adenomas are rare, representing a very small percentage of functioning adenomas. Patients may present with features of hyperthyroidism but on investigation for this they are found to have normal or elevated TSH levels rather than the suppressed levels which would be anticipated in thyrotoxicosis of thyroid origin.

If a TSHoma is suspected, an MR scan of the pituitary gland should be undertaken. Tumours may be either micro-or macroadenomas. Treatment options include surgical excision, radiotherapy or medical treatment. TSHomas may respond well to somatostatin analogues. They can also be more aggressive than other pituitary adenomas and so long-term biochemical and imaging follow-up is appropriate. Radiotherapy is an option which should be considered if the disease is not cured by surgery.

OTHER FUNCTIONING ADENOMAS

Gonadotrophinomas seldom present as functioning tumours. Typically this diagnosis is made on immunohistochemical analysis of a nonfunctioning adenoma following surgery. These tumours will therefore be discussed under nonfunctioning adenomas.

NONFUNCTIONING PITUITARY ADENOMAS

As the name indicates, these tumours do not present with any overt effect of excess hormone release. Their typical presentation is of a space occupying lesion spreading out of the pituitary fossa. In relation to pituitary function, there are key points that are essential in their correct management.

- Identification of associated hypopituitarism. Patients with these lesions may be partially or completely hypopituitary. The classic finding is progressive loss of pituitary hormone secretion with gonadotrophins (LH and FSH) affected first, then GH, TSH and ACTH, but variations do occur. In children, cessation of growth or delayed puberty are the most common presentations. Once clinically suspected, this can be confirmed by measuring plasma cortisol levels, urinary free cortisols, gonadotrophins, GH, testosterone, prolactin (may be elevated in nonfunctioning pituitary adenomas (NFAs), see above) and thyroid function. However the tumour is managed, it is essential to ensure that any hormone deficiencies are corrected for the patient's well-being and before surgery is undertaken.
- Identification of an asymptomatic functioning adenoma. It is particularly important to recognize a prolactinoma, because medical treatment may render surgery unnecessary.

There are a range of other pathologies which arise in and adjacent to the pituitary gland. These are described in Chapter 258, Pituitary tumours: medical and surgical management.

Posterior pituitary function

Diabetes insipidus is caused by lesions of the pituitary gland. The commonest causes are trauma and surgery (see below under Pituitary function in the postoperative period).

VISUAL FIELD ASSESSMENT

- If a patient with a pituitary tumour complains of any visual disturbance, this needs to be fully assessed preoperatively. An ophthalmologist's opinion and documentation of visual fields are important.
- In the presence of a macroadenoma with tumour abutting on the nerves or chiasm, even if there are no ocular symptoms, visual field assessment is essential pre- and postoperatively.
- If there is a microadenoma with no evidence of tumour reaching the nerves or chiasm on imaging and no ocular symptoms, this is unnecessary.

The typical visual field abnormality is a bitemporal superior quadrantanopia or hemianopia, but this will depend on the position of the optic chiasm in relation to the pituitary. The earliest detectable abnormality is loss of perception of a red target. In most cases, the visual field impairment is reversible if detected and treated early.

PITUITARY FUNCTION IN THE POSTOPERATIVE PERIOD

In functioning adenomas, successful surgery should correct the excess of hormone secreted by the adenoma. It may render the patient deficient in other pituitary hormones. It is unlikely to restore hormone levels which were deficient preoperatively.

Hormone assays are used to assess the results of treatment. In microadenomas a resolution of the hormonal excess and persistently normal or low levels of that hormone indicate a cure and are a more accurate method of assessing the results of treatment than imaging. It is essential to test for all the pituitary hormones because the patient may develop a deficiency of any of them. If the pituitary is irradiated, the onset of hypopituitarism may be gradual. Lifelong follow-up is important, as recurrence or hypopituitarism can occur years later.

Patients must have a formal endocrine assessment postoperatively. Our routine is to formally assess all patients fully at approximately one month. Until then, patients are put on physiological doses of hydrocortisone (15–20 mg of hydrocortisone in the morning and 5–10 mg in the afternoon) and should continue to take any other replacement therapy which they needed preoperatively. At one month they have the following:

- a short Synacthen test and only if the patient passes this does she or he stop hydrocortisone;
- in treated Cushing's disease, a plasma cortisol after taking no hydrocortisone for 24 hours;
- in all cases, the range of tests for anterior pituitary function;

- in functioning adenomas, the appropriate test to define whether a cure has been achieved:
  - in Cushing's, a plasma cortisol of less than 30 nmol/L would indicate a cure. Even if normal gland has been left at surgery, it often takes months for normal cells to recover function and so such low levels at one month do not necessarily indicate permanent low levels of ACTH. Results within the normal range (180–550 nmol/L at 9 a.m. and < 130 nmol/L at midnight) may not indicate failure to cure, but are suspicious. Results above the normal range indicate failure. Similarly, urinary free cortisols should be low or normal at this time;
  - in acromegaly, the best assessment is serial measurement of GH through an oral glucose tolerance test and of IGF1. If a fasting growth hormone is below 5 mU/L, it suppresses to less than 2 mU/L with adequate hyperglycaemia and the IGF1 is within normal limits (13–37 nmol/L) the patient is probably cured;[11] [**]
  - in prolactinoma, the serum prolactin should return to normal (60–620 mU/L);
  - in TSHoma, thyroid function tests should reveal a low TSH. The patient may become hypothyroid but still have a low TSH;
- posterior pituitary function does not need formal assessment unless the patient has symptomatic diuresis. If this is the case, diabetes insipidus needs to be diagnosed by a water deprivation test and then treated with DDAVP.

In the early postoperative period, the results for Cushing's disease can be predicted usefully by measuring a plasma cortisol at 72 hours with the patient off all replacement glucocorticoids for 12 hours. A plasma cortisol of less than 30 nmol/L is highly predictive of a surgical cure. In acromegaly, an early measurement of GH is less reliable.

KEY POINTS

- MRI has value and limitations in the diagnosis of pituitary adenomas.
- CT scanning is important for checking bone detail in the sinuses and pituitary fossa.
- Preoperative biochemistry is important in avoiding unnecessary surgery in macroadenomas.
- A multidisciplinary approach with endocrinologists is essential to avoid incorrect diagnosis and optimize management of pituitary tumours.

Best clinical practice

✓ Check serum prolactin levels preoperatively in pituitary macroadenomas.
✓ Prolactinomas respond well to dopamine agents.
✓ Inferior petrosal sinus sampling is essential when there is doubt about the origin of Cushing's syndrome.
✓ Long-term follow-up is essential to avoid missing late recurrence of pituitary adenomas.

Deficiencies in current knowledge and areas for future research

➤ Imaging is developing rapidly. As the new technologies outlined above become more widely available, it is to be hoped that uncertainties in adenoma location should be reduced. The ability to monitor surgical progress intraoperatively is most valuable. These innovations should improve surgical outcomes.
➤ The most difficult syndrome to accurately diagnose and cure is Cushing's. Improvements in the ability to define the precise source of ACTH will allow even more accuracy in identifying which patients should have pituitary surgery and which part of the gland should be removed to cure this otherwise lethal disease.

REFERENCES

* 1. Yamada S. Epidemiology of pituitary tumors. In: Tharpar K, Kovacs K, Scheithauer BW, Lloyd RV (eds). *Diagnosis and management of pituitary tumors.* Totowa, NJ: Humana Press, 2001: 57–69.
2. Hall WA, Luciano MG, Doppman JL, Patronas NJ, Oldfield EH. Pituitary magnetic resonance imaging in normal human volunteers: occult adenomas in the general population. *Annals of Internal Medicine.* 1994; **120**: 817–20.
* 3. Colombo N, Loli P, Vignati F, Scialfa G. MR of corticotropin-secreting pituitary microadenomas. *American Journal of Neuroradiology.* 1994; **15**: 1591–5.
4. Lloyd RV, Chandler WF, McKeever PE, Schteingart DE. The spectrum of ACTH-producing pituitary lesions. *American Journal of Surgical Pathology.* 1986; **10**: 618–26.
5. Schulder M, Carmel PW. Intraoperative magnetic resonance imaging: impact on brain tumor surgery. *Cancer Control.* 2003; **10**: 115–24.
6. Goth MI, Makara GB, Gerendai I. Hypothalamic-pituitary physiology and regulation. In: Tharpar K, Kovacs K, Scheithauer BW, Lloyd RV (eds). *Diagnosis and management of pituitary tumors.* Totowa, NJ: Humana Press, 2001: 41–55.
7. Chatterjee K, Jenkins PJ, Besser GM, Weetman T, Thacker R, Stewart P et al. Endocrine disorders. In: Warrell DA, Cox TM, Firth JD, Benz Jr EJ (eds). *Oxford textbook of medicine,* 4th edn. Oxford: Oxford University Press, 2004: Section 12.
* 8. Colao A, Faggiano A, Pivonello R, Giraldi FP, Cavagnini F, Lombardi G. Inferior petrosal sinus sampling in the differential diagnosis of Cushing's syndrome: results of an Italian multicenter study. *European Journal of Endocrinology.* 2001; **144**: 499–507.
9. Oldfield EH, Girton ME, Doppman JL. Absence of intercavernous venous mixing: evidence supporting lateralization of pituitary microadenomas by venous sampling. *Journal of Clinical Endocrinology and Metabolism.* 1985; **61**: 644–7.
10. Lefournier V, Martinie M, Vasdev A, Bessou P, Passagia JG, Labat-Moleur F et al. Accuracy of bilateral inferior petrosal or cavernous sinuses sampling in predicting the lateralization of Cushing's disease pituitary microadenoma: influence of catheter position and anatomy of venous drainage. *Journal of Clinical Endocrinology and Metabolism.* 2003; **88**: 196–203.
11. Melmed S, Vance ML, Barkan AL, Bengtsson BA, Kleinberg D, Klibanski A et al. Current status and future opportunities for controlling acromegaly. *Pituitary.* 2002; **5**: 185–96.

26

The thyroid gland: anatomy and physiology

JULIAN A McGLASHAN

Introduction	314	Deficiencies in current knowledge and areas for future	
Anatomy of the thyroid gland	314	research	324
Physiology of the thyroid	321	References	324
Key point	324		

SEARCH STRATEGY AND EVIDENCE-BASE

Medline and Embase searches were performed using the key words: thyroid gland, anatomy, histopathology, microstructure, physiology, thyroid hormone and calcitonin. Extensive reference has been made to the extremely comprehensive eighth edition of Werner and Ingbar's classic textbook *The thyroid: a fundamental and clinical text*. This chapter summarizes and reviews the observational studies that relate to anatomy and physiology of the thyroid gland and are therefore levels 3 and 2 evidence.

INTRODUCTION

The aim of this chapter is to provide an overview of the key anatomical and physiological facts which are relevant to surgeons wishing to develop a practice in thyroid surgery and highlight some of the more recent developments of our understanding of thyroid physiology.

The thyroid gland is a bilobed structure situated in the lower anterior neck. It is a highly vascular, reddish-brown organ with two primary endocrine functions: secretion of thyroid hormones, namely thyroxine (T_4) and triiodothyronine (T_3), from follicular cells and calcitonin from parafollicular or C cells. The thyroid hormones ensure that the metabolic demands of the tissues of the body are met by stimulating oxygen consumption and regulating carbohydrate and lipid metabolism. They are also essential for normal growth and maturation. Calcitonin is released rapidly in response to elevated levels of circulating calcium ensuring levels do not fluctuate wildly and thereby helping prevent hypercalcaemia. The thyroid gland itself is not necessary for life but low levels of thyroid hormone (hypothyroidism) can cause severe mental and physical impairment and disability.[1]

An excellent historical review of the key developments in our understanding of the thyroid gland anatomy and function can be found in Sawin.[2] More recent developments have focused on the function and controlling mechanisms at the molecular genetic level.[3, 4] **Table 26.1** provides a summary of the key developments.

ANATOMY OF THE THYROID GLAND

Embryology

In higher vertebrates, including humans, the thyroid develops from fusion of a median anlage with two lateral anlagen, which originate from two distinct regions of the endodermal pharynx.[5] Colloid production starts at 13–14 weeks gestation followed almost immediately by the development of follicles.[6, 7] Thyroxine can be detected in foetal serum at 11–13 weeks.[8]

MEDIAN ANLAGE

The median anlage (**Figure 26.1**) develops from a midline thickening of the ventral surface of the primitive

Table 26.1 Historical summary.

Year	Contribution
BC	Goitres recognized by Chinese and Europeans living in Alps
c. 200BC	Ancient Greeks called the thyroid swelling a bronchocele or tracheal outpouch
c. 1500	Leonardo da Vinci was most likely the first to describe the thyroid gland
1543	Vesalius described the thyroid as a 'laryngeal gland' for lubricating of the vocal cords
1619	Fabricius made the link between the thyroid gland and goitre
1656	Thomas Wharton coined the term 'thyroid' from the Greek meaning 'shield shaped' (referring to its proximity to the thyroid cartilage)
c. 1527/1562	Parcelsus and Platter recognized the clinical significance of goitre and cretinism
1820	Coindet gave potassium iodine to a Swiss patient with goitre and noticed a significant decrease in its size
1825	Parry described thyrotoxicosis without realizing it
1834	Graves described thyrotoxicosis in four patients with goitre and palpitations, one of whom also had exophthalmos, although this was thought to be of cardiac origin
1870s	Myxoedema first recognized but thought to be a neurological or skin disease
1876	Thyroid surgery for goitre introduced by Emil Kocher
1883	Felix Semon first made the link between myxoedema and hypothyroidism
1888	Cretinism, myxoedema and post-thyroidectomy all recognized as being due to one cause, i.e. a loss of thyroid function
1890s	Thyrotoxicosis thought to be due to either excess secretion of a substance or failure of inactivation of a toxin
1891	Murray cured myxoedematous patients with injected extracts of sheep's thyroid gland
1895	Baumann found iodine in the thyroid gland
1897	Tourneaux and Verdun describe the embryological development of the thyroid gland
1914	Edward Kendall isolated thyroxin
1926–7	Harington discovered structure of thyroxine and then synthesized it. However at that time it was too expensive for therapeutic use. Thyroid deficiency and goitre was treated with desiccated thyroid until the 1960s
1952	Pitt-Rivers and Gross in the UK discovered triiodothyronine almost simultaneously with Roche, Lissitsky and Michel in France
1970	Sterling demonstrated the conversion of T_4 to T_3 in normal human subjects

pharynx between the first and second branchial arches adjacent to the developing myocardium.[9, 10] A diverticulum forms from this thickening at approximately the 16th or 17th gestational day. This can be recognized as a small blind pit in the midline between the anterior two-thirds and posterior third of the tongue and is known as the foramen caecum. The diverticulum expands at its distal tip leading to the formation of a bilobed structure. This then migrates into the lower neck anterior to the hyoid bone, laryngeal cartilages and pharyngeal gut. It is pulled into position by the descent of the heart and reaches its final location, immediately anterior to the trachea, in the seventh gestational week. The lumen of the stalk is initially tubular but becomes filled with cords of cells during the seventh to tenth week of gestation but eventually fragments and disappears. Persistence of part of the stalk anywhere between the foramen caecum and thyroid isthmus can result in the development of a thyroglossal duct cyst.[11] When present, the cysts are most commonly found between the hyoid bone and isthmus.[12, 13] Alternatively, and more rarely, thyroid descent may become arrested anywhere along the tract resulting in a lingual thyroid[14] or giving rise to ectopic thyroid tissue in the sublingual, high cervical and mediastinal regions or even within the cardiac endothelium.[5]

LATERAL ANLAGEN: ULTIMOBRANCHIAL BODIES

The two lateral anlagen (**Figure 26.1**), known as the ultimobranchial bodies, are thought to develop as caudal projections from the fourth or fifth pharyngeal pouches. They become separated from them by attenuation and rupture of the common pharyngobranchial duct. The ultimobranchial bodies fuse with the median thyroid anlage by the sixth week of development contributing approximately 10 percent of the mass of the thyroid gland.[15, 16] Rarely, the ultimobranchial bodies can fail to fuse resulting in a true 'lateral thyroid lobe'.

The ultimobranchial bodies also contribute the parafollicular calcitonin-producing cells (C cells). The exact origin of these cells in humans remains controversial although they are thought to be most likely of neural crest origin.[5] Normally, the parafollicular cells migrate to become distributed throughout the gland although they often remain more numerous near the point of fusion between the two anlagen.[7, 17] It is therefore not surprising that medullary carcinomas develop in the central portions of the middle and upper thirds of the thyroid lobes.[18] Lateral thyroid lobes, when present, are also often associated with a greater than normal amount of parafollicular tissue and an increased tendency to become neoplastic.[19]

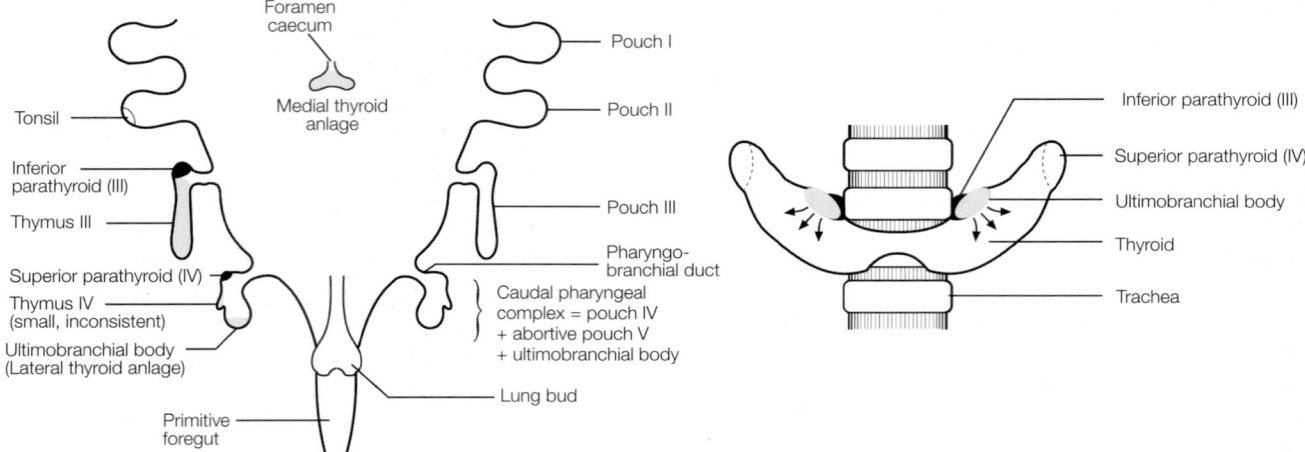

Figure 26.1 Schematic representations of the early development and origin of the follicular and parafollicular (C cells) of the thyroid gland and chief cells of the parathyroid glands.

Macroscopic anatomy

The thyroid gland is the largest endocrine organ in the body weighing between 15 and 25 grams in adulthood and being slightly larger in women. It consists of two lobes joined together by an isthmus (**Figure 26.2**).

Each lobe is pear-shaped measuring approximately 5 cm in length, 3 cm in width and 1.5 cm in depth. Very rarely, one lobe of the thyroid gland fails to develop (more often on the left). The apex of each lobe is narrow and extends beneath the sternothyroid muscle up to its insertion on the oblique line of the thyroid cartilage. The more rounded lower pole extends down to the level of the fourth or fifth tracheal ring and lies lateral to the trachea and oesophagus and medial to the carotid sheath. The isthmus lies immediately caudal to the inferior border of the cricoid cartilage.

A third conical protrusion of varying size, known as the pyramidal lobe, can also be present in up to 50 percent of cases. It represents a distal remnant of the thyroglossal duct and can extend superiorly up to the level of the thyroid cartilage or hyoid bone.[7] Its apex may be replaced by fibrous or fibromuscular tissue when it is then known as the 'levator of the thyroid gland'. Identifying and removing the pyramidal lobe should be part of a routine thyroid lobectomy to avoid leaving functioning thyroid tissue behind.

A lateral or posterior projection of the thyroid lobe, known as the tubercle of Zuckerkandl, can be identified in up to 60 percent of surgical dissections according to Gauger.[20] It is thought to represent the point of embryological fusion of the ultimobranchial body and median anlage. Its surgical importance is reported as being three-fold: (a) the recurrent laryngeal nerve most often runs medial to it; (b) the superior parathyroid gland is usually attached to its cranial aspect; (c) and when enlarged as part of the goitre it can be inadvertently left behind, particularly during a subtotal thyroidectomy.

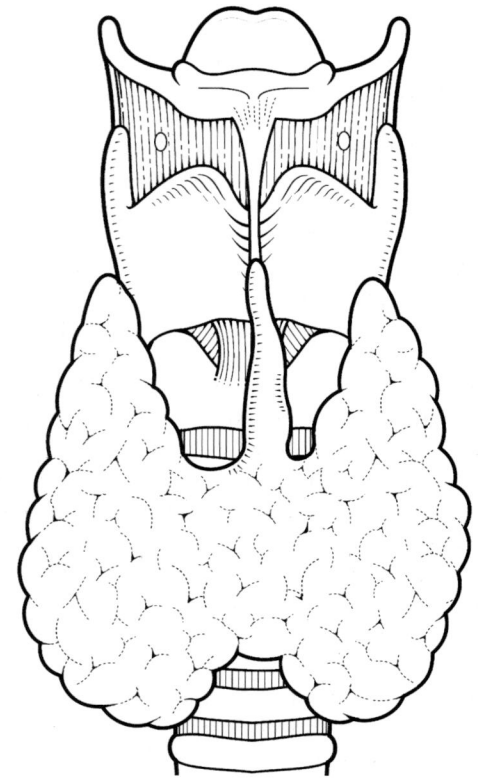

Figure 26.2 Thyroid gland showing relationship to larynx and trachea. In up to 50 percent of cases, a pyramidal lobe ± a fibrous or fibromuscular band may arise from the isthmus and extend a variable distance up to the body of the hyoid.

The thyroid gland is invested in pretracheal fascia, which is part of the deep cervical fascia. Its uppermost attachment is limited by the attachment of the strap muscles (sternothyroid, sternohyoid and omohyoid) to the oblique line on the thyroid cartilage laterally and the hyoid bone more medially. As it passes inferiorly it splits to enclose the thyroid gland, allowing the surrounding structures to slide over the gland. The fascia is not adherent to the thyroid gland except where there are penetrating vessels posteriorly between the isthmus and lower part of the cricoid cartilage down to the fourth tracheal rings. This fixation to the trachea causes the thyroid gland to move up and down on swallowing. The posterior condensation of fascia is known as the lateral ligament of the thyroid or the 'suspensory ligament of Berry'. It is usually penetrated by small blood vessels. During thyroid surgery it must be divided with care and by sharp dissection as the recurrent laryngeal nerve may lay lateral, medial or within the ligament just before it enters the larynx. A further posterior extension of the fascia passes behind the oesophagus allowing the anterior neck structures to glide over the prevertebral fascia and underlying prevertebral muscles on swallowing and neck movements. Laterally, the pretracheal fascia blends with the carotid sheath while inferiorly it passes behind the brachiocephalic veins to blend with the adventitia of the arch of the aorta.

ARTERIAL SUPPLY

The main blood supply of the thyroid gland is from the paired superior and inferior thyroid arteries. In up to 12 percent of cases a thyroidea ima artery may also be present ascending in front of the trachea to end at the isthmus. It most commonly arises from the brachiocephalic artery but it can also originate from the aorta, the right common carotid, subclavian or internal thoracic arteries.

The superior thyroid artery passes antero–inferiorly from its origin on the anterior surface of the external carotid artery just below the level of the greater cornu of the hyoid bone. It lies on the inferior constrictor muscle to reach the superior pole of the thyroid gland where it divides into an anterior and posterior branch. The anterior branch follows the medial margin of the superior lobe to the isthmus to anastomose with its opposite number. Several descending arteries pass from this arcade over the anterior surface of the gland to anastomose with branches from the inferior thyroid artery. The posterior branch descends on the posterior surface of the gland and in 45 percent of cases it joins with the ascending branch of the inferior thyroid artery.[21] Additional lateral branches may also be present (**Figure 26.3**).

The inferior thyroid artery usually arises from the thyrocervical trunk, a branch of the first part of the subclavian artery, although in approximately 15 percent of cases it may come directly off the subclavian artery. It ascends in front of the medial border of the scalenus anterior muscle turning medially in front of the vertebral arteries and then behind the carotid sheath and the sympathetic trunk. It then descends on the anterior surface of the longus colli muscle to the lower border of the thyroid. Before reaching the gland it divides into ascending and descending branches on the posterior border of the gland. The superior parathyroid usually

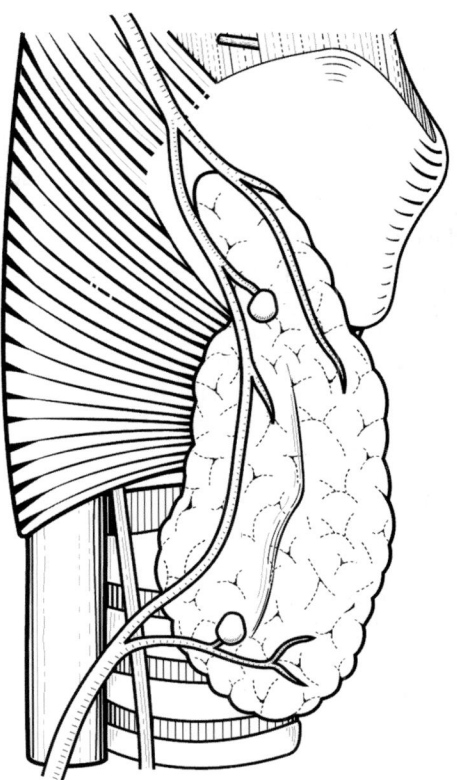

Figure 26.3 Schematic representation showing a common relationship between the superior and inferior thyroid arteries, parathyroid glands and recurrent laryngeal nerve. On the right side the nerve passes behind, between or occasionally in front of the inferior thyroid artery while on the left side it most commonly passes behind the artery.

receives a terminal blood supply, either from its anastomosis with the posterior branch of the superior thyroid or directly from the superior thyroid artery.[21] The inferior parathyroid is also supplied by a terminal branch: this arises from the descending branch as it passes towards the inferior pole to anastomose with its opposite number.

In addition to supplying the thyroid gland, the inferior thyroid artery gives off branches to the trachea, oesophagus and lower part of the pharynx. The inferior laryngeal artery, a branch of the inferior thyroid artery, ascends with the recurrent laryngeal nerve on the trachea to enter the larynx deep to the inferior constrictor muscle.[22] It is often accompanied by a small plexus of veins in the region of the ligament of Berry, especially where the nerve enters the larynx. The vessels invariably have to be divided during thyroid dissection and great care is required with haemostasis to avoid damage to the nerve.

VENOUS DRAINAGE

The veins in the substance of the thyroid and on its surface form a venous plexus and drain via three main groups, namely the superior, middle and inferior thyroid veins. The superior thyroid veins accompany the corresponding artery and drain into the internal jugular or occasionally the facial vein. The middle thyroid veins arise from the lateral surface of the gland near the junction of the middle and lower thirds of the thyroid gland. They may be double or absent. They receive blood from the inferior and antero–lateral part of the gland as well as the larynx and trachea. They most commonly cross the common carotid artery to drain into the internal jugular vein.

Multiple inferior thyroid veins form a plexus on the anterior surface of the trachea on leaving the gland. These usually drain into right and left inferior veins, which in turn drain into their respective brachiocephalic vein in the superior mediastinum. Occasionally these paired inferior veins form a common trunk and drain into the superior vena cava or left brachiocephalic vein.[23]

LYMPHATIC DRAINAGE

The thyroid gland contains a rich network of lymphatics, which drain into several main groups of nodes in the anterior and lateral aspects of the lower neck (**Figure 26.4**). The lateral aspects of the gland drain into the middle and lower jugular nodes (levels III and IV) and those of the posterior triangle (level V). The more medial aspects of the gland also drain into the nodes of the anterior compartment of the neck (level VI), which in turn can drain into those of the upper anterior mediastinum (level VII). From a clinical perspective, levels I and II are rarely involved in metastatic thyroid cancer disease.

NERVES

Although the recurrent laryngeal and external branch of the superior laryngeal nerves do not actually supply the thyroid gland, their close proximity to the gland render them an extremely important consideration during the assessment of thyroid conditions and in thyroid and parathyroid surgery. The recurrent laryngeal nerves (**Figure 26.5**) are branches of the vagus nerve, which supply all the intrinsic muscles of the larynx except the cricothyroid muscle. They also supply sensory fibres to the mucous membrane below the level of the vocal folds and carry afferent fibres from stretch receptors of the intrinsic muscles and other sensory receptors.

On the left side, the nerve leaves the vagus in the mediastinum anterior to the arch of the aorta passing behind the ligamentum arteriosum and then posteriorly under the concavity of the arch before passing superiorly to lie in the tracheo-oesophageal groove. It most usually passes behind the inferior thyroid artery and then posterior to the ligament of Berry before passing under or between the fibres of the cricopharyngeal part of the inferior constrictor (**Figure 26.6a**).[24] At this point it lies

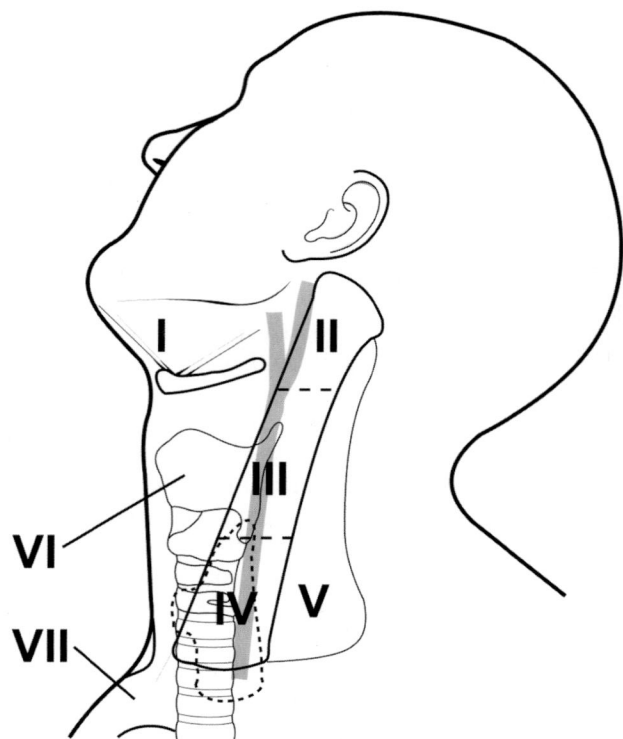

Figure 26.4 Lymphatic drainage of the thyroid gland is predominantly to levels VI, IV and III. In metastatic thyroid cancer, levels V and VII may also be affected. Level II is rarely involved and level I almost never.

immediately behind the capsule of the cricothyroid joint (**Figure 26.6b**).[25, 26] On the right side (**Figure 26.5**), the nerve passes posteriorly looping under the first part of the subclavian artery and then has a more oblique course to the tracheo-oesophageal groove. Its relationship with the inferior thyroid artery is more variable:[25] in order of decreasing frequency it lies behind, between the terminal branches or occasionally superficial to the artery before entering the larynx in a similar fashion to the left.

The recurrent laryngeal nerve is variable in size ranging from 1.5–4 mm in diameter. It can be identified by its whitish appearance, characteristic longitudinal vessel running along its length and its flattened, rounded surface. In up to 39 percent of cases the nerve divides into two (and occasionally up to six) terminal branches between 6 and 35 mm from the cricoid cartilage.[25, 27, 28] Special care is therefore required in order not to damage any of these branches during surgical dissection.

A nonrecurrent laryngeal nerve is found in 0.2–0.4 percent of patients.[29] It tends to be thicker than a normally sited nerve and is usually associated with a vascular anomaly of the subclavian artery on the right side and transposition of the great vessels on the left side.

The external branch of the superior laryngeal nerve, which supplies the cricothyroid muscle, runs parallel to the superior thyroid vessels in approximately 85 percent of

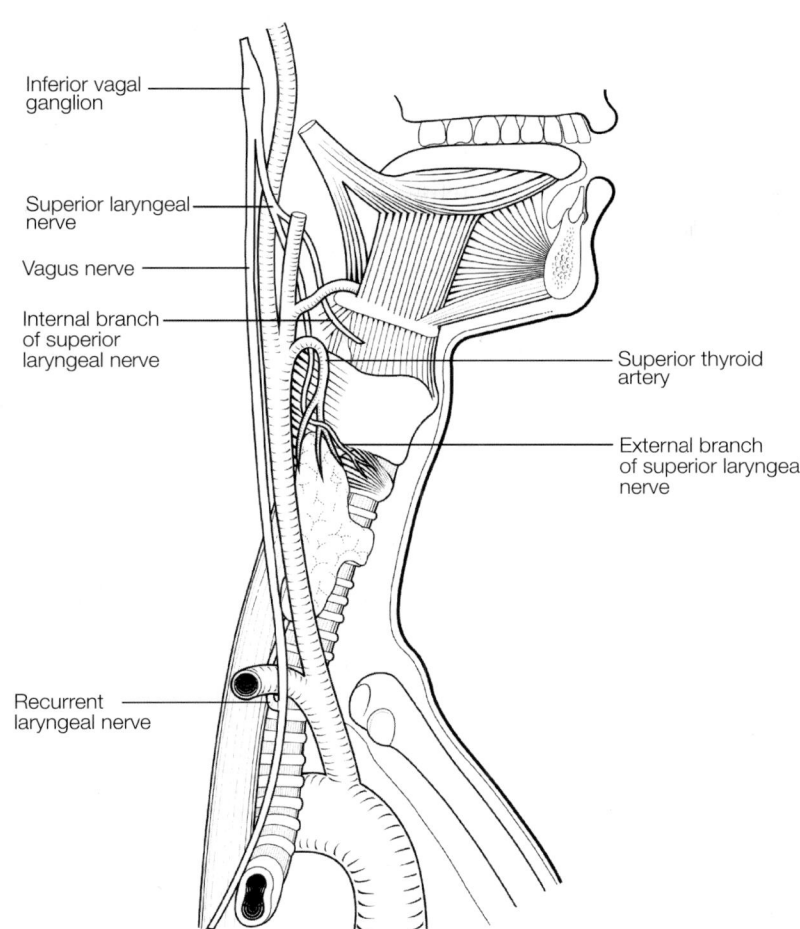

Inferior vagal
ganglion

Superior laryngeal
nerve

Vagus nerve

Internal branch
of superior
laryngeal nerve

Recurrent
laryngeal nerve

Superior thyroid
artery

External branch
of superior laryngeal
nerve

Figure 26.5 The superior laryngeal nerve branches from the inferior vagal ganglion and divides into a sensory internal branch which perforates the thyrohyoid membrane and a motor external branch which supplies the cricothyroid muscle. The external branch is at risk during thyroid surgery as it may be intimately related to the terminal branches of the superior thyroid artery. The recurrent laryngeal nerve arises from the vagus in the mediastinum and has a longer and more vertical course on the left.

cases. Most often it runs medial to the vessels but it can also run partly lateral, pass between the main branches or lie protected within the inferior constrictor muscle.[30, 31, 32, 33] The nerve is probably damaged more often than appreciated and is a major cause of changes in voice quality after thyroid surgery.[34] The nerve is less likely to be damaged if the branches of the vascular pedicle are ligated on the surface of the gland rather than at the main trunk.

The thyroid gland is under the influence of the autonomic system as well as hormonal control. Sympathetic nerve fibres originate from the superior cervical and stellate ganglia and enter the gland along with the main arteries to form plexuses within the connective tissue between the follicles. Parasympathetic fibres have been shown to originate from the nodose and local vagal ganglia in the rat although the pathways in humans are less well understood. In addition, sensory innervation passes to the jugular, trigeminal and cervical dorsal root ganglia. Pharmacological and physiological studies have shown that there are a multitude of active neuropeptides in the thyroid whose function and interaction is not completely understood but they are likely to have a wide range of roles in the regulation of local blood supply, thyroid hormone synthesis and secretion.[16, 35]

Microscopic anatomy

The thyroid gland consists mainly of follicular cells, which are arranged in aggregates one cell thick around a central pool of colloid to form follicles (**Figure 26.7**). The follicles are approximately spherical in shape and between 0.02 and 0.9 mm in diameter.[36] A thyroid lobule consists of 20 to 40 follicles and is supplied by a lobular artery.[37] The follicular cells have the characteristic cytoplasmic features of an endocrine gland in that they have long segments of rough endoplasmic reticulum and a large Golgi apparatus, for synthesizing and packaging protein, and prominent electron-dense lysosomal bodies. The plasma membranes of the apical and basal layers have separate functions and are kept separate by tight junctions, which bind adjacent cells together. This allows the cell to control the storage of the thyroid hormones in the colloid and their release into the circulation.

When the gland is relatively inactive, the cells are flattened and the colloid is abundant, dense and homogenous in appearance. On prolonged and excessive thyroid stimulating hormone (TSH) stimulation, the follicular cells become hypertrophied and hyperplastic and they adopt a more columnar shape. This cellular enlargement is associated with an increase in the

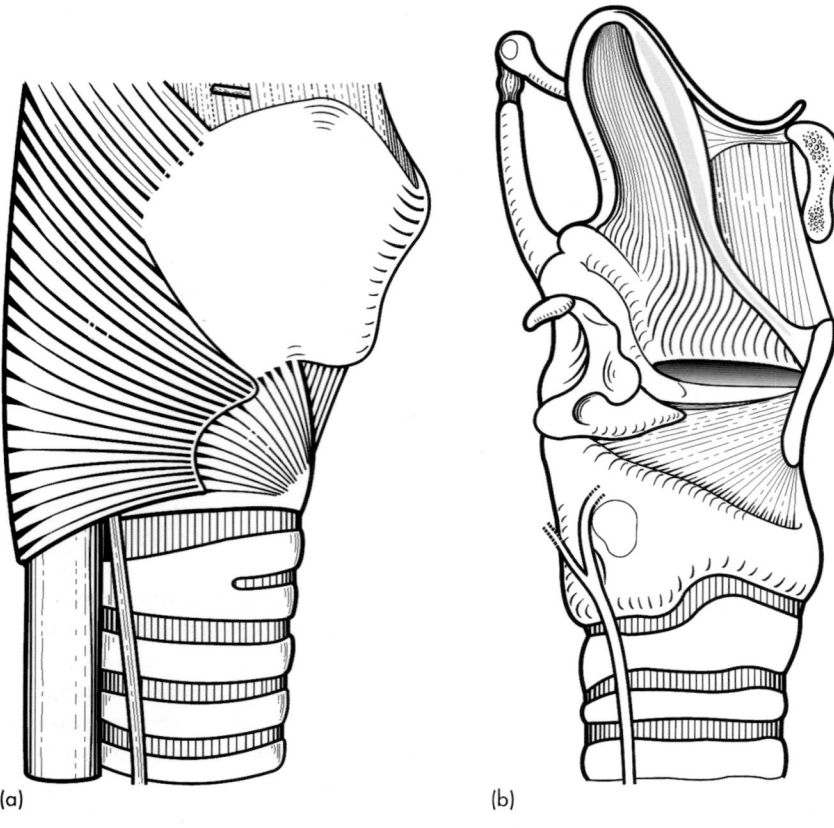

(a)

(b)

Figure 26.6 **(a)** The recurrent laryngeal nerve passing under the lower border of the cricopharyngeal part of the inferior constrictor muscle. **(b)** The right lamina of the thyroid cartilage has been removed with the thyroarytenoid, lateral and posterior cricoarytenoid muscles to show the lateral border of the cricoid cartilage, the lateral aspect of the conus elasticus and the recurrent laryngeal nerve passing posterior to the articular facet of the cricothyroid joint.

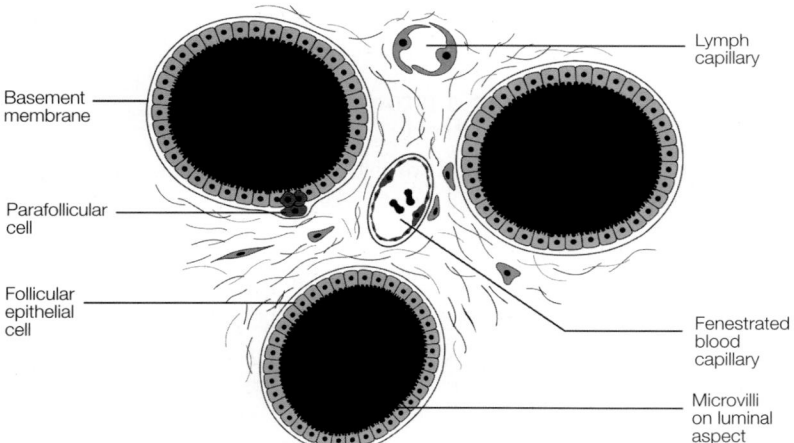

Basement membrane

Parafollicular cell

Follicular epithelial cell

Lymph capillary

Fenestrated blood capillary

Microvilli on luminal aspect

Figure 26.7 The relationship between thyroid follicles and parafollicular cells.

prominence of the intracellular organelles and the development of microvilli on their apical surfaces.[38] The microvilli enable the colloid to be absorbed by endocytosis. This is associated with the development of 'reabsorption lacunae' and a reduction in the size of the follicular lumen. This process is also associated with an overall increase in vascularity of the gland.

Each follicle is invested and interlaced with loose connective tissue (stroma) containing a close-meshed plexus of fenestrated capillaries and expanded lymphatics.[36] The interfollicle connective tissue spaces are relatively large and contain a collagenous matrix,

fibroblasts, unmyelinated nerve fibres with Schwann cells, fat cells, plasma cells, macrophages and lymphocytes.[39, 40] The fibroblasts form a highly organized 'neuro-reticular network' by linking their long, thin, branching cytoplasmic processes. These processes are surrounded by autonomic nerve endings in a similar manner to that found in bone marrow and in the submandibular gland. The presence of CD34-positive antigen on the fibroblasts may mean they play an important role in immune surveillance.[39]

The calcitonin-producing parafollicular cells can be found either singly or in small clumps adjacent to the stromal aspect of the follicular cells and can be recognized by their polygonal or spindle shape, their relatively large size and their 'light' cytoplasm.[41]

PHYSIOLOGY OF THE THYROID

The aim of this section is to provide a brief overview of the physiology of thyroid gland covering formation, storage and secretion of thyroid hormones, their transport to and effect on peripheral tissues and their ultimate metabolism.

Regulation, formation, storage and secretion of thyroid hormones

The formation, synthesis, storage and secretion of thyroid hormones is a complex, highly regulated process under the control of the hypothalamic-pituitary axis (**Figure 26.8**).[42] It is also highly dependent on the availability of iodine.

REGULATION OF THYROID GLAND METABOLISM

The secretion of thyrotropin or TSH is mainly under the influence of thyrotropin-releasing hormone (TRH) which is produced in neurons in the paraventricular nucleus of the hypothalamus of the brain. The TRH is then transported along axons and released into the hypophyseal-portal blood circulation by means of specialized nerve terminals where it is carried directly to the basophilic thyrotrophic cells of the anterior pituitary

gland. TRH, and to some extent α-adrenergic agonists, stimulate TSH secretion which in turn cause an increase in iodide uptake in the thyroid gland and in the cellular activities associated with synthesis and secretion of both the precursor and the circulatory thyroid hormones. The thyroid hormones, together with somatostatin and dopamine, inhibit the function of the thyrotrophs.[43]

Iodine also plays a key role in thyroid physiology and in general has an inhibitory effect on hormonogenesis. By reducing the sensitivity of the thyroid gland to TSH stimulation, it plays an important role in autoregulation of the gland.[44, 45] Iodine in the diet is absorbed from the gastrointestinal tract in the form of inorganic iodide. It is transported in the plasma and erythrocytes and then actively transported into the thyroid and other organs, such as the gastric mucosa, salivary gland, mammary gland, colloid plexus, placenta and skin. Iodide is secreted from these other nonthyroidal organs and then either reabsorbed or lost from the body. Ninety percent of iodide is excreted through the kidneys,[3] the rest being lost in the sweat and faeces (and breast milk).

Selenium is also an essential element necessary for thyroid hormone synthesis and the thyroid gland has the highest content of selenium per gram of tissue of any organ. It is an important constituent of several enzymes found in follicular cells, for example glutathione peroxidases, type I 5-deiodinase, thioredoxin reductase and selenoprotein P.[46] The peroxidases, for example, are responsible for protecting the cells against oxidative damage from by-products of thyroxine metabolism such as hydrogen peroxide (H_2O_2).

THYROID HORMONES

The main hormone secreted by the thyroid gland is 3,5,3′,5′-tetraiodothyronine (thyroxine, T_4). It functions mostly as a prohormone and is deiodinated in the target tissue by iodothyronine 5′-monodeiodinase to the more biologically active form 3,5,3′-triiodothyronine (T_3).[47] Both thyroid hormones are iodinated forms of the amino acid thyronine and contain four or three atoms of iodide, respectively. Twenty to twenty-five percent of the total T_3 production, together with small amounts of reverse triiodothyronine (rT3) and monoiodotyrosine (MIT), are released from the thyroid gland. The biological significance of rT3 and MIT in humans remains unclear.

IODINE TRAPPING

Radioactive iodine (^{131}I) isotope studies have shown that iodide is actively transported from the blood stream into follicular cells through the basal membrane.[48, 49] This is by means of a sodium iodide (Na^+/I^-) symporter whereby two sodium ions are transported for each iodide ion. The inward flux of sodium iodide uptake is stimulated and regulated by TSH in the thyroid gland but not in other

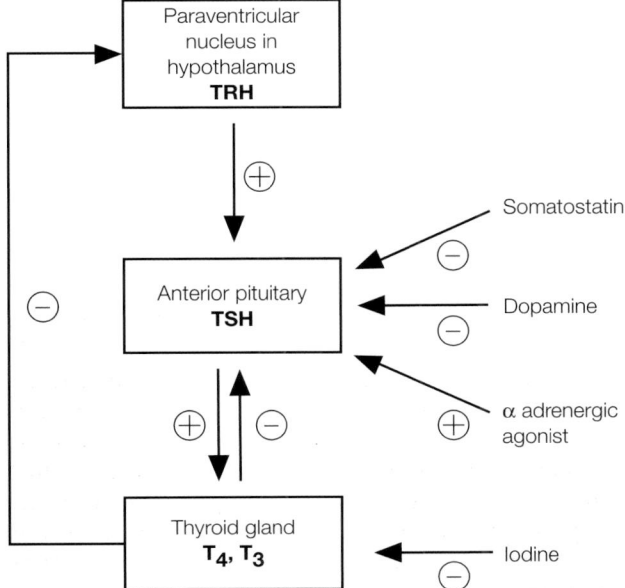

Figure 26.8 Simplified regulatory and biofeedback mechanism of the hypothalamic-pituitary-thyroid axis.

organs that take up iodide. This is not immediate and the presence of the symporter is mostly found in active, cuboidal/columnar form of the cells.[50, 51] It is thought that TSH stimulates increased gene expression and protein synthesis of the Na^+/I^- symporter although there are also intrinsic factors which influence its properties which remain undetermined.[7, 49, 52]

The accumulated iodide in the follicular cells is then transferred to the apical plasma membrane down an electrochemical gradient. TSH stimulation increases adenosine triphosphate (ATP) and ATPase activity at the apex of the cell increasing the efflux of iodide into the colloid down a further electrical gradient.

IODIFICATION OF THYROGLOBULIN

Thyroglobulin is a large alpha-protein and is the major constituent of colloid. It is only synthesized by the follicular cells[53] and, once formed, it is incorporated into apical vesicles for export into the follicular lumen. At the apical membrane thyroid peroxidase uses hydrogen peroxide and iodide to oxidize and organify the thyroglobulin protein in a TSH-sensitive cAMP-mediated process.[4] This creates the bound precursor thyroid hormones, namely MIT and diiodotyrosine (DIT), as well as some T_4 and T_3, where they can be stored until required (**Figure 26.9**).[53]

SECRETION OF THYROID HORMONE

Stimulation of the thyroid gland by TSH leads to small droplets of colloid being taken up into the follicular cells by micropincocytosis to form endosomes or less commonly in bulk as colloid droplets (CD).[54, 55] Both the endosomes and colloid droplets fuse with lysosomes[56] and proteolysis takes place. This results in the release into the cytoplasm of the peptides MIT, DIT, thyroxine and triiodothyronine. MIT and DIT are then rapidly

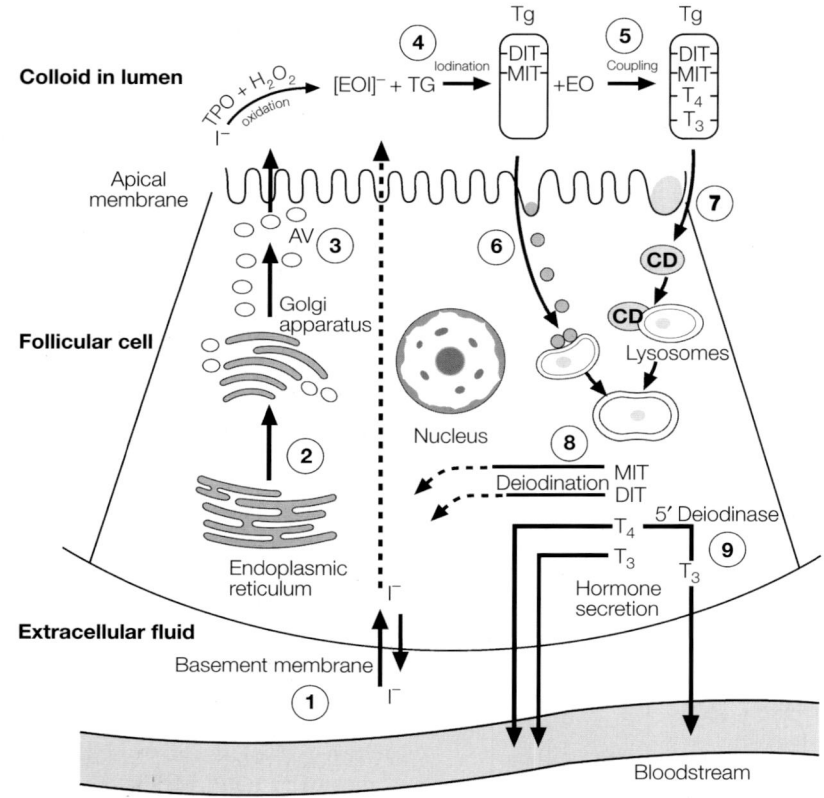

Figure 26.9 Summary of the key steps in the biosynthesis and secretion of thyroid hormone: (1) Iodide is transported by a symporter through the basement membrane of the follicular cell. (2) Polypeptide chains are synthesized on the surface of the endoplasmic reticulum (ER) before being transported into the ER lumen. (3) Dimers are formed and the polypeptide chains are then folded and modelled prior to the addition of carbohydrate units in the Golgi apparatus to form the thyroglobulin (TG) molecules. Newly formed thyroglobulin is then transported to the lumen in apical vesicles (AV). (4) Iodination of thyroglobulin takes place at the apical membrane prior to (5) coupling of iodotyrosyl precursors by thyroperoxidase to form MIT, DIT and small amounts of T_4 and T_3 on the surface of the thyroglobulin molecule. (6) Colloid is absorbed by micropincytosis to form endosomes and also taken into the cell to form colloid droplets. (7) The thyroglobulin in the endosomes and colloid droplets undergoes proteolysis by lysosomic enzymes releasing iodide and DIT and MIT. (8) The iodide is recycled and the MIT and DIT peptides undergo further deiodination by 5′ deiodinase (9) to form T_4 and T_3 which are then released into the bloodstream.

deiodinated by microsomal iodotyrosine deiodinase and iodide is released which is then recycled or excreted from the cell into the circulation. The efflux of iodide from the basolateral aspect of the cell is a regulated Ca^+-dependent process, the details of which have not been fully determined. It is clear, however, that it is different from the apical mechanism as it does not involve cAMP.

Once the thyroid hormones have been released from the thyroglobulin molecule, they are rapidly released from the cell into the circulation although the exact mechanism is not known.[53] Thyroglobulin is mostly degraded although some is recycled back into the lumen and small amounts of both the iodinated and uniodinated forms are also released into the circulation. It can also reach the circulation by being transported from the apical to the basolateral cell membrane within vesicles. Its release into the bloodstream is by a TSH-stimulated process known as transcytosis.[4] The concentration of thyroglobulin in the serum is ultimately determined by the balance between the rate of synthesis and the rate of metabolism by hepatocytes.[57] Serum levels vary from undetectable to 40 ng/mL in normal subjects (**Table 26.2**).[58] They are elevated in newborn infants and also in response to TSH and TRH stimulation, thyroid inflammation, thyrotoxicosis and metastatic thyroid carcinoma.[59]

THYROID HORMONE TRANSPORT PROTEINS

Over 99 percent of the serum thyroid hormones are bound to transport proteins. Although not essential for hormone action, they appear to be required for the smooth functioning of the thyroid gland. They are thought to have three main functions: (1) extrathyroidal storage of T_4 and T_3; (2) buffering and protection against the effect of excessive thyroid hormones; and (3) controlled release of the hormones into the very small free hormone pool (<0.1 percent of serum T_4 and 0.3 percent of T_3) that is made available to peripheral cells.[60] A variety of proteins take part in this transport system including thyroxine-binding globulin (TBG), transthyretin (TTR or T_4-binding prealbumin), albumin and lipoproteins. TBG, TTR and albumin are all produced by hepatocytes.

TBG is one of the minor components of the alpha-globulin family. It carries 70 percent of the circulating

T_4 and T_3 and has the highest affinity of all the serum proteins that bind T_4 and T_3. It is thought that it has no other physiological function other than binding these hormones in contrast to the other major carrying proteins. Transthyretin binds 10–15 percent of the thyroid hormones and is thought to be responsible for the more immediate delivery of the hormones to cells as it dissociates from the hormone more quickly. It forms the major thyroid binding protein in the CSF, where it is produced by the choroid plexus. It is thought, however, that more biologically active thyroid hormone is probably delivered to the central nervous system through the capillary network. Albumin carries a multitude of small molecules including approximately 15–20 percent of the circulating T_4 and T_3 in spite of having a very low affinity for these hormones. Lipoproteins, and in particular high-density lipoproteins, are responsible for carrying 3–6 percent of the thyroid hormones. Fatty acids and other anions, including chloride, reduce the binding of T_4. They may have a special effect in thyroid hormone physiology as the transport proteins are internalized by specific cell-surface receptors.[61]

INTRACELLULAR EFFECTS AND METABOLISM OF THYROID HORMONES

On reaching the target tissue via the circulation, thyroid hormones enter the cell either by diffusion through the plasma membrane or by active or facilitated transport after binding to specific cell surface sites. The thyroid hormone is then transferred to cytosol binding sites and to the 5′-deiodinase on the endoplasmic reticulum (and/or plasma membranes, although this has not been determined for all cell types) where most of the T_4 is deiodinated to form T_3. An equal amount of rT_3 is also formed but its functional significance is uncertain.[59] It may have a regulatory role in thyroid hormone metabolism but has no calorigenic activity and is rapidly deiodinized to DIT (**Table 26.3**).[3, 59]

This intracellular T3 acts by binding to specific nuclear receptors.[62, 63, 64] These receptors are members of the large *c-erbA* superfamily that includes receptors for steroid hormones, vitamin D, retinoic acid, and peroxisomal proliferator activators responsible for regulating the expression of target genes.[65]

A detailed description of the effect of thyroid hormones on the different tissues is beyond the scope of this chapter. Most of the effects of intracellular T_3 are related to the stimulation of O_2 consumption in almost all metabolically active tissues with the exception of the adult brain, testes, uterus, lymph nodes, spleen and anterior pituitary. Increased metabolism is associated with increased nitrogen secretion. Endogenous protein and fat are catabolized, resulting in weight loss if food intake is not increased. High levels of thyroid hormones cause the following: significant skeletal muscle catabolism and

Table 26.2 Typical normal serum levels for thyroid hormones. Local laboratory reference ranges and assay techniques may vary.

	Metric (SI units)
TSH	0.3–4.0 mU/L (~1–15 pM)
T_4	4–11 μg/dL (60–140 nM)
Free T_4	0.7–2.1 ng/dL (10–25 pM)
T_3	75–175 ng/dL (1.1–2.7 nmol/L)
Free T_3	0.2–0.5 ng/dL (0.2–0.7 nM)

Table 26.3 Properties of iodothyronine deiodinase isozymes.

Property	Type I 5′-deiodinase	Type II 5′-deiodinase	5-Deiodinase
Main function	Bioactivation of T_3	Local intracellular bioactivation of T_3	Inactivation and degradation of iodothyronines + recycling of iodide
Substrate preference	$rT_3 \gg T_4 \gg T_3$	$T_4 > T_3$	T_3 (sulphate) $> T_4$
Tissue distribution	Thyroid, kidney, liver, euthyroid CNS	CNS, pituitary, brown adipose fat	Almost every tissue
Subcellular location	Liver: endoplasmic reticulum	Microsomal membranes	Microsomal membranes Liver: endoplasmic reticulum
	Kidney: basolateral membrane		

consequent weakness, hypercalcaemia and a degree of osteoporosis from mobilization of bone protein and a slight rise in body temperature due to the increased heat production. Thyroid hormones also potentiate the effect of growth hormone on the tissues and are essential for normal growth and skeletal development.

Deactivation of the thyroid hormones involves further deiodination by 5-deiodinase into diiodothyronine, monoiodothyronine and thyronine. This pathway is important in the regulation and bioinactivation of the thyroid hormones and the recycling of iodide. Alternatively, the thyroid hormones can be deactivated in the liver by sulphoconjugation by cytosolic sulphotransferases and the products are then excreted in the bile. These are mostly reabsorbed in the enterohepatic circulation although a small amount is lost from the body.

Parafollicular cells (C cells)

Parafollicular cells secrete calcitonin in response to elevated serum levels of calcium or gastrin. A total thyroidectomy does not always abolish calcitonin secretion as it can be produced by other organs, such as the brain, gastrointestinal tract, urinary bladder, thymus and lungs.[66] Calcitonin lowers serum calcium and phosphate levels by inhibiting the osteoclastic resorption of bone and enhancing the excretion of calcium by the kidneys. Its physiological importance is debatable as parathyroid hormone and vitamin D are thought to be more important in calcium haemostasis.[67]

KEY POINT

- Understanding the relationship between the thyroid blood supply and courses of the recurrent laryngeal nerves, external branch of the superior laryngeal nerves and parathyroids is an essential prerequisite for performing thyroid surgery with low morbidity.

Deficiencies in current knowledge and areas for future research

We only have a broad understanding of the the hugely complex intracellular and extracellular control mechanism of thyroid glandular tissue and the mechanisms whereby this homeostasis breaks down in different thyroid diseases, which can often lead to the formation of a goitre. In addition, we need to develop a greater understanding of how the thyroid hormones interact with the end-organ tissue receptors to produce the wide variety of systemic effects. A better understanding of this interaction may lead to compounds being developed that have selectively beneficial effects, such as lowering cholesterol and weight reduction, while avoiding the adverse cardiac effects.

REFERENCES

1. Braverman LE, Utiger RD. Introduction to hypothyroidism. In: Braverman LE, Utiger RD (eds). *Werner and Ingbar's The thyroid*. Philadelphia: Lippincott, Williams and Wilkins, 2000: 719–20.

∗ 2. Sawin CT. The heritage of the thyroid. In: Braverman LE, Utiger RD (eds). *Werner and Ingbar's The thyroid. A fundamental and clinical text*. Philadelphia: Lippincott, Williams and Wilkins, 2000: 3–6.

∗ 3. Cavalieri RR. Iodine metabolism and thyroid physiology: current concepts. *Thyroid*. 1997; **7**: 177–81.

∗ 4. Dunn JT, Dunn AD. Update on intrathyroidal iodine metabolism. *Thyroid*. 2001; **11**: 407–14.

∗ 5. Pintar JE. Normal development of the hypothalamic-pituitary-thyroid axis. In: Braverman LE, Utiger RD (eds). *Werner and Ingbar's The thyroid*. Philadelphia: Lippincott, Williams and Wilkins, 2000: 7–43.

6. Shepard TH. Onset of function in the human fetal thyroid: biochemical and radioautographic studies from organ culture. *Journal of Clinical Endocrinology and Metabolism*. 1967; **27**: 945–58.

7. Capan CC. Anatomy. In: Braverman LE, Utiger RD (eds). *Werner and Ingbar's The thyroid*. Philadelphia: Lippincott, Williams and Wilkins, 2000: 20–51.

8. Ballabio M, Nicolini U, Jowett T, Ruiz de Elvira MC, Ekins RP, Rodeck CH. Maturation of thyroid function in normal human foetuses. *Clinical Endocrinology*. 1989; **31**: 565–71.

* 9. Boyd JD. Development of the thyroid gland. In: Pitt-Rivers R, Trotter WR (eds). *The thyroid*, Vol. 1. Washington DC: Butterworth, 1964: 9–31.

10. Nunez EA, Gershon MD. Development of follicular and parafollicular cells of the mammalian thyroid gland. In: Greenfield LD (ed.). *Thyroid cancer*. West Palm Beach, FL: CRC Press, 1978: 1.

11. Allard RHB. The thyroglossal cyst. *Head and Neck Surgery*. 1982; **5**: 134–6.

12. Josephson GD, Spencer WR, Josephson JS. Thyroglossal duct cyst: the New York Eye and Ear Infirmary experience and a literature review. *Ear, Nose and Throat Journal*. 1998; **77**: 642–4, 646–7, 651.

13. Ewing CA, Kornblut A, Greeley C, Manz H. Presentations of thyroglossal duct cysts in adults. *European Archives of Oto-Rhino-Laryngology*. 1999; **256**: 136–8.

14. Neinas FW, Goman CA, Devine KD, Woolner LB. Lingual thyroid: clinical characteristics of 15 cases. *Annals of Internal Medicine*. 1973; **79**: 205–10.

15. Merida-Velasco JA, Garcia-Garcia JD, Espin-Ferra J, Linares J. Origin of the ultimobranchial body and its colonizing cells in human embryos. *Acta Anatomica*. 1989; **136**: 325–30.

16. Hoyes AD, Kershaw DR. Anatomy and development of the thyroid gland. *Entechnology*. 1985; **64**: 318–33.

17. Gibson W, Croker B, Cox C. C cell populations in normal children and young adults. *Laboratory Investigation*. 1989; **42**: 119–20.

18. Ball DW, Baylin SB, De Bustros AC. Medullary thyroid carcinoma. In: Braverman LE, Utiger RD (eds). *Werner and Ingbar's The thyroid. A fundamental and clinical text*. Philadelphia: Lippincott, Williams and Wilkins, 2000: 930–43.

19. Rogers WM. Normal and anomalous development of the thyroid. In: Wener SC, Ingbar SH (eds). *The thyroid*. Hagerstown, MD: Harper and Row, 1971.

20. Gauger PG, Delbridge LW, Thompson NW, Crummer P, Reeve TS. Incidence and importance of the tubercle of Zuckerkandl in thyroid surgery. *European Journal of Surgery*. 2001; **167**: 249–54.

21. Nobori M, Saiki S, Tanaka N, Harihara Y, Shindo S, Fujimoto Y. Blood supply of the parathyroid gland from the superior thyroid artery. *Surgery*. 1994; **115**: 417–23.

22. Lore JM. Practical anatomical considerations in thyroid tumor surgery. *Archives of Otolaryngology*. 1983; **109**: 568–74.

23. Moriggl B, Pomaroli A. [The openings of the inferior thyroid vein(s)]. *Anatomischer Anzeiger*. 1994; **176**: 389–93.

24. Wafae N, Vieira MC, Vorobieff A. The recurrent laryngeal nerve in relation to the inferior constrictor muscle of the pharynx. *Laryngoscope*. 1991; **101**: 1091–3.

25. Rustad WH. Revised anatomy of the recurrent laryngeal nerves: surgical importance, based on the dissection of 100 cadavers. *Journal of Clinical Endocrinology and Metabolism*. 1954; **14**: 87–96.

26. Williams PL, Warwick R. *Neurology. Gray's anatomy*. Edinburgh: Churchill-Livingstone, 1984: 1080–1.

27. Nemiroff PM, Katz AD. Extralaryngeal divisions of the recurrent laryngeal nerve. *American Journal of Surgery*. 1982; **144**: 466–9.

28. Katz AD, Nemiroff P. Anastamoses and bifurcations of the recurrent laryngeal nerve. Report of 1177 nerves visualized. *American Surgeon*. 1993; **59**: 188–91.

29. Friedman M, Toriumi DM, Grybauskas V, Katz A. Nonrecurrent laryngeal nerves and their clinical significance. *Laryngoscope*. 1986; **96**: 87–90.

30. Lennquist S, Cahlin C, Meds S. The superior laryngeal nerve in thyroid surgery. *Surgery*. 1987; **102**: 999–1008.

31. Cernea CR, Ferraz AR, Nishio S, Dutra Jr. A, Hojaij FC, dos Santos LR. Surgical anatomy of the external branch of the superior laryngeal nerve. *Head and Neck*. 1992; **14**: 380–3.

32. Durham CF, Harrison TS. The surgical anatomy of the superior laryngeal nerve. *Surgery, Gynecology and Obstetrics*. 1964; **118**: 38–44.

33. Moosman DA, De Weese MS. The external laryngeal nerve as related to thyroidectomy. *Surgery, Gynecology and Obstetrics*. 1968; **127**: 1011–6.

34. Kark AE, Kissin MW, Auerbach R, Meikle M. Voice changes after thyroidectomy: Role of the external laryngeal nerve. *British Medical Journal*. 1984; **289**: 1412–5.

35. Grunditz T, Sundler F. Autonomic nervous control: Adrenergic, cholinergic, and peptidergic regulation. In: Braverman LE, Utiger RD (eds). *Werner and Ingbar's The thyroid. A fundamental and clinical text*. Philadelphia: Lippincott-Raven, 1996: 247–53.

* 36. Williams PL, Warwick R. *Endocrine glands: The thyroid gland. Gray's anatomy*. Edinburgh: Churchill-Livingstone, 1984: 1449–53.

37. Klinck GH. Structure of the thyroid. In: Hazard JB, Smith DE (eds). *The thyroid*. Baltimore: Lippincott, Williams and Wilkins, 1964: 1–31.

38. Sobrinho-Simoes M, Johannessen JV. Scanning electron microscopy of the normal human thyroid. *Journal of Submicroscopic Cytology*. 1981; **13**: 209–22.

39. Yamazaki K, Eyden BP. Interfollicular fibroblasts in the human thyroid gland: recognition of a CD34 positive stromal cell network communicated by gap junctions and terminated by autonomic nerve endings. *Journal of Submicroscopic Cytology and Pathology*. 1997; **29**: 461–76.

40. Gnepp DR, Ogorzalek JM, Heffess CS. Fat-containing lesions of the thyroid gland. *American Journal of Surgical Pathology*. 1989; **13**: 605–12.

41. LiVolsi VA. Pathology of thyroid diseases. In: Braverman LE, Utiger RD (eds). *Werner and Ingbar's The thyroid. A fundamental and clinical text.* Philadelphia: Lippincott-Raven, 2000: 488–511.

∗ 42. Dumont JE, Takeuchi A, Lamy F, Gervy-Decoster C, Cochaux P, Roger P *et al.* Thyroid control: an example of a complex cell regulation network. *Advances in Cyclic Nucleotide and Protein Phosphorylation Research.* 1981; **14**: 479–89.

43. Scanlon MF, Toft AD. Regulation of thyrotropin secretion. In: Braverman LE, Utiger RD (eds). *Werner's and Ingbar's The thyroid.* Philadelphia: Lippincott, Williams and Wilkins, 2000: 234–53.

44. Ingbar SH. Autoregulation of the thyroid: The response to iodide excess and depletion. *Mayo Clinic Proceedings.* 1972; **47**: 814–23.

∗ 45. Nagataki S, Yokoyama N. Autoregulation: Effects of iodide. In: Braverman LE, Utiger RD (eds). *The thyroid: A fundamental and clinical text.* Philadelphia: Lippincott-Raven, 1996: 3789–93.

46. Brown KM, Arthur JR. Selenium, selenoproteins and human health: a review. *Public Health Nutrition.* 2001; **4**: 593–9.

∗ 47. Chopra IJ, Sabatino L. Nature and sources of circulating hormones. In: Braverman LE, Utiger RD (eds). *Werner and Ingbar's The thyroid: A fundamental and clinical text.* Philadelphia: Lippincott, Williams and Wilkins, 2000: 121–35.

48. Carrasco N. Iodide transport in the thyroid gland. *Biochimica et Biophysica Acta.* 1993; **1154**: 65–82.

∗ 49. Nilsson M. Molecular and cellular mechanisms of transepithelial iodide transport in the thyroid. [Review] [58 refs]. *Biofactors.* 1999; **10**: 277–85.

50. Jhiang SM, Cho J-Y, Ryu K-Y, DeYoung BR, Smanik PA, McGaughty VR *et al.* An immunohistochemical study of Na^+/I^- symporter in human thyroid tissues and salivary gland. *Endocrinology.* 1998; **139**: 4416–9.

51. Studer H, Derwahl M. Mechanisms of nonneoplastic endocrine hyperplasia-changing concept: a review focused on the thyroid gland. *Endocrine Reviews.* 1995; **16**: 411–26.

52. Kaminsky SM, Levy O, Slavador C. Na + -I-symport activity is present in membrane vesicles from thyrotropin-derived non-I-transporting cultured thyroid cells. *Proceedings of the National Academy of Sciences of the United States of America.* 1994; **91**: 3789–93.

53. Dunn JT, Dunn AD. Thyroglobulin: Chemistry and biosynthesis. In: Braverman LE, Utiger RD (eds). *Werner and Ingbar's The thyroid: A fundamental and clinical text.* Philadelphia: Lippincott-Raven, 2000: 91–104.

54. Siffroi-Fernandez S, Delom F, Nlend MC, Lanet J, Franc JL, Giraud A. Identification of thyroglobulin domain(s) involved in cell-surface binding and endocytosis. *Journal of Endocrinology.* 2001; **170**: 217–26.

55. Taurog AM. Hormone synthesis: Thyroid iodine metabolism. In: Braverman LE, Utiger RD (eds). *Werner and Ingbar's The thyroid.* Philadelphia: Lippincott, Williams and Wilkins, 2000: 61–85.

56. Wetzel BK, Spicer SS, Wollman SH. Changes in fine structure and acid phosphatase localization in rat thyroid cells following thyrotropin administration. *Journal of Cell Biology.* 1965; **25**: 593–618.

57. Spencer CA. Thyroglobulin. In: Braverman LE, Utiger RD (eds). *Werner and Ingbar's The thyroid: A fundamental and clinical text.* Philadelphia: Lippincott-Raven, 1996: 406–15.

58. Van Herle AJ, Uller RP. Elevated serum thyroglobulin: a marker of metastasis in differentiated thyroid carcinoma. *Journal of Clinical Endocrinology and Metabolism.* 1973; **37**: 741–5.

59. Chopra IJ, Sabatino L. Nature and sources of circulating thyroid hormones. In: Braverman LE, Utiger RD (eds). *Werner and Ingbar's The thyroid.* Philadelphia: Lippincott, Williams and Wilkins, 2000: 121–35.

60. Mendel CM. The free hormone hypothesis: A physiologically based mathematical model. *Endocrine Reviews.* 1989; **10**: 232–74.

61. Robbins J. Thyroid hormone transport proteins and the physiology of hormone binding. In: Braverman LE, Utiger RD (eds). *Werner and Ingbar's The thyroid.* Philadelphia: Lippincott, Williams and Wilkins, 2000: 105–20.

62. Oppenheimer JH, Schwartz HL, Surks MI, Koerner D, Dillmann WH. Nuclear receptors and the initiation of thyroid hormone action. *Recent Progress in Hormone Research.* 1977; **32**: 529–65.

63. Brent GA. The molecular basis of thyoid hormone action. *New England Journal of Medicine.* 1994; **331**: 853–74.

64. Leonard JL, Koehrle J. Intracellular pathways of iodothyronine metabolism. In: Braverman LE, Utiger RD (eds). *Werner and Ingbar's The thyroid.* Philadelphia: Lippincott, Williams and Wilkins, 2000: 136–73.

∗ 65. Anderson GW, Mariash CN, Oppenheimer JH. Molecular actions of thyroid hormone. In: Braverman LE, Utiger RD (eds). *Werner and Ingbar's The thyroid.* Philadelphia: Lippincott, Williams and Wilkins, 2000: 174–95.

66. Becker KL, Snider RH, Moore CF, Monoghan KG, Silva OL. Calcitonin in extrathyroidal tissues of man. *Acta Endocrinologica.* 1979; **92**: 746–51.

67. Baran DT. The skeletal system in thyrotoxicosis. In: Braverman LE, Utiger RD (eds). *Werner and Ingbar's The thyroid. A fundamental and clinical text.* Philadelphia: Lippincott, Williams and Wilkins, 2000: 658–66.

27

The thyroid gland: function tests and imaging

SUSAN CLARKE

Introduction	327	Investigation of structural abnormalities with abnormal function	334
Thyroid pathology	330	Conclusion	336
Investigation of abnormal development and structure	332	References	336

SEARCH STRATEGY

Information for this chapter was gathered by searching Medline using the key words thyroid, thyroid function tests, radionuclide scan, thyroid stimulating hormone, thyroxine, endocrine disease.

INTRODUCTION

Development and function

The thyroid gland is a key endocrine organ located in the head and neck region. It develops from the first branchial pouch during foetal development and descends to its normal position in the neck above the suprasternal notch. The path of the gland's descent is marked by the thyroglossal duct. The normal gland is commonly asymmetrical and the asymmetry of its two lobes is enhanced with thyroid enlargement.

The two lobes of the thyroid, connected by the fibrous isthmus, contain follicular cells arranged in a follicular pattern around colloid where thyroid hormones bound to thyroglobulin are stored. The stroma of the thyroid contains fibrocytes and occasional lymphoid cells.

The main function of the gland is the production of thyroxine (T4) and triiodothyronine (T3) by the iodination of tyrosine residues in the thyroglobulin molecule within the thyroid follicular cells. The presence of peroxidase and coupling enzymes is essential for this process, as is an adequate supply of dietary iodine and a functioning NaI symporter system. T4 and T3 remain contained within the thyroglobulin molecule until, under thyroid stimulating hormone (TSH) stimulation, the thyroglobulin containing colloid is endocytosed by the thyroid follicular cells, the resulting endosomes fused with lysosomes containing hydrolases and T4 and T3 released by the hydrolyzation of the thyroglobulin and then secreted into the circulation. It is now believed that little T3 is produced by the normal thyroid, the majority of T3 production (80 percent) occurring in the peripheries by conversion of T4 to T3 through the process of deiodination. Iodine uptake and T4 and T3 release are under the control of the hypothalamus and pituitary gland with a negative feedback system. Thyroid releasing hormone (TRH) and TSH levels rise with falling serum T4 and T3 levels.

T4 and T3 are hormones that are predominantly bound in the serum with T4 conversion to T3 occurring at the peripheries, T3 being the active hormone. In conditions of ill-health and under the influence of certain drugs, such as propanalol, the conversion of T4 to the inactive hormone reverse T3 (rT3) occurs.

The parafollicular or C cells within the thyroid secrete the hormone calcitonin, the function of which is unclear in man.

Disorders of the thyroid may result from developmental failures, abnormalities of hormone production and structural changes which may or may not be

Table 27.1 Biochemical tests in thyroid disease.

	FT4	FT3	TSH	TSI	Anti-TPO	Anti-microsomal	Anti-thyroglobulin	Thyroglobulin	Calcitonin
Euthyroid goitre	Normal	Normal	Normal	Normal	Normal	Normal	Normal	Normal	Normal
Autoimmune thyrotoxicosis	Raised	Raised	Low	Raised	Raised	Normal	Normal	Raised	Normal
Toxic nodule/s	Raised/normal	Raised	Low	Normal	Normal	Normal	Normal	Normal	Normal
Autoimmune thyroiditis	Low	Low	Raised	Normal	Raised	Raised	Raised	Raised	Normal
Viral thyroiditis	Raised	Raised	Low	Normal	Normal	Normal	Normal	Raised	Normal
Ca thyroid	Normal	Normal	Normal	Normal	Normal	Normal	Normal	Raised	Normal
Medullary Ca thyroid	Normal	Normal	Normal	Normal	Normal	Normal	Normal	Normal	Raised

accompanied by changes in function. Blood tests measuring hormone production or the antibodies associated with disordered function may be measured *in vitro* (**Table 27.1**). Structural and local functional changes within the gland may be identified using a variety of imaging techniques (**Table 27.2**).

In vitro tests of thyroid function

The standard tests of thyroid function are widely available. Since only 0.02 percent of T4 and 0.3 percent of T3 circulate in the unbound form, and it is the free hormones that are physiologically active, measurements of free T4 and free T3 levels most accurately indicate a patient's thyroid status.

The single most useful measure of thyroid function is the ultrasensitive measurement of TSH. A normal TSH measurement is a good indicator of normal thyroid function except in the rare situation of pituitary dysfunction. Changes in the TSH level will precede changes in FT4 and FT3 levels and TSH levels above or below the normal range indicate developing or recovering thyroid pathology.

Autoantibodies associated with thyroid pathology may also be measured. Identification of raised serum antibody levels to thyroglobulin, thyroid peroxidase, microsomes and the TSH receptor will significantly faciliate the accurate diagnosis of thyroid disease. The measurements of these antibodies are constantly being refined to avoid cross-reactivity. An excellent review of the interpretation of thyroid function tests is found in the review article of Dyan.[1]

Imaging investigations

ULTRASOUND

Ultrasound (US) can differentiate solid from cystic lesions and can identify cysts as small as 2 mm. It is performed using a 12 MHz transducer that is optimal for high resolution imaging though a 5 MHz transducer may be needed for very large goitres. Colour flow or power Doppler is helpful in assessing vascularity. US coupled with fine needle aspiration cytology (FNAC) provides further information.[2]

Computed tomography

Computed tomography (CT) is used to characterize large thyroid masses, to assess invasion of adjacent structures and identify metastatic nodes in the neck and mediastinum. Collimation of 3–5 mm is used and intravenous contrast medium administered. This should not be given until the thyroid function tests have been measured. The normal thyroid is of higher attenuation than muscle.

Magnetic resonance imaging

Magnetic resonance imaging (MRI) is also used to assess large tumours, especially those with suspected mediastinal extension with 3 mm axial, coronal and sagittal T1 and T2 weighted sequences. Postcontrast fat suppressed sequences may be helpful. The normal thyroid is of low signal on T1 weighted images, relative to muscle and intermediate signal on T2 weighed images. The multiplanar capability is helpful and although the specificity of MRI differs little from CT, the lack of the need for iodinated contrast is an advantage.

Radionuclide imaging

A variety of radiopharmaceuticals are suitable for imaging the thyroid and thyroid pathologies (**Table 27.2**). The radiopharmaceuticals include those that are taken up by the thyroid by normal pathways, such as ^{123}I iodine, ^{131}I iodine and ^{99m}Tc pertechnetate, as well as those that are taken up into pathological processes, such as ^{99m}Tc V dimercapto succinic acid (DMSA). ^{99m}Tc pertechnetate has the advantage of availability and low cost for routine thyroid imaging. The disadvantage is that unlike ^{123}I iodide it is trapped but not organified by the thyroid.[3]

Table 27.2 Imaging investigations in thyroid disease.

	Goitre	Graves	Toxic nodule/s	Viral thyroiditis	Hypothyroidism	Ectopic	Ca thyroid differentiated	Ca thyroid dedifferentiated	MTC	Lymphoma
US	Diffuse/nodular/cystic	Diffuse or micronodular	Solitary or multiple nodules	Diffuse	Diffuse or nodular	No thyroid tissue in neck	Nodular change/thyroid destruction/nodes	Nodular change/thyroid destruction/nodes	Nodular change/thyroid destruction/nodes	Nodular or diffuse
Tc	Diffuse/patchy	Increased	Focal increased	Reduced	Reduced/patchy		Focal reduced	Reduced	Focal reduced	Reduced
^{123}I	Diffuse/patchy	Increased	Focal increased	Reduced	Reduced/patchy		Focal reduced	Reduced	Focal reduced	Reduced
^{123}I + Perchlorate	Normal/discharge				Discharge		Focal discharge	Discharge	Focal discharge	Discharge
^{131}I							Increased in tumour	No uptake in tumour	No uptake in tumour	No uptake in tumour
18FDG		Increased	Increased				Normal/increased	Increased	Normal/increased	Increased
Tc MIBI	Normal						Increased	Increased	Increased	
Tc V DMSA									Increased	
^{111}In octreotide									Increased	Increased
^{123}I MIBG									Increased	
Gallium					Increased					Increased

THYROID PATHOLOGY

A summary of thyroid pathology is provided as follows.

- Developmental disorders:
  - maldescent:
    - lingual;
    - sublingual;
    - subhyoid.
  - maldevelopment:
    - absent thyroid;
    - aplastic, hypoplastic thyroid lobe;
    - thyroglossal cyst.

- Disorders of function:
  - hyperthyroidism:
    - toxic diffuse goitre (Graves' disease);
    - solitary toxic nodule;
    - toxic nodule(s) in nodular goitre (Plummer's disease);
    - subacute viral thyroiditis;
    - iodine induced thyrotoxicosis;
    - post-partum thyroiditis;
    - thyroxine administration;
    - hashitoxicosis (rare);
    - Ca thyroid (rare);
    - TSH secreting pituitary tumours (rare);
    - struma ovarii (rare).
  - hypothyroidism:
    - autoimmune (Hashimoto's thyroiditis);
    - thyroid aplasia (cretinism);
    - radioiodine;
    - x-rays;
    - surgery;
    - pan hypopituitarism;
    - hypothalamic injury or disease.

- Disorder of structure:
  - nodular change:
    - single benign (follicular adenoma, focal Hashimoto's, teratoma);
    - single malignant (follicular, papillary, medullary, metastasis);
    - multiple benign (multinodular);
    - multiple malignant (papillary, medullary);
    - cyst (simple/complex/haemorrhage).
  - diffuse change:
    - sporadic goitre;
    - endemic goitre;
    - dyshormonogenesis;
    - compensatory (following surgery);
    - autoimmune (Hashimoto's thyroiditis);
    - invasive (Riedel's thyroiditis, amyloid, haemochromatosis);
    - malignant (lymphoma).

Developmental disorders

Maldescent of the thyroid is usually detected in childhood following the discovery of an abnormal swelling at the base of the tongue or in the sublingual area. Midline swellings above the normal position of the thyroid may be due to a thyroglossal duct cyst. Most occur at (15 percent) or immediately below (65 percent) the hyoid bone. Suprahyoid cysts occur in only 20 percent of cases.

Structural abnormalities of the thyroid with normal function

A common presentation of patients with thyroid disorders affecting the structure of the gland is the awareness of a nodular or generalized swelling of the thyroid.

DIFFUSE GOITRE

Euthyroid diffuse goitre is not an uncommon finding in women. The thyroid may enlarge during puberty, pregnancy and at the time of the menopause. Women commencing the contraceptive pill may also become aware of thyroid swelling. Although these diffuse swellings of the thyroid are usually transient, some women may have permanent swellings of their thyroid which are not associated with thyroid dysfunction.

Patients with a diffuse goitre and a family history of goitre may have a congenital dyshormonogenesis leading to a partial failure of iodide organification. This is commonly associated with deafness in Pendred's syndrome. Despite the organification defect, these patients are commonly euthyroid.

NODULAR GOITRE

Palpation has proven to be unreliable in accurately assessing the structure of the thyroid, as apparently solitary nodules are frequently part of multinodular change[4] and many ultrasound identified nodules are not palpable. Nodules within the thyroid may be cystic or solid. Cystic lesions may be simple or complex and rapid swelling accompanied by discomfort is usually indicative of haemorrhage. Colloid nodules are a common benign cause of thyroid swelling in patients with multinodular change within the gland.

Adenomas represent 10 percent of thyroid nodules and are either follicular (micro-, normo- or macrofollicular) or nonfollicular. Thyroid cancer is an uncommon malignancy with 900 new cases reported annually in the UK and the histology includes papillary (60–80 percent), follicular (10–18 percent), anaplastic (3–10 percent) and medullary (4–8 percent).

Papillary carcinomas occur in 30–40 year olds and tend to be well differentiated, slow growing with an excellent prognosis and an average size of 1.5 cm. Tumours presenting in older age groups are often poorly differentiated, invade the larynx and oesophagus, and have a poor prognosis. Papillary carcinomas are not uncommonly multifocal and are bilateral in 10 percent of cases. Spread to lymph nodes is common, occurring in up to 70 percent of cases. Follicular carcinomas are commoner in females and have a peak incidence in the fifth decade. They are solitary, slow growing encapsulated tumours and resemble adenomas. The more aggressive tumours extend outside the gland and have a poor prognosis. Lymph node involvement is unusual (5–13 percent) but haematogenous spread to bone, liver and brain is not uncommon. Medullary carcinoma is the most uncommon subtype. It originates from C cells and produces calcitonin. It may either be sporadic (75–90 percent) or familial as part of multiple endocrine neoplasia (MEN) 2a or 2b syndrome, or familial medullary thyroid cancer. The tumours associated with MEN occur in younger patients (mean age 35 years) and are bilateral in 80 percent of MEN 2b, but bilateral in only 20 percent of sporadic cases.

MULTINODULAR GOITRES

Adenomatous or colloid multinodular goitres are common, occurring in 3–5 percent of the general population. Haemorrhage, fibrosis and calcification are found within goitres and the incidence of malignant transformation is approximately 7.5 percent.

Patients with a family history of goitre should be suspected of having dyshormonogenesis. In geographical regions of iodine deficiency, endemic goitre remains common.

Structural abnormalities with abnormal function

HYPERTHYROIDISM

Toxic diffuse goitre (Graves' disease)

This is the commonest cause of thyrotoxicosis in the UK. The clinical picture of a diffuse goitre and dysthyroid eye disease is pathognomonic of Graves' disease but only 50 percent of patients present with dysthyroid eye disease, and dysthyroid eye disease may precede or succeed the development of thyrotoxicosis by up to two years.

Solitary toxic nodule

Clinical examination of the thyroid will frequently determine the presence of a nodule within the thyroid. In the presence of thyrotoxic symptoms, a presumptive diagnosis of solitary toxic nodule can be made. However, this diagnosis requires confirmation with imaging studies as clinically single nodules are not infrequently part

of impalpable multinodular change within the thyroid. Graves' disease in an asymmetrical thyroid may also be mistaken clinically for a unilateral toxic nodule. Similarly, the rare coexistence of thyroid carcinomas in patients with Graves' disease may lead to a misdiagnosis of a solitary toxic nodule if clinical palpation alone is relied upon.

Multiple toxic nodules

The association of clinical thyrotoxicosis in a patient with a palpable multinodular goitre will usually result from the development of one or more autonomous nodules in a multinodular gland. The presence of palpable nodule(s) in a thyrotoxic patient does not confirm a diagnosis of toxic nodular goitre however, as Graves' disease may occur in a multinodular goitre.[5, 6] Since the management of Graves' thyrotoxicosis and toxic nodular disease is different, with Graves' patients usually being offered a prolonged trial of antithyroid medication, the correct diagnosis is essential to ensure optimal management. Similarly, small multinodular goitres with toxic nodules may be difficult to palpate and a misdiagnosis of Graves' disease may be made.

Transient hyperthyroidism

Patients may present with transient episodes of hyperthyroidism associated with transient swellings of the thyroid. Subacute viral thyroiditis or De Quervain's thyroiditis is typically preceded by a viral upper respiratory tract infection followed by acute painful swelling of the thyroid and symptoms of thyrotoxicosis. Whilst the swelling is typically bilateral, unilateral disease has been described. The condition is self-limiting and usually resolves within one month of onset. Post-partum thyroiditis affects 7 percent of women after delivery. Unlike subacute viral thyroiditis, the goitre is painless and is associated with a transient episode of hyperthyroidism usually followed by a short period of hypothyroidism. The condition generally resolves spontaneously although patients may remain permanently hypothyroid after the episode.

Hyperthyroidism associated with cancer of the thyroid

Thyroid cancer is generally characterized by being well differentiated with thyroid follicular cells retaining many of the properties of normal thyroid follicular cells including the ability to take up iodine. Rarely, in patients with disseminated large volume metastatic disease, the bulk of tumour may result in the overproduction of T4 leading to overt thyrotoxicosis. This rare condition is usually associated with widespread bone metastases.

HYPOTHYROIDISM

Hypothyroidism may rarely be congenital associated with agenesis of the thyroid. More commonly, it is associated with the presence of autoantibodies leading to juvenile or adult Hashimoto's thyroiditis. The changes in the structure of the thyroid resulting from the autoimmune condition are generally nodular although the pattern of change may be diffuse, mimicking those seen in Graves' disease. In patients with established Hashimoto's thyroiditis, maintained on adequate replacement doses of thyroxine, a rapid increase in size of the goitre should be investigated urgently as a B cell lymphoma of the thyroid may develop within a Hashimoto's goitre.

INVESTIGATION OF ABNORMAL DEVELOPMENT AND STRUCTURE

In vitro investigations

DEVELOPMENTAL ABNORMALITIES

The most important role of in vitro studies of thyroid function in patients with developmental abnormalities of the thyroid gland, such as a lingual thyroid and thyroglossal cysts, is to confirm normal thyroid function. A TSH value in the middle of the normal range excludes any abnormality of function.

DIFFUSE CHANGE

The history of a patient with a diffuse goitre may often give insight into the cause of the goitre. Recent changes in the pituitary ovarian axis in women or a family history of goitre will direct further investigations. Confirmation of normal thyroid function with a TSH in the middle of the normal range is essential to exclude early structural change preceding overt biochemical changes. A TSH level towards the upper end of the normal range may indicate developing hypothyroidism in a patient with a familial dyshormonogenesis or developing Hashimoto's thyroiditis. A TSH in the lower end of the range may indicate a resolving viral thyroiditis, or developing autoimmune thyrotoxicosis (Graves' disease). Serial measurements of thyroid function are indicated in patients with TSH values at the upper or lower end of the range to determine whether a drift in thyroid function is occurring.

Autoantibody measurements are also indicated to identify covert Hashimoto's thyroiditis with elevation of the antithyroid peroxidase antibody, antimicrosomal antibodies and antithyroglobulin antibodies or early Graves' disease in a patient with raised TSH receptor antibodies.

NODULAR CHANGE

It is essential to determine the biochemical status of any patient presenting with one or more thyroid nodules as part of the diagnostic strategy for assessing nodules.

Normal thyroid function, as evidenced by a normal TSH value, excludes toxic nodular change or conversely, developing Hashimoto's thyroiditis. In patients with a family history of goitre and or hypothyroidism, it is appropriate to measure thyroid autoantibody levels, specifically antithyroid peroxidase antibody and antithyroglobulin antibody. If levels of these antibodies are raised, then as with the patient presenting with a diffuse goitre, the patient is at risk of developing Hashimoto's thyroiditis in the future and requires regular monitoring with thyroid function tests. A low normal TSH value with a low normal FT4 level may occasionally be misinterpreted as 'sick euthyroid syndrome'. A further FT3 measurement may indicate high normal values consistent with a developing autonomous nodule. Serial thyroid function tests together with imaging are indicated.

Any patient with normal thyroid function and a palpable nodule requires urgent further investigation to exclude malignancy as the cause of the nodular change.

Imaging investigations

DEVELOPMENTAL DISORDERS

Maldescent of the thyroid is usually detected in childhood following the discovery of an abnormal swelling at the base of the tongue or in the sublingual area. A ^{99m}Tc thyroid scan will clarify the location of the thyroid and avoid the necessity for biopsy or inadvertent excision of ectopic thyroid tissue. A lingual thyroid is easily identified on CT as a high attenuation mass within the tongue base at the foramen caecum. Midline swellings above the normal position of the thyroid may be investigated using ultrasound, which will determine the cystic nature of a thyroglossal duct cyst. MRI is the best imaging modality for assessment of cradiad extension using T2 weighted sagittal imaging. CT and MRI show a characteristic midline cystic mass nestled within the infrahyoid strap muscles. A ^{99m}Tc thyroid scan will confirm the normal position of the thyroid and the absence of functioning thyroid tissue in the cyst. As ectopic thyroid tissue has a higher incidence of malignant transformation compared with normally situated tissue, excision of such tissue is usually performed.

Disorders of structure

NODULAR CHANGE

Palpation has proven to be unreliable in accurately assessing the structure of the thyroid as apparently solitary nodules are frequently part of multinodular change.[4]

An ultrasound scan of the thyroid in a patient presenting with an apparently solitary nodule will accurately determine whether the nodule is truly solitary, and will also determine the cystic or solid nature of the nodule and facilitate biopsy. Palpable nodules that are identified as cystic on ultrasound can be aspirated under ultrasound guidance and cytology performed on the aspirate. If the cyst reaccumulates, or if there is evidence of a complex cyst, surgery should be performed in view of the risk of malignancy. Rapid onset swellings associated with pain are frequently shown on ultrasound to have the classic appearance of haemorrhage into a cyst with internal debris, septation or both[7] and again this may be confirmed with FNAC.

On ultrasound, microfollicular and nonfollicular adenomas are hypoechoic whereas macrofollicular adenomas are hyperechoic. Most homogeneous hyperechoic lesions are benign but 50 percent of adenomas are isoechoic with a hypoechoic capsule. On colour Doppler, adenomas have a vascular rim and central vascularization is seen in both autonomous adenomas and carcinomas. The features suggestive of a benign adenoma include cystic lesions without solid areas, homogeneous hyperechoic masses, thin hypoechoic rims, multiple lesions and the presence of egg shell calcification. Signs of malignancy include infiltrative margins, papillary solid areas in a cystic lesion, central vascularization, inhomogeneous echo pattern and associated lymphadenopathy.

On CT, follicular adenomas are either solid enhancing masses or have areas of cystic degeneration and calcification.

Papillary carcinomas on ultrasound are hypoechoic with irregular central vascularization and microcalcification. On CT, these tumours are solid with cystic areas and contain punctate or amorphous calcification, while on MRI they are isointense with muscle on T1 and intermediate to high intensity on T2-weighted sequences.[8] Distant metastases to lung and bone occur in 5–7 percent of patients.

Follicular carcinomas on CT and MRI are usually well-defined solid nodules with no cystic component, with the more aggressive showing local invasion. On ultrasound these tumours are iso- or hypoechoic with central vascularization of 90 percent.

Medullary thyroid cancers on CT and MRI are solid with coarse or psammomatous calcification. Local invasion is not uncommon and spread to neck and mediastinal nodes occur in up to 50 percent of cases with distant metastases in liver, lung and bone in 15–25 percent. On ultrasound the lesions are hypoechoic with ill-defined margins and microcalcification.

It is not possible to confidently distinguish between an adenoma and carcinoma on ultrasound and FNAC should be undertaken if there is any doubt. FNAC has been shown to be simple and cost-effective,[9] with reported positive predictive value for malignant disease of 94 percent and a false negative and false positive rate of 2.7 and 5.4 percent, respectively. The role of radionuclide imaging in the diagnosis of the solitary solid nodule is controversial.[10] Whilst fine needle aspiration will usually yield results that guide management, some problems may exist in interpreting the results. Sampling errors may occur in multinodular goitres and it is only the radionuclide scan that will ensure that nonfunctioning nodules are sampled. A follicular lesion will require surgical removal to determine whether the lesion is a benign follicular adenoma or a follicular carcinoma. However, follicular lesions, if 'hot' on radionuclide imaging with ^{99m}Tc or ^{123}I, have a low likelihood of malignancy (less than 4 percent in a review of 4000 patients)[11, 12] and if the TSH value is towards the lower end of the normal range, may safely be kept under observation whilst the TSH level continues to be monitored. If there is no downward trend in the TSH value, then excision should be performed. Solitary solid nodules will also require further investigation with FNAC under US control if the thyroid function tests show no evidence of developing autonomous function with a low normal or abnormally low TSH value in the presence of high normal T4 and/or T3 levels.

Other radiopharmaceuticals have been investigated in an attempt to reduce the number of unnecessary operations performed in patients with follicular lesions. The uptake of both ^{99m}Tc Sestamibi (MIBI) and ^{201}Tl has been assessed and although the uptake of both tracers has been shown to be generally higher in follicular carcinomas than follicular adenomas, there is no clear cut off in the uptake values to distinguish benign from malignant lesions.[13, 14] If malignancy is diagnosed on FNAC, ultrasound, CT or MRI may be used to assess the locoregional lymph nodes prior to surgery. Care should be taken with use of contrast media during CT imaging, as this will block the uptake of subsequent therapy dose of ^{131}I iodine used to ablate remaining thyroid tissue following surgery.

Following the diagnosis of Ca thyroid and the surgical resection of the thyroid and involved lymph nodes, ^{131}I iodine is used to ablate remnant thyroid tissue and then, in tracer doses, to image for recurrent disease.

A whole body scan using ^{131}I iodine as the tracer will usually identify recurrent disease, but it is essential that the TSH level is elevated at the time of administration of radioiodine necessitating the discontinuation of thyroid supplements for a minimum of four weeks for thyroxine and two weeks for triiodothyronine. Recently, an injectable form of recombinant TSH has been licensed for use in Ca thyroid to administer with radioiodine. If the recurrent disease is radioiodine avid on tracer imaging, a therapy dose of radioiodine may by given (5–7 GBq). Radioiodine therapy is continued at six-monthly intervals until the tracer scan clears and the thyroglobulin level falls.

Although iodine-based radionuclides remain the main agents in use for nuclear medicine imaging in the follow-up of differentiated thyroid cancer, there are other radiopharmaceuticals that can be used. Progressive dedifferentiation of a thyroid cancer commonly leads to a loss of iodine-concentrating ability by the tumour cells. In addition, the requirement to discontinue thyroxine or triodothyronine for a period of time prior to iodine imaging may delay imaging in patients who develop new masses. The TSH rise associated with discontinuing thyroid replacement medication may also accelerate tumour growth in aggressive tumours. There is, therefore, a role for alternative imaging agents to localize dedifferentiating tumours and which permit imaging whilst the patient is still on thyroxine. The most useful include [201]thallium, ^{99m}Tc MIBI, ^{99m}Tc tetrofosmin (Myoview) and [18]fluorine fluorodeoxyglucose (FDG)-positron emission tomography (PET).

These agents are used in conjunction with anatomical imaging methods, ultrasound, CT and MRI.

The sensitivities of [201]thallium and ^{99m}Tc tetrofosmin are comparable with that of [131]iodine for detecting distant metastases (0.85, 0.85, 0.78), although [131]iodine is more sensitive that the other two for detecting post-surgical residual thyroid tissue.[15] Scintigraphic imaging with [201]thallium has been thought to reflect the abnormal DNA characteristic of poor prognosis in differentiated thyroid carcinoma. Nakada *et al.* found that [201]thallium uptake was significantly higher in patients with aneuploidic nuclear DNA ($p < 0.01$). These patients went on to exhibit the aggressive clinical behaviour characteristic of metastatic tumours.[16]

When compared to [201]thallium, MIBI has been proved to be clinically more useful in detecting lung, lymph node and bone metastases from differentiated thyroid carcinoma, as image quality is better. The overall sensitivity of the two techniques is not, however, significantly different.[17] The superiority of MIBI in detecting lymph node disease before initial [131]iodine treatment was confirmed by Ng *et al.*[18] who also noted that MIBI is not as sensitive as ^{131}I scanning for thyroid remnants or lung metastases.

Both MIBI and [201]thallium yield high specificity and positive predictive value for residual thyroid cancer in patients with increased risk of recurrence after ^{131}I therapy who have had negative [131]iodine scans. Both imaging agents have been shown to detect residual cancer and cause a change in management in more than half the patients in whom conventional imaging techniques were unreliable.[19]

The main value of [18]fluorine FDG-PET in the management of thyroid carcinoma patients, in common with the other methods above, lies in its ability to demonstrate metastatic sites after negative iodine scanning. Its accuracy is high, especially for cervical lymph nodes where it has proved particularly helpful for directing surgical management. It can also identify metastases in the mediastinum, lungs and bone. Studies on patients with thyroglobulin positive/iodine scan negative disease gave sensitivities of 94 percent[20] and 71 percent[21] for detecting iodine negative disease. The increased metabolic activity of dedifferentiating aggressive

tumours would explain the high [18]fluorine FDG-PET uptake compared with much lower uptake seen in iodine avid tumours.

Patients with medullary thyroid cancer and rising calcitonin levels may be imaged with ultrasound, CT or MRI to localize respectable disease. In some patients, however, the recurrent disease volume is small and radionuclide imaging may be helpful in detecting areas of recurrence (**Table 27.2**). Uptake by ^{123}I meta iodobenzylguanidine (MIBG) will identify patients who may respond to therapy with ^{131}I MIBG.

Multinodular goitres

The appearance of goitres on CT or MRI is variable, depending on the histology, with calcification best seen on CT. On MRI there is variable signal intensity due to fibrosis (low signal on T1 and T2W), colloid (low or high signal on T1, high signal on T2W), blood (variable signal on T1 and T2W) and calcium (low signal).

On ultrasound, a goitre is more echogenic than normal thyroid and as it increases in size it becomes more inhomogeneous with ill-defined posterior borders. It may be difficult to visualize the full extent on ultrasound.

Euthyroid goitres may be imaged by CT or MRI prior to surgery to assess the presence of retrosternal extension and, in patients with pressure symptoms, the degree of tracheal deviation or compression.

Patients with a family history of goitre and suspected dyshormonogenesis may be investigated using a combination of ^{123}I iodine and perchlorate. Failure of organification of [123]iodide occurs and the nonorganified iodine is displaced from the gland when perchlorate is administered.

INVESTIGATION OF STRUCTURAL ABNORMALITIES WITH ABNORMAL FUNCTION

In vitro investigations

AUTOIMMUNE THYROTOXICOSIS (GRAVES' DISEASE)

Patients with Graves' disease usually present with classical symptoms of thyrotoxicosis and the clinical findings of a diffuse goitre. The measurement of thyroid function will confirm elevations of FT4, and occasionally FT3, together with a suppressed TSH level. The size of the goitre often correlates with the severity of the biochemical abnormality. The findings of raised TSH receptor antibody levels (TSHrA or TSI) will confirm the diagnosis in the majority of cases although 10 percent of patients will not demonstrate elevated antibody levels. It is believed that this 10 percent represents a failure of antibody detection and newer assays claim a higher antibody detection rate. Patients who have been treated with antithyroid medication may not have elevated antibody levels as the immunosuppressive action of these agents becomes effective. Thyroid peroxidase antibodies are also elevated in the majority of patients.

TOXIC NODULAR GOITRE

Thyroid function tests will confirm the biochemical status of the patient with a nodular goitre and a clinical suspicion of thyrotoxicosis. Elderly patients or patients with early disease may be asymptomatic however, and any patient with a nodular goitre and a low normal or suppressed TSH is at risk of developing frank thyrotoxicosis and should be regularly monitored. Whilst the classical pattern of elevated FT4 measurements and a suppressed TSH level is the usual finding, some patients have nodules specifically secreting T3 and the FT3 levels will be elevated with normal or even low FT4 levels.

HYPOTHYROID GOITRE

Patients with developing Hashimotos' thyroiditis will usually develop a goitre before the biochemical changes occur. Indeed, in a small percentage of patients, there may be a brief period of thyroid overactivity or 'Hashitoxicosis' before the classical features of hypothyroidism develop. Elevation of the autoantiobodies to thyroid peroxidase (TPO) and thyroglobulin are diagnostic of this condition but antibody elevation and goitrous change may precede the development of thyrotoxicosis by many years. These patients require regular biochemical review and thyroxine replacement commenced when the blood tests start to drift down.

Imaging investigations

HYPERTHYROIDISM

Whilst biochemical tests of thyroid function are the mainstay of identifying the presence of thyrotoxicosis, the underlying pathogenesis may not be diagnosed by blood tests alone. Imaging investigations will give an insight into the functionality and structure of regions of the gland.

Toxic diffuse goitre (Graves' disease)

On ultrasound the gland is moderately enlarged and in 80 percent of patients the gland is diffusely hypoechoic secondary to lymphoctyic infiltration. The gland may appear normal in some patients and in others echogenic nodules are seen within the hypoechoic matrix suggesting Graves' superimposed on a pre-existing nodular goitre. A characteristic pulsatile flow pattern is seen within the gland on colour Doppler ('thyroid inferno'[22]). The volume of the gland will decrease during therapy, as may the vascularity.[23]

Quantitative uptake may be undertaken to measure the trapping function of the thyroid. The 20 minute uptake value for ^{99m}Tc is normally between 0.4 and 4 percent and the two hour uptake of ^{123}I iodide is 20 percent. Patients with untreated toxic diffuse goitre will have trapping values higher than the normal range. The level of uptake corresponds to the severity of the thyrotoxicosis and the level of TSH receptor antibodies.

Solitary toxic nodule

Clinical examination of the thyroid will frequently determine the presence of nodules within the thyroid. However, the presence of palpable nodule(s) in a thyrotoxic patient does not confirm a diagnosis of toxic nodular goitre as Graves' disease may occur in a multinodular goitre and Graves' disease in an asymmetrical thyroid may be mistaken clinically for a unilateral toxic nodule. Since the management of Graves' thyrotoxicosis and toxic nodular disease is different, with Graves' patients usually being offered a prolonged trial of antithyroid medication, the correct diagnosis is essential to ensure optimal management. Similarly, small multinodular goitres with toxic nodules may be difficult to palpate and a misdiagnosis of Graves' disease may be made. Imaging therefore contributes to the diagnosis of the hyperthyroid patient, and ultrasound is used to confirm the presence of a solitary nodule and ensure that appropriate management is instigated.

If a discrete nodule is identified, the ^{99m}Tc or ^{123}I thyroid scan will assess the functionality.[24, 25] The probability of carcinoma in solitary nonfunctioning solid nodules varies from 10 to 25 percent in reported series and FNAC should be performed if such a nodule is demonstrated. The probability of cancer in a single nodule of a multinodular goitre is variably reported as 1–3 percent,[26] or up to 6 percent in other series.[27]

Thyroiditis

If the patient presents with painful swelling of the thyroid or if there is any history of iodine administration, an isotope scan should be performed as soon as possible. In subacute viral thyrodits (De Quervain's), the classical scan pattern of low or absent uptake with biochemical evidence of thyrotoxicosis is diagnostic. The uptake will normalize within four to six weeks after the onset of the illness. With iodine-induced thyrotoxicosis, the low uptake pattern on the scan may persist for many months.

The gland is moderately enlarged on ultrasound with geographical hypoechoic areas that are hypervascular. There may be associated lymphadenopathy.[28]

Hypothyroidism

Hypothyroidism may present with the clinical symptoms of an underactive thyroid or be discovered during investigation for goitre. The swelling of the thyroid during the early phases of Hashimoto's thyroiditis may precede the onset of classical symptoms of hypothyroidism and imaging may be of value in assessing the nature of the goitre.

The radionuclide scan pattern in Hashimoto's thyroiditis ranges from a diffuse pattern of uptake through to discrete nodular change.[29] In the early stages of the disorder the uptake of radioactive tracer is increased as the TSH level rises. As the gland fails functionally, the uptake value falls until eventually there is no uptake and no visualization of the thyroid on a radionuclide scan.

On ultrasound in the subacute phase, the gland is moderately enlarged and hypoechoic and returns to normal after treatment. Occasionally there are hypoechoic areas with echogenic hypervascular septa similar to those seen in Graves' disease. In the chronic phase the thyroid is small or atrophic and hypoechoic with no hypervascularity.

On CT the appearances are nonspecific with variable diffuse enlargement of the thyroid. On T2 weighted MRI, the gland may show increased signal intensity with peripheral lower-intensity bands, which probably represent fibrosis. Rarely, lymphoma may develop in the thyroid gland of a patient with Hashimoto's thyroiditis and present as a rapidly increasing swelling of the thyroid in a patient with known hypothyroidism and the development of lymphadenopathy. A ^{67}Ga citrate scan will identify increased uptake in the developing lymphoma of the thyroid. On ultrasound there are diffuse or focal areas of hypoechogenicity within the enlarged gland with associated lymphadenopathy. Lymphoma is of low attenuation on both unenhanced and enhanced CT scans and hypointense on T1 and T2 weighted MR images. The diagnosis can be confirmed on FNAC. Since these tumours are frequently radiosensitive, accurate diagnosis will spare the patient unnecessary surgery.

CONCLUSION

Whilst the diagnosis of thyroid disease is highly dependent on adequate history taking and clinical examination, biochemical and imaging investigations contribute significantly to the accuracy of the diagnosis and in management planning and patient monitoring.

REFERENCES

1. Dyan CM. Interpretation of thyroid function tests. *Lancet*. 2001; **357**: 619–24.
2. Takashima S, Fukada H, Kobayshi T. Thyroid nodules: clinical effect of ultrasound-guided fine needle aspiration biopsy. *Journal of Clinical Ultrasound*. 1994; **22**: 535–42.
3. Becker D, Charkes ND, Dworkin H, Hurley J, McDougall IR, Price D *et al*. Procedure for thyroid scintigraphy. *Journal of Nuclear Medicine*. 1996; **37**: 1264–6.
4. Brander A, Viikinkoski P, Tuuhea J, Voutilainen L, Kivisaari L. Clinical versus ultrasound examination of the thyroid in common clinical practice. *Journal of Clinical Ultrasound*. 1992; **20**: 37–42.
5. Fogelman I, Cooke SG. Maisey MN The role of thyroid scanning in hyperthyroidism. *European Journal of Nuclear Medicine*. 1986; **11**: 397–400.
6. Lacey NA, Jones A, Clarke SEM. Role of radio nuclide imaging in hyperthyroid patients with no clinical suspicion of nodules. *British Journal of Radiology*. 2001; **74**: 486–9.
7. King AD, Ahuja AT, King W, Metreweli C. The role of ultrasound in the diagnosis of a large, rapidly growing, thyroid mass. *Postgraduate Medical Journal*. 1997; **73**: 412–4.
8. Weber AL, Randolph G, Aksoy FG. The thyroid and parathyroid glands. CT and MR imaging and correlation with pathology and clinical findings. *Radiologic Clinics of North America*. 2000; **38**: 1105–29.
9. Lioe TF, Elliot H, Allen DC, Spence RA. A 3-year audit of thyroid fine needle aspirates. *Cytopathology*. 1998; **9**: 188–92.
10. Lind P. Multi-tracer imaging of thyroid nodules: is there a role in the preoperative assessment of nodular goitre? *European Journal of Nuclear Medicine*. 1999; **26**: 795–8.
11. Ashcraft M, VanHerle A. Management of thyroid nodules. I: History and physical examination, blood tests, X-ray tests, and ultrasonography. *Head and Neck Surgery*. 1981; **3**: 216–27.
12. Ashcraft M, VanHerle A. Management of thyroid nodules. II: Scanning techniques, thyroid suppressive therapy, and fine needle aspiration. *Head and Neck Surgery*. 1981; **3**: 297–322.
13. Kanmaz B, Erdil TY, Yardi OF, Sayman HB, Kabasakal L, Sonmezoglu K *et al*. The role of 99Tcm-tetrofosmin in the evaluation of thyroid nodules. *Nuclear Medicine Communications*. 2000; **21**: 333–9.
14. Kresnik E, Gallowitsch H-J, Mikosch P, Gomez I, Lind P. Technetum-99m-MIBI scintigraphy of thyroid nodules in an endemic goiter area. *Journal of Nuclear Medicine*. 1997; **38**: 62–5.
15. Ünal S, Menda Y, Adalet I, Boztepe H, Ozbey N, Alogol F *et al*. Thallium-201, technetium-99m-tetrofosmin and iodine-131 in detecting differentiated thyroid carcinoma metastases. *Journal of Nuclear Medicine*. 1998; **39**: 1897–902.
16. Nakada K, Katoh C, Morita K, Kanegae K, Tsukamoto E, Shiga T *et al*. Relationship among 201Tl uptake, nuclear DNA content and clinical behavior in metastatic thyroid carcinoma. *Journal of Nuclear Medicine*. 1999; **40**: 963–7.
17. Miyamoto S, Kasagi K, Misaki T, Alam MS, Konshi J. Evaluation of Technetium-99m-MIBI scintigraphy in metastatic differentiated thyroid carcinoma. *Journal of Nuclear Medicine*. 1997; **38**: 352–6.
18. Ng DCE, Sundram FX, Sin AE. 99mTc-Sestamibi and 131I whole-body scintigraphy and initial serum thyroglobulin in

the management of differentiated thyroid carcinoma. *Journal of Nuclear Medicine*. 2000; **41**: 631–5.

19. Seabold JE, Gurll N, Schurrer ME, Aktay R, Kirchner PT. Comparison of 99mTc-methoxyisobutyl isonitrile and 201 Tl scintigraphy for detection of residual thyroid cancer after 131 I ablative therapy. *Journal of Nuclear Medicine*. 1999; **40**: 1434–40.

20. Chung J-K, So Y, Lee JS, Choi CW, Lim SM, Lee DS *et al.* Value of FDG PET in papillary thyroid carcinoma with negative 131I whole-body scan. *Journal of Nuclear Medicine*. 1999; **40**: 986–92.

21. Wang W, Macapinlac H, Larson SM, Yeh SD, Akhurst T, Finn RD *et al.* [18F]-2-Fluoro-2-deoxy-D-glucose positron emission tomography localizes residual thyroid cancer in patients with negative diagnostic 131I whole body scans and elevated serum thyroglobulin levels. *Journal of Clinical Endocrinology and Metabolism*. 1999; **84**: 2291–302.

22. Ralls PW, Mayekawa DS, Lee KP, Colletti PM, Radin DR, Boswell WD *et al.* Color flow Doppler in Graves' disease: thyroid inferno. *American Journal of Roentgenology*. 1982; **150**: 781–3.

23. Castognone D, Rivolta R, Rescalli S, Baldini MI, Tozzi R, Cantalamessa L. Color Doppler sonography in Graves' disease: value in assessing activity and predicting outcome. *American Journal of Roentgenology*. 1996; **166**: 203–7.

24. Beierwaltes WH. Comparison of Tc 99m and I 123 nodules: correlation with pathologic findings. *Journal of Nuclear Medicine*. 1990; **31**: 400–4002.

25. Kusic Z, Becker DV, Saenger EL, Paras P, Gartside P, Wessler T. Comparison of 99mTc and 123 I imaging of thyroid nodules: correlation with pathologic findings. *Journal of Nuclear Medicine*. 1990; **31**: 393–9.

26. Price DC. Radioisotopic evaluation of the thyroid and parathyroids. *Radiologic Clinics of North America*. 1993; **31**: 991–1015.

27. Mathew R, Ali N, Taylor A, Philips Z. Clarke SEM. Thyroid carcinoma in solitary cold nodules, and cold nodules in diffuse toxic and multi-nodular goitres. *Nuclear Medicine Communications*. 2002; **23**: 396–7.

28. Gritzmann N, Koischwitz D, Rettenbacher T. Sonography of the thyroid and parathyroid glands. *Radiologic Clinics of North America*. 2000; **38**: 1131–45.

29. Ramtoola S, Maisey MN, Clarke SEM, Fogelman I. The thyroid scan in Hashimoto's thyroiditis: The great mimic. *Nuclear Medicine Communications*. 1988; **9**: 639–45.

28

The thyroid: nonmalignant disease

LORRAINE M ALBON AND JAYNE A FRANKLYN

Thyrotoxicosis	338	Thyroid disease in pregnancy	358
Best clinical practice	351	Best clinical practice	360
Transient thyrotoxicosis/thyroiditis	351	Nonmalignant euthyroid conditions	360
Key points	353	Key points	363
Subclinical hyperthyroidism	353	Best clinical practice	364
Hypothyroidism	353	Deficiencies in current knowledge and areas for future	
Key points	358	research	364
Best clinical practice	358	References	364

SEARCH STRATEGY

The data in this chapter are supported by a Medline search using the key words hyperthyroidism, thyrotoxicosis, Graves' disease, multinodular goitre, toxic adenoma, nodular thyroid disease, subclinical hyperthyroidism, thyroiditis, hypothyroidism, Hashimoto's thyroiditis, subclinical hypothyroidism. The emphasis is on pathogenesis, diagnosis and treatment.

THYROTOXICOSIS

Epidemiology

Thyrotoxicosis results from an excess of the thyroid hormones, thyroxine (T4) and/or triiodothyronine (T3). It is a common condition occurring eight to ten times more frequently in women than in men in the UK. Its prevalence is approximately 2 percent of the female UK population with an annual incidence of 2 per 1000 women.[1] Primary thyrotoxicosis results from disease of the thyroid itself; secondary thyrotoxicosis results from abnormalities in the anterior pituitary gland, the site of thyroid stimulating hormone (TSH) production. Primary thyrotoxicosis is by far the most common, the majority of cases reflecting either Graves' disease or a 'toxic' nodule occurring singly or as part of a multinodular goitre.

Although often used interchangeably, the terms hyperthyroidism and thyrotoxicosis are not identical.

Hyperthyroidism should be used when hyperfunction of the thyroid gland leads to thyrotoxicosis. **Thyrotoxicosis** is the resulting clinical, physiological and biochemical picture resulting from thyroid hormone excess which may result from a variety of causes. The causes of hyperthyroidism are outlined in **Table 28.1**.

Clinical manifestations of thyroid hormone excess

SYMPTOMS

Patients with florid thyrotoxicosis have an easily recognizable constellation of symptoms and signs, many of which are attributable to sympathetic overactivity. [**/*] They will complain of anxiety, poor concentration and irritability. There may be insomnia despite extreme fatigue. Appetite is increased yet weight may fall as a result of the increase in basal metabolic rate.

Table 28.1 The causes of hyperthyroidism.

Associated with hyperthyroidism	Not associated with hyperthyroidism

Autoimmune conditions
  Graves' disease
  Hashitoxicosis
Autonomous nodules
  Toxic solitary nodule
  Toxic multinodular goitre
  Well differentiated thyroid cancer (very rare)
Pituitary conditions
  TSH-oma
Other conditions
  Trophoblastic tumours (produce HCG with thyrotrophic activity)
	Thyroid inflammation
	  Post-partum thyroiditis
	  De Quervain's (subacute) thyroiditis
	  Drug-induced thyroiditis (amiodarone)
	Exogenous thyroid hormone excess
	  Overtreatment with thyroxine
	  Thyrotoxicosis factitia (use of thyroxine in nonthyroid disease)
	Endogenous thyroid hormone excess
	  Metastatic thyroid carcinoma
	  Struma ovarii (teratoma containing functional thyroid tissue)

Stool frequency is increased yet frank diarrhoea is rare. Heat intolerance and increased perspiration are common complaints, and in women oligo- or amenorrhoea may occur.

In those with modestly elevated circulating thyroid hormones, or in the elderly patient, the symptoms are more subtle. Cardiovascular symptoms may predominate in the elderly, with palpitations, dyspnoea and peripheral oedema occurring commonly. Weight loss in conjunction with depression and agitation can occur, termed 'apathetic hyperthyroidism'.[2]

SIGNS

The clinical features and signs of thyrotoxicosis are summarized in **Table 28.2**. Patients may be agitated and have rapid speech and have warm, moist skin and palmar erythema. The hair may be thin and fine. The eyes may appear staring due to lid retraction and there may be lid lag, due again to sympathetic overactivity. Cardiovascular examination reveals sinus tachycardia or atrial fibrillation and in severe cases there will be signs of cardiac failure. Neurological examination may reveal a fine tremor of the outstretched hands, hyperreflexia and a proximal myopathy. There may be a goitre, the nature of which can give clues as to the aetiology of the thyrotoxicosis.

There may be a single palpable nodule in patients with an autonomously functioning adenoma or a nodular goitre in those with toxic multinodular goitre, and there may be a smooth goitre in Graves' disease (see under Graves' disease). The absence of goitre raises the possibility of exogenous thyroid hormone ingestion or struma ovarii. The thyroid is impalpable in a significant proportion (approximately 30 percent) of those with Graves' disease and toxic nodular hyperthyroidism.

Occasionally, the severity of symptoms and signs of thyroid hormone excess supports the diagnosis of 'thyroid storm', which is a medical emergency.

Table 28.2 Clinical features and signs of thyrotoxicosis.

Clinical features	Patient complaints
Sinus tachycardia, atrial fibrillation	Anxiety, agitation, irritability
Fine tremor of outstretched hands	Fast or irregular heart beat
Warm moist skin, palmar erythema	Fatigue, weakness and breathlessness
Onycholysis	Heat intolerance and increased sweating
Hair loss	Weight loss despite increased appetite
Proximal myopathy, muscle wasting	Increased frequency of defaecation
High output congestive cardiac failure	Irregular or absent periods.
Thyroid bruit	Swollen legs Hair loss and brittle nails

ATRIAL FIBRILLATION AND THYROTOXICOSIS

New onset atrial fibrillation or worsening heart failure may represent the development of hyperthyroidism, and atrial fibrillation complicates thyrotoxicosis in approximately 15 percent of cases. Its incidence rises with age, thus it will appear more prevalent in the elderly in whom cardiac failure or cerebral emboli may be precipitated.

Investigation of suspected thyrotoxicosis

A history and examination suggestive of thyroid overactivity should be investigated prior to initiation of treatment or further investigation. Laboratory investigations in suspected thyrotoxicosis are listed in **Table 28.3**. The single most important test is the measurement of serum TSH. If the TSH is within the normal range then a

Table 28.3 Laboratory investigations in suspected thyrotoxicosis.

Laboratory test	Findings	Comment
Thyroid function tests	Elevated free T4 and/or free T3	
Hormonal assay	Suppressed TSH	Unless TSH-oma/T3 resistance
Immunology	Positive thyroid autoantibodies	Typical of Graves' disease
Biochemistry	Elevated alkaline phosphatase	Elevated calcium
Haematology	Normochromic normocytic anaemia	Long-standing cases
Raised ESR	Subacute thyroiditis	

diagnosis of hyperthyroidism can be ruled out. The exceptions to this rule are rare pituitary causes of thyrotoxicosis such as TSH-oma or syndromes of thyroid hormone resistance. In these cases there may be a modest rise in TSH accompanied by a rise in T3 and T4.

A low TSH is not specific for thyrotoxicosis, and 'nonthyroidal' illness or treatment with a variety of drugs may lower the TSH below the normal range although it is still usually detectable in these circumstances. For these reasons it is preferable to measure the TSH in conjunction with serum T4 and, in specific cases, T3 as well.

In most cases of hyperthyroidism the typical picture is of undetectable serum TSH with elevated serum concentrations of T4 and T3. A low TSH and normal T4 should prompt T3 measurement as 10 percent of cases of thyrotoxicosis are so-called 'T3 toxicosis'. This is most commonly seen in mild cases of toxic nodular hyperthyroidism (either a single autonomous nodule or a multinodular goitre) or early in relapse of Graves' disease.

Specific patterns of thyroid function tests (TFT) are shown in **Table 28.4**.

THE ROLE OF SCINTIGRAPHY IN THE INVESTIGATION OF THYROTOXICOSIS

Although the biochemical diagnosis of thyrotoxicosis is easy to make, the aetiology of the underlying disease may be less clear. In most cases of thyrotoxicosis, a thorough history, examination and laboratory tests will be sufficient to make the diagnosis. In some cases where the aetiology of thyroid hyperfunction is unclear, diagnosis can be aided by the use of scintigraphy (see Chapter 27, The thyroid gland: function tests and imaging). This imaging modality can provide detail on overall thyroid size and

can be used to differentiate between 'hot' and 'cold' areas of increased and decreased function respectively. There are specific scintigraphic appearances associated with different conditions (**Figure 28.1** and **Table 28.5**).

Graves' disease

In iodine-replete parts of the world, the disease known in Europe and the USA as Graves' disease is the most common cause of thyrotoxicosis (**Figure 28.2**). First described in 1835, Graves' disease is a syndrome consisting of hyperthyroidism, moderate goitre, ophthalmopathy and dermopathy. In many patients, hyperthyroidism and goitre are the only features. Signs specific to Graves' disease include:

- diffuse goitre;
- thyroid acropachy (see below);
- ophthalmopathy;
- pretibial myxoedema.

It is more common in women than men in a ratio of over 5:1. Men are often affected later and the disease may be more severe. Its peak incidence is in the twenties and thirties, but it can occur at any age, although is uncommon before puberty. Graves' disease is more common in smokers (whose risk of the disease is almost

Table 28.4 Specific patterns of thyroid function tests.

TSH	T4	T3	Diagnosis
Suppressed	++	++	Primary hyperthyroidism
Suppressed	N	+	T3 toxicosis
Suppressed/low	N	N	Subclinical hyperthyroidism
+/N	+	+	TSH-oma
N	+	Low	Amiodarone effect without overt thyroid dysfunction

Table 28.5 Scintigraphic appearances associated with thyroid disease.

Condition	Scintigraphic appearances
Graves' disease	Increased uptake, homogeneous pattern
	Overall increase in gland size
De Quervain's (subacute) thyroiditis	Low or absent uptake
Thyrotoxicosis factitia	Low uptake
Solitary toxic nodule (solitary adenoma)	Gland may be of normal size
	Solitary area of high uptake
	Uptake in surrounding gland may be suppressed
Toxic nodular goitre	Gland may be enlarged overall
	Patchy areas of high uptake

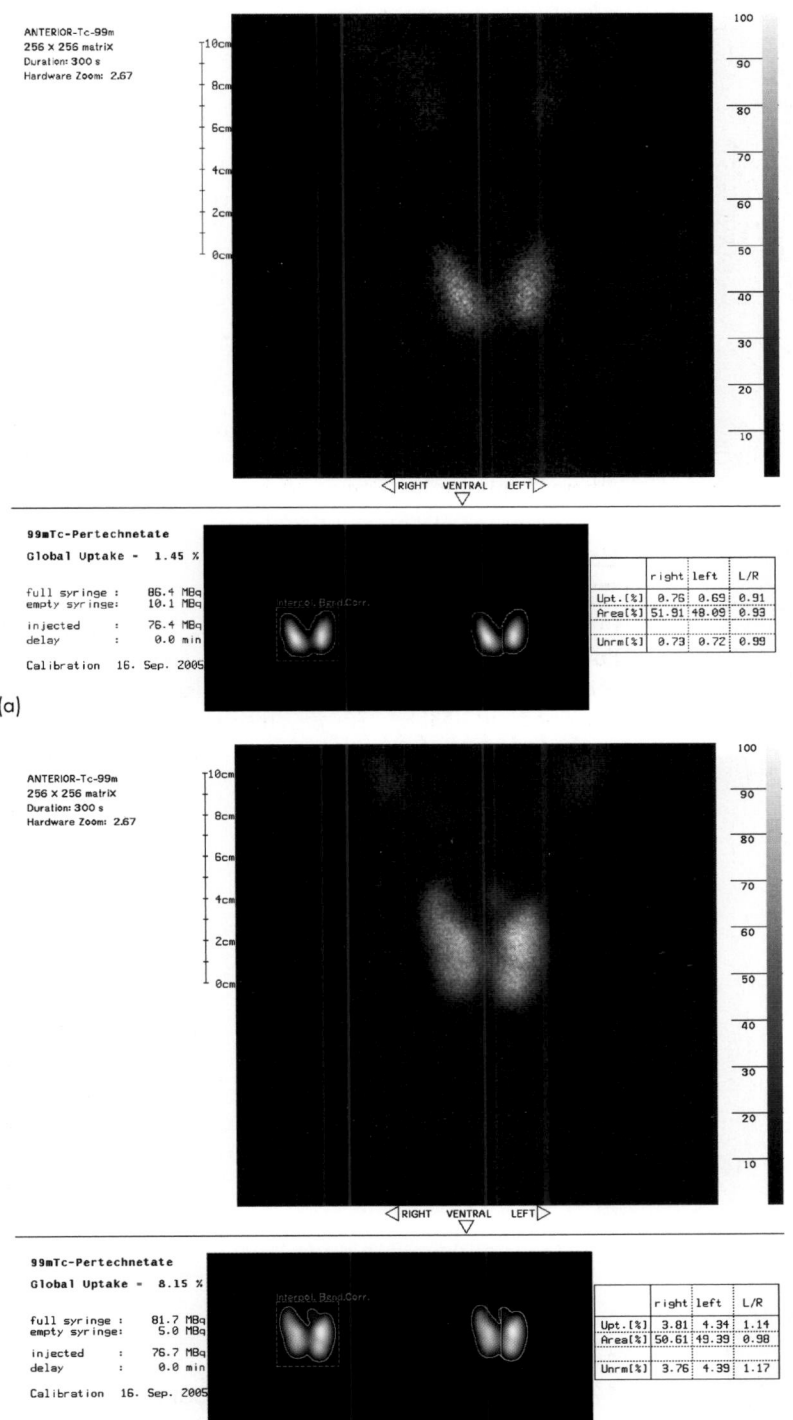

Figure 28.1 Scintigraphic appearances: (a) normal thyroid; (b) Graves' disease with pyramidal lobe (continued over). With kind permission from Dr Q Siraj, Queen Alexandra Hospital, Portsmouth, UK.

doubled) and smoking is an even stronger risk factor for the development of thyroid eye disease.

PATHOGENESIS

Graves' disease is an autoimmune condition and the hyperthyroidism is mediated by autoantibodies to the TSH receptor in thyroid tissue (TSHR-Ab). These bind to the extracellular domain of the TSH receptor causing activation. This stimulates thyroid hormone synthesis and secretion. Increased expression of growth factors such as fibroblast growth factor (FGF) contributes to enlargement of the gland resulting in a diffuse swelling. TSHR-Abs are IgG and are thought to be oligoclonal, unlike thyroid microsomal and thyroglobulin antibodies which are polyclonal. TSHR-Abs are not measured routinely in

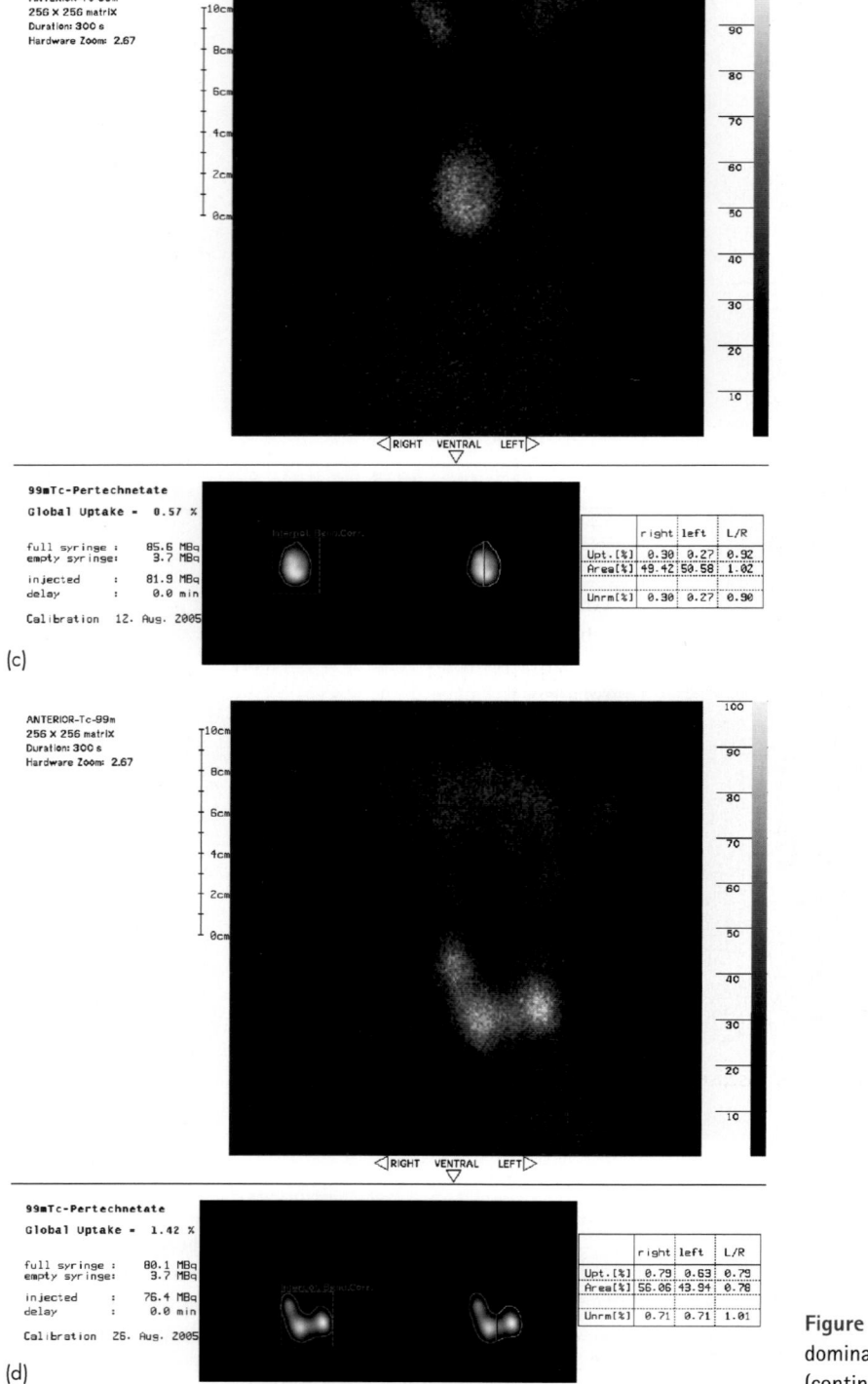

(c)

(d)

Figure 28.1 Scintigraphic appearances: (c) dominant hot nodule; (d) multinodular goitre (continued).

clinical practice as their prevalence varies between different assay systems and their presence or absence does not alter management of the individual (**Figure 28.2**).

Graves' disease tends to run in families, and a high concordance rate in monozygotic twins suggests a genetic contribution to the aetiology. The genetics of Graves' disease is complex with some genes conferring susceptibility, and others protection.[3] It is likely that Graves' is a polygenic disease occurring as a result of the interaction of several genetic loci in association with environmental factors, for example smoking has been suggested to increase risk. Graves' disease may be associated with other diseases mediated by the immune system.

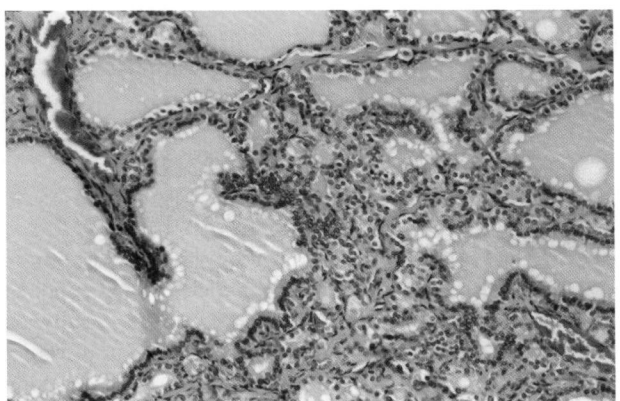

Figure 28.2 Graves' disease. A vascular gland displaying characteristic tortuous, hyperplastic follicles with blunt papillary infoldings. The thryocytes are columnar in outline and there is accentuated marginal vacuolation of stored colloid. (Haematoxylin and eosin, original magnification ×50). With kind permission from Dr Adrian Warfield, University of Birmingham, UK.

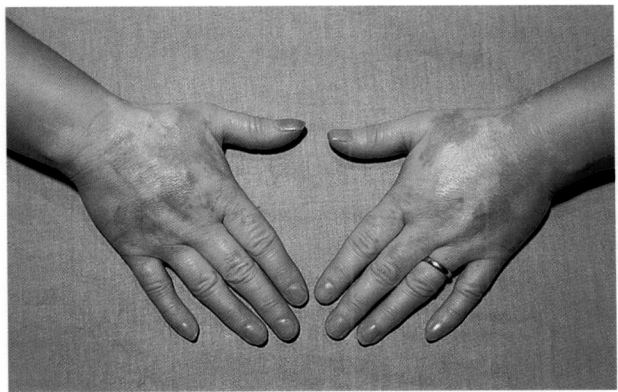

Figure 28.3 Vitiligo in hands of patient with Graves' disease.

In Caucasians, this is especially the HLA-DR3, B8 and CTLA-4 haplotypes. Associated conditions include type 1 diabetes, vitiligo (**Figure 28.3**), coeliac disease, pernicious anaemia and Addison's disease.

CLINICAL MANIFESTATIONS AND NATURAL HISTORY OF GRAVES' DISEASE

Although Graves disease can occur rapidly over a few weeks, in most the onset is gradual and insiduous. Patients exhibit many of the clinical features discussed above but in addition may have extrathyroidal manifestations such as ophthalmopathy (with exophthalmos and conjuctival oedema) and, rarely, dermopathy and acropachy.

A diffuse goitre is present in the majority of cases but its absence does not rule out Graves' disease, as the thyroid may be of normal size in around 3 percent. The goitre is usually symmetrical, there may be an overlying palpable thrill and a bruit may often be heard. The thrill and bruit result from the increased blood flow to the thyroid.

Graves' disease is usually treated with antithyroid medication in the first instance. Whilst adequate therapy is given the disease may be quiescent but may return if compliance diminishes or dosage is inappropriately reduced. As with many autoimmune conditions, Graves' disease is sometimes self-limiting and around 30 percent of patients experience lasting remission after treatment.

THYROID AUTOANTIBODIES

Three thyroid autoantibodies may be measured in clinical practice, those against thyroid peroxidase (TPO), thyroglobulin and the TSH-receptor. In a study of the prevalence and usefulness of thyroid autoantibodies, TPO antibodies were positive in 90 percent of cases of Graves' disease, thyroglobulin antibodies in 49 percent, whilst TSHR-Abs were found only in 45 percent.[4] Thyroid peroxidase antibodies are thus the most commonly measured antibodies in clinical practice.

EXTRA THYROIDAL MANIFESTATIONS OF GRAVES' DISEASE

Dermopathy

This occurs in approximately 5 percent of patients with Graves' disease, almost always accompanied by severe eye disease. Usually occurring over the skin of the shins and known as pretibial myxoedema, it may affect other areas of the body. The skin appears raised, oedematous, nodular and discoloured with a pink or brownish tinge (**Figure 28.4**).

The oedema is nonpitting and usually painless but may itch. It is caused by a build-up of glycosaminoglycans along with a florid lymphocytic infiltrate. Although not usually treated, if severe, fluorinated steroids may be used topically with occlusive dressings.

Acropachy

This is very rare and presents as clubbing of the fingers with subperiosteal new bone formation seen on plain radiograph. Again, thought to arise from glycosaminoglycan accumulation, it occurs in conjunction with ophthalmopathy or dermopathy. There is no treatment.

Thyroid eye disease

Many patients with Graves' disease have involvement of the eyes. Clinically detectable disease is present in around 30 percent, while imaging such as MRI will provide evidence of eye involvement in a much larger proportion. In the majority of cases eye disease is mild; however in some cases it may be severe (**Figure 28.5**). Patients who smoke are

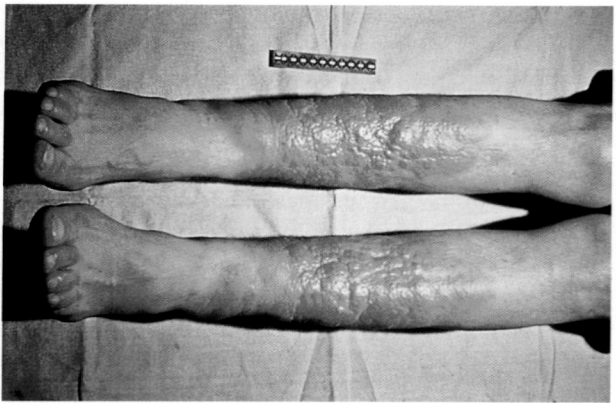

Figure 28.4   Pretibial myxoedema.

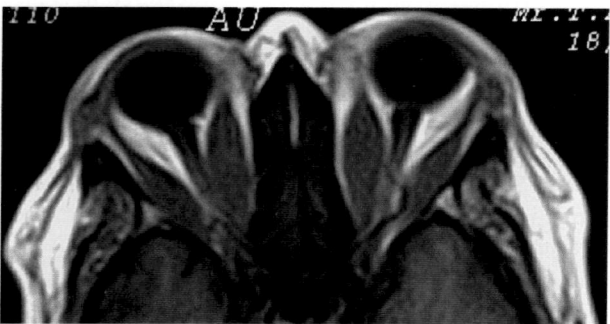

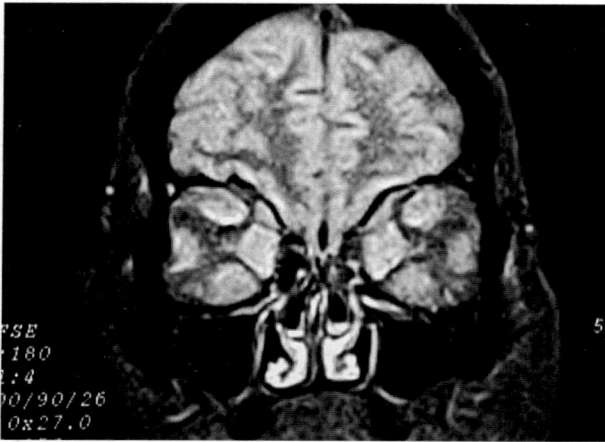

Figure 28.5   Thyroid eye disease: MRI orbits, showing enlarged extraocular muscles. With kind permission from Mr J Uddin, Moorfields Hospital, London, UK.

more likely to suffer eye disease of greater severity that nonsmokers and hypothyroidism may exacerbate it. In approximately three-quarters of cases, Graves' disease will develop either a year before or a year after eye problems begin, but on occasions this period may be longer. In these cases one may falsely conclude that one is looking at a case of 'euthyroid Graves' ophthalmopathy'. At diagnosis, 5 percent of patients are hypothyroid and 5 percent are euthyroid. The ophthalmopathy is characterized by

swelling of the extraocular muscles, proliferation of periorbital fat and late fibrosis leading to muscle tethering. The lesions develop due to an accumulation of glycosaminoglycans and a lymphocytic infiltration of the orbital and retro-orbital tissues.

Clinical features of ophthalmopathy

Early in the disease, patients may complain of irritation in the eyes and a feeling of a foreign body. There may be excessive watering, especially in the wind. As the disease progresses, there may be a change in physical appearance with periorbital oedema and/or a staring expression caused by exophthalmos and/or eyelid retraction. Eyelid retraction may give the false impression of proptosis, though both most often coexist. This may be bi- or unilateral and patients may complain of a feeling of pressure behind the eyes. Even in apparent unilateral cases, one will find evidence of bilateral disease, provided the right imaging techniques are used, such as MRI (**Figure 28.5**) or CT scanning. In the worst cases the eyes may not close fully at night leading to corneal ulceration and scarring. There may be apparent nerve palsies due to infiltration of the extraocular muscles with fat and fibrotic changes.

Signs of thyroid eye disease

Signs of thyroid eye disease include:

- conjunctival oedema;
- periorbital oedema;
- proptosis greater than 22 mm;
- corneal ulceration;
- decreased colour vision;
- conjunctival injection;
- lid retraction and lid lag;
- squint and eye movement problems;
- papilloedema;
- decreasing visual acuity.

Decreasing visual acuity and a loss of colour vision are ominous signs and may be caused by pressure on the optic nerve by the swollen extraocular muscles, or – less commonly – sheer stretch of the optic nerve. Urgent treatment is needed if permanent visual loss is to be avoided; the following symptoms indicate that the patient should be referred to an ophthalmologist as a matter of urgency:

- rapid deterioration in visual acuity;
- decreased colour vision;
- squint and eye movement problems;
- visual acuity of less than 6/18;
- corneal ulceration.

The disease occurs in two phases: a dynamic active phase and a quiescent phase. Unfortunately, even when well-treated and quiescent, patients do not always achieve a return in physical appearance to the premorbid state.

Treatment of thyroid eye disease

For mild disease, often no treatment is necessary. For local discomfort, artificial tears are useful, as is elevation of the head of the bed to reduce oedema. As proptosis and conjuctival oedema worsen, treatment with parenteral or high-dose oral steroids is required for a period of weeks. Radiotherapy is also a treatment option in early and active disease. Ocular nerve palsies need treatment by an experienced surgeon, as multiple operations may be necessary to align eye movements. Optic neuropathy may be treated both medically and surgically (**Figure 28.6**) with high-dose steroids, radiotherapy and orbital decompression having a role.[5]

Toxic multinodular goitre

EPIDEMIOLOGY AND PATHOGENESIS

Although Graves' disease is the commonest cause of thyrotoxicosis, in the elderly, nodular thyroid disease predominates. In all age groups, toxic nodular thyroid disease is more common in areas of the world where iodine is relatively deficient and, like all thyroid disease, is commoner in women than in men. The pathogenesis, aetiology and natural history of the goitre are covered in detail elsewhere, but may progress from diffuse enlargement to the development of one or more nodules. Autonomous function of one or more of these nodules results in thyrotoxicosis.

This may occur spontaneously or as a result of exposure to increased quantities of iodine (e.g. in contrast media), termed the Jod Basedow effect. Due to the long

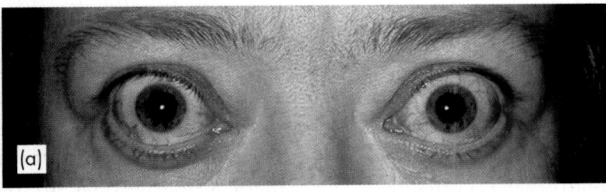
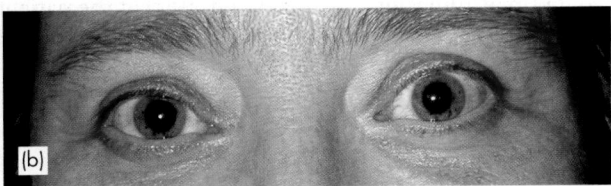

Figure 28.6 Patient with thyroid eye disease and optic neuropathy. (a) Pre-corrective surgery. Note the upper lid retraction, corneal injection, periorbital fat deposition and proptosis. (b) After surgical decompression. With kind permission from Mr J Uddin, Moorfields Hospital, London, UK.

natural history, an elderly patient presenting with a toxic multinodular goitre (MNG) may describe the presence of the goitre many years before the thyrotoxicosis develops.[6]

CLINICAL MANIFESTATIONS OF TOXIC MNG

In general, this diagnosis is observed in an older patient group than those who present with Graves' disease, and the degree of thyroid hyperfunction is typically less marked. For these reasons, the classical clinical symptoms and signs of thyrotoxicosis may not all be present. It is the cardiovascular effects that predominate, these include palpitations, atrial fibrillation and other tachyarrhythmias. In addition, patients with toxic MNG may complain of the presence of a goitre which may be longstanding. There may be dysphagia to solids and dyspnoea especially at night.

Toxic adenoma (Plummer's disease)

EPIDEMIOLOGY AND AETIOLOGY

A single toxic adenoma is a benign tumour autonomously secreting thyroid hormone. This is a rare cause of thyrotoxicosis and in the US accounts for only 2 percent of cases. A mutation in the TSH receptor gene occurs in 20–83 percent[7, 8] of patients with a toxic adenoma. Several point mutations of this gene have been identified, mostly in the transmembrane domain (see **Figure 28.1c**). The mutations are somatic, i.e. not in the germ line, and are therefore not inherited. These mutations result in the TSH receptor being activated, leading to autonomous function not under pituitary control. For this reason, the first biochemical abnormality often seen is suppression of serum TSH with a normal circulating T4 concentration. This is termed 'subclinical hyperthyroidism' and presents a complex problem (see below under Subclinical hyperthyroidism).

CLINICAL MANIFESTATIONS

Patients with a toxic adenoma are often younger than those with a toxic MNG, and present in the fourth or fifth decade. There may be a history of a slowly enlarging neck mass and many will have a palpable nodule. This is not always the case, as the autonomously functioning tissue may be diffuse and in this case the thyrotoxicosis may incorrectly be attributed to Graves' disease. The level of thyroid hyperfunction is again less than is seen in Graves' disease, so the symptoms and signs may not be so florid.

As Graves' disease may be treated differently to toxic MNG or a toxic adenoma correct diagnosis is important. The presence of a high titre of microsomal antibodies is more suggestive of Graves' disease, whilst scintigraphy distinguishes Graves' disease from toxic MNG and single toxic adenoma.

The treatment of thyrotoxicosis

MEDICAL TREATMENT

The initial approach to the hyperthyroid patient is to minimize symptoms (often with a beta-adrenergic blocking drug) and to reduce the synthesis of thyroid hormones. Three modalities of treatment exist: drug therapy, radioiodine treatment and surgery. These are summarized in **Table 28.6**. One randomized controlled trial compared thionamides, radioiodine and surgery in the treatment of hyperthyroidism and concluded that each was as effective at reducing thyroid hormone concentration in six weeks.[9]

DRUG TREATMENT

Antithyroid drugs

The thionamides – carbimazole (or its active metabolite methimazole) and propylthiouracil represent the mainstay of drug treatment of thyrotoxicosis. [***] [Grade B] These drugs block the organification and oxidation of iodide, thus blocking the synthesis of T4 and T3 early in their biosynthetic pathway. They are the most effective and rapid way of reducing circulating thyroid hormone concentration. They may be used in several ways:

- short term in the preparation for definitive treatment with radioiodine or surgery;
- medium term in the hope of inducing remission in Graves' disease;
- long term for control of clinical and biochemical thyroid hormone excess.

Dose regimen

Carbimazole is usually given in a starting dose of 20–30 mg per day in a single dose. Propylthiouracil (PTU) is given in divided doses and 200 mg of PTU is approximately equivalent to 20 mg carbimazole.

Side effects

Side effects can occur with both carbimazole and PTU. The most common side effect is a pruritic rash, which can usually be managed conservatively. Occasionally, the rash necessitates a change from one drug to the other and cross reactivity in this context is typically not a problem. Other relatively minor side effects include fever, urticaria and arthralgia. Mild side effects occur in 1–5 percent of patients. More serious side effects are rare and include development of an antineutrophil cytoplasmic antibody-associated vasculitis (typically associated with PTU) and hepatitis (induced more often by carbimazole than PTU).

The most serious side effect, agranulocytosis, occurs in less than 1 in 1000 patients. Agranulocytosis typically occurs in the first few weeks of treatment and is more common in those taking high doses. For this reason it is essential that all patients are warned (preferably in writing) of the risk of agranulocytosis and that clear instructions are given to present urgently for a full blood count if they develop a fever or sore throat. The agranulocytosis is usually transient and resolves after thionamide withdrawal. Agranulocytosis, along with hepatitis and vasculitis, is an absolute contraindication to the further use of thionamides.

Drug treatment of Graves' disease

Thionamides are used in Graves' disease due to their inhibitory effect on thyroid hormone synthesis and because of a questionable immunomodulatory effect.[10] If an established diagnosis of Graves' disease has been made, then the patient may be offered a full course of thionamide therapy in the hope of inducing remission. Two randomized controlled trials have attempted to define the optimal duration of treatment and concur that treatment should be offered for a period of 12–18 months[11, 12] as shorter courses are associated with higher rates of relapse. Treatment duration is agreed with the patient at the outset, but at any point medication may be stopped if definitive therapy is preferred. Drug doses are titrated according to the serum concentration of T4. This should be measured regularly, ideally every four to six weeks initially, then 8–12 weekly once control is achieved. Serum TSH may remain suppressed in the medium to long term in patients with Graves' disease. Most patients require a maintenance dose of 5–10 mg carbimazole and

Table 28.6 Advantages/disadvantages of treatment modalities for thyrotoxicosis.

Treatment	Advantages	Disadvantages
Thionamides	Rapid symptom relief	Risk of severe side effects
	Inexpensive drugs	Frequent clinic visits
	Chance of remission	Common mild side effects
	No exposure to radioactivity	Long course of treatment
		High chance of relapse
Radioiodine	Definitive treatment	Risk of hypothyroidism
	Outpatient procedure	Radiation protection measures
		Radiation thyroiditis
Surgery	Definitive treatment	Inpatient procedure
	Histological diagnosis	Risk of surgery
		Permanent hypothyroidism
		Risk of hypocalcaemia

50–100 mg PTU. Larger requirements are suggestive of poor compliance.

Efficacy and relapse

Remission rates with this regimen are less than 50 percent,[9] although may be slightly higher in the elderly. Relapse usually occurs within three to six months of thionamide withdrawal, in which case patients should be offered definitive treatment.

Increased likelihood of remission is associated with a small goitre or one that shrinks during therapy, although age and sex appear to be the most important predictors. Remission in men is approximately 20 percent, compared to 40 percent in women, and 33 percent for those less than 40 years of age, compared to 48 percent for those over 40. The ability to accurately predict who will enter remission would be of great benefit but at present is not possible. Once remission has been achieved, cure is likely if the patient remains euthyroid for six months, although a slowly increasing proportion relapses with length of time of follow-up. Relapse may occur after several years; poor prognostic factors for relapse of medically treated Graves' disease include:

- male sex;
- large goitre;
- severe biochemical disease at diagnosis;
- high T3 to T4 ratio;
- young age.[13]

Thionamides alone or 'block and replace'

Although most clinicians use thionamides alone to treat Graves' disease, some prefer the 'block and replace' regimen that uses thionamides to block endogenous thyroid hormone production completely, which is then replaced with thyroxine. Advocates believe this latter approach requires less monitoring and leads to better compliance.

There is no substantial evidence that the block and replace approach has any advantages in terms of remission of Graves' disease. There is clear evidence for increased side effects, some serious, probably related to the higher doses of thionamides required.[14] This regimen is also contraindicated in pregnancy because thionamides cross the placenta more easily than T4, leading to the potential for foetal goitre and hypothyroidism.

Drug treatment of toxic MNG and toxic adenoma

Thionamides do not induce remission or cure of thyrotoxicosis which is due to nodular disease. They may be used in the short term to induce euthyroidism, prior to proceeding to definitive treatment. As the thyrotoxicosis is usually biochemically less severe than Graves' disease, the starting dose of thionamides may be smaller, and if surgery or radioiodine is not appropriate, thionamides can be continued indefinitely.

Adjuncts to antithyroid drugs
Beta-adrenergic blockers

Beta-adrenergic blockers are useful adjuncts to thionamides in the treatment of thyroid hormone excess. They act promptly to reduce the symptoms, such as tremor, palpitations and tachycardia, but should be used cautiously in the elderly where heart failure may be present. Propranolol given three times a day or longer acting beta blockers, such as nadolol and atenolol, are the most widely used.

Anticoagulants

In patients who develop atrial fibrillation, anticoagulation with warfarin should be considered due to the risk of embolic complications. There have been no controlled trials of the use of anticoagulants in thyrotoxic atrial fibrillation (AF) but overwhelming evidence of their efficacy in other settings argues in favour of their use unless clear contraindications exist. Approximately half of those with thyrotoxic AF will revert spontaneously to sinus rhythm; this typically occurs within three months of initiation of antithyroid therapy. For those who remain in AF, joint cardiological management involving specific therapy to restore sinus rhythm may be considered when the patient is euthyroid. Chemical or electrical cardioversion is more likely to restore sinus rhythm in those whose AF is of short duration and in those who have no underlying heart disease.

Radioiodine (iodine–131)
Administration and side effects

Radioiodine generally represents the treatment of choice for hyperthyroidism, either as a first line in Graves' disease, toxic multinodular goitre or toxic adenoma, or as a second line in patients where treatment has failed in those initially treated with a course of thionamides for Graves' disease. [***] [Grade B] Radioiodine is administered orally as sodium I^{131} in capsule form, and may be given in the outpatient department. It is incorporated into thyroid tissue and the beta emissions result in lasting thyroid tissue damage. There is a lag effect with the maximum thyroid ablation occurring over six weeks to four months.

Efficacy and dosage

Radioiodine is the most popular first-line treatment for hyperthyroidism in the USA, with approximately 70 percent of physicians preferring radioiodine to treat Graves' disease.[15] Traditionally less popular in the UK, most large thyroid centres now also advocate radioiodine as the treatment of choice for Graves' disease. Depending on dose, 50–70 percent of patients achieve euthyroidism and shrinkage of goitre around two months after therapy.

The Royal College of Physicians of London recommended that the dose used should be enough to achieve euthyroidism with an acceptable risk of the subsequent development of hypothyroidism.[16] Empirical fixed doses of between 400 and 600 MBq are used to achieve these aims. Studies have attempted to define the optimal radioiodine dose for an individual patient in the hope of avoiding iatrogenic hypothyroidism. Factors such as thyroid size (judged clinically or by imaging), isotope uptake or turnover have been studied. A review of the current literature suggests that measurement of gland size and radioiodine uptake/turnover do not allow effective dose titration. In addition (and in conflict with older literature), it is clear that the dose of radioiodine required to cure toxic nodular hyperthyroidism is not different from that required in Graves' disease in the majority of cases. In iodine-replete countries such as the USA and the UK, doses of between 400 and 600 MBq are commonly used. Some centres give larger doses to men and those with large goitres in whom it is suggested that relative radioiodine resistance may be found.

Larger doses may be preferable in the elderly, especially in those with concomitant heart disease, to be certain of rapid resolution of hyperthyroidism.

Safety

Many patients are concerned about the concept of radiation treatment and perceive that there may be an increased risk of subsequent cancer. Radioiodine has been used for many years, with well-established efficacy. In terms of cancer, long-term safety has been well demonstrated.[17]

In children and adolescents, the thyroid appears to be more sensitive to the effects of radiation and most paediatricians would avoid radioiodine in these cases. National radiation protection policies exist and include measures to avoid contamination of the home or work place with I^{131}, including avoidance of close contact with small children, avoiding sharing utensils and sleeping alone.

Contraindications to radioiodine

Pregnancy is an absolute contraindication to the use of radioiodine due to the risk of ablating foetal thyroid tissue and resulting cretinism. A pregnancy test is necessary before administration of radioiodine and pregnancy should be avoided for four months after treatment to allow for resolution of the effects of transient gonadal radiation. Inadvertent pregnancies may be allowed to proceed to term, albeit with close monitoring. With exposure early in pregnancy there is a theoretical potential late cancer risk due to foetal irradiation, and exposure after 14 weeks may result in thyroid ablation, however, there is little evidence to suggest that birth defects are increased in this group. Radioiodine is also contraindicated in women who are lactating, in young children due to the risk of developing subsequent thyroid carcinoma, and in those who are unable to understand or comply with local radiation protection measures. This latter category excludes the elderly mentally infirm and those who are incontinent of urine.

Pretreatment with antithyroid medication

In those who are young and tolerating hyperthyroidism well, or those with modest elevation of thyroid hormones, radioiodine may be used as a first-line agent, perhaps with the concomitant use of beta-adrenergic blockers for symptom control. In the majority of cases, pretreatment with antithyroid drugs is preferred to make the patient as close to euthyroidism as possible before radioiodine is given. This is because it may take three to four months for radioiodine to induce euthyroidism whereas thionamides act much more quickly.

There may also be a temporary exacerbation of hyperthyroidism as the radiation damage causes follicular destruction and 'dumping' of preformed thyroid hormone into the circulation. Depleting the thyroid hormone stores with thionamides is advisable in the elderly or those with cardiac disease, which may be exacerbated by worsening hyperthyroidism. If pretreatment is necessary, then carbimazole may be preferable to PTU, as there is some evidence to suggest that there is a higher failure rate of a given dose of radioiodine when PTU is used.

Whichever thionamide used must be discontinued shortly before radioiodine administration to allow maximum uptake into the gland. Success rates fall from over 90 percent to under 50 percent if the drug is continued at the time of radioiodine administration.

Most clinicians advise discontinuing thionamides five days to a week before radioiodine is given and many recommend that the drug is restarted afterwards, especially in those with severe disease or who tolerate hyperthyroidism poorly. It may then be tailed off according to measurements of serum T4 concentration.

Side effects

Some patients notice a sore throat or neck tenderness reflecting a radiation thyroiditis, which is thought to occur in around 1 percent of cases. These symptoms are usually mild and transient. As a result of thyroid ablation, the main side effect of radioiodine treatment is hypothyroidism, although the percentage of patients who become so during the first year varies according to the dose of radioiodine used. After the first year, the annual incidence is around 3 percent and seems dose independent.

Follow-up

In the short term, clinical assessment of the patient should be carried out every four to six weeks. In addition to serum TSH, serum T4 concentration should be measured. Measurement of TSH concentration alone may be misleading as it may be suppressed for many months after treatment and does not necessarily imply that relapse is imminent, especially if the patient is clinically euthyroid and the serum T4 concentration is normal. If biochemical hyperthyroidism persists after a six-month period, it is likely that a second (and rarely a third) dose of radioiodine will be necessary, eventual hypothyroidism in these cases being common. Those treated with low-dose radioiodine, males, those with severe hyperthyroidism, and those with a medium to large goitre are less likely to be cured after a single dose of I^{131}.[18]

All patients who have received radioiodine require long-term biochemical follow-up. Effectively achieved with a computerized recall system, this is essential as the incidence of hypothyroidism is significant many years after treatment with radioiodine and, eventually, up to 90 percent may become hypothyroid. Annual measurement of serum TSH is appropriate.

Radioiodine and Graves' disease

Radioiodine is increasingly regarded as the treatment of choice in Graves' disease. In certain groups of patients, such as young women or those with mild disease, a course of thionamide therapy may be appropriate in an attempt to induce remission.

In general, radioiodine may be considered as first line, especially in those whom antithyroid medication is unlikely to result in a cure, for example in young men.

Some attempt to achieve euthyroidism with low-dose radioiodine but there are problems with this approach. Firstly, Graves' may recur in the thyroid remnant resulting in recurrent hyperthyroidism. In addition, uncontrolled hyperthyroidism results in a permanent reduction in bone density, and subclinical hyperthyroidism is a risk factor for AF. As the primary aim is to cure the hyperthyroidism, many physicians give radioiodine in a dose large enough to attain euthyroidism in the majority and to avoid recurrence. A dosage of 4–600 MBq results in euthyroidism in 90 percent of cases but at the expense of around 70 percent hypothyroidism over 20 years.

Radioiodine and ophthalmopathy

Evidence suggests that radioiodine may worsen moderate to severe ophthalmopathy. Studies have shown that the administration of corticosteroids may ameliorate or even prevent the development of ophthalmopathy. Most physicians delay administration of radioiodine until moderate or severe eye disease has been stable for 12 months. Those with mild eye disease are given radioiodine alongside a course of steroid prophylaxis.[19]

Radioiodine and nodular thyroid disease

Radioiodine may be used as the definitive treatment of toxic nodular thyroid disease. It can be used as first-line treatment in those who have mild biochemical hyperthyroidism and who tolerate it well. In the elderly, pretreatment with a thionamide is necessary to rapidly relieve hyperthyroidism prior to administration of radioiodine.

Radioiodine is effective in achieving euthyroidism and, in those with autonomously functioning nodules, hypothyroidism is less common. The autonomously functioning nodule causes TSH suppression, which, in turn, suppresses surrounding thyroid tissue;[20] radioiodine is then preferentially taken up into the nodule with sparing of the rest of the gland. Radioiodine may also cause shrinking of nodular goitres, with a reduction in thyroid size of 45 percent after two years.

Although around 90 percent are cured, those with large goitres or with severe hyperthyroidism may not achieve a cure with a single dose of radioiodine and a subsequent dose may be necessary after six months treatment with antithyroid medication.[21]

SURGERY

Indications for surgery

Although most experts agree that surgery has little part to play in the routine management of thyrotoxicosis, there are instances where partial or subtotal thyroidectomy is a safe and effective treatment for thyroid overactivity. [***] [Grade B] **Table 28.7** lists the indications for thyroid surgery.

Preparation for surgery

Thorough preparation is required to avoid thyroid storm postoperatively, as well as other significant, often cardiovascular complications. 'Thyroid storm' is due to the liberation of preformed thyroid hormone during surgery (see **Table 28.8**). Antithyroid drugs are routinely used prior to surgery to restore euthyroidism and, in addition, propranolol or another beta-adrenergic blocker

Table 28.7 Indications for thyroid surgery.

Indication	Comment
Patient fear/rejection of radioiodine	
Additional nonfunctioning nodule	If carcinoma cannot be excluded
Cosmetically unacceptable goitre	Slow shrinkage occurs with radioiodine
Severe ophthalmopathy and uncontrolled disease	No worsening of ophthalmopathy with surgery
Radiation protection rules cannot be followed	Mothers of infants, incontinent, mentally infirm
Local compressive symptoms (toxic MNG)	Radioiodine will also cause slow shrinkage
Pregnant women with severe side effects to thionomides	
Pregnant women with severe uncontrolled disease	Surgery performed in second trimester
Occasionally for amiodarone-induced thyrotoxicosis	If thionamides/steroids ineffective

Table 28.8 Features and management of extremes of thyroid dysfunction, myxoedema coma and thyroid storm.

Predisposing factors	Features/signs	Treatment	
		General measures	Specific measures
Myxoedema coma	Occurs in elderly patients with hypothyroidism who: • have withdrawn thyroxine; • have a severe concomitant illness; • are inactive, immobile or live in unheated accommodation.	Ideally HDU/ITU • coma; • hypothermia; • bradycardia; • hyponatraemia; • hypoglycaemia; • hypotension.	 • Treat precipitating illness with antibiotics if necessary. • Slow rewarming (0.5°C/h). • Warm humidified oxygen or ventilation if necessary. • Monitor and treat arrhythmias. • Correct hypotension and electrolyte imbalance.	 • T4 300–500 µg via NG tube, then 50–100 µg daily. • If no improvement T3 10 µg i.v. 8 hourly or 25 µg orally. • Hydrocortisone 50–100 mg 6–8 hourly unless hypocortisolism excluded.
Thyroid storm	Develops in hyperthyroid patients with acute infection who: • are post-partum; • have undergone thyroid or nonthyroid surgery; • receive iodine containing contrast agents; • withdraw antithyroid medication.	Rare but life-threatening condition, significant mortality (up to 50%): • severe signs of hyperthyroidism; • fever/hyperpyrexia; • alteration in mental state; • tachycardia or tachyarrhythmias; • vomiting, diarrhoea; • multiorgan failure – cardiac failure, hepatic congestion with hyper-bilirubinaemia and jaundice, dehydration and renal failure.	Best carried out in ITU • Cooling, fluid balance, antibiotics, respiratory support if necessary. • Correction of electrolyte imbalance. • Standard antiarrhythmic therapy. • Anticoagulation if in atrial fibrillation. • Chlorpromazine if agitated.	 • PTU 300 mg 6 hourly via NG tube (PTU blocks T4 to T3 conversion) • Potassium iodide (60 mg 6 hourly via NG) inhibits thyroid hormone release. Start 6 hours after PTU. • Propranolol 160–180 mg in divided doses or by infusion to block adrenergic manifestations. • Prednisolone 60 mg OD may also stop T4 to T3 conversion. • Plasmapheresis may be necessary in refractory cases.

may be required if euthyroidism has not been achieved by the time of operation. In some cases, for example those unable to take antithyroid medication due to serious side effects, it is vital to prevent the release of preformed thyroid hormone. Potassium iodide may be given for three days preoperatively to decrease thyroid secretion and reduce vascularity, during this time bruits disappear and the gland will be firm.

In the past, Lugol's iodine was traditionally used in this respect but is now avoided due to the unpredictable response and its potential for exacerbation rather than improvement in thyrotoxicosis.

Complications of surgery

Complications of thyroidectomy are relatively unusual, as there is universal agreement that those who perform such surgery should be experienced and perform it frequently. The most serious complication is bleeding into the operative site with airway compromise due to haematoma. Immediate evacuation of the clot and ligation of bleeding vessels is required. Damage to the recurrent laryngeal nerve is possible during surgery and vocal cords are checked prior to surgery. Unilateral damage causing some hoarseness usually improves after a few weeks. Bilateral damage is rare, but serious, as stridor develops soon after extubation. The ensuing airway obstruction necessitates a tracheostomy.

Damage to the parathyroid glands may be transient resulting from direct insult or an interruption of blood flow to the glands. The frequency and severity of damage increases with the extent of thyroid surgery and also correlates with the incidence of postoperative hypothyroidism. Transient hypocalcaemia may be seen postoperatively and the patient may be symptomatic with signs of neuromuscular excitability such as Chvostek's sign, Trousseau's sign and carpopedal spasm. Hypocalcaemia typically occurs one to seven days post-surgery; repeated measurement of serum calcium concentration is mandatory in this period, as is close clinical monitoring of the patient for the signs outlined above. Mild hypoparathyroidism may be treated orally with calcium supplements but more severe cases will require intravenous calcium gluconate.

Other complications of thyroidectomy include wound infection and keloid formation.

Surgery and Graves' disease

In most large centres the surgical treatment of choice in Graves' disease is a total thyroidectomy. In expert hands the recurrence rate with this procedure is less that 4 percent but at the expense of hypothyroidism, such that the patients leave hospital on T4 therapy.

Surgery and nodular thyroid disease

Toxic nodular hyperthyroidism may be treated by thyroid lobectomy or excision of a single hot nodule. The adenomas are often easy to excise and there is very little

risk of either recurrence or postoperative hypothyroidism. For patients with a toxic MNG, surgery is appropriate for those with compressive symptoms, such as dysphagia and upper airway obstruction, and for those with a cosmetically unacceptable goitre. Radioiodine may cause shrinkage of the gland and may be preferable in the high-risk patient although the rate of shrinkage is relatively slow.

Best clinical practice

Investigation of thyrotoxicosis

✓ Measure T4, TSH and thyroid autoantibodies in suspected hyperthyroidism. T3 and ESR may be useful.
✓ Ultrasound and nuclear medicine scans should be reserved for specialist use.
✓ Hyperthyroidism due to thyroiditis is often self-limiting. Treat with nonsteroidal anti-inflammatory drugs (NSAID) +/− beta blockers.

Treatment of thyrotoxicosis

✓ Treat hyperthyroidism with antithyroid drugs +/− beta blockers and refer to an endocrinologist.
✓ Warn patients (preferably in writing) of the side effects of thionamides.
✓ 'Block and replace' regimes with both thyroxine and thionamides are of unproven benefit.
✓ Radioiodine is safe and effective but hypothyroidism may result.
✓ Consider radioiodine as first line for the elderly and those with cardiac dysfunction.
✓ Severe Graves' ophthalmopathy is an emergency – refer urgently to an ophthalmologist.
✓ Reserve surgery for toxic multinodular goitre with compressive symptoms, severe eye disease, severe disease in pregnancy and in those who decline radioiodine.

TRANSIENT THYROTOXICOSIS/THYROIDITIS

Transient thyrotoxicosis may occur during the acute phase of thyroiditis. [**] [Grade C] The classification of thyroiditis is confusing but may be divided into those processes in which pain and tenderness develop, and those that do not have pain as a predominant feature (Table 28.9). Generally, the former rarely result in permanent hypothyroidism, but the latter often do.

Subacute (granulomatous/De Quervain's) thyroiditis

De Quervain's, giant cell or subacute thyroiditis is an uncommon cause of transient thyrotoxicosis. The typical

Table 28.9 Classification of thyroiditis.

Associated with pain and tenderness	No association with pain and tenderness	Also known as
Subacute granulomatous thyroiditis (De Quervains')	Subacute lymhocytic thyroiditis	Painless/silent thyroiditis
Infectious thyroiditis Gm+/Gm− organisms Mycobacteria	Occurring postpartum	Post-partum thyroiditis
Radioiodine-induced thyroiditis	Drug induced	Lithium-induced thyroiditis
	Chronic lymphocytic thyroiditis	Hashimoto's thyroiditis
	Occurring post-partum	Post-partum thyroiditis
	Fibrous thyroiditis	Reidel's thyroiditis
	Amiodarone-induced thyroiditis	

patient is female and aged between 40 and 60. Presentation is with pain in the region of the thyroid, often (but not always) with swelling. This is associated with systemic symptoms such as fever, dysphagia and malaise. The pain is a striking feature, may radiate to the ear and is worse on turning the head. On examination there is often swelling of either thyroid lobe, which may be extremely painful to palpate. Signs of thyrotoxicosis may present, such as tachycardia, tremor and irritability. There may also be fever. It can take eight weeks for pain to resolve and a complete resolution is seen in six months. Laboratory tests show raised inflammatory markers, such as erythrocyte sedimentation rate (ESR) and C-reactive protein (CRP), and there may be a normocytic normochromic anaemia.

Thyroid scintigraphy with Tc^{99m} or $I^{125/131}$ shows a complete absence of uptake, although this can also occur with thyrotoxicosis factitia and iodine-induced hyperthyroidism. Histology is characteristic and lends the condition its name, with multinucleate giant cells surrounding a central core of colloid. Initial TFTs show thyrotoxicosis with a suppressed TSH and an elevated serum T4. This reflects destruction of the thyroid follicles by the inflammatory process and release of preformed thyroid hormone.

At 12–16 weeks there may be a hypothyroid phase during which the damaged tissue is unable to generate thyroid hormone. Most patients do not require treatment with thyroxine and most are ultimately euthyroid.[22] Rarely, hypothyroidism may be permanent. Initially, thyroid autoantibodies may be positive but again this is often transient although some retain thyroid autoimmunity for life. The course of subacute thyroiditis is shown in **Figure 28.7**.

Treatment is supportive. Nonsteroidal antiinflammatory drugs such as aspirin and indomethacin are effective analgesics; beta-adrenergic blockers are useful if symptomatic in the thyrotoxic phase. Rarely, the severity may necessitate high-dose steroids (e.g. prednisolone 30–40 mg daily) which are extremely effective in reducing the pain

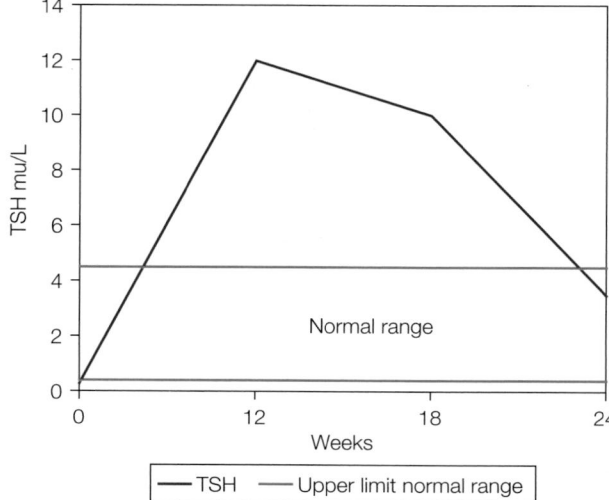

Figure 28.7 Course of subacute thyroiditis.

and swelling but must be withdrawn slowly over some months if the condition is not to recur.

The female preponderance, seasonal incidence, geographical aggregation and raised inflammatory markers have led to a hypothesis of a viral aetiology. Mumps virus, Coxsackie, influenza and adenoviruses have been implicated in the development of the disease although viral role in pathogenesis remains obscure.

Silent/painless thyroiditis

Painless thyroiditis can occur in the early stages of autoimmune thyroiditis. This may lead to mild biochemical hyperthyroidism and occasionally to symptomatic thyrotoxicosis. The thyrotoxicosis is generally mild and raised markers of inflammation are rarely found in contrast to subacute thyroiditis. The thyroid is enlarged in approximately half of the patients and is not painful. Fine needle aspirate reveals the changes associated with Hashimoto's disease and includes extensive lymphocytic infiltrate with plasma cells rather than multinucleate giant cells. Thyroid autoantibodies are often positive.

The duration of the thyrotoxic phase is around eight weeks and symptomatic treatment with beta-adrenergic blockers may be required. There then follows a hypothyroid phase that can last over six months. In most, euthyroidism is eventually restored but permanent hypothyroidism is almost certain to develop over time.

KEY POINTS

- Thyrotoxicosis affects around 2 percent of the female population.
- Signs and symptoms are due to sympathetic overactivity.
- Most thyrotoxicosis is due to Graves' disease but nodular thyroid disease is more common in the elderly.
- Treatment aims to ease symptoms and reduce thyroid hormone synthesis.
- Antithyroid drugs may induce a remission in Graves' disease but not in nodular thyroid disease.
- Radioactive iodine is effective in treating thyrotoxicosis, often at the expense of hypothyroidism.
- Total thyroidectomy may be necessary in some cases.
- Transient thyrotoxicosis may result from thyroiditis.
- Thyrotoxicosis may complicate pregnancy, and post-partum thyroiditis is relatively common.
- Subclinical hyperthyroidism predisposes to atrial fibrillation and may contribute to osteoporosis.

SUBCLINICAL HYPERTHYROIDISM

This is essentially a biochemical diagnosis consisting of an undetectable serum TSH concentration with a normal T4 and T3 concentration. Subclinical hyperthyroidism may be exogenous as a consequence of treatment with thyroxine, or endogenous as a result of nodular thyroid disease or undetected early Graves' disease. Exogenous subclinical hyperthyroidism is by far the largest group with over 20 percent having low TSH values on at least one occasion.[23] In the USA, over 600,000 elderly patients are estimated to be overtreated with thyroxine.

Complications

Potential complications of subclinical hyperthyroidism include a loss of bone mineral density, an increase in risk of AF and cardiovascular disease.

Evidence that subclinical hyperthyroidism is a risk factor for AF is clear, indeed it has been suggested that those aged over 60 with an undetectable TSH have a three-fold increase in relative risk.[24] Low TSH appears to affect long-term survival, since in the elderly population an increased mortality due to cardiovascular causes can be predicted by a single low TSH measurement.[25] There is evidence that subclinical hyperthyroidism is associated with osteoporosis, especially in postmenopausal women,[26] but clear evidence for an increased risk of fracture is lacking.

To treat or not to treat

In 1996, the Royal College of Physicians issued a consensus statement indicating that there was little agreement on whether subclinical hyperthyroidism caused morbidity, and thus the benefits of detecting it remain unclear.[16] Since that time, increasing evidence for associated morbidity and mortality (described above) is leading to the view that intervention (reduction in T4 dosages or consideration of antithyroid medication) is important.

Practically, it is sensible to repeat TFTs on a six monthly basis in those who have endogenous subclinical hyperthyroidism where AF and osteoporosis may have been exacerbated by excess thyroid hormone treatment. As these patients are usually elderly, radioiodine is the treatment of choice unless contraindications exist.

HYPOTHYROIDISM

Hypothyroidism results from insufficient production and secretion of thyroid hormones. This may be due to disturbance within the thyroid gland itself (primary hypothyroidism), or within the hypothalamic-pituitary-thyroid axis (secondary hypothyroidism). The causes of primary and secondary hypothyroidism are summarized in **Table 28.10**. Primary autoimmune hypothyroidism is by far the commonest cause.

The term **myxoedema** is not synonomous with hypothyroidism and refers to the accumulation of glycosaminoglycans occurring in severe hypothyroidism. These hydrophilic substances are deposited within the dermis leading to induration of the skin and the characteristic facial features of hypothyroidism.

Epidemiology

As in other autoimmune conditions, hypothyroidism affects females more commonly than males and its

Table 28.10 Causes of primary and secondary hypothyroidism.

Primary			Secondary	
Associated with goitre (TSH raised, T4 low)	**Not associated with goitre (TSH raised, T4 low)**	**Self-limiting**	**Hypothalamic (TSH low, T4 low)**	**Pituitary (TSH low, T4 low)**
Hashimoto's thyroiditis (chronic thyroiditis)	Atrophic thyroiditis	Transient thyroiditis — Subacute, or silent thyroiditis	Congenital — Lack of TRH	Congenital — Lack of TSH
Iodine deficiency (affects 800 million worldwide)	Iatrogenic, e.g. radioiodine, surgery, neck irradiation	Post-partum thyroiditis	Infiltrative — Sarcoidosis, tuberculosis, primary or metastatic malignancy	Panhypopituitarism — Pituitary tumour, cranial irradiation, infection, inflammation
Inherited defects of biosynthesis	Congenital anomaly, e.g. thyroid agenesis	Iatrogenic — Overtreatment with antithyroid medication	Infective — Encephalitis	
Maternal transmission, e.g. antithyroid agents	Drug induced, e.g. amiodarone, lithium, iodides, phenylbutazone			

incidence peaks in the 40–50 year age group, although it can occur at any age and juvenile hypothyroidism is not uncommon. The prevalence of hypothyroidism is estimated at around 2 percent of adult women and 0.2 percent of men.[1] Primary hypothyroidism accounts for 95 percent of cases with less than 5 percent being due to a lack of TSH.

Neonatal hypothyroidism, which if untreated results in severe intellectual impairment, occurs in around 1 in 4000 births and is routinely screened for in the post-natal period in the UK. At the other end of the spectrum of age, the incidence of hypothyroidism in the elderly is around 5–10 percent in women over 65. The symptoms may be nonspecific or falsely ascribed to increasing age, thus a high index of suspicion should exist in this group of patients and some advocate routine screening for hypothyroidism in the elderly.

Clinical features of hypothyroidism

An insufficiency of thyroid hormone affects almost every organ system in the body and the effects of hypothyroidism can be broadly divided into two: firstly the generalized slowing of all metabolic processes leading to, amongst others, fatigue, cold intolerance and weight gain; secondly, the tissue accumulation of glycosaminoglycans, which leads to characteristic changes such as coarse dry skin, hair loss and doughy peripheral oedema. Manifestations of and laboratory findings in hypothyroidism are listed in **Table 28.11**.

The onset of symptoms may be insidious and go unrecognized, such that severe myxoedema may result. The typical patient complains of lethargy and fatigue, and these complaints, plus the accompanying apathy and listlessness, mean that the ability to work is impaired. There may be a slow increase of weight despite a reduction in appetite and constipation is a common feature. Cold intolerance is typical with the patient wearing layers of clothes at initial consultation.

There may be a husky gruff voice attributed to 'laryngitis' but resulting from oedema of the vocal cords. Women may complain of dry coarse hair and brittle nails. Menstrual periods may be heavy and a desired conception elusive.

Myopathy may cause difficulty in walking upstairs or rising from a chair and numbness and paraesthesia in the hands may develop as carpal tunnel syndrome results from peripheral oedema. Occasionally, neuropsychiatric complications may develop with bizarre behaviour, so-called 'myxoedema madness', although this condition is now uncommon and confined to historical literature, which probably reflects earlier diagnosis and therapy. This is to be distinguished from a myxoedema coma, which is a life-threatening condition often precipitated by infection, trauma or cold and occurring most often in older patients (see **Table 28.8**).

Aetiology of hypothyroidism

CHRONIC AUTOIMMUNE HYPOTHYROIDISM/HASHIMOTO'S THYROIDITIS

This condition is the most common cause of hypothyroidism in areas replete with iodine. It occurs in around 3.5 per 1000 per year in women and less than 1 per 1000 per year in men. It is, in many respects, the archetypal

Table 28.11 Manifestations and laboratory findings in hypothyroidism.

Symptoms	Signs	Laboratory findings
Weakness/fatigue	Pale cool skin	Low serum free T4 concentration
Periorbital oedema	Characteristic facial features	Mild hyponatraemia
Constipation	Peripheral/facial oedema	Usually raised TSH concentration
Myopathy	Bradycardia	Positive thyroid microsomal autoantibodies
Slow/hoarse speech	Slow relaxing tendon reflexes	If TSH concentration suppressed consider central lesion
Menorrhagia	Hoarse voice	Normochromic normocytic anaemia
Coarse dry skin	Goitre	Raised serum cholesterol, triglycerides, LDL
Loss/drying of hair		Lowered HDL (atherogenic lipid profile)
Cold intolerance		Raised serum prolactin
Peripheral oedema		
Carpal tunnel syndrome		
Ovulatory failure		
Pale skin/flush (peaches and cream)		
Coarse facial features		
Decreased appetite with weight gain		
Intellectual impairment		
Neuropsychiatric problems		
Galactorrhoea		

autoimmune condition and is commoner in females, running in families where a history of Graves' disease may feature along with other autoimmune conditions, such as vitiligo, pernicious anaemia, rheumatoid arthritis and type 1 diabetes mellitus. Although it is most common in older women, it can occur in infants as young as two years of age and is the major cause of hypothyroidism in children.

First recognized in 1912, the pathogenesis of the condition is now relatively well understood. Both cell-mediated and humoral factors contribute to the destruction of the thyroid gland. T cell infiltration is pronounced with cellular injury resulting from direct action by cytotoxic T cells.

Although patients have high circulating antibodies to thyroid microsomes and to thyroglobulin, these are not thought to have functional activity. Histologically, the gland is infiltrated with lymphocytes and areas of follicular destruction and fibrosis may be evident. Enlarged epithelial cells with oxyphilic changes in the cytoplasm and Askenazy cells are commonly found in this condition (**Figure 28.8**).

Initially, the thyroid hypofunction may be subclinical, but may become overt with a rate of developing hypothyroidism at a rate of around 5 percent per year. A slowly growing goitre may have been found on examination or noted by the patient or a family member.

The typical goitre is moderate in size and smooth. Although both lobes are affected, the gland may appear asymmetrical. The presence of the goitre may predate the development of overt hypothyroidism and, generally, the goitre remains static or may decrease in size. Some patients present without a palpable goitre and are said to have atrophic autoimmune thyroiditis, which is thought to represent the end point of Hashimoto's thyroiditis.

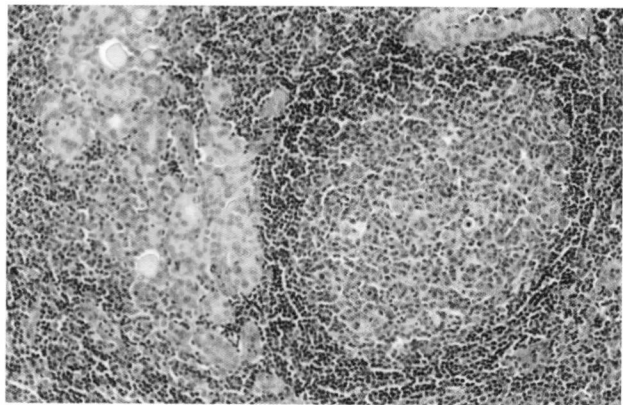

Figure 28.8 Histology of Hashimoto's thyroiditis. There is a dense interstitial lymphocytic infiltrate, with secondary germinal centre formation, enveloping small colloid-depleted follicles. These are lined with plump cuboidal oxyphil (Askanazy or Hurthle) cells possessing characteristic copious pink granular cytoplasm. H&E, original magnification ×50). With kind permission from Adrian Warfield, University of Birmingham, UK.

IATROGENIC HYPOTHYROIDISM

Iatrogenic hypothyroidism may result from surgery, treatment with radioactive iodine and external beam radiotherapy, such as used in lymphoma. Occasionally, hypothyroidism can result from overtreatment of hyperthyroidism with antithyroid medication, but with close monitoring this is not common.

Thyroidectomy

After total thyroidectomy hypothyroidism would be evident without treatment at around two to four weeks postoperatively, thus all patients who have undergone total thyroidectomy commence thyroid hormone replacement before leaving hospital. Hypothyroidism may also result from subtotal thyroidectomy with the majority of patients becoming so within a year of surgery.

Radioiodine therapy

This can lead to transient hypothyroidism resulting from radiation thyroiditis some four to six weeks after treatment, or permanent hypothyroidism may ensue months or years after therapy.

External beam neck irradiation

Radiotherapy given to the neck may result in both hypothyroidism and an increased risk of thyroid malignancy, especially in children and adolescents.

For patients who have had more than 25 Gy there may be a slow onset dose-dependent development of hypothyroidism.[27] Such patients should be carefully monitored for both the hypothyroidism that may initially be subclinical, and for nodular thyroid disease which may herald a thyroid malignancy.

IODINE DEFICIENCY AND THE THYROID

Iodine deficiency is the most common cause of hypothyroidism and goitre worldwide. In 1993, the World Health Organization estimated that 29 percent of the world's population live in areas of iodine deficiency.[28] Around eight million people have some degree of deficiency in iodine intake and 200 million are at high risk. Low iodine intake leads to impaired production and secretion of thyroid hormones, resulting in a raised serum TSH which stimulates thyroid growth. Diets high in goitrogens, such as cassava and some soya beans, can exacerbate the situation. Affecting those living in mountainous areas, it may result in neonatal cretinism, a combination of intellectual impairment, ataxia, coarse facies and deaf mutism. Poor performance and deafness in children can result from marginal iodine deficiency in iodine-deficient regions. Goitres may be present from young adulthood and can enlarge causing obstructive symptoms.

Iodine requirements are around 60–100 μg daily, and in the USA iodine is added to salt giving an intake of around 500 µg, thus goitre due to iodine deficiency is extremely rare. Occasionally seen in Europe where less iodine is added to salt, goitre may also be seen in those migrating from areas where iodine intake is low, such as Pakistan and Bangladesh.

CENTRAL HYPOTHYROIDISM

Lack of hypothalamic thyrotropin releasing hormone (TRH) or pituitary TSH may lead to hypothyroidism, although central hypothyroidism accounts for less than 1 percent of all cases of hypothyroidism. The commonest cause is a tumour in the hypothalamic/pituitary region, isolated TSH or TRH deficiency being very rare. Such central causes may be distinguished from primary hypothyroidism by a normal or low-serum TSH concentration that is inappropriate given a low-serum T3 and T4 concentration. Approximately a third of patients with central hypothyroidism display marginal elevation of TSH which is bioinactive.

Those with a pituitary adenoma may have other features of hypopituitarism, such as hypogonadism and hypoadrenalism, obscuring the symptoms of thyroid hormone deficiency.

Treatment of hypothyroidism

PHARMACOLOGY OF THYROID HORMONE REPLACEMENT

Thyroxine is the drug of choice for the treatment of hypothyroidism. [***] [Grade B] It is absorbed from the upper small bowel with approximately 80 percent efficiency and has a long enough half-life (seven days) to allow for daily or even weekly dosing if compliance is an issue. Thyroxine is a prohormone which is deiodinated in peripheral tissues to the active hormone T3. T3 has a ten-fold higher affinity than T4 for thyroid hormone receptors.

ADMINISTRATION AND MONITORING OF THERAPY

The aim of treatment is to return the patient to a euthyroid state both clinically as judged from symptoms, and biochemically as judged from serum TSH estimations. The average daily dose is around 125 µg daily but variation exists, typical doses required to achieve euthyroidism being 100–150 µg. In those less than 50 years of age with no evidence of ischaemic heart disease, a moderate dose (typically 100 µg) may be started immediately. In older patients, or those with known cardiac disease, a starting dose of 25 µg is prudent due to the risk of exacerbating or precipitating cardiac disease because of the rise in cardiac output associated with initiation of therapy. Increments of 25 µg can be added every four to six weeks until TSH concentrations are within the normal range. Due to the long half-life of thyroxine, four to six weeks should elapse before measuring TSH concentration

after initiating therapy or after dose adjustment. Once stable, serum TSH needs to be checked on an annual basis to ensure ongoing compliance.

In those with central hypothyroidism, it is imperative that hypoadrenalism be excluded before initiating thyroxine therapy. An adrenal crisis may be precipitated if hypoadrenalism is not treated before thyroxine therapy is commenced. In central hypothyroidism, the serum TSH concentration is of no value in monitoring therapy, thus dose adjustments should be made on serum T4 and T3 levels alone.

SITUATIONS REQUIRING ALTERATION OF THYROXINE DOSE

Elderly patients

Thyroxine therapy should be started at a dose of 25–50 µg daily and increased every four weeks until stable. Overtreatment, resulting in a suppressed TSH concentration, should be avoided due to the risk of precipitating atrial fibrillation.

Pregnant women

Women need more thyroid hormone during pregnancy and those with pre-existing hypothyroidism cannot increase T4 and T3 secretion as can normal women. Hypothyroid women need around 40 percent more thyroxine in pregnancy and serum TSH concentration should be measured at least in each trimester throughout the pregnancy and doses titrated accordingly. Most increases are needed in the second and third trimester when the baby is growing faster.

Patients with poor compliance

Due to the long half-life of thyroxine, poorly compliant patients may be witnessed taking seven days of thyroxine once a week.

Patients preferring T3 therapy

Some patients feel that their symptoms of hypothyroidism are not controlled on thyroxine therapy despite normal concentrations of TSH and T4. Some choose to take T3 in addition to or instead of thyroxine, although due to its rapid absorption and short half-life it must be taken three times a day and fluctuations in thyroid hormone levels exist. At present there is little evidence to suggest advantage over T4 therapy and is probably best avoided.[29]

Subclinical hypothyroidism

The term 'subclinical hypothyroidism' is used to describe a state where there is a raised TSH concentration with a normal concentration of T4. It is essentially a biochemical diagnosis. Subclinical hypothyroidism is relatively common with data from population surveys estimating a prevalence of 7–8 percent in women and 2–4 percent in men. The prevalence rises with age to approximately 15 percent in women over 60. It is also more common in those with other autoimmune conditions.

AETIOLOGY

Often this may be clear from the history, for example in those who have previously been treated with radio-active iodine or who have had a subtotal thyroidectomy. The patient may be already known to be hypothyroid and replacement may be suboptimal or compliance an issue.

A history of autoimmune disease, either in the patient or in close relatives, suggests autoimmune (Hashimoto's) thyroid disease. Around 60 percent of women with subclinical hypothyroidism have positive antibodies to thyroid peroxidase in the UK.

Prospective studies have confirmed that those with both positive antibodies and elevated TSH concentration are at risk of developing overt hypothyroidism at the rate of around 5 percent per year,[30] the risks being higher for those aged over 60.

MANAGEMENT

Controversy exists as to who should be treated and at what point, as the risks of inappropriate overtreatment to bone and cardiovascular system have been outlined. Recent guidelines state that apart from the fair data relating raised TSH to cholesterol, data showing clear benefits of treatment are lacking.[31] Many clinicians would treat if there were symptoms, a raised TSH over 10 mU/L and positive autoantibodies, due to the high risk of progression to overt hypothyroidism. For asymptomatic patients with a modestly raised TSH (below 10 mU/L) or with a low or negative titre of microsomal antibodies, retest on a six monthly basis is advised.

KEY POINTS

- Hypothyroidism affects 2 percent of adult women but its prevalence rises with age.
- Symptoms are due to an accumulation of glycosaminoglycans in soft tissues and a general slowing of all body processes.
- Chronic autoimmune (lymphocytic) thyroiditis (Hashimoto's) is the most common cause but iatrogenic hypothyroidism is also common.
- Thyroxine is the treatment of choice and treatment is usually lifelong.
- Instigation of treatment should be cautious in those where cardiac problems may be exacerbated.

Best clinical practice

Investigation of hypothyroidism

- ✓ Measure T4, TSH and thyroid autoantibodies in suspected hypothyroidism.
- ✓ Ultrasound/nuclear medicine scans are not helpful.
- ✓ Refer to an endocrinologist if atypical features or other concerns.

Treatment of hypothyroidism

- ✓ Treat with thyroxine if hypothyroidism confirmed.
- ✓ In the elderly or those with cardiac dysfunction reduce the starting dose.
- ✓ Monitor to ensure TSH remains in the normal range.
- ✓ In hypothyroidism due to pituitary disease TSH is unhelpful. Monitor T4 levels.
- ✓ There is no evidence supporting the use of T3 in addition to or instead of T4.
- ✓ Treat subclinical hyperthyroidism if symptomatic and TSH over ten. If TSH below ten, re-test periodically.

THYROID DISEASE IN PREGNANCY

Hyperthyroid states in pregnancy

POST-PARTUM THYROIDITIS

The immunological changes associated with pregnancy and delivery can affect thyroid status in different ways. Those with pre-existing disease may find symptoms are aggravated or ameliorated at different times during the pregnancy.

Post-partum, around 5 percent of women develop thyroid dysfunction.[32] The risk is higher in those who have positive thyroid antibodies, type 1 diabetes mellitus (25 percent), a family history of thyroid disease or another coexisting autoimmune condition.

Of those who develop post-partum thyroid dysfunction, around one-third have post-partum thyroiditis, with symptoms of thyrotoxicosis at around 12 weeks post-delivery, followed by a period of hypothyroidism at around three to six months. In some women, only the hypothyroid phase is evident and eventually there will be a return to a euthyroid state. Histologically, there is a destructive thyroiditis with a florid lymphocytic infiltrate seen at around 16 weeks in those who are antibody positive. The remainder of patients with post-partum thyroid dysfunction may present with either Graves' disease or Hashimoto's thyroiditis. In those with bio-chemical and clinical thyrotoxicosis developing later than three to six months post-partum, Graves' disease is more likely, and in these cases the hyperthyroidism will be sustained.

Iodine uptake measurements are the investigation of choice and can help to distinguish between post-partum thyroiditis and Graves' disease. The distinction is important, as treatment choices will differ according to the aetiology of thyroid dysfunction. Those with post-partum thyroiditis will show reduced uptake on scintigraphic scanning whereas those with Graves' disease will show elevated uptake. Breast-feeding should be avoided for only 24 hours if ^{99m}Tc is used.

Post-partum thyroiditis may be managed symptomatically with propranolol if necessary but Graves' disease is treated with thionamides. PTU is excreted less than carbimazole into breast milk and is preferred if breast-feeding is continued. Treatment of the hypothyroid phase may be needed in around a third of women and T4 may be necessary for up to 12 months.

Long term, patients who have experienced post-partum thyroiditis are at risk of further episodes in subsequent pregnancies, as well as having a high risk (over 50 percent) of developing long-term hypothyroidism. These women need follow-up with annual TFTs.

TRANSIENT HYPERTHYROIDISM OF HYPEREMESIS GRAVIDARUM

Transient thyrotoxicosis may be seen in cases of hyperemesis gravidarum, the likely mechanism being the raised beta human chorionic gonadotropin (HCG) level. Beta HCG and TSH are glycoproteins consisting of an alpha and beta subunit. The alpha subunit is common to these and other anterior pituitary hormones, whilst the beta subunit is hormone specific. Beta HCG concentrations rise to a peak at 10–12 weeks of pregnancy and then decline.

During this time there is stimulation of the TSH-receptor and increased production of T3 and T4. When HCG is at its highest, 10–20 percent of normal women have low-serum TSH. Women with hyperemesis gravidarum have higher HCG and estradiol concentrations than those without and around 60 percent show a raised serum T4 concentration with a suppressed serum TSH. Management is supportive and antithyroid medication should be avoided.

Thyrotoxicosis associated with hyperemesis can be distinguished from Graves' disease by a negative family history, a lack of any other autoimmune illnesses, negative thyroid antibodies and an absence of physical signs specifically associated with Graves' disease, such as eye signs and a diffuse goitre.

GRAVES' DISEASE IN PREGNANCY

Graves' disease accounts for around 90 percent of cases of thyrotoxicosis observed in pregnancy. Around two in every thousand women are affected. Menstrual irregularities, difficulties in conception and an increased rate of miscarriage are seen in women with thyrotoxicosis and women should be advised to delay pregnancy until euthyroid. Pregnancy in women who are biochemically hyperthyroid is not uncommon, and occasionally Graves' disease develops *de novo* in pregnancy. The diagnosis of thyrotoxicosis may be delayed as symptoms and signs may be wrongly attributed to physiological changes occurring in pregnancy, such as increased metabolic rate, increased cardiac output, heat intolerance and mood changes. Other symptoms may include hyperemesis gravidarum, muscle fatigue and, occasionally, cardiovascular problems such as pregnancy-induced hypertension or high output cardiac failure.

Treatment of thyrotoxicosis in pregnancy aims to achieve rapid biochemical euthyroidism whilst alleviating symptoms. Propranolol may be used as an adjunct but the mainstay of treatment is antithyroid medication, as radioiodine is contraindicated in this situation. PTU is preferred to carbimazole, being more strongly bound to plasma proteins; less drug is delivered to the foetus. In the rare instance of a serious adverse reaction to thionamides, surgery may be performed, preferably in the second trimester.

Joint management with the endocrinologist, obstetrician and paediatrician is important as there is a risk of foetal and neonatal thyrotoxicosis indicated by low birth weight, irritability and tachycardia.

Hypothyroid states in pregnancy

Overt hypothyroidism presenting at conception and in early pregnancy is relatively rare, largely as a result of a combination of anovulation and first trimester abortion which are associated with overt thyroid hormone deficiency. For those women who develop the condition in pregnancy, overt hypothyroidism can have adverse effects on both mother and foetus with increasing risks of pre-eclampsia, placental abruption, low birth weight and an increased perinatal mortality.

Considerable debate and concern surrounds the potential effect of mild or 'subclinical' hypothyroidism, indicated by raised serum TSH with normal free T4 concentrations, or indeed those with slight reductions in free T4 alone. Recent studies have shown mild but statistically significant adverse neuropsychological effects in children born to mothers with raised TSH in the first trimester. One study showed a decreased IQ in children born to mothers where the TSH was greater than the 98th centile, i.e. severe hypothyroidism.[33] Another study has shown a delay in psychomotor functioning in children born to women with T4 levels below the 10th centile at 12 weeks. Many of these neurocognitive deficits may be explained by prematurity or reduced placental function, and these studies have led to debate regarding screening for thyroid dysfunction in pregnant women. Current opinion is that only targeted screening should be undertaken, for example those with a previous or family history of thyroid disease or those with type 1 diabetes mellitus, but this approach may change as the evidence base increases.

TREATMENT OF HYPOTHYROIDISM IN PREGNANCY

During pregnancy, the requirement for thyroid hormone increases for many reasons including weight gain, transfer of T4 to the foetus and the raised concentration of thyroxin binding globulin.

Around three-quarters of women with treated hypothyroidism will need an increased dose during pregnancy, often by around 50 percent and sometimes as early as five weeks gestation. Most clinicians would measure TFTs around four to six weeks gestation, six weeks after any increase in dose of T4 and at least once per trimester. Post-delivery, the dose can be reduced to prepregnancy levels and checked to ensure it was sufficient.

Best clinical practice

✓ Thyroid disease in pregnancy should be jointly managed by an endocrinologist, obstetrician and paediatrician.
✓ Hyperemesis may be associated with transient thyrotoxicosis – treat supportively.
✓ Graves' disease in pregnancy should be treated with thionamides. Propylthiouracil is preferable to carbimazole.
✓ Aim to keep TSH in the normal range in pregnant hypothyroid women. They require frequent TFTs and usually need an increase in thyroxine.
✓ Post partum thyroiditis is common. Measure TFTs and antibodies in symptomatic women. Referral and treatment may be required.

NONMALIGNANT EUTHYROID CONDITIONS

Nodular thyroid disease

EPIDEMIOLOGY AND AETIOLOGY

Nodular thyroid disease describes the presence of a single or multiple nodules within the thyroid gland. These nodules may be palpable or impalpable, functioning or nonfunctioning. Functioning solitary nodules are those that synthesize thyroid hormones autonomously and thus may lead to thyroid hormone excess and symptoms of thyrotoxicosis. Aetiology, diagnosis and management are covered in detail under Thyrotoxicosis.

Thyroid nodules and goitre are very common. Lifetime risk for the development of a palpable nodule is approximately 10 percent, but prevalence may be as high as 50 percent depending on the imaging methods used. Nodules are more frequent in women and prevalence increases with age, exposure to ionizing radiation and iodine intake. The causes of thyroid nodules are listed in **Table 28.12**. The difficulty facing the clinician is to differentiate between the vast majority of benign lesions and the smaller proportion (between 5 and 6 percent) of malignant neoplasms.

In those with thyroid nodules, malignancy is more likely in those below 20 and above 60 years of age, in those with a previous history of neck irradiation and in men (although the majority of nodules occur in women). It is more common in those with a history of Hashimoto's thyroiditis, which is associated with lymphoma, and those with a family history of multiple endocrine neoplasia syndromes 2a and 2b (associated with medullary carcinoma). Those giving a history of a rapidly enlarging painless lesion, dysphonia or dysphagia should be viewed with high clinical suspicion. The factors suggesting malignancy in a thyroid nodule are listed in **Table 28.13**.

MULTINODULAR GOITRE

Data from the Whickam Survey in an iodine-replete region indicated the presence of a small goitre in 8.6 percent, a palpable goitre in 15 percent and a visible goitre in a further 7 percent,[1] the majority of lesions occurring in premenopausal females. TSH and thyroid hormones

Table 28.12 Causes of thyroid nodules.

Benign	Malignant
Colloid cyst	Papillary carcinoma
Simple cyst	Follicular carcinoma
Subacute thyroiditis	Medullary carcinoma
Infection, e.g. TB	Nonthyroidal malignancy
Lymphoma	Metastases
Follicular adenoma	Breast
Hurthle cell adenoma	Renal

Table 28.13 Factors suggesting malignancy in a thyroid nodule.

Highly suspicious	Moderately suspicious
Rapidly enlarging painless mass	Age <20 or >60
Firm or hard lesion	Male gender
Fixation to underlying structures	Solitary nodule
Vocal cord paralysis	Previous head or neck irradiation
Palpable lymphadenopathy	Compression symptoms, cough, dysphagia, dyspnoea
Family history of MEN 2a or 2b	Hashimoto's thyroiditis

did not differ significantly between those with and without goitres. When the same subjects were studied 20 years later, it became evident that the prevalence of goitre had fallen, confirming that a proportion may regress and thus treatment is not always necessary.[30]

Patients may present because the lesion was noticed by themselves, a family member or a health care professional. Many patients are asymptomatic and seek reassurance that all is well. Others may have symptoms suggesting thyroid hyperfunction, the investigation and management of which has previously been outlined. Those with a sizeable goitre may be unhappy with the cosmetic appearance of the lesion or may present with pressure and symptoms such as dysphagia, breathlessness and very occasionally, stridor.

Physical examination should focus on the size and consistency of the goitre with special attention to the presence or absence of dominant nodules, factors suggesting malignancy such as a fixed mass, lymphadenopathy and signs of invasion, such as dysphonia and stridor (**Table 28.13**)

INVESTIGATION OF NODULAR THYROID DISEASE

Modalities of investigation will, to some extent, depend on the clinical situation. For example, a flow volume loop may be appropriate in those with a large goitre and respiratory symptoms, a CT may be appropriate for those in whom a significant retrosternal goitre is suspected.

TFTs, antibody status and calcitonin

TFTs are frequently the first investigations in nodular thyroid disease. Those with suppressed TSH and elevated thyroid hormones should be investigated and treated as outlined previously, and those with a raised TSH and low T4 also treated accordingly. Biochemical investigation is important as fine needle aspiration cytology (FNAC) should not be performed in those with overt hyper- or hypothyroidism as cytological changes may be difficult to interpret in this setting.

TPO antibodies are also often measured but, in the setting of a euthyroid patient with nodular disease, do not add much to management, other than perhaps identify those at risk for developing thyroiditis or Graves' disease as a result of I^{131} therapy.

Serum calcitonin is elevated in medullary carcinoma of the thyroid but is not a cost-effective screening test in all patients with thyroid nodules. Measurement of calcitonin is best reserved for monitoring patients previously diagnosed with medullary thyroid carcinoma or in those in whom there is a high index of suspicion because of a family history.

FNAC

The mainstay of investigation of thyroid nodules, FNAC is safe, quick, cost-effective and has a high degree of diagnostic accuracy. FNAC is an outpatient procedure, best carried out by an experienced operator, with or without local anaesthetic and a 24–27 g needle. Samples should be interpreted by an experienced cytopathologist and may be graded as benign, malignant, suspicious or nondiagnostic. Nondiagnostic samples are obtained in around 15 percent depending on the operator (**Figure 28.9**).

FNAC in expert hands is very reliable, with studies showing overall diagnostic accuracy of between 85 and 100 percent, with specificity for the diagnosis of neoplasia of 72–100 percent and sensitivity of 65–98 percent. In a series of over 800 subjects, accuracy of FNAC was over 95 percent, with a false positive rate for malignancy of 2.3 percent, and a false negative rate of 1.1 percent,[34] rates that have been confirmed by others.[35] An important limitation of FNAC is the inability to distinguish benign from malignant follicular lesions, determining that all such lesions require surgical excision for histological diagnosis. If the patient is managed conservatively, then FNAC is often repeated after three to six months to attempt to further reduce the false negative rate from initial sampling error. Ultrasound has been used to guide FNAC, and in some centres is used routinely, however, the use of ultrasound scanning has not been shown to significantly increase diagnostic accuracy over FNAC guided by palpation.[36] Outcomes of FNAC are shown in **Table 28.14**.

Thyroid scintigraphy

Scintigraphy is of little value in the differentiation between benign and malignant nodular disease. This is because the majority of nodules trap isotope (Tc^{99} or I^{123})

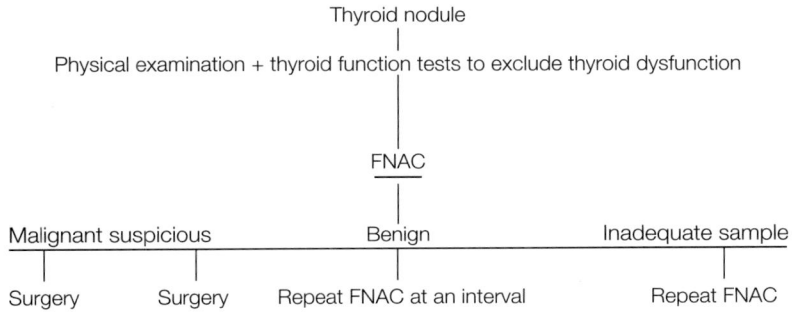

Figure 28.9 Algorithm for investigation of solitary thyroid nodule.

Table 28.14 Outcomes of fine needle aspiration cytology.

Category	Diagnosis	Percentage of samples	Range
Benign	Colloid nodule Hashimoto's thyroiditis	60	53–90
Suspicious	Cellular adenoma Follicular neoplasm Hurthle cell (oxyphilic) change	15–20	5–23
Malignant	Papillary carcinoma Medullary carcinoma Follicular carcinoma Nonthyroidal malignancy	< 10	1–10
	Insufficient/ nondiagnostic sample (can be halved with repeat FNAC)	17	15–20

less well than normal thyroid tissue, so appearing 'cold' on scintigraphy, yet the incidence of cancer in cold nodules is only approximately 10 percent. Scinitgraphy is thus poorly specific for the diagnosis of thyroid neoplasia.

Cost-effectiveness analyses have shown that where scintigraphy precedes FNAC, a delay in diagnosis occurs from 6.9 days from FNAC alone (in clinically euthyroid patients) to 17.7 days, and adds considerably to the cost of investigation.[37] Both the British Thyroid Association and the American Thyroid Association have published guidelines stating that scintigraphy has no role in the routine management of the thyroid nodule.[38, 39]

Ultrasound scanning

Ultrasound scanning has the ability to delineate the anatomy of the thyroid gland and some characteristics may indicate an increased likelihood that a nodule is malignant, for example the presence of microcalcification, hypervascularity and capsular invasion. It also allows the detection of other nodules in a gland where only one is palpable, additional nodules being found in around 40 percent, thought on palpation to harbour a single palpable lesion. The high sensitivity of ultrasonography can, however, lead to an increase in detection of clinically insignificant lesions leading to anxiety and further investigation.

Magnetic resonance imaging and computerised tomography

Both modalities provide high-resolution visualization of the thyroid and adjacent tissues, although do not give additional information about the structure of the thyroid over and above that provided by ultrasonography. Both modalities are useful in the evaluation of large irregular lesions with a suspected retrosternal component but are not considered useful in the evaluation of the presence and degree of tracheal compression due to variations in tracheal diameter with phase of respiration and position of the patient. With a large goitre, a flow volume loop should always be considered, as asymptomatic tracheal compression is not uncommon.

MEDICAL MANAGEMENT OF NODULAR THYROID DISEASE

Nontoxic multinodular goitre

Surgery is the treatment of choice where there is evidence of moderate to severe compressive symptoms, where FNAC of a dominant nodule is suspicious of malignancy, or where the patient prefers surgery for cosmetic reasons.[40]

Medical treatment of goitre involves the administration of radioactive iodine; the other medical option of administration of suppressive thyroid hormone is now considered outdated.

Radioiodine therapy

In those with severe compressive symptoms, a large cosmetically unacceptable goitre, or one where there is any suspicion of malignancy, surgery is the treatment of choice. In some patients, however, surgery is not an option either due to age, frailty or other co-morbid conditions, or because the patient refuses surgery. Medical treatment with thyroxine is unattractive for reasons outlined below. Current evidence supports the view that radioiodine is the treatment of choice in this group of patients.

Studies have found that nearly all patients experience a reduction in goitre size, which can be as much as 60 percent, and that although most shrinkage occurs soon after treatment, reduction in size can continue for some years after treatment. Most patients experience relief from obstructive symptoms with dyspnoea improving in three-quarters of those with the largest goitres, accompanied by an increase in cross-section area of the trachea of 36 percent.[41]

Factors suggesting a favourable outcome include smaller goitres in younger patients, a shorter history of goitre and higher doses of radioiodine. In those with large goitres, large doses of radioiodine may be necessary, which, due to radiation protection legislation, can entail the hospitalization and isolation of the patient. An alternative is to fractionate therapy over a course of some months in an outpatient setting.

Side effects of radioiodine therapy for multinodular goitre

Radiation thyroiditis (neck pain and tenderness) is uncommon, studies suggesting an occurrence of between 3 and 13 percent. Graves' type hyperthyroidism associated with development of TSH receptor antibodies may occur after radioiodine administration and is usually transient.

Occurring in around 5 percent, it is more common in those with high titres of thyroid peroxidase antibodies prior to radioiodine treatment.

Hypothyroidism, either transient or permanent, is not uncommon. The prevalence varies according to the amount of radiation exposure, with figures quoted ranging between 8 and 40 percent at one to two years. The use of multiple fractionated doses of radioiodine may significantly increase the risk of hypothyroidism.

There has been concern over the risk of deterioration in respiratory function in those with tracheal compression after I^{131} administration due to a transient increase in goitre size immediately after therapy. Studies have shown only a small decrease in tracheal cross-sectional area after therapy with no deterioration of inspiratory function. Some recommend the use of prednisolone peri- and post-I^{131} to minimize any risks in those with severe tracheal compression, but there is no evidence base for this practice.[40]

New approaches to radioiodine treatment of nontoxic multinodular goitre

Recombinant TSH may be used in this setting. The logic is that the higher the serum TSH, the greater the stimulus for radioiodine uptake into the goitre and the greater the chance of efficacy with a lower overall dose of radio-iodine. Although preliminary results are encouraging,[42] evidence for efficacy in volume reduction is not yet available, so recombinant TSH is not widely used at present.

Thyroid hormone suppressive therapy

Suppressing TSH secretion in those with goitres may result in a reduction in size of the lesions, as TSH is necessary for goitre development. This practice, first carried out in the late nineteenth century, fell out of favour until the mid-1950s. Although some studies have shown benefit, growth of thyroid nodules or goitres often resumes after discontinuation of thyroxine, meaning therapy may need to be lifelong. Suppressive therapy necessarily induces a state of subclincal hyperthyroidism (suppression of TSH) with risks of AF and reduced bone density, as previously outlined. For this reason, the use of suppressive therapy has been abandoned by most thyroidologists.[40]

Solitary nontoxic nodule

Much of the treatment of the solitary thyroid nodule has been covered elsewhere and is effectively similar to the treatment of multinodular goitre. Surgery remains the treatment of choice in those who desire it for cosmetic reasons, and in those whom malignancy is suspected either on clinical grounds or on the basis of cytological changes suggestive or suspicious of neoplasia. Suppressive therapy with thyroid hormones is not recommended for solitary nodules for reasons previously discussed.

Radioiodine therapy

This is a simple, safe and cost-effective treatment for those with solitary thyroid nodules which take up iodine (hot nodules) and a thyroid volume reduction of 40 percent may be seen after a single dose of I^{131}. Hypothyroidism is relatively rare with a prevalence of around 10 percent at five years and is higher in those with pre-existing thyroid autoimmunity.

Cystic nodules

These comprise around 10–15 percent of solitary thyroid nodules and simple aspiration is the treatment of choice, however, recurrence rates may be as high as 80 percent with larger lesions. For this reason, and the fact that many cysts resolve spontaneously over time, an expectant approach may be taken with small cysts less than 3 mL. Larger ones should be aspirated with FNAC performed on any residual nodule and surgery considered, as around 10 percent of large lesions may harbour thyroid cancer.

Thyroid incidentalomas

These are nodules detected on routine imaging for other conditions, such as Doppler ultrasound of the carotid arteries and CT or MRI of the head and neck. In nodules of less than 1.5 cm the risk of carcinoma is less than 5 percent, and it remains unclear whether incidentally found (and small) nodules require further investigation. If FNAC is contemplated, then ultrasound guidance may be necessary, as the majority of nodules will be impalpable.

New approaches to the management of solitary nodules

In some specialist centres, injection of ethanol into solitary nodules appears to be effective in causing shrinkage due to coagulative necrosis.[43] Problems with this therapy include seepage of ethanol outside the lesion damaging adjacent tissue, a painful rise in pressure inside the nodule and development of thyroid autoimmunity. For these reasons the procedure should be regarded as experimental.

Ethanol can also be injected into cystic lesions and a short-term placebo-controlled study has been promising with success rates for shrinkage of up to 80 percent.[44] Side effects seem less than those seen in injection into a solid lesion but the practice is not yet widespread.

KEY POINTS

- Thyroid nodules are common and occur singly or as part of a multinodular goitre.
- Nodules may function autonomously producing thyroid hormones, a small proportion may be malignant.
- Multinodular goitres may be large and cause compressive symptoms.

- Fine needle aspiration cytology is the investigation of choice in the management of thyroid nodules.
- Surgical excision is necessary where there is any suspicion of malignancy on cytology, for compressive symptoms or cosmesis.
- Medical treatment of multinodular goitre and autonomously functioning nodules with radioiodine is safe and effective.
- Medical treatment of thyroid nodules with thyroxine induces subclinical hyperthyroidism and should be abandonded.

Best clinical practice

✓ Assess thyroid status in patients with nodular thyroid disease clinically and biochemically.
✓ Refer all nodules for further investigation.
✓ Urgent referral if young or older, rapidly enlarging, fixed, invasive or compressive symptoms.
✓ Multinodular goitre causing compressive symptoms should be referred.
✓ Reserve ultrasonography, FNAC and other investigations for specialist use.

Deficiencies in current knowledge and areas for future research

Further work on the long-term sequelae of thyroid disease, both in the foetus and in adulthood, may add to the debate on screening for thyroid dysfunction, especially in women of childbearing age. Research into Graves' disease pathogenesis centres on identifying genes conferring susceptibility and protection from this disease. Already, major progress has been achieved in identifying the role of specific components of the HLA system and other immune regulatory genes such as CTLA-4, which have functional consequences. Better understanding of the genetic mechanisms leading to this autoimmune disorder may lead to targeted therapies for immune modulation. Such understanding may also allow better prediction of treatment outcomes, for example response to antithyroid drugs and hence better tailoring of therapies for individual patients. The ability to predict outcome in Graves' disease would be of immense clinical value.

Current research into Graves' ophthalmopathy attempts to elucidate the precise aetiology of the condition. Newly developed animal models may have a positive impact in this field. Research into new approaches to treating thyroid eye disease has focused on the use of cytokine antagonists, somatostatin and analogues and also on the use of antioxidants;[45] in future it would be expected that double blind trials involving some of these agents may begin.

Importantly, we are beginning to understand the long-term morbidity, and indeed mortality, associated with thyroid dysfunction, largely vascular. This understanding will drive the development of more intensive and effective clinical management strategies and identification of those at particular risk. Future research in nodular thyroid disease will focus on ways of improving the diagnostic pathway to reduce the number of patients undergoing lobectomy for what proves to be benign disease. Current research into ultrasound and colour Doppler criteria for identification of malignancy may have a positive impact. More likely, however, is a major impact of gene expression studies allowing discrimination, perhaps on biopsy specimens, of benign from malignant disease, as well as identification of genetic and molecular markers in resected tumours which will predict potential recurrence and hence the need for intensive therapy.

REFERENCES

1. Tunbridge WM, Evered DC, Hall R, Appleton D, Brewis M, Clark F *et al.* The spectrum of thyroid disease in a community: the Whickham Survey. *Clinical Endocrinology.* 1977; **6**: 481–933.
2. Nordyke RA, Gilbert Jr FL, Harada AS. Graves' disease. Influence of age on clinical findings. *Archives of Internal Medicine.* 1998; **3**: 626–31.
3. Gough SC. The genetics of Graves' disease. *Endocrinology and Metablism Clinics of North America.* 2000; **2**: 255–66.
4. Kumar H, Daykin J, Betteridge J, Holder R, Sheppard MC, Franklyn JA. Prevalence and clinical usefulness of thyroid autoantibodies in different disease states of the thyroid. *Clinical Endocrinology.* 1999; **50**: 679–82.
5. Wiersinga WM, Prummel MF. Graves ophthalmopathy: a rational approach to treatment. *Trends in Endocrinology and Metabolism.* 2002; **7**: 280–7.
 * 6. Vitti P, Rago T, Tonnachera M, Pinvera A. Toxic multinodular goiter in the elderly. *Journal of Clinical Investigation.* 2002; **10**: 16–18.
 * 7. Russo D, Arturi F, Suares HG, Schlumberger M, Du Villard JA, Crocetti U *et al.* Thyrotropin receptor gene alteration in thyroid hyperfunctioning adenomas. *Journal of Clinical Endocrinology and Metabolism.* 1996; **4**: 1548–51.
 * 8. Tonnachera M, Chiovato L, Pincera A, Agretti P, Fiore E, Cetani F *et al.* Hyperfunctioning nodules in toxic multinodular goiters share activating receptor mutations with solitary toxic adenoma. *Journal of Clinical Endocrinology and Metabolism.* 1998; **2**: 492–8.

∗ 9. Torring O, Tallstedt L, Wallin G, Lundell G, Ljunggren JG, Taube A *et al.* Graves' hyperthyroidism: treatment with anti-thyroid drugs, surgery or radioiodine – a prospective randomised study. Thyroid Study Group. *Journal of Clinical Endocrinology and Metabolism.* 1996; **8**: 2986–93.

∗ 10. Franklyn JA. Drug therapy: the management of hyperthyroidism. *New England Journal of Medicine.* 1994; **330**: 1731–8.

∗ 11. Allanic H, Fauchet R, Orgiazzi J. Anti-thyroid drugs and Graves' disease: a prospective randomised evaluation of the efficacy of treatment duration. *Journal of Clinical Endocrinology and Metabolism.* 1990; **3**: 675–9.

12. Maugendre D, Gatel A, Campion L, Massart C, Guilhem I, Lorcy Y *et al.* Anti-thyroid drugs and Graves' disease-prospective randomized assessment of long-term treatment. *Clinical Endocrinology.* 1999; **1**: 127–32.

13. Chowdhury TA, Dyer PH. Clinical, biochemical and immunological characteristics of relapsers and non-relapsers of thyrotoxicosis treated with anti-thyroid drugs. *Journal of Internal Medicine.* 1998; **4**: 293–7.

14. Wiersinga WM. Immunosuppression of Graves' hyperthyroidism – still an elusive goal. *New England Journal of Medicine.* 1996; **334**: 265–6.

15. Wartofsky L, Glinoer D, Solomon B, Nagataki S, Lagasse R, Nagayama Y *et al.* Differences and similarities in the diagnosis and treatment of Graves' disease in Europe, Japan and the United States. *Thyroid.* 1991; **2**: 129–35.

16. Vanderpump MP, Alquist JA, Franklyn JA, Clayton RN. Consensus statement for good practice and audit measures in the management of hypothyroidism and hyperthyroidism. The Research Unit of the Royal College of Physicians of London, the Endocrinology and Diabetes Committee of the Royal College of Physicians of London, and the Society for Endocrinology. *British Medical Journal.* 1996; **7056**: 539–44.

17. Franklyn JA, Maisonneuve P, Sheppard M, Betteridge J, Boyle P. Cancer incidence and mortality after radioiodine treatment for hyperthyroidism: a population-based cohort study. *Lancet.* 1999; **9170**: 2111–5.

∗ 18. Allahabadia A, Daykin J, Sheppard MC, Gough SC, Franklyn JA. Radioiodine treatment of hyperthyroidism – prognostic factors for outcome. *Journal of Clinical Endocrinology and Metabolism.* 2001; **8**: 3611–7.

19. Wiersinga WM, Bartalena L. Epidemiology and prevention of Graves' ophthalmopathy. *Thyroid.* 2002; **10**: 855–60.

20. Nygaard B, Hegedus L, Nielsen KG, Ulriksen P, Hansen JM. Long-term effect of radioactive iodine on thyroid function and size in solitary autonomously functioning toxic thyroid nodules. *Clinical Endocrinology.* 1999; **2**: 197–202.

21. Nygaard B, Hegedus L, Ulriksen P, Nielsen KG, Hansen JM. Radioiodine for multinodular goitre. *Archives of Internal Medicine.* 1999; **12**: 1364–8.

22. Fatourechi V, Anisewzki JP, Fatourechi GZ, Atkinson EJ, Jacobse SG. Clinical features and outcome of subacute thyroiditis in an incidence cohort: Olmsted County, Minnesota, study. *Journal of Clinical Endocrinology and Metabolism.* 2003; **5**: 2100–5.

∗ 23. Parle JV, Franklyn JA, Cross KW, Jones SC, Sheppard MC. Thyroxine prescription in the community: serum thyroid stimulating hormone level assays as an indicator of undertreatment or overtreatment. *British Journal of General Practice.* 1993; **43**: 107–9.

24. Sawin CT, Geller A, Wolf PA, Belanger AJ, Baker E, Bacharach P *et al.* Low serum thyrotropin concentrations as a risk factor for atrial fibrillation in older persons. *New England Journal of Medicine.* 1994; **19**: 1249–52.

25. Parle JV, Maisonneuve P, Sheppard MC, Boyle P, Franklyn JA. Prediction of all-cause mortality in elderly people from one low serum thyrotropin result: a 10 year cohort study. *Lancet.* 2001; **9285**: 861–5.

26. Faber J, Galloe AM. Changes in bone mass during prolonged sub-clinical hyperthyroidism due to L-thyroxine treatment: a meta-analysis. *European Journal of Endocrinology.* 1994; **4**: 350–6.

∗ 27. Hancock SL, Cox RS, McDougall IR. Thyroid diseases after treatment of Hodgkin's disease. *New England Journal of Medicine.* 1991; **9**: 599–605.

28. WHO/UNICEF/ICCIDD. Global prevalence of iodine deficiency disorders. MDIS working paper #1. Micronutrient Deficiency Information System. Geneva. World Health Organisation. 1993.

∗ 29. Bunevicius R, Kazanavicuis G, Zalinkevicius R, Prange Jr AJ. Effects of thyroxine as compared with thyroxine plus triiodothyronine in patients with hypothyroidism. *New England Journal of Medicine.* 1999; **6**: 424–9.

30. Vanderpump MP, Tunbridge WM, French JM, Appleton D, Bates D, Clark F *et al.* The incidence of thyroid disorders in the community: a twenty-year follow-up of the Whickham Survey. *Clinical Endocrinology.* 1995; **1**: 55–68.

31. Surks MI, Ortiz E, Daniels GH, Sawin CT, Col NF, Cobin RH *et al.* Subclinical thyroid disease: scientific review and guidelines for diagnosis and management. *Journal of the American Medical Association.* 2004; **291**: 228–38.

32. Muller AF, Drexhage HE, Berghout A. Postpartum thyroiditis and autoimmune thyroiditis in women of childbearing age: recent insights and consequences for antenatal and post natal care. *Endocrine Reviews.* 2003; **22**: 605–30.

33. Haddow JE, Palomaki GE, Allan WC, Williams JR, Knoght GJ, Gagnon J *et al.* Maternal thyroid deficiency during pregnancy and subsequent neuropsychological development of the child. *New England Journal of Medicine.* 1999; **341**: 549–55.

34. La Rosa GL, Belfiore A, Guiffrida D, Sicurell C, Ippolito O, Russo G *et al.* Evaluation of fine needle aspiration biopsy in the preoperative selection of cold thyroid nodules. *Cancer.* 1991; **67**: 2137–41.

35. Kumar H, Daykin J, Holder R, Watkinson JC, Sheppard MC, Franklyn JA. Gender, clinical findings, and serum thyrotropin measurements in the prediction of thyroid neoplasia in 1005 patients presenting with thyroid enlargement and investigated by fine needle aspiration cytology. *Thyroid.* 1999; **9**: 1105–9.

36. Danese D, Sciaccitano S, Farsetti A, Andreaoli M, Pontecorvi A. Diagnostic accuracy of conventional *vs* sonography-guided fine-needle aspiration biopsy of thyroid nodules. *Thyroid*. 1998; **8**: 15–21.

37. Ortiz R, Hupart KH, DeFesi CR, Surks MI. Effect of early referral to an endocrinologist on efficiency and cost of evaluation and development of treatment plan in patients with thyroid nodules. *Journal of Clinical Endocrinology and Metabolism*. 1998; **11**: 2803–7.

38. Guidelines for the management of thyroid cancer in adults. Joint publication, British Thyroid Association and Royal College of Physicians 2002.

39. Singer PA, Cooper DS, Daniels GH, Ladenson PW, Greenspan FW, Levy EG *et al.* Treatment guidelines for patients with thyroid nodules and well differentiated thyroid cancer. American Thyroid Association. *Archives of Internal Medicine*. 1996; **156**: 2165–72.

40. Hegedus L, Bonemma SJ, Bennedbaek FN. Management of simple nodular goiter: current status and future perspectives. *Endocrine Reviews*. 2003; **24**: 102–32.

41. Huysmans DA, Hermus AR, Corstens FH, Barentsz JD, Kloppenborg PW. Large compressive goitres treated with radioiodine. *Annals of Internal Medicine*. 1994; **121**: 757–62.

42. Huysmans DA, Nieuwlaat W, Erdtsieck J, Schellekens AP, Bus JW, Bravenboer B *et al.* Administration of a single low dose of recombinant human thyrotropin significantly enhances radioidine uptake in nontoxic nodular goitre. *Journal of Clinical Endocrinology and Metabolism*. 2000; **85**: 3592–6.

43. Caraccio N, Goletti O, Lippolis PV, Casolaro A, Cavina E, Miccoli P *et al.* Is percutaneous ethanol injection a useful alternative for the treatment of the cold benign thyroid nodules? Five years experience. *Thyroid*. 1997; **7**: 699–704.

44. Verde G, Papini E, Pacella CM, Galloti C, Delpiano S, Strada S *et al.* Ultrasound guided percutaneous ethanol injection in the treatment of cystic thyroid nodules. *Clinical Endocrinology*. 1994; **41**: 719–24.

45. Bartalena L, Wiersinga WM, Pinchera A. Graves' ophthalmopathy: state of the art and perspectives. *Journal of Endocrinological Investigation*. 2004; **27**: 295–301.

29

The parathyroid glands: anatomy and physiology

MATEEN H ARASTU AND WILLIAM J OWEN†

Introduction	367	Physiology of parathyroid glands	373
Development of parathyroid glands	367	Key points	375
Anatomy of parathyroid glands	369	References	376
Surgical viewpoint	373		

SEARCH STRATEGY AND EVIDENCE-BASE

The data in this chapter are supported by a Medline search using the key words parathyroid glands, anatomy and histology, embryology, physiology, calcium homeostasis, parathyroid hormone. This chapter primarily relies on observational studies and the peer-reviewed literature relating to anatomy and physiology and is therefore level 4 evidence.

INTRODUCTION

The normal parathyroid glands vary in number, location and macroscopic appearance. The principal role of the surgeon in parathyroid surgery is to be able to localize and distinguish diseased from normal parathyroid glands. At present, there are several noninvasive imaging techniques available for aiding the localization of parathyroid tissue. These include high-resolution ultrasound, computed tomography (CT), magnetic resonance imaging (MRI) and dual radioactive isotope scanning (thallium-201/technetium-99m subtraction). However, the precise application of knowledge of the anatomy and embryology of the parathyroid glands is essential to plan an operative strategy and to achieve successful therapy in those patients with parathyroid disease.

Disorders of calcium and bone metabolism are common. Parathyroid hormone (PTH), vitamin D and calcitonin are involved in the maintenance of normal calcium levels by modifying intestinal absorption, renal excretion and bone turnover. A thorough understanding of the physiology and regulation of calcium metabolism is important to the clinician.

DEVELOPMENT OF PARATHYROID GLANDS

The parathyroid glands develop from endodermal cell proliferation of the lateral tips of the third and fourth pharyngeal pouches (**Figure 29.1**).[1, 2, 3] The pouches are divided into solid, dorsal bulbar and hollow, elongated ventral portions.[4] Cell division in the endodermal wall leads to the internal space being obliterated by week six in the embryo. The dorsal aspect of the third pharyngeal pouch forms the inferior parathyroid gland (parathyroid III) and the ventral aspect forms the thymus gland. A duct-like connection exists between the third pharyngeal pouch and the pharyngeal wall which is soon lost, although the connection between the parathyroid and thymic rudiments persists for longer.[5] The persistence of this connection results in the inferior parathyroid gland migrating inferiorly and medially with the developing thymus gland at the end of the fifth gestational week. At the end of the seventh gestational week, the inferior parathyroid gland is located in its normal position dorsal to the inferior aspect of the thyroid lobes (**Figure 29.2a and b**).[6] The inferior parathyroid gland can become adherent to the thyroid capsule at this early stage of

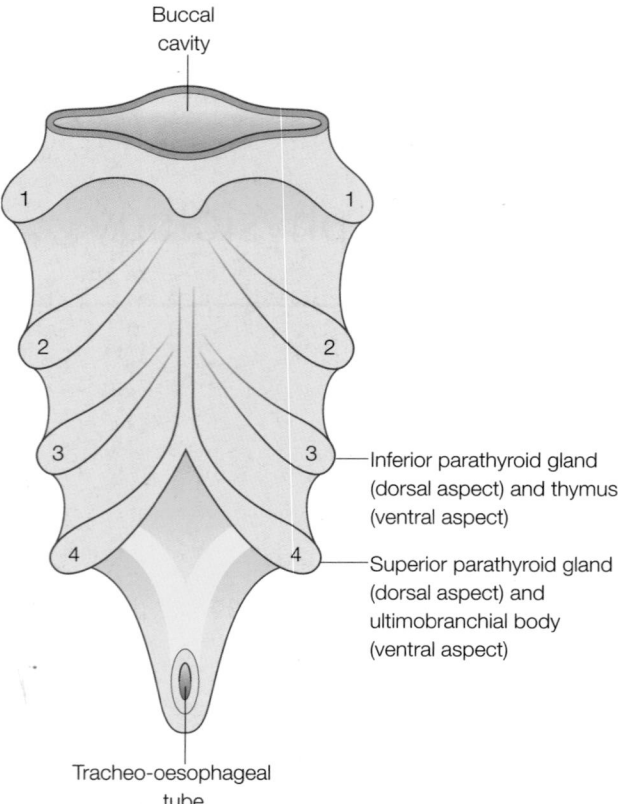

Figure 29.1 Embryology of the parathyroid glands. Schematic posterior view of the pharyngeal arches. Pharyngeal pouches are numbered 1 to 4.

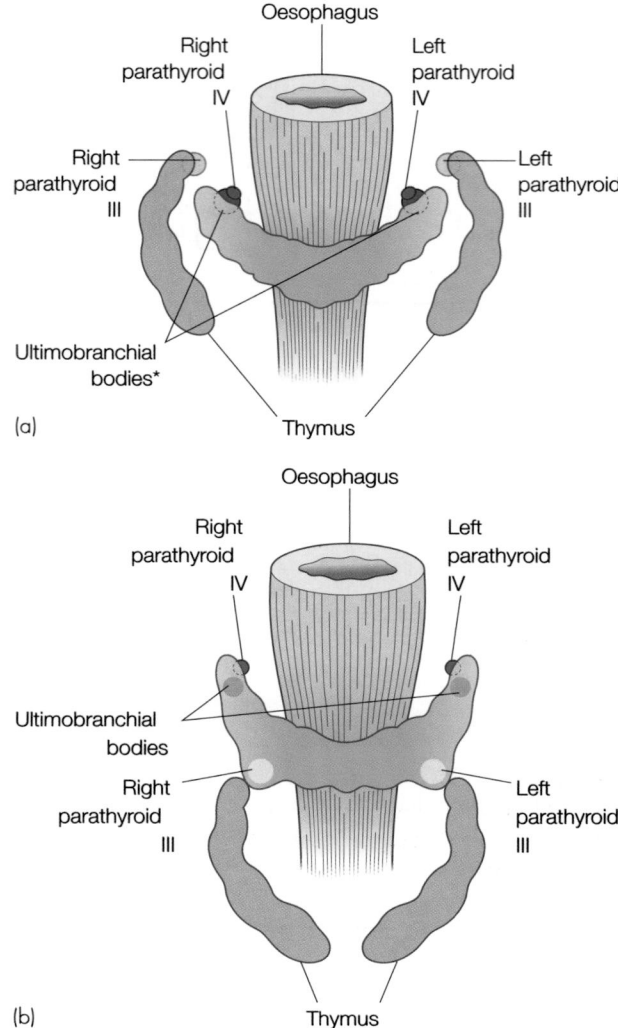

Figure 29.2 Schematic views of shifts in location of parathyroid tissue during embryological development. *Also known as lateral thyroid – contains C (parafollicular) cells.

development. The thymus gland ultimately migrates to the anterior mediastinum.

The dorsal aspect of the fourth pharyngeal pouch forms the superior parathyroid gland (parathyroid IV). The ventral aspect of the pouch and the remnants of the fifth pharyngeal pouch form the ultimobranchial bodies, which form C (parafollicular) cells. The ultimobranchial bodies appear to be analogues of parathyroid tissue and play a role in calcium metabolism with their embryological origin supporting this. The C cells ultimately fuse with the thyroid gland and are sometimes termed the lateral thyroid (**Figure 29.2a and b**).[1]

The superior parathyroid gland begins to migrate caudally and medially at the end of the fifth gestational week to reach its final anatomical position posterior to the lateral thyroid lobes at a point where the inferior thyroid artery enters the gland or at a point of intersection of the artery and the recurrent laryngeal nerve.

The pathway of embryological descent of the superior and inferior parathyroid glands along the thyro-thymic axis is shown in **Figure 29.3**. The superior parathyroid gland is usually located above the inferior thyroid artery and behind the recurrent laryngeal nerve, whereas the inferior gland is usually below the inferior thyroid artery and in front of the

recurrent laryngeal nerve (**Figure 29.4a**). This migration is complete at the end of the seventh gestational week.[6]

The migratory pathways of the parathyroid glands during embryological development result in many variations in their final anatomical location. The caudal migration of the superior parathyroid gland is less in comparison to the migration of the inferior parathyroid gland which is associated with the descent of the thymus gland, thus explaining their paradoxical positioning. This is the reason for the increased proportion of anomalies of position of the inferior parathyroid gland.

There is some controversy regarding the embryological origin of the parathyroid glands from the ectodermal (epipharyngeal) placode. The parathyroid glands have been classified as part of the amine precursor uptake and decarboxylation (APUD) system.[7, 8] Protein SP-1 has been found to be secreted with PTH and is analogous to chromogranine-A found in the suprarenal medulla. In

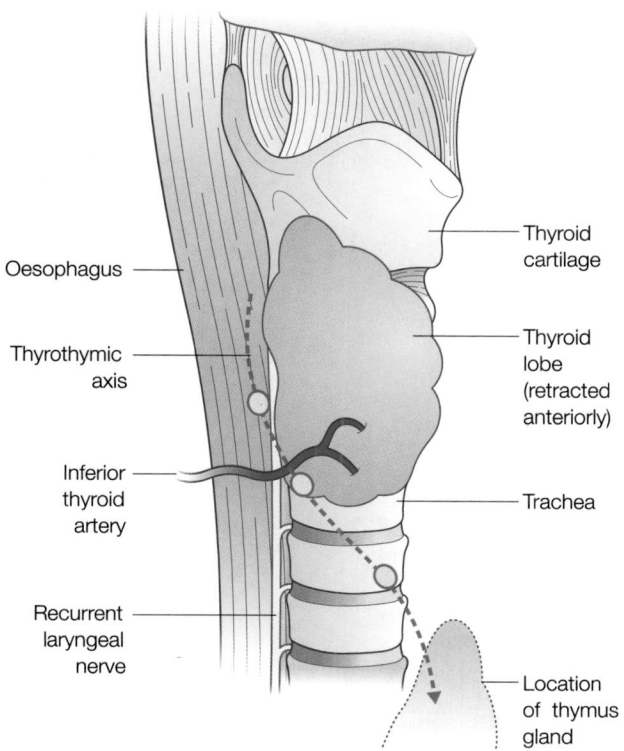

Oesophagus

Thyrothymic axis

Inferior thyroid artery

Recurrent laryngeal nerve

Thyroid cartilage

Thyroid lobe (retracted anteriorly)

Trachea

Location of thymus gland

Figure 29.3 The thyro-thymic axis explains the embryological descent of the parathyroid glands during development and may offer the surgeon a logical pathway to find parathyroid tissue in the neck and superior mediastinum. The majority can be found and identified exploring along the linear thyro-thymic axis. See text for description of anatomy.

addition, pieces of grafted third pharyngeal pouch ectoderm of chick embryos have been shown to develop into distinct parathyroid tissue.[9] In view of the above it would explain the involvement of the parathyroid glands in the multiple endocrine neoplasia (MEN) syndromes (1 and 2). The above references have been cited for those with further interest in the subject.

ANATOMY OF PARATHYROID GLANDS

The parathyroid glands eluded the notice of anatomists until 1850, when Richard Owen described, 'a small, compact, yellow glandular body that was attached to the thyroid at the point where the veins emerged' at the autopsy of a great Indian rhinoceros. The specimen may be seen today in the Hunterian Museum of the Royal College of Surgeons, England. Independently, in 1877 a Swedish anatomist, Ivar Sandström, described the gross anatomy and microscopic appearance of the parathyroid glands in a dog and subsequently in cat, ox, horse and 50 humans. He suggested the name 'glandulae parathyroideae'.[10]

The parathyroid glands vary considerably in number, size, shape, appearance and location.

Number

Typically, there are four parathyroid glands in 80–97 percent of humans.[4] Gilmour[11] dissected 527 autopsy cases, and reported four glands in 80 percent, three in 13 percent, five in 6.1 percent and two in 0.2 percent (one case). Alveryd[12] studied 1405 parathyroid glands (histologically confirmed) from 354 autopsy cases, finding four in 90.6 percent of cases and five in 3.7 percent of cases. Akerström[4] reported from 503 autopsy cases that four glands were found in 84 percent of cases, more than four in 13 percent and only three glands in 3 percent. Cases of three or fewer glands identified strongly suggested that a fourth gland had been missed. In individuals with four or more glands the supernumerary glands were either rudimentary (2 percent cases) or divided (6 percent cases). Supernumerary glands weighing 5 mg or more were found in 5 percent of cases. The clinical significance of supernumerary glands is that they can be a persistent cause of hyperparathyroidism if not located. However, it is uncommon to find patients with fewer than three or more than five glands.

Size

A normal gland usually measures approximately 5 mm in length, 3 mm in width and 1–2 mm in depth, although, there can be considerable variation. Glands as large as 12 mm and as small as 2 mm have been reported.[11] The two lower parathyroid glands are usually heavier than the two upper glands.[13] Reported maximal weights of normal parathyroid glands vary from 8.2 to 78 mg.[13, 14, 15, 16] Gland weights also vary with age and gender, being heavier in males and subjects aged 20–30 years, and lighter in females and subjects aged 70–80 years.[14] There is a correlation between increasing gland weight and body weight ($r^2 = 0.15$).[17] Healthy black subjects have heavier glands than healthy white subjects independent of body weight.[17] Size and weight are regarded as important determinants of parathyroid normality.[11] A parathyroid gland *in situ* is larger because of its degree of vascularity. Confusion can arise as the weight of a gland reported by the pathologist may be lower than what was expected. In clinical practice, a gland weighing greater than 40–50 mg is considered enlarged.

Shape and macroscopic appearance

The inelasticity of the normal parathyroid gland accounts for its variation in shape and contour. Subcapsular glands located at the upper pole of the thyroid gland have a tendency to be flattened, whereas glands in the cricothyroidal and intrathymic regions appear more oval and spherical in shape. Occasionally, a gland is bean, sausage or rod shaped.[14] In contrast, Akerström[4] documented

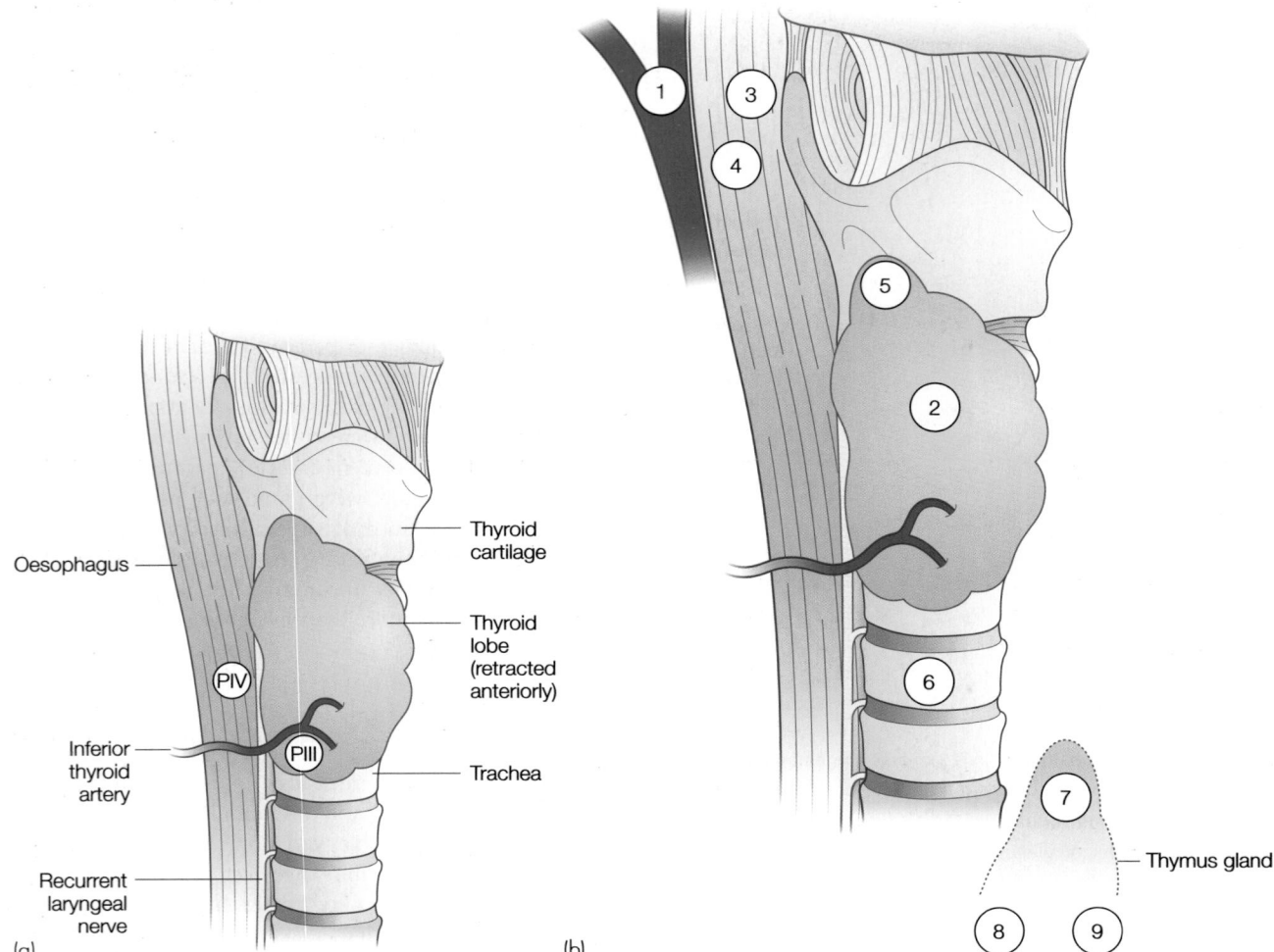

Figure 29.4   (a) Cardinal sites to consider first for parathyroid localization, indicating the relationship of the parathyroid glands to the inferior thyroid artery and recurrent laryngeal nerve. Fixed points: parathyroid IV (PIV) – above inferior thyroid artery and behind recurrent laryngeal nerve. Parathyroid III (PIII) – below inferior thyroid artery and in front of recurrent laryngeal nerve. (b) Abnormal sites for parathyroid glands. 1. Carotid sheath – rare and can cause difficulty unless opened exploring the vagus nerve, carotid artery and internal jugular vein. 2. Intrathroid – rare, but can occur producing recurrent hyperparathyroidism. The majority are subcapsular in location. The clue to exploration is that there is a missing parathyroid gland on that side. In this setting, the surgeon may perform a thyroid lobectomy and find the missing parathyroid gland in the middle of the thyroid. 3. Upper thyroid cartilage. 4. Retropharyngeal/retro-oesophageal. 5. Superior pole of thyroid gland. 6. Paratracheal. 7. Intrathymic. 8. Aortopulmonary window – rare, in these cases a sternotomy needs to be performed and careful excision of the gland in this delicate position. 9. Superior mediastinum.

that the majority of glands were oval, bean shaped or spherical (83 percent of cases), though some glands were elongated (11 percent of cases), bilobed (5 percent of cases) and mutilobed (1 percent of cases). Two para-thyroid glands can appose one another forming a 'kissing pair', but this should not be confused with a bilobed gland. The former has a true cleavage plane and a true capsule throughout, which is absent in a bilobed gland. Failure to recognize this anomaly can result in inaccurate accounting of all glands at operation.

The experienced surgeon can identify a parathyroid gland based on its macroscopic appearance and consistency. The colour varies from a light yellow to a reddish-brown which may be partially surrounded by fat. In rare cases, the glands can appear orange or greenish-yellow and in children a salmon-pink colour is often noted.[18] The yellow tan is attributable to a higher fat content and the salmon-pink colour observed in children is due to a lower fat content. The glands are usually soft and pliable and with a smooth surface. The cut surface of a gland appears vascular and its capsule is often visible.

Other structures in close proximity to the parathyroid glands must be identified by the surgeon. Fat lobules, lymph nodes, thyroid nodules and the tips of the upper cornua of the thymus gland can complicate the identification of the parathyroid glands. The surface of a parathyroid gland is usually not as shiny as that of a fat lobule, but is often surrounded by a fat lobule. Parathyroid tissue is

Table 29.1 An aid to identify a parathyroid gland. Distinguishing features between tissues found in close proximity to the parathyroid glands.

	Parathyroid gland	Lymph node	Fat lobule	Thyroid nodule
Colour	Yellow or reddish-brown Blue if stained with Methylene blue	More translucent appearance than parathyroid tissue	Yellow	Reddish
Consistency	Soft Mobile ('wobbles')	Hard	Soft	Hard
Form (appearance)	Distinct edge/capsule (Like a 'baby spleen') Merge with fat pad	Indistinct Less well demarcated from surrounding fat		Not separable from thyroid gland
Texture	Fine texture/homogenous	Not homogenous		Less homogenous
Vascularity	Minute blood vessels in hilus of gland/vascular	Less vascular	Less vascular	Less vascular

denser than fat and sinks in normal saline, but the latter floats. This helps to differentiate the two types of tissue.[14] A specific finding when parathyroid tissue is cut is that the cut surface oozes, testifying to its marked vascularity and therefore confirming identification. Its appearance is similar to that of other vascular organs, such as the liver or spleen. Whereas fat and lymph nodes are not as vascular as parathyroid tissue when cut, they tend to lose their shape and the thymus gland bleeds very little. However, the definitive identification is performed by a frozen section examination. Identifiable features of parathyroid glands are outlined in **Table 29.1**.

Anatomical location

Great variation exists in the final anatomical location of the parathyroid glands. This is attributed to the complex migratory pathways and embryological development with other glandular tissue, the thymus and thyroid glands.

The superior parathyroid gland is more constant in position compared to the inferior parathyroid gland. It lies posterior to the corresponding upper half of the thyroid lobe, either at the cricothyroid junction or adjacent to the upper pole at a point at which the inferior thyroid artery enters the substance of the thyroid gland.[14] This corresponds to the level of the posterior ring of the cricoid cartilage. This finding was observed in 99 percent of cases dissected by Wang (77 percent at the cricothyroidal junction and 22 percent behind the upper pole of thyroid gland), 92 percent of cases dissected by Gilmour and 80 percent of cases dissected by Akerström.[4, 11, 14] Therefore, this constant anatomical location in the majority of cases provides a useful landmark for the superior glands which are in a circumscribed area above the intersection between the inferior thyroid artery and the recurrent laryngeal nerve. In Wang's study, 22 percent of the glands behind the upper pole of the thyroid were subcapsular (below the thyroid capsule). They were always mobile and demonstrated a fine vascular pedicle,

which originated from the thyroid gland. This is useful in distinguishing these glands from thyroid nodules at operation.

Akerström observed that the glands were often hidden by the connective tissue binding the posterior edge of the thyroid lobe to the pharynx, but the glands remained mobile. Occasionally, the glands were immobile and attached to the thyroid capsule.[4] In 4 percent of cases the superior gland was located more inferiorly, obscured by the inferior thyroid artery, recurrent laryngeal nerve or a protrusion of the thyroid gland (tubercle of Zuckerlandl).[4, 11] More unusual sites have been documented, 2 percent of cases at the upper thyroid pole and 1 percent above the upper thyroid pole. Other ectopic sites found were more posterior in the neck in the retro-pharyngeal or retro-oesophageal space (1 percent of cases).[4] One cause for failure in parathyroid exploration is that the surgeon does not explore the neck far enough posteriorly. If the initial exploration was performed by a less experienced surgeon, re-exploration is relatively simple as this posterior field will not have been entered. Indeed, at post-mortem, experienced pathologists choose to look for the parathyroid glands via a posterior approach starting at the vertebral column and extending anteriorly. This point is vital to the understanding of parathyroid exploration.

The inferior parathyroid glands are more widely distributed. In 81 percent of glands dissected by Wang, and 70 percent in Gilmour's series, the inferior glands were distributed evenly between the lower pole of the thyroid and the thymus gland.[11, 14] Akerström found more than half of the inferior glands were located either inferior, posterior or lateral to the lower pole of the thyroid. Some of the lower glands were situated anteriorly on the lower thyroid lobe (17 percent of cases). Other locations of the inferior glands are inferior to the thyroid in close association with the thyrothymic ligament (fibrous tissue connecting the inferior pole of the thyroid to the superior aspect of the thymus) or within the cervical part of the thymus (26 percent of cases).[4]

The majority of superior mediastinal parathyroid glands can be explored successfully through the neck (98 percent of cases) and it is rare not to be able to reach a thymic parathyroid gland in this way.

Clearly, in the operation of total parathyroidectomy in cases of renal failure, it would be important in this situation to thoroughly explore the superior mediastinum and expose the thymus. This can nearly always be achieved via the cervical route. Sternal split is usually only required in cases where there has been previous retrosternal surgery such as in cases of coronary artery grafting, previous exploration for parathyroid glands in this area or a rare occurrence of ectopic parathyroid tissue in the aortopulmonary window. Rarer sites for an inferior parathyroid gland include an area extending from the carotid bifurcation (due to failure of descent embryologically) to the anterior and posterior mediastinum.[4, 11] Failure to localize parathyroid tissue can also be due to its location within the carotid sheath, which sometimes needs to be explored. Inferior glands which fail to descend are located superiorly to the superior parathyroid glands and usually have remnants of thymic tissue surrounding them which facilitates their identification. Postero–inferior embryonic displacement can result in inferior glands being placed along the recurrent laryngeal nerve and along the lateral border of the oesophagus.[19] Theoretically, however, parathyroid glands can be ectopically located anywhere from the base of the skull to the diaphragm, but in practical terms such cases are rare and usually fit into the previously described scheme for locating parathyroid glands. **Figure 29.4b** illustrates the potential ectopic sites for the parathyroid glands.

Normal parathyroid glands in ectopic locations receive their blood supply from local vessels, for example, the thymic or internal thoracic arteries. Usually, the inferior glands are obscured by fatty or vascular tissue, or lie within the fibrous sheath of the thyroid gland, which makes identification difficult.

Symmetry in position of the superior glands has been documented in 80 percent of cases, in inferior glands in 70 percent of cases and for all four glands 60 percent of cases.[4] Asymmetrical locations of the parathyroid glands have been demonstrated. Three glands were located within the thyroid region and a fourth gland from either side was located within the thymus (13 percent of cases); on one side the superior and inferior glands were located above and below the inferior thyroid artery and recurrent laryngeal nerve intersection, respectively, and on the other side both superior and inferior glands were located below (5 percent cases) or above (2 percent cases) the intersection.[4]

Arterial blood supply

The principal blood supply to the parathyroid glands is from specific ascending glandular branches from parenchymal, muscular or oesophageal branches of the inferior thyroid artery.[20] The inferior thyroid artery is a branch of the thyrocervical trunk, which arises from the first part of the subclavian artery.[21] The artery ascends anterior to the medial border of scalenus anterior and turns medially at the level of the sixth cervical vertebra. At this point, it descends on *longus colli* to the lower border of the thyroid gland. The superior thyroid artery, a branch of the external carotid artery may supply the superior parathyroid gland, but more commonly it receives an independent direct blood supply from the inferior thyroid artery.[22] However, there is considerable controversy about the arterial supply to the superior parathyroid glands. Injected contrast material into the superior thyroid artery of cadavers demonstrated that it supplied the superior parathyroid gland in 98 percent of cases. A distinct anastomosis between the superior and inferior thyroid arteries was seen in 45 percent of cases.[23] Laser Doppler flowmetry has shown that the blood supply to the parathyroid glands is not as dependent upon the inferior thyroid artery as previously suggested.[24] Occlusion of either the inferior or superior thyroid artery decreased blood flow to the parathyroid glands by approximately one-third.

A single artery usually supplies each gland, dividing into several branches before entering the glandular tissue, although sometimes, two or three vessels may supply a gland. The *thyroidea ima* artery and other accessory vessels may contribute to the blood supply but are of less importance. Ectopic parathyroid tissue receives its blood supply locally, as mentioned earlier. Despite vascular anastomoses existing between the thyroid vessels, injury to the vascular supply to the parathyroid gland can result in infarction and necrosis, an important point to note at operation. There have also been reported cases of spontaneous infarction of the parathyroid glands in patients with hypercalcaemia and subsequent resolution.[25, 26, 27]

Venous drainage

The parathyroid gland veins drain via the thyroid venous plexus. The superior and middle thyroid veins drain the upper and central parts of the ipsilateral thyroid and parathyroid glands in that region. The superior thyroid veins are relatively constant in position and always drain into the internal jugular veins, but can communicate with the facial venous system superiorly. The middle thyroid vein's point of entry into the internal jugular vein is variable. The inferior thyroid veins are more variable in position and usually drain into the left brachiocephalic vein.[28, 29] Dunlop showed that the left and right inferior thyroid veins fuse to form a common trunk which drains into the proximal portion of the left brachiocephalic vein in 60 percent of patients. Drainage into the right and distal segment of the left brachiocephalic vein was also documented. In some patients the inferior thyroid veins drained the mediastinum, communicating with the thymic vein. Monchik[30] performed 32 autopsies and demonstrated that the inferior thyroid veins drained separately into the left brachiocephalic vein (25 percent of cases) or formed a common trunk (47 percent of cases). Occasionally, the inferior thyroid venous trunk drained directly into the internal jugular vein. Each parathyroid gland tends to drain ipsilaterally and inferiorly, but contralateral drainage can occur. This results from anastomoses posteriorly with the vertebral venous plexus and anteriorly with the anterior jugular veins, which drain via the transverse cervical vein into the subclavian vein.

Innervation

The nerve supply to the human parathyroid glands is principally adrenergic from the sympathetic system.[31, 32] Sympathetic fibres reach the glands from the superior and middle cervical sympathetic ganglia or via the perivascular plexus of the thyroid gland. The nerves are vasomotor, but not secretomotor, with gland activity controlled by changes in plasma calcium levels.[33] Further evidence for this is that transplanted parathyroid glands function normally.

Microscopic appearance

The parathyroid gland has a thin connective tissue capsule and septae which divide it into lobules. Vascular mesenchyme grows into nodules on the dorsal aspect of the pharyngeal pouches to form a rich capillary network in the parathyroid glands. Chief cells, or principal cells, synthesize PTH and are the predominant cell type in the parathyroid gland of children. There are three types of chief cells, dependent upon the depth of cytoplasmic staining visible on light microscopy, named light, dark and clear cells. The chief cells are organized into columns surrounded by sinusoidal capillaries responsible for transporting PTH from the gland. Chief cells in humans can be divided into active and inactive cells, the latter outnumbering the former by three to one.

A second cell type, the oxyphil cell, becomes apparent before puberty and increases in number with age. Oxyphil (eosinophilic) cells are not thought by some to be involved in the secretion of PTH, but have high concentrations of mitochondria. Rare cases of hyperparathyroidism have been documented with only oxyphil cells present in the excised glands. Excess hormone production stopped when these glands were removed, hence, their probable role in PTH secretion, though the exact role of these cells remains to be elucidated.[34] A third transitional cell has also been described though its exact function is unknown.[35] Connective tissue starts to increase in the glands of young adults. With advancing age the number of fat cells increases and may occupy 60–70 percent of the gland in an elderly adult, with associated decrease in the functional mass of chief cells.

SURGICAL VIEWPOINT

The surgical approach to the parathyroid glands should involve the following important points.

- Is this a normal parathyroid gland? Knowledge of the variations in appearance will aid the surgeon to identify normal parathyroid tissue. Tissue located in the region of the parathyroid glands may be mistaken for parathyroid tissue, especially lymph nodes, fat lobules and thyroid nodules.
- How many parathyroid glands are there? This is variable but it is uncommon for either less than three or more than five glands to be found.
- Where are the parathyroid glands located and what are the possible locations of an aberrant parathyroid gland? Bearing in mind the embryological development and due to the variable extent of their migratory pathways, the surgeon should have a systematic approach to explore the anatomical regions in which the parathyroid glands are likely to be found. The superior parathyroid glands are more constant in their location than the inferior glands. A missing parathyroid gland may be located at an ectopic site more often than the patient having only three glands.

PHYSIOLOGY OF PARATHYROID GLANDS

Calcium homeostasis is mediated by the complex interactions of PTH, an active metabolite of vitamin D, 1,25-dihydroxyvitamin D_3 (1,25-$(OH)_2D_3$) and calcitonin. The average human contains 800–1000 g of calcium, of which 99 percent is skeletal and a small fraction is extracellular. Fifty percent of plasma calcium exists in its free (ionized) form, which is metabolically active and under tight hormonal regulation. The remainder is bound to albumin, and small amounts are bound to pyruvate, citrate and lactate.

PTH

PTH is secreted by chief cells of the parathyroid gland and is essential for the maintenance of life in humans. Essential functions reliant upon tight regulation of serum calcium levels include neural transmission, muscle contraction (and relaxation), exocrine secretion, blood clotting and cellular adhesion. Chief cells can synthesize large amounts and rapidly secrete stored PTH, replicate if chronically stimulated, giving short-, medium- and long-term control of serum calcium levels. PTH is a polypeptide, 84 amino acids long, derived from a precursor molecule of 115 amino acid residues, pre-proPTH. Pre-proPTH has a 25 residue 'pre' signal sequence which, if mutated, results in hypoparathyroidism and a six residue 'pro' sequence with an unknown role.[36, 37] Pre-proPTH is initially cleaved to proPTH (90 amino acids) which ultimately loses six base residues to form PTH. The hormone is cleaved into two major fragments in chief cells and Kuppfer cells of the liver. The biologically active fragment is PTH-(1-34).

The parathyroid glands can react within seconds to secrete PTH, being controlled by circulating levels of ionized calcium. Calcimimetic compounds inhibit PTH secretion in humans.[38] Catecholamines, magnesium and other stimuli can also affect PTH secretion.[39] Calcium-sensing receptors on parathyroid cells determine the extracellular level of serum calcium, controlling PTH secretion. This calcium-sensing receptor is a typical seven-spanning membrane G protein-coupled receptor.[40, 41, 42] Binding of calcium to the receptor causes a conformational change which lowers intracellular cyclic AMP levels and decreases PTH secretion. The dose-response curve for PTH responding to serum calcium levels is sigmoidal. The minimal secretory rate is low but not zero, with the maximal secretory rate representing parathyroid gland reserve. A steady-state occurs lower on the dose-response curve which means the parathyroid gland responds more efficiently to hypocalcaemia than to hypercalcaemia.[43]

PTH blood levels are regulated on a minute to minute basis, but over a longer time period PTH gene expression is regulated.[44] Vitamin D_3 has no effect on PTH secretion *per se* but decreases PTH gene expression.[45] Regulation of PTH gene expression is relevant in patients with renal failure, as low calcium and $1,25-(OH)_2D_3$ levels and uraemic toxins alter calcium homeostasis. Treatment with vitamin D_3 and calcium will increase calcium absorption inhibiting PTH secretion by the parathyroid glands.

Parathyroid cells replicate little in adulthood, but can increase dramatically in number secondary to hypocal-caemia, low levels of vitamin D_3 and neoplasia. Calcium inhibits PTH cell proliferation. An increased cell number secondary to hypocalcaemia is a slow response, but appears to be irreversible, as after renal transplantation persistent hyperparathyroidism can be problematic.

The half-life of PTH is 2 minutes, with 70 percent metabolized in the liver and 20 percent in the kidneys. Less than 1 percent of secreted PTH reaches its target organs.[46] Therefore, PTH blood levels are principally related to the rate of secretion.

Actions of parathyroid hormone

PTH acts on a number of target tissues, mostly increasing the circulating levels of calcium and decreasing phosphate (PO_4^{3-}). The receptor for PTH has been cloned.[47] The receptor is found in the kidney and osteoblasts but not osteoclasts or in the intestine.

PTH plays an important role in the kidney.[48] Almost all calcium in the glomerular filtrate of the kidney is reabsorbed, 65 percent in the proximal convoluted tubule, 20 percent in the thick ascending limb of the loop of Henle and 10 percent in the distal convoluted tubule. Some reabsorption in the thick ascending limb of the loop of Henle and the distal convoluted tubule is PTH dependent, thus helping to increase serum calcium levels. PO_4^{3-} reabsorption occurs in the proximal and distal convoluted tubules and is inhibited by PTH, thus decreasing serum PO_4^{3-}.

PTH stimulates $1,25-(OH)_2D_3$ synthesis in the proximal tubules by activating 25-hydroxyvitamin D-1α-hydoxylase (25-OH-D_3-1α-OHase) and decreases renal 24-hydroxylase activity, the major enzyme involved in the destruction of vitamin D.[49, 50] PTH increases bone resorption by increasing the number and activity of osteoclasts. Despite this relationship, isolated mature osteoclasts cannot respond to PTH, though when cultured with osteoblasts they do so.[51, 52] The mechanism of bone resorption is dependent upon both cell types interacting closely.

Vitamin D

Exposure to ultraviolet irradiation converts the cutaneous precursor of vitamin D, 7-dehydrocholesterol, to vitamin D_3. The degree of skin pigmentation regulates the conversion by influencing the penetration of ultraviolet light. An important source of vitamin D, if exposure to sunlight is limited, is from dietary sources.

Metabolites of vitamin D are fat-soluble compounds which circulate bound to vitamin D-binding protein, and some to albumin. A small fraction of circulating vitamin D is free. Vitamin D is transported to the liver where it is hydroxylated by cytochrome P450 enzyme to form 25-OH-D_3, the major circulating metabolite but which functionally is weak acting. Further hydroxylation occurs in the proximal convoluted tubules of the kidney to form $1,25-(OH)_2D_3$, the main active metabolite. The half-life of $1,25-(OH)_2D_3$ is six to eight hours.

PTH and low PO_4^{3-} levels regulate this second crucial hydroxylation step. Calcitonin, $1,25-(OH)_2D_3$ and calcium decrease the activity of 1α-hydroxylase activity.[53] Animal work has shown that other hormones, including oestrogen, growth hormone and prolactin, increase 1α-hydroxylase activity but the significance of this in humans has not been shown.

$1,25-(OH)_2D_3$ binds to a nuclear receptor and forms a heterodimeric complex with the retinoid-X receptor. This upregulates target genes that control $1,25-(OH)_2D_3$ RNA transcription.[54]

The vitamin D-receptor is expressed by most tissues and regulates cellular differentiation and function in many cell types. Probably the most important physiological function is the regulation of intestinal calcium transport. Calcium is absorbed in the intestine by three pathways: transcellular, vesicular and paracellular transport. The transcellular and vesicular pathways are $1,25-(OH)_2D_3$ dependent. The role of $1,25-(OH)_2D_3$ in the regulation of paracellular transport remains controversial.

1,25-$(OH)_2D_3$ activates osteoblasts which in turn activate osteoclastic-mediated bone resorption. This increases the transport of calcium from the skeletal system to the plasma. Vitamin D-deficient animals have abundant calcium in their bones but cannot mobilize calcium in response to PTH unless 1,25-$(OH)_2D_3$ is administered.[55] Similarly, parathyroidectomized animals cannot mobilize calcium in response to 1,25-$(OH)_2D_3$ unless PTH is administered. Both PTH and 1,25-$(OH)_2D_3$ are required *in vivo*.

1,25-$(OH)_2D_3$ and PTH function in concert in the distal convoluted tubule of the kidney, controlling the reabsorption of the last 1 percent of filtered calcium. This small amount of calcium may be crucial in the fine balance necessary to regulate calcium levels and by further inhibiting PTH secretion by the parathyroid gland.

Parathyroid hormone–related protein

Parathyroid hormone-related protein (PTHrP) was initially discovered to be secreted by some tumour cells contributing to the hypercalcaemia of malignancy. Unlike PTH, it is made by a variety of normal tissues but has little role to play in the normal regulation of calcium levels. PTHrP has a similar structure to PTH and can stimulate PTH receptors as a result. Fortunately, however, PTHrP is not measured by a standard PTH assay, therefore a patient with possible hyperparathyroidism and a raised PTH level suggests primary hyperparathyroidism. PTHrP functions as a hormone, acting on the kidney and bone elevating serum calcium levels.[56] PTHrP acts as a calcitropic hormone during foetal life and lactation, which may be involved in the regulation of calcium levels in breast milk.[57] It is also secreted by a number of normal human tissues, such as skin and hair, and may regulate cell proliferation and differentiation.[58]

Calcitonin

The role of calcitonin in the regulation of human calcium levels is uncertain. It is secreted by the C cells of the thyroid gland and, as mentioned previously, has close embryological origins from the neural crest as the ultimobranchial bodies associated with the development of the superior parathyroid gland.

Calcitonin is a 32 amino acid polypeptide. The calcium-sensing receptor found on parathyroid cells is also found on C cells, and may regulate the release of calcitonin as well as PTH.[59] Somatostatin secreted by C cells inhibits calcitonin release, and 1,25-$(OH)_2D_3$ decreases calcitonin mRNA levels.

Calcitonin impairs osteoclast-mediated bone resorption, but its physiological role in humans is unknown.[60] Long-term administration of exogenous calcitonin has resulted in no physiological abnormalities.[61]

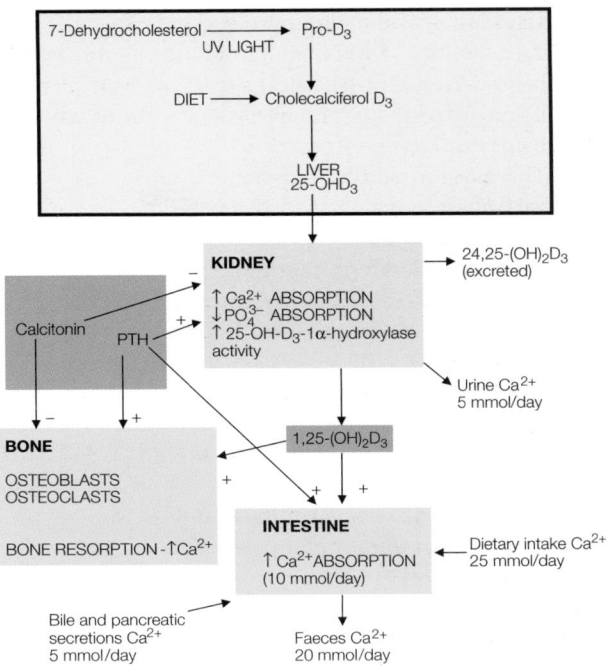

Figure 29.5 Endocrinology of calcium homeostasis. Close interaction between PTH, 1,25-$(OH)_2D_3$ and the kidneys, intestine and skeleton regulating serum calcium levels.

Summary of calcium homeostasis

Serum calcium regulation is controlled within a narrow range by the close interaction of PTH and 1,25-$(OH)_2D_3$. Serum calcium levels regulate hormone secretion and the hormones regulate the production of each other (**Figure 29.5**).

Low serum calcium levels stimulate the parathyroid gland to secrete PTH, which augments 1,25-$(OH)_2D_3$ synthesis by the proximal renal tubules. This increases the renal reabsorption of calcium. 1,25-$(OH)_2D_3$ also increases the efficiency of intestinal calcium absorption by enterocytes. The combined action of PTH and 1, 25-$(OH)_2D_3$ increases serum calcium by inducing osteoclast-mediated bone resorption.

Minimal elevation of serum calcium levels reduces PTH secretion by the parathyroid glands to a minimal amount. The role of calcitonin in humans may inhibit osteoclast-mediated bone resorption to increase osteoblast numbers and decrease osteoclasts.

KEY POINTS

- The inferior parathyroid gland is derived from the third pharyngeal pouch and the superior parathyroid gland from the fourth pharyngeal pouch.
- Embryological descent of the parathyroid glands follows the thyro-thymic axis.

- Usual sites of the parathyroid glands are: superior, above inferior thyroid artery and behind recurrent laryngeal nerve; inferior, below inferior thyroid artery and in front of recurrent laryngeal nerve.
- The inferior parathyroid gland is more variable in position than the superior parathyroid gland.
- A thorough understanding of the embryological development of the parathyroid glands can aid the surgeon when performing a systematic search to localize aberrant parathyroid tissue.
- It is uncommon to find patients with fewer than three or more than five parathyroid glands.
- PTH levels are regulated on a minute to minute basis with a plasma half-life of 2 minutes.
- PTH stimulates bone resorption and 1,25-$(OH)_2D_3$ synthesis in the proximal tubules of the kidney which increases serum calcium levels.
- 1,25-$(OH)_2D_3$ increases calcium absorption from the kidney and also increases bone resorption.
- Bone resorption is dependent upon close interaction between osteoblasts and osteoclasts.
- The exact role of calcitonin in the regulation of human calcium levels remains to be elucidated. It may inhibit osteoclast-mediated bone resorption.

REFERENCES

1. Sedgwick CE, Cady B. Surgery of the thyroid and parathyroid glands. In: Sedgwick CE (eds.) *Major problems in clinical surgery*. Philadelphia: WB Saunders, 1974; 15: 13–8.
2. Gilmour JR. The embryology of the parathyroid glands, the thymus and certain associated rudiments. *Journal of Pathology*. 1937; 45: 507–22.
3. Gray SW, Skandalakis JE, Akin JT. Embryological considerations of thyroid surgery: Developmental anatomy of the thyroid, parathyroids and the recurrent laryngeal nerve. *American Surgeon*. 1976; 42: 621–8.
* 4. Akerström G, Malmaeus J, Bergström R. Surgical anatomy of human parathyroid glands. *Surgery*. 1984; 95: 14–21.
5. Gray H. Embryology and development. In: Collins P (ed.). *Gray's anatomy*. Churchill Livingstone: Edinburgh, 1995: 176–7.
6. Lengelé B, Hamoir M. Anatomy and embryology of the parathyroid glands. *Acta Oto-rhino-laryngologica Belgica*. 2001; 55: 89–93.
7. Pearse AGE, Takor-Takor T. Embryology of the diffuse neuroendocrine system and its relationship to the common peptides. *Federation Proceedings*. 1979; 38: 228–94.
8. Pearse AGE, Takor-Takor T. Neuroendocrine embryology and the APUD concept. *Clinical Endocrinology (Oxford)*. 1976; 5: 2295–445.
9. Mérida-Velasco JA. Experimental study of the origin of the parathyroid glands. *Acta Anatomica*. 1991; 141: 163–9.
10. Organ Jr. CH. The history of parathyroid surgery, 1850-1996: the Excelsior Surgical Society 1998 Edward D Churchill Lecture. *Journal of the American College of Surgeons*. 2000; 191: 284–99.
* 11. Gilmour JR. The gross anatomy of the parathyroid glands. *Journal of Pathology*. 1938; 46: 133–48.
12. Alveryd A. Parathyroid glands in thyroid surgery. I. Anatomy of parathyroid glands. II. Postoperative hypoparathyroidism – identification and autotransplantation of parathyroid glands. *Acta Chirurgica Scandinavica (Supplementum)*. 1968; 389: 1–120.
13. Gilmour JR, Martin WJ. The weight of the parathyroid glands. *Journal of Pathology*. 1937; 44: 431–62.
* 14. Wang C. The anatomic basis of parathyroid surgery. *Annals of Surgery*. 1976; 183: 271–5.
15. Grimelius L, Akerström G, Johanson H, Bergström R. Anatomy and histopathology of human parathyroid gland. *Pathology Annual*. 1981; 16: 1–24.
16. Dufour DR, Wilkerson SY. Factors related to parathyroid weight in normal persons. *Archives of Pathology and Laboratory Medicine*. 1983; 107: 167–72.
17. Ghandur-Mnaymneh L, Cassady J, Hajianpour MA, Pas J, Reiss E. The parathyroid gland in health and disease. *American Journal of Pathology*. 1986; 125: 292–9.
18. Cannoni M, Thomassin JM, Zanaret H, Dessi P, Pech A. Hypoparathyroidism its prevention and the indications and technique for parathyroid autotransplantation. *Acta Oto-rhino-laryngologica Belgica*. 1987; 41: 926–45.
19. Pyrtek LJ, Painter PhL. An anatomical study of the relationships of the parathyroid glands to the recurrent laryngeal nerve. *Surgery, Gynecology and Obstetrics*. 1964; 119: 509–12.
20. Halsted WS, Evans HM. The parathyroid glandules. Their blood supply, and their preservation in operation upon the thyroid gland. *Annals of Surgery*. 1907; 46: 489–506.
21. Gray H. Cardiovascular. In: Gabella G (ed.). *Gray's anatomy*. Churchill Livingstone: Edinburgh, 1995: 1535.
22. Hunt PS, Poole M, Reeve TS. A reappraisal of the surgical anatomy of the thyroid and parathyroid glands. *British Journal of Surgery*. 1968; 55: 63–6.
23. Norbori M, Saiki S, Tanaka N, Harihara Y, Shindo S, Fujimoto Y. Blood supply of the parathyroid gland from the superior thyroid artery. *Surgery*. 1994; 115: 417–23.
24. Johansson K, Ander S, Lennquist S, Smeds S. Human parathyroid blood supply determined by laser-Doppler flowmetry. *World Journal of Surgery*. 1994; 18: 417–21.

25. Hammes M, DeMory A, Sprague SM. Hypocalcaemia in end-stage renal disease: a consequence of spontaneous parathyroid gland infarction. *American Journal of Kidney Diseases.* 1994; **24**: 519–22.

26. Lucas DG, Lockett MA, Cole DJ. Spontaneous infarction of a parathyroid adenoma: two case reports and review of the literature. *American Surgeon.* 2002; **68**: 173–6.

27. McLatchie GR, Morris EW, Forrester A, Fogleman I. Autoparathyroidectomy: a case report. *British Journal of Surgery.* 1979; **66**: 552–3.

28. Dunlop DAB, Papapoulos SE, Lodge RW, Fulton AJ, Kendall BE, O'Riordan JLH. Parathyroid venous sampling: anatomic considerations and results in 95 patients with primary hyperparathyroidism. *British Journal of Radiology.* 1980; **53**: 183–91.

29. Doppman JL, Hammond WG. The anatomic basis of parathyroid venous sampling. *Radiology.* 1970; **95**: 603–10.

30. Monchik JM, Doppman JL, Earll JM, Aurbach GD. Localization of hyperfunctioning parathyroid tissue. Radioimmunoassay of parathyroid hormone on samples from the large veins of the neck and thorax and selectively catheterized thyroid veins. *American Journal of Surgery.* 1975; **129**: 413–20.

31. Norberg K, Persson B, Granberg P. Adrenergic innervation of the human parathyroid glands. *Acta Chirurgica Scandinavica.* 1975; **141**: 319–22.

32. Luts L, Bergenfelz A, Alumets J, Sundler F. Peptide-containing nerve fibres in normal human parathyroid glands in human parathyroid adenomas. *European Journal of Endocrinology.* 1995; **133**: 543–51.

33. Gray H. Diffuse neuroendocrine system. In: Dyson M (ed.). *Gray's anatomy.* Churchill Livingstone: Edinburgh, 1995: 1898.

34. Gray H. Diffuse neuroendocrine system. In: Dyson M (ed.). *Gray's anatomy.* Churchill Livingstone: Edinburgh, 1995: 1897–8.

35. Cinti S, Sbarbati A. Ultrastructure of human parathyroid cells in health and disease. *Microscopy Research and Technique.* 1995; **32**: 164–79.

36. Hendy GN, Krokenberg HM, Potts Jr. JT, Rich A. Nucleotide sequence of cloned cDNAs encoding human preproparathyroid hormone. *Proceedings of the National Academy of Sciences of the United States of America.* 1981; **78**: 7365–9.

37. Wiren KM, Potts Jr. JT, Krokenberg HM. Importance of the propeptide sequence of human preproparathyroid hormone for signal sequence function. *Journal of Biological Chemistry.* 1988; **3**: 19771–7.

38. Heath III H, Sanguinetti EL, Oglesby S, Marriott TB. Inhibition of human parathyroid hormone secretion in vivo by NPS R-568, a calcimimetric drug that targets the parathyroid cell-surface calcium receptor. *Bone.* 1995; **16**: 85S.

39. Brown EM. PTH secretion in vivo and vitro. Regulation by calcium and other secretagogues. *Mineral and Electrolyte Metabolism.* 1982; **8**: 130–50.

40. Brown EM, Herbert SC. Calcium-receptor-regulated parathyroid and renal function. *Bone.* 1997; **20**: 303–9.

41. Chattopadhyay N, Mithal A, Brown EM. The calcium-sensing receptor: A window into the physiology and pathophysiology of mineral ion metabolism. *Endocrine Reviews.* 1996; **17**: 289–307.

42. Brown EM, Gamba G, Riccardi R, Lombardi M, Butters R, Kifor O et al. Cloning and characterisation of an extracellular Ca^{2+}-sensing receptor from bovine parathyroid. *Nature.* 1993; **366**: 575–80.

43. Brown EM. Four-parameter model of the sigmoidal relationship between PTH release and extracellular calcium concentration in normal and abnormal parathyroid tissue. *Journal of Clinical Endocrinology and Metabolism.* 1983; **56**: 572–81.

44. Reis A, Hecht W, Groger R, Bohm I, Cooper DN, Lindenmaier W et al. Cloning and sequence analysis of the human PTH gene region. *Human Genetics.* 1990; **84**: 119–24.

45. Russell J, Lettieri D, Sherwood LM. Supression by 1,25 $(OH)_2 D_3$ of transcription of the pre-proparathyroid hormone gene. *Endocrinology.* 1986; **119**: 2864–6.

46. Rouleau MF, Warshawsky H, Goltzman D. Parathyroid hormone binding in vivo to renal, hepatic, and skeletal tissues of the rat using a radioautographic approach. *Endocrinology.* 1986; **118**: 919–31.

47. Schneider H, Feyen JH, Seuwen K, Movva NR. Cloning and functional expression of a human parathyroid hormone receptor. *European Journal of Pharmacology.* 1993; **246**: 149–55.

48. Friedlander G, Amiel C. Cellular mode of action of parathyroid hormone. *Advances in Nephrology from the Necker Hospital.* 1994; **23**: 265–79.

49. Garabedian M, Holick MF, De Luca HF, Boyle IT. Control of 25-hydroxycholecalciferol metabolism by parathyroid hormone. *Proceedings of the National Academy of Sciences of the United States of America.* 1972; **69**: 1673–6.

50. Shigematsu T, Horiuchi N, Ogura Y, Miyahara T, Suda T. Human parathyroid hormone inhibits renal 24-hydroxylase activity of 25-hydroxyvitamin D_3 by a mechanism involving adenosine 3′,5′-monophosphate in rats. *Endocrinology.* 1986; **118**: 1583–9.

51. McSheehy PMGJ, Chambers TJ. Osteoblastic cells mediate osteoclastic responsiveness to parathyroid hormone. *Endocrinology.* 1986; **118**: 824–8.

52. McSheehy PMGJ, Chambers TJ. Osteoblast-like cells in the presence of parathyroid hormone release soluble factor that stimulates osteoclastic bone resorption. *Endocrinology.* 1986; **119**: 1654–9.

53. Tanaka Y, Deluca HF. The control of 25-hydroxyvitamin D metabolism by inorganic phosphorous. *Archives of Biochemistry and Biophysics.* 1973; **154**: 566–74.

54. Kliewer SA, Umesono K, Mangelsdorf DJ, Evans RM. Retinoid X receptor interacts with nuclear receptors in retinoic acid, thyroid hormone and vitamin D_3 signalling. *Nature.* 1992; **355**: 446–9.

55. Garabedian M, Tanaka Y, Holick MF, De Luca HF. Response of intestinal calcium transport and bone calcium mobilization to 1,25-dihydroxyvitamin D_3 in parathyroidectomized rats. *Endocrinology.* 1974; **94**: 1022–7.

56. Orloff JJ, Wu TL, Stewart AF. Parathyroid hormone-like proteins: biochemical responses and receptor interactions. *Endocrine Reviews.* 1989; **10**: 476–95.

57. Grill V, Hillary J, Ho PMW, Law FM, MacIsaac RJ, MacIsaac IA *et al.* Parathyroid hormone-related protein: a possible endocrine function in lactation. *Clinical Endocrinology.* 1992; **37**: 405–10.

* 58. Philbrick WM, Wysolmerski JJ, Galbraith S, Holt E, Orloff JJ, Yang KH *et al.* Defining the roles of parathyroid hormone-related protein in normal physiology. *Physiological Reviews.* 1996; **76**: 127–73.

59. Garrett JE, Tamir H, Kilfor O, Simin RT, Rogers KV, Mithal A *et al.* Calcitonin-secreting cells of the thyroid express an extracellular calcium receptor gene. *Endocrinology.* 1995; **136**: 5202–11.

60. Chambers TJ, McSheehy PM, Thomson BM, Fuller K. The effect of calcium-regulating hormones and prostaglandins on bone resorption by osteoclasts disaggregated from neonatal rabbit bones. *Endocrinolgy.* 1985; **116**: 234–9.

61. Wimalawansa SJ. Long- and short-term side effects and safety of calcitonin in man: a prospective study. *Calcified Tissue International.* 1993; **52**: 90–3.

30

Parathyroid function tests and imaging

DAVID HOSKING

Normal or appropriate parathyroid function	379	Key points	385
Routine serum and urine biochemistry	379	Best clinical practice	385
Best clinical practice	382	Deficiencies in current knowledge and areas for future	
PTH	382	research	385
Key points	383	References	385
Parathyroid imaging	383		

SEARCH STRATEGY

The data in this chapter are based on a Medline search using the key words parathyroid glands, parathyroid hormone/analysis, radionuclide imaging, sestamibi, ultrasonography, magnetic resonance imaging, tomography/x-ray computed. These were limited to human studies published in the English language.

NORMAL OR APPROPRIATE PARATHYROID FUNCTION

The role of the parathyroid glands is to maintain a level of extracellular and intracellular fluid calcium, magnesium and phosphate which is compatible with normal cellular and neuromuscular function. When evaluating parathyroid function, it is critical to understand the difference between a 'normal' level of parathyroid hormone (PTH) which lies within the age and sex specific reference range and one which is 'appropriate'. For example, after parathyroidectomy for hyperparathyroidism, the concentration of PTH postoperatively may approach the preoperative level as the gland attempts to maintain a normal ECF calcium in the face of a relative excess of bone formation (hungry bone syndrome). Equally, a normal serum PTH concentration in the presence of hypercalcaemia is inappropriate and indicates the presence of primary hyperparathyroidism. As in many other areas of medicine, normal organ function cannot be defined by a single parameter but by a combination of measurements which indicate whether function is appropriate to the needs of homeostasis and can therefore be regarded as 'normal'.

The tools at our disposal include routine measurements of serum and urine calcium, phosphate, magnesium and sodium together with standard tests of renal and hepatic function. Recent development of the two-site immunoassays for 'intact' PTH avoid the confusion caused by circulating, but biologically inactive, peptides while, on occasion, direct stimulatory tests are needed to identify glandular or end organ resistance. However, most errors in the diagnosis of disorders of mineral metabolism are due to poor attention to detail in the history and examination, rather than incorrect interpretation of laboratory data.

ROUTINE SERUM AND URINE BIOCHEMISTRY

Calcium

METHODOLOGY

Total serum calcium comprises the protein bound (40 percent), ionized (48 percent) and the complexed (12 percent) fractions, and most clinical chemistry laboratories will correct the serum concentration for the prevailing level of serum albumin which accounts for 90 percent of the protein binding (with the remainder complexed to globulin).[1] If this is not carried out routinely, a simple correction factor is to add (or subtract) 0.2 mmol/L for every G/L by which the albumin falls below (or exceeds) 40 G/L.

It is the ionized serum calcium which regulates all physiological events but measurements require more care since values vary between methods and type of sample (serum, plasma or heparinized whole blood) which must be collected anaerobically to avoid altered calcium binding due to *ex vivo* changes in pH. Although ionized measurements are seldom used in routine clinical practice, they are of value in profound hypoalbuminaemic states, acid-base disturbances and after massive (citrated) blood transfusion where the use of ion selective electrodes has made this methodology more generally available.

TECHNICAL FACTORS

Serum protein concentration rises with the erect posture which seems to be the major cause of the diurnal variation in total, but not protein corrected, calcium. Serum calcium, unlike phosphate, is little affected by food but may show significant variation in hypoparathyroid patients treated with calcium and vitamin D supplements. The normal reference range for calcium is 2.20–2.60 mmol/L and this can be converted to mg/dL by multiplying by four.

INTERPRETATION

The common causes of hypocalcaemia and hypercalcaemia are set out in **Table 30.1** together with major clinical and biochemical characteristics which allow their separation.

Phosphate

METHODOLOGY

The importance of the measurement of the plasma phosphate is that it can be used as an indirect (but rapidly available) assessment of parathyroid function since it will be low in hyperparathyroidism and high in hypoparathyroidism. Although hypophosphataemia is a feature of hyperparathyroidism, the plasma phosphate is of much less value in the differentiation of the various causes of hypercalcaemia. The level of plasma phosphate rises after the intake of food and has the greatest discriminatory value when measured during fasting. Plasma levels also rise as renal function deteriorates since less phosphate will be filtered by the glomerulus.

TECHNICAL FACTORS

In nonfasting patients, and those with renal impairment, a random plasma phosphate is unreliable and it is necessary to calculate the setting of renal tubular phosphate reabsorption (TmP/GFR). This requires a simultaneous serum and urine sample measured for phosphate and creatinine from which the clearance of phosphate to creatinine can be calculated from:

$$\frac{C_{phosphate}}{C_{creatinine}} = \frac{Up \times [Creatinine]}{Ucreatinine \times [PO_4]}$$

and TmP/GFR read off from a nomogram.[2]

Phosphate moves into cells in response to respiratory alkalosis, the intravenous infusion of glucose, insulin or an increase in adrenaline. Delay in separation of samples or *ex vivo* haemolysis can falsely elevate plasma levels. The normal reference range for plasma phosphate, measured

Table 30.1 Causes of hypocalcaemia and hypercalcaemia.

	Cause	Diagnostic features
Hypocalcaemia	Hypoparathyroidism	Carpopedal spasm, paraesthesiae, fits
		Abnormal body habitus (pseudohypoparathyroidism)
		↑PO_4 ↓PTH (↑PTH in pseudohypoparathyroidism)
	Vitamin D deficiency	Bone pain, proximal myopathy, tetany
		↓PO_4 ↑PTH ↑creatinine (renal failure)
	Hypomagnesaemia	Tetany ↑PO_4 ↓PTH ↓K +
	Acute pancreatitis	Clinical features, ↑amylase
Hypercalcaemia	Hyperparathyroidism	'Stones bones abdominal groans'
		↓PO_4 ↑PTH ± ↑creatinine ± ↑bone turnover
	Malignancy	Clinical features of primary tumour
		↓PO_4 ↓PTH ± ↑creatinine ± ↑liver function
	Milk-alkali syndrome	↑Creatinine ± ↑HCO_3
	Sarcoidosis	Erythema nodosum, hilar adenopathy (CXR)
		↓PTH ± ↑creatinine ± ↑liver function
		Steroid responsive hypercalcaemia

Table 30.2 Causes of hypophosphataemia and hyperphosphataemia.

	Cause	Diagnostic features
Hypophosphataemia	Hyperparathyroidism	Primary: 'stones bones abdominal groans' Secondary: vitamin D deficiency/osteomalacia
	Malignancy	Clinical features of primary tumour ↑Ca ↓PTH ± ↑creatinine ± ↑liver function
	Hypophosphataemic osteomalacia	Short stature, no proximal myopathy Normal Ca PTH ± ↑alkaline phosphatase
Hyperphosphataemia	Hypoparathyroidism	Idiopathic: carpopedal spasm, paraesthesiae, fits Pseudohypoparathyroidism (appearance)
	Renal failure	↓Ca ↑PTH ↑creatinine ± renal bone disease

by automated spectrophotometry, is 0.8–1.4 mmol/L and can be converted to mg/dL by multiplying by 3.1.

INTERPRETATION

The common causes of hypophosphataemia and hyperphosphataemia are set out in **Table 30.2** together with major clinical and biochemical characteristics which allow their separation.

Magnesium

METHODOLOGY

Serum magnesium is also regulated by PTH but unlike calcium, where the stimulus is progressive, the initial increase in PTH which develops as serum magnesium falls is replaced by progressive functional hypoparathyroidism. This makes it important to measure serum magnesium in all hypocalcaemic and hypoparathyroid patients. Like calcium, magnesium in serum is present in an ionized (55 percent), protein bound (30 percent) and complexed (15 percent) form but correction factors are not available causing uncertainty in the interpretation of serum levels in the presence of hypoalbuminaemia. The normal serum concentration, usually measured by automated spectrophotometry, is 0.7–1.0 mmol/L and can be converted to mg/dL by multiplying by 2.4.

TECHNICAL FACTORS

Magnesium is a predominantly intracellular ion and serum concentrations are a poor indicator of magnesium status which is best assessed by a magnesium tolerance test which measures the retention after an intravenous load (0.1 mmol elemental Mg^{2+}/Kg body weight) in 50 mL 5 percent dextrose over four hours. This correlates well with both skeletal muscle content and Mg balance studies[3] in that magnesium-replete individuals excrete >50 percent of the load within 24 hours while those who

are deplete retain >50 percent of the dose; probable deficiency is indicated by an intermediate retention of 25–50 percent.

INTERPRETATION

The common causes of hypomagnesaemia and hypermagnesaemia are set out in **Table 30.3** together with major clinical and biochemical characteristics which allow their separation. Because magnesium deficiency is usually secondary to some other disease, the clinical and biochemical picture is usually dominated by the primary cause. Important clues to the presence of magnesium depletion are the presence of hypokalaemia and hypocalcaemia. Magnesium is needed for the effective tubular reabsorption of potassium, and hypokalaemia in this situation may be resistant to the administration of potassium supplements because of the renal leak. In addition, as magnesium depletion progresses, the initial stimulation of PTH secretion is replaced by progressive functional hypoparathyroidism and the development of hypocalcaemia.

Hypermagnesaemia is an uncommon problem and is usually due to inappropriate rates of infusion particularly where there is renal impairment. [****]

Table 30.3 Causes of hypomagnesaemia and hypermagnesaemia.

Cause	Diagnostic features
Gastrointestinal loss	Malabsorption, prolonged nasogastric suction Acute/chronic diarrhoea
Renal tubular disease	Diuretics, cisplatin, aminoglycosides Inherited defects, chronic renal disease Post-renal transplantation
Alcoholism	
Parathyroid failure or resistance	

Best clinical practice

✓ Parathyroid function needs to be assessed in conjunction with the prevailing levels of calcium, phosphate and magnesium.

✓ Serum calcium must be corrected for serum albumin but need not be measured fasting.

✓ Phosphate is elevated by food and renal failure and in their presence it is necessary to calculate Tmp/GFR.

✓ Magnesium is predominantly intracellular ion and depletion is best assessed from the retention after an intravenous load.

PTH

PTH is secreted as a 1–84 amino acid peptide with a half-life of less than five minutes, but is cleaved both within the parathyroid gland and in the peripheral tissues, such as the liver, to shorter carboxy-terminal peptides which have much longer half-lives. These fragments, together with a larger 7–84 peptide, are eliminated from the serum mainly by glomerular filtration and subsequent tubular degradation.[4] As a consequence, their circulating concentrations are relatively high relative to the biologically active intact hormone.

Current PTH assays in clinical use are based on a two-site immunoradiometric assay (IRMA) using antibodies to the 1–34 region of PTH with another reacting with the 39–84 C-terminal sequence.[5] This technique does not measure biologically inactive C-terminal fragments, is sensitive enough to detect PTH in normal subjects and can distinguish them from patients in whom PTH is suppressed. It completely separates hypercalcaemic patients with hyperparathyroidism from those with malignancy. The assay has precision over a wide range of PTH concentrations and, with a turnaround time of 24 hours, it has proved durable in clinical practice. However, it is clear that as well as measuring 1–84 PTH it also cross-reacts with the 7–84 peptide (N-terminal truncated PTH), and even the more recently developed 'specific' 1–84 assays include a 10–20 percent contribution from 7–84 PTH in normal subjects or patients with primary hyperparathyroidism.[6] This proportion may rise to 35 percent in chronic renal failure but even here there is a close correlation between assays detecting only 1–84 PTH and those that measure fragments as well as intact hormone.[7] The clinical significance of the truncated peptide is uncertain but there is experimental evidence that it may act as an endogenous inhibitor to PTH.[8] At present, there is insufficient evidence that the differences between the assays that measure PTH (1–84) alone and those that also measure the N-terminal truncated peptide influence clinical management and this is also true for most cases of chronic renal failure.[9] [***]

PTH measurements in clinical practice

The major indications for PTH measurement are outlined below.

- Diagnosis of the causes of hypercalcaemia (**Table 30.4**) and hypocalcaemia (**Table 30.5**). The major distinguishing features of these conditions have already been outlined in the sections on calcium, phosphate and magnesium.
- Guide to therapeutic strategies:
  - Management of renal bone disease. It is important to be able to separate adynamic and hyperparathyroid bone disease since their management is different. Adynamic bone disease may be associated with oversuppression of parathyroid function and this is an important constraint to the use of active vitamin D metabolites or anti-resorptive drugs.
  - Adjustment of phosphate therapy in hypophosphataemic osteomalacia. Phosphate supplements are an essential component of treatment but lead to calcium malabsorption,

Table 30.4 PTH concentration in hypercalcaemia.

Concentration	Effect
High	Primary or tertiary hyperparathyroidism
	Familial hypocalciuric hyperparathyroidism
	Lithium
Normal	Primary hyperparathyroidism
	Familial hypocalciuric hyperparathyroidism
	Lithium
Low	Malignancy
	Vitamin D intoxication
	Sarcoidosis
	Immobilization
	Milk-alkali syndrome
	Addison's disease

Table 30.5 PTH concentration in hypocalcaemia.

Concentration	Effect
High	Vitamin D deficiency
	Pseudohypoparathyroidism
	Acute pancreatitis
	'Hungry bone syndrome'
	Post-parathyroidectomy
	Sclerotic metastases
	Acute inhibition of bone resorption
Normal	Functional hypoparathyroidism
	Spurious hypocalcaemia (hypoalbuminaemia)
Low	Hypoparathyroidism
	Magnesium deficiency

secondary hyperparathyroidism and worsening of the phosphate leak. This has to be offset by calcitriol therapy where the dose is adjusted to maintain a normal level of PTH.

– Evaluation of vitamin D nutrition in osteoporosis. Many elderly patients with osteoporosis have an inadequate intake of vitamin D which leads to secondary hyperparathyroidism, increased bone turnover and amplification of their age-related or postmenopausal bone loss. This can be corrected by vitamin D supplementation.

End organ resistance to PTH (pseudohypoparathyroidism)

This is an unusual syndrome expressing the combination of biochemical hypoparathyroidism, an unusual body habitus (Albrights hereditary osteodystrophy: short metacarpals, round face, truncal obesity and basal ganglia calcification) with end organ resistance to the action of PTH leading to secondary hyperparathyroidism. Prior to the introduction of the current two-site PTH assay, this syndrome was usually confirmed by demonstrating an impaired serum or urinary cyclic AMP response to exogenous PTH[10] and this still remains the most reliable way of separating the different variants of this rare syndrome.[11] In practice, the identification of this condition can be made from a combination of the clinical picture, the biochemical features of hypoparathyroidism (and the absence of vitamin D deficiency) in the presence of an elevated PTH. [****/***]

> ### KEY POINTS
>
> - Assays for 1–84 PTH cross-react to some extent (10–20 percent) with an N-terminal 7–84 truncated peptide, but this may not adversely affect the clinical utility of the measurement.
> - Current assays reliably separate hyperparathyroidism from the hypercalcaemia of malignancy.
> - PTH measurements are an integral part of the diagnosis and management of most common metabolic bone diseases.

PARATHYROID IMAGING

The major stimulus for the development of parathyroid imaging, with the required sensitivity and specificity, has been the interest in minimally invasive parathyroidectomy, which is critically dependent on reliable identification of the abnormal gland(s). Two technical options are available.

Dual phase single tracer scintigraphy

This relies on the differential time course of tracer uptake by the thyroid (early at 10 minutes) and parathyroids (late at 120 minutes). The problem is that approximately 30 percent of patients have coincidental thyroid nodules[12] which may have a tracer uptake similar to that of the parathyroid glands (false positive). In contrast, some parathyroid adenomas may show early tracer washout leading to false negative scans, and a comparison of early and late imaging[13] showed that the former had a higher sensitivity (92 percent) than the latter (74 percent). Another option is to combine scintigraphy with ultrasound to separate thyroid and parathyroid nodules.[14]

DUAL ISOTOPE SUBTRACTION SCANS

With this method, a tracer which is only taken up by the thyroid is subtracted from the thyroid/parathyroid sestamibi image using data acquisition which can be either sequential or simultaneous. The latter avoids motion artefact but requires separation of the two tracer energies. ^{123}I is the optimal thyroid scanning agent but is not available on a daily basis from a generator and ^{99m}Tc is an alternative. Use of ^{99m}Tc pertechnetate may give quite high thyroid activity and may obscure the relatively low uptake from a posteriorly placed parathyroid. This can be overcome by the use of oral potassium perchlorate to wash out the ^{99m}Tc pertechnetate from the thyroid.[15]

Choice of tracer

There has also been considerable interest in the choice of tracer for parathyroid imaging. The accuracy of thallium-technetium scanning is dependent on adenoma size[16] and, since it is the small gland that presents the surgical problem, there has been a shift to the use of the more sensitive ^{99m}Tc-sestamibi.[13, 17] In a meta-analysis of 6331 cases scanned with ^{99m}Tc-sestamibi, there was a sensitivity of 90.7 percent and a specificity of 98.8 percent.[18] [***]

The ability to use the same tracer for multiple imaging techniques has stimulated the use of ^{99m}Tc-tetrofosmin, which can also be used in nuclear cardiology. This tracer is unsuitable for dual phase imaging because of poor differential washout between thyroid and parathyroids, but it can be used with dual isotope subtraction scanning. In a direct comparison of ^{99m}Tc-sestamibi and tetrofosmin it was shown that the early differential uptake by thyroid and parathyroids was poorer with tetrofosmin, but the later uptake was superior to sestamibi.[14]

SINGLE PHOTON EMISSION TOMOGRAPHY

Single photon emission tomography (SPET) has the advantage over the planar technique in terms of separation of thyroid and parathyroid images, improved ability to localize ectopic glands, specificity and sensitivity.[14] There have been direct comparisons between planar scanning and SPET which have supported its superiority over both planar dual phase and subtraction techniques[19] although delayed phase SPET may not be optimal.[20] If the technique is available, as it may be in some nuclear cardiology departments, then it does have attractions as a routine parathyroid imaging technique. Otherwise, its main application is in the identification of ectopic parathyroid glands or where there has been a failed neck exploration.

ULTRASOUND, CT AND MRI

Local expertise with ultrasound, CT and MRI may determine its use in a particular centre. Ultrasound is widely available but highly dependent on operator skill, with the result that the reported sensitivity of this technique in parathyroid disease ranges from 30 to 90 percent.[21] Particular limitations of ultrasound are the inability to identify medially situated upper parathyroid glands and those which are intrathyroidal or in the mediastinum. Ultrasound is good for identifying parathyroids behind the thyroid or below the lower poles. Identification of their vascular pedicles by Doppler ultrasound can also help distinguish thyroid and parathyroid adenomas.

CT and MRI find their main role in the localization of mediastinal parathyroid glands. The major limitation with CT is the similar densities of thyroid and parathyroid tissue and, in the neck, MRI may be preferable. Even so, MRI is generally less sensitive and specific than sestamibi scanning.[14]

INTRAOPERATIVE GAMMA PROBE LOCALIZATION AND RAPID PTH ASSAY

In difficult cases, a combination of preoperative scintigraphy, introperative gamma probe gland localization with measurement of tracer content of removed tissue[22] and confirmation by rapid PTH assay may be helpful.[23] In this approach, ^{99m}Tc-sestamibi is administered two to three hours before operation and a hand-held gamma probe is used to localize abnormal parathyroid tissue (> 20 percent above background).[24] A requirement is that the preoperative sestamibi scan has shown the presence of an adenoma (approximately 80 percent of cases), although the gamma probe may be useful where there has been a negative scan in reoperative procedures or where there is an ectopic gland.[25] While helpful, the gamma probe may not provide unique information which will not be available from other modalities, such as the preoperative sestamibi scan. The rapid PTH assay with a turnaround time of 15 minutes does provide additional practical information:

- prediction of clinical cure (decrease in intraoperative PTH >50 percent);[26]
- indicates the probability of multiglandular disease (and the need for a bilateral neck exploration);
- suggests the probability of postoperative hypoparathyroidism and the potential for autografting of removed parathyroid tissue (final PTH below the lower limit of detection).

This approach seems particularly appropriate for specialist centres treating a high proportion of failed or recurrent hyperparathyroidism, but there is no evidence that it is needed for previously untreated primary hyperparathyroidism. [**]

Indications for parathyroid imaging

The need for parathyroid imaging is driven entirely by the interest in limited surgery for hyperparathyroidism. This seems reasonable for a condition which is due to a solitary adenoma in almost 90 percent of patients.[18] Minimally invasive parathyroidectomy offers the prospect of shorter operation times under local anaesthetic as day cases[27] with potential cost savings and may follow the trend in other areas by being driven by patient preference. The need here is to identify cases with a single adenoma, since those with hyperplasia, multigland disease or abnormal neck anatomy (goitre, previous neck surgery or irradiation) will need a bilateral operation, which remains the 'gold standard' against which newer approaches are judged. A recent meta-analysis suggested that 87 percent of patients with sporadic primary hyperparathyroidism would be candidates for a unilateral parathyroidectomy.[18] However, while a recent systematic review of minimally invasive parathyroidectomy suggested that it may have an advantage over the bilateral exploration, the confidence intervals were wide and there may have been bias due to rigorous case selection.[28]

There is general agreement that patients with failed or recurrent hyperparathyroidism require detailed preoperative imaging, and this approach is increasingly being extended to the previously untreated case since localization of the adenoma allows unilateral operation which is of shorter duration. However, the experienced parathyroid surgeon has a better than 90 percent probability of success compared to the 80 percent identification rate of sestamibi and may well find the small gland missed by scanning.[29] The conventional bilateral surgical approach of identifying all the parathyroid glands may succeed where scanning may fail if there are asymmetrically enlarged glands and only the largest adenoma is identified. [***]

KEY POINTS

- No single test of parathyroid function is diagnostic.
- Measurement of serum calcium, phosphate, magnesium and PTH are the main tests of function.
- The two-site IRMA for intact PTH is reliable and discriminatory.
- Misdiagnosis of calcium disorders is usually due to lack of attention to history and examination rather than incorrect interpretation of laboratory tests.
- Intraoperative measurement of PTH may facilitate management.
- ^{99m}Tc-sestamibi parathyroid imaging has high sensitivity and specificity. It is increasingly used to identify a solitary adenoma and facilitate unilateral parathyroidectomy.
- Ultrasound, CT and MRI may help in the localization of ectopic glands.

Best clinical practice

- ✓ Dual phase single tracer scintigraphy or dual isotope subtraction scans are the method of choice for the identification of a parathyroid adenoma.
- ✓ ^{99m}Tc-sestamibi scanning has 90 percent sensitivity and almost 99 percent specificity for a solitary parathyroid adenoma.
- ✓ SPET, ultrasound, CT and MRI may have a place where there is local expertise but they are less sensitive and specific.
- ✓ Rapid PTH assays with a turnround time of 15 minutes provide important additional information during parathyroidectomy.

Deficiencies in current knowledge and areas for future research

- ➤ Refinements in the assays for PTH are needed to eliminate cross reactivity with peptide fragments. This would be important in better defining changes in parathyroid function in disease states since this would influence both diagnostic precision and facilitate management. Such assays would need validation over a wide range of disease states including renal failure.
- ➤ Although sestamibi scanning is now well established, its use in the management of primary

hyperparathyroidism is dependent on careful case selection to eliminate possible cases of hyperplasia or multiple adenomata. Development of an imaging technique which was able to distinguish multiple parathyroid glands from the normal or adenomatous thyroid would greatly increase the scope of preoperative gland localization.

REFERENCES

* 1. Portale AA. Blood calcium, phosphorus, and magnesium. In: Favus MJ (ed.). *Primer on the metabolic bone diseases and disorders of mineral metabolism.* Philadelphia: Lippincott Williams and Wilkins, 1999: 115–8.

2. Walton RJ, Bijvoet OLM. Nomogram for derivation of renal threshold phosphate concentration. *Lancet.* 1975; **2**: 309–10.

3. Rude RK. Magnesium metabolism and deficiency. *Endocrinology and Metabolism Clinics of North America.* 1993; **22**: 377–95.

4. Lepage R, Roy L, Brossard JH, Rousseau L, Dorais C, Lazure C *et al.* A non-(1-84) PTH circulating fragment interferes significantly with intact PTH measurement by commercial assaysin uraemic samples. *Clinical Chemistry.* 1998; **44**: 805–9.

* 5. Nussbaum SR, Zahradnik RJ, Lavigne JR, Brennan GL, Nozawa-Ung K, Kim LY *et al.* Highly sensitive two-site immunoradiometric assay of parathyrin and its clinical utility in evaluating patients with hypercalcemia. *Clinical Chemistry.* 1987; **33**: 1364–7.

6. Brossard JH, Lepage R, Cardinal H, Roy L, Rousseau L, Dorais C *et al.* Influence of glomerular filtration rate on non-(1-84) parathyroid hormone (PTH) detected by intact PTH assays. *Clinical Chemistry.* 2000; **46**: 697–703.

7. Gao P, Scheibel S, D'Amour P, John MR, Rao SD, Schmidt-Gayk H *et al.* Development of a novel immunoradiometric assay exclusively for biologically active whole parathyroid hormone 1-84: implications for improvement of accurate assessment of parathyroid function. *Journal of Bone and Mineral Research.* 2001; **16**: 605–14.

8. Slatopolsky E, Finch J, Clay P, Martin D, Sicard G, Singer G *et al.* A novel mechanism for skeletal resistance in uremia. *Kidney International.* 2000; **58**: 753–61.

* 9. Blumsohn A, Hadari AA. Parathyroid hormone: what are we measuring and does it matter? *Annals of Clinical Biochemistry.* 2002; **39**: 169–72.

10. Chase LR, Melson GL, Aurbach GD. Pseudohypo-parathyroidism: Defective excretion of 3'5' -AMP in response to parathyroid hormone. *Journal of Clinical Investigation.* 1969; **48**: 1832–44.

11. Levine MA. Pseudohypoparathyroidism: from bedside to bench and back. *Journal of Bone and Mineral Research.* 1999; **14**: 1255–60.

12. Hinde E, Melliere D, Jeanguillaume C, Perlemuter L, Chehade F, Galle P. Parathyroid imaging using

simultaneous double-window recording of technetium-99m-sestamibi and iodine-123. *Journal of Nuclear Medicine.* 1998; **39**: 1100–5.

13. Carty SE, Worsey J, Virji MA, Brown ML, Watson CG. Concise parathyroidectomy: the impact of preoperative SPECT 99mTc sestamibi scanning and intra-operative quick parathormone assay. *Surgery.* 1997; **122**: 1107–16.

* 14. Giordano A, Rubello D, Casara D. New trends in parathyroid scintigraphy. *European Journal of Nuclear Medicine.* 2001; **28**: 1409–20.

15. Rubello D, Saladini G, Casara D, Borsato N, Toniato A, Piotto A *et al.* Parathyroid imaging with pertechnetate plus perchlorate/MIBI subtraction scintigraphy. A fast and effective technique. *Clinical Nuclear Medicine.* 2000; **25**: 527–31.

16. Tsukamoto E, Russell CF, Ferguson WR, Laird JD. The role of preoperative thallium-technetium subtraction scintigraphy in the surgical management of patients with solitary parathyroid adenoma. *Clinical Radiology.* 1995; **50**: 677–80.

17. Borley NR, Collins RE, O'Doherty M, Coakley A. Technetium-99m sestamibi parathyroid localisation is accurate enough for scan-directed unilateral neck exploration. *British Journal of Surgery.* 1996; **83**: 989–91.

* 18. Denham DW, Norman J. Cost-effectiveness of preoperative sestamibi scan for primary hyperparathyroidism is dependent solely upon the surgeon's choice of operative procedure. *Journal of the American College of Surgeons.* 1998; **186**: 293–305.

19. Gallowitsch HJ, Mikosch P, Kresnik E, Gomez I, Lind P. Technetium-99m- tetrofosmin parathyroid imaging: results with double-phase study and SPECT in primary and secondary hyperparathyroidism. *Investigative Radiology.* 1997; **32**: 459–65.

20. Chen CC, Holder LE, Scovill WA, Tehan AM, Gann DS. Comparison of parathyroid imaging with technetium-99m-pertechnetate/sestamibi subtraction, double-phase technetium-99m-sestamibi and technetium-99m-

sestamibi SPECT. *Journal of Nuclear Medicine.* 1997; **38**: 834–9.

21. Mitchell BK, Merrell RC, Kinder BK. Localization studies in patients with hyperparathyroidism. *Surgical Clinics of North America.* 1995; **75**: 483–98.

22. Norman JG, Jaffray CE, Chheda H. The false-positive parathyroid sestamibi: A real or percieved problem and a case for radioguided parathyroidectomy. *Annals of Surgery.* 2000; **231**: 31–7.

23. Irvin 3rd. GL, Molinari AS, Figueroa C, Carneiro DM. Improved success rate in reoperative parathyroidectomy with intraoperative PTH assay. *Annals of Surgery.* 1999; **229**: 874–8.

24. Goldstein RE, Blevins L, Delbeke D, Martin WH. Effect of minimally invasive radioguided parathyroidectomy on efficacy, length of stay, and costs in the management of primary hyperparathyroidism. *Annals of Surgery.* 2000; **231**: 732–42.

25. Dackiw APB, Sussman JJ, Fritsche HA, Delpassand ES, Stanford P, Hoff A *et al.* Relative contributions of technetium Tc 99m sestamibi scintigraphy, intraoperative gamma probe detection, and rapid parathyroid hormone assay to the surgical management of hyperparathyroidism. *Archives of Surgery.* 2000; **135**: 550–7.

26. Garner SC, Leight Jr. GS. Initial experience with intraoperative PTH determinations in the surgical management of 130 cases of primary hyperparathyroidism. *Surgery.* 1999; **126**: 1132–7.

27. Vogel LM, Lucas R, Czako P. Unilateral parathyroid exploration. *American Surgeon.* 1998; **64**: 693–6.

* 28. Reeve TS, Babidge WJ, Parkyn RF, Edis AJ, Delbridge LW, Devitt *et al.* Minimally invasive surgery for primary hyperparathyroidism: systematic review. *Archives of Surgery.* 2000; **135**: 481–7.

29. McIntyre RC, Ridgway EC. Sestamibi: opening a new era of parathyroid surgical procedures. *Endocrine Practice.* 1998; **4**: 241–4.

31

Parathyroid dysfunction: medical and surgical therapy

E DINAKARA BABU, BILL FLEMING AND JA LYNN

Normal parathyroid glands	387	Best clinical practice	396
Genetics of hyperparathyroidism	388	Deficiencies in current knowledge and areas for future	
Primary hyperparathyroidism	389	research	396
Secondary and tertiary HPT	395	References	396
Key points	396		

SEARCH STRATEGY

The data in this chapter are supported by a Medline search using the key words parathyroid glands, hyperparathyroidism, hypercalcaemia and parathyroid carcinoma. Further relevant articles were obtained by manual screening of the reference lists of selected papers.

NORMAL PARATHYROID GLANDS

Anatomy

The parathyroid glands are best identified by their relationship to the plane of the recurrent laryngeal nerve: superior glands posterior and inferior glands anterior to this plane. There are four glands in 87 percent of patients, five in 6 percent and six in 0.5 percent, but up to ten have been reported in one individual, which may in fact represent chief-cell hyperplasia. In less than 1 percent of cases only three glands are identified.[1, 2] There is also positional symmetry to the upper parathyroid glands in 80 percent of cases and to the inferior glands in 70 percent of cases.

Embryology

Parathyroid glands are formed during the fifth week of intrauterine life. Superior glands develop from the fourth pharyngeal pouch and are found at the junction of the upper and middle third of the posterior surface of the thyroid gland, near the cricothyroid junction in 80 percent of cases. The importance of this position is its proximity to the point where the recurrent laryngeal nerve enters the larynx. In 15 percent they are found on the posterior surface of the thyroid, while 3 percent are to be found in retro-oesophageal, retrolaryngeal or retro-pharyngeal positions and, finally, 1 percent lie above the thyroid upper pole.

Inferior glands develop from the third pharyngeal pouch and are closely related to the developing thymus (thyrothymic ligament). The inferior glands take a longer and more variable migration through the neck, with a more widespread final resting position and ectopic glands potentially anywhere from the carotid bifurcation down to the pericardium. The inferior glands are at the lower pole of the thyroid in 50 percent of cases, within the thymus or the thyrothymic ligament in 25 percent, while approximately 10 percent are more lateral and 10 percent lie on or next to the trachea.

Physiology

Parathyroid glands are composed of chief and oxyphil cells, and secrete parathyroid hormone (PTH), which plays a major role in calcium metabolism either by directly acting on the bone or indirectly through vitamin D. Calcium ion homeostasis is maintained by a complex of hormones and different organ systems, controlled by PTH, vitamin D and calcitonin.

PTH

PTH is synthesized and secreted by the chief cells in response to a fall in extracellular calcium concentrations. PTH is secreted in an episodic manner as pre-pro and pro-PTH, before being cleaved into fragments within the chief cells and in the Kuppfer cells of the liver. The 1–34 N-terminal fragment is the biologically active form of PTH, which has a half-life of PTH of around five minutes.

Parathyroid and C–cells utilize a calcium sensing receptor (CaR), which senses the level of extracellular calcium to determine the secretion of PTH and calcitonin (see below). PTH acts on target tissues by binding to PTH receptors on the cell surface. Three PTH receptors have been described to date with PTH-1 being the most important mediator of PTH and parathyroid hormone-related peptide (PTHrP) actions on calcium homeostasis.[3] In bone, PTH induces bone resorption by indirectly acting on osteoclast cells to increase their number and activity. It acts via the PTH-1 receptor primarily on osteoblasts, which release a cytokine that acts on the osteoclasts.

In the kidney PTH acts via the PTH-1 receptor to decrease calcium excretion by increasing the reabsorption of calcium in the distal convoluted tubule. It also increases phosphate excretion and stimulates production of calcitriol, the active form of 1,25 dihydroxycholecalciferol (vitamin D) in the proximal convoluted tubule. This PTH-induced increase in calcitriol has an effect on the intestine which results in enhanced gut absorption of calcium.

PTHrP

PTHrP closely resembles PTH and is an important mediator regulating the hypercalcaemia of malignancy. It acts via all three PTH receptors, and the PTH-2 receptor will only bind PTHrP. The normal physiological role for PTHrP appears to be in the foetus, where it facilitates placental mineral transport.

VITAMIN D

1,25-dihydroxy-vitamin D is a fat-soluble compound, synthesized in the skin from its precursor 7-dehydro-cholestrol by the action of sunlight, and is also derived from plant ergosterol in the diet. It is transported to the liver where it is converted to the major circulating metabolite 25-hydroxycholecalciferol. A further hydroxylation to the active form 1,25-dihydroxycholecalciferol takes place in the kidney, under the control of PTH and calcitonin. Vitamin D exerts its action through specific receptors present in the cell nucleus in bone and gut.

CALCITONIN

Calcitonin is a hormone secreted by the parafollicular cells of the thyroid, with a half-life of ten minutes. Calcitonin reduces the serum calcium level by its effect on specific cell surface receptors on osteoclasts and on the proximal convoluted tubules. The exact physiological role of calcitonin remains uncertain however, as patients with high circulating calcitonin levels in medullary carcinoma of the thyroid do not have any disorder of calcium homeostasis.

CALCITONIN GENE–RELATED PEPTIDE

Calcitonin gene-related peptide (CGRP) is the product of the same gene that directs the synthesis of calcitonin, and is found in thyroid, pituitary, pancreas and adrenal medulla. Its exact role is unknown.

OTHER HORMONES

Other hormones that affect calcium metabolism are only important in times of greater calcium need, such as during growth, pregnancy and lactation. These are growth hormone, oestrogens, corticosteroids, thyroxine and insulin. [***/**]

GENETICS OF HYPERPARATHYROIDISM

Most of the parathyroid disorders are due to genetic abnormalities and have a familial tendency. These genetic disorders are due to a defect in either PTH or the PTH receptors producing either hyper or hypoparathyroidism.[4]

Parathyroid tumours are either sporadic or inherited as a part of a multiple endocrine neoplasia (MEN) syndrome. They are produced by overexpression of PRAD-1 and RET gene or due to inactivation of the MEN 1 gene, retinoblastoma (RB) gene, and the gene on chromosome 1b.

PRAD-1

Parathyroid adenoma-1, or PRAD-1, is a gene on chromosome 11 that controls the cell cycle. Overexpression of PRAD-1, resulting in overexpression of the regulatory protein cyclin D1, is responsible for at least 50 percent of sporadic parathyroid adenomas.

MENIN

The MEN-1, or MENIN, gene is a tumour suppressor gene located on chromosome 11q13. Somatic mutations of this gene cause MEN-1, but are found in approximately 25 percent of sporadic parathyroid adenomas. MEN-1 is characterized by parathyroid, pancreatic islet cell and pituitary tumours, with 95 percent having hyperparathyroidism (HPT) due to parathyroid tumours. There are over 250 different mutations of the MENIN gene found in the kindred of MEN-1 patients, and 90–95 percent of MEN-1 patients have demonstrable mutations.

RET protooncogene

The cRET, or MEN-2, gene is a protooncogene located on chromosome 10. Mutations of this gene result in MEN-2, which has two subtypes. MEN-2A is the more common type, characterized by medullary carcinoma of the thyroid, phaeochromocytoma and parathyroid tumours, but the latter are only present in 20 percent, reflecting the lower virulence of the multiglandular disease. MEN-2B is characterized by medullary carcinoma of the thyroid and phaeochromocytoma, marfanoid features and mucosal neuromas, but without parathyroid tumours. The cRET genetic mutation is found in 90 percent of patients, so that mutational analysis of the cRET gene is useful in the screening and management of first-degree relatives.

RB gene

The RB gene is a tumour suppressor gene present on chromosome 13q14. Allelic deletion of the RB gene is found in parathyroid tumours, especially in parathyroid carcinoma, so that with the presence of abnormal RB protein staining may play an important role in differentiating benign and malignant parathyroid disease.

Gene on chromosome 1b

This is a protooncogene located on the chromosome 1q21–q31, and mutation of this gene is found in 40 percent of sporadic parathyroid adenomas. In the hereditary form there is an association with a family history of mandibular and maxillary tumours, Wilm's tumour and adult nephroblastoma, as well as an increased risk of parathyroid cancer.

Gene on chromosome Xp11

This is a tumour suppressor gene, which may play an important role in the refractory secondary HPT seen in chronic renal failure. Hyperplasia of parathyroid glands in these patients is due to monoclonal mechanisms and produces nodular hyperplasia.

Gene for CaR

The calcium sensing receptor has a key role in the calcium-mediated regulation of PTH secretion, parathyroid cellular proliferation and probably the mRNA levels of pre-proPTH.[3] Inactivating mutations of this gene produce two types of hypercalcaemic disorders that reset the 'set-point' of calcium-mediated PTH secretion. Heterozygous mutations result in familial hypocalciuric hypercalcaemia (FHH), with a mild, generally asymptomatic hypercalcaemia. Individuals with homozygous mutations have parathyroid glands with much more marked calcium resistance, presenting with neonatal severe hyperparathyroidism (NSHPT) and profound hypercalcaemia and HPT.

PTH–receptor gene

This gene is located on chromosome 3 and activated mutation of this gene results in Jansen's disease. It is an autosomal dominant disorder characterized by dwarfism, hypercalcaemia and hypophosphataemia, with normal or undetectable serum PTH. William's syndrome is an autosomal dominant disorder, with a genetic defect located on chromosome 7, characterized by infantile hypercalcaemia, supravalvular aortic stenosis, psychomotor retardation and elfin facies.

PRIMARY HYPERPARATHYROIDISM

Hyperparathyroidism can be caused by primary parathyroid gland dysfunction or by a variety of secondary causes that lower calcium levels or raise phosphate levels. Hypoparathyroidism is usually a complication of thyroid surgery, from removal or damage to parathyroid glands. Its presentation and management are discussed in Chapter 28, The thyroid: nonmalignant disease.

Normally, PTH secretion is exceedingly sensitive to changes in serum calcium, with PTH changes occurring within seconds, sequentially and graded.[3] The immediate effect of lowered calcium is the release of preformed PTH from secretory vesicles, followed by a decrease in the degradation of PTH in the parathyroid cell, so that more intact hormone is released. If the stimulus persists then there is an upregulation of the expression of pre-proPTH mRNA. If the stimulus lasts for an extensive period of time, then parathyroid chief cells begin to proliferate within days (as in chronic renal failure). In primary hyperparathyroidism (pHPT) this sensitive feedback mechanism is lost.

Diagnosis

Diagnosis of pHPT is made when there is a high serum calcium, with an abnormally high or nonsuppressed PTH level. Occasionally, it may be difficult to identify milder forms of pHPT, as PTH is not released at an even rate, so repeated measurements of serum PTH and calcium may be required to make a biochemical diagnosis.

pHPT occurs in two forms, as nonfamilial or sporadic in 95 percent, and as familial or hereditary in 5 percent. In the hereditary form, pHPT may be a part of one of the MEN syndromes.

Incidence

The exact incidence of pHPT is unknown, but is increasing with the use of multichannel autoanalysers picking up hypercalcaemia more often. Overall, the incidence in men is around 0.3 percent, and in women 1–3 percent, but in autopsy examination this sex discrepancy disappears, perhaps reflecting the more likely diagnosis in women being screened for osteoporosis. In women, the incidence rises with age and could be as high as 1 in 500, with a rate of 2.6 percent in women aged between 55 and 75 years.[5]

Pathology

The aetiology of primary HPT is unknown, but radiotherapy to the head and neck during childhood can predispose to either adenoma or hyperplasia.[6] The pathology of pHPT is adenoma in 80 percent, hyperplasia in 15–20 percent and carcinoma in 1 percent of patients.

ADENOMA

Parathyroid adenomas are usually solitary, with the other glands showing evidence of suppressed activity. Double or multiple adenomas may occur occasionally, but more likely are misdiagnosed hyperplasia. Parathyroid tumour more often affects the lower glands than the upper glands, and intrathymic and intrathyroidal adenomas are not uncommon.

The adenomas are generally ovoid, soft, reddish-brown tumours, usually a little darker than the normal glands. Microscopically, they are characterized by varying compositions of chief, clear and oxyphil cells, with chief-cell adenoma by far the most common. Parathyroid adenomas generally exhibit a peripheral rim of condensed normal parathyroid tissue, separated by a slender capsule.

HYPERPLASIA

Parathyroid hyperplasia affects more than one gland, as a result of an increase in parathyroid parenchyma. The enlarged glands are rounded or grossly lobulated, and grey-brown in colour, but the process may not involve all glands or involve them uniformly.

Microscopically, primary chief-cell or nodular hyperplasia is the predominant finding, but a multiplicity of cell types can be found. Nodular chief-cell hyperplasia is the characteristic pathology of the parathyroids in MEN-1 syndrome.

CARCINOMA

Parathyroid carcinomas are nearly always functioning tumours and account for approximately 1 percent of cases of pHPT, usually with a very high serum calcium and PTH. These tumours are often large and clinically palpable, usually greater than 2 cm in size, and appear firm, greyish-white and adherent to adjacent structures.

Microscopically, carcinoma shows features of malignancy, such as invasion of the capsule, vascular invasion, marked fibrosis with nodule formation, focal areas of necrosis, cellular atypia and a high mitotic rate. Chief and oxyphil cells are predominantly seen. Flow cytometry studies show that an aberrant ploidy pattern is associated with a bad prognosis. It is extremely difficult for the pathologist to make the diagnosis at frozen and paraffin section. Parathyroid carcinoma spreads by local invasion and lymphatic permeation, and distant metastasis occurs to lung, liver and bones. Treatment involves en bloc resection of parathyroid and adjacent structures, including ipsilateral thyroid lobectomy and node dissection. [**]

Clinical features

In asymptomatic, ambulatory patients, over 80 percent of patients with hypercalcaemia will have pHPT, but this falls to less than a third in symptomatic and/or hospitalized patients. More often in this hospital group, severe symptomatic hypercalcaemia is caused by malignant disease. The majority of patients with pHPT have no symptoms or only mild symptoms, and are picked up on biochemical screening for another reason. Symptomatic presentation due to hypercalcaemia with the classical rhyme of bones, stones, abdominal groans and psychic moans is extremely rare.

MUSCULOSKELETAL

The most common symptoms are muscular weakness, bone and joint pain; fatigue and lethargy are very common. Patients have reduced bone mineral density, but the severe form of bone disease known as osteitis fibrosa cystica is extremely rare in developed countries. Parathyroidectomy leads to incomplete improvement of bone density, but does improve muscle function and relieves the feeling of tiredness.

RENAL

The usual symptoms are renal and ureteric stones; renal failure and nephrocalcinosis are extremely rare. Parathyroidectomy lowers the frequency of recurrent stones.

GASTROINTESTINAL

Abdominal pain can arise from chronic constipation, but the linkage between peptic ulceration, pancreatitis and pHPT is controversial. Improvement of symptoms after parathyroidectomy is unpredictable.

PSYCHOLOGICAL

Prospective analyses have suggested that even apparently asymptomatic patients with pHPT may have psychiatric symptoms, which can be reversed by active treatment.[7] Anxiety and depression, lassitude, dementia and loss of concentration or memory are the common symptoms. Parathyroidectomy reverses the dementia-like symptoms in the elderly population, and significant improvements can be made in other symptoms.[8]

METABOLIC 'SYNDROME'

pHPT is associated with a metabolic syndrome which carries an increased risk of premature death, even in mild hypercalcaemia, and increases with the extent of hypercalcaemia.

Diabetes mellitus and an impaired glucose tolerance can be seen due to peripheral insulin resistance. Blood lipid levels show a decrease in high-density lipoprotein (HDL) and low-density lipoprotein (LDL) levels and a rise in very low-density lipoprotein (VLDL) levels. Cardiovascular disorders, such as hypertension, left ventricular hypertrophy and valvular calcification, are known to be associated with pHPT. Many of these effects can be reversed or improved after parathyroidectomy. [****/**]

Investigations for HPT

pHPT is responsible for over 80 percent of cases of asymptomatic hypercalcaemia in the ambulatory population, but accounts for only 20 percent in the symptomatic or hospitalized population with hypercalcaemia.

BIOCHEMICAL

The common biochemical tests performed are plasma calcium, albumin, vitamin D and intact PTH. Measurements may have to be repeated due to the episodic secretion of PTH, which can result in normocalcaemic periods. A 24 hour urine collection for calcium will help to exclude FHH and lithium as causes of hypercalcaemia.

Complementary tests that may be helpful to support the diagnosis are plasma phosphate, creatinine and magnesium.

LOCALIZATION STUDIES

Preoperative localization of parathyroid tumours can locate abnormal glands in 80–85 percent of cases, which allows minimally invasive techniques to be used, with the potential for operation under local anaesthesia. Typically, localization is achieved by a combination of high-resolution ultrasound and ^{99m}Tc-sestamibi scan. Other investigations, such as selective angiography and venous sampling, CT and MRI will be needed if a second or subsequent operation is being planned.

Ultrasound

Ultrasound is cheap, noninvasive and can be used intraoperatively. Parathyroid adenoma is typically sonolucent (**Figure 31.1**) and colour Doppler will demonstrate the presence of an arterial signal at the vascular pole.[9] Ultrasound can only be used to locate adenomas in the neck, with a sensitivity of around 85 percent in the unexplored neck, dropping to 40 percent in patients who have had a previous exploration.

Sestamibi scintiscan

Parathyroid adenoma concentrates ^{99m}Tc-labelled sestamibi because of the higher number of metabolically active mitochondria (**Figure 31.2**). It can be used to locate glands in either the neck or mediastinum with or without the addition of single photon emission computerized tomography (SPECT). Scanning can detect 87 percent of solitary adenomas, 55 percent of abnormal glands in patients with multiglandular disease and 75 percent of persistent or recurrent lesions in the previously explored neck.[10] Diffuse hyperplasia will often lead to a negative scan as the parathyroid glands are less mitochondria-rich.

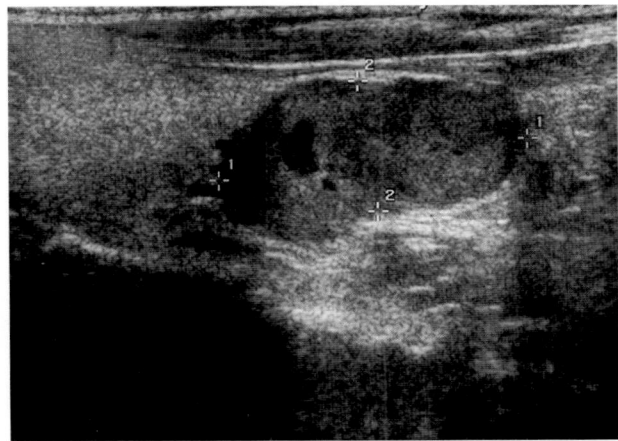

Figure 31.1 Ultrasound of a typical parathyroid adenoma.

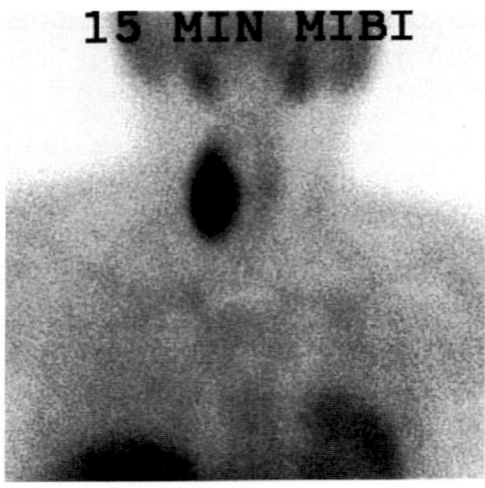

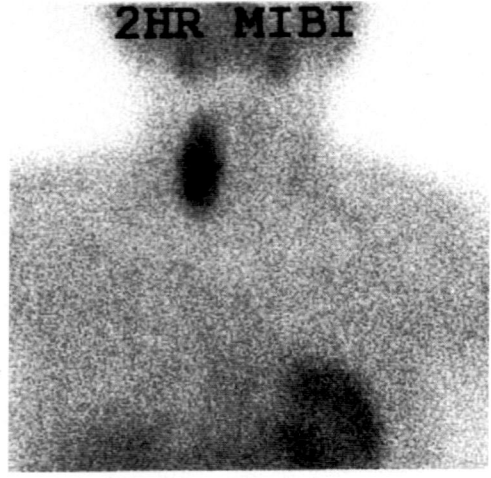

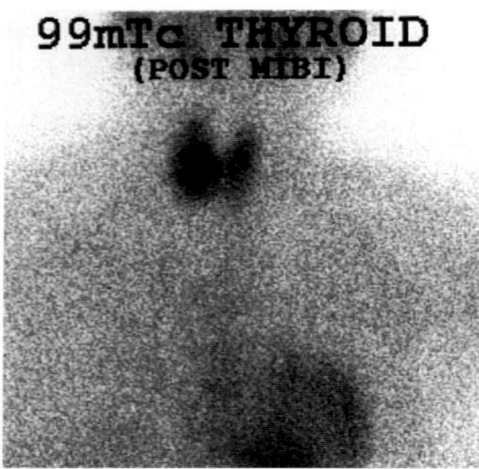

Figure 31.2 Sestamibi scan showing right inferior parathyroid adenoma.

Selective venous sampling and angiography

In the patient who has had a previous failed exploration, perhaps due to a mediastinal adenoma, more invasive investigative measures may be needed in addition to sestamibi scan and ultrasound. Selective angiography will

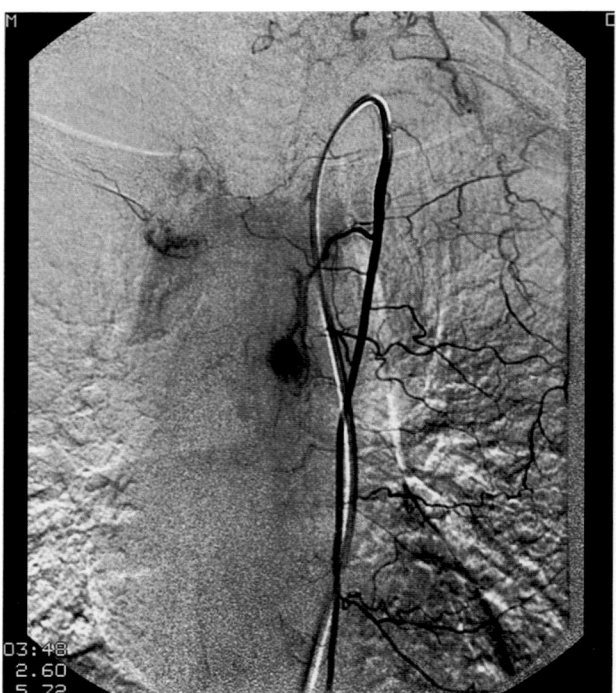

Figure 31.3 Selective arteriogram showing a mediastinal parathyroid adenoma.

usually identify the missed gland, with a sensitivity of 90–95 percent, especially when combined with venous sampling for parathyroid hormone assay (**Figure 31.3**). Almost all enlarged glands are hypervascular, with a distinctive angiographic 'blush', resulting in a low false-positive rate.

Computed tomography and magnetic resonance imaging

Thin-slice computed tomography (CT) will visualize ectopic parathyroids in the anterior mediastinum, where ultrasound cannot see. CT and magnetic resonance imaging (MRI) have a sensitivity of 75–85 percent in an unexplored neck, which decreases to 45 percent for CT after previous surgery, but remains more accurate (50–75 percent) with MRI.

Positron emission tomography scanning

11C-methionine positron emission tomography (PET) is clinically useful in highly preselected patients with recurrent pHPT, as well as in secondary and tertiary HPT, with a sensitivity of 83 percent, a specificity of 100 percent and an accuracy of 88 percent in successfully locating parathyroid adenomas.[11, 12]

Indications for surgery

SYMPTOMATIC

All patients with symptomatic pHPT should have parathyroidectomy. The advantages of the operation are:

- relief of muscle pain, lethargy and weakness;
- improvement in bone pain and the bone disease of hypercalcaemia;
- reduction in incidence of renal stones;
- improvement in psychiatric symptoms;
- reversal of many of the symptoms of 'metabolic syndrome'.

ASYMPTOMATIC

Opinions differ as to the correct management of patients without symptoms; however, the NIH Consensus Development Conference held in 1990 provided some guidelines.[13] Patients with levels of calcium above 3.00 mmol/L should have parathyroidectomy with or without symptoms. Patients with mild HPT (calcium 2.85–3.00 mmol/L) should have surgery if any of the following criteria are fulfilled:

- creatinine clearance reduced by at least 30 percent;
- urine calcium excretion above 400 mg/24 hours;
- bone mass two standard deviations below that of age and sex-matched persons;
- age below 50 years;
- recent history of kidney stones;
- apparent neuromuscular or psychiatric symptoms;
- medical surveillance undesirable or unsuitable.

However, despite these guidelines, the authors feel that parathyroidectomy should be recommended for all patients with hypercalcaemia and pHPT, for the following reasons:

- the difficulty of determining symptoms preoperatively (especially psychiatric symptoms), that may be alleviated by surgery;
- approximately 50 percent of conservatively-treated asymptomatic patients become symptomatic;
- 6 percent develop renal stones, 5 percent develop bone disease and 5 percent develop psychological problems;[14]
- the present evidence shows untreated asymptomatic patients have increased mortality due to cardiovascular disease;[15]
- minimally invasive surgery under local anaesthesia is now possible;
- low rate of complications of parathyroidectomy in experienced hands;
- high rate of postoperative cure in experienced hands.

Management of pHPT

MEDICAL THERAPY OF HYPERCALCAEMIA

The treatment of pHPT is predominantly surgical. Prior to surgery, the medical treatment of hypercalcaemia will depend on its severity. The main aim is to reduce hypercalcaemia as rapidly as possible and then to diagnose the underlying cause. Mild (<3.0 mmol/L) to moderate (3–3.5 mmol/L) hypercalcaemia can generally be managed on an outpatient basis, whereas severe (>3.5 mmol/L) hypercalcaemia requires more vigorous inpatient treatment.

Acute treatment of hypercalcaemia involves rehydration with i.v. normal saline, diuretics and the use of bisphosphanates intravenously, such as pamidronate. Longer-term treatment requires maintenance of adequate hydration, a low calcium diet, oral bisphosphanates and parathyroidectomy if pHPT is present.[16] An alternative for the future may be the use of a calcimimetic drug to interact with the calcium receptor on the parathyroid cell, decreasing serum PTH and ionized calcium concentrations.[17] [***/**]

SURGICAL STRATEGIES

Conventional parathyroidectomy

Bilateral neck exploration in the conventional operation allows access to all four glands and the ability to diagnose hyperplasia, double adenoma and microadenoma that might be missed by minimally invasive techniques.[18] Frozen section biopsy is useful in confirming parathyroid tissue, but differentiating adenoma from hyperplasia is only 60 percent reliable at frozen section and is better achieved by the assessment of an experienced surgeon.[19]

While exploring the parathyroid glands, it is essential to understand the following principles.

- The normal parathyroid gland tends to be approximately 5 mm in size, and can be seen to move independently within its fascial layer.
- Parathyroids tend to be symmetrically placed on each side.
- Most parathyroid glands are situated in the normal anatomical position, medial to the carotid arteries;
- superior glands are located behind the plane of the recurrent laryngeal nerve usually above the inferior thyroid pedicle (**Figure 31.4**).
- Inferior glands are found in front of the plane of the recurrent nerve, usually below the inferior thyroid pedicle, but their position is more variable.

Missing superior gland

Eighty percent of upper glands lie in a 2 cm radius 1 cm above the intersection of the inferior thyroid pedicle and the recurrent nerve (**Figure 31.5**). If not found there, it may help to divide the superior part of the sternothyroid muscle and/or take down the superior pole of the thyroid to improve exposure. It may be that a large adenoma has descended into the tracheo-oesophageal groove, so a search behind the oesophagus, higher in the retropharyngeal space and down into the posterior mediastinum should be made.

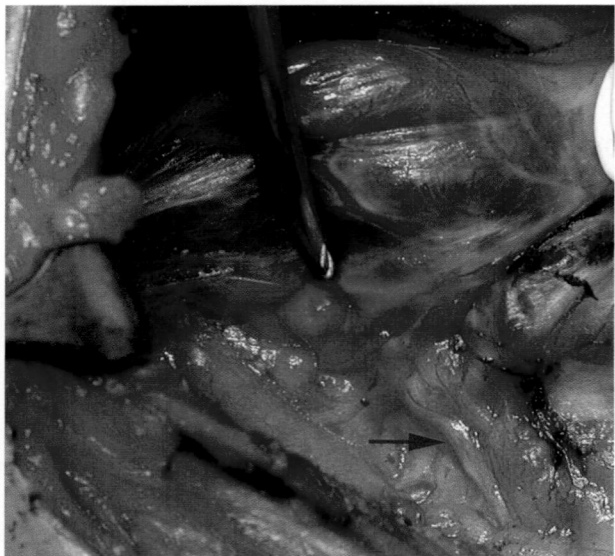

Figure 31.4 Normal right upper parathyroid gland (at tip of metal forceps) in front of the plane of the recurrent laryngeal nerve (blue arrow).

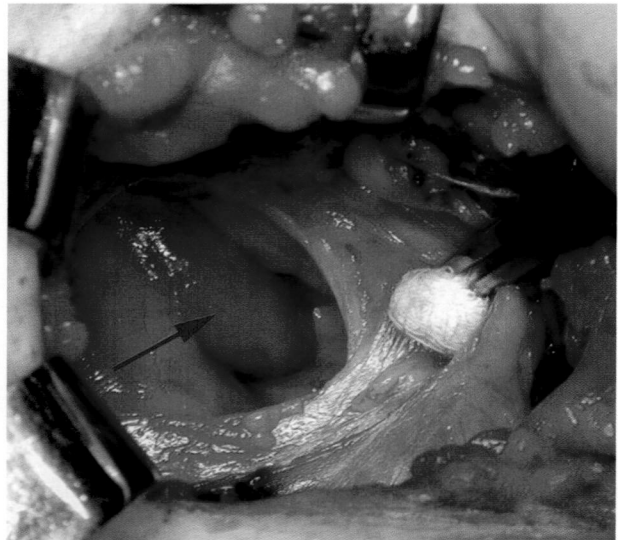

Figure 31.5 Right upper parathyroid adenoma in tracheo-oesophageal groove (blue arrow).

Missing inferior gland

Most commonly, the inferior gland is found within a 1 cm radius of the lower pole of the thyroid, but its position is more variable than the upper gland. If the inferior gland is missing, a thymectomy should be performed which may reveal the adenoma lying within the gland (**Figure 31.6**). The surgeon should also consider an undescended inferior parathyroid, particularly if the ipsilateral thymus is absent from its normal position. The carotid sheath should be opened and explored from the hyoid to the thoracic inlet, and consideration also given to a possible intrathyroidal adenoma.

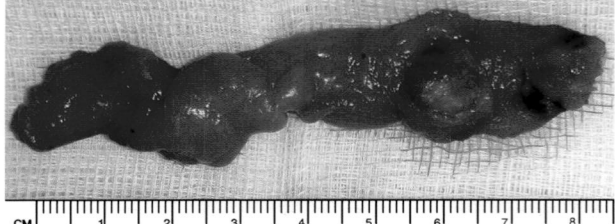

Figure 31.6 Parathyroid adenoma in thymus.

Indication for mediastinal exploration

If four normal glands have been found, the neck should be closed and a reassessment made of the original diagnosis. Further dissection at this point places the blood supply of the remaining parathyroids at risk, as well as increasing the potential for recurrent nerve damage. Post-operatively, the patient should be reinvestigated, including selective venous sampling.

Less than 1 percent of patients need a mediastinotomy as the majority of mediastinal lesions are actually in the thymus, which can be safely removed from the neck. The advantages of staging mediastinal surgery as a second procedure are:

- dissection in the neck may disrupt an adenoma's blood supply, turning an apparently negative exploration into a successful result;
- the pathologist may identify parathyroid tissue, for example in the thymus, which was missed at operation;
- there is an opportunity to reconfirm or change the diagnosis;
- angiographic ablation can be performed for inaccessible mediastinal glands.

Scan-directed minimally invasive open parathyroidectomy

The technique of scan-directed minimally invasive open parathyroidectomy (MIP) has rapidly gained favour with the advent of accurate preoperative localization techniques, which allow a targeted approach to the adenoma, minimizing dissection and potential complications.[20] The parathyroid adenoma is localized by sestamibi scan and ultrasound, and only the area identified is explored, either under general or local anaesthesia. Access is either through a small lateral transverse incision, or one made along the medial border of the sternocleidomastoid muscle. Ideally, the success of MIP should be confirmed by measurement of intraoperative PTH.[21] If scans are concordant, then MIP should cure between 92 and 95 percent of patients. [***/**]

Radio-guided parathyroidectomy

Radio-guided parathyroidectomy, popularized by Norman and Chheda,[22] relies on uptake into the adenoma of ^{99m}Tc-labelled sestamibi given two hours before operation, then a hand-held gamma probe is used intraoperatively. Focused dissection is performed in the area of highest activity and the radioactive gland is removed. The main disadvantages are cost and the organizational difficulties of arranging and timing of the scan before operation. [**]

Video–assisted and endoscopic parathyroidectomy

Minimally invasive video-assisted (MIVAP) and endoscopic parathyroidectomy are more recent techniques that result in a smaller scar in the neck and a quicker recovery, but at the expense of longer operating times and higher costs. Endoscopic parathyroidectomy uses gas insufflation and several 3 mm ports in the neck. Miccoli et al.[23, 24] modified this operation, substituting a gasless, video-assisted approach, in combination with intraoperative PTH measurement. Ikeda et al.[25] have gone even further to remove the scars from the neck by approaching the parathyroid tumour via an axillary or a submammary approach. [****/***]

Results of parathyroidectomy

CURE RATE

Many patients will require post-operative calcium and vitamin D supplementation until the suppressed glands recover their function. At the first operation, more than 95 percent of pHPT patients will be cured, with 83 percent of those requiring reoperation. The outcome is significantly dependent on how many parathyroidectomies are carried out by a given surgeon per year, with higher failure rates for those performing less than 15 cases per year.[26]

COMPLICATIONS

The post-operative complication rate is under 1 percent after primary operations and less than 5 percent after reoperative surgery, with a mortality rate well below 1 percent. Approximately 8 percent of primary operations for pHPT result in recurrent or persistent disease, this is higher in multigland disease and particularly the MEN syndromes, where it may be as high as 40 percent.

PERSISTENT OR RECURRENT HPT

Persistent HPT is defined as the presence of hypercalcaemia in the immediate postoperative period or within six months. Recurrent HPT is defined as the return of hypercalcaemia after six months of post-operative normocalcaemia or hypocalcaemia, which is caused by inadequate resection of diseased glands, such as regrowth of residual, unresected, hyperplastic gland after subtotal parathyroidectomy, incomplete resection of an adenoma, rupture and spillage of parathyroid cells (parathymomatosis) or recurrence of parathyroid carcinoma.[27]

Patients with persistent or recurrent HPT need to be reinvestigated more vigorously and the diagnosis reconfirmed prior to any second operation. Mild asymptomatic or normocalcaemic HPT may not need reoperation at all, but symptomatic patients with high serum calcium and renal or bony disease will need a second exploration.

Reoperations may be relatively uncomplicated, but generally are technically difficult, with a high complication rate and low success rate in inexperienced hands. Injury to the recurrent laryngeal nerve and permanent hypoparathyroidism occur in 8 percent of patients. The technique involves a 'back door' approach to a focused dissection of the abnormal area identified at reinvestigation. The sites of missed adenoma are in the normal positions in 40 percent, posterior superior mediastinum in 30 percent, intrathymic in 15 percent, posterior midline in 5 percent, mediastinal in 5 percent, intrathyroidal in 2 percent and other areas 3 percent. Mediastinal glands are usually found around the aortic arch, superior vena cava and aorto–pulmonary window.[28]

SECONDARY AND TERTIARY HPT

Secondary HPT is caused by hypocalcaemia or phosphate retention, typically seen in chronic renal failure. Less common causes are vitamin D deficiency and lithium ingestion.

Chronic renal failure causes hyperphosphataemia and hypocalcaemia stimulating diffuse hyperplasia of all four glands and a rise in serum PTH. Prolonged stimulation of parathyroid glands results in nodular hyperplasia from monoclonal cell proliferation and a decrease in vitamin D receptor and CaR density. This results in resistance to medical treatment.[29]

In tertiary HPT, one of the hyperplastic nodules becomes autonomous due to alteration in PTH-gene transcription, resulting in hypercalcaemia and raised PTH similar to pHPT.

Medical treatment

The primary treatment of secondary and tertiary HPT is predominantly medical, through management of chronic renal failure by medical manipulation of phosphate levels and peritoneal or haemodialysis. Renal transplantation usually cures secondary HPT.

Parathyroidectomy

Twenty-eight percent of renal patients on dialysis have secondary HPT, and 10 percent of patients who have had successful renal transplantation develop either secondary or tertiary HPT. These patients will generally need surgical parathyroidectomy.

There are a number of different surgical strategies available: total parathyroidectomy, with or without autotransplantation, and subtotal parathyroidectomy. Some endocrine surgeons prefer subtotal parathyroidectomy, removing three-and-a-half glands, but it is extremely difficult to judge the correct amount of parathyroid tissue to achieve normocalcaemia. In addition, graft-dependent recurrence occurs in up to 75 percent of patients on dialysis who have had autotransplantation, and 10 percent develop graft failure with hypocalcaemia.[30] For this reason, the authors favour total parathyroidectomy and transcervical thymectomy. [****/***/**]

KEY POINTS

- Primary hyperparathyroidism and malignancy are responsible for 90 percent of hypercalcaemia.
- Eighty percent of pHPT is due to single gland disease.
- Sestamibi and ultrasound localization allows unilateral exploration of the neck.
- Intraoperative quick PTH assay is an essential tool.
- Management of secondary HPT is difficult.
- Parathyroid carcinoma is rare; when suspected will require en bloc excision with ipsilateral thyroidectomy.

Best clinical practice

✓ The approach to pHPT is the same as for any endocrine condition, following five basic principles: confirmation of endocrine diagnosis; localization of the tumour or tumours; ensuring the patient is biochemically safe for surgery; deciding necessity for operation; choosing a suitable procedure.

✓ Minimal diagnostic investigations:
  – biochemical tests: calcium, PTH, vitamin D and 24 hour urine calcium;
  – localization studies: ultrasound, sestamibi scan;
  – before reoperation: CT or MRI, PET and selective venous sampling and angiography. [****/***/**]

✓ Indications for parathyroidectomy:
  – symptomatic hypercalcaemia;
  – asymptomatic hypercalcaemia with: calcium >3 mmol/L; calcium <3 mmol/L with renal disease, bone disease, young age (<50 years) or 'metabolic syndrome'. [Grade A/B]

✓ Plan of parathyroid exploration:
  – find recurrent laryngeal nerve;

– look for upper parathyroid (2 cm radius from 1 cm above intersection of RLN and ITA);
– missing upper: look tracheo-oesophageal groove, retro-oesophageal and retropharyngeal spaces;
– look for lower parathyroid (inferior thyroid pole to thymus);
– missing lower: perform thymectomy, look in carotid sheath;
– consider thyroid lobectomy;
– stop, then reassess diagnosis and consider mediastinal exploration. [****/***/**]

✓ Revision parathyroid surgery. Recurrent or persistent HPT requires:
  – reinvestigation to confirm diagnosis and localize tumour;
  – more invasive investigation, for example selective venous sampling;
  – assess need for surgery;
  – 'back door' approach between sternocleidomastoid and strap muscles;
  – focused exploration in identified area, with meticulous dissection. [***/**]

Deficiencies in current knowledge and areas for future research

The main problem in primary hyperparathyroidism is separating multiple gland disease from single gland disease. If accurately detected, single gland disease can be easily managed by minimally invasive techniques, either open, video-assisted or endoscopically, with the potential for operation under local anaesthetic. Thus, there is a great need for an accurate scan that will separate single from multiple gland disease.

Our wish list for the future would therefore be:

➤ more accurate forms of scanning;
➤ a preoperative method of separating carcinoma of the parathyroid from benign disease;
➤ effective, long-acting inhibitors of PTH secretion by either hyperplastic glands or adenomas, such as calcimimetic drugs;
➤ a more effective way of controlling preoperative hypercalcaemia without the inherent risk of post-operative hungry bone disease.

REFERENCES

1. Akerstrom G, Malmaeus J, Bergstrom R. Surgical anatomy of human parathyroid glands. *Surgery.* 1984; 95: 14–21.

2. Randolph GW, Urken ML. Surgical management of primary hyperparathyroidism. In: Randolph GW (ed.). *Surgery of the thyroid and parathyroid glands.* Philadelphia, USA: Elsevier Science, 2003: 507–28.

∗ 3. Mithal AM, Brown EM. An overview of extracellular calcium homeostasis and the roles of the CaR in parathyroid and C-cells. In: Chattopadhyay N, Brown EM (eds). *Calcium-sensing receptor.* Boston, USA: Kluwer Academic Publishers, 2003: 1–27.

∗ 4. Thakker RV. Molecular genetics of parathyroid disease. *Current Opinion in Endocrinology and Diabetes.* 1996; **3**: 521–8.

5. Lundgren E, Rastad J, Thurfjell E, Akerstrom G, Ljunghall S. Population-based screening for primary hyperparathyroidism with serum calcium and parathyroid hormone values in menopausal women. *Surgery.* 1997; **121**: 287–94.

6. Tezelman S, Rodriguez JM, Shen W, Siperstein AE, Duh QY, Clark OH. Primary hyperparathyroidism in patients who have received radiation therapy and in patients who have not received radiation therapy. *Journal of the American College of Surgeons.* 1995; **180**: 81–7.

7. Rastad J, Joborn C, Akerstrom G, Ljunghall S. Incidence, type and severity of psychic symptoms in patients with sporadic primary hyperparathyroidism. *Journal of Endocrinological Investigation.* 1992; **15**: 149–56.

8. Solomon BL, Schaaf M, Smallridge RC. Psychologic symptoms before and after parathyroid surgery. *American Journal of Medicine.* 1994; **96**: 101–6.

9. Mazzeo S, Caramella D, Marcocci C, Lonzi S, Cambi L, Miccoli P *et al.* Contrast-enhanced color Doppler ultrasonography in suspected parathyroid lesions. *Acta Radiologica.* 2000; **41**: 412–6.

10. Pattou F, Huglo D, Proye C. Radionuclide scanning in parathyroid diseases. *British Journal of Surgery.* 1998; **85**: 1605–16.

11. Otto D, Boerner AR, Hofmann M, Brunkhorst T, Meyer GJ, Petrich T *et al.* Pre-operative localization of hyperfunctional parathyroid tissue with 11C-methionine PET. *European Journal of Nuclear Medicine and Molecular Imaging.* 2004; **31**: 1405–12.

12. Beggs AD, Hain SF. Localization of parathyroid adenomas using 11C-methionine positron emission tomography. *Nuclear Medicine Communications.* 2005; **26**: 133–6.

∗ 13. Consensus Development Conference Panel: Diagnosis and management of asymptomatic primary hyperparathyroidism. Consensus development conference statement. *Annals of Internal Medicine.* 1991; **114**: 593–7.

14. Scholz DA, Purnell DC. Asymptomatic primary hyperparathyroidism: 10 year prospective study. *Mayo Clinic Proceedings.* 1981; **56**: 473–8.

15. Dahlberg K, Brodin LA, Juhlin-Dannfelt A, Farnebo LO. Cardiac function in primary hyperparathyroidism before and after operation: an echocardiographic study. *The European Journal of Surgery.* 1996; **162**: 171–6.

16. Swan JW, Stevenson JC. The medical management of hypercalcaemia. In: Lynn J, Bloom SR (eds). *Surgical endocrinology.* Oxford: Butterworth-Heinemann, 1997: 341–50.

∗ 17. Silverberg SJ, Bone III HG, Marriott TB, Locker FG, Thys-Jacobs S, Dziem G *et al.* Short-term inhibition of parathyroid hormone secretion by a calcium-receptor agonist in patients with primary hyperparathyroidism. *New England Journal of Medicine.* 1997; **337**: 1506–10.

18. Ogilvie JB, Clark OH. Parathyroid surgery: we still need traditional and selective approaches. *Journal of Endocrinological Investigation.* 2000; **28**: 566–9.

19. Saxe A, Baier R, Raile R, Tesluk H, Toreson W. The role of the pathologist in the surgical treatment of hyperparathyroidism. *Surgery, Gynecology and Obstetrics.* 1985; **161**: 101–5.

∗ 20. Carty S, Worsey M, Virji M, Brown ML, Watson CG. Concise parathyroidectomy. The impact of preoperative SPECT 99mTc sestamibi scanning and intraoperative quick parathormone assay. *Surgery.* 1997; **122**: 1107–16.

21. Gupta VK, Yeh KA, Burke GJ, Wei JP. 99m-Technetium sestamibi localized solitary parathyroid adenoma as an indication for limited unilateral surgical exploration. *American Journal of Surgery.* 1998; **176**: 409–12.

22. Norman J, Chheda H. Minimally invasive parathyroidectomy facilitated by intraoperative nuclear mapping. *Surgery.* 1997; **122**: 998–1004.

23. Miccoli P, Bendinelli C, Vignali E, Mazzeo S, Cecchini GM, Pinchera A *et al.* Endoscopic parathyroidectomy: report of initial experience. *Surgery.* 1998; **124**: 1077–80.

24. Miccoli P, Bendinelli C, Berti P, Vignali E, Pinchera A, Marcocci C. Video-assisted versus conventional parathyroidectomy in primary hyperparathyroidism: a prospective randomized study. *Surgery.* 1999; **126**: 1117–22.

25. Ikeda Y, Takami H, Sasaki Y, Kan S, Niimi M. Endoscopic neck surgery by the axillary approach. *Journal of the American College of Surgeons.* 2000; **191**: 336–40.

26. Sosa JA, Powe NR, Levine MA, Udelsman R, Zeiger MA. Profile of a clinical practice: thresholds for surgery and surgical outcomes for patients with primary hyperparathyroidism: a national survey of endocrine surgeons. *Journal of Clinical Endocrinology and Metabolism.* 1998; **83**: 2658–65.

27. Carty SE, Norton JA. Management of patients with persistent or recurrent primary hyperparathyroidism. *Journal of Clinical Endocrinology and Metabolism.* 1991; **15**: 716–23.

28. Gaz RD. Revision parathyroid surgery. In: Randolph GW (ed.). *Surgery of the thyroid and parathyroid glands.* Philadelphia, USA: Elsevier Science, 2003: 564–70.

29. Hruska KA, Teitelbaum SL. Renal osteodystrophy. *New England Journal of Medicine.* 1995; **333**: 166–74.

30. Rothmund M, Wagner PK, Schark C. Subtotal parathyroidectomy versus total parathyroidectomy and autotransplantation in secondary hyperparathyroidism: A randomized trial. *Journal of Clinical Endocrinology and Metabolism.* 1991; **15**: 745–50.

32

Head and neck manifestations of endocrine disease

JONATHAN M MORGAN AND THOMAS McCAFFREY

Introduction	398	Pancreatic islet cell disease	401
Pituitary disease	399	Pregnancy and gonadal disease	402
Thyroid disease	399	Key points	403
Adrenal disease	401	References	403
Parathyroid disease	401		

SEARCH STRATEGY AND EVIDENCE-BASE

Information for this chapter was gathered by searching Medline using the key words head and neck, endocrine disease, as well as using the specific disease names. Due to the nature of the context of this chapter, studies cited here are predominantly retrospective and/or observational, unless specifically stated in the body of the text, and therefore fall into evidence levels 3 and 4.

INTRODUCTION

Although endocrine disorders usually produce symptoms and findings that are primarily systemic, specific and localized manifestations of endocrine disease may occur early or predominantly in the head and neck region. Awareness of these presentations may lead to the early diagnosis of the underlying endocrine disease. This chapter presents the symptoms and findings in the head and neck that are caused by changes in hormone levels or endocrine disease. We begin with perturbations of the hormones produced in the pituitary, then progress to the thyroid, adrenals, pancreas and gonads. We should also note that altered physiologic states, including pregnancy, and paraendocrine diseases are defined by changes in hormone levels. These changes in physiologic states are also seen in the head and neck region and are addressed in this chapter.

The regulation of the endocrine system is based upon a basic principle of negative and positive feedback loops. The complex interactions of the endocrine system are beyond the scope of this text and we would refer you to an endocrinology text for a more complete description.

The feedback mechanism begins with neuroendocrine regulation. The hypothalamus produces chemical mediators (growth hormone-releasing hormone (GHRH), leuteinizing hormone-releasing hormone (LHRH), thyrotropin-releasing hormone (TRH), corticotropin-releasing hormone (CRH) and dopamine (prolactin inhibiting hormone.) These mediators travel via a portal system to the anterior pituitary and in turn regulate the release of growth hormone (GH), leuteinizing hormone (LH) and follicle-stimulating hormone (FSH), thyroid-stimulating hormone (TSH), adrenocorticotropic hormone (ACTH) and prolactin. The hypothalamus also produces vasopressin and oxytocin and these are stored in the posterior pituitary. The main feedback loop continues from the hormones of the anterior pituitary to the three target endocrine glands, the gonads, adrenal cortex and the thyroid, these in turn produce an additional set of hormones that effect multiple glands and organ systems. There are many possible mechanisms that can cause a disturbance in this feedback loop. The result of these disturbances being a real or apparent increase or decrease of hormone levels, which in turn cause the signs and symptoms of endocrine disease. Hypothalamic disease can cause hypopituitarism and all of the associated symptoms, although typically head and neck manifestations are rare in diseases of the hypothalamus.

PITUITARY DISEASE

Diseases of the anterior pituitary can result in the production of many different hormones, although otolaryngologic manifestations are rare. The exception is acromegaly, or the overproduction of GH (somatotropin). The overproduction of GH prior to epiphyseal closure results in gigantism. Acromegaly is an insidious chronic debilitating disease. This is a rare disease with a prevalence of 50–70 cases per million and an incidence of 3–4 per million per year.

The disease presents most frequently in middle age and has no predilection for men or women. Facial features are well documented. **Table 32.1** documents all of the head and neck manifestations. The pathophysiology of increased GH is the result of pituitary adenomas (in almost all cases). Typically, the tumour is found laterally in the sella, where somatotrophs are abundant. However, rare cases have been reported of tumours along the migration line of Rathke's pouch, including the sphenoid sinus and the parapharyngeal space.[7]

Regional symptoms secondary to either mass effect of direct extension of pituitary adenomas most commonly present with blurred vision and visual field defects. (**Figure 32.1**). However, several pathways of extension of invasive adenomas have been defined:[8]

- pharyngeal extension via the floor of the sella and sphenoid sinus;
- hypothalamic extension via the floor of the third ventricle;
- temporal extension;
- invasion of the cavernous sinus and associated cranial nerves;
- posterior subtentorial extension involving the third, fourth and fifth nerves;
- frontal extension.

Extension of the tumour into the middle ear and external auditory canal is a very rare presentation.[9] Another rare

presentation of invasive pituitary adenomas is nasal obstruction.[10] These tumours are typically diagnosed by transnasal biopsy of the mass.

THYROID DISEASE

The thyroid is also under the control of the hypothalamic-pituitary axis. Hypothyroidism is caused by many processes including the following: thyroid agenesis, surgical removal (thyroidectomy and laryngectomy), therapeutic irradiation (I^{131} or external radiation), autoimmune (Hashimoto's) thyroiditis, replacement by cancer or other disease, post-thyroiditis (acute or subacute), inhibition of thyroid hormone synthesis, iodine deficiency, excess iodine in susceptible patients, antithyroid drugs, inherited enzyme defects and post-partum. The incidence of hypothyroidism increases with age, and affects women four- to six-times as frequently as men. It occurs at all ages but gradually rises with age and peaks at 40–60 years. Up to 5 percent of persons older than age 65 have clinically overt hypothyroidism, whereas 15 percent have subclinical hypothyroidism marked only by serum TSH elevations. General symptoms include weakness, dry and coarse skin, myxedema and pallor. The hair of these

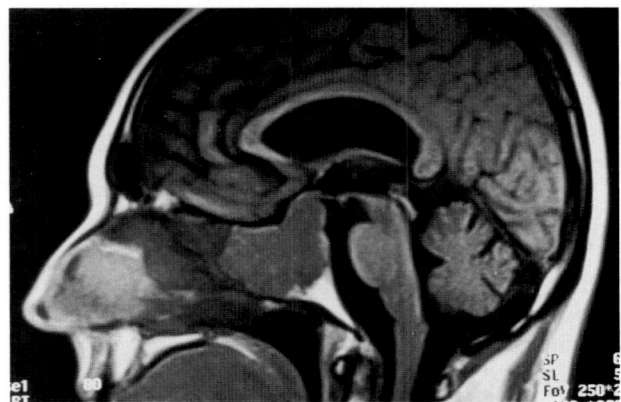

Figure 32.1 MR scan showing a pituitary adenoma impinging on the optic chiasm and extending into the sphenoid sinus.

Table 32.1 Signs and symptoms of acromegaly manifested in the head and neck.

General	Oral	Nasal	Laryngeal
Headaches	Enlarged tongue	Sinus congestion	Hoarseness
Visual field changes	Malocclusion	Rhinorrhoea	Decreases vocal pitch
Prognathism[1]	Mandibular protrusion	Enlarged paranasal sinuses[3]	Asymmetric enlargement of epiglottis, aryepiglottic folds, false and true vocal cords
Obstructive sleep apnoea[2]			Cricoarytenoid arthritis[4]
Coarse facial features			Vocal cord paresis/paralysis[5]
Oily skin			Airway obstruction[6]
Soft tissue and bony enlargement			

patients may be dry and fine, and they may suffer from alopecia. A classic symptom of hypothyroidism is the loss of the outer third of the eyebrows, also known as Queen Anne's eyebrows.

Vocal manifestations include hoarseness and a generalized slow speech rate. These patients may exhibit a low pitch and decreased vocal clarity. It was first postulated that this was due to central oedema of the vagal nuclei. Ritter noted that there was retention of proteinaceous fluid, high in mucopolysaccharides within the mucosa of the larynx in rats rendered hypothyroid by treatment with either propothiouracil, or radioactive I[131].[11]

Rhinitis is a common complaint of patients with hypothyroidism. There is a correlation between hypothyroidism and rhinitis, however, no clear definition of the pathophysiology has been elucidated. Proetz[12, 13] assessed 130 hypothyroid patients and found nasal congestion, rhinorrhea, pale wet nasal mucosa, as well as rarely a dry red ('chapped') mucosa. Mucosal biopsy revealed nonspecific inflammatory changes only. In a study of 66 hypothyroid patients, Gupta[14] described symptoms of nasal stuffiness in 64 percent and increased colds and rhinorrhea in 55 percent. Rhinoscopy revealed pale, boggy mucosa in 41 percent and erythematous dry mucosa in 27 percent. Biopsies of 16 patients showed increased submucosal acid mucopolysaccharide ground substance and glandular hypertrophy. In general, symptoms of nonallergic rhinitis are common for patients with hypothyroidism. However, undiagnosed hypothyroidism among patients with uncomplicated rhinitis is very low.[15, 16] Therefore, tests of thyroid function of patients with nonallergic rhinitis should be reserved for patients with other systemic symptoms of hypothyroidism.[17] [Grade D]

Vestibular and otologic symptoms of hypothyroidsim include vertigo, hearing loss and pruritic external auditory canals; the latter has been postulated to be due to the decrease of cerumen production. As many as two-thirds of patients with hypothyroidism suffer from vertigo. The attacks are typically mild and brief and are not associated with changes in ENG or hearing loss.[18] These patients can also experience hearing loss. Although this is much more common in congenital disease, approximately 30–40 percent of patients with myxoedema suffer from bilateral sensorineural hearing loss. These patients can also experience conductive losses secondary to Eustachian tube mucosal oedema.[19]

Congenital hypothroidism (cretinism) is a rare disease with a higher incidence in the underdeveloped nations. Head and neck manifestations of affected children are puffy face, yellowish skin, flat nose and enlarged tongue that can protrude from an open mouth. Fontanels and sutures may be widened, and the child's cry is hoarse. A goitre is characteristic of endemic cretinism, but the sporadic type caused by thyroid agenesis or dysgenesis typically has no palpable thyroid. Sensorineural hearing loss is progressive and responds to early treatment with thyroid hormone replacement. Bilateral sensorineural

hearing loss is more common in endemic cretinism, whereas sporadic cretinism tends to exhibit either a conductive, mixed or sensorineural hearing loss.[20]

Pendred's syndrome is an autosomal recessive disorder that is characterized by a goitre and progressive sensorineural hearing loss. The children are typically euthyroid and have an abnormal perchlorate discharge. The hearing loss is more pronounced in higher frequencies and recruitment is present, indicating a lesion of the cochlea. This syndrome results from an inborn defect in thyroid hormone synthesis, a peroxidase defect in iodine metabolism.

Graves' disease and toxic nodular goitre account for more than 90 percent of hyperthyroidism and thyrotoxicosis, both more common in women. Graves' disease is classically manifested by an infiltrative opthalmopathy (**Figure 32.2**). This is a lymphocytic inflammatory reaction that infiltrates the extraocular muscles and orbital fat; the fibroblasts proliferate and deposit glycosaminoglycans, predominately hyaluronic acid.[21] As enlargement of orbital muscle and fat progresses, the bony walls of the orbit will not allow any increase in volume, therefore proptosis occurs. With an average orbital volume of 26 mL in healthy adults, an increase of only 4 mL in the volume of the orbital contents will result in 6 mm of proptosis. As the proptosis progresses, the protective mechanisms of the cornea are diminished. This can cause exposure, desiccation, irritation and, ultimately, ulceration and blindness if not treated. The inflammatory reaction in turn evokes a deposition of collagen into the extraocular muscles and this results in a restrictive opthalmoplegia. Optic nerve involvement as a result of compression at the orbital apex by the enlarged extraocular muscles[22] is another later finding in Graves' disease.

Lid lag and the appearance of a 'stare' are ocular manifestations of thyrotoxicosis and are often seen in the earliest forms of Graves' disease. This is the result of an increased sympathetic sensitivity to catecholamines.[23] Generalized tremors are common in patients with thyrotoxicosis. In the head and neck these manifest as fine tremors of the lips and the tongue (more evident when it is protruding[24]). Vocal changes are often noted in these patients as well. Although no true dysphonia is noted, there is a tremulous voice that is a result of the increased respiratory rate and the resultant decreased vital

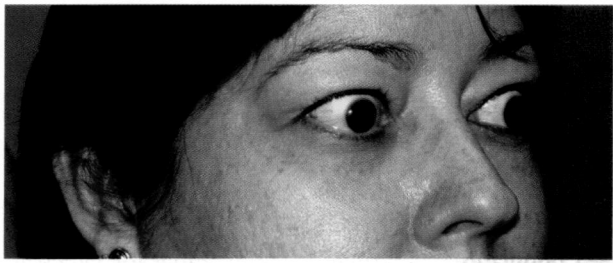

Figure 32.2 A patient with Graves' opthalmopathy showing proptosis and lid retraction characteristic of this condition.

capacity.[25] Less common manifestations are osteoporosis of the mandible and maxilla and dark pigment deposits in the buccal mucosa.

Goitre, or neck masses, are very common in patients with thyrotoxicosis, as well as thyroid neoplasia. Neoplasia will be addressed in another chapter in this text, however, it should be noted that dysphagia, hoarseness, haemoptysis and haematemesis are all common symptoms and should alert the otolaryngologist to possible thyroid neoplasia.

ADRENAL DISEASE

Of the diseases of the adrenal gland, or disease processes that cause perturbations in the hormones produced within the adrenal gland, Cushing's syndrome/disease is the one with the most significant head and neck manifestations. Common causes of Cushing's syndrome/disease include adrenal hyperplasia, adrenal adenoma/carcinoma, ectopic production of ACTH and iatrogenic causes. A rare cause of ectopic production of ACTH is medullary thyroid carcinoma (MTC). These tumours have demonstrable adrenocorticotropin immunoreactivity and can release adrenocorticotropin. Classic signs of this disease are central obesity and 'moon' faces. Androgen excess causes acne and hirsutism. Patients with Cushing's disease are at an increased risk of infectious diseases, oral candidiasis is a common problem. Generalized muscle weakness (steroid myopathy) can cause difficulties with phonation and deglutition. In contrast to Cushing's disease, adrenocortical insufficiency (Addison's disease) has oral mucosal hyperpigmentation and generalized muscle weakness that results in vocal weakness.

PARATHYROID DISEASE

Patients with hypoparathyroidism display many common head and neck signs and symptoms. The patients who suffer from hypoparathyroidism and resulting hypocalcaemia complain of perioral tingling and numbness. Hoarseness, aphonia and stridor are the typical vocal manifestations of laryngospasm seen with tetani. Chvostek's sign is also commonly seen with tetani (however, as many as 10 percent of normal patients will have a positive sign). Chvostek's sign is elicited by percussing over the facial nerve, anterior to the tragus. Facial muscle twitching is a positive response. Long-term hypocalcaemia can cause enamel defects and hypoplasia of the teeth.

Hyperparathyroidism and resulting hypercalcaemia is most often caused by parathyroid adenoma (in the ambulatory population), or malignancy (in the hospitalized population), although the differential for hypercalcaemia is long and getting longer. Classically, this disease process manifests as 'stones' (renalithiasis), 'bones' (bone pain, with demineralization often seen in the skull), 'groans' (GI distress) and 'psychiatric overtones' (emotional changes including abnormal mentation). Osteitis fibrosis cystica or 'brown tumours' consisting of osteoblasts, osteoclasts and fibrous tissue are occasionally seen in the mandible and maxilla. In a small study, Simpson noted that auditory dysfunction, in three cases, and aphonia, in two cases, were reversed after removal of parathyroid adenomas.[26] He postulated that the high calcium ion concentration inhibited neural synaptic transmission, causing both of these symptoms.

Hyperparathyroidism also has a genetic component: multiple endocrine neoplasia (MEN) syndromes. MEN 1 (Wermer's syndrome) includes pituitary adenoma/hyperplasia, parathyroid adenoma/hyperplasia and pancreatic islet cell hyperplasia/adenoma/carcinoma. MEN 2A (Sipple syndrome) includes MTC, pheochromocytoma and parathyroid hyperplasia/adenoma. The MEN syndromes are inherited as autosomal dominant traits, therefore a family history is important to ascertain and decide if further work-up is necessary. Hyperparathyroidism is often the first manifestation of MEN 1 and usually appears after the patient reaches 18 years of age.

PANCREATIC ISLET CELL DISEASE

Diabetes mellitus (DM) is a disease that is caused by inadequate action of insulin, due to either resistance of end organs due to obesity reducing the insulin receptors on insulin responsive cells (type 2), or reduced levels of insulin due to autoimmune response to beta cells of the pancreas triggered by infection (type 1). Type 1 typically presents in patients under age 25 in 0.2–0.5 percent of the population, with no predilection for men or women. There is only a 50 percent concordance in identical twins. Prevalence of type 2 is 2–4 percent, and usually occurs in patients older than 40. There is a slight predilection for women. There is also a 100 percent concordance rate in identical twins. Head and neck manifestations of type 1 and type 2 diabetes are identical, and we will discuss these as a unit. Chronic manifestations of DM are secondary to micro and macrovascular disease, neuropathies (including peripheral, autonomic radiculopathy and mononeuropathy) as well as immunodeficiency secondary to impaired leukocyte/phagocyte function.[27] [***]

General considerations for otolaryngologists as surgeons revolve around the immunodeficiency and the decreased ability of diabetics to heal their surgical wounds and their increased susceptibility to infection. This should be considered prior to operating and glycaemic control should be optimized during the perioperative period. [Grade B]

The ocular findings of DM include diabetic retinopathy where venous dilatation leads to full-blown exudates and haemorrhage in the retina and vitreous body. Haemorrhages in the conjunctiva and iris result in glycogen deposits, as well as depigmentation and neovascularization. Abnormal lens function leads to cataract formation. Mononeuropathy in the head and neck can be a presenting sign of DM. Bell's palsy has a high comorbidity with DM. In a retrospective study, 45 percent of patients between the ages of 10 and 19 who presented with Bell's palsy had DM, and in a series of 130 patients with DM, 66 percent presented with Bell's palsy.[28] Other neuropathies of the cranial nerves can result in unilateral vocal cord paralysis, dysphagia and dysphonia. Laryngeal nerve sections of moderate to severe diabetics showed segmental demyelination, axonal degeneration and concentric proliferation of Schwann cells.[29]

Neuropathies affecting all other cranial nerves (with the exception of the olfactory and hypoglossal) have been documented in DM. Retrospective studies also show that as many as 50 percent of patients with diabetes have some manifestations of auditory dysfunction, and analysis of diabetic temporal bones has been found to contain PAS-positive lesions of the capillaries in the stria vascularis.[30] This is the same lesion seen in Kimmelstiel–Wilson disease (diabetic nephropathy). Animal studies of auditory brainstem responses (ABRs) have also shown significant prolongation of wave I as well as an elevation in the ABR threshold in diabetic rats.[31]

Equilibrium disorders are also very common for diabetics. Aetiologies for disequilibrium include peripheral neuropathy, direct toxicity of the vestibular end organ and fluctuations in glucose concentrations in the cerebral circulation. Diabetics routinely have abnormal electronystagmography and dynamic posturography. In a recent animal study, diabetic rats were shown to have prolonged latency and decreased amplitude of the first wave of the vestibular evoked potentials (VEPs). These parameters of the first wave have been shown to correlate with vestibular end-organ function.[4]

Diabetics are particularly prone to certain infections. Malignant otitis externa, commonly due to *Pseudomonas aeruginosa*, typically presents in the older diabetic with severe otalgia, otorrhoea, fever and leukocytosis. Granulation tissue at the bony-cartilagenous junction is a classic sign, and cranial nerve findings including facial nerve paralysis, as well as involvement of V, X, XI, XII are all poor prognostic indicators. Disease may spread beyond the external auditory canal and cause osteitis, chondritis and osteomyelitis of the temporal bone. Intracranial extension and death are possible if treatment is not thorough. Early cases are responsive to oral floroquinolones and meticulous and frequent debridements under the binocular microscope, more advanced cases require hospitalization and i.v. anti-*Pseudomonas* antibiotics and possible surgical debridement. [Grade B/C]

Another infection particular to diabetics and other imunocompromised hosts is invasive fungal sinusitis (rhinocerebral mucormycosis) (**Figure 32.3**). Presentation

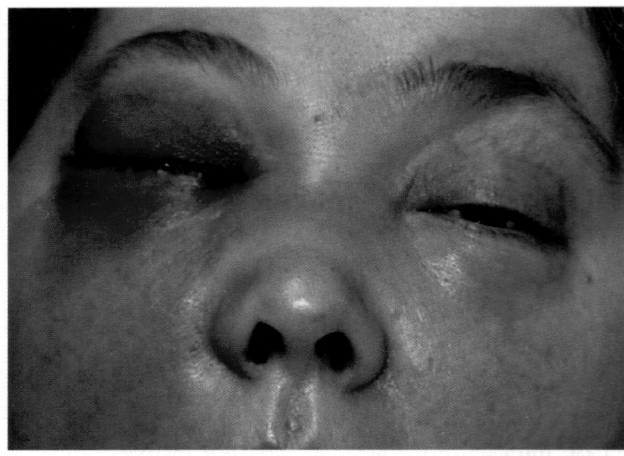

Figure 32.3 A diabetic patient with invasive fungal sinusitis involving the paranasal sinuses and orbit.

in the immunocompromised patient includes fever and localization of symptoms to the paranasal sinus area, such as orbital swelling, facial pain or nasal congestion. Physical examination may show necrosis of the nasal mucosa, indicative of mucormycosis and, in rare situations, actual hyphae. However, typical examination findings are indistinguishable from nonfungal causes of sinusitis. Anaesthesia of the nasal mucosa or cheeks, independent of topical anaesthetics, is suspicious for mucormycosis. The oral cavity always should be examined for invasion through the hard palate from the sinuses. Changes seen on sinus CT or plain radiographs are usually nonspecific and usually indistinguishable from bacterial sinusitis, although they may show bony erosion or soft-tissue invasion. Biopsy and culture are critical to making the diagnosis. Appropriate antifungal therapy and aggressive surgical debridement should be initiated as soon as possible.

PREGNANCY AND GONADAL DISEASE

The most common head and neck complaints during pregnancy are nasal obstruction and rhinorrhoea, typically serious and frequently accompanied by postnasal drip. Physical examination reveals hyperaemic mucosa with marked oedema and hypersecretory states. This is most common during the second and third trimesters and tends to continue for the duration of the pregnancy. Typically, resolution occurs within one week of parturition. Approximately 15–30 percent of pregnant females suffer from these symptoms.[32] Although some patients have pre-existing allergic rhinitis, vasomotor rhinitis or sinus disease, and pregnancy merely exacerbates these conditions, many patients who do not have these underlying problems also suffer from this. The exact pathophysiology is not understood. It is clear that there are direct influences of oestrogens on the nasal mucosa and resulting airflow, however no correlation has been shown between estradiol levels and nasal symptomatology.[33] [***]

Animals given oestrogen over a period of weeks to months show histologic changes of the mucosa, including proliferation of squamous metaplasia with increases in the cornification of the epithelium and a decrease in the number of cilia and goblet cells. Diffuse glandular hyperplasia with increased secretory activity of the acini was also seen. Vascular changes included endothelial proliferation and capillary and arteriolar swelling.[34] [***]

Symptomatic patients versus asymptomatic pregnant patients showed increased activity of succinic dehydrogenase indicative of increased secretory activity, and an increase in alkaline phosphatase concentration indicative of increased vascularity and a transfer of metabolites across plasma membranes.[35] The reasons why some women are symptomatic and others are not is not clearly understood.

Another common problem during pregnancy is an inflammatory gingival hyperplasia caused by increased gingival reactivity to local irritants. Typically seen in the patient's first trimester and commonly maintained until termination of the pregnancy, it may evolve into a 'pregnancy tumour' of the gingival. Biopsies of these have shown to be pyogenic granuloma. Menopause may be associated with several oral manifestations; the most common are desquamative gingivitis and generalized atrophic alterations of the oral mucosa.

Kallmen's syndrome and Turner's syndrome are two syndromes pertaining to the reproductive organs that deserve mention here. Kallmen's syndrome (hypogonadotropic hypogonadism) has two inheritance patterns: the first is X-linked recessive and the second is autosomal dominant with variable expressivity. The syndrome consists of gonadotropin deficiency secondary to LHRH deficiency in association with anosmia. This is often diagnosed when males fail to achieve puberty. There are variable degrees of dysnosmia and even female carriers are shown to have decreased olfactory ability. Studies have shown that some of these patients have no olfactory bulb and stalks, while others have varying degrees of malformation of the olfactory epithelium (ranging from complete intact epithelium to complete agenesis). Other head and neck manifestations sometimes seen are midline facial deformities including cleft palate and deafness.

Turner's syndrome (gonadal dysgenesis) is characterized by an XO karyotype and occurs in 1 in 2500–10,000 live female births. This disease presents in females with gonadal dysgenesis, short stature and often a webbed neck and/or shield chest. Sensorineural, conductive or mixed hearing loss, which may be progressive, is often an early sign of Turner's syndrome in prepubertal females. These patients can also have a high arching palate, epicanthal folds and low-set ears.

KEY POINTS

- General awareness of endocrine disorders can aid in their early diagnosis as head and neck manifestations are often the presenting signs or symptoms.
- Patients with DM often complain of many common head and neck symptoms; this includes cranial neuropathies, sensorineural hearing loss and vestibular dysfunction.
- Patients with DM are susceptible to unique and invasive infections including malignant otitis externa and invasive fungal sinusitis.
- Pregnancy should be considered as a cause of rhinorrhea in the child-bearing age woman.
- Thyroid perturbations are often associated with abnormal function of the larynx, causing changes in pitch and clarity of speech, the nose, causing rhinitis, and the inner ear, causing vertigo and hearing loss.

REFERENCES

1. Maceri DR. Head and neck manifestations of endocrine disease. *Otolaryngologic Clinics of North America*. 1986; **19**: 171–80.
2. Melmed S. Acromegaly. *New England Journal of Medicine*. 1990; **322**: 966–77.
3. Daughaday WH. The adenohypophysis. In: Williams RH (ed.). *Textbook of endocrinology*. Philadelphia: WB Saunders, 1981: 31–79.
* 4. Lucente FE. Endocrine problems in otolaryngology. *Annals of Otology, Rhinology, and Laryngology*. 1973; **82**: 131–7.
5. Grotting JK, Pemberton J. Fixation of the vocal cords in acromegaly. *Archives of Otolaryngology*. 1950; **52**: 608–17.
6. Jackson C. Acromegaly of the larynx. *Journal of the American Medical Association*. 1918; **71**: 1787–9.
7. Sano T, Asa SL, Kovacs K. Growth hormone-releasing hormone-producing tumors: clinical, biochemical and morphological manifestations. *Endocrine Reviews*. 1988; **9**: 357–9.
8. Jefferson G. Extrasellar extension of pituitary adenomas. *Proceedings of the Royal Society of Medicine*. 1940; **33**: 433–58.
9. Rowe PJW, Jones TK. Malignant adenoma with extensive skull destruction. *Radiology*. 1966; **86**: 532–4.
10. Dent JA, Rickhuss PK. Invasive pituitary adenoma presenting with nasal obstruction. *Journal of Laryngology and Otology*. 1989; **103**: 605–9.
* 11. Ritter FN. The effects of hypothyroidism upon the ear, nose and throat. *Laryngoscope*. 1967; **78**: 1427–79.
12. Proetz AW. The thyroid and the nose. *Annals of Otology, Rhinology, and Laryngology*. 1947; **56**: 328–33.

13. Proetz AW. Further observations of the effect of thyroid insufficiency on the nasal mucosa. *Laryngoscope*. 1950; **60**: 627–33.

14. Gupta OP, Bhatia MS, Agarival MS, Mehrorta MD, Mishr SK. Nasal, pharyngeal, and laryngeal manifestations of hypothyroidism. *Ear Nose and Throat Journal*. 1977; **56**: 10–22.

15. Proctor DF, Andersen IB. *The nose: upper airway physiology and the atmospheric environment*. Amsterdam: Elsevier Biomedical Press, 1982: 207.

16. Settipane GA, Klein DE. Nonallergic rhinitis: the domography of eosinophils, nasal smear, blood total eosinophil counts, and IgE levels. *Allergy Proceedings*. 1985; **6**: 363–6.

∗ 17. Gustafson RO, Knops JL. In: McCaffrey TV (ed.). *Effect of thyroid disease, pituitary disease, and pregnancy on the nasal airway: systemic disease and the nasal airway*. New York: Thieme Medical Publishers, 1993: 120–30.

18. Bhatia PL, Gupta OP, Agrawal MK, Mishr SK. Audiological and vestibular function tests in hypothyroidism. *Laryngoscope*. 1977; **87**: 2082–9.

19. Debruyne F, Vanderschueren-Lodeweyckx M, Bastijns P. Hearing in congenital hypothyroidism. *Audiology*. 1983; **22**: 404–9.

20. Fraser GR. Association of congenital deafness with goiter (Pendred's syndrome): a study of 207 families. *Annals of Human Genetics*. 1965; **28**: 201–49.

21. Sergott RC, Glasner JS. Graves' ophthalmopathy: a clinical, immunologic review. *Survey of Ophthalmology*. 1981; **26**: 1–21.

22. Neigel JM, Rootman J, Belkin RI, Nugent RA, Drance SM, Beattie SW *et al*. Dysthyroid optic neuropathy: the crowded orbital apex syndrome. *Ophthalmology*. 1988; **95**: 1515–21.

23. Calcaterra TC, Thompson JW. Antral-ethmoidal decompression of the orbit in Graves' disease: 10-year experience. *Laryngoscope*. 1980; **90**: 1941–9.

24. Burke H. Endocrine aspects of otolaryngology. *Laryngoscope*. 1968; **78**: 857–62.

25. Maceri D. Head and neck manifestations of endocrine disease. *Otolaryngologic Clinics of North America*. 1986; **19**: 171–80.

26. Simpson JA. Aphonia and deafness in hyperparathyroidism. *British Medical Journal*. 1954; **1**: 494–6.

∗ 27. Drachman RH, Root RH, Wood WB. Studies on the effect of experimental nonketotic diabetes mellitus on antibacterial defense. *Journal of Experimental Medicine*. 1966; **124**: 227–40.

28. Korezyn A. Bell's palsy and diabetes mellitus. *Lancet*. 1971; **1**: 108–10.

∗ 29. Schechter GL, Kostianovsky M. Vocal cord paralysis in diabetes mellitus. *Transactions-American Academy of Ophthalmology and Otolaryngology*. 1972; **76**: 729–40.

30. Igarashi M. Pathology of the inner ear end organs. In: Minkler J (ed.). *Pathology of the nervous system*. New York: McGraw Hill, 1972.

31. Perez R, Ziv E, Freeman S, Sichel JY, Sohmer H. Vestibular end-organ impairment in an animal model of type 2 diabetes mellitus. *Laryngoscope*. 2001; **111**: 110–3.

∗ 32. Mabry RL. Rhinitis of pregnancy. *Southern Medical Journal*. 1986; **79**: 965–71.

33. Bende M, Hallgarde M, Sjogren U, Uvnas-Moberg K. Nasal congestion during pregnancy. *Clinical Otolaryngology and Allied Sciences*. 1989; **14**: 385–7.

34. Helmi AM, El-Ghazzawi IF, Mandour MA, Shehata MA. The effect of estrogen on the nasal respiratory mucosa. *Journal of Laryngology and Otology*. 1975; **89**: 1229–41.

35. Toppozado H, Michaels L, Toppozado M, El-Ghazzawi I, Talaat M, Elwany S. The human respiratory nasal mucosa in pregnancy. *Journal of Laryngology and Otology*. 1982; **96**: 613–26.

PART 7

PHARMACOTHERAPEUTICS

EDITED BY MARTIN J BURTON

33 Drug administration and monitoring   407
    Geraldine Gallagher

34 Corticosteroids in otolaryngology   418
    Niels Mygind and Jens Thomsen

35 Drug therapy in otology   429
    Wendy Smith and Martin Burton

36 Drug therapy in rhinology   436
    Wendy Smith and Grant Bates

37 Drug therapy in laryngology and head and neck surgery   446
    Wendy Smith and Rogan Corbridge

33

Drug administration and monitoring

GERALDINE GALLAGHER

Introduction   407
Drug development   407
Drug administration   408
Drug pharmacology   409
Monitoring of drug therapy   412
Adverse drug reactions   414
Drug prescribing in special treatment groups   415
Key points   416
Best clinical practice   416
Deficiencies in current knowledge and areas for future research   416
References   416

SEARCH STRATEGY

The information in this chapter is supported by a PubMed search using the key words drug regulation and development, drug bioavailability, clinical pharmacokinetics and pharmacodynamics, drug compliance and monitoring, and adverse drug reactions.

INTRODUCTION

In clinical ear, nose and throat (ENT) practice, therapeutic decision making has become increasingly complex, particularly in the realm of drug prescribing. The increasing range of possible interventions and the changing expectations of patients have been accompanied by a dramatic rise in the number of drugs available. In 1932, the British Pharmacopoeia listed 213 medical products. By 2001, this figure had increased to 2760.

For clinicians, these factors have created a personal responsibility: we are now required to assess the relevant published evidence, to make a balanced therapeutic decision and to evaluate the outcome of that decision. Ideally, each drug prescription for a patient should be an individualized therapeutic plan which maximizes the clinical benefit and the patient's well-being while achieving the lowest toxicity and the lowest cost. To implement such a logical approach to drug therapy, a number of steps are known to be important. The clinician must:

- make an accurate diagnosis;
- understand the pathophysiology of the disease;
- have a good knowledge of the therapeutic options;
- select treatment: either no drug or an optimum drug and dosing schedule;
- monitor the effect of treatment and decide a therapeutic end point;
- maintain a 'therapeutic alliance' with the patient.

In this chapter, the aim is to discuss the regulatory mechanisms involved in drug control and to examine the factors which influence the therapeutic options for individual patients. In essence, the chapter sets out the principles involved in rational prescribing.

DRUG DEVELOPMENT

The discovery and development of a drug can take 15 years or more and involves many steps. Once a chemical with a potential therapeutic effect has been identified, a series of investigations in animals and humans is carried out to check whether the chemical is effective and whether it is safe to use. The first step in the development of a drug is to establish its pharmacokinetic and toxic profile in animals. Three stages of trials in humans establish its potential for the treatment of disease. Phase I studies are primarily concerned with assessing a drug's safety, and are typically carried out on a small number of healthy volunteers, investigating the side effects as the dose increases. Phase II studies test for efficacy and may involve up to several hundred patients in a randomized, controlled trial. Finally, in phase III, most drugs are ideally entered into a randomized, double-blind, controlled trial involving several hundred to several thousand people, giving a more thorough understanding of the effectiveness, benefits and range of possible adverse reactions compared to an existing drug or placebo.

In the UK, once a drug has been successfully trialled, the pharmaceutical company applies to the Committee on Safety of Medicines (CSM) for a licence to launch the drug into the market. When a licence is received, the drug then joins the range of therapeutic options available to the clinician.

Drug regulatory systems

In most countries, a drug cannot be made legally available until a government-sponsored regulatory body has reviewed its safety and efficacy. This system was put in place in the UK in 1968 as a consequence of the thalidomide tragedy. Prior to this, there was no body in the UK which could prevent the marketing of a new medicinal product. Thalidomide was launched in Britain in 1958 as a sedative/hypnotic and for use in morning sickness. By 1961, however, it became clear that its use in early pregnancy was causally related to a congenital abnormality where the long bones in babies failed to develop. Around 1000 deformed babies were born in Britain as a result and around 10,000 worldwide. Following this tragedy, the Committee on Safety of Drugs was established, later to become the CSM following the Medicines Act of 1968. The CSM is an independent group of 34 clinicians, pharmacologists, toxicologists and pharmacists plus two lay appointees who advise the licensing authority (the health and agriculture ministers) on medicinal products. Adverse drug reactions are reported to the CSM by individual doctors, using a voluntary yellow card system. Although the voluntary system has yielded some impressive regulatory decisions, there is evidence that adverse reactions are significantly under-reported.[1,2,3]

In 1995, the European Union (EU) established the European Agency for the Evaluation of Medicinal Products (EMEA). This body coordinates the scientific evaluation of the safety, quality and efficacy of medicinal products for use throughout the EU. EMEA employs a system of 'mutual recognition' of drug authorizations already granted by individual member states. In addition, EMEA provides a centralized European evaluation for new drugs and all decisions agreed under this new system are binding on member states.

Herbal medicines are largely outside the current regulatory systems. Used by 80 percent of the world's population and an increasing number of patients and practitioners in Europe and North America, herbal medicines include homeopathic, traditional herbal, Ayurvedic, naturopathic and native medicines. Most products are still unregulated, but in the UK, adverse reactions to Chinese and herbal medicine are reported to the CSM. The most comprehensive current regulatory system and information resource is provided by the German 'Commission E' monographs.

DRUG ADMINISTRATION

Following diagnosis of the disease and a decision to choose drug therapy, the clinician has to select an appropriate drug and decide the mode of administration. There is a wealth of information available about licensed drugs, including recommendations on delivery methods, dosage and dosage frequency, as well as information on known adverse effects. In considering the mode of administration, it is important for the clinician to assimilate and understand this information in order to select the best options for the individual patient.

Delivery methods

When a drug is used therapeutically the aim is to achieve an adequate concentration at the site of action and to maintain that concentration for as long as the effect is required. 'Systemic bioavailability' is a term used to describe the proportion of administered drug that reaches the systemic circulation and is available for distribution to the receptor site. The method of administration is a major determinant of bioavailability.

When a drug is given intravenously, the total dose enters the systemic circulation. This method achieves 100 percent bioavailability. However, use is limited by the constraints of venous access and issues of safety.

When a drug is given orally, the bioavailability depends on the extent of absorption from the gut and the metabolic activity of the liver as the drug circulates following absorption, known as the 'first pass effect'. This effect can substantially reduce the bioavailability of a drug. Most drugs are given orally and are therefore subject to 'first pass'.

Transnasal, sublingual, buccal and rectal formulations all avoid the first pass effect. The bioavailability depends only on the absorption across the mucosa. This mechanism may become an important consideration in some circumstances. For example, prochlorperazine in the buccal form may help a patient suffering an acute labyrinthine attack in the presence of nausea and vomiting.

Transdermal formulations in the form of patches are absorbed through the skin and enter the systemic circulation directly. Absorption depends on lipid solubility and a concentration gradient being established across the dermis. Only some drugs are successful, one example being transdermal hyoscine for the treatment of motion sickness.

Intramuscular and subcutaneous preparations are limited in number because the absorption of drugs given by these routes is variable and often unpredictable, hindering their usefulness. Special consideration has to be given to the formulation of the drug and to the site of application. Drugs given intramuscularly are given into the deltoid muscle rather than gluteal, as absorption in the former is much more rapid due to the higher vascularity. A reduction in the rate of local absorption can be achieved, for example, by the use of adrenaline in combination with local anaesthetics administered subcutaneously, causing local vasoconstriction. Important subcutaneous preparations include heparin and insulin.

DRUG PHARMACOLOGY

The biological activity of a drug, whether therapeutic or toxic, is proportional to the concentration of the drug at the receptor site and the persistence of the drug's effect is directly related to the length of time the drug remains at the receptor site. Therefore, the biological activity of a drug is dependent on the rate and completeness of its absorption, distribution, metabolism and elimination. Within ENT practice, getting a drug to a receptor site can either be by direct application to that site (as with nasal antihistamines), or by administration via a site remote from the target (as with oral antihistamines in the case of allergic rhinitis). Whatever the method used, the drug must then diffuse across several membranes (absorption), distribute into a variety of tissues and fluids (distribution), be subject to a wide array of metabolizing enzymes

(metabolism) and finally be eliminated from the body (elimination).

Pharmacokinetics is the study of the rate of drug movement into and through body tissues. This information will help predict the time course and magnitude of the drug effect. The pharmacokinetics of a drug can be studied by regular analysis of plasma and urine samples following its administration, giving quantitative assessment of the rate of drug movement, metabolism and elimination. Plasma concentration is not necessarily the same as tissue concentration, but accurately reflects it in most therapeutic regimens and for practical clinical purposes is taken to be the same.

The study of the underlying mechanism of action of the drug at the receptor site and the resultant biological response is known as pharmacodynamics. Variations in this biological response due to genetically determined factors is known as pharmacogenetics.

Pharmacokinetics and clinical practice

Pharmacokinetics is the key factor in deciding on drug formulation and dosing frequency. To understand why, it is necessary to look at how drug concentration in the plasma (and by implication, at the receptor site) changes with time. After a drug is administered to the body in any form, the concentration of the drug in the plasma rises in keeping with absorption, then falls as a result of distribution, metabolism and elimination. **Figure 33.1** shows a typical profile of drug concentration in nasal tissue following instillation of nasal drops. The curve contains three features of interest.

C_{max} This is the maximum level of drug in the plasma after a single administration (reflecting the maximum level of drug in the tissue). C_{max} dictates the initial therapeutic and toxic responses. Most drug applications aim to have C_{max} falling within the therapeutic range. The position of C_{max} along the time-axis reflects the rate at which the drug becomes bioavailable.

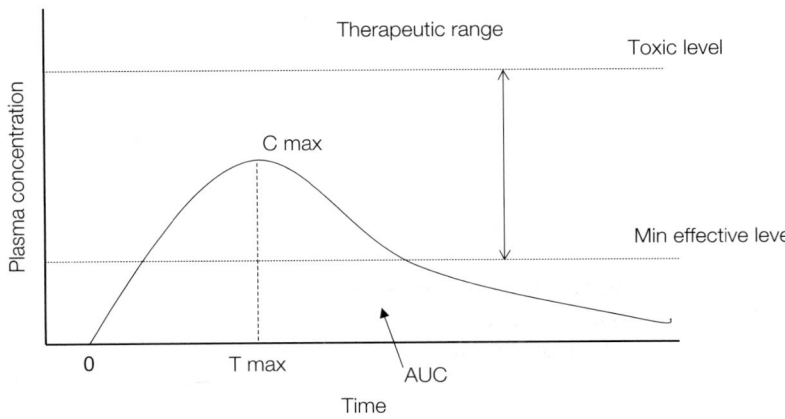

Figure 33.1 Change in drug concentrations in the plasma/tissue following nasal administration.

T_{max} This is the time taken to reach the maximum level of drug in the tissue.

Area under the curve The area under the curve (AUC) is a measure of the total amount of drug absorbed from a single dose. The bioavailability of the drug – that is, amount instilled versus amount absorbed – can be computed from the AUC.

Choosing the drug formulation

Figure 33.2 shows two curves representing the theoretical plasma/tissue concentration over time, following oral administration of equal doses of the same drug using different formulations. The total bioavailability, as indicated by the AUC, is the same in each case. However, the rate at which the drug becomes available depends on the formulation. For drugs such as analgesics, where a rapid plasma concentration is required after single dosing, choice of formulation may therefore be very important. For example, a soluble Diclofenac formulation giving a curve A would be preferable in the treatment of acute pain (such as postoperative tonsillectomy) rather than an enteric-coated formulation giving rise to a curve B. However, the latter would be more useful in the long-term treatment of chronic pain or for an antiinflammatory effect, allowing a reduction in the frequency of administration.

Deciding on dosing frequency

The frequency with which drugs are administered is governed by the rate at which they are metabolized and by the rate of clearance of the unmetabolized drug by the body. The overall rate of loss of the drug is described as the half-life ($t_{1/2}$): the time for the plasma concentration to fall to one half of the maximum value. The half-life in turn dictates the timing interval for delivering the second and subsequent doses; the recommended interval equals the half-life of the drug. The resultant plasma level shows a series of peaks and troughs as in **Figure 33.3**. The peak and trough levels rise over time because each subsequent dose given at $t_{1/2}$ is additional to the quantity of the drug left behind from the earlier administration. Eventually, the size of the fall in plasma concentration after the peak equals the preceding rise and a steady state is reached. At steady state, the amount of drug eliminated from the body in a single dose interval is the same as the amount which enters it. Strictly speaking it is not a true steady state because the plasma concentration fluctuates. However, for practical purposes, a steady state is reached within a finite number of doses, usually between four and six. The concentration of drug in the plasma after multiple doses will be greater than the single dose, C_{max}, but at all times should be within the therapeutic range.

If the half-life is long and it takes several days to reach a steady state, then an initial loading dose can be prescribed to overcome the delay in establishing the therapeutic effect. In **Figure 33.4**, a standard oral regime (Oral regime A) should ideally maintain a therapeutic plasma range throughout the drug administration. It can be seen that shortening the dosing interval and giving the drug more frequently (Oral regime B) may result in toxic plasma levels. Furthermore, a decrease in the dosing frequency could result in a subtherapeutic effect.

Choice of dosing interval is therefore extremely important in achieving and maintaining therapeutic effectiveness with minimal toxicity.

Metabolism

Most drug metabolism occurs in the liver, but can occur elsewhere, for example in the lungs and kidneys. The end result is inactivation of the drug. The enzymatic processes involved in drug metabolism are described as phases I and II.

Phase I involves chemical alteration of the basic structure of the drug by a number of versatile groups of enzymes in the liver, one of the most important being

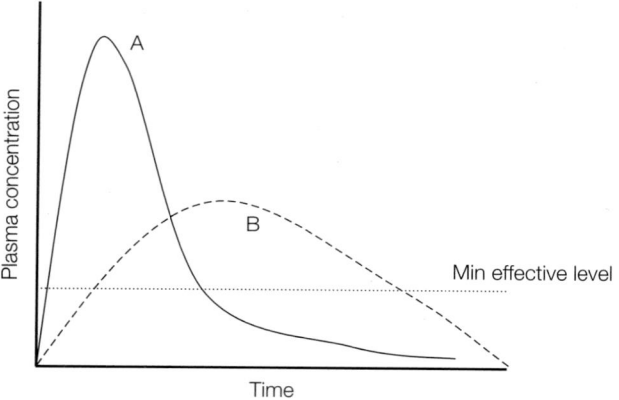

Figure 33.2 Drug bioavailability curves for differing formulations.

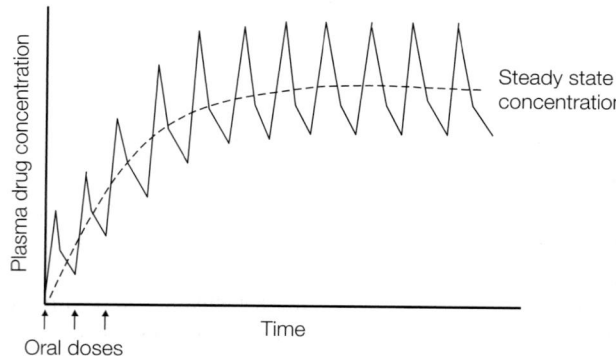

Figure 33.3 Achieving steady state concentration following initiation of oral therapy.

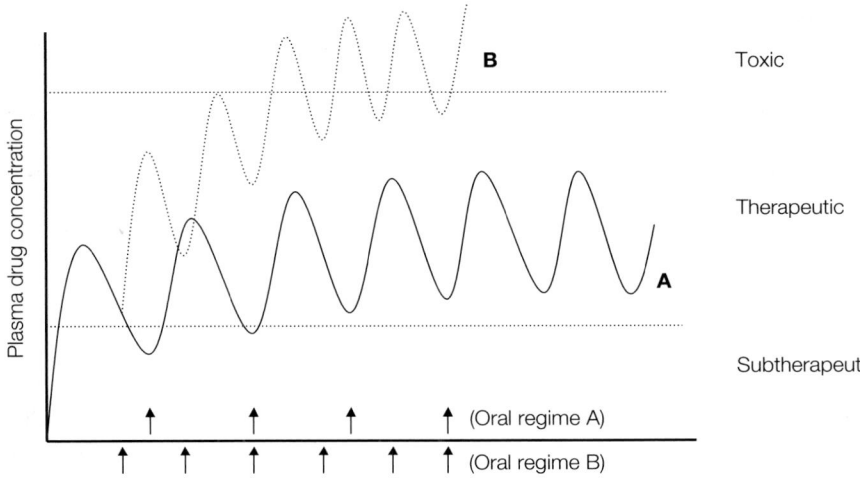

Figure 33.4 Drug concentration in plasma/tissue following change in dosing schedule.

cytochrome P-450. Cytochrome P-450 consists of a large number of genetically related enzymes. (The name is derived from the fact that a light wavelength of 450 nm is absorbed by the enzymes.) Where a patient is on two or more drugs, competition between the drugs for attachment to cytochrome P-450 can result in a rise in the concentration of one of these drugs to a toxic level.

This problem has been experienced in ENT in the past, due to a practice of coprescribing antihistamines, such as terfenadine, with macrolide antibiotics, such as erythromycin. Erythromycin competes with terfenadine for a binding site, and will then inhibit the isoenzyme within the P-450 system that degrades terfenadine. This leads to toxic levels of terfenadine resulting in a characteristic pattern of ventricular tachycardia known as torsades de pointes, which is potentially fatal.

Phase II metabolism introduces hydrophilic molecules to the drug resulting in end products which are water soluble and can more easily be eliminated from the body.

Drug elimination

This overwhelmingly takes place through kidney excretion. Minor routes include lungs, breast milk, sweat and tears.

Pharmacodynamics and clinical practice

Pharmacodynamics are the key factor in determining which drug and dosing schedule to prescribe. When a drug is administered, it enters the pharmacokinetic process and eventually reaches its target tissue. The next stage, the pharmacodynamic stage, will lead to a therapeutic effect. This stage involves attachment of the drug to receptors. Receptors are proteins situated either in the cell membranes or within the cellular cytoplasm of target organs. For each receptor there is a specific group of

ligands (either drugs or endogenous substances) that can bind to the receptor and produce pharmacological effects.

There are two types of ligands of interest in ENT prescribing – agonists and antagonists. Agonists are ligands that bind to a receptor, stimulate it and produce a response. The drugs ephedrine and hyoscine are examples. Antagonists are ligands that bind to a receptor and thereby prevent an endogenous agonist from binding to and stimulating the receptor. The drugs ipratropium bromide and cetirizine hydrochloride are examples.

The intensity of the therapeutic response that drugs produce, through agonist or antagonist activity, can be plotted against the dosage. Most drugs produce graded dose-related effects and **Figure 33.5** is a dose–response curve for two similar analgesics (A and B) used in clinical ENT practice.

There are a number of important points to note in the figure.

- A log conversion is used for dosage to allow a greater range of dosage to be represented.
- There is a straight line relationship between log dose and response over a large part of the curve which allows easier comparison of drugs with similar therapeutic actions.
- There is a 'therapeutic range' within which most patients will achieve a therapeutic effect. The recommended dosing schedule for drugs is based on the median effective dose or ED_{50}, which is the dose effective for 50 percent of the population studied. For drug A, the therapeutic range is between 8 and 25 mg and the ED_{50} is 15 mg.
- There is a ceiling effect represented by the plateau, beyond which increasing the dose achieves no increase in the therapeutic effect.
- The potency of a drug, a term often used by pharmaceutical companies in their marketing, describes where the curve lies along the x-axis. So, in **Figure 33.5**, drug A is more potent than drug B: less

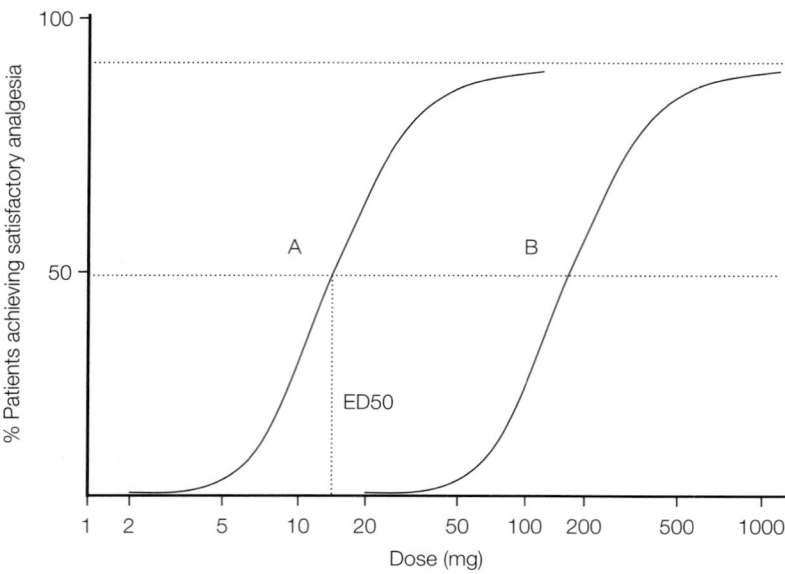

Figure 33.5 Dose response curves for analgesic drugs A and B.

of A is needed for a given therapeutic effect. A difference in potency is not an important issue in itself, unless the actual volume or mass to be given is so large that it causes difficulty in administration, or the drugs differ significantly in cost.

- The therapeutic index is a measure of the safety of a drug. It is the ratio of the dose producing the desired therapeutic effect, to the dose which produces a toxic effect. A low therapeutic index indicates a potentially dangerous drug. In **Figure 33.5**, the therapeutic index is represented by the slope of the curve. If the slope is steep, then increasing the dosage by a small amount can increase the effect to levels where toxic side effects can occur.

We have now seen how a drug formulation and drug pharmacokinetics affect the bioavailability and how pharmacodynamics relate to a therapeutic response. The next step in the therapeutic process is to monitor the therapeutic response.

Pharmacogenetics

From the previous discussion on pharmacokinetics and pharmacodynamics, it can be seen that the resultant therapeutic response to a drug could be modified by genetic factors at many different stages of the pharmacological process, from transit through the body to effector action. Sensitivity to succinyl choline is one example of an inherited autosomal recessive trait. Administration of this drug during anaesthesia in patients carrying this trait can lead to prolonged periods of apnoea, which may result in unplanned mechanical ventilation. In these patients, the cholinesterase enzyme which converts succinyl choline to succinyl monocholine has altered properties resulting either in an unexpected

sensitivity to the drug or on occasions an abnormal resistance to its effects. Biochemical variations can occur unpredictably with many drugs, giving rise to occasional idiosyncratic responses. Often these genetic variations are undetected and the effects misinterpreted.

MONITORING OF DRUG THERAPY

Once a drug regime is decided and treatment is underway, it is important to monitor the effect of the treatment and provide feedback to the patient. As well as gauging the therapeutic effect of the drug, monitoring is essential to identify adverse drug reactions.

Methods of monitoring

These fall into one of three categories.

1. **Physical monitoring**. Certain medical problems lend themselves to serial physical measurements to assess the effects of treatment, for example blood pressure in hypertensive patients, forced expiratory volume in asthmatic patients or the extent of nodal disease in lymphoma.
2. **Patient self-monitoring**. This is probably the most common type of monitoring in use in ENT practice. Patients report back on their changing symptomatology following a trial of therapy. Because such reports are subjective, problems arise in quantifying the improvement or deterioration in symptoms. It is therefore often difficult to decide whether change of dosage is required unless the expected outcome of therapy is the complete alleviation of symptoms. Short of this aim, using a written record of a problem

list and setting intermediate goals for therapy can be of help.

3. **Plasma concentration monitoring**. This method gives objective measurements of the bioavailability of the drug and reflects the tissue concentration. In clinical practice, such monitoring is important mainly for those drugs with a low therapeutic index (that is, a high risk of toxicity). Examples include aminoglycosides, antiarrythmics, cytotoxic therapy and anticoagulants. Plasma monitoring is also used in cases of therapeutic failure, for example anticonvulsant treatment, to establish an objective level of compliance with the treatment regime. It can be used in a medicolegal context to ascertain the plasma level of recreational or illegal drugs, and is of course essential during clinical pharmacological trials.

Monitoring and compliance

Meaningful monitoring of the therapeutic effect of a drug depends on the compliance of the patient. In clinical terms, compliance is defined as the extent to which a patient's actual history of taking medication corresponds to the prescribed treatment.[4] Many factors are involved in noncompliance. They include failure to take a prescription to the pharmacy, failure to follow the doctor's instructions, taking an incorrect dose, taking the medication erratically, stopping the treatment too early or even failure to attend for follow-up appointments. Whatever the factor, noncompliance or poor compliance is a constant and complex issue which causes major problems in the delivery of health care.

Noncompliance adversely affects:

- the clinical outcome of prescribed regimes;
- the effectiveness of healthcare budgets;
- the conclusions drawn from clinical research, especially drug trials.

The rational prescription of medication is the most common intervention in primary care and thus forms a large part of the health care costs. Poor compliance with prescribed treatment can have a major impact on clinical outcome, especially if the drug is needed to maintain vital physiological functions. This pattern is often seen with cardiac or hypertensive medication. It is also a problem in established preventative health care programmes, for example aspirin for patients with atherosclerotic disease.

Drug trials rely on an intention-to-treat analysis and unless specifically structured, do not reliably account for the effects of poor compliance. Thus results are analysed on the basis of the treatment to which the patients were assigned, regardless of whether the drugs were actually taken. This approach has created a number of problems, including biased estimates of the effectiveness of some drugs. Compliance is difficult to measure, but studies suggest that poor compliance is to be expected in 30–50 percent of all patients, irrespective of their disease or prognosis.[5,6,7] If this extrapolation were applied to drug trials, then the sample size would often need to be increased five-fold in order to yield the same number of 'complying' patients as for a sample where 100 percent compliance is assured.

Numerous methods of measuring compliance have been introduced, such as patient diaries and blister packs. These depend on the patient being motivated and truthful. Newer methods such as microelectromechanical systems (MEMS) are at present used only during research trials. MEMS are devices containing microchips which are attached to a bottle and are stimulated on opening the bottle. They record the number of times the patient opens the bottle – not necessarily when the patient takes the medication. Although much research has been carried out on compliance over the last three decades, no single factor or group of factors has emerged as the dominant influence on compliance. Therefore, few if any changes introduced into therapeutic regimes have led to a significant improvement in compliance. One of the reasons for the lack of progress in compliance research may be the difficulty in achieving meaningful input from patients themselves.[8]

Factors affecting compliance

NATURE OF THE TREATMENT

It has been shown that poor compliance is related to the duration of the treatment, with long-term therapies being most problematic. Other factors related to low compliance are the number of medications prescribed and the frequency of administration. The more frequently patients have to take a drug, the less likely they are to take it, and the more drugs they are prescribed the lower the overall compliance.[9]

THE TYPE OF ILLNESS

Low compliance is universally associated with psychiatric disorders and the more symptoms reported, the lower the compliance. Elderly patients with memory disorders have difficulty following complex instructions and this contributes to poor compliance. Disability can also be a factor, with patients finding difficulty in managing tablet containers. On the other hand, high compliance is found in patients who are severely disabled, and in young children, probably due to increased supervision by health care workers and parents.

BEHAVIOURAL ISSUES

Patients have been shown to have poor compliance if they are unsure about their diagnosis, if they are asymptomatic, if there is a significant time lag between taking the drug and its effect, or if they fear the adverse effects. There may also be social or physical reasons why they do not pick up their medication from the pharmacy – for example, financial difficulties or mobility problems – in addition to the everyday inconveniences involved in carrying or taking medication.

BEHAVIOUR OF THE DOCTOR

Compliance appears to be related to the quality of the interaction between the patient and the doctor. The enthusiasm and confidence with which treatment is prescribed has been shown to influence compliance, as does the frequency of interaction and the duration of medical appointments.

Methods of improving compliance

Research has shown that compliant patients generally have better clinical outcomes than noncompliant patients. Therefore measures aimed at improving patients' understanding of their illness, their treatment and their doctor's instructions, should improve compliance.

Supervised administration of tablets and practical aids, such as blister packs and dosage counters, do help to improve compliance.

It is advisable to develop a menu of compliance-enhancing strategies that can then be tailored to the individual patient. Examples include:

- involving the patient in determining the treatment goal;
- reducing the complexity of the treatment;
- tailoring the treatment to the patient's lifestyle;
- using reminders to the patient;
- encouraging family support;
- informing the patient about possible side effects;
- monitoring compliance;
- giving the patient feedback.

The patient's input is now considered such an important aspect of compliance that the Royal Pharmaceutical Society of Great Britain has changed its terminology from compliance to concordance.[10] At the centre of the concordance model is the patient as decision maker, with professional support forming a cornerstone of the medical treatment.

ADVERSE DRUG REACTIONS

Adverse drug reactions are 'unwanted effects of drugs occurring at therapeutic doses'. They may be due either to toxic effects or to side effects. A toxic effect is an adverse effect that arises because of an exaggeration of the therapeutic action and is therefore dose related. A side effect is an adverse effect that arises through a pharmacodynamic action other than that which produces a therapeutic effect; such effect may or may not be dose related. It is estimated that up to 5 percent of hospital admissions per year are due to adverse reactions, mostly dose related.[11, 12] [****] More than 10,000 hospital beds in the UK are constantly occupied by sufferers, at a cost to the National Health Service (NHS) of up to £1 billion per year.

Adverse drug reactions can be classified as:

- non-dose related;
- dose related;
- long-term effects;
- drug interactions.

Non–dose-related adverse reactions

These are caused by allergic responses to drugs and are unrelated to the drug's therapeutic action or dosage. The ability to mount an allergic response may be inherited or may arise spontaneously. Allergic reactions are subdivided into four types:

1. **Type 1 reactions (anaphylactic):** The drug couples to cell-bound IgE leading to release of immune mediators. Type 1 reactions are caused by antibiotics such as penicillin, nonsteroidal antiinflammatory drugs such as indomethacin, plus other chemicals such as iodinated contrast media used in radiography.
2. **Type 2 reactions (cytotoxic):** The drug engages with a protein on the surface of cells, in particular hepatocytes and blood cells. Together they form a surface antigen which attracts and binds circulating IgE or subclasses of IgG, resulting in complement fixation and cell lysis. Examples of drugs causing this reaction are penicillin, heparin and methyldopa.
3. **Type 3 reactions (immune complex):** The drug binds directly to circulating IgG or IgM. The resulting immunoglobin–drug complex becomes trapped in small capillaries, causing release of complement with destruction of the underlying capillary endothelium. Drugs causing type 3 reactions include penicillin, aspirin and cephalosporins.
4. **Type 4 reactions (cell mediated):** The drug binds to Langerhans or dendritic cells in the skin. Together, they sensitize T lymphocytes resulting in an inflammatory response. Examples are contact dermatitis due to latex, topical antibiotics or antifungal drugs.

PSEUDOALLERGIC REACTIONS

'Pseudoallergy' is a term applied to reactions that clinically resemble allergic reactions, but for which no underlying immunological basis can be currently established. For example, aspirin and nonsteroidal anti-inflammatory drugs can trigger asthma attacks in patients who have coexisting nasal polyposis and asthma.

Dose–related adverse reactions

Dose-related adverse reactions are a consequence of the drug's normal therapeutic effects. They may be due to inaccurate prescribing or to inadvertent administration. They may on occasions result from a change in the generic formulation of a drug which can in turn lead to an increase in its bioavailability. This can be critical for drugs with a low therapeutic index and can be a risk when using different generic formulations. An example occurred in Australia with the drug phenytoin. The drug diluent was changed from calcium sulphate to lactose, resulting in toxic effects and death.

Dose-related adverse reactions can also be related to pharmacokinetic or pharmacodynamic variation among individuals. Such variation can be genetic in origin, as seen in a Gaussian distribution, where some patients display toxic effects with even a small 'normal' dose of a drug.

Variation in patients' responses may also be caused by disease such as cirrhosis or by environmental factors such as smoking, diet or alcohol consumption.

Long–term therapy causing adverse reactions

Some drugs cause adverse reactions which only develop after a prolonged period of treatment. The adverse reaction may or may not be reversible on stopping the treatment. For example, a patient may develop drug tolerance. This is a state of decreased responsiveness to a drug and can be seen following prolonged application of ephedrine nasal drops. Ephedrine causes release of noradrenalin from sympathetic nerve endings but leads to its depletion in prolonged treatment. Another example is the development of abnormal facial movements with neuroleptic drugs, such as chlorpromazine. Both these reactions are reversible on stopping the drugs.

Some long-term therapies result in irreversible adverse reactions. A well-known example is hypothyroidism occurring many years after treatment with radioactive iodine. Other irreversible adverse affects are more serious, for example, the increased risk of bladder cancer in patients taking cyclophosphamide.

Adverse reactions caused by drug interactions

When two drugs are present one may alter the effects of the other and the interaction may produce an adverse drug reaction. Drug interactions are responsible for about 7 percent of all adverse drug reactions. The drugs most likely to produce harmful interactions are those with a steep dose–response curve and therefore a low therapeutic index. The adverse reactions may arise from many different causes, such as stimulation or inhibition of metabolism, as in the case of terfenadine and erythromycin (see above under Metabolism) or through altering renal function, thereby effecting drug elimination.

DRUG PRESCRIBING IN SPECIAL TREATMENT GROUPS

Drugs are prescribed because of their potential to benefit the patient, but in every case this is accompanied by the risk of adverse effects. This risk is greater during certain stages of life: pregnancy, childhood, old age and also in certain diseases such as hepatic or renal failure.

Pregnancy

In pregnancy, total body water increases by 6–8 L, resulting in a fall in the concentration of plasma albumin. For drugs that bind to albumin (such as anticonvulsants) the result is an increase in the free drug fraction. At the same time, the high level of endogenous progesterone during pregnancy stimulates hepatic enzymes and renal blood flow increases, which can lead to rapid clearance of drugs excreted by the kidney. In addition, there is a risk to the foetus from drugs crossing the placenta, leading to spontaneous abortion, foetal abnormalities or behavioural abnormalities.

Neonatal, infancy and childhood

In the neonatal and infancy period, major physiological changes take place in the respiratory, cardiovascular and renal systems which have important implications for drug therapy. The childhood period lasts from 1 to 12 years, and when prescribing drugs for children it is important to remember that they are not 'miniature adults'. Research suggests the incidence of adverse drug reactions occurring in hospitalized children is as high as 9.5 percent.[13, 14]

Old age

Equally, in later years, there is a pattern of change in the physiological functioning of the body with age which can affect drug pharmacokinetics and pharmacodynamics. Greater numbers of drugs are prescribed in the elderly and the resulting polypharmacy increases the risk of drug interactions. If there is a concomitant disease such as hepatic or renal failure, then drug pharmacology is even further affected due to decreased metabolism and elimination. These cumulative factors can have profound results: it has been estimated up to 18 percent of deaths in the elderly are related to adverse drug reactions.[15]

Renal and hepatic failure

The treatment of patients with renal or hepatic failure is outside the scope of this chapter. It is important to recognize that the kidney is often a major determinant of drug kinetics, drug efficacy and drug toxicity. Renal function must be considered in the planning of any therapeutic strategy. As discussed above, the liver plays a major role in the pharmacodynamics of almost all drugs. In the event of liver failure, the metabolism of a drug may be radically altered, resulting in toxic levels, leading to adverse effects. Liver function must be taken into consideration when prescribing and appropriate rational therapeutic strategies implemented.

KEY POINTS

- The drug prescription should
  - maximize clinical benefit;
  - maximize patient well-being;
  - achieve lowest toxicity;
  - achieve lowest cost.
- The method of administration of a drug is the major determinant of drug bioavailability at the target organ.
- The plasma half-life of a drug determines the dosing frequency.
- The choice of dose interval is important in achieving and maintaining a steady state of therapeutic effectiveness and minimal toxicity.
- Most drugs are metabolized in the liver.
- Virtually all drugs are excreted via the kidney.
- If a drug has a narrow therapeutic range, ineffective dosing or drug toxicity are more likely to occur.
- The recommended dosing schedule for a drug is based on the median effective dose for 50 percent of the population, the ED_{50}.
- Poor compliance with prescribed treatments has a major negative impact on clinical outcomes.
- A therapeutic concordance model places the patient at the centre, as a decision maker, with surrounding professional support.
- Adverse drug reactions account for 5 percent of all hospital admissions.

Best clinical practice

✓ In monitoring the effect of a drug, the use of a written symptom list and the setting of intermediate treatment goals can be effective.

✓ The quality of the interaction between patient and doctor has a significant effect on prescription compliance.

✓ A menu of compliance-enhancing strategies should be devised for individual patients.

Deficiencies in current knowledge and areas for future research

➤ In clinical practice, ENT surgeons use a range of oral medication, topical medication, sprays, drops and inhalers. Thus, for ENT, the mechanisms of drug administration and drug absorption are particularly important. However, fundamental absorption issues such as the patterns of the mucosal distribution of nasally administered drugs, both in health and disease, are still incomplete.

➤ Further study may lead to improvements in the delivery systems for drugs to the nasal mucosa, with enhanced absorption and clinical effect.

➤ Patient compliance with prescribed medication and the related issue of the identification and recording of adverse drug reactions are problems shared by all medical specialities, but progress on specific ENT solutions to these problems should be sought.

➤ Respiratory medicine, ophthalmology and ENT all share the need for better mechanisms to assess the dose delivery of sprays, drops and inhalers. More work is required before reliable, effective and affordable mechanisms can emerge.

➤ The next edition of *Scott-Brown's otorhinolaryngology, head and neck surgery* may well see progress in:
  - mapping the distribution and absorption of nasal drugs in health and disease;
  - understanding the factors affecting patient compliance and identifying proven strategies for improvement;
  - progress towards an effective and comprehensive reporting system for adverse drug reactions (ADR);
  - the continued development towards optimal drug delivery systems for ENT mucosal administration.

REFERENCES

1. Smith CC, Bennett PM, Pearce HM, Harrison PI, Reynolds DJ, Aronson JK *et al*. Adverse drug reactions in a hospital general medical unit meriting notification to the Committee on safety of Medicines. *British Journal of Clinical Pharmacology*. 1996; **42**: 423–9.

2. Heeley E, Riley J, Layton D, Wilton LV, Shakir SA. Prescription-event monitoring and reporting of adverse drug reactions. *Lancet.* 2001; **358**: 1872–3.

3. Eland IA, Belton KJ, van Grootheest AC, Meiners AP, Rawlins MD, Stricker BH. Attitudinal survey of voluntary reporting of adverse drug reactions. *British Journal of Clinical Pharmacology.* 1999; **48**: 623–7.

4. Haynes RB. Introduction. In: Haynes RB, Taylor DW, Sackett DL (eds). *Compliance in Health Care.* Baltimore: The Johns Hopkins University Press, 1979: 1–7.

5. Lassen LC. Patient compliance in general practice. *Scandinavian Journal of Primary Health Care.* 1989; **7**: 179–80.

6. Griffith S. A review of the factors associated with compliance and the taking of prescribed medicines. *British Journal of General Practice.* 1990; **40**: 114–6.

7. Dunbar-Jacob J, Mortimer-Stephens MK. Treatment adherence in chronic disease. *Journal of Clinical Epidemiology.* 2001; **54**: S57–60 (Review).

8. Donovan JL. Patient decision making. The missing ingredient in compliance research. *International Journal of Technology Assessment in Health Care.* 1995; **11**: 443–55 (Review).

∗ 9. Vermeire E, Hearnshaw H, Van Royen P, Denekens J. Patient adherence to treatment: three decades of research. A comprehensive review. *Journal of Clinical Pharmacy and Therapeutics.* 2001; **26**: 331–42 (Review).

Major review of literature on factors affecting patient compliance.

10. Royal Pharmaceutical Society of Great Britain. *From compliance to concordance: towards shared goals in medicine taking.* London: Royal Pharmaceutical Society of Great Britain, 1997.

11. Lagnaoui R, Moore N, Fach J, Longy-Boursier M, Begaud B. Adverse drug reactions in a department of systemic diseases-oriented internal medicine: prevalence, incidence, direct cost and avoidability. *European Journal of Clinical Pharmacology.* 2000; **56**: 181–6.

∗ 12. Lazaron J, Pomeranz BH, Corey PN. Incidence of adverse drug reactions in hospitalized patients. A meta-analysis of prospective studies. *Journal of the American Medical Association.* 1998; **279**: 1200–5.

13. Weiss J, Krebs S, Hoffmann C, Werner U, Neubert A, Brune K et al. Survey of adverse drug reactions on a paediatric ward: a strategy for early and detailed detection. *Pediatrics.* 2002; **110**: 254–7.

14. Impicciatore P, Choonara I, Clarkson A, Provasid, Pandolfini C, Bonati M. Incidence of adverse drug reactions in paediatric in/out patients: a systematic review and meta-analysis of prospective studies. *British Journal of Clinical Pharmacology.* 2001; **52**: 77–83.

15. Beijer HJ, de Blaey CJ. Hospitalisations caused by adverse drug reactions (ADR): a meta-analysis of observational studies. *Pharmacy World and Science.* 2002; **24**: 46–54.

34

Corticosteroids in otolaryngology

NIELS MYGIND AND JENS THOMSEN

Pharmacodynamics	418	Mononucleosis	422
Pharmacokinetics	418	Croup	422
Side effects	419	External otitis	422
Allergic rhinitis	419	Secretory otitis media	423
Idiopathic rhinitis (perennial nonallergic noninfectious rhinitis)	420	Acute otitis media	423
		Chronic otitis media	423
Rhinitis medicamentosa	421	Sudden deafness	423
Infectious rhinitis (common cold)	421	Menière's disease	423
Nasal polyposis	421	Facial palsy	424
Hyposmia and anosmia	421	Sarcoidosis	424
Sinusitis	421	Wegener's granulomatosis	424
Angioedema	421	Key points	424
Adenoids	422	Best clinical practice	424
Pharyngitis	422	Deficiencies in current knowledge and areas for future research	425
Epiglottitis	422		
Tonsillectomy	422	References	425

SEARCH STRATEGY

The data in this chapter are supported by a Medline search using the key words corticosteroids and the specific diseases cited throughout the text.

PHARMACODYNAMICS

Corticosteroids (CS) are small, lipophilic molecules that readily diffuse across the cell membrane into the cytoplasm, where they bind to the glucocorticoid receptor.[1] The CS–glucocorticoid receptor complex interacts with proteins that serve as transcription factors. This results in a reduced synthesis of inflammatory cytokines and subsequently in a reduced number and activity of inflammatory cells in inflamed tissue. Due to this mode of action, there is a time delay between the administration and the clinical activity of CS. However, studies have shown that the clinical effect of an intranasal CS starts as early as three hours after application.[2]

The density of CS molecules at receptor sites in the surface epithelium, lamina propria, blood vessels, circulating cells and the bone marrow varies markedly between topically and systemically administered drugs. This difference in target cell accessibility to CS has an influence on the effect of topical versus systemic therapy. In the nose, for example, topical treatment is most effective on itching and sneezing, while systemic treatment is most effective on blockage and anosmia.

PHARMACOKINETICS

Intravenous corticosteroids

One hour is gained when a CS is given intravenously instead of orally. Methylprednisolone or dexamethasone are preferred, as they have a minimal minerallocorticoid effect. When adrenal insufficiency is suspected in a patient on long-term oral treatment, hydrocortisone is the drug of choice.

Oral corticosteroids

Prednisolone is, in principle, preferred to prednisone, which is an inactive prodrug, metabolized to prednisolone in the liver. Dexamethasone is more potent and has minimal minerallocorticoid effects.

Intramuscular depot–injection of corticosteroids

When a depot-injection, e.g. methylprednisolone acetate, is given the maximum CS effect on the hypothalamic–pituitary–adrenal (HPA)-axis, measured by its effect on the plasma cortisol level, occurs after three days and the effect lasts for up to three weeks.[3] The CS dose in one injection of 80 mg methylprednisolone corresponds to about 100 mg prednisolone orally.

Intranasal corticosteroids

When an aqueous spray is used, 50 percent is deposited in the nostril and in the nonciliated anterior part of the nose, while 50 percent will reach the ciliated mucous membrane, where it is either absorbed or removed by mucociliary clearance within 30 minutes.[4] Intranasal CS are not deactivated locally and it has to be assumed that the active drug is also absorbed once it reaches the inflammatory cells. Thus, only the dosage which has been absorbed to the nasal mucosa will have an antiinflammatory effect. The measured bioavailability, demonstrated by routine tests, depends upon the CS molecule used. Highly lipophilic molecules, such as fluticasone propionate and mometasone furoate, have a large tissue distribution volume, while less lipophilic molecules, such as beclomethasone dipropionate and budesonide, are quickly absorbed into the circulation.[5] Consequently, highly lipophilic drugs have a long elimination time, while the less lipophilic drugs have a shorter elimination time. Use of these drugs for 10–30 years has shown that both types of drug have a minimal systemic effect without a risk of clinical side effects, when used once daily in the morning at the recommended dosage.

SIDE EFFECTS

Systemic corticosteroids

The side effects from long-term systemic CS therapy are well known. However, side effects following treatment for two to three weeks are few and minor,[3] unless treatment is given to patients with diabetes or glaucoma.

Intranasal corticosteroids

When nasal CS is first sprayed into a hyperreactive nose, it can result in sneezing. Patients should be encouraged to continue treatment, as this symptom usually disappears after a few days.[6] The condition is more a symptom of the disease than a true side effect.

A sensation of dryness in the nostrils, associated with slight blood-stained crusts, is frequently encountered, but it does not seem to worsen during long-term treatment. Usually patients can continue therapy if they reduce the dosage, use the medication only once daily and use a neutral lotion in the nostril. The patient should be told to return for examination if frequent bleeding or crusting develops. Rarely, treatment has to be temporarily stopped because of epistaxis. In very rare cases, a septal perforation can develop during treatment.[7]

Studies have shown that long-term treatment with an intranasal CS has no effect on the growth rate in children, when the drug is given once in the morning in an ordinary recommended dose, i.e. half the adult dose.[8, 9] However, one study has indicated a slight effect on growth, when a high adult dose is given twice daily.[10] Long-term studies of inhaled CS have shown that although there might be a temporary growth inhibition, the children will reach normal final height.[11] Consequently, the risk of a reduced final height from correct nasal medication seems negligible.

Theoretically, even a small systemically active dose of CS, given for a prolonged period of time, may give an increased risk of osteoporosis and cataract. Although studies have not shown such adverse effects from intranasal CS treatment,[12] a small risk cannot be completely excluded.

Corticosteroid ear drops

There is no risk of systemic side effects from this very small CS dose. It is unknown whether ear drops can reach the middle ear mucosa and whether this implies a risk of side effects, but it seems highly unlikely. Theoretically, long-term use may cause atrophy of the skin in the external ear canal.

ALLERGIC RHINITIS

As rhinitis is a disease confined to 0.1 percent of the body weight, local intranasal treatment is, in principle, preferable to systemic treatment.

Intranasal corticosteroids

Since the introduction of beclomethasone dipropionate in 1973, a series of other molecules has been developed and marketed (flunisolide, budesonide, fluticasone propionate, mometasone furoate, triamcinolone acetonide). As these drugs do not differ significantly with regard to effect and risk of side effects, it is recommended to choose the cheapest drug. The drug is usually given as an aqueous spray. In some countries, budesonide is also available as a powder (Turbuhaler) and fluticasone propionate as nose drops.

The clinical effect has been demonstrated in more than 100 placebo-controlled studies.[13, 14, 15, 16] [****] The effect on the nasal symptoms is pronounced. It begins after a few hours and the maximum effect is achieved after several days. When treatment is stopped, the effect disappears over a number of days.

The effect is equally good on all nasal symptoms (sneezing, rhinorrhea, blockage). A series of placebo-controlled studies has clearly shown intranasal CS to be more effective on nasal symptoms than oral and intranasal antihistamines, especially on nasal blockage.[17, 18] [****]

Treatment is usually started with a daily dose equivalent to 400 μg beclomethasone dipropionate in an adult. When control of symptoms has been achieved, dose reduction can be attempted. A study has shown that even 64 μg budesonide is more effective that placebo.[2] In some patients, continuous treatment can be replaced by periodic treatment for two to four weeks.[19]

Some physicians are reluctant to prescribe topical nasal CS in children because of concern about long-term systemic and local adverse effects. However, used for 30 years, topical nasal CS have resulted in virtually no adverse reports. Consequently, these agents may be used in children with persistent moderate to severe allergic rhinitis, particularly when nasal blockage is a pronounced symptom. The dosage is half the adult dose or less and the medication is given once daily in the morning. In our opinion, allergic rhinitis in children is more often undertreated than overtreated. It is the task of the clinician to balance the minimal theoretical risk of side effects against the increased quality of life for a child who can breathe again through the nose and be rid of disturbing itching, sneezing and runny nose.

Pregnancy is not a contraindication as intranasal CS treatment has not been associated with any teratogenic or adverse effects. However, as there are no adequate and well-controlled studies in pregnant women for any drug, treatment should be used only if the expected benefit justifies the potential risk to the foetus.

Systemic corticosteroids

Treatment can be given to adults either orally or as an intramuscular injection of a slow-release formulation.

There is no reason to believe that these two therapies have different therapeutic indices.

Surprisingly, there is only a single placebo-controlled study of oral CS (three different doses of methylprednisolone given three times daily). The study showed an effect on nasal blockage at 6 mg (equipotent to 7.5 mg prednisolone) and on blockage and rhinorrhoea at 24 mg (30 mg prednisolone).[3] [***/**] Three placebo-controlled studies of a depot-injection have shown a marked effect on nasal blockage, lasting for more than four weeks, but merely a mild to moderate effect on sneezing and rhinorrhea.[3] [***]

The treatment can be added, when an intranasal CS is insufficient. However, there are no studies to demonstrate added efficacy of these two types of CS administration. [*] The optimum dose of oral CS is not known. The CS dose of a depot-injection (e.g. 80 mg methylprednisolone acetate) corresponds to 100 mg prednisolone.

Systemic CS treatment should not be given to children, pregnant women or to patients with diabetes mellitus, severe osteoporosis, glaucoma or cataract.

The risk of side effects from a short-term, two- to three-week treatment is very small and should be balanced against the benefits of therapy.

IDIOPATHIC RHINITIS (PERENNIAL NONALLERGIC NONINFECTIOUS RHINITIS)

It is more difficult to treat perennial rhinitis than simple hay fever. Tarlo et al.[20] found that only 54 percent of patients with perennial rhinitis achieved acceptable symptomatic improvement from a CS spray. However, after administration of short-term oral prednisone, 73 percent of the patients obtained moderate or marked symptomatic improvement from topical treatment. In severe cases, it would be advisable to conduct a therapeutic trial with short-term systemic CS, when the effect of nasal CS is insufficient.

In patients suffering from idiopathic rhinitis, intranasal CS have shown a significant effect in most,[20, 21, 22, 23] but not in all studies.[24]

The general impression, supported by a few small studies,[25, 26] is that the treatment is particularly effective when nasal eosinophilia is present. However, a recent large study of idiopathic rhinitis has shown equal efficacy in patients with and without nasal eosinophilia.[23] While the effect is marked in patients with eosinophil-dominated inflammation and intolerance to acetylsalicylic acid,[27] the effect in other cases of idiopathic rhinitis cannot be predicted. It would be advisable to conduct a one-month therapeutic trial with intranasal CS in all patients with persistent idiopathic rhinitis. [***]

RHINITIS MEDICAMENTOSA

A placebo-controlled study of topical CS in rhinitis medicamentosa has shown that patients on intranasal CS have a faster onset of symptom reduction and of improvement of mucosal swelling,[28] indicating that an adequate treatment of such patients consists of a combination of vasoconstrictor withdrawal and a topical CS to alleviate the withdrawal symptoms. Another study has shown an effect of intranasal CS on oxymethazoline-induced rebound congestion.[29] A short course of intranasal CS is recommended, when a vasoconstrictor is withdrawn. [***]

INFECTIOUS RHINITIS (COMMON COLD)

The common cold is a virus-induced inflammation, characterized by neutrophil accumulation in the nasal mucous membrane. Theoretically, a clinical effect could be expected from an antiinflammatory CS. However, at least two placebo-controlled trials have failed to show any effect.[30,31] Thus, CS are highly effective in eosinophil-dominated inflammation and allergy, but not in neutrophil-dominated inflammation and infection. CS are not recommended for the treatment of common cold. [***]

NASAL POLYPOSIS

The aetiology of nasal polyps is unknown. Eosinophils are commonly found in polyps, but the association with allergy appears to be coincidental. Topical CS treatment reduces nasal symptoms, polyp size and the number of recurrences after polypectomy. [****] A short course of systemic CS may help combat obstruction, improve intranasal spray distribution, improve the sense of smell and facilitate intranasal surgery. [***] Management of patients with severe polyposis is still unsatisfactory but it has been improved by the combination of long-term topical CS, short-term systemic CS and surgery, as described in Chapter 121, Nasal polyposis.

HYPOSMIA AND ANOSMIA

Hyposmia is a common finding in patients with allergic rhinitis, especially when the disease is chronic. Severe hyposmia or anosmia frequently occurs in nasal polyposis. While intranasal CS treatment has a beneficial effect on this symptom in allergic rhinitis, the effect in polyposis is poor. Systemic CS are invariably effective, but the effect is short-lasting.[32]

A short course of systemic CS can be used occasionally, when olfactory dysfunction impairs the quality of life in patients with nasal polyposis and when it is indicated to make a distinction between a potentially reversible (rhinitis, polyposis) and an irreversible (viral respiratory infection, toxic chemical exposure, head trauma) olfactory dysfunction. [***]

SINUSITIS

Clinically it is difficult to define sinusitis, especially in those patients with chronic disease where a distinction needs to be made between the symptoms of rhinitis and those of sinusitis.[33] Information received from studying the patient's symptoms and the imaging examination may not agree. Based on a CT scan, a simple common cold is, as a rule, sinusitis, and patients with nasal polyposis invariably show sinusitis on imaging, whether they have sinusitis symptoms or not.

In patients known to be steroid responders, an antirhinitis effect may masquerade as an antisinusitis effect. Therefore, the inclusion of some steroid responders (nasal polyposis, perennial eosinophilic rhinitis, acetylsalicylic acid intolerance) in sinusitis studies may give a false-positive result.

While a few small studies of intranasal CS treatment of acute exacerbations in patients with chronic recurrent sinusitis have been negative,[34,35,36,37] two recent large placebo-controlled studies have been more positive, showing a significant effect on symptoms, but not on imaging.[38,39]

At present, an unqualified recommendation for the use of intranasal CS treatment for chronic recurrent sinusitis cannot be made. However, a therapeutic trial for three months could be made in selected patients. [***]

As a nasal spray will not reach the sinuses nor the middle meatus, with the openings to the paranasal sinuses, it seems possible that a short course of systemic CS may be effective, but placebo-controlled studies have not been performed. [*]

In conclusion, many clinicians believe that intranasal CS are important in the treatment of sinusitis. However, only scant controlled studies support this conjuncture and the use of CS remains controversial.

ANGIOEDEMA

Due to their antiinflammatory and antioedema effects, systemic CS, in conjunction with epinephrine and antihistmine, are generally used in the treatment of angioedema involving the mouth, throat and the upper respiratory tract[40] and as such should be considered an acceptable treatment.[41] However, this practice is not supported by any placebo-controlled study, which are unlikely to be undertaken. [**/*]

ADENOIDS

Lymphocytes are sensitive to CS and, by mucociliary clearance, a nasal spray will be carried to the adenoidal region. There has been only one placebo-controlled study of intranasal CS treatment of children with adenoidal hypertrophy. This study, involving only 17 children, showed a highly significant and long-lasting effect on both adenoid/choanal ration and symptom scores.[42] Further studies are warranted before this treatment can be recommended. [***/**]

PHARYNGITIS

A single placebo-controlled study of an intramuscular CS injection has shown an improvement of pain score in adults with severe pharyngitis.[43] However, in our opinion, this does not justify the use of CS in pharyngitis in general, but it may be tried in selected cases with severe and threatening oedema, compromising breathing. [***/**]

EPIGLOTTITIS

There is a remarkable absence of documentation of the use of CS in acute epiglottitis. Due to the severity of this condition, placebo-controlled studies should not be carried out. However, such investigations should be undertaken, since it is common practice in intensive care units to use CS in patients with severe oedema. [*]

TONSILLECTOMY

Tonsillectomy is one of the most commonly performed surgical procedures. The effect of a single preoperative intravenous dose of CS (dexamethasone, 0.15–1.0 mg/kg) has been studied in a number of placebo-controlled trials. A recent meta-analysis of randomized studies found that the effect is clinically relevant with regard to nausea, vomiting and intake of solid food on the first post-operative day.[44] Given the frequency of tonsillectomy, the relative safety and low cost of a single injection of CS, and the reduction in postoperative morbidity, the authors recommend routine use of a single intravenous dose during paediatric tonsillectomy. In contrast to the above studies, Palme et al.[45] concluded that a seven-day course of CS plays a limited role in patients' recovery from tonsillectomy.

We find that the use of CS in tonsillectomy is open for debate and reference should be made to an article expounding the merits of CS use[46] and another against their use.[47] [****]

MONONUCLEOSIS

In upper airway obstruction due to infectious mononucleosis, it is tempting to resort to some antioedematous drug treatment. The use of CS in this disease is not investigated in any larger study, not to mention any meta-analysis. Tynell et al.[48] demonstrated that acyclovir combined with prednisolone inhibited oropharyngeal Epstein–Barr virus (EBV) replication without affecting the duration of clinical symptoms or development of EBV-specific cellular immunity, while Brandfonbrener et al.[49] found a more beneficial effect, although the results were not striking. Furthermore, there is one report of presumably CS-induced lethal disseminated intravascular coagulation and hepatic necrosis.[50] We must conclude that the use of CS in EBV infection is still a moot point. [**/*]

CROUP

Croup (acute laryngotracheobronchitis) is a frequent disease in children. It is characterized by hoarseness, a dry barking cough and inspiratory stridor. These symptoms occur as a result of oedema in the larynx and trachea due to a viral infection. The disease is usually benign and self-limiting, but it may be the cause of death due to sudden obstruction of the airways.

There is ample evidence from randomized, placebo-controlled trials, summarized by a meta-analysis[51] that CS are effective in croup. [****] Symptoms are improved as early as six hours and for up to at least 12 hours. There is no demonstrable effect after 24 hours. Dexamethasone (orally or intramuscularly) has been evaluated in 17 trials and nebulized budesonide in nine studies.

In most studies, dexamethasone has been given as a single dose of 0.3 mg/kg. This is a high dose, corresponding to 150 mg prednisolone in an adult. However, the risk of side effects from a single dose is very small.

In mild to moderate cases, it is preferable to start treatment at home with a palatable soluble CS (e.g. betamethasone tablets dissolved in a drink). In hospitalized patients, treatment is usually given as an intramuscular injection of dexamethasone (0.3 mg/kg). If available, nebulized budesonide can be used instead (2 mg).

EXTERNAL OTITIS

The symptoms of external otitis vary considerably based on whether the otitis is caused by slight eczema or severe inflammation caused by a bacterial infection. Consequently, the standard treatment is either CS alone, antimicrobial agents alone or a combination of the two. Considering the widespread use of CS ear drops, there is a remarkable absence of placebo-controlled studies. Only one study[52] has demonstrated a significant effect of budesonide compared to placebo. This CS molecule is, however, not marketed as ear drops. Several animal studies have been published demonstrating the availability of an animal model for studying external otitis.[53, 54] In these studies the potency of the CS is discussed and it is most likely that the commonly used CS, hydrocortisone, is too weak to have the desired effect. Further controlled studies are needed. [**]

It is strange that perforation in the drum is listed as a contraindication for using ear drops containing CS. This must be a misconception, since litres of steroid-containing ear drops have been poured into middle ears without causing any inner ear damage, and we believe this warning is not based on solid evidence.

SECRETORY OTITIS MEDIA

secretory otitis media (SOM) is one of the most frequent diseases in childhood. The demonstration of or the rejection of the efficacy of CS is therefore of utmost importance. It is likely that the addition of systemic CS to an antibiotic treatment has a beneficial effect upon the status of the middle ear.[55, 56, 57, 58] On the other hand, Lambert[59] and Macknin and Jones[60] could not demonstrate any effect of either prednisone or dexamethasone.

In a Cochrane review,[61] it was concluded that there is evidence that CS combined with an antibiotic leads to a faster resolution of SOM in the short term. However, there is no evidence for a long-term benefit from treating hearing loss-associated SOM with either oral or topical nasal CS. These treatments are therefore not recommended at the present time. [***]

Considering the possibility that SOM is indeed a bacterial infection, it cannot be ignored that CS inhibit the development of endotoxin-induced otitis media with effusion as demonstrated by Baggett et al.[62] This adds to the confusion, but stresses the need for additional controlled studies.

ACUTE OTITIS MEDIA

From a theoretical point of view, only systemic CS administration can be taken into consideration. In children with tympanostomy tubes, who experience a bout of acute otitis media, with discharge through the tubes, a borderline effect of oral prednisolone has been suggested.[63] Apart from this report, there is no evidence supporting the notion that CS are of any value in the treatment of this disease entity, and such treatment is not to be recommended. [**/*]

CHRONIC OTITIS MEDIA

As with acute otitis media, evidence for supporting the notion that CS have a place in the treatment in chronic suppurative otitis media is scarce. Using monkeys inoculated with *Pseudomonas aeruginosa* in the middle ear, it was found that dexamethasone enhanced the efficacy of tobramycin,[64] whereas a 0.2 percent solution of ciprofloxacin was as effective as a combination preparation with CS.[65] Further placebo-controlled studies are needed to shed light on this issue, and for the present time CS treatment in suppurative otitis media is not recommended. [**/*]

SUDDEN DEAFNESS

Sudden deafness or idiopathic sudden sensorineural hearing loss (ISSNHL) is an abrupt sensorineural hearing loss of at least 30 dB in at least three contiguous audiometric frequencies, variably defined as developing in 12 hours or less,[66] 24 hours or less[67] or in 3 days or less.[68] In making the diagnosis of ISSNHL, identifiable causes of hearing loss should be excluded and the patient should not have a history of previous fluctuations of hearing. The most commonly proposed hypotheses for the aetiology of ISSNHL include disturbance of labyrinthine blood circulation, subclinical viral labyrinthitis, spontaneous labyrinthine membrane rupture and autoimmune pathogenesis.[67] Among the postulated aetiologies of ISSNHL, autoimmunity and perhaps viral infection may be ameliorated by steroids.

The documentation for an effect of CS is poor. A number of publications claim a beneficial effect of CS,[69, 70, 71, 72] while others have come to the opposite conclusion.[73, 74, 75, 76] A Medline search[77] came to the conclusion that no concensus existed on the effective treatment of ISSNHL.

At this point we will refrain from recommending systemic use of CS in patients with ISSNHL. [***/**] However, recent developments have rendered it possible to deliver CS directly at the round window membrane, resulting in a much higher concentration of CS in the inner ear fluids. Anecdotal reports show that such delivery results in hearing improvement in patients who had no benefit from systemic CS prior to the intratympanic, round window application.[78]

MENIÈRE'S DISEASE

Treatment of Menière's disease is hampered by the erratic course of the disease. Oral CS is one treatment that is heralded as being effective. To date, there are no existing controlled studies proving that systemic CS have any effect upon the course of the disease. In recent years, intratympanic CS application has been suggested as an effective treatment; however, the only existing randomized double-blind study[79] concludes that intratympanic administration of dexamethasone showed no benefit over placebo. New delivery systems are now available, resulting in a more specific delivery of the drug to the inner ear. While there are only anecdotal reports of the efficacy, we cannot rule out a possible effect. However, at the present time we cannot recommend either systemic or intratympanic use of CS in Menière's disease. [**/*]

FACIAL PALSY

Bell's palsy, also known as idiopathic facial nerve paralysis (IFNP) is the most common cause of facial paralysis. IFNP results in facial motor dysfunction, the degree of which ranges from minor weakness to complete paralysis. Treatment is aimed at improving recovery of facial function and the prevention of neural degeneration and its associated complications. Of the multiple treatment modalities evaluated over the past three decades, CS therapy has become the most widely accepted. However, despite the widespread clinical acceptance of CS therapy for IFNP, the efficacy of this therapy has not been clearly demonstrated in the literature.

In this age of meta-analysis and Cochrane database systemic reviews, the confusion about the efficacy of CS in the treatment of INFP is striking. A meta-analysis including 47 trials[80] came to the conclusion that there is a statistically significant benefit for complete IFNP patients treated with a total prednisone dose equivalent to 400 mg or more started within seven days of onset of paresis. It is, however, remarkable among the 47 trials used to reach this conclusion that only three met the criteria for a randomized controlled trial. In contrast to this meta-analysis, a Cochrane database systemic review[81] came to the opposite conclusion that the available evidence from randomized controlled trials does not show significant benefit from treating Bell's palsy with CS. More randomized controlled trials with a greater number of patients are needed to determine reliably whether there is real benefit (or harm) from the use of CS therapy in patients with Bell's palsy. Also in this review, only three trials met the requirements of a randomized controlled trial. These trials were not the same as the trials used in the meta-analysis of Ramsey et al.[80]

We must conclude that using CS for IFNP is still a moot point and further placebo-controlled, blinded randomized studies are required before a recommendation for CS therapy can be made. [***]

SARCOIDOSIS

Nasosinal involvement is rare in patients with sarcoidosis and exceptionally rare as an isolated disease manifestation.[82] In the absence of controlled trials, the efficacy of CS needs to be deduced from pulmonary studies. [**]

Only five randomized controlled trials of CS treatment (prednisolone 15–40 mg/day) for pulmonary sarcoidosis were identified in a meta-analysis.[83] Oral steroids improved the chest x-ray, symptoms and lung function (diffusion capacity) over 6–24 months. There are no data beyond two years.

In a consensus report,[84] it was concluded that oral CS is an effective short-term therapy, but it is not known whether the treatment alters the natural history of the disease. It is recommended to start with prednisolone 20–40 mg/day. Among steroid responders, the dose is slowly tapered to 5–10 mg/day. Treatment should be continued for a minimum of 12 months.

Oral CS will probably relieve the discomfort of nasosinal sarcoidosis, but the symptoms need to be severe in order to balance the expected side effects from long-term treatment.

WEGENER'S GRANULOMATOSIS

Combined therapy with cyclophosphamide and systemic CS for remission induction in Wegener's granulomatosis is a well-established and generally recommended treatment.[85] [*] Placebo-controlled trials have not been performed.

KEY POINTS

- Corticosteroids are widely used in otolaryngology and especially in rhinology.
- Topical nasal steroids are safe and effective.
- The risk of side effects from short-term systemic steroids is small.

Best clinical practice

✓ Allergic rhinitis, idiopathic rhinitis and nasal polyposis are best treated with an intranasal CS, when necessary with a supplement of a short course of systemic CS.

✓ A short course of systemic CS can be tried in anosmia.

✓ The role of intranasal CS in chronic sinusitis remains controversial.

✓ Systemic CS are often used for angioedema and epiglottitis, but the effect is unproven.

✓ CS for adenoids and for pharyngitis cannot be recommended at present.

- ✓ The use of a short course of systemic CS in tonsillectomy is open for debate.
- ✓ A single dosage of systemic CS has a proven effect in croup and prompt treatment, either orally or intravenously, is recommended.
- ✓ CS ear drops alone or in combination with an antibiotic has a well-established, but poorly documented, place in the treatment of external otitis.
- ✓ A short course of systemic CS for otitis media with effusion may be helpful, but a recommendation awaits further controlled studies.
- ✓ At present, CS are not to be recommended for acute otitis media, chronic otitis media, sudden deafness, Menière's disease and facial palsy.
- ✓ Systemic CS must be used for Wegener's granulomatosis in spite of a lack of controlled evidence.

Deficiencies in current knowledge and areas for future research

- ➤ Systemic CS are often used for a variety of diseases. However, the treatment is often not evidence based and there is a striking lack of placebo-controlled studies and in particular of dose–effect studies.
- ➤ In severe allergic rhinitis, a short course of systemic CS is often used, but the optimal dosage has not been defined.
- ➤ Intranasal CS are effective in some, but not all, cases of idiopathic rhinitis. Could responsiveness be predicted by local eosinophila or by another inflammatory marker?
- ➤ The role of intranasal CS in subgroups of chronic sinusitis needs to be defined by placebo-controlled studies. Are systemic CS effective?
- ➤ Placebo-controlled studies of intranasal CS treatment for enlarged adenoids in children are warranted.
- ➤ There are no placebo-controlled studies of the effect of systemic CS in angioedema, in epiglottitis and in mononucleosis.
- ➤ We need studies of whether more than a single dose of systemic CS is indicated in croup.
- ➤ CS ear drops alone or in combination with an antibiotic for external otitis media are remarkably poorly documented. A study with one formulation used in one ear and placebo/another formulation in the other ear would be easy to perform.
- ➤ The usefulness of intranasal and of systemic CS for otitis media with effusion needs a detailed analysis in placebo-controlled studies.

REFERENCES

1. Mygind N, Nielsen LP, Hoffman H-J, Shukla A, Blumberga G, Jacobi H. Mode of action of intranasal corticosteroids. *Journal of Allergy and Clinical Immunology.* 2001; **108**: S16–25.
2. Day JH, Briscoe MP, Rafeiro E, Ellis AK, Pettersson E, Åkerlund A. Onset of action of intranasal budesonide (Rhinocort Aqua) in seasonal allergic rhinitis in a controlled exposure model. *Journal of Allergy and Clinical Immunology.* 2000; **105**: 489–94.
3. Mygind N, Laursen LC, Dahl M. Systemic corticosteroid treatment for seasonal allergic rhinitis: a common but poorly documented therapy. *Allergy.* 2000; **55**: 11–5.
4. Newman SP, Morén F, Clarke SW. Deposition pattern of nasal sprays in man. *Rhinology.* 1988; **26**: 111–20.
5. Szefler SJ. Pharmakokinetics of intranasal corticosteroids. *Journal of Allergy and Clinical Immunology.* 2001; **108**: S26–31.
6. Toft A, Whil J-Å, Taxman J, Mygind N. Double-blind comparison between beclomethasone dipropionate as aerosol and as powder in patients with nasal polyposis. *Clinical Allergy.* 1982; **12**: 391–401.
7. Cervin A, Andersson M. Intranasal steroids and septum perforation – an overlooked complication. *Rhinology.* 1998; **36**: 128–32.
8. Scenkel EJ, Skinner DP, Bronsky EA, Miller D, Pearlman DS, Rooklin A. et al. Absence of growth retardation in children with perennial allergic rhinitis after one year of treatment with mometasone furoate nasal spray. *Pediatrics.* 2000; **105**: E22.
9. Möller C, Ahlström H, Henricson K-Å, Malmqvist L-Å, Åkerlund A, Hildebrand H. Safety of nasal budesonide in the long-term treatment of children with perennial rhinitis. *Clinical and Experimental Allergy.* 2003; **33**: 816–22.
10. Skoner DP, Rachelefsky GS, Meltzer EO, Chervinsky P, Morris RM, Storms WW et al. Detection of growth suppression in children during treatment with intranasal beclomethasone dipropionate. *Pediatrics.* 2000; **105**: E23.
11. Agertoft L, Pedersen S. Effect of long-term treatment with inhaled budesonide on adult height in children with asthma. *New England Journal of Medicine.* 2000; **343**: 1064–9.
12. Derby L, Maier WS. Risk of cataract among users of intranasal corticosteroids. *Journal of Allergy and Clinical Immunology.* 2000; **105**: 912–6.
13. Lund VJ, Aaronson D, Bousquet J, Durham SR, Mygind N et al. International consensus report on the diagnosis and management of rhinitis. *Allergy.* 1994; **49**: 1–34.
14. van Cauwenberge P, Bachert C, Passalacqua G, Bousquet J, Mygind N, Durham SR et al. Consensus statement on the treatment of allergic rhinitis. *Allergy.* 2000; **55**: 116–34.
15. Bousquet J, van Cauwenberge P, Khaltaev N. Aria Workshop Group and the World Health Organization. Allergic rhinitis and its impact on asthma. *Journal of Allergy and Clinical Immunology.* 2001; **108**: S147–333.

16. Nielsen LP, Mygind N, Dahl R. Intranasal corticosteroids for allergic rhinitis. *Drugs*. 2001; **61**: 1563–79.

17. Stempel DA, Thomas M. Treatment of allergic rhinitis: an evidence-based evaluation of nasal corticosteroids versus nonsedating antihistamines. *American Journal of Management Care*. 1998; **4**: 89–96.

18. Weiner JM, Abramson MJ, Puy RM. Intranasal corticosteroids versus oral H1 receptor antagonists in allergic rhinitis: systemic review of randomised controlled trials. *British Medical Journal*. 1998; **317**: 624–9.

19. Rinne J, Simola M, Malmberg H, Haathela T. Early treatment of perennial rhinitis with budesonide or cetirizine and its effect on long-term outcome. *Journal of Allergy and Clinical Immunology*. 2002; **109**: 426–32.

20. Tarlo SM, Cockroft DW, Dolovich J, Hargreave FE. Beclomethasone dipropionate aerosol in perennial rhinitis. *Journal of Allergy and Clinical Immunology*. 1977; **59**: 232–6.

21. Hansen I, Mygind N. Local effect of intranasal beclomethasone dipropionate aerosol in perennial rhinitis. *Acta Allergologica*. 1974; **29**: 281–7.

22. Lindkvist N, Balle V, Karma P, Karja K, Lindstrom D, Makinen J *et al*. Long term safety and efficacy of budesonide nasal aerosol in perennial rhinitis – 12 month multicenter study. *Allergy*. 1986; **41**: 179–86.

23. Webb DR, Meltzer EO, Finn Jr AF, Rickard KA, Pepsin PJ, Westlund R *et al*. Intranasal fluticasone propionate is effective for perennial nonallergic rhinitis with and without eosinophilia. *Annals of Allergy, Asthma and Immunology*. 2002; **88**: 385–90.

24. Lundblad L, Sipilä P, Farstad T, Drozdziewicz D. Mometasone furoate nasal spray in the treatment of perennial non-allergic rhinitis: a Nordic multicenter, randomised, double-blind, placebo-controlled study. *Acta Oto-laryngologica*. 2001; **121**: 505–9.

25. Small P, Black M, Frenkiel S. Effect of treatment with beclomethasone dipropionate in subpopulations of perennial rhinitis patients. *Journal of Allergy and Clinical Immunology*. 1982; **70**: 78–82.

26. Feiss G, Welch M, Meltzer E, Alderfer V, Smith J. The predictive value of nasal eosinophilia for therapeutic response to intranasal corticosteroid treatment in perennial allergic rhinitis. *Journal of Allergy and Clinical Immunology*. 1992; **89**: 209 (Abstr.).

27. Mastalerz L, Milewski M, Duplago M, Nizankowska E, Szczeklik A. Intranasal fluticasone propionate for chronic eosinophilic rhinitis in patients with aspirin-induced asthma. *Allergy*. 1997; **52**: 895–900.

28. Hallén H, Enerdal J, Graf P. Fluticasone propionate nasal spray is more effective and has a faster onset of action than placebo in treatment of rhinitis medicamentosa. *Clinical and Experimental Allergy*. 1997; **27**: 552–8.

29. Ferguson BJ, Paramaesvaran S, Rubinstein E. A study of the effect of nasal steroid sprays in perennial allergic rhinitis patients with rhinitis medicamentosa. *Otolaryngology and Head and Neck Surgery*. 2001; **125**: 253–60.

30. Farr BM, Gwaltney Jr JM, Hendley JO, Hayden FG, Naclerio RM, McBride T *et al*. A randomised controlled trial of glucocorticoid prophylaxis against experimental rhinovirus infection. *Journal of Infectious Diseases*. 1990; **162**: 1173–7.

31. Puhakka T, Makela MJ, Malmström K, Uhari M, Savolainen J, Terho EO *et al*. The common cold: effect of intranasal fluticasone propionate treatment. *Journal of Allergy and Clinical Immunology*. 1998; **101**: 726–31.

32. Seiden AM, Duncan HJ. The diagnosis of a conductive olfactory loss. *Laryngoscope*. 2001; **111**: 9–14.

33. Kaliner MA, Osguthorpe JD, Fireman P, Anon J, Georgitis J, Davis ML *et al*. Sinusitis: bench to bedside. *Journal of Allergy and Clinical Immunology*. 1997; **99**: S829–48.

34. Qvarnberg Y, Kantola O, Salo J, Toivanen M, Valtonen H, Vuori E. Influence of topical steroid treatment on maxillary sinusitis. *Rhinology*. 1992; **30**: 103–12.

35. Meltzer EO, Busse WW, Druce HM, Metzger WJ, Mitchell DO, Selner J *et al*. Assessment of flunisolide nasal spray versus placebo as an adjunct to antibiotic treatment of sinusitis. *Journal of Allergy and Clinical Immunology*. 1992; **89**: 301.

36. Meltzer EO, Orgel HA, Backhaus JW, Busse WW, Druce HM, Metzger WJ *et al*. Intranasal flunisolide spray as an adjunct to oral antibiotic therapy for sinusitis. *Journal of Allergy and Clinical Immunology*. 1993; **92**: 812–23.

37. Parikh A, Scadding GK, Darby Y, Baker RC. Topical corticosteroids in chronic rhinosinusitis. *Rhinology*. 2001; **39**: 75–9.

38. Meltzer EO, Charous BL, Busse WW, Zinreich SJ, Lorber RR, Danzig MR. Added relief in the treatment of acute recurrent sinusitis with adjunctive mometasone furoate nasal spray. *Journal of Allergy and Clinical Immunology*. 2000; **106**: 630–7.

39. Dolor RJ, Witsell DL, Hellkamp AS, Williams Jr JW, Califf RM, Simel DL. Comparison of cefuroxime with and without intranasal fluticasone propionate for the treatment of rhinosinusitis. *Journal of the American Medical Association*. 2001; **286**: 3097–105.

40. Kaplan AP. Chronic urticaria and angioedema. *New England Journal of Medicine*. 2002; **346**: 175–9.

41. Shah UK, Jacobs IN. Pediatric angioedema: ten years' experience. *Arch Otolaryngology and Head and Neck Surgery*. 1999; **125**: 791–5.

42. Demain J, Goetz DW. Pediatric adenoidal hypertrophy and nasal obstruction: reduction with aqueous nasal beclomethasone. *Pediatrics*. 1995; **95**: 355–64.

43. O'Brian JF, Falk JL. Dexamethasone as adjuvant for severe acute pharyngitis. *Annals of Emergency Medicine*. 1993; **22**: 212–5.

44. Steward DL, Welge JA, Myer CM. Do steroids reduce morbidity of tonsillectomy? Meta-analysis of randomised trials. *Laryngoscope*. 2001; **111**: 1712–8.

45. Palme CE, Tomasevic P, Pohl DV. Evaluating the effects of oral prednisolone on recovery after tonsillectomy: a prospective double blind randomised trial. *Laryngoscope*. 2000; **110**: 2000–4.

46. Heathley DG. Perioperative intravenous steroid treatment and tonsillectomy. *Archives of Otolaryngology and Head and Neck Surgery.* 2001; **127**: 1007–8.

47. Shott SR. Tonsillectomy and postoperative vomiting. Do steroids really work? *Archives of Otolaryngology and Head and Neck Surgery.* 2001; **127**: 1009–10.

48. Tynell E, Aurelius E, Brandell A, Julander I, Wood M, Yao QY et al. Acyclovir and prednisolone treatment of acute infectious mononucleosis: a multicenter, double-blind, placebo-controlled study. *Journal of Infectious Diseases.* 1996; **174**: 324–31.

49. Brandfonbrener A, Epstein A, Wu S, Phair J. Corticoid treatment in Epstein–Barr virus infection. Effect on lymphocyte class, subset, and response to early antigen. *Archives of Internal Medicine.* 1986; **146**: 337–9.

50. Shane SA, Wollman M, Claassen D. Herpes simplex dissemination following glucocorticoids for upper airway obstruction in an adolescent girl. *Pediatric Emergency Care.* 1994; **10**: 160–2.

51. Ausejo M, Saenz A, Pham BK, Kellner JD, Johnson DW, Moher D. The effectiveness of glucocorticosteroids in treating croup: metaanalysis. *British Medical Journal.* 1999; **341**: 595–600.

52. Jacobsson S, Karlsson G, Rigner P, Sanner E, Schrewlius C. Clinical efficacy of budesonide in the treatment of eczematous external otitis. *European Archives of Otorhinolaryngology.* 1991; **248**: 246–9.

53. Engard P, Hellstrom S. An animal model for external otitis. *European Archives of Otorhinolaryngology.* 1997; **254**: 115–9.

54. Engard P, Hellstrom S. A topical steroid without an antibiotic cures external otitis efficiently: a study in an animal model. *European Archives of Otorhinolaryngology.* 2001; **258**: 287–91.

55. Tracy JM, Demain JG, Hoffman KM, Goetz DW. Intranasal beclomethasone as an adjunct to treatment of chronic middle ear effusion. *Annals of Allergy, Asthma and Immunology.* 1998; **80**: 198–206.

56. Rosenfeld RM, Mandel EM, Bluestone CD. Systemic steroids for otitis media with effusion in children. *Archives of Otolaryngology and Head and Neck Surgery.* 1992; **117**: 984–9.

57. Hemlin C, Carenfelt C, Papatziamos G. Single dose of betamethasone in combined medical treatment of secretory media. *Annals of Otology, Rhinology, and Laryngology.* 1997; **106**: 359–63.

58. Zocconi E. Antibiotics and contisone in the treatment of otitis media with effusion. *Pediatria Medica e Chirurgica.* 1994; **16**: 273–5.

59. Lambert PR. Oral steroid therapy for chronic middle ear persusion: a double-blind crossover study. *Otolaryngology – Head and Neck Surgery.* 1986; **95**: 193–9.

60. Macknin ML, Jones PK. Oral dexamethasone for treatment of persistent middle ear effusion. *Pediatrics.* 1985; **75**: 329–35.

61. Butler CC, van Der Voort JH. Oral or topical nasal steroids for hearing loss associated with otitis media with effusion in children. Cochrane Database of Systematic Reviews 2000: CD001935.

62. Baggett HZ, Prazma J, Rose AS, Llane AP, Pillsbury 3rd HC. The role of glucocorticoids in endotoxin-mediated otitis media with effusion. *Archives of Otolaryngology and Head and Neck Surgery.* 1997; **123**: 41–6.

63. Ruohola A, Heikkinen T, Jero J, Puhakka T, Juven T, Narkio-Makel M et al. Oral prednisolone is an effective adjuvant therapy for acute otitis media with discharge through tympanostomy tubes. *Journal of Pediatrics.* 1999; **134**: 459–63.

64. Alper CM, Dohar JE, Gulhan M, Ozunlu A, Bagger-Sjobak D, Hebd PA et al. Treatment of chronic suppurative otitis media with topical tobramycin and dexamethasone. *Archives of Otolaryngology and Head and Neck Surgery.* 2000; **126**: 165–73.

65. Miro N. Controlled multicenter study on chronic suppurative otitis media treated with topical applications of ciprofloxacin 0.2 percent solution in single-dose containers or combination of polymyxin B, neomycin, and hydrocortisone suspension. *Otolaryngology and Head and Neck Surgery.* 2000; **123**: 617–23.

66. Mattox DE, Lyles A. Idiopathic sudden sensorineural hearing loss. *American Journal of Otology.* 1989; **10**: 242–7.

67. Stokroos RF. Summary and conclusions. In: Stokroos RJ (ed.). *Idiopathic sudden sensorineural hearing loss.* Groningen: Van Denderen BV, 1997: 99–104.

68. Wilson WR, Byl FM, Laird N. The efficacy of steroids in the treatment of idiopathic sudden hearing loss. *Archives of Otolaryngology.* 1980; **106**: 772–6.

69. Alexiou C, Arnold W, Fauser C, Schratzenstaller B, Gloddek B, Fuhrmann S et al. Sudden sensorineural hearing loss: does application of glucocorticosteroids make sense? *Archives of Otolaryngology and Head and Neck Surgery.* 2001; **127**: 253–8.

70. Chandrasekhar SS. Intratympanic dexamethasone for sudden sensorineural hearing loss: clinical and laboratory evaluation. *Otology and Neurotology.* 2001; **22**: 18–23.

71. Parnes LS, Sun AH, Freeman DJ. Cortisteroid pharmacokinetics in the inner ear fluids: an animal study followed by clinical evaluation. *Laryngoscope.* 1999; **109**: 1–17.

72. Moskowitz D, Lee KJ, Smith HW. Steroid use in sensorineural hearing loss. *Laryngoscope.* 1984; **94**: 664–6.

73. Kitajiri S, Tabuchi K, Hiraumi H, Hirose T. Is corticosteroid therapy effective for sudden-onset sensorineural hearing loss at lower frequencies? *Archives of Otolaryngology and Head and Neck Surgery.* 2002; **128**: 365–7.

74. Cinamon U, Bendet E, Kronenberg J. Steroids, carbogen or placebo for sudden hearing loss: a prospective double-blind study. *European Archives of Otorhinolaryngology.* 2001; **258**: 477–80.

75. Minoda R, Masuyama K, Habu K, Yumoto E. Initial steroid hormone dose in treatment of idiopathic sudden deafness. *American Journal of Otology.* 2000; **21**: 819–25.

76. Wilkins SA, Mattox DE, Lyles A. Evaluation of a 'shotgun' regimen for sudden hearing loss. *Otolaryngology and Head and Neck Surgery.* 1987; **97**: 474–80.

77. Haberkamp TJ, Tanyeri HM. Management of idiopathic sudden sensorineural hearing loss. *American Journal of Otology.* 1999; **20**: 587–92.

78. Kopke RD, Hoffer ME, Wester D, O'Leary MJ, Jackson RL. Targeted topical steroid therapy in sudden sensorineural hearing loss. *Otology and Neurotology.* 2001; **22**: 475–9.

79. Silverstein H, Isaacson JE, Olds MJ, Rowan PT, Rosenberg S. Dexamethasone inner ear perfusion for the treatment of Meniere's disease: a prospective, randomized, double-blind, cross-over trial. *American Journal of Otology.* 1998; **19**: 196–201.

80. Ramsey MJ, DerSimonian R, Holtel MR, Burgess LPA. Corticosteroid treatment for idiopathic facial nerve paralysis: a meta-analysis. *Laryngoscope.* 2000; **110**: 335–41.

81. Salinas RS, Alvarez G, Alvarez MI, Ferreira J. Corticosteroids for Bell's palsy (idiopathic facial paralysis). Cochrane Database of Systematic Reviews 2002: CD001942.

82. Wilson R, Lund V, Sweatman M, Mackay IS, Mitchell DN. Upper respiratory tract involvement in sarcoidosis and its management. *European Respiratory Journal.* 1988; **1**: 269–72.

83. Paramothayan NS, Jones PW. Corticosteroids for pulmonary sarcoidosis. Cochrane Database of Systematic Reviews. 2000: CD001114.

84. Costabel U, Hunninghake GW. ATS/WASOG statement on sarcoidosis. *European Respiratory Journal.* 1999; **14**: 735–7.

85. Langford CA, Sneller MC. Update on the diagnosis and treatment of Wegener's granulomatosis. *Advances in Internal Medicine.* 2001; **46**: 177–206.

35

Drug therapy in otology

WENDY SMITH AND MARTIN BURTON

Introduction	429	Key points	434
Topical ear preparations	429	Best clinical practice	435
Preparations used in the management of vertigo	433	Deficiencies in current knowledge and areas for future	
Drugs used in sudden sensorineural hearing loss	434	research	435
Sodium fluoride treatment in otosclerosis	434	References	435

SEARCH STRATEGY

The data in this chapter are supported by a Medline search using the key words otitis externa, ear drops, antibiotics, betahistine, gentamicin, Menières, acyclovir and sodium fluoride.

INTRODUCTION

Medicines are commonly prescribed in the management of otological diseases. Whilst the efficacy of some treatments may be uncertain, it is important to understand how these drugs act, their indications, contraindications and side effects. This chapter discusses these factors in relation to a number of specific types of otological medications.

TOPICAL EAR PREPARATIONS

Eardrops are solutions or suspensions of medicaments in water, glycerol, diluted alcohol, propylene glycol or other suitable solvent for instillation into the ear. A solution comprises a solute (drug) dissolved in the solvent whereas a suspension consists of an insoluble drug distributed in a liquid. Some preparations used in otology are also used as eye or nose drops. Since these drops are in multiple-application containers, the vehicle contains a bactericidal and fungicidal agent such as benzalkonium chloride (0.01 percent). Other adjuvants in ear and eye drops include buffers such as sodium metabisulphite and disodium

edetate. The buffers are used to maintain the pH to minimize breakdown of the active constituents or to increase comfort for the patient. Both sodium metabisulphite and disodium edetate are effective at retarding oxidation reactions and the latter can enhance the bactericidal activity of benzalkonium chloride and chlorhexidine acetate. Information on excipients contained in drops is found in the British National Formulary or its equivalent. This information is useful since some patients may be allergic to topical ear medication and this allergy may not be to the primary constituent but to the excipients.

Ear drops are dispensed in coloured fluted glass bottles with a plastic screw cap incorporating a glass dropper tube and rubber teat, or, more commonly, in plastic squeeze bottles fitted with a plastic cap incorporating a dropper device. Such containers are designed to prevent light degradation of the contents.

Some ear preparations are available as creams or ointments where the antimicrobial and/or antiinflammatory substance is prepared in a suitable base such as liquid paraffin, wool fat and yellow soft paraffin. Both are semisolid preparations but in a cream the base is absorbed into the skin, whereas in an ointment only the medication is absorbed from the greasy base. In general, ointments are useful in dry scaly conditions whereas creams can also be used in weeping skin conditions.

Again, warnings that the preparation contains lanolin (wool fat) are useful since some patients are allergic to lanolin.

Topical ear preparations for inflammatory and infective conditions

INDICATIONS

A number of topical ear preparations in the form of drops or ointments are available for the treatment of otitis externa and discharging mastoid cavities. Many are also used in discharging ears with a perforated tympanic membrane or ears with a grommet *in situ*. In this latter situation this is an unlicensed indication for the use of many of these preparations. Manufacturers' data sheets continue to state that even plain steroid drops are contra-indicated in the presence of a perforation. In chronic suppurative otitis media, it has been shown that aural toilet and topical antibiotics, especially a quinolone, is effective in resolving otorrhoea and eradicating bacteria from the middle ear. Topical antibiotic preparations are more effective than oral preparations and the addition of oral therapy to topical antibiotics confers no greater benefit than the latter used alone (see Chapter 34, Corticosteroids in otolaryngology).[1]

SPECIFIC PREPARATIONS

Acetic acid 2 percent has antifungal and antibacterial properties and can be used to treat mild otitis externa. Aluminium acetate is an astringent that can be applied as drops or onto a gauze wick. An astringent is an agent which causes shrinkage or constriction and is usually applied topically. The hydroscopic effect reduces oedema in the inflamed ear canal, opening the meatus. Aluminium acetate has a tendency to form crystals in the ear. Regular aural toilette is required to remove both the crystals that form as well as the debris produced by the inflammatory process. This treatment can be safely used in pregnancy. Boric acid has been used in the past for its weak fungistatic and bacteriostatic activity and is used as a mild disinfectant in lotions, ointments and powders in concentrations of up to 5 percent. It is absorbed through damaged skin and may cause systemic toxicity. Acute and chronic toxicity can occur, presenting with gastrointestinal disturbance, rash, central nervous system and renal involvement that may result in death. Slow excretion of boric acid can lead to cumulative toxicity during repeated use.

Some preparations contain only a steroid and are used in eczematous otitis externa. The steroid reduces inflammatory swelling and helps control irritation. The steroid stimulates the synthesis of lipocortin in leukocytes. This protein inhibits phospholipase A_2 that reduces the formation of arachidonic acid, the precursor of many inflammatory mediators. Betamethasone sodium phosphate (Betnesol®) and prednisolone sodium phosphate (Predsol®) are steroids available as ear drops. These steroids are combined with anti-infective agents for use in the management of infected otitis externa. Other steroids found in combination with anti-infective drugs include dexamethasone (Otomize® – with neomycin and glacial acetic acid, Sofradex® – with framycetin sulphate and gramicidin), flumetasone pivalate (Locorten-Vioform® – with flumetasone pivolate and clioquinol), hydrocortisone acetate (Gentisone HC® – with gentamicin, Neo-Cortef® – with neomycin sulphate) and triamcinolone acetonide (Audicort® – with neomycin undecanoate and Tri-Adcortyl Otic® – with gramicidin, neomycin and nystatin). Clioquinol (found in Locorten-Vioform) is an 8-hydroxyquinolone with both antibacterial and antifungal properties and is useful when a mixed infection is suspected. The other antibiotics included in ear preparations are framycetin sulphate, gentamicin and neomycin sulphate which are all aminoglycosides. They are bactericidal, inhibiting microbial protein synthesis and are effective against aerobic Gram-negative bacteria. Bacteria may acquire resistance via plasmids against one aminoglycoside but these bacteria rarely exhibit resistance to other aminoglycosides. This accounts for the benefit in changing the ear drops if the otitis externa fails to respond to one preparation.

Some of these preparations are available as ear sprays (Otomize) and there is some evidence that these cover the external meatus more effectively than traditional ear drops[2] and are easier for the elderly to apply. However, in some clinical situations, drops are more likely to reach the infected and inflamed parts of the external ear, middle ear or mastoid cavity at which treatment is aimed. Prolonged use of antibiotic/steroid preparations may sensitize the skin and may lead to fungal infections.

Clotrimazole is an azole derivative with a broad-spectrum antifungal activity that acts by inhibiting ergosterol synthesis in the fungal cell membrane. At lower concentrations, clotrimazole merely inhibits fungal growth but at higher concentrations, fungi are killed by clotrimazole action causing direct membrane damage. Increasingly, ciprofloxacin eye drops are used as ear drops in the management of *Pseudomonas* spp. ear infections. This is an unlicensed use in the UK where licensed ciprofloxacin ear drops are unavailable. Ciprofloxacin drops have been used widely in the rest of Europe, North America and beyond.

CONTRAINDICATIONS

The use of preparations containing only a steroid is contraindicated in untreated infections since the immunosuppressive effect of corticosteroids may exacerbate the infection. More controversial is the use of preparations with anti-infective agents in the presence of a perforated tympanic membrane because of the potential for ototoxicity.

SIDE EFFECTS

The most common side effects with these preparations are hypersensitivity reactions and local irritation, burning and itching.

The use of anti–infective ear drops in the presence of a tympanic membrane perforation

The product licences do not permit the use of anti-infective ear drops in ears with perforated tympanic membranes as a result of cochlear damage that occurred when such drops were instilled into guinea pig ears.[3,4] These authors recognize that the round window niche in humans is relatively deep and often protected by a pseudomembrane whilst in the guinea pig the round window is completely exposed. In patients with active chronic suppurative otitis media there is no evidence that the use of these ear drops causes sensorineural deafness. (see Chapter 34, Corticosteroids in otolaryngology).[5,6,7]

Topical ear preparations for removal of ear wax

Many cerumenolytics, including oils and aqueous preparations, are available to soften wax prior to syringing or to disintegrate or disperse the wax, to avoid the need for syringing altogether. Burton and Dorée[8] undertook a systematic review and found eight clinical trials. All had a small number of participants, and most were of poor methodological quality. The review concluded that there is insufficient evidence to favour any one particular cerumenolytic. Water and sodium chloride 0.9 percent seem to be as effective as any proprietary agent. Sodium bicarbonate 5 percent ear drops, olive or almond oil ear drops are also safe and inexpensive although their effectiveness has not been evaluated in randomized controlled trials. If the wax is impacted, these drops can be used twice a day for a few days prior to syringing. Some proprietary preparations contain organic solvents (chlorbutanol, paradichlorobenzene) that may cause irritation to the meatal skin. The rational for inclusion of these ingredients in the preparations is not clear and the vehicle alone is often effective.

SYSTEMIC ANTIBIOTICS

Indications

Systemic antibiotics are prescribed in the otological conditions of acute otitis media (AOM), cellulitis associated with furunculosis, otitis externa and perichondritis.

In AOM, the use of antibiotics is controversial. Galsziou et al.[9] found that antibiotic usage in AOM in children varied from 31 percent in the Netherlands to 98 percent in the USA and Australia. Their Cochrane review concluded that antibiotics provide a small benefit, however, since most cases resolve spontaneously, this benefit must be weighed against possible adverse reactions. Seventeen children must be treated to prevent one child from having pain after two days. Antibiotic treatment may play an important role in reducing the risk of mastoiditis in populations where it is more common. If antibiotics are used, amoxicillin appears to be the first-line treatment, with erythromycin in those who are penicillin sensitive. Should treatment fail, second-line agents include co-amoxiclav and cephalosporins.

Conservative management of acute mastoiditis (without subperiosteal abscess) has been adopted since a third of patients will settle in 24–48 hours with intravenous antibiotics.[10,11,12]

Flucloxacillin is the antibiotic of choice in treating cellulitis due to Staphylococcus. Penicillin V is used in erysipelas due to Streptococcus.

Ciprofloxacin is the drug of choice in malignant otitis externa and is also used in treating perichondritis due to *Pseudomonas aeruginosa*.

Mechanisms of actions

The penicillins have a bactericidal action, inhibiting cell wall synthesis by preventing the formation of peptidoglycan cross-bridges. The penicillinase-resistant penicillins, flucloxacillin, cloxacillin and methicillin, are semisynthetic penicillins, resistant to penicillinase by virtue of an isoxazolyl group on R_1. Many bacterial β-lactamases are inhibited by clavulanic acid, and a mixture of this inhibitor with amoxicillin(co-amoxiclav) is available. The cephalosporins are also bactericidal. They contain a β-lactam ring and their mechanism of action is similar to the penicillins.

The macrolides, for example erythromycin, act by inhibiting bacterial protein synthesis. It binds to the 50s bacterial ribosome subunit inhibiting translocation.

Metronidazole was initially used in protozoal infections but was found to be very effective against anaerobic bacteria. The drug is reduced to active metabolites that interfere with nucleic acid function. Ciprofloxacin is a fluroquinolone and acts on both stationary and dividing bacteria by inhibiting DNA gyrase, an enzyme that compresses the bacterial DNA into supercoils. Cell death is thought to occur as a result of the unwinding of the supercoils.

Antibacterial spectrum

Table 35.1 demonstrates the antibacterial spectrum of the various antibiotics. The penicillinase-sensitive penicillins have a greater spectrum of activity than the β-lactamase resistant drugs, but the combination of clavulanic acid with amoxycillin enables protection of the β-lactam ring, allowing this essential part of the penicillin molecule to remain active.

Table 35.1 The antibacterial spectrum of antibiotics.

Penicillins	Antibacterial spectrum
Benzylpenicillin and phenoxymethylpenicillin	Streptococcal, non β-lactamase producing staphylococcal, pneumococcal, clostridial infection, meningococcal, gonococcal, spirochaetes (syphilis), anthrax, actinomycosis
Ampicillin and amoxycillin	As above and *Strep. faecalis*, most *Haemophillus influenzae* and many coliforms
Methicillin, cloxacillin, flucloxacillin	Similar to penicillin but less active. Stable to staphylococcal β-lactamase
Carbenicillin and ticarcillin	Similar to amoxyillin and in addition activity to *Ps. aeruginosa*, most *Proteus* spp. and against bacteroides
Mezlocillin, azlocillin, piperacillin	Similar to ticarcillin and in addition to *Klebsiella* spp. and greater activity against pseudomonads
Mecillinam	Coliforms, little activity against Gram-positive bacteria

Cephalosporins	Antibacterial spectrum
First generation: cephaloridine, cephalothin, cephalexin, cephradine and cephazolin	Broad spectrum EXCEPT against *Strep. faecalis*, *Ps. aeruginosa*, *H. influenzae* and *Bacteroides* spp. Staphylococcus is sensitive, except for MRSA
Second generation: cefuroxime, cefamandole, cefoxitin	Broad spectrum with stability against β-lactamases. Active against *H. influenzae* and *Bacteroides* spp. but less activity against staphylococcus
Third generation: cefotaxime, latamoxef, ceftazidime, cefsulodin	As for second generation but also active against *Ps. aeruginosa*
Erythromycin	See penicillins but also active against *H. influenzae*, *Bord. Pertussis*, *Bacteroides* spp., *Campylobacter* spp. *Legionella pneumophilia*, *Mycoplasma pneumoniae* and *Chlamydiae*
Sulphonamides and trimethoprim: co-trimoxazole	Broad, active against Gram-positive and -negative bacteria except *Ps. aeruginosa*
Aminoglycosides: gentamicin, tobramycin, netilmicin, amikacin, kanamycin and neomycin	Coliforms, *Ps. aeruginosa* and staphylococci; streptomycin; mycobacteria
Vancomycin	Staphylococci including MRSA, streptococci and clostridia
Tetracyclines: tetracycline, chlortetracycline, oxytetracycline, doxycycline, minocycline	Broad; Gram-positive and -negative bacteria, brucellae, *M. pneumoniae*, rickettsia, *Coxiella burneti* and *Chlamydiae*. Some resistance to *Strep. pyogenes*, pneumococci and *H. influenzae*. *Ps. aeruginosa* and *Proteus* spp. resistant
Metronidazole	Anaerobic bacteria and protozoa
Ciprofloxacin	Broad; Gram-negative bacteria including *Ps. aeruginosa*, staphylococci including MRSA, streptococci less sensitive
Monobactams: aztreonam	Narrow, active against aerobic Gram-negative bacteria (less sensitive to *Ps. aeruginosa*)

Dosage

Specific dosage recommendations can be found in the British National Formulary. Phenoxypenicillin, amoxycillin and flucloxacillin have better oral absorption than ampicillin but all should be taken at least 30 minutes before food since they are destroyed, to some extent, by gastric acid. The penicillins have good penetration to most tissues but poor entry to CSF (overcome by giving higher doses intravenously). Dosage modification is required in patients with severe renal failure.

Ciprofloxacin can achieve high concentrations in bone and soft tissue, even after oral administration. A dosage of 1.5 g daily over a period of 6–12 weeks has been recommended in the treatment of malignant otitis externa.[13, 14]

Contraindictions

In all cases the prescribing of these drugs is contraindicated when the patient is known to be allergic to the ingredients or related compounds. Immediate hypersensitivity to penicillins occurs in 0.05 percent of patients, the severity of which ranges from urticaria or wheezing to a life-threatening anaphylactic response. Less than 5 percent of patients may develop a delayed hypersensitivity response to penicillins, usually a rash. Occasionally, haemolytic anaemia, leukopenia and interstitial nephritis may occur. There is a 10 percent hypersensitivity crossover with cephalosporins.

Precautions

The prolonged use of antibiotics may result in superinfection with nonsusceptible organisms. There is no evidence that the penicillins, cephalosporins or erythromycin are hazardous in pregnancy but metronidazole should be avoided in high dosages and ciprofloxacin must be avoided in all trimesters of pregnany. Antibiotics are secreted into breast milk and ciprofloxacin should be avoided in lactation. Other antibiotics, such as the penicillins and cephalosporins, are secreted into the breast milk but may not be harmful to the infant. Antibiotics, such as the cephalosporins and ciprofloxacin, cleared by the kidneys may require dosage adjustments in patients with renal impairment. Similarly, antibiotics metabolized by the liver, for example erythromycin, may require dosage adjustments or be avoided in patients with liver failure.

Interactions

Before prescribing a specific medication, the reader is advised to check for interactions in, for example, The British National Formulary. Antibiotics may lead to oral contraceptive failure, probably because of diminished enterohepatic circulation. The anticoagulant effect of warfarin is affected by the penicillins, macrolides, metronidazole and quinolones.

Erythromycin interacts with some antihistamines and cisapride, resulting in cardiac arrythmias. It also increases the plasma level of a number of drugs.

Metronidazole produces a disulfiram-like reaction with alcohol. Acetaldehyde accumulates in the body producing facial flushing, headaches, palpitations, nausea and vomiting.

Indigestion, iron or zinc therapies must not be taken within two hours of ciprofloxacin since absorption of this antibiotic is significantly affected.

Side effects

Most antibiotics may produce diarrhoea, rashes, blood disorders, nausea and vomiting. Ampicillin and amoxycillin have a unique adverse effect, comprising a rash, in up to 90 percent of patients with mononucleosis or chronic lymphocytic leukaemia. Reversible hearing loss has been reported with erythromycin. Angioneurotic oedema and anaphylaxis are, fortunately, relatively rare.

PREPARATIONS USED IN THE MANAGEMENT OF VERTIGO

Betahistine

Betahistine hydrochloride is commonly prescribed in the management of vertigo, usually when associated with Menière's disease or syndrome.

Betahistine is thought to reduce the endolymphatic pressure through improved microvascular circulation in the stria vascularis of the cochlear[15] or by inhibiting activity of the vestibular nuclei.[16]

There is insufficient evidence from high quality randomized trials to say whether or not betahistine has any effect on Menières.[17] It may reduce vertigo, and possibly tinnitus, but does not seem to influence the hearing loss.

Betahistine should be used with caution in patients with asthma, a history of peptic ulcer disease, in pregnancy and breastfeeding. It is contraindicated in patients with phaeochromocytoma. The side effects include gastrointestinal disturbance, headaches, rashes and pruritis, however, these are uncommon. Betahistine is prescribed initially at 16 mg three times a day, a maintenance dose of 24–48 mg has been recommended.

Dopamine antagonists

Prochlorperazine (Stemetil®) is a dopamine antagonist and acts centrally by blocking the chemoreceptor trigger zone and thereby blocking the vomiting centre. The vomiting centre also has afferent input from the vestibular apparatus. This region has a high concentration of muscarinic receptors and histamine H_1-receptors.

Prochloperazine belongs to group three of the phenothiazines. This means it has less sedative effects, fewer antimuscarinic effects but more pronounced extrapyramidal side effects when compared to the other phenothiazine groups.

Prochloperazine is available as tablets, syrup, effervescent sachets, injection, suppositories and as a buccal preparation (Buccastem®). These last two preparations are useful because patients using prochlorperazine often vomit and fail to absorb the orally ingested form. The oral dosage varies from 5 mg three times a day increasing to 30 mg daily.

Antihistamines

The antihistamines are competitive antagonists of histamine at H_1-receptors, and their main action is on the vomiting centre rather than on the chemoreceptor trigger zone. They have weak anticholinergic effects and may occasionally produce a dry mouth and blurred vision. Drowsiness, occasional insomnia and euphoria are side effects which have been reported. These central effects are accentuated with alcohol. Cinnarazine (Stugeron®) and cyclizine (Valoid®) are less sedating than promethazine teoclate (Avomine®). Cinnarizine has been used in the prophylaxis and treatment of Menières at a dosage of 30 mg three times a day. Cyclizine may be given in the acute attack orally or parentally at a dosage of 50 mg three times a day.

Gentamicin therapy in Menières disease

Intratympanic gentamicin therapy was described by Beck and Schmidt[18] in 1978 and has been used both in Canada and the UK. Since its introduction, a variety of gentamicin dosage regimens and methods of administration have been developed and remain in clinical practice. These range from injection through the tympanic membrane, through a grommet or via intratympanic or round window catheters.

Other medical treatment for Menière's disease

The use of salt restriction and diuretic therapy (hydro-chlorothiazide, acetazolamide and co-triamterzide 50/25 (Dyazide®) are aimed at reducing the accumulation of endolymph. Although a study with Dyazide showed a reduction in vestibular symptoms, there was no effect on hearing loss or tinnitus. Acetazolamide may initially increase the hydrops and Brookes and Booth[19] concluded that this drug has no place in treating Menière's disease. Steroids and immunological therapy have also been proposed by those who believe that a disorder of the immune system underlies Menière's disease or syndrome.

DRUGS USED IN SUDDEN SENSORINEURAL HEARING LOSS

Corticosteroids

Steroids are commonly used in patients with sudden sensorineural hearing loss (SSNHL), but evidence for their effectiveness is lacking. There are several alternative dosage regimes when a 'short reducing course' of steroids are required. One such consists of enteric-coated prednisolone, 60 mg on the first day, 50 mg on the second day, 40 mg daily for three days, 30 mg daily for three days and a further reduction so that therapy is discontinued after three weeks. The action, side effects, etc. are discussed in Chapter 34, Corticosteroids in otolaryngology.

Acyclovir

Acyclovir (acycloguanosine) is an antiviral agent active against herpesviruses and is prescribed in patients with Ramsay Hunt syndrome (herpes zoster oticus). It acts by inhibiting nucleic acid synthesis. Herpes simplex and varicella zoster contain a thymidine kinase that converts the acyclovir to a monophosphate that is then phosphorylated by the host cell enzymes of acycloguanosine triphosphate that inhibits viral DNA polymerase and viral DNA syntheses. Selectivity for infected cells is achieved since the DNA polymerase of herpesvirus has a much greater affinity for the activated drug than the cellular DNA polymerase.

Acyclovir may be administered orally at a dosage of 800 mg five times a day for five days. If treatment is commenced prior to 72 hours after the onset of the rash, acyclovir may shorten the rash duration and acute symptoms and reduce the incidence of post-herpetic neuralgia.[20] Acyclovir should be used with caution in patients with renal impairment or who are pregnant or breastfeeding. Side effects include nausea, vomiting, gastrointestinal disturbances, rash, photosensitivity and, rarely, hepatitis, acute renal failure and neurological

reactions (see British National Formulary[21] for further details).

SODIUM FLUORIDE TREATMENT IN OTOSCLEROSIS

Sodium fluoride has been used for 35 years in an attempt to slow down or arrest sensorineural hearing loss in patients with stapedial otosclerosis or after stapedectomy. It has also been used in patients with 'pure' cochlear otosclerosis.

Sodium fluoride is an enzyme inhibitor and reduces osteoclastic bone resorption. The clinical benefit of sodium fluoride is controversial. Causse et al.[22] found that in 'otospongiosis-otosclerosis', sodium fluoride influenced the underlying bony changes in the labyrinth so as to arrest or prevent the onset of hearing loss. In their prospective clinical double-blind, placebo-controlled study of 95 patients, Bretlau et al.[23] found that there was a statistically worse deterioration of hearing loss in the placebo group than in the active treated (40 mg sodium fluoride daily) group. Further work by Colletti[24] showed benefit in 50 percent of patients five years after a two-year treatment with sodium fluoride (dosages up to 16 mg/day). Deka et al.[25] suggested the use of Florical at a dosage of two capsules three times a day in active cochlear otospongiosis. Their study showed that variation in absorption occurs with the use of different preparation and also amongst individuals.

The side effects of sodium fluoride need to be considered. In a prospective case-controlled study of ten patients with otosclerosis receiving sodium fluoride 30 mg/day and matched healthy volunteers, Das et al.[26] found a high incidence (70 percent) of dyspeptic symptoms in those taking sodium fluoride, as well as histological and electron microscopic abnormalities.

KEY POINTS

- Topical ear preparations can be used for a limited period in discharging ears with a perforated tympanic membrane or a grommet in situ.
- The use of topical ear preparations containing a steroid only is contraindicated in untreated infections since the immunosuppressive action of the corticosteroid may exacerbate the infection.
- Flucloxacillin is the antibiotic of choice in cellulitis due to Staphyloccus. Penicillin V is used in erysipelas due to Streptococcus. Ciprofloxacin is the antibiotic of choice in malignant otitis externa.

Best clinical practice

✓ Before prescribing, ensure that the patient is not known to be allergic to the medicine or adjuvants (such as the preservatives).

✓ Ensure medication does not interact with patient's established medication or medical conditions.

✓ Prescribe medicines at the lowest dose for the shortest time that is effective.

✓ Review whether medication is still required.

Deficiencies in current knowledge and areas for future research

➤ There is insufficient evidence to favour any one particular cerumenolytic and a randomized controlled trial may be useful to determine the most clinically and cost-effective preparations for this purpose.

➤ There is insufficient evidence from high-quality randomized trials to determine whether betahistine, diuretics, steroids and immune therapy have any effect in Menière's disease.

REFERENCES

1. Acuin J, Smith A, Mackenzie I. Interventions for chronic suppurative otitis media. The Cochrane Library, Issue 2, Oxford Update Software, 2002.

2. Mcgarry GW, Swan IRC. Endoscopic photographic comparison of drug delivery by ear drops and by aerosol spray. *Clinical Otolaryngology*. 1992; 17: 359–60.

3. Kohonen A, Tarkanen J. Cochlea damage by ototoxic antibiotics by intratympanic application. *Acta Otolaryngologica*. 1969; 68: 90–7.

4. Brummett RE, Harris RF, Lindgren JA. Detection of ototoxicity from drugs applied topically to the middle ear space. *Laryngoscope*. 1976; 86: 1177–87.

5. Browning GG, Gatehouse S, Calder IT. Medical management of active chronic otitis media: a control study. *Journal of Laryngology and Otology*. 1988; 102: 491–5.

6. Fairbanks DNF. Anti-microbial therapy for chronic otits media. *Annals of Otology, Rhinology, and Laryngology*. 1981; 90: 58–62.

7. Phillips JS, Yung MW, Burton M, Swan IRC for the Clinical Audit and Practice Advisory Group, British Association of Otolaryngologists – Head and Neck Surgeons (ENT-UK). *Use of aminoglycoside-containing ear drops in the presence of a perforation: evidence review and ENT-UK consensus statement* (in press).

8. Burton MJ, Dorée CJ. Ear drops for the removal of ear wax (Cochrane Review). In: The Cochrane Library, Issue 3, Chichester, UK: John Wiley and Sons, Ltd, 2004.

9. Galsziou PP, Del Mar CB, Sanders SL, Hayem M. Antibiotics for acute otitis media in children. The Cochrane Library, Issue 2, Oxford Update Software, 2002.

10. Rubin JS, Wei WI. Acute mastoiditis: a review of 34 patients. *Laryngoscope*. 1985; 95: 963–5.

11. Ogle JW, Lauer BA. Acute mastoiditis. Diagnosis and complications. *American Journal of Diseases of Children*. 1986; 140: 1178–82.

12. Nadal S, Herrmann P, Baumann A, Fanconi A. Acute mastoiditis: clinical, microbiological, and therapeutic aspects. *European Journal of Paediatrics*. 1990; 149: 560–4.

13. Brody T, Pasak ML. The fluoroquinolones. *Americal Journal of Otology*. 1991; 17: 902–4.

14. Levenson MJ, Parisier SC, Dolitsky J, Bindra G. Ciprofloxacin: drug of choice in the treatment of malignant external otitis. *Laryngoscope*. 1991; 101: 821–84.

15. Martinez DM. The effect of Serc on the circulation of the inner ear in experimental animals. *Acta Otolaryngologica*. 1972; Suppl 305: 29–46.

16. Timmerman H. Pharmacotherapy of vertigo: any news to be expected? *Acta Otolaryngologica*, 1994; Suppl 573: 28–32.

17. James AL, Burton MJ. Betahistine for Menieres disease or syndrome. The Cochrane Library, Issue 2, Oxford Update Software, 2002.

18. Beck C, Schmidt CL. 10 years experience with intratympanically applied streptomycin (gentamicin) in the therapy of morbus Meniere. *Archives of Otorhinolaryngology*. 1978; 221: 149–52.

19. Brookes GB, Booth JB. Oral acetazolamide in Menieres disease. *Journal of Laryngology and Otology*. 1984; 98: 1087–95.

20. Collier J. Acyclovir in general practice. *Drug and Therapeutics Bulletin*. 1992; 30: 101–4.

* 21. British National Formulary 43. March 2002.

22. Causse JR, Causse JB, Uriel J, Berges J, Shambaugh Jr. GE, Bretlau P. Sodium fluoride therapy. *American Journal of Otolaryngology*. 1993; 14: 482–90.

23. Bretlau P, Causse J, Causse JB, Hansen HJ, Johnsen NJ, Salomon G. Otospongiosis and sodium fluoride. A blind experimental and clinical evaluation of the effect of sodium fluoride treatment in patients with otospongiosis. *Annals of Otology, Rhinology and Laryngology*. 1985; 94: 103–7.

24. Colletti V, Fiorino FG. Effect of sodium fluoride on early stages of otosclerosis. *American Journal of Otolaryngology*. 1991; 12: 195–8.

25. Deka RC, Kacker SK, Shambaugh Jr GE. Intestinal absorption of fluoride preparations. *Laryngoscope*. 1978; 88: 1918–21.

26. Das TK, Susheela AK, Gupta IP, Dasarathy S, Tandon RK. Toxic effects of chronic fluoride ingestion on the upper gastrointestinal tract. *Journal of Clinical Gastroenterology*. 1994; 18: 194–9.

36

Drug therapy in rhinology

WENDY SMITH AND GRANT BATES

Introduction	436	Related topics	442
Treatment of rhinosinusitis with corticosteroids	436	Key points	443
Treatment of rhinosinusitis with antibiotics	438	Best clinical practice	444
Treatment of rhinosinusitis with other medicines	439	Deficiencies in current knowledge and areas for future	
Medication that may improve the immune response	441	research	444
Nasal and antral irrigation with saline	441	References	444
Antileukotrienes	441	Further reading	445
Agents used to block the parasympathetic nervous system	442		

SEARCH STRATEGY

The data in this chapter are supported by a Medline search using the key words acute rhinosinusitis, intermittent rhinosinusitis, chronic rhinosinusitis, persistent rhinosinusitis, fungal rhinosinusitis and medical treatment. The chapter has also relied on a review produced by the European Academy of Allergology and Clinical Immunology (EAACI) that was published as a supplement by *Rhinology* in March 2005.

INTRODUCTION

This chapter covers the medical treatment of all forms of rhinosinusitis. The most effective drugs for managing rhinosinusitis are corticosteroids and antibiotics. The majority of this chapter discusses these two major groups of medication. A separate section is devoted to other medicines that are used in the management of rhinosinusitis. Finally, other medical treatments used in rhinology are discussed under Related topics.

Rhinosinusitis is a significant health problem which reduces the quality of life for individuals and places a large financial burden on society. Effective medical treatment is available for allergic rhinosinusitis and infective rhinosinusitis. The evidence for the effectiveness of medical treatment of rhinosinusitis has been reviewed by the European Academy of Allergology and Clinical Immunology (EAACI) and the authors of this chapter have relied on the EAACI review.[1]

Rhinosinusitis is an inflammatory process involving the mucosa of the nose and one or more of the sinuses.

Factors that contribute to the inflammation include mucociliary impairment, bacterial infection, allergy, swelling of the mucosa for other reasons and mechanical obstruction. It is recognized that inflammation around the osteomeatal complex is of particular importance in causing rhinosinusitis. Drug therapy in the treatment of rhinosinusitis is aimed at reducing the factors causing inflammation with the additional aim of ensuring adequate ventilation through the osteomeatal complex.

Acute rhinosinusitis is now known as intermittent rhinosinusitis and the term chronic rhinosinusitis has been replaced by persistent rhinosinusitis (PRS).

TREATMENT OF RHINOSINUSITIS WITH CORTICOSTEROIDS

Topically administered glucocorticoids have improved the treatment of rhinosinusitis and asthma. The efficacy of glucocorticoids may partly depend on their ability to reduce the viability and activation of eosinophils and, in addition, to reduce the secretion of chemotactic cytokines by the nasal mucosa. The biological action of glucocorticoids is mediated through activation of intracellular glucocorticoid receptors that are expressed in many tissues and cells.

Intermittent rhinosinusitis without nasal polyps

There are a number of high-quality studies where intranasal steroids have been used as an additional treatment to antibiotics, but at present there are no studies where topical nasal steroids have been compared to antibiotics as a single treatment for intermittent rhinosinusitis. Studies are now underway but the results have yet to be published. In published studies, where either a placebo or a topical steroid has been added to antibiotic treatment for intermittent rhinosinusitis, the results generally show that the patients who were treated with a topical corticosteroid improved more rapidly than when the antibiotic was combined with placebo. A representative study is that conducted by Meltzer et al.[2] Mometasone furoate 400 µg a day, was given to 200 patients and placebo to 207 patients, all of whom had intermittent rhinosinusitis. All patients were also treated with amoxicillin clavulanate potassium for 21 days. The symptom score, which considered congestion, facial pain, headache and rhinorrhoea, improved significantly in the mometasone group. The effect was most obvious after 16 days treatment and no side effects were seen. [****]

Gehanno et al.[3] looked at the effectiveness of systemic steroids in the treatment of intermittent rhinosinusitis. Eight milligrams of prednisolone was given three times a day for five days as an adjunct to ten days treatment with amoxicillin clavulanate potassium in patients with intermittent rhinosinusitis. The diagnostic criteria consisted of facial pain, purulent nasal discharge, purulent secretions from the middle meatus, together with opacities on CT scan. The conclusion was that there was no difference in the therapeutic outcome at day 14 between the steroid group and the placebo group, although four days after initiating treatment, the headache and facial pain was significantly less in the steroid group. [****]

Persistent rhinosinusitis without nasal polyps

The majority of studies have compared the effects of topical steroid versus placebo as an adjunctive treatment to antibiotics. Two large trials of 407 and 967 patients, respectively, found that mometasone furoate produced a significant improvement in symptom score over the placebo. In one study,[4] topical steroid did not help the symptom of post-nasal drip but it did in the second study.[5] In both these studies there was no statistical

difference in the CT findings of the treatment group compared with placebo.

A recent multicentre double-blind placebo-controlled randomized trial of 134 patients with persistent rhinosinusitis took a different approach in that topical budesonide was compared against placebo after all the patients had received and had not been cured by two weeks of antibiotics. The treatment period was for 20 weeks and the topical steroid produced a significant reduction in nasal congestion and discharge scores and improved the patient's sense of smell when compared with placebo. Peak nasal and inspiratory flows also significantly improved in both allergic and nonallergic patients.[6] [****]

Persistent rhinosinusitis with nasal polyps: topical steroids

In patients with persistent rhinosinusitis and nasal polyps the studies have tended to consider the effectiveness of the treatment on the rhinitic symptoms and then, as a separate outcome measure, the effect of the treatment on the size of the polyps. In a landmark paper published in 1979, Mygind et al.[7] showed that beclomethasone dipropionate (BDP), at a dose of 400 µg daily for three weeks, reduced nasal symptoms in 19 patients with nasal polyps when compared to a controlled group of 16 patients treated with a placebo aerosol. There was no reduction in the size of the polyps during this short treatment period. [****]

Subsequent studies in which a topical steroid has been compared to placebo in patients with persistent rhinosinusitis and nasal polyposis, have generally shown that the topical steroid is more effective than placebo in reducing the patient's symptoms and, in particular, the symptom of nasal blockage. In approximately half of the reported studies an improvement in the sense of smell occurred and, again, in approximately half the studies the topical steroid also reduced the size of the polyps. The treatment interval in the various studies varied from between 3 and 120 weeks. [****/***]

A comprehensive study compared fluticasone propionate, 400 µg daily, with BDP 400 µg daily and with topical placebo over a 12-week period in a double-blind randomized parallel group that was conducted in a single centre study.[8] The symptom score was significantly improved in the fluticasone group and the nasal cavity volume improved in both active treatment groups when measured with acoustic rhinometry. The peak nasal and inspiratory flow also improved in both active groups but the improvement was quicker in the FP group. After 12 weeks there was no difference statistically in the symptoms between the two active groups. [****]

In conclusion, therefore, there is good evidence that topical corticosteroids improve the symptoms associated with nasal polyps, in particular nasal blockage, nasal secretions and sneezing, and in some patients they are effective at improving the sense of smell. In the majority of patients, but not all, topical corticosteroids also appeared to reduce the size of the nasal polyps, provided they were used for several weeks.

Persistent rhinosinusitis with nasal polyps: systemic steroids

There are no studies on treatment with systemic steroids alone in patients with nasal polyps. Topical steroids have always been given as well. Placebo-controlled studies are also lacking but there is a clinical acceptance that systemic steroids have a significant effect on the symptoms of nasal polyposis. [*]

In one study, oral prednisolone was given in doses of 60 mg daily to 25 patients with severe nasal polyposis for four days and, for each of the following 12 days, the dose was reduced by 5 mg daily. Antibiotics and antacids were also given. Seventy-two percent of patients experienced a symptom improvement due to the involution of polyps and in 52 percent of patients an improvement was seen on the CT. The symptoms of nasal obstruction and the sense of smell were improved. The findings of this study support the general clinical impression that systemic steroids are highly effective in treating a patient's symptoms when the patient is actually taking the systemic steroid. Unfortunately, the beneficial effects seem to be lost once the steroid is stopped.[9] [**]

There have been anecdotal reports of injecting corticosteroid directly into the polyp or into the inferior turbinate. There is no evidence to support this treatment and there have been case reports of blindness following intranasal injection of steroid, and so this method is not to be recommended.

The postoperative treatment of patients with chronic rhinosinusitis and nasal polyps with steroids

To date, there have been six studies into the effectiveness of topical steroids against a placebo and their ability to prevent recurrence of nasal polyps. Topical steroids do reduce the recurrence rate of nasal polyps after nasal polyp surgery. To quote from two of the representative studies, Karlsson and Rundcrantz[10] treated 20 patients with BDP and 20 were followed with no treatment after polyp surgery. The follow-up period was for 30 months. After six months, there was a statistically significant difference between the groups in favour of BDP and its effect increased during the study period over the next 30 months.

Hartwig et al.[11] used budesonide six months after polypectomy in a double-blind parallel group on 73 patients. In the budesonide group, 'polyp' scores were

significantly lower than in the controls after three and six months. Interestingly, this difference was only significant for patients with recurrent nasal polyposis and not those who had had a polypectomy operation for the first time. [****]

TREATMENT OF RHINOSINUSITIS WITH ANTIBIOTICS

The exact incidence of rhinosinusitis within populations is not known but it is a common condition for which antibiotics are frequently prescribed. According to the National Ambulatory Medical Care Survey in the USA, rhinosinusitis is the fifth most common diagnosis for which antibiotics are prescribed, accounting for 9 and 21 percent of all paediatric and adult antibiotic prescriptions, respectively, written in 2002.[12]

Intermittent (acute) acquired rhinosinusitis

There are more than 2000 studies in the literature concerning the effect of antibiotic treatment on intermittent sinusitis. However, only 49 studies met the appropriate criteria for inclusion in a systematic review in the Cochrane Library. These criteria included placebo control, appropriate statistical analysis and sufficient sample size, together with an adequate description of clinical improvements or success rates.[13] Amongst these 49 studies, major comparisons were between antibiotic versus control; the newer nonpenicillin antibiotics (macrolides) versus penicillins, and finally the amoxicillin/clavulanate versus other extended spectrum antibiotics. Most trials were conducted within ENT departments and only 20 of the 40 trials were double-blinded. [****/***]

In the studies looking at antibiotic versus control, in general, both penicillin and amoxicillin were more likely to effect a cure than placebo, typical figures being an 82 percent cure for amoxicillin against a 68 percent cure for placebo.[13]

When comparisons were made between the newer nonpencillins (cephalosporins, macrolides, minocycline) versus penicillins (amoxicillin and penicillin V), no significant differences were shown. The rates of cure or improvement appeared to be 84 percent for both antibiotic classes. Drop-outs due to adverse effects were infrequent and there was no significant difference between the two groups of antibiotics. Sixteen trials involving 4818 patients compared newer nonpenicillin antibiotics (macrolide or cephalosporin) to amoxicillin/clavulanate. Rates for cure or improvement were 72.7 and 72.9 percent for the newer nonpenicillins and amoxicillin/clavulanate, respectively. Drop-out rates due to adverse effects were significantly lower for the cephalosporin antibiotics. Relapse rates within one month of successful therapy did not differ between the groups.

Six trials, of which three were double-blinded, involving 1067 patients, compared a tetracycline (doxycycline, tetracycline, minocycline) to a heterogeneous group of antibiotics (folate, cephalosporin, macrolide, amoxicillin) and no relevant differences were found.

The Cochrane reviewers[13] concluded that for intermittent rhinosinusitis, confirmed radiologically, current evidence is limited but supports the use of penicillin or amoxicillin for 14–17 days. [****/***] In the Cochrane review, local differences in susceptibility of microorganisms to antibiotics used were not acknowledged, although it is known that resistance patterns of predominant pathogens, such as *Streptococcus pneumoniae*, *Haemophilus influenzae* and *Moraxella catarrhalis*, vary considerably.[14] The prevalence and degree of antibacterial resistance in common respiratory pathogens is also increasing worldwide, presumably because of the increase in antibiotic consumption. The choice of which antibiotic is used will not be the same in all regions. The selection may depend on local resistance patterns and the disease aetiology.

Antibiotic treatment for persistent rhinosinusitis

It is significantly more difficult to evaluate the efficacy of antibiotic treatment in PRS compared to intermittent rhinosinusitis because of the difficulties of defining the clinical diagnosis of PRS in the literature. In many studies there is no radiological diagnosis and, therefore, data supporting the use of antibiotics in persistent rhinosinusitis is limited and there are no randomized placebo-controlled clinical trials.

In a double-blinded prospective study by Legent et al.,[15] 251 adult patients with PRS were treated with ciprofloxacin or amoxicillin/clavulanic acid for nine days. Only 141 of the 251 patients had positive bacterial cultures from the middle meatus at the beginning of the study. At the end of the treatment period, the nasal discharge disappeared in 60 percent of the patients in the ciprofloxacin group and 56 percent of those in the amoxicillin/clavulanic acid group. The clinical cure and bacteriological eradication rates were 59 and 89 percent for ciprofloxacin versus 51 and 91 percent for amoxicillin/clavulanic acid, respectively. The differences were not significant. [***]

There is some evidence that long-term treatment with low-dose macrolide antibiotics may be effective in treating patients with PRS that has not been cured by surgery or corticosteroid treatment. In animal studies, macrolides have been shown to increase mucociliary transport and reduce goblet cell secretion. There is evidence *in vitro*, as well as clinical experience, that macrolides reduce the virulence and tissue damage caused

by chronic bacterial colonization without actually eradicating the bacteria.

Clinical studies have shown that long-term treatment with macrolide antibiotics increases ciliary function.[16] In a prospective randomized controlled trial (RCT), 90 patients with polypoid and nonpolypoid PRS were randomized to oral macrolide (erythromycin) for three months, or endoscopic sinus surgery, and the patients were followed for over a year. The outcome measures included a symptom score, the SNOT 22, the SF 36, nitrous oxide levels, acoustic rhinometry, saccharine clearance times and nasal endoscopy. Both the medical and surgical treatment of PRS significantly improved almost all the subjective and objective parameters with no significant difference between the two groups, or between polypoid and nonpolypoid PRS, except for the increase in total nasal volume which was greater following surgery.[16]

To summarize, for persistent rhinosinusitis, there are no placebo-controlled studies on the effectiveness of antibiotic treatment. Studies comparing different antibiotics did not show any significant difference between ciprofloxacin versus amoxicillin/clavulanic acid. The few available prospective studies showed a positive effect on the patient's symptoms in 56–95 percent of patients. [***]

Long-term low-dose macrolide treatment may be of use if surgery and/or steroids have failed. Placebo-controlled studies should be performed to establish the efficacy of macrolides if this treatment is to be accepted in the future. There is also an urgent need for randomized placebo-controlled studies to investigate the effectiveness of antibiotics in general for persistent rhinosinusitis.

TREATMENT OF RHINOSINUSITIS WITH OTHER MEDICINES

Decongestants

After corticosteroids and antibiotics, the medications that are perceived to be most useful for treating rhinosinusitis are decongestants. The rationale behind the use of decongestants is to improve sinus ventilation and drainage. Radiological studies show that topical decongestants markedly reduce the size of the inferior and middle turbinates and improve osteomeatal complex patency.[17]

Experimental studies suggest that topical decongestants (zylometazoline and oxymetazoline) have a beneficial antiinflammatory action that is caused by decreasing nitric oxide synthetase.[18] A controlled clinical trial showed that there was improved mucociliary clearance *in vivo* after two weeks of oxymetazoline for persistent bacterial rhinosinusitis when compared to fluticasone and hypertonic saline. The clinical course of the disease between the three groups, however, was not significantly indifferent.[19] [***]

Topical decongestants are also recommended for individuals who have problems clearing their ears while flying or diving. The decongestants are all alpha adrenergic agonists and act on the two types of alpha receptor, one of which controls the venous capacitance vessels of the nasal tissues which are responsible for erectile function, and the other alpha receptors which mediate contraction of arterioles that supply the mucosa. [*]

Ephedrine nasal drops (0.5 and 1 percent) are the weakest of the sympathomimetic preparations, whilst oxymetazoline and zylometazoline are more potent and cause intense vasoconstriction. The rebound effect that occurs after the vasoconstriction wears off is more likely to occur with the potent decongestants and, generally, patients should be advised not to use topical decongestant for more than ten days. In patients who become addicted to decongestant drops or sprays, there is a risk of developing rhinitis medicamentosa and, in this condition, the nasal mucosa becomes permanently damaged.

One preparation combines the steroid dexamethasone isonicotinate with the sympathomimetic tramazoline hydrochloride (Dexa-Rhinaspray Duo). The spray is promoted for the treatment of allergic rhinitis. The suggestion is that the decongestant allows better mucosal access for the steroid. Clinical experience suggests that this is a useful spray. [*] The use of all sympathomimetic preparations is contraindicated in patients on monoamine oxidase inhibitors (MAOIs) and they should be used with caution in patients with hypertension, hyperthyroidism, cardiovascular disease, diabetes mellitus and closed angle glaucoma, and in infants of less than three months of age.

The use of decongestants for persistent rhinosinusitis has not been evaluated in any RCTs. There are no controlled trials to test the efficacy of decongestants for the treatment of nasal polyps.

Systemic decongestants appear to be less effective than local preparations but rebound nasal congestion on withdrawal of the drug does not arise. Pseudo-ephedrine is available over the counter in the UK, both in tablet form and as a linctus. There is little evidence to support the use of systemic decongestants in the treatment of rhinosinusitis.

Mucolytics

The rationale for using mucolytics in the treatment of rhinosinusitis is that they may reduce the viscosity of the nasal secretions. There is minimal evidence to support the use of mucolytics in the treatment of rhinosinusitis. In one paediatric study, an RCT did not prove a bomhexine to be superior to saline inhalation for children with PRS.[20] [****]

Antihistamines

These can be used both orally and as a nasal spray. Clinical experience suggests that they reduce rhinorrhoea, sneezing and itching, but have little effect on nasal obstruction. There is no evidence that antihistamines reduce or abolish the symptoms of the common cold. The nonsedating antihistamines, acrivastine (Semprex), cetirizine hydrochloride (Zirtek), desloratadine (Neoclarityn), fexofenadine hydrochloride (Telfast) and terfenadine (Triludan) cause less sedation and psychomotor impairment because they penetrate the blood–brain barrier to a lesser degree than the older type of antihistamines. Terfenadine, however, was found to be associated with hazardous arrhythmias. The side effects of antihistamines include hypotension, hypersensitivity reactions, extrapyramidal effect, dizziness, blood disorders and liver dysfunction.

In the treatment of intermittent rhinosinusitis, the beneficial effect of loratadine (the predecessor of desloratadine) for patients with allergic rhinitis was confirmed in a multicentre randomized double-blind placebo-controlled trial. Patients receiving loratadine as an adjunct to antibiotic treatment suffered significantly less sneezing and obstruction on daily visual analogue scale (VAS) scores.[21] [****]

In PRS, there is little evidence that antihistamines are effective. However, they are often prescribed for patients with PRS, particularly in the USA. There are no controlled trials evaluating such treatment.

Sprays such as azelastine hydrochloride (Rhinolast) and levocabastine (Livostin) are topical antihistamines that are promoted for use in allergic rhinitis. Topical antihistamines are considered less effective than topical steroids and good evidence to support their use is lacking.

Sodium cromoglicate

Sodium cromoglicate is available as a 4 percent aqueous nasal spray (Rynacrom) and a 2 percent nasal spray (Vividrin), and it is also combined with xylometazoline (Rynacrom) and is promoted for prophylactic use in allergic rhinitis. Depending on the preparation, it needs to be taken either four or six times a day. Its mechanism of action is debatable; it was originally thought to act by preventing mediator release from mast cells. However, agents subsequently developed with this property do not demonstrate the same anti-asthmatic affects as cromoglicate. There is some evidence that cromoglicate depresses the exaggerated neuronal reflexes generated by irritant receptor stimulation. The side effects are few and include local irritation and transient bronchospasm. It may have a role in the treatment of allergic rhinitis in children but the fact that it needs to be taken several times a day means that compliance is low. [**]

Antimycotics

There is increased interest in the role of fungi as a possible cause for the various types of rhinosinusitis. Antimycotics can be used topically and systemically and as an adjunct to sinus surgery in the treatment of allergic rhinosinusitis, invasive fungal rhinosinusitis and conventional intermittent rhinosinusitis.

Surgery is considered the first-line treatment for allergic fungal rhinosinusitis,[22] and surgery and systemic antimycotics are used in the treatment of invasive fungal rhinosinusitis.[23] Although the use of antimycotics in the treatment of allergic fungal rhinosinusitis has not been tested in controlled trials, a high dose of postoperative itraconazole, combined with oral and topical steroids in a cohort of 139 patients with allergic fungal rhinosinusitis, reduced the need for revision surgery.[24] [**] The optimum medical treatment for invasive fungal sinusitis is not known because the available evidence comes from small series and case reports which do not meet the criteria for a meta-analysis. [**/*]

A group of researchers from the Mayo Clinic produced the hypothesis that persistent rhinosinusitis may arise because of a local immune response to fungi that are present in nasal and sinus secretions.[25] Given the correct equipment, fungi can be detected in nasal secretions in virtually all patients with PRS, but also in a controlled disease-free population. As yet, there is no definitive proof that fungi are involved in the aetiology of the inflammatory response in some patients. One double-blind placebo-controlled trial has looked at this in 60 patients with PRS, giving them topical treatment with amphotericin B, comparing this with saline douching.[26] Radiological and subjective scores were actually worse in the treatment group; however this is an area of considerable interest and further randomized controlled trials are awaited. [****]

MEDICATION THAT MAY IMPROVE THE IMMUNE RESPONSE

It is thought that an altered immune response to bacterial infection or fungal infection may be responsible for some of the episodes of recurrent rhinosinusitis. With resistance to antibiotic treatment increasing, there is interest in medications that may alter the immune response.

Bacterial lysate preparations

Bacterial lysate preparations, e.g. ribosomal fractions of *Klebsiella pneumoniae*, *Streptococcus pneumoniae*, *Streptococcus pyogenes* and *Haemophilus influenzae*, have been tested against placebo in three multicentre placebo-controlled trials and the evidence from these studies

suggested that this type of therapy may reduce the need for antibiotics in the treatment of PRS.[27, 28, 29] [****]

Treatment with more expensive agents that either stimulate or modulate the immune system, e.g. recombinant human granulocyte colony stimulating factor, have been tested in a randomized controlled trial in a group of patients with PRS that were refractory to other types of treatment. The studies showed there was no significant improvement with this expensive treatment. [****]

A pilot study has looked at treatment with gamma interferon and it suggested that this treatment may be beneficial in treating resistant PRS but the number of patients was small.[30] [**]

NASAL AND ANTRAL IRRIGATION WITH SALINE

Saline irrigation

A number of randomized controlled trials have tested nasal irrigation with isotonic or hypertonic saline in the treatment of intermittent and persistent rhinosinusitis. In these randomized trials, modalities of application of the saline or hypertonic saline are compared. The evidence is that nasal washout with isotonic or hypertonic saline is beneficial in alleviating symptoms and improves endoscopic findings in patients with PRS. Irrigation with saline has also shown to significantly improve nasal mucociliary clearance, as measured by saccharine tests in healthy volunteers.[31] [***]

ANTILEUKOTRIENES

The role of leukotrienes in the pathogenesis of bronchial asthma has been well documented and increased levels of these mediators have been detected in patients with rhinosinusitis and nasal polyps. Antileukotrienes have been evaluated in the treatment of asthmatics, especially in those with the aspirin-induced asthma (ASA) triad.

When seasonal allergic rhinitis was considered, antileukotrienes were not found to be superior to placebo in reducing symptom scores in a randomized controlled trial.[32] [****]

For patients with PRS and nasal polyps, one study looked at antileukotriene treatment in 36 patients and found that when antileukotrienes were added to standard treatment regimes, there was a significant reduction in symptom score.[33] [***]

Two other studies support the use of antileukotriene treatment as an adjunct to standard treatment in patients with nasal polyps, asthma and aspirin intolerance.[34, 35] [**]

Aspirin desensitization

This treatment has been used in patients with nasal polyps. A case-controlled trial of treatment with lysine aspirin to one nostril and placebo to the other in 13 patients with bilateral nasal polyposis, resulted in delayed polyp recurrence on the lysine aspirin-treated side.[36] [***] A large randomized controlled trial is underway at the Royal National Throat, Nose and Ear Hospital in London.

AGENTS USED TO BLOCK THE PARASYMPATHETIC NERVOUS SYSTEM

Ipratropium bromide (Rinatec) is a muscarinic receptor antagonist and therefore blocks the parasympathetic nervous system. In theory, it should be effective in anyone with a wet dripping nose due to parasympathetic overactivity. In practice, it is effective for some elderly men with a dripping nose. It does not have any other clinical use and there are side effects which include a dry mouth, epistaxis and dryness of the nose. [*]

RELATED TOPICS

Preparation of the nasal mucosa prior to surgery

Cocaine solution (5 or 10 percent) or cocaine paste (25 percent) has been used to prepare the nose prior to surgery for over 100 years. The majority of rhinologists believe it to be the most effective way of ensuring good operating conditions. As with all local anaesthetic techniques, leaving sufficient time for the drug to work is paramount. The application of Moffat's solution by a spray (**Figure 36.1**) is one method of preparing the nose and it is sensible to do this immediately after the induction of anaesthesia.

Moffat's solution consists of 2 mL of 5 percent cocaine, 1 mL of 1:1000 adrenalin and a small amount of bicarbonate solution. In order to avoid systemic effects, the maximum dose recommended for application to the nasal mucosa in fit adults is 1.5 mg/kg. Colouring the cocaine solution with pink dye reduces the risk of it being mistaken for other drugs in the anaesthetic room.

Antifungal agents used in rhinology

Fungal infections may be superficial or systemic. Antifungal agents can be classified into polyenes, fluocytosine, imidazoles and triazoles. The polyenes, amphotericin and

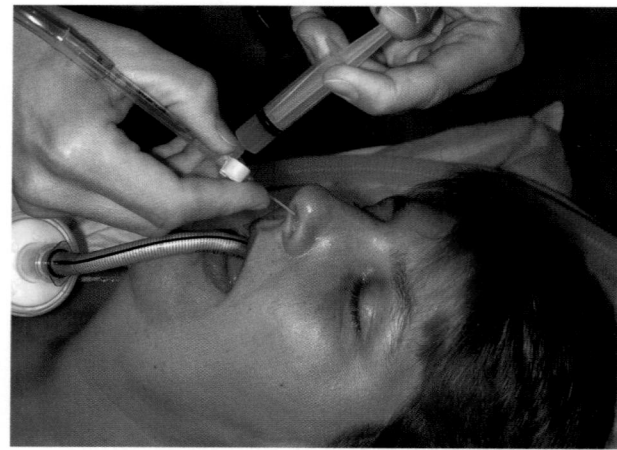

Figure 36.1   The application of Moffat's solution by a spray.

nystatin interact with ergosterol in the fungal cell membrane. Pores are formed through which the fungal cell contents are lost. Selectivity is obtained since the human cell membrane contains mostly cholesterol rather than ergosterol.

Amphotericin has a wide spectrum of activity and is used parentally in severe systemic infections since oral absorption is poor. Side effects are common and include nausea and fevers. Renal impairment can occur but is reversible if detected early. Liposomal amphotericin is significantly less toxic but is more expensive. It is likely that it will become the agent of choice. Nystatin is used principally for *Candida albicans* infections of the skin and mucosal membranes.

Flucytosine is given orally or intravenously to treat systemic candidiasis or cryptococcal infections, often in combination with amphotericin to prevent resistance. Flucytosine is converted in fungal cells to flurouracil which inhibits DNA synthesis.

The imidazoles, miconazole, ketoconazole and clotrimazole, are mostly used to treat topical infections. They are broad-spectrum antifungals that prevent ergosterol synthesis. Ketoconazole is better absorbed by mouth than the other imidazoles but it has been associated with fatal hepatotoxicity.

The triazoles include fluconazole and itraconazole and both can be given orally and parentally. Itraconazole is active against Aspergillus but has been associated with heptatoxicity.

Vestibulitis

Noninfective vestibulitis may be treated by applying vaseline or a mild topical corticosteroid to the vestibule. In the presence of infection, however, an antibiotic ointment should be applied and the infective agent is usually *Staphylococcus aureus*. Two preparations are available in the UK, a combination of chlorhexidine and neomycin (Naseptin) and mupirocin (Bactroban nasal). The latter is used as a second-line agent for the eradication of methicillin-resistant *Staphylococcus aureus* (MRSA). The ointment is applied three times a day for five days and a swab is taken two days later to determine whether MRSA has been successfully eradicated. Naseptin, when it is used, should be applied four times a day for ten days to treat an infection. It is important to remember that naseptin includes arachis (peanut) oil and this should therefore not be used in patients who have an allergy to peanuts. Naseptin is also contraindicated in pregnancy.

Hereditary familial telangiectasia

The epistaxis associated with hereditary familial telangiectasia (HFT) is difficult to treat and a variety of medical and surgical treatments have been tried. Systemic and topical oestrogen provoke squamous metaplasia of the epithelium and in this way provide a protective coat over the blood vessels. Ethinyloestradiol may be used under supervision for the treatment of HFT in women. The side effects include nausea, fluid retention and thrombosis. It is not popular in men because of the gynaecomastia it induces.

Atrophic rhinitis

Atrophic rhinitis is characterized by a dry crusting mucosa, nasal obstruction and a foul smell. Steam inhalation and humidification are useful, as is nasal douching with saline. A 25 percent glucose in glycerine solution appears to restore some moisture to the nasal mucosa. [*] To prepare the solution, 75 g of glycerine is gently warmed to which 25 g of glucose is added and the mixture stirred until the glucose has dissolved. After bottling, the drops have a three-month life span. The drops can be used several times a day and provide some relief to this distressing condition.

METHODS OF ADMINISTERING TOPICAL NASAL PREPARATIONS

Nasal sprays: If two sprays are to be administered to each nostril, one spray should be directed upwards and the other backwards whilst the patient does not breath or breaths in gently.

The best position for administering nasal drops is head-down as in **Figure 36.2.**

- If betamethasone drops are used it is difficult for the patient to put two drops only into each nostril. In order to establish an exact dose of betnesol drops, they can be decanted into an empty cophenylcaine spray bottle and the patient instructed to put one

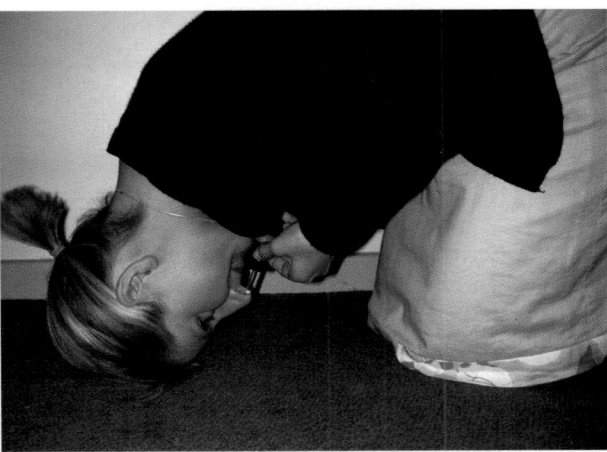

Figure 36.2   The best position for administering steroid drops.

spray in each nostril once daily. One spray is equivalent to two drops.
- Topical steroid drops (fluticasone or betamethasone) give a higher systemic dose (approximately equivalent to 2 mg of prednisolone daily) than the topical steroid sprays (triamcinolone acetonide – nasacort at 55 μg per spray, mometasone furoate – nasonex at 50 μg per spray).
- Fluticasone propionate nasules (400 μg) can be used to increase the topical dose of steroid. One nasule is shared between each nostril once daily; thus the dose given is precisely known.

KEY POINTS

- Rhinosinusitis is one of the most common health care problems. It diminishes patients' quality of life and consumes resources.
- Corticosteroids and antibiotics are effective treatments for rhinosinusitis.
- Topical decongestants are a useful adjunct.
- Antihistamines reduce rhinorrhoea, sneezing and itching but not nasal obstruction.
- Antimucolytics are indicated for invasive fungal rhinosinusitis and their role may extend to other types of rhinosinusitis in the future.
- Saline irrigation of the nose is an effective treatment for rhinosinusitis.
- Antileukotrienes, used as an adjunct, work in 50 percent of patients with the ASA triad.
- Topical aspirin desensitization may improve nasal obstruction in PRS with and without polyps. Further trials are underway.
- Topical cocaine remains the best way to prepare the nose for surgery.

Best clinical practice

✓ Topical steroids improve the symptoms associated with nasal polyps and reduce the recurrence rate of nasal polyps after surgery.

✓ The best position for administering steroid drops is head-down (**Figure 36.2**).

✓ One way of introducing cocaine into the nose is by spraying Moffat's solution (cocaine and adrenalin) into the nose immediately after induction of anaesthesia, increasing the chances of obtaining a 'bloodless surgical field'.

✓ Before prescribing naseptin, ensure the patient is not allergic to peanuts.

Deficiencies in current knowledge and areas for future research

➤ Topical steroids reduce the recurrence rate of nasal polyps following surgery and antileukotrienes help 50 percent of patients with the ASA triad, but there is yet to be an effective long-lasting medical polypectomy.

➤ The optimum length of treatment with topical steroids is yet to be established with the different clinical scenarios. The role of fungi in the aetiology of rhinosinusitis has yet to be clarified. The current role of systemic and topical antifungal medication may be extended in the future.

➤ Placebo-controlled trials are required to study the effectiveness of antibiotics for persistent rhinosinusitis. Currently, there is considerable interest in macrolide antibiotics.

➤ It is not known why some patients with rhinosinusitis develop polyps and others do not.

REFERENCES

* 1. Fokkens W, Lund V, Bachert C, Clement P, Hellings P, Jones N et al. European position paper on rhinosinusitis and nasal polyps. *Rhinology.* 2005; 27–46.

2. Meltzer EO, Orgel HA, Backhaus JW, Busse WW, Druce HM, Metzger WJ et al. Intranasal flunisolide spray as an adjunct to oral antibiotic therapy for sinusitis. *Journal of Allergy and Clinical Immunology.* 1993; **92**: 812–23.

3. Gehanno P, Beauvillain C, Bobin S, Chobaut JC, Desaülty A, Dubreuil C et al. Short therapy with amoxicillin-clavulanate and corticosteroids in acute sinusitis: results of a multicentre study in adults. *Scandinavian Journal of Infectious Diseases.* 2000; **32**: 679–84.

4. Meltzer EO, Charous BL, Busse WW, Zinreich SJ, Lorber RR, Danzig MR. Added relief in the treatment of acute recurrent sinusitis with adjunctive Mometasone furoate nasal spray. The Nasonex Sinusitis Group. *Journal of Allergy and Clinical Immunology.* 2000; **106**: 630–7.

5. Nayak AS, Settipane GA, Pedinoff A, Charous BL, Meltzer EO, Busse WW et al. Effective dose range of Mometasone furoate nasal spray in the treatment of acute rhinosinusitis. *Annals of Allergy, Asthma and Immunology.* 2002; **89**: 271–8.

* 6. Lund VJ, Black JH, Szabo LZ, Schrewelius C, Akerlund A. Efficacy and tolerability of budesonide aqueous nasal spray in chronic rhinosinusitis patients. *Rhinology.* 2004; **42**: 57–62.

7. Mygind N, Pedersen CB, Prytz S, Sorensen H. Treatment of nasal polyps with intranasal Beclomethasone dipropionate aerosol. *Clinical Allergy.* 1975; **5**: 159–64.

8. Keith P, Nieminen J, Hollingworth K, Dolovich J. Efficacy and tolerability of Fluticasone propionate nasal drops 400 microgram once daily compared with placebo for the treatment of bilateral polyposis in adults. *Clinical and Experimental Allergy.* 2000; **39**: 1460–8.

9. van Camp C, Clement PA. Results of oral steroid treatment in nasal polyposis. *Rhinology.* 1994; **32**: 5–9.

10. Karlsson G, Rundcrantz H. A randomized trial of intranasal Beclomethasone dipropionate after polypectomy. *Rhinology.* 1982; **20**: 144–8.

11. Hartwig S, Linden M, Laurent C, Vargo AK, Lindqvist N. Budesonide nasal spray as prophylactic treatment after polypectomy (a double blind clinical trial). *Journal of Laryngology and Otology.* 1988; **102**: 148–51.

12. Anon JB, Jacobs MR, Poole MD, Ambrose PG, Benninger MS, Hadley JA et al. Antimicrobial treatment guidelines for acute bacterial rhinosinusitis. *Otolaryngology and Head and Neck Surgery.* 2004; **130**: 1–45.

* 13. Williams Jr. JW, Aguilar C, Cornell J, Chiquette E, Dolor RJ, Makela M et al. Antibiotics for acute maxillary sinusitis (Cochrane review). Cochrane Database of Systematic Reviews 2003(4).

14. Hoban D, Felmingham D. The PROTEKT surveillance study: antimicrobial susceptibility of Haemophilus influenzae and Moraxella catarrhalis from community-acquired respiratory tract infections. *Journal of Antimicrobial Chemotherapy.* 2002; **59**: 49–59.

15. Legent F, Bordure P, Beauvillain C, Berche P. A double-blind comparison of ciprofloxacin and amoxycillin/clavulanic acid in the treatment of chronic sinusitis. *Chemotherapy.* 1994; **40**: 8–15.

* 16. Ragab SM, Lund VJ, Scadding G. Evaluation of the medical and surgical treatment of chronic rhinosinusitis: a prospective, randomised, controlled trial. *Laryngoscope.* 2004; **114**: 923–30.

17. Stringer SP, Mancuso AA, Avino AJ. Effect of a topical vasoconstrictor on computed tomography of paranasal sinus disease. *Laryngoscope.* 1993; **103**: 6–9.

18. Westerveld GJ, Voss HP, van der Hee RM, de Haan-Koelewijn GJ, den Hartog GJ, Scheeren RA et al. Inhibition of nitric oxide synthase by nasal decongestants. *European Respiratory Journal.* 2000; **16**: 437–44.

19. Inanli S, Ozturk O, Korkmaz M, Tutkun A, Batman C. The effects of topical agents of fluticasone propionate, oxymetazoline, and 3% and 0.9% sodium chloride solutions on mucociliary clearance in the therapy of acute bacterial rhinosinusitis in vivo. *Laryngoscope.* 2002; **112**: 320–5.

20. Van Bever HP, Bosmans J, Stevens WJ. Nebulization treatment with saline compared to bromhexine in treating chronic sinusitis in asthmatic children. *Allergy.* 1987; **42**: 33–6.

21. Braun JJ, Alabert JP, Michel FB, Quiniou M, Rat C, Cougnard J *et al.* Adjunct effect of loratadine in the treatment of acute sinusitis in patients with allergic rhinitis. *Allergy.* 1997; **52**: 650–5.

22. Schubert MS. Medical treatment of allergic fungal sinusitis. *Annals of Allergy, Asthma and Immunology.* 2000; **85**: 90–7; quiz 97–101.

23. Kuhn FA, Javer AR. Allergic fungal rhinosinusitis: perioperative management, prevention of recurrence, and role of steroids and antifungal agents. *Otolaryngologic Clinics of North America.* 2000; **33**: 419–33.

24. Rains 3rd BM, Mineck CW. Treatment of allergic fungal sinusitis with high-dose itraconazole. *American Journal of Rhinology.* 2003; **17**: 1–8.

25. Ponikau JU, Sherris DA, Kern EB, Homburger HA, Frigas E, Gaffey TA *et al.* The diagnosis and incidence of allergic fungal sinusitis. *Mayo Clinic Proceedings.* 1999; **74**: 877–84.

26. Weschta M, Rimek D, Formanek M, Polzehi D, Podbielski A, Riechelmann H. Topical antifungal treatment of chronic rhinosinusitis with nasal polyps: a randomized, double-blind clinical trial. *Journal of Allergy and Clinical Immunology.* 2004; **113**: 1122–8.

27. Habermann W, Zimmermann K, Skarabis H, Kunze R, Rusch V. [Reduction of acute recurrence in patients with chronic recurrent hypertrophic sinusitis by treatment with a bacterial immunostimulant (Enterococcus faecalis Bacteriae of human origin]. *Arzneimittelforschung.* 2002; **52**: 622–7.

28. Serrano E, Demanez JP, Morgon A, Chastang V, Van Cauwenberge P. Effectiveness of ribosomal fractions of Klebsiella pneumoniae, Streptococcus pneumoniae, Streptococcus pyogenes, Haemophilus influenzae and the membrane fraction of Kp (Ribomunyl) in the prevention of clinical recurrences of infectious rhinitis. Results of a multicenter double-blind placebo-controlled study. *European Archives of Otorhinolaryngology.* 1997; **254**: 372–5.

29. Heintz B, Schlenter WW, Kirsten R, Nelson K. Clinical efficacy of Broncho-Vaxom in adult patients with chronic purulent sinusitis – a multi-centric, placebo-controlled, double-blind study. *International Journal of Clinical Pharmacology, Therapy and Toxicology.* 1989; **27**: 530–4.

30. Jyonouchi H, Sun S, Kelly A, Rimell FL. Effects of exogenous interferon gamma on patients with treatment-resistant chronic rhinosinusitis and dysregulated interferon gamma production: a pilot study. *Archives of Otolaryngology – Head and Neck Surgery.* 2003; **129**: 563–9.

31. Talbot AR, Herr TM, Parsons DS. Mucociliary clearance and buffered hypertonic saline solution. *Laryngoscope.* 1997; **107**: 500–3.

32. Pullerits T, Praks L, Skoogh BE, Ani R, Lotvall J. Randomized placebo-controlled study comparing a leukotriene receptor antagonist and a nasal gluco-corticoid in seasonal allergic rhinitis. *American Journal of Respiratory and Critical Care Medicine.* 1999; **159**: 1814–8.

33. Parnes SM, Chuma AV. Acute effects of antileukotrienes on sinonasal polyposis and sinusitis. *Ear, Nose and Throat Journal.* 2000; **79**: 18–20, 24–5.

34. Ulualp SO, Sterman BM, Toohill RJ. Antileukotriene therapy for the relief of sinus symptoms in aspirin triad disease. *Ear, Nose and Throat Journal.* 1999; **78**: 604–6, 613, passim.

35. Ragab S, Parikh A, Darby YC, Scadding GK. An open audit of montelukast, a leukotriene receptor antagonist, in nasal polyposis associated with asthma. *Clinical and Experimental Allergy.* 2001; **31**: 1385–91.

36. Scadding GK, Hassab M, Darby YC, Lund VJ, Freedman A. Intranasal lysine aspirin in recurrent nasal polyposis. *Clinical Otolaryngology.* 1995; **20**: 561–3.

FURTHER READING

British Society for Allergy and Clinical Immunology, ENT Sub-Committee. *Rhinitis Management Guidelines*, 3rd edn. London: Martin Dunitz.

European Academy of Allergology and Clinical Immunology. European position paper on rhinosinusitis and nasal polyps. *Rhinology Supplement.* 2005; **18**: 1–87.

37

Drug therapy in laryngology and head and neck surgery

WENDY SMITH AND ROGAN CORBRIDGE

Introduction	446	Use of botulinum toxins in spasmodic dystonia	449
Anticoagulants	446	Collagen injection of paralysed vocal cords	450
Antibiotics	448	Drugs used in thyroid disease including the management	
Preparations used to irrigate wounds	448	of hypocalcaemia	450
Local anaesthetic sprays and lozenges	448	Treatment of reflux oesophagitis	451
Mouthwashes	448	Chemotherapeutic agents	452
Throat lozenges and pastilles	448	Management of fungating wounds	453
Solutions, suspensions and syrups	448	Key points	453
Treatment of dry mouth	449	Best clinical practice	453
Cough medicines	449	References	453
Management of stridor	449	Further reading	453
Drug therapy in angioneurotic oedema	449		

SEARCH STRATEGY

The data in this chapter are supported by a Medline search using the key words anticoagulant, antibiotic prophylaxis, and head and neck surgery. This chapter relied on the medicines listed in the *British National Formulary*.[1]

INTRODUCTION

The laryngologist and head and neck surgeon prescribes medicines for prophylactic purposes, for example antibiotics and anticoagulants, as well as for therapeutic use in the management of infections, immune conditions and voice/throat problems. An appreciation of the pharmacology, preparations available, side effects and contraindications is required for appropriate and safe prescribing. This chapter addresses these matters.

ANTICOAGULANTS

The perioperative management of patients taking anticoagulants may be complex and should be considered on an individual patient basis, taking into account the increased risk of haemorrhagic complications in that procedure with the risk of thromboembolism if the anticoagulation therapy was stopped. Where necessary, involvement of the haematology/medical teams is advised.

The anticoagulant drugs heparin and warfarin are widely used in the prevention and treatment of venous thrombosis and embolism perioperatively. Anticoagulants should not be used where there is a history of haemorrhagic disorders, peptic ulcer disease, severe hypertension and severe liver disease. **Figure 37.1** illustrates the clotting pathway and the action of heparin and oral anticoagulants.

Heparin is a family of mucopolysaccharides with a molecular weight of 4000–30,000. The molecules are attached to a protein backbone consisting entirely of

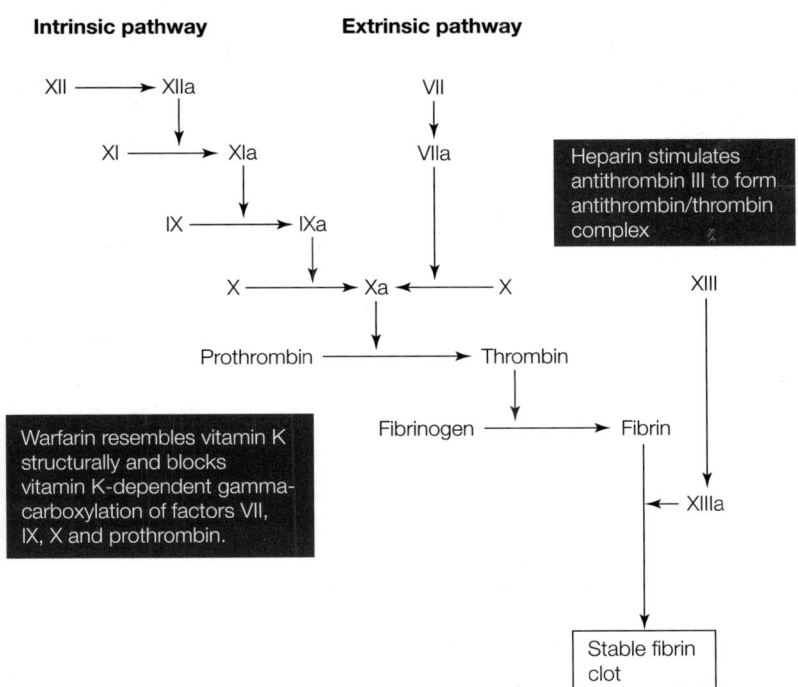

Intrinsic pathway

Extrinsic pathway

Heparin stimulates antithrombin III to form antithrombin/thrombin complex

Warfarin resembles vitamin K structurally and blocks vitamin K-dependent gamma-carboxylation of factors VII, IX, X and prothrombin.

Figure 37.1 The clotting pathway and the mechanism of action of heparin and oral anticoagulants.

serine and glycine residues. Heparin is found in mast cells, in plasma and in the endothelial cell layer of blood vessels. This highly acidic substance is extracted from beef lung or hog intestinal mucosa for therapeutic use. Heparin's main action is preventing fibrin formation by interacting with the protease inhibitor antithrombin III enhancing (by 1000-fold) the binding of antithrombin III with thrombin. In addition, the heparin–antithrombin III complex has inhibitory effects on factors IXa, Xa, XIa and XIIa.

Heparin is not absorbed from the gastrointestinal mucosa because of its charge and large molecular weight; therefore it must be given intravenously or by subcutaneous injection. Intramuscular injection is avoided to prevent haematoma formation. The onset of action of heparin is immediate and it has a half-life of 40–90 minutes. It is inactivated by heparinase in the liver and platelet factor IV released from activated platelets may also have a role.

When used for prophylaxis of deep vein thrombosis in surgery, 5000 units of heparin should be given two hours before surgery, then 8–12 hourly for seven days or until the patient is ambulant. Monitoring is not required in this situation but when used to treat a thrombosis, a regime of 5000 units intravenously followed by 15–25 units/kg/hour intravenous infusion or 15,000 units 12 hourly necessitates monitoring of the thrombin time, which should be increased by a factor of two to three.

Low molecular weight heparins (certoparin, dalteparin, enoxaparin, reviparin and tinzaparin) are also effective in the prophylaxis of venous thromboembolism and their once daily subcutaneous administration is more convenient. These can also be used to treat deep vein thrombosis and monitoring is not required.

Platelet counts should be measured in patients receiving heparin since thrombocytopenia (an immune reaction) may occur but this does not usually happen until six to ten days after the start of treatment. Should thrombocytopenia, or a 50 percent reduction of the platelet count occur, and further anticoagulation is required, patients should be given the heparinoid, danaparoid, or the hirudin, lepirudin.

Heparin inhibits aldosterone and may result in hyperkalaemia, especially in patients with diabetes mellitus, chronic renal failure, acidosis, raised plasma potassium or those taking potassium-sparing drugs.

The oral anticoagulants prevent the reduction of vitamin K that is required as an active cofactor of carboxylase in factors II, VII, IX and X. The effect on fibrin formation depends upon the balance between the decreased rate of carboxylation and the unaltered rate of degradation of factors already carboxylated. Warfarin has a half-life of 40 hours and a duration of action between two and six days. It takes at least 48–72 hours for the anticoagulant effect to develop fully and so heparin is also used initially when an immediate anticoagulant effect is required. Warfarin is the most commonly prescribed oral anticoagulant; nicoumalone and phenindione are rarely used. The drugs are metabolized by the mixed function oxidases in the liver.

Monitoring of the prothrombin time (usually reported as the international normalized ratio (INR) is required and dose adjustments made accordingly. Target INR values (usually between two and four) are detailed in the British National Formulary. The INR can be dramatically altered by co-prescribing other medication and the reader is again directed to the British National Formulary[1] prior to co-prescribing.

ANTIBIOTICS

Antibiotics are commonly prescribed prophylactically, even in so-called clean operations. The use of antibiotics post-tonsillectomy has failed to show a reduction in the secondary haemorrhage rate but may reduce pain at day five postoperatively.[2,3] Where there is no violation of mucosa, no preoperative inflammation and no drain, the incidence of wound infection in the head and neck is 2 percent. In surgery such as laryngectomy, prophylactic antibiotics with a broad spectrum are used to prevent wound infections. A preoperative dose (given to allow a high tissue level at the time of surgery) and three post-operative doses of a cephalosporin and metronidazole are suitable. Violaris and Bridger, using a cephalosporin at eight hours preoperatively with the premedication and three doses eight hourly postoperatively, reduced the development of pharyngocutaneous fistulae.[4] Johansen et al.[5] found prophylactic metronidazole resulted in a highly significant decrease in the frequency of post-operative fistulae.

Antibiotic prophylaxis is also necessary in patients with artificial heart valves or cardiac valve disease. Local policies may vary but amoxicillin 3 g orally or 1 g intramuscularly can be given one hour before surgery and six hours postoperatively.

The choice of antibiotic to treat an established infection is initially on a 'best guess' policy based on the probable pathogen until swab results and sensitivities become available.

PREPARATIONS USED TO IRRIGATE WOUNDS

Before closing a wound following tumour excision it has been recommended that it should first be washed out well. Stell and Maran[6] describe the use of Savlon, hydrogen peroxide and sterile water as suitable solutions since it appears that the mechanical process of washing rather than the lytic action on the cells is important. They recommend the use of at least 1 L of solution. In a xenograft model of tumour-cell wound contamination, Allegretto et al.[7] found that irrigation with water, saline or gemcitabine delayed tumour development: the latter two improved rates of long-term disease control.

LOCAL ANAESTHETIC SPRAYS AND LOZENGES

These preparations are used to desensitize the mouth and pharynx prior to examination, investigation or treatment. Lidocaine (lignocaine) is effectively absorbed from mucous membranes and is available as a pump spray as a 10 percent solution (maximum dose is 20 sprays in pharynx, larynx or trachea) and more commonly as a topical 4 percent solution (maximum dose is 7.5 mL). Benzocaine is a neutral, water-insoluble local anaesthetic of low potency and is only used for surface anaesthesia in noninflamed tissue in the mouth and pharynx. It is available in lozenges and sprays, sometimes combined with antiseptics. Sensitization may occur and there is little evidence for the benefit in using these combined preparations. Patients should be advised not to eat or drink until the numbness has worn off. Lidocaine belongs to the amide class, benzocaine to the ester class of local anaesthetics. Both bind to a receptor on the sodium channel in the axon preventing the opening of the channels, thereby preventing depolarization of the nerve. In overdosage, cardiac toxicity can occur.

MOUTHWASHES

Mouthwashes are usually aqueous solutions in a con-centrated form of substances with deodorant, antiseptic, local anaesthetic or astringent properties. Sometimes they should be diluted before use. They have a mechanical cleansing action. Hydrogen peroxide mouthwash is a 6 percent solution and 15 mL should be diluted in half a tumblerful of warm water two to three times daily. It contains an oxidizing agent and is useful in the treatment of acute ulcerative gingivitis. It froths in contact with oral debris, thereby having a mechanical cleansing effect, hence its use in the management of secondary tonsillect-omy haemorrhages. Chlorhexidine gluconate, used when toothbrushing is not possible or in combating oral infection, inhibits plaque formation on teeth but has the side effect of causing reversible brown staining of the teeth.

THROAT LOZENGES AND PASTILLES

Lozenges and pastilles are both used to deliver medica-ments for local effect, either to soothe or treat infections. Lozenges consist of medicaments incorporated into a flavoured base that dissolves or disintegrates slowly in the mouth. They are prepared either by moulding and cutting or by compression. Colours, flavours and sweetening agents may be incorporated. Heavy compression is used to ensure slow disintegration in the mouth.

Pastilles consist of medicaments in a base containing gelatin and glycerol or a mixture of acacia and sucrose. Sodium benzoate and citric acid monohydrate may be used as a preservative and antioxidant, respectively. Flavourings such as lemon oil may be incorporated.

SOLUTIONS, SUSPENSIONS AND SYRUPS

Solutions are liquid preparations containing one or more soluble ingredients, usually dissolved in water. They may be used internally, externally or for instilling into body cavities and may be sterile or unsterilized depending on the application. Solutions given orally usually result in rapid absorption. Problems with solubility, taste and stability may prevent this formulation being available for a particular drug.

Suspensions are formulations in which the drug does not dissolve in the solvent but is distributed within it. It usually provides a more rapid dispersion and dissolution of the drug when compared to tablets and capsules so long as the drug has a suitable particle size and does not settle or cake on storage. The primary particle size may grow due to the action of surfactants, emulsifiers and other adjuvants.

Syrups are concentrated aqueous solutions of sucrose or other sugars to which medicaments or flavourings are added. Glycerol, sorbitol and polyhydric alcohols may be added to reduce the rate of crystallization of sucrose and to increase the solubility of other ingredients. Growth of microorganisms is usually retarded by sucrose concentrations greater than 65 percent w/w.

TREATMENT OF DRY MOUTH

Artificial saliva can be useful to relieve dry mouth resulting from radiotherapy or diseases affecting the salivary glands. These preparations should be of neutral pH and contain electrolytes approximating to the composition of saliva. These preparations are available as oral sprays, lozenges and pastilles. Pilocarpine (Salagen) is a muscarinic and can stimulate any residual salivary gland function. Side effects relate to the muscarinic action and its use is contraindicated in those with significant respiratory and cardiovascular disease, angle-closure glaucoma, pregnancy and breastfeeding.

COUGH MEDICINES

These are divided into cough suppressants and the expectorant and demulcent cough preparations. After excluding an underlying cause of a cough, such as asthma and gastro-oesophageal reflux, cough suppressants may be used. It is thought that these drugs act by an ill-defined central action in the nervous system and may depress the 'cough centre' in the brain stem. The narcotic analgesics are effective as antitussives in sub-analgesic doses. Codeine phosphate is useful for dry or painful coughs but it also inhibits the secretion and mucociliary clearance of sputum, is constipating and dependence can develop. Pholcodine (related to codeine) and dextromethorphan (a non-narcotic, nonanalgesic) have lesser side effects. Over the counter preparations include sedating antihistamines, such as diphenhydramine, and may work by causing drowsiness.

There is no evidence that expectorants (ammonium chloride, ipecacuanha and squill) are effective at promoting expulsion of bronchial secretions. Their action is

more placebo. Demulcent cough preparations may relieve a dry irritating cough by virtue of the fact that they contain a syrup or glycerol that has a soothing effect. Simple linctus (a sugar-free preparation is also available) is harmless and inexpensive.

MANAGEMENT OF STRIDOR

The treatment required depends upon the cause and severity of the stridor. Heliox is useful in an acute situation but antibiotics, adrenaline, steroids and antihistamines may be required, as may surgery.

Helium is a colourless, odourless, tasteless gas that when mixed, one volume of helium to two volumes of air, diffuses more rapidly than air itself. Breathing such a mixture requires less effort and an air–helium mixture or a mixture of 21 volumes of oxygen and 79 volumes of helium (Heliox) has been used in the management of stridor.

DRUG THERAPY IN ANGIONEUROTIC OEDEMA

Swelling of the face and lips, and occasionally of the larynx, occurs in angioneurotic oedema of allergic origin. Antihistamines and corticosteroids are prescribed and, if life-threatening, 1 mL/1:1000 adrenaline can be administered subcutaneously. The nonallergic type results from a serum deficiency of the C1 esterase inhibitor protein. An acute attack is treated with an intravenous injection of 36,000 units of C1 esterase inhibitor protein. This can also be given prior to surgery for prophylaxis. Long-term prophylaxis is achieved with epsilon aminocaproic acid or its derivative tranexamic acid or with androgen methyltestosterone or its derivative danazol. These stimulate the production of C1 esterase inhibitor protein.

USE OF BOTULINUM TOXINS IN SPASMODIC DYSTONIA

Botulinum is available as botulinum A toxin–haemagglutinin complex (Botox, Dysport) and botulinum B toxin (NeuroBloc). The dosage is specific to each individual preparation and therefore the product literature must be consulted prior to use. In laryngeal dystonia, localization of the involved muscles and confirmation of correct needle position can be achieved by electromyographic guidance. The effect of botulinum toxin is observed within a few days. Patients may initially have worsening of their voice, dysphagia with the potential for aspiration and occasionally airway compromise. Improvement is seen two weeks post-injections and the effects of treatment may last for three to six months.

Botulinum toxin is contraindicated in patients known to be hypersensitive to ingredients, bleeding disorders, pregnancy and lactation, concurrent or potential amino-glycoside or spectinomycin administration (neuromuscular blockade is enhanced). It should not be used in patients with generalized muscle disorders such as myasthenia gravis. No information is available on its use in patients with renal or hepatic impairment. Adrenaline should be available in case anaphylaxis occurs.

COLLAGEN INJECTION OF PARALYSED VOCAL CORDS

As a result of Teflon injection being unavailable in the UK, collagen (Contigen) is now used to medialize paralysed vocal cords. It is a purified bovine dermal gluteraldehy-decross-linked collagen and has been used in genuine stress incontinence. A skin test (0.1 mL collagen and lignocaine, injected intradermally into the volar surface of the forearm) should be carried out four weeks prior to the treatment. Many patients requiring this treatment have a short life expectancy and so a compromise with the skin test performed only a week prior to vocal cord injection is practised. A positive response is defined as erythema, induration, tenderness or swelling with or without purities, persisting for more than six hours or first appearing more than 24 hours after the injection.

The use of collagen injection is contraindicated in patients hypersensitive to the ingredients, with a positive skin test, in pregnancy and lactation and in patients with autoimmune disease or a history of multiple severe allergies.

DRUGS USED IN THYROID DISEASE INCLUDING THE MANAGEMENT OF HYPOCALCAEMIA

Thyroid hormones

The two preparations levothyroxine sodium/thyroxine sodium (Eltroxin) and liothyronine sodium (Tertroxin) are available for use in the management of hypothyroidism, diffuse nontoxic goitre, Hashimoto's thyroiditis and thyroid carcinoma. Levothyroxine sodium (thyroxine sodium) is used for maintenance therapy, usually as a single dose before breakfast. The initial dose is 50–100 μg daily increasing at two to three week intervals by 25–50 μg increments until normal metabolism is obtained. In the elderly, patients with cardiac insufficiency or severe hypothyroidism, the initial dose is 25 μg, increased by 25 μg every four weeks until normal metabolism is achieved. The usual maintenance dose is 100–200 μg, the higher dose is used to suppress T4 in thyroid carcinoma.

Liothyronine has a shorter half-life with a more rapid onset of action and shorter duration of action. Twenty micrograms of liothyronine is equivalent to 100 μg of thyroxine sodium. It can also be given intravenously. A pretherapy ECG should be performed since hypothyroidism can produce changes resembling ischaemia. The starting dose is 10–20 μg every eight hours. The usual maintenance dose is 60 μg daily in three divided doses. Sometimes it is co-administered with carbimazole to treat thyrotoxicosis. It may be used in severe hypothyroid states when a rapid response is required and is used in patients awaiting radioactive iodine scan following thyroid surgery. The latter enables patients to remain euthyroid in this interval period and patients need to stop liothyronine only two days prior to the scan.

These thyroid hormones must be used with caution in patients with hypertension, diabetes mellitus and insipidus, cardiovascular disorders, angina, the elderly, lactation, pregnancy (especially the first trimester) and in adrenal insufficiency. Interactions include sucralfate, phenylbutazone, warfarin, carbamazepine, phenytoin, rifampicin, barbiturates and propranolol. The side effects of arrythmias, insomnia, tremor, palpitations, sweating, weight loss, thyroid crisis, vomiting, diarrhoea and headache have been reported.

Drugs used in hyperthyroidism

Antithyroid drugs are used for hyperthyroidism either preoperatively or for long-term management. Carbimazole (Neo-Mercazole) is the most commonly used in the UK; propyluracil is used in patients sensitive to carbimazole. Both are thionamides containing a thiocarbamide group ($S = C–N$) that is essential for their activity. Carbimazole is rapidly converted to methimazole *in vivo*. Methimazole is available in the USA. Thioamides prevent the synthesis of thyroid hormones by competitive inhibition of I^- to I^2 by peroxidase and also block the coupling of the iodotyrosine, especially in forming diiodothyronine. More controversial is the possibility that the thionamides have immunosuppressive properties. These drugs are administered orally and accumulate within the thyroid gland. Their delayed onset of action of three to four weeks results from the need of preformed hormones to be depleted first.

The main concern with thionamides is the development of neutropenia and agranulocytosis. Carbimazole has an incidence of causing agranulocytosis in 0.1 percent of patients; propylthiouracil has an incidence of four times this (explaining the preference for carbimazole in the UK).

The Committee on Safety of Medicines recommends that:

- patients should be asked to report symptoms and signs suggestive of infection, especially sore throat;
- a white blood count should be performed if there is any clinical evidence of infection;
- the drug should be stopped promptly if there is clinical or laboratory evidence of neutropenia.

Iodine is used as an adjunct to antithyroid drugs in the preoperative management of thyrotoxicosis. An aqueous iodine oral solution (Lugol's solution) is given at a dose of 0.1–0.3 mL three times a day, taken well diluted with water or milk. Patients may develop flu-like symptoms, headache, rashes, insomnia, lacrimation, conjunctivitis, laryngitis and bronchitis. It must be used with caution in pregnancy and be avoided in lactation.

Drugs used in hypocalcaemia

Following thyroid or parathyroid surgery, patients may develop hypoparathyroidism either temporarily or permanently. Parathormone is the most important regulator of the extracellular calcium concentration. Hypocalcaemic tetany is initially managed by an initial intravenous injection of 10 mL 10 percent calcium gluconate followed by a continuous infusion of 40 mL daily or oral calcium with careful monitoring of the plasma calcium concentration. Bradycardia, arrhythmias and irritation after intravenous injection may occur as can gastrointestinal disturbances after oral administration. Failure to obtain and maintain a corrected calcium concentration within the normal range with calcium supplements alone necessitates the additional administration of a vitamin D preparation. **Figure 37.2** demonstrates the control of calcium plasma concentration by vitamin D. Vitamin D is a prohormone, metabolized to hormones that increase intestinal absorption of calcium, mobilize calcium from bone and inhibit renal excretion. The hypocalcaemia of hypoparathyroidism often requires doses of up to 2.5 mg (1,000,000 units) calciferol daily. Calcifediol is the main derivative of liver hydroxylation and this is further hydroxylated in the kidney to the potent calcitriol. The latter step is regulated by parathyroid hormone. A synthetic derivative of vitamin D commonly prescribed in hypoparathyroidism is alfacalcidiol.

TREATMENT OF REFLUX OESOPHAGITIS

Initial treatment depends on the severity of the symptoms and treatment response. Antacids and alginates alone may be used for mild symptoms. The alginates are said to form a raft on the surface of the stomach's contents to reduce reflux and protect the oesophageal mucosa.

Histamine H_2 receptor antagonists (cimetidine, famotidine, nizatidine and ranitidine) block the action of histamine on the parietal cells and reduce acid secretion. They should be used with caution in patients with liver or renal disease, in pregnancy and breastfeeding. Side effects include diarrhoea, altered liver function tests, rashes and, more rarely, hypersensitivity reactions, A V block and blood dyscrasias. Cimetidine has been reported to cause gynaecomastia and it binds to cytochrome P-450 reducing the hepatic metabolism of drugs such as warfarin.

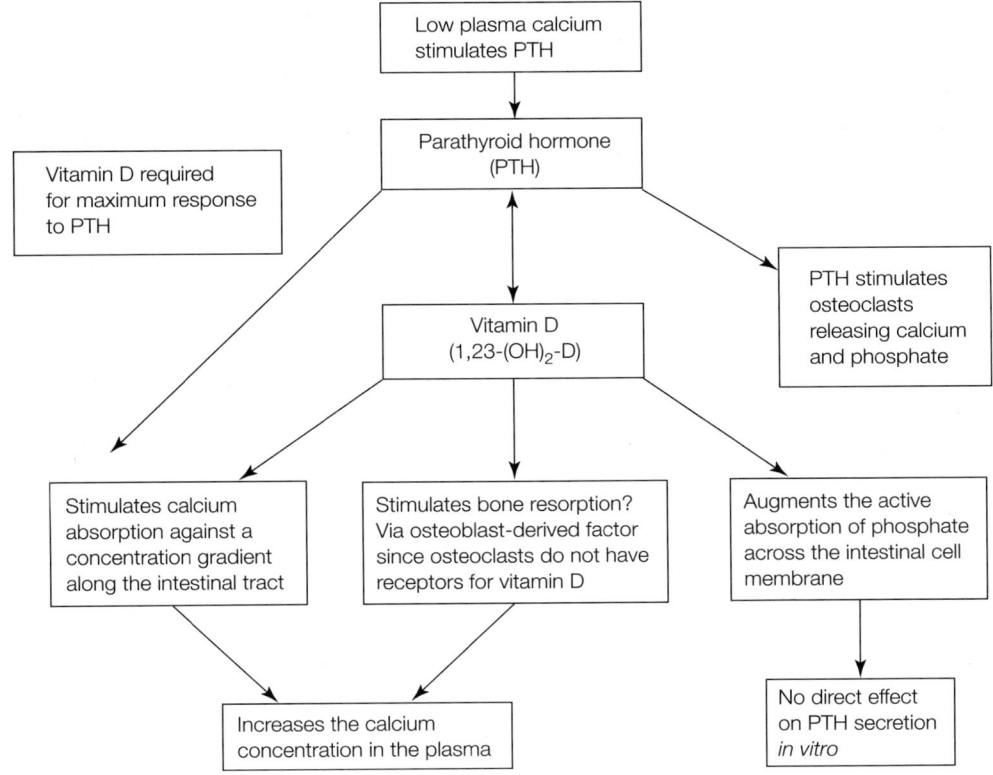

Figure 37.2 Calcium homeostasis and the role of Vitamin D.

The proton pump inhibitors (omeprazole, esomeprazole, lansoprazole, pantoprazole and rabeprazole sodium) react with sulphydryl groups in the H^+/K^+ ATPase (proton pump) responsible for the transportation of H^+ ions out of the parietal cells.

CHEMOTHERAPEUTIC AGENTS

These drugs are used either alone or in combination with surgery and/or radiotherapy with the aim to cure or palliate a cancer. They inhibit the mechanisms of cell proliferation and rely upon malignant tumours having a greater proportion of cells undergoing division than in normal proliferating cells, especially in the bone marrow, gastrointestinal mucosa and in hair follicles.

Chemotherapeutic agents are classified with respect to their site of action, as demonstrated in **Figure 37.3**.

Alkylating agents (mustine, cyclophosphamide, chlorambucil, cisplatin and busulphan) cross-link the two strands of the double helix of DNA. The antibiotics actinomycin D, doxorubicin, mitomycin, mithramycin and bleomycin interact with the DNA preventing RNA production. DNA synthesis is prevented by a group of antimetabolites (methotrexate, flurouracil, mercaptopurine and thioguanine) that prevent purine or pyrimidine synthesis. The vinca alkaloids (vincristine and vinblastine) bind to the microtubular proteins inhibiting mitosis. Glucocorticoids are included in regimes since they inhibit cell division by interfering with DNA synthesis.

Side effects such as nausea and vomiting, intestinal ulceration, diarrhoea, alopecia and bone marrow suppression are common but may become life-threatening.

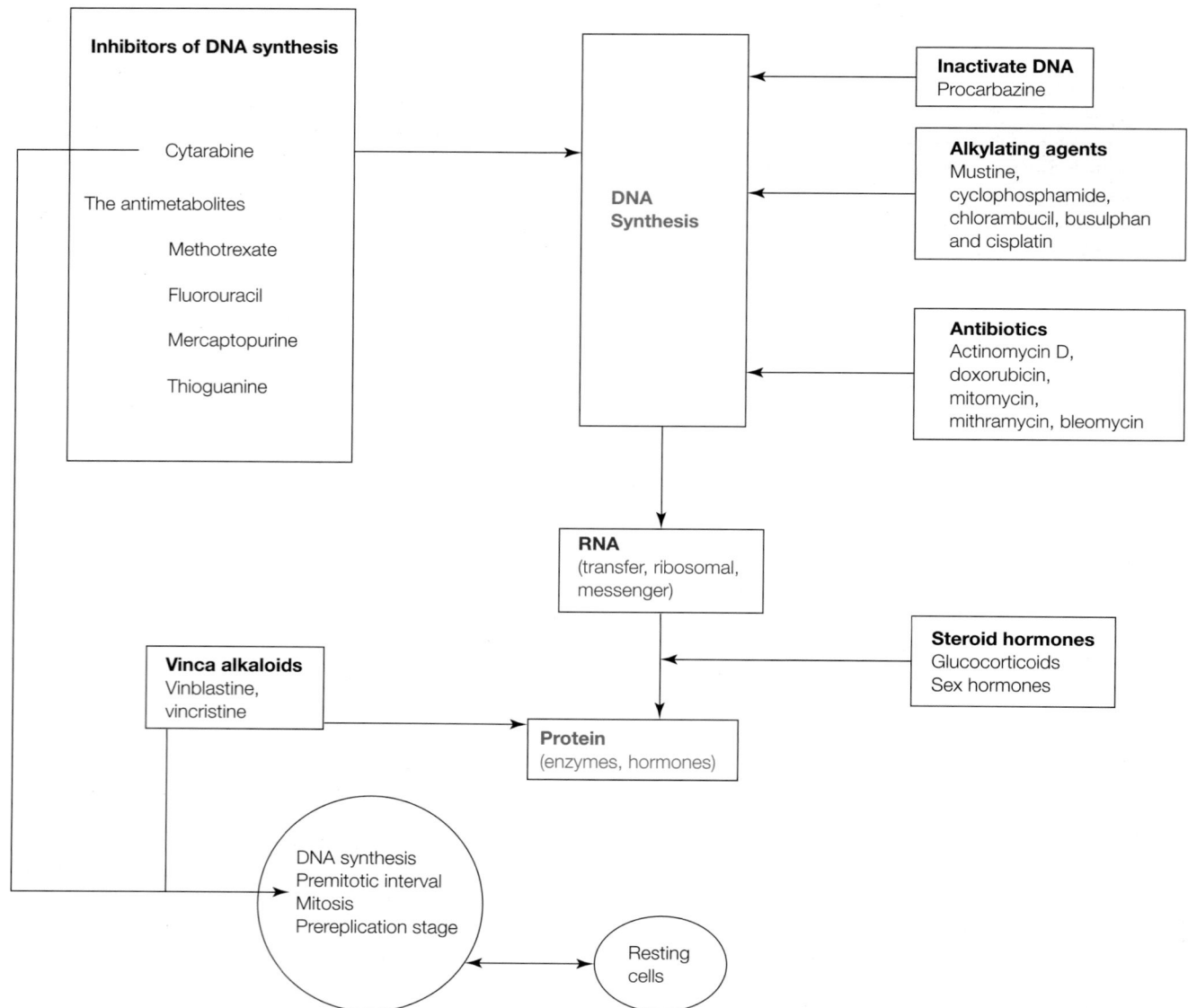

Figure 37.3   Site of action of chemotherapy.

MANAGEMENT OF FUNGATING WOUNDS

Charcoal dressings have been used to help combact malodorous fungating tumours. When this fails, topical metronidazole gel (Anabact or Metrotop) can be applied to the cleaned wound once or twice a day and covered with a nonadherent dressing. The metronidazole has antimicrobial activity against the anaerobes likely to be responsible for the odour.

Alginate dressings may stop bleeding from fungating wounds and, if moistened prior to a dressing change, the risk of bleeding at this time can be reduced.

KEY POINTS

- Perioperative antibiotics have not been shown to reduce bleeding rates after tonsillectomy but may reduce pain.
- The use of perioperative cephalosporins and metronidazole reduce the rates of fistula formation in head and neck operations.
- Pilocarpine (used in the treatment of dry mouth) is contraindicated in patients with significant respiratory/cardiovascular disease, glaucoma, pregnancy or breastfeeding.
- Rarely, carbimazole can cause agranulocytosis.
- Botulinum is available as botulinum A toxin–haemogglutinin complex and botulinum B toxin. It is important to realize that the dosage is specific to each preparation.

Best clinical practice

- ✓ The starting or stopping of anticoagulants should be in accordance with guidance from the haematologist and medical colleagues, taking into account other prescribed medications which may interact.
- ✓ Platelet counts should be monitored in patients on heparin to detect any thrombocytopenia.
- ✓ Cefuroxime and metronidazole should be given at induction and for at least three postoperative doses in head and neck procedures where the mucosa is breached.
- ✓ Heliox is easier to breath than air and buys useful time in patients with stridor, however, it is important to take additional steps to treat the underlying cause and to secure the airway.
- ✓ First-line treatment of angioneurotic oedema consists of intravenous antihistamines and steroids with nebulized or subcutaneous adrenaline.

- ✓ In order to avoid severe hypersensitivity reactions, preoperative test injections of collagen are necessary where this is used to perform vocal cord medialization.

REFERENCES

* 1. British National Formulary 42. British Medical Association and Royal Pharmaceutical Society of Great Britain. 2005, chapter 12.
2. Lee WC, Duignan MC, Walsh RM, McRae-Moore JR. An audit of prophylactic antibiotic treatment following tonsillectomy in children. *Journal of Laryngology and Otology*. 1996; **110**: 357–9.
3. Telian SA, Handler SD, Fleisher GR, Baranak CC, Wetmore RF, Potsic WP. The effect of antibiotic therapy on recovery after tonsillectomy in children. A controlled study. *Archives of Otolayngology and Head and Neck Surgery*. 1986; **112**: 610–5.
4. Violaris N, Bridger M. Prophylactic antibiotics and post laryngectomy pharyngocutaneous fistulae. *Journal of Laryngology and Otology*. 1990; **104**: 225–8.
5. Johansen LV, Overgaard J, Elbrrond O. Pharyngo-cutaneous fistulae after laryngectomy. Influence of previous radiotherapy and prophylactic metronidazole. *Cancer*. 1988; **61**: 673–8.
6. Watkinson JC, Gaze MN, Wilson JA (eds). *Stell and Maran's Head and Neck Surgery*, 4th edn. London: Arnold, 2000: 55–6.
7. Allegretto M, Selkaly H, Mackay JR. Intraoperative saline and gemcitabine irrigation improves tumour control in human squamous cell carcinoma-contaminated surgical wounds. *Journal of Otolaryngology*. 2001; **30**: 121–5.

FURTHER READING

Doctors.net.uk eFormulary.
Hardman JG, Limbird LE, Molinoff PB, Ruddon RW, Gilman AG (eds). *The pharmacological basis of therapeutics*, 9th edn. New York: McGraw-Hill.
Johnson JT, Myers EN, Thearle PB, Sigler BA, Schramm Jr. VL. Antimicrobial prophylaxis for contaminated head and neck surgery. *Laryngoscope*. 1984; **94**: 46–51.
Lambert HP, O'Grady FW (eds). *Antibiotic and chemotherapy*, 6th edn. Churchill Livingstone, 1992.
Lund W (ed.). *Pharmaceutical codex principles and practice of pharmaceutics*, 12th edn. Pharmaceutical Press, 1994.
Rang HP, Dale MM. *Pharmacology*. Churchill Livingstone, 1990.

PART 8

PERIOPERATIVE MANAGEMENT

EDITED BY MARTIN J BURTON

38 Preparation of the patient for surgery		457
Adrian Pearce		
39 Recognition and management of the difficult airway		467
Adrian Pearce		
40 Adult anaesthesia		488
Andrew D Farmery and Jaideep J Pandit		
41 Paediatric anaesthesia		507
Alistair Cranston		
42 Adult critical care		526
Gavin G Lavery		
43 Paediatric intensive care		542
Helen Allen and Rob Ross Russell		

38

Preparation of the patient for surgery

ADRIAN PEARCE

Patient pathway	457	Planning and scheduling of theatre time and	
Preoperative assessment	458	postoperative care	464
Preoperative tests	460	Preparation on the day of surgery	465
Explanation of, and written consent for, planned surgery	461	Key points	465
Explanation of, and consent for, anaesthesia	462	Best clinical practice	465
Consideration of venous thromboembolism prophylaxis	463	References	466
Consideration of special requirements	464		

SEARCH STRATEGY

This included recent publications in scientific journals, from professional bodies and the UK Department of Health, using key words such as consent, suitability for day surgery, preoperative assessment, preoperative preparation and venous thromboembolism prevention.

PATIENT PATHWAY

The patient pathway describes the 'route' taken by a patient from initial referral to regaining health. A pathway includes processes and documentation, and should be amenable to audit and external review. Generally, the surgeon makes a broad judgement at the time of seeing the patient as to whether or not the patient is fit for surgery. The in-hospital segment of the pathway begins here and, within the confines of a busy clinic, the patient requiring surgery should be placed into one of five routes:

1. day surgery;
2. inpatient, scheduled admission within a few weeks;
3. inpatient, elective surgery, fit patient;
4. planned inpatient but requiring prior medical/anaesthetic review;
5. immediate admission.

Suitability for day or ambulatory surgery

It is helpful to be able to refer to guidelines about which patients are suitable for day surgery in a particular hospital. The National Health Service Modernisation Agency published its recommendations[1] and advice on day surgery in December 2002. Traditional criteria for suitability are outlined in **Table 38.1**.

Table 38.1 Factors indicating suitability for day surgery.

Factors indicating suitability	
Patient	Access to a telephone
	Responsible adult available for the first 24 hours
	GP back-up
	Travelling distance home/day unit <1 hour
	Escort to collect
	Suitable home circumstances
Surgical	Peripheral surgery
	Duration of surgery <2 hours
	Limited blood loss
	No wound drain
	Early resumption of oral intake fluid/food
Anaesthetic	No previous or predicted serious anaesthetic problems
	Post-operative pain control with oral agents only

There are a number of conditions which either exclude day surgery or require considerable thought:

- body mass index (BMI, mass kg/height m^2) > 35–40;
- diastolic blood pressure BP > 100 mmHg, systolic > 170 mmHg;
- moderate/severe cardiorespiratory disease;
- patients on haemodialysis;
- advanced liver disease;
- some neuromuscular disorders such as myasthenia;
- opioid dependency if pain relief likely to be difficult;
- limited mouth opening or difficult intubation.

The head and neck surgical procedures recommended in the original Audit Commission basket of day surgery procedures 1990 were myringotomy with or without grommets, submucous resection, reduction of nasal fractures and operation for bat ears. A revised list was proposed by the British Association of Day Surgery (BADS)[2] in 1999 which added tonsillectomy in children. BADS also suggested a number of procedures of which it felt that 50 percent should be possible as day cases – submandibular gland excision, partial thyroidectomy, superficial parotidectomy, rhinoplasty, tympanoplasty and dentoalveolar surgery. In 2000, the Audit Commission prepared a list or basket of 25 operations suitable for day surgery which included myringotomy, tonsillectomy, submucous resection, reduction of nasal fractures and correction of bat ears. The Healthcare Commission's latest acute hospital portfolio review[3] on day surgery was published in July 2005.

Failure of the initial broad screening will direct the patient into the wrong pathway and may lead to substantial delays or frustration and patient harm. It is the pathway of medical/anaesthetic review prior to surgery that is particularly testing since it involves initial detection of problem patients, sending them for review, initiating treatment as required and waiting for optimal response before admission for surgery. It is clear that perioperative mortality is reduced by preoperative optimization, particularly of cardiac and respiratory disease.[4]

PREOPERATIVE ASSESSMENT

The general health of the patient is assessed to determine whether it can be improved, whether the risk of surgery is worthwhile and to determine the site of perioperative care and the assessment includes:

- problems with previous surgery;
- personal or family problems with anaesthesia;
- cardiovascular system, usual BP;
- respiratory system;
- other diseases;
- bleeding/clotting tendencies;
- assessment of difficulty with airway management;

- presence of significant gastro-oesophageal reflux;
- problems with venous thromboembolism;
- likelihood of postoperative nausea/vomiting (PONV);
- difficulties with pain control;
- medications, allergy, weight;
- smoking, alcohol and recreational drugs;
- current or prior drug dependency;
- home/family circumstances.

A structured form covers the relevant areas, improves data capture,[5] aids assessment and can be used by nurse specialists.

Problems detected at preadmission clinics are quite varied and need to be resolved before admission. Monoamine oxidase inhibitors present opportunities for serious drug reactions and some anaesthetists feel they should be changed, if possible, to other classes of antidepressants. Special needs patients may require intricate arrangements to attend for surgery on a particular date.

Previous problems with anaesthesia/surgery

Notable problems are a history of latex allergy, anaphylaxis to an anaesthetic agent, artificial colloid or antibiotic, difficult or failed intubation, pulmonary aspiration, post-operative nausea or vomiting, awareness, prolonged action of suxamethonium due to plasma cholinesterase deficiency, malignant hyperpyrexia or unexpected admission to a high dependency or intensive care unit. Elective surgery should be postponed until the nature of the previous incident has been fully understood.

Cardiovascular disease

Relevant conditions are systemic hypertension, valvular disease, arrythmias, angina (**Table 38.2**), myocardial infarction, ventricular failure, dyspnoea (**Table 38.3**), cerebro- or renovascular disease and presence of an

Table 38.2 New York Heart Association (NYHA) classification of angina.

Classification	
0	No angina
1	No limitation of ordinary physical activity. Angina caused by strenuous or rapid, prolonged exertion
2	Slight limitation of normal activity, e.g. angina with rapid walking, climbing stairs, emotional stress
3	Marked limitation of normal activity, e.g. angina on one flight of stairs, but comfortable at rest
4	Incapacitation with angina on mildest effort or at rest

Table 38.3 Dyspnoea grading.

Grade	
0	No dyspnoea whilst walking on level at normal pace
1	Mild, restricted by speed of walking, not distance (OK if I take my time...)
2	Moderate, specific outdoor limitation (Stop after a certain distance...)
3	Marked dyspnoea on mild indoor exertion
4	Dyspnoea at rest

Table 38.4 Clinical predictors of increased perioperative cardiac risk.

Severity	Clinical predictor
Major	
Unstable coronary syndromes	Acute or recent MI (<4 weeks)
	Unstable or severe angina
Decompensated heart failure	
Significant arryhthmias	High grade AV block
	Symptomatic ventricular with underlying heart disease
	Supraventricular with fast ventricular rate
Severe valvular disease	
Intermediate	
Mild angina	
Previous MI by history or Q waves	
Compensated or prior heart failure	
Diabetes mellitus (particularly insulin dependent)	
Renal insufficiency	
Minor	
Advanced age	
Abnormal ECG	
Rhythm other than sinus	
Low functional capacity (unable to climb one flight of stairs)	
History of stroke	
Uncontrolled systemic hypertension	

implanted pacemaker or defibrillator. The recent recommendations[6] of the American College of Cardiology/American Heart Association (ACC/AHA) for perioperative cardiovascular evaluation give the following advice.

- Hypertension with systolic blood pressure greater than or equal to 180 mmHg and diastolic greater than or equal to 110 mmHg should be controlled before surgery. Usually, an effective regimen can be achieved within several days to weeks. With urgent surgery, agents can be administered that allow effective control within hours. Beta blockers are particularly attractive agents.
- Valvular disease. Symptomatic stenotic lesions are associated with high risk and consideration should be given to valvotomy or valve replacement prior to elective surgery. Mild regurgitant valve disease appears to be tolerated well but optimal medical therapy and monitoring should be employed.
- The presence of arrythmias or cardiac conduction defects should provoke a careful evaluation for underlying cardiopulmonary disease, but the indications for antiarrhythmic therapy or pacing are identical to those in the nonoperative setting. Frequent ventricular extrasystoles are not associated with an increased risk of nonfatal myocardial infarction (MI) or cardiac death.
- Pacemakers should be checked for correct functioning, preferably by a pacemaker clinic, and implantable defibrillators should be turned off immediately before surgery and on again postoperatively.

Risk indices[7] have been developed over the years and, generally, coronary artery disease, heart failure, cerebrovascular disease, elevated creatinine, insulin-dependent diabetes and high-risk surgery have all been associated with increased perioperative cardiac morbidity. Age is another risk factor[8] with the overall 30-day mortality associated with surgery and anaesthesia rising from 2.2 percent (age 60–69) to 8.4 percent (age >90 years). The ACC/AHA recommendations place risk factors into three categories of predictors (**Table 38.4**) and provide three levels of surgery-specific risk with head and neck surgery in the intermediate group.

Areas of particular concern are the evaluation of the degree of myocardial ischaemia and function.[9]

Assessment of coronary artery disease generally involves history, an exercise ECG, followed where necessary by coronary angiography. Angiography may indicate coronary stenosis amenable to stenting or severe disease requiring coronary grafting. Medical treatment of angina is usually with aspirin or clopidogrel, nitrates, beta blockers, calcium channel antagonists or angiotensin-converting enzyme (ACE) inhibitors. Whilst patients with mild, infrequent, stable angina and normal exercise tolerance do not require any additional investigation, it is generally useful to seek cardiological opinion preoperatively for:

- patients with new onset angina who are not on treatment or under review;
- patients with increasing frequency of angina;
- patients with NYHA class 3 or 4 angina.

Heart failure is a serious condition and generally should be evaluated in all patients before surgery. Relevant history is of limited exercise tolerance, dyspnoea, orthopnoea, paroxysmal nocturnal dyspnoea and ankle oedema. Medical therapy involves frusemide, spirono-lactone, ACE inhibitors and good control of hypertension or arrhythmias. The best investigation is echocardiography which will demonstrate size of chambers, wall thickness, wall motion, valve function and allow an estimate of ejection fraction. Ejection fraction refers to the proportion of left ventricular blood volume ejected during ventricular contraction. The normal value is 60–65 percent and values below 35–40 percent are significantly reduced and require a raised level of perioperative cardiovascular monitoring. Other investigations look at myocardial perfusion during stress; poorly perfused areas during stress may return to normal on resting (indicating ischaemia) or remain poorly perfused (infarction).

Patients with valvular disease, prosthetic valves or cardiomyopathy are at risk of bacterial endocarditis and should receive antibiotic prophylaxis. The current recommendation for most head and neck surgery under general anaesthesia is for amoxycillin 1 g and gentamicin 120 mg intravenously at induction.

Patients with mechanical prosthetic valves, or with some cardiomyopathies or atrial fibrillation, may be anticoagulated with warfarin. These patients require admission three to four days before surgery so that warfarin may be discontinued and anticoagulation continued with a heparin infusion at an initial rate of 1000 IU/hour adjusted according to the activated partial thromboplastin time (APTT). Aspirin therapy affects platelet function irreversibly and is a contraindication to surgery if small degrees of platelet dysfunction are unacceptable (e.g. neurosurgery). The drug should be stopped, if required, for one month prior to surgery.

Respiratory disease

Common conditions are chronic bronchitis, emphysema, chronic obstructive airway disease and asthma. Generally, a patient with known, mild, stable disease under review by the GP or respiratory department will not need special preoperative assessment. Medical therapy involves inhaled or oral bronchodilators, inhaled or oral steroids, inhaled anticholinergic agents and inhaled agents influencing local immune function. The disease severity can be gauged by history of exercise capability, number of attacks, requirement for admission to hospital or ITU, need for ventilation, requirement for home support or domiciliary oxygen, chest x-ray and respiratory function testing. Asthmatic patients often know their normal peak flow measurement and this is a simple test to carry out. A respiratory physician and anaesthetic review should be sought for patients with respiratory disease who:

- have limited exercise capability;
- have required hospital admission, particularly ventilation;
- are nearly housebound by respiratory symptoms;
- have deteriorating symptoms or signs;
- require home oxygen therapy.

All patients should be advised to stop smoking.

PREOPERATIVE TESTS

Recommendations come from the American Society of Anesthesiologists (ASA) Task Force[10] on preanesthesia evaluation and the Association of Anaesthetists of Great Britain and Ireland.[11] Preoperative tests may be routine (a test ordered in the absence of specific clinical indication or purpose) or indicated (ordered for a specific clinical indication or purpose). A consensus view has been reached that preoperative tests may be ordered on a selective basis for purposes of guiding or optimizing perioperative management, but should not be ordered routinely. The Association of Anaesthetists of Great Britain and Ireland states that 'Blanket routine preoperative investigations are inefficient, expensive and unnecessary'.

Written guidelines are, therefore, hospital or department-based and should be discussed during induction of new department members. All patients should undergo 'dipstick' urinalysis for blood, glucose and protein, and pregnancy testing should be offered to relevant patients. Audiometry should be undertaken on all patients undergoing surgery on the middle ear, and vocal cord function visualized when surgery might damage the recurrent laryngeal nerve. Reasonable guidelines for preoperative tests in adult patients undergoing head and neck surgery are:

- haemoglobin in all females, males aged over 40 years and in any patient in whom blood grouping will be undertaken;
- urea and electrolytes in all patients over 40 years or when indicated by disease process or medication;
- clotting studies when indicated by history;
- sickle cell testing in all patients of African or Afro-Caribbean origin;
- pregnancy testing when pregnancy is possible;
- blood grouping (group and save) in patients with a normal preoperative haemoglobin and an anticipated blood loss of 10–15 percent blood volume (blood volume 70 mL/kg in adult), and all patients who have had a previous blood transfusion in case of the presence of antibodies;
- blood grouping and cross-matching in all patients with an expected blood loss in excess of 15 percent blood volume (>750 mL in the average adult) or at significant risk of sudden severe haemorrhage. The number of blood units requested for a particular surgical procedure should follow written guidelines drawn up in consultation with the Hospital Transfusion Committee;

- electrocardiography in any patient with cardiovascular disease or in asymptomatic patients aged over 60–70 years;
- chest x-ray in patients with signs or symptoms of cardiac, respiratory or multisystem disease referable to the chest.

National Institute for Clinical Excellence guidelines on preoperative tests

The National Institute for Clinical Excellence (NICE)[12] produced its recommendations for the use of routine preoperative tests for elective surgery in June 2003. These are guidelines arising from expert opinion using a consensus development process and the clinical experience of the guideline development group. Specific recommendations are made according to:

- grade of surgery 1–4 (minor, intermediate, major, major+);
- ASA status 1–3 (**Table 38.5**);
- cardiovascular, respiratory or renal comorbidity;
- age of patient.

Recommendations are made for chest x-ray, ECG, full blood count, haemostasis, renal function, random glucose, urine analysis, blood gases, lung function, sickle cell and pregnancy testing. A wall-chart or booklet shows individual recommendations as green (test recommended), red (test not recommended) and yellow (consider this test). **Table 38.6** refers to a patient undergoing intermediate or grade 2 surgery (e.g. tonsillectomy) who is ASA 2 with co-morbidity from cardiovascular disease (perhaps well-controlled, mild hypertension). **Table 38.7** refers to a patient undergoing major or grade 3 surgery (e.g. thyroidectomy) who is classed as ASA 3 with co-morbidity from cardiovascular disease. Unfortunately, many recommendations are 'yellow' and individual hospitals or departments are still required to produce their own guidelines. Without these, unnecessary tests will continue to be ordered 'just in case' they are required by the anaesthetist or surgeon. Staff undertaking clinical preoperative assessments should discuss with patients which tests are recommended, what they involve and the possible implications of an abnormal result. Doctors or nurses ordering the tests should write in the notes that they have discussed the recommended tests and their implications with the patient, who should be informed of the results of the tests.

EXPLANATION OF, AND WRITTEN CONSENT FOR, PLANNED SURGERY

Valid consent to treatment is central in all forms of health care, from providing personal care to undertaking major surgery. In the UK, in accordance with the NHS Plan, the Department of Health instituted substantial changes in consent in 2001. The seminal document is 'Good practice in consent implementation guide' available on www.doh.gov.uk/consent.

Consent is a patient's agreement for a health professional to provide care. Seeking consent indicates the

Table 38.5 Physical status grading of American Society of Anesthesiologists.

Grade	Physical status
Grade 1	Normal healthy patient without any clinically important co-morbidity
Grade 2	Patient with a mild systemic disease
Grade 3	Patient with one (or more) severe systemic disease which does not present a constant threat to life
Grade 4	Patient with systemic disease processes which present a constant threat to life
Grade 5	Patient not expected to survive more than 24 hours

Table 38.6 Tests recommended by NICE for intermediate surgery in ASA 2 patient with cardiovascular co-morbidity.

Test	Age (years)			
	≥16 to <40	≥40 to <60	≥60 to <80	≥80
Chest x-ray	?	?	?	?
ECG	Yes	Yes	Yes	Yes
Full blood count	?	?	?	?
Haemostasis	No	No	No	No
Renal function	?	?	Yes	Yes
Random glucose	No	No	No	No
Urine analysis	?	?	?	?
Blood gases	No	No	No	No
Lung function	No	No	No	No

?, local decision required.

Table 38.7 Tests recommended by NICE for major surgery in ASA 3 patient with cardiovascular co-morbidity.

Test	Age (years)			
	≥16 to <40	≥40 to <60	≥60 to <80	≥80
Chest x-ray	?	?	?	?
ECG	Yes	Yes	Yes	Yes
Full blood count	Yes	Yes	Yes	Yes
Haemostasis	?	?	?	?
Renal function	Yes	Yes	Yes	Yes
Random glucose	No	No	No	No
Urine analysis	?	?	?	?
Blood gases	?	?	?	?
Lung function	No	No	No	No

?, local decision required.

whole process of information provision, discussion and decision-making. When a patient formally gives their consent to a particular intervention, this is only the end point of the consent process.

Patients may indicate consent nonverbally (for example by presenting their ear for examination in outpatients), orally or in writing. For the consent to be valid, the patient must:

• be competent to take the particular decision:
• have received sufficient information to take it;
• not be acting under duress.

When an adult patient lacks the mental capacity (either temporarily or permanently) to give or withhold consent for themselves, no one else can give consent on their behalf.

It is good practice to gain written consent if:

• the treatment or procedure is complex or involves significant risks;
• the procedure involves general/regional anaesthesia or sedation;
• providing clinical care is not the primary purpose of the procedure;
• there may be significant consequences for the patient's employment, social or personal life;
• the treatment is part of an approved project or programme of research.

In the UK, standard forms are used in all NHS hospitals. Four differing forms are available to cover:

1. adult patients undergoing surgery who are competent to consent;
2. parental agreement for a child or young person;
3. adult patients undergoing treatment or procedures where the patient is expected to remain alert and an anaesthetist is not involved
4. when an adult patient is unable to consent.

For an adult patient, the consent process begins with the provision of information to the patient and discussion of treatment options and oral agreement may be reached that particular surgery is appropriate. When written consent is appropriate, the patient should be familiar with the contents of their consent form before they arrive for the procedure and should have received a copy of the page documenting the decision-making process. They may be invited to sign the form at any appropriate time before the procedure – in outpatients, preadmission clinic or when they arrive for treatment. A member of the health care team must check immediately before treatment that the patient has no concerns and that their condition has not changed. Patients must not be under duress to give valid consent and patients should not be expected to give consent when already changed for theatre or, indeed, in the anaesthetic room.

EXPLANATION OF, AND CONSENT FOR, ANAESTHESIA

It is the duty of the anaesthetist to gain consent for anaesthesia, but specific written consent for anaesthesia is not required in the UK. Each patient should receive a general leaflet about anaesthesia in outpatients. This allows the patient time to consider the issues surrounding provision of anaesthesia. Discussion between the anaesthetist and patient addresses (as relevant):

• previous anaesthetic problems;
• likely difficulties or risks in provision of anaesthesia for the planned surgery;
• local versus general anaesthesia;
• general conduct of general anaesthesia and recovery;
• intravenous fluids;
• blood transfusion;
• pain relief;
• control of nausea/vomiting;

- urinary catheterization;
- nasogastric tube insertion;
- placement of arterial and central venous lines.

Patient anxieties are generally to do with death, brain damage, awareness, loss of control, memory loss, pain control, nausea or vomiting and needle insertion.[13] Premedication with either an anxiolytic or analgesic is discussed and written as required. In the UK it is possible that the preoperative anaesthetic visit will occur only minutes before planned surgery but a better arrangement exists in France. Here, all patients must be seen in an outpatient anaesthetic clinic before surgery. This gives time for proper preoperative assessment, preoperative preparation and discussion of anaesthetic options.

Acute pain management plans

Individual plans for postoperative pain management should be formulated with the patient in the preoperative period. In the intraoperative period virtually all patients undergoing head and neck surgery receive intravenous opioids and, where possible, incisions should be infiltrated with a long-acting local anaesthetic such as bupivacaine 0.5 percent (maximum dosage 2 mg/kg) before the end of surgery. Early postoperative pain may be treated by intravenous opioid, often morphine in 2 mg increments every five minutes to a total of 10 mg, administered by the recovery nurse or doctor. Simple oral analgesia in adults, such as paracetamol 1 g six hourly and ibuprofen 400 mg six hourly, should be prescribed regularly. If oral administration is not possible, drugs may be given parenterally, by suppository or via a nasogastric tube. Initiation of analgesia by suppository (such as diclofenac 100 mg) towards the end of surgery is common, provided that the patient has consented to this.

More severe pain may be treated in the ward by regular dihydrocodeine 30 mg six hourly or morphine given by the oral or intramuscular route. If it is expected that the patient will require regular morphine, this is best given by patient-controlled analgesia (PCA) in which the patient receives a small dose of morphine intravenously on pressing a button. Preoperative instruction in the use of a PCA machine may be given by the anaesthetist, ward nurse or member of the acute pain team. The acute pain team consists usually of nurses, doctors and pharmacists and provides the lead in the generation of acute pain guidelines and management. The expertise of the acute pain team should be sought preoperatively in any patient in whom postoperative pain is likely to be difficult to manage, particularly those on preoperative opioids for medical or nonmedical reasons. Epidural analgesia is not suitable for surgery in the head and neck territory, but is useful to cover abdominal surgery when this is required to mobilize the bowel for major reconstructions. Acute pain guidelines usually detail the analgesic solution to be used via the epidural route and the appropriate level of postoperative care.

CONSIDERATION OF VENOUS THROMBOEMBOLISM PROPHYLAXIS

Venous thromboembolism (VTE) is one complication among hospital inpatients and contributes to longer hospital stays, morbidity and mortality. Recent recommendations arise from the Seventh ACCP Conference on Antithrombotic and Thrombolytic Therapy[14] in 2004. Risk factors and conditions predisposing to VTE are:

- history of previous VTE;
- prolonged immobility or confinement to bed;
- lower limb, pelvic or abdominal operations;
- trauma particularly of pelvis or acute spinal injury;
- obesity;
- major medical illnesses, such as MI, ischaemic stroke, cardiac failure and acute respiratory failure;
- oestrogen use, such as oral contraception or hormone replacement therapy;
- cancer, especially metastatic adenocarcinoma
- age >40 years;
- acquired hypercoaguable states, such as lupus anticoagulant and antiphospholipid antibodies, hyperhomocysteinaemia, dysfibrinogenaemia and myeloproliferative disorders;
- inherited hypercoaguable states, such as activated protein C resistance, protein C or S deficiency, antithrombin deficiency or prothrombin gene mutation.

All patients undergoing surgery should be placed in a risk stratification for VTE, with particular importance attached to identifying the high- and very high-risk patient. Expert haematological assessment is required when acquired or inherited hypercoaguable states are suspected.

- **Low risk.** Uncomplicated surgery in patients aged <40 years with minimal immobility postoperatively and no risk factors.
- **Moderate risk.** Any surgery in patients aged 40–60 years, major surgery in patients <40 years and no other risk factors, minor surgery with one or more risk factors.
- **High risk.** Major surgery in patients >60 years, major surgery in patients aged 40–60 years with one or more risk factors.
- **Very high risk.** Major surgery in patients >40 years with previous VTE, cancer or known hypercoaguable state.

An appropriate strategy for the prevention of VTE should be formulated for each patient and written guidelines should exist in each department. The preventative measures which have been shown to reduce the incidence of VTE are early mobilization, compression elastic stockings, pneumatic intermittent calf compression which provides rhythmic external compression of the lower limb or calf to a pressure of 35–40 mmHg for ten seconds every minute, low-dose unfractionated heparin (LDUH) and low molecular weight heparin (LMWH). LMWH has the advantages over LDUH of once daily dosage and lower incidence of heparin-induced thrombocytopenia, but is more expensive. Comparative studies of LDUH and LMWH have shown a broadly similar efficacy but comparisons are hampered by the dosage and timing. LDUH is usually given as 5000 units 8–12 hourly and LMWH may be given in low doses (<3400 anti-Xa IU daily) or high doses (>3400 antiXa IU daily). High-dose LMWH appears to be associated with more surgical bleeding problems.

Unfortunately, little data exist on preventative measures in head and neck patients exclusively and data appropriate to groups may not benefit an individual patient. Surgery itself in the head and neck territory is considered low risk and there is the additional perceived problem of heparin causing minor, but surgically troubling, bleeding. This may cause difficulty during microscopic surgery or surgery near the skull base or brain, or result in an increase in incidence of wound haematoma.

A reasonable strategy for VTE prophylaxis in head and neck patients might be:

- **Low risk patients.** No specific prophylaxis other than early ambulation.
- **Moderate risk patients.** Either LMWH <3400 U daily, LDUH 12 hourly, compression elastic stockings or intermittent pneumatic compression. Each alone is better than no prophylaxis.
- **High risk patients.** LDUH eight hourly, or LMWH >3400 U daily plus compression stockings, or compression stockings and intermittent calf compression if anticoagulation considered inadvisable.
- **Very high risk.** LDUH eight hourly or LMWH >3400 U daily plus compression stockings and intermittent pneumatic compression.

CONSIDERATION OF SPECIAL REQUIREMENTS

Patients undergoing surgery in the head and neck region may lose, temporarily or permanently, sensation or motor activity in the distribution of the cranial nerves. Particularly important from a patient's perspective are the loss of communication arising from impairment of hearing, speech or vision, disabling sensation such as vertigo through vestibular dysfunction or alteration to normal activity such as eating, drinking or breathing. Patients who will be unable to speak postoperatively require a plan for communication, such as a bell to attract attention, prepared cards indicating common needs, pen and paper or the use of hand-signals. For those patients undergoing laryngectomy, the preoperative period is the appropriate time to discuss voice reconstruction options and for the patient to meet the speech therapist and another patient who has undergone, and recovered from, similar surgery.

The disease process or nature of surgery may interfere with nutrition. Failure of adequate nutrition may lead to morbidity and mortality through infection, failure of wound healing and gross catabolism. Nutrition may be provided orally, through a nasogastric tube, via a percutaneous or open gastrostomy, via an open feeding jejunostomy or intravenously. The enteral route is superior in all regards to the intravenous route and should be used whenever possible. Poorly nourished patients require preoperative supplementation and there is some evidence that a week of enteral (but not parenteral) nutrition improves outcome. A feeding gastrostomy or jejunostomy can be placed in a planned manner at the time of extensive surgery to cover postoperative feeding.

Patients in whom the small or large bowel is required for surgical reconstruction of the upper GI tract may require bowel preparation with a low residue diet or intravenous fluids and laxatives.

PLANNING AND SCHEDULING OF THEATRE TIME AND POSTOPERATIVE CARE

The Confidential Enquiry into Postoperative Deaths (CEPOD)[15] process identifies patients as being **elective** when the surgery can be planned for the convenience of the patient and surgeon, **scheduled** when admission will be prioritized within a few weeks of initial referral, **urgent** indicating an unplanned admission where resuscitation can be achieved before theatre and **emergency** in which surgery is required coexistent with resuscitation. A better scheme starts by indicating whether the patient is listed or unlisted, since the classification of CEPOD urgent or emergency is not always understood or useful.

The operating theatre list should be presented to theatre reception in the manner required within that hospital. Generally, a theatre list should contain the patients' name, hospital number, date of birth or age and planned surgery. The side of surgery should be recorded as left or right. Some hospitals use the Office for Population Censuses and Surveys (OPCS) or Read codes. The first patients on a list are generally children in ascending age, or shorter operations before longer ones or patients with diseases such as diabetes. Patients with latex allergy must be scheduled first to allow correct preparation of the operating theatre. Scheduling problems should be resolved by discussion between the surgeon, anaesthetist and theatre sister. Some patients will require a planned extended stay in Recovery, or admission to HDU/ITU. Generally, this will be for longer, major procedures, when ventilation is required postoperatively, when the airway is at risk or if extended patient monitoring is required for cardiorespiratory disease. The bed should be booked as soon as surgery is planned for a particular date. Patients should know about the plans for the immediate recovery period (which may change) and may benefit from seeing the HDU/ITU preoperatively or talking to a nurse from the unit.

PREPARATION ON THE DAY OF SURGERY

It should be possible to estimate a provisional time of surgery and preparation aims to make certain that the patient is ready when the theatre calls for the patient. Most units use a form with tick boxes to cover the areas of baseline blood pressure, heart rate, weight, allergies, false or capped teeth, patient's wrist band present, consent form signed, notes and x-rays present, investigations present, blood cross-matched, time of last oral intake and details of premedication. The side and site of surgery should be indicated with an indelible marker by the surgeon who reviews the patient on the day.

Oral intake

Patients should not eat or drink prior to anaesthesia to reduce the risk of aspiration of gastric contents. The Association of Anaesthetists of Great Britain and Ireland recommends the following fasting periods which are now generally accepted:[16]

- six hours for solid food, infant formula or other milk;
- four hours for breast milk;
- two hours for clear nonparticulate and noncarbonated fluids.

There is no evidence that safety is improved by extending these fasting times. Some patients should not be left for long periods without fluids and consideration should be given to intravenous fluid administration. These include elderly or sick patients, children, those undergoing bowel preparation and breastfeeding mothers.

Medication

Generally, all regular medication should be given on the day of surgery unless specifically crossed off by the anaesthetist or surgeon. It is particularly important to give cardiac medication for angina, hypertension or arrythmia. Diuretics are often omitted. Diabetic medication needs to be specifically addressed by the anaesthetist but generally tablets are not given on the morning of surgery and insulin given in either a reduced dosage subcutaneously with a covering intravenous infusion of 5 percent dextrose, or as a sliding scale. In a sliding scale the

patient receives a constant dextrose infusion such as dextrose 4 percent with saline 0.18 percent (with potassium 20 mmol in 1000 mL bag) at 100 mL/h and an insulin infusion adjusted one to two hourly according to blood glucose. There is some evidence that tight control of glucose to a range of 4–6 mmol/L is beneficial. Some oral medication, for example nitrates, may be prescribed as a transdermal preparation. Patients on oral steroids require an additional dose parenterally, either 50 mg hydrocortisone intravenously 8–12 hourly or an infusion of 150–200 mg/24 h.

KEY POINTS

- Consider day surgery where possible.
- Assess the risk of operation/anaesthesia.
- Moderate or severe cardiorespiratory disease requires medical/anaesthetic review.
- Routine preoperative tests are expensive and unnecessary.
- Valid, written consent required for most surgery.
- Consider venous thromboembolism prevention.
- Book HDU/ITU bed (if required) as soon as date of surgery known.
- Patients presenting for ENT surgery may be of either gender and of any age, with general health at any point between fit and moribund, for elective, scheduled or emergency surgery lasting between a few minutes and many hours. Perioperative care may need to be appropriate for minor surgery such as insertion of grommets as a day case or extensive head and neck surgery requiring intensive care.

Best clinical practice

✓ The patient should be directed into the correct pathway as soon as surgery is contemplated, and sufficient oral and written information given to inform the patient and initiate the consent process.
✓ Attendance at a preadmission clinic a few weeks before surgery allows a full history and examination to be taken, leading to the identification of any medical, anaesthetic or personal problems. This is particularly important when the interval between scheduling and admission for surgery is more than a few months.
✓ The requirement for specific preoperative blood tests, investigations and blood cross-matching should be agreed by the whole team and produced in a written

form which is available to doctors and nurses involved in preoperative preparation.

✓ Preoperative assessment of the problem patient by an anaesthetist, preferably the one who will be involved, is valuable and should be easy to arrange.

✓ Preoperative tests taken at preadmission should be reviewed before the admission for surgery so that abnormalities can either be treated in time or the patient rescheduled.

✓ Notify the acute pain team of any patient in whom postoperative pain control is likely to be difficult, particularly those with opioid dependency or on a drug withdrawal programme.

REFERENCES

1. www.archive.modern.nhs.uk/scripts/ default.asp?site_id=28&tid=8100
2. BADS. *BADS Directory of procedures.* London: BADS, 2006.
3. www.healthcarecommission.org.uk/ serviceproviderinformation/reviewsandinspections/ acutehospitalportfoliohomepage.cfm
4. Prause G, Ratzenhofer-Komenda B, Smolle-Juettner F, Krenn H, Pojer H, Toller W *et al.* Operations on patients deemed "unfit for operation and anaesthesia": what are the consequences? *Acta Anaesthesiology Scandinavica.* 1998; **42**: 316–22.
5. Ausset S, Bouaziz H, Brosseau M, Kinirons B, Benhamou D. Improvement of information gained from the pre-anaesthetic visit through a quality assurance programme. *British Journal of Anaesthesia.* 2002; **88**: 280–3.
* 6. ACC/AHA guideline update for perioperative cardiovascular evaluation for non-cardiac surgery – executive summary. *Anesthesia Analgesia.* 2002; **94**: 1052–64.
7. Goldman L, Caldera DL, Nussbaum SR. Multifactorial index of cardiac risk in non-cardiac surgical procedures. *New England Journal Medicine.* 1977; **297**: 845–50.
8. Jin F, Chung F. Minimizing perioperative adverse events in the elderly. *British Journal of Anaesthesia.* 2001; **87**: 608–24.
* 9. Mangano DT. Assessment of the patient with cardiac disease. An anesthesiologist's paradigm. *Anesthesiology.* 1999; **91**: 1521–6.
* 10. American Society of Anesthesiologists Task Force on Preanesthesia Evaluation. Practice advisory for preanesthesia evaluation. *Anesthesiology.* 2002; **96**: 485–96.
11. Preoperative assessment – the role of the anaesthetist. The Association of Anaesthetists of Great Britain and Ireland, November 2001. www.aagbi.org
12. National Institute for Clinical Excellence, MidCity Place, 71 High Holborn, London WC1 V 6NA or www.nice.org.uk
13. Matthey P, Finucane BT, Finegan BA. The attitude of the general public towards preoperative assessment and risks associated with general anaesthesia. *Canadian Journal of Anaesthesia.* 2001; **48**: 333–9.
* 14. Geerts WH, Pineo GF, Heit JA, Bergqvist D, Lassen MR, Colwell CW *et al.* Prevention of venous thromboembolism: the seventh ACCP conference on antithrombotic and thrombolytic therapy. *Chest.* 2004; **126**: 338–400.
15. www.ncepod.org.uk
16. Soreide E, Eriksson LI, Hirlekar G, Eriksson H, Henneberg SW, Sandin R *et al.* Preoperative fasting guidelines: an update. *Acta Anaesthesiologica Scandinavica.* 2005; **49**: 1041–7.

39

Recognition and management of the difficult airway

ADRIAN PEARCE

Definitions	467	Obstructed airway	477
Prevalence	468	Extubation and recovery	483
Evaluation	468	Follow-up	484
Prediction of difficulty	471	Key points	485
Strategy	472	Best clinical practice	485
Alternative techniques for tracheal intubation	473	Deficiencies in current knowledge and areas for future	
Role of the classic LM	475	research	485
Failed ventilation and emergency cricothyrotomy	476	References	486

SEARCH STRATEGY

The data in this chapter are supported by a PubMed search using the key words difficult intubation, difficult airway, obstructed airway.

DEFINITIONS

The difficult airway is the clinical situation in which a practitioner experiences difficulty with adequate maintenance and/or protection of the airway. Three airway devices are in common use – the face mask, laryngeal mask and tracheal tube – and each offers a different level of airway protection and maintenance. A cuffed tracheal tube offers the highest level and for this reason is prominent in airway management plans in head and neck surgery.

Two broad airway problems can be defined, difficult ventilation and difficult intubation. Difficult mask ventilation was defined by the American Society of Anesthesiologists (ASA)[1] as the inability to maintain the oxygen saturations above 90 percent by face mask inflation with 100 percent inspired oxygen or to reverse signs of inadequate ventilation. Oxygen stores in the body are exhausted within a few minutes and difficult or failed ventilation will rapidly result in morbidity or mortality

from hypoxaemia. Difficult intubation was defined by the ASA as the inability to complete tracheal intubation within three attempts at direct laryngoscopy or within ten minutes. Provided that face mask ventilation is possible, failed tracheal intubation by itself should not result in hypoxaemia unless the failure of airway protection leads to gross airway soiling from gastric contents or blood. Unfortunately, failed tracheal intubation is, in clinical practice, associated with the problems of unrecognized oesophageal intubation, damage to the airway and hypoxaemia.

Difficult intubation may be defined by the number of attempts at direct laryngoscopy or time to achieve intubation, but also by the view of the laryngeal structures seen at direct laryngoscopy. Cormack and Lehane[2] described the commonly used classification of the best view of laryngeal structures seen at direct laryngoscopy. Grade 1 is visualization of the entire laryngeal aperture, grade II is visualization of the posterior portion of the laryngeal aperture, grade III is visualization of the epiglottis only and grade IV is no view of any laryngeal structures. Difficult laryngoscopy (and therefore difficult intubation) indicates that it is not possible to see any portion of the vocal cords (grade III/IV) after multiple attempts at conventional direct laryngoscopy.[3] A final method of defining difficult intubation is through the need for specialized equipment, often taken as requiring an intubation device other than the standard Macintosh or straight-blade laryngoscope. This has some practical significance because when an anaesthetist fails to intubate by direct laryngoscopy (equipment present in each operating theatre) it is often necessary to use equipment from a difficult intubation trolley located centrally in a theatre complex.

Difficult direct laryngoscopy is only one cause of difficulty with intubation. It may be easy to visualize the larynx but intubation is unsuccessful because the larynx, subglottis or trachea are abnormally narrowed or distorted.

PREVALENCE

Both difficult intubation and difficult ventilation are uncommon. The prevalence of Cormack and Lehane laryngoscopic grade III is 1.5 percent in the general population. Requiring more than three attempts at direct laryngoscopy occurs in approximately 0.4 percent patients and the average anaesthetist will abandon intubation in approximately 1:2500 general surgical patients. In 1200 consecutive ENT and general surgical patients the overall prevalence of difficult intubation (defined as requiring specialist equipment) was 4.2 percent.[4] The highest prevalence was 12.3 percent in ENT cancer surgery, 3.5 percent in ENT noncancer surgery and 2.0 percent in general surgical patients. This confirms the clinical impression that difficult intubation is more common in patients undergoing head and neck surgery, particularly in those patients following extensive surgery, flap reconstruction and postoperative radiotherapy or with an obstructed airway. [**]

It is difficult to know the precise prevalence of difficult face mask ventilation. Catastrophic failure leading to serious morbidity or mortality is generally quoted as 1:10,000–1:100,00. However, in any large series, a number of problem patients are identified preoperatively and do not receive a general anaesthetic. A North American study involved 18,500 patients of whom 18,200 were intubated under general anaesthesia with 1.8 percent requiring more than two attempts at direct laryngoscopy and no patient being impossible to mask ventilate.[5] Approximately 300 patients underwent awake intubation and it is this group of patients that is likely to contain those who would have proved difficult to ventilate if anaesthetized. A study of 1502 patients determined a prevalence of difficult mask ventilation of 5 percent but the definition used was that the anaesthetist considered the difficulty was clinically

relevant and could have led to potential problems if mask ventilation had to be maintained for a longer period.[6]

EVALUATION

The aim of airway management is to adequately maintain and protect the airway by use of the face mask, laryngeal mask or tracheal intubation, and preoperative evaluation seeks to initially determine which airway device is required and whether there will be any difficulties in the use or insertion of it. The face mask provides no airway protection and is little used in anaesthesia for head and neck surgery, except for operations such as insertion of grommets. The decision as to whether to use the laryngeal mask or tracheal intubation is taken after considering such factors as the length of surgery, surgical access, requirement for positive pressure ventilation and risk of airway soiling from either blood, pus, cerebrospinal fluid or gastric contents.

The airway may be evaluated according to the scheme outlined in **Table 39.1**.

History

The anaesthetic or hospital notes may indicate previously encountered difficulty with airway management. The patient may pass on verbal or written information from a previous anaesthetist that they are difficult, or difficulty may be inferred from a history of displaced front teeth, bruised lips, excessive sore throat or an unexpected stay in ITU. Past surgery or radiotherapy, or the current surgical condition, may be relevant if it affects the head, neck or mediastinum. A number of medical conditions, such as rheumatoid arthritis, obstructive sleep apnoea and acromegaly, have some association with difficult airway management. In a prospective study of 128 patients with acromegaly, laryngoscopy was difficult (laryngoscopic view grade III) in 10 percent.[7] This indicates that the prevalence is six to eight times higher than in normal patients but 90 percent of acromegalics are still easy to intubate. [**] There are a number of congenital

Table 39.1 Scheme for evaluation of the airway.

Evaluation	
History	Previous airway difficulty
	Previous surgery
	Current surgical condition
	Current medical condition
Examination	General
	Specific predictive tests
Investigations	MR imaging
	CT imaging
	Flow-volume loop
	Flexible nasendoscopy

conditions, such as Treacher-Collins and Pierre-Robin, in which airway management, particularly intubation, is often difficult. **Figure 39.1** illustrates a patient with Hunter's syndrome in which abnormal mucopolysaccharide is deposited in the tissues. Characteristically, he was difficult to intubate for a tonsillectomy to alleviate obstructive sleep apnoea and required an emergency tracheostomy in the recovery period. He is pictured in his late teens when his original standard tracheostomy tube had been replaced by one designed to circumvent lower tracheal and carinal deposits. This T-Y silastic stent passes from just below the vocal cords into each main bronchus (an inverted Y shape) with a limb passing out through the tracheostomy (the T component).

Examination

General examination of the patient looks for the features in the following list and the practitioner may be alerted to possible difficulties by various findings:

- trauma, burn, swelling, infection, scarring, haematoma of the mouth, tongue, larynx, trachea or neck;
- large tongue, receding jaw, high-arched palate, prominent upper incisors, short thick neck, large breasts, microstomia, fixed larynx, impalpable

cricothyroid membrane, limited mouth opening, limited head/neck movements;
- voice change, shortness of breath, stridor, inability to lie down.

A number of these factors, such as the appreciation of a short neck or receding jaw (**Figure 39.2**), are subjective. This does not diminish their importance since professional judgements may often be subjective. However, there is a vast literature on prediction of difficult intubation by specific or objective tests. A number have been introduced and the five tests most commonly used are gape, jaw slide, thyromental distance, Mallampati and atlanto-occipital movement.

GAPE

Gape is the measurement of maximal mouth opening and is usually expressed as interincisor distance in finger-breadths or centimetres. Normal values are 3 fb or 5 cm. A mouth opening of 2 fb is limited and 1 fb is severely limited making direct laryngoscopy very difficult. It is difficult to insert a laryngeal mask when the gape is less than 1–1.5 cm (**Figure 39.3**).

JAW SLIDE OR MANDIBULAR PROTRUSION

Functions are graded as follows: class A if the lower jaw can be protruded beyond the top teeth; class B if the lower

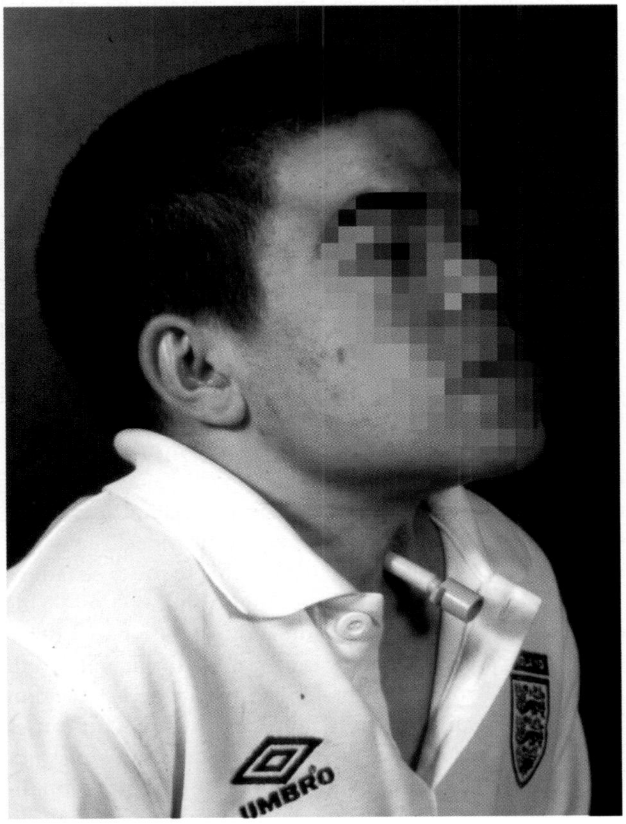

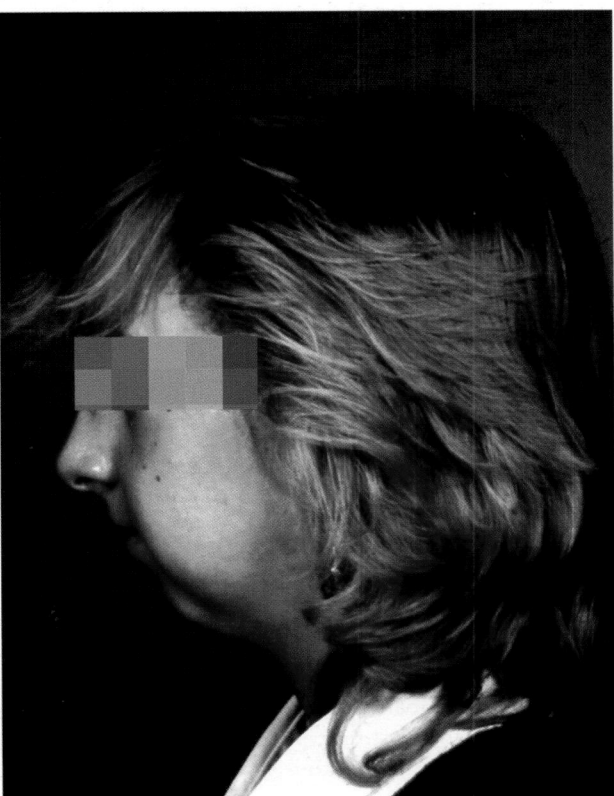

Figure 39.1   Mucopolysaccharidosis (Hunter's syndrome).

Figure 39.2   Receding jaw.

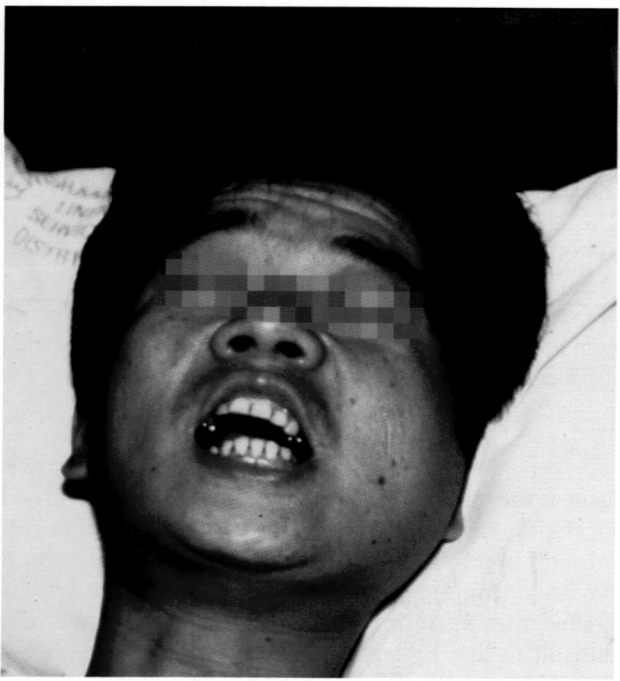

Figure 39.3 Limited mouth opening due to dental abscess.

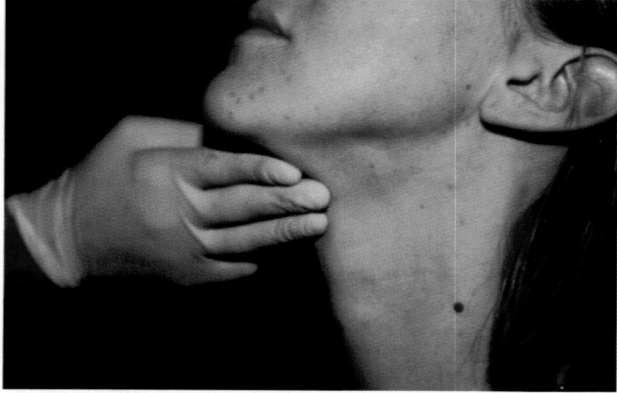

Figure 39.4 A normal thyromental distance.

teeth can only reach the top teeth; and class C if the lower teeth will not reach the top teeth. The value of testing this function is that, in intubation by direct laryngoscopy, the lower jaw must slide forward. In some scoring systems, mouth opening and jaw slide are combined, the greatest difficulty indicated by a gape of <3.5 cm and class C jaw slide. Another method of testing mandibular protrusion is the upper lip bite test[8] in which the patient demonstrates how much of the upper lip may be covered by the lower incisors. Class 1 indicates 'biting' above the vermilion line, class 2 below the vermilion line and class 3 inability to bite the upper lip.

THYROMENTAL DISTANCE

This measurement, described by Patil, is from the mentum to thyroid notch in full neck extension. The normal measurement is 6–7 cm or 3 fb (**Figure 39.4**). A short distance (2 fb) indicates a 'high' larynx and difficult direct laryngoscopy.

MALLAMPATI

Mallampati's contribution was a test to assess oropharyngeal space. The test asks a seated patient to open their mouth fully and extend the tongue maximally. The practitioner notes which posterior pharyngeal structures are visible. Mallampati described only three grades: class 1 indicates that the posterior pharyngeal wall, fauces and uvula are visible; class 2 indicates that only a part of the fauces, posterior wall and uvula are visible; and class 3 indicates that the tongue meets the palate. Samsoon and

Young arbitrarily introduced a subdivision of class 3 (tongue against soft palate) and class 4 (tongue meets hard palate).

ATLANTO-OCCIPITAL MOVEMENT

Optimal head and neck positioning for direct laryngoscopy requires cervical spine flexion and almost maximal extension of the head on the spine. A simple clinical test to look at atlanto-occipital movement is for the clinician to ask the patient to flex their neck maximally and then nod; the observer's hand placed posteriorly on the neck makes certain that the nodding motion is at the level of the cranium on the upper cervical vertebrae. Atlanto-occipital extension may be clinically graded as normal or reduced or measured and the normal value is 35°.

Investigations

Plain x-rays may demonstrate abnormalities, such as enlargement of the retropharyngeal space (**Figure 39.5**), a swollen epiglottis, tracheal deviation or narrowing, a radio-opaque foreign body or obstructive emphysema suggesting a ball-valve obstruction in the relevant bronchus. However, imaging of the whole airway by CT or MR scan is better and will show narrowing or distortion and allow planning of airway instrumentation. Flexible nasendoscopy under topical anaesthesia is extremely useful in delineating supra- or glottic pathology, and a longer flexible fibrescope can inspect the whole respiratory tract although generally this requires sedation.

Another useful test is the flow-volume loop. This expresses flow during expiration and inspiration as a function of lung volume. Airflow is measured during inhalation from residual volume to total lung capacity and exhalation back to residual volume. Extrathoracic obstruction causes limitation of inspiratory flow whilst intrathoracic obstruction causes limitation in expiratory flow. Limitation in expiratory flow is particularly noticeable because the highest flow-rates are usually present in peak expiration.

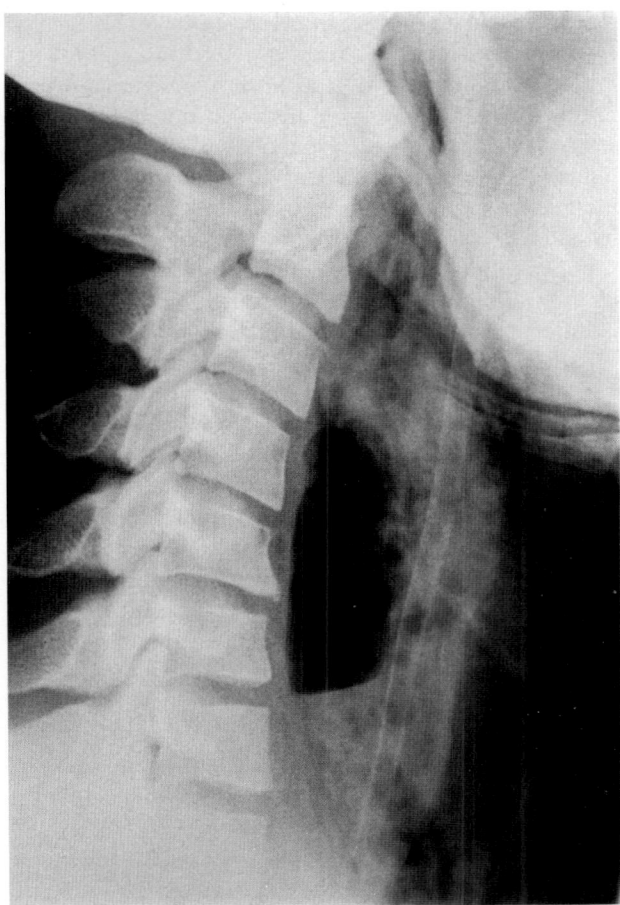

Figure 39.5 Retropharyngeal abscess.

PREDICTION OF DIFFICULTY

The practitioner forms a professional judgement as to whether airway management plans need to be altered from that carried out normally. It is easy to be definite or accurate in prediction when there are 'barn-door' abnormalities in the past anaesthetic history, past surgical history, examination and current disease process or from imaging. Examples would be a known history of failed intubation, presentation with breathing difficulty or stridor, absent mouth opening or previous head and neck reconstructive surgery. In a study of 181 patients with pharyngolaryngeal disease,[9] the single most predictive factor of difficult intubation was a tumour in the supraglottic region. In a study of 320 patients with a goitre undergoing thyroid surgery,[10] the presence of tracheal compression, presence of dyspnoea or a cancerous goitre were the three major predictive factors. [**]

However, when there are no abnormalities in the anaesthetic, medical or surgical history, the presenting disease process does not affect the head, neck or mediastinum and the patient does not 'look' difficult, then it is not possible to predict difficulty accurately.

Most attention has been on predicting difficult direct laryngoscopy using various specific or predictive tests (described above), combination of tests and scoring systems. All are imperfect and the reason is partly the low prevalence of difficult intubation. Test sensitivity indicates the ability of the test to label a difficult patient as difficult, test specificity the ability to label a normal patient as normal and the positive predictive value (PPV) is the proportion of patients found to be difficult out of all patients predicted by that test to be difficult. **Table 39.2** shows values of test sensitivity, specificity and PPV for various tests. It can be seen that an individual test, such as Mallampati, has a low PPV indicating that most patients predicted to be difficult will, in fact, be normal. A study comparing the upper lip bite test with the Mallampati in 1425 patients concluded that 'both tests are poor predictors as single screening tests'.[11] The more tests that are abnormal increases the likelihood that the patient will be difficult to intubate.

Another approach is to produce a score from consideration of various predictive tests, with appropriate weighting. In Wilson et al.'s risk sum,[12] five aspects of examination are used – weight, head and neck movement, jaw movement, receding mandible and buck teeth. Each factor is allocated a score of 0, 1 or 2 depending on severity. Wilson's group suggested that a total score of 2 or more would provide a sensitivity of 75 percent and specificity of 85 percent. These figures may appear to be good but one-quarter of difficult patients will be missed and there will be 1500 false alarms per 10,000 patients. A more recent French study[4] produced a scoring system involving seven factors – previous difficult intubation, pathologies associated with difficult intubation, clinical symptoms of airway pathology, interincisor gap and mandibular luxation, thyromental distance, maximum range of head and neck movement and Mallampati. The maximum score is 48 and a score of 11 provided the best level of sensitivity and specificity.

The subject of prediction of difficulty is fraught with difficulties arising from studies with small numbers of patients, definitions, curious mathematics and inappropriate conclusions. The topic has been elegantly examined in an editorial which provides a review of the mathematics and an extensive list of references.[13] A recent meta-analysis of bedside screening tests for predicting difficult intubation in apparently normal patients concludes that they have limited value.[14] [**]

Table 39.2 Test sensitivity, specificity and positive predictive value from the literature and reference 13.[13]

Test	Sensitivity %	Specificity %	PPV %
Thyromental	65–91	81–82	8–15
Mallampati	42–56	81–84	4–21
Wilson risk sum	42–55	86–92	6–9
Mouth opening	26–47	94–95	7–25
Neck movement	10–17	98	8–30

It must be remembered that the objective tests aim only to predict difficult direct laryngoscopy when the tongue has a normal compliance and the respiratory tract is normal. Fixation or restricted movement of the tongue was thought to be the direct cause of failed conventional intubation in a series of five patients[15] and an abnormality, such as a vallecular cyst, may be symptomless and will not be predicted but may cause great problems with airway management.[16] A number of patients who had been found to be unexpectedly difficult to intubate were reviewed and it was discovered that they all had lingual tonsillar hypertrophy.[17]

Airway evaluation is an essential part of preoperative assessment. It may be rewarded by the detection of severe or obvious problems that necessitate a change from 'normal' management. When there are no obvious problems, evaluation is imperfect and safe airway management in all circumstances depends on the adoption of an airway strategy that is able to respond to unexpected difficulty with intubation or oxygenation.

STRATEGY

The recommendations of the ASA on management of the airway[1, 3] promoted the five-step linear model of evaluation of the airway, preparation for difficulty, strategy at intubation, strategy at extubation and follow-up. The ASA difficult airway algorithm presents an overall scheme of planning airway management and a recent version[18] is shown in **Figure 39.6**. The algorithm indicates that airway difficulty may be predicted or unexpected and, in the unexpected limb, attention must first address oxygenation before employing alternative means of intubation. Strategy indicates a combination of plans, also known as plan A/plan B at both initial instrumentation of the airway (induction or intubation) and at the end of surgery (eduction or extubation). Each plan at the start of anaesthesia addresses ventilation of the patient, the abolition of laryngeal reflexes (if required), the airway device and method of insertion, and the abolition of patient distress. The default strategy when intubation is required is shown in **Table 39.3**. During intubation, there is no ventilation and the patient is oxygenated by intermittent face mask ventilation. Laryngeal reflexes are abolished by muscle relaxation, patient distress is overcome by general anaesthesia and intubation is by optimal direct laryngoscopy. The components of optimal direct laryngoscopy are optimal head and neck position, muscle relaxation, external laryngeal manipulation, laryngoscope blade length/design and use of the gum-elastic bougie. The bougie is the most useful

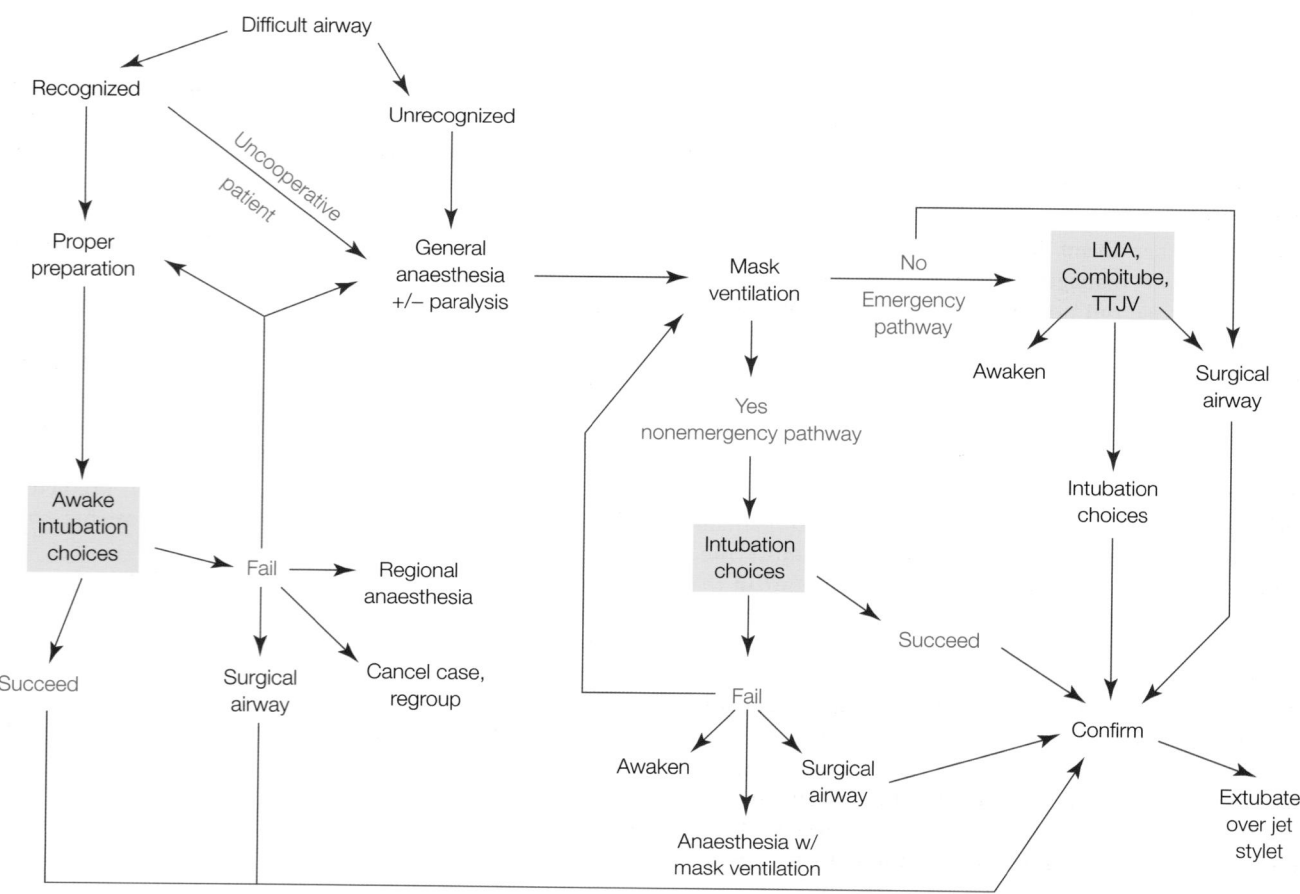

Figure 39.6 ASA difficult airway algorithm. Redrawn from ref. 18, with permission.

Table 39.3 Default airway strategy for intubation.

	Plan A	Plan B
Means of ventilation	Face mask inflation	Failed ventilation
Abolition of laryngeal reflexes	Muscle relaxation	Muscle relaxation
Device/technique for intubation	Optimal direct laryngoscopy	Failed intubation
Control of patient distress	General anaesthesia	General anaesthesia

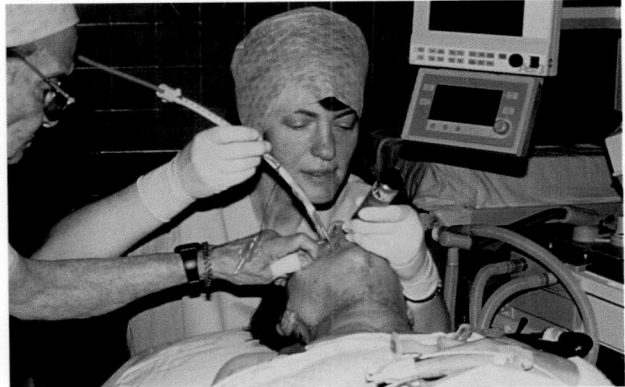

Figure 39.7 The gum-elastic bougie is a very effective aid to intubation.

'low-tech' device (**Figure 39.7**) and it proved successful in 80 percent of the unexpected difficult intubations in one series of 11,257 intubations.[19] Its correct use during attempted direct laryngoscopy is by placement through the glottis, either blindly or by educated guess, confirming placement by feeling the tracheal rings and hold-up at 25 cm when the bougie contacts the carina, followed by railroading the tracheal tube with the laryngoscope still *in situ*.

The components of optimal direct laryngoscopy indicate that a limited number of attempts are possible, perhaps to change the length of blade, use the bougie or apply external laryngeal pressure. However, generally, no more than three attempts should be made and recent evidence in 2833 critically ill patients indicates increased morbidity with more than two attempts.[20] The correct decision is to acknowledge 'failed intubation' and abandon plan A. Within default strategy, plan B addresses both failed ventilation and failed intubation by using alternative techniques. In response to the request by the Royal College of Anaesthetists for the display in each hospital of strategies to combat unexpected failed intubation and/or failed ventilation, the Difficult Airway Society (www.das.uk.com) has produced guidelines and flowcharts for the UK.[21] [*]

ALTERNATIVE TECHNIQUES FOR TRACHEAL INTUBATION

When intubation by direct laryngoscopy fails, a number of alternative techniques should be considered.

Other laryngoscope blade design

The Macintosh curved design is the blade most commonly used by anaesthetists. However, it has a lower success rate than straight blade direct laryngoscopy by the right paraglossal approach. Recently, a British enthusiast, John Henderson, has designed his own straight blade and makes a good case for the reintroduction of the straight blade into mainstream anaesthesia.[22] It is a similar technique to that employed by head and neck surgeons, and there seems to be little reason that anaesthetists and surgeons should view the larynx by differing techniques. Another blade, originally invented by McCoy, employs a lever to increase markedly the angulation of the tip (**Figure 39.8**). A number of direct laryngoscopy blades have been introduced over the years incorporating prisms or mirrors to try and provide an indirect view of the larynx but these have not become mainstream devices.

Rigid fibrescopes

Two notable rigid fibrescopes, Upsherscope (**Figure 39.9**) and Bullard, have been introduced. A fibreoptic viewing bundle is incorporated into a rigid curved blade. The tracheal tube is loaded into or onto the device, the blade is introduced into the pharynx and is then positioned under fibreoptic vision. When the tip of the scope has been positioned directly in front of the larynx, the tracheal tube is passed out of its guiding channel or over an introducer into the trachea. The Bullard appears to be the more popular device and has the support of a Canadian consensus group.[23] The device is expensive, training is required and it has not become widely popular in the UK.

Flexible fibrescopes

Tracheal intubation using the flexible fibrescope was first described in 1967 by Peter Murphy,[24] an anaesthetic senior registrar working at the National Hospital, Queen Square, London, and flexible intubating fibrescopes have been commercially available for over 20 years. Several textbooks[25, 26] are concerned solely with the technique. A standard adult intubating fibrescope has a length of 60 cm and a nominal external diameter of 4 mm. Its narrow diameter allows it to pass through the nose or mouth, its flexibility allows it to conform to the anatomy of the patient, the working channel can be used to instil local anaesthesia, oxygen or to pass wires in the antero- or

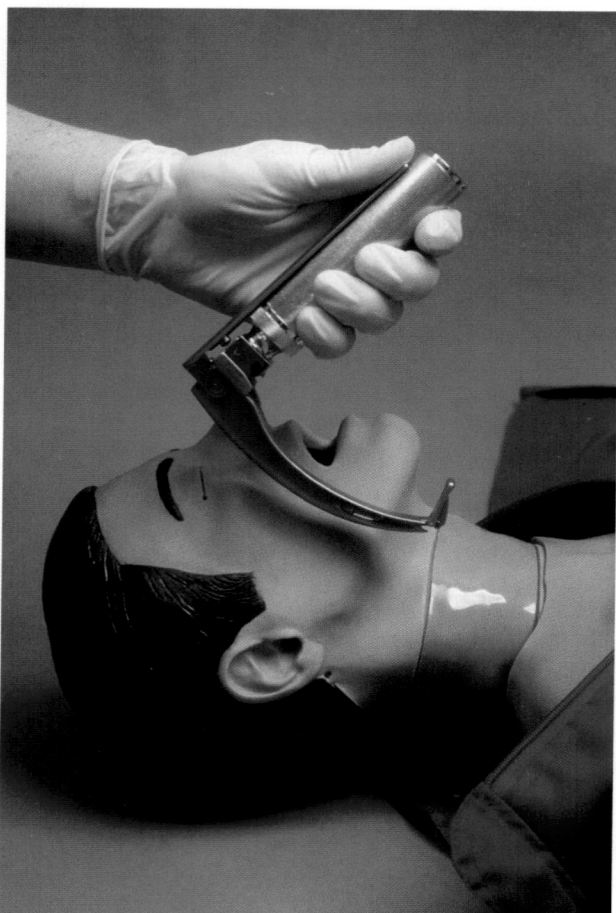

Figure 39.8   McCoy blade with a hinged tip.

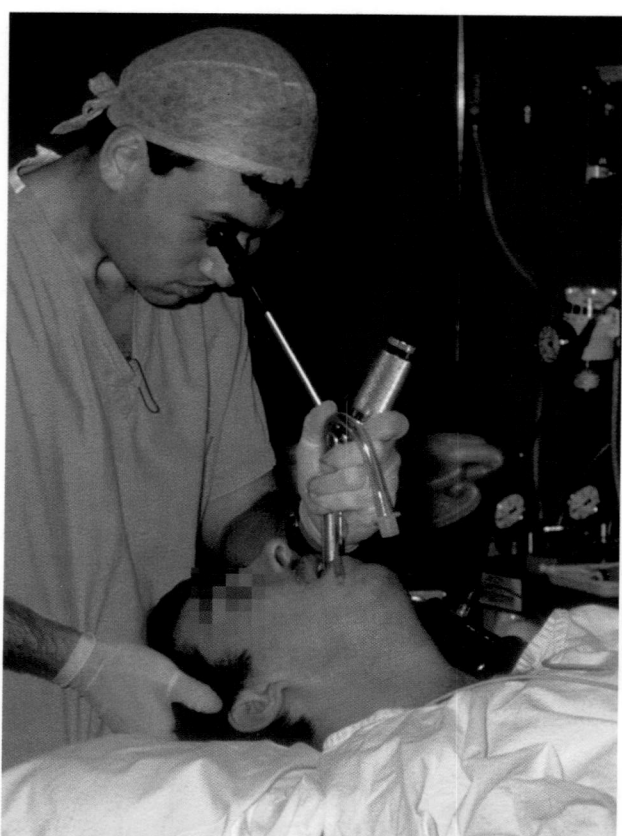

Figure 39.9   Using the Upsherscope.

retrograde direction to aid intubation, the technique is visual and can be used to confirm correct positioning of the tube in the trachea. It is fairly easy to use anaesthetic breathing system connectors or attachments which allow concurrent ventilation of the patient during intubation, or specially adapted airways to make oral intubation easier. It is not surprising that such an instrument has become the safest and most successful technique of intubation. A Swiss study[27] examines the results of 13,248 intubations from one hospital in which the fibrescope is used widely as the primary or back-up intubation technique. The failed intubation rate was 0.045 percent. [**] Ovassapian[28] gives figures of 98.4 percent success rate in over 2,000 fibreoptic intubations. The complication rate is extremely low.

Fibre-endoscopic skills appear in the core competencies for trainee anaesthetists and include visual inspection of the respiratory tract for diagnostic purposes and placement of double lumen tracheal tubes. The problems associated with the intubating fibrescope are that some skill is necessary, the device is expensive and repays careful handling, and disinfection requires chemical agents. There has been particular concern over the inability of cold sterilizing agents to destroy prions. The recommendation from the Department of Health is that a register should be maintained such that all patients treated with an individual fibrescope can be traced easily.

Intubating laryngeal mask airway

The intubating laryngeal mask was devised by Brain and introduced in 1999. The intubating laryngeal mask airway (ILMA) kit (**Figure 39.10**) differs from the classic laryngeal mask (LM) in several ways. The stem is a rigid highly curved metal tube with a handle, there is an epiglottic elevator bar, a ramp at the junction of the stem and bowl directs the tube appropriately and it is supplied with a special wire-spiral tracheal tube with novel bevel. The described technique of intubation in the anaesthetized, paralyzed patient is for the mask to be placed and the patient ventilated through it. Mask placement appears to be easy provided the mouth opening is more than 2 cm. The tracheal tube is inserted through the stem and advanced slowly without force. As the tip of the tube emerges from the stem, it lifts the epiglottic elevator bar and the route is now clear for the tube to be advanced into the trachea. This blind intubation has a success rate of 95 percent or so if two to three manipulations of mask position and tube advancement are allowed. A fibreoptic modification can be used which allows a visually guided technique and would seem to be preferable. In the largest

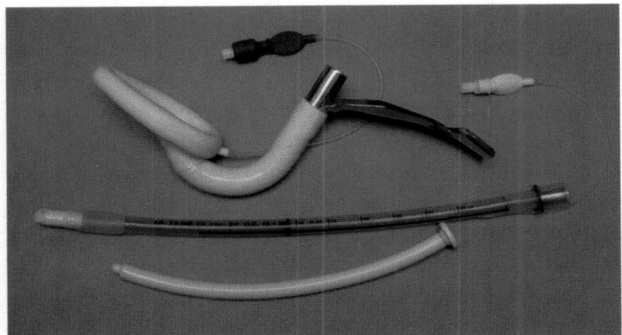

Figure 39.10 Components of the intubating laryngeal mask airway.

series of difficult intubations published so far,[29] the ILMA was used in 254 patients with a known difficult airway, including 50 patients with airway distortion due to tumour, surgery or radiotherapy. The successful intubation rate was 96.5 percent with a blind technique and 100 percent when used with the fibrescope. [**] Another North American study[30] compared intubation by the ILMA in anaesthetized patients with awake fibre-optic intubation in 38 patients with suspected difficult intubation and found them both to be 100 percent successful.

Lighted stylets

The technique of transillumination of the neck to guide oro- or nasotracheal intubation was described first in 1959. A lighted stylet[31] uses the principle of transillumination and takes advantage of the anterior or superficial location of the trachea. A number of commercially available devices have been produced over the years and the most recent, the Trachlight, appears to be the most successful. The tracheal tube is loaded onto the stylet which has a distal bulb, and the stylet is shaped into a hockey-stick. The lighted stylet is introduced into the oropharynx from the side and brought into the midline. The tip of the lightwand is passed around the tongue and a bright, well-circumscribed circle of light seen externally at the level of the hyoid indicates that the tip lies in the vallecula. The tube is advanced into the trachea without resistance. In one large series of anticipated difficult intubation, successful Trachlight use by the inventor resulted in intubation in 99 percent patients with a mean time of 26 seconds.

ROLE OF THE CLASSIC LM

The classic LM is the most successful of all supraglottic airway devices for maintenance of the airway. In one study of over 11,000 patients, the incidence of failed placement was 1:600 patients. It is, of course, designed for maintenance of the airway in planned, elective surgery. It

Table 39.4 Role of the classic LM in difficult airway management.

Role of the classic LM	
As the desired airway device	
Instead of a tracheal tube	
Rescue device in failed ventilation	
Conduit during emergence	
Conduit for fibre-endoscopy of the airway	
Conduit for intubation:	Blind
	Bougie
	Fibreoptic-guided bougie
	Fibreoptic
	Aintree catheter

has the advantages, when compared with tracheal intubation, of easier placement, no requirement for muscle relaxation and is tolerated *in situ* by the awakening patient. The major disadvantages are that it does not offer the same level of airway protection as a cuffed tracheal tube against gross gastric regurgitation and it does not traverse the larynx, so is no protection against airway occlusion by glottic or infraglottic pathology. It has, however, proved to be a very useful device in difficult airway management and appears in several places in airway algorithms (**Table 39.4**).

Intubation via the LM

In normal use, the LM should be seated in close proximity to the vocal cords and it is not surprising that it can provide a route for passage of a tracheal tube. There are five methods for this (**Table 39.4**). A size 6.0 mm will pass through the stem/connector of a size three or four LM and a size 7.0 mm tube will pass through the size five LM. Blind placement, in which the tube is lubricated and advanced blindly, has a success rate of only 50–90 percent and passing a bougie through the LM first has an even lower success rate. Techniques under vision have appreciably higher success rates and flexible fibreoptic techniques are particular useful. The fibrescope may be used to guide placement of a bougie into the trachea with intubation occurring over the bougie.

Fibreoptic-assisted techniques are useful because they are visually guided (**Figure 39.11**). The core technique is to insert the LM, load a 6.0 mm tube onto the fibrescope, pass the fibrescope into the trachea through the stem of the LM and slide the well-lubricated tube into the trachea. It is also possible to ventilate an anaesthetized patient through the LM whilst intubation is in progress. This introduces the concept of the laryngeal mask as a dedicated airway,[32] 'a device used for maintenance of

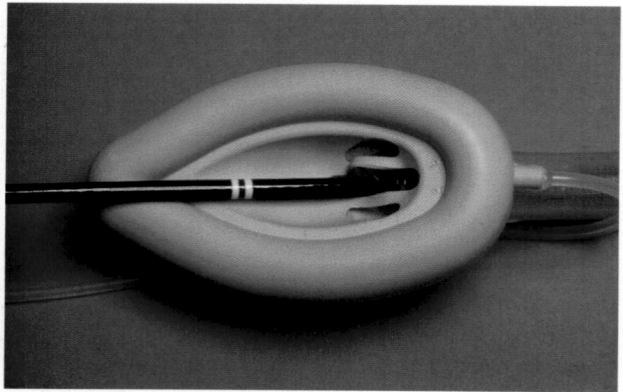

Figure 39.11 The laryngeal mask is a good conduit for fibreoptic intubation.

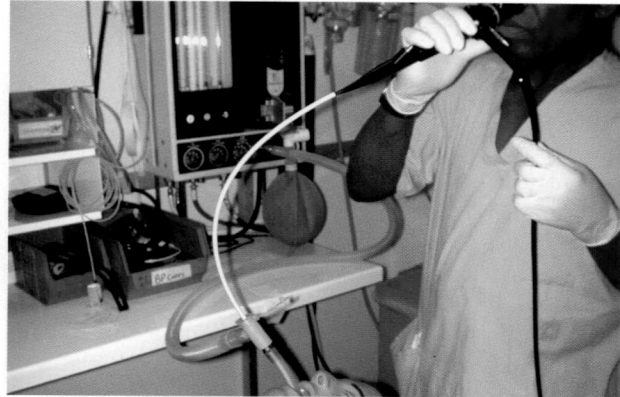

Figure 39.12 Aintree catheter – a hollow bougie inserted over a fibrescope.

the airway whilst other airway interventions (e.g. intubation) are in progress'. Development of this concept led to the design of the Aintree catheter,[33] a hollow bougie which may be placed over the fibrescope and inserted through the LM into the trachea (**Figure 39.12**). Effectively, the technique places a hollow bougie under vision into the airway, over which a tracheal tube is railroaded.

FAILED VENTILATION AND EMERGENCY CRICOTHYROTOMY

Failed ventilation refers to the situation where a patient has been anaesthetized and muscle relaxants administered but it is not possible to provide positive pressure ventilation by use of the face mask and oral airway. A prepared sequence of steps should commence to provide rescue oxygenation as quickly as possible. Bag/mask ventilation in which two hands are used to try to maintain airway patency and another hand squeezes the anaesthetic reservoir bag should be followed by insertion of a classic LM. This may prove life-saving and must

always be considered. If oxygenation cannot be achieved by face mask or LM, it may be worthwhile attempting intubation by direct laryngoscopy. This must be a brief attempt only and must not delay oxygenation by the next step. Airway deaths, unfortunately, often involve prolonged fruitless attempts to intubate when oxygenation is the immediate necessity. When the anaesthetized patient cannot be oxygenated by face mask or LM, and tracheal intubation is not possible, emergency oxygenation should be attempted directly into the respiratory tract below the level of the vocal cords. Anaesthetists generally use the cricothyroid membrane (CTM) which has a number of desirable properties:

- superficial;
- easy landmarks to locate;
- present in most patients;
- rarely calcifies;
- relatively avascular;
- wide enough to accept 6.0 mm tube;
- inferior to vocal cords;
- cricoid ring holds airway open;
- posterior lamina protects back wall.

There are three types of cricothyrotomy as detailed in the following sections.[34]

Needle or small cannula cricothyrotomy

A narrow-calibre rigid needle or flexible cannula is inserted through the CTM in a caudad direction. In adults, an appropriate size is 14 G with an internal diameter of 2 mm (**Figure 39.13**). The resistance to flow through such a calibre is high and this has implications for inspiration and expiration; in inspiration, adequate gas flows cannot be obtained by the pressures generated within a standard anaesthetic breathing system and exhalation of 500 mL takes >30 seconds. Inspiratory gas flows of 500 mL/s require oxygen at a pressure of 2–4 bar supplied by a Sanders injector (**Figure 39.14**). The Sanders injector attaches to the 4 bar (400 kPa, 4 atmospheres) oxygen pipeline and has a hand-operated lever to control gas flow during inspiration. Exhalation occurs through the upper airway and particular attention must be taken to ensure that this happens, otherwise airway pressures rise and pulmonary barotrauma develops. A needle cricothyrotomy is a temporary measure and consideration must be given to creation of a tracheostomy in relevant circumstances. It is possible for ventilation via needle cricothyrotomy to be used in the planned elective or urgent case. **Figure 39.15** shows a patient whose partial denture had fallen into the pharynx in such a position that the larynx was obscured. The cricothyrotomy needle was placed in the awake patient and its correct position in the trachea confirmed by aspiration of free air and attachment of the capnograph to show an appropriate trace. Following intravenous anaesthesia and

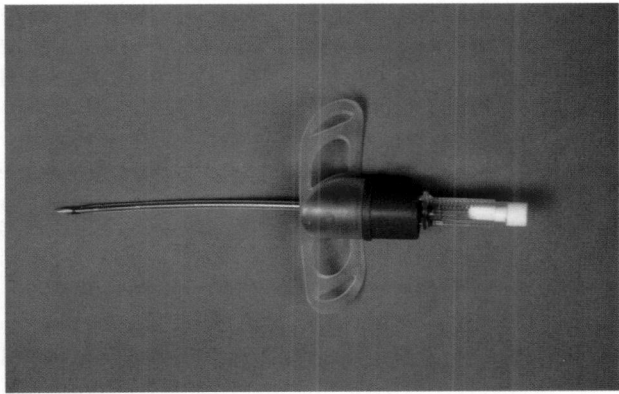

Figure 39.13   Ravussin style cricothyrotomy cannula.

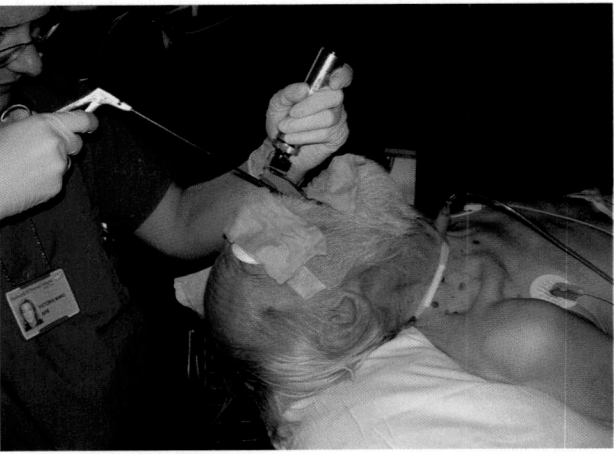

Figure 39.15   Planned use of transtracheal jet ventilation.

Surgical cricothyrotomy

The technique is to make a 3 cm midline incision in the skin followed by a horizontal stab incision in the inferior part of the cricothyroid membrane. The incision is spread horizontally and vertically and a 6 mm tube is inserted. The complication rate was 40 percent in one series of 38 emergency surgical cricothyrotomies. Misplacement and bleeding requiring ligation of vessels were the most common problem. A more rapid four-step technique has been described[35] in which a single horizontal incision is made through the skin and cricothyroid membrane together. In a cadaver study, emergency physicians compared the standard and rapid technique. The rapid technique was faster than the standard 43 versus 134 seconds, but the complication rate was higher. The horizontal incison through the skin may cause more haemorrhage. A cricothyrotomy tube should not be left in place for more than a few days and conversion to tracheostomy prevents the complications of dysphonia and subglottic stenosis.

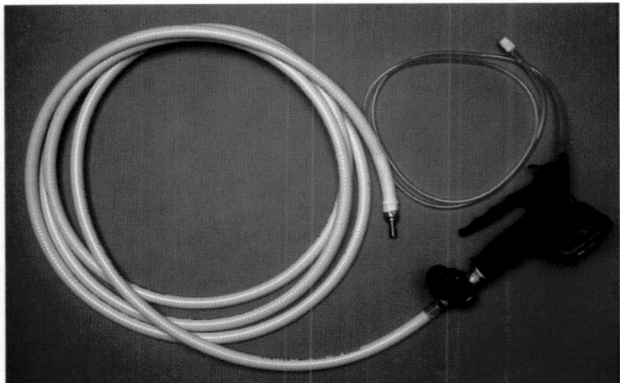

Figure 39.14   Sanders injector.

muscle relaxation, the Sanders technique of intermittent application of high pressure oxygen provided adequate oxygenation and ventilation. Exhalation through the upper airway was unobstructed.

Large cannula cricothyrotomy

A purpose-built cannula with an internal diameter of >4 mm allows adequate inspiratory gas flows with the pressures generated by the standard breathing system and exhalation of 500 mL takes approximately 5–6 seconds. This is an advantage because there is no requirement for high pressure oxygen. It is easy to attach the capnograph to the circuit for confirmation of correct positioning within the trachea, and to suction the respiratory tract. Exhalation occurs through the cannula, even in the presence of complete upper airway obstruction. The cannula may be a cannula-over-needle or a Seldinger-type dilatational device. Cannula-over-needle devices place an uncuffed tube whereas the Melker Seldinger device allows positioning of a 6.0 mm cuffed tube. There are advantages in placing a cuffed tube in allowing controlled positive pressure ventilation and protecting the airway.

OBSTRUCTED AIRWAY

The obstructed airway[36] is one in which the primary symptoms or signs are due to narrowing or distortion of the airway. There are two broad clinical presentations. In acute obstruction (**Figure 39.16**), a previously normal person develops problems over a matter of minutes or hours. The aetiology is usually one of inhaled foreign body or abnormal fluid accumulation, such as blood, pus or oedema. Typical clinical scenarios are infections in the head and neck, postoperative haematoma, and airway swelling secondary to anaphylaxis or angiotensin-converting enzyme inhibitors. The rapidity of onset produces prominent signs of difficulty with breathing and the patients may present in extremis. Imaging of the airway by x-ray, CT or MR scan is often inappropriate because

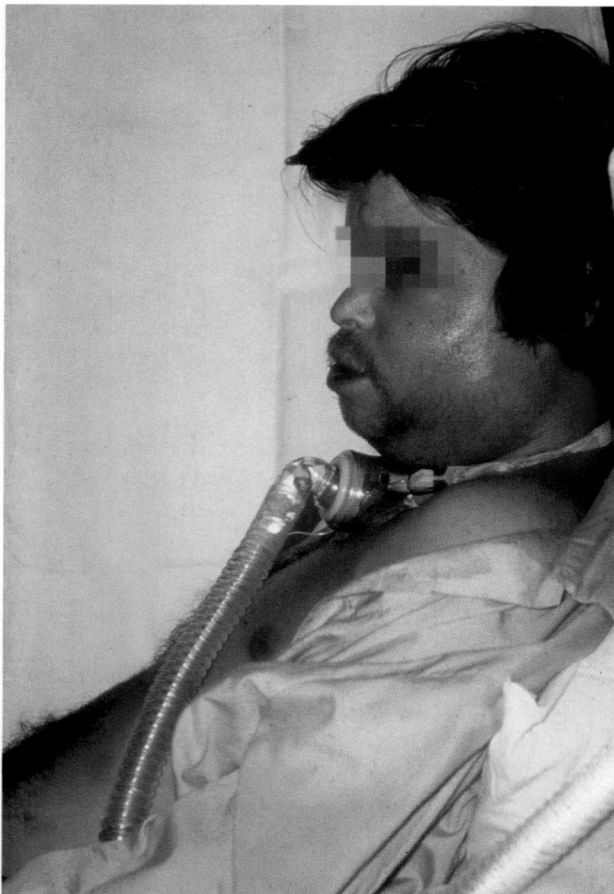

Figure 39.16   Patient with Ludwig's angina.

the patient may be unable to adopt the necessary position to complete the procedure and the radiology suite is not an appropriate location for a patient with a deteriorating airway. The management of acute obstruction includes 100 percent oxygen by face mask, trial of administration of heliox, nebulized adrenaline (epinephrine) if oedema is prominent, drainage of pus, tracheal intubation or emergency cricothyrotomy or tracheostomy. Heliox is a combination of oxygen 21 percent and helium 79 percent and is three times less dense than air because of the low atomic weight of helium (4) compared with nitrogen (14). In airway obstruction, turbulent gas flow is inversely proportional to the square root of density and the use of heliox improves gas flow in turbulent conditions and also promotes laminar flow. It is suggested also that carbon dioxide molecules diffuse four to five times faster through heliox than an equivalent oxygen–nitrogen mixture and this may enhance carbon dioxide excretion in the airway.

In chronic obstruction, the airway pathology has developed over a period of weeks or months and is usually due to growth of tissue or to scarring. The slow onset allows development of enlarged intercostal muscle mass and patients can tolerate a very significantly narrowed airway without symptoms. Generally, a patient will not be dyspnoeic at rest until the airway is narrowed

to <5 mm diameter, although they are likely to be short of breath on exercise. The slower time course of obstruction allows complete imaging of the airway and controlled intervention. Appropriate imaging in the stable, chronic condition is through flexible nasendoscopy and CT or MR imaging of the entire airway. Flow-volume loops may be helpful in detecting that a patient's problem is large airway narrowing and not truly pulmonary, or assessing the degree of tracheal narrowing before planning surgery.

Evaluation of the obstructed airway seeks to define the degree of obstruction, likely site, rapidity of onset and likely time course of deterioration by history, examination and special investigations. The history from the relative or patient usually indicates whether this is acute, chronic or acute-on-chronic. Specific symptoms/signs in airway obstruction are degree of difficulty with breathing, stridor (noisy breathing) and phase of respiration of any stridor. Stridor indicates that the airway is narrowed to <50 percent normal diameter, but this degree of airway narrowing is not always accompanied by stridor. Expiratory stridor indicates an infraglottic problem and inspiratory stridor a supra or glottic aetiology. There may be a positional aspect to the difficulty with breathing and patients may be more comfortable in the sitting or lateral position. Voice change and difficulty with swallowing may indicate the site or extent of disease, and pyrexia or sepsis indicates an infective component. Unilateral reduction in breath sounds in the chest indicate specific bronchial obstruction. With progressive obstruction, signs of ineffective ventilation and poor gas exchange are present. These include agitation, anxiety, confusion, restlessness and depressed level of consciousness. Increased work of breathing is indicated by a high respiratory rate, use of accessory muscles of respiration, flaring nostrils, sweating and tachycardia. Oximetry is not a good monitor of work of breathing and normal oxygen saturation does not indicate that all is well. In severe acute obstruction with untrained respiratory muscles, exhaustion occurs relatively quickly with a resulting decrease in effective minute ventilation, hypoxaemia, bradycardia and death.

Management strategy in the obstructed airway

The Confidential Enquiry into Perioperative Deaths (CEPOD) report[37] 1996/97 examined 30 patients who had died within 30 days of surgery for management of lesions in the upper airway or who presented with stridor. In most cases death was due to the underlying disease process but in some cases difficulties with maintenance of the airway led to death in the operating theatre or recovery unit. Brief case scenarios are given in the report and one describes a 76 year-old patient with fixed cervical spine flexion (due to rheumatoid arthritis) and a retrosternal goitre. After induction of anaesthesia with thiopentone and muscle relaxation with suxamethonium, the patient proved impossible to intubate and mask ventilate adequately. An emergency tracheostomy proved difficult and cardiac arrest occurred in theatre.

The surgical and anaesthetic assessors made several good recommendations. The patients should be seen by the consultant surgeon and anaesthetist who consider carefully the plan for securing the airway. Imaging of the airway should be obtained, if possible, to allow delineation of whether the airway is narrowed at supraglottic, glottic or infraglottic level. Airway strategy should include a primary and back-up plan with coherence between the individual plans. If a long-acting muscle relaxant is used in plan A, plan B cannot rely on a patient 'waking-up'. If a surgical tracheostomy is the back-up plan, anaesthesia should start in the operating theatre with the equipment, surgeon and theatre team immediately ready – it is foolish to start anaesthesia in the anaesthetic room and scramble into theatre when plan A fails. [*]

There has been much discussion in the anaesthetic literature about provision of anaesthesia in the presence of the abnormal airway but general agreement that classification according to the site of obstruction is helpful. Currently, the terms used by anaesthetists are not as precise as the ones used by surgeons to localize tumours.

'SUPRAGLOTTIC' OBSTRUCTION

In 'supraglottic' obstruction the obstruction is above or superior to the glottis and the glottic aperture is of normal dimensions. An example would be a base of tongue tumour (**Figure 39.17**), although clearly this is not truly a supraglottic structure in disease terminology. Direct laryngoscopy is likely to prove difficult and may cause bleeding if the blade contacts the tumour. It may also prove difficult to ventilate by face mask following induction of general anaesthesia. In this circumstance it is helpful to retain spontaneous respiration and to use an alternative means of intubation. Awake fibreoptic intubation (**Figure 39.18**) by the nasal or oral route has much

to recommend it[38] and was used successfully in a series of 26 adult patients with deep neck infections including classical Ludwig's angina.[39] [**]

Awake intubation is a misnomer because it is very difficult to intubate a truly awake patient. The more correct term is tracheal intubation under topical anaesthesia with conscious sedation. It has a very good record of safety in airway management because the patient maintains their own airway and continues with spontaneous respiration until the airway is secure. It is possible for the patient to adopt a change in position, such as sitting up, and to aid intubation by protruding their tongue, vocalizing or taking deep breaths. There are a number of intubation techniques in an awake patient, such as oral direct laryngoscopy, blind intubation through the nose, through the classic or intubating laryngeal masks or a retrograde wire technique. Awake fibreoptic intubation appears to be the best technique, combining awake intubation with a visually guided method of both inspecting and intubating the airway, applying local anaesthesia to the airway and confirming correct positioning of the tube within the trachea. Fibreoptic intubation is generally easier in the awake rather than anaesthetized, paralysed patient because airway patency is maintained, the airway opens and closes with respiration and the flow of gas indicates the route to the larynx.

There are a number of specific practical steps and attention to detail is required. Premedication may be employed if there is no airway embarrassment, but should be avoided if there are symptoms or signs of airway obstruction. An antisialogogue is important and absence of secretions allows earlier and more profound topical anaesthesia, and easier fibre-endoscopy. Preoperative

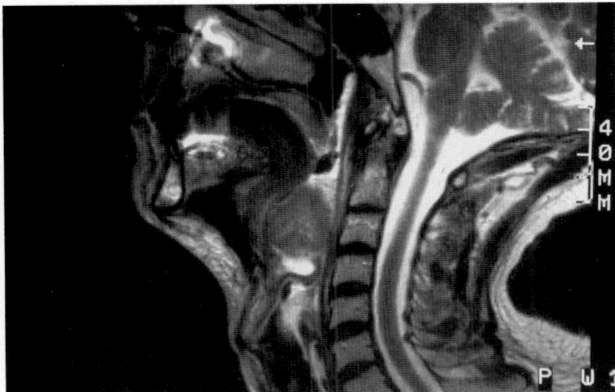

Figure 39.17 Magnetic resonance image of tongue base tumour.

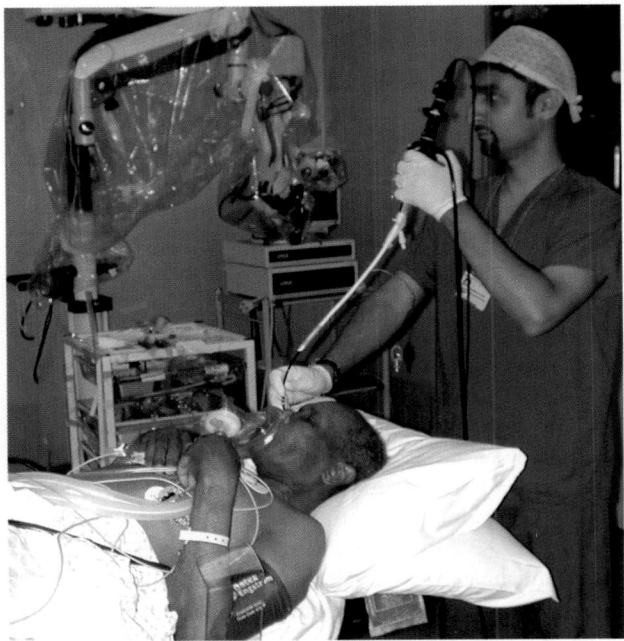

Figure 39.18 Awake fibreoptic intubation.

intramuscular atropine 0.6 mg, hyoscine 0.4 mg or glycopyrrolate 0.4 mg are suitable but it is common to administer glycopyrrolate 0.2–0.4 mg intravenously as soon as the patient arrives in the operating room.

Sedation aims to provide a comfortable patient who maintains spontaneous respiration, airway patency and verbal contact. Small incremental doses of a benzodiazepine and opioid are administered, taking care not to produce oversedation. Typical total doses are midazolam 1–5 mg and fentanyl 25–100 μg. Both drugs have a peak onset of five minutes and a specific antagonist (flumazenil and naloxone, respectively). Benzodiazepines cause relaxation of genioglossus and destabilization of the airway and opioids are associated with central respiratory depression so neither drug is benign. However, appropriate doses produce a compliant patient who is not unduly upset by airway topicalization or instrumentation, and is usually amnesic. Propofol, an anaesthetic agent, provides sedation at subhypnotic concentrations and is particularly useful when given by target-controlled infusion. Target controlled infusion (TCI) devices are sophisticated syringe pumps which incorporate a pharmacokinetic model of the relevant drug. The operator enters the age and weight of the patient and the desired blood level. The TCI pump calculates and delivers the appropriate bolus dose to reach the required blood level and the subsequent infusion required to maintain it. Appropriate starting blood levels for propofol are 0.5–1.0 μg/mL. Remifentanil, an ultrashort-acting opioid, may also be used by TCI and is gaining a reputation as a useful opioid for awake intubation. If the nasal route is chosen for intubation, a topical vasoconstrictor should be applied. This may be xylometazoline or ephedrine 0.5 percent drops or cocaine (3 mL 5 percent), which produces both vasoconstriction and topical anaesthesia.

Topical anaesthesia may be provided by:

• nebulization;
• translaryngeal administration;
• specific nerve blocks;
• transendoscopic administration.

Nebulization sounds attractive but use of the technology which provides particles for alveolar deposition of drug (e.g. salbutamol nebulizer), may lead to disappointing results partly because the particles are too small but also because a large amount of the drug escapes to the atmosphere. High-drug concentrations may be effective and nebulized lignocaine 10 percent in a dose of 6 mg/kg has been described as effective. A useful variant is the production of a larger droplet size produced during inspiration. This manual spray-and-inhale technique employs a 22 g Venflon attached to a constant oxygen flowrate of 1–2 L/min. Small increments of lignocaine 4 percent are injected through the port of the cannula and coordinated with inspiration. One spray-and-inhale regime is to use 3 mL lignocaine 4 percent with ephedrine 15 mg to the nose, wait three minutes and apply the second 3 mL lignocaine 4 percent, asking the patient to inspire deeply and slowly through the nose. The droplets are inhaled and deposited onto the larynx and trachea. After a three minute wait, a further 3 mL lignocaine 4 percent is nebulized during slow forced inspiration. Maximum lignocaine dosage should be 9 mg/kg.

Translaryngeal administration has a long history of safe use. A study reviewing 17,500 administrations reported only six noteworthy complications.[40] A 22 G cannula or needle is passed through the cricothyroid membrane or trachea and 3–4 mL lignocaine 4 percent is injected preferably at end-expiration. The injection provokes a short period of intense coughing which distributes the drug to the glottis and above. The experimental addition of methylene blue to the local anaesthetic shows staining of the superior aspect of the vocal cords in 95 percent of patients.

Appropriate specific nerve blocks are of the superior laryngeal and glossopharyngeal nerves. The internal branch of the superior laryngeal nerve supplies sensation to the under surface of the epiglottis and the superior surface of the vocal cords. It may be blocked on each side as it traverses the thyrohyoid membrane. Extension of the head and neck aids identification of the hyoid and thyroid cartilages. A 22 G needle is placed inferiorly to the greater horn of the hyoid, passed into the membrane and 2 mL lignocaine 2 percent is injected. The glossopharyngeal nerve supplies sensation to the posterior third of the tongue, superior part of the epiglottis, lateral pharyngeal wall and inferior surface of the soft palate. The nerve may be blocked behind the anterior pillar of the tonsillar fossa. With full mouth opening the tongue is grasped and pulled to the contralateral side. A 20 G spinal needle is inserted to a depth of 5 mm into the base of the anterior tonsillar pillar at the level of the reflection onto the tongue, and 2 mL lignocaine 2 percent injected. Bilateral glossopharyngeal nerve blocks will abolish the gag reflex and allow greater manipulation in the oropharynx or direct laryngoscopy, perhaps when placing a large double lumen tube. These specific nerve blocks are not performed routinely.

Transendoscopic administration of lignocaine 4 percent through the working channel of the intubating fibrescope is an extremely effective means of applying local anaesthetic to the airway under vision. This spray-as-you-go technique is highly favoured and noninvasive. The intubating fibrescopes have connectors for injection but an easier alternative is to place an epidural catheter, cut to produce one terminal hole, substantially into the working channel (**Figure 39.19**). Aliquots of lignocaine 4 percent to a maximum dose of 9 mg/kg are administered.

It is helpful for the fibrescope to be attached to a CCTV system, particularly for training. An appropriate size tracheal tube is loaded onto the fibrescope and the scope is introduced under vision into the mouth or more patent nostril. The fibrescope is advanced without

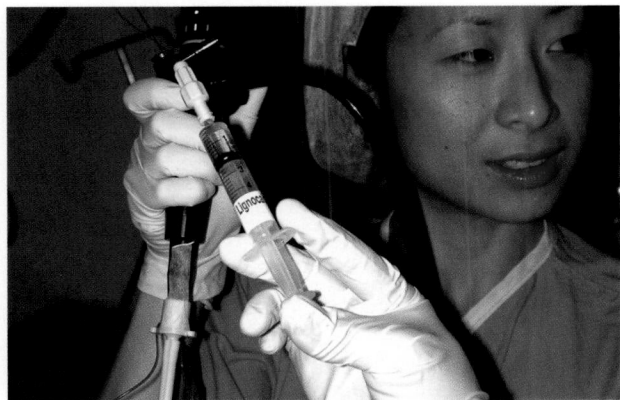

Figure 39.19 Injection of lignocaine through an epidural catheter inserted into working channel of fibrescope.

touching the mucosa until the vocal cords are seen. Additional local anaesthetic may be applied before the fibrescope is advanced to the carina. The tube is advanced or railroaded over the fibrescope. This may be difficult because the bevel impinges on the larynx. Use of a small diameter tube and rotation of the tube minimize this problem.

Awake fibreoptic intubation may be difficult when the airway anatomy is abnormal and when there is blood or secretions in the airway. An illustrative case scenario indicates some of the pitfalls in management. An adult patient underwent removal of a fishbone impacted in the lower pharynx/upper oesophagus. Three days later the patient was pyrexial, with a sore throat, unable to swallow and with limited mouth opening. A lateral x-ray of the neck showed a retropharyngeal abscess. The patient was seen by two anaesthetic trainees who did not inform the consultant on call. They decided on an awake fibreoptic intubation but administered too much sedation. In a deteriorating situation with a semirousable patient they attempted nasal fibreoptic orotracheal intubation (FOI) with the patient supine. They were unsuccessful and were moved aside by the consultant surgeon who managed to intubate the patient fibreoptically with the patient sitting, leaning forward on the edge of the operating table. Mistakes made here include failure to appreciate the seriousness of the condition and to inform a consultant, failure to realize that awake nasal FOI in the supine position would be difficult in the presence of retropharyngeal swelling and failure to realize that airway patency would be compromised by any sedation.

PERIGLOTTIC/GLOTTIC OBSTRUCTION

In these situations it may be difficult to visualize the vocal cords by direct laryngoscopy and the glottic aperture may be significantly narrowed or distorted. Much lively discussion is evident over the correct anaesthetic technique. When awake fibreoptic intubation is used, it allows visualization of the airway but becomes less useful

in the patient with stridor due to glottic narrowing. The fibrescope has little rigidity to 'push' through a narrow hole and attempts to do this may precipitate bleeding and oedema. If the scope is passed through a small hole, the airway is completely obstructed for a short time and patients feel uncomfortable at this stage. There have been a few reports[41, 42] of destabilization of the airway by applanaesthetic agent to the airway and this is a reminder of the need to work at all times in the correct environment for immediate activation of the preformulated back-up plan. Awake fibreoptic intubation is, therefore, a technique which should always be considered but may not be suitable. It is not appropriate when adequate operator skill is not present, in children and uncooperative adults and in the opinion of some anaesthetists when stridor is present.

Mason and Fielder[43] argue that the correct anaesthetic technique in the presence of stridor due to periglottic/glottic pathology is inhalational induction of general anaesthesia. [*] This permits a gradual onset of anaesthesia and maintains spontaneous respiration, even at a depth of anaesthesia appropriate for direct laryngoscopy and intubation. The maintenance of spontaneous respiration is viewed as highly desirable with supraglottic airway obstruction. A typical case scenario would be a child with epiglottitis and, in a survey of college tutors in the UK, 98 percent of anaesthetists would choose this form of anaesthesia. The face mask is applied to the patient who is in the most comfortable position (sitting if necessary) and 100 percent oxygen administered for a few minutes. The volatile agent is administered in increasing concentrations until a surgical level of anaesthesia is obtained. The agent commonly used initially is either halothane or sevoflurane and both drugs are nonirritant so do not provoke coughing. The speed of onset of anaesthesia is inversely proportional to the blood–gas solubility and is therefore faster with sevoflurane (0.6) than halothane (2.4). However, it is more difficult to establish sufficient depth of anaesthesia to instrument the airway with sevoflurane and it has a more rapid offset than halothane. Halothane may be associated with increased cardiac rhythm irritability and is now difficult to obtain in the UK. It is usual, therefore, to start with sevoflurane but change over to isoflurane which does permit adequate levels of anaesthesia.

It is not an easy anaesthetic to administer in the presence of stridor and requires a sanguine anaesthetist. There may be periods of increasing obstruction due to glottic irritability or change in position. Generally, there should be no change in the position of the anaesthetist's hands or the face mask and no attempt in light planes of anaesthesia to provide positive pressure ventilation. Insertion of an oral airway is risky but there may be benefit in a nasopharyngeal airway, although it is perhaps useful to have applied a vasoconstrictor to the nasal mucosa first. Glottic irritability is confined to light planes of anaesthesia and should resolve, although induction may take much longer than normal because of the reduced alveolar ventilation. When an adequate depth of anaesthesia is reached, which may take 20 minutes, direct laryngoscopy is undertaken. The view may be quite abnormal and it may be necessary to press on the chest and observe the egress of bubbles to detect the glottis. A small tube will be needed and the use of a bougie should be considered. If intubation is not possible, the face mask is reapplied and a tracheostomy undertaken. Plan B must be formulated and ready so that anaesthesia is induced in the operating theatre with the surgeon scrubbed and ready to undertake tracheostomy.

It is apparent that the safety of any approach is the combination of plans and the close cooperative working of the surgeon, anaesthetist and theatre team. In the common scenario of a known obstructing glottic tumour which requires initial histology and debulking, it is possible to construct a primary plan of (in the operating theatre) preoxygenation, followed by intravenous induction and rapid muscle relaxation. Direct laryngoscopy using a bougie and size 5.0 mm microlaryngeal tube is attempted. If it is unsuccessful, the surgeon is in the best situation to undertake tracheostomy – the patient is as well oxygenated as possible, unconscious and remains still. This technique is logical and popular but appears 'heretical' since it abolishes spontaneous respiration. However, it illustrates that safety lies in the combination of plans rather than any particular plan A, that the site of obstruction requires plans which are specific for that level of obstruction and the safety which arises from the close working of experienced surgeon and anaesthetist.

There is an increasing evidence-base to the practice of planned prior placement of a transtracheal ventilation catheter under local anaesthesia and using this as a route for oxygenation and ventilation during intubation attempts under general anaesthesia. The technique was used in 11 patients over 22 months in one institution with great success.[44] [**]

TRACHEOSTOMY UNDER LOCAL ANAESTHESIA

This should be considered in any patient with an obstructed airway. It is particularly appropriate as the primary plan when the disease process is a large friable mass or abscess in the supraglottis or glottis and intubation attempts may destabilize or compromise the airway. There are differences between countries and between surgeon–anaesthetist pairs as to when the patient undergoes traditional intubation in the awake or anaesthetized state or awake tracheostomy. Elements within the decision making are the availability of a skilled fibre-endoscopist, the ability of the patient to cooperate with the procedure and adopt a suitable position, the pretracheal anatomy and the likely time for resolution of the disease process. It may be a very difficult procedure in patients with short stocky necks, a previous tracheostomy or post-radiotherapy with respiratory distress.

Tracheostomy under local anaesthesia is undertaken in the operating theatre with the patient breathing oxygen or heliox, monitored by noninvasive blood pressure, ECG and pulse oximetry with intravenous access. A semisitting position with a roll under the shoulders and neck extension is ideal. Generally, reassurance is given to the patient but intravenous sedation is not required and should be used cautiously. Restlessness during the procedure may be due to hypoxia, hypercarbia or an inability to breathe in that position. Sedation may destabilize the airway leading to sudden hypoxia and loss of consciousness. The anaesthetist must be prepared for the back-up plan if the patient deteriorates. Placement of a cricothyrotomy needle at the outset may be useful when it is known that the pathology is supraglottic. The cricothyrotomy needle does not interfere with a surgical tracheostomy and can be used to provide oxygenation. If the patient becomes so restless that the surgeon is unable to operate, consideration should be given to providing general anaesthesia and oxygenation through the needle.

Another option in the distressed patient is to provide sedation/anaesthesia by addition of a volatile anaesthetic agent, such as sevoflurane, to the breathing system with 100 percent oxygen. At best, the airway proves to be adequate enough to allow a surgical plane of anaesthesia to be reached and the tracheostomy is undertaken in a relatively unhurried fashion on 100 percent oxygen/sevoflurane by face mask. At worst, the airway deteriorates with the onset of sedation/anaesthesia but the patient stops moving and a rapid emergency tracheostomy can be undertaken. In a rapid tracheostomy, the surgeon enters the airway with one or two incisions and a small cuffed microlaryngeal or armoured tube size 5.0–6.0 mm is inserted. Once the patient has been stabilized, a more measured exploration of the neck and fashioning of a formal tracheostomy may be undertaken.

It is important to verify that the tube is within the trachea before ventilation starts otherwise gas may be forced into the mediastinal tissues. Signs of correct placement when undertaking a tracheostomy under local anaesthesia (with the patient breathing spontaneously) are firstly regular respiratory movement of the reservoir bag of the anaesthetic breathing system connected to the tracheostomy tube, and the presence of six successive breath-related carbon dioxide traces on the capnograph. If no carbon dioxide is detected in the breathing system, inflation of the cuff of the tracheal tube or tracheostomy and connection of the capnograph to the breathing system should be checked first. If both are correct, failure to detect carbon dioxide indicates that the tube is not in the airway. When an emergency tracheostomy is undertaken in an apnoeic patient, the confirmatory signs of anaesthetic bag movement and capnography can be obtained only by applying a number of positive pressure breaths. If the tube is not within the trachea, these positive pressure breaths into the mediastinum may prove deleterious. An alternative confirmatory device in these circumstances, although not widely used, is the oesophageal detector device. The principle is simple and takes advantage of the structural differences between the oesophagus and trachea. In the original version described by Wee in 1988, an empty 60 mL syringe is attached to the 15 mm connector of the inserted tracheal tube and aspiration attempted. Aspiration of air is not possible if the tube is in the oesophagus because the mucosa is 'sucked' over the end of the tube, whereas the more rigid cartilaginous structure of the trachea allows free aspiration of air. The syringe can be replaced by a self-inflating bulb with a volume of approximately 75 mL and in this version the bulb is squeezed flat before being attached to the inserted tube. If the bulb reinflates immediately, the tube is in the trachea and if the bulb does not reinflate the tube is in a false passage or the oesophagus.

SUBGLOTTIC AND MIDTRACHEAL OBSTRUCTION

Imaging is particularly useful in delineating the length of narrowing, the diameter of the airway at its narrowest and that sufficient distance is present inferiorly to the obstruction to permit the cuff of a tracheal tube to be positioned above the carina. The obstruction may arise from external pressure, such as a retrosternal goitre or other mediastinal mass, from a mass arising from the trachea, from an inflammatory condition such as Wegener's granulomatosis, from previous surgery or from damage due to prolonged intubation. The type of narrowing may range from a short subglottic stenosis due to previous prolonged intubation to a narrowing of several centimetres in the midtrachea due to tumour. In the presence of stridor, the principles of management vary according to whether it can be bypassed by tracheostomy. This will be true for subglottic disease but the CEPOD assessors noted that in two patients it had been difficult to bypass a mid/low

tracheal lesion with a standard length tracheostomy tube. Awake fibreoptic intubation has a role in management of trachea narrowing, allowing inspection of the airway and confirmation that the tip of the tracheal tube has passed beyond the obstruction. Rigid bronchoscopy is an extremely effective means of managing these patients.

LOW TRACHEAL OBSTRUCTION

Narrowing of the lower trachea or carina presents great difficulty. The anaesthetic literature contains case reports of failed airway maintenance leading to death.[45] This characteristically occurs after induction of general anaesthesia or muscle relaxation when, presumably due to loss of muscle tone, airway patency is lost. Tracheal intubation may not provide an adequate airway because the obstruction is beyond the tip of the tube. Occasionally, the presence of carinal obstruction is not known and anaesthetic induction, intubation or indeed extubation may result in unexpected disaster. When imaging has provided good preoperative localization of obstruction, a number of options may be used. Rigid bronchoscopy is invaluable and will often provide a route for ventilation (**Figure 39.20**). The rigid bronchoscope may also act as a guide to therapy, such as lasering of a tumour or introduction of a tracheobronchial stent. Surgical resection of carinal lesions requires specialist anaesthetic techniques including jet ventilation and undertaking surgery during cardiopulmonary bypass.

EXTUBATION AND RECOVERY

At the end of surgery a decision is made as to where and when the airway device should be removed. There is little problem with removal of a laryngeal mask. This is usually tolerated well by a patient until they are awake. Tracheal intubation is common in head and neck surgery due to

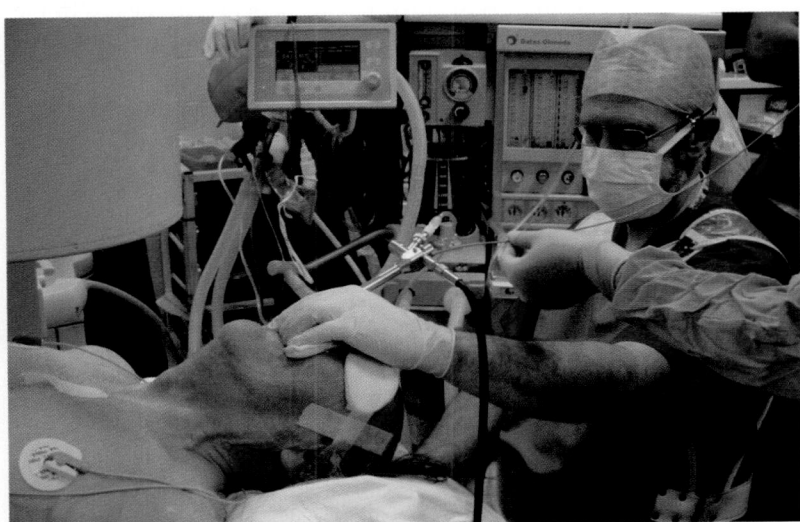

Figure 39.20 Rigid bronchoscopy used for ventilation and conduit for tracheal stent.

the constraints of providing clear operative fields for the surgeon and maintaining a secure airway to the distal trachea. Extubation requires as much thought, and gives rise to as much difficulty, as intubation. Transient difficulties with oxygen saturations are common due to coughing, breath-holding and laryngospasm, particularly in children. Extubation problems may arise in those patients who were difficult to intubate and those who were not difficult to intubate but in whom surgery has affected the airway.

Default strategy at extubation when no difficulty is expected is for the anaesthetist to remove any pharyngeal packs, suction the pharynx under direct vision, administer 100 percent oxygen, antagonize residual neuromuscular blockade and consider whether to remove the tube in the anaesthetized or awake state. After extubation, 100 percent oxygen is administered by face mask and the patient observed by the anaesthetist until it is clear that the patient is safe to go to the post-anaesthetic care unit (Recovery).

In the patient with a normal airway who was difficult to intubate, it is prudent to make certain that oxygen stores are maximal and to extubate in the awake state. Lung oxygen stores can be considered maximal when the end-tidal (i.e. alveolar) oxygen is 91 percent. This may take at least five minutes of breathing 100 percent oxygen or longer if nitrous oxide has been used. Awake extubation refers to removal of the tracheal tube when the person has opened their eyes and is able to obey commands. An additional option is to assess the leak around the tube before removal. This may be carried out by applying positive pressure to the tube, deflating the cuff and listening for egress of gas around the tube, or alternatively occluding the tube in spontaneous respiration and making certain that inspiration can occur around the tube. Failure of a leak test indicates that the tube is a very tight fit within the airway and an inadequate air passage may be left after extubation.

In the patient with an abnormal airway, either present preoperatively or due to surgery, consideration should be given to keeping the tracheal tube *in situ* for 24–48 hours until any airway oedema subsides. The patient should be nursed in a high-dependency unit with an appropriate level of sedation to avoid inadvertent removal of the tube. In some circumstances it is appropriate to perform a tracheostomy to provide a secure airway in the first few postoperative days.

Extubation of the high-risk airway requires a strategy. Awake extubation after maximal oxygenation in the presence of an anaesthetist in a well-equipped environment may be a good plan A, but what happens if it fails? The situation rapidly becomes critical with a struggling, hypoxic patient possibly with blood in the oropharynx. One possibility is to extubate over a thin bougie and to leave the bougie in the airway for a period until it is certain that the patient is coping satisfactorily. The bougie acts as a guide if reintubation is required and, if it is hollow, may be used for emergency oxygenation.

Problems may arise in the Recovery unit or postoperatively on the ward. Of most concern is postoperative bleeding following carotid endarterectomy or removal of a parapharyngeal mass. The physical presence of a mass of blood may compress the airway itself but also induces mucosal oedema, perhaps by impairment of lymphatic drainage. The deterioration of the airway may be very dramatic and necessitate emergency cricothyrotomy or tracheostomy as part of resuscitation. In a dire situation it is always worth fitting an LM. It is helpful to open the wound and evacuate the blood clot and this may provide temporary improvement. The patient is returned to theatre for surgical exploration. Intubation should take place with the patient breathing spontaneously, if possible. This may be by awake intubation or with inhalational anaesthesia. Blood in the pharynx may impair the view and the first response is to try suctioning. An LM may cover the larynx and provide some respite before being used as a conduit for intubation. Emergency tracheostomy may be required (**Figure 39.21**). In this patient, drainage of a peritonsillar abscess had been undertaken with intubation by awake fibreoptic intubation. The patient had been extubated and returned to Recovery. Approximately 45 minutes later, the patient developed severe breathing difficulties and was returned immediately to the operating theatre. Awake intubation was not possible due to soiling of the airway, the patient was too restless to adopt a position suitable for formal tracheostomy and, in a deteriorating situation, the surgeon managed to carry out a rapid emergency tracheostomy.

FOLLOW-UP

Following difficulties with airway management, a certain scheme should be followed. An account of the problem and management should be written in the anaesthetic record and in the hospital notes. The patient needs to be reviewed clinically to detect and treat any morbidity, an explanation is required for the patient with details of the problem encountered and management, and a written

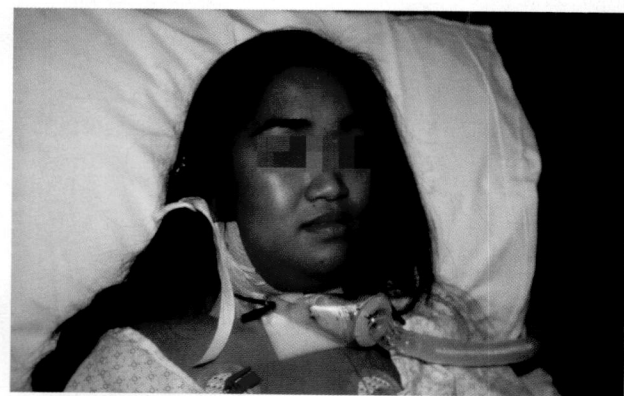

Figure 39.21 Post-extubation emergency tracheostomy.

account should be sent to the patient with a copy to their general practitioner.[46] If the problem with airway management is likely to be recurrent with subsequent anaesthetics, consideration should be given to the patient registering with Medic Alert and wearing a bracelet or to registering the patient with the difficult airway database supported by the Difficult Airway Society. [*]

Immediate morbidity or mortality from difficult airway management arise from the effects of severe hypoxia, hypercarbia or cardiovascular responses, from failure to adequately protect the airway leading to aspiration and from physical trauma to the airway during attempts at intubation or resuscitation. Airway damage may occur even when airway management has not been notably difficult. Valuable information can be obtained from detailed analysis of the medical information contained in insurance reports, once claims for negligence have been settled or closed. In an analysis of such closed claims in North America,[47] 6 percent of 4460 claims were for airway injury. The most frequent sites of injury were the larynx (33 percent), pharynx (19 percent) and oesophagus (18 percent). Approximately 20 percent of laryngeal injuries were associated with difficult intubation and included granuloma formation, arytenoid dislocation and hoarseness. Injuries to the pharynx and oesophagus had a much stronger association with difficult airway management. Half of all pharyngeal injuries and 68 percent of pharyngeal perforations were associated with difficult intubation.

There were five deaths in the pharyngeal injury claims and all involved perforation and the development of mediastinitis. The oesophageal injuries involved a significantly greater proportion of females and patients older than 60 years than the other sites and oesophageal perforation involved difficult intubation in 67 percent of claims. Oesophageal injuries were the most severe and were associated with a poor outcome with 19 percent mortality. Pharyngo-oesophageal perforation is a serious condition (overall mortality 25 percent) and risk factors include difficult intubation, emergency intubation and intubation by inexperienced personnel. Perforation may also be caused by passage of a nasogastric tube. The triad of surgical emphysema, chest pain and pyrexia should be sought and treatment with antibiotics, limitation of oral intake and surgical review initiated as soon as possible. In the closed claims study, surgical emphysema was only evident in 56 percent of patients and the diagnosis was sometimes delayed. It is suggested that treatment within 24 hours improves outcome. [*]

- Evaluation of the airway is imperfect and may fail to predict difficulty.
- Airway obstruction may be acute or chronic.
- Imaging of the airway is essential, when possible, to delineate the level of obstruction.
- Airway strategy means a primary plan A and back-up plan B.
- The anaesthetic room is an inappropriate location for plan A if plan B is a surgical tracheostomy.
- Pharyngo-oesophageal perforation due to intubation attempts has a high mortality and needs early detection and treatment.

Best clinical practice

- ✓ All patients should undergo airway evaluation as part of preoperative assessment.
- ✓ Strategy must cover unexpected failed intubation and failed ventilation.
- ✓ The LM is a versatile airway device and should always be available.
- ✓ Decisions about management of the obstructed airway are made by senior anaesthetists and surgeons.
- ✓ Awake fibreoptic intubation and tracheostomy under local anaesthesia should be considered in the obstructed airway.
- ✓ Maintenance of spontaneous respiration is recommended when general anaesthesia is employed in the presence of upper airway obstruction.
- ✓ Consider placement of a transtracheal ventilation catheter prior to inducing general anaesthesia in the difficult upper airway.
- ✓ Always confirm correct placement of the tube in the trachea.
- ✓ A strategy is required for extubation.
- ✓ Follow-up is important to detect and treat morbidity caused by airway management.

KEY POINTS

- The difficult airway is an important feature in head and neck surgery.
- Difficult intubation and difficult mask ventilation are different entities.

Deficiencies in current knowledge and areas for future research

- ➤ Unified surgical and anaesthetic terms describing the location of disease pathology in the airway.
- ➤ Randomized comparative studies of anaesthetic techniques in management of the obstructed airway.
- ➤ National collection of serious adverse incidents resulting from airway management in head and neck disease.

➤ National audit of attempts at emergency cricothyrotomy.

➤ Annual publication of circumstances of death within 28 days of surgery for the obstructed airway.

REFERENCES

1. Caplan RA, Benumof JL, Berry FA, Blitt CD, Bode RH, Cheney FW *et al*. A practice guideline for management of the difficult airway. *Anesthesiology*. 1993; **78**: 597–602.

2. Cormack RS, Lehane J. Difficult tracheal intubation in obstetrics. *Anaesthesia*. 1984; **39**: 1105–11.

* 3. Practice guidelines for management of the difficult airway. An updated report by the American Society of Anesthesiologists Task Force on management of the difficult airway. *Anesthesiology*. 2003; **98**: 1269–77. *Definitions and national evidence-based practice guidelines from USA.*

4. Arne J, Descoins P, Fusciardi J, Ingrand P, Ferrier B, Boudigues D *et al*. Preoperative assessment for difficult intubation in general and ENT surgery: predictive value of a clinical multivariate risk index. *British Journal of Anaesthesia*. 1998; **80**: 140–6.

5. Rose DK, Cohen MM. The airway: problems and prediction in 18,500 patients. *Canadian Journal of Anaesthesiology*. 1994; **41**: 372–83.

6. Langeron O, Masso E, Huraux C, Guggiari M, Bianchi A, Coriat P *et al*. Prediction of difficult mask ventilation. *Anesthesiology*. 2000; **92**: 1229–36.

7. Schmitt H, Buchfelder M, Radespiel-Troger M, Fahlbusch R. Difficult intubation in acromegalic patients. *Anesthesiology*. 2000; **93**: 110–4.

8. Khan ZH, Kashfi A, Ebrahimkhani E. A comparison of the upper lip bite test (a simple new technique) with modified Mallampati classification in predicting difficulty in endotracheal intubation: a prospective blinded study. *Anesthesia and Analgesia*. 2003; **96**: 595–9.

9. Ayuso MA, Sala X, Luis M, Carbo JM. Predicting difficult orotracheal intubation in pharyngo-laryngeal disease: preliminary results of a composite index. *Canadian Journal of Anaesthesia*. 2003; **50**: 81–5.

10. Bouaggad A, Nejmi SE, Bouderka MA, Abbassi O. Prediction of difficult tracheal intubation in thyroid surgery. *Anesthesia and Analgesia*. 2004; **99**: 603–6.

11. Eberhart LH, Arndt C, Cierpka T, Schwanekamp J, Wulf H, Putzke C. The reliability and validity of the upper lip bite test compared with the Mallampati classification to predict difficult laryngoscopy: an external prospective evaluation. *Anesthesia and Analgesia*. 2005; **101**: 284–9.

12. Wilson ME, Spiegelhalter D, Robertson JA, Lesser P. Predicting difficult intubation. *British Journal of Anaesthesia*. 1988; **61**: 211–6.

13. Yentis SM. Predicting difficult intubation – worthwhile exercise or pointless ritual. *Anaesthesia*. 2002; **57**: 105–9.

* 14. Shiga T, Wajima Z, Inoue T, Sakamato A. Predicting difficult intubation in apparently normal patients: a meta-analysis of bedside screening test performance. *Anesthesiology*. 2005; **103**: 429–37. *Excellent reference list and analysis of predictive power of individual tests.*

15. Rosenstock C, Kristensen MS. Decreased tongue mobility – an explanation for difficult endotracheal intubation? *Acta Anaesthesiologica Scandinavica*. 2005; **49**: 92–945.

16. Kamble VA, Lilly RB, Gross JB. Unanticipated difficult intubation as a result of an asymptomatic vallecular cyst. *Anesthesiology*. 1999; **91**: 872–3.

17. Ovassapian A, Glassenberg R, Rendel GI, Klock A, Mesnick PS, Klafta JM. The unexpected difficult airway and lingual tonsillar hyperplasia: a case series and review of the literature. *Anesthesiology*. 2002; **97**: 124–32.

18. Benumof JL. Laryngeal mask airway and the ASA difficult airway algorithm. *Anesthesiology*. 1996; **84**: 686–99.

19. Combes X, Le Roux B, Suen P, Dumerat M, Motamed C, Sauvat S *et al*. Unanticipated difficult airway in anesthetized patients. Prospective validation of a management algorithm. *Anesthesiology*. 2004; **100**: 1146–50.

20. Mort TC. Emergency tracheal intubation: complications associated with repeated laryngoscopic attempts. *Anesthesia and Analgesia*. 2004; **99**: 607–13.

* 21. Henderson JJ, Popat MT, Latto IP, Pearce AC. Difficult Airway Society guidelines for management of the unanticipated difficult intubation. *Anaesthesia*. 2004; **59**: 675–94. *Excellent reference list and national airway management guidelines from the UK.*

22. Henderson JJ. The use of paraglossal straight blade laryngoscopy in difficult tracheal intubation. *Anaesthesia*. 1997; **52**: 552–60.

23. Crosby ET, Cooper RM, Douglas MJ, Doyle DJ, Hung OR, Labrecque P *et al*. The unanticipated difficult airway with recommendations for management. *Canadian Journal of Anaesthesiology*. 1998; **45**: 757–76.

24. Murphy P. A fibre-optic endoscope used for nasal intubation. *Anaesthesia*. 1967; **22**: 489–91.

25. Popat M. *Practical fibreoptic intubation*. Oxford: Butterworth Heinemann, 2001 ISBN 0 7506 4496 6.

26. Hawkins N. *Fibreoptic intubation*. London: Greenwich Medical Media, 2000 ISBN 1 84110 060 9.

27. Heidegger T, Gerig HJ, Ulrich B, Kreienbuhl G. Validation of a simple algorithm for tracheal intubation: daily practice is the key to success in emergencies - an analysis of 13,248 intubations. *Anesthesia and Analgesia*. 2001; **92**: 517–22.

28. Ovassapian A. *Fiberoptic endoscopy and the difficult airway*. Lippincott-Raven, 1996 ISBN 0 7817 0272 0.

29. Ferson DZ, Rosenblatt WH, Johansen MJ, Osborn I, Ovassapian A. use of the intubating LMA-Fastrach in 254 patients with difficult-to-manage airways. *Anesthesiology*. 2001; **95**: 1175–81.

30. Joo HS, Kapoor S, Rose K, Naik VN. The intubating laryngeal mask airway after induction of general anesthesia versus awake fiberoptic intubation in patients with difficult airways. *Anesthesia and Analgesia*. 2001; **92**: 1342–6.

31. Davis L, Cook-Sather SD, Schreiner MS. Lighted stylet tracheal intubation: a review. *Anesthesia and Analgesia*. 2000; **90**: 745–56.

32. Charters P, O'Sullivan E. The dedicated airway: a review of the concept and an update of current practice. *Anaesthesia*. 1999; **54**: 778–86.

33. Atherton DP, O'Sullivan E, Lowe D, Charters P. A ventilation-exchange bougie for fibreoptic intubations with the laryngeal mask airway. *Anaesthesia*. 1996; **51**: 1123–6.

34. Vanner R. Emergency cricothyrotomy. *Current Anaesthesia and Critical Care*. 2001; **12**: 238–43.

35. Brofeldt BT, Panacek EA, Richards JR. An easy cricothyrotomy approach: the rapid four-step technique. *Academic Emergency Medicine*. 1996; **3**: 1060–3.

36. Popat M, Dudnikov S. Management of the obstructed upper airway. *Current Anaesthesia and Critical Care*. 2001; **12**: 225–30.

37. National Confidential Enquiry into Patient Outcome and Death. 1996/97 Report. London: NCEPOD, cited April 07. Available from: http://www.ncepod.org.uk/sum96.htm#32

38. Woodall N. Awake intubation. *Current Anaesthesia and Critical Care*. 2001; **12**: 218–24.

39. Ovassapian A, Tuncbilek M, Weitzel EK, Joshi CW. Airway management in adult patients with deep neck infections: a case series and review of the literature. *Anesthesia and Analgesia*. 2005; **100**: 585–9.

40. Gold MI, Buechel DR. Translaryngeal anesthesia: a review. *Anesthesiology*. 1959; **20**: 181–5.

41. Shaw IC, Welchew EA, Harrison BJ, Michael S. Complete airway obstruction during awake fibreoptic intubation. *Anaesthesia*. 1997; **52**: 582–5.

42. Ho AM, Chung DC, To EW, Karmakar MK. Total airway obstruction during local anesthesia in a non-sedated patient with a compromised airway. *Canadian Journal of Anaesthesia*. 2004; **51**: 838–41.

43. Mason RA, Fielder CP. The obstructed airway in head and neck surgery. *Anaesthesia*. 1999; **54**: 625–8.

44. Gerig HJ, Schnider T, Heidegger T. Prophylactic percutaneous transtracheal catheterisation in the management of patients with anticipated difficult airways: a case series. *Anaesthesia*. 2005; **60**: 801–5.

45. Goh MH, Liu XY, Goh YS. Anterior mediastinal masses: an anaesthetic challenge. *Anaesthesia*. 1999; **54**: 670–4.

46. Barron FA, Ball DR, Jefferson P, Norrie J. Airway alerts. How UK anaesthetists organise, document and communicate difficult airway management. *Anaesthesia*. 2003; **58**: 73–7.

∗ 47. Domino KB, Posner KL, Caplan RA, Cheney FW. Airway injury during anesthesia. *Anesthesiology*. 1999; **91**: 1703–11. *Analysis of closed claims in USA.*

40

Adult anaesthesia

ANDREW D FARMERY AND JAIDEEP J PANDIT

Principles of general anaesthesia	488		Anaesthetic technique and principles for specific ENT	
Premedication	489		operations	500
Key points	490		Salivary gland surgery	503
Anaesthetic agents	490		Nasal and sinus surgery	503
Key points	491		Laryngeal microsurgery and laryngoscopy	503
Inhalational agents	491		Laser surgery	503
Key points	491		Key points	505
Devices used in airway management	492		Best clinical practice	505
Key points	495		Deficiencies in current practice and areas for future	
Conduct of anaesthesia: principles guiding induction of			research	505
anaesthesia	495		References	506
Monitoring in anaesthesia	496			

SEARCH STRATEGY AND EVIDENCE-BASE

The search strategy for the evidence in the chapter was by Medline search of the key words anaesthesia, ear, nose, throat and maxillofacial, and combinations of the words. Reference lists of retrieved papers were searched manually as were reference lists of standard text (listed in the reference list at the end of the chapter).

As is the case with anaesthesia in general the evidence levels are largely from observational, nonexperimental, noncontrolled studies or expert opinion (i.e. levels 3 and 4), or in the case of clinical evidence from low-quality case-controlled/cohort studies or clinical series and expert opinion (i.e. grades C and D). This arises purely due to the paucity of randomized controlled trials or metaanalyses of the common questions covered in this chapter.

PRINCIPLES OF GENERAL ANAESTHESIA

Anaesthesia is a relatively modern specialty. Before the mid-nineteenth century, the scope of operative surgery was small. The advent of anaesthesia, however, facilitated a revolution in surgical practice. Although anaesthetic techniques have changed considerably since this time, the basic principles that underpin the practice have changed little. Modern anaesthetic practice encompasses many things, including perioperative system support, monitoring, postoperative intensive care and pain relief. However, the roots of anaesthetic practice lie in the simple requirement to **facilitate successful surgery**. The main aims to this end are summarized in the triad of surgical anaesthesia below:

1. to abolish consciousness, implicit and explicit memory (= hypnosis);
2. to prevent movement (= akinesia);
3. to obtund the subconscious response to pain, stress and trauma (= analgesia).

These are both functional and humanitarian aims. The principal benefit to the pioneering surgeon was the abolition of movement in their patients, so now for the first time, subtle and delicate procedures could successfully be undertaken. The abolition of consciousness and recall is a clear humanitarian benefit to the patient, and the obtunding of the response to pain produces better operating conditions as well as having other advantages.

Early anaesthesia, to some extent, achieved all three of these aims with a single agent, namely ether. Given in sufficient dosage, ether could produce surgical anaesthesia achieving hypnosis, akinesia and, to some extent, analgesia. The drawback with this kind of 'single-agent anaesthesia' was that the doses of ether required to achieve all these was often perilously high.

In contrast, modern anaesthesia tackles the triad of anaesthesia using a combination of drugs or agents to satisfy each of the aims separately. This has become known as 'balanced anaesthesia' and is depicted in **Figure 40.1**.

In balanced anaesthesia, the 'anaesthetic vapour' (such as halothane or isoflurane) is used merely to depress cognitive function and provide the element of 'hypnosis'. This is achieved at relatively low concentrations; far below those required to achieve akinesia and analgesia and far below concentrations associated with respiratory depression and cardiovascular collapse.

The element of analgesia is provided by specific drugs (such as the opioid fentanyl or the opiate morphine), or by supplemental use of regional or local anaesthetic blocks.

This combination of hypnotic and analgesic drugs may be sufficient also to provide akinesia, i.e. to abolish movement in response to stimulus, and yet the patient may still breath spontaneously. However, there are occasions when it is desirable to abolish all movement and to relax the tone in all skeletal muscle, for example to facilitate endotracheal intubation and permit mechanical ventilation. This can be achieved by specific drugs which block the neuromuscular junction and paralyse skeletal muscle such as atracurium or vecuronium. When the element of akinesia is provided in this way, it is possible to reduce the doses of hynotic and analgesic drugs yet further. So by judicious use of hypnotics, analgesics and muscle relaxation, a state of balanced anaesthesia can be achieved in which the dose of anaesthetic agent is a fraction of that which would be required if it were used as a sole agent.

PREMEDICATION

Until relatively recently, premedicant drugs were used religiously and routinely as an accompaniment to general anaesthesia. This habit probably stemmed from the necessity of using such drugs when ether inhalation was standard practice.

The need for anxiolysis

Induction of anaesthesia by inhalation of ether and chloroform was a lengthy process, and many patients still have unpleasant memories of it. As these experiences entered the folklore, patients often became more anxious about their impending anaesthetic than their surgery.

The need for an antisialogogue

In addition, inhalation of the early anaesthetic agents produced copious secretions which was not only undesirable to the ENT surgeon, but also made spontaneous respiration via a face mask a challenge for the anaesthetist.

The need for an antiemetic

Ether is a particularly potent emetic. Even modern volatile agents can contribute to postoperative nausea and vomiting.

The need for an opiate

In modern anaesthesia, rapidly acting, lipid soluble synthetic opioids can be used to produce desired levels of analgesia with precision. By contrast, the traditional opiates (morphine, omnopon, etc.) used in early anaesthesia have a slow onset of action and so were best given an hour or so before the onset of surgery to ensure adequate analgesia. Such opiates were not usually given intraoperatively in any significant dose because, since most patients breathed spontaneously via face masks, any depression of respiration was considered undesirable.

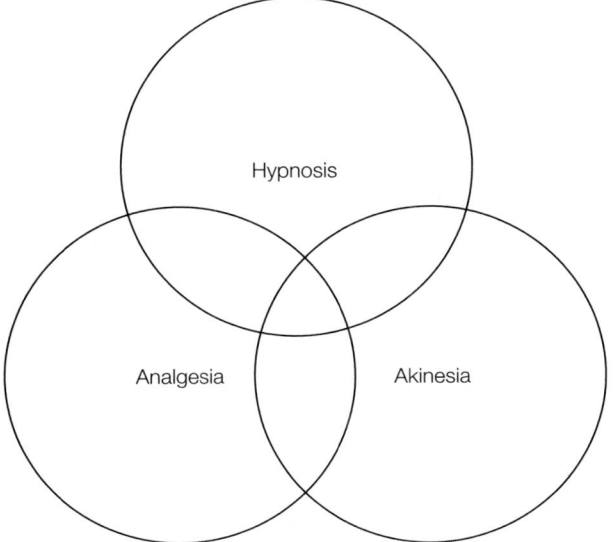

Figure 40.1 Balanced anaesthesia.

Table 40.1   Modern premedicant drugs.

Analgesics		Gastric alkalinizers	Prokinetics/antiemetics	Anxiolytics
NSAIDs	Paracetamol			
NSAIDs are widely used in the perioperative period. They are remarkably effective and relatively safe when used in healthy patients for a short duration. Although many preparations can be given rectally, they are well absorbed from the stomach and best, and most economically, given orally if possible	This is a safe and effective analgesic which can be given orally with an NSAID one hour preoperatively	Aspiration of even small volumes of acid gastric fluid can produce severe respiratory complications. All patients with a history of gastro-oesophageal reflux should receive prophylactic treatment to reduce gastric acidity. Many anaesthetists would routinely do this for all patients H_2 blockers, e.g. ranitidine Proton pump inhibitors, e.g. omeprazole Sodium citrate. This is a 'buffer' which mops up acid and is given, if indicated, immediately pre-induction.	Metoclopramide is a dopamine antagonist, which increases gastric motility and emptying and has antiemetic properties. The evidence is not clear whether the benefits of such drugs justify their prophylactic use	The best anxiolysis is provided by good communication between doctor and patient. Well-informed and reassured patients will seldom require pharmacological anxiolysis. Where indicated, it is usually provided by oral drugs, e.g. benzodiazepines such as temazepam

The combination of intramuscular omnopon and scopolamine ('om and scop') was for many years the 'pre-med' of choice for adult anaesthesia, since it combined analgesia, anxiolysis, antiemesis and the drying of secretions.

Modern anaesthetic drugs and techniques are now so finely honed that the traditional 'pre-med' is rarely required and is seldom used. However, in some cases premedication with other drugs is indicated (see **Table 40.1**).[1]

> **KEY POINTS**
>
> - Sedative premedication is seldom used in modern anaesthetic practice, especially as day-case surgery is increasing.
> - Pre-emptive analgesia (from simple agents such as nonsteroidal antiinflammatory drugs (NSAIDs) and paracetamol) are usefully given preoperatively to provide early postoperative pain relief.

> - Antiemetic and antacid prophylaxis can usefully be given preoperatively to high-risk patients.

ANAESTHETIC AGENTS

Intravenous agents

Intravenous (i.v.) anaesthetic agents can be used to induce and/or to maintain anaesthesia, although they are more commonly used for induction alone. For many years, the barbiturate thiopentone dominated this class of drugs. However, by far the most commonly used i.v. induction agent in the western world is propofol, which is a derivative of phenol. Most induction agents are extremely lipid soluble, and this accounts for their rapid onset of action, since they are delivered to the brain with a high blood flow and diffuse into it (the brain being principally lipid) with ease. Plasma levels then fall rapidly. This is not due to rapid metabolism, but rather because the drug redistributes (via the large cerebral blood flow) to other lipid-rich tissues with lower blood flows. Metabolic clearance accounts for a much slower 'background' elimination of drug and reduction in the brain-drug levels.

Propofol is so lipid soluble that it cannot easily be dissolved in aqueous media. For this reason it is prepared as a lipid emulsion and this accounts for its milky appearance.

As well as being used for induction, propofol can be infused intravenously to maintain anaesthesia. This is an increasingly popular technique and can be associated with more rapid clear-headed recovery and a reduction in postoperative nausea. Like most anaesthetic agents, thiopentone and propofol are associated with a fall in blood pressure mediated by a number of mechanisms, including reduction in central sympathetic vasomotor tone and reduction in cardiac contractility. These features are particularly marked in the elderly and patients who are hypovolaemic and dehydrated.

> **KEY POINTS**
>
> - Intravenous induction agents owe their rapid onset and offset of action to rapid diffusion across the blood–brain barrier due to their high lipid solubility.
> - Hepatic clearance is moderately slow, and does not play a significant part in the return of consciousness after a bolus dose of intravenous agent.

INHALATIONAL AGENTS

Inhalational or 'volatile' agents may be used for induction and/or maintenance of anaesthesia, although they are more commonly used for maintenance alone. The historical archetype is 'ether' (actually diethyl ether) but the more commonly used modern agents such as isoflurane and sevoflurane are also ethers (halogenated methyl-ethyl ethers). Like the intravenous agents, the volatile agents are lipid soluble: the higher the lipid solubility, the higher the potency. Modern agents are extremely lipid soluble and so their potency is sufficiently high to require only 1 or 2 percent concentration in the inspired gas to induce anaesthesia. The depth of anaesthesia is determined by the partial pressure (i.e. the effective concentration) of the volatile agent in the brain. Since the brain is in equilibrium with the arterial blood, and the latter is in equilibrium with the alveolar gas, then the depth of anaesthesia should be determined by the partial pressure (or concentration) of volatile agent in the alveoli. Given that we can easily measure the

concentration of anaesthetic vapours in the alveoli (i.e. in the expired breath), we can therefore reliably determine and estimate the anaesthetic depth with precision and confidence. In contrast, we have no means of doing this for i.v. agents.

Volatile agents can also be used to induce anaesthesia, and some do so more quickly than others. We have already stated that the depth of anaesthesia is determined by the partial pressure of the agent in the alveoli/blood/brain. In the blood, only molecules that are not in solution contribute to the partial pressure. As soon as a molecule of gas or vapour enters solution in the blood, it is effectively 'hidden' and no longer contributes to the partial pressure. This is analogous to the absorbency of a sponge. When water is absorbed into the sponge it no longer contributes to its external 'wetness'. A large volume of water will need to be added to a highly absorbent sponge before it contributes to its external wetness, whereas only a small volume needs to be added to a poorly absorbent sponge before it appears wet.

So, for agents which are highly soluble in blood (such as traditional ether or halothane), the partial pressure in the blood will be slow to rise because almost as fast as the molecules of gas diffuse across the lung into the blood, they enter solution and are effectively hidden, thus failing to contribute to the partial pressure. Conversely, modern agents, such as sevoflurane, have a low blood solubility. As these molecules enter the bloodstream, only a few enter solution, the remainder do not, and therefore contribute to the partial pressure in the blood. Consequently, the arterial partial pressure rises and equilibrates rapidly with the alveolar gas. In turn, the high partial pressure in the arterial blood equilibrates with the brain and induction occurs rapidly. In summary, modern agents have a high lipid solubility (and hence high potency) and low blood solubility (and hence allow rapid induction).[2]

The sections above outline the drugs that can be used to induce and maintain anaesthesia. The following section outlines how anaesthetic technique is planned for some common or important ENT operations, with a particular emphasis on management of the patient's airway. One of the hallmarks of anaesthesia for ENT surgery is the concept of the 'shared airway': the surgeon operates in the same anatomical region as the anaesthesia airway devices are situated. Therefore, the detailed properties of the airway device selected and precise conduct of anaesthesia are particularly important to ENT surgery as compared with many other types of surgery.

> **KEY POINTS**
>
> - Older agents (ether, halothane) have high solubility in blood and therefore a slow onset and offset of action.

- Modern agents (sevoflurane, desflurane) have low solubility in blood and therefore rapid onset and offset of action.
- Because of our ability to measure vapour concentrations in the expired breath, adequate depth of anaesthesia can be determined with confidence.

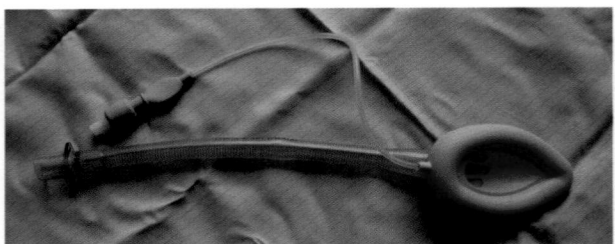

Figure 40.2   Laryngeal mask airway.

DEVICES USED IN AIRWAY MANAGEMENT

The simple face mask

Induction of anaesthesia invariably results in a degree of collapse of the upper airway resulting in airway obstruction. This is largely due to the reduction in tone of the pharyngeal dilator muscles and genioglossus. These muscles are innervated by the efferent outflow of the 'respiratory centre', and tone varies cyclically in much the same way as does the diaphragm under the command of the phrenic nerve. Drugs that depress the respiratory centre and have a tendency to produce a 'central' apnoea, also by this mechanism, have a tendency to produce an 'obstructive' apnoea. Central and obstructive apnoeas are therefore inextricably linked, and cannot adequately be categorized as separate entities.[3]

If neuromuscular blocking drugs are also used, then spontaneous ventilation is abolished completely. All these factors require the use of devices that give both anatomical support to the upper airway and also facilitate ventilation. Perhaps the simplest means of achieving these aims is a face mask which, when connected to a suitable supply of oxygen and/or anaesthetic gas, may be used to support the airway manually or (if spontaneous ventilation is absent) allow hand-ventilation of the patient's lungs. Problems with the face mask technique are that it does not allow good surgical access to the face, head or airway; it requires that one or both of the anaesthetist's hands are occupied in airway maintenance and active ventilation of the patient's lungs can be often inefficient (i.e. not all the tidal volume administered to the patient enters the lungs, and some is lost as a 'leak').

Supraglottic airway devices

A range of supraglottic airway devices (SADs) have been developed which reduce some of these problems. In general, these are tubes (often with inflatable distal components to 'hold' the airway in place) that lie in the oropharynx, above the level of the glottis. The device most commonly used is the laryngeal mask airway and others include the cuffed oropharyngeal airway and the Proseal™ laryngeal mask (**Figure 40.2**). SADs allow spontaneous breathing and, similar to the face mask technique, facilitate active ventilation by hand. However, since SADs lie above the glottic opening and do not seal it, there is a risk that prolonged positive pressure ventilation of the lungs (for example, if the SAD is connected to a mechanical ventilator) may cause air to enter the oesophagus and stomach. If gastric fluid should then regurgitate, SADs will not completely protect the airway from lung soiling. There is currently a debate concerning the role of some SAD devices in positive pressure ventilation, and some authorities argue that their use during positive pressure ventilation is, in fact, justified.[4]

Tracheal tubes

There is a range of tracheal tubes available (**Figure 40.3**). These tubes lie in the trachea and (usually) have a small cuff at the distal end, whose purpose it is to protect the airway from soiling (for example by blood or regurgitant gastric contents) and to improve the efficiency of ventilation by minimizing leaks. Tracheal tubes vary in shape, size and the material from which they are made, and these factors are important in relation to their specific use.

CUFFED VERSUS UNCUFFED TUBES

Generally speaking, cuffed tubes are used in adult anaesthesia, and 'plain' or uncuffed tubes are used in prepubertal children for the following reason. In adults, the narrowest part of the larynx is at the level of the vocal cords, and so if a tube can be passed between the cords, one can be confident that at any point distal to the vocal cords, the tube will be sitting loosely and will not be wedged-in, causing epithelial damage. The high-volume, low-pressure cuff can be inflated to provide a loose seal at this level. In children however, the narrowest part of the larynx is at the level of the cricoid cartilage and not at the vocal cords. It is, therefore, quite possible to pass a tracheal tube which is small enough to pass through the cords with ease, but which may be wedged-in at the level of the cricoid, and this may cause epithelial oedema or necrosis at this level. This is particularly problematic in small airways because any further reduction in calibre in an already small airway produces a disproportionately

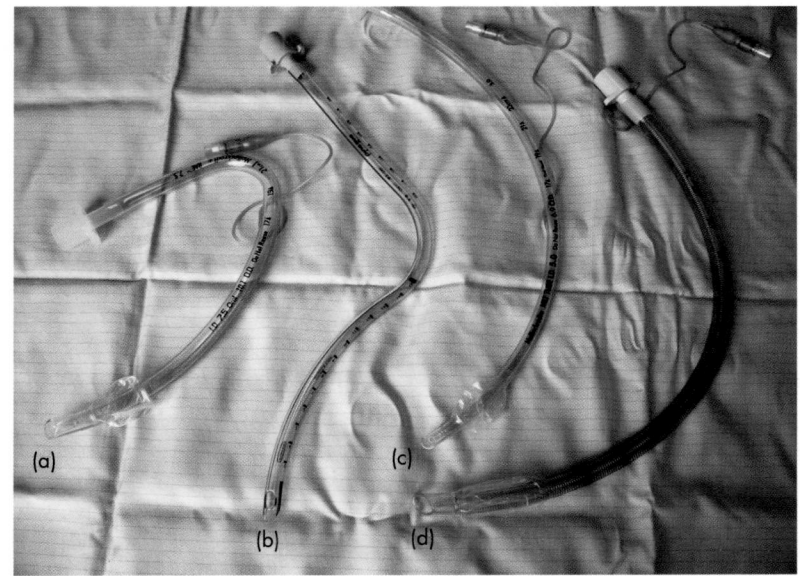

Figure 40.3 Tracheal tubes. (a) A cuffed RAE tube. The tube is preformed in a 'south-facing' curve so that the anaesthetic breathing system passes out of the way of the surgical field; (b) a 'north-facing' RAE tracheal tube; useful if the anaesthetist and the breathing system are 'north' of the patient's head and the surgeon is working from the 'south'; (c) a microlaryngeal tube. This has an internal diameter of 5 mm and is sufficiently narrow to allow the vocal cords to be inspected during panendoscopies; (d) a reinforced tracheal tube. Note the metallic spiral in the wall of the tube that allows it to be bent in any direction without kinking the lumen.

greater increase in airflow resistance, since this is inversely related to the fourth power of the airway radius.

In order to confirm that the tracheal tube is sitting loosely at all points in the larynx, plain tubes are used and one deliberately seeks to allow a small leak. This should be audible on inflation of the chest under positive pressure and excludes the possibility that the tube is exerting any circumferential pressure on the laryngeal epithelium at its narrowest point. The disadvantages of having this small leak is that ventilation may not be as efficient and the lower airway is not definitively secured and protected from soiling from above. For this reason, if the type of surgery permits, the laryngeal inlet can be packed with damp ribbon gauze.

Since tracheal tubes form a sealed conduit into the trachea, they are primarily used when the patient is paralysed and requires positive pressure ventilation (there is no risk of blowing air into the stomach). It is indeed possible to allow the patient to breathe spontaneously through a tracheal tube, but since the glottis and trachea are richly innervated, deep anaesthesia is required to prevent the patient from reflex coughing. The doses required to achieve this may lead to dose-related side effects (as described above). Whereas most SAD devices can be used effectively after relatively short periods of training, the techniques used by the anaesthetist to insert a tracheal tube are more specialized and are described in more detail in Chapter 39, Recognition and management of the difficult airway. Tracheal tubes may be passed either orally or nasally, and these routes are important and can depend upon the type of surgery performed (for example, a nasotracheal tube facilitates better surgical access for dental surgery, but is clearly a hindrance during operations on the nose).

Regardless of which airway device is selected, it is vital that there is constant communication between surgeon and anaesthetist regarding the other's needs during surgery (and also at the stage of planning an operation). The airway device must not hinder the surgical process because of its size or shape; it must be properly secured in place to prevent dislodgement during head movement by the surgeon; and the direction of the airway device shaft must be appropriate to the operation. Use of surgical gags and props may compress the airway device, so the anaesthetist must be vigilant about the patency of the airway. Airway obstruction may occur not only during induction of anaesthesia, but also after extubation of the trachea or recovery and it is often especially important that the surgeon is present in the operating room at extubation.

Factors influencing choice of device in airway management

In general terms, patient factors and surgical factors dictate the choice of which of the above devices is used in anaesthetic airway management.

PATIENT FACTORS INFLUENCING CHOICE OF AIRWAY DEVICE

There are a number of factors or signs in the patient which would suggest to most anaesthetists that a tracheal tube (with the patient consequently artificially ventilated), rather than a SAD device (with the patient breathing spontaneously), should best be used.

Gastro-oesophageal reflux

Hiatus hernia, peptic ulcer disease, symptomatic reflux, pregnancy, recent ingestion of solids or particulate liquids, abdominal sepsis or injury all predispose to regurgitaton of gastric contents during induction of anaesthesia. Tracheal intubation (as part of a 'rapid sequence' induction of anaesthesia) would minimize the risk of lung soiling.

Obesity

Obese patients do not always find it easy to breathe when lying supine, even when awake. This difficulty is exacerbated when anaesthetized, and artificial positive pressure ventilation (necessitating tracheal intubation) is therefore often necessary.

Patients with known or anticipated difficult airway

In any patient whose trachea is known or anticipated to be difficult to intubate, it is reasonable to formulate a plan to intubate the trachea during induction of anaesthesia and so achieve a definitive, 'secured airway' in the patient before surgery begins. While it is also acceptable (and sometimes necessary should tracheal intubation fail) to use a SAD device, the problem is that should tracheal intubation subsequently be necessary urgently during the course of surgery, this might be difficult or impossible to achieve in a short space of time.

SURGICAL FACTORS INFLUENCING CHOICE OF AIRWAY DEVICE

A number of surgical requirements reasonably influence the choice of airway device.

Factors related to the 'shared airway'

For certain operations, it is necessary for the surgeon to have an unobstructed view of the relevant anatomy. Most SAD devices (as a result of the large distal cuff) do not permit a good view of structures distal to the oropharynx. Thus, for almost all periglottic, laryngeal and subglottic operations, a tracheal tube is more suitable or necessary. SAD devices may, however, be used for operations related to the tonsils, anterior tongue, nose, teeth and ears without obstructing the surgical field.

Laser surgery

Standard (polyvinyl chloride) tracheal tubes are not laser-resistant and may ignite if struck by the laser beam. A number of specialized tracheal tubes have been developed which are more laser-resistant. The materials used include various metals, Teflon and ceramics. Some recent work suggests that the flexible laryngeal mask airway is also suitably laser-resistant and, if used in the presence of laser, its distal cuff should be filled with saline (or methylene blue dye so that rupture can be easily detected). Anaesthesia for laser surgery is further discussed below under Laser surgery.

Requirement for neuromuscular blockade

For certain operations (for example abdominal surgery) it is necessary that the patient's muscles are fully flaccid to facilitate surgery. This is best achieved by use of neuromuscular blocking drugs. Since these also paralyse spontaneous ventilation, artificial mechanical ventilation is required; an endotracheal tube is most commonly used to facilitate this. While strict muscle relaxation of the degree needed in abdominal surgery is rarely required in ENT surgery, there are some operations in which it is desirable to minimize risk of the patient moving, coughing or swallowing (for example skull base surgery, any ENT operation in combination with neurosurgery or pharyngeal surgery). This is most reliably achieved by using neuromuscular blocking drugs.

Neuromuscular blockade and facial nerve monitoring

For certain ENT operations, such as vestibular schwannoma resection, middle ear, mastoid and parotid surgery, it is necessary that the surgeon is able to monitor the integrity of the facial nerve and minimize the risk of damaging it during surgery. For this purpose, needle electrodes are placed in the orbicularis oculi and oris muscles that detect EMG potentials generated in these muscles as a result of surgical or electrical stimulation of the facial nerve. The electrical activity evoked in these muscles is amplified and converted into an audible signal by the monitor. By this means, the surgeon is warned of the impending proximity of the nerve should he be unaware of its precise position, and can use the sound signal to moderate his handling of the nerve in those situations where this is necessary. At the completion of surgery the electrical integrity of the nerve can be assessed by proximal stimulation. In addition, it is possible to identify the site of a neuropraxia and, by varying the intensity of the stimulating current, assess its severity. A block that can be overcome by increasing the stimulation current is probably not as bad as one that cannot. Obviously, it is impossible to monitor facial nerve activity in the presence of complete neuromuscular blockade. Partial blockade can be overcome by decreasing the stimulation frequency from 30 to 3 Hz, but information derived in this state may be unreliable.

From the anaesthetic standpoint, if direct nerve monitoring is necessary, it is advisable to avoid long-acting neuromuscular blocking drugs altogether during surgery. If tracheal intubation is required, it is possible to use a short-acting muscle relaxant to facilitate intubation on the premise that the effect will have worn off by the time monitoring is required by the surgeon. Offset of muscle relaxation should be confirmed by using a peripheral nerve stimulator to stimulate the ulnar nerve (**Figure 40.4**) and feeling forceful contraction of adductor pollicis. Alternatively, intubation may be accomplished without muscle relaxants by administration of high doses of opioids or volatile anaesthetic agents. An infusion of remifentanil, a very potent and ultra-short acting opioid, often produces good conditions for intubation and allows stable levels of anaesthesia during surgery. In some cases it will be possible to avoid intubation by the use of a supraglottic airway device. It is good practice to test the correct assembly and functioning of the facial nerve

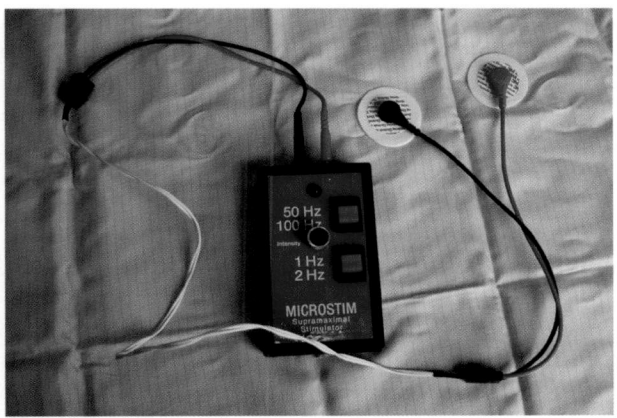

Figure 40.4 A peripheral nerve stimulator. This passes a supramaximal (>50 mA) stimulus transcutaneously over the desired motor nerve, typically the ulnar nerve at the wrist, in order to assess the degree of neuromuscular block.

monitoring system before surgery by using the peripheral nerve stimulator. A short burst of tetanic stimulation applied over the facial nerve in front of the ear should produce visible contractions of the muscles and both visual and audible alerts from the monitor.

Postoperative plan

After some major operations of the head and neck (for example for tumour) involving free flap transfer, it is conventional for the postoperative plan to include admission to an intensive care unit for a period of artificial ventilation, which itself would require the presence of a tracheal tube. This plan might also be necessary if the patient has certain medical conditions (for example poor lung function).

KEY POINTS

- Anaesthesia and loss of consciousness result in reduced tone in the pharyngeal dilators and posterior displacement of the tongue.
- The oropharnyx behaves as a Starling resistor: airflow is critically dependent on pharyngeal tone and transmural pressure.
- Maintaining the airway manually with a simple bag and mask is an important clinical skill.

CONDUCT OF ANAESTHESIA: PRINCIPLES GUIDING INDUCTION OF ANAESTHESIA

Preoxygenation

It is usual to allow a patient to breathe 100 percent oxygen via a face mask for a period of approximately two to three minutes before the induction of anaesthesia. This process in known as preoxygenation and has a number of theoretical and real advantages. Perhaps counter-intuitively, breathing 100 percent oxygen in this way does not increase the oxygen content of the blood at all. This is because, for most patients, the arterial blood is almost fully saturated with oxygen even when breathing room air, so breathing oxygen cannot really improve on this. The purpose of this manoeuvre is rather to 'de-nitrogenate' the gas within the lungs. This increases the mass of oxygen within the alveolar compartment, which serves as a reservoir during a subsequent apnoea, and markedly delays the rate of desaturation during this period. An alternative technique for preoxygenation is to allow the patient to take three successive vital capacity breaths of 100 percent oxygen. For a resting lung volume of 2 L, and tidal breaths of 2 L, the alveolar oxygen concentration should rise from 16 percent on breath zero, to approximately 60 percent on breath one, 80 percent on breath two and 90 percent on breath three.[5, 6]

Intravenous induction

Perhaps the commonest mode of induction of anaesthesia is by i.v. injection (using one of the drugs listed in the above section, but most commonly probably propofol). This route rapidly induces anaesthesia. The advantage of this is that there is little or no 'stage of hyperexcitability'. This is a stage just before deep anaesthesia is attained, in which the patient may be paradoxically excitable and there is tongue-biting, vomiting and laryngeal spasm (see below under Inhalational induction). The aim is to titrate the intravenous administration of drug, slowly, according to the observed effect. Injudicious dosing of intravenous induction agents invariably causes loss of spontaneous ventilation, so at least for a period of time after induction (and for longer if neuromuscular blocking drugs are used) the anaesthetist must be confident of maintaining ventilation, using any or all of the means described above. If, therefore, there is any doubt on the part of the anaesthetist that s/he is able to maintain ventilation, then even the most carefully administered i.v. induction is probably not the safest means of inducing anaesthesia. The details and nature of these doubts (i.e. the ability to predict a patient who is difficult to intubate or ventilate) are discussed in Chapter 39, Recognition and management of the difficult airway.

If the use of neuromuscular blocking drugs is planned, it is important that the anaesthetist is satisfied that s/he can, if necessary, ventilate the patient with a bag and mask before such drugs are given. The precaution ensures that if for some reason the trachea cannot be intubated, then ventilation can at least be achieved with a bag and mask until spontaneous ventilation resumes.

Rapid sequence induction

This is a special form of i.v. induction that is employed to secure the airway with a tracheal tube, and so protect it from soiling, as quickly as possible. It is particularly indicated in emergency surgery where a patient may have a full stomach or a hiatus hernia with active reflux. It may also be considered where there is bleeding (as in post-tonsillectomy bleeding). In a rapid sequence induction we appear to break all the rules detailed above. Here, the induction is not slow, nor the dose titrated to effect so as to minimize the risk of apnoea, airway collapse and obstruction, but rather, a predetermined dose of i.v. agent is given rapidly as a bolus.

The muscle relaxant rule is also broken. In the rapid sequence induction we do not test our ability to ventilate the patient with a bag and mask before given neuromuscular blockers, but rather, give a dose of suxamethonium (or other rapidly acting drug) immediately following injection of the induction agent. This adds an extra burden of responsibility on the anaesthetist to be able to intubate the trachea, since we have chosen to neglect our 'escape plan'.

As soon as consciousness is seen to fall, the anaesthetic assistant applies 'cricoid pressure' to the larynx. Empirically, it is found that if a force of 40 N (4 kg weight) is applied to the cricoid cartilage using the finger and thumb, the posterior part of the cricoid cartilage will compress the oesophagus posteriorly against the C6 cervical vertebral body and so prevent passive spillage of gastric contents. Laryngoscopy and intubation are now undertaken in the usual manner.

Inhalational induction

An alternative means of inducing anaesthesia is by inhalational induction, using one of the vapours discussed above (most commonly either sevoflurane or halothane). Anaesthesia in children, who may be frightened of intravenous cannulation, is often induced in this manner. Historically, this was the first method of induction. One advantage of the technique is that it is theoretically a 'controlled' means of induction. If, during the course of inhalational induction, the patient's upper airway collapses and the patient's breathing becomes obstructed, then no further anaesthetic vapour can enter the lungs. The patient begins to wake up and thereby the upper airway tone and breathing are restored. For this reason, it has been advocated as the technique of choice in a case of upper airway obstruction and stridor (for example due to supraglottic tumour). Unlike an i.v. induction, therefore, inhalational induction may be used even when the anaesthetist has doubts about the ability to intubate the trachea or maintain ventilation. However, there are some practical disadvantages. First, because

induction is slow, there is a danger that the stage of excitability is prolonged. Second, should collapse of the upper airway occur during inhalational induction then not only anaesthetic vapour, but also oxygen is prevented from reaching the lungs. Thus, inhalational induction may not be as safe or controlled as may be claimed.

Induction after securing the airway

Certain patients, especially those whose tracheas are predicted to be difficult to intubate, are subjected to techniques that achieve tracheal intubation with the patient awake or sedated, with anaesthetic induction occurring only after the airway is secured. These methods are discussed further in Chapter 39, Recognition and management of the difficult airway. The methods may also include planned awake tracheostomy under local anaesthesia.

MONITORING IN ANAESTHESIA

Derived from the Latin *monere* – to warn, monitoring is used to describe measurements whose prime purpose is to 'warn' of imminent (possibly injurious) events, and allow action to be taken to avoid them, or moderate their effect. The Association of Anaesthetists of Great Britain and Ireland publishes guidelines for minimum monitoring standards, and these are reviewed from time to time. Undoubtedly, the most important 'monitor' is the very presence of an anaesthetist throughout the duration of anaesthesia who can synthesize information derived from clinical observation, and specialized devices.

Basic intraoperative monitoring

ECG

Continuous single-lead ECG recording is universally used. Electrical activity of the heart gives no information about pump function and circulation. Its purpose is to detect the development of dysrhythmias and/or myocardial ischaemia.

Lead II configuration is best for rhythm disturbances (AF, heart block, asystole, VT, VF) since this lead shows the presence (or absence) of P waves best. The CM_5 configuration is best for detecting myocardial ischaemia, (ST depression, T wave inversion) (see **Figure 40.5**).

PULSE OXIMETRY

These devices shine red light through an extremity, usually a finger, and measure the absorbance of this transmitted light by substances in its path. Clearly, there will be a number of substances which absorb and/or

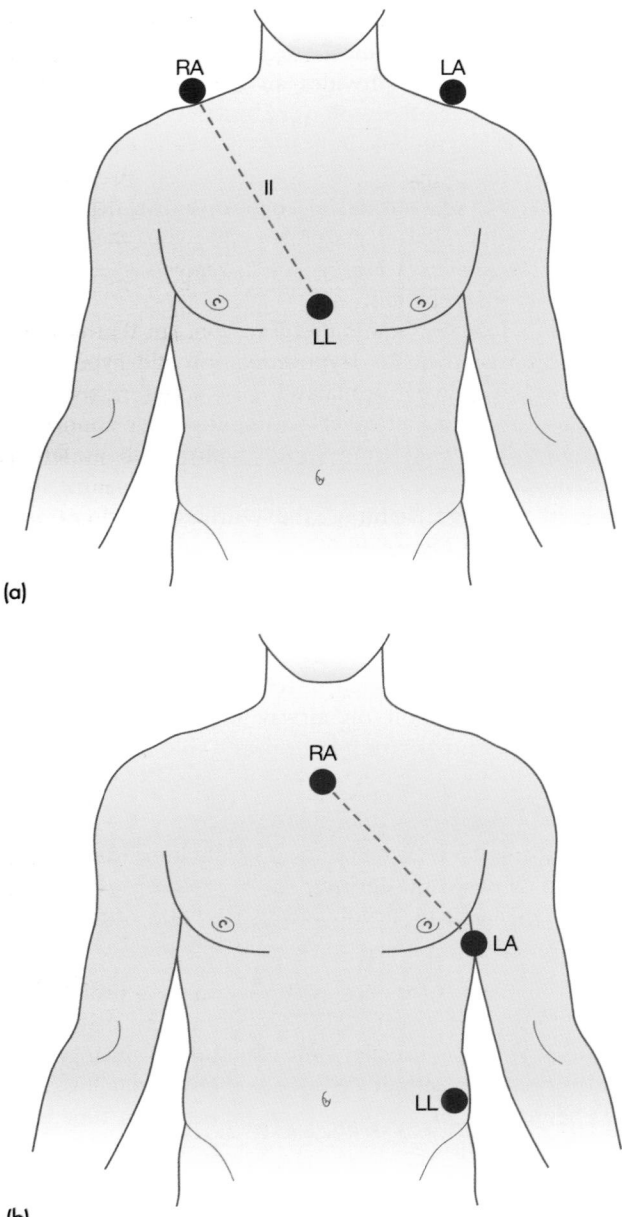

Figure 40.5 (a) For standard lead connection, the right arm lead is placed on the right shoulder, the left arm lead on the left shoulder, and the left leg lead is placed centrally to form an equilateral triangle. Selection of 'lead II' on the monitor will connect leads RA to the negative terminal and LL to the positive terminal. Lead LA acts as an earth lead. (b) For CM$_5$ configuration, lead RA is placed on the central manubrium and lead LA at the V5 position in the anterior axillary line. The monitor is set to display 'lead I', which connects RA to the negative terminal and LA to the positive terminal. Lead LL is earth/ground/indifferent and its placement is not critical.

scatter this light energy, including arterial haemoglobin, venous haemoglobin, skin, bone and nail-bed. However, in addition to the background absorbance, there will be a component that varies throughout the cardiac cycle, and this pulsatile absorbance is due to the added volume of arterial blood which enters during (or shortly after) systole. If this pulsatile signal is subtracted from the background signal we achieve an arterial absorbance signal that is wholly accounted for by the composition of arterial blood. The red light comprises two different wavelengths and these are absorbed by deoxygenated and oxygenated haemoglobin to different degrees. The relative absorbances of these wavelengths are used to calculate the proportions of oxygenated and deoxygenated haemoglobin, yielding a percentage SpO$_2$.

The pulse oximeter monitors oxygenation but **not** ventilation. This is an extremely important concept when considering high-risk patients nursed on the ward and recovery area. Patients breathing supplemental oxygen may still be pink, despite being virtually apnoeic (i.e. imminent respiratory arrest). Pulse oximeters must not be relied upon to monitor the adequacy of ventilation in patients who are at risk of respiratory depression or obstruction.

In addition, pulse plethysmography (the pulsatile waveform display shown on the pulse oximeter) gives a beat-to-beat indication of circulation, which is the electronic equivalent of keeping one's finger on the pulse at all times. This has become an invaluable tool.

BLOOD PRESSURE

Automatic noninvasive blood pressure

Automatic noninvasive blood pressure (NIBP) uses the principle of oscillotonometry applied to an inflatable cuff around the arm. This principle differs from the more familiar auscultatory method. The mean blood pressure measured by oscillotonometry is reasonably accurate. Systolic and particularly the diastolic values are less so. These automatic NIBP devices have gained widespread acceptance because they are safe and easy to use. They can be set to take measurements every few minutes and produce a printed chart, which is useful for detecting trends in theatre or the high dependency area.

NIBP measurement has a number of disadvantages. Firstly, its readings, even if taken frequently, are 'intermittent' and so do not allow one to detect sudden circulatory collapse. NIBP measurements tends to overestimate low pressures, and underestimate high pressures. It is often impossible to get any reading from patients who are 'shocked' and peripherally shut down.

Invasive monitoring of blood pressure

Invasive monitoring of blood pressure (IBP) can be measured by siting a cannula in a suitable artery, usually the radial. This has the advantage of allowing beat-to-beat blood pressure measurement, which allows extremely rapid changes to be detected almost in real time. The IBP monitor allows the arterial 'waveform' to be displayed on screen. The morphology of this waveform (e.g. the rate of upstroke, pulse pressure, presence 'pulsus paradoxus' with respiration) provides useful information on circulatory and vasotonic status. Having an arterial cannula *in situ* also permits easy and regular blood gas sampling. IBP measurements are reliable and accurate in both high and low pressure states. Disadvantages are few, but include the fact that siting such cannulae can be fiddly, and the disposables are relatively expensive. There is a very small risk of thrombosis, distal ischaemia and infection.

GAS ANALYSIS

Inspired oxygen fraction (F_iO_2)

It is axiomatic that oxygen is vital for safe anaesthesia. However, since it is odourless and colourless it is not straightforward to know how much is being given to a patient, or more worryingly, whether any is being given at all! Deaths still occur due to administration of gas devoid of oxygen, either by inadvertently giving pure nitrous oxide or carbon dioxide, or as a result of an error in gas pipeline connections. It is therefore vital that the labelled identity of the gas in a cylinder or pipeline is not relied upon, but that the composition of gases as they leave the anaesthetic machine and enter the patient's airway is monitored. This is usually carried out by means of continuous aspiration of a sample of gas from the airway into a rapid gas analyser which can display the concentration of inspired and expired oxygen breath-by-breath. Most analysers are also capable of monitoring other gas, such as CO_2 and anaesthetic gases and vapours.

Inspired/end–tidal anaesthetic agent concentration

By sampling the concentration (or partial pressure) of anaesthetic vapours in the expired breath, one can estimate the anaesthetic partial pressure in the alveolar gas and hence the arterial blood and brain. This is a very reliable way of monitoring anaesthetic depth because the dose-response curves (or more accurately the partial pressure-response curves) for these agents show very little interindividual variation. So, for example, if the end-tidal concentration of isoflurane is 1 percent, we can be extremely confident that for all patients, anaesthetic depth is adequate and there will be no danger of 'conscious awareness'.

Inspired and expired PCO_2

Inspired CO_2 should be zero or near zero. Rising inspired CO_2 concentrations indicate that the patient is rebreathing exhaled breath and this usually results from a faulty breathing circuit or inadequate gas supply from the anaesthetic machine.

Expired PCO_2, and its waveform, is one of the most important monitors in anaesthesia. The term 'end-tidal' refers to the concentration at the very end of expiration

and this is taken to represent alveolar gas. The 'capnogram' (a graphical representation of expired PCO_2 versus time) provides an enormous amount of information on cardiorespiratory function. It is one of the earliest and most robust indicators of whether the trachea or oesophagus has been intubated. The presence of expired CO_2 and a normal 'alveolar waveform' definitively confirms endotracheal placement. Likewise, the absence of an alveolar waveform is strongly suggestive of oesophageal intubation.

The end-tidal PCO_2 is useful to confirm that alveolar ventilation is adequate. Hypoventilation and hyperventilation result in hypercapnia and hypocapnia, respectively. Clues to a number of other cardiopulmonary abnormalities can be gained from capnography, such as falling cardiac output, pulmonary embolus, V/Q maldistribution, the patient 'fighting' the ventilator. See example capnograms in **Figure 40.6**.

AIRWAY PRESSURE, TIDAL VOLUME

If patients are ventilated mechanically, the ventilator provides information on airway pressure and expired volume. Pressure is required to pass a volume of gas into the lungs. Two separate processes contribute to this pressure:

1. the compliance (or elastance) of the lung (the springiness of the spring);
2. the resistance to airflow (the narrowness of the tubes).

The compliance of the lungs is not usually a problem in most theatre cases (cf. ITU cases). Sudden changes in airway pressure usually indicate sudden changes in resistance (for example, sudden onset of bronchospasm in anaphylaxis, or kinking of the endotracheal tube by a Boyle Davis gag).

TEMPERATURE

Patients tend to get cold during surgery. This is because of:

- heat at loss to the environment (cold theatre, naked body, exposed body cavities);
- altered homeothermic mechanisms under anaesthesia.

This is bad for a number of practical and theoretical reasons. Hypothermia delays wound healing, depresses immunity, adversely affects skin integrity (so prone to pressure sores) and adversely affects coagulation.

Temperature is usually measured with an oro- or nasopharyngeal thermister. Rectal and intravascular varieties also exist. Our aim is to maintain normothermia by means of warm air convection blankets (e.g. Bair-Hugger[TM]) and by using an intravenous fluid warmer if the need for large volumes of fluid is anticipated.

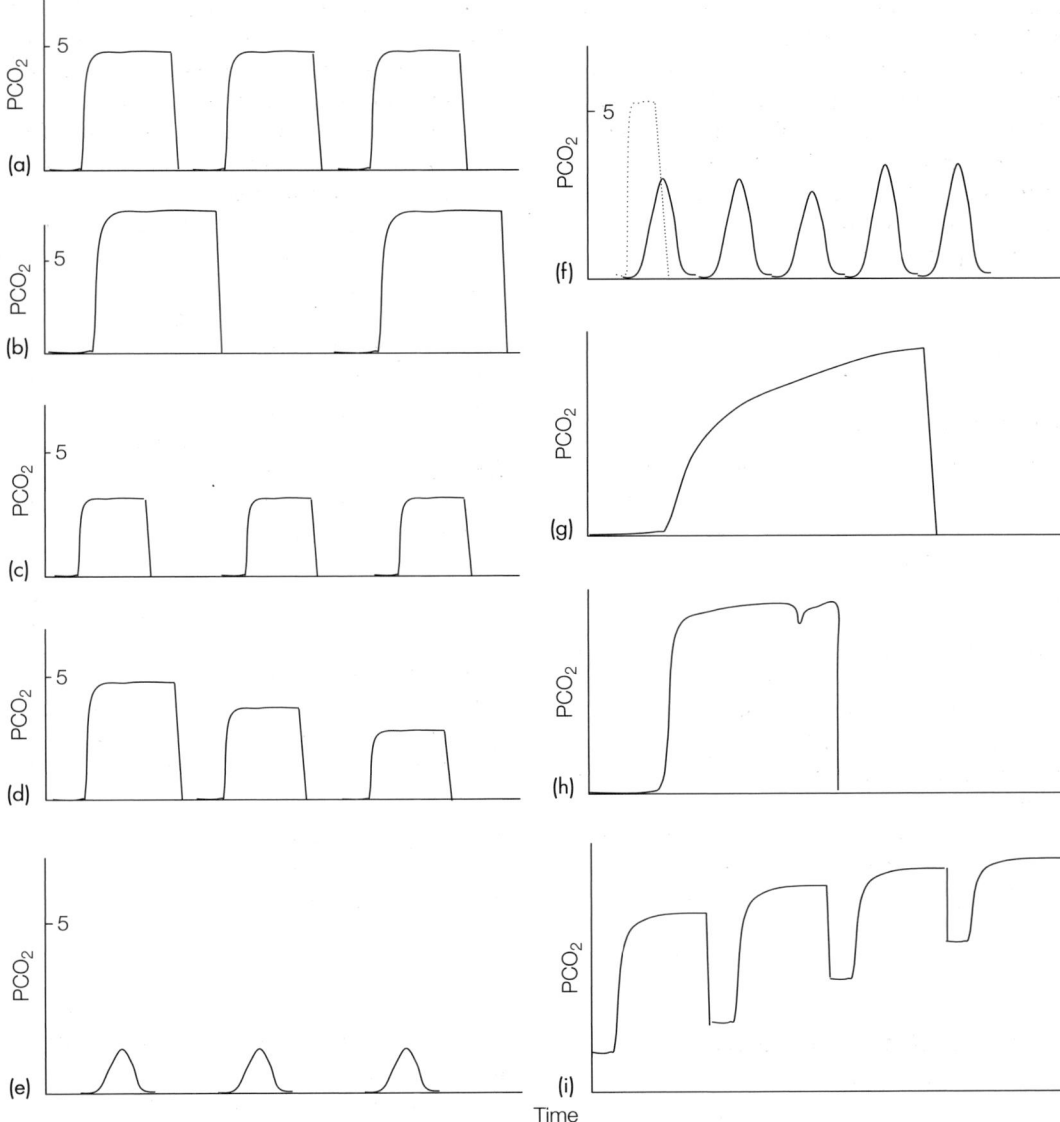

Time

Figure 40.6 Example capnograms: (a) Normal capnogram series. Note: regularity of ventilatory cycle, flat alveolar plateaux, normal PACO2 value, zero inspired PCO$_2$. (b) Hypoventilation. Shape of capnogram is normal, and alveolar plateau preserved, so airway flow must be normal. The likely cause is bradypnoea due to opiates. (c) Hyperventilation. Note that respiratory rate is normal so it is likely that the patient is being overventilated (tidal volume too great). Another rarer cause would be systemic shock with poor venous return. (d) Sudden fall in PCO$_2$ despite no change in ventilation. Causes: Pulmonary embolus (clot or air); circulatory arrest. (e) Loss of normal morphology. Small blips indicate insufficient alveolar gas is making it as far as the sample probe (at the lips). This is either because the tidal volume is very small (only just exceeding the dead space), or there is some upper airway obstruction which is physically hindering gas efflux on the final part of its journey from larynx to lips. In the case of ventilation via a face mask, this could indicate air leak from a poor seal, i.e. ventilation may be normal, but alveolar gas is not sampled properly because of the poor face mask seal. (f) Tachypnia. Rapid respiration is normal in babies. In adults, it may indicate inadequate anaesthesia or analgesia. In this example, the 'response time' of the analyser is not rapid enough to measure the true capnogram at this respiratory rate, so it appears as a series of rapid blips, the peaks of which do not represent true capnogram (dotted). (g) V/Q mismatch/lower airway obstruction. Note the sloping alveolar 'plateau'. Alveolar gas is not homogeneous. Low-resistance units, by definition, are well ventilated and have a low PCO$_2$, and because they are low-resistance, they empty first. High resistance units are poorly ventilated and have a high PCO$_2$. Because they are slow to empty, they dominate the latter part of expiration. This is classically seen in COAD and asthma. (h) 'Curare notch'. The notch in the alveolar plateau indicates that a patient may be trying to breathe in at this point (i.e. to fight against the ventilator). It usually means that the muscle relaxant is starting to wear off, this should be checked with the peripheral nerve stimulator before giving further doses. (i) Rebreathing/inadequate fresh gas supply. Here, the inspired PCO$_2$ is not zero. Some degree of 'rebreathing' is occurring as breathing in and out of a paper bag. The usual reason is failure of the gas supply from the anaesthetic machine to the breathing circuit. The patient's expired gas is not washed away by fresh gas, and so it ends up being rebreathed at the next inspiration.

CENTRAL VENOUS PRESSURE/PULMONARY ARTERY WEDGE PRESSURE/CARDIAC OUTPUT/TRANSOESOPHAGEAL ECHOCARDIOGRAPHY

This is **not** routine monitoring, but is used in situations where indicated either by:

- the patient's preoperative medical condition, e.g. left ventricular failure, sepsis;
- the surgery is likely to produce significant deviations in these parameters, e.g. large blood loss or compression of the mediastinum and great vessels.

The aim is to detect and correct changes in left and/or right ventricular preload, afterload or contractility indicated by changes in venous and pulmonary pressures, arterial pressure and cardiac output. Transoesophageal echocardiography (TOE) is particularly useful as it provides information on ventricular volume rather than pressure.

MONITORING OF NEUROMUSCULAR FUNCTION

The problems of neuromuscular blockade in the context of facial nerve monitoring in middle ear and parotid surgery has been discussed.

In general, the anaesthetist monitors the adequacy or completeness of neuromuscular blockade by means of a peripheral nerve stimulator. This comprises two adhesive electrodes placed over a convenient peripheral nerve (usually the ulnar) by which current pulses of around 50 mA are passed. These pulses provoke a visible, palpable and unfatiguable twitch in the relevant muscles in the unparalysed patient. In the completely paralysed patient, no twitches are palpable. For degrees of paralysis between these extremes, a reduction in twitch amplitude (relative to the unparalysed twitch) is observed and, more particularly, a diminution in twitch amplitude with each successive impulse is seen, which is characteristic of the nondepolarizing (curare-like) neuromuscular blockers. It is important to remember that the ability to elicit palpable twitches is a crude test of neuromuscular function, in contrast to the facial nerve monitor used by the ENT surgeon, which detects microvolts of EMG activity, rather than gross movement. It is possible for patients to be moderately but adequately blocked from the anaesthetic perspective, but satisfactorily unblocked from the per-spective of facial nerve monitoring. The important point here is that if this approach is used, the surgeon, as well as the anaesthetist, needs to be aware of it.

INDICES OF ANAESTHETIC DEPTH: EEG/AEP/BIS

A number of devices that measure and process EEG signals are available for estimating anaesthetic depth during surgery. In addition, auditory evoked potentials can be used since increasing anaesthetic depth increases the latency and reduces the amplitude of the early cortical responses. Knowledge of anaesthetic depth is important

for clinical and medico–legal purposes. For patients breathing spontaneously, i.e. not paralysed, 'awareness' under anaesthesia is very unlikely because if such patients became 'light', they would indicate this by moving or coughing, long before awareness supervened. In paralysed patients however, such early warning signs are absent. This is not routine monitoring.

ANAESTHETIC TECHNIQUE AND PRINCIPLES FOR SPECIFIC ENT OPERATIONS

The above sections indicate the broad principles used to determine choice of anaesthetic drugs, airway device and mode of induction. We now turn to some specific operations in ENT surgery and outline the relevant anaesthetic considerations.

Tonsillectomy and adenoidectomy

The most common reason for this operation is chronic or recurrent infection, and it is usually carried out in children. Thus, the incidence of upper respiratory tract infection on day of surgery is common, often requiring postponement of the operation. Extremely anxious children may need sedation on the ward using oral midazolam 0.5–1 mg/kg, and may need inhalational induction of anaesthesia, but this is rare. Most children, however, accept local anaesthetic cream (EMLA or Ametop) which facilitates i.v. cannulation and induction. It is usual for parents to be present during induction. Other reasons for the operation include: as part of treatment for sleep apnoea syndrome or snoring; excision biopsy for suspected malignancy; or peritonsillar abscess. These operations are usually performed in adults.

AIRWAY MANAGEMENT

Most anaesthetists would probably choose to intubate the trachea because this secures the airway and facilitates ventilation more definitively. Commonly a 'preformed' tracheal tube is used, such as an RAE tube (**Figure 40.3**). This tube is designed such that its outside end (which connects to the breathing circuit) points 'south' naturally (i.e. sits under the Boyle Davies gag) without having to be bent. The act of bending tubes usually results in kinking and obstruction. An alternative tube is a reinforced tube, whose shaft is flexible and kink resistant. An integral metallic spiral provides this protection from external compression and kinking (**Figure 40.3**). Since tonsillec-tomy is mostly carried out in children, uncuffed or 'plain' tracheal tubes are mostly used. This means that the lower airway is not definitively sealed and protected from soiling by blood. In addition, the laryngeal inlet cannot easily be sealed with a throat-pack (as would be done in other types of surgery) because this would most likely obscure the surgical field. The anaesthetist therefore relies on the surgeon to prevent blood from entering the larynx by careful haemostasis and use of suction.

It is now relatively common for the flexible, reinforced version of the LMA to be used, as it is suggested that the inflated cuff, which sits around the outside of the laryngeal inlet, acts as an effective barrier to lung soiling. The reinforced LMA has a narrower tube portion which is not only kink resistant and sits under the Boyle Davies gag, but also obscures the surgical view less than the standard LMA. Whichever airway device is used, care should be taken that it remains patent during surgery, especially at the point where the Boyle Davis gag is placed (**Figure 40.7**).

MAINTENANCE

The traditional technique, with a number of advantages, is to use a volatile anaesthetic agent and to allow the patient to breathe spontaneously. In this technique, after induction of anaesthesia, a short-acting muscle relaxant such as suxamethonium or mivacurium is used to facilitate tracheal intubation. Spontaneous respiration will soon resume and the patient allowed to breathe a mixture of oxygen and nitrous oxide with the addition of a volatile agent such as isoflurane or sevoflurane. As discussed above, a relatively deep plane of anaesthesia will be required for the patient to tolerate the tracheal tube without coughing. Analgesia may be provided by an opioid, and titrated such that respiration is not depressed.

EXTUBATION/RECOVERY

At the end of the case, the laryngeal inlet is examined with the aid of a Macintosh laryngoscope and gently suctioned to confirm that haemostasis is secure. The patient is positioned in the lateral position, with a pillow placed under the upper chest and the head tilted down so that any blood or secretions will drain without soiling the airway. The patient, still breathing spontaneously, is then extubated at the peak of inspiration, still under a 'deep' plane of anaesthesia. The subsequent expiration should clear any small quantity of blood or secretions from the laryngeal inlet, and respiration should continue unimpeded and without coughing. The patient is then transferred to the recovery ward where, with modern fast onset/offset agents, the volatile agent will soon be washed-out, and consciousness return.

THE POSTOPERATIVE BLEEDING TONSIL

This is a serious complication. Anaesthesia and surgery may be necessary after appropriate fluid and volume resuscitation. The patient (especially a child) may have swallowed most of the blood and must be treated as a high risk for regurgitation and aspiration. At the same time, the trachea may be difficult to intubate due to the presence of blood in the oropharynx and oedema from the recent surgery. The options for anaesthetic induction are either a standard 'rapid sequence' intravenous technique (probably favoured by most anaesthetists), or a careful inhalational induction with the patient in the head down, lateral position. There must be good communication between the teams: the surgeon must be prepared to establish an emergency surgical airway or tracheostomy should tracheal intubation fail.

Ear surgery

Surgery on the external ear is performed for a variety of reconstructive or cosmetic reasons. Surgery on the middle ear is performed to restore hearing, eliminate infection, treat cholesteatoma or, rarely, for neoplasm.

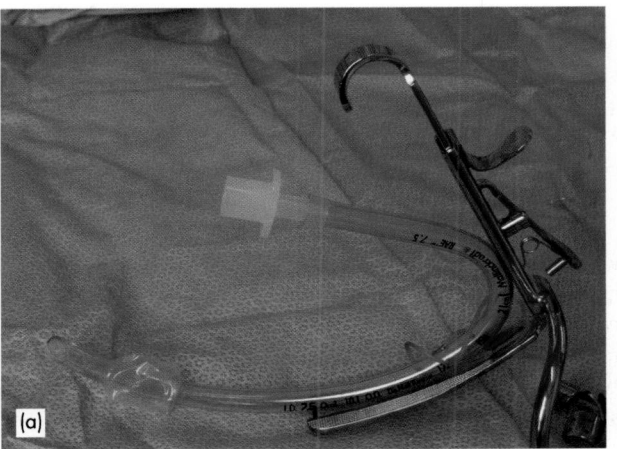

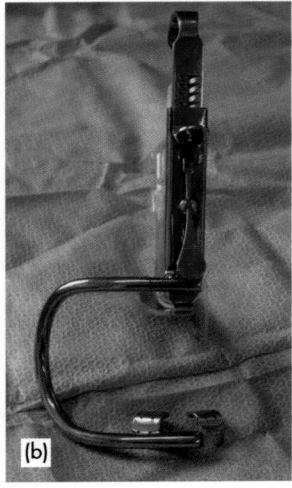

Figure 40.7 The relative positions of: (a) the tracheal tube; and (b) the tonsillectomy (Boyle Davis) gag. Note how the blade retracts the tongue and the tube upwards.

The main anaesthetic implication is that the head must be turned so that the ear on which the operation occurs is turned upward. It is one instance in ENT surgery when, strictly speaking, the airway is not 'shared' and so anaesthetic considerations, rather than surgical considerations, predominate in choice of airway or anaesthetic drugs. However, where tympanoplasty, tympanomeatal flaps, stepedotomy or stapedectomy is performed, it is advisable to avoid nitrous oxide. Nitrous oxide (due to its relative solubility) enters the middle ear cavity at a rate faster than nitrogen (the ambient gas in the air) leaves the space: consequently, there is a rise in middle ear pressure which can displace the structures being operated on. Myringotomy (grommet) surgery, is usually a very short operation in children and any suitable anaesthetic technique may be employed.

More invasive operations of the ear include exploratory middle ear surgery and mastoidectomy. The surgical approach is often by a post-auricular approach, through the mastoid. The main consideration is that the facial nerve needs to be monitored during surgery (see above under Monitoring of neuromuscular function).

HYPOTENSIVE ANAESTHESIA

In certain operations, notably major ear surgery, special techniques are employed to improve the view of the surgical field by minimizing bleeding. These techniques have become collectively known as 'hypotensive anaesthesia' although they comprise a number of other approaches in addition to hypotension.

Blood in the surgical field may arise from arterial, capillary or venous bleeding. Arterial bleeding is directly proportional to mean arterial blood pressure (MABP), which is governed by the following relationship:

$$MABP = \text{cardiac output} \times \text{peripheral vascular resistance}$$
$$= (\text{stroke volume} \times \text{heart rate}) \times \text{peripheral vascular resistance}$$

A reduction in stroke volume (via a reduction in contractility) and a reduction in heart rate can be achieved by β blockade. A reduction in peripheral vascular resistance can be achieved (via vasodilatation) with alpha blocking drugs (such as phentolamine) or increased concentrations of volatile anaesthetic agents.

Capillary bleeding depends on local flow in the capillary bed, which in turn is dependent on upstream arterial pressure and downstream venous tone, in addition to local metabolic factors. Capillary bleeding can be moderated by the use of locally infiltrated adrenaline (although the systemic effects of this will transiently confound the anaesthetist's attempts to control blood pressure) and by reduction in arterial and venous PCO_2 by hyperventilation.

A reduction in venous tone and backpressure will reduce both capillary and venous bleeding. Venous tone can be moderated by the use of intravenous nitrates, and positioning can reduce the hydrostatic venous pressure, for example a 25° head up tilt can be employed in middle ear surgery.

In young healthy patients, blood flow to vital organs such as the brain, kidney and heart is regulated such that it remains constant despite variations in perfusion pressure. This autoregulation occurs within a mean arterial pressure range of 60–160 mmHg. At pressures below 60 mmHg mean, blood flow becomes 'pressure dependent' and will diminish with diminishing pressure, (see **Figure 40.8**).

For such patients, MABP may safely be lowered to 60 mmHg without diminution of vital organ blood flow. Even at pressures lower still, a modest reduction in organ blood flow is unlikely to be clinically significant since there is little metabolic demand under these basal conditions.

However, in elderly patients, and particularly those with systemic hypertension or coronary artery disease, the imposition of deliberate hypotension should not be undertaken lightly. In systemic hypertension, the normal autoregulation curve (shown in **Figure 40.8**) is shifted to the right, and so even moderate degrees of induced hypotension may produce pressure-dependent flow and reduce vital organ perfusion. The 're-setting' of these autoregulatory mechanisms is time-dependent and may take several weeks to normalize after a hypertensive

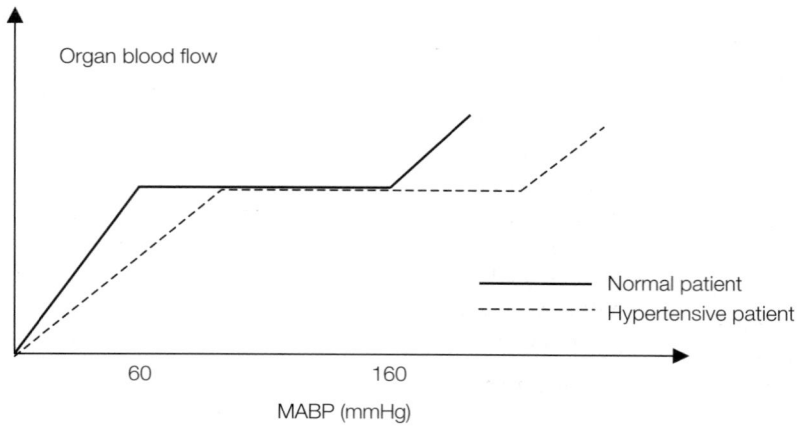

Organ blood flow

———— Normal patient

------- Hypertensive patient

60   160

MABP (mmHg)

Figure 40.8 Autoregulation curve.

patient is started on antihypertensive therapy. It is for this reason that it is unwise to embark on anaesthesia in hypertensive patients, even though we can quite easily and quickly achieve systolic and diastolic blood-pressure values that are in the normal range. The second group of patients in whom induced hypotension should be effected with caution are those with coronary or cerebrovascular disease. The arterial pressure just downstream of a stenosis may be 20 or more mmHg lower than the upstream (or systemic) arterial pressure. So, whilst a mean systemic pressure of 60 mmHg may be adequate for the majority of an arteriopathic patient's organ systems, such a pressure may only generate 40 mmHg of pressure downstream of a fixed stenosis, thus producing a diminished and pressure-dependent flow with a risk of myocardial ischaemia or cerebral thrombosis.[7]

SALIVARY GLAND SURGERY

Parotidectomy and removal of submandibular gland may be performed for tumour, stone or chronic infection. Any suitable anaesthetic technique may be used, but the facial nerve may need to be monitored.

NASAL AND SINUS SURGERY

Nasal surgery is performed for cosmetic or functional restoration of the nasal airway, and includes operations such as septoplasty (operations to the nasal septum), rhinoplasty (operations to remodel the nasal contour), turbinectomy or these combined. Sinus surgery is performed to eliminate infection, polyps or neoplastic conditions of the sinuses, and the goal is to provide aeration of the sinuses so that secretion can drain adequately into the nasopharynx. The operations are usually performed in young adults.

Anaesthetic considerations for all these operations are similar. An oral (as opposed to nasal) airway device is necessary (usually a tracheal tube in combination with a gauze throat pack to collect any blood which trickles from the nose). Nasal bleeding is often minimized by surgical application of cocaine mixtures to the nose before the operation begins. At the end of surgery, the patient's nose is usually packed, so a good oral airway should be established to allow the patient to breathe spontaneously.

LARYNGEAL MICROSURGERY AND LARYNGOSCOPY

These operations are performed for diagnostic or therapeutic purposes and may be combined with an examination of the pharynx, oesophagus or bronchial tree. Often, lasers are used to treat isolated lesions of the larynx.

Because of the rigid nature of the laryngoscope, a small size (6 mm internal diameter or less) tracheal tube (a microlaryngeal tube) is commonly employed, and if lasers are to be used, an appropriate laser-resistant type is needed. This type of tracheal tube is sufficiently flexible and long that it does not interfere with the surgical field, although good communication is needed between surgeon and anaesthetist throughout the procedure. The operation is usually relatively short, but laryngospasm or postoperative airway obstruction due to oedema of the vocal cords may occur. The risk of this may be minimized if steroids (for example dexamethasone 8 mg intravenously) are used peroperatively.

LASER SURGERY

The use of laser, especially for laryngeal microsurgery, has become widespread. Lasers are also used for stapedectomy, tympanoplasty, turbinate surgery and oropharyngeal surgery. There are various types of laser (CO_2, Nd:Yag, KTP; all named after the source of substrate for the laser beam). It is important to know the general properties of the laser beam that is being used. The Nd:Yag laser (yttrium-aluminium-garnet) was introduced in the 1980s, and its main advantage over CO_2 laser is that it can be delivered by means of an easily handled flexible fibreoptic light cable. It has more coagulative but less cutting ability than a CO_2 laser. The KTP laser is a variant of the Nd:Yag, in which the laser beam is passed through a potassium titanyl phosphate crystal. Lasers can produce either a parallel or divergent beam. Parallel beams impart much greater power densities to the tissues they strike than divergent beams. The greatest concern during use of lasers is the possibility of uncontrolled combustion of either tissues or extraneous materials (including airway devices) if accidentally struck for prolonged periods by the laser beam. A fire in the patient's airway is serious and is often fatal. The steps shown under Best clinical practice are reasonable precautions to minimize this risk.[8]

Bronchoscopy

Rigid bronchoscopy is performed for a variety of reasons, including inhaled foreign body, diagnosis of endobronchial lesions, and staging of disease prior to pulmonary resection. The type of patient who presents for this procedure can therefore be extremely variable, from a small child to an elderly smoker with severe lung disease. An important anaesthetic consideration is that the large rigid bronchoscope competes for space with anaesthetic devices within the trachea itself (**Figure 40.9**). Pulmonary ventilation needs to continue during the procedure and this can be achieved in the following ways:

- Using a small tracheal tube, though the risk is that the bronchoscope may dislodge this.

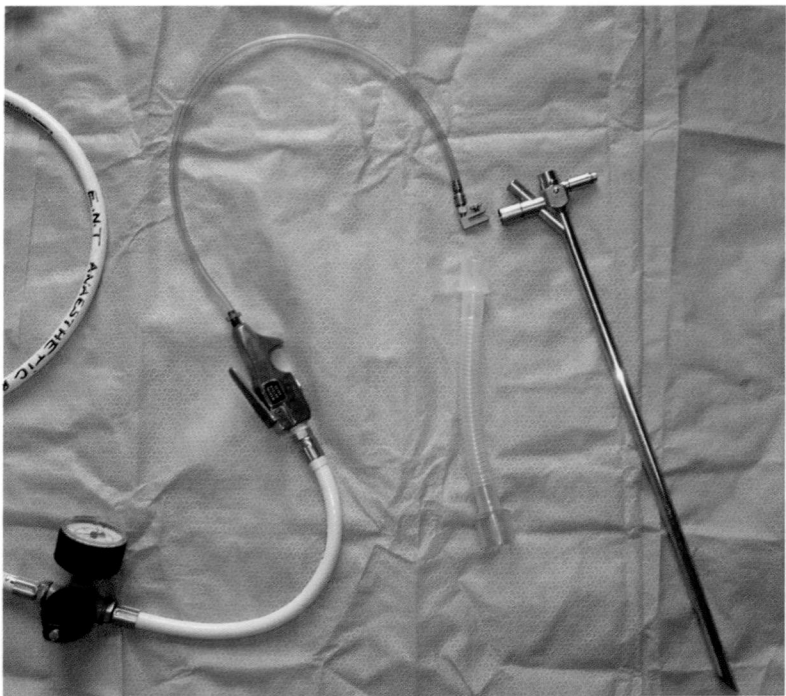

Figure 40.9 A Sanders injector and rigid bronchoscope. High-pressure oxygen is fed from the regulator to a jet orifice, which clips or screws loosely onto a sideport of the rigid bronchoscope. The jet is controlled by the hand trigger. Note that the connection of the jet orifice to the sideport is not sealed and there is considerable leak so the patient is not exposed to the full pressure of the injector, but rather room air is entrained into the scope by the jetting oxygen. Note also how the conventional anaesthetic circuit can also be attached (without leak) to the sideport to allow conventional ventilation (although the leak at the level of the bronchoscope and the vocal cords may make ventilation in this way difficult).

- Using the technique of 'apnoeic oxygenation'. This involves oxygenating the patient's lungs with 100 percent oxygen until the lung volume is depleted of nitrogen and effectively full of oxygen and no other gas. All airway devices are removed save for a small catheter, which insufflates oxygen into the oropharynx. The surgeon is then allowed to proceed with bronchoscopy with the patient apnoeic. Because of the relatively low rate of basal oxygen consumption, and the continued minimal delivery of oxygen via the catheter, it is theoretically possible to continue oxygenation indefinitely. However, the duration of the procedure is limited by the accumulation of carbon dioxide (active pulmonary ventilation is necessary for its removal). This accumulates in the patient's blood at a rate of approximately 0.5 kPa per minute, which limits the safe time of apnoea to approximately ten minutes.
- Employing a method known as 'jet ventilation' using a Sanders injector (**Figure 40.9**). This injector is essentially a pressure relief valve and tubing, one end of which is attached directly to the high pressure (4 bar) oxygen pressure supply on the anaesthetic machine. The other end of the tubing is attached to the rigid bronchoscope. Opening the injector blows oxygen at high pressure into the lungs and inflates them. Because of the high pressures involved, such injectors can be extremely dangerous to use without training. After injection of oxygen, sufficient time must then be allowed for air to leave the lungs (passive expiration).

- Some bronchoscopes have a side-port (Racine adaptor) which allows the standard anaesthetic/oxygen tubing to be attached: the anaesthetist can hand-ventilate the patient's lungs in a conventional manner using this attachment during bronchoscopy (**Figure 40.9**).

Since the anaesthetic management for rigid bronchoscopy is varied and relatively specialized, good communication between anaesthetist and surgeon is essential.

Laryngectomy

This is normally performed for tumour of the larynx. A total laryngectomy involves removal of all tissues from the valecula (and sometimes base of tongue) to the second or third tracheal rings. Occasionally, the thyroid gland also needs to be removed. The pharynx is closed in a T-shape, and the trachea is brought out to the skin as an end-tracheostomy (so no special tube is required long term to maintain airway patency). There are variations of this operation. A supraglottic laryngectomy involves resection of all tissue from the base of tongue to the vocal cords (which are left intact). The strap muscles are also preserved. A temporary tracheostomy is required post-operatively. A hemilaryngectomy involves removal of the epiglottis and just one half of the larynx (including one true and false vocal cord).

The main anaesthetic considerations are usually:

- the preoperative state of the patient;
- tracheal intubation during anaesthetic induction;
- changes of airway device during surgery.

PREOPERATIVE PATIENT STATE

Laryngeal tumours commonly occur in elderly smokers, so there may be considerable coexistent cardiovascular and respiratory disease which the anaesthetist needs to manage during surgery. There may need to be a preoperative plan to optimize any coexistent medical conditions and additional monitoring (for example invasive arterial pressures and central venous monitoring) may be necessary during surgery. If lung function is particularly poor, the plan may include a period of elective postoperative ventilation in intensive care.

TRACHEAL INTUBATION

The presence of a laryngeal tumour may make conventional tracheal intubation difficult, and specialized techniques may be necessary (for example awake intubation) during induction of anaesthesia. These are further discussed in Chapter 39, Recognition and management of the difficult airway.

AIRWAY DURING SURGERY

The operation might begin with the patient's trachea intubated with a standard (Magill) orotracheal tube. As surgery proceeds, this may (for reasons of surgical access) need to be exchanged for a tracheal tube which is inserted directly percutaneously into the trachea and shaped to lie against the neck, pointing caudally (for example Montandi tube, reinforced flexible tube or RAE tube). Finally, as the permanent end-tracheostomy is fashioned, all tracheal tubes will be removed. Thus, the anaesthetist needs to have ready a number of sterile airway devices, sterile connectors and tubing which often need to be sited directly by the surgeon. Close communication is clearly necessary.[9]

KEY POINTS

- Anaesthesia for ENT surgery epitomizes the quintessentially anaesthetic 'art' of airway mastery.
- It requires a unique dialogue between surgeon and anaesthetist who share the same territory. As such it requires, perhaps more than any other branch of surgery, an understanding of, and respect for each others contribution towards a common end.

Tonsillectomy and adenoidectomy

- The airway may be maintained by either insertion of a tracheal tube, or with a laryngeal mask. The choice is down to operator preference.

- The return to theatre of a bleeding tonsil poses special problems for the anaesthetist due to the probability of a full stomach and obscured laryngoscopy.

Ear surgery

- Moderate hypotension may help to reduce bleeding in the surgical field.
- It requires a multimodal approach rather than the use of a single agent or technique.
- It should be used with caution in patients with uncontrolled hypertension, cerebrovascular or ischaemic heart disease.

Best clinical practice

Laser surgery

✓ The surgeon should exercise caution and avoid any direct strikes to the airway device. This risk might be minimized during oral surgery if a Boyle Davis gag without the Doughty modification is used, thus protecting the shaft of most airway devices. If the Doughty modification is used, then the shaft of the airway device might be protected using damp gauzes or swabs.

✓ The minimum power output of the laser should be used and the duration of laser strike limited. It has been found that the risk of combustion increases with duration of strike at the same power.

✓ Both oxygen and nitrous oxide support combustion. Ideally, a mixture of oxygen (perhaps limited to no greater than 30 percent) mixed with air should be used to ventilate the patient's lungs during anaesthesia, to minimize the risk of combustion.

✓ Cuffs of tracheal and SAD devices are more vulnerable to laser strike than are the shafts of these devices. Therefore, the cuffs should be filled with saline (or coloured water) rather than air. This protects them, to some extent, from combustion with laser strike; it slows any deflation of the cuff after strike; it aids, to some extent, in preventing spread of any fire; and the leak of fluid allows the surgeon to see that the cuff has been ruptured.

Deficiencies in current practice and areas for future research

The scope for research in anaesthesia is huge. At the most fundamental level, it is not known how anaesthetic drugs induce unconsciousness and research in this field will span neurophysiology as well as, perhaps, psychology. Of more immediate relevance to anaesthesia in the context of head and neck surgery are the following areas:

➤ Drug developments
  – In particular, the search continues for anaesthetic drugs that have minimal effects on the cardiovascular and respiratory systems. It is expected that such drugs will possess a better safety profile, with fewer adverse cardio-respiratory side effects.
  – The search for drugs that minimize – or treat – postoperative nausea and vomiting is also important. While not addressing life-saving issues, this area of research certainly aims to improve quality of life, and also costs, since delayed discharge from hospital due to nausea/vomiting is an important cause of additional costs to a healthcare organization.
➤ Airway management. Current techniques for airway management in those patients who present particular difficulties (especially common in head and neck surgery) involve relatively expensive items of equipment such as fibreoptic endoscopes, and also require additional training in their use by experts who are proficient in managing these difficult cases. It would be desirable to introduce a technique – or equipment – which is both low-cost and which requires minimal expertise in its use to maintain an airway. However, developing such devices or techniques will require far more understanding of the reasons underlying the concept of the 'difficult airway' than we have at present.
➤ Reducing blood loss and blood replacement. Anaesthetic techniques that help minimize blood loss during surgery (such as 'hypotensive anaesthesia' in which the patient's blood pressure is held at low levels) require further research. This research also involves developments in more precise monitoring of

the circulation. Related to this are areas of research in artificial haemoglobins or haemoglobin substitutes designed to minimize the transfusion of blood and so reduce the attendant risks.

REFERENCES

1. Baker L. Premedicant drugs. In: Wilson I, Allman KG (eds). *Oxford Handbook of Anaesthesia*, 2nd edn. Oxford: Oxford University Press, 2006.
* 2. Smith G. Inhalational anaesthetic agents. In: Aitkenhead AR, Rowbotham DJ, Smith G (eds). *Textbook of Anaesthesia*, 4th edn. London: Churchill Livingstone, 2001.
* 3. Farmery AD. Physics and physiology. In: Calder I, Pearce A (eds). *Core Topics in Airway Management*. Cambridge: Cambridge University Press, 2005.
* 4. Cook TM. Supraglottic airway devices. In: Calder I, Pearce A (eds). *Core Topics in Airway Management*. Cambridge: Cambridge University Press, 2005.
5. Farmery AD. Physiology of apnoea and hypoxia. In: Calder I, Pearce A (eds). *Core Topics in Airway Management*. Cambridge: Cambridge University Press, 2005: Chapter 2.
6. Pandit JJ, Duncan T, Robbin PA. Total oxygen uptake with two maximal breathing techniques: a physiologic study of preoxygenation. *Anesthesiology*. 2003; **99**: 841–6.
7. Dodds C. Hypotensive anaesthesia. In: Aitkenhead AR, Rowbotham DJ, Smith G (eds). *Textbook of Anaesthesia*, 4th edn. London: Churchill Livingstone, 2001.
8. Pandit JJ, Chambers P, O'Malley S. KTP laser-resistant properties of the reinforced laryngeal mask airway. *British Journal of Anaesthesia*. 1997; **78**: 594–600.
* 9. Roberts F. ENT surgery. In: Wilson I, Allman KG (eds). *Oxford Handbook of Anaesthesia*, 2nd edn. Oxford: Oxford University Press, 2006.

41

Paediatric anaesthesia

ALISTAIR CRANSTON

Introduction	507	Key points	522
Preoperative assessment	508	References	522
Equipment and techniques	510	Further reading	525
Specific surgical procedures	513		

INTRODUCTION

This chapter is intended to provide an overview of the principles of anaesthetic care for children in general, with specific reference to ear, nose and throat (ENT) surgery. The introductory section briefly deals with the organization of services for paediatric surgery and anaesthesia. This is followed by a consideration of preoperative factors, including physical assessment, preoperative fasting and premedication. The third section of the chapter addresses the equipment and skills necessary for the safe conduct of anaesthesia in children, with a particular emphasis on management of the airway. Induction of anaesthesia and physiological monitoring during anaesthesia are also covered in this section. The final section comprises an account of anaesthetic considerations and conduct for specific operative procedures commonly encountered in paediatric ENT surgery.

Ear, nose and throat surgery accounts for a significant percentage of all paediatric surgical procedures and provides the basis of many anaesthetists' experience with children. Many of these procedures are undertaken in centres where little or no other paediatric surgery is encountered. Whilst the majority of such operations are minor and of short duration, the nature of some ENT surgical procedures, particularly those involving the airway, require considerable expertise and experience. The development of cooperation and understanding between surgeon and anaesthetist is of enormous importance when undertaking such procedures.

Fundamental to the delivery of a safe, high-quality anaesthetic service for children is a suitably trained anaesthetist with continuing paediatric experience. Such an individual, however, must work in an environment with appropriate facilities and support if the reasonable expectations of children and their carers are to be met. The UK Department of Health defined the requirements for such a service in *The Welfare of Children and Young People in Hospital*.[1] There has been debate concerning who, where and what constitutes best practice in the delivery of surgical services for children, addressing such issues as training, ongoing experience and the merits of caring for children in a specialist paediatric centre as opposed to a general hospital environment.[2, 3, 4] The majority of children presenting for surgical treatment in the UK have been cared for in the district hospital environment and there is no reason why most children should not be treated outside specialist centres if standards can be maintained.

The 1989 National Confidential Enquiry into Perioperative Deaths reviewed the surgical and anaesthetic care of children in hospital.[5] The report highlighted the problems of 'occasional paediatric practice' and that the outcome of surgery and anaesthesia for children is related to experience. Numerous changes, which have required considerable reorganization in service delivery for children, have been recommended. It is increasingly the case that surgeons, anaesthetists and others are now working to defined values and standards and are organizing and auditing paediatric surgical services in a way that has led to a better defined and improved service for children.

PREOPERATIVE ASSESSMENT

Preoperative assessment for surgery involves an exchange of information between anaesthetist, child and carers that addresses three important issues vital to the conduct of a safe and satisfactory procedure. The first objective is to establish the nature of the procedure and to determine that the child is fit for surgery. Additionally, anatomical or physiological factors that may be specific to the condition to be treated or represent an unrelated disease process should be identified. Information obtained here will inform the development of the optimal anaesthetic care plan and may prompt further investigation or treatment before the procedure is undertaken. Thirdly, establishment of a rapport with children and their carers based on honesty and trust is vital to allay anxiety.

Psychological preparation for anaesthesia and surgery

For many children and their carers, the psychological disruption attendant upon a surgical procedure is at least as disturbing as the effects of the operation itself. Anaesthesia is particularly likely to contribute to emotional disturbance and so the conduct of pre-anaesthetic preparation is of great importance. Care should be taken to understand and address the concerns of both the child and their parents simply but truthfully. An understanding of age-specific responses to stress and the provision of a dedicated, child-friendly environment are important to consider when preparing children for surgery.

Day case surgery

The majority of minor ENT surgical procedures are undertaken on a day-stay basis, which affords an effective use of resources and has advantages for the child and their family. Pre-admission assessment of children, often nurse-led and employing questionnaire screening, speeds the admission process, limits wastage of operating time and reduces preventable cancellation on the day of surgery.

Physical examination

All children receive a full physical examination before anaesthesia and surgery, with emphasis placed on respiratory and cardiovascular systems. A careful assessment of the airway, including mouth opening, loose dentition and nasal obstruction is important to anticipate difficulties in airway management during anaesthesia.

Attention should also be paid to coexisting anomalies or disease that may require modifications of the anaesthetic technique or particular precautions to be taken.

Respiratory assessment

Airway and respiratory complications are the most common causes of peri-anaesthetic morbidity in children. Children presenting for ENT surgical procedures frequently exhibit concurrent or associated respiratory disease, emphasizing the importance of thorough preoperative evaluation.

Healthy children, in particular infants and toddlers, have a significantly greater risk of respiratory complications than do healthy adults.[6] This is predominantly related to maturational aspects of the respiratory system and the effects of anaesthesia on active mechanisms that help to maintain lung volume and functional residual capacity in infants and small children. In addition, stimulation of vagal airway receptors tends to increase the incidence of laryngospasm and apnoea in infants.

The inherent predisposition of small children to respiratory complications is compounded by the frequency of upper respiratory tract disturbances in the ENT surgical population and the decision to proceed with or defer surgery in a child with signs of an upper respiratory tract infection (URTI) presents a common dilemma. The features of URTI associated with anaesthetic complications may be difficult to define and the decision to proceed or not is often based on personal experience and a hierarchy of symptoms. Two recent studies[7, 8] have examined the incidence of and risk factors for adverse respiratory events in children with URTI. These studies suggest that many children with acute or recent URTI can undergo minor elective procedures such as myringotomy safely. The variables most likely to predict an adverse event are outlined in **Table 41.1**.

Asthma is common in childhood and there is a perception that the prevalence is increasing. Optimization of maintenance medication may be required prior to surgery but, in the absence of significant bronchospasm or intercurrent respiratory infection, most children can be safely managed with attention to the avoidance of anaesthetic agents likely to provoke histamine release.

Upper airway obstruction is frequent in paediatric ENT patients and evaluation of the cause and severity is important both in terms of airway management during anaesthesia and in determining the risk of airway difficulties in the postoperative period. Adenotonsillar hypertrophy is the most common cause of upper airway obstruction but others, notably congenital and acquired anomalies of the jaw, nasal and oral airways and larynx as well as craniofacial anomalies, particularly of the midface, are also encountered in this population. In addition, children with other conditions, such as Down's syndrome or neuromuscular disease, may develop airway

Table 41.1 Disease and anaesthetic factors likely to predict an adverse event in children with URTI.[7, 8]

Patient factors	Anaesthetic factors
Parental report of a 'cold'	Tracheal intubation versus face mask or LMA
Presence of a productive cough	Lack of anticholinesterase administration
Passive smoke exposure	Thiopentone or halothane induction versus propofol or sevoflurane
Presence of snoring	Surgery involving the airway
Presence of nasal congestion	

obstruction in the presence of relatively mild degrees of hypertrophy.

Although minor airway obstruction and benign snoring are common in children and do not usually pose particular risks, more severe airway obstruction may cause obstructive sleep apnoea syndrome (OSAS) and may predispose to significant airway compromise in the postoperative period. Preoperative OSAS, characterized by disturbed sleep with snoring, apnoeic pauses and hypoxia, in children undergoing adenotonsillectomy is a risk factor for postoperative respiratory compromise,[9, 10] and prediction of those most at risk is the subject of extensive studies.[11, 12, 13, 14]

Preoperative fasting

Preoperative fasting has long been considered essential for elective surgery. Prolonged fasting, however, does not reduce the aspiration risk during anaesthesia and current practice has focused on reduction of starvation times and a greater appreciation of other risk factors for regurgitation and aspiration of gastric contents.[15] The current practice in most centres for elective surgery, summarized in **Table 41.2**, is based on ensuring minimal residual gastric volume at induction of anaesthesia and avoiding patient distress and potential under hydration associated with prolonged starvation.

This practice is supported by studies in children and infants[16, 17, 18] and appears to improve the preoperative experience of children and parents.[19] In children undergoing emergency procedures, however, a full six-hour fasting period may be considered necessary, unless the urgency of the surgery dictates otherwise and anaesthesia is conducted assuming that the child has a full stomach.

Premedication

Pharmacological premedication in paediatric practice remains a controversial subject. The routine use of premedicant schedules has largely been abandoned in favour of an individualized approach with specific goals in mind. Although the general trend has been a reduction in premedication and certainly in the use of

Table 41.2 Minimum preoperative fasting times in infants and children for elective surgery.

	Clear fluids	Breast milk	Formula or cow's milk	Solids
Children	2 hours	–	6 hours	6 hours
Infants	2 hours	4 hours	6 hours	6 hours

intramuscular agents, topical local anaesthetics, sedative agents and anticholinergics are still widely used.

The topical local anaesthetic agents EMLA cream[20] and Ametop gel[21] are effective in reducing the pain of venepuncture and in facilitating intravenous induction. Although effective, in some children the anticipation of an unpleasant experience may outweigh the benefits afforded.

The value of sedative premedication is questionable for many children and is certainly no substitute for sympathetic psychological preparation. Historically, many classes of drugs have been used for this purpose but currently benzodiazepines and particularly Midazolam administered orally or, less frequently, intranasally, are the most popular agents.[22] Midazolam affords anxiolysis and amnesia and its elimination half-life of two hours makes it suitable for use in day-case or inpatient procedures. Timing of premedication is important, maximal effect being within 30 minutes of oral administration.

Preoperative administration of anticholinergic agents, particularly Atropine, has long been considered best practice in paediatric anaesthesia, especially in infants. Newer anaesthetic agents and techniques have modified this approach and there has been a general decline in the use of anticholinergic premedication,[23, 24] although some still advocate its routine use.[25] Procedures involving the pharynx or airway and ophthalmic operations are particularly likely to provoke vagal reflexes and many anaesthetists continue to use anticholinergics in these cases.

There is an increasing trend in paediatric anaesthesia to prescribe simple analgesic or antiinflammatory drugs, such as paracetamol, preoperatively to children undergoing minor procedures. In appropriate dosage (30–40 mg/kg), this appears to be effective in reducing the use of postoperative opiate analgesia with its attendant problems of nausea and vomiting[26] and is safe in terms of residual gastric volume at induction of anaesthesia.[27]

EQUIPMENT AND TECHNIQUES

Equipment for paediatric anaesthesia

Historically, anaesthetists dealing with children were faced with the task of adapting equipment designed for adult use and using their ingenuity to produce results that were at best mediocre by modern standards. Significant advances in technology and the understanding of paediatric physiology now make it unacceptable to consider anaesthesia for children without a full range of equipment designed specifically for that purpose. Most anaesthesia departments now have a designated 'lead' for paediatric anaesthesia with particular responsibility for the procurement and maintenance of appropriate equipment.

Paediatric breathing systems

The observations of Phillip Ayre[28] in 1937 on the effects of using a closed breathing system designed for adults in infants led him to develop the T-piece system with minimal dead space and resistance to breathing and a continuous supply of oxygen close to the airway. The Jackson Rees modification of this system[29] described in 1950 remains popular with many anaesthetists despite many subsequent advances (**Figure 41.1**).

The classification of anaesthetic breathing systems and an understanding of their functional characteristics[30, 31] has allowed the development of a number of different systems appropriate for paediatric use.[32, 33] Other considerations, such as reduction of atmospheric pollution by inhalational agents and the economic use of newer, expensive inhalation agents, have further influenced development.

Airway management equipment

Much of the morbidity in anaesthetized children is related to airway difficulties, and safe management of the airway

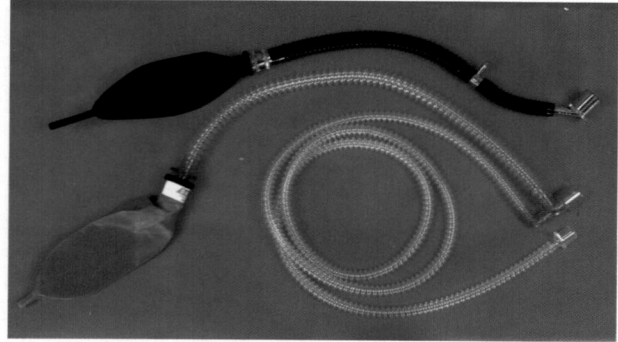

Figure 41.1 'T' piece breathing systems. Original system with metal connector and rubber hoses (above). Modern single use system (below).

is, perhaps, the most important aspect of paediatric anaesthesia. This is particularly the case in many ENT procedures where surgery involves a 'shared airway' between surgeon and anaesthetist. Notwithstanding the huge range of airway devices available, the anaesthetist's most important assets are sound basic airway management skills and an understanding of the anatomy and physiology of the paediatric airway. Equipment choices for airway maintenance during anaesthesia are a face mask with or without an oral or nasopharyngeal airway, a laryngeal mask airway, a tracheal tube or a more complex method such as tracheostomy.

Face masks are used during spontaneous breathing for short procedures, such as myringotomy and for pre-oxygenation and inhalational induction of anaesthesia. Ideally, they should be nonthreatening, easy to apply and achieve a good seal with minimal pressure on the face. Clear plastic face masks with cushioned rims are available in appropriate shapes and sizes for children of all ages and fulfil these requirements in all respects. Most of these are latex-free and some are available with 'flavour' impregnated rims, which may be helpful during inhalational induction.

The laryngeal mask airway (LMA)[34] introduced in the mid-1980s has greatly assisted in the management of both the routine and the difficult airway. Although originally developed for adults, LMAs are now available in sizes suitable for use in children of all ages, including neonates (**Table 41.3**).

Laryngeal masks are particularly useful in many ENT procedures, allowing adequate surgical access whilst avoiding intubation of the trachea. The reinforced LMA, which has a kink-resistant flexometallic oropharyngeal tube, is commonly used in head and neck surgery (**Figure 41.2**). As well as its extensive use in routine anaesthetic practice, the LMA is increasingly being used as an adjunct to fibrescopic examination and intubation of the paediatric airway.

Tracheal intubation remains the standard for airway maintenance during many procedures. The anatomical features of the child's airway influencing tube selection are well known[36] and hinge on the nature of the cricoid ring. Generally, a tracheal tube of the largest possible

Table 41.3 LMA sizes for paediatric patients.

Patient weight (kg)	Suggested laryngeal mask size
Less than 5	1
5–10	1.5
10–20	2
20–30	2.5
Not chosen by weight	3
Not chosen by weight	4
Not chosen by weight	5

Adapted from Ref. 35, with permission.

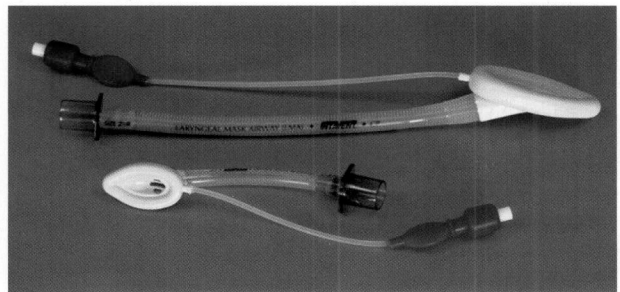

Figure 41.2 LMAs. Reinforced airway (top) and standard airway (bottom).

internal diameter should be chosen to minimize resistance to gas flow and avoid an excessive leak around the tube. It is important, however, to avoid inserting too large a tube, which may cause mucosal damage with the attendant risks of post-extubation airway difficulties.

Uncuffed, disposable polyvinyl chloride (PVC) tubes are available in a wide range of internal diameters and are commonly used in children under eight years of age. Although there is considerable individual variation, it is generally the case that a child's age, rather than height, weight or other characteristics, correlates best with the optimal tube diameter. Numerous formulae to help choose the correct diameter have been proposed of which the most often quoted (for uncuffed PVC tubes) is:[37]

$$\text{Internal diameter (mm)} = \frac{\text{Age (years)}}{3}$$
$$+ 3.75 \text{ (for children under six years of age)}$$

$$\text{Internal diameter (mm)} = \frac{\text{Age (years)}}{4}$$
$$+ 4.5 \text{ (for children over six years of age)}.$$

(It should be noted that tubes are sized according to the internal diameter and that there may be some variation in the external diameter depending on the manufacturer and style of tube.) Below the age of two years, this guide is not reliable and the use of any formula must be modified by individual considerations. The length of the tracheal tube is similarly important, the distance between the vocal cords and the carina being age- and height-dependent. Endobronchial intubation is a common hazard and the effect of flexion or extension of the neck in some procedures must be considered. The following formulae have been suggested as a guide to tube length:

$$\text{Length} = \text{Age (years)}/2$$
$$+ 12 \text{ (cm) for orotracheal intubation}$$

$$\text{Length} = \text{Age (years)}/2$$
$$+ 15 \text{ (cm) for nasotracheal intubation.}$$

As for tube diameter, these formulae are useful guides but correct tube position must be confirmed by careful auscultation, capnography and, if necessary, a chest x-ray.

In older children approaching puberty, cuffed endotracheal tubes are used, reflecting the anatomical development of the airway.

Despite concerns about the potential for mucosal damage, the use of cuffed tubes (with high volume, low pressure cuffs) is increasing in younger children and even newborns.[38] Provided that adjustments are made to size calculations and that the reduced margin of safety for endobronchial intubation[39] is appreciated, this has been shown to be safe and may afford advantages in terms of gas leak and environmental pollution and may reduce the need for repeat intubation if an incorrect tube size is selected.

Endotracheal tubes are available in a variety of materials, although the use of PVC and silicone rubber is now almost universal with the exception of tubes designed for laser procedures, discussed under Laser endoscopy. Similarly, a range of configurations has been developed (**Figure 41.3**). Preformed tubes, such as the 'south-facing' Ring, Adair, Eluyn (RAE) tube,[40] 'north-facing' nasal tubes or armoured tubes may be of particular benefit in head and neck procedures, allowing security of fixation with less interference in the surgical field than standard tubes.

A huge range of laryngoscopes and blades is available. Anatomical considerations and, to some extent personal choice, determine the most appropriate blade to use. In general, the relatively cephalad position of the infant larynx and the long epiglottis makes intubation easier with a straight-bladed instrument and these are often used in children under six months of age. Mackintosh pattern curved blades used in older children are positioned in the vallecula and indirectly lift the epiglottis. Vagal innervation of the posterior epiglottis makes bradycardia a potential hazard of the use of a straight-bladed technique. Various blade designs, with different cross sections and shapes, are produced, as well as different blade lengths. Not infrequently, failure to position and stabilize the head correctly can lead to intubation difficulties. Attention to basic details such as this should be assured before resorting to additional equipment.

Bougies or introducers over which a tube can be advanced are often helpful but care must be taken to avoid trauma to the larynx or trachea. In situations where anatomical abnormalities present particular problems, the use of a fibreoptic technique is often successful provided the operator is trained and practised in the use of such equipment.

Vascular access

Secure access to the circulation is mandatory for all children undergoing anaesthesia. Intravenous access should be obtained before induction of anaesthesia in emergencies, where fluid resuscitation is necessary or when an intravenous induction of anaesthesia is planned.

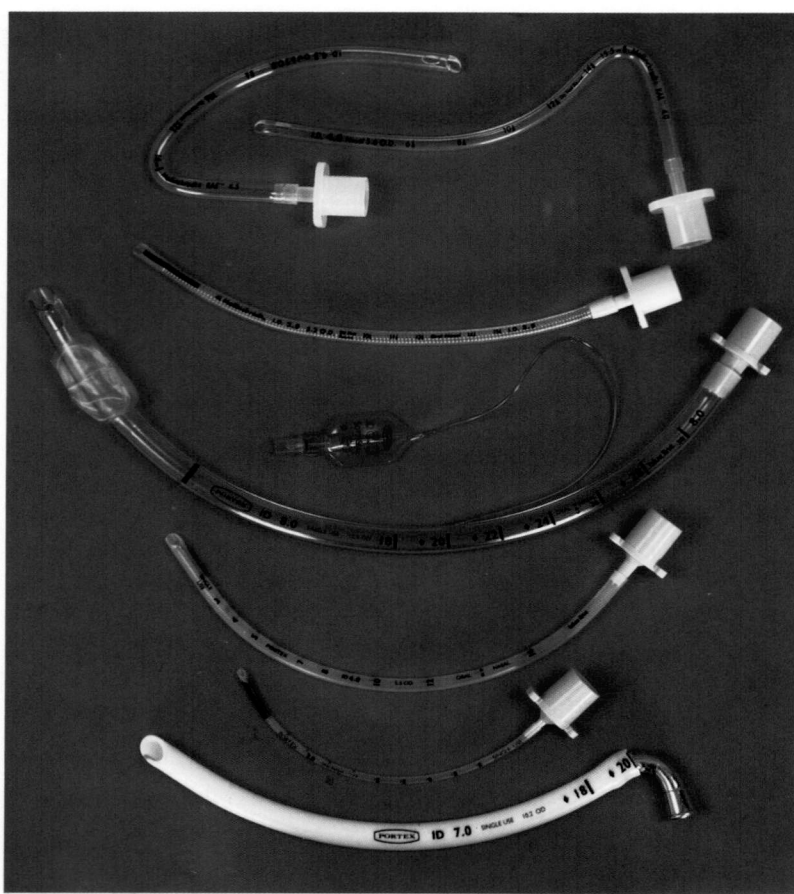

Figure 41.3 Endotracheal tube patterns. From above; 'RAE' north and south facing, armoured uncuffed, cuffed and uncuffed pvc, Portex 'Ivory' for nasal intubation with metal 'Magill' connector.

The use of topical local anaesthetic creams (see under Premedication) is increasingly common in paediatric practice and has led to an increase in the use of intravenous induction of anaesthesia in children of all ages.

Intravenous cannulae are available in a range of designs and size, generally made from inert materials such as Teflon, polyurethane or silicone. Appropriate sites for cannulation depend on the age of the child.[41] Following cannulation, secure fixation should be ensured and attention taken to ensure access to the cannula after positioning and draping for surgery.

In some situations, central venous or arterial cannulation may be necessary. Such interventions should not be undertaken lightly and performed only by those trained in the appropriate techniques.

Heat conservation

Control of body temperature is an important consideration in paediatric surgical patients. Most children become hypothermic to some degree unless active measures are taken to avoid this. Hypothermia results partly from environmental exposure but more importantly from anaesthesia-induced failure of thermoregulatory control.

Even a modest reduction in body temperature may be undesirable; consequently measurement of body temperature and active measures to conserve heat should be a standard part of paediatric anaesthetic practice.

General anaesthesia inhibits normal thermoregulatory mechanisms and superimposed heat loss to the environment predominantly radiant in nature increases the likelihood of hypothermia. Different body tissues have different temperatures and measurements are usually described as 'core' or 'peripheral'. Measurement of core temperature is of greatest clinical importance and thermocouple or thermistor thermometers are widely available. Common sites for core temperature measurement, such as the nasopharynx, distal oesophagus or tympanic membrane, may be inappropriate during ENT surgery!

Avoiding unnecessary exposure of the child is a simple, but effective, method of reducing heat loss, the area of skin covered being more important than the material used. In particular, the large surface area of the head in infants should remain covered if possible. Similarly raising the ambient temperature will help, although the temperature required to maintain normothermia in neonates (c. 26 °C) can create uncomfortable working conditions in the operating theatre. Hence, maintenance of the room temperature at a comfortable level and warming the microclimate around the child is more usual practice.

A number of warming devices are available, but forced warm-air convective blankets appear to be the most effective and are commonly used in paediatric practice.[42] When active warming devices are used, temperature monitoring is mandatory to guard against unintentional hyperthermia.

Induction of anaesthesia

The transition from an awake to an anaesthetized state creates a number of physiological changes, with potentially hazardous consequences. It is the responsibility of the anaesthetist to conduct a safe induction of anaesthesia whilst maintaining a calm and unhurried manner that will reassure the child and, commonly, accompanying parents and carers. Immediately before induction of anaesthesia, patient identity, preparation and consent for all procedures should be confirmed. The function of any anaesthetic and ancillary equipment should be checked and the availability of appropriate drugs and, importantly, skilled assistance should be assured.

Parental presence during the induction of anaesthesia is now the norm in UK paediatric practice and is generally agreed by both anaesthetists and parents to be helpful. The anxiety felt by many parents should not be underestimated and it is important that accompanying their child is a choice rather than compulsory.

The changes that accompany induction of anaesthesia necessitate careful monitoring, both by clinical observation and through the use of physiological monitoring devices. It is often possible to apply monitoring equipment prior to the induction of anaesthesia and pulse oximetry is viewed as essential in this respect. ECG and blood pressure monitoring are desirable, but may be deferred until after induction in healthy children.

Inhalational induction of anaesthesia has been the mainstay in paediatric anaesthesia and remains in common use. The development of agents such as Sevoflurane, with low blood gas solubility (hence rapid induction), less cardiovascular depression than older agents and a less pungent odour has allowed smoother and more rapid anaesthesia.[43] The use of topical anaesthetic creams and the availability of fine gauge cannulae have similarly improved the acceptance of intravenous anaesthesia in children.

Frequently, the choice of induction technique is of no great clinical significance and is often influenced by personal preference, either on the part of the anaesthetist or the child. However, clinical considerations may influence the choice of technique, for example in the child with a difficult or partially obstructed airway most anaesthetists regard an inhalational technique as the safest, allowing the maintenance of spontaneous respiration.

Physiological monitoring during anaesthesia

Modern anaesthesia is expected to provide optimal conditions for surgical interventions whilst ensuring patient safety, minimizing morbidity and mortality. Advances in the last 20 years have allowed the development of equipment that provides almost instantaneous detection of physiological changes, particularly respiratory and cardiovascular, which has greatly enhanced the safety of paediatric anaesthesia. Minimum standards for monitoring during anaesthesia[44, 45] have been widely adopted, although it must be appreciated that increasing reliance on complex electronic equipment, which may fail, should assist rather than replace basic clinical monitoring and that interpretation of information must be guided by the individual clinical situation.

Routine patient monitoring includes ECG, pulse oximetry, blood pressure measurement and capnography. The importance of temperature monitoring, particularly in infants, is mentioned under Heat conservation. Routine monitoring, particularly of respiratory function and oxygenation should be continued during recovery from anaesthesia. Unfortunately, monitoring the effect of anaesthetic agents on the brain is difficult and although methods based on processed EEG signals may be used,[46] these may be cumbersome and impractical in routine clinical practice. Monitoring of neuromuscular blockade is advisable, particularly in neonates or during prolonged procedures, primarily to ensure adequate recovery from relaxants at the end of surgery. During some procedures, for example parotid surgery, the surgical team may rely on stimulation of the facial nerve to avoid damage to this structure. In such surgery, monitoring of neuromuscular transmission is of particular relevance to ensure a muscular response to nerve stimulation. In some situations, patient or procedure considerations may merit more complex or invasive monitoring such as central venous pressure, direct arterial pressure, blood gas estimation or cardiac output measurement.

SPECIFIC SURGICAL PROCEDURES

The principles of preoperative preparation and conduct of anaesthesia described under Preoperative assessment outline the general approach to the paediatric surgical patient. Whilst these are applicable to all procedures, specific surgical operations may require the use of particular techniques to allow adequate surgical access and to ensure patient safety and comfort.

Operations on the ear

MYRINGOTOMY AND GROMMET INSERTION

Ventilation of the middle ear in children is a common procedure usually performed on a day case or outpatient basis. The majority of patients are satisfactorily managed with a standard inhalation or intravenous induction of anaesthesia and airway maintenance with an LMA provides good operating conditions[47] and may have some advantages over a simple face mask technique.[48] Despite the potential for nitrous oxide to increase middle ear pressure, its use is widespread for grommet insertion and has not been associated with increased postoperative vomiting.[49] Paracetamol or nonsteroidal antiinflammatory agents afford adequate postoperative analgesia in most patients.[50, 51] Modification of anaesthetic technique or overnight hospital admission may be necessary in grommet insertion cases in a significant minority of children with underlying conditions (such as palatal clefting, craniofacial or chromosomal anomalies) or with coexisting adenoidal hypertrophy and potential airway difficulties.

CONGENITAL EAR DEFECTS

Congenital defects of the ear may necessitate surgical intervention to reconstruct the external ear or for the implantation of bone-anchored hearing aids. Whilst the surgery is superficial and rarely of prolonged duration, the association of ear defects with other dysmorphic features of the face and mandible (particularly Treacher Collins and hemifacial microsomia syndromes) may pose significant anaesthetic concerns. These may include difficulties in visualizing the larynx and tracheal intubation[52, 53] and careful assessment and planning of airway management are essential. Scrutiny of previous anaesthetic records can provide valuable information regarding airway management strategies. Fortunately, unless mouth opening is very severely limited, the LMA often allows adequate airway maintenance for these patients.[54] If tracheal intubation is necessary, a full range of equipment to assist in the management of difficult intubation and experienced assistance is essential.

MIDDLE EAR EXPLORATION, MASTOIDECTOMY, MYRINGOPLASTY, COCHLEAR IMPLANTATION

Anaesthesia for middle ear surgery requires an appreciation of the conditions necessary for successful microsurgery including a quiet, bloodless field, the influence that nitrous oxide may have on a tympanic graft and, in some procedures, the importance of preservation of the facial nerve.

Although adequate conditions may be achieved with a number of different anaesthetic techniques, common to them all is attention to detail. Careful preparation and judicious use of premedication will aid a smooth induction of anaesthesia avoiding hypertension and tachycardia. Subsequently, the avoidance of airway obstruction and minimizing mean airway pressure will help reduce venous bleeding which is often

more troublesome than arterial bleeding. When positioning the child for surgery, a 15 to 20° head-up tilt is helpful to reduce venous congestion, provided that compression of the neck, chest and abdomen is also avoided.

The rapidity with which depth of anaesthesia can be altered with modern inhalational or intravenous agents such as Desflurane and Remifentanil means that hypotensive agents are rarely required.

Tracheal intubation and controlled ventilation is a common technique for middle ear surgery, although the use of a reinforced LMA may reduce the potential for airway complications at the end of surgery. Clearly, avoidance of coughing, laryngospasm and straining at the end of surgery is equally important as at induction of anaesthesia.

The solubility of nitrous oxide allows its diffusion into and out of air-filled spaces more rapidly than air leading to an increase in volume of the space, or an increase in pressure in noncompliant spaces such as the middle ear. Thus, pressure in the intact middle ear increases during nitrous oxide anaesthesia.[55] When nitrous oxide is discontinued, pressure falls as nitrous oxide diffuses out faster than air diffuses in. These pressure changes may distort or displace a tympanic graft and so nitrous oxide should be discontinued before the middle ear is closed.

The proximity of the facial nerve to the surgical field in some middle ear procedures demands careful monitoring to avoid nerve damage. A nerve stimulator may be used in the surgical field to identify branches of the facial nerve. It is important that the anaesthetist is aware of this and monitors the effect of any neuromuscular relaxant agents used.

The anaesthetic considerations for cochlear implantation are essentially the same as for other middle ear surgery although surgery, particularly if bilateral, may be prolonged. Profound sensorineural hearing loss may be associated with other features of relevance to the anaesthetist. For example, the prolongation of the QT interval in the Jervell and Lange-Nielsen syndrome presents a daunting challenge.[56]

Operations on the nose, nasopharynx and pharynx

CHOANAL ATRESIA

Bilateral occlusion of the posterior nares may cause acute respiratory distress in the neonatal period and maintenance of a patent oral airway or, sometimes, endotracheal intubation is necessary until surgical intervention is undertaken. Repeated anaesthesia may be required for nasal dilatation and restenting during early infancy. In some cases, the cytotoxic agent Mitomycin C may be topically applied following nasal dilatation[57] and great care should be taken to avoid exposure of surgical, anaesthetic and theatre staff.

ADENOIDECTOMY AND TONSILLECTOMY

Adenotonsillectomy remains one of the most common paediatric surgical procedures and comprises much of many anaesthetists' paediatric practice. Although often considered a routine procedure, a minority of patients with severe upper airway obstruction from adenotonsillar hypertrophy present stern challenges for even the most experienced anaesthetist. Considerable variation in pre-, intra- and postoperative management of children undergoing adenotonsillectomy exists and controversies abound.

Preoperative assessment is informed by the indication for adenotonsillectomy and, as indicated above, identification of children with OSAS is of great importance when planning intra and postoperative care. Although largely a clinical diagnosis, sleep studies with pulse oximetry and cardiological assessment may be required in children with severe or longstanding symptoms. Prediction of postoperative apnoea and hypoxia in children with severe OSAS will necessitate careful observation with pulse oximetry, supplemental oxygen and occasionally airway support.[11, 12] Particular difficulties may be expected in younger children under three years old[13] and those with other congenital or acquired anomalies. Routine preoperative coagulation testing for healthy children is not generally indicated unless a history of bleeding tendency is suspected.[58]

Factors dictating an appropriate anaesthetic technique include the preoperative and expected postoperative degree of airway compromise, airway security during surgery, postoperative pain relief and control of nausea and vomiting, postoperative bleeding and the proposed duration of hospital stay. In addition, recent concerns regarding the potential transmission of prion disease (variant Creutzfeld Jakob disease) have, in the UK, determined anaesthetic technique to some extent.

In children with significant obstructive symptoms induction of anaesthesia may precipitate severe obstruction, which can usually be improved by continuous positive airway pressure (CPAP) and the insertion of an oropharyngeal airway. In such patients, a technique employing endotracheal intubation, ventilation and minimal opiate use affords good operative conditions and an awake child at the end of surgery. Careful postoperative observation with supplemental oxygen therapy and sometimes nasophayngeal airway support or even tracheal intubation may be needed in the most severely obstructed patients. Particular attention should be directed to the care of such children on the first postoperative night.

Protection of the airway from blood and tissue debris is essential during surgery. To achieve this, most anaesthetists employ endotracheal intubation or the reinforced LMA. Tracheal intubation, usually with a

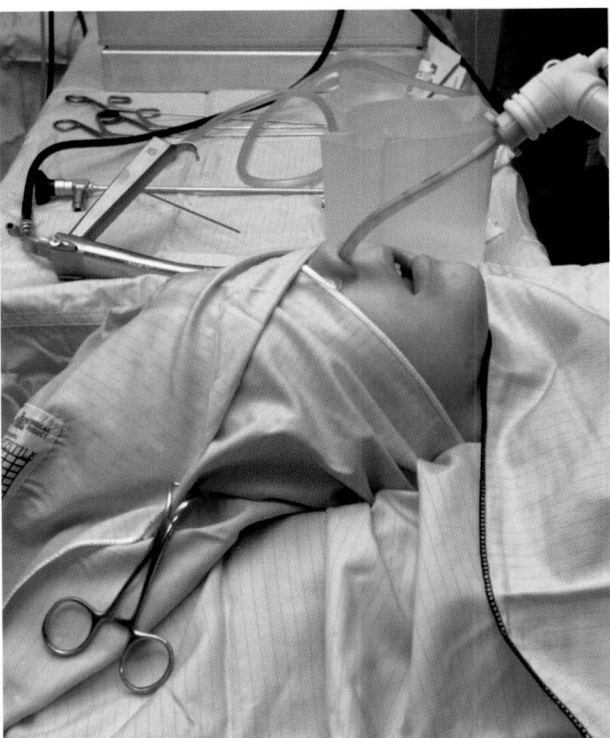

Figure 41.4 Insufflation of oxygen and volatile anaesthetic agent via nasopharyngeal tube.

preformed plastic RAE pattern tube[40] (see **Figure 41.4**) has been the mainstay of airway management prior to the introduction of the reinforced LMA and is usually satisfactory for both surgeon and anaesthetist. Potential problems inherent in the fixed length of such tubes are well known and occasionally difficulties may be encountered with compression from the mouth gag, particularly if the gag is short or opened excessively. These difficulties are more likely with small tube sizes (less than 4.5 mm internal diameter) as is the potential for 'wedging' of the tube in the gag blade and accidental extubation of the patient when removing the gag.[59]

The reinforced LMA has been widely used for tonsillectomy[60, 61] and may have some advantages over tracheal intubation. Placement of the mask does not require the use of muscle relaxants, creates a seal that protects the larynx from blood and debris and can be left in place to secure the airway until protective reflexes have returned. Use of the LMA requires full surgical cooperation and may necessitate particular care when positioning the mouth gag. Difficulties with surgical access[62] may preclude the use of the LMA, particularly in smaller children (less than 15 kg) or when other complicating factors are present. A meta-analysis of the use of LMA in tonsillectomy concludes that this is a safe alternative to intubation provided full cooperation between surgeon and anaesthetist is ensured.[63]

Analgesia following adenotonsillectomy in children has been achieved by a variety of means, most of which

Table 41.4 Suggested doses of paracetamol and NSAIDs in children.

	Loading dose (mg/kg)	Maintenance dose (mg/kg)	Dose interval (hours)	Maximum daily dose (mg/kg/24 h)
Oral paracetamol	20	15–20	4–6	90
Rectal paracetamol	30	20	6–8	90
Oral ibuprofen	5	4–10	6–8	20
Oral diclofenac	N/A	1	8–12	3
Rectal diclofenac	N/A	1	8–12	150 mg/day

Reproduced from Ref. 64, with permission.

involve a combination of paracetamol and nonsteroidal antiinflammatory drugs (NSAIDs), often with the addition of low-dose opioids such as codeine phosphate. The combination of paracetamol and codeine has long been used in paediatric practice and appears to be effective. Many anaesthetists use intravenous opioid drugs such as fentanyl or morphine intraoperatively, although this may increase postoperative nausea and vomiting and caution is advocated in the presence of severe obstructive symptoms. There has been much debate regarding the efficacy and safety of varying doses and routes of administration of both paracetamol and NSAIDs in children. A suggested dosage schedule is indicated (**Table 41.4**) based on the Royal College of Paediatrics and Child Health (RCPCH) guidelines.[64]

Guidelines for the use of NSAIDs in the perioperative period based on a structured literature review have been issued by the Royal College of Anaesthetists.[65] There is good evidence for the analgesic efficacy of NSAIDs compared with opioids after adenotonsillectomy, although a risk of increased bleeding has been shown in some studies. The guidelines suggest that NSAIDs (but not paracetamol) be avoided in children with proven asthma, particularly if associated with nasal polyps, severe eczema or atopy, although most anaesthetists believe that it is reasonable to use NSAIDs in asthmatic children in whom previous exposure to these drugs has been uncomplicated. Studies published since this review are generally supportive of the analgesic benefits of NSAIDs although are not conclusive on the issue of increased bleeding risk.[66, 67, 68] A recent systematic review concluded that the use of NSAIDs in paediatric tonsillectomy did not cause any increase in bleeding requiring a return to theatre and that there was less nausea and vomiting when NSAIDs were used compared to other analgesics.[69] It has been suggested that the surgical technique employed during tonsillectomy may influence postoperative pain although the evidence for this is conflicting.[70, 71, 72] Similarly, the infiltration of the tonsillar bed with local anaesthetic agents is advocated by some authors,[73, 74] whilst a systematic review of this practice concludes that there is no evidence that postoperative pain control is improved.[75]

Nausea and vomiting following adenotonsillectomy is a significant problem in terms of patient comfort and satisfaction and may delay discharge of children undergoing day care. The 5-hydroxytryptamine antagonists ondansetron and tropisetron are effective in reducing postoperative nausea and vomiting either alone or in combination with dexamethasone.[76, 77]

Primary haemorrhage requiring surgical intervention in the first few hours following adenotonsillectomy is an uncommon (0.5–1 percent) but potentially life-threatening event that requires immediate attention. Blood loss is often difficult to estimate but clinical signs of tachycardia, pallor and reduced capillary refill should prompt intervention. Blood pressure is usually maintained in children until 25 percent or more of circulating volume has been lost and hypotension is a late and very worrying sign. Rapid volume replacement with crystalloid or colloid solutions should be instituted and hypovolaemia corrected whilst a theatre is prepared for surgery. During this time, blood is cross-matched and a full blood count and a coagulation screen performed.

The anaesthetic approach to a bleeding post-tonsillectomy patient must address the problems presented by the potential for regurgitation of swallowed blood together with active bleeding obscuring the view at laryngoscopy. Although opinions differ, most anaesthetists would favour a rapid sequence intravenous induction of anaesthesia with preoxygenation and cricoid pressure with the patient in a head down position on the operating table. In addition to the usual anaesthetic equipment, a back-up suction device and tracheal tubes smaller than that used at the original procedure should be to hand.

Following the provision of a secure airway, close cardiovascular monitoring and further fluid or blood transfusion are undertaken during surgery. The stomach should be emptied via a wide bore nasogastric tube and extubation should be performed with the child awake in a lateral, head down position. A postnasal pack placed to stem bleeding from the adenoid bed is poorly tolerated by younger children and may necessitate sedation and intubation in an intensive care unit until the pack is removed.

Adenotonsillectomy is now frequently performed on a day stay basis, particularly in North America, and appears safe provided that careful selection criteria and meticulous operative techniques are followed. Strict observation in the postoperative period, usually for four to six hours postoperatively, is ensured and clear instructions issued for homecare and support following discharge. Despite an increase in day care tonsillectomy in the UK, many patients remain in hospital overnight, as much for social and organizational reasons as for clinical indications.

In recent years, the potential for transmission of vCJD via surgical equipment has prompted the UK Department of Health to implement improvements in decontamination procedures for surgical instruments, as advised by the Spongiform Encephalopathy Advisory Committee (SEAC).[78] In addition, adenotonsillectomy was identified as a procedure suitable to pilot the use of single use equipment as patients are generally young, a limited number of instruments are used and patient safety was unlikely to be compromised. Disposable surgical and anaesthetic equipment was introduced in 2001, but increased reports of adverse incidents prompted a withdrawal of the directive in December of that year. Although the return to reusable equipment was applied to anaesthetic and surgical equipment, it was subsequently decided, presumably on the basis of relative risk, that this change did not apply to anaesthetic equipment.[79] Currently then, anaesthetic equipment placed in the mouth or respiratory tract during tonsillectomy must be disposable or covered by a disposable protective sheath.

Airway endoscopy procedures

Anaesthesia for children undergoing airway endoscopy procedures requires an understanding of the medical condition and likely airway pathology, an appreciation of the surgical requirements for the procedure and the functions, hazards and limitations of bronchoscopic and laser equipment, close cooperation between all members of the theatre team and, not infrequently, a degree of ingenuity and adaptation.

DIAGNOSTIC AIRWAY ENDOSCOPY

Infants and children presenting for diagnostic laryngoscopy and bronchoscopy usually exhibit some degree of airway obstruction, stridor being the most frequent presenting feature. In many cases, a careful history of the onset and features of the obstruction will suggest a likely cause. Investigations, including chest and neck x-rays, barium swallow studies, respiratory function studies (although these are often difficult and unreliable in small infants) may further assist diagnosis.

Preoperative information is useful but preparation should be made for unexpected findings and a clear appreciation of the requirements of the surgeon and a cooperative approach are essential to allow accurate diagnosis to be made safely.

The anaesthetic technique must afford assessment of both fixed and dynamic elements of the airway whilst ensuring airway maintenance and adequate oxygenation and ventilation of the child. An unobstructed view of laryngeal, tracheal and bronchial structures is necessary in a still, spontaneously breathing patient. Depth of anaesthesia must be sufficient to control the intense stimulation associated with laryngoscopy but also allow assessment of vocal cord and cricoarytenoid function without laryngospasm in the almost awake patient.

It is essential that a clear understanding exists between anaesthetist, surgeon and operating theatre personnel as to the conduct of the procedure. A range of airway equipment and experienced assistance should be available and all staff should be familiar with the assembly and use of bronchoscopic equipment. Sedative premedication is usually avoided in children with airway obstruction although may be useful in carefully selected patients (for instance frequent attenders) if anxiety is likely to worsen existing airway obstruction. Despite the general reduction in the use of anticholinergic premedication in children, most anaesthetists continue to use these agents in airway endoscopy procedures. The benefits include control of secretions, reducing the incidence of breath holding and laryngospasm, attenuation of vagal responses to airway instrumentation and deep inhalational anaesthesia, as well as more effective topical anaesthesia of the larynx.[80] Traditionally, atropine has been used preoperatively for this purpose, either orally or intramuscularly, and certainly is effective. The unpleasant sequelae of this practice for the child (i.m. injection, dry mouth, and diplopia) should be considered and many anaesthetists now employ intravenous atropine or glycopyrrolate at the time of induction of anaesthesia. The technique most commonly employed for diagnostic airway examination involves a volatile anaesthetic agent in combination with topical anaesthesia of the larynx. Maintenance of spontaneous ventilation, certainly until it is established that positive pressure ventilation is possible, is paramount and, in general, an inhalational induction is recommended using 100 percent oxygen and an increasing concentration of volatile agent. Historically, halothane has been the agent of choice but is increasingly being superseded by sevoflurane, which affords a more rapid induction. Debate continues over the place of halothane in paediatric anaesthesia,[81] although its availability and cost mean that it is still widely used worldwide.

Airway obstruction prolongs the induction of anaesthesia and gentle assistance of ventilation with the application of CPAP may speed the process and improve gas exchange. Intravenous access, if not already secured, is obtained and depth of anaesthesia increased. Some anaesthetists choose to intubate the trachea following induction of anaesthesia, affording airway security for transfer to theatre and setting up of equipment. Intubation, however, may be difficult and muscle relaxants should not be used to facilitate this unless positive pressure ventilation is shown to be possible. Others avoid this to allow a surgical view of the unsullied larynx. If intubation is performed at this point, the nasotracheal route is convenient, allowing the tube to be withdrawn into the nasopharynx for endoscopy.

Topical anaesthesia of the larynx, commonly using lignocaine, is an essential component of the anaesthetic technique to reduce coughing and laryngospasm and to allow assessment of vocal cord and cricoarytenoid function at very light planes of anaesthesia and during awakening. Although there are some concerns that topical anaesthesia may produce subtle changes in glottic function, and one study reports exaggeration of the magnitude of the signs of laryngomalacia in sedated children undergoing flexible bronchoscopy,[82] the benefits outweigh these considerations.

The glottis, vallecula and trachea are anaesthetized, usually by the application of lignocaine spray. There is considerable risk of laryngospasm during spontaneous ventilation and often a short-acting muscle relaxant is used if intubation has not been performed. It appears, however, that the use of relatively dilute (2 percent lignocaine) solutions without preservative and flavourings found in multi-use metered dose sprays, significantly reduces the risk of laryngospasm (personal observation). Systemic effects from absorption of local anaesthetic agents from the mucosa may occur and it is recommended that dosage is limited to 4–5 mg/kg.

During the examination of the airway, spontaneous ventilation is maintained and anaesthesia is continued by insufflation of oxygen and a volatile agent, usually via a tracheal tube placed in the nasopharynx (**Figure 41.4**). This 'open' technique is well established, allows spontaneous ventilation to be maintained and has the merit of simplicity. Of major concern, however, is contamination of the working environment with volatile anaesthetic agents and occupational exposure of theatre personnel to concentrations considerably higher than currently recommended health regulation guidelines permit.[83] Alternative techniques for maintenance of anaesthesia, using intravenous agents such as propofol in place of volatile agents, are well described[84] and increasingly employed, even in small infants.

If intubation is not undertaken during anaesthetic induction this might form part of the examination to 'size' the larynx and subglottis allowing documentation of any stenotic lesions based on the external diameter of the endotracheal tube. This information is important when serial examinations are undertaken and also extremely useful anaesthetic information should the child present for other surgical procedures. At the end of the procedure the patient is allowed to waken with the laryngoscope in the vallecula to assess vocal cord function fully.

Careful monitoring of cardiovascular and respiratory function is imperative during endoscopy procedures and it is important that the operator, as well as the anaesthetist, are aware of any changes, particularly hypoxia or hypoventilation that may necessitate interruption of the examination or urgent intubation of the trachea. In this respect pulse oximetry with an audible tone and a camera allowing the anaesthetist to view the surgical field are particularly helpful in promoting patient safety.

Following the examination, careful observation and continued monitoring is necessary as instrumentation may exacerbate the pre-existing airway problems. Although infrequently necessary, facilities for immediate tracheal intubation should be at hand. Humidified oxygen is often used during the recovery phase and nebulized adrenaline may be useful if airway oedema is suspected. If topical anaesthesia has been applied to the larynx, oral fluids should be withheld for one to two hours postoperatively. Many anaesthetists administer intravenous steroids such as dexamethasone to children undergoing these procedures in an attempt to reduce the development of oedema. Although evidence suggests that this may reduce post-extubation stridor in children and reintubation rates in neonates in intensive care units,[85] the value of steroids during airway endoscopy is questionable. Limiting the number and duration of airway instrumentations and ensuring that appropriate calibre endoscopes are used is probably of greater importance.

BRONCHOSCOPY

Anaesthetic considerations and techniques for rigid bronchoscopy are essentially the same as for diagnostic laryngoscopy. The use of Storz scopes with Hopkins telescopic rods is almost universal (**Figure 41.5**) affording excellent optical quality and ease of anaesthetic delivery via a side arm that allows connection to the anaesthetic breathing system.

Insertion of the telescope effectively closes the system allowing ventilation of the trachea, although there is a considerable resistance to airflow, particularly with small scopes, and assisted ventilation is often required in infants. Occasionally, it is necessary to withdraw the telescope temporarily to allow adequate oxygenation or ventilation.

Adequate topical anaesthesia of the lower airways is often difficult to achieve and coughing may be a problem when the scope is advanced to the carina and beyond,

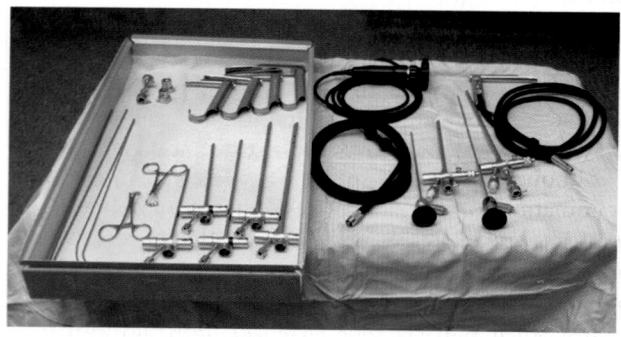

Figure 41.5 'Storz' bronchoscopy equipment.

despite deep anaesthesia. Intermittent neuromuscular blockade may be used, provided adequate ventilation via the bronchoscope is assured, but this may preclude a full dynamic assessment of the lower airways. As in laryngoscopy, constant communication and cooperation between surgeon and anaesthetist is essential.

Fibreoptic bronchoscopes may also be used to evaluate the upper and lower airways,[86] increasingly so with the availability of ultra-thin scopes suitable for use in infants. Although the procedure may be performed under sedation, anaesthesia may be necessary. The use of an LMA through which the bronchoscope is passed allows safe airway management whilst affording easy passage and manoeuvring of the fibrescope.[87]

FOREIGN BODY REMOVAL

Removal of an inhaled foreign body is a common indication for bronchoscopy in toddlers. Foreign body inhalation may precipitate acute airway obstruction and require urgent intervention or, more commonly, presentation may be delayed if a small object that passes beyond the main bronchi is inhaled. The conduct of anaesthesia is largely the same as for diagnostic endoscopy although the procedure may be prolonged and require multiple instrumentation of the airway. A spontaneous respiration technique, as described above, is frequently employed with volatile or intravenous anaesthetic agents. Some advocate controlled ventilation via the bronchoscope with neuromuscular blockade although caution should be exercised if a tracheal foreign body is likely to produce distal air trapping.[88] Whatever anaesthetic technique is employed, both anaesthetist and endoscopist should be aware of the potential difficulties involved. Airway inflammation and oedema, particularly when an organic foreign body is present, exacerbated by prolonged instrumentation and if removal is difficult, merits careful observation and follow up.

Operative procedures of the airway

Advances in microscope and laser technology have allowed the development of operative procedures on the paediatric airway that require particular attention from the anaesthetist. Frequently, patients with varying degrees of airway obstruction undergo repeated procedures and the special risks associated with the use of lasers must be taken into account.

Although the techniques described for diagnostic examination of the airway are satisfactory for many surgical procedures, alternative methods for airway management have been employed with varying degrees of success. The simplest of these involves intubation with a small tracheal tube that can be withdrawn into the nasopharynx when surgical access is impeded and

anaesthesia is continued with insufflation of oxygen and volatile agents as described above. Intermittent apnoeic oxygenation is a modification of this technique using neuromuscular blockade and intravenous maintenance of anaesthesia. Following a period of ventilation, the endotracheal tube is withdrawn to allow surgical access and reinserted repeatedly to allow intermittent ventilation, surgery being interrupted for this. Although successful and safe provided that close monitoring and a cooperative approach are ensured, infants tolerate only short periods of apnoea and repeated intubation may traumatize the airway.

Venturi jet ventilation involves entrainment of air produced by the delivery of high pressure gas boluses from a cannula attached to the suspension laryngoscope[89] or placed in the trachea. Muscle paralysis is maintained and ventilation monitored by observation of chest movement. Great care is taken to ensure that the cannula is correctly aligned and unobstructed at all times as gastric distension or direct injury to the airway from the high pressure jet may occur. This technique is not suitable when there is significant obstruction at glottic level as serious barotrauma may result. Trans-tracheal high frequency jet ventilation uses a similar principle where ventilation is provided by a high frequency jet ventilator via a cannula inserted percutaneously into the trachea via the cricothyroid membrane.[90] The driving pressure is similar or less than that used during conventional ventilation, reducing the risk of barotrauma, and the technique is suitable for use when there is significant obstruction at laryngeal level. Injuries such as extensive surgical emphysema may occur if the catheter is misplaced and a special jet ventilator is required. Use of these techniques will allow adequate anaesthetic and surgical conditions for the majority of procedures. In some children, however, the degree of airway obstruction may necessitate tracheostomy for treatment to be undertaken safely. The availability of tracheostomy equipment and the ability to secure the airway rapidly is mandatory when undertaking laryngeal surgery in children.

Laser endoscopy

Use of the carbon dioxide and other laser technology is well established for the treatment of laryngeal papillomatosis and other lesions of the larynx and trachea in children.[91] The hazards of laser use (see Chapter 58, Laser principles in otolaryngology, head and neck surgery) must be appreciated by all theatre personnel and strict guidelines followed during laser activation.

Apart from general considerations, the major difficulty with laser surgery is safe airway management and the avoidance of airway fires caused by ignition of non-metallic materials. The choice of anaesthetic technique

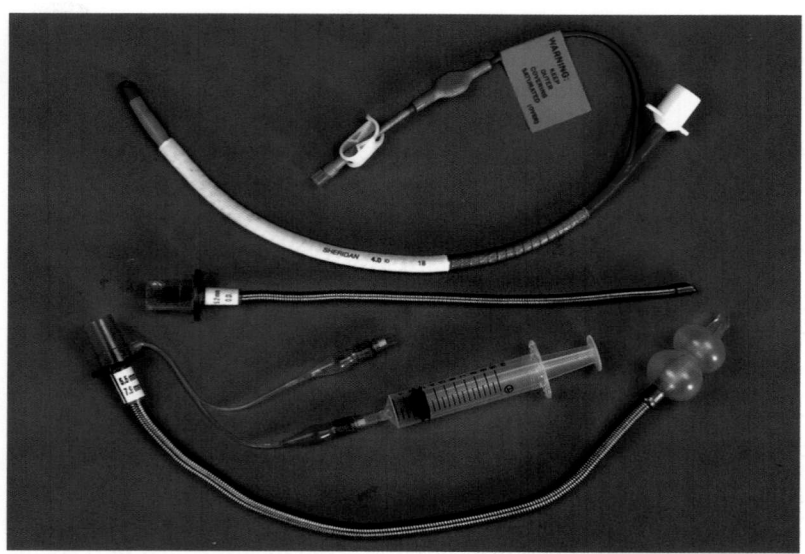

Figure 41.6 Laser endotracheal tubes. 'Lasertrach' copper wound red rubber tube (above), 'Laserflex' uncuffed and double-cuffed tubes (below).

will depend on the lesion being treated, patient size and, to some extent, the preferences of surgeon and anaesthetist. Often a tubeless technique with insufflation of oxygen via a nasal catheter and maintenance of anaesthesia with volatile or intravenous agents is satisfactory, safe and reduces the risk of mishaps. This technique is widely employed and appears safe and efficient for children undergoing treatment of recurrent laryngeal papillomatosis.[92] Although concerns have been raised about the use of high oxygen concentrations in the presence of laser energy, many children require this to avoid hypoxia and, provided all sources of combustion are avoided, the risk appears minimal.

If tracheal intubation is necessary, disposable metal or foil protected tubes are available in a range of sizes down to 3 mm internal diameter (**Figure 41.6**). All of these tubes, however, are either lined with PVC or have a rubber core and so there is a small risk of ignition. Cuffs on the larger tubes are also made from PVC or rubber and should be filled with saline rather than air. The construction of these tubes is such that the external diameter is large when compared to a standard tube of the same internal diameter and care should be taken to avoid trauma to the airway. In children with a tracheostomy, the tube should be removed or replaced with a metal tube before the laser is activated. Similarly, if trans-tracheal jet ventilation is used, the cannulae should be metallic.

Although every effort is made to reduce the risk of ignition, prompt action is required in the event of an airway fire to minimize the damage. Any combustible material should immediately be removed and oxygen delivery stopped. The fire should be extinguished with saline or water and ventilation resumed by mask. A thorough and careful examination of the airway is performed to assess damage and formulate a management plan that may include prolonged intubation or urgent tracheostomy.[93]

ARYEPIGLOTTOPLASTY

Laryngomalacia is a common indication for laryngoscopy in infants and aryepiglottoplasty may be indicated. Following diagnostic endoscopy, anaesthesia can be continued with an insufflation technique or, commonly, a nasotracheal tube is inserted.[94] The child can be extubated at the end of surgery and although careful observation is necessary, postoperative problems are rare. Some surgeons prefer to use the carbon dioxide laser rather than microlaryngeal instruments for supraglottoplasty, in which case full laser precautions are necessary.

LARYNGEAL CYSTS

Laryngeal cysts are uncommon but may give rise to intermittent airway obstruction. Anaesthetic considerations are essentially the same as for any other cause of upper airway problem, although positive pressure ventilation may be impossible if the cyst produces a ball-valve obstruction to the larynx. Although intubation is usually possible, urgent aspiration of the cyst may be required if the larynx is completely obscured. Following definitive deroofing, extubation and recovery are usually uneventful.

LARYNGEAL CLEFTS

Posterior deficiency of interarytenoid tissue may prevent complete glottic closure and result in repeated episodes of aspiration and recurrent pulmonary problems. This may be attributed to other pathology frequently present in these infants. Minor clefts may be closed by direct suture using a microlaryngeal technique under orotracheal anaesthesia. Long clefts are associated with significant morbidity and mortality and usually require tracheostomy and gastrostomy for pulmonary protection.

Anaesthetic and surgical management of these patients is complex and repeated procedures may be necessary.

Laryngotracheal stenosis and reconstruction

ANTERIOR CRICOID SPLIT

Cricoid split procedures are usually undertaken in neonates (often premature) with mild stenosis of the cricoid ring. These infants frequently present as extubation failures following a period of neonatal intubation and ventilation. Endotracheal intubation and positive pressure ventilation are continued during the procedure and, following laryngofissure, a larger sized tube is placed to stent the larynx for five to ten days postoperatively. The tip of the tube must be positioned distal to the split and securely fixed. Postoperatively, meticulous intensive care management is required to ensure that reintubation, which may cause extensive damage, is avoided. Should extubation fail following a cricoid split, tracheostomy is usually necessary.

LARYNGOTRACHEAL RECONSTRUCTION

Reconstructive procedures on the larynx usually involve laryngofissure and interposition of an anterior and/or posterior cartilage graft to widen the lumen. The procedure may be single-stage, following which the larynx is stented with an endotracheal tube for a short period postoperatively or as a staged procedure if a tracheostomy has already been performed to secure the airway.

The anaesthetic technique for the single-stage procedure is as for cricoid split and postoperative management in an intensive care environment is essential to ensure tube patency and minimize laryngeal trauma. A similar technique is employed when treating suprastomal collapse in patients with a tracheostomy.

To allow surgical access the head is extended and the existing tracheostomy tube is replaced with a reinforced tube that can be sutured or taped to the chest during surgery. If possible, a cuffed tube is used to avoid tracheal soiling with blood and debris and also to prevent anaesthetic gas leakage via the opened airway. Dilation of the tracheostome may be necessary to allow insertion of an appropriate calibre endotracheal tube. In smaller patients the cuff may impinge into the surgical site or a risk of endobronchial intubation may necessitate the fashioning of a shortened preformed tube. In this case, leakage of anaesthetic gases may make adequate ventilation of the patient difficult at some stages of the procedure and close monitoring of gas exchange is vital. However the trachea is managed, constant vigilance is required to maintain airway patency and avert displacement of the tube during surgical manipulations.

If an anterior costal cartilage graft is taken, the possibility of a pneumothorax must be recognized. Significant pain may also result from the graft site and infiltration with local anaesthetic agents and postoperative opioid analgesia are often required. A chest x-ray is essential at the end of the procedure to exclude a pneumothorax. Postoperatively, airway secretions are increased and aspiration may occur if the stent causes glottic incompetence.

Tracheostomy

Many children undergoing tracheostomy are intubated and anaesthesia is continued via the existing tracheal tube. Initially, spontaneous ventilation and topical anaesthesia of the larynx may be advised if it is proposed to extubate the child for a brief examination of the airway before reintubation and tracheostome formation. In the unintubated child, inhalational induction of anaesthesia is usual, followed by intubation with an appropriate sized endotracheal tube. A range of tubes should be available if subglottic stenosis is present, the smallest Portex tube having an internal diameter of 2 mm. Occasionally, a pinhole subglottic airway will preclude intubation even with the smallest tube in which case an LMA or face mask with spontaneous ventilation may prove an adequate technique.

Before surgery an appropriate sterile breathing system and connectors should be selected and the ability to connect the tracheostomy tube to the breathing system is checked. Secure intravenous access and full cardiovascular and respiratory monitoring are essential during the procedure and attention should be paid to temperature maintenance, particularly in small babies. Surgical drapes should be placed in such a way that immediate access to the endotracheal tube is assured should airway difficulties occur during surgery.

The child is ventilated with 100 percent oxygen prior to tracheal incision and under direct vision the tip of the tracheal tube is withdrawn to allow insertion of the tracheostomy tube. The tube should not be removed from the larynx until correct placement of the tracheostomy is checked, to allow reinsertion should difficulty be experienced in tracheostomy insertion. Anaesthesia is continued via the tracheostomy using a sterile connector and breathing system passed out from the surgical field. Careful inspection of chest wall movement, chest auscultatation, oxygen saturation and end tidal carbon dioxide measurement are imperative to assure correct placement of the tracheostomy tube.

At the end of surgery, the tracheostomy tube is secured with ties or tapes and careful suction of the pharynx and tracheostomy tube is performed. If tracheal 'stay' sutures have been placed in the tracheal wall, these should be carefully marked and instructions issued for the management of accidental tube dislodgement.

KEY POINTS

- ENT surgery provides the core of many anaesthetists' paediatric practice.
- Local organization of surgical services for children is in a state of flux.
- Careful preoperative assessment and preparation is vital for the safe conduct of anaesthesia.
- Relatively recent advances in technology and understanding of paediatric physiology have led to significant improvements in anaesthetic practice.
- Attention to detail, particularly regarding airway management, is essential.
- Close cooperation between anaesthetist and surgeon and a mutual understanding of the problems faced by each affords better care for patients.
- Objective evidence to support clinical practice in paediatric anaesthesia is limited.

REFERENCES

1. Department of Health. *Welfare of children and young people in hospital.* London: HMSO, 1991.
2. McNichol R. Paediatric anaesthesia – who should do it? The view from the specialist hospital. *Anaesthesia.* 1997; **52**: 513–5.
3. Rollin A-M. Paediatric anaesthesia – who should do it? The view from the district general hospital. *Anaesthesia.* 1997; **52**: 515–6.
4. The Report of a Joint Working Group. *The transfer of infants and children for surgery.* London: British Paediatric Association, 1993.
5. Campling EA, Devlin HB, Lunn JN. *The report of the confidential enquiry into perioperative deaths 1989.* London: NCEPOD, Royal College of Surgeons of England, 1990.
6. Holzman RS. Morbidity and mortality in pediatric anesthesia. *Pediatric Clinics of North America.* 1994; **41**: 239–56.
7. Tait AR, Malviya S, Voepel-Lewis T, Munro HM, Siewert M, Pandit UA. Risk factors for perioperative adverse events in children with upper respiratory tract infections. *Anesthesiology.* 2001; **95**: 299–306.
8. Parnis SJ, Barker DS, Van Der Walt JH. Clinical predictors of anaesthetic complications in children with respiratory tract infections. *Paediatric Anaesthesia.* 2001; **11**: 29–40.
9. Biavatti MJ, Manning SC, Phillips DL. Predictive factors for respiratory complications after tonsillectomy and adenoidectomy in children. *Archives of Otolaryngology and Head and Neck Surgery.* 1997; **123**: 517–21.
10. Gerber ME, O'Connor DM, Adler E, Myer 3rd CM. Selected risk factors in pediatric adenotonsillectomy. *Archives of Otolaryngology and Head and Neck Surgery.* 1997; **123**: 116–7.
11. Rosen GM, Muckle RP, Mahowald MW, Goding GS, Ullevig C. Postoperative respiratory compromise in children with obstructive sleep apnea syndrome: can it be anticipated? *Pediatrics.* 1994; **93**: 784–8.
12. Wilson K, Lakheeram I, Morielli A, Brouillette R, Brown K. Can assessment for obstructive sleep apnea help predict postadenotonsillectomy respiratory complications? *Anesthesiology.* 2002; **96**: 313–22.
13. McColley SA, April MM, Carroll JL, Naclerio RM, Loughlin GM. Respiratory compromise after adenotonsillectomy in children with obstructive sleep apnea. *Archives of Otolaryngology and Head and Neck Surgery.* 1992; **118**: 940–3.
14. Helfaer MA, McColley SA, Pyzick PL, Tunkel DE, Nichols DG, Baroody FM *et al.* Polysomnography after adenotonsillectomy in mild pediatric obstructive sleep apnea. *Critical Care Medicine.* 1996; **24**: 1323–7.
15. Phillips S, Daborn AK, Hatch DJ. Preoperative fasting for paediatric anaesthesia. *British Journal of Anaesthesia.* 1994; **73**: 529–36.
16. Splinter WM, Steward DA, Muir JG. The effect of preoperative apple juice on gastric contents, thirst and hunger in children. *Canadian Journal of Anaesthesia.* 1989; **36**: 55–8.
17. Litman RS, Wu CL, Quinlivan JK. Gastric volume and pH in infants fed clear fluids and breast milk prior to surgery. *Anesthesia and Analgesia.* 1994; **79**: 482–5.
18. Meakin G, Dugnall AE, Addison GM. Effects of fasting and oral premedication on the pH and volume of gastric aspirate in children. *British Journal of Anaesthesia.* 1987; **59**: 678–82.
19. Schreiner MS, Triebwasser A, Keon TP. Ingestion of liquids compared with preoperative fasting in pediatric outpatients. *Anesthesiology.* 1990; **72**: 593–7.
20. Gajraj NM, Pennant JH, Watcha MF. Eutectic mixture of local anaesthetics (EMLA[R]) cream. *Anesthesia and Analgesia.* 1994; **78**: 574–83.
21. Lawson RA, Smart NS, Morton NS. Evaluation of an amethocaine gel preparation for percutaneous analgesia before venous cannulation in children. *British Journal of Anaesthesia.* 1995; **75**: 282–5.
22. Kain ZN, Mayes LC, Bell C, Weisman S, Hofstadter MB, Rimar S. Premedication in the United States: a status report. *Anesthesia and Analgesia.* 1997; **84**: 427–32.
23. Parnis SJ, Van Der Walt JH. A national survey of atropine use by Australian anaesthetists. *Anaesthesia and Intensive Care.* 1994; **22**: 61–5.
24. Rautakorpi P, Manner T, Kanto J. A survey of current usage of anticholinergic drugs in paediatric anaesthesia in Finland. *Acta Anaesthesiologica Scandinavia.* 1999; **43**: 1057–9.
25. Shaw CA, Kelleher AA, Gill CP, Murdoch LJ, Stables RH, Black AE. Comparison of the incidence of complications at

induction and emergence in infants receiving oral atropine vs. no premedication. *British Journal of Anaesthesia.* 2000; **84**: 174–8.

26. Korpela R, Korvenoja P, Meretoja OA. Morphine-sparing effect of acetaminophen in pediatric day case surgery. *Anesthesiology.* 1999; **91**: 442–7.

27. Anderson BJ, Rees SG, Liley A, Stewart AW, Wardill MJ. Effect of preoperative paracetamol on gastric volumes and pH in children. *Paediatric Anaesthesia.* 1999; **9**: 203–7.

28. Ayre P. Endotracheal anesthesia for babies with special reference to hare-lip and cleft palate operations. *Anesthesia and Analgesia.* 1937; **16**: 330–3.

29. Jackson Rees G. Anaesthesia in the newborn. *British Medical Journal.* 1950; **2**: 1419–22.

30. Conway CM. Anaesthetic breathing systems. *British Journal of Anaesthesia.* 1985; **57**: 649–57.

31. Miller DM. Breathing systems reclassified. *Anaesthesia and Intensive Care.* 1995; **27**: 281–3.

32. Moyle JTB, Davey A, Ward C. *Ward's anaesthetic equipment*, 4th edn. London: W B Saunders, 1997.

33. Meakin G, Perkins RJ. Anaesthetic breathing systems for children. *Paediatric Anaesthesia.* 1996; **6**: 346.

34. Brain AIJ. The development of the laryngeal mask – a brief history of the invention, early clinical work from which the laryngeal mask evolved. *European Journal of Anaesthesiology.* 1991; **4**: 5–17.

35. Brimbacombe JA, Brain AIJ, Barry AM (ed.). *The laryngeal mask airway instruction manual*, 3rd edn. Maidenhead: Intavent Research, 1996.

36. Eckenhoff JE. Some anatomic considerations of the infant larynx influencing endotracheal anaesthesia. *Anesthesiology.* 1951; **12**: 401–10.

37. Penlington GN. Endotracheal tube sizes for children. *Anaesthesia.* 1974; **29**: 494.

38. Khine HH, Corddry DH, Kettrick RG, Martin TM, McCloskey JJ, Rose JB *et al.* Comparison of cuffed and uncuffed endotracheal tubes in young children during general anesthesia. *Anesthesiology.* 1997; **86**: 627–31.

39. Ho AM-H, Aun CST, Karmakar MK. The margin of safety associated with the use of cuffed paediatric endotracheal tubes. *Anaesthesia.* 2002; **57**: 173–5.

40. Ring WH, Adair JC, Elwyn RA. A new pediatric endotracheal tube. *Anesthesia and Analgesia.* 1974; **54**: 273–4.

41. Murdoch L, Bingham R. Venous cannulation in infants and small children. *British Journal of Hospital Medicine.* 1990; **44**: 405–7.

42. Russell SH, Freeman JW. Prevention of hypothermia during orthotopic liver transplantation: comparison of three intraoperative warming methods. *British Journal of Anaesthesia.* 1995; **74**: 415–8.

43. Kataria B, Epstein R, Bailey A, Schmits M, Backus WW, Schoeck D *et al.* A comparison of sevoflurane to halothane in paediatric surgical patients: results of a multicentre international study. *Paediatric Anaesthesia.* 1996; **6**: 283–92.

44. *Recommendations for standards of monitoring during anaesthesia and recovery.* London: Association of Anaesthetists of Great Britain, Ireland, 1994.

45. American Society of Anesthesiologists. *Standards for basic anesthetic monitoring.* In: ASA Directory of Members. Park Ridge, IL: American Society of Anesthesiologists, 1994: 735–6.

46. Denman WT, Swanson EL, Rosow D, Ezbicki K, Connors PD, Rosow CE. Pediatric evaluation of the Bispectral Index (BIS) monitor and correlation of BIS with end-tidal sevoflurane concentration in infants and children. *Anesthesia and Analgesia.* 2000; **90**: 872–7.

47. Johnston DF, Wrigley SR, Robb PJ, Jones HE. The laryngeal mask airway in paediatric anaesthesia. *Anaesthesia.* 1990; **45**: 924–7.

48. Watcha MF, Garner FT, White PF, Lusk R. Laryngeal mask airway vs. face mask and Guedel airway during paediatric myringotomy. *Archives of Otolaryngology and Head and Neck Surgery.* 1994; **120**: 877–80.

49. Splinter WM, Roberts DJ, Rhine EJ, MacNeill HB, Komocar L. Nitrous oxide does not increase vomiting in children after myringotomy. *Canadian Journal of Anaesthesia.* 1995; **42**: 263–6.

50. Bennie RE, Boehringer LA, McMahon S, Allen H, Dierdorf SF. Postoperative analgesia with preoperative oral ibuprofen or acetaminophen in children undergoing myringotomy. *Paediatric Anaesthesia.* 1997; **7**: 399–403.

51. Tan CL, Tan S. Diclofenac or paracetamol for analgesia in paediatric myringotomy outpatients. *Anaesthesia and Intensive Care.* 2002; **30**: 55–9.

52. Nargozian C, Ririe DG, Bennun RD, Mulliken JB. Hemifacial microsomia: anatomical prediction of difficult intubation. *Paediatric Anaesthesia.* 1999; **9**: 393–8.

53. Uezono S, Holzman RS, Goto T, Nakata Y, Nagata S, Morita S. Prediction of difficult airway in school-aged patients with microtia. *Paediatric Anaesthesia.* 2001; **11**: 409–13.

54. Jones SE, Dickson U, Moriarty A. Anaesthesia for insertion of bone-anchored hearing aids in children: a 7-year audit. *Anaesthesia.* 2001; **56**: 777–80.

55. Thomsen KA, Terkildsen K, Arnfred I. Middle ear pressure variations during anesthesia. *Archives of Otolaryngology.* 1965; **82**: 609.

56. Green JD, Schuh MJ, Maddern BR, Haymond J, Helffrich RA. Cochlear Implantation in Jervell and Lange-Nielsen syndrome. *Annals of Otology Rhinology and Laryngology Supplement.* 2000; **185**: 27–8.

57. Prasad M, Ward RF, April MM, Bent JP, Froehlich P. Topical mitomycin as an adjunct to choanal atresia repair. *Archives of Otolaryngology and Head and Neck Surgery.* 2002; **128**: 398–400.

58. Asaf T, Reuveni H, Yermiahu T, Leiberman A, Gurman G, Porat A *et al.* The need for routine pre-operative coagulation screening tests (prothrombin time PT/partial thromboplastin time PTT) for healthy children undergoing elective tonsillectomy and/or adenoidectomy. *International Journal of Pediatric Otorhinolaryngology.* 2001; **61**: 217–22.

59. Wood P. Difficulty in extubation. *Anaesthesia*. 1987; **42**: 220.

60. Williams PJ, Bailey PM. Comparison of the reinforced laryngeal mask airway and tracheal intubation for adenotonsillectomy. *British Journal of Anaesthesia*. 1993; **70**: 30–3.

61. Webster AC, Morley Forster PK, Dain S, Ganapathy S, Ruby R, Au A *et al*. Anaesthesia for adenotonsillectomy: a comparison between endotracheal intubation and the armoured laryngeal mask airway. *Canadian Journal of Anaesthesia*. 1993; **40**: 1171–7.

62. Hern JD, Jayaraj SM, Sidhu VS, Almeyda JS, O'Neill G, Tolley NS. The laryngeal mask airway in tonsillectomy: the surgeon's perspective. *Clinical Otolaryngology*. 2000; **25**: 240.

63. Kretz FJ, Reimann B, Stelzner J, Heumann H, Lange-Stumpf U. The laryngeal mask in pediatric adenotonsillectomy. A meta-analysis of medical studies. *Anaesthetist*. 2000; **49**: 706–12.

64. Southall DP. (ed.). *Prevention and control of pain in children*. A Manual for Healthcare Professionals. Report of the working party of the Royal College of Paediatrics and Child Health. London: BMJ Publications; 1997.

65. Royal College of Anaesthetists. *Guidelines for the use of non-steroidal anti-inflammatory drugs in the perioperative period*. London: Royal College of Anaesthetists, 1998.

66. Harley EH, Dattalo RA. Ibuprofen for tonsillectomy pain in children: efficacy and complications. *Archives of Otolaryngology and Head and Neck Surgery*. 1998; **119**: 492–6.

67. Romsing J, Ostergaard D, Walther-Larsen S, Valentin N. Analgesic efficacy and safety of preoperative versus postoperative ketorolac in paediatric tonsillectomy. *Acta Anaesthesiologica Scandinavia*. 1998; **42**: 770–5.

68. Splinter WM, Rhine EJ, Roberts DW, Reid CW, MacNeill HB. Preoperative ketorolac increases bleeding after tonsillectomy in children. *Canadian Journal of Anaesthesia*. 1996; **43**: 560–3.

69. Cardwell M, Siviter G, Smith A. Non-steroidal anti-inflammatory drugs and perioperative bleeding in paediatric tonsillectomy. *Cochrane Database of Systematic Reviews*. 2005 (2) CD003591.

70. Atallah N, Kumar M, Hilali A, Hickey S. Post-operative pain in tonsillectomy: bipolar electrodissection technique vs. dissection ligation technique. A double-blind randomised prospective trial. *Journal of Laryngology and Otology*. 2000; **114**: 667–70.

71. Nunez DA, Provan J, Crawford M. Postoperative tonsillectomy pain in paediatric patients: electrocautery (hot) vs. cold dissection and snare tonsillectomy – a randomised trial. *Archives of Otolaryngology and Head and Neck Surgery*. 2000; **126**: 837–41.

72. Temple RH, Timms MS. Paediatric coblation tonsillectomy. *International Journal of Pediatric Otorhinolaryngology*. 2001; **61**: 195–8.

73. Giannoni C, White S, Enneking FK, Morey T. Ropivacaine with or without clonidine improves pediatric tonsillectomy pain. *Archives of Otolaryngology and Head and Neck Surgery*. 2001; **127**: 1265–70.

74. Hung T, Moore-Gillon V, Hern J, Hinton A, Patel N. Topical bupivacaine in paediatric day-case tonsillectomy: a prospective randomised controlled trial. *Journal of Laryngology and Otology*. 2002; **116**: 33–6.

75. Hollis LJ, Burton MJ, Millar JM. Perioperative local anaesthesia for reducing pain following tonsillectomy (Cochrane Review). In: *The Cochrane Library*, Issue 2 2003. Oxford: Update Software.

76. Morton NS, Camu F, Dorman T, Knudsen KE, Kvalsvik O, Nellgard P *et al*. Ondansetron reduces nausea and vomiting after paediatric adenotonsillectomy. *Paediatric Anaesthesia*. 1997; **7**: 37–45.

77. Holt R, Rask P, Coulthard KP, Sinclair M, Roberts G, Van Der Walt J *et al*. Tropisetron plus dexamethasone is more effective than tropisetron alone for the prevention of postoperative nausea and vomiting in children undergoing tonsillectomy. *Paediatric Anaesthesia*. 2000; **10**: 181–8.

78. Department of Health. *£200 million for NHS equipment to protect patients against possible variant CJD risk*. London: Department of Health, press release January 4, 2001.

79. The Royal College of Anaesthetists. *Anaesthesia equipment and tonsillectomy*. London: Royal College of Anaesthetists, press release April 2, 2002.

80. Whittet HB, Hayward AW, Battersby E. Plasma lignocaine levels during paediatric endoscopy of the upper respiratory tract. Relationship with mucosal moistness. *Anaesthesia*. 1988; **43**: 439–42.

81. Wark H. Is there still a place for halothane in paediatric anaesthesia? *Paediatric Anaesthesia*. 1997; **7**: 359–61.

82. Nielson DW, Ku PL, Egger M. Topical lidocaine exaggerates laryngomalacia during flexible bronchoscopy. *American Journal of Respiratory, Critical Care Medicine*. 2000; **161**: 147–51.

83. Westphal K, Strouhal U, Kessler P, Schneider J. Workplace contamination from sevoflurane. Concentration measurement during bronchoscopy in children. *Anaesthetist*. 1997; **46**: 677–82.

84. Thaung MK, Balakrishnan A. A modified technique of tubeless anaesthesia for microlaryngoscopy and bronchoscopy in young children with stridor. *Paediatric Anaesthesia*. 1998; **8**: 201–4.

85. Markovitz BP, Randolph AG. Corticosteroids for the prevention and treatment of post-extubation stridor in neonates, children and adults (Cochrane Review). In: *The Cochrane Library*, 1, 2002. Oxford: Update Software.

86. Wood RE. Spelunking in the pediatric airways: explorations with the flexible fibreoptic broncho-scope. *Pediatric Clinics of North America*. 1984; **31**: 785–99.

87. Bandla HP, Smith DE, Kiernan MP. Laryngeal mask airway facilitated fibreoptic bronchoscopy in infants. *Canadian Journal of Anaesthesia*. 1997; **44**: 1242–7.

88. Holzman RS, Mancuso TJ. *Point/counterpoint. spontaneous vs. controlled ventilation for suspected airway foreign body.* In: Society for Pediatric Anesthesia, Summer 2001 newsletter.
89. Grasl MC, Donner A, Schragl E, Aloy A. Tubeless laryngotracheal surgery in infants and children. *Laryngoscope.* 1997; **107**: 277–81.
90. Depierraz B, Ravussin P, Brossard E, Monnier P. Percutaneous transtracheal jet ventilation for paediatric endoscopic laser treatment of laryngeal and subglottic lesions. *Canadian Journal of Anaesthesia.* 1994; **41**: 1200–7.
91. Rimell FL. Pediatric laser bronchoscopy. *International Anesthesiology Clinics.* 1997; **35**: 107–3.
92. Stern Y, McCall JE, Willging JP, Mueller KL, Cotton RT. Spontaneous respiration anesthesia for respiratory papillomatosis. *Annals of Otology Rhinology and Laryngology.* 2000; **109**: 72–6.
93. McCall JE. Anesthetic techniques with laser endoscopy. In: Myer 3rd CM, Cotton RT, Shott SR (eds). *The pediatric airway: an interdisciplinary approach.* Philadelphia: JB Lippincott, 1995.
94. Baxter MR. Congenital laryngomalacia. *Canadian Journal of Anaesthesia.* 1994; **41**: 322–9.

FURTHER READING

∗ Myer CM, Cotton RT, Shott SR (eds). *The pediatric airway. An interdisciplinary approach.* Philadelphia: JB Lippincott, 1995.
∗ Sumner E, Hatch DJ (eds). *Paediatric anaesthesia*, 2nd edn. London: Arnold, 2000.
∗ Gregory GA (ed.). *Pediatric anesthesia*, 3rd edn. New York: Churchill Livingstone, 1994.
∗ Baum VC, O' Flaherty JE (eds). *Anesthesia for genetic, metabolic and dysmorphic syndromes of childhood.* Philadelphia: Lippincott Williams, Wilkins, 1999.
∗ Katz J, Steward D (eds.) *Anesthesia and uncommon pediatric diseases*, 2nd edn. Philadelphia: W. B. Saunders, 1993.
∗ Cote CJ, Todres DI, Ryan JF, Goudsouzian NG (eds). *A practice of anesthesia for infants and children*, 3rd edn. Philadelphia: W. B. Saunders, 2001.

42

Adult critical care

GAVIN G LAVERY

Introduction   526
Definition of ICU, high dependency unit and critical care   526
Staffing, structure and role of ICU and HDU   527
Organ system support   527
Interface between critical care and ENT   533

Severe sepsis/SIRS   534
Recent evidenced-based strategies in critical care   535
End of life issues   536
References   537

INTRODUCTION

The development of the intensive care unit (ICU) and intensive care medicine (ICM) has been driven by advances in medicine/surgery, the need to treat acute illness in an older, sicker population and increased public expectation. The origin of the ICU (which is the official term now used in the UK in preference to ITU – intensive therapy unit) is usually attributed to the large Danish polio epidemic in 1952, when there were insufficient 'iron lungs' available to provide respiratory support to the victims. Mortality was decreased significantly by the use of life support techniques previously only applied in the operating theatre. Techniques such as positive pressure ventilation required the constant attendance of medical and nursing staff and therefore these patients were brought together in a specific area of the hospital. Since then, increasingly complex medical problems have been successfully managed due to the increasing ability of the ICU to take over the role of a failing (or failed) organ system until recovery occurs.

DEFINITION OF ICU, HIGH DEPENDENCY UNIT AND CRITICAL CARE

As explained above, the ICU is a geographically defined area in the hospital which utilizes specialized personnel and equipment to provide care for the critically ill.

Indications for admission to ICU are:[1]

- patient requiring (or likely to require) mechanical ventilation;
- patients requiring the support of two or more systems;
- patients with significant chronic impairment in one or more organ systems who require support for an acute reversible failure of another organ system.

Patients with no chance of survival due to irreversible disease should not normally be admitted to ICU. The admission of those whose survival would result in an 'unacceptable quality of life' may also be unwise. However, since such issues revolve around subjective judgement and opinions, it is recommended that such cases be considered by very senior and experienced staff before ICU admission is granted (or denied).

The high dependency unit (HDU) may be defined as an area for patients requiring more intensive observation, treatment and/or nursing care than can normally be provided on a general ward.[2] Such units would not normally accept patients requiring mechanical ventilation for more than a few hours. Costs and staffing of such units are significantly less than that of ICU since the usual nurse:patient ratio is 1:2 or 1:3. It has a role as a 'step-down' unit providing an appropriate level of care for ICU patients who have reached a level of function which makes further ICU management unnecessary, but who are still too ill/unstable for care in a general ward. The HDU may also provide a 'step up' facility for patients who are too unstable to be safely treated at general ward level. An HDU should ideally be adjacent to (or in a designated area within) an ICU and have strong clinical and managerial links with the ICU. Some ICUs have a mixed caseload of both ICU- and HDU-type patients and would not be viable if delivering only ICU support. Thus the management of illness in ICU and HDU can be seen as a continuum and the term 'critical care' is now used to cover this.[3]

STAFFING, STRUCTURE AND ROLE OF ICU AND HDU

It is no longer appropriate to view the ICU solely as a place where patients receive mechanical ventilation. The ICU should possess the means to support all the major organ systems including circulatory support, haemodialysis and other forms of renal support, nutritional support and the ability to treat coagulation disorders, severe infection and metabolic derangement.

ICU should gather in one area equipment, technical expertise and a high concentration of appropriately trained nursing staff which cannot be duplicated elsewhere in the hospital. Although ICU is always one of the most expensive areas for patient treatment (£1200–2500 STG/day), every hospital expected to treat severe acute illness requires this capability. Concentrating resources in one area is the most cost effective way to do this.

Patient management in ICU requires a team approach. Medical and nursing staff are the basis of this team but it also includes technical, physiotherapy and dietetic staff in addition to the input of radiology, bacteriology and other laboratory-based personnel. To weld this group together requires a medical director who has specific training and an ongoing interest in critical care and who spends the bulk (if not all) of his/her clinical time there.[4] The other senior medical and nursing staff should also be specifically trained and be focused on critical care.

Medical responsibility for the patients in ICU varies from unit to unit and between medical systems. At one extreme, treatment is dictated by the referring service at all times. This is usually inappropriate since the people making decisions concerning treatment do not see the patient continuously and may not see 'all the pieces in the jigsaw'. Conversely, in some units all clinical decisions are taken by the ICU medical staff without any reference to the referring service. This may work and is a common model in Australia. At worst, however, it may lead to professional friction, poor staff relations and poor care. Many well-run units steer a middle path in which the decisions are made by the ICU team after discussion with the other relevant clinicians/support services.

An ICU should be large enough to ensure that it is never empty since this would result in the staff being deployed elsewhere and the unit being unable to respond quickly to clinical needs. Therefore, a *minimum* of six bed spaces has been recommended. The average size of ICUs in many countries has been increasing as demand increases and units of 20+ beds are now commonplace. ICU requires a high nurse:patient ratio – 1:1 is viewed as appropriate within the UK.[4] To achieve this, each bed requires approximately 6.5–7.0 nurses to cover shifts, weekends, holidays, sick and study leave. In addition, each unit needs 24-hour resident medical cover, i.e. a doctor who has no other clinical committments, present physically in the unit at all times. Likewise, there must be 24 hour technical back-up available rapidly. Most units also have their own 'in house' laboratory which provides blood gas analysis (at least) and measurement of blood/plasma electrolytes, glucose, lactate, osmolarity and some drug levels.

ORGAN SYSTEM SUPPORT

A substantial part of the benefit of ICU admission is due to attention to detail with immediate intervention and correction of deranged physiology. In ICU or HDU, patients have continuous monitoring of vital signs, frequent blood gas analyses, frequent checks on haematology and biochemistry, hourly calculations of fluid balance and trained staff immediately to hand 24 hours a day. This ability to have real time information about a patient's condition and to make appropriate changes in management/support is the hallmark of good critical care. Clinical management often involves initiation of or adjustment to organ support. We will now briefly consider some of the commonest forms of organ support in critical care.

Respiratory support

At its simplest, this may involve the use of high concentrations of well-humidified (warm) oxygen delivered via standard or continuous positive airway pressure (CPAP) mask in conjunction with aggressive regular physiotherapy. However, in ICU rather than HDU, it is likely to involve tracheal intubation and mechanical (positive pressure) ventilation.

In health, the work of breathing (WOB) accounts for only 2–3 percent of total oxygen consumption. With respiratory disease, required minute volume may quadruple, lung compliance is decreased and the efficiency of chest wall movements is reduced. The result is that WOB may require more than 20 percent of total oxygen consumption and precipitate tissue hypoxia and cardiac failure. WOB cannot be easily quantified but is associated with the clinical findings of increased respiratory rate, sweating, tachycardia and the use of accessory muscles of respiration. Following assessment, a patient with respiratory difficulties may receive one or more of the following.

- Increased concentration of inspired oxygen by means of a well applied face mask, with a reservoir bag, high oxygen flow (12–15 L/min) and initiation of pulse oximetry. A patient with oxygen saturations below 90 percent, particularly with appreciably increased work of breathing, may require transfer to ICU or HDU.
- CPAP, applied via a tightly fitting face mask or hood and a suitable circuit with oxygen enriched air.
- Tracheal intubation, with maintenance of spontaneous respiration, usually via the oral route (with or without CPAP). Indications for tracheal intubation are as follows:
  - protection of the airway;
  - long-term correction/prevention of airway obstruction;
  - to facilitate positive pressure ventilation;
  - to facilitate broncho-pulmonary toilet.
    - This approach is useful when airway patency is in question or when removal of bronchial secretions is difficult. However, tracheal intubation alone may be of minimal clinical benefit in many cases since it does not address the problem of increased WOB.
- Mechanical ventilation (MV). The general indications for institution of mechanical ventilation are:
  - depressed respiratory drive;
  - inefficient respiratory effort/increased work of breathing;
  - abnormal pulmonary physiology.
    - More specifically the need for mechanical ventilation is often associated with one or more of the following findings:
  - $PaO_2 < 6$ kPa on 60 percent inspired oxygen;
  - $PaCO_2 > 8$ kPa with pH < 7.2;
  - evolving respiratory fatigue;
  - cardiovascular decompensation;
  - recent major/prolonged surgery;
  - multiple organ dysfunction.

Much of the benefit of MV is that it can completely abolish WOB since the patient may not have to initiate any spontaneous breaths. Unlike spontaneous respiration, MV requires the generation of positive intrathoracic pressure which may produce ventilator-induced lung injury (VILI) due to the effects of pressure (barotrauma) or lung stretch (volutrauma).[5] Positive intrathoracic pressure may also reduce venous return to the heart and thus precipitate hypotension – particularly in the hypovolaemic patient. Modern ICU ventilators, with many different modes of ventilation,[6] strive to reduce the complications of positive pressure ventilation, but there is no scientific evidence that any specific mode of ventilation is superior.

WEANING FROM MECHANICAL VENTILATION

This is a programme of gradual reduction in respiratory support which is specifically intended to (eventually) result in the patient breathing spontaneously (without any outside support) 24 hours/day. It suggests that the original cause of acute respiratory failure has been controlled or eradicated. Weaning may be achieved over a matter of hours, days or (occasionally) weeks. It is usually achieved by gradually reducing the support supplied by the mode of ventilation being used. There is no convincing evidence for one mode of ventilation being superior to others as a method of weaning, although pressure support weaning has gained converts in recent years. ICU patients who have had short periods of ventilation (24–48 hours) may wean perfectly well by being taken off ventilation abruptly to breathe spontaneously on a CPAP circuit (T-piece weaning).[7]

Cardiovascular support

The primary function of the circulation is to transport oxygen, nutients, carbon dioxide and other waste products to and from cells. This requires adequate amounts of haemoglobin and oxygen and appropriate cardiac output/perfusion. The latter depends on circulating volume (preload), cardiac contractility and the vascular tone in the arterial/arteriolar system (afterload).

Normally, arterial blood (100 percent saturated with oxygen) contains approximately 20 mL O_2/100 mL. With a normal adult cardiac output of 5000 mL/min, this gives a total oxygen delivery to the tissues of 1000 mL O_2/min. Resting healthy adults use approximately 250 mL O_2/min, i.e. the extraction ratio is only 25 percent and venous blood is (on average) 75 percent saturated with O_2 (15 mL/100 mL blood). There is, therefore, a large safety margin regarding the balance between O_2 supply and O_2 demand in health. This safety margin is felt to be eroded or absent in critical illness due to increased metabolic rate and decreased efficiency at the cellular level in utilizing available O_2. Shock can be defined as inadequate perfusion (or O_2 delivery) for the needs of the tissue resulting in cellular hypoxia. Shoemaker et al.[8] suggested that, since O_2 delivery does not keep up with increased tissue demand in critically ill patients, augmentation of O_2 supply by increasing cardiac output would lead to greater, beneficial tissue O_2 consumption. Although his specific targets (cardiac index > 4.5 L/m²/min, O_2 delivery > 600 mL/m²/min and O_2 consumption > 170 mL/m²/min) have declined in popularity,[9] the principle of maintaining good tissue oxygenation is the foundation of cardiovascular support. For this reason, the end-points of cardiovascular resuscitation are not based on heart rate and blood pressure, but on flow related clinical parameters such as capillary refill, urinary output, serial measurement of arterial lactate or plasma bicarbonate and objective measures of cardiac index (cardiac output/ body surface area).

MONITORING OF CARDIAC INDEX AND PERFUSION

Perfusion can be assessed clinically using the clinical parameters above.[10] In many situations, such serial assessments are all that is required. In a minority of cases, the severity of illness or the number of organ dysfunctions mean that more objective measures of cardiac function blood flow and perfusion are required.

The cardiac index (CI) may be measured noninvasively using ultrasound probes, either placed in the oesophagus behind the left atrium or in the suprasternal notch. A pulsed Doppler shift technique allows the measurement of flow velocity and (since the cross-sectional area of the aorta is also measured) the flow/unit time. Difficulties may arise in maintaining a good probe position. Transthoracic impedance plethysmography assesses CI by measuring the change in voltage across the chest in response to a high frequency current (usually 100 kHz). Changes in transthoracic resistance are assumed to be due to changes in blood volume which reflects cardiac filling and emptying. Unfortunately, the correlation between results obtained using the above techniques and the gold standard (invasive) technique is variable.

Invasive measurement of CI requires the placement of a catheter in the pulmonary artery. The principle use to measure CI is the reverse Fick principle. Short bursts of an electrical microcurrent is used to cause a heating effect in the plasma. Quantifying the resultant change in blood temperature allows continuous measurement of CI. It is important to balance the risks of insertion of insertion of a pulmonary artery catheter (PAC) with the benefit obtained. Changes in management prompted by information obtained from PACs has been shown to result in improved outcome in shocked patients who were not responding to standard therapy.[11] In contrast, failure to use PACs (and the information they provide) appropriately has been shown to be associated with poorer outcomes[12] and the risk of infection increases with time *in situ*.[13] When it is no longer providing information which is being used to make clinical decisions, a PAC should be removed. The use of PAC has decreased in recent years and this trend is unlikely to change. The largest clinical study on the use of the PAC found no evidence of benefit or harm associated with its use.[14] Increasingly, clinicians are using less invasive methods of measuring cardiac index at the bedside, e.g. (1) oesophageal Doppler and (2) lithium indicator dilution and pulse power analysis.

FLUID THERAPY – WHAT TYPE OF FLUID SHOULD WE USE?

All forms of shock, except cardiogenic shock, involve either true or relative hypovolaemia. Thus, expanding the blood volume by administration of fluids is the first step in cardiovascular resuscitation. The controversy regarding crystalloid or colloid fluid resuscitation has raged in the literature for decades.[15, 16, 17] Fortunately, most clinicians are not so extreme in their views and use a mixture of crystalloid and colloid fluids. Some points seem beyond argument:

- colloids are more expensive than crystalloids;
- colloids may cause anaphylactoid reactions (rarely);
- the use of either solution in initial resuscitation allows blood to be used more effectively and safely later in the patient's care;
- colloids are more time-efficient at restoring intravascular volume;
- plasma oncotic pressure is better maintained with colloid – this may or may not clinically advantageous.

The most important point in resuscitation is to ensure that the patient has received adequate fluid. This will often mean transfusing three to four times the volume of blood lost when using crystalloid replacement or one and a half to two times the volume lost using colloid. When appropriate, filling pressures and/or cardiac index should be measured using a central venous line or PAC. Many studies have suggested that resuscitation to supranormal levels of CI and tissue oxygen delivery may improve survival.[8, 18] Even if global perfusion appears satisfactory, regional hypoperfusion may exist, particularly in the splanchnic bed.[19, 20]

The best clinical guide to good organ perfusion is a urinary output of at least 1 mL/kg/hour without the influence of diuretics or hyperglycaemia. Oliguria is an important clinical sign of hypovolaemia and should frequently lead to a fluid challenge and not administration of a loop diuretic. The sequelae of persistent hypovolaemia are tissue hypoxia, multiple organ dysfunction and death. The sequelae of fluid overload (congestive cardiac failure, pulmonary oedema) may carry a lower associated mortality.

INOTROPES

Inotropes are agents which increase the force of myocardial contraction by a direct effect on the myocardium. Those used clinically are administered intravenously by continuous (accurately controlled) infusion and most are catecholamines or their synthetic analogues. The use of dopamine, for many years the most widely used inotrope, has declined due to doubts about its supposed dose-dependent effects,[21, 22] and concerns about endocrine and immunosuppressant side effects.[23]

The choice of inotrope is often determined not by its inotropic effects but by its other effects – either desirable or undesirable.[24] Often a major consideration is whether the drug is being given to improve arterial pressure or improve tissue perfusion. Dobutamine is an inotrope and vasodilator and is the preferred inotrope in many instances. It is a drug which improves perfusion although it has minimal and unpredictable effects on arterial pressure. It is often used in association with noradrenaline.

Adrenaline may improve perfusion and/or pressure and is sometimes used as a single agent in the treatment of septic shock. However, its unpredictable mix of alpha and beta adrenergic receptor stimulation and its potential to produce cardiac arrhythmias is a drawback. Noradrenaline also stimulates both alpha and beta adrenergic receptors but is particularly potent at alpha-receptors, thus it is an inotrope with vasoconstrictor effects. It will raise blood pressure and is often used to treat the hypotension associated with the generalized vasodilatation of severe sepsis/septic shock. It is often used in association with dobutamine in sepsis as dobutamine augments cardiac contractility in the face of sepsis-induced depression and the increased afterload due to noradrenaline.

The importance of the splanchnic circulation has raised interest in dopexamine. This dopamine analogue predominantly stimulates dopamine and beta-adrenergic receptors. It is a (weak) inotrope, vasodilator and (possibly) increases splanchnic blood flow. Studies have claimed that dopexamine beneficially improves oxygen flux in the postoperative period[25] and that it promotes better colonic mucosal perfusion,[26] though this has been questioned by other work.[27] A multicentre trial failed to show any outcome benefit from the use of dopexamine.[28]

The manipulation of the cardiovascular system should follow a logical sequence. In general this sequence is

1. Is the cardiac output adequate? An inadequate cardiac output is suggested by hypotension, oliguria, cold peripheries, an elevated plasma lactate.
2. Is the low cardiac output due to hypovolaernia or poor myocardial function? Central venous pressure (CVP) measurement may be useful. A very low value (0–4 mmHg) suggests hypovolaemia and the CVP trend will guide fluid replacement. A high CVP (> 15 mmHg) suggests a cardiogenic (pump) problem which may improve with dobutamine (5–20 µg/kg/min).
3. The use of a PAC will give much greater information and should be considered whenever intelligent manipulations based on CVP measurements has failed to produce improvement.
4. Patients with sepsis have rapidly changing haemodynamic profiles. Invasive monitoring with appropriate pharmacological support should be initiated early in patients with septicaemia/septic shock.

Renal support

There are many factors associated with the development of acute renal failure (ARF) in the critically ill patient. These often coexist and are summarized in **Table 42.1**. Common pharmacological causes of ARF are high doses of some radiological contrast media, toxic plasma levels of some antibiotics, e.g. the aminoglycosides, the use of nonsteroidal antiinflammatory agents, cyclosporin A and antimitotics, e.g. cis-platinum and methotrexate.[29] As the understanding of the pathophysiology has advanced, strategies have been developed which might reduce the incidence of ARF. Adequate fluid replacement guided by central venous or pulmonary artery pressure, adequate blood transfusion, attention to oxygen transport and early nutritional support may all be important. The use of dopexamine (0.5–1.0 µg/kg/min) may increase renal blood flow and promote urine flow. Although such a strategy is often used in at-risk patients, there is no objective evidence that it prevents ARF. Previously, dopamine (2–3 µg/kg/min) was thought to have the same effect but the evidence for its potential benefit is now viewed as less convincing. Many clinicians now use n-acetyl cysteine as a pretreatment which may mitigate the renotoxic effects of radiological contrast.

Indications for renal replacement therapy (dialysis) can be summarized as the presence of hyperkalaemia, fluid overload, metabolic acidosis and a high plasma level of urea and creatinine. The absolute values of the latter which trigger the decision to dialyse varies between centres.

Until recent years, haemodialysis (HD) was usually performed for a three or four hour session on a daily or alternate day basis. Originally performed through surgical or plastic arteriovenous connections, short-term HD is now usually achieved using a double lumen catheter inserted in a large vein, e.g. subclavian or femoral. ICUs are increasingly performing continuous HD (often termed CRRT – continous renal replacement therapy) over a 24 hour period.[30, 31] This produces less cardiovascular instability as fluid and electrolyte shifts occur more gradually. The disadvantages are increased costs, need for continuous heparinization and the need for ICU staff training. No satisfactory comparison of these techniques has been performed, although there is evidence that CRRT produces normalization of plasma electrolytes, etc., more quickly than HD.[32] Although there is some suggestion of better outcome with CRRT,[31] this has been refuted by other studies.[33]

Nutritional support

Simple starvation leads to the exhaustion of glycogen stores within 48 hours and an increase in glucose production from amino acids derived from breakdown of body proteins (gluconeogenesis). The glucose provided is used to fuel the brain and red blood cells which cannot normally utilize other substrate. This produces a rate of body protein breakdown which would be life-threatening if unchecked. Fortunately, in persistent uncomplicated starvation, the body switches to fat as the predominant energy source and the brain adapts to

Table 42.1 Causes of acute renal dysfunction.

Renal dysfunction	Cause
Pre-renal dysfunction	
Decrease in blood volume	Haemorrhage
	Dehydration
	Burns
	GI losses (vomiting/diarrhoea)
	Renal losses (diuretics, diabetes insipidus, adrenal insufficiency)
Decrease in effective blood volume	Cardiogenic shock
(Renal hypoperfusion)	Liver disease with ascites
	Hypoalbuminaemia
	Pancreatitis
	Peritonitis
	Hypercalcaemia
	Catecholamines
	Cyclosporine
	Amphotericin B
	Cyclooxygenase inhibition
	Angiotensin-converting enzyme inhibitors
	Renal artery stenosis/occlusion
	Hyperviscosity syndromes
Intrinsic renal dysfunction	
	Glomerulonephritis
	Vasculitis
	Acute tubular necrosis (ischaemia, drugs/toxins, pigments)
	Interstitial nephritis (antibiotics, NSAIDs, ACE inhibitors)
	Pyelonephritis
	Infiltration (sarcoidosis, lymphoma, leukaemia)
	Radiation nephritis
Post renal dysfunction	
	Papillary necrosis
	Ureteric obstruction (stone, tumour, retroperitoneal fibrosis)
	Bladder obstruction (tumour, prostatic enlargement, neurogenic dydfunction)
	Urethral stricture
	Posterior urethral valves
	Phimosis

use ketones as a metabolic fuel, thus allowing gluconeo-genesis to slow.[34] Unfortunately, in critical illness (particularly when complicated by sepsis), gluconeogenesis is not suppressed and this has to be fuelled by rapid protein breakdown – the so-called hypermetabolic or hypercatabolic state in which the body is subject to a process which has been termed 'autocannibalism'. Such protein breakdown has significant deleterious effects on organ function and outcome. By providing exogamous glucose, amino acids and other nutrients, we hope to modify this process.

Enteral nutrition (EN) is nutritionally, immunologically and metabolically superior to feeding using the total parenteral nutrition (TPN) route. The present preference for EN could be justified on the basis that it is less expensive, does not require central venous cannulation with its attendant complications and is less likely to produce fluid overload, hyperglycaemia or hypophosphataemia. To fully appreciate the superiority of EN, we should consider the effects of critical illness and lack of luminal nutrients on the gastrointestinal tract.

The mucosal cells of the gastrointestinal (GI) tract have one of the highest turnover rates of any body tissue. An intact gut mucosa requires a balance between cell renewal and exfoliation. Its prime function is to allow the controlled absorption of nutrients while providing a barrier to the passage of toxins and bacteria from the lumen of the gut into the portal circulation. Barrier function is due to a series of elements: the intact mucosal layer, tight junctions between cells, lymphocytes, macrophages and neutrophils in the submucosa and Peyer's patches and gut-generated IgA. The absence of nutrients within the gut lumen appear to compromise both gut mucosal health and barrier function.

Moore and colleagues[35] published a meta-analysis of eight studies comparing EN and TPN in surgical patients. Infective complications were significantly less in EN groups, with lower incidences of pneumonia, intra-abdominal abscesses and (not unexpectedly) catheter sepsis. It should be stressed that, even when catheter-related sepsis is excluded, TPN is associated with a significantly higher incidence of infective complications than EN. In animals, EN is associated with less intestinal mucosal atrophy, liver dysfunction, bacterial transloca-tion, greater immunocompetence and better survival after a variety of systemic insults.

TIMING AND METHOD OF DELIVERING EN

Which clinical findings tell us when we might introduce enteral feeding? The presence of bowel sounds, though comforting, is irrelevant. Many patients with no bowel sounds may tolerate and absorb nasogastric feeds. In contrast, gastric stasis, leading to high aspirates and vomiting, may occur even when bowel sounds are present. Often, a low nasogastric aspirate (< 250–300 mL in 24 hours) is the most appropriate prompt to initiate feeding. The common problem of gastric stasis may require the increasing use of feeding (surgical) jejunostomy tubes and the selective use of nasoduodenal or nasojejunal tubes. Persuading feeding tubes to negotiate the pyloric canal and remain in position can be a problem. Endoscopic guidance or fluoroscopy are useful – the latter having a 95 percent success rate – but may be logistically difficult in critically ill patients. With such strategies it is possible to feed patients via the enteral route within 24 hours of major surgery. Graham and colleagues,[36] in a controlled trial, showed that aggressive early jejunal feeding was associated with fewer infective complications and a shorter ICU and hospital stay than standard nasogastric feeding in head injured patients.

EN is usually administered by continuous infusion into the GI tract. This reduces GI side effects but may lead to increased Gram-negative colonization of the upper GI tract. Stopping enteral infusion for four hours to permit a (bactericidal) decrease in intragastric pH has been suggested as a strategy to reduce the incidence of Gram-negative pulmonary infection.[37] However, an extensive systematic review, while confirming the superiority of early EN over TPN, could not make recommendations regarding composition of feed, bolus versus infusion feeding and many other issues.[38] When patients have suffered a prolonged period of poor nutrition, initiation of feeding may produce severe hypophosphataemia and other electrolytic disturbances which may lead to acute respiratory failure, cardiac dysfunction and neurological problems – the so-called refeeding syndrome.[39] The daily maintenance requirements vary between patients and at different stages of their illness. Typical daily values for ICU patients are shown in **Table 42.2**.

Table 42.2 Typical daily fluid, electrolyte and nutritional requirements in critical illness.

Variable	Requirement
Water	35–40 mL/kg
Sodium	1–1.5 mmol/kg
Potassium	0.6–0.8 mmol/kg
Calories	20–30 kcal/kg
Nitrogen	0.2–0.3 g/kg (increased in severe illness)
Calorie:nitrogen ratio	150:1 (moderate illness)
	100:1 (sepsis/MODS/hypercatabolism)

IMMUNONUTRITION

Immunonutrition seeks to use nutrients to modify the immunological response to illness and injury. Potential immunonutrients given by the enteral route include glutamine, arginine, omega-3 fatty acids and nucleotides. Glutamine and omega-3 fatty acids have also been administered parenterally. Their potential role is the preservation of cellular immune function and to benefi-cially alter the production of inflammatory mediators.

Glutamine is required both as a primary fuel and in the synthesis of nucleotide precursors by the immune system. It appears to be conditionally essential in the critically ill. Despite a large reserve, excessive demand for glutamine in such patients may cause glutamine defi-ciency, resulting in decreased intestinal integrity and cellular immune function.[40] Administration of parenteral glutamine has been associated with improved outcome in intensive care patients and patients having major elective abdominal surgery.[41, 42]

In a small study, the use of enteral glutamine in burns patients was found to reduce the incidence of positive blood cultures and mortality but, puzzlingly, had no effect on length of care or polymorph phagocytosis.[43] A well-designed large study of enteral glutamine in ICU patients failed to show any benefit in terms of incidence of severe sepsis, death or a number of other secondary outcomes.[44] The Canadian Critical Care Group systematic review recommended glutamine in critically ill burns and trauma patients, but did not recommend the addition of arginine to EN.[38]

An enteral feed rich in omega-3 fatty acids has been shown to decrease the requirement for supplemental oxygen, the period of ventilatory support, ICU length of stay and new organ failure in patients with moderate or severe acute respiratory distress syndrome.[45] The same group has more recently studied the mechanism of the improvement in pulmonary function and found a decrease in indices of alveolar membrane protein permeability and reduced levels of IL-8, leukotiene B4 and neutrophils in broncho-alveolar lavage fluid in patients fed on an enteral feed containing omega-3 fatty acids and enhanced antioxidants.[46] Parenteral omega-3 fatty acids show immune benefits and antiinflammatory effects but no effect on infection rate or mortality in surgical patients.[47]

Galban et al.[48] showed a reduction in mortality in critically ill patients with sepsis receiving immunonutrition, but benefit was confined to those with relatively low illness severity. Another study showed significantly increased mortality in critically ill patients receiving immunonutrition, an effect that was more pronounced in patients with sepsis.[49]

The most recent meta-analysis found that the use of immunonutrition reduced infections and hospital stay, particularly in surgical (rather than critically ill) patients.[50] Despite these apparent benefits of immunonutrition, none (of three) meta-analyses have identified a significant effect on mortality, either globally or across any patient grouping.[50, 51, 52]

INTERFACE BETWEEN CRITICAL CARE AND ENT

Postoperative care after surgery

Like other surgical specialties, ENT may refer patients for critical care management following (and occasionally prior to) elective or emergency surgery. This may be due to:

- the nature of the acute illness (e.g. major haemorrhage with shock after tonsillectomy or acute mastoiditis/sinusitis with signs of intracranial infection);
- the nature of the surgery (e.g. major head and neck surgery after which airway swelling and respiratory compromise might be expected in the postoperative period;
- patient factors (e.g. severe cardiac or respiratory disease in a patient requiring prolonged and/or extensive surgery).

Often, several of these factors coexist. In such cases the critical care phase may last just one to two days, or may be much longer – particularly in patients with severe cardio-respiratory disease in whom weaning from mechanical ventilation may be difficult. The development of severe infection or systemic inflammatory response syndrome (SIRS) is relatively frequent during critical illness and may lead to the development of multiple organ dysfunction syndrome (MODS) and, potentially, an increased length of stay (LOS) in ICU, morbidity and mortality. Good communication between the ICU staff, ENT staff and the relatives is important, particularly if this phase of care is prolonged and/or complications occur.

Post–head/neck trauma

The management of injuries to the head, face or neck may require ENT surgical intervention, either in the acute phase or after many days in ICU/HDU. Early intervention may be required after major vascular or airway injury. Treatment of nasal injury or the drainage of blood-filled sinuses may be required later in the management of such patients. The assessment of actual or possible injury to the tympanic membrane or other parts of the auditory mechanism may also be required.

Management of the difficult airway

There are two common clinical scenarios. First, acute management of partial or complete airway obstruction. This is often in cases were it is suspected that tracheal intubation will be difficult or impossible. Airway obstruction may occur at any level:

- supralaryngeal – tumour, infection, anaphylaxis;
- laryngeal – infections, tumours, surgery, anaphalaxis;
- infralaryngeal – tumour, infection, tracheomalacia, subglottic stenosis.

The techniques required will vary. In many cases, the role of the ENT surgeon will merely be to observe, providing back-up to the anaesthetic staff in the (rare) event that tracheal intubation is not achieved. It is important, however, that ENT expertise is immediately available, as attempts to intubate the trachea may lead to increase swelling/inflammation and worsen airway obstruction. When ENT intervention is required, this may be to facilitate tracheal intubation via the oral route (e.g. use of an anterior commissure laryngoscope). In other cases, tracheostomy or cricothyroidotomy may be required. In cases where tumour or infection/abscess is the basis for the airway obstruction, resection/debulking of tumour or evacuation of an abscess cavity may be carried out after the airway problem has been resolved.

The second common clinical scenario is the late management of patients with continuing need for tracheal intubation. This is usually managed by tracheostomy. It should be remembered that since many tracheostomies are now performed as a bedside, percutaneous procedure, referral to ENT suggests the procedure is expected to be difficult, often due to anatomical factors or coagulation disorders. The indications for late tracheostomy is usually due to the need for prolonged tracheal intubation for the following reasons:

- failure (or predicted failure) to wean from mechanical intubation;
- lack of airway protection (bulbar palsy, cord dysfunction, coma);
- need for tracheobronchial toilet (decreased level of consciousness).

Assessment of cord function

In patients with problems concerning airway patency/ stridor, inability to cough effectively or suspected (repeated) pulmonary aspiration, ENT may be asked to rule out vocal cord dysfunction. This may be required after surgery on the thyroid, parathyroid or nearby structures when recurrent laryngeal nerve injury may occur. Some neck, mediastinal and apical lung tumours may also produce dysfunction of the recurrent laryngeal nerve. Assessment usually involves visualizing the cords (without neuromuscular blockade) either using a fibreoptic or rigid bronchoscope. The former may be carried out in ICU as a bedside procedure.

Investigation of source of sepsis

Attempts to identify an occult source of severe or recurrent sepsis is a common process in ICU. After exclusion of the usual sites by culturing blood/sputum/urine/cerebrospinal fluid (CSF), imaging the chest and abdomen and removing invasive lines, the question of sinus infection must be ruled out. Since most ICU patients have feeding and/or other tubes passing through the nasal passages, they are predisposed to retention and superinfection of sinus secretions. This may be particularly so after head and facial trauma when there may have been bleeding into the sinus cavities. In such circumstances, ENT services may be asked to perform antral lavage to provide material for culture and remove a nidus of infection.

SEVERE SEPSIS/SIRS

The triggering of the inflammatory response is designed to be (and usually is) protective. The usual trigger is invasion by microorganisms (infection) and is termed sepsis. However, tissue damage from trauma, burns or major surgery may also act as the trigger to this inflammatory response, in which case it is termed systemic inflammatory response syndrome (SIRS). Both SIRS and severe sepsis may lead to septic shock whose clinical manifestations include hypotension, tachycardia, pyrexia and warm flushed peripheries. The early cardiovascular changes can be summarized by stating that there is peripheral vasodilatation with an elevated cardiac index, low arterial pressure and low filling pressures. Younger patients with more cardiac reserve may well not become hypotensive due to their ability to substantially increase cardiac index. The criteria for SIRS, sepsis and severe sepsis are well established, as are the definitions of severe sepsis and sepsis with shock.[53]

Management should include restoration of circulating volume, correction of tissue hypoxia and prevention of avoidable insults to organ function and has been well described elsewhere.[54, 55] Good infection control policies and practices have been shown to reduce nosocomial infection rates.[56] Early treatment of sepsis with appropriate antimicrobial therapy has been shown to improve survival in critical illness.[57, 58]

Resuscitation

The aggressive infusion of colloid and/or crystalloid under the guidance of central venous or pulmonary artery occlusion pressures will stabilize the condition in many patients. Should it prove impossible to attain an adequate blood pressure, then the problem is usually one of profound vasodilatation. In such cases a controlled infusion of a vasoconstrictor, such as noradrenaline or phenylephrine, may restore pressure and return coronary perfusion to normal. Vasoconstrictors are often used in conjunction with dobutamine to sustain cardiac contractility and general perfusion. When using noradrenaline in this way, it may be desirable to use a means of quantifying cardiac output and global perfusion (e.g. pulmonary artery catheter) to ensure that excessive vasoconstriction does not take place. Even this does not give any guide to the flow through regional capillary networks.

The guiding principles of haemodynamic manipulations in SIRS/solidus sepsis are:

- restore normovolaemia;
- commence dobutamine;
- use the smallest dose of noradrenaline which is compatible with acceptable blood pressure;
- augment cardiac contractility if required (e.g. dobutamine);
- check haemodynamic status by serial measures of arterial lactate and/or measurement of cardiac index.

Even with the above measures, a minority of patients remain grossly vasodilated, hypotensive and may die of refractory cardiovascular failure. Others improve haemodynamically with the above measures only to die later following the development of acute lung injury, renal dysfunction and other manifestations of SIRS/sepsis-induced multiple organ dysfunction syndrome (MODS).

Antimicrobials

Antibiotics should be administered as soon as possible. At this point the nature of the microorganisms concerned is unknown. Therefore, it is common currently standard practice to use double or even triple antibiotic therapy to cover all possible causative organisms. Fungi should not be forgotten as possible causative agents, especially in patients who have been on long-term broad spectrum antibacterial agents. The next step is to identify and remove potential sources of sepsis. Wounds should be examined and probed if necessary. All intravascular lines and the urinary catheter should be changed.

Investigating the source of infection

The source of sepsis is often obvious. In other cases, however, full examination fails to reveal a problem. This group of patients needs persistent investigation. Initial cultures should be taken from blood, sputum, urine, CSF and any surgical drains, if possible before the administration of antibiotics. A chest x-ray may reveal any pulmonary infection and/or the presence of fluid in the pleural cavity. If the latter is present, then a diagnostic tap and/or drainage via a chest drain will be necessary. If cultures, x-ray and clinical examination are unrewarding, the location of an occult source of sepsis may lie in the abdominal cavity (including the pelvis) or the intracranial space or the paranasal sinuses.

These possibilities can be narrowed further by ENT endoscopy or double antral punctures and lumbar puncture. The abdominal cavity can be assessed noninvasively in several ways using ultrasound scan, CT scan or labelled white cell scan. After all three of these investigations have been performed and repeated, there should be an 80 percent 'pick up' rate for septic foci within the abdomen/pelvis.[59] Once located, a septic focus may be obliterated either by radiologically guided percutaneous drainage or by surgical laparotomy. There is still an indication for the investigative laparotomy which will occasionally find a lesion previously missed by other forms of investigation. Laparotomy may need to be repeated after an interval before all sources of sepsis can be excluded.

RECENT EVIDENCED-BASED STRATEGIES IN CRITICAL CARE

Rigid glycaemic control

Hyperglycaemia is commonly associated with critical illness and has been considered an adaptive response to ensure an energy source for brain cells and erythrocytes. However, high titres of insulin-like growth factor binding protein 1 are associated with decreased insulin production and increased mortality.[60] The use of insulin infusion in over 1500 (mainly surgical) ICU patients to maintain blood glucose in the (low) normal range (4.4–6.1 mmol/L) showed a significant benefit over conventional treatment (mortality rates of 4.6 and 8.0 percent, respectively).[61] This benefit was most pronounced with prolonged ICU stay (≥ 5 days). Although this effect might have been due to other effects of insulin, e.g. on plasma free fatty acids, further work has suggested control of blood glucose and not the dose of insulin used, was the factor conferring survival advantage.[62]

Target haemoglobin levels/blood transfusion

Anaemia is common in critical illness for many reasons, including a blunted erythropoietin response to acute anaemia.[63, 64] The first issue is whether or not this anaemia is harmful? Studies would indicate that moderate anaemia is potentially beneficial[65, 66] and that red cell transfusion to maintain a higher than necessary level of haemoglobin may be detrimental.[67, 68] What is unclear is whether the harmful factor is a relatively higher level of haemoglobin or the transfusion of donated stored allogeneic blood. While exogenous erythropoietin has been shown to reduce transfusion requirements and result in increased haemoglobin concentration in critically ill patients,[69] we should not assume that this will necessarily lead to improved outcome.

We need to develop appropriate triggers for transfusion which maximize the potential advantage of anaemia and also reduce the need for allogeneic red cell transfusion with its well-known risks. Other strategies, such as use of blood conservation policies or devices, should be investigated,[70] although there is little evidence to date that the latter are effective.[71, 72]

Early goal-directed therapy

The underlying principle of early goal-directed therapy (EDGT) is that the early resuscitation of patients with severe haemodynamic compromise may be incomplete if blood pressure is used as the end-point (see under Cardiovascular support above). This may leave many patients with 'normal vital signs' but occult shock with ongoing tissue hypoperfusion/hypoxia and increased risk of subsequent organ failure. The EGDT approach uses fluid/blood transfusion and dobutamine and perfusion related parameters as the end-points of resuscitation. Specifically, central venous oxygen saturation ($ScvO_2$) is monitored via a central venous line. EGDT commenced in the emergency room has been shown to reduce mortality in patients with severe sepsis.[73]

Low tidal volume ventilation

Excessive positive pressure and/or lung stretch has been linked to VILI as discussed under Respiratory support. This may be due to production of inflammatory mediators promoted by use of higher tidal volume ventilation.[74, 75] Clinical studies have suggested that limiting the tidal volume and/or the ventilatory pressure improves outcome in patients with acute lung injury.[76, 77] Hence, there is an increasing tendency to use low tidal volume (6–8 mL/kg) rather than the more traditional 10–12 mL/kg for MV in critical illness. However, methodological differences[78] mean it is difficult to compare studies and some work suggests increased morbidity and poorer outcome with a low tidal volume/low inflation pressure strategy.[79]

Activated protein C

Sepsis, decreased protein C levels and high mortality have been linked,[80, 81] while infusion of activated protein C has been shown to improve survival in animals infused with live coliforms.[82] Use of recombinant human activated protein C (APC) in severe sepsis has been shown to achieve an absolute reduction in mortality of 6.1 percent and has an even greater benefit in those patients with associated multiple organ failure (absolute mortality reduction 7.4 percent).[83] Although the anticoagulant, profibrinolytic and antiinflammatory (reduction in IL-6) actions of APC are known, its beneficial effects in severe sepsis are still not fully explained.

Steroids

Critical illness can unmask and even cause a relative failure in adrenal function. The adrenal gland is vital in the adaptive response to critical illness. It produces glucocortoids (cortisol) and mineralocorticoids from the cortex of the gland and catecholamines from the medulla. It is common in ICU to use catecholamines to support the circulation. However, glucocorticoids are often avoided because of their side effects and so unrecognized adrenal dysfunction may lead to life-threatening cortisol deficiency. Predisposing factors include major surgery, trauma, coagulopathy, but particularly severe sepsis.[84] The clinical manifestations of the condition are hypotension unresponsive to treatment and other relatively nonspecific findings such as electrolyte abnormalities (hyperkalaemia, hyponatraemia) and generalized weakness which are common in the ICU population.

Although investigation of the use of steroids in severe sepsis has produced well over 100 papers, there have been few methodologically rigorous studies.[85] Relative adrenal insufficiency may exist in ≥ 50 percent of patients with septic shock which is refractory to inotropic support.[86] Patients with sepsis exhibit reduced plasma cortisol binding and decreased glucocorticoid receptor binding.[87, 88]

Two studies seemed to confirm that moderate doses of steroid in patients with septic shock improved responsiveness to catecholamines.[89, 90] This prompted a multicentre French trial using a seven day course of moderate dose (200–300 mg/day) hydrocortisone and fludrocortisone in patients whose adrenal function was assessed using an ACTH stimulation test.[91] Relative adrenal insufficiency was found in 229 of 300 subjects. In this subgroup, 115 received steroids and 114 placebo. The mortality rates were 63 and 53 percent, respectively ($p < 0.023$). In ACTH responders, steroids had no survival advantage, nor excess attributable mortality. A subsequent cross-over study showed hydrocortisone restored haemodynamic stability in critically ill patients with septic shock and promoted an antiinflammatory, but not immunosuppressed, state.[92] Diagnosis of relative adrenal insufficiency requires a high index of suspicion and blunted response to an ACTH or Synacthen stimulation test.[84] Treatment is by steroid replacement during the stressed period – 100 mg of hydrocortisone six hourly is a widely used regime.

END OF LIFE ISSUES

Communication with relatives

Critical care patients are often unaware of their ICU stay until they are almost ready for discharge. Their relatives often bear a heavy emotional burden, their degree of confusion and helplessness made greater by the complexity and the seriousness of the clinical situation. This may be compounded by the numbers of doctors, nurses and clinical teams involved and the length of time the patient may remain in a life-threatening state. It should be remembered that even a short 'routine' admission to ICU is one of the most stressful events ever experienced by most families.

Relatives' stress can be reduced by reducing the number of staff through whom they receive information. Interviews with relatives should occur in a quiet, private and comfortable counselling room adjacent to the ICU. An individual's interpersonal skills and personality will have a significant influence on their approach and success in counselling relatives. The experience of others, however, can give valuable lessons. These include:

- always sit down when talking to relatives (this may mean sitting on the floor when dealing with a large family) otherwise you may appear unfriendly or in a rush;
- always introduce yourself and any other accompanying member of staff. If possible, bring the patient's bedside nurse;
- know before you enter the room who will be there and their relationship to the patient;
- check the patient's name (including first name), age and address. Remind yourself of the date of hospital and ICU admission and other details of the case. It is advisable to have the clinical notes with you;
- start your delivery with a question such as 'Before I update you, can I ask what *you* understand the position to be?' This achieves several goals. You find out what is already known. You will therefore be able to judge whether the family are inappropriately optimistic or pessimistic. They will focus on the issues which they feel are important or which most worry them. This will allow you time to tailor your information to bring them up to date and (hopefully) correct any misconceptions. You are also able to judge the degree of understanding within the family and the level at which to pitch your discussion.

In cases involving multiple clinical teams there is an increased danger of families receiving 'mixed messages' and being further distressed and confused. It may be helpful, at an early interview, to point out that each clinician involved will tend to focus on their own particular area/role and that the ICU staff are in the best position to give an overall view of the patient's condition and short-term prognosis.

Limitation of treatment

Limitation in this context means to either withhold or withdraw one or more treatments from a patient – presumably because in the view of those clinicians making such a decision, the treatment(s) are not in the patient's best interest. In ICU, this usually means that the patient has no prospect of survival (irrespective of the treatment offered) or that survival would be unacceptable (in terms of quality of life). The latter needs to be considered very carefully since quality of life is a subjective judgement. Although withholding or withdrawing treatment do not differ ethically, some feel that withdrawal is more difficult as the cessation of treatment appears to be more closely associated with death than withholding, when the progression of disease appears to cause the death of an individual. The opposing view is that having started a treatment and then withdrawn it, we are in a better position to know that it was a futile intervention and one which was not going to alter outcome.

Potential difficulties arise because of the clash of ethical and legal principles, medical policies and the emotional responses of both relatives and ICU staff in a situation where the views of the patient are often unknown and unobtainable. Such problems are always more difficult in the ICU environment where many kinds of organ support are made possible by medical technology. Mostly, such interventions are totally appropriate. Occasionally they are obviously inappropriate. However, it is when there is disagreement on appropriateness of treatment that problems may arise and a structured approach to decision making is required.[93]

Although limitation of treatment is common in ICU,[94] doctors, nurses and the public differ in their view of who should have input into such decisions.[95] Doctors and nurses in ICU may also disagree on how to conduct end-of-life decision-making and who should be involved.[96] If limitation of treatment is to be acceptable in ICU, the conduct surrounding such orders (often termed do not resuscitate (DNR) orders) should adhere to the following.

- DNR orders should be made in concert by several of the most senior ICU clinicians. The process should include consultation with other members of the ICU team. The views of the next-of-kin should be sought but it should be made clear that they are not being asked to make the decision.
- Such decisions should be indicated by a written, unambiguous entry in the patients clinical notes.
- The relatives and other clinical services involved should be informed of the decision before it is initiated.
- The decision should be reviewed and (if appropriate) renewed every day.

Effective communication and a caring and open approach will prevent and/or resolve many of the problems which may arise in an 'end-of-life' situation.

REFERENCES

1. Department of Health. *Report of the Working Group on Guidelines on admission to and discharge from the intensive care and high dependency units.* London: Department of Health, 1996.
2. Association of Anaesthetists of Great Britain and Ireland. *The high dependency unit. Acute care for the future.* London: AAGBI, 1991.
3. Department of Health. *Comprehensive critical care. A review of adult critical care services.* London: Department of Health, 2000.
4. Intensive Care Society. *Standards for intensive care units.* London: Intensive Care Society, 1997.
5. Gattinoni L, Caironi P, Carlesso E. How to ventilate patients with acute lung injury and acute respiratory distress syndrome. *Current Opinion in Critical Care.* 2005; **11**: 69–76.
6. Tobin MJ. Current concepts, Mechanical ventilation. *New England Journal of Medicine.* 1994; **330**: 1056–61.
7. Esteban A, Alia I, Gordo F, Fernandez R, Solsona JF, Vallverdu I et al. Extubation outcome after spontaneous breathing trials with T-tube or pressure support ventilation. The Spanish Lung Failure Collaborative Group. *American Journal of Respiratory and Critical Care Medicine.* 1997; **156**: 459–65.
8. Shoemaker WC, Appel PL, Kram HB, Waxman K, Lee T-S. Prospective trial of supranormal values of survivors as therapeutic goals in high-risk surgical patients. *Chest.* 1988; **94**: 1176–86.
9. Russell JA, Phang PT. The oxygen delivery/consumption controversy: approaches to management of the critically ill. *American Journal of Respiratory and Critical Care Medicine.* 1994; **149**: 533–7.
10. Shephard JN, Brecker SJ, Evans TW. Bedside assessment of myocardial performance in the critically ill. *Intensive Care Medicine.* 1994; **20**: 513–21.
11. Mimoz O, Rauss A, Rekik N, Brun-Buisson C, Lemaire F, Brochard L. Pulmonary artery catheterization in critically ill patients: a prospective analysis of outcome changes associated with catheter-prompted changes in therapy. *Critical Care Medicine.* 1994; **22**: 573–9.
12. Connors AF, Speroff T, Dawson NV, Thomas C, Harrell FE, Wagner D et al. The effectiveness of right heart catheterization in the initial care of critically ill patients. *Journal of the American Medical Association.* 1996; **276**: 889–97.
13. Mermel LA, and Maki DG. Infectious complications of Swan-Ganz pulmonary artery catheters. *American Journal*

of Respiratory and Critical Care Medicine. 1994; **149**: 1020–36.

14. Harvey S, Harison DA, Singer M, Ashcroft J, Jones CM, Elbourne D et al. Assessment of the clinical effectiveness of pulmonary artery catheters in management of patients in intensive care (PAC-man): a randomised controlled trial. *Lancet.* 2005; **366**: 472–7.

15. Ross AD, Angaran DM. Colloids vs crystalloids – a continuing controversy. *Drug Intelligence and Clinical Pharmacy.* 1984; **18**: 202–12.

16. Shoemaker WC, Schlucter M, Hopkins JA, Appel PE, Schwartz S, Chang PC. Comparison of the relative effectiveness of colloids and crystalloids in emergency resuscitation. *American Journal of Surgery.* 1981; **142**: 7381.

17. Hillman K. Colloid versus crystalloid fluid therapy in the critically ill. *Intensive and Critical Care Digest.* 1986; **5**: 7–9.

18. Edwards JD, Brown GCS, Nightingale P, Slater RM, Faragher EB. Use of survivors' cardiorespiratory values as therapeutic goals in septic shock. *Critical Care Medicine.* 1989; **17**: 1098–103.

19. Gottlieb ME, Sarfeh IJ, Stratton H, Goldman ML, Newell JC, Shah DM. Hepatic perfusion and splanchnic oxygen consumption in patients postinjury. *Journal of Trauma.* 1983; **2**: 836–43.

20. Edouard AR, Degremont A-C, Durantaeu J, Pussard E, Berdeaux A, Samii K. Heterogeneous regional vascular responses to simulated transient hypovolaemia in man. *Intensive Care Medicine.* 1994; **20**: 414–20.

21. Baldwin L, Henderson A, Hickman P. Effect of postoperative low-dose dopamine on renal function after elective major vascular surgery. *Annals of Internal Medicine.* 1994; **120**: 744–7.

22. Thompson BT, Cockrill RA. Renal dose dopamine: a siren's song? *Lancet.* 1994; **344**: 7–8.

23. Van den Berghe G, de Zegher F, Lauwers P, Veldhuis JD. Growth hormone secretion in critical illness: effect of dopamine. *Journal of Clinical Endocrinology and Metabolism.* 1994; **79**: 41–6.

24. Lavery GG, McMurray TJ. Inotropic drugs. In: McCaughey W, Clarke RSJ, Fee JPH, Wallace WFM (eds). *Anaesthetic physiology and pharmacology.* Edinburgh: Churchill-Livingstone, 1997: Chapter 34.

25. Boyd O, Grounds RM, Bennett ED. The use of dopexamine hydrochloride to increase oxygen delivery postoperatively. *Anesthesia and Analgesia.* 1993; **76**: 372–6.

26. Baguneid MS, Welch M, Bukhari M, Fulford PE, Howe M, Bigley G et al. Randomized study to evaluate the effect of a perioperative infusion of dopexamine on colonic mucosal ischemia after aortic surgery. *Journal of Vascular Surgery.* 2001; **33**: 758–63.

27. McGinley J, Lynch L, Hubbard K, McCoy D, Cunningham AJ. Dopexamine hydrochloride does not modify hemodynamic response or tissue oxygenation or gut permeability during abdominal aortic surgery. *Canadian Journal of Anaesthesia.* 2001; **48**: 238–44.

28. Takala J, Meier-Hellmann A, Eddleston J, Hulstaert P, Sramek V. Effect of dopexamine on outcome after major abdominal surgery: a prospective, randomized, controlled multicenter study. European Multicenter Study Group on Dopexamine in Major Abdominal Surgery. *Critical Care Medicine.* 2000; **28**: 3417–23.

29. Parsons V. Recent advances in the management of acute renal failure. In: Ledinghan MI (eds). *Recent advances in critical care medicine,* Vol. 3. Edinburgh: Churchill Livingstone, 1980.

30. Bellomo R, Ronco C. Continuous haemofiltration in the intensive care unit. *Critical Care.* 2000; **4**: 339–45.

31. Kellum JA, Angus DC, Johnson JP, Leblanc M, Griffin M, Ramakrishnan N et al. Continuous versus intermittent renal replacement therapy: a meta-analysis. *Intensive Care Medicine.* 2002; **28**: 29–37.

32. Uchino S, Bellomo R, Ronco C. Intermittent versus continuous renal replacement therapy in the ICU: impact on electrolyte and acid-base balance. *Intensive Care Medicine.* 2001; **27**: 1037–43.

33. Tonelli M, Manns B, Feller-Kopman D. Acute renal failure in the intensive care unit: a systematic review of the impact of dialytic modality on mortality and renal recovery. *American Journal of Kidney Diseases.* 2002; **40**: 875–85.

34. Meguid MM, Collier MD, Howard U. Uncomplicated and stressed starvation. *Surgical Clinics of North America.* 1981; **61**: 529–43.

35. Moore FA, Feliciano DV, Andrassy RJ, McArdle AH, Booth FV et al. Early enteral feeding, compared with parenteral, reduces post-operative septic complications. *Annals of Surgery.* 1992; **216**: 172–83.

36. Graham TW, Zadronzy DB, Harrington T. The benefits of early jejunal hyperalimentation in the head-injured patient. *Neurosurgery.* 1989; **25**: 729–35.

37. Lee B, Chang RWS, Jacobs S. Intermittent nasogastric feeding: a simple and effective method to reduce pneumonia among ventilated ICU patients. *Clinical Intensive Care.* 1990; **1**: 100–2.

38. Heyland DK, Dhaliwal R, Drover JW, Gramlich L, Dodek P. Canadian Critical Care Clinical Practice Guidelines Committee. Canadian clinical practice guidelines for nutrition support in mechanically ventilated, critically ill adult patients. *Journal of Parenteral and Enteral Nutrition.* 2003; **27**: 355–73.

39. Crook MA, Hally V, Panteli JV. The importance of the refeeding syndrome. *Nutrition.* 2001; **7**: 632–7.

40. Andrews FJ, Griffiths RD. Glutamine: essential for immune nutrition in the critically ill. *British Journal of Nutrition.* 2002; **87**: 3–8.

41. Griffiths RD, Allen KD, Andrews FJ, Jones C. Infection, multiple organ failure, and survival in the intensive care unit: influence of glutamine-supplemented parenteral nutrition on acquired infection. *Nutrition.* 2002; **18**: 546–52.

42. Jian ZM, Cao JD, Zhu XG, Zhao WX, Yu JC et al. The impact of alanyl-glutamine on clinical safety, nitrogen balance, intestinal permeability, and clinical outcome in postoperative patients: a randomized,double-blind, controlled study of 120 patients. *Journal of Parenteral and Enteral Nutrition*. 1999; **23**: S62–6.

43. Garrel D, Patenaude J, Nedelec B, Samson L, Dorais J, Champoux J et al. Decreased mortality and infectious morbidity in adult burn patients given enteral glutamine supplements: a prospective, controlled, randomized clinical trial. *Critical Care Medicine*. 2003; **31**: 2444–9.

44. Hall JC, Dobb G, Hall J, de Sousa R, Brennan L, McCauley R. A prospective randomized trial of enteral glutamine in critical illness. *Intensive Care Medicine*. 2003; **29**: 1710–6.

45. Gadek JE, DeMichele SJ, Karlstad MD, Pacht ER, Donahoe M, Albertson TE et al. Effect of enteral feeding with eicosapentaenoic acid, γ-linolenic acid, and antioxidants in patients with acute respiratory distress syndrome. *Critical Care Medicine*. 1999; **27**: 1409–20.

46. Pacht ER, DeMichele SJ, Nelson JL, Hart J, Wennberg AK, Gadek JE. Enteral nutrition with eicosapentaenoic acid, gamma-linolenic acid, and antioxidants reduces alveolar inflammatory mediators and protein influx in patients with acute respiratory distress syndrome. *Critical Care Medicine*. 2003; **31**: 491–500.

47. Weiss G, Meyer F, Matthies B, Pross M, Koenig W, Lippert H. Immunomodulation by perioperative administration of n-3 fatty acids. *British Journal of Nutrition*. 2002; **87**: 89–94.

48. Galban C, Montejo JC, Mesejo A, Marco P, Celaya S, Sanchez-Segura JM et al. An immune-enhancing diet reduces mortality rate and episodes of bacteremia in septic intensive care unit patients. *Critical Care Medicine*. 2000; **28**: 643–8.

49. Bertolini G, Iapichino G, Radrizzani D, Facchini R, Simini B, Bruzzone P et al. Early enteral immunonutrition in patients with severe sepsis: results of an interim analysis of a randomized multicentre clinical trial. *Intensive Care Medicine*. 2003; **29**: 834–40.

50. Heyland DK, Novak F, Drover JW, Jain M, Su X, Suchner U. Should immunonutrition become routine in critically ill patients? A systematic review of the evidence. *Journal of the American Medical Association*. 2001; **286**: 944–53.

51. Beale RJ, Bryg DJ, Bihari DJ. Immunonutrition in the critically ill: a systematic review of clinical outcome. *Critical Care Medicine*. 1999; **27**: 2799–805.

52. Heys SD, Walker LG, Smith I, Eremin O. Enteral nutritional supplementation with key nutrients in patients with critical illness and cancer – a meta-analysis of randomized controlled clinical trials. *Annals of Surgery*. 1999; **229**: 467–77.

53. American College of Chest Physicians/Society of Critical Care Medicine. Consensus Conference: definitions for sepsis and organ failure and guidelines for the use of innovative therapies in sepsis. *Critical Care Medicine*. 1992; **20**: 864–74.

54. Guidelines for the management of severe sepsis and septic shock. The International Sepsis Forum. *Intensive Care Medicine*. 2001; **27**: S1–134.

55. Task Force of the American College of Critical Care Medicine Society of Critical Care Medicine. Practice parameters for hemodynamic support of sepsis in adult patients in sepsis. *Critical Care Medicine*. 1999; **27**: 639–60.

56. Misset B, Timsit JF, Dumay MF, Garrouste M, Chalfine A, Flouriot I et al. A continuous quality-improvement program reduces nosocomial infection rates in the ICU. *Intensive Care Medicine*. 2003; **30**: 395–400.

57. Harbarth S, Garbino J, Pugin J, Romand JA, Lew D, Pittet D. Inappropriate initial antimicrobial therapy and its effect on survival in a clinical trial of immunomodulating therapy for severe sepsis. *American Journal of Medicine*. 2003; **115**: 529–35.

58. Kollef MH. The importance of appropriate initial antibiotic therapy for hospital-acquired infections. *American Journal of Medicine*. 2003; **115**: 582–4.

59. Hinsdale JG, Jaffe BM. Reoperation for intra-abdorninal sepsis. *Annals of Surgery*. 1984; **199**: 31–6.

60. Van den Berghe G, Wouters P, Weekers F, Mohan S, Baxter RC, Veldhuis JD et al. Reactivation of pituitary hormone release and metabolic improvement by infusion of growth hormone-releasing peptide and thyrotropin-releasing hormone in patients with protracted critical illness. *Journal of Clinical Endocrinology and Metabolism*. 1999; **84**: 1311–23.

61. Van den Berghe G, Wouters P, Weekers F, Verwaest C, Bruyninckx F, Schetz M et al. Intensive insulin therapy in the critically ill patients. *New England Journal of Medicine*. 2001; **345**: 1359–67.

62. Van den Berghe G, Wouters PJ, Bouillon R, Weekers F, Verwaest C, Schetz M et al. Outcome benefit of intensive insulin therapy in the critically ill: Insulin dose versus glycemic control. *Critical Care Medicine*. 2003; **31**: 359–66.

63. Corwin HL, Surgenor SD, Gettinger A. Transfusion practice in the critically ill. *Critical Care Medicine*. 2003; **31**: S668–71.

64. Krafte-Jacobs B, Levetown ML, Bray GL, Ruttimann UE, Pollack MM. Erythropoietin response to critical illness. *Critical Care Medicine*. 1994; **22**: 821–6.

65. Hebert PC, Wells G, Blajchman MA, Marshall J, Martin C, Pagliarello G et al. A multicenter, randomized, controlled clinical trial of transfusion requirements in critical care. Transfusion Requirements in Critical Care Investigators, Canadian Critical Care Trials Group. *New England Journal of Medicine*. 1999; **340**: 409–17.

66. Hebert PC, Yetisir E, Martin C, Blajchman MA, Wells G, Marshall J et al. Transfusion Requirements in Critical Care Investigators for the Canadian Critical Care Trials Group. Is a low transfusion threshold safe in critically ill patients with cardiovascular diseases? *Critical Care Medicine*. 2001; **29**: 227–34.

67. Corwin HL, Gettinger A, Pearl RG, Fink MP, Levy MM, Abraham E et al. The CRIT Study: Anemia and blood transfusion in the critically ill – Current clinical practice in the United States. Critical Care Medicine. 2004; 32: 39–52.

68. Vincent JL, Baron JF, Reinhart K, Gattinoni L, Thijs L, Webb A et al. ABC (Anemia and Blood Transfusion in Critical Care) Investigators. Anemia and blood transfusion in critically ill patients. Journal of the American Medical Association. 2002; 288: 1499–507.

69. Corwin HL, Gettinger A, Pearl RG, Fink MP, Levy MM, Shapiro MJ et al. EPO Critical Care Trials Group. Efficacy of recombinant human erythropoietin in critically ill patients: a randomized controlled trial. Journal of the American Medical Association. 2002; 288: 2827–35.

70. Fowler RA, Berenson M. Blood conservation in the intensive care unit. Critical Care Medicine. 2003; 31: S715–20.

71. MacIsaac CM, Presneill JJ, Boyce CA, Byron KL, Cade JF. The influence of a blood conserving device on anaemia in intensive care patients. Anaesthesia and Intensive Care. 2003; 31: 653–7.

72. Thorpe S, Thomas AN. The use of a blood conservation pressure transducer system in critically ill patients. Anaesthesia. 2000; 55: 27–31.

73. Rivers E, Nguyen B, Havstad S, Ressler J, Muzzin A, Knoblich B et al. Early Goal-Directed Therapy Collaborative Group. Early goal-directed therapy in the treatment of severe sepsis and septic shock. New England Journal of Medicine. 2001; 345: 1368–77.

74. Parsons PE, Eisner MD, Thompson BT, Matthay MA, Ancukiewiez M, Bernard GR et al. Lower tidal volume ventilation and plasma cytokine markers of inflammation in patients with acute lung injury. Critical Care Medicine. 33: 1–6.

75. Ranieri VM, Suter PM, Tortorella C, De Tullio R, Dayer JM, Brienza A et al. Effect of mechanical ventilation on inflammatory mediators in patients with acute respiratory distress syndrome: a randomized controlled trial. Journal of the American Medical Association. 1999; 282: 54–61.

76. Amato MB, Barbas CS, Medeiros DM, Magaldi RB, Schettino GP, Lorenzi-Filho G et al. Effect of a protective-ventilation strategy on mortality in the acute respiratory distress syndrome. New England Journal of Medicine. 1998; 338: 347–54.

77. The Acute Respiratory Distress Syndrome Network. Ventilation with lower tidal volumes as compared with traditional tidal volumes for acute lung injury and the acute respiratory distress syndrome. New England Journal of Medicine. 2000; 342: 1301–8.

78. Petrucci N, Iacovelli W. Ventilation with lower tidal volumes versus traditional tidal volumes in adults for acute lung injury and acute respiratory distress syndrome. Cochrane Database of Systematic Reviews. 2004: CD003844.

79. Stewart TE, Meade MO, Cook DJ, Granton JT, Hodder RV, Lapinsky SE et al. Evaluation of a ventilation strategy to prevent barotrauma in patients at high risk for acute respiratory distress syndrome. Pressure- and Volume-Limited Ventilation Strategy Group. New England Journal of Medicine. 1998; 338: 355–61.

80. Yan SB, Helterbrand JD, Hartman DL, Wright TJ, Bernard GR. Low levels of protein C are associated with poor outcomes in severe sepsis. Chest. 2001; 120: 915–22.

81. Mesters RM, Helterbrand J, Utterback BG, Yan B, Chao YB, Fernandez JA et al. Prognostic value of protein C concentrations in neutropenic patients at high risk of severe septic complications. Critical Care Medicine. 2000; 28: 2209–16.

82. Taylor Jr. FB, Chang A, Esmon CT, D'Angelo A, Vigano-D'Angelo S, Blick KE. Protein C prevents the coagulopathic and lethal effects of Escherichia coli infusion in the baboon. Journal of Clinical Investigation. 1987; 79: 918–25.

83. Bernard GR, Vincent JL, Laterre PF, LaRosa SP, Dhainaut JF, Lopez-Rodriguez A et al. Recombinant Human Protein C Worldwide Evaluation in Severe Sepsis (PROWESS) Study Group: Efficacy and safety of recombinant human activated protein C for severe sepsis. New England Journal of Medicine. 2001; 344: 699–709.

84. Oelkers W. Adrenal insufficiency. New England Journal of Medicine. 1996; 335: 1206–12.

85. Cronin L, Cook DJ, Carlet J, Heyland DK, King D, Lansang MA et al. Corticosteroid treatment for sepsis: a critical appraisal and meta-analysis of the literature. Critical Care Medicine. 1995; 23: 1430–9.

86. Annane D, Sébille V, Troché G, Raphael JC, Gajdos P, Bellissant E. A 3-level prognostic classification in septic shock based on cortisol levels and cortisol response to corticotropin. Journal of the American Medical Association. 2000; 283: 1038–45.

87. Beishuizen A, Thijs LG, Vermes I. Patterns of corticosteroid-binding globulin and the free cortisol index during septic shock and multitrauma. Intensive Care Medicine. 2001; 27: 1584–91.

88. Koo DJ, Jackman D, Chaudry IH, Wang P. Adrenal insufficiency during the late stage of polymicrobial sepsis. Critical Care Medicine. 2001; 29: 618–22.

89. Briegel J, Forst H, Haller M, Schelling G, Kilger E, Kuprat G et al. Stress doses of hydrocortisone reverse hyperdynamic septic shock: a prospective, randomized, double-blinded, single-center study. Critical Care Medicine. 1999; 27: 723–32.

90. Bollaert PE, Fieux F, Charpentier C, Levy B. Baseline cortisol levels, cortisol response to corticotropin, and prognosis in late septic shock. Shock. 2003; 19: 13–5.

91. Annane D, Sebille V, Charpentier C, Bollaert PE, Francois B, Korach JM et al. Effect of treatment with low doses of hydrocortisone and fludrocortisone on mortality in patients with septic shock. Journal of the American Medical Association. 2002; 288: 862–71.

92. Keh D, Boehnke T, Weber-Cartens S, Schulz C, Ahlers O, Bercker S et al. Immunologic and hemodynamic effects of 'low-dose' hydrocortisone in septic shock: a double-blind,

randomized, placebo-controlled, crossover study. *American Journal of Respiratory and Critical Care Medicine.* 2003; **167**: 512–20.

93. Levack P. Live and let die? A structured approach to decision-making about resuscitation. *British Journal of Anaesthesia.* 2002; **89**: 683–6.

94. Prendergast TJ, Claessens MT, Luce JM. A national survey of end-of-life care for critically ill patients. *American Journal of Respiratory and Critical Care Medicine.* 1998; **158**: 1163–7.

95. Sjokvist P, Nilstun T, Svantesson M, Berggren L. Withdrawal of life support – who should decide? Differences in attitudes among the general public, nurses and physicians. *Intensive Care Medicine.* 1999; **25**: 949–54.

96. Ferrand E, Lemaire F, Regnier B, Kuteifan K, Badet M, Asfar P *et al.* Discrepancies between perceptions by physicians and nursing staff of intensive care unit end-of-life decisions. *American Journal of Respiratory and Critical Care Medicine.* 2003; **167**: 1310–5.

43

Paediatric intensive care

HELEN ALLEN AND ROB ROSS RUSSELL

Introduction	542	Key points	547
General principles	542	Best clinical practice	547
ENT emergencies in PICU	544	Deficiencies in current knowledge and areas for future	
Major surgery	546	research	548
Summary	547	References	548

SEARCH STRATEGY

Data for this chapter are mostly generic management strategies for children in intensive care. The data were gathered through reference to standard texts on paediatric intensive care, notably *Textbook of pediatric intensive care*[1] and *Fluid balance and volume resuscitation for beginners*.[2] Specific information on ENT trauma in children was obtained through PubMed using the key words laryngeal trauma and laryngeal injury, limiting the search to children 0–18. This revealed 65 review articles of which five were found relevant and scrutinized. Information on bronchoscopy was located on PubMed using the key words fibreoptic bronchoscopy and intensive care, limiting the search to children 0–18. This only yielded two papers (one from 1980), but searching on the related links button located a number of relevant articles.

INTRODUCTION

Children are liable to present acutely with ENT pathologies, many of which are specific to the paediatric population and may require intensive care management. Those children undergoing major ENT surgery also frequently require admission to a paediatric intensive care unit in the postoperative period. This chapter aims to outline the general management principles of ENT patients within the paediatric intensive care setting. Important differences in the anatomy and physiology of children compared to adults are reviewed. A systematic approach to evaluation of children admitted to the paediatric intensive care unit (PICU) is outlined, together with general principles of fluid and analgesia management in children. Specific issues relating to the care of the major paediatric emergencies, as well as the postoperative management of patients undergoing major ENT surgical procedures, are discussed. Finally, indications and

procedures for performing bronchoscopy within the unit are detailed.

GENERAL PRINCIPLES

Anatomical and physiological considerations

Care of the paediatric patient requires an understanding of the anatomy and physiology of children, which have some important differences from adulthood.

Anatomically, the child has quite different body proportions and shape. The head of the infant and small child is proportionately larger, accounting for nearly 10 percent of body surface area, compared to the 3.5 percent in adults. The neck of a child is shorter, and these two factors tend to increase neck flexion, particularly in the emergency setting. A relatively large tongue and small mandible can make access to the airway difficult.

Table 43.1 Physiological parameters at different ages.

Age	Heart rate (bpm)	Respiratory rate (bpm)	Mean BP (mmHg)
Newborn	110–140	50–60	50–60
1 year	90–110	30–40	70–90
2–5 years	75–90	25–30	80–100
5–12 years	60–90	20–25	90–110
>12 years	50–80	15–20	100–120

In all young children the epiglottis is rounded ('horseshoe shape') and the larynx sits high (opposite the third cervical vertebra, compared to the fifth or sixth in an adult) and anterior. The larynx itself is conical, unlike the cylindrical adult larynx, and the narrowest part lies at the cricoid cartilage. Finally, the tracheal cartilage is often less rigid than in adults, and may compress if the neck is overextended.[3]

Infants (up to approximately six months old) are also obligate nasal breathers. When this is combined with the relatively small airways and risk of mucous obstruction, airway compromise is common. Between three and six years of age, tonsillar and adenoidal hypertrophy further contribute to airway obstruction.

Physiologically, there are also substantial and important differences. Respiratory muscle function is affected by the position of the ribs in infants, which lie perpendicular to the spine rather than running caudally as they do in adults. This makes the diaphragm the only effective inspiratory muscle. Infants and children have a faster respiratory rate than adults (see **Table 43.1**), which is partly related to an increased metabolic rate. In infants, increased chest wall compliance can increase the work of breathing substantially.

In the cardiovascular system, a limited stroke volume causes a faster heart rate in children, and they also display a lower mean blood pressure. Their response to cardiovascular stress is limited, and cardiac output can only be increased significantly by increasing the heart rate, hence tachycardia is common.

Evaluation

Admission of a child into the PICU is a difficult and important moment in the child's care. The care of the child is transferred to a new team of doctors and nurses, and the family are moved to a new and stressful environment. It is essential that this handover is careful and complete. Ideally, there should be a face to face handover between the medical and nursing teams involved in the care. The background history, current problems and care plan should be clearly documented.

The family of the child need to be included in this handover. Where the admission is planned, families

should be offered the chance to visit the intensive care unit prior to the surgery so that they have met some of the staff and seen the environment. There should be an area for them to stay in while procedures are being carried out and they need regular updates from medical and nursing staff on progress.

The doctors admitting the child also need to evaluate the child carefully on admission. This should follow standard 'ABC' rules, assessing the airway, breathing and circulation. Issues of fluid balance (including any feeding plan), analgesia, sedation and blood tests should also be clarified (**Table 43.2**).

Fluid management

Although the principles of fluid balance in children are the same as in adults, there are a number of complicating factors that make life more difficult for the junior doctor. The first and most obvious is an unfortunate tendency for children to grow! Any fluids that need to be given are therefore based on the child's weight or occasionally the body surface area. Metabolic requirements, including insensible water loss, vary with age and this must be taken into consideration.

The distribution of fluids between compartments is different for adults and children, and an understanding of this difference is important in deciding on appropriate volumes and types of fluid. The infant has approximately one-third of their body weight as interstitial fluid – twice as much as in an adult. Consequently, fluids constitute approximately 75 percent of body weight in infancy, compared to 60 percent in the adult.

THE NEWBORN INFANT

The full-term infant requires approximately 150 mL/kg per day of fluid (although less in the first few days of life). Of this, approximately 30 mL/kg will be accounted for by insensible losses. Normal fluid intake is entirely as milk, which provides both fluid and nutrition for the first few months of life. Fluid requirements (per kg) gradually

Table 43.2 Issues to be considered on admission of a child to PICU.

	Issues to consider
Airway	Clear? ET tube position? ET tube secured properly?
Breathing	Air entry? Ventilation adequate?
Circulation	Peripheral perfusion? Adequate access?
Fluids	Drug infusions? Adequate sugar? Urine output?
Analgesia/ sedation	Pain control AND sedation adequate? Paralysis needed?
Tests	Blood gas? Electrolytes? FBC?

Table 43.3 Fluid and electrolyte requirements at different ages.

Age	Daily fluid requirements	Sodium/potassium requirements
1 day	60 mL/kg	2–3 mmol/kg/day
5 days	150 mL/kg	2 mmol/kg/day
1 month	120 mL/kg	1–2 mmol/kg/day
6 months	110 mL/kg	
1 year	100 mL/kg	
Over 1 year	1000 mL for first 10 kg, 500 ml for next 10 kg then 20–25 mL/kg for rest of body weight	

reduce thereafter, as shown in **Table 43.3**. It should be emphasized that these requirements are based on normal needs and that they frequently need adjustment in disease.

Electrolyte requirements will also vary with age, although not so dramatically as fluid volume. In the infant, immature renal function increases the salt requirements, and 3 mmol/kg of sodium and potassium are usually required daily. In older children this falls to approximately 2 mmol/kg/day of each ion. Calcium, magnesium and other ions are broadly given in the same (per kg) dose as in adults.

Glucose requirements are critical, especially in young children. The daily calorie requirement of infants is approximately 100 kcal/kg, more than double that in adults. Maintenance of adequate glucose levels in infants is critically important and hypoglycaemia (even for short periods) can cause permanent brain damage. In infants and small children, enough glucose must be given to maintain blood glucose levels.

THE UNWELL CHILD

Fluid requirements following surgery can be quite variable. In most units, children are started on a regime restricting their input to approximately two-thirds normal requirements. This is especially true if oral feeds are not to be used and fluids are being given intravenously. Intravenous fluids should be chosen with care. Recently, concerns have been raised about the use of hypotonic fluids (especially 0.18 percent saline) as this tends to induce hyponatraemia which can cause substantial problems including seizures and indeed death.[4, 5] Solutions containing adequate sodium (such as 0.45 percent saline, 2.5 percent dextrose) are therefore recommended. Whatever regime is used, it needs to be remembered that children are prone to become dehydrated or fluid overloaded quite rapidly and need to be monitored carefully. In infants especially, blood glucose levels need to be measured regularly (up to four hourly). [**/*]

Analgesia

Appropriate analgesia needs to balance the sedative and respiratory suppressive effects of opiates against the need for good pain control. Oral paracetamol, or other nonsteroidal antiinflammatory drugs (NSAIDs) may often be adequate, but opiates (e.g. morphine) may be needed. An infusion (e.g. morphine at 10–30 µg/kg/hour) is easily administered. In older children, patient controlled analgesia (PCA) pumps are helpful. Background rates (e.g. morphine at 10 µg/kg/hour) with boluses as needed (e.g. morphine 10 µg/kg up to hourly) is often a good combination but should be discussed with the anaesthetist involved. Sedation may also be needed for patients in the PICU, especially if ventilated or undergoing painful procedures. Units vary between using infusions (e.g. midazolam 50–250 µg/kg/hour) or boluses (e.g. midazolam 0.1 mg/kg, p.r.n. up to four hourly). Current trends favour intermittent bolus dosage as this reduces total sedative load, but patients need close observation to avoid distress. [*]

ENT EMERGENCIES IN PICU

Trauma

All trauma cases, including those who have sustained craniofacial trauma, should be managed acutely according to advanced life support guidelines,[3] with immediate evaluation and management of airway, breathing and circulation. Cases of blunt laryngeal trauma are rare. They may occur if a child is unrestrained in a car involved in a road traffic accident if they hit the dashboard when the head and neck are in a hyperextended position. In children presenting with laryngotracheal injuries in the absence of such a history, the possibility of nonaccidental injury with a direct blow to the anterior neck should be considered as a possible aetiology.

A protocol for the management of acute laryngeal trauma was devised and published by Schaefer in 1982.[6] This advocates immediate protection of the airway by emergency tracheostomy for all but the most minor of cases, with endoscopy to evaluate the injuries. In patients with moderate injuries, the degree of traumatic damage can be further assessed using CT scanning once the airway has been protected by tracheostomy. In cases where the injuries are severe, open exploration is recommended. [**/*]

Upper airway obstruction

The small cross-sectional area and conical shape of the paediatric airway renders children particularly susceptible to upper airway obstruction. A relatively small reduction in the radius of the airway through mucosal oedema, secretions or a foreign body, results in a significant increase in airway resistance (resistance α diameter).[6] Stridor on inspiration is indicative of upper airway obstruction. In children where severe upper airway obstruction is suspected as a diagnosis, it is imperative to avoid all invasive procedures and aspects of the examination liable to distress the child as this may precipitate complete upper airway occlusion. Children should be kept warm and calm while experienced anaesthetic and surgical staff are brought together. Examination can then be undertaken in a controlled manner. A full examination of the child is also needed at a convenient point. Birthmarks, and especially haemangiomas (which may indicate a laryngeal lesion), should be recorded. If a child is dysmorphic, a genetic opinion may help identify a syndrome that may have airway implications.

EPIGLOTTITIS

The advent of the Hib vaccine and its inclusion in childhood immunization schedules to protect them against *Haemophilus influenzae* type B infections, has led to a marked decline in the incidence of epiglottitis so that it is now a rare condition. However, occasional cases do still occur in unimmunized children or in those in whom the vaccine has failed. Clinical presentation is with a toxic child who is stridulous and drooling.

The priority of immediate management is to secure the airway by intubation or, in extreme cases, emergency tracheostomy. They will then remain ventilated in intensive care whilst receiving treatment with intravenous antibiotics (third generation cephalosporin) until the epiglottic swelling has been reduced, usually within 24–36 hours.[7] [*]

CROUP

Acute viral laryngotracheobronchitis (viral croup) is the most common cause of stridor in children and the vast majority of patients can be managed either at home or on the general paediatric wards. Only the most severe cases require admission to a high dependency unit (HDU) or PICU.

In such cases, short-term relief of the upper airway obstruction can be achieved by nebulizing epinephrine (1 mL/kg of 1:1000 up to 5 mL maximum dose) with oxygen. Steroids, either in the form of nebulized budesonide or systemic dexamethasone or prednisolone, can be given to reduce the upper airway inflammation. A very small minority of children with croup require intubation to protect their airway (<5 percent), but the administration of systemic steroids to this group of patients has been shown to reduce both the duration of intubation and the need for reintubation (**Table 43.4**).[8]

Table 43.4 Features of croup versus epiglottitis.

	Croup	Epiglottitis
Age	1–3 years	2–7 years
Cause	Parainfluenza viruses	*H. influenzae*
Prodrome	1–2 days coryza	Hours
		Sore throat
		Dysphagia
Fever	<38°C	>38°C
Appearance	Lethargic	Pale and toxic
		Drooling and dysphagic
		Sits with neck extended
Stridor	Barking cough	Muffled stridor
	Loud stridor	Stertorous breathing
Hypoxia	Unusual	Frequent
Severity	<3% hospitalized cases require intubation	All require intubation

In all children with stridor, the consideration of other diagnoses, such as a postpharyngeal abscess, needs to be undertaken. [****/***/**/*]

Bacterial tracheitis

Bacterial tracheitis, or pseudomembranous croup, is much less common than viral croup but it is potentially life threatening and the majority of patients will require intubation to secure their airway whilst receiving treatment with intravenous antibiotics. The pathogens are usually *Staphylococcus aureus* or *Streptococci*, which infect the tracheal mucosa causing necrosis and the production of purulent secretions that may occlude the upper airway. Clinically, a child with bacterial tracheitis is septic with a high fever, croupy cough and progressive signs of upper airway obstruction.

Foreign body inhalation

A history of possible foreign body inhalation can usually be elicited, but in the absence of such information it should be suspected as a cause if there is sudden onset of stridor and upper airway obstruction with no history of preceding fever or illness. It occurs most commonly in children between the ages of one and three years, with foodstuffs being the usual cause.

In such cases, if the child presents with increasing dyspnoea, apnoea or loss of consciousness which has not responded to simple airway opening manoeuvres, then the advanced paediatric life support guidelines for management of a choking child should be instituted.[3] In an older child the Heimlich manoeuvre can safely be attempted or, if the child is unconscious and supine, abdominal thrusts may be equally effective at dislodging the foreign body.

The foreign body may in some cases pass through the larynx and become lodged lower down in the bronchial tree. As discussed earlier, the larynx in the prepubertal child is conical, and objects passing the vocal cords can lodge at the level of the cricoid.[3] It is essential that one does not use blind finger sweeps in the mouth for the foreign body as this may push it tighter into the larynx.[3] Objects may also pass right into the lungs. On clinical examination there may be unilateral wheezing, reduced air entry on one side or signs suggestive of unilateral lung collapse. A chest x-ray may show hyperinflation of the affected lung with mediastinal shift due to the foreign body causing gas trapping on expiration, or alternatively lung collapse. These patients require a general anaesthetic for rigid bronchoscopic removal of the foreign body and may need a period of ventilation on the PICU afterwards. [**/*]

MAJOR SURGERY

Craniofacial surgery and cleft lip and palate

Children who undergo craniofacial surgery or a cleft lip or palate repair, may require admission to a PICU or HDU, particularly if there is a risk of the airway becoming compromised by postoperative swelling. If the child returns from theatre ventilated, sedation and analgesia need to be maintained for the whole period of ventilation. A partially sedated child may struggle with an endotracheal tube (ETT) *in situ*, and this may damage a palatal or laryngeal repair. It may be necessary to paralyze the child once they are adequately sedated. This is often best carried out with short-acting anaesthetic agents, particularly when there is a planned extubation, as this will allow the child to be woken promptly. With longer-acting drugs there may be accumulation of the drug, and a period of suboptimal sedation/wakefulness as it is metabolized.

Other important considerations include the use of orogastric rather than nasogastric tubes, best sited under direct vision at the time of the operation, as nasogastric tubes can traumatize a palate repair. Nursing staff should be aware not to perform blind oropharyngeal suction with a rigid Yankaeur sucker, but should use a soft wide bore flexible suction catheter to remove visible secretions only. Infection, particularly with streptococcus, can be devastating to palatal repairs. As well as careful nursing and cleanliness, patients should not be nursed close to other children who may be carrying pathogens. [*]

Surgery of the nose and upper airway

Patients who have surgery to the nose rarely require an admission to PICU in the postoperative period. If they do,

then the general principles of evaluation and management should be applied. The exception may be with infants who require surgery for choanal atresia/stenosis. In these children, maintaining a patent nasal stent may require close nursing observation for the first few days.

Those undergoing surgery to the upper airway are, however, frequently admitted to PICU for a period after the operation due to the high risk of developing upper airway obstruction as oedema evolves around the site of surgery. This includes operations for laryngeal reconstruction, but also for more minor procedures such as aryepiglottoplasty. It is therefore important to ensure that a PICU/HDU bed is available for the patient before proceeding with surgery. Children who have major upper airway surgery, such as laryngotracheal reconstruction, are electively ventilated for a period of five to seven days after the operation to allow the oedema to resolve before the ETT is removed. In these patients, sedation and analgesia are again critical (see Craniofacial surgery and cleft lip and palate). Paralysis is usually used in this patient group to prevent trauma to the site of surgery and exacerbation of upper airway oedema due to movement of the ETT whilst *in situ*. Close observation of cardiovascular parameters in paralyzed patients will detect tachycardia and hypertension suggestive of inadequate sedation or pain underneath the paralysis. It is important that a significant leak is allowed to develop around the ETT before extubation is attempted as this may signify that the postoperative oedema is resolving and that extubation is more likely to be successful. [*]

Laryngeal surgery and tracheostomy

Managing a tracheostomy in the PICU involves the management of the newly formed stoma, care of an established tracheostomy and training requirements for families looking after long-term tracheostomies.

In the first week after a tracheostomy is formed, the airway is dependent on the tracheostomy stent (i.e. the tube) to maintain the airway open. Loss of the stent over this period can allow the airway to close, and the reinsertion of a tube through an immature tracheostomy can be difficult, as the tracheal opening can be obscured (especially in obese patients) and the tube can easily be passed into the wrong plane. This results in obstruction of the airway and ventilation of the tissues of the neck. For the first week, a new tracheostomy should therefore be carefully secured. In our unit, stay sutures are attached to the edges of the trachea at surgery, allowing the trachea to be brought up to the surface of the neck in an emergency and thus facilitating tube reinsertion.[9] A tracheal dilator and spare tracheostomy tubes (of the same size and one size smaller) should be kept at the bedside.

If a tracheostomy tube does become dislodged in this period and cannot easily be reinserted, then (assuming the larynx permits this) a conventional endotracheal tube should be put in through the mouth or nose to secure the airway. This allows a measured replacement of the tracheostomy tube either in the PICU or in theatre.

Following the first tracheostomy tube change (usually at seven to ten days), the tracheostomy is more secure. Care of an established stoma involves the establishment of routine tube changes, tape care and training for the carers (where appropriate). The development of difficulties with tube insertion or of bleeding should raise the possibility of granulation formation.

Parents who are to go home with a child who has a tracheostomy will need careful training. As well as confidence in tube and tape changes, training in resuscitation is necessary, as is an ability to perform adequate tracheal suction. Preparation of equipment and provision of support at home may take many weeks to organize. [*]

Bronchoscopy in PICU

FIBREOPTIC BRONCHOSCOPY

This is a very useful technique, as it is extremely simple to pass a fibreoptic scope through an ETT and directly into the lung. Its advantages include simplicity and access. The scope can visualize all lobes of the lung and identify both static (e.g. mucous plugs) and dynamic (e.g. broncho-malacia) problems. The disadvantages include a narrow suction channel that blocks easily, and the inability to effectively ventilate through the scope. The latter can be circumvented if the scope is passed through a rubber valve in the ETT, allowing continued ventilation around the scope, but is difficult if the diameter of the scope is close to that of the ETT.

RIGID BRONCHOSCOPY

This technique is much more effective at removing debris from the airway, and may be easier to use in the very unstable patient as ventilation can be continued through the scope during the procedure.

There are several indications for either fibreoptic or rigid bronchoscopy in PICU:

- *Persistent collapse of lobe/lung.* Ventilated children may develop complete collapse of a lung, usually secondary to blockage of the major airways with secretions and mucous plugs. This can lead to major ventilatory problems with shunting. Fibreoptic bronchoscopy down the ETT can often identify the degree of blockage but a rigid bronchoscope may be needed to clear thick secretions.
- *Assessment of malacia.* Clinical tracheo- or bronchomalacia may be difficult to confirm. Flexible bronchoscopy may help locate the site and degree of weakness, but needs to be carried out with the patient self-ventilating as positive pressure ventilation can stent the airway open artificially.

- *Assisted intubations.* In particularly difficult airways, a flexible bronchoscope or laryngoscope can be extremely useful in locating the airway. By threading an ETT over the scope prior to entering the airway, the ETT can then be placed into the correct position.
- *Collection of bronchoalveolar lavage fluid.* In patients who develop severe lung disease, and particularly in patients who are immunosuppressed, the diagnosis of lung pathogens can be very difficult. Bronchoalveolar lavage may be very useful in this situation. It can either be carried out 'blind'[10] by passing a nasogastric tube into the lungs, washing in a small volume of 0.9 percent saline, and then aspirating, or using a fibreoptic scope to direct the lavage to a particular part of the lung. [**/*]

SUMMARY

Whilst principles of care for children are similar to those of adults, there must be careful consideration of the different physiological responses seen in children and how they vary with age. Some ENT procedures are also very specific to the younger age group, and in units which are not undertaking paediatric surgery frequently, well maintained guidelines for the care of this group of patients is essential.

KEY POINTS

- Foreign body inhalation should be suspected in any child with unexplained stridor or respiratory symptoms.
- Paediatric anatomy and physiology is significantly different from adults.
- Fluid and electrolyte prescriptions for children must be adapted to the individual and calculated according to weight.
- Frequent monitoring and adjustments of fluid and electrolyte prescriptions are required.
- All patients with suspected epiglottitis require intubation.
- Trauma and infection are the greatest threats to palate repairs.
- Good evidence to support clinical practice in the PICU is limited.

Best clinical practice

General Principles

✓ Anatomical and physiological differences between adults and children need to be recognized.

✓ Fluid and electrolyte administration must be age-and weight-appropriate.

✓ Appreciation of family carers and their involvement is essential.

ENT emergencies in PICU

✓ Laryngeal trauma in children usually requires a tracheostomy.

✓ Epiglottitis is now rare in the UK following the introduction of the Hib vaccination.

✓ Foreign body inhalation is an important, if uncommon, cause of acute respiratory symptoms in children.

Major surgery

✓ Paralysis may be needed following palatal surgery to avoid damage from a struggling child.

✓ Infection is a major cause of palatal breakdown in children following surgery.

✓ Flexible bronchoscopy in children can clear secretions, but the size of the bronchoscope limits its suctioning ability.

✓ Suspected foreign bodies should be removed through a rigid bronchoscope.

Deficiencies in current knowledge and areas for future research

Many of the clinical practices on PICU have evolved through sharing of experience rather than being substantiated by medical evidence or clinical trials and the potential for research projects aimed at providing evidence to support or refute current practices is huge. However, in reality there are significant practical limitations to undertaking such research, for example the ethics of research in children, difficulties in obtaining parental consent for entry into trials, and recruiting sufficient numbers of patients to achieve adequate power. Much of current research focuses on establishing optimal sedation and analgesia regimes for intensive care patients.

REFERENCES

1. Rogers MC, Nichols DG (eds). *Textbook of pediatric intensive care*, 3rd edn. Baltimore, MD: Lippincott Williams and Wilkins, 1996.

2. Park GR, Roe PG. *Fluid balance and volume resuscitation for beginners.* London: Greenwich Medical Media Ltd, 2000.

3. Advanced Life Support Group. *Advanced paediatric life support.* London: BMJ Publishing Group, 2000.

4. Berleur MP, Dahan A, Murat I, Hazebroucq G. Perioperative infusions in paediatric patients: rationale for using Ringer-lactate solution with low dextrose concentration. *Journal of Clinical Pharmacy and Therapeutics.* 2003; **28**: 31–40.

5. Bohn D. Problems associated with intravenous fluid administration in children: do we have the right solutions? *Current Opinion in Pediatrics.* 2000; **12**: 217–21.

6. Schaefer SD. Primary management of laryngeal trauma. *Annals of Otology, Rhinology, and Laryngology.* 1982; **91**: 399–402.

7. Damm M, Eckel HE, Jungehulsing M, Roth B. Management of acute inflammatory childhood stridor. *Otolaryngology and Head and Neck Surgery.* 1999; **121**: 633–8.

8. Stannard W, O'Callaghan C. Management of croup. *Paediatric Drugs.* 2002; **4**: 231–40.

9. Burke A. The advantages of stay sutures with tracheostomy. *Annals of the Royal College of Surgeons of England.* 1981; **63**: 426–8.

10. Ashton MR. 'Blind' bronchoalveolar lavage. *Lancet.* 1992; **340**: 1104.

PART 9

SAFE AND EFFECTIVE PRACTICE

EDITED BY MARTIN J BURTON

44 Training, accreditation and the maintenance of skills   551
   Paul O'Flynn
45 Communication and the medical consultation   559
   Damian Gardner-Thorpe and Richard Canter
46 Clinical governance: Improving the quality of patient care   568
   Debbie Wall, Patrick J Bradley and Aidan Halligan
47 Medical ethics   581
   Katherine Wasson
48 Medical jurisprudence and otorhinolaryngology   594
   Maurice Hawthorne and Desmond Watson

Training, accreditation and the maintenance of skills

PAUL O'FLYNN

Introduction	551	Guidance for surgeons on appraisal and revalidation: specialty-specific guidance for ear, nose and throat surgeons	556
Ear, nose and throat surgical training in the UK	552		
Continuing professional development and the maintenance of skills	553	References	558

INTRODUCTION

Over the past 20 years, surgical practice has changed almost beyond recognition. Ear, nose and throat (ENT) surgery, and particularly rhinology and rhinological surgery, are excellent examples of this. The technical aspects of surgery have changed as the materials, investigations and instruments available have evolved. Techniques have radically changed as completely new approaches have developed.

A simple illustration of this is the use of rigid endoscopes in nasal and sinus surgery, both for diagnostic and therapeutic purposes. Prior to the mid-1980s, almost all sinus surgery was undertaken using a headlamp. At that time, the illumination was relatively poor and access to parts of the nose and sinuses restricted. In the 1980s, a number of surgeons started to see the benefit of using the illumination and magnification of the operating microscope to deal with sinus disease. However, within a few years rigid endoscopes became increasingly available and in less than ten years entered widespread use in the USA, UK and Europe. This change from relatively crude surgery to accurate dissection, based on ever-improving imaging and now image-guided systems, has entirely changed our knowledge and practice.

The concepts that underpin our understanding of sinus disease have changed. A far greater emphasis is placed on medical, allergic and immunological aspects, as well as the relationship between the upper and the lower airway.

The transition described above has not been without problems. In both endoscopic sinus surgery and laparoscopic surgery, overenthusiasm for the method with inadequate training has lead to serious adverse outcomes. The need for structured training was recognized even for experienced surgeons. This change in technology and the rapidly expanding availability of computerized tomography (CT) scanning, giving the surgeon far more information about what they could expect to find anatomically and pathologically in the sinuses, has driven a need for on-going training for established practitioners and new curriculum for trainees. The Hill Surgical Workshop at the Royal College of Surgeons was one response to this need.

Surgeons today, both trainees and experienced, have to continue to acquire substantial new knowledge, new diagnostic skills and new technical skills throughout their career. We, as surgeons, have a duty to do this.[1]

All these technical matters need to be seen within the broader context of change. The public, patients, legislators, healthcare professionals and the Government have all started to voice 'needs' within the healthcare system. Public confidence was shaken by the actions of Dr Shipman and the apparent lack of scrutiny of them.[2] 'Disasters', such as the cases highlighted in Bristol, where well-meaning surgeons fell below an acceptable standard, and the subsequent reports and inquiries have heightened the public taste for scrutiny of the medial professions.[3]

Patients, in general, want to be fully informed before consenting to a surgical procedure and we as surgeons are bound by the requirements of *Good surgical practice* to obtain informed consent.[4]

The issues surrounding consent are in themselves highly complex and outside the scope of this chapter, but highlight yet another change. A good doctor–patient relationship is a fundamental part of the care of a surgical patient. Some surgeons have an innate 'skill' of communication, others simply do not. Attention to this aspect of the surgeons overall ability is now well recognized and is assessed and examined in both the MRCS and Intercollegiate FRCS examinations. Good hand–eye coordination is not sufficient to make a modern surgeon.

The Royal College of Physicians and Surgeons of Canada published a substantial document in 1996 subtitled 'Skills for the new millennium' in which seven 'roles' were described as being important in a medical practitioner.[5] The precise mixture of the roles and the extent to which they are relevant will vary from specialty to specialty and will be dependent on the stage of development of the practitioner, but to some extent all roles will be relevant to some degree in every practitioner. The roles defined are:

- medical expert;
- communicator;
- collaborator;
- manager;
- health advocate;
- scholar;
- professional.

Methods of evaluating these areas are also suggested.

The role of medical education, training and revalidation can be seen as a broad development of various roles largely defined by (though not exclusively) the list above.

EAR, NOSE AND THROAT SURGICAL TRAINING IN THE UK

Historic perspective

Until the mid-1990s, surgical training in the UK, and largely in those countries associated with the Commonwealth, had been based on an apprenticeship model. This tradition has assumed that over time the apprentice (young surgeon) would:

- acquire knowledge relevant to their particular specialization;
- develop clinical skills;
- gain exposure to conditions and diseases and understand their natural history and standard treatment;
- see complications and their resolution.

Over time, the novice would gain experience, skill and knowledge to ultimately master his or her specialty. The range of skills and knowledge acquired would be tested by examination and in-training assessment. In the UK, this individual would then progress to positions that are more senior and ultimately become a consultant 'master practitioner'. The cycle would then continue with the consultant training young surgeons and handing on skills and knowledge.

The mark of a consultant surgeon is the ability to 'practice independently'. The real meaning of this phrase is not well defined and does not fit well with the likely organization of the surgical professions in the future where 'team working' is much more emphasized.[6] One view of the organization of surgical teams involves groups of specialists in the generality of an area of surgery 'where team members work within a closely defined range of skills', rather like aircrew. Pilots cannot change between levels of competence or types of aircraft without demonstrating competence and usually after specific training.

The apprenticeship model, despite considerable criticism, served the UK well. The following are the principle advantages of this system:

- it is not time constrained, therefore the apprentice can learn at his or her own pace;
- training is close to the 'coal face', so that common conditions are seen and treated frequently;
- a close working relationship often develops between master and apprentice, helping with ongoing personal and professional development.

Critics of this system point to a number of weaknesses, including:

- the system fails to meet changing the needs of the profession;
- progress to more senior positions depends on availability of such a post and the degree of competition at that time;
- criteria against which to measure competency are generally lacking;
- poor trainer–trainee relationships could lead to underperformance.

Prior to the Calman Report, a typical career pathway in otolaryngology could be summarized as follows:

1. medical school (five to six years) to obtain medical degree. Provisional registration with the General Medical Council (GMC);
2. pre-registration house officer (one year), full registration with GMC;
3. senior house officer (approximately two to three years) including time spent in non-ENT posts such as general surgery, plastics, neurosurgery and accident and emergency. Obtain Primary FRCS (examination in anatomy, pathology and physiology);
4. registrar in otolaryngology (approximately three years). Entry into post by competitive interview. Obtain FRCS in otolaryngology during tenure;
5. senior registrar (approximately three years). Entry into post by competitive interview;
6. Maintain log book. Obtain Certificate of Completion of Higher Surgical Training;
7. consultant post. Competitive interview. Virtually permanent tenure.

Although the tenure of each post was fixed, the time in that grade was not. There was an imbalance in the numbers of posts available and a bottleneck between registrar and senior registrar grades. Over time, the UK system led to excessively long periods of 'training'. In some specialties, so few consultant posts were available that experienced and able trainees were stuck in the senior registrar grade for many years. This situation failed to satisfy the needs of the National Health Service or the trainees. European Working time legislation[7] and the 'New deal on junior doctors' hours'[8] have forced a rethink of UK training.

The Calman Report

In the early 1990s, Sir Kenneth Calman, as Chief Medical Officer, set up a working party that produced a report on the future direction of training.[9] As part of the implementation of that report the grades of registrar and senior registrar were merged into the specialist registrar grade between 1995 and 1997. The new grade had protected training time and was not to be seen as part of service provision. Other features of the grade were to be a defined curriculum with clearer educational objectives and assessment. Protected training time has been widely implemented. Specialist registrars, however, remain important service providers. The bottleneck is now at the senior house officer (SHO) level. In ENT, the specialist registrar grade is tenable for six years; after this time, trainees 'fall off' the training scheme whether or not there is a post available or suitable for them. After four years of higher surgical training and satisfactory in-training assessments, trainees sit the Intercollegiate FRCS in Otolaryngology.

Current and future training in otolaryngology/ head and neck surgery

At the time of writing, further changes to training are in the pipeline. The Chief Medical Officer, Sir Liam Donaldson, has published *Unfinished business*[10] and *Modernising medical careers*.[11] The Working Time Directive continues to bite, reducing the hours available for training further.

In the current proposals, the senior house officer grade is to be abolished and the preregistration house officer time replaced by two post-graduate foundation years. The remaining period of specialty training will be confined to six years:

1. medical qualification;
2. two years' post-graduate training – foundation years;
3. specialist registrar – six years' specialty training based on new curriculum. Specialty-specific

MRCS after two years. FRCS (Otolaryngology) towards the end of the training period;
4. specialist in generality of ENT.

At present, there is no consensus as to the precise nature of what a specialist in this context will be or be able to do. 'Working in teams within a defined range of competencies' is the phase currently used. This is very different from 'independent practice'.

Terms such as 'emergency safe' have been widely adopted. Emergency safe in all aspects of ENT represents a high level of training. To deal with adult and paediatric airway problems, acute middle ear disease and orbital cellulitis and even severe nose bleeds requires a wide range of skills. There is no clarity about provision for super-specialized training in areas such as otology, paediatrics, skull base and head and neck surgery.

Curriculum development project

Under the auspices of the Surgical Royal Colleges, each specialty has been working on curriculum development. The new curriculum is much more explicit than any previous attempt and contains standards, criteria and assessment modalities. The ENT curriculum is near completion. The curriculum covers both generic and specialist skills. Using *Good surgical practice*[4] as a guide, the following generic skills are specified and assessed:

- good clinical care;
- communication skills;
- maintaining good medical practice;
- maintaining trust;
- working with colleagues;
- teaching and training.

For example, communication skills have a specified objective and the appropriate knowledge, skills, attitudes and means of assessment are explicit.

Table 44.1 shows an example of the curriculum document relating to ENT communication skills. In the specialty-specific parts of the curriculum, a similar approach is applied and the knowledge, skills, professional attributes and assessment are specified. In addition, an indication of the depth of the ability or knowledge at each stage in training is given, where (1) is introductory level and (4) is advanced. **Table 44.2** shows an example of the paediatric ENT curriculum document.[12]

CONTINUING PROFESSIONAL DEVELOPMENT AND THE MAINTENANCE OF SKILLS

All practitioners are obliged to keep up to date and monitor their performance. These obligations are laid out

Table 44.1 ENT communication skills. Objective: To communicate effectively with patients, relatives and colleagues in the different spheres of clinical practice.

Circumstance	Knowledge	Skills	Attitudes	Assessment
Within a consultation	Structuring the interview by identifying the concerns of patients and, where applicable, parents of paediatric patients	Active listening: Appropriate use of different question types. Use language appropriate for developmental stage of child. Check patients and where appropriate parents and child's understanding. Avoid jargon. Appropriate use of interpreters	Demonstrate empathy with patients and family. Be aware of importance of utilizing these skills. Be aware of importance of involving patients and parents in decisions. Offering choices. Respecting other views	Observed practice on ward rounds (teaching and business). Theatre practice and 'on-take'. Progress and outcomes recorded in trainer's report. Might include attendance at taught course
Breaking bad news	Structuring the interview and organizing setting. Normal process of bereavement and associated behaviours. Awareness of local policy on organ donation procedures and role of transplant coordinators	As above with emphasis on the avoidance of jargon. Encourage questions. Appropriate manner, avoiding undue optimism or pessimism	Demonstrate empathy sensitivity and honesty	Observed involvement in the clinical setting. Might include attendance at taught course. Information forwarded to trainer's report
With colleagues	How and when to communicate effectively with other members of the care team, including the use of handover rounds	To outline clinical case concisely. Identifying patients' and parents' concerns	Be aware of who requires information and expected level of detail. The contribution others can make to clinical decisions	Observed practice in clinical setting. Information forwarded to trainer's report
Complaints	Awareness of local policy for dealing with complaints	Deal with complaints in oral and written communication. Contribute where required to local complaints procedure	Demonstrate honesty and sensitivity in dealing with complaints	Observed practice and review of complaints with trainee as part of appraisal process

in detail in *Good medical practice* and *Good surgical practice*. The key points are:

- 'you must maintain the standard of your performance by keeping your knowledge and skills up-to-date throughout your working life';[1]
- 'all surgeons must maintain their knowledge base and performance by fulfilling the continuing professional development (CPD) requirements of the Senate of Surgery and registering this with their college'.[4]

There are European and UK policy and frameworks for CPD.[13, 14] The Senate of Surgery expects that all surgical staff, other than those in training, will participate in CPD. This includes substantive and locum consultants, associate specialists and staff grades.

Requirements for continuing professional development

The minimum requirement for CPD in the UK is 50 credits per annum. One credit represents one hour of activity. CPD is viewed over a five-year cycle. Full- and part-time practitioners require full CPD (not *pro rata*).

Table 44.2 Management of common paediatric conditions.

Subject/topic	Knowledge	Clinical skills	Relevant professional skills	Assessment
Neck masses in infants and children	The embryology and anatomy of the neck with particular reference to the thyroid gland and branchial arch structures[4]	Elicit clinical history and signs. Be able to deduce a differential diagnosis and formulate strategy to reach final diagnosis	Be able to advise the patient and parents of the treatment options[4]	Knowledge-based assessment
	Understanding of the classification of neck masses[4]	Able to examine the oral cavity, oropharynx and neck[4]		Clinical assessment in out patients
	Awareness of the various hypotheses relating to the aetiology of neck masses[4]	Be able to perform excision of thyroglossal and branchial cleft cysts competently[4]	Discuss risks and potential benefits, potential complications and obtain informed consent[4]	Supervised operating, including pre- and postoperative patient management
	Understand the principles of the medical and surgical management of neck masses and their complications[4]	Recognize rarer causes of neck masses, such as first arch abnormalities, tumours, e.g. lymphomas, granulomatous conditions and lymphangiomas[3]	Be aware of specific issues that relate to the management of children in hospital[4]	Evidence of attendance on course dealing with issues relating to the surgical child

To understand the aetiology, presenting signs, symptoms and management of common paediatric ORL conditions. This module gives some indication of the breadth and depth of required knowledge and surgical skills. The list should not be considered to be fully inclusive or exhaustive.

A number of categories of CPD exist, the principle ones being internal and external. Practitioners need to participate in a mix of activities, such as outlined below:

- 25 external credits: for example, attendance at courses or conferences for which CPD credits have been awarded;
- 25 internal credits:
  - 10 hospital-based activities: for example, teaching rounds, pathology and radiology meetings;
  - 10 independent study: reading journals, writing papers;
  - 5 audit: contributing to and attendance at meetings.

At the time of writing, no CPD return has been checked, validated or audited. There is no policing of the system. The number of returns completed overall has been unsatisfactory, 63 percent in 2000. ENT surgeons have done better with returns of approximately 70 percent. Of the returns received by the Surgical Royal Colleges, little more than a half meet all the requirements.

Table 44.3 indicates the categories and amount of continuing medical education (CME) required by the Surgical Royal Colleges. Table 44.4 summarizes the CPD returns held by the Royal College of Surgeons of England in ENT and surgeons in general.

Accreditation of continuing professional development points

The system for conferring CME credits is as follows. Applications are made to either the Surgical Royal College or specialist association. The application form requires basic details of the course or conference content. There is an obligation on the course organizer to keep an attendance register and to collect feedback from the participants. Credits are awarded, on behalf of the British Association of Otolaryngologists – Head and Neck Surgeons, by the Chair of the Education and Training Committee. Feedback from the course is then collected. Despite the current lack of supervision and enforcement,

Table 44.3 Annual continual professional development (CPD) requirements.

Division of CPD activity		Annual requirement
Internal CPD, hospital-based		
A	Postgraduate meetings	Minimum 10 CPD credits
B	Research meetings	
C	Journal clubs	
D	Other CPD	
Internal CPD		
E	Independent study	Minimum 10 CPD credits
Internal CPD		
F	Clinical audit	Minimum 5 CPD credits
External CPD, meetings and courses		
G	External meetings	Minimum 25 CPD credits
H	External courses	
I	Distance learning	
J	Postgraduate examinations work	
K	Visiting another unit	

Internal CPD (A–F) = 25 CPD credits, external CPD (G–K) = 25 CPD credits. Fifty credits per annum are in line with European and US norms. However, it is unclear why this number was chosen. In educational terms, the quality and appropriateness of CPD is considered more important than the quantity.

Table 44.4 Continuing professional development participation 2000–2001.

	2000	2001
No. surgeons registered for CPD		
All	5342.0	5888.0
ENT	579	573
Percentage of returns received		
All	63	60
ENT	71	72
Percentage of those returned who achieved (all)	46	46
Minimum CPD requirements for ENT	52	48

Note. As of February 2003, there are 719 ENT surgeons registered for CPD with the Senate of Surgery of Great Britain and Ireland, 80% of these are consultant ENT surgeons, 20% are non-consultant career-grade (NCCG) doctors.

all surgeons would be well advised to ensure that their CPD affairs are in order. These credits are reviewed at annual appraisals for National Health Service (NHS) consultants.

A review of applications for CPD credits to the British Association of Otolaryngologists over a six-month period is shown in **Table 44.5**.

Table 44.5 CME points awarded by BAO-HNS for applications received between October 2003 and April 2004.

	Points awarded
Number of events	32
Number of days	73
Number of points awarded	375
Average points per day	5.14

GUIDANCE FOR SURGEONS ON APPRAISAL AND REVALIDATION: SPECIALTY-SPECIFIC GUIDANCE FOR EAR, NOSE AND THROAT SURGEONS

The Joint Committee on Continuing Professional Development, chaired by Professor Graham T. Layer (reporting to Senate) is reviewing the system of CPD. New methods of registration and monitoring are likely. As part of this overhaul, specialty-specific guidelines are being drawn up. These specialty-specific guidelines should be read in conjunction with the parent generic document.

Good clinical care

DEFINITION

The ENT surgeon possesses a defined body of knowledge and skills within the area of the head and neck. These are used to collect and interpret data, make appropriate clinical decisions and carry out diagnostic and therapeutic procedures within the boundaries of their expertise. Their care is characterized by up-to-date, ethical clinical practice and effective communication with patients, other health workers and the community.

INDIVIDUAL STANDARDS

- Demonstrate diagnostic and therapeutic skills for ethical and effective patient care in the area of the head and neck.
- Access and apply relevant information to clinical practice.
- Demonstrate effective consultation services with respect to patient care and education.
- Establish therapeutic relationship with patients/ families.

PRESENTING YOUR EVIDENCE

- Demonstrate awareness and application of good practice guidelines such as those produced by the British Association of Otorhinolaryngologists – Head and Neck Surgeons (BAO-HNS) (vestibular schwannoma, head and neck cancer documents

available on www.entuk.org) and others, e.g. *Good practice in cosmetic surgery.*
- Proof of involvement in audit, including national audit, if appropriate, e.g. National Sino-nasal Audit, National Prospective Tonsillectomy Audit.

Maintaining good surgical practice

DEFINITION

The ENT surgeon recognizes the need to constantly review activity and ensure that part of their regular CPD focusses on the generality of ENT, as well as on their own area of subspecialization.

INDIVIDUAL STANDARDS

- Attendance at annual general meeting of BAO-HNS (or equivalent body) at least every other year (home or abroad).
- Attendance at subspecialty professional surgical meeting at least every other year (home or abroad).
- Attendance at practical skills revision workshop, perhaps every five years.
- Involvement in regular audit meetings on a local/regional basis with involvement in national audit/attendance at national audit meeting every five years.
- If involved in teaching, attendance at 'Training the trainers' or equivalent course.
- Attendance at a critical appraisal course or equivalent.
- Regular review of a relevant journal, e.g. *Clinical Otolaryngology*, *Journal of Laryngology and Otology* or equivalent journal.

DEMONSTRATING YOUR EVIDENCE

- Certificates of attendance at courses.
- Copies of published articles, book chapters, etc.
- Guidelines written.
- Logbooks.

Teaching/training

DEFINITION

ENT surgeons have a responsibility for the training of students, trainees and other members of the healthcare team (including staff working in audiology, speech and language departments).

INDIVIDUAL STANDARDS

- Help others define learning needs and directions for development.
- Provide constructive feedback.

- Demonstrate an understanding of preferred learning methods in dealing with students and trainees.

DEMONSTRATING YOUR EVIDENCE

- Summary of formal teaching activities.
- Results of feedback from trainees on the effectiveness of teaching/training.

Relationship with patients

DEFINITION

Communication skills are essential for the functioning of an ENT surgeon and are necessary for obtaining information from, and conveying information to, patients and their families.

INDIVIDUAL STANDARDS

- Ability to establish and maintain rapport with patient characterized by understanding, trust, empathy and confidentiality.
- Ability to inform and counsel a patient in a sensitive and respectful manner, while fostering understanding, discussion and the patient's active participation in decisions about their care.

DEMONSTRATING YOUR EVIDENCE

- Evidence of involvement of patient groups when composing guidelines/information leaflets.
- Summary of complaints/letters of thanks.

Working with colleagues

DEFINITION

It is essential for an ENT surgeon to be able to collaborate effectively with a multidisciplinary team of expert health professionals for provision of optimal patient care.

INDIVIDUAL STANDARDS

- A collaborative approach includes the ability to recognize the limits of personal expertise, understand the roles and expertise of other individuals involved and explicitly integrate the opinions of those individuals into the management plan.
- Contributing effectively to other interdisciplinary activities implies the ability to recognize team members' areas of expertise, respect the opinions and roles of individual team members, contribute to healthy team development and conflict resolution, and contribute his/her own expertise to the team's task.

DEMONSTRATING YOUR EVIDENCE

- Evidence of involvement in multidisciplinary team meetings/clinics, e.g. head and neck oncology clinics, voice clinics, etc.
- Evidence of liaising with colleagues regarding emergency on-call cover, cover for absence, etc.

Probity, health and managerial

See generic continuing professional development document.

Future directions for training and revalidation

Surgery and its practice are evolving. The needs of society are changing and the pace of this change is accelerating. The modern surgeon has to respond to this situation. The demands on trainees and established surgeons will continue to grow. Resources will always be restricted. We will have to train the next generation of surgeons in considerably less time than at present. Ahead lies a simple choice between depth and breadth of training. Few will ever be able to acquire the full range of skills and experience of their predecessors. Those embarking on a surgical career will become 'specialists' in a shorter time. They are likely to have a proscribed range of skills and will from time to time need to demonstrate their on-going competency. Assessment of competence and demonstration of on-going performance requires considerable effort. One needs to determine precisely what is to be tested, devise ways to do so, ensure consistent assessment and determine appropriate standards.[15]

Revalidation of specialists and consultants may take many formats: bench top models, observation of practice, formal examinations or peer reviews. Whatever method is used, most surgeons will 'pass' the test. If they do not, then there is either something wrong with the test or the service will collapse. The General Medical Council is currently considering what form revalidation will take.[16] In the future, a doctor will need to be registered, but will also need a licence to practise. The licence will be subject to revalidation. Revalidation will be possible by two routes, an appraisal route open to those working in a hospital or academic environment and an independent route in which the practitioner will have to demonstrate evidence of adopting the standards of *Good medical practice* and undertaking continuing medical and professional development. Revalidation is due to commence in 2005.

REFERENCES

1. General Medical Council. *Good medical practice.* London: General Medical Council, May, 2001.
2. The Shipman Inquiry. Chair Dame Janet Smith. First report, July, 2002.
3. The Inquiry into the Management of Care of Children Receiving Complex Heart Surgery at the Bristol Royal Infirmary. Chair Professor Ian Kennedy, July, 2002.
4. The Royal College of Surgeons of England. *Good surgical practice.* London: The Royal College of Surgeons of England, September, 2002.
5. Skills for the New Millennium: Report of the Societal Needs Working Group. The Royal College of Physicians and Surgeons of Canada's Canadian Medical Education Directions for Specialists 2000 Project. September, 1996.
6. Consultant Surgeons. *Teamworking in surgical practice.* The Senate of Surgery of Great Britain and Ireland, May, 2000.
7. European Working Time Directive, No. 93/104/EC. Council of the European Union.
8. Department of Health. *New deal for junior doctors.* London: Department for Health, 1991.
9. Department of Health. *A guide to specialist training.* London: Department of Health, 1993.
10. Department of Health. *Unfinished business: proposals for the reform of the SHO grade.* London: Department of Health, 2002.
11. Department of Health. *Modernising medical careers.* London: Department of Health, 2003.
12. ENT Curriculum Document. *Work in progress by SAC in otolaryngology.* Chair: Mr Kevin Gibbin, 2004.
13. Academy of Medical Royal Colleges. *A framework for continuing professional development.* London: Academy of Medical Royal Colleges, February, 2002.
14. European Union of Medical Specialists. *Basel declaration and policy on continuing professional development.* UEMS (European Union of Medical Specialists), October, 2001.
15. The Royal College of Surgeons of England and Smith and Nephew Foundation. *Surgical competence, challenges of assessment in training and practice.* London: The Royal College of Surgeons of England, 1999.
16. General Medical Council. *A licence to practise and revalidation.* London: The General Medical Council, 2003.

45

Communication and the medical consultation

DAMIAN GARDNER-THORPE AND RICHARD CANTER

Introduction	559	Conclusions	566
The biomedical approach to patient care	559	Key points	566
The patient-centred approach	560	References	567
Core communication skills	564		

INTRODUCTION

Every day of our working lives we rely upon communication skills to build up relationships with our patients and colleagues. These core clinical skills are undeniably important in establishing trust and rapport with those who come to us for help and advice. To understand the increasing importance of communication skills, it is helpful to consider the way in which healthcare delivery has altered within western culture. The traditional biomedical approach to healthcare, which defines illness largely in terms of abnormal anatomy and physiology, has become outmoded because of its failure to recognize the full emotional cost of illness and the wider effects of disease upon the individual. The patient-centred approach to healthcare tackles the problem by focussing upon the patient's perspective.

There is, of course, an additional reason why the otolaryngologist takes a particular interest in communication issues. Whilst most of us are able to take our primary senses for granted, a proportion of our patients live with significant hearing loss or speech impairment, and this imparts upon us a special responsibility to remain sensitive to these differences without underestimating the ability of our patients to adapt to their unique environment. Just as our patients experience frustration in some clinical encounters, we too become aware of communication difficulties when our usual channels of conversation are blocked. To meet the challenge, we must acknowledge and accept our role in difficult encounters and devise strategies to meet them.[1]

In this chapter, we discuss the traditional biomedical approach, its limitations in maintaining a balanced consultation and the concept of patient-centred care. We hope to explore aspects of the consultation, which present particular challenges, and to understand the patient's perspective to generate a better awareness of our own behaviour in difficult clinical encounters.

THE BIOMEDICAL APPROACH TO PATIENT CARE

Over 50 years ago, Parsons examined the relationship between doctors and patients in order to describe their roles within society in the context of the prevailing attitudes towards healthcare.[2] Most patients accepted their responsibility to overcome illness as soon as possible, to seek professional advice from their doctor and to cooperate willingly with any advice offered. The doctor was expected to apply his or her knowledge and specialist skills to affect a cure. The doctor had a duty to act in the interests of the patient before his or her own and to adopt an emotionally detached and professional manner. In return for this, he or she was granted the right to enquire into intimate areas of personal life, to perform physical examinations and to assume a position of authority in relation to the patient. Whilst these values are still recognizable, the majority of patients now expect a very different style of healthcare and doctors have learnt to modify their traditional practice to meet an increased demand for a mutualistic approach to the consultation.

Intrigued by the changing face of healthcare, Byrne and Long[3] tape-recorded over 2500 general practice consultations and analysed the behaviour of the doctors and the patients. They identified two extreme consultation styles, which they labelled 'patient-centred' and 'doctor-centred'. The patient-centred approach avoids an authoritarian style and encourages the patient to take a pro-active part in the consultation. Key aspects of this include listening, moments of reflection, facilitation and the use of silence, but were found in no more than one quarter of the taped consultations. One characteristic of a doctor-centred relationship is the frequency with which the doctor will interrupt a patient's account of their illness. In a patient-centred encounter, the patient is encouraged to participate actively in the consultation whilst the doctor provides 'expert' knowledge, contextualizes appropriate management options and facilitates decision-making.

Other investigators have identified more sophisticated models of doctor–patient experiences. One such model describes four categories of interaction reflecting the balance of power that exists within a consultation. These categories are paternalism, consumerism, mutuality and default (**Figure 45.1**).[4]

Paternalism describes a traditional model of a passive patient and a dominant physician. This relationship is generally outmoded, but can offer significant support to frightened or anxious patients who derive comfort in such a traditional doctor–*parent* figure. Paternalism is especially important when patients are sick and vulnerable. It is of interest that when they are ill, physicians themselves prefer to hand over responsibility for their care to their colleagues and are most comfortable with a paternalistic model.[5] However, they have usually chosen their attending physician with care.

A consumerist approach is one where the power relationship is reversed and the patient takes a more pro-active role in the consultation. The doctor adopts a passive role and accedes to the patient's requests, for example for a prescription, procedure or second opinion. Although the model at first sight espouses patient control, it may also reveal situations where the doctor is reliant upon the patient for goodwill or financial settlement. There are some groups in society, including the young, the better educated and those with previous experience of unhappy consultations, who are more likely to confront the doctor's traditional authority and expect a consumerist approach.

A default situation occurs when neither doctor nor patient takes a lead in the consultation. This situation arises when the patient adopts an overly passive style and the doctor fails to assume control. This inevitably leads to a lack of direction and purpose in the encounter.

Mutuality exists when the physician brings their experience and expertise to the consultation, the patient brings his or her expectations, feelings and symptoms, and both parties participate in a joint venture to explore the possible outcomes and treatment options. Mutuality succeeds because of shared decision-making responsibility and because of a willingness of both parties to adhere to any agreed plan. The style has been described as a 'contractual' approach to patient care because within this arrangement the patient is free to seek care elsewhere when his or her expectations are not satisfied, and the doctor may withdraw from the relationship when patient requests are considered inappropriate, ethically untenable or impossible to meet.

Of course it is possible, indeed likely, that more than one model will be employed during a course of treatment. At the outset, when investigations need to be performed and the diagnosis made, a paternalistic model may be appropriate. This is particularly the case when patients are anxious, for example if there is the possibility of cancer. Later, when treatment options are discussed, a model of consumerism or mutuality would be more appropriate. There is a case for negotiating these different models of consultation style with the patient. The physician may therefore suggest that to begin with he or she 'takes over the running of the care', but later when treatment options are to be discussed, he or she will switch to a more mutualistic consultation style.

THE PATIENT-CENTRED APPROACH

There are several aspects of the consultation which we might wish to consider in the context of the evolution of the patient-centred approach. These include issues of power, an understanding of basic ethical principles and the factors which determine compliance. A basic understanding of these may help to understand why communication sometimes fails.

Issues of power

Doctors, perhaps subconsciously, control the behaviour of their patients. Sometimes the reverse is also true. The balance of 'power' depends upon several patient factors including the extent of the patient's medical knowledge and their capacity to choose between options. Nevertheless, an appreciation of power dynamics helps avoid the risk of applying unintentional or unjustified influence on our patients.

	Low physician control	High physician control
Low patient control	Default	Paternalism
High patient control	Consumerism	Mutuality

Figure 45.1 Consultation styles resulting from the level of interaction between the patient and the doctor. Redrawn from Ref. 4, with permission from Sage Publications.

To understand the role of power in the clinical encounter, let us define power as the means by which A gets B to do something, where A might be the doctor and B might be the patient.

Power is exerted upon patients in several ways. The most obvious form is expert power, in which a doctor exerts influence by virtue of his or her possession of specialist knowledge. Expert power is rarely used alone, but is instead exercised in conjunction with other forms of power including power of legitimacy (power devolved to a doctor from the Royal Colleges or the General Medical Council), coercive power, charismatic power and of course the offer of rewards, including relief of symptoms.[6] Most clinicians exercise these elements of power to suit their consultation style and to achieve a degree of patient compliance. Nevertheless, this is a simple model of power and it is not that helpful in understanding power in the clinical encounter.

Lukes[7] produced a generalized model of power that does shed light on the clinical situation. He saw power as operating in three dimensions: first dimensional power is when A forces B to do something, the second is that in which A controls the agenda in any interaction with B and the third dimension, in which A controls the world view of B.

So how does this power model apply to the clinical encounter?

First dimensional power is analogous to coercive power. It might be exercised appropriately in emergency situations, in certain acute psychiatric states or when patients are extremely distressed or anxious and do not wish to debate alternative choices. First dimensional power is frequently exercised in the emergency arena, for example, when a stridulous patient is told that he needs a tracheostomy or a patient with a brisk epistaxis is told that he must undergo immediate nasal packing, even if the treatment itself causes agitation or distress.

Second dimensional power is exercised when the doctor deliberately steers conversation towards or away from certain topics in order to influence final outcome. Patient choice will be biased because of a selective presentation of information. This may happen when consultation time is limited or when doctors make it difficult for patients to ask questions in clinic. Second dimensional power may also result from the increasing reliance upon guidelines and protocols which dictate outcome goals without offering any flexibility for alternative options within the process of the consultation. It also includes the power to silence or make it difficult for the patient to ask certain questions.

Third dimensional power is harder to appreciate. It manifests itself when a doctor constructs for his or her patient a world view of disease and treatment. The patient believes he or she moves autonomously, but is in fact under the influence of the flow of medical knowledge as presented by the doctor. Consider for a moment the situation faced by a patient with malignant disease of the larynx, who has to make choices about the treatment options of palliation, radiotherapy, chemotherapy, surgery or various combinations of each. The encounter is framed within a definition of malignant disease in a conventional biomedical model. A discussion follows, looking at the effectiveness of each of these treatment options, based upon the physician's understanding of results reported in the medical literature together with his or her experience of previous cases. The patient is apparently free to choose, but these choices have been shaped and polished by the manner in which they have been presented.

The biomedical world view can be demonstrated quite easily, because within a conventional biomedical framework model there would be no place for herbal medicine, acupuncture, osteopathy or any other of the many complementary medical alternatives. Indeed, when these issues are raised within a conventional medical consultation, they are frequently problematic.

An ethical framework

An ethical framework is required to place the patient's interests at the centre of the decision-making process. Because of the imbalances that exist between doctors and patients, not only in terms of power but also in terms of knowledge and skills, there is a very real benefit in having a set of principles, sanctioned by society, to guide the doctor in making the best decisions with or on behalf of his or her patients. Such ethical principles have existed since Hippocratic times and have evolved through history in response to novel treatments, new dilemmas and changing attitudes within society.

The most widely employed ethical framework is the four principle framework, or *Principlism*. It comprises a simple, logical and culturally sensitive approach to ethical problems and is useful for most clinical situations where there is a difficult conflict of interest. The four components are autonomy, justice, beneficence and nonmaleficence.[8]

The first of these, autonomy, is the capacity to think and to have freedom to act upon these free thoughts without let or hindrance. Autonomy empowers patients to make decisions for themselves. Full self-determination is not possible within the constraints of a civilized society as we cannot each expect to live according to our own personal rules. Instead we must act within the rules of society and exercise our right to autonomy within cultural boundaries and the laws of the land. In the context of the medical consultation, the individual's right to autonomy should be respected as long as it does not adversely affect other members of the community. This means that the patient has the absolute right, in almost all situations, to choose their preferred treatment and be free to reject any intervention without prejudice. There are, of course, situations where the patient delegates his or her autonomy to the doctor – 'You decide for me, doctor' – in which case the doctor must defer to the basic Hippocratic principles of beneficence (doing what is good) and nonmaleficence (not doing that which is harmful).

Situations exist where the doctor bypasses the principle of autonomy. Usually this results from the patient's lack of capacity to exercise autonomy resulting from immaturity, disability or disease, but it also happens when the individual's actions impinge upon the well-being of others and in this instance the doctor must consider the rules of justice. Nevertheless, it follows that we need to be honest and open with our patients, consult them before we do things to them, keep patient information confidentially and respect a patient's right to choose what is and what is not done to them whenever possible.

Beneficence and nonmaleficence are the oldest two principles. Beneficence is the duty to do that which is best for the patient – even if this is at some personal cost to the doctor. Beneficent traits include basic qualities of a doctor including friendliness, good manners and good time-keeping. Nonmaleficence is the duty to do no harm. However, it is all too easy to envisage a situation where an intervention has the potential to improve an outcome, but only with the risk of serious side effects. We are responsible for considering the best option for our patients, 'all things considered'.

We run into difficulties, especially in the modern technological world of medicine, when we cause harm to our patients through an intention to do well. Although the principle of nonmaleficence tempers us in our decision-making process, we must try to avoid the tendency towards inappropriate paternalism in deciding the best management option for our patients – to do so takes choice away from patients and risks a breach in the duty of autonomy. Consider this in the context of another, perhaps more traditional approach where arrogance is held as a virtue, preferable indeed to the virtue of humility: 'if you agree that the physician's primary function is to make the patient feel better, a certain amount of authoritarianism, paternalism and domination are the essence of the physician's effectiveness'.[9]

Justice, or a 'just' distribution of health care resource focusses upon making fair decisions when there are competing claims. Justice is particularly important in rationed health care systems where available services are shared out among many individuals. Doctors are some-times responsible for deciding how to share out these resources, which include their time and skills, as well as expensive investigations and treatments, and this may not necessarily mean being even-handed to every patient.

Compliance

Compliance has been defined as the 'extent to which the patient's behaviour coincides with medical or other health care advice' and applies equally to lifestyle advice,

accepting prescription medication and following advice to undergo surgery.[10] Amongst doctors, there is perhaps a naive expectation that patients should comply with their advice, though in practice it is hard to determine the reasons why patients do not act upon guidance.

Not surprisingly, there is increasing interest in the factors which underpin compliance. The three prime factors are believed to be a good understanding of advice, a high level of satisfaction and an ability to recall information handed over by the clinician.

While it is clear that compliance depends upon a good level of understanding between doctor and patient, there is a tendency for health care providers to overestimate the patient's medical knowledge. When a group of patients were asked to describe the approximate position of vital organs within the body, fewer than one-fifth were able to locate the stomach and fewer than half knew where to find the heart or liver.[11, 12]

Medical jargon is often confusing and despite our best intentions we frequently lapse into a technical vocabulary which patients cannot comprehend. The word vertigo means very different things to different individuals and the ear, nose and throat (ENT) specialist will also be aware of the imprecise usage of this term throughout the profession. We need to be sure that patients understand our definition of terms and that we appreciate their use of descriptive language too. One straightforward way to check the level of this understanding is to ask patients to repeat back in simple terms their interpretation of the situation.

Some expressions run the risk of trivializing the serious nature of a medical problem, for example 'just pop on the couch' or 'we'll just have a quick look at your ear'. Nevertheless, we need to remain sensitive to the patient's level of understanding and contextualize our language according to patients' individual needs. There are circumstances where rapport is strengthened by setting out a clear agenda at the start of a consultation, by explaining, for example that we may interrupt in order to focus on to particular aspects of a history. An example of this might be during a consultation for 'dizziness' where a fastidious approach to history taking is required to reach a reliable differential diagnosis.

The capacity for information recall varies greatly between individuals. The factors which influence recall include the volume and complexity of the message, as well as the impact that it has upon the individual. Evidence from primary care suggests that surprisingly little factual information is retained by the patient following the end of the consultation. For example, in one study over a third of patients failed to recall the name of their prescription medicine and a quarter failed to appreciate the duration of the course of their medication.[13] Given the particular importance of accurate information transfer in surgical specialties, one approach to reinforce handover of knowledge is to dictate the clinic letter in the presence of the patient, in plain and unambiguous English, and to offer the patient a copy for his or her own records.

A number of interesting cognitive factors explain how patients behave in particular health settings. Heuristics are 'rules of thumb' which explain patterns of behaviour, for example in relation to perception of risk or threat from disease. Weinstein[14] coined the term 'unrealistic optimism' to account for the observation that individuals tend to underestimate the risk of a threat to which they are specifically vulnerable. He tested the popular belief that people think themselves invulnerable, by demonstrating in a group of college students a systemic error in estimating personal risk from negative and positive threats. For example, the students overestimated their chances of enjoying their first job or owning their own home, but underestimated their risk of contracting a venereal disease, having a drink problem or getting lung cancer. Their misguided perceptions result from a complex interplay of factors including differing egocentric biases, personal experiences and stereotyped beliefs. Other heuristics influence susceptibility judgements; for example, the tendency for individuals to overestimate their personal risk from less likely causes of death, but to underestimate the risk from more common ones.[15] An appreciation of risk perception is especially pertinent to those taking informed consent for surgery.

Simple and effective techniques for increasing compliance include provision of written information, keeping explanations simple, repeating important points and the judicious use of follow-up appointments. We should remember too that patients tend to recall the first and last pieces of information that they receive – the primacy and recency effects.[12, 16]

Consultation models

In accepting the validity of the patient-centred approach, we can consider basic consultation theories which help explain the decision-making process from the patient's perspective. A number of these models overlap the field of health psychology and explore the role of the patient's motivation, health beliefs and the factors which underpin compliance.

Within the traditional paternalistic encounter, the consultation essentially involves the transfer of knowledge from expert to lay person. Whilst there may be many straightforward medical complaints where psychological and emotional components are less important, it is increasingly recognized that patient compliance and

satisfaction improve when the doctor contextualizes the disease within a more holistic approach.

Byrne and Long[3] outlined the essence of the doctor-centred relationship, largely analogous to the 'paternalistic' approach (**Figure 45.2**).

Pendleton *et al.*[17] devised a patient-centred model which encourages the doctor to explore the patient's ideas, concerns and expectations and to frame the consultation in a problem-solving approach. One vital tenet of Pendleton's model is the maintenance of a healthy doctor–patient relationship:

- define the reasons for the patient's attendance;
- consider other problems (including risk factors for current complaint);
- negotiate the correct course of management of each of the presenting problems;
- achieve a shared understanding of the problem – both doctor and patient;
- involve the patient in management and encourage patient responsibility for care;
- use resources and time efficiently;
- establish and maintain a healthy doctor–patient relationship.

Neighbour,[18] in perhaps the most widely used patient-centred model, espouses an appreciation of subtle clues in the consultation, verbal and nonverbal. The model establishes good doctor–patient rapport and helps the clinician identify and address underlying concerns. This elegant model uniquely recognizes the importance of the role of the doctor and reminds the clinician of his personal risk of stress, anxiety and burn-out:

- **connecting**: where the doctor establishes rapport;
- **summarizing**: clarification of the patient's reason for attendance;
- **handing over**: joint negotiation of the correct course of management;
- **safety netting**: managing uncertainty and planning for the unexpected;
- **housekeeping**: staying in touch with emotions and awareness of burn-out.

While none of these consultation models provides a comprehensive or universally reliable guide to a successful outcome, each has its place in dealing with difficult clinical encounters. Through the evolution of consultation modelling there has been a gradual shift towards a patient-centred emphasis which is likely to be

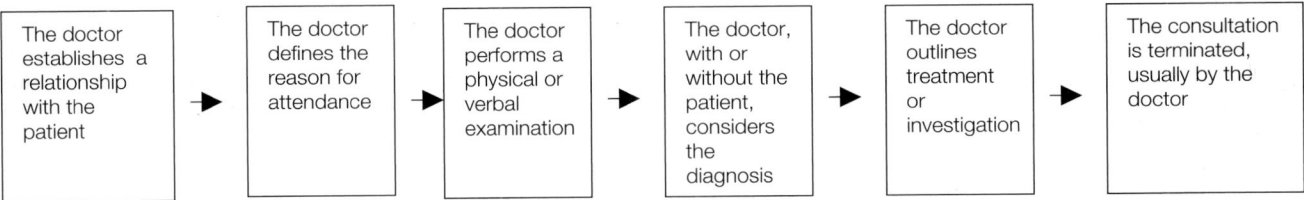

Figure 45.2 The traditional doctor-centred model. Redrawn from Ref. 3, with permission from HMSO.

the trend, at least for the current generation of healthcare providers.

CORE COMMUNICATION SKILLS

In an encounter between two individuals, it is said that less than 35 percent of the contact is established through verbal means, whilst 65 percent or more is conveyed through nonverbal cues including facial expression and eye contact.[19] Patients are particularly sensitive to nonverbal cues from their doctors, but doctors are often unaware of their influence in this respect. It is important to recognize the importance of subtle behavioural cues which are highly influential in determining the direction of the consultation and the subsequent outcome.

It is obvious that our patients are likely to prefer a more relaxed consulting environment. Since nonverbal methods of communication include the use of eye contact and body language, we may consider how these are influential in the consulting room. These factors include the layout of furniture, the relative positions of doctor and patient and the distance between them. A relaxed interaction is more likely when chairs are positioned at the same height to ensure good eye contact. A desk represents a potential barrier between the doctor and patient and may be an important factor in limiting the free flow of conversation. In one interesting experiment, the influence of the desk was analysed during consultations between a cardiologist and his patients. On alternate days the cardiologist removed the desk from his consulting room to assess the impact upon nonverbal cues and body language. When the desk was absent, more than half of all patients sat back and relaxed, but when the doctor was positioned behind the desk fewer than one in ten assumed a relaxed body posture and this corresponded with a drop in the level of meaningful interaction between the two.[19]

Knapp[20] looked into the importance of seating configurations in more detail, not only in the context of the medical encounter but also for its significance in business meetings and any other number of social occasions. He identified four independent seating positions for any interaction: the corner position, the cooperative position, the competitive-defensive position and the independent position (**Figure 45.3**).

In the corner position, two individuals are positioned in such a way that the corner of the desk intervenes. It usually results in casual friendly conversation. It allows unlimited eye contact and a full appreciation of gesture. The corner of the desk behaves as a partial barrier but does not intrude as a territorial division. The cooperative position differs from the corner position by the absence of any barrier and a straight face-to-face seating posture. Whilst this favours a mutualistic relationship, a number of individuals feel threatened by the lack of a firm boundary.

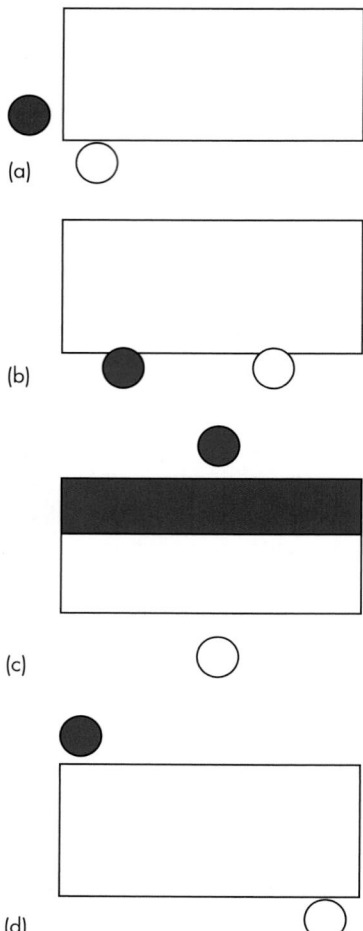

Figure 45.3 Examples of seat and desk arrangements. (a) The corner position; (b) The cooperative position; (c) The competitive–defensive position (the territorial line); (d) The independent position. Redrawn from Ref. 20, with permission.

In the competitive-defensive position, the desk constitutes a firm physical barrier. Not only does this prevent intimacy, but it may create competition for control of the consultation. An imaginary territorial line is evident between the doctor and patient. In contradistinction, the independent position is adopted by those who want to avoid interaction, just as people do when they sit in a library or on a train. This style would clearly be alien to a sensitive medical encounter and cannot be recommended!

Listening is of course a core communication skill in clinical medicine, though little attention is paid to its full importance. Burnard[21] describes three levels of listening. The first is at the linguistic level, comprising an understanding of words, phrases and metaphors. The second level is paralinguistic, where the listener takes cues from timing, volume, pitch and accent including the use of 'umms' and 'ahhs' in the fluency of speech. The third level is an appreciation of facial expression, gesture, touch, body position, proximity of doctor and patient, body movement and eye contact.

The first level involves the content of speech without any emotional connection. Second level skills allow the doctor to develop a 'free floating' attention, observing patient cues other than words alone. At the third level, the doctor maintains a 'free floating' attention whilst noticing paralinguistic features and nonverbal cues, as well as noting his own internal thoughts, sensations and feelings. Watkins[22] describes this as 'resonance' between doctor and patient, whereby information determined from the history is weighted according to nonverbal cues and is characterized in such a way that any underlying anxieties are exposed and addressed.

Eye contact serves many functions, and used appropriately, establishes trust, demonstrates integrity, controls the level of intimacy and assists in information transfer. The comfortable level of eye contact depends on the context of the consultation, the physical distance between the participants and their degree of familiarity. An appropriate distance between the doctor and patient is hard to gauge, but it has been established that as distance is reduced, many start to feel uncomfortable, and a distance of less than 30 cm produces tension in most individuals.[23]

Frustrating encounters

Notwithstanding our best attempts to construct the ideal consultation, each and every doctor encounters patients from time to time who provoke an inner sense of frustration or irritation, and this may be for no discernable reason. These patients have been identified within the general practice setting as 'heart-sink' patients. While general practitioners are more likely to see their patients repeatedly, the same emotional response to patients is encountered by doctors within hospital practice, especially when patients return with new symptoms on repeated occasions or when they fail to respond to treatment. One interesting aspect of this problem is that a heart-sink patient to one is not necessarily a heart-sink to another. This is explained by understanding that frustration is produced by both doctor- and patient-related factors, and probably represents a generalized failure of the doctor–patient interaction at a fundamental level. Of the many factors involved in a heart-sink encounter, doctor factors not surprisingly include low job satisfaction, the perception of an excessive workload and a lack of training or experience in counselling or communication skills.[24]

The heart-sink may be avoided by improved communication strategies, including a commitment to the ongoing development of consultation skills and identification of situations which cause stress. A number of special skills exist to combat the heart-sink encounter including a 'holding strategy' for listening and understanding the patient's problems without feeling the need to tackle all issues in one sitting.

Breaking bad news to patients

Sharing bad news with our patients is a difficult task to do well, so it is a little surprising that so often this has been the responsibility of relatively inexperienced members of a surgical team. A number of simple techniques may help to undertake this more sensitively. Some appear obvious, such as planning the consultation in advance, checking the facts and avoiding interruptions to ensure privacy. Breaking bad news can take a significant amount of time and it is important to avoid being rushed. We need to use simple straightforward language and avoid jargon. Many patients value the invitation to bring a relative or close friend for support, though we should be clear in establishing the nature of the relationship in order to understand how the news will impact upon them as well.

Nonverbal messages are as important as verbal ones. Patients need to be given sufficient time for silence, tears or anger. Even when the future looks bleak, be careful in using the phrase 'nothing can be done' since there are always ways of encouraging hope in any dire situation. Nevertheless, it is equally important to admit when we do not know the answers to difficult questions, such as life expectancy after a diagnosis of terminal disease. Most patients value the offer of ongoing support and follow up is especially valuable.

Dealing with loss

Surgical patients inevitably experience concerns about the potential disfigurement and loss of function which result from our actions. We have a clear duty to address these issues in appropriate depth. Within our specialty, patients undergo radical neck surgery, lose the functions of speech, swallowing, balance and the ability to hear properly. Perhaps not surprisingly, those who cope less well with loss of body function are those with a history of premorbid anxiety or depression, and these are factors that are easy to overlook in a busy consultation.[25] Consequently, a professional assessment of mental health may be a helpful part of preoperative planning for some of these patients prior to major surgery.

The reaction to a loss of function depends upon many complex factors. A sudden unexpected loss may magnify shock and increase difficulty in coping, and our colleagues in primary care will testify to the longer-term consequences of mental health problems after serious disease. Doctors are advised to be honest and frank to their patients in the early stages of disease, especially when there is little hope for recovery.

There are circumstances in which patients are disenfranchised from their normal pattern of grief and these include elements described as hidden and concealed losses. Hidden loss takes place when patients are unable to share their experiences with even close friends or relatives, perhaps because of the shame of human immunodeficiency virus (HIV) or because of religious or social stigma. Concealed loss happens when relatives or doctors fail to share information with patients because of a misplaced belief, often with good intentions, that the patient cannot cope with bad news. This rationale for concealment is usually poorly grounded and an opportunity to come to terms with reality may be missed. Many patients have a remarkable capacity to adapt to bad news and may become angry if they later learn that information has been withheld.[26]

Whether consciously or unconsciously, avoiding grief can lead to difficult outcomes both for doctors and for patients. While doctors are conditioned to remain calm in adversity, they often experience difficulty describing their emotions once a stressful situation has passed. Those who learn to express their emotions report greater satisfaction at work and presumably function better as doctors.[26]

Loss of hearing

The limitations caused by hearing loss depend greatly on the age of onset and on the extent of any residual function. Prelingual deafness is that in which impairment of hearing predates language acquisition and by definition necessitates development of communication skills by alternative means. It is misleading to consider prelingual deafness a loss of function without considering the rich alternative language skills that arise through the use of sign language. The visual–spatial axis of sign language may be developed in the first few years of life, during the critical period of language assimilation, to the same extent as the more common linguistic route. The distinction between truly deaf individuals and those who become deafened later in life is important. Properly nurtured, the congenitally deaf individual is able to develop normal communication skills within the deaf community without any requirement for the spoken word, whereas the individual who encounters hearing loss after normal development suffers an immeasurable handicap without augmentation or alternative aids.

THE DEAF COMMUNITY

Absence of hearing does not necessarily correspond to handicap. Deaf communities thrive throughout the world, enjoying their unique cultural existence with a vibrant and expressive language. Different forms of sign have developed across the world independent of spoken language.

In 2003, the UK Government formally recognized British sign language (BSL) as a language in its own right, banishing the fallacy that it represents a rudimentary translation of spoken English. The ruling affords BSL the status of a native British language, equal to Welsh or Scots Gaelic as a minority language. As many as 70,000 people in the UK communicate in BSL, a rich and complex language employing hand shapes, facial expressions and body language within defined spatial boundaries.

To understand the importance of this landmark recognition, one must recall the bigotry and persecution experienced by generations of deaf individuals, many of whom were forced to learn to vocalize language and suppress their natural tendency to sign during the critical time of language acquisition.

Our role as health care providers is to encourage and respect the autonomy of the deaf community and to assist with technological innovation or general professional services, when required.

ACQUIRED HEARING LOSS

In routine practice we frequently encounter patients with acquired hearing loss. There are a number of simple methods for improving communication within the consultation. Slow, deliberate speech of adequate volume in a room with low ambient noise will assist those with a modest hearing loss. A face-to-face position and clear enunciation of words enables lip reading in those with longstanding loss. Other simple but underused communication aids include diagrams, models and picture boards.

CONCLUSIONS

There has been a cultural shift in the way in which doctors and patients interact and this has resulted in the evolution of the patient-centred approach to health care. Despite this, there are many elements of the consultation which are difficult to recognize, including issues of empowerment. Since our prime responsibility is to act in our patients' best interests, it is important for us to understand the ways in which we influence our patients, whether consciously or not. We also need to recognize our own feelings and anxieties when we deal with difficult situations and to appreciate the particular difficulties which arise when we deal with patients with sensory deficit. To learn good communication techniques takes time and experience and inviting feedback from patients should be encouraged rather than feared. It is a useful idea to encourage feedback from patients either during or at the end of the consultation. As the old saying goes 'asking saves a lot of guesswork'.

KEY POINTS

- The traditional approach to the consultation is being superseded by a more patient-centred ethos.
- Power dynamics play an important but often unappreciated role in the doctor–patient encounter.

- The four-principle framework is comprised of beneficence, nonmaleficence, autonomy and justice.
- Compliance is related to the level of patient understanding, patient satisfaction and recall.
- Consultation models offer a technique for understanding the doctor–patient encounter.
- Listening to patients is an underused clinical skill.
- Most doctors experience heart-sink situations at some point – it is important to recognize the signs.
- Remember the grief reaction: denial, anger, despair and acceptance.
- Simple techniques, such as models and diagrams, are highly effective methods of communication.

REFERENCES

1. Fitzgerald RG, Parkes M. Coping with loss – blindness and loss of other sensory and cognitive functions. *British Medical Journal.* 1998; **316**: 1160–3.
2. Parsons T. *The social system.* Glencoe, IL: Free Press, 1951.
3. Byrne PS, Long BEL. *Doctors talking to patients.* London: HMSO, 1976.
* 4. Stewart M, Roter D (eds). *Communicating with medical patients.* London: Sage, 1989.
5. Ende J, Kazis L, Ash A, Moskowitz MA. Measuring patients desire for autonomy: Decision making and information seeking preferences among medical patients. *Journal of General Internal Medicine.* 1989; **4**: 23–30.
6. French JR, Raven B. The bases of social power. In: Cartwright D (eds). *Studies in social power.* Ann Arbor: University of Michigan Press, 1959: 150–67.
7. Lukes S. *Power: A radical view.* London: British Sociological Association, Macmillan Press, 1974.
8. Beauchamp TL, Childress JF. *Principles of biomedical ethics,* 5th edn. Oxford: Oxford University Press, 2001.
9. Ingelfinger FJ. Arrogance. *New England Journal of Medicine.* 1980; **303**: 1507–11.
10. Haynes RB, Sackett DL, Taylor DW. *Compliance in health care.* Baltimore: Johns Hopkins University Press, 1979.
11. Ley P. Professional non-compliance: a neglected problem. *British Journal of Clinical Psychology.* 1981; **20**: 151–4.
12. Ley P. Improving patients understanding, recall, satisfaction, and compliance. In: Broome A (ed.). *Health psychology.* London: Chapman and Hall, 1989.
13. Bain DJ. Patient knowledge and the content of the consultation in general practice. *Medical Education.* 1977; **5**: 347–50.
14. Weinstein ND. Unrealistic optimism about future life events. *Journal of Personality and Social Psychology.* 1980; **39**: 806–20.
15. Slovic P, Fischoff B, Lichtenstein S. Behavioural decision theory. *Annual Review of Psychology.* 1977; **28**: 1–39.
16. Ley P, Morris LA. Psychological aspects of written information for patients. In: Rachman S (eds). *Contributions to medical psychology.* Oxford: Pergamon Press, 1984: 117–49.
* 17. Pendleton D, Schofield T, Tate P, Havelock P. *The consultation: Developing doctor–patient communication.* Oxford: Oxford University Press, 1984.
18. Neighbour R. *The inner Consultation: How to develop an effective and intuitive consulting style.* Lancaster: MTP Press, 1987.
19. Pietroni P. Language and communication in general practice. In: Tanner B (ed.). *Communication in the general practice surgery.* London: Hodder and Stoughton, 1976.
20. Knapp M. *Non-verbal communication in human interaction,* 2nd edn. New York: Holt, Rhinehart and Winston, 1978.
21. Burnard P. *Effective communication skills for health professionals: Therapy in practice no. 28.* London: Chapman and Hall, 1992.
22. Watkins J. *The therapeutic self.* New York: Human Sciences Press, 1978.
23. Argyle M, Dean J. Eye-contact, distance and affiliation. *Sociometry.* 1965; **28**: 289–304.
24. Mathers N, Jones N, Hannay D. Heartsink patients: A study of their general practitioners. *British Journal of General Practice.* 1995; **45**: 293–6.
25. Maguire P, Parkes CM. Coping with loss – surgery and loss of body parts. *British Medical Journal.* 1998; **316**: 1086–8.
26. Parkes CM. Facing loss. *British Medical Journal.* 1998; **316**: 1521–4.
27. Butler C, Evans M. The heart sink patient revisited. *British Journal of General Practice.* 1999; **49**: 230–3.
28. Crichton EF, Smith DL, Demanuele F. Patients' recall of medication information. *Drug Intelligence and Clinical Pharmacy.* 1978; **12**: 591–9.

46

Clinical governance: Improving the quality of patient care

DEBBIE WALL, PATRICK J BRADLEY AND AIDAN HALLIGAN

Introduction	568	Good practice case studies	576
What is clinical governance?	569	Conclusion	578
Why clinical governance?	570	Note	578
Setting standards for delivery on quality	571	Key points	578
Patient and public involvement	574	References	578
The NHS Clinical Governance Support Team	575	Further reading	580
Multidisciplinary teamworking	576		

INTRODUCTION

John Shaw is a 45-year-old ear, nose and throat (ENT) consultant and has spent the last eight years working in the ENT unit of a large London hospital. During that time, he has rarely questioned the way that he communicates with his National Health Service (NHS) patients or reflected on his attitude towards the other health care professionals who work with him. John's behaviour at directorate meetings is proof positive that at least one of the consultants' unwritten rules has survived the new millennium: 'Turn up, do the work, don't get noticed!' After all, if John maintains his distance, does the job he's always done and doesn't stick his head above the parapet, he will avoid getting sucked into management issues.

The multidisciplinary team (MDT) that John says he's part of is 'multidisciplinary' and a 'team' in name only. In reality, team members are neither accountable to each other for their clinical practice nor do they work together in a multidisciplinary way. They are a group of individuals who share the occasional clinical meeting. The consultants themselves work in silos, in separate clinics, rarely coming together to coordinate patient care – although they often treat the same patients. If you asked John, he would not know whether his practice varied from Sarah's across the corridor or whether he was making different decisions about treatment of the same patient.

Recently, John had a 'near miss' when he divided a facial nerve trunk during a parotidectomy. Even though he had resutured the injury at the time, he felt that it was better that he kept this complication to himself. He knew from past experience that if he reported it, he would be blamed. Similarly, he did not want his mistakes exposed to colleagues through his department's new system of multidisciplinary audit. After all, it may draw attention to deficiencies in his surgical experience and patient selection for surgery, and he would in all probability be held responsible. What's more, audit threatened to interfere with his clinical work and generally took up too much of his time.

Things had been like this in ENT as long as John could remember. The service was under pressure from all sides: long waiting lists, lack of funding, insufficient resources, including incompatible information technology systems and too few consultants to provide the modern service expected. As far as John Shaw is concerned, he does the best that he can for his patients under the circumstances. He does not hear nor want to hear of any complaints, so he assumes that his patients must be satisfied with their treatment and care. Mind you, he has never asked them.

John feels that people and the system always want more from him, always want changes to the historic order of things. He has become more sceptical about anything labelled modernization or innovation, because he has seen it all before: too many initiatives come and go in the NHS.

A few years ago John's hospital was involved in a clinical governance review. The Commission for Health Improvement (CHI) undertook reviews of clinical governance arrangements in NHS organizations throughout England and Wales until April 2004, when it was replaced by the Commission for Healthcare Audit and Inspection (Healthcare Commission (HC)) (www.healthcarecommission.org.uk).

Clinical governance is one initiative that has not come and gone. The clinical director continues to emphasize it within the department. What exactly is clinical governance to people like him working hands on with patients? The definition he has seen says that it is:

> A framework through which NHS organisations are accountable for continually improving the quality of their services and safeguarding high standards of care by creating an environment in which excellence in clinical care will flourish.[1]

But, what does that mean for the way that he works in the unit?

WHAT IS CLINICAL GOVERNANCE?

'People can't grasp that clinical governance is an integral part of your job – it's just what you're doing.' These words from a clinician show an awareness that clinical governance is a unifying concept; it brings together the aspects of

care implicit in the work of any health professional or support worker who day-in, day-out strives to ensure that the service they offer patients is safe, and of the highest quality that they are able to provide.

Clinical governance is not just about risk management. In an organization where it is fully integrated, there are not only effective processes for identifying and managing risk; there are clear lines of accountability; there is alignment of processes with systems and behaviours (**Figure 46.1**). In the clinical governance organization:

- patients come first;
- care is delivered with the highest standards of patient safety;
- clinicians work collaboratively, in multidisciplinary teams;
- there are clear lines of communication between staff;
- staff, regardless of their position, feel valued, included, listened to and empowered;
- there is regular clinical audit of services;
- clinical decisions are supported by research evidence;
- patients' complaints and clinical errors are reviewed and acted upon;
- there are professional development opportunities through education and training;
- staff have access to current information technology systems;
- data and information are used effectively to review service quality and support decisions and processes;
- the organizational culture is open, questioning and blame-free;

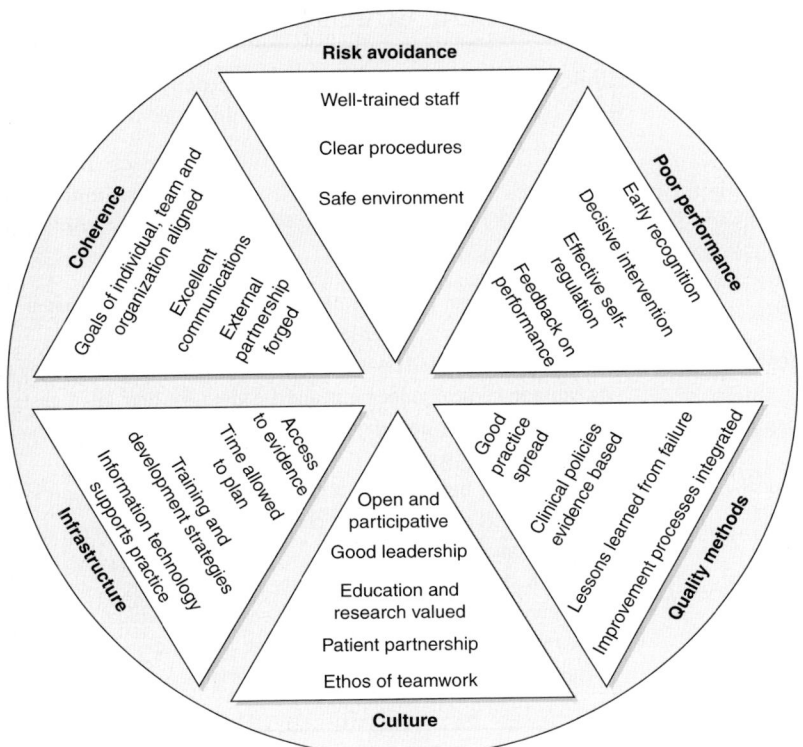

Figure 46.1 Integrating approaches of clinical governance. Redrawn with permission from Ref. 1.

- clinical governance is high on the corporate agenda;
- there is strong leadership throughout the organization.

An organization where clinical governance is mainstream would be able to provide support for clinicians like John Shaw where it is needed. This would enable them to be more accountable for the care they deliver, to re-examine their ways of working and to reflect on whether changes in their attitude and behaviour would not only benefit their relationships with colleagues, but place patient rather than professional concerns at the centre of their thinking.

However, developing an organizational culture, where staff feel they can freely report and learn from their mistakes, does not happen overnight. NHS trust chief executives and clinical governance leads have identified cultural difficulties as a major barrier impeding the successful implementation of clinical governance and there is much scope for improvement in communications between trust boards and clinical teams.[2] For clinical governance to be fully integrated throughout local NHS organizations, such barriers need to be overcome, but this is not easy if individuals are defensive about their clinical performance and continue to relate to others in ways that maintain hierarchies between professional groups.[3]

Hackett et al.[4] have identified three features of organizational life which need to be tackled by chief executives if a successful clinical governance framework is to be established: culture, leadership of changes to introduce the systems and dealing with established networks of power. They also state that any effort to implement clinical governance must ensure that consultant medical staff, as the key organizational stakeholders, are carried with the change, since the chances of success are limited if they are not 'signed up' to the process, its aims and values. (This point also applies to the NHS programme for information technology, *Connecting for Health*. It has been widely reported that the programme has had difficulty in winning over the very clinicians who will apply new IT systems in the future, because they have not been fully engaged from the outset of the programme.)[5] The values of clinicians and their managers may well differ and without constructive dialogue, this may affect doctors' attitudes towards clinical governance arrangements in their hospitals (see **Table 46.1**):

> The clinician's traditional values...professional autonomy, the focus on individual patients, the desire for self-regulation, and the role of evidence-based practice...Those of managers: the emphasis on populations, the need for public accountability, the preoccupation with systems and the allocation of resources...we should not pretend there are no differences between the way that doctors and managers see the world.[6]

The goal however, whether doctor or manager, should be a common one: continuous improvement in the quality and safety of care for patients and for those who use health services.

The required change in organizational culture to make clinical governance mainstream is movement towards a 'learning organization'.[7] This means that NHS organizations learn from their mistakes, including adverse incidents and near misses;[8] that the results of clinical audit are widely shared and acted upon; that evidence-based practice is encouraged and that staff themselves are encouraged to learn and develop their skills as healthcare professionals.

WHY CLINICAL GOVERNANCE?

Clinical governance sits within a national quality framework which drives, supports and reinforces the

Table 46.1 Clinical governance: barriers to implementation in trusts.

Behavioural	Cultural
Reluctance of professions to change 'yet again'	Concern that clinical time will be invested in clinical governance (CG) systems at the expense of patient care
'Why bother' syndrome – created by lack of suitable evidence-based guidelines combined with lack of time locally	Belief that systems based on evidence, guidelines and protocols may discourage clinical judgement and freedom for individual cases
Resistance to CG systems as another vehicle for managerialism of professions	CG as a management agenda to improve performance by reducing or controlling costs
Absence of good clinical leadership in some specialities locally and resources to invest in a satisfactory output	Perceived tension between the mechanisms for self-regulation by doctors and the management culture of accountability, hierarchy and control
Erosion of powerbases: Threat to power, prestige and status of internal stakeholders in organization	Reticence to share CG systems outputs with the public as this will undermine professions, clinical services and individual doctors
	Incident reporting undermined by increase in litigation and the culture of medicine which emphasizes professional autonomy, collegiality and self-regulation

Adapted from Ref. 4.

introduction and implementation of local NHS clinical governance activities. Before explaining what systems have been established to improve standards of treatment and care, and monitor and inspect the quality of services provided, it is necessary to establish why it was felt necessary to introduce clinical governance in the NHS – a public service where for years the notion of 'quality' was implicit. The recruitment of well-trained staff, good facilities and equipment were considered synonymous with high standards of patient care (see **Table 46.2**). *The NHS Plan*[20] and *Delivering the NHS Plan*[21] further emphasized the importance of successful implementation of quality structures and mechanisms to help reinforce the NHS quality strategy. A range of national structures and mechanisms was established to develop national standards, provide effective monitoring and inspection of progress and ensure local delivery of this national policy for high quality health care. Clinical governance is central to the delivery of this strategy and provides the framework by which local organizations work to improve and assure the quality and safety of clinical services for patients.[18]

SETTING STANDARDS FOR DELIVERY ON QUALITY

Standards are the cornerstone of quality assurance. The National Service Frameworks (NSF), the National Institute for Health and Clinical Excellence (NICE) and healthcare standards are instrumental in establishing and maintaining them across the NHS. One of the key aims of the Health Care Standards Unit (HCSU) is to develop standards for better health (SfBH).[22, 23] These 24 core standards and the optional developmental standards, describe the level of quality that health care organizations, including foundation trusts, and private and voluntary providers, are expected to meet. All NHS organizations in England are required to take them into account when developing, providing and commissioning healthcare.

They are grouped into seven domains including safety, governance, patient focus and accessible and responsive care. The standards are grounded in clinical governance as is demonstrated by the outcome specified for 'governance':

> Managerial and clinical leadership and accountability, as well as the organisation's culture, systems and working practices ensure that probity, quality assurance, quality improvement and patient safety are central components of all the activities of the health care organisation.[24]

National Service Frameworks are considered part of the developmental standards of SfBH, and the NHS and local authorities need to demonstrate they are progressing towards achieving the service quality described in them too. NSFs were launched in April 1998, as a rolling programme of national standards designed to address unacceptable variations in health services. They identify key interventions for particular services or care groups. By

Table 46.2 Clinical governance: a brief history.

Date	Event
1948	NHS founded: In its first 40 years, quality improvement initiatives had mixed success; efforts to improve the quality of patient care remained fragmented and disparate.
1980s	Managers and policy-makers tried to apply industry-based approaches of total quality management (TQM) and continuous quality improvement (CQI).[9] Initiatives not widely accepted within health service organizations.
Early 1990s	Medical and clinical audit introduced, but criticized as being dominated by medical professions. Benefits not readily apparent to the wider health service or to patients.[10]
End of 1990s	Public confidence in the NHS undermined and serious doubts raised about the quality of care available to patients. A series of clinical and organizational failures, included bone tumour diagnosis in Birmingham, UK, and paediatric cardiac surgery at the Bristol Royal Infirmary.[11, 12]
	Small number of clinicians continued to practise, while their poor performance and professional conduct was tolerated by colleagues and went unchallenged by regulatory bodies.[13, 14]
	Urgent action required to systematically address the quality and safety of patient care across all NHS organizations. Systems and processes were failing when credible individuals were able to do incredible things to patients to whom they had a duty of care.[15]
1997	The NHS policy paper, *The new NHS modern, dependable* was published.[16]
1998	The consultation document, *A first class service: Quality in the new NHS* was published.[17]
1999	NHS Executive Health Service Circular, *Clinical governance: Quality in the new NHS* was published.[18]
1999	Health Act[19] made 'quality' a legal duty and introduced corporate accountability for clinical and organizational performance across the NHS.
	The concept of clinical governance was introduced and implemented.
	Every NHS Trust chief executive became ultimately responsible for assuring the quality of healthcare services provided by their organization

2006, there were NSFs for mental health, coronary heart disease, older people (including stroke), paediatric intensive care, children, diabetes, long-term conditions, cancer and renal services.[25]

Other standards are produced by the Medical Royal Colleges and the General Medical Council, while guidelines and advice specific to ENT are issued through organizations, such as the British Association of Otorhinolaryngologists, Head and Neck Surgeons (BAOHNS), the British Association of Head and Neck Oncologists (BAHNO) and the Department of Health (www.entuk.org; www.bahno.org.uk/bulletin.htm; www.dh.gov.uk).

A nationwide body, the National Institute for Health and Clinical Excellence (NICE), was set up in 1999 for the appraisal of new and existing health treatments (for example, drugs and medical devices).[26] NICE provides guidance on clinical procedures and develops clinical guidelines for disease management. For example, in June 2006, guidance was published on the use of the ultrasonic scalpel in tonsillectomies and in July, on tonsillectomy using laser.[27, 28] NICE also uses evidence about clinical effectiveness and cost effectiveness to inform decisions in the health sector.

Seven national collaborating centres have been established by NICE; one of which helps develop clinical guidelines and service guidance for the NHS in England and Wales on cancer treatment and care, including head and neck cancer. Guideline development groups are composed of doctors, other health professionals and patient/carer representatives.[29] The Healthcare Commission sponsors a head and neck cancer audit, part of the National Clinical Audit Support Programme (NCASP). The aim is to deliver risk-adjusted, clinical audit data for head and neck cancer treatment centres in England through the Data for Head and Neck Oncology (DAHNO) audit service.[30] Clinical audit is an important component of clinical governance. In 2006, the Chief Medical Officer cited clinical audit as one of a number of quality improvement methods necessary to ensure good clinical governance and a valuable tool for clinical engagement in quality asssurance and improvement. However, he also acknowledged that not only does it fall short of its potential (it needs 're-energizing' locally), but there are concerns about the lack of mechanisms for findings of local clinical audits to be systematized into national service improvements.[31] Head and neck cancer services are receiving local feedback reports from the DAHNO with the intention that collecting these data will enable comparative analyses to be made of cancer services across England and the identification of those areas where the quality of patient care could be improved.

Monitoring and inspecting clinical governance

As part of the greater emphasis on quality assurance and improvement, and patient safety in healthcare, a monitoring and inspection system was put in place in November 1999 to independently regulate NHS performance in England and Wales. The Commission for Health Improvement placed the clinical governance arrangements of all NHS trusts under its scrutiny and completed clinical governance reports on each trust. CHI review teams looked at the effectiveness of the policies, systems and processes an organization put in place to deliver clinical governance, gathered data on patient care and gained the views of staff, patients and carers. It also conducted investigations into serious service failures, including the unacceptable performance and behaviour of individual clinicians. NHS employers may initially refer a poorly performing doctor to the National Clinical Assessment Service (NCAS) which assesses concerns about doctors and offers advice (www.ncas.nhs.uk).

In 2003, CHI became responsible for publishing NHS performance ratings. All NHS trusts were rated from zero to three stars based on data collated by CHI, including each trust's clinical governance report. These star ratings were replaced by an annual health check in 2005 after an independent body with statutory powers, the Healthcare Commission superseded CHI.

Under the 'health check', each NHS Trust Board in England is required to produce an annual report in which it rates the extent to which its services meets the 24 core standards of SfBH.[32] This annual rating of performance has two parts: one looks at the quality of services available to patients and the public; the other at trusts' management of finance and other resources. The system is one of self-assessments, although the focus on the quality of an organization's leadership and management and other key elements of clinical governance are retained.

The Healthcare Commission has made the interests, welfare and experiences of patients paramount among its concerns and adopted a patient-centred approach to improvement in the quality of the NHS and independent healthcare. It has an integrated approach to assessing the standards of services provided for patients and carers and its remit concentrates the functions of what were several organizations, into one. This includes:

- coordinating inspection by registering and inspecting private and voluntary healthcare services, including private hospitals and exclusively private doctors;
- national studies of the efficiency, effectiveness and economy of healthcare;
- production of clinical audit tools to support clinicians in their local clinical governance and audit activities;
- independent assessments of patient complaints and arrangements in place for promoting public health;
- joint inspections of integrated health and social care services with the Commission for Social Care Inspection (CSCI) (from 2008, the HC and CSCI will merge);
- working with the Mental Health Act Commission to assess the provision of care in mental health (the

Healthcare Commission is expected to take over many of its functions in 2007);
- surveys of patients' and users' experiences of healthcare.

The National Patient Safety Agency

Clinical governance has been recognized as a key driver in improving the safety culture within NHS trusts.[33] The National Patient Safety Agency (NPSA)[34] was set up in 2001 to build a safer NHS, promoting an open and fair culture in which patient safety incidents and 'near misses' from across the NHS would be reported, collected and acted on to improve the quality and safety of care for patients. The NPSA also aims to initiate preventative measures so healthcare organizations nationally can learn from these reports, as well as from the mistakes and problems that affect patients' satisfaction. Although most information is extracted from existing local risk management systems, an online form allows health professionals across England and Wales to report directly to the system and retain anonymity.

The agency's work also includes safety aspects of hospital design, cleanliness and food, as well as having responsibility for research ethics committees and the National Clinical Assessment Service.

By early 2005, all NHS trusts were linked to an NPSA National Reporting and Learning System (NRLS), although by 2006 the lack of timely deliverance of the system was the subject of a number of critical reports.[33, 35] There remained a lack of accurate information on serious incidents and deaths; at least 35 trusts had not submitted data and trusts were provided with only limited feedback and solutions to reduce serious incidents. Few trusts formally evaluated their safety culture so incidents were not being seen as opportunities for learning that prevent reoccurrence.

These findings were reiterated in the Chief Medical Officer's proposals for doctors' regulation and patient safety. By 2006, the systematic attempts to improve adverse event detection were still 'in their infancy' and events were still not reported by healthcare workers because of fear of blame.[36] Not only was under-reporting of incidents still a problem, but doctors were less likely to report an incident than other staff groups. The Healthcare Commission's 2006 report on the state of healthcare also expressed concern that there was no reliable information nationally about the avoidable deaths of patients and about serious injuries. It is, therefore, to work with the NPSA and others to improve the collection, analysis and action around reported patient safety incidents.[37]

Assuring the quality of a doctor's practice

The General Medical Council (GMC) is the regulatory body for doctors who work in the UK. It sets the educational requirements for entry on to the medical register and the professional standards expected of doctors once they are on it. These professional standards are made explicit in *Good medical practice*,[38] which describes the principles of good practice and standards of competence, care and conduct expected of doctors in all aspects of their professional work. Serious failure to follow the guidance will put registration at risk.

At the time of writing the GMC is undergoing the most extensive reform of medical regulation since it was founded in 1858. Part of these reforms is intended to ensure that clinical governance systems are joined up and effective through the maintenance of high standards of professional practice and patient protection. The GMC oversees the quality assurance of standards of practice. It is the duty of doctors to promote patient safety and to take part in systems of quality assurance and quality improvement,[38] that is, to participate in activities related to clinical governance. The GMC, however, has been the subject of mounting criticism over its inability to adequately safeguard high standards of patient safety and care.[39] A number of investigations into the practice of individual doctors, culminating in Dame Janet Smith's inquiry reports into the murders committed by Dr Harold Shipman, showed both a 'past culture of inaction' and a 'conspiracy of silence', whereby well-known concerns about a doctor were denied or avoided and the interests of the patient were subordinated to other considerations.[40]

The concerns expressed in the fifth report of the inquiry[41] led to the postponement of the launch of doctors' revalidation (a system, including annual appraisal, to enable doctors to have their licence to practise renewed every five years) – and the commissioning of the *Good doctors, safer patients* report. The latter report advocated a new approach to promoting and assuring good medical practice and to protecting patients from bad practice. A radical reshaping of the role, structure and functions of the GMC was proposed with increased lay representation and public accountability. The report also recommended that educational and standard-setting bodies for doctors be given a more formal role in medical regulation. Among the needs it addresses are to:

- design an effective interface between local healthcare systems for assuring good clinical governance and patient safety and the system of regulating the practice of individual doctors;
- introduce an effective system of regular assessment of doctors' practice which overcomes the weaknesses in earlier revalidation proposals;
- create standards of medical practice that are transparent and capable of assessment;
- develop methods of assessment that can measure a doctor's performance against a predetermined standard;
- reduce the climate of blame, retribution and disciplinary action that usually attends poor medical

performance and introduce stronger elements of prevention and earlier recognition of problems, retraining and rehabilitation;

- eliminate situations where poor practice is not recognized and acted upon because of adverse organizational culture and weak local clinical governance.[42]

Future measures will be implemented within a developing environment which recognizes that, inevitably, even good doctors make errors, which encourages open discussion and honesty about performance of individuals and clinical teams and which recognizes the importance of professional accountability for delivering care that is safe for patients and of high quality. Such an environment, in which weaknesses can be identified and individuals can be helped to learn and improve, rather than be blamed, may offer the best chance for sustained quality.

Underpinning all of the above is the maintenance of clinicians' professional knowledge and skills through professional development, improved access to information and communication technology and evidence-based research to support patient treatment and care.

Good medical practice also stipulates that it is the duty of a doctor to put the care of patients first, to listen and respect their views and to respect the rights of patients to be fully involved in their care. Relationships with patients should be based upon openness, trust, good communication, politeness, honesty and consideration.

PATIENT AND PUBLIC INVOLVEMENT

The NHS of the past 'has been characterised by paternalistic providers and compliant patients'.[43] Clinical governance, however, aims to change this and put the patient at the centre of delivery of their care.

Robinson and Dixon[43] acknowledged the changes of culture occurring in the NHS. Over the last decade, there has been a radical change in public knowledge and attitudes towards health. As healthcare consumers, patients have expectations that: information will be readily available about the service they are being offered; their consent will be gained prior to treatment; they will be respected; and they will be genuinely involved in services.

In 2003, the Isaacs Report provided evidence that as part of medical research programmes undertaken in Manchester, UK (1985–1997), the organs and tissues of hundreds of people were retained from coroners' post-mortems and community mortuaries without relatives' knowledge or consent. These practices were carried out in the belief that they were 'in the public interest'.[44] Practices carried out 'for the public', but without their consent are no longer acceptable. Seeking consent is an essential feature of good clinical practice.

The availability of health information for patients is due, in no small part, to the internet. Many patients and

carers in the UK and elsewhere have access to an ever increasing number of public-friendly health websites. As people become more knowledgeable, they are more able to make informed choices about their care and gain recognition from healthcare professionals that the patient is a partner in making treatment choices and not simply a passive recipient who takes what they are given.

In January 2003, a statutory duty was placed on every NHS organization to involve and consult patients and the public in the ongoing planning and provision of NHS services.[45] The NHS Community Health Councils, representing patient and public interest in the NHS, were replaced by Patient Public Involvement Forums, designed to give the public a voice in decisions that affect their health and that of their community. These provide a useful contact point for health professionals who seek public involvement and representation, for example when planning and designing new ENT services. In addition, Patient Advice and Liaison Services (PALS) were introduced in trusts for 'on the spot' support to patients, carers and their families with concerns relating to their care and treatment, and to provide information on the NHS complaints procedure.

The Commission for Patient and Public Involvement in Health (CPPIH) set up in January 2003 to support and manage the patient forums, and the forums themselves, are to be replaced by Local Involvement Networks (LINks), to be established for every local authority with social service responsibilities. *A stronger local voice*[46] sets out these plans for the future of patient and public involvement (PPI), giving people a greater say in health and social care service provision, consultation about changes to services and about design of new services.

In addition, the NHS Centre for Involvement was established in 2006 as a 'one-stop shop' for information and advice on PPI.[47] This aims to support the development of local PPI networks for professionals, patients and the public by providing practical resources and information. In order to promote, lead and support sustained patient and public involvement across the NHS, it will work with PPI advocates from diverse sectors of the community including from PPI forums (whilst they continue), voluntary and community organizations, statutory authorities and local authority Overview and Scrutiny Committees (OSCs). (The latter scrutinize the activities of organizations that provide local health and social care services to see whether services are appropriate to local needs.) The OSCs should be consulted if there are major changes or variations to health services in the community, and, subject to legislation, will be encouraged to focus their attention on the work of commissioners of services.

Patient and public involvement in ENT

The care of patients is the primary concern of a good doctor.[38] In head and neck surgery, as across all specialties, if patients are to be at the centre of care, then professionals need to be accountable not only to their colleagues, their professional colleges and associations, but directly to the patients themselves. The BAOHNS guidance on clinical governance goes as far as to state, 'Clinicians should hold themselves accountable to their patients first and their profession second.'[48]

Patient-centred care in ENT involves:

- working well with other professional groups and disciplines across health and social care, to meet patient needs as a whole;
- openly exploring treatment options with patients, including patients' preferences and personal circumstances;
- involving patients and carers in decision-making;
- responding to patients' needs for clear information about their care and understanding of what the treatment process involves:
- listening to patients and carers and answering their questions honestly, directly and sensitively;
- recording at every stage of the care process;
- communicating diagnosis and treatment decisions quickly to the patient's general practitioner (GP) and to other professionals involved in their care;
- involving patients and the public in all aspects of monitoring and developing the service.

An example of patient involvement in service development concerns cancer care standards used by clinicians. Birchall et al.[49] involved 40 head and neck cancer patients and 18 carers in a series of focus group meetings. They showed that although participants' views differed substantially from the professionals, the patients generated information that translated into improvements in existing national, professionally derived, standards of care for head and neck cancer (2000 national consensus standards).

The above patients' views may have differed from those of professionals, but differences may also occur when patients, carers and the public are asked what should be done to improve health services. A team of health professionals on a Clinical Governance Development Programme sought patients' and carers' views about the service they provided and how it could be improved. They did this through interviews, questionnaires and workshops. Repeatedly, patients and carers came up with the same concerns about the hospital environment, in particular the state of the waiting room and a lack of decent drink facilities. The team of professionals were perplexed by the responses they received because they expected patients and carers to be concerned about the same things as staff, that is, the clinical aspects of care.

Similarly, when the public were surveyed about the assessment of doctors for Good doctors, safer patients,[50] they wanted a doctor's assessment to go beyond their technical skills and whether or not the doctor was up to date. They placed a high value on interpersonal qualities such as communication, respect, affording patients dignity and involving patients in treatment decisions.

Understanding that patients and carers are likely to have a different viewpoint about what constitutes high quality and safe services is key to effective clinical governance in ENT, as in all services.

THE NHS CLINICAL GOVERNANCE SUPPORT TEAM

The team of health professionals in the hospital environment example above was attending a programme run by the NHS Clinical Governance Support Team (CGST).[51] The CGST was set up in 1999 to help implement and embed clinical governance in the NHS at a local level and support the delivery of high quality, patient-centred care. It also aims to improve awareness and understanding of clinical governance across and throughout NHS organizations, by acting as a focus of expertise, advice and information on clinical governance.

Until 2005, much of the CGST's work focused on delivering a series of national development programmes and activities designed for multidisciplinary healthcare teams and the board teams of NHS trust organizations.[52] The CGST's earliest activity was to establish a Clinical Governance Development Programme that supported multidisciplinary teams of frontline NHS staff to review their local services and to implement changes in healthcare quality for patients and for staff. In addition, there were programmes for trust boards to ensure that strategic leadership and clinical governance were high on the board's agenda, and a programme, utilizing learning from the aviation industry, to establish effective team-based working through training 'team coaches'. A website at www.appraisalsupport.nhs.uk was also established to provide appraisal support and a discussion forum for all doctors, regardless of specialty. This developed out of an earlier general practitioner appraisal programme which trained GPs across England as appraisers. The CGST continues to be a source of expertise on patient and carer involvement for frontline NHS staff and supports more effective means of engaging patients and communities in their local services.

In 2006, the work of the Clinical Governance Support Team became the subject of review. Its main development programmes ceased in 2005, although two modular e-learning programmes were established for community pharmacists and primary care managers. The CGST also worked to follow up the clinical governance aspects of the Shipman Inquiry[41] and to support medical appraisal and revalidation for all doctors.[53] Two further workstreams provided customized support to referred NHS organizations operating under challenging circumstances and worked with a small number of trusts to identify 'known' leaders and establish a team of people with the skills to drive though clinical governance improvement projects.

Developing teams and supporting the way that they function as units has been an important aspect of CGST work. Team development continues to be a difficult task in the NHS, especially where there have been barriers between different professional groups, multiple lines of management, perceived status differentials and a lack of organizational systems and structures for supporting and managing teams of people working together. ENT is a specialty that often brings people together to work in multidisciplinary and multiprofessional ways involving, for example, oncologists, audiometricians, maxillofacial surgeons, speech and language therapists, and so on. A poorly functioning team can not only undermine clinical performance, but also compromise the safety of the patients in its care.

MULTIDISCIPLINARY TEAMWORKING

The philosophy of clinical governance has patient safety at its very core. Delivering care that is both high quality and patient-centred must, of necessity, also be safe.

Poor team-working can endanger patient safety[54, 55] and put patients' lives at risk,[56] whereas effective teamworking has been linked to lower patient mortality.[57] As treatment programmes become more complex, patient safety is ever more dependent on the effective, collaborative working of multidisciplinary teams.

Good medical practice recognizes that most doctors work in teams with colleagues from other professions, that the skills and contributions of colleagues must be respected, communication must be effective and that team roles and responsibilities should be understood by both colleagues and patients.[38]

Modern healthcare is increasingly complex and requires coordinated and integrated delivery, none more so than in the treatment of cancer patients, where care can be poorly coordinated and confusing for those patients who experience both a wide range of services and different professionals involved in their care pathway.[58]

Multidisciplinary team-based working is a way of tackling this potential fragmentation of patient care. There is growing evidence that it makes a critical contribution to the delivery of effective, innovative and safe healthcare in the NHS.[54, 57]

The 1995 Calman-Hine Report on Cancer Care supported the widespread establishment of multidisciplinary teamworking across all cancer professions to address patients' needs from diagnosis onwards. The underlying principles for cancer services developed in the report were based on high quality, localized, accessible and patient-centred care. A follow-up review of the implementation of the Calman Report showed that of a sample of 22 trusts/hospitals visited, MDTs who reported as meeting regularly, usually using case notes, were increasingly the norm in cancer care. However, differences between the nine common cancers were highlighted.

Whilst 85 percent of breast cancer teams regularly met to review patients, only 45 percent of head and neck MDTs did so.[59]

Birchall *et al.*'s 2003 study[58] identified a shift towards multidisciplinary teamworking in head and neck cancer in the UK, although there was some indication of differing work patterns within teams, multiple teams in the same hospital and overlapping teams. This begs the question, what is a team? Many practising head and neck surgeons consider themselves to be working in teams, but what passes as a team, particularly a MDT, may be neither multidisciplinary nor a team.

Mohrman *et al.*[60] have defined a team as:

> … a group of individuals who work together to produce products or deliver services for which they are mutually accountable. The team members share goals and are held mutually accountable for meeting them, they are interdependent in their accomplishment, and they affect the result through their interactions with one another. Because the team is held collectively accountable, the work of integrating with one another is included among the responsibilities of each member.

Case study 1 illustrates the benefits for the patient, their carers and the professionals involved, of making a 'team' in a head and neck cancer clinic in a NHS trust in England (a team more like John Shaw's) into an effective, well-functioning MDT. Working from a multidisciplinary combined oncology clinic or team has many advantages, including:

- increased continuity of patient care;
- reduced multiple appointments with different professionals;
- increased professional knowledge and understanding through pooled expertise;
- development of professional peer support and communication;
- cost-effective use of time and resources;
- individual consultants being accountable and not working in isolation;
- decisions being audited and treatment aligned with agreed procedures;
- reduced likelihood that mistakes and errors are hidden and will reoccur.

GOOD PRACTICE CASE STUDIES

Case study 1: Making the team multidisciplinary

Case study 1 illustrates part of a broad portfolio of clinical governance activities being undertaken in local organizations across the NHS to improve patient safety and care.

HOW THINGS WERE

- A typical head and neck cancer team was made up of single surgeons (e.g. ENT, maxillofacial, plastic) who worked surgically alone, with occasional help from colleagues.
- Surgeons referred patients to radiotherapists for radiotherapy after surgery, or if unable to perform surgery, for radiotherapy.
- Patients were clinically treated in parallel rooms at best, in different hospitals at worst.
- Clinicians ran different clinics and were largely unaware of colleagues' activities.
- Managers tried to encourage more multidisciplinary activity (as recommended by the NHS Cancer Plan, 2000[61]). They initially suggested the team met at lunchtime to minimize the effect on clinical activity.
- Minimal equipment for viewing radiology images and histopathology specimens was available at such sessions and there was 'no regular room availability' to accommodate such meetings.

WHAT WAS DONE

- Some specialists work across specialties and locations and MDT meetings are often difficult to schedule outside normal clinical working hours.
- Most clinicians attended an 'old style' weekly combined head and neck clinic for one to several hours. They decided to have the MDT meeting as a part of the normal head and neck clinic and discuss problem and new patients.
- Patients who had been discussed or who had previously agreed a combined treatment to include radiotherapy would be seen following the MDT meeting, in a combined clinical MDT environment.

WHAT HAPPENS NOW

- The MDT meeting has a planned structure and is executed 'like clockwork'.
- The MDT usually meets in a room in the radiology suite. A move closer to the clinic is planned, to improve transit time from the MDT meeting to the MDT clinic.
- The case for each patient (most are recently diagnosed) is presented by each team leader to an audience of peers and medical students.
- Clinical pictures prior to biopsy, radiology and pathology are shown and each patient's management is openly discussed.
- The diverse group assembled may include surgeons, pathologists, radiologists, physiotherapists, dieticians, speech and language therapists, Macmillan nurses, the pain management team and social workers.
- A consensus is recommended and agreed prior to the patient's treatment.

- The team attending the patient now 'sing to the same hymn sheet'.
- Younger members of staff can seek advice and discuss patient care.
- Allied health professionals attend weekly meetings in increasing numbers.
- A clinic nurse coordinator was appointed to ensure that histopathology and x-ray results are available on the day, that patients have been informed that their case will be discussed and that they can attend the subsequent clinic.
- Patients are no longer inconvenienced by a time delay in decision planning. Only new patients, planned postoperative patients and more difficult patient cases are seen in a 'controlled environment'.

> It has been agreed that in such a clinic environment, we agree on one principle: that we need a combination of good communication and effective team working to get results.
>
> Consultant

Case study 2: Improved pathways for children with grommets

As the second case study shows, by addressing the needs of patients when building services, and considering how their journey through the care pathway may be reduced, it is possible to make changes which not only improve the patient experience, but improve the experience of healthcare professionals too.

HOW THINGS WERE

- A child with grommets inserted as treatment for secretory otitis media (glue ear) was examined by the ENT consultant about six weeks after surgery.
- The consultant checked that the grommets were still in position and infection had not set in, before sending the child to the audiologist for a hearing test.
- There were follow-up visits to the consultant to check the grommets; each required a test to ensure hearing gain had been maintained.
- The audiometrician or audiological scientist was not involved in the patient's examination or party to the consultation.

WHAT HAPPENS NOW

- Despite some resistance to change, a new process was implemented.
- The audiologist runs a clinic in parallel with the consultant, examines the child, takes a history from

the parent, performs and interprets the post-grommet insertion hearing test.

- If results are normal, an audiometrician or an audiological scientist recommends further management of the child following agreed practice guidelines. This allows for direct patient/parent feedback there and then.
- If hearing is abnormal, the consultant can see and review the patient at the same session – sometimes even in the audiology booth.
- If the grommets have been rejected, the tympanic membrane is intact and hearing is satisfactory, the child is discharged back into the care of their family doctor.
- The new process means at least two visits to the doctor are cut out; clinic slots that can be reused, so that new patients can be seen sooner.

CONCLUSION

Standards for better health reiterated that 'quality' is at the forefront of the agenda for the NHS and for private and voluntary providers of NHS care.[23] Clinical governance is integral to this agenda, but is in need of further development if it is to be effective. In 2006, the chief medical officer stated that:

> The culture of clinical governance needs to be spread to more local NHS organizations, there needs to be more consistent adherence to best practice standards and guidelines; more information on quality of care should be available to patients; and more effective and timely learning from adverse events needs to take place.[62]

The fundamental challenge in implementing clinical governance is to achieve this culture, which for many requires a transformation of ways of working, of attitudes towards others and of systems at the level of local NHS organizations.

Clinical governance invites the re-examination of traditional ways of working within health services. It questions existing professional, organizational and cultural boundaries. It questions individuals like John Shaw, since, when appropriately applied, it is a way of working and a way of rethinking professionalism and partnership with patients. The appeal and impact of clinical governance lies in a 'whole systems' approach to improving the quality of patient care. It is essential for organizations to have effective systems and processes in place for clinical governance to be delivered, but these alone are not sufficient. Organizations are only as good as the people who work in them. The true mark of successful implementation is when clinical governance is embedded to the extent of it being 'the way we work around here'.

NOTE

The information in this chapter, particularly with regard to the work of the NHS Clinical Governance Support Team and other national bodies associated with delivering the quality and safety agenda, is subject to change beyond 2007, following a period of review. However, the principles of good clinical governance remain applicable to all involved in continually improving patient safety and care.

For the latest clinical governance information, see the CGST website at www.cgsupport.nhs.uk.

KEY POINTS

- It is the duty of a doctor to promote patient safety and take part in systems of quality assurance and improvement.
- Clinical governance provides the framework by which NHS organizations work to improve and assure the quality and safety of clinical services.
- It is supported by systems established to improve standards and to monitor and inspect the quality of services for patients.
- Clinical governance puts the patient rather than the professional at the centre of care.
- A national Clinical Governance Support Team helps implement and embed clinical governance in the NHS.
- A poorly functioning team can undermine clinical performance and compromise patient safety.
- Multidisciplinary team-based working makes a critical contribution to the delivery of effective, innovative and safe healthcare.

REFERENCES

* 1. Scally G, Donaldson LJ. Clinical governance and the drive for quality improvement in the new NHS in England. *British Medical Journal.* 1998; **317**: 61–5.
2. National Audit Office, Report by the Comptroller and Auditor General. *Achieving Improvements through Clinical Governance: A Progress Report on Implementation by NHS Trusts.* HC105 Session 2002–2003. London: The Stationery Office, September 2003, cited November 29, 2006. Available from: www.nao.gov.uk.
3. Bradley PJ. The culture of consultant hospital doctors and the difficulties of implementing change – The introduction of clinical governance. MBA thesis, University of Nottingham, unpublished, 2002.

4. Hackett M, Lilford R, Jordan J. Clinical governance: Culture, leadership and power – The key to changing attitudes and behaviours in trusts. *International Journal of Health Care Quality Assurance*. 1999; **123**: 98–104.

5. National Audit Office, Department of Health. Report by the Comptroller and Auditor General. *The National Programme for IT in the NHS*. HC 1173 Session 2005–2006. London: The Stationery Office, 16 June 2006, cited November 29, 2006. Available from: www.nao.gov.uk.

6. Edwards N, Marshall M, McLellan A, Abbasi K. Doctors and managers: A problem without a solution? No, a constructive dialogue is emerging. *British Medical Journal*. 2003; **326**: 609–10.

7. Garside P. The learning organisation: A necessary setting for improving care? *Quality in Health Care*. 1999; **8**: 211–2.

8. Department of Health. *An organisation with a memory*. London: The Stationery Office, 2000.

9. Deming WE. *Out of the crisis*. Cambridge: Cambridge University Press, 1986.

10. Thomson RG, Donaldson LJ. Medical audit and the wider quality debate. *Journal of Public Health Medicine*. 1990; **12**: 149–51.

11. Malcolm AJ. Enquiry into the bone tumour service based at the Royal Orthopaedic Hospital. Birmingham: Birmingham Health Authority, 1995.

∗ 12. Kennedy I. Learning from Bristol: The report of the public inquiry into children's heart surgery at the Bristol Royal Infirmary 1984–1995. London: The Stationery Office, July 2001: Command Paper 5207-1, cited November 29, 2006. Available from: www.bristol-inquiry.org.uk.

13. Dyer C. Obstetrician accused of committing a series of surgical blunders. *British Medical Journal*. 1998; **317**: 767.

14. Roach JO. Management blamed over consultant's malpractice. *British Medical Journal*. 2000; **320**: 1557.

15. Commission for Health Improvement. *Investigation into issues arising from the case of Loughborough GP Peter Green*. London: The Stationery Office, 2001.

∗ 16. Department of Health. *The new NHS: Modern dependable*. London: The Stationery Office, 1997(Cm 3807).

∗ 17. Department of Health. *A first class Service – Quality in the new NHS*. London: Department of Health, September, 1998.

∗ 18. NHS Executive Health Service Circular. Clinical Governance: Quality in the new NHS. Department of Health, 16 March 1999: 65.

∗ 19. The Health Act. *Chapter c8*. London: The Stationery Office, 1999.

∗ 20. Department of Health. *The NHS Plan: A plan for investment. A plan for reform*. London: The Stationery Office, July, 2000, Command paper 4818-1.

21. Department of Health. *Delivering the NHS Plan*. London: The Stationery Office, 2002, circular.

22. Health Care Standards Unit, cited November 29, 2006. Available from: www.hcsu.org.uk.

∗ 23. Department of Health. *Standards for Better Health*. Department of Health, April, 2006.

24. Department of Health. *Standards for Better Health*. Department of Health, April, 2006: 12.

25. National Service Frameworks, cited November 29, 2006. Available from:www.nelh.nhs.uk/nsf/.

26. National Institute for Health and Clinical Excellence, cited November 29, 2006. Available from: www.nice.org.uk.

27. NICE. Tonsillectomy using ultrasonic scalpel. IP Guidance No. IPG178. Published guidance 28 June 2006, cited November 29, 2006. www.nice.org.uk/page.aspx?o=IP_242.

28. NICE. Tonsillectomy using laser. IP Guidance No. IPG186. Published guidance 26 July 2006, cited November 29, 2006. www.nice.org.uk/page.aspx?o=IP_57.

29. National Collaborating Centre for Cancer (NCC-C), cited November 29, 2006. Available from: www.wales.nhs.uk/sites3/home.cfm?orgid=432.

30. The National Clinical Audit Support Programme's Head and Neck Cancer Audit, cited November 29, 2006. Available from: www.icservices.nhs.uk/ncasp/pages/audit_topics/DAHNO/default.asp?om=m1.

∗ 31. Chief Medical Officer. *Good doctors, safer patients. Proposals to strengthen the system to assure and improve the performance of doctors and to protect the safety of patients*. London: Department of Health, 2006: 15.

32. Healthcare Commission NHS Performance Ratings 2005/2006. October 12, 2006, cited November 29, 2006. Available from: http://annualhealthcheckratings.healthcarecommission.org.uk.

33. National Audit Office. *A safer place for patients: Learning to improve patient safety*. HC 456 Session, 2005–2006. London: The Stationery Office, November 2005: 2, cited November 29, 2006. Available from: www.nao.org.uk.

34. The National Patient Safety Agency, cited November 29, 2006. Available from: www.npsa.nhs.uk.

35. House of Commons Committee of Public Accounts. *A safer place for patients: Learning to improve patient safety*. Fifty-first report of session 2005–2006, HC 831, London: The Stationery Office. 6 July 2006.

36. Chief Medical Officer. *Good doctors, safer patients. Proposals to strengthen the system to assure and improve the performance of doctors and to protect the safety of patients*. London: Department of Health, 2006: 30.

37. Commission for Healthcare Audit and Inspection. *State of healthcare 2006*. October, 2006.

38. General Medical Council. *Good medical practice*, 2006, cited November 29, 2006. Available from: www.gmc-uk.org/guidance/good_medical_practice/index.asp.

39. Dyer O. GMC regrets failure to act on police warning about gynaecologist. *British Medical Journal*. 2004; **328**: 1035.

40. Chief Medical Officer. *Good doctors, safer patients. Proposals to strengthen the system to assure and improve the performance of doctors and to protect the safety of patients*. London: Department of Health, 2006: 3.

* 41. Smith, Dame J. *The Shipman Inquiry Fifth Report: Safeguarding patients: Lessons from the past – Proposals for the future.* London: The Stationery Office, 2004.

42. Chief Medical Officer. *Good doctors, safer patients. Proposals to strengthen the system to assure and improve the performance of doctors and to protect the safety of patients.* London: Department of Health, 2006: xiii/xiv.

43. Robinson R, Dixon A. *Completing the Course. Health to 2010.* Fabian Ideas 605. London: Fabian Society, 2002: 53.

44. Department of Health. *Isaacs Report: The investigation of events that followed the death of Cyril Mark Isaacs.* London: The Stationery Office, 2003.

45. Department of Health. *Strengthening accountability: Involving patients and the public.* Policy Guidance, Section 11 of the Health and Social Care Act 2001. February, 2003.

46. Department of Health. *A stronger local voice: A framework for creating a stronger local voice in the development of health and social services.* July, 2006.

47. The NHS Centre for Involvement, cited November 29, 2006. Available from: www.nhscentreforinvolvement.nhs.uk.

48. BAOHNS. *Clinical governance and the role of BAOHNS.* London: British Association of Otorhinolaryngologists – Head and Neck Surgeons, 2000.

49. Birchall M, Richardson A, Lee L. Eliciting views of patients with head and neck cancer and carers on professionally derived standards of care. *British Medical Journal.* 2002; 324: 1–5.

50. Chief Medical Officer. *Good doctors, safer patients. Proposals to strengthen the system to assure and improve the performance of doctors and to protect the safety of patients.* London: Department of Health, 2006: 144.

* 51. NHS Clinical Governance Support Team, cited November 29, 2006. Available from: www.cgsupport.nhs.uk.

52. Fine words into action: Learning from the first five years of the NHS Clinical Governance Support Team. *Clinical Governance: An International Journal.* 2006; 11.

53. NHS Clinical Governance Support Team Expert Group. *Assuring the quality of medical appraisal,* cited November 29, 2006. Available from: www.cgsupport.nhs.uk/About_CG/Resources/CG_Publications/CG_Guides/.

54. NCEPOD. *Functioning as a team? The 2002 Report of the National Confidential Enquiry into Perioperative Deaths* (Executive Summary), 2002 London: NCEPOD. Available from: www.ncepod.org.uk/pdf/2002/02sum.pdf.

55. West MA, Borrill C, Dawson J, Scully J, Carter M, Anelay S et al. The link between the management of employees and patient mortality in acute hospitals. *International Journal of Human Resource Management.* 2002; 13: 1299–1310.

56. Mayor S. Poor team work is killing patients. *British Medical Journal.* 2002; 325: 1129.

* 57. Borrill CS, Carletta J, Carter AJ, Dawson JF, Garrod S, Rees A et al. *The Effectiveness of Health Care Teams in the National Health Service - Report.* Universities of Aston, Glasgow, Edinburgh, Leeds and Sheffield, 2000, cited November 29, 2006. Available from: http://homepages.inf.ed.ac.uk/jeanc/DOH-final-report.pdf

58. Birchall M, Brown PM, Browne J. The organisation of head and neck oncology services in the UK: the Royal College of Surgeons of England and British Association of Head and Neck Oncologists' preliminary multidisciplinary head and neck oncology audit. Annals of the Royal College of Surgeons of England 2003; 85:154-157.

59. Commission for Health Improvement and the Audit Commission. *NHS Cancer Care in England and Wales. National Service Frameworks Assessments No. 1.* London: The Stationery Office, 2001.

60. Mohrman SA, Cohen SG, Mohrman Jr. AM. *Designing team-based organisations.* San Francisco: Jossey-Bass, 1995.

61. Department of Health. *The NHS Cancer Plan: A plan for investment, a plan for reform.* London: Department of Health, 2000.

62. Chief Medical Officer. *Good doctors, safer patients. Proposals to strengthen the system to assure and improve the performance of doctors and to protect the safety of patients.* London: Department of Health, 2006: 31.

FURTHER READING

Clinical governance and ENT resources

Clinical Audit Support Centre. www.clinicalanditsupport.com.
Copeland G A Practical Handbook for Clinical Audit, NHS Clinical Governance Support Team, March 2005. http://www.cgsupport.nhs.uk/About_CG/Resources/CG_Publications/CG_Guides/.
ENT and Audiology Services site replacing *Action on* ENT, http://www.wise.nhs.uk/cmsWISE/Clinical+Themes/ent-audiology/services.htm.
ENT and Audiology Specialist Library at National Library for Health, www.library.nhs.uk/ent.
King's Fund library resources (search term, clinical governance), www.kingsfund.org.uk.
Modernisation Agency Action on ENT Good Practice Guide, 2002, www.institute.nhs.uk/Products/ActiononENTGoodPracticeGuide.htm.
Modernisation Agency Action on ENT Top 10 Tips, 10 July 2006, www.institute.nhs.uk/Products/ActiononENTTop10Tips.htm.
Modernisation Agency Improvement Leaders' Guides, www.wise.nhs.uk/cmswise/default.htm.
NHS Clinical Governance Support Team, www.cgsupport.nhs.uk.
Pre-operative tests guidelines for ENT, www.entuk.org/publications.
Royal Society of Medicine Clinical Governance Bulletin, www.clinical-governance.com.
Supporting Doctors Appraisal forum and website, www.appraisalsupport.nhs.uk.

47

Medical ethics

KATHERINE WASSON

Introduction: Why do we need medical ethics?	581	Research ethics	588
The doctor–patient relationship	581	Resource allocation	589
Duties and responsibilities of doctors	582	Conclusions	591
Bases for medical ethics and moral decision-making	583	Key points	591
Ethical issues in practice	585	Best clinical practice	592
Confidentiality	586	References	592
Stopping treatment	587		

SEARCH STRATEGY

The data in this chapter are supported by a Medline search using the key words medical ethics, bioethics, duties and responsibilities, consent, refusal, confidentiality, withholding and withdrawing treatment, resource allocation and research ethics.

INTRODUCTION: WHY DO WE NEED MEDICAL ETHICS?

We live in a multifaith, multicultural society. In this pluralist context there is a lack of moral consensus. People do not necessarily share a common moral outlook and determining what is right and wrong is based on a variety of different values and value systems. Not only do different individuals hold different moral views, e.g. an atheist and a Muslim, but one person may draw on different and even contradictory moral values in him/herself, e.g. naturalism and a technological imperative. In medicine, these differences lead to disagreement both in practice and theory between doctors, other professionals, patients, families and institutions. Difficult cases highlight the differences in moral perspectives and pose challenges for determining a 'best' or 'right' way forward.

In response to these difficulties, theoretical ethics provides a framework for approaching complex dilemmas and difficult decisions. Ethics does not provide easy answers to difficult problems, but it offers a clear structure and more consistent means of making moral decisions. On the practical level, ethics is not something which is outside medicine, but it is an integral part of doctors' daily practice, whether in relation to gaining a patient's consent, observing confidentiality or using professional judgement to assess areas such as best interests. It offers critical analysis of difficult issues and guidance in making decisions in practice.

THE DOCTOR–PATIENT RELATIONSHIP

The doctor–patient relationship is the context within which many medical ethical dilemmas arise. In the UK and other countries, there has been a general shift from paternalism towards consumerism in medicine. Patients are less willing to accept what the doctor says without question and are more likely to pressurize doctors to do what they wish. Doctors are seen as 'need-meeters' who can and should dispense a pill or offer a treatment for every ailment. This poses difficult decisions for doctors in balancing what patients need, want and even demand.

Along with this shift towards consumerism has come an increasing emphasis on individual autonomy and 'rights'. Patients' rights have been enshrined in the Patients' Charter (and the Human Rights Act 1998). This is partly a reaction against the paternalism of medicine where 'doctor knows best' and takes little note of patients' choice, desires or preferences regarding treatment. Respecting patient autonomy is now recognized as a fundamental principle in medical ethics.[1]

Rather than watching the pendulum swing from one extreme to the other, a balance can be struck between paternalism and consumerism. Both the doctor and patient have valuable input to provide in any medical consultation. A partnership model allows for the patient to provide information about his/her own body and symptoms, as well as personal choices and preferences, while the doctor brings his/her knowledge, skills, expertise and experience to the individual case.[2] Together they are able to determine the best way forward for this particular patient. This partnership model requires good communication on both sides and recognizes the role of duties and responsibilities in medicine.

DUTIES AND RESPONSIBILITIES OF DOCTORS

Duties and responsibilities of doctors go back as far as the Hippocratic Oath and are set out in professional codes of conduct.[3, 4, 5] These codes highlight both the positive and negative duties doctors have to their patients, colleagues, institutions and wider society. Duties and responsibilities are fundamental to the practice of medicine and include nonmaleficence, beneficence, respect for autonomy and justice.[1]

Doctors have a negative duty of nonmaleficence, or doing no harm, to patients. Both professionally and ethically doctors have a responsibility not to harm their patients. A doctor may harm his/her patient by being negligent or not following correct medical procedures. Yet, it is difficult to uphold nonmaleficence in its literal sense as doctors may inflict initial harm on patients in order to achieve good in the end. This is not doctors being negligent or unethical in their practice. Patients who undergo head and neck surgery experience initial harm and pain, but the aim is to bring about cure from disease. This harm is unavoidable and if doctors could cure the patient through other, less harmful, means then they would. The long-term benefits of cure outweigh the short-term detriments of medical intervention. The intention and motivation of the doctor, as well as the results of a treatment, are crucial in assessing the harm done to patients. Some degree of harm may be unavoidable in order to cure a patient and justifiable if the good done is expected to outweigh the harm.

The danger is that nonmaleficence may be simply defensive. In contrast, beneficence is proactive and is about doing good to patients. Not only are doctors to refrain from harming their patients whenever possible, but they also have a duty to do good to them. The most obvious way of fulfilling this duty is to cure a patient of his/her illness, disease or dis-ease and restore him/her to full health. Cure is not possible in all cases. Both doctors and patients should recognize the reality and the limits of medicine. In some cases, limiting the harm done by a disease or illness may be the best doctors are able to do. Beneficence extends beyond cure and includes caring for patients and treating them with respect and dignity.

Part of doing good to patients involves respecting their autonomy. Autonomy literally means self-rule and is understood as self-determination and choice. In health care, respecting autonomy generally means allowing patients the freedom to make decisions for themselves, even if doctors disagree with those choices. A patient might refuse curative maxillofacial surgery because of the degree of disfigurement caused even though doctors advocate it.

In modern western societies, the autonomy of individuals is frequently emphasized. The ability and freedom to make our own choices is paramount. This carries over into health care too. Considerations of autonomy highlight at least two points within medicine. The first is that patients are not the only people who possess autonomy. Doctors, nurses and other professionals also have autonomy which can and is exercised. For example, a doctor cannot be forced to give a treatment against his/her professional judgement. The second is that in any society or community, individual autonomy is always limited. Autonomy is limited if there is a risk of, or actual, harm to oneself or others. If a patient is suicidal, he/she can be sectioned to avoid harming him/herself. If a patient attempted to attack someone on the hospital ward, then his/her autonomy would be restricted to prevent harming others. For all of us within health care and society more generally, autonomy is limited. Legislation in dealing with the threat of infectious diseases shows that an individual's freedom and autonomy can be limited if the risk to others is great.

Part of doing good to patients and respecting their autonomy involves being just. Doctors have a duty to treat individual patients fairly and equally. This means treating similar cases in similar ways and dissimilar cases in dissimilar ways. Both types of justice ensure there is a minimum standard of consistency in interactions with all patients.[6] Fairness and equality do not allow doctors to discriminate against patients based on clinically irrelevant factors, e.g. religion, race, sex. Doctors not only have to weigh up considerations of justice in relation to individual patients, but also between all of their patients.

These key responsibilities of nonmaleficence, beneficence, respect for autonomy and justice are four of the fundamental principles in medical ethics and practice. In recent years these have been seen as the key principles that provide the foundation for doctors' duties in medical ethics. It can be argued that other ethical duties are significant in medicine. That these principles are necessary in medicine is generally agreed, but whether they are sufficient is debated.[7]

In looking beyond these four principles, doctors also have a duty to care. This duty is fundamental to each and every interaction a doctor has with patients. It is the basis from which doctors begin and carry out their work. For the doctor, this involves looking after patients to the best of his/her ability and applying his/her knowledge, expertise and skills to care for the patient.

Part of this duty to care includes protecting the best interests of the patient. Doctors have a responsibility to act in the best interests of their patients. This does not mean that doctors make decisions about best interests without reference to or discussion with the patient. Yet, deciding what is in the best interests of the patient may not be straightforward depending on how and when best interests are defined and who defines them, e.g. doctor, patient, relatives or other professionals. Doctors may not agree whether surgery, radiotherapy or chemotherapy is in the best interests of a child with a neck tumour and the patient and parents may also have differing views.

When examining the duties of doctors, there may be a problem over who defines best interest and how it is defined. There is also a difficulty when different duties and responsibilities conflict, e.g. nonmaleficence and beneficence. Analyzing how to proceed and which responsibilities take priority are key questions in medical practice. A hierarchy of duties may be required to clarify priorities and aid decisions in practice. For example, it might be argued that doing no harm is more important than doing good and that the duty of care is fundamental to all interactions with patients.

BASES FOR MEDICAL ETHICS AND MORAL DECISION-MAKING

Individuals make and assess moral decisions on different bases. These form the foundations of our view of what is 'right' and 'wrong'. At their root, such decisions can be primarily based on principles, consequences or virtues or some combination of these.

Principle-based morality

Deontological morality is based on principles. It deals with what we ought to do; that moral obligation arises from fundamental ethical principles. Whenever people use principles to make decisions, it is important to ask, 'from where do these principles come?' There are various sources from which doctors and patients draw moral principles.

NATURE/NATURALISM

Naturalism argues that by looking at and reflecting on nature moral truths or principles can be discerned. This includes both the natural world and nature of human beings.[8] In the nature of things and the nature of people, there are moral principles which reason can discern. Goodness and badness are natural features of the world and people. By observing the way the world is and people are, we can see morality in the nature of things and people.[9] This is closely tied to what we regard as 'normal' function. Where there is damage to the head or neck, the aim of surgical intervention is to restore normal function and enable the natural processes to function without impediment.

Yet, people have different ideas and conceptions of what is 'natural'. These different views may conflict. In fact, doctors often try to put right things that have gone wrong in nature. Medicine struggles against the ravages of nature and tries to prevent natural disease from harming people. It is also clear that medicine and surgery are in a crucial sense fighting against natural disease and breakdown. Determining what is natural, and the implications of a naturalistic moral view, may not be straightforward.

RELIGIOUS MORALITY

Religion also provides a key source of moral principles. Christianity, Islam, Judaism, Buddhism and Hinduism all teach certain fundamental moral precepts.[10] These are usually enshrined in moral and religious codes such as the Koran and the Ten Commandments. There may be debate about whether such principles are independently valid or dependent on being a follower of a particular religion, but the problem for medicine is whether the different religions all support the same principles or whether they are fundamentally different. At first glance, the Jehovah's Witness refusal of blood transfusions is very different from the ready acceptance of life-saving treatments by other religious groups. Different religions seem to offer different moral principles.

KANT

The philosopher Immanuel Kant also emphasized the role of principles in his highly influential contribution to moral thinking. For Kant, morality is about asking, 'What ought I do?'[10] In response, he tried to identify fundamental principles, or maxims, of action that all people ought to adopt. The key moral principle is the Categorical Imperative, which states 'Act only on the maxim through which you can at the same time will that it be a universal law.'[11] The key test for moral principles is whether they are universalizable, i.e. anyone in the same moral situation would necessarily make the same choice. This is a check against begging the question in your own favour or being biased. Essentially, medical treatment ought to be given to every individual without bias.

For Kant, morality involves respect for people. This respect is based on the intrinsic worth and dignity of human-beings. He requires that we treat humanity, whether ourselves or any other, never simply as a means, but also always as an end.[12] People are ends in themselves. We cannot do medical experiments on people for the benefit of future generations without their consent. That would be using people for some other end than for their own good. Kant's ethics involves moral duties, which apply to ourselves and others. He argues that we have positive and negative moral duties. There are both things we should do as well as those we should avoid, e.g. doctors doing good and not harming patients.

Any morality based on principles may run into difficulties when different moral principles, like duties, conflict. Kant's approach is no exception here. Deciding between principles is often problematic and Kant does not provide a clear way forward. Principles are one key aspect of morality and moral decision-making, but morality also can be based on consequences.

Consequence-based morality

Morality based on consequences is called teleological morality. A consequentialist approach argues that morality should and does focus on the potential outcomes of our choices and actions, particularly in terms of what will happen if we do something against doing nothing at all.

UTILITARIANISM

Utilitarianism is the most well known of consequentialist theories, particularly in health care. It is a moral theory concerned with social reform and it argues that society should adopt laws which make people happy and avoid pain. At the heart of utilitarianism is the Greatest Happiness Principle (GHP), which states that morality is about achieving the greatest happiness for the greatest number of people. If this is the case, then we must have some way of measuring happiness or pleasure. To this end, Jeremy Bentham developed a pleasure calculus.[8, 13] It includes:

- duration: how long it lasts;
- intensity: how intense it is;
- propinquity: how near it is;
- extent: how widely it covers;
- certainty: how sure we are it will come;
- purity: how free from pain it is;
- fecundity: how much it will lead to more pleasure.

In Bentham's version of utilitarianism, the pleasure or pain of one person, if particularly acute, could outweigh that of many others. To counteract the implicit lack of justice in Bentham's theory, John Stuart Mill introduced the notion of fairness.[14] In assessing pleasure or pain in society, each person should count for one and not more than one. This was an attempt to ensure that the pleasure and pain of each person was weighed fairly against that of others.

Even with the inclusion of justice and fairness, utilitarianism poses difficulties when making moral decisions. One is the danger that the minority will have to sacrifice or forego pleasure for the happiness of the majority and that increasing pleasure may be given a greater moral importance than preventing pain. This view would give equal moral weight to giving people a thrill and alleviating pain. Such critique is particularly important for doctors who are confronted with people who are suffering from illness, disease and in pain.

Underlying utilitarianism, and all consequentialist theories, is a focus on the ends rather than the means of moral choices. But do the ends always justify the means or are there some means which are wrong or immoral in and of themselves and cannot be justified even if they achieve a good end? This question is important in medicine where doctors are weighing up the potential benefits and burdens of treatment. Either doctors or patients may think that the means of achieving a potentially good end are not acceptable, as in the case of some cancer treatments. One critique of a morality based on consequences is that it is difficult to predict, nonetheless control, the consequences of our actions. Doctors are faced with this challenge on a daily basis when treating patients. What they intend to achieve may significantly differ from the end result.

Both morality based on consequences and principles pose problems for doctors. Morality involves an examination of both, but requires more.

Virtue-based morality

In recent moral theory, there have been moves away from a morality primarily based on principles or consequences. The emphasis has shifted toward an appeal to virtues,[15] harking back to Aristotle and Aquinas. Virtue theory focusses on growing virtuous people and asks, 'What is a good person?' It seeks to identify certain qualities and characteristics of a good person and to foster these in individuals. The way that these characteristics are grown and developed in people is in the context of a community.

We may ask, 'What makes a good doctor?' The list of qualities might include having specific scientific knowledge (of disease and illness, as well as treatments), professional expertise and skills, being caring, compassionate, a good communicator and wise. This would affect the selection criteria of would-be medical students.

Then we should ask how these qualities or virtues of a good doctor would be fostered. This would take place within the professional community which trains medical students and newly qualified doctors. Teaching, training and practice are all crucial in the development and fostering of the virtues of a good doctor.

The picture painted in virtue theory is very optimistic. It may not be easy to agree on the characteristics of a good person or good doctor, far less to foster them. Virtue theory does not provide clarity about what to do when these characteristics conflict. In the end, it can seem highly optimistic about how virtuous people really are and how easy it would be to encourage and grow a virtuous person, as well as the nature and role of community in that process.

In examining three approaches to morality, based on principles, consequences or virtues, we have seen that all three harbour difficulties. Perhaps a more balanced view of morality should incorporate considerations of all three – recognizing that principles offer fundamental grounds for making moral decisions, but these cannot and should not be taken without weighing up the potential consequences of any decision. This should all happen within the context of trying to foster the development of virtuous doctors who will be able to make 'good' and 'right' decisions in practice, based on who they are rather than primarily on decision-making processes.

ETHICAL ISSUES IN PRACTICE

Three approaches to making moral decisions – principles, consequences and virtues – have been examined within the context of the doctor–patient relationship, as well as duties and responsibilities. It is helpful to consider the specific ethical issues in medicine and how we might approach them, rather than simply analyzing the theories of ethics. These include consent and refusal, confidentiality, stopping treatment, ethical issues in research and resource allocation.

Consent and refusal

Consent is fundamental to any and every interaction between doctors and patients. By its nature, gaining and giving consent is a process, not a one-off decision, and patients must be free to change their minds at any point. Consent may be implicit or explicit. A patient may give implicit, or implied, consent by indicating nonverbally that he/she is happy to participate in a procedure, for example holding out his/her arm to have blood taken or opening his/her mouth to have the throat checked. Alternatively, consent may be explicitly stated in verbal or written form. Consent forms provide evidence that a particular process has taken place, but serve only as a minimum standard for recording consent, as they do not

guarantee the quality of communication or level of patient understanding.

The normal standard in medicine is fully informed, valid consent given by a patient who is mentally competent. The 'fully informed' part of consent involves the patient being given all relevant information regarding the treatment options and potential consequences of having against not having a particular treatment. In the UK, doctors should provide the competent patient with as much information as he/she needs or desires to make an informed decision.[16] This will vary from patient to patient and doctors are required to use their professional judgement about the degree of detail regarding benefits, risks and burdens in each case. They should assume patients wish to be well informed and use a 'prudent patient' standard.[16] This is in sharp contrast to the United States where doctors must make clear any and every known risk, regardless of its likelihood. When attempting to gain fully informed consent, doctors face the challenge of providing sufficient information for a patient to make a decision and telling the truth about the potential risks, over and against allowing patients to keep hope.

To be valid, consent must be freely given, ensuring that patients are free from any improper, undue pressure from doctors or other professionals. How, when and by whom information is given to patients about potential treatment or nontreatment options can have a significant impact on the decisions made. If the consultant emphasizes a particular option as the best course, the patient may be more likely to agree to it. Patients need time to digest the information given to them, ask questions, consult others and weigh up different options.

There are some instances in which (as well as groups of patients for whom) gaining valid consent is a more ethically and practically difficult process. In emergency situations, where patients cannot give consent or refuse treatment, doctors are obliged to act in the best interests of the patient. They have both a legal and ethical duty to take measures to secure the patient's life and health. These may be short-term interventions that then enable the patient to recover sufficiently to make longer-term decisions about further treatment for him/herself.

For children in the UK, the legal age of consent is 16 years. While the general standard is that parental consent should be sought for medical interventions with children under 16, children should be encouraged to participate in their care and health professionals should act as their advocates.[17] Sometimes, children and young people under 16 may have the capacity to give valid consent. A doctor can give treatment without parental consent if he/she judges the young person to be 'Gillick competent' and it is in the patient's interests.[17, 18] The former involves assessing whether the child or young person understands the consequences of having against not having a particular treatment or intervention. In reality, the degree of competence required is proportional to the weightiness of the decision. A 13-year-old might be deemed competent to consent to a tonsillectomy, but not brain surgery.

Individuals who enter the armed forces agree to give up a degree of their individual autonomy and freedoms in the interests of the unit as a whole. They may be called on to put their life and/or health at risk for the good of the service and country. Prisoners also forfeit their autonomy and are less free to give or refuse consent, in particular with respect to intimate body searches. Both groups are still entitled to a high ethical standard of medical care and doctors have the same professional and ethical duties to these patients as others.[19, 20]

Some patients may be incompetent or lack capacity to make choices and decisions for themselves.[21] Patients who are mentally impaired or disordered or handicapped may lack sufficient understanding of the nature, purpose, risks and benefits of a proposed treatment to give valid consent. In England, Wales and Northern Ireland, no-one can legally give consent on behalf of a competent adult.[21, 22] In Scotland, people over the age of 16 may appoint a proxy decision-maker to give consent or refuse treatment for them if they become incapacitated.[23] Doctors should not assume that these patients are incompetent without seeking to engage with them and discern the level of competence. Such patients should be encouraged to participate in decisions about their care whenever possible.

Refusal is at the heart of consent. Patients are free to refuse any treatment or intervention at any time. An adult Jehovah's Witness may refuse a life-saving blood transfusion. If a doctor attempts to treat this patient in the face of a valid refusal, he/she can be charged with assault or battery. Valid refusal requires the patient understands the significance of his/her choice and its implications. The ethical basis for this is respect for autonomy. Patients are free to make their own choices regarding their health care and can even refuse life-saving treatment, regardless of whether doctors agree with them or not. Because of the potential significance of refusing treatment, in reality a refusal requires a higher degree of competency than consent to treatment. Good practice means doctors strive to ensure the patient fully understands the implications of his/her refusal. It should be carefully documented to safeguard the doctor.

Gaining fully informed, valid consent or exploring refusal highlight ethical issues in medical practice. Along with confidentiality, they are fundamental starting points for the doctor–patient relationship and any treatment.

CONFIDENTIALITY

Doctors have a duty to protect patient confidentiality and privacy. Confidentiality matters because it is a key basis for trust between the doctor and patient. In practice, understanding what confidentiality means may vary. Patients may think that in telling their doctor something in confidence it will not be discussed with anyone else. They may not realize that doctors not only talk to each other and other professionals about particular cases, but the number of health professionals who have access to their 'confidential' medical notes.

Confidentiality involves issues both of truth-telling and disclosure. Doctors have a positive duty to tell the truth to patients and a negative duty not to lie. Without these duties, patients cannot be certain whether to trust what their doctor tells them. Patients expect doctors to give them information and advice which is true and accurate. Not telling patients the truth fundamentally undermines this trust and means that patients' confidence in what their doctor says is eroded.

One argument for not telling patients the truth is that it is sometimes in their best interests. A doctor may decide not to tell a woman with a malignant tumour of the neck that she has cancer. The rationale may be that it would be too upsetting for her. This attitude is paternalistic and assumes that the doctor knows better than the patient how she will cope with the news. If this patient asks for information about her diagnosis, doctors have an obligation to be clear and truthful.

A more difficult area is where patients do not directly enquire about their diagnosis. How much information should doctors give and how detailed should it be? Is it acceptable to be 'economical with the truth'? Information about diagnosis or prognosis should not be forced on patients if they do not want it, but that differs from doctors denying them the opportunity to have this information or patients being given an inaccurate or misleading account of their condition.

There are appropriate and inappropriate ways of telling the truth to patients. A woman with motor neurone disease went to see her general practitioner (GP). She had concerns about her death and wanted to know what would happen to her. The doctor told her she would eventually choke to death. The woman then had recurring nightmares where she would wake up choking. This doctor told the truth, but in a way which was insensitive and inappropriate. There is a balance to be struck between answering questions truthfully and being sensitive to the patient's situation and anxieties.

Any disclosure of information about the patient's condition must be given to him/her first. Doctors should make sure the information and its significance is clear to the patient. Doctors must balance the disclosure of all relevant information to the patient with being sensitive to what the patient does or does not want to know. Patients are free to indicate they do not wish to know certain information, but they should be given the option to decline.

Sometimes relatives believe that they have a 'right' to know details of the patient's condition and pressurize doctors to tell them. Doctors have an ethical duty to protect patient confidentiality and privacy and not to disclose information to relatives without the explicit consent of the patient. Even though it may put doctors in a difficult position with relatives, patients are entitled to expect doctors not to disclose information about their medical condition to relatives.

There are times when doctors need to consult colleagues about a patient's condition. It is ethically acceptable to share relevant information, even if confidential, in order to determine what care or treatment options are in the best interests of the patient. Good practice ensures that the patient is aware of these discussions and disclosures and the reasons for them. When working in a team, patient information may need to be shared to ensure good and consistent care is delivered. Disclosure at these times should be on a 'need to know' basis and differs from disclosing confidential information which is not relevant to the clinical situation, e.g. the patient's sexual orientation or family situation.

There are some instances where patient confidentiality can be broken without his/her consent. Under the Public Health (Control of Diseases) Act 1984 in England and Wales and the Infectious Diseases (Notification) Act 1889 in Scotland, doctors are under a legal obligation to report notifiable diseases to the appropriate authority.[24, 25] Ideally, this should be done with the patient's full knowledge and consent and every effort made to encourage the patient to comply. If a patient refuses to agree to the notification, the doctor has a legal and ethical duty to report the disease for the protection of the wider public.

Disclosure in the case of HIV/AIDS poses particularly difficult ethical issues. On the one hand, doctors have to weigh up the potential harm done to patients from disclosing their HIV status against the potential risk of infection to others, like health care professionals or sexual partners. If patients perceive that confidentiality will not be kept, then they may not come forward for testing and treatment. Every effort should be made to encourage the patient to disclose this information him/herself. If this is unsuccessful, disclosure may take place if a doctor believes a specific person, including a sexual partner, is being placed at 'serious and identifiable risk' of becoming infected.[24, 25, 26]

Data protection and medical records

The Data Protection Act 1984 provides protection of personal information held by others, e.g. medical records on computer. Personal information given for one purpose cannot then be used for a different purpose without consent. The use and handling of this information is restricted. The Act also allows people to have access to personal data at reasonable intervals. Patients can request to have access to their medical notes and read what has been written about them. This has altered both the style and content of what doctors write in the medical notes and the use of medical records for research.

Protecting patient confidentiality and information ensures that trust is maintained between the doctor and patient. When there is a risk of harm to others, doctors may have a duty to break confidentiality. This should be carefully weighed, the British Medical Association or the Medical Defence Union should be consulted and the facts clearly communicated to the patient. The discussions and rationale for breeching confidentiality should be documented.

STOPPING TREATMENT

Withholding and withdrawing treatment

One of the most difficult areas for doctors is deciding when to stop active treatment for an individual patient. There are tensions between whether and when to begin and stop treatment. Whether to withhold or withdraw a medical treatment or intervention, such as chemotherapy, artificial feeding or hydration, can be a contentious area for doctors, other health professionals, patients and relatives. Weighing up the benefits and burdens of treatment, assessing best interests and quality of life are necessary features of such judgements.[27]

Whether to begin or withhold a treatment is the first phase in this debate. Judgements about withholding treatment should be based on the best available evidence and the individual patient's condition. If the likely burdens and risks of treatment outweigh the potential benefits, the doctor may judge the treatment to be futile. There is much debate about what constitutes futile treatment and who decides, as doctors' and patients' interpretations of futility may differ. In the literature, the generally accepted definition of a futile treatment is one that has less than a 1 percent chance of success.[28, 29]

If a treatment has been started, there may come a point where doctors believe it should be stopped. The British Medical Association (BMA) document *Withholding and withdrawing life-prolonging medical treatment* offers guidance for doctors in making these decisions. It states that although prolonging a patient's life usually provides a health benefit, doctors are not obliged to prolong life at all costs with no reference to burdens of treatment or quality of life. If a treatment fails or ceases to provide a net benefit for a patient, the justification for providing it is removed and the treatment may, ethically and legally, be withheld or withdrawn (pp. 1–2).[30]

In practice, doctors may find it more difficult to withdraw than to withhold treatment. To prevent situations where patients are denied treatments which might be beneficial because doctors think it will be too difficult to withdraw at a later stage, the BMA has argued, 'Although emotionally it may be easier to withhold treatment than to withdraw that which has been started, there are no legal, or necessary morally relevant, differences between the two actions.'[30] This view is debated.[31] Philosophically, it can be argued that withdrawing treatment is more like an action (doing something) than an omission (refraining from doing something) and so has a different moral weight and significance.[32] Regardless of where one sits within this philosophical debate, in practice there will be cases where it is appropriate to stop or withdraw treatment. Doctors are justified in withdrawing treatment and this does not constitute euthanasia. If treatment is withdrawn and 'nature takes its course', it is the disease which brings about the patient's death, not the doctor.

In the UK, the Tony Bland case has become crucial to the debate about withholding and withdrawing treatment. He was a young man who was seriously injured in the Hillsborough football disaster and was in a persistent vegetative state (PVS). After four years, the doctor and family wanted to remove the nasal-gastric tube through which Tony was being fed. They appealed to the coroner, under whose protection all of the Hillsborough victims were placed, who asserted that he would charge the doctor with murder if he stopped feeding Tony. The case eventually went to the House of Lords and two key rulings were given.[33] First, the Law Lords ruled that artificial feeding was now a medical treatment and, therefore, could be withdrawn. Second, because Tony was in PVS it was not in his best interests to be kept in PVS. Both judgements have been debated and raised issues of withholding and withdrawing treatment among the wider public.

In reaching a decision about whether to withhold or withdraw treatment, good medical practice elicits and incorporates the patient's views and that of the relatives, provided the patient has given permission for that discussion to take place. If doctors are recommending that treatment be withheld or withdrawn, clear rationale and justifications should be communicated to the patient and recorded in the notes. Patients are free to request treatments and some demand particular interventions, but doctors are not obliged to give treatments against their clinical judgement.

Clinical judgements to withdraw treatment should consider futility, best interests and quality of life issues. Doctors have a duty to act in and protect the best interests of their patients. When making treatment or nontreatment decisions, good practice will involve competent patients in that process. For the incompetent patient, the views of the relatives should be sought to ascertain what the patient would have wanted, but doctors are under no legal obligation to do as the relatives wish. Ultimately, the doctor must act in a way which he/she thinks will be in the best interests of the patient. If the patient is a child below the age of consent, then the parents' views are crucial in deciding what constitutes best interests. Even when the child may be deemed competent to consent or refuse treatment, good practice would include the parents in that decision whenever possible.

Similar issues are raised when attempting to assess quality of life. Doctors will have some view of what constitutes a reasonable quality of life, but this may be very different from the patient's view. Competent patients should be given the opportunity to express their view of quality of life issues. For incompetent patients, the relatives should be consulted about the patient's views, but ultimately doctors must make a decision which they believe to be in the best interest of the patient.

RESEARCH ETHICS

Good medical practice relies on a solid knowledge base. This requires good research. The government's emphasis on 'evidence-based medicine' has led to the creation of the National Institute for Clinical Excellence (NICE), which monitors the quality of clinical practice. The rationale for treatments and techniques should be supported by research results and not simply past practice. Research is needed to continue to improve practice and develop new techniques and treatments. However, medical research raises ethical questions for doctors, researchers, patients and the wider community. The nature, content and process of research merit ethical, clinical and scientific scrutiny.

Research can cover a broad range of activities. It can involve tracking a specific genetic disorder in the population or developing a new surgical intervention for hearing impairment. A key aspect of scientific research is that it tests a thesis or hypothesis and that the results are testable and repeatable.[34] If the results cannot be tested or duplicated, there is reason to be sceptical about the research. Peer review is an integral and necessary part of all scientific research. This provides a level of scrutiny for the claims and results of research. For a new technique, intervention or therapy to become a standard treatment, researchers must convince their peers of its merits.

A key question in setting up any research study is who will benefit from it? Therapeutic research is intended to benefit the subject, or patient, directly. Nontherapeutic research does not benefit the individual subject, but aims to contribute to medical knowledge and may benefit others in the future.[35] Whether the development of innovative treatment should be categorized as research or an extension of usual practice is debated. On the one hand, if the digression is small and focussed on the individual patient's situation then it may be justifiable and the innovation may be seen as a useful byproduct of effectively treating an individual patient. On the other hand, such innovation may be seen as 'trial and error' which is ethically and scientifically unacceptable and puts patients at risk because the procedures are not monitored or scrutinized sufficiently or at all.[35, 36]

The process of setting up a medical research study involves obtaining ethical approval from the local research ethics committee (LREC). They were introduced to help weigh up the potential benefits and risks of research for individuals and society. LRECs examine the scientific quality of the protocol, whether the investigators are competent and facilities adequate, possible hazards, measures for providing information and seeking consent, adequate compensation arrangements regarding harm from the trial, methods of recruitment, payment to investigators, and storage and use of subject-identifiable information.[35] For multicentre trials, multicentre regional ethics committee (MRECs) have been instituted both to speed the process of ethical assessment and to prevent duplication.

According to the BMA,[17] although there is no legal requirement for researchers to obtain ethical approval for a study, it is almost impossible to get funding and becoming increasing difficult to publish results without it. These committees examine the nature, purpose and process of proposed studies with consent processes being the subject of particular scrutiny.

Consent to participate in research must be valid and freely given. According to the Declaration of Helsinki (1964), subjects must be 'adequately informed of the aims, methods, anticipated benefits and potential hazards of the study and the discomfort it may entail'. Participants need information about the positives and negatives of any study and the alternatives before being able to give valid consent.

For minors and children, the same guidelines apply to consenting to take part in research as for treatment. Parental consent should be sought if the child is under 18 years, but it should not override refusal by a competent child. In UK law, parents cannot give consent for a child for procedures which are of no particular benefit and may carry a risk of harm, or refuse treatment which would be in the child's best interests, e.g. a life-saving blood transfusion.[37, 38] Great care is taken in research on vulnerable groups, such as psychiatric patients.

Voluntariness is a key element in consenting to research. Subjects must not be pressurized in any way to take part and they must be free to refuse before or at any time during a study without this impacting on their basic care and treatment. This can be difficult, as doctors are in a position of power and may pressurize subjects unintentionally. Subjects may feel guilty if they refuse to participate or fear that a refusal will negatively affect their care. To avoid this situation, recruitment of subjects should be undertaken by someone other than the person carrying out the research, e.g. a research nurse who explains the options.[36] It should be made clear to subjects that a refusal will not be counted against them by their doctor. Written information for subjects and their GPs is particularly important.

Randomized control trials (RCT) are viewed by many as the gold standard for medical research, but are criticized by others.[36] This method randomly allocates participants into different groups who then receive different treatments. It enables researchers to compare different interventions and determine which one produces the most beneficial results. If they are double-blinded, then neither the participant nor researcher knows which subjects are given the different interventions. This approach attempts to remove bias from the research. Yet, it also removes choice regarding treatment options from the participant and raises ethical concerns.

The use of placebos in research has come under scrutiny as it denies some subjects the potential benefits of the intervention. It is no longer considered ethical to use placebos if there are known treatments which may offer some benefit to the subject.[39] Whether or not placebos should be used to test the effectiveness of an existing treatment, where no other exists, is still debated.[40]

Research also raises ethical concerns about confidentiality and the handling of medical records and information. To undertake a study, participants medical records may become available to a number of people other than the doctor, research team or practice. The means of protecting confidentiality both during the course of the study and future use of the findings must be addressed. The BMA[17] states that whenever patient-identifiable information is used, a medically qualified person should be identified to ensure the information is handled correctly and confidentiality is protected.

A vital part of good research is that it offers some benefit to the individual or society, that consent is freely given on the basis of detailed information, that confidentiality of patient-identifiable information is protected and that the research constitutes good science which is ethically sound.

To improve treatments, develop new techniques and interventions, medicine must rigorously assess current practice. This should not be at the expense of subjects' health, life or conditions or without careful consideration of the risks and benefits and ethical issues involved. These should be clearly explained to participants and they should be given the option to consent or refuse to participate.

Whether and how much money should be given towards research raises ethical questions of resource allocation.

RESOURCE ALLOCATION

Regardless of the specialty or setting (National Health Service (NHS) or private sector), the issue of limited resources is a reality for doctors. They face multiple pressures from patients, relatives, colleagues, management and Departments of Health, and doctors must make choices about how they spend their time, energy and money.

Levels of allocation

Resource allocation happens on different levels. In macro-allocation, central government divides its resources between areas such as health care, education and defence. Monies given to health care are then allocated between different hospitals trusts, primary care trusts and regional health authorities that distribute among primary, secondary and tertiary care. Micro-allocation includes decisions about treatment options, staffing levels and how much each service or department spends on research and administration.

NEEDS

For doctors on the front line, there is a tension between meeting the needs of individual patients and assessing the cost to the wider community. Assessing patient need is a key part of determining treatment options. Who defines needs and how are they defined? Abraham Maslow argued that there is a hierarchy of humans needs, ranging from physiological and safety needs to self-actualization (the ability to fulfil oneself and realize one's full potential). He also claimed that people seek to have lower level needs met first before focussing on higher level needs.[41] Basic needs are those things universally required by all people to survive, such as food, water and shelter. Nonbasic needs are not required for survival, but contribute to our psychological, social and spiritual well-being.[42] Within the context of limited resources, doctors may have to focus on the most urgent and pressing basic needs before addressing other needs.

PREFERENCES, DESIRES AND WANTS

Patients have a wide variety of health needs, but they also have desires and preferences about their treatment options. With the move away from paternalism, patients are less willing to do what the doctor tells them without question. Patients can and do communicate what they want and may also place demands on doctors for particular treatments or drugs; for example, parents who insist their child be given grommets for their ears. Of course, sometimes patients want things they do not need, such as cosmetic surgery, and need things they do not want, such as chemotherapy. There is a danger that doctors give in to pressure from patients and the most demanding patients get what they want, while others do not.

RIGHTS CLAIMS

Sometimes patient demands are based on 'rights'. Claims to rights have become a common part of modern Western culture. In medicine, the Patient's Charter and the

Human Rights Act (1998) have raised the notion of rights and correlative expectations in the public consciousness. When confronted with rights claims, doctors need to decipher what kind of rights are involved and whether or not they have a duty to fulfil them.

Legal rights provide a minimum standard of protection from harm for all people in a society. If anyone breaches another person's legal rights, then he/she can be taken to court and prosecuted. In medicine, if a doctor is negligent and harms a patient then he/she may be struck off or even sent to prison. Doctors and patients have clear duties to uphold and respect legal rights.

In contrast, the duties and responsibilities doctors have in relation to human rights are less clear. The Human Rights Act (1998) includes both the 'right to life' (Article 2) and a right to be free from 'inhuman or degrading treatment' (Article 3). These may conflict in medicine, particularly when considering issues such as 'do not attempt resuscitation' orders or whether or not to switch off the ventilator for an unconscious patient in the intensive therapy unit (ITU). How doctors are to make decisions in light of human rights, particularly when they conflict, is not clear.

ENTITLEMENTS

Arguably, a more useful means of approaching rights, expectations and duties is to focus on entitlements. To what are patients entitled in health care? In the UK, people are entitled to access the NHS and receive good quality care and appropriate treatment. Patients are not necessarily entitled to any and every treatment they want or demand. Doctors have a responsibility to provide care, but should only supply treatment which is likely to be successful, unlikely to cause harm and there are sufficient resources.

Doctors should be clear about the extent of their duties and recognize that these may vary depending on the type of rights involved. Patients also have responsibilities which include giving their doctor all information relevant to their condition and wherever possible not needlessly endangering their own health.

Patients do pressurize doctors based on needs, desires and rights and doctors must make decisions about how best to allocate their resources. These factors should be weighted against considerations of justice.

CONSIDERATIONS OF JUSTICE

One key moral basis for making and assessing allocation decisions is that of justice. Justice as fairness, equality and equity all have an impact on medical and health care. Fairness requires that a universal and uniform standard of treatment is provided for all.[43] It requires consistency in the way people are treated. To be fair, two patients with the same condition should have access to the same types of services and care and be given the same treatment options.

Equality, like fairness, provides a minimum standard of consistency in treating people. It requires that similar cases are treated in similar ways and dissimilar cases are treated in dissimilar ways. Equality seeks to eliminate discrimination based on inappropriate grounds such as race or religious belief. Inequality exists where similar cases are treated in different ways. When allocating resources, doctors should be consistent in their dealings with patients and not allow discrimination based on clinically irrelevant factors to determine those decisions.

Although equality and fairness highlight important principles of justice and offer protection for individuals because of their focus on uniform treatment, they do not necessarily allow for differences in individual cases to be weighed sufficiently. In contrast, equity allows for differences in treatment between individuals, but these are permitted only for morally justifiable reasons.[44] It recognizes that giving people equal consideration is not the same as identical treatment.[45] A diversion from the normal standard of fairness and equality must be both justified and justifiable. Inequity exists where differences in treatment are not morally justified. If two patients have the same congenital abnormality of the ear and one is offered surgery and the other is not based on their economic class this would not be justifiable. Doctors must be able to provide a clear rationale for their decisions to the patient, relatives, other colleagues, management, government and wider public. The process and basis for these decisions should be communicated to the patient at the time and recorded in the notes.

When weighing up how best to use resources, doctors have to balance the needs, wants, rights and entitlements of the individual patient with their own duties and responsibilities to that individual and the wider community. This involves considerations of justice as fairness, equality and equity.

CONCLUSIONS

Doctors experience increasing pressure on their time, skills and resources. Daily, they are faced with difficult decisions, whether in relation to consent, confidentiality or withholding and withdrawing treatment. The moral basis on which they weigh up and make such decisions is crucial to their own practice and the delivery of patient care.

In our pluralist society, it may not be clear how and on what basis such decisions are made. Disagreements between doctors and patients, relatives and other colleagues can and do arise when confronted with moral choices and decisions. Reflecting on the specific ethical grounds for such decisions provides a more consistent framework for approaching such decisions. Whether they involve principles, consequences, virtue theory or a combination of these, ethical frameworks must be applied in practice. How they are applied may be seen in light of the doctor's duty to care for his/her patients and protecting patients' best interests, which involves non-maleficence, beneficence, being just and respecting autonomy. All of these must be weighed and prioritized in the context of the doctor–patient relationship where both parties bring particular knowledge and skills to the decision.

When this relationship breaks down and some consensus about a moral dilemma cannot be reached, there is an increasing tendency to retreat to law to sort it out. This leads to polarization of the parties involved and defensive medicine as doctors seek to protect themselves rather than put the best interests of the patient first. The law can be a blunt instrument, serves as a minimum standard and addresses legal, not ethical, questions.

As one way to avoid this retreat to law and in order to resist practising defensively, doctors should be increasing their moral awareness. Addressing ethical dilemmas within medical practice and discussing them with patients and relatives is one means of avoiding ending up in the courts. Doctors should be able to justify their decisions ethically and be clear about the moral basis on which they were made. Such justifications may have to be given to patients, families, colleagues, management, the government and wider society. With increasing pressure from the media, it is important that doctors offer a moral, as well as clinical, justification for their decisions.

As medical science and technology continue to advance, ethical challenges will continue to be faced within medicine. Encouraging healthy debate and dialogue within the medical profession and good communication with patients, relatives and colleagues can help avoid defensive practice and legal battles. Doctors should be encouraged to reflect on the moral basis for their decisions, while being aware of the different moral perspectives and values of patient and relatives, and look for some common ground and shared values in the midst of disagreement rather than focussing solely on the differences.

KEY POINTS

- Medical ethics is necessary as part of good clinical practice in dealing with patients, families, colleagues and institutions.
- The doctor–patient relationship is characterized by partnership and good communication.
- The good doctor fulfils the duty of care, acting in the best interests of patients,

respecting their autonomy and acting justly.

- Good medical moral decision-making draws on principles, consequences and medical virtues.
- Consent and refusal of treatment are based on competence, the giving of full information, understanding of its significance and freedom of choice.
- Confidentiality is both legally and morally required, except in extreme circumstances.
- Withdrawing and withholding treatment is both clinically and morally permissible in situations of futility and in the best interests of the patient.
- Careful allocation of limited resources means clear setting of priorities and acting fairly, equitably and equally.
- The conduct of research is subject to strict ethical guidelines to safeguard the patient/participant and the researcher.

Best clinical practice

✓ In all dealings with patients, families and colleagues, doctors should recognize the need for high moral standards.
✓ Doctors and patients should both act in partnership.
✓ The patient's autonomy should be respected, while recognizing autonomy has limits.
✓ Good communication with colleagues and patients is vital.
✓ Doctors should not only do no harm, do good, act justly and maximize autonomy, but also have a duty of care and to act in the best interests of patients.
✓ Doctors should be able to recognize the need for and make moral decisions on the basis of principles, consequences and medical virtues.
✓ Consent and refusal are part of a process based on competence, full information, understanding of its significance and free choice.
✓ Confidentiality must be respected, unless legally required to be broken.
✓ Withholding and withdrawing treatment may be appropriate when the situation is futile and it is in the best interests of the patient.
✓ Resources should be allocated fairly and equitably.
✓ Research should be conducted ethically with good clinical and statistical grounds, consent, protection of confidentiality and communication.

REFERENCES

* 1. Beauchamp TL, Childress JF. *Principles in biomedical ethics*, 5th edn. Oxford: Oxford University Press, 2001. *This text provides a good grounding in the theory of medical ethics and the four key principles.*
2. Cook ED. Choice and consent. In: *Patients' choice: A consumer's guide to medical practice*. London: Spire, 1993: 18–21.
* 3. British Medical Association. *Rights and responsibilities of doctors*, 2nd edn. London: British Medical Association, 1992. *In this text, the BMA outlines carefully multiple duties of doctors and offers guidance for ethical practice in relation to issues such as consent and refusal, confidentiality, stopping treatment, resource allocation and research.*
4. General Medical Council. *Duties of a doctor*. London: General Medical Council, 1995.
* 5. British Medical Association. *Medical ethics today: The BMA's handbook of ethics and law*, 2nd edn. London: BMJ Publishing, 2004. *This offers useful guidance on a range of clinical and ethical issues for doctors including consent, confidentiality, stopping treatment, resource allocation and research.*
6. Wasson K. Ethical arguments for providing palliative care to non-cancer patients. *International Journal of Palliative Nursing*. 2000; **6**: 66–70.
7. Takala T. What is wrong with global bioethics? On the limitations of the four principles approach. *Cambridge Quarterly of Healthcare Ethics*. 2001; **10**: 72–7.
* 8. Cook ED. The values that surround us. In: *The moral maze*. London: SPCK, 1983: 21–4. *David Cook provides an accessible and clear explanation of different approaches to morality as well as one framework for approaching such decisions.*
* 9. Wasson K, Cook ED. Morality in medicine: Five approaches to ethics. *CME Bulletin of Palliative Medicine*. 2001; **2**: 6–10. *This provides a concise overview of five approaches to ethics in medicine-principles, consequences, relativism, reductionism and virtue theory.*
10. O'Neill O. Kantian ethics. In: Singer P (ed.). *A companion to ethics*. Oxford: Blackwell, 1993: 175–85.
11. Paton HJ. *The moral law: Kant's groundwork of the metaphysics of morals*. London: Hutchinson, 1961.
12. Kant I. *The foundations of the metaphysics of morals*. Translated by Beck LW. London and New York: MacMillan, 1985.
13. Bentham J. A fragment on government and introduction to the principles of morals and legislation. Harrison W (ed.). Oxford: Basil Blackwell, 1948.
14. Mill JS. *Utilitarianism, liberty, representative government*. London: Dent, 1954.
15. MacIntyre A. *After virtue: A study in moral theory*, 2nd edn. Notre Dame: Notre Dame University Press, 1984.
16. British Medical Association. Consent and refusal. In: *Medical ethics today: Its practice and philosophy*. London: British Medical Association, 1993: 10.

17. British Medical Association. Consent and refusal: Children and young people. *Medical ethics today: The BMA's handbook of ethics and law*, 2nd edn. London: BMJ Publishing, 2004: 131–64.

18. British Medical Association. Children and young people. In: *Medical ethics today: Its practice and philosophy.* London: British Medical Association, 1993: 78.

19. British Medical Association. Chapter 16, Doctors with dual obligations and Chapter 17, Doctors working in custodial settings. In: *Medical ethics today: The BMA's handbook of ethics and law*, 2nd edn. London: BMJ Publishing Group, 2004: 565–601 and 602–47.

20. British Medical Association. Chapter 1, Consent and refusal and Chapter 9, Doctors with dual obligations. In: *Medical ethics today: Its practice and philosophy.* London: BMA, 1993: 21–22, 245–54.

21. British Medical Association. Treatment without consent: Incapacitated adults and compulsory treatment. In: *Medical ethics today: Its practice and philosophy*, 2nd edn. London: British Medical Association, 2004: 99–126.

22. British Medical Association. Mental health. In: *Rights and responsibilities of doctors*, 2nd edn. London: British Medical Association, 1992: 99.

23. Adults with Incapacity (Scotland) Act 2000.

24. British Medical Association. Confidentiality. In: *Rights and responsibilities of doctors*, 2nd edn. London: British Medical Association, 1992: 41–3.

25. British Medical Association. Confidentiality. In: *Medical ethics today: The BMA's handbook of ethics and law*, 2nd edn. London: British Medical Association, 2004: 173.

26. General Medical Council. *HIV infection and AIDS.* London: General Medical Council, 1988.

27. British Medical Association. Caring for patients at the end of life. In: *Medical ethics today: The BMA's handbook of ethics and law*, 2nd edn. London: British Medical Association, 2004: 351–87.

28. Schneiderman LJ, Jecker NS, Jonsen AR. Medical futility: Its meaning and ethical implications. *Annals of Internal Medicine.* 1990; **112**: 949–54.

29. Schneiderman LJ, Jecker NS, Jonsen AR. Medical futility: Responses to critiques. *Annals of Internal Medicine.* 1996; **125**: 669–74.

30. British Medical Association. *Withholding and withdrawing life-prolonging medical treatment.* London: British Medical Association, 1999.

31. Rhymes JA, McCullough LB, Luchi RJ, Teasdale TA, Wilson N. Withdrawing very low-burden interventions in chronically ill patients. *Journal of the American Medical Association.* 2000; **283**: 1061–3.

32. Cook ED. Stopping treatment. In: *Patients' choice: A consumer's guide to medical practice.* London: Spire, 1993: 125–6.

33. Airedale NHS v Bland (1993) AC 789.

34. Cook ED. Research. In: *Patients' choice: A consumer's guide to medical practice.* London: Spire, 1993: 191.

35. British Medical Association. Research and innovative treatment. In: *Medical ethics today: The BMA's handbook of ethics and law*, 2nd edn. London: British Medical Association, 2004: 489–90.

36. British Medical Association. Research. In: *Medical ethics today: Its practice and philosophy.* London: British Medical Association, 1993: 198–9.

37. Medical Research Council. *The ethical conduct of research on children.* London: Medical Research Council, 1991.

38. British Medical Association. Accessed on June 30, 2005, www.bma.org.uk/ap.nsf/Content/ Parental#Consentfrompeoplewithparental

39. Michels KB, Rothman KJ. Update on unethical use of placebos in randomised trials. *Bioethics.* 2003; **17**: 188–204.

40. Rothman KJ, Michels KB, Baum M. For and against: Declaration of Helsinki should be strengthened. *British Medical Journal.* 2000; **321**: 442–5.

41. Maslow A. *Motivation and personality*, 3rd edn. Revised by Frager R, Fadiman J, Reynolds C, Cox R. New York: Harper and Row, 1987.

42. Wasson K. Resource allocation. *Christian Medical Fellowship File 17.* London: Christian Medical Fellowship, 2002.

43. Rawls J. *A theory of justice.* Cambridge: Belknap and Harvard University Press, 1971.

44. Downie RS, Telfer E. *Caring and curing: A philosophy of medicine and social work.* New York and London: Methuen, 1980.

45. Outka G. Social justice and equal access to health care. In: Lammers SE, Verhey A (ed.). *On moral medicine: Theological perspectives in medical ethics.* Grand Rapids: Eerdmans, 1987: 632–43.

48

Medical jurisprudence and otorhinolaryngology

MAURICE HAWTHORNE AND DESMOND WATSON

Introduction	594	Performance and complaints	605
Tort	595	The Human Rights Act	606
Negligence	595	The criminal law	607
Consent	600	The future	609
Confidentiality	602	Key points	610
The coroner	602	References	610
The role of the expert	603		

INTRODUCTION

When these authors were first appointed as consultant otolaryngologists, the closest contact with the legal process that they envisaged was the writing of expert witness reports in personal injury cases. Along with this was a realization that there was a small chance that these reports might lead to a court appearance as an expert witness. The regional health authorities and later hospital trusts had by then been forced to accept vicarious liability for the actions of the consultants they employed so the only other contact that apparently was possible was the result of a claim alleging negligence in private practice. Although this event was feared by most consultants, the chances of a successful claim were and still remain low. The last decade and a half has seen some changes in how claims of clinical negligence are decided but the developments in other fields such as consent, confidentiality and clinical performance have been much more significant. The medical profession in general has twice been put in the spotlight by very major events which were subject to intense media interest: the Bristol Royal Infirmary Inquiry into unacceptable complication rates in the paediatric cardiac surgery unit and the trial of Harold Shipman who was convicted of murdering an unknown number of his patients have changed the way that the public views the medical profession. The response from politicians has been to try to tighten the legal framework in which doctors practise so that the public can be reassured that it can never happen again.

The law in England differs slightly from that in Scotland and Northern Ireland but most of the principles are the same. The first major subdivision is into criminal law and civil law. In criminal law, the state prosecutes an individual or an organization (the defendant) alleging breach of a law or statute. If the case is proven, the individual or organization is subject to a sentence, often a fine or a custodial term of some kind. In civil law, one individual or organization (now known as the claimant, formerly the plaintiff) brings a suit for damages against a defendant and seeks damages from that defendant. Ideally, the damages would exactly redress the loss suffered by the claimant. For instance, a claimant proved to have been swindled out of his car by a defendant might be happy merely to have his car back. In medical negligence cases, it is manifestly impossible to restore negligently caused losses so the damages are monetary. There are three important forms of monetary damages in clinical negligence: general, special and punitive or exemplary.

General damages are those awarded to compensate the successful claimant for pain and suffering. Special damages are those awarded to take account of loss of income, special nursing needs, etc., arising from the negligence. Punitive damages are exactly what they say they are: damages awarded to the claimant to punish the negligent defendant. These are similar in a way to a fine in criminal cases but are not awarded in clinical negligence cases in the UK where most defendants have insurance to cover any damages awarded against them.

Civil and criminal jurisdictions differ in two other important ways: in the standard of proof required and in the influence of statutes. In criminal cases, the standard of proof is 'beyond reasonable doubt' which is often taken to imply a probability of guilt of at least 95 percent. In civil cases the standard of proof is 'on the balance of probabilities' which means greater than 50 percent probability. This figure leads to some apparently illogical conclusions in the field of causation where it has been argued that, as far as the law is concerned, a 5 percent five-year survival is identical to a 49 percent five-year survival (so no compensation should be paid even if negligence is proven) but completely different from 51 percent five-year survival. The view of the House of Lords, the highest legal authority in England and Wales, on this subject is awaited.

The source of the criminal law is founded in the common law and on statutes passed by Parliament and, more recently, European law. Statutes, precedent and European legislation state what actions constitute criminal behaviour. In the course of a criminal trial, counsel may well cite a precedent of what has been said and what decisions were made by courts in the past in similar cases. In a civil trial, there may be no statute that has any relevance to the questions to be decided so the decisions are based almost entirely on what happened in previous cases. This is referred to as the common law. The common law is in a state of continuous development as civil cases are tried by high courts, such as the Court of Appeal and the House of Lords, which can introduce subtle changes in decisions that then become the common law. Much argument may then occur as to what exactly their Lordships meant. Was what they said in a previous case relevant to the one currently being tried? Even more debatable is whether or not the important remark was part of a judgement or some sort of subjunctive aside to the judgement in the form of 'if this case had been similar to case A then I would have decided as follows'. The next section of the chapter (see under Causation below) illustrates exactly how one word in a judgement can be important when the case referred to as Bolitho[1] is considered.

Besides major sections devoted to clinical negligence and the duties of an expert medical witness, this chapter examines the two most common questions asked of a medical indemnity organization's helpline: consent and the doctor's duty of confidentiality. The criminal law and the role of the coroner as they are likely to apply to surgeons in their professional activities are discussed. The duties of a consultant surgeon as a doctor and the mechanisms that are or shortly will be in place to ensure that these are complied with are described and the additional duties of that consultant as a trainer is also mentioned.

TORT

Before discussing clinical negligence and consent issues, it is relevant to review the legal principle on which these are largely based. This is the law of tort or wrong done by one party to another. The two forms of tort that are relevant to surgeons are negligence and assault and battery.

There are four essential elements of the legal tort of negligence:

1. there must be a duty of care;
2. there must be a breach of that duty;
3. harm must have occurred;
4. the breach must have caused the harm.

Negligence occurs when party A is considered to owe a duty of care to party B, to have breached that duty and, as a result, harm has come to B. It must be shown that A could reasonably have foreseen that the breach might cause the harm. For instance, a driver travelling quickly on a country road should have it in mind that there might be a cyclist just around the corner. A second important aspect of negligence on which many clinical negligence cases fail is causation. This works on the so-called 'but for' test. It must be proved that, 'but for' the breach of duty by the defendant, the damage suffered by the claimant would not have occurred.

It is perhaps a surprise to many people that assault and battery are sources of both civil and criminal litigation. Assault is the threat of physical violence and battery is any unlawful touching or physical contact of one person by another. The law makes an exception for ordinary day-to-day contact such as occurs in a bus queue or when handing over change for a newspaper but this does not apply to medical examination. Only with consent (which will be discussed further under Consent below) does a medical examination become lawful. Without consent, approaching a patient with a shining Lack's tongue depressor at the ready is an assault and using it to depress the tongue is a battery. Although the act of opening the mouth probably implies consent, the patient has the option of lodging a civil claim alleging battery or even of reporting a possible criminal battery to the police. It is important to note that civil actions for battery, unlike those for negligence, do not require that there has been any harm. Patients seeking damages for lack of adequate consent can sue either in negligence (where the 'but for' test applies but consent must be truly informed) or in battery (where causation is not an issue but a much less rigorous consent is enough to refute the allegations).

NEGLIGENCE

Standard of skill and care

In deciding negligence the claimant must establish four things.

1. A duty of care was owed to the claimant.
2. There has been a breach of that duty.

3. Damage has occurred to the claimant.
4. The breach must have caused the damage.

To establish a duty it is necessary for a doctor/patient relationship to be in existence. There is no Good Samaritan law in the UK, and doctors only have a legal responsibility to people they have agreed to treat. In general practice the agreement arises by virtue of accepting a patient onto one's list. In a hospital setting, the agreement either arises out of the doctor's Terms and Conditions of Employment, or with private patients, as a result of contract.

Patients tend to be seen by several different doctors and, therefore, the question: 'who owes the duty of care?' may be a pertinent one. In the National Health Service (NHS), the employing authority will usually be named as first defendant as it would be liable to pay damages arising from any successful action by virtue of the principle of vicarious liability. Individual doctors may then be named as subsequent defendants.

An unresolved issue is who should be sued if a patient is placed on a waiting list, but suffers additional damage in the time it takes to receive a first appointment? Is the defendant the referring GP, or the Authority, or NHS Trust at whose clinic the patient is awaiting an appointment?

The standard of care is that of the reasonably skilled and experienced doctor. The appropriate test, known as the Bolam (*Bolam* v. *Friern Hospital Management Committee*) test,[2] states that it is:

the standard of the ordinary skilled man exercising and professing to have that special skill. A man need not possess the highest expert skill; it is well-established law that it is sufficient if he exercises the ordinary skill of an ordinary competent man exercising that particular art.

The standard of care relates to the specialty in which the doctor practices. A GP will not be required to possess the skills of a specialist. An inexperienced doctor cannot rely on his lack of experience as a defence to alleged negligence (*Wilsher* v. *Essex Area Health Authority*).[3] However, a junior doctor may discharge his duty by seeking the help of a superior.

While a doctor is under a duty to keep himself appraised of developments in his area, this is subject to the bounds of reasonableness. Failure to read one article, which might have prevented the negligent act, could be excusable, while failure to be aware of new techniques that have become widespread may be inexcusable (*Crawford* v. *Board of Governors of the Charing Cross Hospital*).[4]

A doctor will not be negligent simply because he acted in a way that another doctor would not have done. The Bolam test establishes that a man is not negligent if he is acting in accordance with a practice merely because there is a body of medical opinion which would take a contrary view, provided there is a reasonable body of opinion which supports the practice. A body of opinion must consist of at least two people. This statement has recently been qualified by the case referred to as Bolitho (*Bolitho* v. *City and Hackney Health Authority*).[1]

Causation

In Bolitho, a registrar in paediatrics was accepted to be in breach of her duty of care by failing to visit an infant with breathing difficulties. Her defence was that, given the clinical circumstances at the time she should have visited, she would not have intubated the infant. The Court of Appeal had found that the failure to attend the infant constituted negligence. The House of Lords heard opposite expert opinions, one asserting that there was a body of opinion that would undoubtedly have intubated in those circumstances and the other that there was also a responsible body of opinion that would not have intubated. Their Lordships then reversed the judgement saying that the defendant's assertion that she would not have intubated, a practice supported by a reasonable body of opinion, meant that on the balance of probabilities the brain damage would have occurred even if the registrar had visited. The causal link from the failure to discharge her duty of care by visiting the patient to the harm suffered was therefore broken so no negligence could be proved.

Bolitho is important because it clearly brings Bolam into the field of causation and also because of the dissenting judgement of Lord Browne-Wilkinson. Referring to the reasonable body of medical opinion that would allow a Bolam-based defence, he said 'The use of these adjectives – responsible, reasonable and respectable – all show that the court has to be satisfied that the exponents of the body of opinion relied on can demonstrate that such opinion has a **logical** basis' (our emphasis). Later in judgement he qualified this by saying, 'it will very seldom be right for a judge to reach the conclusion that views genuinely held by a competent medical expert are unreasonable'. It is not yet clear how these comments will be used as precedents for future cases but they certainly will be. An example might be the practice of stripping all the mucosa from a vocal cord in Reinke's oedema. There is certainly a body of expert opinion that would condone the practice but, in view of our knowledge of the physiology of the superficial lamina propria, is it logical to operate in this way and can that body of expert opinion be considered responsible?

Proof of medical negligence

The onus lies upon the claimant to prove that the surgeon's negligent treatment caused the injury. It is not sufficient simply to prove that the surgeon's actions were reprehensible or even reckless if the claimant cannot go on to show that their injury is directly attributable to the surgeon's poor performance. Hence, while it was clear that a casualty officer was in breach of his duty of care when he failed to examine a patient attending his department with the obvious signs of poisoning, there was a complete defence (*Barnett* v. *Chelsea & Kensington Hospital*)[5] when it was shown that there was no antidote to the poison taken by the patient. This is similar to the reasoning in Bolitho above, although that case was much more complicated than Barnett. In Barnett, it was a straightforward and uncontested statement that the workmen who had accidentally ingested arsenic in their tea were doomed whether or not they received medical attention. In Bolitho the courts had to decide whether or not, on balance of probabilities, the hypoxic brain damage would have occurred even if the registrar had visited the child.

The standard to which the claimant must prove his case is on the balance of probabilities. This means that the claimant must show that his version of events and expert analysis are more likely to be true than those put forward by the defence. If the case for each side is evenly balanced then the claimant will fail. Hence, where a patient suffers a nerve palsy that could equally have been due to negligence, or could have occurred as an inherent risk of the operation even when performed with proper skill and care, the claimant's case will fail in the absence of some item of evidence to tip the scales in favour of negligence (*Ashcroft* v. *Mersey Regional Health Authority*).[6]

An apparent reversal of the burden of proof can occur where the likelihood of negligence is so obvious that it 'speaks for itself' (*res ipsa loquitur*). In other words, a defendant may find that he is obliged at least to provide an explanation of the patient's injury that is consistent with reasonable care having been taken, even where the claimant has no positive evidence of negligence, where:

- there is no evidence as to how or why the accident occurred;
- the accident is such that it would not occur without negligence;
- the defendant is proved to have been in control of the situation in which the accident occurred.[7]

The doctrine first evolved in simple personal injury cases concerning falling objects (*Scott* v. *London & St Katherine's Docks*,[8] *Byrne* v. *Boadle*[9] and *Pope* v. *St Helen's Theatre*[10]), but has obvious attractions to a claimant in a medical case, where there may well be very real uncertainty as to how an injury came about, and where the often unconscious patient is entirely under the control of the medical team. Despite the fact that it is often pleaded, in England the doctrine has more often been conceded than litigated in medical cases, and so its ambit is unclear.[11] In practice the courts are reluctant to apply a doctrine derived from the relatively simple 'bumps and thumps' of stevedoring to the complex issues of causation found in medical litigation. It has been said:

> The human body is not a container filled with a material whose performance can be predictably charted.... because of this medical science has not yet reached the stage where the law ought to presume that a patient must come out of an operation as well or better than when he went into it.[12]
>
> (*Girard* v. *Royal Columbian Hospital*)

Thus, as a matter of law, the onus of proving negligence will almost always fall on the claimant, although in cases where there is a strong and obvious inference of negligence from the very facts themselves (e.g. a retained swab (*Mahon* v. *Osborne*)[13] or where the claimant woke from his anaesthetic with the septic finger still attached and an adjacent one in the bucket[14]) the defence may well find that onus discharged unless they are able to provide some alternative theory, not involving negligence, to answer the claimant's case.

Damages

A claimant having established negligence, and having proved injury as a consequence, the question turns to the assessment of the compensation to be paid. The court must award a sum of money that will, as nearly as possible, put the injured person in the same position as he would have been had he not been injured (*Livingstone* v. *Rawyards Coal Company*).[15] In some jurisdictions (notably the USA) an element of punitive damages may be awarded. Such an approach has been rejected in England and Wales (*Kralj* v. *McGrath*)[16] and the rest of the UK for mere inadvertent negligence. The argument is based on mens rea being present before the claimant can be given a monetary award by way of punishing the defendant.

Damages are broadly classified into two categories.

GENERAL DAMAGES

These include damages for pain, suffering and loss of amenity. This is the aspect of the claimant's loss which is not ascertainable by a mathematical calculation of economic loss and, in the past, was determined by a jury (*Ward* v. *James*).[17] Juries were effectively abolished in personal injury trials in the mid-1960s. While the level of general damages will depend on the claimant's circumstances, and the suffering which the particular injury has caused the individual, a general bracket for a particular injury will be determined with reference to awards (adjusted for inflation) from previously decided cases. Obviously, it is impossible to 'compensate' someone for loss of a limb or for a life of continual pain so the awards are essentially conventional figures. As a guide, the current conventional figure for injuries of the utmost severity is between £120,000 and £150,000, and so injuries of lesser significance will be a proportion of that 'maximum'. In a recent case in Teeside (*Levitt* v. *Hartlepool Area Health Authority*),[18] a minor born deaf was awarded £50,000 general damages (adjusting for inflation in 2003 this would probably be £60,000), which included her total hearing loss.

SPECIAL DAMAGES

These are the specific 'out-of-pocket' monetary expenses and losses which the claimant has incurred up until the date of the trial. These will include loss of earnings, medical expenses, travel costs and the cost of any special equipment consequent upon the injury. Often there will be a claim for losses expected in the future. (Future loss is technically an item of general damages as its assessment is uncertain and it was formerly a matter for the jury to determine. As a matter of practice, the calculation of future loss is inseparable from that of past loss, many of the same arguments rehearsed in both, and one flows naturally to the other.) The amount of money at issue will depend almost exclusively on the particular circumstances of the claimant (*Lim* v. *Camden Health Authority*),[19] guided by the principle that a claimant should only recover what he has lost as a result of the injury. He must prove that his expenditure was (or will be) reasonably necessary, and that his needs cannot be met more cheaply by other reasonable means.

As a rule, English law seeks to compensate a claimant by way of a single lump sum award. This creates obvious problems where a claimant is likely to remain unemployed or requires continuing care for many years in the future. The only certain result is that the claimant will be either under- or overcompensated, depending on how circumstances unfold. This problem has not been solved, but ameliorated in certain cases. Where a claimant suffers a condition that may deteriorate significantly in the future, rather than receive a small sum to represent the risk, they can apply for an order for 'Provisional Damages', which leaves it open to the claimant to come back to court at a later date.[20]

In very large claims where the claimant's life expectancy will determine the level of the award, the risk can be borne by an insurance company by the purchase of an annuity. This is known as a 'Structured Settlement'.

Dealing with medical negligence claims

What happens when a surgeon is sued?[21] The Civil Procedure Rules 1998[22] are considered below. They require that, in cases of clinical disputes, a pre-action protocol be followed. This sets procedures and time limits for various stages of the process of being sued. There are also recommendations for Trusts about how they should respond to a claim and what processes should be in place to ensure that they are able to respond in an appropriate and timely way. In effect, the pre-action protocol will penalize a Trust which has such a poor clinical governance structure that it is unable to respond to a claim in a relatively short time.

What the individual consultant surgeon will experience if his patient sues him alleging negligence will differ in some ways depending whether the patient was a private patient or an NHS patient. The first stage of the proceedings is the same: the patient, having found some means of financial support for his or her claim against the health care provider (a matter outside the remit of this chapter but considerably more difficult than formerly) will request, via a solicitor, release of notes. In private practice, the consultant will need to release these notes himself and is wise to check with his anaesthetist, the private hospital and other doctors involved in the secondary care that they will do the same. The consultant would be most unwise at this stage if he did not inform his medical indemnity organization and seek their help and advice. If the case is an NHS one, the matter must be referred to the Trust's legal department immediately. If the clinical governance system in the Trust is working well, there is a good chance that the events have already been reported to the legal section via an incident form and that contemporaneous statements have already been taken and filed in preparation for a potential claim. Alternatively, the claimant may have already used the NHS complaints' procedure so all the statements from that will be available. A Trust is vicariously liable for the actions of its employees and so the legal department should take over all further responses to solicitors and communication with the defendant legal team. Both Trusts and independent practitioners have 40 days to provide the copy medical records and failure to meet this deadline will prejudice any defence.

The potential claimant's solicitors will now obtain an expert report on the medical records with examination of their client if appropriate and can decide whether or not the claim has merit. If it has, they will serve a letter of claim on the health care provider setting out a summary of facts, the main allegations of negligence, description of injuries and an outline of losses. This may include an offer to settle. The defendant organization or individual must provide a reasoned answer within three months of receipt.

In addition, the defendant's solicitors will be concerned to obtain guidance from experts swiftly and, once received, be able to form an initial view about whether or not the claim is defensible. The assessment of a claim at this stage will be facilitated by recent rule changes which have been made concerning the conduct of personal injury actions, including medical negligence litigation. These changes require that at the time of service of a writ, a claimant must also submit a medical report setting out the claimant's condition and prognosis, together with a Schedule of Special Damages said to result from any alleged negligence. Traditionally, such information was not available until much later in the litigation process. The change has resulted in a defendant's solicitors being able to assess the potential value of a claimant's claim at an early stage. Accordingly, following that initial expert opinion, a settlement can be proposed early in the proceedings on behalf of the otolaryngologist, if appropriate.

If settlement is desired but cannot be negotiated between the solicitors, then the solicitors acting for the otolaryngologist may try to settle the claim by what is known as a 'payment into court'. In making a payment into court, the defendant can make an assessment of the damages which might be awarded in due course at trial, if negligence is established. If the trial judge awards a sum higher than the level of the payment in, the claimant will receive his or her costs in the usual way. If, however, the sum awarded is the same or a lesser sum then, as a general rule, all costs of the action, including the defendant's costs after the payment into court, must be borne by the claimant. The claimant has 21 days to decide whether or not to accept the payment in. Thereafter the costs conservancies will operate. In cases where the claimant is legally aided, this device is of more limited assistance to a defendant. In other circumstances, there may well be a strong incentive to a claimant to accept a payment into court through fear of being prejudiced on costs in this way.

Following the service of a defence, in response to allegations contained in the statement of claim, both parties may raise requests for further information about their respective pleadings, and the claimant may choose to file a reply to the defence.

Directions concerning the conduct of a claim will be given by the court, usually after the pleadings are completed. In the High Court, a formal hearing will take place to consider these directions, but in personal injury actions brought in the County Court, a series of so-called automatic directions is given by the court. These are rarely, if ever, appropriate in medical negligence cases and it is therefore usual for the parties to apply to the court for specific directions to be given. These directions will provide for, among other things, the disclosure of witness statements as to fact and expert reports. In the past, in medical negligence actions, neither expert reports nor witness statements were disclosed by one party to another. Only at trial would the nature of the respective cases become clear. However, as a result of recent cases and changes in the procedural rules, expert reports and witness statements must now be disclosed, and this will be ordered by the court at a directions hearing. It is usual for witness statements to be disclosed, followed shortly thereafter by expert reports, in order that experts can consider this information available from the other side in preparing the report. The exchange of both statements and reports gives a further opportunity for review of the case, both by claimant and medical defendant. At this stage the claimant may realize that the claim is weak and the case may be discontinued. Equally, the defence may feel that the case is not defensible and settlement negotiations or a payment into court may follow.

TRIAL AND PREPARATION FOR TRIAL

If the exchange of witness statements and expert reports does not promote the settlement of a claim, then the case proceeds towards trial. In medical negligence actions, a fixed date for trial will usually be given by the court because of the significant number of clinicians who may have to make themselves available, either as experts or as witnesses of fact.

By way of preparation for trial, both parties should arrange conferences with counsel in order to review the case in detail, and ensure all preparations are complete. If the defence considers that the case should be settled, or there are certain aspects of the case where a defendant may be vulnerable, a payment into court may be made. The payment in may be limited to those aspects of the claim where the defendant could be found liable. The claimant has 21 days within which to accept the payment in before the penalty of costs starts to run. As a significant proportion of the costs of an action result from the trial itself, the defendants are usually anxious to make any payment into court before 21 days in advance of the trial. Thereafter bundles of documents must be prepared for use in the court by all parties, which will include the pleadings, medical records, witness statements and expert reports.

A proportion of cases are settled literally at the doors of the court, the last opportunity for compromise before further significant costs of trial are incurred.

If no compromise can be reached, the trial will commence with an explanation of the case to the judge by counsel for the claimant, setting out the relevant events and the nature of the allegations. The claimant's counsel will then call witnesses of fact, usually followed then by expert witnesses. Each witness will be cross-examined in turn by the defence, and then re-examined by claimant's counsel if necessary. When the claimant's evidence has been called, the defence case is then put in the same way, and usually in the same order.

The trial judge may allow variation in this order of evidence, particularly in complex cases, so that witnesses for both sides are called first, to be followed then by experts. This will allow experts to hear all the evidence of fact before giving a final opinion. However, the present arrangements for disclosure of witness statements make such variation rare.

At the conclusion of the case, the judge will usually hear submissions from counsel on the law to be applied and the appropriate level of damages to be awarded if the claimant is successful. It is usual then for the judge to reserve judgement, to be delivered at a later day, as most negligence cases are complex and will require some consideration. Once judgement is given, and if the claimant is successful, the judge will indicate the level of damages to be awarded. Only at that stage is the judge informed about any payment into court which may have been made, and the costs to be awarded can then be considered.

FUNDING OF NEGLIGENCE CLAIMS

Otolaryngologists may well have been concerned at the possibility that medical negligence actions in England and Wales will follow the pattern of the USA, and that the perceived increase in the number of actions here may continue. However, with the reduction in the eligibility for legal aid, many actions which would have been funded by legal aid in the past will now have to be funded privately. The introduction of contingency or conditional fees is unlikely to assist all those who are no longer eligible for legal aid. As an incentive for the claimant's solicitor, the conditional fee system[23] will allow the solicitor to claim twice the rate of fees they might have otherwise obtained in a successful action. There is a risk that the solicitor might receive no payment at all if the case is unsuccessful. As suggested above, solicitors acting for patients are therefore likely to take on fewer claims,[24] concentrating on those where liability is obvious and can be quickly established. The result is likely to be that there will be no significant increase in the number of medical negligence actions in the short term. Indeed, it is possible that there will be a reduction at the expense of patients who might otherwise have had successful claims for compensation.

CONSENT

Much medical litigation is caused by the practitioner's failure to disclose adequate information about the risks inherent in a given procedure. Common law recognizes the principle that every person has the right to have his bodily integrity respected. There is a presumption that a person should not be exposed to risk unless he has voluntarily accepted that risk, based on adequate information and adequate comprehension.

Obtaining consent to carry out an operation is necessary to avoid three sorts of legal jeopardy. The first and second arise because any touching of another person is a potential battery. (Assault is the threat of causing physical injury. An unconscious person can be battered but cannot be assaulted.) This means that, in very exceptional circumstances, a surgeon performing an operation without consent may be prosecuted in the criminal courts for alleged criminal battery. A more likely

outcome of such surgery is a civil case seeking damages for the tort (or wrong) of battery. There is no need to show that anything went wrong with the surgery, merely that it was carried out without valid consent. The third, and much the most likely legal outcome regarding consent, is that the claimant tries to show that he was not warned of the risks of a proposed therapy that resulted in harm and that, had he been warned of those risks, he would have refused the treatment. An example might be a patient with a dead ear after a competently performed stapedotomy who was not warned of that risk before surgery. He may well be able to claim damages from the surgeon because he can say that 'but for' the surgeon's failure to warn of the risk, he would not have undergone the surgery. It is immediately obvious that any careful surgeon must record what potential adverse outcomes of a proposed operation have been discussed with a patient. If it is not recorded in the notes, courts have become sceptical of a statement such as 'it is my usual practice to warn of these risks'.

The question of how much information must be given to the patient will vary from situation to situation, but is generally set by the professional standard according to the Bolam test, with doctors being arbiters of how much information should be given. This means that, in the example above, if the defendant surgeon could assemble a respectable body of opinion whose practice would not be to warn of the risk of dead ear, his conduct did not breach a duty of care. Notably, in England and Wales, there is no notion of informed consent, as in the USA, whereby the amount of information to be disclosed is dictated by what a patient would want to know.

This is modified to a degree by the case of Sidaway (*Sidaway* v. *Board of Governors of the Bethlem Royal Hospital*)[25] in which the House of Lords held that where the proposed treatment involved a substantial risk of grave or adverse consequences such that, notwithstanding any practice to the contrary, a patient's right to decide whether to consent to the treatment was so obvious that no prudent medical man could fail to warn of the risk (save in emergency or some other sound clinical reason for nondisclosure), then it would be negligent not to warn. To continue the example above, the claimant could argue that total deafness in one ear is such a disability that any reasonable patient would wish to be told about it preoperatively.

Accordingly, the right of the doctor (acting in accordance with a reasonable body of medical opinion) to decide what the individual patient should be told remains enshrined in English case law. Such medical paternalism, which may be in the best interest of some of our patients, is currently and repeatedly being questioned. The doctor should realise that in Sidaway when the question 'is informed consent a part of English law?' was put to the five law lords, the answer was not unanimous. Scarman said 'Yes', Diplock said 'No' and Bridge, Keith and Templeman said 'Yes with reservations'.

In assessing which material risks should be mentioned, doctors should consider the degree of probability of the risk materializing and seriousness of possible injury if it does. A risk, even if it is a mere possibility, should be disclosed if its occurrence would cause serious circumstances (*Hopp* v. *Lepp*).[26] Medical evidence will be necessary for the court to assess the degree of probability and the seriousness. A further medical factor upon which expert evidence will also be required is to assess the character of the risk, i.e. is this risk common to all surgery or is it specific to the particular operation? Special risks inherent in a recommended operation are more likely to be material.

The legal standard of disclosure required in response to direct questions is also set by the professional standard (*Blyth* v. *Bloomsbury Health Authority*).[27] Although the amount of information given must depend upon the circumstances, as a general proposition it is governed by the Bolam test (supra).

In Australia, the doctrine of informed consent has gone one stage further from Sidaway where the reasonable patient was considered the arbiter of what risks should or should not be disclosed preoperatively. In *Rogers* v. *Whittaker*,[28] it is clear that the risks that must be disclosed are those that affect that one patient and not the generality of reasonable patients. To take the stapedotomy analogy one last stage further, few surgeons would warn of a dead ear risk of 1 in 2000 operations and probably the reasonable patient would be unlikely to want to know that this was a complication as it is so unlikely. The question arises of whether the patient having that operation on an only hearing ear might view the risk differently and want to be aware of it in making a decision.

Who can give consent?

There are three categories of patient described in the Department of Health Reference Guide to Consent for Examination or Treatment: the adult with capacity to consent; the adult without capacity to consent; and children and young people.

CHILDREN

Section 8(1) of the Family Law Reform Act 1969 provides that a person over 16 may give a valid consent to medical treatment as though he was an adult. As regards children under 16, the general principle is that laid down in the Gillick (*Gillick* v. *West Norfolk and Wisbech Area Health Authority*) case,[29] that the parental right to determine whether or not a child under 16 should have medical treatment terminates when the child achieves a significant understanding and intelligence to enable him or her to understand fully what is proposed. Until such time, the parents, or others acting in loco parentis, may give their consent or refusal to medical treatment. Recent case law suggests that it may still be possible to treat a seemingly competent child who is refusing to give consent, providing someone else with the capacity to consent provides consent on the child's behalf (In re R, and in re W).[30, 31]

MENTALLY INCOMPETENT PATIENTS

Where a patient is unable to provide consent on his or her own behalf by reason of mental incapacity, no one else, including a court, may give consent on that person's behalf. The doctrine of necessity, however, permits a doctor to lawfully operate on or give other treatment to adult incompetent patients, provided that the treatment is in their best interest, either to save their lives or to ensure improvement in their physical or mental health (Re F).[32]

JEHOVAH'S WITNESSES

Certain groups of patients, including Jehovah's Witnesses, may refuse to receive blood transfusions or other life-saving therapies. The Court of Appeal has affirmed patients' rights to refuse medical treatment, even if this will result in their death; nevertheless, for such a refusal to be effective, the court must be satisfied that at the time of refusal the patient's capacity is not diminished by illness or medication or given on the basis of false assumptions or misinformation. In the case of Re T,[33] Lord Donaldson said:

> An adult patient who suffers from no mental incapacity has an absolute right to choose whether to consent to medical treatment, to refuse it or to choose one rather than another of the treatments being offered.

A decision to refuse medical treatment does not have to be sensible, obviously rational or well considered, and in the case of a competent patient, the doctor cannot override the patient's wishes because he believes it to be in the patient's best interests.

OTHER SPECIAL GROUPS

Pregnant women, patients who are human immunodeficiency virus positive or suffering from acquired immunodeficiency syndrome and the elderly do not represent special categories for the purposes of consent. Although the amount of information which has to be given to a patient varies from case to case, a decision to withhold information solely on paternalistic grounds that it may deter the patient from accepting the therapy may not be justified in law.

CONFIDENTIALITY

Doctors are well aware of their duty, originally stated in the Hippocratic oath, of confidentiality. What is often not appreciated is the common law and statutory basis of this duty and the circumstances in which confidential information may legally be revealed. There is a common law duty placed upon professionals to guard confidential information. A patient may sue a doctor through the civil courts if there is alleged to have been damage as a result of breach of confidentiality. The Data Protection Act (1997) places a statutory duty on anyone who holds patient identifiable data (in any form) to guard and release that information under strict controls. Any surgeon who keeps any sort of patient identifiable information at his residence (where his employer's blanket registration under the act will probably not apply) and who is not registered with the data commissioner breaches the provisions of the act. It is particularly important to note in this context that, if disclosure is properly requested, it is an offence to fail to disclose ALL of the records, both computerized and manual.

The second statute that obliges surgeons to care for information appropriately is the Human Rights Act (1998). This enshrines in UK law the sixth clause of the European Convention on Human Rights granting citizens an absolute right to privacy and to family life.

There are a number of instances in which confidential information can be released. The first is with the consent of the patient. This is sometimes implied consent such as applies when a GP releases confidential information in a referral to a consultant (and so to both secretaries). On other occasions, there needs to be expressed consent, for instance in release of information to insurers when a holiday must be cancelled. Sometimes a doctor is obliged to release information. The statutory examples concern the Terrorism Act 2000, the Abortion Act 1967 and the infectious diseases regulations. A court has power to require disclosure of records and there are several cases where disclosure is appropriate in the public interest. These are to protect the rights of others, such as reporting to prevent or detect serious crime or to prevent suspected child abuse and in reports to the Driver and Vehicle Licensing Authority. In all cases of this nature where the disclosure is not governed by the Data Protection Act, the information released must be no more than that necessary to comply with the public duty. A surgeon with any doubt as to how to resolve the conflict between duties of confidentiality and the public interest is well advised to consult his or her medical indemnity organization and to ensure that the final decision is one with which a responsible body of medical opinion would concur (Bolam).

The situation after the death of the patient is different. Doctors have a duty to disclose on death certificates and to national confidential enquiries as well as to the police and courts, especially the coroner. Data protection no longer applies and the relevant statute is the Access to Health Records Act 1990. This clarifies that executors or, failing them, next of kin can consent to release of medical records. It appears that anyone with a legitimate claim to view the record can see that part of the record that is relevant.

THE CORONER

By the time this chapter is published, it is likely that the changes in the role of the coroner will be clearer. For some time, there has been unease about exactly what coroners are expected to do but the moves to reform have been hastened by the Shipman case and the subsequent inquiry.

Harold Shipman, a general practitioner, was found guilty of murdering a large number of his patients. For a number of successive years, the local coroner received considerably greater numbers of reported deaths of patients of Dr Shipman than of any other local GP. Despite this, no alarm bells appear to have rung and Dr Shipman's murderous activities continued unabated. The Shipman Inquiries which followed the criminal trial have recently been completed and they seem likely to make wide-ranging recommendations about the role of the coroner and the General Medical Council (GMC). There is also an independent inquiry into the office of coroner which may possibly arrive at a different conclusion.

As things stand at present, the coroner for a particular area is appointed by the Crown and is usually a lawyer. There are a few medical coroners but these are less prevalent than previously. The coroner has a number of duties of which the investigation of certain deaths is the one relevant to this chapter. In the course of these investigations, the coroner has wide powers to call or subpoena witnesses and to make whatever investigation he sees fit to establish the facts relevant to the death. The equivalent officer in Scotland, the Procurator Fiscal, has similar powers, which may be even wider.

When the coroner is mentioned, most doctors ask three questions: what deaths must be reported to the coroner; what verdicts can be brought and will these criticize the doctor; what must I do if required to write a report for or appear before the coroner?

The following deaths must be reported to the coroner:

- violent or unnatural death;
- death in custody (even if the prisoner was licensed on leave to attend the hospital);
- death where no doctor is able to issue a death certificate.

Most jurisdictions also have local agreements about the reporting of deaths within a certain period after hospital admission and after surgical procedures. Coroners usually wish to know about deaths from notifiable diseases, industrial diseases and those in receipt of war pensions.

The range of verdicts that the coroner can return is surprisingly limited. The coroner's court is (in theory at least) not adversarial and no finger of blame should be pointed by the court. The coroner's remit is to establish the identity of the deceased, the time and place of death and the mode of death. Although death due to gross neglect is an acceptable verdict, death due to negligence is not. In practice, of course, the family of the deceased and their lawyers may use the proceedings of the coroner's court to assess whether or not an action in negligence is likely to succeed.

What about the surgeon called upon to provide a report to the coroner? The first piece of advice would be for the surgeon to contact his or her defence organization for support. The report itself should be factual and full and directed to a nonmedical audience. The report should not contain opinion but just facts. In particular, a report to a coroner should never contain the words 'negligent' or 'negligence'. Not only are these a matter of opinion and not fact, but they also have special well-defined meanings for lawyers that may not be apparent to doctors.

In most cases, the report will be all that the coroner needs and the doctor will not be required to appear. If the coroner feels that the evidence that the doctor can give may be crucial to his investigations, then he will summon the doctor to the inquest. Sometimes the family of the deceased will see this as their opportunity to confront the doctor who they see as the source of their grief. To be fair, sometimes the process works well, the family see that the doctor is not some kind of ogre and the resentment fades. Even if this does not occur, the coroner should ensure that the family do not persecute the doctor and that the proceedings remain directed towards establishing the who, when, where and how but not why the deceased perished.

If the doctor anticipates a difficult inquest, he may be accompanied by legal assistance but the solicitor may not answer for him nor is there any cross-examination of the other side. Defence organizations can advise the doctor but there is always a risk that the presence of a legal advisor will make the family (and the coroner) suspect that some sort of cover-up is being attempted.

Doctors summoned to the coroner's court need to follow the usual rules of court appearances – dress smartly but conservatively and do show appropriate respect to the coroner. Bring the notes or fair copies and copies of the reports already supplied and read them through before the case opens. Remember that the doctor is a witness and not an advocate or defendant and so there is no problem in asking for a question to be repeated or for a pause while the notes are consulted before answering.

THE ROLE OF THE EXPERT

An expert medical witness is instructed by either the defence or the claimant to give his or her opinion on the medical matters pertinent to the case to the court. This evidence is different from that of a material witness who is asked for the facts. The expert's job is to interpret the facts for the court. In simple terms, it is 'to give impartial advice and opinion'. Many otolaryngologists will be called upon to give expert opinion on personal injury cases where neither the claimant nor the defendant is a clinician. The many reports on noise-induced hearing loss that have been written by otolaryngologists are a form of written expert testimony in just such personal injury cases. A few otolaryngologists will be asked to prepare reports that assist courts in deciding clinical negligence claims and the special circumstances that pertain to these are discussed below.

Until the Civil Procedure Rules 1998 came into force, experts were retained by either the claimant or defendant's side and to some extent this remains the case. In theory, an expert's report would be the same whether he was instructed by the solicitors of the claimant or those of the defendant. The 1998 Rules have made it clear that the duty of an expert, whether he is expecting to be paid by the defendant or by the claimant, is to produce for the court an unbiased opinion. The 1998 Rules encourage a court, where practical, to appoint a single joint expert to produce such an opinion. They also give direction about exchange of reports, communication between and with experts and the expert's right to ask the court for directions.

In practice, the expert's evidence is usually contained in a report and it is rare for an expert to have to appear in court. The form and content of an expert report were previously based upon a well-known civil case.

In the Ikarian Reefer (*National Justice Compania Naviesa SA* v. *Prudential Assurance Company Ltd, The Ikarian Reefer*),[34] Mr Justice Cresswell stated that he considered that a misunderstanding on the part of some of the expert witnesses had taken place concerning their duties and responsibilities which had contributed to the length of the trial. Although this was a shipping case, the seven duties and responsibilities laid down have equal validity for medical experts.

1. Expert evidence presented to the court should be, and should be seen to be, the independent product of the expert uninfluenced as to form or content by the exigencies of litigation.
2. Independent assistance should be provided to the court by way of objective unbiased opinion regarding matters within the expertise of the expert witness. (An expert witness should never assume the role of advocate.)
3. Facts or assumptions upon which the opinion was based should be stated together with material facts which could detract from the concluded opinion.
4. An expert witness should make it clear when a question or issue fell outside his expertise.
5. If the opinion was not properly researched because it was considered that insufficient data was available then that had to be stated with an indication that the opinion was provisional. If the

witness could not assert that the report contained the truth, the whole truth and nothing but the truth, then that qualification should be stated on the report.

6. If after exchange of reports an expert witness changed his mind on a material matter then the change of view should be communicated to the other side through legal representatives without delay and when appropriate to the court.

7. Photographs, plans, survey reports and other documents referred to in the expert evidence had to be provided to the other side at the same time as exchange of reports.

More recently, the Civil Procedure Rules have modified these directions. The expert should obtain the Civil Procedure Rules Chapter 35 and read sections 1.1 through to 1.6, which is too extensive to reproduce here.

Before writing a report the expert should be aware of what the solicitor requires. Reports usually refer to one or more of the following six areas which are:

1. An initial statement on the possible merits of an allegation for a claimant before notes and other evidence are obtained.
2. Liability.
3. Causation.
4. Current condition.
5. Prognosis.
6. Expert opinion on an area of medicine.

A quote should be given on the cost of the report in advance. Lawyers may have no concept of the cost in time and research to answer what to them may be the most simple of questions. The solicitor will not be pleased to receive a report of 100 pages with detailed bibliography costing £2,000 when the damages sought are only £500 for a relatively minor event.

The report should be double spaced and typed on A4 paper. Each sheet should have the name of the claimant or defendant typed in the top right-hand corner and be separately numbered. It is also helpful to number the paragraphs. The names of the parties should be stated as should the requesting solicitor or insurance company. It is inadvisable to use the word 'negligent' in the report. Negligence may be implied by using phrases such as 'falling below an acceptable standard' or 'followed a course of action that could not be supported by any body of medical opinion'. Phrases such as 'reckless action' or 'flagrant disregard' may have a special meaning and lead to criminal charges rather than a civil case.

There is always the possibility that the credentials of the expert will be tested in court. It is extremely unwise for the expert to step outside his field. Should he be forced to comment outside his field of expertise he should add the rider that he is speaking only as an average medical practitioner. The expert will need to be au fait with up-to-date research in his own field.

The medical expert in clinical negligence

The medical expert retained in a case of medical negligence is usually asked to elucidate the areas of medical contention within a case. He needs to be aware of the various views on current practice even if these views are held by a minority of doctors, provided always that the minority is a reasonable one and that the practices supported are logical (Bolitho). Although the temptation is to be an arbitrator of medical colleagues, in court, this is the province of the judge. Nevertheless, the expert will be asked to comment as to whether the claimant's complaint has merit. When acting for the defence the expert will inevitably come across cases where defence is impossible. Here it is the expert's duty to advise that a speedy settlement be made to the aggrieved patient. This will have the secondary benefit of avoiding a colleague's professional shortcomings being exposed to public criticism in court. Rarely, some doctors expect their colleagues to defend them whatever the circumstances. Hence, being an expert can lead to criticism or alienation by colleagues.

Medical negligence cases can take an inordinate amount of time. Not only may the expert have to inspect all the records, examine the claimant and prepare reports, he will have to do research, attend meetings with solicitors and counsel and attend court. A single case may, in unusual circumstances, take up to 100 hours of time or more. The expert should never take on a case if he cannot afford the time.

Subsection 1.6 of the practice direction requires that experts comply with the relevant approved expert's protocol. As might be expected, there is a detailed pre-action protocol for the resolution of clinical disputes. Although this is aimed primarily at the legal profession, it is required reading for any doctors involved in providing expert testimony in clinical negligence cases. In particular, the times allowed by the court for the completion of various stages of the claim and the defence are clearly stated.

The doctor as an expert witness in court

The purpose of expert opinion given in court is to persuade the judge that one side of a case has greater merit than the other. It is the judge who will decide between the two sides of the argument. The expert should not be tempted to usurp the role of the judge for this may do untold damage to his own side or at the very least earn a rebuke which may undermine his confidence.

In court, the expert should wear conservative clothes. Evidence should be given in a straightforward, unequivocal manner. A personal view may be represented especially in response to a direct question but should always be tempered with information about acceptable alternative practice and opinion. He should always be prepared to concede points if it is appropriate to do so, and not to adhere rigidly to one view when that cannot be sustained. The expert often has difficult concepts to convey to the judge. The expert should not hesitate to use pictures, models or even video to illustrate a point but should avoid being seen as a flamboyant 'show off' lest he discredits himself by not giving due respect to the court.

The usual course of examining a witness in court is that the barrister for the side calling the witness will examine that witness and try to anticipate and pre-empt difficult questions from the other side. Counsel for the opposing side will then cross-examine the witness and may attempt to undermine the evidence given by the expert or the standing of the expert in his profession. Above all, the expert must not see this as a personal insult lest he should lose his temper and hence his dignity. After this potentially hostile cross-examination, the first barrister is permitted to re-examine the witness and try, if necessary, to restore the faith of the judge in that witness.

PERFORMANCE AND COMPLAINTS

Besides using the legal system to sue a surgeon in tort, patients have recourse to a number of mechanisms to resolve concerns about how they have been treated or managed. Some of these mechanisms have the potential to involve doctors in disciplinary or performance investigations so the two elements are considered together. A patient or a family unhappy with the outcome of a surgical process can of course sue in the tort of negligence but this is expensive and will succeed in only a few cases. Another option is a complaint to the Trust employing the surgeon. Trusts are obliged to have a complaints procedure and the patient is entitled to a prompt reply from the chief executive. In practice, the time limits are so tight that especially when the complaint is a complex clinical one (rather than the more usual gripes about hospital food or parking for visitors) the first reply is a form letter. Following this the complaint should be answered point by point with an apology if appropriate. If this is rejected by the patient then the complaint is passed to a convenor (usually a nonexecutive director of the Trust) whose job is to decide whether or not to convene an interim review panel to try to resolve the matter. This should be done only if, in the convener's view, there is no other way to resolve the complaint and there is a good chance that the panel will achieve such a resolution. The convener also sets the terms of reference of this investigation. A glance at the advice to conveners on this suggests that this structure was neither well thought out nor transparently nonpartisan. Conveners who refuse to sanction further investigation are seen as agents of the Trust that they work for. Aggrieved patients tend to see the narrow terms of reference that may be required to allow the review panel to function as further evidence of attempts to quash legitimate complaints. Some patients turn at this stage to clinical negligence proceedings; as soon as this happens, the complaints process ceases. The independent review panel will in time produce a report to the complainant, the complained against and the Trust chief executive. The chief executive must then report to the complainant what action has been taken. Among the possible actions are Trust disciplinary procedures or report of a doctor to the GMC. Before considering what threats the GMC poses to surgeons, the Health Service Commissioner must be mentioned. This officer, also referred to as the ombudsman, can review the decisions of the convenor not to set up an independent review. There may also be grounds for appeal to the ombudsman if there are problems with the terms of reference or the conduct of the independent review. Following general dissatisfaction with the process and especially the role of the convenor, there has been a process of consultation followed by a report on how the system might be improved. If the legislation goes through to put this report into practice, then the convenor will disappear and the follow-up to failed local resolution will be the Healthcare Commission.

If the investigation of a complaint leads to further investigation of the conduct or performance of a doctor, there are a number of forms that this can take. One is an internal investigation by the doctor's Trust. Although there are regulations that govern the conduct of such investigations, there is such a variety of approaches that this chapter cannot be dogmatic. It is clear that a Trust must not unjustifiably suspend a doctor pending investigation and then drag its heels in the investigation. There may well be a case against the trust under the Human Rights Act (1998) and the doctor is probably best advised to consult his or her defence organization.

Two new organizations may put a doctor's reputation or right to practise in jeopardy. These are National Patient Safety Agency (NPSA) including the National Clinical Assessment Authority (NCAA) and the Healthcare Commission. The Healthcare Commission arose out of Commission for Healthcare Audit and Inspection which arose from the Commission for Healthcare Improvement (CHI). The NCAA will deal with concerns about the performance of individual doctors by investigating problems and arranging performance assessments where necessary. Memoranda of understanding have been agreed between the NCAA and both CHI and the GMC so it is clear that a suggestion of deficient performance or conduct uncovered by one of the three organizations may well be reported to the other two.

The organization that these newer groups feed to and which has disciplinary control over doctors in the UK is the GMC. This organization has a statutory duty to maintain standards and ensure that doctors registered with the GMC do not endanger the public. The GMC is bedevilled by lots of committees with similar acronyms but there are basically three routes through the system. The first stage is usually the reporting to the GMC by a Trust, by a member of the public, by another doctor or the NCAA.

Increasingly, the GMC is looking at reports in the media which suggest poor performance or conduct and initiating proceedings on the basis of these. The complaint is screened and the decision made to reject it at this stage or to refer it on for investigation. The screener decides which of the three routes: health, conduct or performance is the most appropriate.

Health procedures are aimed to rehabilitate the ill doctor whose illness is affecting his or her work. The four stages of the process are initial assessment, medical examination, medical supervision and health committee action. The possible outcomes are suspension, conditional continued registration to practise or a decision that the doctor is fit to practise without conditions. The performance procedures act where there is 'a departure from good professional practice . . . sufficiently serious to call into question a doctor's registration'. Referrals are examined and the doctor is likely to be asked to have a performance assessment. If he or she refuses, the Assessment Referral Committee may order an assessment. The case coordinator uses the outcome of the assessment process to decide that: no further action is required; counselling or training is required; or the case is so serious or the doctor has refused assessment or to agree to retraining such that referral to the Committee on Professional Performance is required. This committee can leave the surgeon's registration intact, impose conditions or suspend or erase. The third channel through the processes of the GMC is the conduct procedures. Here the first relevant filter is the Preliminary Proceedings Committee (PPC). The PPC meets in private and can clear the doctor; refer into the health process; advise or warn the doctor; or refer to the Professional Conduct Committee (PCC). A PCC hearing is, to all intents and purposes, a court of law with a panel, advised by a legal assessor, sitting in judgement. The GMC and the doctor can be represented by barristers if necessary and, unlike the health process, the tone is adversarial. The PCC can postpone a decision and can admonish, suspend or erase the doctor. Sometimes the case is dismissed or the doctor's continued registration is made conditional. Formerly, outcomes of all three processes could be appealed to the judicial committee of the Privy Council but now appeals are heard by the High Court.

Recently, the government has established the Commission for the Regulation of Healthcare Professionals. If it is felt that a decision of the GMC has been too lenient then it is envisaged that the decision can be overturned by this commission in the interests of protecting the public.

There is one more committee of the GMC which is important when the question of a doctor's continuing practice is in doubt. This is the Interim Orders Committee (IOC) to which a doctor may be referred at the start of any of the three processes. The IOC has powers to impose conditions and to suspend a doctor while the other committees are deliberating. The rationale of the committee is to protect the public from a doubtful doctor while the full process is completed and a fully argued decision of one of the full committees is reached.

All that you have just read about above concerning the GMC is very soon likely to be history. After the Shipman Inquiries a White Paper, *Trust Assurance and Safety – The Regulation of Health Professionals in the 21st Century* was published on February 21, 2007. The Privy Council has extended the term of the 19 elected medical members of the GMC due to stand down on June 30, 2007 until December 31, 2008. This White Paper has several radical proposals which are listed below.

- Doing away with the current standard of proof in fitness to practise cases and replacing it with the civil standard of proof.
- Establishment of an independent body to adjudicate on fitness to practise cases.
- Revalidation will have two parts – relicensing and recertification (which will apply to those on the specialist register and GPs.

The establishment of GMC affiliates to assist employers and the NHS deal with complaints at a local level.

THE HUMAN RIGHTS ACT

Perhaps the two most potentially influential recent statutes affecting surgeons are the Data Protection Act (DPA) (1998) and the Human Rights Act (HRA) (1998). The first of these is discussed under the heading of confidentiality where its effects, although far-reaching, are relatively easy to predict. The effects of the HRA are potentially much more profound but are still being discovered and untangled by current legal cases. In a way this is curious since the HRA formally enshrines in UK legislation, the European Convention on Human Rights.

The European Convention on Human Rights

Many people understand this convention to be a product of the European Community and compliance with it to be a condition of membership. In reality it is a convention to which the UK government signed up in the 1950s. The requirement until the HRA became law was that national legislation should be interpreted in accordance with the convention. The HRA enshrines the rights defined in the convention in UK law, allowing UK citizens to claim in UK courts that their rights have been breached and seek damages or perhaps a stay of criminal proceedings.

A number of rights are described in the HRA and these are divided into qualified and absolute rights. The ones of most relevance to otolaryngologists are numbers 2, 3, 6 and 8.

Article 2 states the right to life. There are a number of ways in which this is relevant. Perhaps this is another route by which the family of a dead patient may seek redress if there is the suggestion that the death occurred due to corporate or individual error. The verdicts that are open to a coroner are discussed under The criminal law below, but, as described, this important field is changing. The coroner is a public body under the terms of the HRA and so must ensure that verdicts are in line with that act. Will we soon see a verdict of death in contravention of Article 2 of the European Convention on Human Rights returned as a halfway house between death by misadventure and unlawful killing? What would be the consequences for a subsequent negligence claim? If the strong lobby seeking to legalize assisted suicide in certain circumstances is successful, how will this sit with the right to life? It is not clear in the legislation how a patient can personally renounce his or her rights under Article 2.

Article 3 is the right not to be subject to torture or to inhumane or degrading treatment or punishment. This appears to influence the facilities that must be made available by hospitals for the care of patients as well as powerful implications for the whole consent process. Surely it will not be long before a Trust is sued by a patient alleging that the wait on a trolley for 24 hours in casualty constituted inhumane or degrading treatment. There is also a suggestion that the coroner will have to pay regard to Article 3 as well if, in his view, there was inhumane and degrading treatment leading to a death.

There are two other articles with relevance to otolaryngologists: Articles 6 and 8. These two interact with each other when the question of GMC and other legal and paralegal proceedings are considered. Article 6 affirms the right of all citizens to a fair and timely trial. A magistrate in the UK has already stayed a prosecution because he judged that the prosecution had taken an unreasonably long time to bring the case to trial. As the defendant was a doctor and now leaves the criminal court without even having been tried, let alone convicted, it is possible that this judgement will profoundly affect his treatment by the GMC.

Since GMC committees are trials within the meaning of the HRA, they are subject to exactly the same legal liabilities as courts and coroners. It is here that Article 6 may begin to conflict with Article 8, which grants the right to respect for private and family life. Consider the position of a surgeon seeking to refute at the GMC committee on professional performance an allegation that there is a consistent pattern of poor professional competence. In order to defend himself and to liaise with his professional advisers (solicitors and counsel), he would surely need access to the notes of the patients that he cared for and to whom he may have given substandard care. Also, the GMC might wish to call the patients as material witnesses to the substandard care. At present,

there is no obligation on a patient, unwittingly a witness at a GMC committee, to grant consent to release of his or her confidential information to either the doctor or the GMC. The patient has rights under the DPA to know what is being done with his or her data and, except in certain circumstances, to withhold consent for release of that information. The exceptions do not seem to apply to GMC proceedings. Surely a patient who found out that a Trust had divulged notes to a surgeon and his legal advisors or to the GMC, in pursuit of a fair trial, could bring action under both the HRA and the DPA. Perhaps also, a patient or even a doctor other than the one being investigated, obliged by subpoena to attend a GMC hearing as a witness and subsequently hounded by the press, can argue that no respect has been shown to his or her privacy.

The whole question of how the HRA (1998) will affect surgeons is under active consideration at present. The only guarantee in this field is that lawyers will continue to use the act to push the common law in new and unusual directions.

THE CRIMINAL LAW

Otolaryngologists rarely face criminal proceedings in connection with medical practice, but mention should be made concerning two types of criminal offence which may flow from medical treatment.

Involuntary manslaughter

In recent years, an increasing number of doctors have faced the prospect of prosecution following the deaths of their patients, allegedly as the result of medical malpractice. The English law relating to involuntary manslaughter has been in a confused state, and clarification has only very recently been provided by the Court of Appeal. Traditionally, the test for involuntary manslaughter has been one of gross negligence. In the words of the then Lord Chief Justice, Lord Hewart, in the case of *R* v. *Bateman*,[35] in order to establish criminal liability the facts must be such that 'the negligence of the accused went beyond a mere matter of compensation between subjects and showed such a disregard for life and safety of others as to amount to a crime against the state and conduct deserving of punishment'. Adjectives such as 'gross', 'wicked' and 'criminal' were used to describe the degree of negligence required. This is effectively something of a 'gut reaction' test for the jury. In a crime of this nature, it is arguably best left open to the jury to make the determination of criminality.

An attempt was made to further define gross negligence by the House of Lords case of *Andrews* v. *DPP*.[36] In that instance, 'recklessness' was considered to be the adjective which most closely described the concept. In this way, the House of Lords was endeavouring to ascribe as guilty states of mind the appreciation of risk, coupled with a determination to run it, or the wilful indifference to the question of whether such a risk existed. However, 'mere inadvertence' was not considered to merit criminal responsibility.

The test was thrown into confusion in 1981 as a result of decisions in two cases (*R v. Caldwell* and *R v. Lawrence*)[37, 38] by the House of Lords which redefined the concept of 'recklessness'. The cases concerned the offences of criminal damage and causing death by reckless driving. It was determined that the defendant would be reckless if his action created an obvious and serious risk (to a victim in the case of manslaughter) and the defendant either appreciated the risk but went on to run it or failed to appreciate the risk. This test has been criticized as being unduly harsh. It allows no realistic explanation of the defendant's state of mind to be put forward. Thus, a doctor under pressure, perhaps through overwork and being asked to perform tasks which he or she should not otherwise have been required to do, would have no opportunity to explain those circumstances as part of defence. The mere fact that an obvious and serious risk had been created to the patient, as a result of which the patient had died, would be sufficient to secure a conviction.

The test was applied in a case of motor manslaughter (*R v. Seymour*)[39] by the House of Lords in 1983. Thereafter, however, there was significant confusion as to whether the case should extend to all cases as an involuntary manslaughter. As a result, in some cases involving doctors charged with involuntary manslaughter the traditional test of gross negligence was applied, in others the new harsh formulation for recklessness was considered appropriate. In yet other cases, attempts were made to combine the two tests.

This unsatisfactory situation has been resolved to a degree by the case of *R v. Prentice and Sulliman*.[40] The case involved two junior doctors, Dr Prentice being a pre-registration House Officer who, as part of the chemotherapy treatment, injected vincristine intrathecally in error. As the Court of Appeal observed, the mitigating circumstances in relation to both doctors were many, but a version of the recklessness test was put to the jury, resulting in their convictions. These were quashed by the Court of Appeal (*R v. Prentice and Sulliman*)[41] on the basis that the test of recklessness was not appropriate for cases of involuntary manslaughter where a breach of duty is concerned, particularly for cases involving doctors, where the court observed: 'Often there is a high degree of danger to the deceased's health, not created by the defendant, and pre-existing risks to the patient's health is what causes the defendant to assume the duty of care with consent. His intervention will often be in situations of emergency.' The traditional test for gross negligence was preferred.

The court set out the matters which need to be established for a prosecution of manslaughter, namely the existence of a duty of care, the breach of the duty causing death and gross negligence which the jury considers justifies criminal conviction. The Court of Appeal went on to set out various states of mind which it considered could probably lead the jury to making a finding of gross negligence.

- Indifference to an obvious risk of injury to health.
- Actual foresight of a risk coupled with the determination nevertheless to run it.
- An appreciation of the risk, coupled with an intention to avoid it but also coupled with such a high degree of negligence in the attempted avoidance as the jury considers justifies conviction.
- Inattention to or failure to avert a serious risk which goes beyond mere inadvertence in respect of an obvious and important matter which the defendant's duty demanded he should address.

The first three states of mind are not unduly onerous. The fourth, however, may present particular problems to medical practitioners. Medical treatment generally may be considered to amount to an obvious and important matter. Further, many serious risks are inherent in treating patients and, accordingly, medical practitioners remain in danger of falling foul of the criminal law relating to manslaughter. At the conclusion of the judgement of the Court of Appeal in the case of Drs Prentice and Sulliman, the court expressed the view that the Law Commissioners should look at the law in relation to involuntary manslaughter as a matter of urgency, and thus modifications may be made to this area of the law in the near future.[42]

In Canada,[42] manslaughter may be committed where a doctor causes the death of a patient by, among other things, criminal negligence which may be committed where someone under a duty shows a wanton or reckless disregard for the lives or safety of others. The precise meaning of 'wanton or reckless disregard' is in doubt. In a recent case (*R v. Tutton and Tutton*)[43] the Supreme Court of Canada was divided between those who considered that a defendant should have an intention to run a prohibited risk, or a wilful blindness to the risk, and those who considered that a marked and substantial departure from a standard of behaviour expected of a reasonably prudent individual would suffice. This dilemma is similar to that recently addressed by the Court of Appeal in this jurisdiction in the case of Drs Prentice and Sulliman.

In New Zealand (*R v. Yogasakaran*),[44] the test for manslaughter is that of mere negligence, and a breach of the civil standard of care resulting in the death of a patient is all that is required. Similarly in Greece, the offence under the Greek Criminal Code[45] is of causing death by negligence, mere civil negligence being sufficient. The charge is often seen as a precursor to civil proceedings, where a victim's family may make complaint to prosecuting authorities, effectively as part of the bargaining process for compensation.

Assault, battery and bodily harm

Charges of assault and battery are considered very infrequently by the prosecuting authorities in this jurisdiction in relation to medical practitioners. Courts are reluctant to consider actions in tort for battery arising out of a failure to obtain consent, let alone criminal charges. Very few doctors will intend to inflict harm on a patient, the overall aim being to provide some form of therapeutic benefit. However, where the clinician performs a procedure which goes substantially beyond that to which the patient has consented and that is known to the clinician, or the clinician is reckless as to whether or not the patient's consent will authorize the procedure actually performed then such an offence may be made out, even if of therapeutic benefit. In circumstances where surgical intervention takes place, an offence of greater seriousness than mere assault may result, for example, assault occasioning grievous bodily harm.

THE FUTURE

It is without doubt that the shift in emphasis is away from the doctor and towards patients' rights. This can clearly be seen in a very recent landmark case (*Chester* v. *Afshar*)[46] heard by the House of Lords. Carole Chester agreed to undergo lumbar surgery on the advice of Mr Afshar, a neurosurgeon. She suffered partial paralysis. The judge found that Mr Afshar had not performed the surgery negligently but had failed to warn her of the partial paralysis inherent in the operation. The judge found that she would not have undergone the operation had she been warned but at the time would have sought further advice before deciding on what to do.

'Lord Hope of Craighead said that the claimant could not succeed on conventional causation principles since she did not assert that, if informed, she would never have undergone the surgery and since the defendant's failure neither affected the risk which eventuated nor was the effective cause of her injury. However the causation issue was to be addressed by reference to the scope of the defendant's duty, namely to advise his patient of the disadvantages and dangers of the treatment he proposed; that duty was closely connected with the need for the patient's consent and was central to her right to exercise an informed choice as to whether and, if so, when and from whom to receive the treatment. The function of the law was to enable rights to be vindicated and to provide remedies when duties had been breached. Unless that was done the duty was a hollow one, stripped of practical force and devoid of content. The injury the claimant sustained was within the scope of that duty and might, on policy grounds, be regarded as having been caused, in the legal sense, by the defendant's breach. Accordingly justice required that the claimant be afforded the remedy she sought.' Lord Steyn and Lord Walker of Gestingthorpe delivered concurring opinions; Lord Bingham and Lord Hoffmann disagreed so the defendant lost his appeal to the House of Lords.

Clearly this has a major impact for no longer does the patient have to state that they would not have had the surgery if they had been aware of all the risks but it is now sufficient for the patient to argue that they would have sought further advice. This has increased pressure on ensuring that specific risks are warned and the warning is recorded. It is now no longer good enough just to record that risks have been explained for a case to be defended where consent is a core issue.

Punitive (exemplary) damages are not normally awarded in jurisdictions of the UK and Australasia but in 2002 the Privy Council heard the case of *A* v. *Botrill*[47] from New Zealand. This case involved the wholesale misreading of cervical smears by a private pathologist in Gisborne, New Zealand. Between 1990 and 1994 he examined four smears from Mrs A. After Mrs A had a radical hysterectomy for invasive cancer the smears were reviewed and all four slides had been misread or misreported. Mrs A made a successful claim for accident compensation. Disciplinary proceedings against Dr Botrill found him guilty of conduct unbecoming of a medical practitioner. Mrs A then brought court proceedings claiming exemplary damages. Justice Young dismissed the action applying the principle 'exemplary damages may be awarded, but only if the level of negligence is so high that it amounts to outrageous and flagrant disregard for the plaintiff's safety, meriting condemnation and punishment'.

Two events then occurred: Mrs A found another ten women whose slides had been misread and there was public concern about smear reporting in the Gisborne area. This led to a review of Dr Botrill's slides in Sydney which showed that Dr Botrill's false reporting rate was 50 percent or higher. In the light of the new evidence Mrs A applied for a retrial which was granted. Dr Botrill then appealed this decision and his appeal was successful. Mrs A sought leave to appeal to the Privy Council which was granted. The argument for Mrs A was that cases of reprehensible wrong doing which are totally unacceptable to the community but arise from inadvertent negligence should not be put beyond the reach of exemplary damages. Dr Botrill's argument was that there was no conscious, outrageous and flagrant disregard for the plaintiff's safety. The Privy Council agreed with Mrs A and allowed her appeal on a majority decision.

Although this is a New Zealand case it now brings the possibility of punitive damages for reprehensible wrong-doing even if there was no flagrant disregard of risk. It seems that now inadvertent negligence may lead to exemplary damages in selected cases of the worst kind of professional practice.

KEY POINTS

- Clinical negligence is a matter for civil law.
- Damages awarded are general and special.
- The standard or proof is 'on the balance of probabilities'.
- There are four essential elements of the legal tort of negligence:
  - there must be a duty of care;
  - there must be a breach of that duty;
  - harm must have occurred;
  - the breach must have caused the harm.
- The standard of care is that of the reasonably skilled and experienced doctor.
- ' It will very seldom be right for a judge to reach the conclusion that views genuinely held by a competent medical expert are unreasonable.'
- If the case for each side is evenly balanced then the claimant will fail.
- The court must award a sum of money that will, as nearly as possible, put the injured person in the same position as he would have been had he not been injured.
- The result of the introduction of contingency fees is likely to be that there will be no significant increase in the number of medical negligence actions in the short term.
- Where a proposed treatment involves a substantial risk of grave or adverse consequences such that, notwithstanding any practice to the contrary, a patient's right to decide whether to consent to the treatment was so obvious that no prudent medical man could fail to warn of the risk, then it would be negligent not to warn.
- The parental right to determine whether or not a child under 16 should have medical treatment terminates when the child achieves a significant understanding and intelligence to enable him or her to understand fully what is proposed.
- 'An adult patient who suffers from no mental incapacity has an absolute right to choose whether to consent to medical treatment, to refuse it or to choose one rather than another of the treatments being offered.'
- Any surgeon who keeps any sort of patient identifiable information at his residence and who is not registered with the data commissioner breaches the provisions of the DPA.
- The coroner's remit is to establish the identity of the deceased, the time and place of death and the mode of death.
- Articles 2, 3, 6 and 8 of the HRA are those most relevant to surgeons.
- Modifications to the law on involuntary manslaughter are awaited; currently the traditional description of gross negligence resulting in death usually applies.

REFERENCES

1. *Bolitho* v. *City and Hackney Health Authority* [1997] Weekly Law Report 151.
2. *Bolam* v. *Friern Hospital Management Committee* [1957] 1 Weekly Law Reports 582.
3. *Wilsher* v. *Essex Area Health Authority* [1988] 1 All England Reports 871, House of Lords.
4. *Crawford* v. *Board of Governors of Charing Cross Hospital* [1953] Times Law Reports, 8 December 1953, Court of Appeal.
5. *Barnett* v. *Chelsea & Kensington Hospital* [1968] 1 All England Reports 1068.
6. *Ashcroft* v. *Mersey Regional Health Authority* [1985] 2 All England Reports 96.
7. Picard E. Legal liability of doctors and hospitals in Canada. In: Kennedy I, Grubb A (eds). *Medical law: text and materials*. London: Butterworths, 1989: 423.
8. *Scott* v. *London & St. Katherine's Docks* [1865] 3 Hurlstone & Coltman's Exchequer Reports 596 ExCh (sugar bags).
9. *Byrne* v. *Boadle* [1863] 2 Hurlstone & Coltman's Exchequer Reports 722 (a barrel of flour).
10. *Pope* v. *St. Helen's Theatre* [1947] Kings Bench 30 (the ceiling of a theatre).
11. M.A.M.S. Leigh. Res ipse Loquitur: What does it mean? Medical Defence Union Journal. 1993; 9: 66.
12. *Girard* v. *Royal Columbian Hospital* [1976] 6 Dominion Law Reports (3d) 676.
13. *Mahon* v. *Osborne* [1939] 2 Kings Bench 1450.
14. Personal correspondence.
15. *Livingston* v. *Rawyards Coal Company* [1880] 5 Appeal Cases 25 @ 39, House of Lords per Lord Blackburn.
16. *Kralj* v. *McGrath* [1986] All England Law Reports 54.
17. *Ward* v. *James* [1965] 2 All England Reports 563, Court of Appeal.
18. *Levitt* v. *Hartlepool Area Health Authority* (1993) (Unreported).
19. *Lim* v. *Camden Health Authority* [1979] 2 All England Reports 910, House of Lords, per Lord Scarman.
20. Rules of the Supreme Court: Order 37 Rules 7–10.
21. See generally the Rules of the Supreme Court and the County Court Practice for Procedure.
22. Civil Procedure Rules 1998.
23. S.58 Courts and Legal Services Act 1990.
24. Preliminary results of the Law Society Survey of Personal Injury Specialists. LS Gaz, 29 September 1993: 3.

25. *Sidaway* v. *Board of Governors of the Bethlem Royal Hospital* [1985] Appeal Cases 871, House of Lords.
26. *Hopp* v. *Lepp* [1979] 112 Dominion Law Reports 3d 67.
27. *Blyth* v. *Bloomsbury Health Authority* [1993] 4 Medical Law Reports, Court of Appeal.
28. *Rogers* v. *Whitaker* [1993] 4 Medical Law Reports 79, High Court of Australia.
29. *Gillick* v. *West Norfolk and Wisbech Area Health Authority* [1986] Appeal Cases 112, [1985] 3 All England Reports 402, House of Lords.
30. In re R [1991] 4 All England Reports 177, Court of Appeal.
31. In re W [1992] 3 Weekly Law Reports 758.
32. Re F [1990] 2 Appeal Cases 1, House of Lords.
33. In re T (Adult: Refusal of treatment) [1992] 3 Weekly Law Reports 783.
34. *National Justice Compania Naviera SA* v. *Prudential Assurance Company Ltd. (Ikarian Reefer)* [1993] Times Law Reports, 3rd March 1993.
35. *R* v. *Bateman* [1925] 19 Criminal Appeal Reports 8, Court of Appeal.
36. *Andrews* v. *DPP* [1937] Appeal Cases 576, PC.
37. *R* v. *Caldwell* [1982] Appeal Cases 341, House of Lords.
38. *R* v. *Lawrence* [1982] Appeal Cases 510, House of Lords.
39. *R* v. *Seymour* [1983] 2 Appeal Cases 493, House of Lords.
40. *R* v. *Prentice and Sulliman* (unreported November 1, 1991, Owen J).
41. *R* v. *Prentice and Sulliman* [1993] 4 All England Reports 935, Court of Appeal.
42. The Annotated Tremear's Criminal Code 1992, Sections 219, 220, 222.
43. *R* v. *Tutton and Tutton* [1989] 48 Canadian Criminal Cases (3d) 129, Canadian Supreme Court.
44. *R* v. *Yogasakaran* [1990] 1 New Zealand Law Reports 399, New Zealand Court of Appeal.
45. Article 302 Greek Penal Code.
46. *Chester* v. *Afshar* [2004] Appeal Cases 41, House of Lords
47. *A* v. *Botrill* [2002] UKPC 44.

PART 10

INTERPRETATION AND MANAGEMENT OF DATA

EDITED BY MARTIN J BURTON

49 Epidemiology   615
   Jan HP van der Meulen and David A Lowe

50 Outcomes research   633
   Iain RC Swan

51 Evidence-based medicine   645
   Martin J Burton

52 Critical appraisal skills   649
   Martin Dawes

Epidemiology

JAN HP VAN DER MEULEN AND DAVID A LOWE

Introduction	615	Choosing the study design	624
What is epidemiology?	616	Key points	630
'Streams' of epidemiology	616	Acknowledgements	631
The 'anatomy' and 'physiology' of epidemiological research	618	References	631

INTRODUCTION

This chapter presents epidemiology as a methodological discipline that provides important principles for clinical and health services research. It introduces the 'determinant–occurrence relationship' as a key epidemiological concept. On the basis of this concept, we will demonstrate how epidemiological methods and techniques can be used to address a wide range of questions. This chapter is intended to inform those who want to read the medical literature and evaluate research evidence. In other words, it has been written especially with the needs of the 'consumers' of research in mind.

We will concentrate on the choice of a study design for different types of research questions with the ultimate aim of developing a study that produces results that are relatively precise (free of random error) and accurate (free of systematic error or bias). An additional consideration is that the study needs to be efficient (affordable in terms of time and money). Strengths and weaknesses of study designs will be discussed as much as possible on the basis of examples related to diseases of the ear, nose and throat.

This chapter is not based on a specific literature search strategy. It amalgamates information and points of view as can be found in major textbooks and reviews of epidemiology, methods of health services research and evidence-based clinical practice.

Example: the indication for tonsillectomy

Simple, but well-designed, epidemiological research can be of great importance for clinical practice. A recent systematic review indicated that the effectiveness of tonsillectomy is uncertain,[1] and in turn, that the indications for tonsillectomy are controversial. Nevertheless, tonsillectomy is one of the commonest surgical procedures carried out in children as well as in adults.

In the 1930s, an estimated 200,000 were performed annually in England and Wales, a huge number compared to an annual number of approximately 40,000 in the year 2000. In the pre-war period, tonsillectomy had become popular to the point of being fashionable, and there was marked variation in its frequency according to geographical location, social class and sex.[2] It was estimated that at least 85 children lost their lives each year as a direct result of tonsillectomy.

Another study carried out in the 1940s demonstrated that there was great uncertainty about effectiveness and indications,[3] as cited in a book by Sackett and coworkers.[4] Among 389 eleven-year-old schoolchildren with intact tonsils examined by a group of clinicians, tonsillectomy was recommended in 174 (45 percent). A second opinion was requested in the 215 schoolchildren for whom tonsillectomy was not recommended, and tonsillectomy was recommended for 99 (46 percent). The remaining 116 children, in whom on the two previous occasions tonsillectomy was not recommended, were then examined for the third time, and tonsillectomy was recommended in 51 (44 percent) of them. The most remarkable finding is that tonsillectomy was recommended in each of the three cycles for approximately 45 percent of the children.

These historical examples illustrate that uncertainty about diagnostic and management decisions can lead to overtreatment, which may have serious consequences for patients. Given the fact that there is still no high-quality evidence on the effectiveness of tonsillectomy more than 50 years later, the same problem may still exist, albeit to a lesser extent. The only published study on the effectiveness of tonsillectomy that could be included in one systematic review studied 91 children and was affected by important baseline differences in the characteristics of the surgical and the control group.[1] It is obvious that this kind of clinical uncertainty can only be solved by epidemiological evidence of high quality.

WHAT IS EPIDEMIOLOGY?

Epidemiology is a relative young discipline, but during its short life many definitions of epidemiology have emerged.[5] Many of these describe epidemiology in terms of its subject matter. The perhaps most frequently cited definition in this context states that epidemiology is the study of the distribution and determinants of disease frequency in human populations.[6] These three closely related components – distribution, determinants and frequency – encompass many epidemiological principles and methods.[7] For example, an epidemiological study that would fit perfectly within this definition is that of the frequency of head and neck cancer in a certain geographical area. This study could also consider the distribution of the disease among different subgroups. The determinants of disease occurrence would then derive from these two.

Although this definition has its merits in that it covers many epidemiological studies, some of which attracted large media attention (for example, smoking and lung cancer, cholesterol and heart disease, effect of diethylstilbestrol on offspring, unprotected sex and the acquired immune deficiency syndrome), a growing number of epidemiologists feel that the above-cited definition does not cover their work. The reason is that the subject matter of what can be considered epidemiological studies has become rather heterogeneous. Attempts to produce a definition of epidemiology based upon its subject matter therefore produce confusion rather than clarity.

The concept of the determinant–occurrence relationship

In the last two decades, an alternative definition has arisen that defines epidemiology as a discipline that studies the functional relationship between the occurrence of disease (or related health outcomes) and its determinants.[8] This may seem a trivial step, but this focus on the concept of the 'determinant–occurrence relationship' rather than the subject matter has considerably broadened the scope of epidemiology in medicine.

One of the major reasons why epidemiology has gained such far-reaching importance lies in the nature of medical knowledge. Medical knowledge is, to a large extent, derived from the experience obtained in groups of similar patients. Medicine is therefore an empirical science, and many of the empirical relationships in medicine can be considered as determinant–occurrence relationships. It is especially this realization on the basis of which epidemiology has become a basic science in medicine.

Epidemiology as a methodological discipline

An alternative approach to clarify the definition of epidemiology is to consider it as a methodological discipline. From this perspective, the subject of epidemiological inquiry is not so much the determinants of the occurrence of disease and other health outcomes, but the principles and methods for the study of determinant–occurrence relationships.

As a methodological discipline, epidemiology allows a large number of different questions to be answered. As explained earlier, it may play a role in describing the distribution of health and disease in a population. Who is affected? Where and when does this health problem occur? Why does it occur in a particular population?

However, other questions can be considered as well. Once a health problem occurs, epidemiology also provides methods for monitoring the course and outcome of a health problem. What is the outcome of the health problem? It may answer questions regarding the outcomes of interventions. Is intervention A more effective than intervention B? How well does a diagnostic test distinguish between people with and without the target disorder?

Epidemiological research is also essential for the assessment of the burden of disease and the need for health services and evaluation of the access to services. How much suffering does this health problem cause in a population? How many people need a certain intervention? Who uses the intervention? What factors explain differences in health care use?

'STREAMS' OF EPIDEMIOLOGY

Given the extension of the boundaries of epidemiology – based on the introduction of the determinant–occurrence relationship as the key epidemiological concept and the realization that epidemiological principles provide the methodological underpinning for the study of a wide range of questions – one can recognize several 'streams' of epidemiological research. These streams differ largely according to the types of questions they address, but they share most of the methodological concepts and principles.

Classical epidemiology

The first stream of research is 'classical epidemiology', sometimes referred to as 'aetiological epidemiology' or 'risk factor epidemiology', of which the ultimate goal is 'the elaboration of causes that can explain patterns of disease occurrence'.[5] The geographical distribution of a disease, the variations in its frequency over time, and the special characteristics of people affected by it, are typical objects of study.

There is often a natural progression in this type of epidemiological research.[7] First, there is a concern about the possible influence of a particular factor on the occurrence of disease. This suspicion can have many origins – clinical practice, laboratory research, theoretical speculation – but it often arises from examination of disease distributions, and leads to the formulation of a specific hypothesis about its causes. It can then be further explored in studies of individuals that include an appropriate comparison group. A systematic collection and analysis of data may reveal that a statistical association exists. It is then essential to assess whether random errors or systematic errors might be responsible for the findings. Finally, a judgement needs to be made about whether an observed association represents a cause–effect relationship.

An otolaryngological example of this type of epidemiological research is the study of the distribution of head and neck cancers and the association of the occurrence of this disease with traditional risk factors such as diet, smoking and drinking habits or socioeconomic status. Another more specific example is the testing of the hypothesis that there is a link between human papillomavirus and the occurrence of a subset of these cancers. The result of aetiological research may guide the first steps towards the development of primary prevention that keeps disease from occurring at all.

However, the reductionist nature of classical epidemiology has been criticized. It has been argued that epidemiological studies often ignore 'the interdependence of multiple agents and how human populations become exposed and susceptible to them'.[9] Epidemiological research that focuses on the effect of risk factors measurable at the level of the individual neglects the population context and the social and cultural determinants that act at population level.

Clinical epidemiology

The second stream of research is 'clinical epidemiology'. The adjective 'clinical' is added because clinical epidemiology 'seeks to answer clinical questions and to guide clinical decision making with the best available evidence'.[10] Clinicians are mainly concerned with problems of individual patients. It may seem paradoxical that results of epidemiological studies that are derived from groups of patients should be applicable to the problems of individual patients. It is obvious, however, that this is because the best evidence to solve a clinical problem is derived from the experience of a large number of similar patients.

Advocates of evidence-based medicine have addressed this paradox directly. They state that clinicians need to carry out 'the particularization, to the individual patient, of our prior experiences (both as individual clinicians and collectively) with groups of similar patients'.[4] A good clinician should therefore use the best available external evidence together with his own unsystematic clinical experience and intuition – based on a blend of knowledge derived from anatomy, physiology and other basic sciences.[11] Evidence alone is never sufficient to make a clinical decision. Decision-makers always trade the benefits and risks, inconvenience and costs associated with alternative management strategies, and in doing so should especially consider the patients' values and preferences.

The significance of the definition of epidemiology as a methodological discipline that addresses determinant–occurrence relationships is based on the reach of the concept of determinant–occurrence relationships in itself. If one considers the presence of disease as the outcome and the diagnostic information as the determinant, then this represents a diagnostic problem. The object of study is, in this case, the functional relationship between diagnostic information and the presence of disease. If one considers the occurrence of a disease or a health-related event in the future as the outcome and the presence of certain patient characteristics as the determinants, then this represents a prognostic problem. One of these patient characteristics can be the use of a specific therapy, and in that case, this represents a therapeutic problem. In the latter case however, to achieve accurate results the 'ceteris paribus principle' – the condition that all other determinants are equal – is a fundamental notion that we will explicitly address under Randomized controlled trials.

A study of the diagnostic accuracy of fine-needle aspiration as a test for malignant disease in patients with nodular thyroid disease is an otolaryngological example of diagnostic research. The influence of the age of patients with an oropharyngeal carcinoma on long-term survival constitutes a prognostic research question. The effect that early surgery compared with watchful waiting for glue-ear has on language development in preschool children represents a therapeutic research question.

Epidemiology and health services and public health research

Epidemiology is also one of the core disciplines of health services research and public health. Whereas classical epidemiology and clinical epidemiology focus largely on determinants of health and disease and related conditions in individuals, health services research is more directed towards questions addressing the quality and organization of health care systems and public health research towards the health and health care problems in communities. One could consider this as a third stream of epidemiological research.

Important questions for health services research are those that address the variations in processes and outcomes of health care services, as well as the determinants of these variations. Research in public health may be concerned with the influence of environmental factors, socioeconomic conditions and health services on health in the community. It will be clear by now that many of these questions take the form of determinant–occurrence relationships, which again confirms the crucial role of an epidemiological approach.

A study comparing the outcome of thyroid surgery performed by experienced surgeons and surgeons in training is an example of an epidemiological study directly addressing a determinant of the quality of otolaryngological care.[12] Another example is a study of the impact that the publication of a guideline on the treatment of persistent glue-ear in children had on the rate of surgery.[13] A systematic review of studies addressing the effectiveness of screening young children to undergo early treatment for glue-ear is a third example of public health research.[14]

THE 'ANATOMY' AND 'PHYSIOLOGY' OF EPIDEMIOLOGICAL RESEARCH

We cannot discuss the different study designs before we have examined what epidemiological research is made up of and how it works. The easiest way to do this is to describe the components of a study protocol and the way results are used to draw inferences from the study results about the truth in the universe. The following sections are based largely on the introductory chapters of a recent book by Hulley and colleagues about designing clinical research.[15]

Essential components of a protocol for an epidemiological study

A research protocol is a document that provides all essential details of a study. A protocol is necessary for guiding all the decisions that need to be made in the course of the study. The process of writing a protocol itself helps the investigator to enhance the scientific rigour and efficiency of the project. Most research involves teamwork and a written document ensures that all members know how the study should be implemented and what they are expected to contribute. A good protocol provides answers to a number of essential questions.

WHAT QUESTION WILL THE STUDY ADDRESS?

The research question defines what you want to achieve. Many experienced researchers will agree that formulating

a question that can be translated into a feasible and valid study can be surprisingly hard. What often happens is that instead of a 'research question', a 'topic' is formulated. 'Framing' the research question is the first step for every new project, of which the importance cannot be overestimated. Conversely, many studies fail not so much because the study design is flawed or the execution of study is poor, but because the question was not formulated adequately in the first place.

An otolaryngological example of such a 'topic' that needs further research is the concern about the rising complication rate after tonsillectomy in the UK. It is clear that we need to provide more detail and structure before we are able to formulate a relevant and answerable 'research question'. The concept of the determinant–occurrence relationship may provide some guidance in this context. In other words, we need to be specific about what outcomes we want to study as well as what determinants we want to consider. Finally, we need to specify the target population, the kind of people for whom the study should provide answers.

In epidemiological research, a good research question therefore has three components. It should define:

1. the target population;
2. the comparison or control group, at least if there is any;
3. the outcome(s) of interest.

An example of a 'good' research question for a study addressing the complication rates after tonsillectomy could be: 'In patients undergoing tonsillectomy because of recurrent tonsillitis, does the use of the bipolar diathermy forceps increase the occurrence of tonsil bleeds severe enough to require return to theatre in the first 28 days after surgery, compared to other tonsillectomy dissection types?' Admittedly, this is a rather convoluted sentence, and is only given here to illustrate how the three components of a research question can be covered in one question. In practice, the question will be shortened to 'Does bipolar diathermy increase the haemorrhage rate after tonsillectomy', but in that case the details that define the target population, the comparison and the outcome of interest need to be provided separately.

WHY IS THE STUDY QUESTION IMPORTANT?

Good epidemiological research should also pass the 'so what' test. In the Introduction or Background section of a protocol, it should be argued that answering the research question will provide a significant contribution to our state of knowledge or, in other words, add to what is already known about the problem. It is therefore important to be on top of the published literature before developing a study. It should also be clear that the results of the proposed study will help to resolve current uncertainties, which may lead to new scientific understanding and influence clinical and public health policies.

It is often 'scholarship' that will identify the gaps in the current knowledge and how these can be addressed in an optimal way by learning from the work of others. For example, a recent systematic review of the literature on the effect of tonsillectomy in patients with chronic or recurrent tonsillitis concluded a lack of evidence to guide decision making for this surgical intervention in adults or children.[1] More importantly in this context, the authors of the systematic review also concluded on the basis of the results of their review that future trials should address the effectiveness of tonsillectomy in subgroups according to age, severity and disease frequency, and that patients should be followed up for at least one year to assess outcomes such as general well-being, behaviour, growth, sleep and eating patterns in addition to severity and frequency of infections. These conclusions based upon a systematic review provide powerful arguments for the direction of future research.

HOW IS THE STUDY STRUCTURED?

Choosing the study design is a complex issue. The actual choice depends strongly on the research question. The study should be designed in such a way that it produces results that are relatively precise (free of random error) and accurate (free of systematic error or bias). An additional consideration is that the study needs to be efficient (affordable in terms of time and money).

A simplistic 'taxonomy' of study designs, presented in **Figure 49.1**, shows that two fundamental decisions have to be made. First, the investigators have to decide whether they want to assign the determinants themselves in an 'experimental study', or whether they want to examine events as nature takes its course in an 'observational study'. Second, if an observational study design is chosen,

the next step is to decide whether the study needs a comparison or control group. If so, the study is often called 'analytical'. If not, it is a 'descriptive' study. Descriptive studies are often used as a first step into a new area of study – the scientific 'toe in the water',[15] and followed by analytical studies to answer questions that can address determinant–occurrence relationships.

A more detailed presentation of study designs follows under Choosing the study design.

WHO ARE THE STUDY SUBJECTS AND HOW WILL THEY BE SELECTED AND RECRUITED?

A good choice of the study subjects ensures that the results of the study will accurately represent what is going on in the population of interest, the target population, the set of people best suited to the research question (for example, patients with early laryngeal squamous cell carcinoma for a study comparing radiotherapy and surgery for laryngeal cancer). The protocol must also specify the study sample, which is the subset of the target population available for study (for example, all consecutive patients with this disease condition referred to a regional head and neck cancer centre in a defined period of time). The study sample should be a subset of the target population that can be studied at an acceptable cost and is large enough to control random error and representative enough to control systematic error.

In many cases, controlling both random error and systematic error sets conflicting demands, which is sometimes referred to as the 'precision–bias' dilemma. For example, a study that aims to evaluate the usefulness of the endoscope compared to the headlamp for sinonasal surgery should carefully consider which patients to include. It is highly likely that the results of the study

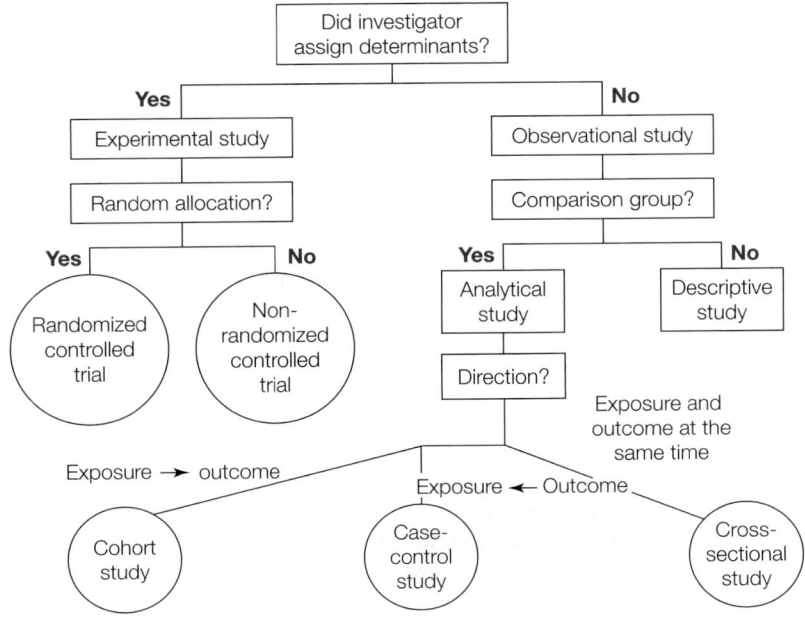

Figure 49.1 Algorithm for classification of types of clinical research. Reproduced from Ref. 16, with permission from Elsevier.

will differ according to the extent of the surgery. The comparison might be most relevant for patients who undergo surgery for procedures around the middle meatus and the anterior ethmoid. Including patients who undergo only simple polypectomy, who comprise approximately 50 percent of the total number of patients who undergo a form of sinonasal surgery, may seem an attractive option because it will double the size of the study. However, including these patients will diminish the extent to which the study sample represents the population for which the research question is of interest.

In an ideal world without practical and financial limitations, we would study the entire target population. Often, if not always, the target population is too large and the study will be carried out in a sample. Earlier, we gave as an example the study comparing radiotherapy and surgery for early laryngeal carcinoma that was carried out in consecutive patients visiting a regional centre in a defined period of time. This type of sampling, including patients that are easily accessible to the investigator, is called 'convenience sampling'. It is very frequently used in clinical research. It has obvious advantages in terms of costs and logistics, but its drawback is that it might not sufficiently represent the target population. Consecutive sampling, including without interruption all accessible people, is especially useful in this context given that it reduces the possibility that selection either by the investigators or self-selection by the subjects influences the results. Probability sampling is the gold standard for ensuring that the study sample is representative of the target population, except for the effect of chance variation. There are several probability-sampling methods. With simple random sampling, every individual in a population has the same chance of being included. However, in some cases, a form of stratified sampling (random sampling with a known sample size within subgroups) is desirable. For a study of patient satisfaction of patients visiting an otolaryngology outpatient clinic, for example, the investigators may wish to divide patients in 'strata' according to their diagnosis or the procedure that was being carried out, and then sample specified numbers from each stratum.

The choices made about the selection of the study subjects (the intended sample) are important as they have an impact on the extent to which the study findings can be generalized. The sampling procedures can affect the generalizability of the results in a number of ways. First, the actual sample might be different from the intended sample. For example, people who were eligible for the study might have refused, and people who participated might be different (more or less healthy, dependent on the study context) from those who did not. Second, the study sample should be sufficiently similar to the target population. For example, the 'spectrum' of disease in patients with laryngeal squamous cell cancer might differ from one centre to the next, and in turn the effects of radiotherapy and cancer might differ as well. Third, the

investigator must form an opinion about whether the results can be generalized to people outside the target population. In terms of our example, do radiotherapy and surgery have similar effects in other countries, in patients with more advanced disease, or in patients who are on average older or younger? This will always be a subjective judgement that depends on findings in other studies, more general scientific knowledge, and what is sometimes called 'a feeling for the organism'. It is not a yes-or-no decision, and may trigger debate among experts. This debate may be informed by the study itself if the study population is diverse enough to explore the constancy of effects in different subgroups within the study.

WHAT MEASUREMENTS WILL BE MADE?

The quality of a study depends on how well the variables measured in the study represent the phenomena of interest. Another concern is how the variables of interest can be measured as precisely (free of random error) and accurately (free of systematic error) as possible without making the study unreasonably expensive.

It is important to have some understanding about the types of variables that are encountered in epidemiological research, and how they can be measured. Any variable can be considered to be of one of two basic types: continuous variables and categorical variables. This distinction determines the way in which these variables should be measured as well as analysed. As a general rule, with categorical variables, the analysis will involve a description or comparison of the proportion of subjects falling into the various categories. With continuous variables, the descriptions or comparisons are most often presented in terms of average values or medians if the sample is small and the average value is considered to be inappropriate to describe the 'midpoint' of the variable's distribution.

Theoretically, continuous variables can take all possible values on a continuum along a specific range. Many clinical parameters are continuous. Variables, such as blood pressure, body weight, body temperature, are not restricted to particular values and are only limited by the accuracy and precision of the measuring procedures. The units in which a continuous variable is expressed specify a uniform difference along the entire length of the scale. A difference in blood pressure of 10 mmHg has the same interpretation irrespective of whether it occurs at the lower or the upper end of the blood pressure scale.

Discrete variables can only take certain numerical values – in most cases only integers (whole numbers). If discrete variables have a considerable number of possible values, they can often be treated as if they were continuous. Examples of these 'quasi-continuous' variables are counts (such as the number of cigarettes smoked, number of episodes of acute tonsillitis in last year, or number of days spent in hospital) or scores on 'clinimetric scales' (such as the 20-item Sino-Nasal Outcome Test) that measures symptom severity of sinonasal conditions on a scale with discrete values ranging from 0 (no symptoms) to 100 (very severe symptoms)[17] or the Epworth Sleepiness Scales, used in patients with obstructive sleep apnoea, that can take discrete values from 0 (no daytime sleepiness) to 24 (very severe daytime sleepiness).[18] Strictly speaking, considering scores on a clinimetric scale as continuous is somewhat problematic, as the interpretation of a difference of one unit may vary along the length of the scale. For example, does an increase from five to ten on the Epworth Sleepiness Score correspond to an increase from 15 to 20?

Phenomena that cannot be measured quantitatively can often be measured by classifying them into categories, and then counting the number of subjects that fall within the defined categories. In its simplest form, there are only two categories (such as man/woman, or dead/alive), and these variables are called dichotomous or binary variables. When there are more than two possible categories, the variables are termed poly- or multichotomous variables. Polychotomous variables can be further classified into those that are ordered, called ordinal variables, and those that are not, called nominal variables. Socioeconomic status, ASA grades describing fitness to undergo surgery,[19] and degree of pain are examples of the former, and race, marital status, and blood type are examples of the latter.

As a general rule, continuous variables are more 'informative' than categorical variables. It is therefore advisable to use continuous variables as much as possible. For example, 'body temperature' as a continuous variable should be preferred to a categorical variable dividing patients into those with a temperature below and above a certain threshold.

Good measurements are precise and accurate. There are largely three sources of random and systematic error: (1) variability due to the observer; (2) variability due to the subject; and (3) variability due to the instrument used.

A number of strategies can be followed to increase simultaneously both precision and accuracy of the measurements. First, the measurement procedures should be standardized and clearly described in the study protocol. Second, those who are involved in taking the measurements should be trained and their performance monitored in the course of the study. Third, the measurements should be carefully chosen in terms of what is known about their performance. Fourth, calibration procedures should be carried out against a 'gold standard'. This is especially essential for mechanical devices such as weighing scales, thermometers and blood pressure measuring devices. Furthermore, a simple and rather effective approach to increase measurement precision is to repeat the measurements and to use the mean of two or more observations. The latter approach is commonly used in studies measuring blood pressure. An important approach to reduce systematic error is blinding, which conceals information about determinants, or in some cases outcomes, to the observers and/or subjects. This reduces the possibility that the observers or the study subjects distort the overall accuracy of the measurements, consciously or unconsciously. Blinding, however, does not ensure overall accuracy of the measurements, but it may eliminate 'differential bias' that affects one study group more than another. Blinding is especially relevant for measurements that incorporate some subjective judgement. For example, a study comparing early surgery with watchful waiting for glue-ear in pre-school children used a tester of language development who was unaware of what treatment the children had received.[20]

HOW WILL THE RESULTS BE ANALYSED?

The main statistical methods that are going to be used to analyse the results should be defined in the study protocol. Choosing the statistical methods after the results have become available will increase the likelihood of finding associations between determinants and outcome on the basis of chance alone.

An important element of the analysis plan is the description of how the outcome variable is going to be analysed. For example, a trial on early surgery for glue-ear that measured language development with the Reynell development language scales (a test of expressive language and verbal comprehension abilities in children aged six months to six years) could analyse the Reynell data as a continuous variable.[20] Conversely, it could define groups with normal language development and with delayed language development by dichotomizing the Reynell data, and use this categorical variable as the main outcome measure.

If a categorical variable is used as the outcome measure, the 'denominator problem' should be considered. **Figure 49.2** summarizes the questions that have to be answered in this respect. The first question asks whether the numerator is going to be included in the denominator. If the answer is yes, the next question is whether time is included in the denominator or not.

Let us first consider the case when the numerator is included in the denominator, but time is not. A first example of this would be a measure of the occurrence of sensorineural hearing loss in neonates. One could simply report the proportion of neonates with hearing loss: the numerator would be the number of neonates with hearing loss and the denominator would be the total number of neonates included in the study. This proportion is often referred to as prevalence. A second example would be a measure of the occurrence of head and neck cancer in people, initially free of the disease, who developed the disease within a specified time period. The numerator would be the number of subjects who developed the disease during follow up and the denominator would be the total number of subjects at the beginning of the study. This proportion is often referred to as cumulative incidence. Suppose that 1000 smokers are followed up

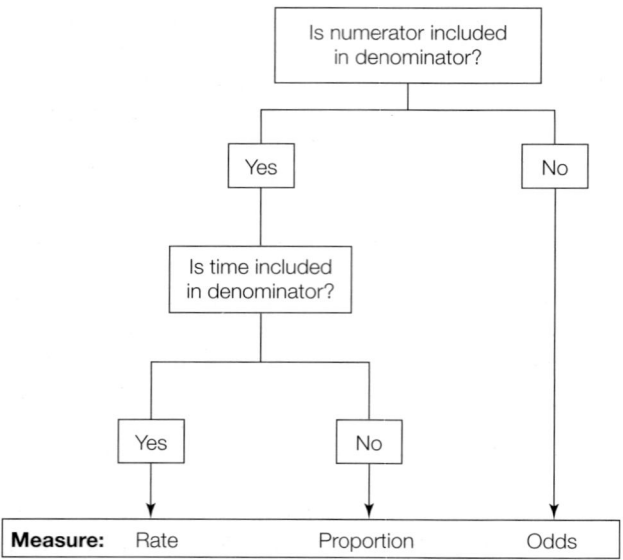

Figure 49.2 Algorithm for distinguishing rates, proportions and odds. Adapted from Ref. 16, with permission from Elsevier.

during five years and that 15 develop head and neck cancer, the cumulative incidence would be 1.5 percent.

The calculation of a proportion as an estimate of disease occurrence, as described above, assumes that the entire study sample has been followed up for the specified time period. This is often not the case. Some subjects might enter the study later, and others might be lost to follow up. An alternative way of measuring outcomes that takes these varying follow-up time periods into account is to include time in the denominator. The numerator would be exactly the same as for proportions, but the sum of the time that each individual was followed up and at risk of becoming a case would be used as the denominator. In this case, an incidence rate (also called incidence density, force of morbidity/mortality, hazard) could be calculated that is equal to the number of people who develop cancer divided by the total person-time at risk during follow up. For example, on the basis of the previous example of the occurrence of head and neck cancer in smokers, one could have expressed the incidence rate of cancer as approximately three cases per 1000 people per year (or 15 divided by approximately 5×1000 years of person-time at risk). Because the incidence is very low, a simple relationship holds: cumulative incidence $\approx$ incidence $\times$ average follow-up time.

Many epidemiological studies report, in some form or other, outcomes expressed as 'odds'. It is important to distinguish odds from probability. A probability can be estimated as the proportion of people in whom a particular characteristic, such as the presence of disease, is present. The larger the group of people under study, the better the observed proportion of people with the disease reflects the 'true' probability. Odds, on the other hand, represents the ratio of two complementary probabilities.

Table 49.1 'Outcome odds ratios' and 'determinant odds ratios' – fictitious example of complication rates after tonsillectomy.

Dissection instruments used	Postoperative complication				
	Yes		No		Total
Bipolar diathermy	36	*a*	264	*b*	300	*a* + *b*
Other	24	*c*	676	*d*	700	*c* + *d*
Total	60	*a* + *c*	940	*b* + *d*	1000

For example, if the probability of disease is 0.20, then the odds are $0.20\%/0.80 = 1:4 = 0.25$. Another way of calculating the odds is by dividing the number of subjects with the characteristic by the number without it. In other words, the numerator is not included in the denominator (see **Figure 49.2**).

Most frequently, it is not the odds itself that is reported in epidemiological studies, but the odds ratio – the ratio of odds in different groups. This can be the 'outcome odds ratio', or the ratio of the odds of the outcome of interest in the group with the determinant to the odds of the outcome in the group without the determinant. Conversely, this can also be the 'determinant odds ratio', or the odds of the determinant in the group with the outcome compared to the odds of the determinant in the group without the outcome of interest. One reason why epidemiologists find odds ratios so attractive is that 'outcome odds ratios' are equivalent to 'determinant odds ratios', which is a fact used in the analysis of case–control studies (see Case–control studies). For example, **Table 49.1** presents fictitious findings of a study on risk factors for postoperative complications after tonsillectomy. The outcome odds ratio is the same as the determinant odds ratio, which can be easily understood as both odds ratios simplify to the 'cross product' of the cell frequencies of a 2×2 table. The 'outcome odds ratio' can be calculated as

$$\frac{\frac{a}{a+b} / \frac{b}{a+b}}{\frac{c}{c+d} / \frac{d}{c+d}} = \frac{a/b}{c/d} = \frac{a \times d}{b \times c} = \frac{36 \times 676}{24 \times 264} = 3.8.$$

Similarly, the 'determinant odds ratio' can be calculated as

$$\frac{\frac{a}{a+c} / \frac{c}{a+c}}{\frac{b}{b+d} / \frac{d}{b+d}} = \frac{a/c}{b/d} = \frac{a \times d}{b \times c} = 3.8.$$

When a dichotomous outcome variable is used (for example, alive/dead, or disease present/absent) 'risk differences' and 'risk ratios' are commonly used as 'measures of effect'.[10] The 'risk' in this circumstance can represent 'prevalence', 'cumulative incidence', 'incidence' or even 'odds', as described above. One might ask, 'What is the additional risk of head and neck cancer in people who smoke, over and above that in people who do not?' The answer to this question is obviously a risk difference. In a previous fictitious example, we supposed that we followed up 1000 smokers for a period of five years and that we found that 15 of them developed head and neck cancer. The cumulative incidence of cancer in this group is therefore 1.5 percent. We can also suppose that we did the same in 1000 nonsmokers and that we found cancer in seven of them. The cumulative incidence in non-smokers is 0.7 percent. The risk difference attributable to smoking is therefore 0.8 percent (= 1.5–0.7 percent). On the other hand, one might ask, 'How many times are smokers more likely to get head and neck cancer compared to nonsmokers?' Following our example, we could calculate the risk ratio as 2.1 (= 1.5 percent/ 0.7 percent). In other words, smokers are approximately twice as likely to develop head and neck cancer over a five-year period as nonsmokers. This risk ratio does not tell us anything about the magnitude of the risk difference. Even for large risk ratios, the risk difference might be quite small if the outcome is uncommon. As a rule of thumb, risk differences are more meaningful as a measure of effect in clinical situations, because it represents the actual additional probability in those exposed. On the other hand, relative risks are more meaningful as effect measures of a causal relationship in aetiological studies.

HOW LARGE IS THE STUDY GOING TO BE?

A major problem of many studies is that the study size is too small. Small studies lead to imprecise results. Small studies often increase, rather than reduce, the scientific and clinical uncertainty in a specific area. Although one might argue that small studies have a value of their own because they might be included in a systematic review and meta-analysis, which would mimic the results of a larger study, it should be the goal of every study to include a number of subjects that would in itself produce 'meaningful' results. A considerably less frequent problem is that of a study that is larger than necessary to be meaningful. Larger studies are more difficult to carry out and may be more costly than necessary. The most important issue in this context is of course to determine what can be considered meaningful.

How can the appropriate size of a study be determined? This question is most commonly answered on the basis of a statistical 'sample size calculation'. Although the answer of a sample size calculation is exact (for example, the number of subjects to be included in a study), in many cases it depends on a number of rather subjective choices. The way that the sample size of study is to be calculated depends on whether it is an analytical study (study with a comparison or control group) or a descriptive study.

For analytical studies, a research hypothesis should be formulated that further refines the study question. This hypothesis sets out the basis for statistical significance testing. Because this hypothesis guides the statistical analysis, it should be simple (addressing one determinant

or comparison and the occurrence of one outcome) and specific (defining unambiguously the target population, the control and comparison group, and the outcome of interest). For the purpose of statistical significance testing, this hypothesis should be given in the form of a 'null hypothesis' that states that there is no association between the determinant and the outcome. A statistical test helps to estimate the probability that an association observed in a study is due to chance (the 'p-value'). The 'alternative hypothesis' states that there is such an association. Sometimes, a distinction is made between one-sided and two-sided hypotheses. Two-sided hypotheses state only that an association exists between determinant and outcome, whereas one-side hypotheses specify the direction of the association. For example, the null-hypothesis of a study comparing early surgery with watchful waiting for glue-ear in pre-school children could be that there is no difference in the language development in the two treatment groups. The one-sided null hypothesis would state that language development with early surgery is poorer than with watchful waiting. One-sided p-values are appropriate in selected circumstances, when only one direction of the association is important. One-sided p-values may seem attractive as, generally speaking, with a one-sided significance test the p-value would be half the size of that with a two-sided test, but, on the other hand, if the results of the study would suggest that the language development is indeed poorer with surgery, then this would produce a large p-value as it is likely to observe a result like that given that the null-hypothesis (language development with surgery is poorer) is true. For this reason, it is convention to use two-sided hypotheses when planning the size of a study as well as two-sided p-values when analysing the results, unless there are well-argued reasons for the contrary.

When developing a study protocol for an analytical study, the investigator does not know the size of the effect that the determinant of interest has on the outcome, as one of the objectives of the study is to estimate it. For example, the investigators of the study of the effect that early surgery has on language development in children with glue-ear had to decide the smallest effect of surgery that in their view would be of clinical importance. This quantity is often called effect size or target difference. Determining this effect size is the most arbitrary step in a sample size calculation. The smaller the effect size, the larger the study needs to be, other things being equal. Previous studies could help to make a guess about what can be expected, but they do not provide any guidance about what is an important difference and what is not.

Before a sample size can be calculated, two further arbitrary choices need to be made. First, the 'alpha level' or 'significance level' has to be chosen that defines the cut-off point for the p-value – conventionally 0.05 – to classify a result either as 'significant' (if p-value $\leq$ cut-off), in which case the null hypothesis is rejected, or as 'not significant' (if p-value $>$ cut-off), in which case the null hypothesis is not rejected. Second, the 'power' of the significance test has to be chosen – commonly used values are 0.80 or 0.90 – that defines the probability to obtain a significant result if we assume that the defined effect size or target difference would be the 'true effect' or 'true difference'.

Finally, and only if a continuous outcome variable is going to be analysed, a measure of the variability (spread) of that outcome – standard deviation or variance – is needed. The greater the variability in the outcome variable among the subjects, the more difficult it will be to demonstrate a difference between two groups, and the larger the study needs to be.

The required sample size can be obtained on the basis of the above-described ingredients either by using the formulae presented in statistical textbooks, from published tables or by using commonly available statistical software packages. The ingredients and the formulae for study size are purely technical. They do not take into account the value of the information obtained in the study. The most important decision is to determine the 'right balance' between the value of greater precision in study results against the greater costs. Essentially, this decision boils down to a cost–benefit analysis in which the benefits are more difficult to quantify than the costs.

For descriptive studies, concepts such as null hypothesis, effect size, alpha level and power do not apply. Instead, descriptive statistics, such as means and proportions, are presented. The sample size of descriptive studies depends on how precise the investigator wants these descriptive statistics to be. Confidence intervals, such as 95 or 99 percent confidence intervals, are commonly used to represent the precision of the estimates. For example, a study of the five-year survival after surgical treatment in 228 patients with hypopharynx carcinoma found that the survival was 27.2 percent with a 95 percent confidence interval ranging from 21.5 to 33.5 percent.[21] This interval indicates that we can be 95 percent confident (which can be considered more or less the same as saying that there is 95 percent chance) that the 'true' five-year survival probability lies within this interval. When estimating the sample size for descriptive studies, the investigator specifies the desired width of the confidence interval, and the sample size derives from that and can be read from tables or obtained from statistical software packages. This approach can be followed for any type of descriptive variable for which confidence intervals can be calculated.

CHOOSING THE STUDY DESIGN

The taxonomy of study designs presented in **Figure 49.1** provides a simple decision aid for choosing the most appropriate design. A number of questions have to be answered with the ultimate goal being to create an affordable study that provides results that are relatively precise (free of random error) and accurate (free of systematic error or bias). A first distinction that has to be made is that between studies in which the investigator actively assigns the determinants (experimental studies) or those in which this is not the case (observational studies). A second distinction that has to be made is that between observational studies that do or do not have a comparison or control group. If so, the study is called analytical, if not, descriptive.

The following sections are largely based on a series of short essays on clinical research published in the *Lancet*,[16] and chapters of recent books about designing clinical research by Hulley and colleagues[12] and clinical epidemiology.[10] We start this section by describing observational studies and will end with the description of experimental studies (randomized controlled trials).

Minimizing bias and confounding

We have indicated earlier that the precision of study results depends mainly on two factors: the size of the study design and the methods used to obtain the measurements. Furthermore, a study should be designed in such a way that it avoids systematic error or bias. A great number of different types of bias have been documented but it is not a major simplification to consider all these types of biases in three categories: selection bias, information bias and confounding.

To examine whether selection bias would introduce systematic error in the study results, two questions need to be answered: 'Do the sample of study subjects sufficiently represent the population of interest?' and 'Are the groups that are going to be compared similar in all important respects apart from the determinant(s) of interest?' The first question is especially relevant when designing a randomized controlled trial, because trials usually enrol patients who tend to be different (often healthier) from the target population and the results tend to overestimate the effects compared to what they would be in routine practice. This contributes to the differences between the efficacy of a therapy observed in the highly controlled circumstances in selected clinical settings and the effectiveness of a treatment in actual practice. The second question refers directly to the comparability of the groups. In other words, do the groups differ importantly aside from the comparison that is being studied?

Information bias results from incorrect information about the determinant or the outcome or both. The important question that has to be answered is: 'Has information been gathered in the same way?' In cohort studies (see Cohort studies), information about the outcome should be obtained in the same way for those with and without the determinants under consideration. Also, those who collect the information about the outcome should be unaware of ('blind to') the determinant status of the subjects as much as possible. In case–control studies (see below), information about the determinant status should be collected in the same way for cases and controls.

Confounding occurs when two determinants or risk factors are associated with each other. In that case, the effect of one is confounded with, or distorted by, the effect of the other. Confounding can occur because of selection bias, by chance, or because the two determinants are really associated in nature. Selection bias and confounding are not mutually exclusive, but they are often presented differently as they represent problems at different stages in a study. Selection bias is an issue when the sampling procedures for patients are determined during the design phase of a study, whereas confounding is an issue to consider during the analysis phase.

Often in the same study more than one bias operates, as in the following example. Imagine a study that compared the effect that surgical and nonsurgical management had on speech and language development in children with persistent otitis media with effusion. In this example, selection bias could have been present if the children who received surgical treatment came from a different background and had parents who were on average of higher socioeconomic status, or if they had a family history of chronic ear infection. Information bias could have occurred because the assessment of language development might have been influenced by the fact that those who were applying and interpreting the speech and language tests knew the treatment the children had received. Finally, the conclusion that surgical treatment improved speech and language development might have been the result of confounding if the children who received surgical treatment had had more serious or more frequent ear infections. The latter bias is often referred to as 'confounding by clinical indication'.

When designing studies, investigators should try as much as possible to rule out bias. The concerns about bias need to be thought through very carefully. This relates directly to the three components of a good research question, and these components should be represented adequately in the study design. First, the study sample should adequately represent the target population. Second, the measurement of the determinants should adequately represent the comparison of interest. Third, the measurements of the outcomes should adequately represent the outcome(s) of interest.

When confounding is anticipated, the investigator should consider design and analysis strategies to control its influence on the outcomes. The simplest approach in the design phase is restriction or specification. For example, investigators could decide to include only nonsmokers in a study on the effect of human papillomavirus and oropharyngeal cancer. The disadvantage of this strategy is that it reduces recruitment and prohibits generalization of the results to smokers. Another potential approach in the design phase is matching which means that subjects with matching values for the confounding variables are included. This can be done individually (pair wise matching) or in groups (frequency matching). However, the use of matching has many disadvantages. The recruitment process can become rather cumbersome. Special analytical techniques are required that represent the fact that the subjects are not sampled independently. There is also the danger of overmatching – matching on the basis of a variable that is not a confounder, which would reduce the study's power. Given these disadvantages, matching should be avoided if other strategies could provide sufficient control for confounding.

In the analysis phase, the investigator can use either stratification or adjustment. Stratification ensures that the analysis compares like with like, first by comparing subjects within a group (or stratum) of subjects with similar values of one or more confounding variables and then, in a second step, by calculating an overall estimate by pooling the stratum-specific results. The most important disadvantage of this approach is the limited number of variables that can be controlled for. Adjustment on the basis of a statistical multivariate model does not suffer from this limitation, but its effects depend on the adequacy of the model fit. Both approaches depend on the completeness, precision and accuracy of the measurements of the confounders.

Observational studies

DESCRIPTIVE STUDIES

Descriptive studies can describe the experience in only one individual, a case report, or a report on a series of individual cases, the case-series report. Case series are the most frequently published studies in surgery. An important function of descriptive studies is that they can describe the distribution of diseases or disease-related conditions and events in a specified population.

Good descriptive research should address the five 'W' questions – who, what, why, when and where, although as soon as these questions are addressed on the basis of the data, the distinction between descriptive studies (no comparison) and analytical studies (comparison between groups essential) starts to disappear, but a distinctive characteristic of descriptive studies is that they cannot directly quantify the risk that can be attributed to a specific determinant. For example, a series of three cases was published recently of perichondritis of the pinna as a result of 'high' ear piercing, and was used to focus attention on the risks of body piercing.[22] The study also presented the increasing trend in the number of hospital admissions for perichondritis of the pinna in the UK and Wales from approximately 600 in 1990–1991 to approximately 1200 in 1997–1998. The latter is an example of a surveillance study, which is another important type of descriptive study. A surveillance study is an ongoing and systematic collection, analysis and interpretation of health data essential to the planning, implementation and evaluation of health services and public health practice. The fact that this particular descriptive study cannot quantify the attributable risk might not be a weakness as most cases of perichondritis of the pinna may be due to piercing practices in the first place.

The strength of descriptive studies is that they often use existing data and thus are inexpensive and efficient to carry out. Furthermore, few ethical limitations exist. The disadvantages are that there is a danger of over-interpretation. For example, in early 2001 the UK government recommended that single-use instruments should be used for adenotonsillectomy to minimize the risk of transmission of variant Creutzfeldt-Jacob disease (vCJD). In the course of the same year, suspicion was raised about the postoperative haemorrhage rate. It was thought that the increase in the haemorrhage rate was due to the poor quality of the single-use instruments and, in late 2001, the UK government recommended the reintroduction of reusable instruments. The need to consider alternative explanations arose later as more detailed analyses of hospital admission data revealed that there also had been a gradual increase in the post-tonsillectomy complication rate from 3.9 percent in 1995–1996 to 7.3 percent in 2000–2001 (unpublished data, Van der Meulen JHP, 2003).

Analytical studies

An important distinction that is often made with respect to observational studies that are analytical is whether the determinants and outcomes relate to phenomena that occur at the same time. If so, it is called a cross-sectional study. If not, it is either a cohort study (looking forward in time from determinant to outcome) or a case–control study (looking backward from outcome to determinant).

CROSS-SECTIONAL STUDIES

The single most important characteristic of cross-sectional studies is that the determinant(s) as well as the outcome(s) measured occur at the same time, and that there is no follow-up period. Cross-sectional designs are very well suited to describe the prevalence of health and disease-related conditions and their distribution patterns. For example, a study was carried out in 864 school children in the UK to investigate the effect of parental smoking on middle ear disease.[23] Data on parental smoking were collected with a questionnaire and glue-ear was considered to be present in children with a flat tympanogram. The study identified 82 cases in total, 45 in the 407 households with at least one smoker and 37 in the 457 households with no smokers, and a risk ratio of 1.4 (= 11.0 percent/8.1 percent, with a 95 percent confidence interval ranging from 0.9 to 2.1) could be calculated.

The major strengths of cross-sectional studies is that they examine the presence or absence of an outcome and determinant at the same time. Cross-sectional studies are therefore fast, relatively cheap, and there is no 'loss to follow-up'. A major disadvantage of cross-sectional studies is that they provide only a snap shot of complicated temporal relationships between determinant and outcome. Parental smoking, for example, is likely to be persistent, but chronic middle ear infection in children is an intermittent disease. As a consequence, causal relationships are difficult to establish with cross-sectional studies. For the same reasons, they are not suitable for producing information on prognosis or the natural history of a condition.

Studies of the accuracy of diagnostic tests are a special case of cross-sectional studies. A key feature of such studies is that the diagnostic test results and 'gold standard information' or reference test results about the presence or absence of the conditions of interest are collected at the same time. The subjects should have both undergone the diagnostic test in question (for example, ultrasound-guided fine-needle aspiration to diagnose malignant disease in patients with nodular thyroid disease), as well as the reference test (histology after surgical resection). The results of one test should not be available to those who are carrying out the other. In terms of the example, the pathologist examining the surgical specimen should be 'blind' to the results of the fine needle aspiration. Another important criterion for a valid evaluation of the diagnostic accuracy is that the diagnostic test is evaluated in 'an appropriate spectrum of patients' (such as those in whom we would use it in practice).

The accuracy of a diagnostic test, a measure of how well the test results help to distinguish between individuals with and individuals without the disease or target disorder, is often expressed in terms of sensitivity and specificity. However, it is important to realize that this is, in most cases, a simplified representation of the diagnostic accuracy. Sensitivity and specificity can only be calculated for a test with dichotomous results, often called 'positive' if the result suggests that the disease is present and 'negative' if it suggests that disease is absent. The sensitivity is estimated as the proportion of individuals with the disease who have a positive test result. The specificity corresponds to the proportion of individuals without the disease who have a negative test result. The sensitivity and specificity of a 'perfect' test are 100 percent. The sum of the sensitivity and specificity is sometimes used as a single measure of the diagnostic accuracy. The sum of the sensitivity and specificity for a 'worthless' test, a test that would perform no better than tossing a coin, is expected to be 100 percent and for a perfect test 200 percent.

In many cases, however, relying on sensitivity and specificity as measures of diagnostic accuracy is too simplistic. For example, many tests, if not all, have more than two possible outcomes, and dichotomizing the results in a positive and a negative test result reduces the amount of diagnostic information that a test can provide. Furthermore, if one would like to dichotomize the test results, it is not immediately obvious what the cut-off value between positive and negative results should be. Lastly, the actual aim of performing a diagnostic test is not to distinguish between individuals with and without the disease, but to identify those individuals for whom the expected benefit of treatment outweighs the expected harm. This indicates that the classic diagnostic 'stepping-stone approach', jumping from signs and symptoms to diagnosis and then from diagnosis to treatment, is rather artificial in many cases. This should be reflected in studies assessing diagnostic tests. They should focus on clinical effectiveness (effect on patient outcomes) rather than on diagnostic accuracy alone (for a comprehensive review of methods for the evaluation of diagnostic technologies, see Knottnerus.[24])

COHORT STUDIES

Cohort studies follow groups of individuals over time. The word 'cohort' originates from the Latin word for a group of 300 to 600 soldiers in a Roman legion. This is appropriate as the same rule applies for epidemiological cohorts as once for Roman cohorts: if a person joins a cohort, he will be a member of that cohort forever, which emphasizes the need for the completeness of follow up. Most follow-up studies are analytical (comparing the occurrence of outcomes according to presence or absence of certain determinants), but they can be descriptive as well.

The design of many cohort studies is relatively straightforward. A group of people is assembled, none of whom have experienced the outcome of interest, but all of whom could experience it. On study entry, people may be classified according to the determinants of interest. These people are then observed over time to see in which of them the outcome of interest occurs. Despite this simple design, the terminology used to describe these studies can be confusing. For example, terms such as 'longitudinal study', 'prospective study' or 'incidence study' are often used interchangeably. The only real problematic issues in this respect is the use of the term 'prospective study', as cohort studies can consider data that are collected prospectively as well as retrospectively.

The terms 'retrospective' and 'prospective' refer to the way that the data have been collected rather than to the study design. The essential characteristic of prospective data collection is that data are being collected on determinants and outcomes that manifest themselves after the establishment of a study protocol. In all other situations, the data collection should be considered to be retrospective. Retrospective data collection can be based on data recorded in the past for other purposes or on the memory of the study subjects, investigators or other parties. It is obvious that the precision and accuracy of prospectively collected data can be expected to be better than retrospectively collected data. Cohort studies can be based entirely on retrospective data (using retrospective data on both the determinants and the outcome), based entirely on prospective data (using prospective data on both the determinants and the outcome), or based on a mix of retrospective data on determinants and prospective data on the outcome.

Cohort studies have many attractive features. They are the best way of ascertaining the incidence of a disease or health-related event or condition, as well as the natural history of a disorder. They also provide insight into the temporal order of determinants and outcome, which strengthens the inferences that can be made about whether an observed risk factor is a cause of the outcome. Furthermore, multiple outcomes can be considered which is especially relevant if cohort studies are compared with case–control studies (see Case–control studies). However, the dangers of considering multiple outcomes are also obvious since testing many hypotheses may lead to misleading results. Lastly, prospective cohort studies are especially valuable for the study of fatal diseases, or more general studies of the occurrence of disease-related conditions with a short duration. When these kind of conditions are studied retrospectively, the observed occurrences may be an under-representation of all occurrences.

The major drawback of cohort studies is that they are relatively expensive and therefore an inefficient way to study rare outcomes. Cohort studies become more efficient as the outcomes become more common. Another disadvantage for cohort studies that collect outcome prospectively is that the results may not be available for a long time. A prospective study of the effect of passive smoking on the head and neck cancer incidence may take more than ten years to come up with relevant results.

However, not all prospective cohort studies need to take a very long time to complete. A cohort study could be used, for example, to study the risk factors for complications after tonsillectomy. Such a study could prospectively collect patient characteristics as well as data on surgical technique, instruments used and experience of the surgeons. Every patient could be followed up for a certain period, say one month, and the occurrence of complications could be registered. Such a study would provide insight into the incidence of complications – it might even distinguish between primary haemorrhage, secondary haemorrhage as well as infection, and also in the way this incidence depends on relevant risk factors.

CASE–CONTROL STUDIES

Case–control studies can be considered as 'research in reverse'.[16] Many epidemiologists consider them as one of the most important tools in their armamentarium. The design of case–control studies can be appreciated by again considering the example of the study on risk factors for complications after tonsillectomy. For this study, we could also use a case–control design. All the patients who experience a complication in the first month after surgery could be considered as 'cases', and patients without postoperative complications as 'controls'. The investigators then have to look back in time to find data on the patient's risk factors that were present at the time of surgery.

The essential feature of a case–control study is that not all controls need to be included but that a selection would suffice. Many case–control studies include only one control for each case, whereas others included more but hardly ever more than four or five. The reason that the number of included controls per case is seldom higher is that including more controls will have only a small effect on the power of the study and on the precision of the estimates ('law of diminishing returns'). The fact that only information has to be collected for a selection of the controls makes that, in many circumstances, case–control studies are the most efficient design in terms of time, effort and therefore money. Hence, case–control studies are especially relevant if the occurrence of the outcome of interest is low. However, if the frequency of the determinant of interest is low, case–control studies might become inefficient. For example, if the frequency of a certain risk factor of post-tonsillectomy complications is low, investigators have to examine many cases and controls to find some who have been exposed. Some have advocated a 'rule of thumb' stating that cohorts are more efficient than case–control studies if the occurrence of the outcome is more frequent than that of the determinant and *vice versa*.

Unlike cohort studies, case–control studies cannot produce an estimate of the occurrence of the outcome of interest since we lack information about the denominator. A case–control study of post-tonsillectomy complications will neither provide information on how many patients underwent the operation nor on what their risk factors were. The relevant effect measure that a case–control study can provide is the odds ratio for a determinant, derived from the proportions in cases and in controls (more precisely, the odds) in whom the determinant is present. Earlier, we referred to this odds ratio as the 'determinant odds ratio'. This determinant odds ratio is equivalent to the 'outcome odds ratio' and the odds ratio obtained from a case–control study can therefore be used as a measure of relative risk.

The advantage of case–control studies (efficiency in time, effort and money) comes at a price however, because two methodological issues may introduce major systematic errors: selecting the control group and obtaining information about the determinants. The selection of cases is relatively straightforward provided that the definition of the outcome being studied (the 'case definition') is clear. The selection of the control group is more problematic. Two criteria need to be met. First,

controls should be representative of the population at risk of becoming cases. In other words, the controls should have been selected as cases had they developed the disease or outcome of interest themselves. Second, selection of the cases should be independent of the determinant(s) being investigated. Therefore, a case–control study of risk factors for post-tonsillectomy haemorrhage should include as controls only patients who underwent a tonsillectomy themselves. Furthermore, it seems inappropriate to select as controls all patients who underwent a tonsillectomy immediately after patients who developed complications. If that were the case, it would be very likely that the same surgeon using the same technique and the same type of instruments treated these patients. It is left as an exercise for the reader to decide what an appropriate strategy to select controls would be.

RANDOMIZED CONTROLLED TRIALS

Randomized controlled trials are cohort studies with prospective data collection. Their distinctive feature is that they use a random allocation scheme to assign the determinant. With randomization, you can expect that the prognostic characteristics of the randomized groups or 'arms' of the trial are similar except for differences due to chance variation. Randomization eliminates the influence of both known and unknown confounders that are present at the time of randomization. Without randomized treatment allocation, it cannot be excluded and is in practice very likely that imbalances in prognostic factors between the groups occur that are the result of selection bias – a type of bias often called 'confounding by clinical indication'.

The ethical argument in favour of a random process deciding what intervention patients receive is that there is equipoise, or a state of genuine uncertainty on the part of the clinical investigator regarding the comparative merits of each intervention. If there is genuine uncertainty about which treatment is best, it is not possible to recommend one over the other which justifies that a random process decides. The problem is, however, that equipoise depends on subjective judgements and that therefore experts may disagree. Furthermore, preferences of patients or those who are candidates to receive the intervention have to be taken into account. The process of informed consent should address all these issues to ensure that patients can evaluate the potential risks and benefits of the study from their own perspective before they agree to participate.

It is important that the randomization process is 'concealed' from the investigators who include the participants into the trial. Proper allocation concealment requires that the investigators do not know the arm to which a participant will be allocated until the participant has definitively been recruited and included in the study. Concealment of the randomization is the only way to prevent the investigators influencing the balance of the prognostic characteristics between the groups that are being compared. For example, prior knowledge of the next allocation may allow investigators to exclude certain candidate participants from the trial because they are perceived to be allocated to an inappropriate group. More directly, the investigators may try to influence the order of inclusion. Concealment of treatment allocation is so important that with inadequate concealment a randomized controlled trial should be considered nonrandomized. Empirical studies have shown that trials with inadequate concealment overestimate the treatment effect by as much as 40 percent on average.

Another important feature of many randomized controlled trials is the use of a form of blinding, which prevents the participants and the investigators who are in contact with the participants from being aware of which treatment has been offered. Blinding can help to prevent bias in a number of ways. First, if participants do not know what treatment they are receiving, it is less likely that their perceptions and expectations of the treatment that they receive can influence their compliance and the physical and psychological response to the intervention. For example, most patients expect that a new treatment is better than an existing one. Second, blinding investigators is important, as this would prevent them consciously or unconsciously managing the participants in the trials differently. Also, their attitude towards the treatment can influence how patients respond to the treatment. Third, blinding participants and investigators will prevent outcomes from being assessed differently. The terms 'single-blind' and 'double-blind' are often used to indicate trials in which only the participants or both the participants and the investigators are blinded.

Double blinding is impossible in almost all surgical trials. To avoid biased management, the investigators should then try to standardize other potential treatments as much as possible. Approaches to minimize biased assessment of outcomes could include the use of a third party who is unaware of the treatment originally given. When blinded assessment is not possible, one should try as much as possible to use 'hard outcomes' (based on measurements resistant to bias). Another alternative includes the use of standardized outcome measurement scales that can be completed by the participant. This approach is likely to produce less biased outcomes than the judgement of an investigator.

Many people also consider the use of a placebo treatment as an essential feature of a randomized controlled trial. Placebo treatment is a form of treatment indistinguishable from the 'active treatment' under study, but it does not have a specific known mechanism to influence a patient's health. Blinding often requires the use of placebo treatment. Apart from that, the choice whether to use placebo treatment depends on the question that the trial tries to answer. First, if the question is whether intervention A is better than intervention B, then it is obvious that one should compare the effects of

A and B with each other and not against placebo treatment. Second, if the question is whether intervention A is better than no treatment at all, the answers may be different for researchers and clinicians. Researchers are likely to be more interested in the specific effects – effects that can be attributed to the 'active component' of an intervention. Clinicians are likely to be more interested in the combined effects of the active and placebo components. On the other hand, it is always useful to know what part of the total effect is due to the active component and what part to the placebo when balancing the potential benefits against potential harms and costs, which are likely to differ between the active and placebo components. It is obvious that placebo treatment is rarely an option for randomized controlled trials in surgery. For example, in a trial comparing tonsillectomy with nonsurgical management, it would require a form of 'sham surgery' to provide a placebo treatment. It is left to the reader to decide what the advantages and disadvantages of using such a form of placebo treatment in this context would be.

If a substantial number of participants do not receive the study interventions, do not comply with the study protocol or are lost to follow up, the trial is likely to be underpowered and its results biased. Strategies to maximize compliance and follow up should therefore be an integral part of every trial protocol. An obvious strategy is to make participation in a trial as convenient, painless and enjoyable as possible. Some trials have a 'run-in period' that can be used to 'screen out' patients who may not adhere to the study protocol and the follow-up procedures. It is essential to ascertain that compliance and completeness of follow up do not differ between the trial arms as this could lead to biased estimates of the effects of the interventions.

The results of trials can be analysed in two ways. First, the comparison of the intervention can be carried out according to the intervention to which the patients were randomized ('intention-to-treat' analysis) or according to the treatment they actually received ('per protocol' analysis). The advantage of an intention-to-treat analysis is that the question that is being addressed corresponds exactly with the one clinicians and patients try to answer in clinical practice. The disadvantage is that if many patients do not receive the treatment they were randomized to, this would obscure the difference between the trial arms. Per protocol analysis, on the other hand, addresses which intervention is better more directly. With this form of analysis, the treatments are being compared according to the treatments that the patients actually received. The problem with this approach is that if many patients do not receive the treatment to which they were randomized, the study no longer represents an experimental study.

The analysis should focus on a single outcome – often referred to as the 'primary endpoint' – to avoid the problems of interpreting the outcome of multiple hypothesis tests. This primary endpoint should also be used for the power calculation in the design phase of the trial. It is often desirable to consider a number of secondary endpoints – outcomes that represent different aspects of the outcome of interest – to provide a more detailed picture of the effects of the interventions under study. For example, a randomized controlled trial of tonsillectomy and nonsurgical management could consider the reduction in the number of episodes of tonsillitis or sore throat as primary endpoint, but could also collect information on postoperative complications, reduction in time off work and reduction in the use of certain drugs, such as analgesics and antibiotics.

Subgroup analyses are comparisons between randomized groups in a subset of the patients with specific characteristics. The most important question that subgroup analyses try to answer is whether the effect measure is different in different subgroups by carrying out a statistical test for interaction (or 'effect modification'). For example, one could investigate – when analysing the results of the trial on tonsillectomy – whether the effects of tonsillectomy on recurrence of tonsillitis are different in children younger than five years compared to children of five years and older.

Subgroup analyses can be dangerous and misleading, but they can also provide an important extra insight into the generalizability of the results. One danger arises from the fact that multiple comparisons are carried out, which increases the risk of producing false–positive results. To avoid this risk, only a limited number of subgroup analyses should be carried out and they should be specified in the study protocol, in other words, before the results of the trial are known and on the basis of patients characteristics that are measured before randomization. Furthermore, the actual number of subgroup analyses carried out should be reported. Another approach to minimize the risk of false-positive results is to reduce the significance level of the statistical tests for interaction (for example, from the conventional 0.05 to 0.05 divided by the number of tests carried out as specified by the Bonferroni method). A further danger is the limited power of the subgroup analyses, because the group size is, by definition, smaller than that of the original trial population.

An important problem of randomized controlled trials is that of generalizability. Most trials are carried out in highly controlled conditions in a selected group of patients. Their results therefore provide evidence about the efficacy of an intervention (does the treatment work under ideal circumstances?) and not about the effectiveness (does the treatment work in actual practice?). It depends on the question that needs to be answered as to what extent the design of a trial should focus on efficacy or on effectiveness. An explanatory trial (addressing the efficacy question) is needed in the early stage of a new intervention. However, a pragmatic trial (addressing the effectiveness question that aims to create study conditions that reflect as much as possible actual practice when effectiveness is more important) is more appropriate to answer whether an intervention should be included in the 'repertoire' of available services.

It is obvious that not all questions about the effectiveness of surgical procedures can be addressed with a randomized controlled trial.[25] A number of obstacles have been identified that make randomized controlled trials inappropriate (outcome of interest relatively rare, relevant outcomes far in the future, or randomization affecting the effectiveness of a procedure), impossible (refusal of clinicians or patients to participate, ethical obstacles), or inadequate (low generalizability of experimental studies).[26] If the obstacles are insurmountable, carefully designed observational studies should be considered.

Concluding remarks

This chapter introduces the 'determinant–occurrence relationship' as a key concept for medical research, and epidemiology as a methodological discipline with immediate relevance for otolaryngological research. A basic understanding of epidemiological principles is therefore essential for all people who are involved in clinical research and desirable for all clinicians who want to read the medical literature critically.

We have only presented a broad picture of epidemiological concepts and principles, but it will be clear to the reader that studies vary according to the likelihood that their results are accurate (free of systematic error) and precise (random error). For this reason, a 'hierarchy of evidence' has been suggested.[11] For therapeutic issues, this hierarchy ranges from well-conducted randomized controlled trials at the top – preferably summarized in a systematic review and meta-analysis – to case-reports and expert opinion at the bottom (used throughout this book). For diagnostic and prognostic issues, very different hierarchies are necessary. These hierarchies of evidence are not absolute. If the therapeutic effects are very large in comparison to the potential effects of bias – for example, effects of insulin in ketoacidosis – a description of a series of cases may already provide compelling evidence. Nevertheless, it should be a leading principle that users of research try to look for the best available evidence from this hierarchy.

KEY POINTS

- Epidemiology is a methodological discipline. Epidemiological concepts and principles will help to design empirical studies that are relatively precise (free of random error), accurate (free of systematic error or bias) and efficient (affordable in terms of time and money).

- The 'determinant–occurrence relationship' is a key epidemiological concept, and many clinical research questions can be 'framed' as determinant–occurrence relationships.
- Epidemiological studies can be distinguished into experimental studies (investigators assign the determinants themselves, e.g. randomized controlled trial) and observational studies (investigators examine events as nature takes its course). Observational studies without a comparison or control group are called descriptive studies.
- A research protocol is a document that provides all essential details of a study. It should contain information on:
  - research question;
  - study design;
  - selection and recruitment of the subjects;
  - measurements;
  - statistical analysis;
  - sample size calculation.

A 'hierarchy of evidence' has been suggested on the basis of the likelihood that results are accurate and precise. For therapeutic issues, this hierarchy ranges from well-conducted randomized controlled trials at the top – preferably summarized in a systematic review and meta-analysis – to case-reports at the bottom.

ACKNOWLEDGEMENTS

Jan van der Meulen is supported by a National Public Health Career Scientific Award, Department of Health, NHS R&D, UK. David Lowe was supported by a project grant from the Department of Health, UK.

REFERENCES

1. Burton MJ, Towler B, Glasziou P. Tonsillectomy versus non-surgical treatment for chronic/recurrent acute tonsillitis (Cochrane Review). In: The Cochrane Library, Issue 1, Oxford: Update Software, 2003.

2. Glover JA. The incidence of tonsillectomy in school children. *Proceedings of the Royal Society of Medicine.* 1938; **21**: 1219–36.

3. Bakwin H. Pseudodoxia pediatrica. *New England Journal of Medicine.* 1945; **232**: 691–7.

4. Sackett DL, Haynes RB, Guyatt GH, Tugwell P. *Clinical epidemiology: a basic science for clinical medicine.* Boston: Little Brown, 1985.

* 5. Rothman KJ, Greenland S. *Modern epidemiology.* Philadelphia: Lippincott Williams & Wilkins, 1998. *Comprehensive and up-to-date textbook that can be used as a reference source for epidemiological principles and concepts.*

6. MacMahon B, Pugh TF. *Epidemiology: principles and methods.* Boston: Little Brown, 1970.

7. Hennekens CH, Buring JE. *Epidemiology in medicine.* Philadelphia: Lippincott Williams and Wilkins, 1987.

8. Miettinen OS. *Theoretical epidemiology: principles of occurrence research in medicine.* John Wiley and Sons, 1985.

9. Loomis D, Wing S. Is molecular epidemiology a germ theory for the end of the twentieth century. *International Journal of Epidemiology.* 1990; **19**: 1–3.

* 10. Fletcher RH, Fletcher S, Wagner EH. *Clinical epidemiology: the essentials.* Philadelphia: Lippincott Williams & Wilkins, 1996. *Accessible and well-written book focussing on methods and techniques for clinical epidemiology.*

11. Guyatt G, Haynes B, Jaeschke R, Cook D, Greenhalgh T, Meade M *et al.* Introduction: the philosophy of evidence-based medicine. In: Guyatt G, Rennie D (eds). *Users' guides to the medical literature: essentials of evidence-based clinical practice.* Chicago: AMA Press, 2002.

12. Manolidis S, Takashima M, Kirby M, Scarlett M. Thyroid surgery: a comparison of outcomes between experts and surgeons in training. *Otolaryngology and Head and Neck Surgery.* 2001; **125**: 30–3.

13. Mason J, Freemantle N, Browning G. Impact of effective health care bulletin on treatment of persistent glue ear in children: time series analysis. *British Medical Journal.* 2001; **323**: 1096–7.

14. Butler CC, Van der Linden MK, MacMillan H, Van der Wouden JC. Screening children in the first four years of life to undergo early treatment for otitis media with effusion (Cochrane Review). In: The Cochrane Library, Issue 3, Oxford: Update Software 2003.

* 15. Hulley SB, Cummings SR, Browner WS, Grady D, Hearst N, Newman TB. *Designing clinical research.* Philadelphia: Lippincott Williams & Wilkins, 2001. *A readable book designed to help beginning investigators to get started in the world of clinical research. The authors have tried to keep it simple and have used numerous examples to explain the options for the design and implementation of clinical epidemiological studies.*

16. Grimes DA, Schulz KF. An overview of clinical research: the lay of the land. *Lancet.* 2002; **359**: 57–61.

17. Piccirillo JF, Merritt Jr. MG, Richards ML. Psychometric and clinimetric validity of the 20-Item Sino-Nasal Outcome Test (SNOT-20). *Otolaryngology and Head and Neck Surgery.* 2002; **126**: 41–7.

18. Johns MW. A new method for measuring daytime sleepineess: the Epworth Sleepiness Scale. *Sleep.* 1991; **14**: 540–5.

19. http://www.asahq.org/clinical/physicalstatus.htm, accessed September 2003.

20. Maw R, Wilks J, Harvey I, Peters TJ, Golding J. Early surgery compared with watchful waiting for glue ear and effect on language development in preschool children: a randomised trial. *Lancet.* 1999; **353**: 960–3.

21. Eckel HE, Staar S, Volling P, Sittel C, Damm M, Jungehuelsing M. Surgical treatment for hypopharynx carcinoma: feasibility, mortality, and results. *Otolaryngology and Head and Neck Surgery.* 2001; **124**: 561–9.

22. Hanif J, Frosh A, Marnane C, Ghufoor K, Rivron R, Sandhu G. Lesson of the week: 'High' ear piercing and the rising incidence of perichondritis of the pinna. *British Medical Journal.* 2001; **322**: 906–7.

23. Strachan DP. Impedance tympanometry and the home environment in seven-year-old children. *Journal of Laryngology and Otology.* 1990; **104**: 4–8.

24. Knottnerus JA (ed.). *The evidence base of clinical diagnosis.* London: BMJ Books, 2002.

25. McCulloch P, Taylor I, Sasako M, Lovett B, Griffin D. Randomised trials in surgery: problems and possible solutions. *British Medical Journal.* 2002; **324**: 1448–51.

26. Black N. Why we need observational studies to evaluate the effectiveness of health care. *British Medical Journal.* 1996; **312**: 1215–8.

50

Outcomes research

IAIN RC SWAN

Introduction	633	How to choose patient-based outcome measure	641
What are patient-based outcome measures?	634	Which generic instrument?	642
Why use patient-based outcome measures in research?	634	Key points	642
Assessment of patient-based outcome measures	634	Deficiencies in current knowledge and areas for future	
Types of patient-based outcome measure	637	research	642
Generic instruments	637	References	642
Specific instruments	640		

SEARCH STRATEGY

The aim of this chapter is to explain the background to patient-based outcomes research. There is a vast literature on this subject, so there was no formal literature search. The emphasis is on instruments relevant to otolaryngology. The instruments described are simply examples for the reader. The author does not suggest that these are the best instruments in their subject area.

INTRODUCTION

Clinical outcomes research examines the outcomes of treatment or of disease. Traditionally, outcomes of medical care are based on clinical observations or laboratory measurements. While these measures provide useful information for the clinician, they are often of limited interest to patients. There is often poor correlation between clinical outcomes and functional capacity and well-being which are the areas of most interest to the patient. There has been increasing recognition that traditional measures need to be complemented by some measure reflecting the impact of the intervention on the patient in terms of health status and health-related quality of life. These terms refer to experiences of illness such as pain, fatigue, disability and broader aspects of the individual's physical, emotional and social well-being. Medicine, in particular surgery, formerly had the principal objective of reducing mortality and morbidity. These objectives are usually straightforward to assess.

Nowadays, a large proportion of clinical practice is either cancer or chronic disease. There has been little improvement for some time in survival in cancer while treatments often have associated side effects and functional impairment which significantly affect the patient's quality of life. There is an increasing prevalence of chronic diseases with an ageing society and here the aims of treatment are to arrest or reverse decline in function.[1] These factors have led to an increased interest in patient-based outcome measures.

At the same time, increased attention is being given to patients' opinions and wishes in relation to their health. Patients should be involved in decisions about their treatment. To contribute usefully, they need information about the outcomes of treatment, not just in terms of surgical results but in terms of the possible effects on their quality of life. Financial resources limit health care around the world, and increasingly the distribution of these resources is influenced by the benefits perceived by patients, their carers and society as a whole.

WHAT ARE PATIENT-BASED OUTCOME MEASURES?

Patient-based outcome measures are, in general, questionnaires that ask patients about their perception of their health. Usually, these instruments are made up of a number of items or questions. These items are linked in a number of domains or dimensions. A domain refers to an area of behaviour or experience, such as mobility, self-care, depression, pain, social functioning and general well-being. Many questionnaires focus on physical function, such as ability to walk, climb stairs, wash and dress themselves. Others ask about the impact of health on various areas of an individual's life, such as ability to socialize with members of their family and friends. These are aspects of health-related quality of life (HRQoL). Overall quality of life is influenced by many factors other than health, such as social, financial and physical factors. Patient-based outcome measures assess only one aspect of quality of life and are not measures of overall quality of life.

Patient-based outcome measures assess some aspect of the patient's subjective experience of health and the consequences of illness – and of treatment. As these experiences are those of an individual patient with an individual personality and lifestyle, they cannot be objectively verified. This point is sometimes raised as a criticism of patient-based outcome measures, but it should be borne in mind that many clinician-based outcomes are the subjective opinion of the clinician.

WHY USE PATIENT-BASED OUTCOME MEASURES IN RESEARCH?

In the early days of research, few if any studies included an assessment of health-related quality of life. It is increasingly argued now that clinical trials should include patient-based outcome measures except where it is clear that these are not relevant outcomes. The UK Medical Research Council (MRC), the European Organisation for Research and Treatment of Cancer (EORTC) and the National Cancer Institute of Canada (NCIC) all have policies stating that the likely impact on quality of life should be assessed, or justification provided for not doing so.[2] Patient-based outcome measures have been used as the primary outcome measure in randomized controlled trials in many areas including cancer and heart disease. They are also useful in providing evidence of the overall value of a treatment in a way that allows comparison with other treatments in the same area or in other areas.

Patient-based outcome measures are particularly relevant in otolaryngology. Head and neck cancer forms a small proportion of our patients, but a much larger proportion of our clinical workload. The majority of our patients do not have a life-threatening condition and the morbidity is small. Most of our patients simply want us to make them feel better. In many cases we do not have reliable, objective clinical measures to assess the outcome of treatment. To justify our treatment we need patient-based outcome measures to demonstrate the efficacy of treatment – improvement in HRQoL. We also need patient-based outcome measures to demonstrate the effects of these non-life-threatening conditions on HRQoL.

Even when we have objective measures, e.g. closure of a tympanic membrane in myringoplasty, we often know little about the effects on HRQoL. There are also occasions where there is disagreement between clinical measures of success and HRQoL outcomes, e.g. septal surgery for deviated nasal septums. It is likely that the results from one of the measures are unreliable or that they are measuring different things – the validity of both measures should be questioned.

ASSESSMENT OF PATIENT-BASED OUTCOME MEASURES

There are eight criteria that should be applied to patient-based outcome measures: appropriateness, validity, reliability, responsiveness, precision, interpretability, acceptability and feasibility[3] (**Table 50.1**). There are few patient-based outcome measures for which there is sufficient evidence to allow judgement on all of these criteria.

Appropriateness

The first and most fundamental question when selecting a patient-based outcome measure is how to identify one

Table 50.1 Assessment of patient-based outcome measures.

Criterion	Meaning
Appropriateness	Does the content of the instrument match the intended purpose of the trial?
Validity	Does the instrument measure what it claims to measure?
Reliability	Does the instrument produce the same results when repeated in the same population?
Responsiveness	Does the measure detect clinically meaningful changes in the patient condition?
Precision	Can the instrument detect small differences between patient groups?
Interpretability	Can results from the measure be interpreted clinically and are they relevant?
Acceptability	Is the format of the instrument and the questions acceptable to the planned subjects?
Feasibility	Is it feasible to use this instrument in this setting with these subjects?

that is appropriate to the aims of the particular trial. The aims of the trial, the patient group being studied, the type of treatment and the relevant quality of life questions should be carefully considered. The instrument should measure aspects of patients' lives that patients consider important, and should not omit aspects of HRQoL that are important to the patients in the trial.[4] Clinicians often think that they know what aspects of HRQoL are important to patients. Many studies have demonstrated, however, that patients' views often differ from clinicians'. The most effective way of establishing the importance to patients is asking patients their views. A list of aspects of HRQoL can be drawn up by clinicians and patients. A group of patients can then be asked which of these items are problems for them and how important these items are. This is the method commonly used in creating the patient-based outcome measures which are widely used, such as the Medical Outcome Study Short-Form 36-Item Health Survey (SF-36).

The purpose of the trial must be specified precisely in order to select an instrument that fits that purpose. In many studies, the rationale for selection of outcome measures is not clear. Careful consideration of content and relevance of a questionnaire to the purpose of the trial should be given. The instrument selected must be as relevant to the health problem and the proposed intervention as possible.

It is often recommended that one generic and one disease-specific instrument be used in a trial to increase the likelihood of appropriate assessment of outcomes.

Validity

The validity of a measure is an assessment of the extent to which it measures what it claims to measure. Validity is not a fixed property of a measure, but is assessed in relation to a specific purpose and setting.[5] It is, therefore, meaningless to refer to a validated outcome measure, as many reports do. Evidence of validity of an outcome measure in one situation does not mean that there will be adequate validity in another research setting.

This apparently simple property depends on a range of different types of evidence, including how the content was chosen and its relationship to other variables. There are several different ways of assessing validity of a patient-based outcome measure. No single set of observations is likely to determine validity, so assessment of validity in relation to a specific trial is not straightforward.

CRITERION VALIDITY

Criterion validity is the correlation of a measure with an objective or 'gold standard' measure. As gold standard measures rarely exist in assessment of quality of life, criterion validity is rarely relevant in patient-based

outcome measures, and validity is judged by a more indirect assessment of content and construct validity. It can be assessed when a shorter version of an instrument is used to predict the results of a full-length version.

FACE AND CONTENT VALIDITY

Face and content validity are among the most relevant issues for the use of patient-based outcome measures in clinical trials. They address whether items clearly address the intended subject matter and whether the range of aspects is adequately covered. They are explained by Guyatt et al.:[6] 'Face validity examines whether an instrument appears to be measuring what it is intended to measure, and content validity examines the extent to which the domain of interest is comprehensively sampled by the items or questions in the instrument.' In other words, does the questionnaire look right and does it cover the right things? Face and content validity are mainly based on careful examination of the content of the instrument and qualitative judgement rather than statistical criteria. Evidence of how the questionnaire was initially developed is useful. Questionnaires with good validity are constructed in phases with involvement of patients with experience of the particular health problem. The content of poor questionnaires is chosen by 'experts'.

CONSTRUCT VALIDITY

Construct validity is also very relevant but is a quantitative assessment of the relationship of a construct to other variables. A construct is a theoretical idea about the domain to be measured. For example, patients with hearing disability should have poorer audiometric thresholds. Many patient-based outcome measures are multidimensional: they assess, for example, physical, psychological and social aspects of an illness. Those questions related to psychological aspects should correlate with each other much more than with questions assessing physical function. The internal structure of such instruments is established by construct validation, most commonly factor analysis. For a detailed discussion of assessment of construct validity, the reader is referred to Fitzpatrick et al.[3]

Reliability

Reliability is the reproducibility and internal consistency of an instrument. It assesses the extent to which the instrument is free from random error. It is essential to establish that any changes observed in a trial are due to the treatment and not to problems in the measuring instrument. As the random error increases, the size of the sample required to produce an accurate result increases.

REPRODUCIBILITY

Reproducibility is the degree to which an instrument gives the same results on repeated applications with the same subjects, and is also known as the test–retest reliability. An instrument should produce the same, or very similar, results on two or more administrations. This should be relatively straightforward to assess, but care must be taken with the time interval between tests. Repeat measurements should be far enough apart in time for the subject to forget their earlier answers, but not so far apart that their health status might have changed. This is commonly reported as a correlation coefficient. However, a correlation coefficient measures the strength of association between two measures and not the extent of agreement.[7] Bland and Altman[7] recommend plotting the scores from the two tests graphically which is certainly a simpler method than a statistical comparison of repeated scores.

INTERNAL CONSISTENCY

More than one question is usually used to measure one domain in a questionnaire because several related observations will produce a more reliable estimate than one. Individual questions in a domain should correlate highly with each other and with the total score for questions in that domain. This is the internal consistency of a patient-based outcome measure. The correlation is often measured using Cronbach's alpha.[8, 9] If all the questions in a domain are the same, Cronbach's alpha will be 1, while if there is no relationship alpha will be 0. If the correlation is too high, it is likely that the questions are addressing a very narrow aspect of an attribute and some items may be redundant which then reduces the content validity. It is therefore suggested that Cronbach's alpha should be between 0.7 and 0.9.[10]

Responsiveness to change

Responsiveness is the ability of an instrument to detect clinically important change, even if that change is small.[11] This is sometimes called sensitivity to change but the term sensitivity has other, more general uses. It is particularly important in clinical trials when changes might correspond to therapeutic effects of treatment. An instrument can be both reliable and valid but not responsive to change.

There are several statistical methods of assessing responsiveness. The simplest method is to compare change scores for an instrument over time with changes in another variable or variables. The other variable should preferably be an objective indicator, such as a physiological measurement or a clinician-based outcome measure.

An alternative method of assessing responsiveness is calculation of the effect size in a given clinical situation. This is the size of change in a measure between assessments, for example before and after treatment, compared with the variability of scores for that measure on one assessment. The effect size is defined as the mean change in a variable divided by the standard deviation of that variable.[12] [**/*] The effect size can then be expressed in standardized units that allow comparisons with other outcome measures. It has been suggested that effect sizes can be used to assess the size of change in a study arm: an effect size of 0.2 is small, 0.5 is medium and 0.8 or greater is a large change.[12] [**/*]

Other more complex statistical measures of responsiveness are described by Fitzpatrick et al.[3]

One of the main limitations on the responsiveness of an instrument is when the wording of questions does not allow reporting of very good or very poor health states: ceiling and floor effects. Subjects with initial high scores may not show any improvement following effective treatment and those with initial poor scores may not show any deterioration when their clinical situation deteriorates.

As with validity, evidence of responsiveness in one situation does not mean that there will be adequate responsiveness in another research setting.

Precision or sensitivity

The preferred term is precision as sensitivity has a number of other uses in research. Precision is the ability of the instrument to reflect true differences in health states. As clinical trials often aim to detect small differences between patient groups, precision is a desirable capability.

One of the main influences on the precision of an instrument is the format of the answers. The simplest answers are 'yes' or 'no', but they do not allow any assessment of difficulty or severity. The most commonly used graded response is a Likert scale, such as:

1. very satisfied;
2. satisfied;
3. neither satisfied or dissatisfied;
4. dissatisfied;
5. very dissatisfied.

There is some evidence that using seven response categories rather than five increases precision, though this is rarely used.

The main alternative to a Likert scale is a visual analogue scale, where patients can mark any point on a line to represent their answer. Though this would appear to offer more precision, comparison studies of Likert scales and visual analogue scales have found no advantage of visual analogue scales. In addition, it appears that visual analogue scales are less acceptable to many patients who find it difficult to translate their feelings into numbers.

Patients' responses in patient-based outcome measures are generally converted into numerical values for statistical analysis. Most instruments use simple ordinal values, for example one to five (or seven) for a Likert scale, which are capable of less precision. However, the majority of published reports of health status measures use parametric statistical analysis that is appropriate for interval scales,[13] though the interval between one and two (very satisfied and satisfied) may not be the same as between four and five (dissatisfied and very dissatisfied).

Some patient-based outcome measures use an explicitly derived weighting system for responses. The weights can be assigned by a panel of patients and health professionals, for example the Nottingham Health Profile,[14] or be based on preference measurements obtained from a random sample of the general population, such as the Health Utilities Index (HUI).[15, 16] The fact that weighted scoring systems appear to be much more exact with their scoring suggests that they might be more precise, but this may well be deceptive. Several studies have compared weighted and ordinal scoring systems and have not shown any significant difference in precision between these two methods of scoring.

Ceiling and floor effects may influence scores of instruments. Some patient-based outcome measures do not include questions that would identify very poor levels of health, so all patients with poor health have similar scores and further deterioration will not be identified. Sometimes patients with minor health problems will be scored as having excellent health so treatment of their problem will not result in any improvement in score.

One other important factor in precision is bias. This can be reduced by general aspects of study design, such as making assessments blind to intervention. In many cases it is not possible to keep the patient blind to which treatment arm of a trial he is in, so his judgement of outcomes may be influenced.

Patient-based outcome measures may therefore vary in how precisely their scores relate to underlying distributions of patients' health status. Researchers need to carefully consider factors that might influence precision. The degree of precision required of a patient-based outcome measure will depend on other aspects of trial design such as sample size and the expected differences between arms of the trial.

Interpretability

Can results from the measure be interpreted clinically and are they relevant? The interpretability of an instrument is concerned with how meaningful are the baseline scores or a change in scores. Clinically important changes in scores can be estimated by comparison with clinical or laboratory tests in the same patient group. Representative data are available from the general population for some widely used instruments such as the HUI (see under Utility measures) and the SF-36. The scores from the trial patients can be compared with the means and standard deviations for the general population. A significant change in the score in the trial could be set at one and a half standard deviations from the population mean.[10]

Acceptability

Clearly it is essential that the format of the instrument and the questions are acceptable to patients. An instrument should not cause distress to patients or be difficult to understand. In general, shorter instruments are more acceptable to patients. The instructions to patients should make it very clear that their answers will not influence their treatment. Acceptability is also important in order to obtain high response rates to questionnaires to make results of trials easier to interpret, more generalizeable and less prone to bias due to nonresponse. When choosing an instrument, it is useful to know if the instrument has been used in similar settings before.

Ideally, acceptability of an instrument should be directly tested at the design stage by seeking the views of patients. Subsequently, evidence of acceptability can be found in patient response rates.

Feasibility

The feasibility of an instrument is dependent on the time available for its completion and the staff available to help with its completion, either by interviewing patients or explaining the instrument to patients. The data collected have to be entered onto a computer and the time required and ease of entering has to be considered. The measure must be short enough to be completed or administered in the intended setting and with the types of patients and families involved in the trial. This is one of the criteria of patient-based outcome measures that can usually be easily judged by investigators in the research setting. If in doubt, feasibility can be assessed by piloting the study methods.

TYPES OF PATIENT-BASED OUTCOME MEASURE

There are two basic types of patient-based outcome measures: generic and specific. Generic instruments access multidimensional health profiles, overall medical condition and personal function. Specific instruments focus on the problems found in individual diseases, disabilities and patient groups.[11] Within each of these categories there are different types of instruments (**Table 50.2**).

GENERIC INSTRUMENTS

Generic instruments are designed to access a broad range of aspects of health status and the consequences of illness

Table 50.2 Types of patient-based outcome measures.

Category	Type	Example
Generic	Health profile	SF-36, Sickness Impact Profile, Nottingham Health Profile, Glasgow Benefit Inventory
	Utility	Health Utilities Index (HUI), EQ-5D
Specific	Disease specific	Dizziness Handicap Inventory (DHI)
	Site specific	Sino-Nasal Outcome Test (SNOT-20)
	Dimension specific	McGill Pain Questionnaire

Table 50.3 Examples of the use of the SF-36 in otolaryngology.

ORL condition	Reference
Chronic rhinosinusitis	van Agthoven et al.,[20] Gliklich and Metson,[21] Piccirillo et al.[22] [***/**]
Chronic otitis media	Nadol et al.[23] [**]
Dysphonia	MacKenzie et al.[24] [****]
Laryngeal cancer	Stewart et al.[25] [**]
Meniere's disease	Smith and Pyle[26] [**]
Rhinoplasty and otoplasty	Klassen et al.[27] [**]

and therefore to be relevant to a wide range of patient groups and conditions. The advantage of generic instruments is that they can be used for a broad range of health problems and this enables comparisons across different groups of patients with diverse conditions. Because of their broad range of content and general applicability, such instruments have been used to assess the health of samples from the general population. Such data have been used to generate normative values across populations with which other groups of patients with specific health problems can be compared. Since generic instruments are used more often than specific instruments, there are usually more data available regarding their reliability and validity.

As generic questionnaires cover a broad range of aspects of health status, many items may be irrelevant to a particular condition. These items result in a wide range of scores which are not relevant to the condition being studied. As there are few questions relevant to a specific condition, the instrument may be insensitive to changes that might occur as a result of treatment for that condition.

Health profile

SF-36

The most commonly used health profile instrument is the SF-36.[17, 18] [**] The SF-36 is a 36-item, self-completed questionnaire which measures health status in eight dimensions: physical functioning, role limitations due to physical problems, role limitations due to emotional problems, social functioning, mental health, energy and vitality, pain and general perceptions of health. It can be completed by the patient in less than ten minutes. Responses are summed to give a score for each dimension: physical component summary (PCS) and mental component summary (MCS).[19] It has been used in a wide variety of patient groups and conditions, including many otorhinolaryngological conditions (**Table 50.3**). Data from trial subjects can be compared with normative data for the population.[28] Garratt et al.[29] identified 408 papers

which included aspects of development and evaluation of the SF-36 over a ten-year period (1990–1999). It can also be used in a reduced 12-item version which is a subset of the original SF-36.[30] [***] However, the larger instrument gives more reliable estimates of individual levels of health and is therefore the better choice of instrument in small studies.

Recently, Brazier et al.[31] derived from the SF-36 a preference-based single index measure, the SF-6D, to make the instrument more useful in evaluations of cost-effectiveness (see Utility measures below and in **Table 50.3**). This weighted scoring model could potentially be applied to any SF-36 data set. However, initial validation studies demonstrated some inconsistencies and further assessment of the scoring model is required.[32] [**]

SICKNESS IMPACT PROFILE

The Sickness Impact Profile (SIP) is a general health-status questionnaire comprising 136 questions answered as either 'yes' or 'no'.[33] [***] They are grouped into twelve categories: walking, body care and movement, mobility, social interaction, alertness behaviour, emotional behaviour, communication, sleep and rest, eating, home management, recreational activities and work. Each item is weighted, and the scores of all answered questions are combined. There are twelve category scores, two summary scores (physical and psychosocial) and a total score. The scores are standardized and range from 0 to 100 points, with 100 indicating the poorest function. The test–retest reliability and internal consistency are high and it has good content and construct validity.[33] [***] It is, however, a long questionnaire and is usually administered by interview. Its acceptability and feasibility in a trial must be carefully considered.

NOTTINGHAM HEALTH PROFILE

The Nottingham Health Profile is a generic, self-administered questionnaire designed to measure perceived physical, social and emotional health problems.[14, 34] An initial pool of statements was collected from patients at interview and from this pool 38 items were chosen relating to six dimensions: physical mobility, pain, social isolation, emotional reaction, energy and sleep. The scores can be compared with the average scores in a population matched for gender and age.

GLASGOW BENEFIT INVENTORY

As other generic instruments are often insensitive to the nonacute disorders generally seen in an ORL clinic, the Glasgow Benefit Inventory (GBI) was developed for use in patients with otolaryngological conditions.[35] [**] The GBI is a post-intervention questionnaire that assesses the effects of interventions on the health status of patient, rather than the actual health status. The GBI has 18 items in three domains: psychological, social and physical well-being. Rather than attempt to assess the difference between before and after treatment measures, it asks directly about the change in health status resulting from treatment. It is likely, therefore, to be more sensitive to such change than two separate instruments before and after intervention. In addition, compliance will be significantly higher because patients are only required to complete one questionnaire. The response to each question is based on a five-point Likert scale, for example: 'Since your *operation/intervention*, have you found it easier or harder to deal with company?' The words in italics (*operation/intervention*) in each question are replaced by words appropriate to the intervention of interest. Responses are scored using a weighted scale from a population sample to give a score between −100 and +100.

The GBI has been used to assess the benefit experienced by patients following various treatments (**Table 50.4**). Details of the questionnaire and its use can be found at www.ihr.gla.ac.uk.

Utility measures

Multi-attribute utility measures access a broad range of aspects of health status, like other generic instruments, but have a particular form of numerical weighting or valuation of health states. Utility measures have been developed from economics and decision theory in order to provide an estimate of individual patients' overall

Table 50.4 Examples of the use of the GBI.

ORL intervention	Reference
Bone-anchored hearing aids	Dutt et al.[36]
Vestibular schwannoma surgery	Fahy et al. 2002[37] [**]
Speech therapy for dysphonia	Wilson et al.[38] [**]
Rhinoplasty	McKiernan et al.[39] [**]
Tonsillectomy	Bhattacharyya et al.[40] [**]
Surgery for snoring	Banerjee and Dempster[41] [***/**]

preferences for different health states. They are scored as a single number between 1 (full health) and 0 (death). The weighted scoring method is based on preference measurements obtained from samples of a general population. They are asked to value different aspects of health as defined by the instrument using one of a number of valuation techniques, most commonly standard gamble, time trade off and visual analogue scales (see Brazier et al.,[42] for explanation).

Utility scores reflect the health status and value of that health status to the patient. As utility measures are scored as a single value, they do not define individual dimensions of health that contribute to the individual's overall sense of well-being. They are relatively insensitive to small but relevant changes in health and are therefore more suited to studies of large populations.

There are several health utility measures that have been widely used. Brazier et al.[42] carried out an extensive review of these and recommended the HUI and the EuroQol (EQ-5D) as the instruments of choice.

HUI

The HUI-I evolved from studies in neonatal intensive care.[43] [**] A second version (HUI-II) was developed to assess outcomes in long-term survivors of childhood cancer, but is suitable for use in a wider range of children.[15] Though it is claimed to be a generic instrument, its content is explicitly aimed at children with questions specifically aimed at developmental age.

The HUI-II was revised to make it more relevant to an adult population. The HUI-III assesses nine aspects of health status: vision, hearing, speech, ambulation, dexterity, emotion, cognition, self-care and pain.[44] It has 15 questions with four to six available responses for each and is easy for patients to complete. The HUI-III has been used in a wide variety of clinical studies and has been shown to be reliable and responsive.[45] It is one of the few generic patient-based outcome measures which specifically assesses hearing and speech and is therefore potentially useful in many areas of otolaryngology. Normative data have been collected from large populations and, from these data, weighted scoring scales have been devised.[16] It has been used in a cost–utility study of cochlear implants[46] and in the UK cochlear implant study.[47] [***]

EQ-5D

The EQ-5D is a self-completed questionnaire with five dimensions: mobility, self-care, usual activities, pain/discomfort and anxiety/depression.[48] It is easy to complete and is very acceptable to patients. Responses can be scored using a weighted scale from a large general population sample.[49] It is very brief with only five questions with three levels of response for each. Brazier et al.[42] compared the EQ-5D and the SF-36 in a survey of 1980 adults and found the EQ-5D to be less sensitive.

However, it was originally intended to complement other forms of health-related quality of life measures. It has been widely used and its test–retest reliability is good.[50]

SPECIFIC INSTRUMENTS

Disease- or condition-specific

The aim of these instruments is to provide the patient's perception of the problems related to a specific disease or condition. It should be remembered that disease may have a broad impact on the patient's life. To make these instruments comprehensive, a detailed survey of patients suffering from the condition should be conducted when developing the instrument. They may also not detect problems associated with a disease and its treatment that have not been anticipated by the developers if patients have not been involved in the planning. As all of the questions are developed specifically to assess a particular health problem, the content should be very relevant for use in studies of that condition: high validity. They are more likely to detect changes that occur in that particular condition as there should be few if any irrelevant questions: high responsiveness. They are also more acceptable to patients as the relevance of the questions to their condition is obvious so completion rates should be high.

The major disadvantage of disease-specific instruments is that they do not allow comparison to be made with other patient groups with other diseases or conditions. Such comparisons require generic instruments designed for use with any health problem, and for this reason it is often useful to combine a specific instrument with a generic one.

VERTIGO

The Dizziness Handicap Inventory (DHI) is a 25-item questionnaire designed to measure the self-perceived disability and handicap caused by dizziness or imbalance.[51] [**] They reported good internal consistency and test–retest repeatability. The questions were grouped in three domains of functional, emotional and physical aspects of dizziness with three possible answers to each question: yes, sometimes and no. The questions were selected from an initial bank of 37 questions chosen from the case histories of patients. They take a clinical perspective of disability and handicap in daily activities and therefore content validity should be carefully inspected before choosing this instrument for use in a trial. It is preferable to have more input from patients in the selection of items to include in a questionnaire (see Face and content validity above). This instrument has been widely used in studies of imbalance in general.

The Vertigo Handicap Questionnaire (VHQ) was developed from patients' accounts of the problems that they experienced with vertigo.[52] [**] It has 25 questions about restriction of physical and social activities and emotional distress, each scored on a five-point Likert scale. It has good reliability and validity but has not been widely used.

HEARING

There are many instruments that have been developed for use in audiology. Assessing hearing disability has one major difference from assessing most other disabilities in otolaryngology – there is a gold standard – pure-tone audiometry. One of the most widely used measures is the Hearing Handicap Inventory for the Elderly (HHIE).[53] [**] This instrument has been shown to have good face and content validity.[54] [***]

While there are reliable tools for measuring hearing, assessment of the efficacy of hearing aid provision and comparison of benefits from different prescription strategies are heavily reliant on patient-based outcome measures. The HHIE has been used for this purpose,[55] but it has been shown to have poor precision when changes in the HHIE were compared with changes in the Speech Intelligibility Index when using a hearing aid.[56] [**] This is probably because the HHIE predominantly assesses the emotional and psychological response to hearing impairment. The Glasgow Hearing Aid Benefit Profile (GHABP) was developed as a measure of hearing disability and the benefit obtained from the use of a hearing aid.[57] It assesses unaided disability, handicap, benefit from a hearing aid, residual disability and patient satisfaction in eight listening situations – four specified and four chosen by the patient. It has good validity in assessing the outcome of hearing aid fitting, high test–retest repeatability and good patient acceptability. It is now used as one of the primary outcome measures in the National Health Service (NHS) programme of modernizing hearing aid services in England. Details of the questionnaire and its use can be found at www.ihr.gla.ac.uk.

OTITIS MEDIA

The OM6 was developed for use in children with recurrent acute otitis media and otitis media with effusion.[58] [**] Six domains (physical suffering, hearing loss, speech impairment, emotional distress, activity limitation, caregiver concerns) are each addressed by a single question. Test–retest repeatability was high, and responsiveness was demonstrated by a significant change in scores after surgery for ventilation tube insertion.[59] [**] The criterion validity has been questioned, however, in that it does not correlate well with other markers of disease severity, such as audiometry and severity of symptoms of recurrent acute otitis media.[60] Kubba et al.[60] suggested that the instrument lacks precision as it does not differentiate between children with otitis media and others with sore throats.

CANCER

The European Organization for Research and Treatment of Cancer Quality of Life Study Group developed the EORTC QLQ-C30 as an instrument of 30 items for use in international trials in cancer.[61] [***] Further modules have been developed which can be added to the core instrument to provide assessment of specific cancers, for example head and neck cancer.[62] [**] This allows collection of data for comparison across cancer groups and additional data that are particularly relevant to specific cancers.

Site-specific

These instruments contain items that are particularly relevant to patients having treatment for a specific region of the body and should be sensitive to changes experienced by patients following treatment in that region. They are particularly useful in otolaryngology and have the advantage that patient groups are not limited to a specific disease classification. They thus allow comparison of patients with similar symptoms but different pathology. Because they have a narrow focus, they are unlikely to detect any change in broader aspects of health or quality of life following intervention.

SINONASAL DISEASE

Many patient-based outcome measures have been designed for use in sinonasal disease. The 20-item Sino-Nasal Outcome Test (SNOT-20)[63] is a modification of the previously used 31-item Rhinosinusitis Outcome Measure (RSOM-31).[22] [**] The 20 questions refer to specific sinonasal symptoms and some general health questions. It has good internal consistency (Cronbach's alpha 0.9), and showed good responsiveness to change. Face and content validity seemed good and the construct validity was high when compared with clinical assessment of disease. Test–retest scores were highly correlated ($r = 0.9$) though this measures the association between tests rather than repeatability (see Reproducibility above). Piccirillo et al.[63] report the SNOT-20 to be a valid outcome measure in their particular research setting. The questionnaire is easily completed by the patient and acceptability is high. [**]

VOICE

There is no generally accepted objective test to serve as a 'gold standard' for the assessment of voice disorders. Various questionnaires have been developed for evaluation of the consequences of dysphonia. The Voice Handicap Index (VHI) was designed to assess the self-perceived effect on quality of life of voice disorders.[64] It is a 30-item questionnaire divided into three subscales: functional handicap, emotional handicap and physical handicap. The questions use a five-point Likert scale. It has been used to assess the impact of a number of voice disorders, including vocal cord polyps, cord palsy, spasmodic dysphonia and functional disorders. Its construct validity has been confirmed by comparing its subscales with appropriate subscales of the SF-36 in assessment of the health-related quality of life in patients after treatment for laryngeal cancer.[25] [**] Significant improvements in VHI scores occurred after treatment of spasmodic dysphonia with botulinum toxin.[65] [**]

Dimension-specific

These instruments assess one specific aspect of health status. The most commonly assessed dimension is psychological well-being. Another common dimension, more relevant to otolaryngology, is pain. The McGill Pain Questionnaire is one of the most widely used measures of pain severity for both clinical and research purposes.[66] It comprises 20 subclasses of pain descriptors that provide pain severity scores across sensory–discriminative, motivational–affective and cognitive–evaluative dimensions. It has been found to have good short-term repeatability in chronic pain conditions, and it discriminates well between different types of pain syndromes. A short form of the McGill Pain Questionnaire has been developed.[67] [***/**] It is highly correlated with the original longer version and has comparable sensitivity. It may be a useful instrument in situations in which the standard questionnaire takes too long to administer.

The advantage of dimension-specific instruments is that they provide a more detailed assessment in the area of concern than is possible in more general instruments. They are perhaps most useful in a study where they are used in combination with another instrument.[20] [***]

HOW TO CHOOSE PATIENT-BASED OUTCOME MEASURE

The choice of patient-based outcome measure depends on the purpose of the study. To assess the effects on health-related quality of life of a disease or condition, a generic instrument is required. Specific instruments are of little value as they do not allow comparison with other conditions. A specific instrument may provide additional information by assessing the severity of the disease if no objective measure is available, for example in tinnitus. Comparison of the scores from the specific instrument with the generic instrument may be valuable.

If the aim of the study is to assess the efficacy of treatment, it is usually recommended that two instruments be combined, a generic and a specific instrument. The two different measures are likely to produce complementary evidence. A disease-specific measure will be more responsive to the main effects of intervention, and therefore produce the evidence most relevant to the clinician. A generic measure may allow comparisons across interventions and disease groups, but is likely to be relatively insensitive to the effects of the intervention. It is possible, however, that the additional burden on the patient may reduce overall compliance, especially if there is overlap between questions in the two instruments.

WHICH GENERIC INSTRUMENT?

Acceptability to the patient and feasibility of completing the questionnaires are obviously important. The time required to complete the commonly used instruments varies. The HUI Mark II takes three minutes, the SF-36 ten minutes and the SIP 20 minutes.[68] [**]

Appropriateness depends on the study. Utility measures are, in general, only appropriate for studies with large numbers of subjects. Small studies would probably be better to choose a generic health status questionnaire. Some generic instruments have been shown to be better than others in assessing patient with particular problems. Edelman et al.[68] reported that the HUI was better used for evaluating relatively healthy populations because of some floor effects, while the SIP was better for more severely ill populations as their study patients were grouped at the healthy end of the scale. Other authors have similarly reported that the SIP has ceiling effects.[69, 70, 71] [***/**]

A careful evaluation of reports of the use of these instruments in similar patient groups and study settings should be carried out before making a final choice. In the absence of this, the SF-36 appears to be the safest choice. The HUI Mark III is suitable for large studies and has the advantage for otolaryngology research of including items about hearing and speech.

KEY POINTS

- Patient-based outcome measures assess the patient's subjective experience of illness and of treatment.
- Generic instruments access a broad range of aspects of health status and enable comparisons across different groups of patients with diverse conditions.
- Specific instruments are more sensitive to the effects of specific diseases or conditions, but do not allow comparison to be made with other patient groups with other diseases or conditions.
- It is often useful to combine a specific instrument with a generic instrument.

Deficiencies in current knowledge and areas for future research

Development of a valid and acceptable patient-based outcome measure takes a great deal of time and effort. Large numbers of subjects are needed as development requires several stages. Patient involvement in the selection of items is essential. There have been many patient-based outcome measures that have been reported once and never used again. On the other hand, the currently available and widely used patient-based outcome measures are not ideal. We need better ones.

REFERENCES

1. van den Bos GAM, Limburg LCM. Public health and chronic diseases. *European Journal of Public Health.* 1995; **5**: 1–2.

* 2. Fayers PM, Hopwood P, Harvey A, Girling DJ, Machin D, Stephens R. Quality of life assessment in clinical trials–guidelines and a checklist for protocol writers: the U.K. Medical Research Council experience. MRC Cancer Trials Office. *European Journal of Cancer.* 1997; **33**: 20–8. *Good advice from authors with experience of reviewing grant applications submitted to the MRC.*

* 3. Fitzpatrick R, Davey C, Buxton MJ, Jones DR. Evaluating patient-based outcome measures for use in clinical trials. *Health Technology Assessment (Winchester, England).* 1998; **2**: i–iv, 1–74. *Extensive review of the literature to describe the range of patient-based outcome measures available and the criteria for selecting an instrument for use in a trial.*

4. Guyatt GH, Cook DJ. Health status, quality of life, and the individual. *Journal of the American Medical Association.* 1994; **272**: 630–1.

5. Jenkinson C. Evaluating the efficacy of medical treatment: possibilities and limitations. *Social Science and Medicine.* 1995; **41**: 1395–401.

6. Guyatt GH, Feeny DH, Patrick DL. Measuring health-related quality of life. *Annals of Internal Medicine.* 1993; **118**: 622–9.

7. Bland JM, Altman DG. Statistical methods for assessing agreement between two methods of clinical measurement. *Lancet.* 1986; **1**: 307–10.

8. Cronbach LJ. Coefficient alpha and the internal structure of tests. *Psychometrika.* 1951; **16**: 297–334.

9. Bland JM, Altman DG. Cronbach's alpha. *British Medical Journal.* 1997; **314**: 572.

* 10. Streiner DL, Norman GR. *Health Measurement Scales: a practical guide to their development and use.* Oxford: Oxford University Press, 1995. *An invaluable practical guide for those who wish to develop a new patient-based outcome measure. Very good and readable explanation of theory behind these instruments.*

11. Guyatt GH, Veldhuyzen van Zanten SJO, Feeny DH, Patrick DL. Measuring quality of life in clinical trials: a taxonomy and review. *Canadian Medical Association Journal.* 1989; **140**: 1441–8.

12. Kazis LE, Anderson JJ, Meenan RF. Effect sizes for interpreting changes in health status. *Medical Care.* 1989; **27**: S178–89.

13. Coste J, Fermanian J, Venot A. Methodological and statistical problems in the construction of composite measurement scales: a survey of six medical and epidemiological journals. *Statistics in Medicine.* 1995; **14**: 331–45.

14. Hunt SM, McEwen J, McKenna SP. Measuring health status: a new tool for clinicians and epidemiologists. *Journal of the Royal College of General Practitioners.* 1985; **35**: 185–8.

15. Feeny D, Furlong W, Boyle M, Torrance GW. Multi-attribute health status classification systems. *Health Utilities Index. PharmacoEconomics.* 1995; **7**: 490–502.

16. Feeny D, Furlong W, Torrance GW, Goldsmith CH, Zhu Z, DePauw S *et al.* Multiattribute and single-attribute utility functions for the health utilities index mark 3 system. *Medical Care.* 2002; **40**: 113–28.

17. Ware Jr. JE, Sherbourne CD. The MOS 36-item short-form health survey (SF-36). I. Conceptual framework and item selection. *Medical Care.* 1992; **30**: 473–83.

18. McHorney CA, Ware Jr. JE, Raczek AE. The MOS 36-Item Short-Form Health Survey (SF-36): II. Psychometric and clinical tests of validity in measuring physical and mental health constructs. *Medical Care.* 1993; **31**: 247–63.

19. Ware JE. *SF-36 Physical and mental health summary scales: a user's manual.* Boston: Health Assessment Lab. New England Medical Center, 1994.

20. van Agthoven M, Fokkens WJ, van de Merwe JP, Marijke van Bolhuis E, Uyl-de Groot CA, Busschbach JJ. Quality of life of patients with refractory chronic rhinosinusitis: effects of filgrastim treatment. *American Journal of Rhinology.* 2001; **15**: 231–7.

21. Gliklich RE, Metson R. Techniques for outcomes research in chronic sinusitis. *Laryngoscope.* 1995; **105**: 387–90.

22. Piccirillo JF, Edwards D, Haiduk A, Yonan C, Thawley SE. Psychometric and clinimetric validity of the 31-item Rhinosinusitis Outcome Measure (RSOM-31). *American Journal of Rhinology.* 1995; **9**: 297–306.

23. Nadol Jr. JB, Staecker H, Gliklich RE. Outcomes assessment for chronic otitis media: the Chronic Ear Survey. *Laryngoscope.* 2000; **110**: 32–5.

24. MacKenzie K, Millar A, Wilson JA, Sellars C, Deary IJ. Is voice therapy an effective treatment for dysphonia? A randomised controlled trial. *British Medical Journal.* 2001; **323**: 658–61.

25. Stewart MG, Chen AY, Stach CB. Outcomes analysis of voice and quality of life in patients with laryngeal cancer. *Archives of Otolaryngology – Head and Neck Surgery.* 1998; **124**: 143–8.

26. Smith DR, Pyle GM. Outcome-based assessment of endolymphatic sac surgery for Meniere's disease. *Laryngoscope.* 1997; **107**: 1210–6.

27. Klassen A, Jenkinson C, Fitzpatrick R, Goodacre T. Patients' health related quality of life before and after aesthetic surgery. *British Journal of Plastic Surgery.* 1996; **49**: 433–8.

28. Jenkinson C, Coulter A, Wright L. Short form 36 (SF36) health survey questionnaire: normative data for adults of working age. *British Medical Journal.* 1993; **306**: 1437–40.

29. Garratt A, Schmidt L, Mackintosh A, Fitzpatrick R. Quality of life measurement: bibliographic study of patient assessed health outcome measures. *British Medical Journal.* 2002; **324**: 1417.

30. Ware Jr. J, Kosinski M, Keller SD. A 12-Item Short-Form Health Survey: construction of scales and preliminary tests of reliability and validity. *Medical Care.* 1996; **34**: 220–33.

31. Brazier J, Usherwood T, Harper R, Thomas K. Deriving a preference-based single index from the UK SF-36 Health Survey. *Journal of Clinical Epidemiology.* 1998; **51**: 1115–28.

32. Brazier J, Roberts J, Deverill M. The estimation of a preference-based measure of health from the SF-36. *Journal of Health Economics.* 2002; **21**: 271–92.

33. Bergner M, Bobbitt RA, Carter WB, Gilson BS. The Sickness Impact Profile: development and final revision of a health status measure. *Medical Care.* 1981; **19**: 787–805.

34. Hunt SM, McKenna SP, McEwen J, Backett EM, Williams J, Papp E. A quantitative approach to perceived health status: a validation study. *Journal of Epidemiology and Community Health.* 1980; **34**: 281–6.

35. Robinson K, Gatehouse S, Browning GG. Measuring patient benefit from otorhinolaryngological surgery and therapy. *Annals of Otology, Rhinology and Laryngology.* 1996; **105**: 415–22.

36. Dutt SN, McDermott AL, Jelbert A, Reid AP, Proops DW. The Glasgow benefit inventory in the evaluation of patient satisfaction with the bone-anchored hearing aid: quality of life issues. *Journal of Laryngology and Otology – Supplement.* 2002; **28**: 7–14.

37. Fahy C, Nikolopoulos TP, O'Donoghue GM. Acoustic neuroma surgery and tinnitus. *European Archives of Oto-Rhino-Laryngology.* 2002; **259**: 299–301.

38. Wilson JA, Deary IJ, Millar A, Mackenzie K. The quality of life impact of dysphonia. *Clinical Otolaryngology and Allied Sciences.* 2002; **27**: 179–82.

39. McKiernan DC, Banfield G, Kumar R, Hinton AE. Patient benefit from functional and cosmetic rhinoplasty. *Clinical Otolaryngology and Allied Sciences.* 2001; **26**: 50–2.

40. Bhattacharyya N, Kepnes LJ, Shapiro J. Efficacy and quality-of-life impact of adult tonsillectomy. *Archives of Otolaryngology – Head and Neck Surgery.* 2001; **127**: 1347–50.

41. Banerjee A, Dempster JH. Laser palatoplasty: evaluation of patient benefit using the Glasgow benefit inventory. *Journal of Laryngology and Otology.* 2000; **114**: 601–4.

42. Brazier J, Deverill M, Green C, Harper R, Booth A. A review of the use of health status measures in economic evaluation. *Health Technology Assessment (Winchester, England).* 1999; **3**: i–iv, 1–164.

43. Torrance GW, Boyle MH, Horwood SP. Application of multi-attribute utility theory to measure social preferences for health states. *Operations Research*. 1982; **30**: 1043–69.

44. Torrance GW, Furlong W, Feeny D, Boyle M. Multi-attribute preference functions. Health Utilities Index. *Pharmacoeconomics*. 1995; **7**: 503–20.

45. Furlong WJ, Feeny DH, Torrance GW, Barr RD. The Health Utilities Index (HUI) system for assessing health-related quality of life in clinical studies. *Annals of Medicine*. 2001; **33**: 375–84.

46. Palmer CS, Niparko JK, Wyatt JR, Rothman M, de Lissovoy G. A prospective study of the cost-utility of the multi-channel cochlear implant. *Archives of Otolaryngology – Head and Neck Surgery*. 1999; **125**: 1221–8.

47. Barton GR, Summerfield AQ, Marshall DH, Bloor KE. On behalf of the POCIA Collaboration. *Choice of instrument for measuring the gain in utility from cochlear implantation*. Oxford: Health Economics Study Group, 2001.

48. EuroQol Group. EuroQol – a new facility for the measurement of health-related quality of life. *The EuroQol Group. Health Policy*. 1990; **16**: 199–208.

49. MVH Group. *The measurement and valuation of health: final report on the modelling of valuation tariffs*. York: Centre for Health Economics, University of York, 1995.

50. Brooks R. EuroQol: the current state of play. *Health Policy*. 1996; **37**: 53–72.

51. Jacobson GP, Newman CW. The development of the Dizziness Handicap Inventory. *Archives of Otolaryngology – Head and Neck Surgery*. 1990; **116**: 424–7.

52. Yardley L, Putman J. Quantitative analysis of factors contributing to handicap and distress in vertiginous patients: a questionnaire study. *Clinical Otolaryngology and Allied Sciences*. 1992; **17**: 231–6.

53. Ventry IM, Weinstein BE. The hearing handicap inventory for the elderly: a new tool. *Ear and Hearing*. 1982; **3**: 128–34.

54. Weinstein BE, Spitzer JB, Ventry IM. Test-retest reliability of the Hearing Handicap Inventory for the Elderly. *Ear and Hearing*. 1986; **7**: 295–9.

55. Newman CW, Weinstein BE. The Hearing Handicap Inventory for the Elderly as a measure of hearing aid benefit. *Ear and Hearing*. 1988; **9**: 81–5.

56. Gatehouse S. Outcome measures for the evaluation of adult hearing aid fittings and services. Scientific and Technical Report to the Department of Health. MRC Institute of Hearing Research, Glasgow, 1997.

57. Gatehouse S. Glasgow Hearing Aid Benefit Profile: derivation and validation of a client-centred outcome measure for hearing aid services. *Journal of American Academy of Audiology*. 1999; **10**: 80–103.

58. Rosenfeld RM, Goldsmith AJ, Tetlus L, Balzano A. Quality of life for children with otitis media. *Archives of Otolaryngology – Head and Neck Surgery*. 1997; **123**: 1049–54.

59. Rosenfeld RM, Bhaya MH, Bower CM, Brookhouser PE, Casselbrant ML, Chan KH et al. Impact of tympanostomy tubes on child quality of life. *Archives of Otolaryngology – Head and Neck Surgery*. 2000; **126**: 585–92.

60. Kubba H, Swan IRC, Gatehouse S. How appropriate is the OM6 as a discriminative instrument in children with otitis media? *Archives of Otolaryngology – Head and Neck Surgery*. 2004; **130**: 705–9.

61. Aaronson NK, Ahmedzai S, Bergman B, Bullinger M, Cull A, Duez NJ et al. The European Organization for Research and Treatment of Cancer QLQ-C30: a quality-of-life instrument for use in international clinical trials in oncology. *Journal of the National Cancer Institute*. 1993; **85**: 365–76.

62. Bjordal K, Ahlner-Elmqvist M, Tollesson E, Jensen AB, Razavi D, Maher EJ et al. Development of a European Organization for Research and Treatment of Cancer (EORTC) questionnaire module to be used in quality of life assessments in head and neck cancer patients. EORTC Quality of Life Study Group. *Acta Oncologica*. 1994; **33**: 879–85.

63. Piccirillo JF, Merritt Jr. MG, Richards ML. Psychometric and clinimetric validity of the 20-Item Sino-Nasal Outcome Test (SNOT-20). *Otolaryngology – Head and Neck Surgery*. 2002; **126**: 41–7.

64. Jacobson BH, Johnson A, Grywalski C, Silbergleit A, Jacobson G, Benninger MS. The Voice Handicap Index (VHI): development and validation. *American Journal of Speech and Language Pathology*. 1997; **6**: 66–70.

65. Rosen CA, Murry T, Zinn A, Zullo T, Sonbolian M. Voice handicap index change following treatment of voice disorders. *Journal of Voice*. 2000; **14**: 619–23.

66. Melzack R. The McGill Pain Questionnaire: major properties and scoring methods. *Pain*. 1975; **1**: 277–99.

67. Melzack R. The short-form McGill Pain Questionnaire. *Pain*. 1987; **30**: 191–7.

68. Edelman D, Williams GR, Rothman M, Samsa GP. A comparison of three health status measures in primary care outpatients. *Journal of General Internal Medicine*. 1999; **14**: 759–62.

69. Andresen EM, Rothenberg BM, Panzer R, Katz P, McDermott MP. Selecting a generic measure of health-related quality of life for use among older adults. A comparison of candidate instruments. *Evaluation and the Health Professions*. 1998; **21**: 244–64.

* 70. Coons SJ, Rao S, Keininger DL, Hays RD. A comparative review of generic quality-of-life instruments. *Pharmacoeconomics*. 2000; **17**: 13–35. *Good reviews of the three most widely used generic instruments: the SF-36, the Nottingham Health Profile and the Sickness Impact Profile.*

* 71. De Korte J, Mombers FM, Sprangers MA, Bos JD. The suitability of quality-of-life questionnaires for psoriasis research: a systematic literature review. *Archives of Dermatology*. 2002; **138**: 1221–7. *Good reviews of the three most widely used generic instruments: the SF-36, the Nottingham Health Profile and the Sickness Impact Profile.*

51

Evidence-based medicine

MARTIN J BURTON

Introduction	645		Conclusion	648
Definition of EBM	645		Key points	648
The application of EBM	647		References	648

INTRODUCTION

Doctors want to give their patients the best treatment they can, i.e. the treatment that is most likely to help the individual patient in front of them. The idea behind evidence-based medicine (EBM) is that healthcare practitioners should only use (prescribe, recommend, implement) therapies that have been proven to be effective, and should not use unproven therapies that may be ineffective at best or, at worst, actually harmful. By 'harmful' we do not necessarily mean 'fatal' or even imply that the harm is serious. Any outcome which disadvantages the patient – their health, lifestyle, even their wallet or purse – might be considered as a harm, or, if not strictly a harm, a factor to be balanced against any benefit which is accrued as a result of the treatment.

The reader may ask – 'so what's new?' Surely the approach described has been at the heart of medical treatment for centuries. It has been suggested that rather than thinking of the pre-EBM era as being unscientific, we should refer to the present as a time in which we make 'better use of evidence in medicine'. The paternalistic and authoritarian approach that characterized much of medical practice in the past should be replaced by one which acknowledges uncertainty more explicitly, and which operates within a defined framework and with a set of rules for the weighing of scientific evidence.

In 1995, Davidoff et al.[1] listed five linked ideas in which EBM is rooted.

1. Clinical decisions should be based on the best available scientific evidence;
2. The clinical problem – rather than habits or protocols – should determine the type of evidence to be sought;
3. Identifying the best evidence means using epidemiological and biostatistical ways of thinking;
4. Conclusions derived from identifying and critically appraising evidence are useful only if put into action in managing patients or making healthcare decisions;
5. Performance should be constantly evaluated.

DEFINITION OF EBM

The most familiar definition of EBM was coined by Sackett and his colleagues in 1996: 'Evidence-based medicine is the conscientious, explicit and judicious use of current best evidence in making decisions about the care of individual patients'.[2] This concise statement contains many, but not all, the important features of EBM. Before unpacking this description on EBM, it is worth recalling that 'EBM... can be seen as a tool, and tools can be used for good and for ill'.[3] It is important that the user knows how to use the tool correctly and does not use it unwisely or inappropriately.

Conscientious

The conscientious otolaryngologist wants to 'do the right thing' for his patient – to do more good than harm. He should also want to do this in the right way. In other words, to 'do things right' – do them better, more efficiently, etc. Muir Gray refers to this practice as 'doing the right things right'.[4] The term 'conscientious' also brings to mind a certain carefulness and attention to detail. These characteristics are clearly a requisite for high quality surgery and many practitioners hone and practice their surgical skills in order to improve them. The same diligence with which they do this, the same desire to master their craft, should be directed to acquiring the skills of critical appraisal and data synthesis necessary to practise EBM successfully.

Explicit

Openness and transparency are features of the modern health service in the UK. They are also key elements of rigorous science – prerequisites for allowing experimental work to be evaluated and replicated. One of the principles underlying evidence-based practice is that the methods used are clearly stated and, whenever possible, are stated *a priori*. This explicitness allows others to evaluate and criticize the methods used and, when appropriate, to make the necessary changes to allow the quality of the work to be improved.

Evidence-based practice explicitly evaluates the strength of the evidence underlying a particular intervention or recommendation. By critically appraising a study, specific questions can be answered about the validity of the evidence it contains. How good is it? Can we really believe the results? How certain (or, more usually, uncertain) are we about the results?

This notion of explicitness extends to consideration of issues of uncertainty. In the past, otolaryngologists, like many other physicians, may have found being open and explicit about the uncertainty which surrounds much medical practice, difficult. They have found sharing this with their patients even more so. As new concepts of doctor–patient partnerships (in distinction to doctor–patient relationships) have developed, this approach has become untenable. In the modern health service 'doctors have the difficult task of explaining the nature of uncertainty and risk in the practice of today's scientific medicine'.[5]

Judicious

The use of the term 'judicious' reminds us that clinical practice must be rooted in considered opinions and sensible decisions. In other words, the evidence has been evaluated and 'weighed', benefits being considered and balanced against harms. Common sense has not been ignored. It is a truism to say 'evidence is necessary but not sufficient'. It needs to be integrated with patient's preferences (of which more below), economic constraints, organizational factors relating to the delivering healthcare organization and ethical obligations. All this is also to be considered in the context of social responsibility and resource allocation prioritization.

Current best evidence

It may once have been possible for the conscientious otolaryngologist to keep their knowledge comprehensive and up-to-date by reading a few journals every month and going to occasional conferences. In the twenty-first century it is impossible. There are now in excess of two million articles per year published in the biomedical press. The internet has resulted in an explosion of knowledge sources which must be acknowledged, even if the quality of their contents is at times uncertain. Whereas once this knowledge was available only to the select few, now it is available to everyone – doctor, patient, carer and healthcare provider.

Whilst this 'sea change in the availability of knowledge offers a tremendous opportunity for the health professions to engage the public in taking an interest in and responsibility for their own health ... for some medical practitioners, and indeed for some members of other health professions, this democracy in information access can pose troubling questions. How does one negotiate differences in the interpretation of medical evidence between doctor and patients? How does one signal which evidence is reliable and which is not? How does one offer advice in the face of lack of evidence?'[5]

The practitioner of EBM needs to be able to locate the evidence relating to the clinical question or questions posed by the patient in front of him, and then assess its quality to determine if it is the 'best' – and most appropriate – available. In Chapter 52, Critical appraisal skills, Martin Dawes discusses the concept of levels of evidence; suffice it to say at this stage that practitioners need to be aware that just because something is written in a distinguished journal, it does not mean that this represents absolute scientific truth. In the same way that EBM challenges '**eminence** based medicine' (the concept that age, authority and seniority *per se* bring with them an inevitable certainty of valid clinical truth), it also challenges a presumption that published studies are always well designed, well conducted and well reported.

Concepts of publishing have changed in recent years, but paper-based journals and textbooks continue to be produced, and the best ones can form a starting point for the clinician's enquiries. However, it is likely that greater use will be made of electronic resources and in particular electronic databases such as MEDLINE and EMBASE.

Assistance in identifying and searching appropriate databases is often available from hospital librarians and information specialists. There are a number of electronic resources which house material that has already been assembled, appraised and included because of its methodological quality and can provide a 'short cut' to 'best evidence'. These include the Cochrane Central Register of Controlled Trials (CENTRAL), part of *The Cochrane Library*, the ENT and Audiology Library of the National Library for Health and Clinical Evidence, published by the BMJ publishing group (**Table 51.1**).

Table 51.1 Evidence-based resources.

Resource	Web address
General	
Centre for Evidence-Based Medicine, Oxford	www.cebm.net/
The Cochrane Collaboration	www.cochrane.org
PubMed (MEDLINE provided by the US National Library of Medicine)	www.ncbi.nlm.nih.gov/ entrez
Clinical Evidence (BMJ Group publication)	www.clinicalevidence.com
Evidence-Based On-Call	www.eboncall.org/
Otolaryngology	
ENT and Audiology Library of National Library for Health	www.library.nhs.uk/ent
Cochrane ENT Disorders Group	www.cochrane-ent.org

Making decisions about the care of individual patients

The original definition of EBM focuses on individual patients, yet EBM is often criticized because the evidence that its practitioners use is derived from groups or populations. The opponents of EBM constantly emphasize their interest in the individual in front of them. The questions they should be asking are these: is my patient so different from those patients who have been evaluated in well-conducted scientific studies that the valid results demonstrating that the treatment is likely to be effective do not apply to them? Or, when studies do show a treatment to be effective, can I be certain that my patient is so different that I would reasonably expect them to respond positively, and without any harms of that treatment outweighing the benefits?

Sackett's definition might be criticized for the use of the phrase 'making decisions'. This suggests that the doctor is making the decision on behalf of the patient. It might be considered more appropriate for the patient to make the decision with the help and assistance of the doctor. Equally, the definition says nothing of the integration of the management options with the patient's values and beliefs. These must always play an important part in the decision-making process. The following modified definition of EBM is proposed:

> Evidence-based medicine is the conscientious, explicit and judicious use of current best evidence in helping individual patients to make healthcare decisions that respect their personal values and beliefs.

THE APPLICATION OF EBM

Since its original description and definition, the role of EBM has been extended from the individual patient to groups and populations of patients. It has become an integral part of modern healthcare practice. However, it is not without its critics and a number of particular issues merit consideration.

EBM has its limitations and these must be recognized. Unfortunately, over-zealous and enthusiastic promotion and practice, which ignores the underlying methodologies or loses focus on individual patients, can lead it into disrepute. It has been said that EBM provides 'a natural environment' for the randomized controlled trial (RCT). The attentive reader will note that this is the first mention of RCTs. Whilst it is true that these help provide the highest 'level' of evidence, they are certainly not a *sine qua non* for the practice of EBM. Indeed, it has been argued that the focus on RCTs may provide a 'selective imbalance' in the nature of the evidence available. For example, it is far more likely that there will be RCT evidence available about pharmacological interventions, compared with complex behavioural interventions, physical therapy, surgery, etc. This reflects the fact that a large amount of 'effort' (including commercial funding and support) is likely to have been put into generating this evidence and the outcomes are often more easily quantifiable.[6] As a result, pharmacological treatments for a condition may appear to be 'evidence-based' because high quality evidence does exist, whereas nonpharmacological treatments (which may in fact be as, or more, effective) are seen as being nonevidence based, simply because they have not been evaluated by RCTs. The greater availability of evidence for certain types of intervention reflects biases in the research agenda. This is produced by several factors but includes the lack of a mechanism whereby the agenda can be set by the health needs of communities.

EBM has been criticized for focusing too much on 'mainstream' medicine. It is undoubtedly true that there is more, and generally better quality, evidence available about traditional medical interventions. However, one advantage of the arrival of EBM has been that those who promote 'complementary' medicine understand the nature of the rules by which the effectiveness of these therapies will be judged. As a result, there are increasing numbers of systematic reviews and RCTs of interventions in the field of complementary medicine.

In addition to embracing the involvement of complementary practitioners, EBM-oriented organizations, such as the Cochrane Collaboration, have tried to widen and encourage participation by consumers. This involvement, in parallel with the explicit involvement of patients in making their own healthcare choices, has helped engage and empower patients in a way that should increase both their confidence in, and compliance with,[5] treatment. Conversely, this has been seen as a threat to the professional autonomy of doctors and a challenge to their therapeutic freedom. Unsurprisingly, the challenge to the 'paternalistic and authoritarian nature of much medical practice' has been resisted in some quarters. Interestingly, a recent Royal College of Physicians Working Party which examined issues of medical professionalism,[5] suggested the abandonment of the word autonomy from the definition of a professional, not least because the word can be open to misinterpretation. Too often the word suggests 'an appeal to personal authority – that is, the right to pursue a practice that is entirely self-generated'. Whereas 'the doctor should tailor his or her care to the expressed needs of the patient in the light of reliable scientific evidence'.

CONCLUSION

The EBM era is characterized by the better use of evidence in medical practice. Finding that evidence, appraising it and integrating it into the advice given to individual patients is a key part of modern medical practice. Otolaryngologists should apply themselves to the study of EBM methodologies with the same perseverance and diligence as they give to the acquisition of their surgical skills.

KEY POINTS

- Evidence-based medicine is a key component of modern medical practice.
- Evidence is necessary but not sufficient.
- All otolaryngologists should acquire the fundamental skills of searching, appraising and synthesizing required to practice EBM and should do so with the same diligence they apply to learning surgical skills.

REFERENCES

1. Davidoff F, Haybes B, Sackett D, Smith R. Evidence based medicine. *British Medical Journal*. 1995; **310**: 1085–6.
2. Sackett DL, Rosenberg WMC, Gray JAM, Haynes RB, Richardson WS. Evidence-based medicine: what it is and what it isn't. *British Medical Journal*. 1996; **312**: 71–2.
3. Hope T. Evidence based medicine and ethics. *Journal of Medical Ethics*. 1995; **21**: 259–60.
4. Gray JAM. *Evidence-based healthcare*. London: Churchill Livingstone, 1997.
5. Royal College of Physicians. Doctors in Society. *Medical professionalism in a changing world*. London: Royal College of Physicians. Retrieved 18 March 2007, from www.rcplondon.ac.uk/pubs/books/docinsoc/docinsoc.pdf 2005.
6. ter Meulen R, Biller-Andorno N, Lenk C, Lie RK. *Evidence-based practice in medicine and healthcare*. Berlin: Springer, 2005.

52

Critical appraisal skills

MARTIN DAWES

Why do we need critical appraisal?	649	Appraising therapy articles	658
Tips for practising evidence-based health care	650	Appraising systematic reviews	661
Basics of critical appraisal	651	Key points	665
Forming answerable questions	652	Appendix	665
Appraising diagnosis articles	654	References	668

WHY DO WE NEED CRITICAL APPRAISAL?

Evidence-based practice (EBP) begins and ends with patients. We can harm patients by giving inaccurate information about prognosis, make assumptions about diagnostic test results that are false, give therapy that is ineffective or harmful, or fail to give effective therapy. The only way to prevent this happening is to ensure that we have the most up to date knowledge available so that we can share that information with patients.

There were 27 randomized control trials published last year just about otitis media. There is no possibility that by reading a couple of journals per week and attending postgraduate seminars that doctors will be able to keep up to date with everything that is important that may affect their patients. EBP starts with the clinician accepting that there is uncertainty about what we do and that sometimes (when that uncertainty occurs frequently or when it is important) we should search for the latest knowledge. Pragmatically, what we do at present is ask colleagues. The flaw with this is the inability to assess the quality of the evidence that is presented to you by your colleague. Does this matter? If the question is important or frequent then yes, it does matter.

Research evidence can be approached from two angles. The first is the clinician who wants to undertake research and the second is the clinician who wants an answer to a clinical question. The latter wants to know what to believe. Is it the randomized trial, or the case series or case–control trial? What papers should they look for to answer their question?

Levels of evidence have been proposed to help clinicians identify trials most likely to yield the 'truth'

and associated with these are grades of recommendation (see the tables in the Appendix to this chapter). For questions about the efficacy of a therapy, these state that a systematic review of homogenous trials is likely to be the most believable evidence.

The process of EBP therefore requires that one searches for the best evidence. For therapeutic decisions, this is usually going to be a systematic review where the authors have searched for and combined, where appropriate, the data from the randomized control trials on that topic. It has the advantage of doing the hard work for you as well as this combination of data in the form of a meta-analysis. Systematic reviews are important as they include the data from all the trials up to that date. It is this that is important and is the hard work. A normal search for papers to be included in the review will often produce a list of more than a thousand papers, and all the titles and abstracts must be read to select relevant articles. The full text of these relevant articles must then be obtained (in itself a time-consuming and expensive task) and read to ensure they meet the selection criteria. The data then have to be independently abstracted from the selected articles. Undertaking a valid, well carried out systematic review is no easy task, but is essential for clinicians to determine the latest evidence.

Once a trial or trials have been found that seems to answer your question, one has to check three things. Is the study valid? What are the results? Can these be applied to my patients?

The need to check for validity seems, on the surface, to be bizarre. Surely this is what journals should be doing. That assumption is correct but in reality the job of a journal is primarily to make a profit. Therefore one will find articles with flawed trials in even the most highly cited journals.[1]

Journals started as the diaries of researchers. These were then passed around colleagues so that the information could be shared. The development of trials and the assessment of bias are subsequent to that descriptive era. What we are now faced with are seemingly complex long papers with obscure statistical analyses. The scenario is no different to a medical student facing their first anatomy class. By reading around the subject and by practice, one is able to quickly identify key anatomical structures. The same is true of reading scientific articles. One can learn certain aspects of trial design very quickly to be able to assess whether an appropriate design was used for a certain research question. The journal *Evidence Based Medicine* critically appraises the literature from over 100 journals. However, it only includes a few that are likely to change the way you think about a problem or change the way you practise. Sadly for the other articles, we must appraise them ourselves.

The need to assess the methodology of individual trials is extremely important. In large systematic reviews of the same clinical outcome with the same therapy, researchers have compared the results of those trials that were randomized and those that were not randomized. There are some large differences in certain studies that are more than one would expect by chance. One cannot always say that randomized trials show less effect than nonrandomized trials.[2]

However, it is not enough to accept that a trial is believable at face value. There is now overwhelming evidence that trial methodology has a major influence on the results of therapeutic trials.[2, 3] Concealment of randomization, masking and randomization itself are three main components of randomized trial design. The numbers of patients involved in the study and their follow up are the other key features.

If there is not concealment of randomization, this may exaggerate the efficacy of the treatment by as much as 30 percent more than trials where there is adequate concealment. Surprisingly, perhaps of lesser importance is blinding (masking) – the doctor looking after the patient, or the patient themselves, knowing whether they are giving (being given) the experimental or placebo treatment. If there is no blinding, the results may exaggerate the effectiveness of the treatment by 15 percent. If less than 80 percent of patients are followed up, one cannot tell what is happening and the results become meaningless.

To assess a study there are checklists (see the **Figures** in the Appendix to this chapter), some of which have now been incorporated into computer programmes such as that found at the Centre for Evidence-Based Medicine website (www.cebm.net) that enable health professionals to appraise the quality of the evidence for themselves.

Systematic reviews therefore need to assess the individual validity of the trials that are included. If they do not assess whether there was concealed randomization,

for example, then you, the reader, may be given incorrect information. Assessing the quality of a randomized controlled trial may be carried out using a Jadad score or other systems.[4] Despite the Quorom statement[5] setting out how systematic reviews should be presented, their quality may be poor.[6]

For systematic reviews, effective transparent searches and defined inclusion and exclusion criteria are important. The homogeneity (similarity) of the studies is also critical in determining whether a meta-analysis of the data is appropriate. The meta-analysis (combination of the results of the individual trials) is usually only appropriate when there is clinical and methodological homogeneity (that is, the methods and clinical outcomes and starting points are similar). In addition, the results must be put into context of present formats of care.

The need to understand how trials may come to the 'wrong' conclusion is as important as understating the treatment itself. Clearly, all this may be daunting to a busy clinician so there are sensible short cuts. Always start by looking at evidence that has already been appraised such as that in *Evidence Based Medicine* and *Clinical Evidence*. The essential part of effective clinical practice is to continue to ask questions.

We need to make sure that what we do is based on the soundest evidence possible. If the only evidence is experiential and anecdotal then that is perfectly satisfactory. However, if there is a systematic review of randomized control trials that all point to an alternative treatment being more effective then that should only be ignored at your patients' peril.

TIPS FOR PRACTISING EVIDENCE–BASED HEALTH CARE

Tip 1: Ask questions

Try making one question per patient. Select one question because:

- There is likely to be an answer.
- The question has arisen more than once or is important;
  - use a sticky label or write down the patient's name;
  - record briefly the problem for example 'chronic obstructive pulmonary disease';
  - write down the question, for example 'are steroids an effective treatment (mortality and morbidity)?';
  - put them in your pocket and look at them at the end of the week.

Tip 2: Searching

- Search one question regularly: every two weeks, every month or every quarter!

- Conduct your search in a logical order:
  – clinical evidence;
  – journal EBM;
  – Cochrane;
  – Medline.

Often you will find too few articles, or that the articles you do find are not in your library or will take a long time to obtain. Sometimes you will find too many articles and a systematic review is needed. Unless you have time and the question is desperately important, pass and move on to the next question – let someone else answer this one!

Appraise only the article(s) that answers your question, have the highest level of evidence and are readily available.

Tip 3: Appraisal

- Look for letters about the article in subsequent issues of the journal.
- Appraise with others until confident.
- Appraise using worksheets or using software, for example CATmaker.
- Mark (highlight) on the printed article where you found the important data.
- Get someone else to check it for you.

Tip 4: Share your knowledge

- Try sharing uncertainty with your colleagues.
- Discuss your questions with colleagues (maybe they have already answered them).
- Find fault with the article(s) rather than your colleagues.

BASICS OF CRITICAL APPRAISAL

Read the abstract

Assuming you have three or four articles to appraise, how should you start? First read the abstract. Read it briefly trying to gain an overview firstly of the methods used and secondly the results. For example, a parent brings in a child referred by their GP for recurrent epistaxis but is worried about surgery (describing cautery in dramatic terms) and wonders whether a cream used by a friend's child might help (Naseptin). You make a note of this and later formulate the question 'In children with recurrent epistaxis, is Naseptin effective, compared with placebo, at reducing attacks of epistaxis?' and find this paper.[7] The abstract is available on line. It takes a minute or two to read through the abstract:

> Epistaxis is common in children. Trials show antiseptic cream is as effective as cautery, but it is not known whether either is better than no treatment. We wished to know the efficacy of cream in children with recurrent epistaxis. The design was a single-blind, prospective, randomized controlled trial set in the otolaryngology clinic in a children's hospital.
>
> The participants were 103 children referred by their general practitioner for recurrent epistaxis. Excluded were those with suspected tumours, bleeding disorders or allergies to constituents of the cream. Referral letters were randomized to treatment and no treatment groups.
>
> Treatment was antiseptic cream to the nose twice daily for four weeks, which was prescribed by the general practitioner before clinic attendance. All children were given an appointment for eight weeks after randomization.
>
> The main outcome measures were the proportion of children in each group with no epistaxis in the four weeks preceding clinic review. Complete data were available for 88 (85 percent) of the children. Of the treatment group, 26/47 (55 percent) had no epistaxis in the four weeks before the clinic appointment. Of the controls, 12/41 (29 percent) had no epistaxis over the four weeks. This is a relative risk reduction of 47 percent for persistent bleeding (95 percent CI 9–69 percent) and an absolute risk reduction of 26 percent (95 percent CI 12–40 percent), giving a number needed to treat of 3.8 (95 percent CI 2.5–8.5).
>
> We conclude that antiseptic cream is an effective treatment for recurrent epistaxis in children.

The format of any abstract should be similar to this. If there is a complex description of the trial that is confusing, ask yourself why? Is it because the authors are hiding an overall negative result or is it really a necessary peculiar design?

So, in this study there were 103 patients with epistaxis in a single blind randomized controlled trial with various outcomes described and a promising result overall.

Does the paper answer the question you are asking?

This is a qualitative judgement that you must make on reading the abstract. If it is the highest level of evidence (systematic review) and it deals specifically with your question then you are home and dry (apart from having to critically appraise the review!). Often though this is not the case, in which case you must look for individual randomized controlled trials that address the specific outcomes relevant to your patient.

Find answers to the validity questions using a checklist for the relevant study

It is very much easier to read an article when you know what you are looking for. The same occurs when an experienced doctor finds it easier to filter the enormous number of questions and signs they can ask or examine for, and homes in on specific areas they think are relevant. This ability to put the patient's symptoms quickly into context is the key to skilful practice. In exactly the same way, learning what to look for in a research article is key. When teaching medical students, we give exactly the same list of questions that are shown below. This gives them focus and they will work through an article in ten minutes answering all the validity questions.

The first place to check for validity questions about the methods employed is, not surprisingly, in the methods section of the paper. However, you will frequently find certain elements of the methodology may be mentioned in the introduction, results or even the discussion. So if you cannot find out, for example, the rate of follow up in the methods, then scan the rest of the text for the answer.

What sort of research design is the trial?

You may have to resort to checking the methods section of the paper to obtain this. This was a randomized control trial with single blinding.

Assess the level of bias

At this stage one has all the methodology neatly summarized. For example, in this paper there were some problems with follow up. They had data available on 88 of the 103 patients randomized, but 15 of these were assessed by telephone. This introduces an element of bias that may reduce the validity. If this was less than 80 percent then really the trial is so severely compromised that one cannot make any interpretation of the result. If there is not concealed randomization (see under Concealed randomization) then the results *may* overestimate the effectiveness by 30 percent. So, assessing bias is the art of appraisal. In the end you have to decide whether the effect of the treatment demonstrated is likely, taking into consideration the level of bias, to translate into benefit in your patient.

Translate the results into something clinically meaningful

If the article talks about risk reduction, how does that translate into my patient? A frequent term used now is numbers needed to treat. This puts the effect into the context of the patient and lets them decide whether the benefit is worth the trouble or potential side effect.

How can I implement this?

Does this help my practice either by reinforcing what I know and making me more confident or does it change my practice. If it is the latter, how am I going to go about implementing that change?

The numbers

The most frequent fear expressed is that of the statistics. How can I tell whether these were the correct statistics to be used? I tackle this obliquely. First, ask yourself what is likely to be a beneficial outcome for your patients. Is a reduction in mortality of 1 percent enough for this invasive procedure, or should it be 5 percent? This is by far the most important feature of the results. If the trial was designed to establish a benefit that you regard as clinically insignificant then you can stop reading!

Let us assume you settle for a 5 percent reduction in mortality, for example. The results of the trial say that this was achieved. The statistical test is there to show you that this difference was very unlikely to have occurred by chance in two ways. First, that the difference observed in this trial was unlikely to have happened by chance (p value) and, second, if this trial were repeated 100 times, 95 percent of the trials would have shown a similar result (confidence interval). How they determine the p value (i.e. with a Student t test or a chi-square is beyond the scope of this article but a quick tip is to check the letters written in response to the article because if the article is in a major journal, statisticians will be quick to point out the incorrect use of statistics). In our experience, there is much less use of incorrect statistical tests than there is of poor trial methodology.

To summarize, check that the difference is clinically significant and did not occur by chance.

Summary

Critical appraisal is a logical way of assessing the likely truth of a piece of research, evaluating the results in terms of individual patient care, and then assessing the whole and determining whether it is useful for your practice. It combines some knowledge of trial design, a small amount of basic arithmetic and some qualitative judgements.

FORMING ANSWERABLE QUESTIONS

The reason we do not usually ask questions is they are so difficult to answer. This was clearly illustrated in the *Hitchhiker's Guide to the Galaxy* when the super computer gave the answer '42' to the Ultimate Question of Life, the Universe, and Everything.[8] The people asking the question were horrified and angry. The computer calmly suggested that, instead of panicking, they should go back and consider the question and that he would of course help them do this. Clearly, this is an extreme example of where the question has been so badly formed that the answer is meaningless.

I see a patient with diabetes. Their control had been haphazard and they had had repeated HbA1C's performed over the last year. Their control seems better now but the HBA1c test is expensive to perform. I wonder how effective is blood glucose at monitoring diabetes. I do a search for 'blood glucose' and 'diabetes mellitus' and turn up 25,000 articles.

I went wrong in two places. You may have spotted that my search was unstructured; the search terms were so vague that I was unable to generate a manageable list of relevant items. However, this arose partly because of the unfocused nature of my question. I want to know how 'effective' the test is. What do I mean by that? If it is negative does that rule out poor control – or if it is positive (high) does that mean they have poor control. In my case it is the former that really is of interest.

We could have gone to a textbook and read thoroughly about diabetes, but we do not have the time, and textbooks are often many years out of date. There are many questions that arise from any consultation and being human we can only deal with those that are most important. In this case it may have been 'diabetic control'. However if I was a medical student and wanted just to know more about diabetes, then a textbook is an excellent place to start. For understanding more about therapy in general, a resource such as *Clinical Evidence*[9] is extremely valuable (*Clinical Evidence* cites all the evidence from which therapeautic recommendations are made). This form of enquiry is termed a 'background question' or one that helps the person understand the problem in general. This in contrast to what is being discussed here, which are termed 'foreground questions' or decision-making questions. As a student, one asks mainly background questions but as one's experience with a condition increases and the clinical need for decision-making increases, the proportion of background questions fall as the foreground questions rise (**Figure 52.1**).

My question now is: 'In diabetics, is fasting blood glucose (compared with HBA1c) effective at excluding poor diabetic control?[10] (a fasting blood glucose <7.8 rules out poor glycaemic control).

The query is becoming better but the first part is still vague. Perhaps I should enter something about non-insulin dependent diabetics. By structuring a question the answer may be found more efficiently.[11] It is therefore important to try to break the question down into several parts:

- patient and problem;
- intervention (or diagnostic test);
- comparison intervention (optional);
- outcomes (PICO).

Patient and problem

The first part is to identify the problem or the patient. Some health care problems are not always about patients! For example, an administrator may want to know whether having acute medical beds in a temporary holding ward next to the accident and emergency department is any better than having conventional acute medical wards in the hospital. Make sure at this stage in the question you are describing the problem or patients that you see. However, if one is too specific at this stage you may miss some important evidence and there is a balance to be struck between obtaining evidence about exactly your group of patients and obtaining all the evidence about all groups of patients.

Intervention

The intervention is equally important. It may in fact be a postponement of an action, such as an operation. In patients with abdominal pain lasting less than 12 hours, does an additional 24-hour delay before referral to hospital alter outcome? Most interventions are more straightforward, such as types of dressings, drug therapies or counselling. Alternatively, they can be about the provision of differing environmental factors, such as the décor of waiting rooms or dealing with the way in which information is given to patients, i.e. positively or negatively.[12]

The intervention can be a diagnostic test. However, specify whether you are trying to detect or exclude a disease.

Comparison intervention

Sometimes, there is a comparison of the intervention. For example, one might seek papers comparing the use of an active compound compared with either a placebo or

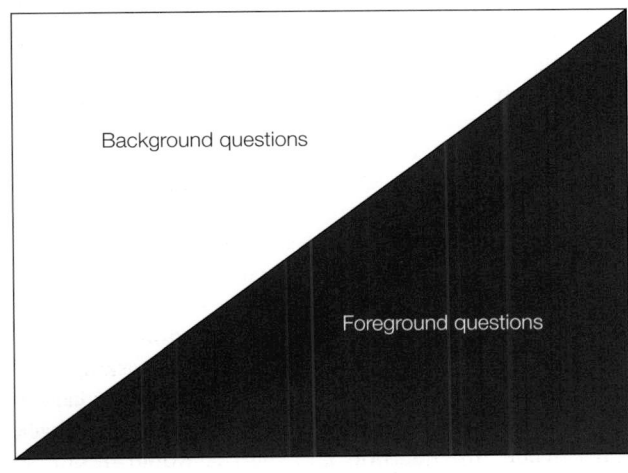

Figure 52.1 Foreground and background questions.

another active drug. Considering whether you are looking for comparative studies will help when searching for that evidence. You may be comparing one diagnostic test against another.

Outcomes

Outcome measures are particularly important when considering the question. It is worth spending some time working out exactly what it is you want. In serious diseases it is often easy to concentrate on the mortality and miss the important aspects of morbidity. For example, the use of toxic chemotherapies for cancer may affect both aspects. This is also the time when it is important to know what outcome is relevant to the patient. In Menière's, deafness and tinnitus may occur but the patient may only really be interested in controlling one problem as a priority. The search should primarily focus on that outcome.

Type of question

Once we have created a question, it is helpful to think about what type of question you are asking, as this will affect where you look for the answer and what type of research you can expect to provide the answer. For example, although randomized controlled trials (RCTs) are a very valid type of study, it would be unethical to perform an RCT on harm (would you volunteer for the exposure arm of such a study?). Questions about harm should look for different types of research, such as case–control studies or cohort studies.

APPRAISING DIAGNOSIS ARTICLES

Diagnoses are usually made through interpreting and combining information from a combination of the clinical history, examination findings and the results of investigations, such as blood tests and x-rays. An important component of evidence-based health care is working out how useful these different pieces of information are in making a diagnosis. For example, if you test a patient's urine and find protein in it, how likely is it that this represents kidney disease? A test result needs to be interpreted in the light of how accurate you think the test is, and what you already know about the patient.

In making a diagnosis you are consciously (or subconsciously) weighing up probabilities. Each question you ask or each observation changes those probabilities. For example, if a patient limps in then there is a probability of arthritis being the cause of the limp. If the patient is 70 years of age, the probability is higher than if the patient is 30. The age of the patient is a diagnostic test, either increasing or decreasing the probability. It is

essential that when contemplating a test that the person requesting the test has some idea of the probability of the diagnosis. They will also need to decide whether the test is helping them exclude or include the diagnosis. Finally, they need to know what is the likely probability of the diagnosis after a positive or a negative result.

What is meant by test accuracy? Accuracy is a description of how well the test diagnoses and excludes the disease when the result is positive or negative (see under What are the results).

Sensitivity reflects the ability of a test to identify people who have disease and specificity reflects the ability of the test to identify 'normality', or people who do not have disease. So this means that tests with very high sensitivities and specificities can be extremely useful at either excluding or including a diagnosis. In primary care some of our time is spent seeing the worried well. These are patients who present with symptoms caused by a mild or self-limiting disease but are naturally worried that it may be something more serious. In these cases we want to use tests that mainly exclude disease. In hospital we are seeing people who are ill and we quickly want to make a diagnosis (including disease).

To see an example of how high sensitivity and specificity values of a test can be used in clinical practice, let us consider how general practitioners deal with patients with a sore throat. We see many sore throats in general practice and it would be useful to know whether a new 'rapid test' could be useful in helping diagnose bacterial sore throats.[13] I selected this particular paper for illustrative purposes rather than it being the 'best' level of evidence.

This paper was about better diagnosis of throat infections in general practice. Four features of patients were determined:

1. fever $\geq 38°C$;
2. lack of cough;
3. tonsillar exudates;
4. anterior cervical lymphadenopathy.

Five hundred and fifty-eight patients older than 11 years presenting with sore throat were swabbed and examined for these features. They all also had a rapid streptococcal antigen detection test for detecting group-A B-haemolytic streptococcus (GABHS).

The next step was to go through the paper checking for validity.

Is the study valid?

- *Did the authors answer the question?* The question is often found at the end of the introduction section of the paper. Some authors leave you guessing as to what the original question might have been. If the paper does not have a clear question, it cannot give any clear answer, so you can save yourself time by moving on to the next paper. You should also consider whether the research question is relevant to your clinical question.

- *What were the characteristics of the groups?* This would contain some description about the numbers of patients, their race and gender, age and any other features that are pertinent to the study.
- *Is it clear how the test was carried out?* To be able to apply the results of the study to your own clinical practice, you need to be confident that the test is performed in the same way in your setting, as it was in the study. What was the test undertaken? How was it done and by whom? Was it a multi-level test (i.e. a serum level) with different thresholds?
- *Is the test result reproducible?* This is essentially asking whether you obtain the same result if different people carry out the test, or if the test is carried out at different times on the same person.
- *Was the reference standard (gold standard) appropriate?* To start with, we need to find out how the study found out how the 'truth' really was about patients. That is to say, how did the investigators know whether or not someone really had a disease? To do this, they will have needed some reference standard test (or series of tests) which they know 'always' tells the truth.
- *Were the reference standard and the diagnostic test interpreted blind and independently of each other?* If the study investigators know the result of the reference standard test, this might influence their interpretation of the diagnostic test and *vice versa.*
- *Was the reference standard applied to all patients?* Ideally, both the test being evaluated and the reference standard should be carried out on all patients in the study. There may be a temptation, for example, if the test under investigation proves positive, not to bother administering the reference standard test. In many cases, the reference standard test may be invasive and may expose the patient to some risk and/or discomfort. While it would usually be ethical to use such a test on a patient in whom one had grounds to suspect that it might be positive, it would not be ethical if one thought that the test would be negative (i.e. if the diagnostic test being evaluated had been negative). Therefore, when reading the paper, you need to find out whether the reference standard was applied to all patients, and if it was not look at what steps the investigators took to find out what the 'truth' was in patients who did not have the reference test.
- *Was the test evaluated on an appropriate spectrum of patients?* Another complication is that a test may perform differently depending upon the sort of patients on whom it is carried out. For example, the more severe is a disease, the easier it tends to be to detect. Thus, you might find that testing for bacterial sore throats might be 'better' at detecting infection when evaluated in patients who attend an ENT clinic, than in those attending family practice. These may be because people with chronic disease who attend an ENT clinic will be more symptomatic and have more bacteria in general, making it easier to detect. This problem is referred to as spectrum bias. A test is going to perform better in terms of detecting people with disease if it is used to identify it in people in whom the disease is more severe, or advanced. Similarly, the test will produce more false–positive results if it is carried out on patients with other diseases that might mimic the disease that is being tested for.

The issue to consider when appraising a paper is whether the test was evaluated on the typical sort of patients in whom the test would be carried out in real life.

The optimal study method for the assessment of a diagnostic test is a cohort study evaluating the test in a group of patients thought to be at risk of having the disease. A less valid alternative method that has been used is a case–control study. The latter method studies patients known to have the disease and control patients without the disease. The performance of the test in the two groups is compared. This sort of study has been shown to overestimate the effectiveness of the diagnostic tests.[14]

What are the results?

In an ideal world, a positive test would mean that someone has disease, and a negative test would mean they do not have disease. Unfortunately, this is rarely the case. When a test is carried out, there are four possible outcomes:

1. The test can correctly detect disease that is present (a true positive result).
2. The test can detect disease when it is really absent (a false–positive result).
3. The test can correctly identify that someone does not have the disease (a true negative result).
4. The test can identify someone as being free of a disease when it is really present (a false–negative result).

These possible outcomes are illustrated in **Table 52.1**.

Given that a test may potentially mislead us if we obtain a false–positive or a false–negative result, we need to have some way of characterizing how accurate the test really is (**Table 52.2**). What does this mean? The high specificity means that there were very few people (16) out of the 375 people who did not have GABHS. So that means (using some reverse logic) that if the rapid test was positive (going across the row), by inference they almost certainly have the disease.

We can simplify this to say that in tests with high **specificities**, where the result is **positive**, it rules the diagnosis **in**. The mnemonic for this is **SpPIn**.

Table 52.1 Possible outcomes of a diagnostic test.

Test result	'Truth'		
	Disease present	Disease absent	Totals
Positive	a	b	a + b
	True positive	False positive	
Negative	c	d	c + d
	False negative	True negative	
Totals	a + c	b + d	a + b + c + d

Sensitivity = a/(a + c) Positive predictive value = a/(a + b).
Specificity = d/(b + d) Negative predictive value = d/(c + d).
Prevalence = (a + c)/(a + b + c + d).
Accuracy = a + d/a + b + c + d.

Table 52.2 Results of rapid test screening for group-A B-haemolytic streptococcus (GABHS) in patients with sore throat.

	'Truth'		
	GABHS+ve	GABHS − ve	Totals
Positive	119	16	135
Negative	64	359	423
Totals	211	375	558

Sensitivity = 119/211 = 65%.
Specificity = 359/375 = 96%.
Positive predictive value = 119/135 = 88%.
Negative predictive value = 359/423 = 85%.
Prevalence = 211/558 = 33%.
Accuracy = 478/558 = 85%.

In tests with high **sensitivities** and the test is **negative** then it rules **out** the disease. So the mnemonic for this is **SnNOut**. Clearly it is not 100 percent accurate at excluding (that would only happen if the sensitivity was 100 percent). How you take that finding and put it into practice depends on the severity of the disease as well as the other symptoms and signs that indicate the pretest probability of the disease.

In reality, patients who are well where you are trying to exclude disease need tests with high sensitivities (primary care). Patients who are ill need tests with high specificities to determine the cause of the illness. This is an oversimplification of the process of diagnosis but is helpful in terms of remembering what tests do.

Often, of course, we are faced with tests whose sensitivity and specificity are not so high that we can use the test to rule in or rule out a disorder. For such cases, we need a measure of a particular test result's ability to predict the presence or absence of disease.

We might think that this is provided by the positive and negative predictive values (for positive and negative results, respectively). However, in practice we find that these values can change depending on the prevalence of the target disorder amongst the test population: if the

Table 52.3 Potential results of rapid test screening for GABHS in patients with sore throat in an imaginary low prevalence setting.

	'Truth'		
	GABHS+ve	GABHS − ve	Totals
Positive	12	16	28
Negative	6	359	365
Totals	18	375	393

Sensitivity = 67%.
Specificity = 96%.
Positive predictive value = 43%.
Negative predictive value = 98%.
Prevalence = 4.5%.

disorder is more common, the positive predictive value will be higher and the negative predictive value lower.

For example, if the results are as follows with a much lower prevalence (**Table 52.3**). The sensitivity remains similar and the specificity is the same but the positive predictive value drops considerably. Now the test only has a 50:50 chance of detecting someone with disease. You can see how the prevalence will sometimes significantly alter the effectiveness of a test. It is important to always consider the setting before recommending tests that perform well in an alternative health care setting.

However, since sensitivity and specificity are not affected by disease prevalence, we can combine them to create a combined measure of the efficacy of a particular test result. This can be thought of as, for a given test result, the likelihood that a patient with the disorder would yield that test results compared to the likelihood that a patient without the disorder would yield that same test result. This is the likelihood ratio (LR). As a rule of thumb, for positive test results, an LR of ten or above shows that the test result is good at ruling in disease; for negative test results, an LR of 0.1 or less shows that the test result is good at ruling out disease.

Two additional benefits of the LR are that they can be used to generate specific post-test probabilities for your patient and that, where we have multiple independent tests, the LRs can be multiplied together to yield a much more powerful test.

The prevalence of GABHS was 33 percent. If the test is positive it is very likely they have GABHS, but what about if it is negative?

What I can do though is work out the likelihood ratios:

Likelihood ratio (+ve result)
$$= \frac{\text{Sensitivity}}{(100\% - \text{specificity})} = \frac{0.65}{(1 - 0.96)} = 16.25$$

Likelihood ratio (−ve result)
$$= \frac{(100\% - \text{sensitivity})}{\text{specificity}} = \frac{(1 - 0.65)}{0.96} = 0.36$$

Figure 52.2 shows the nomogram for likelihood ratios. To use the nomogram I have drawn a line from the pretest probability of 33 percent through 16 (on the likelihood ratio line) to obtain a post-test probability of approximately 90 percent if the result is positive and through 0.36 (roughly) to obtain a post-test probability of approximately 12 percent if the result is negative.

But what if our patient has a lower pretest probability? For example, this might be a patient with only a 20 percent pretest probability. Using a ruler, see what their post-test probability would be. The nomogram lets you quickly see the implications of a positive or negative result in terms of post-test probability.

Will the results help my patient?

ARE THE RESULTS RELEVANT TO YOUR PATIENT?

So far, we have considered how to interpret results of tests for your patients. However, it may be that you feel that the results of studies carried out to assess the accuracy of the test are not generalizeable (or relevant) to your setting, or you may consider that it would not be helpful to your patient to perform the test.

GENERALIZABILITY TO YOUR SETTING

One aspect to consider is whether the assessment(s) that have been carried out of test validity are applicable to your setting. We have already seen how predictive value is dependent upon prevalence, so the predictive value of a test in one setting is usually not the same in another setting. Sensitivity and specificity (and likelihood ratios) are not dependent on prevalence, but they can vary according to the type of patients on which the test is carried out. The sensitivity of a test will depend upon the severity of disease in the population being tested. The more advanced or severe the disease, the more likely the test is to identify it.

The specificity of a test will depend upon the prevalence of other diseases in the population that might lead to false–positive results. The more that other diseases are present, the more likely a false–positive result.

A second aspect to consider is whether the test is carried out the same way in your setting as it was in the study. Some diagnostic tests depend upon the skill of the person carrying out the test, and the skill of the people interpreting the test result. Tests may be carried out in different ways, and it is important to know that it is carried out the same way in your local hospital or laboratory as it was in the study which evaluated the test.

WILL IT HELP YOUR PATIENT?

One way to think about whether or not to perform the test is whether it will influence the management of the

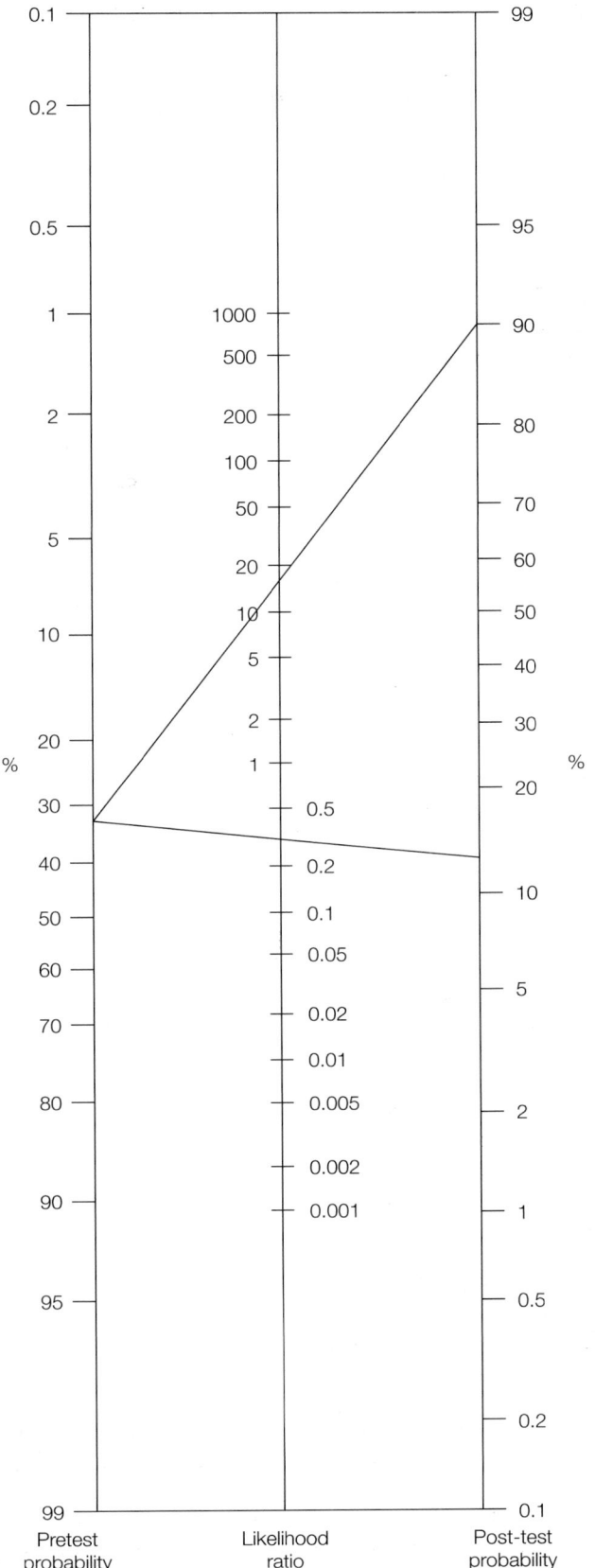

Figure 52.2 Nomogram for likelihood ratios.

patient or groups of patients you are likely to see. If you think that a disease is unlikely in a particular patient, it may be that if you carried out the test and it was positive, you would still think that the disease was unlikely, so it would not influence your management. Conversely, if you think that a disease is likely in a given patient, it may be that a negative test result would not stop you treating the patient, since you would still think that the disease is likely whatever the test result. Putting this in terms of pre- and post-test probabilities, in the first instance the pretest probability of disease is so low, that even with a positive test result, the post-test probability will be less than 50 percent. In the second instance, the pretest probability of disease is so high that even with a negative test result, the post-test probability will be more than 50 percent.

In practice, knowledge about the accuracy of diagnostic tests will perhaps be most useful when planning protocols or guidelines to manage particular groups of patients.

Summary

An evidence-based approach to deciding whether a test is effective for your patient involves the following steps:

- frame the clinical question;
- search for evidence concerning the accuracy of the test;
- assess the methods used to determine the accuracy of the test;
- find out the likelihood ratios for the test;
- estimate the pretest probability of disease in your patient;
- apply the likelihood ratios to this pretest probability using the nomogram to determine what the post-test probability would be for different possible test results;
- decide whether or not to perform the test on the basis of your assessment of whether it will influence the care of the patient, and the patient's attitude to different possible outcomes.

APPRAISING THERAPY ARTICLES

When we are required to answer a question about therapy, the identification of information from an article is not straightforward. The layout is frequently different depending on the journal you are reading. One is often relying on the editorial board of the journal, as well as the people who reviewed the article, to have ensured the quality of the article. There may be confusing statistics that make interpretation of the data seem difficult. These problems seem to be very daunting when one is trying to identify information that may affect the care of a patient. These following questions will help you identify the real validity of the therapy article.

- *Is the study valid?* Did the authors answer the question? For this example I shall be using the Kubba paper[7] on Naseptin and epistaxis. The abstract of this article is shown under Read the abstract. Kubba *et al.*[7] have answered their question about the effectiveness of Naseptin in epistaxis. They state clearly how they did this and what they used to determine 'effective'.
- *What were the characteristics of the groups?* This would contain some description about the numbers of patients, their race and gender, age and any other features that are pertinent to the study. This is usually found in Table 1 in most papers but in this case is described in the protocol part of the subjects and methods section.
- *Are the comparison groups similar?* To determine whether bias has occurred in the selection procedure, certain potentially relevant characteristics of the two populations should be displayed in tabular form. Usually these include age, sex, duration of illness and other demographic and functional characteristics. This is covered in the first paragraph of the results section of this paper. There were more boys than girls, but the age and duration of history were the same in both groups. Is it likely that girls and boys would differ in response? The aim is not to find if there are statistical differences between the two groups but to find whether thare are clinically significant differences. You as a clinician reader should judge whether you think the differences are clinically significant.
- *What was the treatment?* In this case it was either Naseptin or nothing. They describe clearly the reasons for not using a placebo.

Equal treatment

The groups in the trial were treated equally throughout apart from the experimental intervention. It should be clear from the article that, for example, there were no co-interventions that were applied to one group but not the other, or more frequent or detailed assessments on one group compared to the other.

Placebo control

Patients do better if they think they are receiving a treatment than if they do not, even if the treatment is an inactive substance: the placebo effect is a widely accepted potential bias in trials. A placebo is an inactive treatment that is given so that the patient does not know whether he or she has been given the active treatment; the control group in a trial will often receive a placebo treatment so that this effect is equal in both groups. Patients in both groups of the trial should not know whether or not they are receiving the active therapy. However there is a twist in the tail – one can have a placebo-controlled trial where the patients are having active treatments in both arms of the study in addition to the new treatment or the placebo. So the term 'placebo-controlled trial' does not exclude the use of active treatments (as long as both groups get the same).

Follow up

There are three major aspects to assessing the follow up of trials:

1. Did so many patients drop out of the trial that its results are in doubt?
2. Was the study long enough to allow outcomes to become manifest?
3. Were patients analysed in the groups to which they were originally assigned (intention-to-treat)?

Drop-out rates

A good clinical trial requires the complete follow up of patients in both the control and experimental groups. If less than 80 percent of patients are adequately followed up then the results may be invalid. In this study they had problems and had to phone subjects as they did not attend the outpatient clinic. They talk about this weakness of the study in the discussion. Does it invalidate the study?

Length of study

The length of the study is critical in determining the clinical significance of the results. For a disease of short duration, such as an acute infectious disease, the period of the study need only be long enough to cover the course of that infection. Where the disease is more progressive and lengthy then the duration of the study needs to reflect that. The question that the research is trying to answer will also be helpful in deciding the appropriate length of the study.

Intention-to-treat

Because anything that happens after randomization can affect the chances that a patient in a trial has an event, it is important that all patients are analysed in the groups to which they were randomized. This is an essential prerequisite for valid evidence about therapy. For example, it has been repeatedly shown that patients who do and do not take their study medicine have very different outcomes, even when the study medicine they have been prescribed is a placebo. The correct form of analysis, in which patients are analysed in the groups to which they were assigned, is called 'intention-to-treat' analysis.

Were the groups randomized?

The major reason for randomization is to prevent bias. The largest potential cause of bias in research about effectiveness of an intervention, is if the patients allocated to the treatment group are different from those allocated to the control group in a way that might influence outcome. To reduce this bias as much as possible, the decision as to which treatment a patient receives should be determined by random allocation. Why is this important?

There could be any number of confounding variables that affect a given situation, some of which we know about, but also others that our knowledge of human physiology has not yet uncovered. Randomization is important because it spreads all confounding variables evenly amongst the study groups, even the ones we do not know about.

CONCEALED RANDOMIZATION

As a supplementary point, clinicians who are recruiting patients into a trial may consciously or unconsciously distort the balance between groups if they know the treatments that will be given to patients. For this reason, it is preferable that the randomization list be concealed from the clinicians. The amount of impact the lack of concealment may have is larger than if the trial was not blinded. If there is inadequate concealment, the size of the effect may be overemphasized by as much as 30 percent.

BLINDING

It is also important that, if possible, both clinician and patient be 'blind' to whether or not they are receiving treatment. Lack of blinding may lead to exaggeration of the effectiveness of the therapy by as much as 20 percent.[3]

Outcome measures

To determine the impact of an intervention on patient health, one needs to define clearly the outcome that needs to be measured. This sounds straightforward enough but can take up a larger amount of the preparation time of the research. An outcome measure is any feature that is recorded to determine the progression of the disease or problem being studied. In this paper a comprehensive questionnaire was used to determine outcomes.

What are the results?

- How large is the treatment effect?
- How precise is the estimate of the treatment effect?

In any clinical therapeutic study there are three explanations for the observed effect:

1. the effect of the treatment.
2. chance variation between the two groups.
3. bias.

Good research will explicitly endeavour to reduce the effects of chance and bias by using special designs, as we have seen.

NUMBERS NEEDED TO TREAT

The most common approach is to describe the effect of a drug in terms of the risk reduction. The risk is usually of continuing to have, for example, pain or an event. When evaluating a paper on a therapeutic manoeuvre, it is possible to establish its clinical effectiveness by determining the proportion of patients receiving treatment who gain benefit.

From the paper the following results are drawn:

This simple statement obscures the fact that identifying the correct table in the paper and then obtaining the correct figures from it is often not as easy as it sounds. This is one of the parts of appraisal that it is often useful to share with others to ensure you have the correct data.

From **Table 52.4** it can be seen that 47 patients were assigned to the active treatment (or experimental) group and 41 to the watchful waiting (or control) group. There were a total of 50 children with epistaxis; 21 occurred in the experimental group and 29 in the control group.

EVENT RATES

It is important to set some standard methods of describing this data. In therapy, we start by converting the numbers of patients into event rates. In the control group, 29 out of 41 patients had epistaxis. This may be presented as an event rate of $(29/41) = 0.71$. So the control

Table 52.4 Results of a trial of Naseptin against watchful waiting in stopping epistaxis in children.

	Epistaxis	No epistaxis for four weeks	Total
Active treatment (Naseptin)	21	26	47
Watchful waiting	29	12	41
Total	50	38	88

event rate (CER) is 0.71 (this number is also the risk of epistaxis in the control group, and corresponds to a percentage risk of 71 percent).

In the experimental treatment group there were 21 children with epistaxis out of 47 children. The experimental event rate (EER) was therefore 0.44 (44 percent). Now that we have these numbers we can start working with them.

RELATIVE RISK

One way of combining the event rates is to use relative risk (RR). Here, we make a ratio of the two risks to show which group has a higher or lower risk. The relative risk is calculated by dividing the risk of having epistaxis in the treatment group by the risk of the control group $= 0.44/0.71 = 0.62$. This means that the risk of epistaxis continuing with Naseptin was 0.62 (or 62 percent) of the risk without Naspetin.

Relative risk reduction

It is also possible to show the extent of the benefit compared to the original risk by calculating the relative risk reduction (RRR). This is similar to relative risk, except that we take the difference in risk between the two groups and divide that by the control group's risk:

$$RRR = \frac{CER - EER}{CER} = \frac{0.71 - 0.44}{0.71} = 0.38$$

RRRs are often presented as percentages.

The RRR means that the treatment reduced the risk of continued nosebleeds by 38 percent relative to that occurring in this control population (the RRR given by the authors is for persistent bleeding whereas I have calculated for cessation of bleeding). This is a large risk reduction in a population that are all bleeding. But what if it was an RRR for primary stroke reduction where the events are far fewer? So the RRR has to be judged against the prevalence of the outcome we want to prevent.

Absolute risk reduction

The absolute risk is that 71 percent of individuals in the placebo group had nose bleeds and that 44 percent of the treatment group had nosebleeds. The difference (absolute risk reduction (ARR)) between these gives us another view of the effectiveness of the treatment. The ARR of this therapy is 0.27 (CER–EER = $0.71 - 0.44$).

ARR = CER − EER

Consider 100 people given this treatment. We would expect 27 less children to have epistaxis if this group were given Naseptin than if they were not. We can convert this into how many people we would need to treat to prevent one child continuing to have epistaxis. This number is the reciprocal of the ARR. In this example $1/0.27 = 3.7$. Therefore, to prevent a child continuing to have epistaxis we need to treat four people. This is the number needed to treat (NNT). It is more useful than relative measures because, as well as measuring the benefit of a therapy, it also represents the baseline risk and the absolute benefit you can expect from the therapy.

NNT = 1/ARR

Sometimes, papers will present their results in the form of NNTs, as in this one which is very helpful, but often they do not, and prefer to present risk ratios (perhaps not surprisingly, since these tend to make beneficial results look more spectacular) or similar measures. You will often be required to calculate NNTs from the data in the study. Fortunately, the arithmetic is fairly straightforward. Some other examples of NNTs are included in Bandolier (http://www.jr2.ox.ac.uk/bandolier/band50/b50-8.html).

This is a small study and like the relative risk there is a confidence interval around the NNT (to calculate this[15] it is easier to use software (www.ebm.net). Also, there is the 'believability' issue of a relatively small trial. This is where the clinical judgement comes in – would you use this treatment based on 100 patients?

Will the results help my patient?

- Can the results be applied to my patient?
- Were all clinically relevant outcomes considered?
- Are the benefits worth the harms and costs?

Given that your patient was not in the trial and may not even have been eligible for it (due to age, sex, co-morbidity, disease severity or for a host of other sociodemographic, biologic or clinical reasons), how can you extrapolate from the external evidence to your individual patient? (We use the term 'extrapolate' here, although this might more accurately be described as 'particularizing' the results of a trial (which looks at a generic population) to your particular patient.) This requires that you apply some of your knowledge of human biology and clinical experience to answer the question: 'Is my patient so different from those in the trial that its results cannot help me make my treatment decision?'

HOW MUCH BENEFIT CAN YOU EXPECT FOR YOUR PATIENT?

Given that you have decided that your patient is sufficiently similar to those in the study for the effect to be applicable, the next questions is how much? Here is one way of going about this.

f Method

First estimate, as a decimal fraction, your patient's risk compared to the control group from the study. Thus, if your patient is twice as susceptible as those in the trial, $f = 0.2$; if half as susceptible, $f = 0.5$. As long as the treatment produces a constant RRR across a range of susceptibilities, the NNT for your patient is simply the

trial's reported NNT divided by f. (This is a big assumption and we are only beginning to learn when assuming a constant RRR is appropriate (for numerous medical treatments such as antihypertensive drugs) and inappropriate (for some operations such as carotid endarterectomy, where the RRR rises with increasing susceptibility). So, in the above example, we might assign an f of 0.7 (70 percent chance of having epistaxis to the control group of subjects), which would yield an NNT of $(3.7/0.7) = 5$.

INCORPORATING YOUR PATIENT'S VALUES AND PREFERENCES

What does your patient think? Have you talked to them about their personal preferences, concerns and expectations? Here, we must try to determine whether the outcome of the therapy actually serves the values and preferences of the patient. Many factors can come into play, not least the difficulty of representing them. Sometimes, the situation may be very clear-cut or demand immediate action. For example, in a patient having a heart attack, the value of survival and the preference for a simple, low-risk intervention such as aspirin, given the efficacy of this regimen, usually makes this decision quickly agreed and acted upon. In other cases, the answer may take weeks and several visits to sort out, such as in choosing between radiation and adjuvant chemotherapy for stage II carcinoma of the breast.

These questions are perhaps the most important, yet have the least written about them in this chapter. That is because they are also the most complex and depend to a great extent on the clinical situation.

Summary

An evidence-based approach to deciding whether a therapy is effective for your patient involves the following steps.

1. Frame the clinical question.
2. Search for evidence concerning the accuracy of the test.
3. Assess the methods used to carry out the trial of the therapy.
4. Determine the NNT of the therapy.
5. Decide whether the NNT can apply to your patient, and estimate a particularized NNT.
6. Incorporate your patient's values and preferences in to deciding on a course of action.

APPRAISING SYSTEMATIC REVIEWS

What happens when there is more than one randomized control trial on the same treatment or diagnostic test? In this case you want to look for a paper that has combined these trials together.

What you need here is a systematic review, a publication that collects all of the evidence in a particular area and summarizes it. More formally, a systematic review is 'a review of a clearly formulated question that uses systematic and explicit methods to identify, select and critically appraise relevant research, and to collect and analyse data from studies that are included in the review. Statistical methods may or may not be used to analyse and summarise the results of the included studies.'

This section will look at how you appraise studies that search for all research on a specific question and in some way combine it.

You may be familiar with the narrative reviews traditionally found in many journals. Normally someone, usually an expert, looks at the evidence in a certain area. Mulrow[16] argues that traditional reviews do not routinely use systematic methods to identify, assess and synthesize information. Thus, normally there is no methods section for the actual conduct of the review. The reader then has no way of knowing whether the review is based on a systematic review of the evidence, or on a collection of papers that the author has found in a less systematic way and thus the evidence presented may not be complete. There is a need for systematic reviews of the evidence. This needs to be undertaken in just as rigorous a way as any primary piece of research, with a clear question and explicit methods for all stages of the process, such that another person could replicate the review. Three key features of such a review are:

1. a strenuous effort to locate all original reports on the topic of interest;
2. critical evaluation of the reports;
3. conclusions are drawn based on a synthesis of studies which meet preset quality criteria.

When synthesizing results, a meta-analysis may be undertaken. This is 'the use of statistical techniques in a systematic review to integrate the results of the included studies', which means that the authors have attempted to synthesize the different results into one overall statistic.

Where can you find systematic reviews?

Systematic reviews have been published in a variety of journals, and in addition the Cochrane Collaboration provides an important resource in this area. The Cochrane Collaboration is an international collaboration that is committed to 'preparing, maintaining and disseminating systematic reviews of the effects of health care'. It promotes and publishes the Cochrane Library (http://www.cochrane.org). This contains the Cochrane Database of Systematic Reviews. These reviews have a prespecified protocol, where every stage of the process of undertaking the review is made explicit.

Sections covered in a protocol include background, objectives, criteria for considering studies for the review (including types of participants, types of interventions, types of outcome measure, types of study), search strategy for identification of studies, study selection, methodological quality assessment, data extraction, meta-analysis, the comparisons to be made, subgroup analysis and sensitivity analysis to be undertaken. The point to note here is that all these aspects of the protocol are set out before the review is undertaken.

Many of the systematic reviews so far completed are based on evidence of effectiveness of an intervention from RCTs.

Is the review valid

In this section we will focus on systematic reviews of therapy. Of course, systematic reviews exist for other types of research.[17]

- *What databases and other sources did the authors of this review search?* The paper should give a comprehensive account of the sources consulted in the search for relevant papers, and the search strategy used to find them. Since standard databases fail to correctly index up to half of published trials, and negative trials are less likely to be published in the first place, the search strategy should include hand searching of journals and searching for unpublished literature. Other questions to ask yourself about the search strategy are: Have any obvious databases been missed? Did the authors check the reference lists of articles and of textbooks? Did they contact experts (to obtain their list of references checked for completeness and to attempt to find out about ongoing or unpublished research)? Search terms used are also important – has an obvious medical subject heading (MeSH) (a standard thesaurus for medical indexing) term been missed or is there another term they have not used? For example, when searching for papers looking at care of the elderly, use of the term 'senior' in the North American literature may be overlooked. Searching should include languages other than English. Unpublished data are useful to include because studies with significant results are more likely to be published than studies without significant results, known as publication bias. For example, research which is carried out by non-English language teams is more likely to be published in English if it shows a strong result in favour of an intervention than if it shows a negative or indifferent result.
- *How the studies were selected – eligibility criteria?* You should look for a statement of how the trial's validity was assessed, using criteria such as those in the therapy guides. It is particularly reassuring when two or more investigators applied these criteria

independently and achieved good agreement in their results. You need to know what criteria were used to select the research. This should include who the study participants were, what was done and what outcomes were assessed. A point to consider is that the narrower the inclusion criteria, the less generalizeable are the results. However, this needs to be balanced with using very broad inclusion criteria, when heterogeneity becomes an issue. Such studies may cover a wide range of patients and/or interventions and/or outcomes and the justification for then combining these differing groups comes into question. The importance of a clear statement of inclusion criteria is that studies should be selected on the basis of these criteria (that is, any study that matches these criteria is included) rather than selecting the study on the basis of the results.

- *How were the data abstracted?* Data are usually obtained by two individuals working separately (independently) and then compared later. Often the data are not available within the paper and there may be a statement about obtaining the raw data from the authors.
- *Is there a description of the quality of each trial?* A table of the studies meeting the inclusion criteria should include some data on the validity checks itemized in the section on randomized control trials.[4]
- *Were the results consistent from study to study?* Although we might expect some variation from study to study, we would be concerned if some trials confidently concluded a beneficial effect of the therapy, while others confidently concluded harmful or no effects. Unless this heterogeneity can be explained to your satisfaction (such as by differences in patients, dosage or duration of treatment), this should lead you to be very cautious about believing any overall conclusion about efficacy from the review.

Statistical heterogeneity exists when there is greater variation between the results than is likely due to chance. The chi-square statistic on which they are based has on average a value equal to its degrees of freedom. Values much larger than the degrees of freedom suggest a smaller p value and thus significant statistical heterogeneity. This means greater variation exists between the studies than is likely by chance alone. One might then conclude that the studies are so different that it makes no sense to combine them. Since this test of heterogeneity is described as having a low power, a nonsignificant test cannot be interpreted as evidence of homogeneity. The aim of the authors should be to clearly describe the influences of specific clinical differences between the studies, rather than purely relying on an overall statistical test of heterogeneity.

Clinical and statistical heterogeneity need to be distinguished. Clinical heterogeneity refers to differences between settings, patients, techniques and outcomes, which might lead you to suggest it does not make sense to combine the data.

What are the results?

Terms that you will probably come across when looking at systematic reviews include odds ratios, relative risks, weighted mean differences and fixed and random effects, amongst others.

BINARY OR CONTINUOUS DATA

The type of data will dictate what you see when you look at a meta-analysis:

- binary data (for example, an event rate: something that happens or it does not, such as myocardial infarction, stroke, improved/not improved) is usually combined using odds ratios;
- continuous data (for example, numbers of days, peak expiratory flow rate) are combined using differences in mean values for treatment and control groups (weighted mean differences (WMD)) when units of measurement are the same (for example, all using the same anxiety scale), or standardized mean differences when units of measurement differ (for example, using a variety of anxiety scales, where one numerical value could mean very different things, depending on the scale used). Here, the difference in means is divided by the pooled standard deviation.

Thus when you look at a meta-analysis, you will see odds ratios or relative risks and/or weighted mean differences or standardized mean differences, depending on the outcomes measures that have been used in the included studies.

ODDS RATIO

Odds are another way of describing risk. The odds of an event are the probability of it occurring compared to the probability of it not occurring. We cannot do a randomized control trial to assess whether gastrooesophageal reflux disease (GERD) may be associated with laryngeal neoplasm. However, we can do a case–control study looking at people with and without cancer.[18]

We do not know the incidence of laryngeal cancer in the population from this study as they took cases with cancer and compared them to controls, but we can work out the odds (**Table 52.5**). For GERD, the odds of having cancer is $731/1315 = 0.555$. This clearly is not the risk in the general population! The odds of having laryngeal cancer in non-GERD patients was 0.237. The odds ratio was $0.555/0.237 = 2.3$. So patients with GERD in this study had 2.3 times the odds of having laryngeal carcinoma. This was unadjusted for the other major risk factor of smoking. In large studies, odds ratios approximate risk ratio.

Table 52.5 Prevalence of gastrooesophageal reflux disease (GERD) in a case control study of patients with and without laryngeal cancer.

	GERD	No GERD
Laryngeal cancer	731	7497
No laryngeal cancer	1315	31,597
Total	2046	39,094

Clearly, as in randomized controlled trials with risk reduction, unless we know the baseline risk it is impossible to put odds ratios into context. A number needed to treat can be derived from an odds ratio but remember that many assumptions have been made in that process and treat them with some caution.

Many systematic reviews use odds ratios to represent differences between treatment and control groups. Relative risk and absolute risk reduction may also be used to express these sorts of differences, as we have already seen.

WHAT DO ODDS RATIOS USED IN A META-ANALYSIS LOOK LIKE?

The square box or 'blob' on the Forrest Plot (which is sometimes known colloquially as a 'blobogram') (**Figure 52.3**) is the individual study effect (technically referred to as the point estimate), with its associated confidence interval as lines either side of that box (technically known as the interval estimate). Sometimes the size of the box may

vary to reflect the weight that particular study is given, with larger boxes representing higher weighting. Lower weighted studies are usually those with smaller samples and large confidence intervals. The overall or summary effect (from combining or pooling the studies) is usually depicted as a diamond. Since patients may respond differently to treatment, this pooling may need to be supplanted by summarizing evidence along multiple covariates of interest. Thus, although one overall number is appealing in its simplicity, it may oversimplify a more complex situation.

An odds ratio of one on a linear scale means there is no difference between the experimental and control group. This value of one is the line down the middle of the figure (sometimes with the wording 'favours treatment' on one side and 'favours control' on the other). If the confidence interval does *not* cross the line, it means that there is a 95 percent chance that there is a true difference between the groups. That is, that there is a significant difference on that particular outcome between the intervention and control groups. If the confidence interval does cross this vertical line labelled '1' it means that any difference in that outcome between the treatments could have occurred by chance (that is, there are no statistically significant differences). It may be that a very wide confidence interval is due to a very small sample size, and it would reduce with more people in the study. A 95 percent confidence interval covers likely results from a set of similar studies. It therefore provides a more realistic view of what will happen in practice than a point estimate, because it takes potential variability into account.

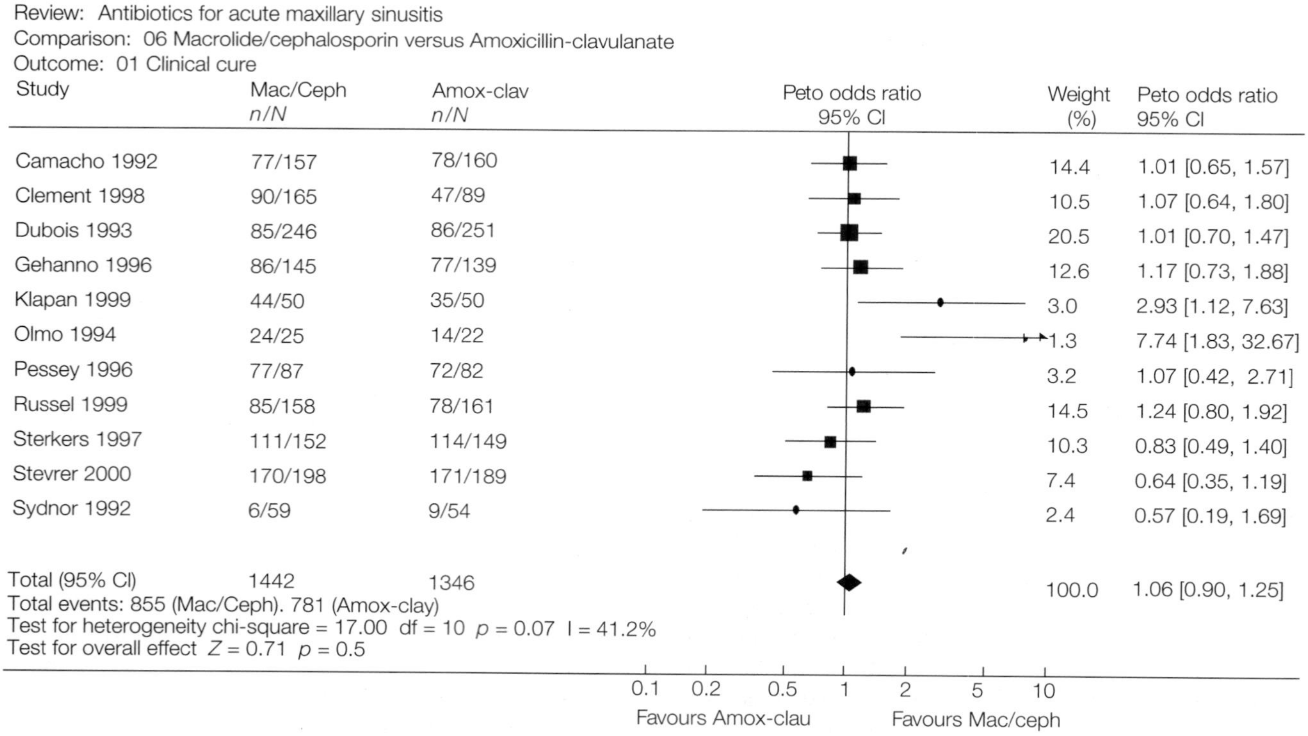

Review: Antibiotics for acute maxillary sinusitis
Comparison: 06 Macrolide/cephalosporin versus Amoxicillin-clavulanate
Outcome: 01 Clinical cure

Study	Mac/Ceph n/N	Amox-clav n/N	Peto odds ratio 95% CI	Weight (%)	Peto odds ratio 95% CI
Camacho 1992	77/157	78/160		14.4	1.01 [0.65, 1.57]
Clement 1998	90/165	47/89		10.5	1.07 [0.64, 1.80]
Dubois 1993	85/246	86/251		20.5	1.01 [0.70, 1.47]
Gehanno 1996	86/145	77/139		12.6	1.17 [0.73, 1.88]
Klapan 1999	44/50	35/50		3.0	2.93 [1.12, 7.63]
Olmo 1994	24/25	14/22		1.3	7.74 [1.83, 32.67]
Pessey 1996	77/87	72/82		3.2	1.07 [0.42, 2.71]
Russel 1999	85/158	78/161		14.5	1.24 [0.80, 1.92]
Sterkers 1997	111/152	114/149		10.3	0.83 [0.49, 1.40]
Stevrer 2000	170/198	171/189		7.4	0.64 [0.35, 1.19]
Sydnor 1992	6/59	9/54		2.4	0.57 [0.19, 1.69]
Total (95% CI)	1442	1346		100.0	1.06 [0.90, 1.25]

Total events: 855 (Mac/Ceph), 781 (Amox-clav)
Test for heterogeneity chi-square = 17.00 df = 10 $p = 0.07$ I = 41.2%
Test for overall effect $Z = 0.71$ $p = 0.5$

0.1   0.2   0.5   1   2   5   10
Favours Amox-clau   Favours Mac/ceph

Figure 52.3 A Forrest plot. Redrawn from Ref. 19, with permission.

It is worth noting that a lack of evidence for an intervention is not the same as evidence of a lack of effect.

HOW PRECISE ARE THE RESULTS?

This is asking whether there are any confidence intervals used, so the reader can see the range of values around the effect size, where in one is 95 percent confidence that the 'true' effect would lie. The *Cochrane handbook* (1998), section 6.1, defines precision as 'a measure of the likelihood of random errors. It is reflected in the confidence interval around the estimate of effect from each study ... more precise results are given more weight'. Thus the more precise the results, the narrower (smaller) the confidence interval. NNTs can be calculated from the odds ratios (see Appendix). However, these should be treated with caution as they can oversimplify.

WILL THE RESULTS HELP ME IN CARING FOR MY PATIENTS?

- *Can the results be applied to my patient care?* How similar are the patients you care for to those included in the review? The wider the type of patients included in the review, the more likely you are to feel the results may apply across a range of different patients. However, it is sometimes a difficult decision to know whether, for example, something that works on men will be equally effective on women, or something that works in younger people will work in the same way in older people. Subgroup analysis may be one way of addressing this concern, although there are concerns with this approach.
- *Were all clinically important outcomes considered?* What is clinically important can depend on your perspective. Sometimes, whilst factors such as bone density may be included in a review to assess the effectiveness of certain orthopaedic procedures, it may be some other outcome, such as ability to get to the shops, that needs to be considered as this sort of outcome may be crucial from the patient's perspective.
- *Are the benefits worth the harms and costs?* This may cover a range of factors, such as benefit of early treatment following a positive cervical smear versus the harms of high anxiety. Or it may be the benefits of a chemotherapeutic agent versus its unpleasant side effects. An economic evaluation may be included.

What is sometimes difficult using a set of criteria like this, is that you end up with a variety of no's or can't tell's in answer to the questions you pose. It is sometimes difficult to decide when a review is 'too bad' to give you any confidence in the findings. Perhaps one pragmatic approach would be that when you have several 'no's' or 'can't tell's' you are more wary about the validity and robustness of the review's findings. What this does illustrate is that, like undertaking a systematic review, critically appraising these reviews is not an exact science,

but there are many subjective decisions along the way. Just like undertaking a systematic review, making explicit your decisions in the critical appraisal is therefore very important.

Although a systematic review can provide you with high quality evidence, clinical experience and patient preferences are an important part of evidence-based medicine. It may be that even high quality evidence does not apply to a particular patient. Similarly, Cochrane reviews do not include recommendations, as reviewers cannot know the local situation or the patient, and this is the province of the health professional caring for the patient.

KEY POINTS

Appraising diagnosis articles

- Criteria for validity of diagnosis trials: was there a reference standard, was it appropriate and was it applied blind, independently and to all patients?
- Appropriate spectrum of patients; clear and reproducible description of test, follow up, intention-to-treat.
- Outcome measures.
- Measures of the accuracy of diagnostic tests: sensitivity, specificity, positive predictive value negative predictive value, likelihood ratios.
- Applying the results to your patient: pre- and post-test probability, SpPin and SnNout.

Appraising therapy articles

- Criteria for validity of therapy trials: randomization, blinding, placebo control, equal treatment, follow up, intention-to-treat, outcome measures.
- Measures of the importance of the results of therapy trials: risk, event rates, NNTs.

Appraising systematic reviews

- Criteria for validity of systematic reviews: search for relevant trials, assessment of included trials' quality, heterogeneity.
- Measures of the importance of the results: risk, event rates, NNTs, odd ratios.

APPENDIX

Levels of evidence

Table 52.6 provides a breakdown of the types of research that answers questions on therapy, prognosis, diagnosis, differential diagnosis or prevalence and economic studies.

Table 52.6 Levels of evidence.

Level	Therapy/prevention, aetiology/harm	Prognosis	Diagnosis	Differential diagnosis/symptom prevalence study	Economic and decision analyses
1a	SR (with homogeneity)[a] of RCTs	SR (with homogeneity)[a] of inception cohort studies; CDR[b] validated in different populations	SR (with homogeneity)[a] of Level 1 diagnostic studies; CDR[b] with 1b studies from different clinical centres	SR (with homogeneity)[a] of prospective cohort studies	SR (with homogeneity)[a] of level 1 economic studies
1b	Individual RCT (with narrow Confidence interval)[c]	Individual inception cohort study with >80% follow-up; CDR[b] validated in a single population	Validating[k] cohort study with good[h] reference standards; or CDR[b] tested within one clinical centre	Prospective cohort study with good follow-up[c]	Analysis based on clinically sensible costs or alternatives; systematic review(s) of the evidence; and including multi-way sensitivity analyses
1c	All or none[d]	All or none case-series	Absolute SpPins and SnNouts[g]	All or none case-series	Absolute better-value or worse-value analyses[j]
2a	SR (with homogeneity)[a] of cohort studies	SR (with homogeneity)[a] of either retrospective cohort studies or untreated control groups in RCTs	SR (with homogeneity)[a] of Level >2 diagnostic studies	SR (with homogeneity)[a] of 2b and better studies	SR (with homogeneity)[a] of level >2 economic studies
2b	Individual cohort study (including low quality RCT; e.g., <80% follow-up)	Retrospective cohort study or follow-up of untreated control patients in an RCT; Derivation of CDR[b] or validated on split-sample[f] only	Exploratory[k] cohort study with good[i] reference standards; CDR[b] after derivation, or validated only on split-sample[f] or databases	Retrospective cohort study, or poor follow-up	Analysis based on clinically sensible costs or alternatives; limited review(s) of the evidence, or single studies; and including multi-way sensitivity analyses
2c	'Outcomes' research; Ecological studies	'Outcomes' research		Ecological studies	Audit or outcomes research
3a	SR (with homogeneity)[a] of case-control studies		SR (with homogeneity)[a] of 3b and better studies	SR (with homogeneity)[a] of 3b and better studies	SR (with homogeneity)[a] of 3b and better studies
3b	Individual case-control study		Nonconsecutive study; or without consistently applied reference standards	Nonconsecutive cohort study, or very limited population	Analysis based on limited alternatives or costs, poor quality estimates of data, but including sensitivity analyses incorporating clinically sensible variations

	Case-series (and poor quality cohort and case–control studies)[e]	Case-series (and poor quality prognostic cohort studies)[l]	Case–control study, poor or nonindependent reference standard	Case-series or superseded reference standards	Analysis with no sensitivity analysis
4					
5	Expert opinion without explicit critical appraisal, or based on physiology, bench research or 'first principles'	Expert opinion without explicit critical appraisal, or based on physiology, bench research or 'first principles'	Expert opinion without explicit critical appraisal, or based on physiology, bench research or 'first principles'	Expert opinion without explicit critical appraisal, or based on physiology, bench research or 'first principles'	Expert opinion without explicit critical appraisal, or based on economic theory or 'first principles'

The levels of evidence used throughout this book are as stated in the prelims on the How to use this book page. These are very similar to the five levels given in this table, except that Levels 3 and 4 of the system described in this table are equivalent to Level 3, and Level 5 (expert opinion) is equivalent to Level 4 in the system used in this book.

Produced by Bob Phillips, Chris Ball, Dave Sackett, Doug Badenoch, Sharon Straus, Brian Haynes and Martin Dawes since November 1998.

Users can add a minus sign '−' to denote the level of that fails to provide a conclusive answer because of:

* EITHER a single result with a wide confidence interval (such that, for example, an ARR in an RCT is not statistically significant but whose confidence intervals fail to exclude clinically important benefit or harm).
* OR a systematic review with troublesome (and statistically significant) heterogeneity.
* Such evidence is inconclusive, and therefore can only generate Grade D recommendations.

[a] By homogeneity we mean a systematic review that is free of worrisome variations (heterogeneity) in the directions and degrees of results between individual studies. Not all systematic reviews with statistically significant heterogeneity need be worrisome, and not all worrisome heterogeneity need be statistically significant. As noted above, studies displaying worrisome heterogeneity should be tagged with a '−' at the end of their designated level.

[b] Clinical decision rule. (These are algorithms or scoring systems which lead to a prognostic estimation or a diagnostic category.)

[c] Good follow-up in a differential diagnosis study is >80%, with adequate time for alternative diagnoses to emerge (e.g. one to six months acute, one to five years chronic).

[d] Met when all patients died before the Rx became available, but some now survive on it; or when some patients died before the Rx became available, but none now die on it.

[e] By poor quality cohort study we mean one that failed to clearly define comparison groups and/or failed to measure exposures and outcomes in the same (preferably blinded), objective way in both exposed and nonexposed individuals and/or failed to identify or appropriately control known confounders and/or failed to carry out a sufficiently long and complete follow-up of patients. By poor quality case–control study we mean one that failed to clearly define comparison groups and/or failed to measure exposures and outcomes in the same (preferably blinded), objective way in both cases and controls and/or failed to identify or appropriately control known confounders.

[f] Split-sample validation is achieved by collecting all the information in a single tranche, then artificially dividing this into 'derivation' and 'validation' samples.

[g] An 'Absolute SpPin' is a diagnostic finding whose Specificity is so high that a Positive result rules-in the diagnosis. An 'Absolute SnNout' is a diagnostic finding whose Sensitivity is so high that a Negative result rules-out the diagnosis.

[h] Good, better, bad and worse refer to the comparisons between treatments in terms of their clinical risks and benefits.

[i] Good reference standards are independent of the test, and applied blindly or objectively to applied to all patients. Poor reference standards are haphazardly applied, but still independent of the test. Use of a nonindependent reference standard (where the 'test' is included in the 'reference', or where the 'testing' affects the 'reference') implies a level 4 study.

[j] Better-value treatments are clearly as good but cheaper, or better at the same or reduced cost. Worse-value treatments are as good and more expensive, or worse and the equally or more expensive.

[k] Validating studies test the quality of a specific diagnostic test, based on prior evidence. An exploratory study collects information and trawls the data (e.g. using a regression analysis) to find which factors are 'significant'.

[l] By poor quality prognostic cohort study we mean one in which sampling was biased in favour of patients who already had the target outcome, or the measurement of outcomes was accomplished in <80% of study patients, or outcomes were determined in an unblinded, nonobjective way, or there was no correction for confounding factors.

Table 52.7 Grades of recommendation.

A	Consistent level 1 studies
B	Consistent level 2 or 3 studies or extrapolations from level 1 studies
C	Level 4 studies or extrapolations from level 2 or 3 studies
D	Level 5 evidence or troublingly inconsistent or inconclusive studies of any level

'Extrapolations' are where data are used in a situation that has potentially clinically important differences than the original study situation.

For each type of research a level of evidence is shown. This helps the reader identify the likely validity of the research. It does not mean that all systematic reviews are 'better' than randomized controlled trials. It should be used more as a pointer for searching and then a guide to the likely level of evidence. If one has a therapeutic question then looking for a systematic review first is logical. If there is no review then one next looks for a randomized controlled trial, etc.

If there is no trial evidence then consensus statements becomes the highest level of evidence answering that question. This just makes the grade of recommendation D rather than A if there was a systematic review. The grades of recommendations vary from country to country and organization to organization and should only be considered as a guide (**Table 52.7**).

Worksheets

The worksheets shown in **Figures 52.4, 52.5** and **52.6** can be used to appraise a randomized controlled trial, a diagnostic study or a systematic review. They are aide memoirs about the items to look for in a paper when appraising the validity, identifying the results and assessing the applicability.

They can be used in journal clubs or in other settings when an important new paper is being discussed. The data from these checklists can be entered into software to make your own electronic database of critical appraisals and saved as web pages or text documents.

REFERENCES

1. Kraaijenhagen RA, Haverkamp D, Koopman MM, Prandoni P, Piovella F, Buller HR. Travel and risk of venous thrombosis. *Lancet*. 2000; **356**: 1492–3.
2. Ioannidis JP, Haidich AB, Pappa M, Pantazis N, Kokori SI, Tektonidou MG *et al*. Comparison of evidence of treatment effects in randomized and nonrandomized studies. *Journal of the American Medical Association*. 2001; **286**: 821–30.
3. Juni P, Altman DG, Egger M. Systematic reviews in health care: Assessing the quality of controlled clinical trials. *British Medical Journal*. 2001; **323**: 42–6.
4. Moher D, Jadad AR, Nichol G, Penman M, Tugwell P, Walsh S. Assessing the quality of randomized controlled trials: an annotated bibliography of scales and checklists. *Controlled Clinical Trials*. 1995; **16**: 62–73.
5. Moher D, Cook DJ, Eastwood S, Olkin I, Rennie D, Stroup DF. Improving the quality of reports of meta-analyses of randomised controlled trials: the QUOROM statement. *Onkologie*. 2000; **23**: 597–602.
6. Shea B, Moher D, Graham I, Pham B, Tugwell P. A comparison of the quality of Cochrane reviews and systematic reviews published in paper-based journals. *Evaluation and the Health Professions*. 2002; **25**: 116–29.
7. Kubba H, MacAndie C, Botma M, Robison J, O'Donnell M, Robertson G *et al*. A prospective, single-blind, randomized controlled trial of antiseptic cream for recurrent epistaxis in childhood. *Clinical Otolaryngology*. 2001; **26**: 465–8.
8. Adams D. *Life, the universe, and everything. The hitchhiker's guide to the galaxy*, Vol. 3. Isbn: ISBN- 0-330-26738-8. London: Millenium (Orion), 1994.
9. BMJ Publishing Group Limited. *Clinical evidence*. www.clinicalevidence.com/
10. Bouma M, Dekker JH, van Eijk JT, Schellevis FG, Kriegsman DM, Heine RJ. Metabolic control and morbidity of type 2 diabetic patients in a general practice network. *Family Practice*. 1999; **16**: 402–6.
11. Booth A, O'Rourke AJ, Ford NJ. Structuring the pre-search reference interview: a useful technique for handling clinical questions. *Bulletin of the Medical Library Association*. 2000; **88**: 239–46.
12. Thomas KB. General practice consultations: is there any point in being positive? *British Medical Journal (Clinical Research Ed.)*. 1987; **294**: 1200–2.
13. Dagnelie CF, Bartelink ML, van der Graaf Y, Goessens W, de Melker RA. Towards a better diagnosis of throat infections (with group A beta-haemolytic streptococcus) in general practice. *British Journal of General Practice*. 1998; **48**: 959–62.
14. Lijmer JG, Mol BW, Heisterkamp S, Bonsel JG, Prins MH, van der Meulen JH *et al*. Empirical evidence of design-related bias in studies of diagnostic tests. *Journal of the American Medical Association*. 1999; **282**: 1061–6.
15. Bender R. Calculating confidence intervals for the number needed to treat. *Controlled Clinical Trials*. 2001; **22**: 102–10.
16. Mulrow CD. The medical review article: state of the science. *Annals of Internal Medicine*. 1987; **106**: 485–8.
17. Oxman AD, Cook DJ, Guyatt GH. Users' guides to the medical literature. VI. How to use an overview. Evidence-Based Medicine Working Group. *Journal of the American Medical Association*. 1994; **272**: 1367–71.
18. El-Serag HB, Hepworth EJ, Lee P, Sonnenberg A. Gastroesophageal reflux disease is a risk factor for laryngeal and pharyngeal cancer. *American Journal of Gastroenterology*. 2001; **96**: 2013–8.
19. Williams Jr. JW, Aguilar C, Cornell J, Chiquette E, Dolor RJ, Makela M *et al*. Antibiotics for acute maxillary sinusitis. *Cochrane Database of Systematic Reviews*. 2003; **2**: CD000243.

The answer:

Are the results of this single preventive or therapeutic trial valid?

PICO QUESTION	
Search terms used	
Databases searched to find this article	
Citation of article	
Why did you select this article(s)?	
Did the authors answer the question?	
1. What were the characteristics of the patients?	
2. Were the groups similar at the start of the trial?	
3. Aside from the experimental treatment, were the groups treated equally?	
4. What was the treatment and what was it compared against (placebo?)	
5a. Was the assignment of patients to treatments randomized? 5b. and was the randomization list concealed	
6a. Were all patients who entered the trial followed up at its conclusion? 6b. and were they analyzed in the groups to which they were randomized? (Intention to treat)	
7. Were patients and clinicians kept 'blind' to which treatment was being received?	
8. Was the length of study appropriate?	

Are the valid results of this randomized trial important?

YOUR CALCULATIONS:

		Absolute risk reduction (ARR)	Number needed to treat (NNT)	Relative risk reduction (RRR)
Control group rate (CER)	Experimental Group Rate (EER)	CER−EER	1/ARR	ARR/CER

95% Confidence Interval (CI) on an NNT = 1/(limits on the CI of its ARR) =

$$+/-1.96 \sqrt{\frac{CER \times (1-CER)}{No. \text{ of control pts.}} + \frac{EER \times (1-EER)}{No. \text{ of exp. pts.}}} =$$

Can you apply this valid, important evidence about a treatment in caring for your patient?

Do these results apply to your patient?	
Is your patient so different from those in the trial that its results can not help you?	
How great would the potential benefit of therapy actually be for your individual patient?	
Method I: f	Risk of the outcome in your patient, relative to patients in the trial. expressed as a decimal: _____ NNT/F = _____/_____ = _____ (NNT for patients like yours)

Are your patient's values and preferences satisfied by the regimen and its consequences?

Do your patient and you have a clear assessment of their values and preferences?	
Are they met by this regimen and its consequences?	

Figure 52.4 Randomized control trial worksheet.

The Answer:

Are the results of this diagnostic study valid?

PICO QUESTION	
Search terms used	
Databases searched to find this article	
Citation of article	
Why did you select this article(s)	
Did the authors answer the question?	
1. What were the characteristics of the patients?	
2a. New diagnostic test description. Is it clear how the test was carried out? 2b. Is the test reproducible in your setting?	
3a. Gold standard description. 3b. Was there an independent, blind comparison with a reference ('gold') standard of diagnosis?	
4. Was the reference standard applied regardless of the diagnostic test result?	
6. Was the diagnostic test evaluated in an appropriate spectrum of patients (like those in whom it would be used in practice)?	

YOUR CALCULATIONS:

		Target disorder		Totals
		Present	Absent	
Diagnostic test result	Positive	a	b	a + b
	Negative	c	d	c + d
	Totals	a + c	b + d1770	a + b + c + d

Sensitivity = a/(a + c) =
Specificity = d/(b + d) =
Likelihood ratio for a positive test result = LR+ = sens/(1–spec) =
Likelihood ratio for a negative test result = LR– = (1–sens)/spec =
Positive predictive value = a/(a + b) =
Negative predictive value = d/(c + d) =
Pretest probability (prevalence) = (a + c)/(a + b + c + d) =
Pretest-odds = prevalence/(1–prevalence) =
Post-test odds = Pretest odds x likelihood ratio =
Post-test probability = post-test odds/(post-test odds + 1) =

Can you apply this valid, important evidence about a diagnostic test in caring for your patient?

Is the diagnostic test available, affordable, accurate and precise in your setting?	
Can you generate a clinically sensible estimate of your patient's pretest probability (from practice data, from personal experience, from the report itself, or from clinical speculation)	
Will the resulting post-test probabilities affect your management and help your patient? (Could it move you across a test-treatment threshold?; Would your patient be a willing partner in carrying it out?)	
Would the consequences of the test help your patient?	

Additional notes:

Figure 52.5 Diagnosis worksheet.

The Answer:

Are the results of this systematic review of therapy valid?

PICO QUESTION	
Search terms used	
Databases searched to find this article	
Citation of article	
Why did you select this article(s)	
Did the authors answer the question?	
1. What databases and other sources did the authors of this review search?	
2. What were their eligibility criteria (inclusion and exclusion) for papers in this study? Do these seem appropriate?	
3. Was their independent data extraction of the results by the reviewers (then compared later)	
4. Is there a description of the quality of each trial included?	
5. Were the results consistent from study to study? (Homogeneous)	

Are the valid results of this systematic review important?

What was the odds ratio?	
What was the control group rate (PEER)	

Can you apply this valid, important evidence from a systematic review in caring for your patient?

Do these results apply to your patient?	
Is your patient so different from those in the overview that its results can not help you? How great would the potential benefit of therapy actually be for your individual patient?	
To calculate the NNT for any OR and PEER $$NNT = \frac{1 - (PEER * (1 - OR))}{(1 - PEER) * PEER * (1 - OR)}$$ Or use calculator from www.cebm.net	

Are your patient's values and preferences satisfied by the regimen and its consequences?

Do your patient and you have a clear assessment of their values and preferences?
Are they met by this regimen and its consequences?
Should you believe apparent qualitative differences in the efficacy of therapy in some subgroups of patients? Only if you can say 'yes' to all of the following:
Do they really make biologic and clinical sense?
Is the qualitative difference both clinically (beneficial for some but useless or harmful for others) and statistically significant?
Was this difference hypothesized before the study began (rather than the product of dredging the data), and has it been confirmed in other, independent studies?
Was this one of just a few subgroup analyses carried out in this study?

Additional notes:

Figure 52.6 Systematic review (of therapy) worksheet.

PART 11

RECENT ADVANCES IN TECHNOLOGY

EDITED BY MARTIN J BURTON

53 Functional magnetic resonance imaging: Principles and illustrative applications for otolaryngology   675
   Paul M Matthews

54 Positron emission tomography and integrated PET/computed tomography   684
   Wai Lup Wong

55 Image-guided surgery, 3D planning and reconstruction   701
   Ghassan Alusi and Michael Gleeson

56 Ultrasound in ear, nose and throat practice   711
   Keshthra Satchithananda and Paul S Sidhu

57 Interventional techniques   731
   James V Byrne

58 Laser principles in otolaryngology, head and neck surgery   742
   Brian JG Bingham

59 Electrophysiology and monitoring   748
   Patrick R Axon and David M Baguley

60 Optical coherence tomography   755
   Mariah Hahn and Brett E Bouma

61 Contact endoscopy   762
   Mario Andrea and Oscar Dias

Functional magnetic resonance imaging: Principles and illustrative applications for otolaryngology

PAUL M MATTHEWS

Introduction	675	Conclusions	681
The physiological basis for blood oxygenation level-dependent functional magnetic resonance imaging	677	Key points	681
		Best clinical practice	682
Practical details	678	Current deficiencies and suggestions for future research	682
Illustrative applications of functional magnetic resonance imaging	679	References	682

SEARCH STRATEGY

The data in this chapter are supported by a PubMed search using the key words functional brain imaging and hearing, restricted to humans.

INTRODUCTION

Functional magnetic resonance imaging (fMRI) has become one of the most versatile tools in cognitive neuroscience. Using blood oxygenation level-dependent (BOLD) fMRI, grey matter regions active during sensory, motor and cognitive activity can be defined based on the accompanying local increase in blood flow and oxygenation. Increasing numbers of applications to basic questions in auditory physiology have been reported. Now, there is the exciting potential for clinical use of the methodology.

An overview of functional brain imaging methods

Functional brain imaging includes any of a broad range of techniques by which physiological changes accompanying brain activity can be followed. For example, neuronal depolarization can be monitored using electroencephalography (EEG) or magnetoencephalography (MEG). The energy-requiring metabolic changes in neurons and glia that accompany neurotransmitter release and reuptake and receptor occupancy can be measured using positron emission tomography (PET). Currently, the most commonly used functional brain imaging technique is fMRI. Functional magnetic resonance imaging is sensitive to the increase in local blood flow with neuronal activation. These changes in blood flow can be measured directly using perfusion MRI.[1] However, as the increase in total oxygen delivery exceeds the increase in oxygen utilization, another fMRI method, BOLD fMRI, can also be used. In BOLD fMRI the imaging contrast arises as a consequence of the higher ratio of oxy- to deoxy-haemoglobin in local capillaries and draining venules with brain activity.[2] While the neuronal events thus are only indirectly observed, the method is widely exploited because of its sensitivity, relatively low cost and ease of examination and the lack of recognized risks.

The different functional brain imaging methods have different temporal and spatial resolutions. Methods that

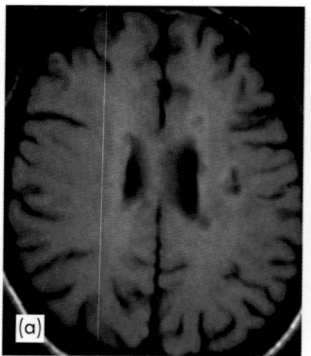 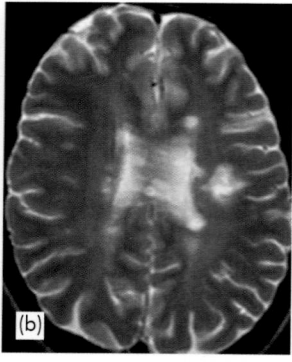 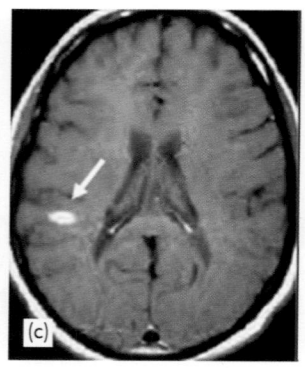 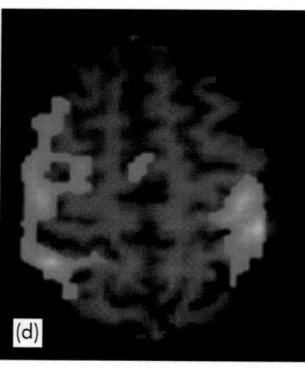

Figure 53.1 Different forms of contrast can be generated using MRI, identifying structural and functional differences across normal or pathological brains. **(a)** T1-weighted contrast in the brain of a patient with multiple sclerosis, showing brain tissue as brighter signal and cerebrospinal fluid (CSF) (or areas of tissue matrix destruction) darker. **(b)** T2-weighted contrast in the brain of a patient with multiple sclerosis. Here CSF is bright as are regions of inflammation with its associated oedema. **(c)** A contrast-enhanced T1-weighted image from the brain of a patient with multiple sclerosis. A region of acute inflammation with loss of an intact blood-brain barrier allows leak of the gadolinium-DTPA contrast agent into the brain parenchyma, enhancing the signal intensity locally (arrow). **(d)** BOLD fMRI contrast defines the hand region of the primary sensorimotor cortex during a simple hand movement. The colours represent the statistical significance of signal enhancement during the active vs. the rest phases.

map the transient brain electrical dipoles generated by neuronal depolarization (e.g. EEG) or the associated magnetic dipoles (MEG) define the underlying cortical neuronal events in real time (10–100 msec), but offer relatively poor spatial resolution (on the order of a centimetre or more). PET methods require relatively long acquisition times (tens of seconds) and give moderately high spatial resolution (5–15 mm). Functional magnetic resonance imaging provides information on the increases in blood flow accompanying neuronal activation with potentially rather higher spatial resolution (approximately 1–10 mm), but has a temporal resolution limited by the haemodynamic changes, which are made slower (several seconds) than the neuronal response (milliseconds).

Generation of image contrast in functional magnetic resonance imaging

Let us consider the problem of developing contrast between different tissues in greater detail. How is a difference in signal intensity (image contrast) generated between regions of brain that are 'active' and those that are at 'rest' in fMRI?

Once the nuclear spins in the tissue are excited by a radiofrequency pulse, they can return (or 'relax') to a low energy state by emission of energy. It is this energy, the frequency of which is made to be spatially variable, that is detected in MRI. The rate at which the emissions decay is determined by interactions with the environment. As local (i.e. on a molecular and cellular level) environments for water molecules vary across a heterogeneous tissue such as the brain, this so-called 'relaxation rate' also varies. The MRI image can be made sensitive to this by

varying the interpulse delay or 'TR' in a pulse sequence. A 'T1-weighted' clinical scan generates image contrast using this principle (**Figure 53.1**). However, while useful for differentiating grey from white matter, this alone does not distinguish 'active' from 'resting' brain. Some functional information can be introduced by scanning after injection of an MRI contrast agent (e.g. gadolinium DTPA), which can define vessels or regions around vessels that become more permeable to small molecules with inflammation, infarction or tumours by changing the local with relaxation time. However, while the first functional imaging was performed in this way,[1] it remains a cumbersome technique for most applications.

In tissue, huge numbers of spins are being observed simultaneously (in the brain for example, there are more than 4×10^{19} water protons/mm^3). Even in a small tissue region, each of the nuclei has a different relation to other molecules and experiences a slightly different, varying local magnetic field. These shifting fields allow an exchange of energy between the nuclei spins. This leads to a faster loss of the net signal from all of the nuclei together. This is described by the so-called 'spin–spin' or T2 relaxation time. The T2 is an intrinsic property of nuclei in a particular chemical environment that accounts for the contrast (generated by changing the imaging parameter 'TE') in a 'T2-weighted' MRI image. While T2 differences are useful for defining differences in, for example, water content between different brain regions (**Figure 53.1**), they also tell us nothing directly about brain function.

However, a related phenomenon provides the answer. The rate of decay of signal is faster if there are local (i.e. on a molecular scale) magnetic field variations that the molecules can diffuse through over the time course of a single TE. As molecules move through different magnetic fields, their resonance frequencies change (although only slightly), lowering the coherence of the nuclear spins. This leads to more rapid decay of the net signal. In the presence of local magnetic field inhomogeneities the rate of signal decay is expressed by the T2* relaxation time. In regions of rapidly changing local magnetic fields (e.g. in tissue adjacent to a blood vessel filled predominantly with paramagnetic deoxyhaemoglobin), the T2* can be substantially shorter than the T2. This mechanism determines the dramatic signal contrast provided by blood breakdown products in tissue for clinical MRI. It is also the mechanism underlying generation of BOLD fMRI images (**Figure 53.1**).

THE PHYSIOLOGICAL BASIS FOR BLOOD OXYGENATION LEVEL–DEPENDENT FUNCTIONAL MAGNETIC RESONANCE IMAGING

Mechanisms of haemodynamic change

The locally increased blood flow with brain activation is a consequence of increased energy utilization at the synapse.[3, 4] Several processes contribute to this, including increased energy utilization in adjacent astrocytes with the uptake of the excitatory neurotransmitter, glutamate, depolarization of the post-synaptic membrane and subsequent spike discharges.[5] However, there is not a simple relationship between increased energy utilization and increased blood flow or BOLD fMRI contrast.

'Metabolic' functional imaging techniques, such as BOLD fMRI, can identify activation-related changes in grey matter (where the synapses are found), but not in the white matter. It is important to emphasize that results should be interpreted primarily in terms of synaptic activity, rather than neuronal activity directly.[6] Because of the lack of a fixed relationship between synaptic energy utilization and neuronal firing, as well as the large number of potentially interacting processes generating the signal, caution should be taken in trying to relate the magnitude of the BOLD response quantitatively to neuronal discharge rate.

Coupling of haemodynamic changes to neuronal activation

Multiple mechanisms contribute to the control of blood flow to the brain and the precise way in which blood flow is coupled to increased metabolic demands with synaptic activity. Nitric oxide (primarily from neuronal nitric oxide synthase) may be the most important chemical signal responsible for local increases in perfusion with neuronal activation and the cerebral vasodilatory response to hypercapnia, but a variety of factors would also

contribute, including K^+ release with neuronal depolarization and H^+ and adenosine release. Locally generated eicosanoids (e.g. prostacyclin)[7] and circulating factors (e.g. norepinephrine, serotonin) can modulate blood flow regulation, as can some drugs in common use (e.g. theophylline or scopolamine, inhibit the haemodynamic response to neuronal activation).[8, 9] Neuronal-haemodynamic coupling can change with age,[10] although the changes after maturity are modest.[11]

Perfusion functional magnetic resonance imaging

The most direct approach to measuring functional activation with MRI would be to directly define the changes in perfusion (or the associated small increase in local increase in blood volume) with the accompanying neuronal activation. The first functional MRI studies did just this using a paramagnetic MRI contrast agent to follow changes in local blood volume with increased activation.[1]

While technically challenging, a more attractive approach to measuring functional activation changes from direct perfusion measurements is to use noninvasive arterial 'spin-tagging' (**Figure 53.2**).[12, 13, 14] Arterial spin-tagging methods use radiofrequency pulses from the MRI system itself to transiently 'label' flowing blood without the need for an exogenous contrast agent. Unfortunately, the sensitivity of this approach is low, which limits its applicability at present.

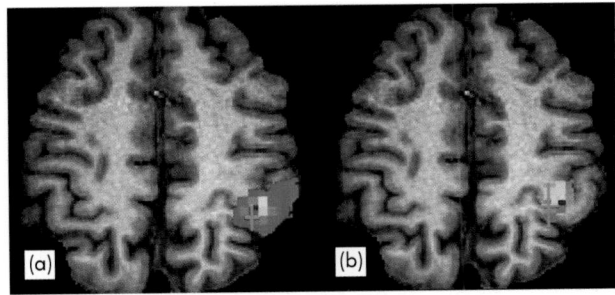

Figure 53.2 Both perfusion MRI and BOLD fMRI can be used to define regions active during brain activity. In this study, the subject alternately moved the right hand in flexion-extension or kept it at rest. The hemodynamic response with brain activation in the left primary sensorimotor cortex is shown using: **(a)** BOLD fMRI; and **(b)** arterial spin tagging (ASL) perfusion imaging. Similar regions are active, although the perfusion method is less sensitive (giving a smaller activation region. The green target shows the mean and standard deviation (in the plane of the image) of activation centres of gravity with respect to the large sulcal draining vein (blue) identified by MR venography in the same experiment. Images were prepared by Dr. T. Tjandra, FMRIB Centre, Oxford.

How is blood oxygenation level–dependent contrast generated?

The most robust and widely used fMRI method is BOLD fMRI. In BOLD fMRI the image signal contrast arises from changes in T2* generated with differences in local 'magnetic susceptibility', an index of the extent to which an applied magnetic field is distorted as it interacts with a material, as blood oxygenation changes. Normal blood can be considered simply as a concentrated solution of haemoglobin (10–15 g haemoglobin/100 cm^3). When bound to oxygen, haemoglobin is diamagnetic, while deoxygenated haemoglobin is paramagnetic. Magnetic flux is reduced in diamagnetic materials, i.e. the applied magnetic field is repelled. Paramagnetic materials, in contrast, have an increased magnetic flux, i.e. the applied magnetic field is attracted into the material. A change in haemoglobin oxygenation therefore leads to changes in the local distortions of a magnetic field applied to it. 'Gradient echo' MR images of a cat brain show signal loss around blood vessels when the animal is made hypoxic, for example.[2] More local changes in blood oxygenation, from the increase in the ratio of oxy- to deoxy-haemoglobin specifically in a region of increased blood flow with brain activation, give rise to small local increases in signal intensity.

PRACTICAL DETAILS

Design of functional magnetic resonance imaging studies

Methods such as PET provide an absolute measure of tissue metabolism. In contrast, BOLD fMRI can be used only for determining relative signal intensity changes associated with different cognitive states during a single imaging session. The most time-efficient approach for comparing brain responses in different states during the imaging experiment is the 'block' design.[15] This design uses relatively long, alternating periods (e.g. 30 s), during each of which a discrete cognitive state is maintained. In the simplest form, there may only be two such states, a 'rest' and an 'active' state (although 'rest' is defined only with respect to the specific activity being considered). These are alternated through the experiment in order to ensure that signal variations from small changes in scanner sensitivity, patient movement or changes in attention have a similar impact on the signal responses associated with each of the different states.

However, it can become difficult to control a cognitive state precisely for the relatively long periods of each block. A 'rest' state is rarely a true rest, as mental events are difficult to constrain in a subject who is not engaged in a specific task. Some types of stimuli (particularly sensory stimuli) may show rapid habituation (a particular problem in studies of olfaction, for example).[16] Some cognitive tasks simply may not be amenable to a block design. For example, an 'oddball' paradigm (in which the reaction to an unexpected stimulus is probed) cannot be adapted to a classical 'block' design directly.

An alternative approach is so-called single-event fMRI,[17] in which data are acquired while discrete stimuli or responses are given. Results from many trials are then averaged together to give a measurable response. This is a potentially powerful approach, as it allows considerable flexibility for study of responses to individual or periodically presented stimuli, but it demands relative longer acquisition times than the block design.

A related approach is to present stimuli in a periodic fashion and then to map responses in terms of their phase relative to that of the stimulus presentation. This was used first for study of the visual cortex, which is organized functionally in multiple retinotopic maps arranged according to increasing eccentricity and polar angle. Because it is effectively a difference mapping procedure,[18] the edge contrast between adjacent functional regions is emphasized.[19] Tonotopy in the auditory system has been mapped using a similar strategy.[20]

Analysis of functional magnetic resonance imaging studies

The raw BOLD fMRI data can be acquired over periods as short as a few minutes. If the approach to analysis is well defined, near 'real-time' viewing of final statistical maps of activation is possible (although in research applications exploratory analyses may take substantial periods of time!). The basic problem in analysis of functional imaging experiments is to identify voxels that show signal changes varying with the changing brain states of interest across the serially acquired images. This is a challenging problem for fMRI data because the signal changes are small (leading to potential false-negatives or type II errors) and the number of voxels simultaneously interrogated across the imaged volume is very large (giving potential false-positives or type I errors).

One of the potentially most significant artifacts for fMRI that distinguishes it from other functional imaging techniques is its extreme susceptibility to motion from movements either of the whole head or even the brain alone (e.g. with the respiratory or cardiac cycles).[21] Effects of small head movements can be reduced by mathematically realigning the brain volumes after the data are first acquired, but larger movements can degrade image quality irrecoverably. This may be a particular confound in studies of patients who may be less comfortable in the magnet environment.

After optimization of the signal-to-noise by digital filtering, analysis of the time course by comparison of the signal of both models of the 'baseline' and 'active' states must be performed. There are many valid ways of

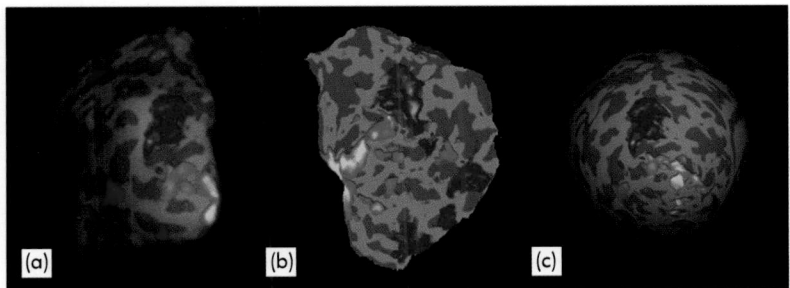

Figure 53.3 New forms of representation of brain activation patterns can make the spatial relationships easier to appreciate. All three images here reflect visual cortex activation associated with watching a flashing checkboard. A 'model-free' analysis using independent components analysis was performed, which distinguishes between the primary visual cortex (orange) and the motion-sensitive, MT cortex (blue). (a) Inflated brain representation; (b) flattened brain representation; (c) spherical brain representation. Images were prepared by Drs S. Smith and C. Beckmann (FMRIB Centre, Oxford, UK) using MELODIC (www.fmrib.ox.ac.uk/fsl) for analysis and the Freesurfer (Athinoula Martinos Imaging Centre, Massachusetts General Hospital NMR Centre, Boston) for representation.

performing statistical comparisons between signals in images acquired during different brain states. A simple approach is to generate a map of the t-statistic for changes on a voxel-by-voxel basis and use this to identify voxels with significance levels exceeding a chosen significance threshold (e.g. $t > 3$, which might correspond in a particular case to $p < 0.01$). A related approach is to correlate the time course of signal change in each voxel with a model time course based on the expected response, which again can be used to generate a t-statistic change.

Valid statistical inference from the image time course data is complicated by the fact that large numbers of voxels are being assessed simultaneously for changes. The significance level must be corrected for the number of truly independent comparisons that are being made. For example, if 10,000 independent voxels are being tested and a threshold for significance of change in each of the individual voxels of $p = 0.05$ is chosen, then 500 ($= 0.05 \times 10,000$) would be 'active' by chance alone! The significance threshold therefore must be made more stringent in proportion to the number of independent comparisons. Fortunately, because observations of immediately neighbouring regions are not really independent, the correction factor is reduced.

There are now a number of software packages produced by academic centres that include a full set of tools for analysis of fMRI data (e.g. FEAT (www.fmri.ox.ac.uk/fsl), SPM (www.fil.ion.ucl.ac.uk/spm/) or AFNI (www.cc.nih.gov/cip/ip_packages/ip_packages.html#afni)).

Neuroanatomical interpretation of functional data for groups of subjects: Use of a common brain space

A strength of fMRI is that it is sensitive enough to allow observations to be made even in individual subjects. Nonetheless, averaging results from studies of many subjects is often useful for identifying areas of activation

common to many members of the group. This can be used to define the 'normal' pattern of behaviour as a basis for detecting pathological patterns in patients, for example. Averaging between brains is possible with the use of a 'common' brain space, a canonical brain shape that can be related easily to the variable anatomy of individuals. The most well-known common brain space was developed by Talairach as a simple geometric parcellation of a single brain according to major anatomical landmarks.[22] This has been extended into a probabilistic framework.[23] More abstract representations of spatial variations in activation across the brain are possible using, for example, flattened representations, produced by computationally unfolding the cortex (**Figure 53.3**).[24, 25, 26] Other representations using standard geometric shapes for which coordinate systems (which allow relative positions of activations to be described precisely) are derived readily and that demand less distortion (e.g. a sphere) are also possible.[27]

ILLUSTRATIVE APPLICATIONS OF FUNCTIONAL MAGNETIC RESONANCE IMAGING

Applications of fMRI are growing rapidly and potentially have relevance to several aspects of otolaryngology. Here, applications to selected issues in hearing research are described to illustrate the range of problems that can be studied using the technique.

Imaging the normal auditory system

Functional magnetic resonance imaging has already contributed important information concerning the organization of the human auditory cortex, directly demonstrating parallels with the functional organization of the auditory brain in animals that previously were only assumed.[28] For example, tonotopic representations in the human primary auditory cortex comparable to those identified electrophysiologically in animals have been demonstrated using fMRI.[29] Differences between humans and other species have also begun to be defined. Animal studies, for example, have not demonstrated evidence for differences in cortical organization reflecting the sound level of the stimulus, while evidence for this level of representation of 'sound space' has been found in humans.[28]

One of the most striking areas of difference between humans and animals lies in the relative hemispheric specialization for auditory signal processing. Microelectrode studies in animals have consistently demonstrated a simple contralateral dominance for processing, similar with monoaural stimulation to either of the two ears. In contrast, recent fMRI studies have provided evidence for left hemispheric dominance for this process in humans even for pure tones (Devlin *et al.*, unpublished observations) (**Figure 53.4a** and **b**). This lateralization for pure tone processing may be central to understanding the specialization of the left hemisphere for language.

In auditory language processing, a left hemisphere dominance has long been recognized. This can be made clear with functional imaging by appropriate choice of contrasts of auditory tasks during the imaging study. Processing associated specifically with language intelligibility is strongly left-lateralized, for example, but this is made apparent only when an unintelligible control ('rest') stimulus of identical auditory complexity is contrasted (**Figure 53.4**).[30]

Development of function in the brain may also be studied with these techniques. While the demands for prolonged stationary periods in the unusual environment of the scanner probably preclude direct application of the technique to very young children while awake, responses in primary sensory systems, including audition, can be studied even under conditions of anaesthesia.[31]

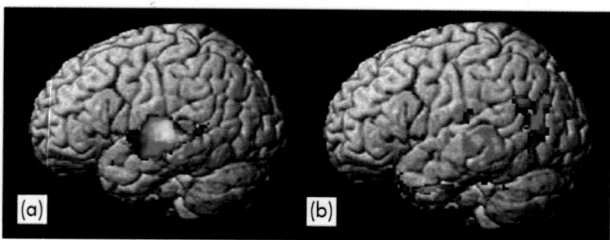

Figure 53.4 Functional imaging of audition. A 'sparse-sampling' protocol was used for analysis of auditory and language cortex activation by fMRI. Intelligible vs. unintelligible speech matched for acoustic characteristics were used. Both images show the left hemisphere for a group average activation map. (a) Activation primarily in the region of Heschl's gyrus with acoustic stimulation. (b) Activation primarily in more posterior, language-related regions with presentation of intelligible speech. Images courtesy of Dr. C. Narain and Dr. S. Scott (FMRIB Centre, Oxford).

As described earlier in this chapter, one of the general problems with the use of fMRI to study auditory processing is the noise of the imaging itself. Use of paradigms such as 'sparse sampling' (in which the stimuli are presented during quiet periods, with only intermittent sampling) avoid this problem, but are highly time-inefficient. An intriguing alternative approach that can be used with deaf patients is electrical stimulation via cochlear implants. This strategy poses technical challenges because of magnetic susceptibility image artifacts from the metal and safety concerns regarding the potential for current generation in the wires with gradient switching. However, with proper shielding of the stimulation cables, any induced currents can be reduced to levels below the acoustic perceptual threshold for cochlear implant subjects. In a recent report, stimulation of different intracochlear electrodes was associated with distinct cortical activations, consistent with the known tonotopical organization of the auditory cortex.[32]

Defining functional relations between brain regions

An important aspect of fMRI studies is the ability to define potentially interacting regions across broad regions of the brain. This ability to discriminate anatomically specific processing regions sets it apart from electrophysiological methods such as evoked potential studies. Functional magnetic resonance imaging has recently been used to probe the ways in which the brain processes identity and spatial information in sound.[33] In one study, participants had to match two sounds either for pitch or spatial location. Relative to location, pitch processing generated greater activation in the auditory cortex and the inferior frontal gyrus. Conversely, the task of recognizing location generated greater activation in posterior temporal cortex, parietal cortex and the superior frontal sulcus. The specialized auditory processing streams in the human brain implied by these differences are analogous to the 'what' and 'where' segregation of visual information processing, suggesting common modes of information organization.

Another general area of interest catalyzed by functional brain imaging has been understanding the functions of the cerebellum, classically thought of simply as a motor centre. Data now show that the cerebellum is involved in a broad range of tasks (perceptual, as well as motor) that demand representations of temporal information. Temporal sequencing plays an important role in auditory perception. Consistent with this hypothesis, bilateral injury to the cerebellar hemispheres can compromise the ability to make distinctions between words whose differences are determined by the closure time, a purely temporal measure of the lengths of pauses within words. To test for cerebellar involvement with this function, subjects were studied by fMRI to contrast patterns of brain activation during word discriminations made possible by variations in relative timing or the sound of central consonants.[34] The timing categorization selectively activated the right cerebellar cortex (Crus I) and the prefrontal lobe (anterior to Broca's area), while the sound categorization preferentially activated the supratemporal plane of the dominant hemisphere. This suggests that representation of the temporal structure of speech sound sequences is the crucial aspect of cerebellar involvement in cognitive tasks involving auditory comprehension.

Imaging plasticity

Short-term plasticity or 'learning' has become a particularly fruitful area of fMRI-based research. One example of this is in responses to an 'oddball' tone.[35] Brain responses elicited to pure tones of 950 Hz (standard) with occasional deviant tones of 952, 954 and 958 Hz were measured before and one week after subjects had been trained in these frequency discriminations. Frequency discrimination improved after the training session for some subjects (T +), but not for others (T −). Haemodynamic responses in the auditory cortex comprising the planum temporale, planum polare and sulcus temporalis superior significantly decreased during training, but only for the T + group. The results suggest that there is a short-term, plastic reorganization of cortical representations specifically for the trained frequencies.

Auditory reafferentation by cochlear implants (CI) offers a unique opportunity to study longer-term auditory plastic changes taking place at up to the supra- or polymodal organizational level.[36] One functional magnetic resonance imaging study investigated the impact of early auditory deprivation and use of a visuospatial language (American sign language (ASL)) on the organization of neural systems important in visual motion processing by comparing hearing controls with deaf and hearing native signers.[37] Participants monitored images of moving dots under different conditions of spatial and featural attention. Recruitment of the motion-selective brain visual-processing area, known as MT in hearing controls, was greater when attention was directed centrally and when the task was to detect motion features, confirming previous reports that the motion network is selectively modulated by different aspects of attention. More importantly, marked differences in the recruitment of motion-related areas as a function of early experience were observed. First, the lateralization of MT was found to shift toward the left hemisphere in early signers, suggesting that early exposure to ASL is associated with a greater reliance on the left MT. Second, whereas the two hearing populations displayed more MT activation under central than peripheral attention, the opposite pattern was observed in deaf signers, indicating enhanced recruitment of MT during peripheral attention after early deafness. Third, deaf signers (but not subjects with

normal hearing), displayed increased activation of the posterior parietal cortex, supporting the view that parietal functions are modified after early auditory deprivation. Finally, attention to motion lead to enhanced recruitment of the posterior superior temporal sulcus only in deaf signers, establishing for the first time in humans that this polymodal area is modified after early sensory deprivation.

Imaging drug responses

The ability to monitor changing responses of subjects over several examinations makes fMRI potentially attractive for studying the effects of drugs. Cholinergic blockade is known to attenuate conditioning-related neuronal responses in the human auditory cortex. One recent study investigated the effects of cholinergic enhancement on experience-dependent responses in the auditory cortex.[38] The cholinesterase inhibitor physostigmine, or a placebo control, were continuously infused into healthy young volunteers, during a conditioning protocol conducted while fMRI data were being acquired. Volunteers were presented with two tones, one of which (CS +) was paired with an electrical shock, while the other was always presented without the shock (CS −). Conditioning-related fMRI activations were found in the left auditory cortex during placebo administration, but not with physostigmine. Analysis showed that this absence of conditioning-related activation with physostigmine administration was due to enhanced responses to CS − with physostigmine relative to placebo. The study report concluded that increases in cholinergic activity in the auditory cortex enhances processing of behaviourally irrelevant stimuli and that attenuates differential conditioning-related cortical activations.

CONCLUSIONS

Functional magnetic resonance imaging is already a major tool for cognitive neuroscience research. Studies can be performed on single subjects and in all current high-field MRI systems. With a growing appreciation for interpretation of the data, fMRI can also be expected to provide new clinical strategies for establishing diagnosis and prognosis and in treatment monitoring.

KEY POINTS

- Functional magnetic resonance imaging is currently the most commonly used functional brain imaging technique.
- With blood oxygenation level dependent fMRI, image contrast arises as a consequence

of the higher ratio of oxy- to deoxy-haemoglobin in local capillaries and draining venules with brain activity.

- Functional magnetic resonance imaging thus has a spatial (approximately 1–10 mm) and temporal resolution determined by the haemodynamic changes accompanying neuronal activity.
- Results should be interpreted primarily in terms of synaptic activity, rather than neuronal firing directly.
- Coupling between the neuronal and haemodynamic changes is complex and BOLD fMRI provides a measure of only relative synaptic activity.
- Applications of fMRI are growing rapidly and potentially have relevance to several aspects of otolaryngology.

Best clinical practice

A rigorous evaluation of fMRI as a tool for clinical decision-making has not been performed. While encouraging preliminary evidence has been presented in applications such as localization of functional tissue and lateralization of language and memory activity in preoperative surgical planning, there is little information with which to judge the validity and informativeness of data outside specific research contexts. However, the techniques are promising in several areas and active, clinically based research to test the possible utility in decision-making should be encouraged.

At this point, fMRI may be best regarded as experimental in a clinical context and the data derived from it should not be used independently to provide primary information for clinical decision-making.

Current deficiencies and suggestions for future research

There are several areas of current research that should provide the new clinical imaging strategies of the future. Some of these can be highlighted here to give a vision of what is to come.

MRI is highly versatile and can be used to generate contrast relevant to brain function based on phenomenon other than perfusion or BOLD. It may be possible to detect local distortions in MRI signal induced by the transient magnetic fields generated with neuronal depolarization, for example. New approaches to analysis of fMRI are addressing the problem of developing more

accurate models for the haemodynamic response. The better this is defined, the greater the potential sensitivity of the method. Several research groups are working to develop approaches that make no assumptions about the timing or nature of the haemodynamic response. Successful work in this area would allow brain activity to be defined independent of information regarding stimuli or behaviour. These developments and rapidly growing experience are fuelling an increasingly confident application of the technique to complex clinical problems, such as those related to understanding decision-making, motivation and emotion, as well as more sensitively studying changes in brain functions over time.

REFERENCES

1. Belliveau JW, Kennedy Jr. DN, McKinstry RC, Buchbinder BR, Weisskoff RM, Cohen MS et al. Functional mapping of the human visual cortex by magnetic resonance imaging. Science. 1991; 254: 716–9.
2. Ogawa S, Lee TM, Kay AR, Tank DW. Brain magnetic resonance imaging with contrast dependent on blood oxygenation. Proceedings of the National Academy of Sciences of the United States of America. 1990; 87: 9868–72.
3. Duncan GE, Stumpf WE. Brain activity patterns: assessment by high resolution autoradiographic imaging of radiolabeled 2-deoxyglucose and glucose uptake. Progress in Neurobiology. 1991; 37: 365–82.
4. Duncan GE, Stumpf WE, Pilgrim C. Cerebral metabolic mapping at the cellular level with dry-mount autoradiography of [3H]2-deoxyglucose. Brain Research. 1987; 401: 43–9.
5. Attwell D, Laughlin SB. An energy budget for signaling in the grey matter of the brain. Journal of Cerebral Blood Flow and Metabolism. 2001; 21: 1133–45.
6. Logothetis NK, Pauls J, Augath M, Trinath T, Oeltermann A. Neurophysiological investigation of the basis of the fMRI signal. Nature. 2001; 412: 150–7.
7. Kuschinsky W. Coupling of function metabolism and blood flow in the brain. Neurosurgical Review. 1991; 14: 163–8.
8. Dirnagl U, Niwa K, Lindauer U, Villringer A. Coupling of cerebral blood flow to neuronal activation: role of adenosine and nitric oxide. American Journal of Physiology. 1994; 267: H296–H301.
9. Ogawa S, Menon RS, Tank DW, Kim SG, Merkle H, Ellermann JM et al. Functional brain mapping by blood oxygenation level-dependent contrast magnetic resonance imaging. A comparison of signal characteristics with a biophysical model. Biophysical Journal. 1993; 64: 803–12.
10. Meek JH, Firbank M, Elwell CE, Atkinson J, Braddick O, Wyatt JS. Regional hemodynamic responses to visual

stimulation in awake infants. *Pediatric Research*. 1998; **43**: 840–3.

11. Hock C, Muller-Spahn F, Schuh-Hofer S, Hofmann M, Dirnagl U, Villringer A. Age dependency of changes in cerebral hemoglobin oxygenation during brain activation: A near-infrared spectroscopy study. *Journal of Cerebral Blood Flow and Metabolism*. 1995; **15**: 1103–8.

12. Detre JA, Zhang W, Roberts DA, Silva AC, Williams DS, Grandis DJ *et al*. Tissue specific perfusion imaging using arterial spin labeling. *NMR in Biomedicine*. 1994; **7**: 75–82.

13. Wong EC, Buxton RB, Frank LR. Implementation of quantitative perfusion imaging techniques for functional brain mapping using pulsed arterial spin labeling. *NMR in Biomedicine*. 1997; **10**: 237–49.

14. Kim SG, Tsekos NV, Ashe J. Multi-slice perfusion-based functional MRI using the FAIR technique: Comparison of CBF and BOLD effects. *NMR in Biomedicine*. 1997; **10**: 191–6.

15. Friston KJ, Zarahn E, Josephs O, Henson RN, Dale AM. Stochastic designs in event-related fMRI. *Neurolmage*. 1999; **10**: 607–19.

16. Sobel N, Prabhakaran V, Desmond JE, Glover GH, Goode RL, Sullivan EV *et al*. Sniffing and smelling: Separate subsystems in the human olfactory cortex. *Nature*. 1998; **392**: 282–6.

17. Buckner RL, Bandettini PA, O'Craven KM, Savoy RL, Petersen SE, Raichle ME *et al*. Detection of cortical activation during averaged single trials of a cognitive task using functional magnetic resonance imaging. *Proceedings of the National Academy of Sciences of the United States of America*. 1996; **93**: 14878–83.

18. Grinvald A, Slovin H, Vanzetta I. Non-invasive visualization of cortical columns by fMRI. *Nature Neuroscience*. 2000; **3**: 105–7.

19. Sereno MI, Dale AM, Reppas JB, Kwong KK, Belliveau JW, Brady TJ *et al*. Functional MRI reveals borders of multiple visual areas in humans. *Science*. 1995; **268**: 889–93.

20. Servos P, Zacks J, Rumelhart DE, Glover GH. Somatotopy of the human arm using fMRI. *Neuroreport*. 1998; **9**: 605–9.

21. Liepert J, Tegenthoff M, Malin JP. Changes of cortical motor area size during immobilization. *Electroencephalogr. Clinical Neurophysiology*. 1995; **97**: 382–6.

22. Talairach J, Tournoux P. *Coplanar stereotactic atlas of the human brain: 3-dimensional system, and approach to cerebral imaging*. Stuttgart, New York: George Thieme Verlag, 1988.

23. Collins DL, Neelin P, Peters TM, Evans AC. Automatic 3D intersubject registration of MR volumetric data in standardized Talairach space. *Journal of Computer Assisted Tomography*. 1994; **18**: 192–205.

24. Van Essen DC, Drury HA. Structural and functional analyses of human cerebral cortex using a surface-based atlas. *Journal of Neuroscience*. 1997; **17**: 7079–102.

25. Van Essen DC, Drury HA, Joshi S, Miller MI. Functional and structural mapping of human cerebral cortex: solutions are in the surfaces. *Proceedings of the National Academy of Sciences of the United States of America*. 1998; **95**: 788–95.

26. Dale AM, Fischl B, Sereno MI. Cortical surface-based analysis. I. Segmentation and surface reconstruction. *Neurolmage*. 1999; **9**: 179–94.

27. Fischl B, Sereno MI, Dale AM. Cortical surface-based analysis. II: Inflation, flattening, and a surface-based coordinate system. *Neurolmage*. 1999; **9**: 195–207.

28. Palmer AR, Summerfield AQ. Microelectrode and neuroimaging studies of central auditory function. *British Medical Bulletin*. 2002; **63**: 95–105.

29. Guimaraes AR, Melcher JR, Talavage TM, Baker JR, Ledden P, Rosen BR *et al*. Imaging subcortical auditory activity in humans. *Human Brain Mapping*. 1998; **6**: 33–41.

30. Scott SK, Blank CC, Rosen S, Wise RJ. Identification of a pathway for intelligible speech in the left temporal lobe. *Brain*. 2000; **123**: 2400–6.

31. Altman NR, Bernal B. Brain activation in sedated children: auditory and visual functional MR imaging. *Radiology*. 2001; **221**: 56–63.

32. Lazeyras F, Boex C, Sigrist A, Seghier ML, Cosendai G, Terrier F *et al*. Functional MRI of auditory cortex activated by multisite electrical stimulation of the cochlea. *Neurolmage*. 2002; **17**: 1010–7.

33. Alain C, Arnott SR, Hevenor S, Graham S, Grady CL. 'What' and 'where' in the human auditory system. *Proceedings of the National Academy of Sciences of the United States of America*. 2001; **98**: 12301–6.

34. Mathiak K, Hertrich I, Grodd W, Ackermann H. Cerebellum and speech perception: a functional magnetic resonance imaging study. *Journal of Cognitive Neuroscience*. 2002; **14**: 902–12.

35. Jancke L, Gaab N, Wustenberg T, Scheich H, Heinze HJ. Short-term functional plasticity in the human auditory cortex: an fMRI study. Brain research. *Cognitive Brain Research*. 2001; **12**: 479–85.

36. Giraud AL, Truy E, Frackowiak R. Imaging plasticity in cochlear implant patients. *Audiology and Neuro-otology*. 2001; **6**: 381–93.

37. Bavelier D, Brozinsky C, Tomann A, Mitchell T, Neville H, Liu G. Impact of early deafness and early exposure to sign language on the cerebral organization for motion processing. *Journal of Neuroscience*. 2001; **21**: 8931–42.

38. Thiel CM, Bentley P, Dolan RJ. Effects of cholinergic enhancement on conditioning-related responses in human auditory cortex. *European Journal of Neuroscience*. 2002; **16**: 2199–206.

Positron emission tomography and integrated PET/ computed tomography

WAI LUP WONG

Principles of PET   684
Squamous cell carcinoma   686
Occult primary tumours   691
Other malignant tumours   692
Indeterminate pulmonary lesions   694
Alternative imaging methods for FDG uptake   694
Radiotracers other than FDG   696
Nononcological applications   696

Integrated PET/CT   696
Key points   696
Best clinical practice   696
Deficiencies in current knowledge and areas for future
　　research   697
Acknowledgements   697
References   697

SEARCH STRATEGY

This chapter is supported by literature obtained by electronic searches of four biomedical databases (Medline, Embase, Cochrane Library, PubMed) using combinations of key words including PET, PET-CT, integrated PET/CT, FDG, positron emission tomography, tomography emission computed, fluoro-deoxyglucose F18, head and neck, cancer, thyroid cancer, staging, nodal metastases, occult primary, recurrence, surveillance, coincidence imaging and gamma camera. Studies were also sought from hand searches of head and neck surgery and other relevant journals, and scanning the reference lists of relevant articles. In this discussion, PET refers to a full ring bismuth germinate PET system.

PRINCIPLES OF PET

Computed tomography (CT), magnetic resonance (MR) and ultrasound produce anatomical images, whereas positron emission tomography (PET) provides a means of identifying pathology based on altered tissue metabolism. This functional imaging technique relies on a radioactive molecule (radiotracer) that decays with positron emission. The radiotracer is given intravenously to the patient and is taken into cells. The cell recognizes it as being 'foreign' and as a consequence it is trapped early in its metabolic pathway. Malignant cells trap more radiotracer compared with nonmalignant cells. The local radiotracer concentration can be measured *in vivo* since

these unstable radiotracers decay by positron emission. Positrons travel a short distance in tissue before colliding with electrons. When they collide, the annihilation reaction results in two photons also known as gamma rays of 511 kilo electron volts (keV) each emitted at approximately 180° to each other. The photons are detected by opposing detectors. A computer reassembles these signals into images that represent radiotracer uptake in the part of the body scanned (**Figure 54.1a,b**).

One of the main strengths of PET is the ability to perform quantitative studies. Absolute quantification is not often carried out in clinical practice as it is complicated to obtain and can demand direct arterial blood sampling. The standardized uptake value (SUV),

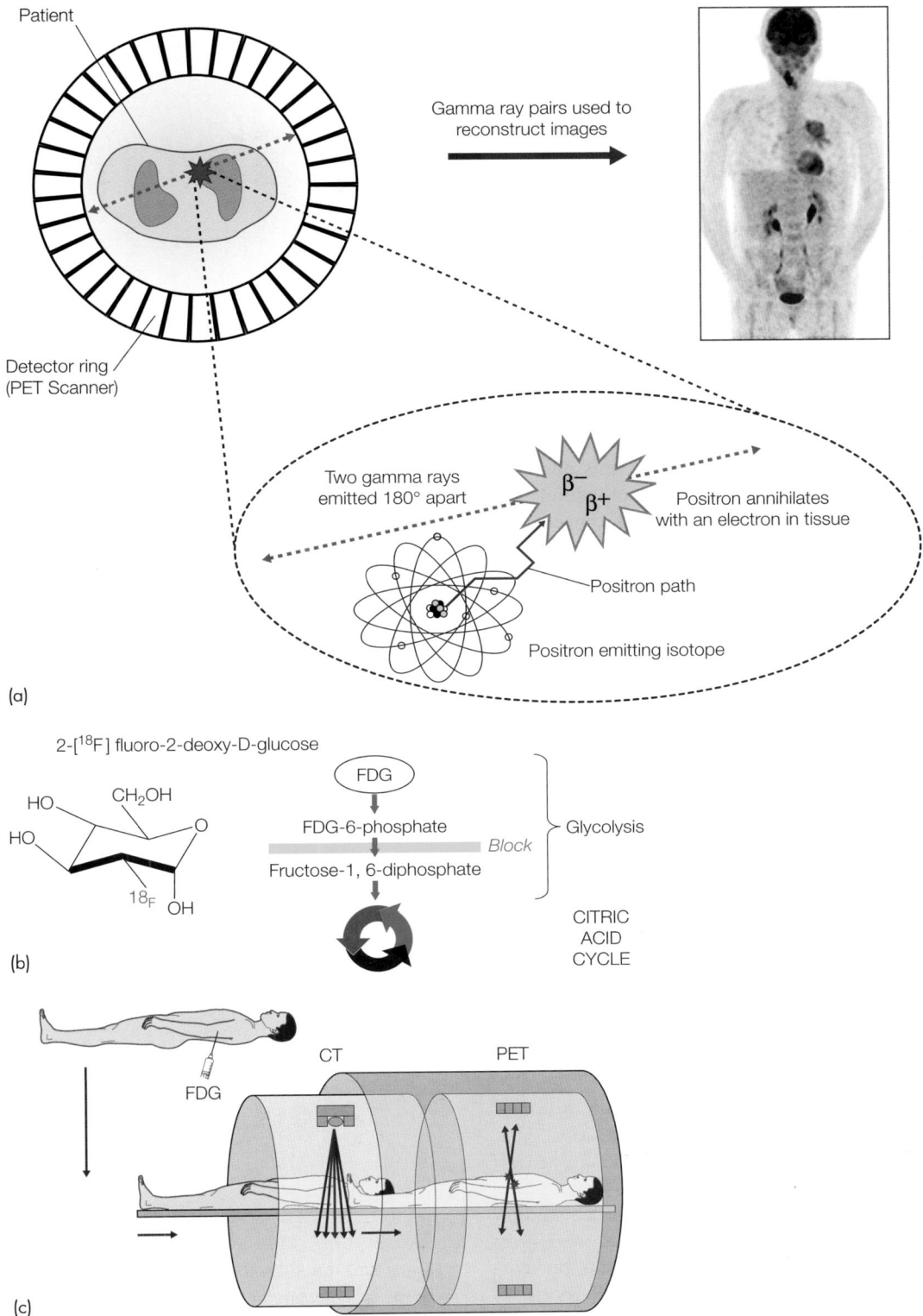

Figure 54.1 **(a)** The principles of PET imaging. Projection FDG–PET shows a patient with a primary bronchogenic carcinoma with extensive bony and cutaneous deposits. **(b)** Schematic representation of FDG metabolism. **(c)** Schematic representation of scanning with integrated PET/CT. The radiation burden is equivalent to two whole body diagnostic CTs. The CT is usually obtained using a low-voltage technique with no intravenous contrast given, but it is of diagnostic quality for detecting pulmonary metastases. Courtesy of Dr Bal Sanghera, Mount Vernon Hospital.

which provides a semiquantitative index of radiotracer uptake is widely used in clinical PET:

$$\frac{\text{Tracer uptake (MBq/mL)}}{\text{Administered activity (MBq)/(patient weight (kg)} \times 1000)}$$

PET images lack anatomical detail, which can be overcome by combining PET with CT/MR using software techniques (registration). With 2-[18F] fluoro-2-deoxy-D-glucose (FDG), these techniques are most robust in the cranium, extracranial head and neck and pelvis.[1]

Depending on the radiotracer used, different aspects of tissue metabolism can be measured, such as distribution of blood flow, oxygen utilization and protein synthesis. The overwhelming majority of clinical studies are in conjunction with an analogue of glucose, 2-[18F] fluoro-2-deoxy-D-glucose, which reflects glucose metabolism. Cancer cells have a greater avidity for glucose than normal cells. Otto Warburg and colleagues[2] made this observation in the 1920s. FDG can be used to exploit the differences in glucose metabolism between cancer cells and normal cells.

2-[18F] fluoro-2-deoxy-D-glucose–positron emission tomography (FDG-PET) has been used effectively for imaging of a variety of malignancies including breast, lung, colorectal, oesophageal cancer, brain tumours, malignant melanoma and lymphoma.[3] Seifert and others demonstrated that head and neck cancers take up FDG, an observation which was subsequently confirmed by other studies.[4]

SQUAMOUS CELL CARCINOMA

Primary disease

STAGING

FDG-PET can detect the majority of clinically visible primary tumours.[1, 5] The ability of FDG-PET to detect clinically visible lesions is of limited clinical use, but can be useful for more precisely delineating the primary tumour where submucosal extension of disease is a feature, such as in post-cricoid carcinoma and tracheal carcinoma (**Figure 54.2**).

Drawing from the cumulative results of three studies which included 2004 nodes correlated with resection specimens, FDG-PET had a sensitivity of 90 percent (200/222), specificity 94 percent (1666/1782), positive predictive value (PPV) 63 percent (200/316), negative predictive value (NPV) 99 percent (1666/1688).[6, 5, 7] With regard to 'neck sides', from the summed data of 280 neck dissections, FDG-PET had a sensitivity of 82 percent (96/117), specificity 80 percent (130/163), PPV 74 percent (96/129), NPV 86 percent (130/151) and accuracy 81 percent (226/280).[5, 7, 8, 9, 10, 11] Encouragingly,

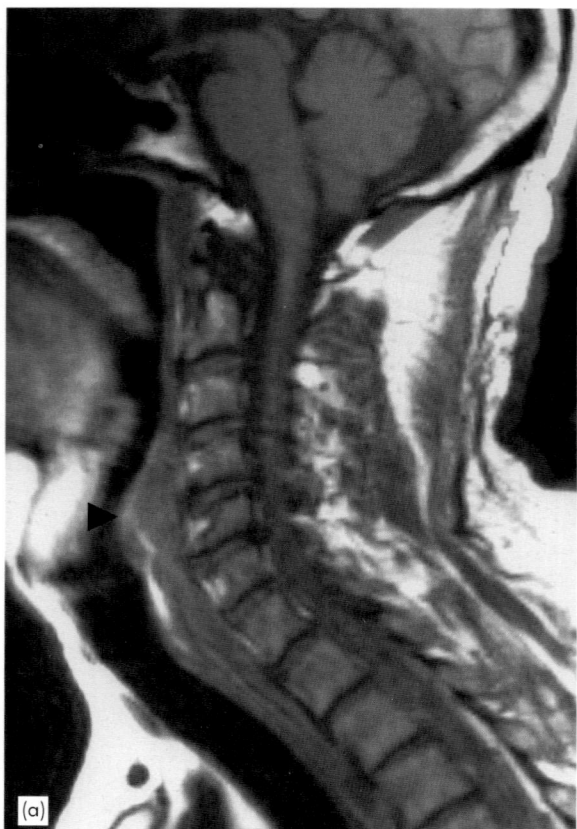

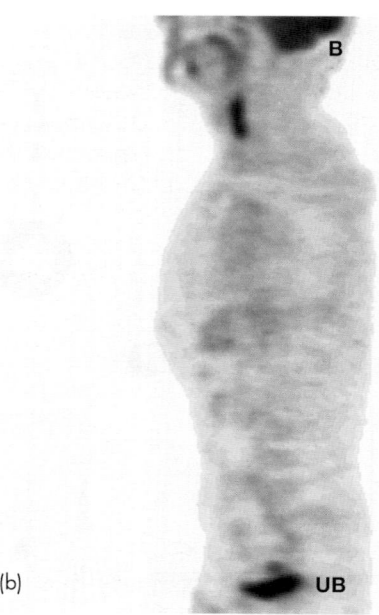

Figure 54.2 A 59-year-old man with a post-cricoid SCC. MR suggested more extensive disease than suspected on clinical assessment. **(a)** Sagittal T1-weighted MR scan demonstrates an intermediate signal intensity mass in the post-cricoid region (arrowhead). **(b)** FDG-PET sagittal image shows the post-cricoid SCC (arrowheads). The extent of disease seen on FDG-PET was in agreement with the MR. B, physiological uptake in brain; UB, normal activity in bladder as FDG is excreted via the kidneys through the bladder.

FDG-PET detected contralateral neck metastases, but it is unclear how many of these were unsuspected prior to FDG-PET.[6, 5, 7, 8, 12] All studies show a high NPV but this may be overestimated because not all patients had radical neck dissections. Preliminary results suggest that FDG-PET is at least as effective as conventional imaging, if not more so, at staging the neck.[6, 5, 7, 8, 9, 13, 14] However, the additional information gained from FDG-PET compared with other imaging is unclear. In a prospective study which included 100 neck sides, colour-coded duplex ultrasonography (CCDU) was as accurate as FDG-PET for detecting nodal disease, with similar sensitivity and specificity.[14] In accessible areas, namely levels I–VI, CCDU especially when combined with fine needle aspiration cytological examination (FNAC) may well prove to be as accurate as FDG-PET.[15] However, CCDU will not detect retropharyngeal and mediastinal nodal disease.

What is clear from the literature is that FDG-PET cannot consistently detect subclinical disease and so does not obviate elective treatment of the neck.[5, 7, 11, 12] It can have a role to play in those patients with equivocal nodal disease following conventional assessment. In patients with high risk of neck metastases, a positive scan will be highly indicative of neck nodal disease and the detection of contralateral or bilateral nodal disease can be particularly useful in this group of patients (**Figure 54.3**). Conversely, a patient with low risk of nodal metastases and a negative FDG-PET is most unlikely to have neck nodal disease (**Figure 54.4**).

In patients with advanced disease in the head and neck (stage III/IV), FDG-PET is potentially useful for detecting occult mediastinal nodal disease.[16] Distant metastatic disease in patients presenting with head and neck cancer is unusual and limits the use of FDG-PET as a screening test. However, it may have a role in those patients with a high risk of distant metastases, e.g. locally advanced nasopharyngeal cancer.[17]

Detection of synchronous malignancies

The cumulative incidence of a second malignancy following head and neck cancer is up to 15 percent. Fewer than half will have a detectable synchronous primary malignancy and almost half will be detected by a thorough clinical assessment and a further number by chest CT. So, the pick-up rate of FDG-PET at the time of primary diagnosis is likely to be 2–3 percent, substantiated by one study of 56 patients where it detected one occult lung cancer, a case finding yield of 2 percent.[18] FDG-PET has the advantage over other imaging modalities as it can scan the entire body for disease, which is often not possible with other techniques. The low rate of synchronous malignancy perhaps does not justify routine screening.

OTHER COMMENTS

Pilot studies suggest that pretreatment FDG-PET can be useful as an independent predictor of treatment response and also subsequent prognosis.[19, 20, 21, 22, 23] If these results can be substantiated, it will allow the clinician to identify patients where a more aggressive treatment approach should be considered. [***/**]

Recurrent/residual disease

PRIMARY SITE

A recent survey of the literature identified 10 relevant studies where FDG-PET was used to assess recurrent/residual disease and where there was pathological confirmation of the positive FDG-PET findings and follow-up of at least six months for negative FDG-PET results. The sensitivity of FDG-PET varied between 71 and 100 percent, the specificity between 85 and 100 percent, PPV between 64 and 100 percent, NPV between 60 and 100 percent and accuracy between 78 and 100 percent.[13, 14, 24, 25, 26, 27, 28, 29, 30, 31] The varying results are a reflection not only of the small number of patients in each study, 8 to 43 patients, but also the various different clinical situations where FDG-PET was used.

The challenging clinical issue is the detection of recurrent disease when it is still amenable to curative salvage treatment. Prospective studies that have focussed on patients who become symptomatic during follow-up show FDG-PET to be effective and superior to CT/MR in this area.[13, 14, 24, 29, 30] Cumulatively, these studies included 215 patients, 218 FDG-PET scans and an analysis of 226 anatomical sites. FDG-PET distinguished between recurrent disease and treatment sequelae at the primary site with an overall sensitivity of 88 percent (102/116), specificity 83 percent (91/110), PPV 85 percent (102/121), NPV 87 percent (91/105) and accuracy 85 percent (193/226).[13, 14, 24, 25, 26, 27, 28, 29, 30, 31] In a group of 38 patients where FDG-PET was used to differentiate between post-irradiation laryngeal recurrent cancer from laryngeal oedema, it achieved a correct diagnosis in 79 percent and was superior to CT (61 percent) and clinical assessment (43 percent).[30]

FDG-PET is potentially useful as a surveillance tool for patients with high risk of relapse. In one study, in 10/10 patients FDG-PET accurately detected the presence of recurrent disease despite negative or equivocal MR and indeterminate clinical examinations.[25] In a prospective study of 30 advanced head and neck cancer (stage III/1V) patients with FDG-PET performed 2 and 10 months after completion of therapy, FDG-PET detected all 16 recurrences which occurred during the first year post-treatment. In five of these 16 patients, FDG-PET was the only technique which detected the recurrences, four at the primary site and one patient with lung metastases.[32]

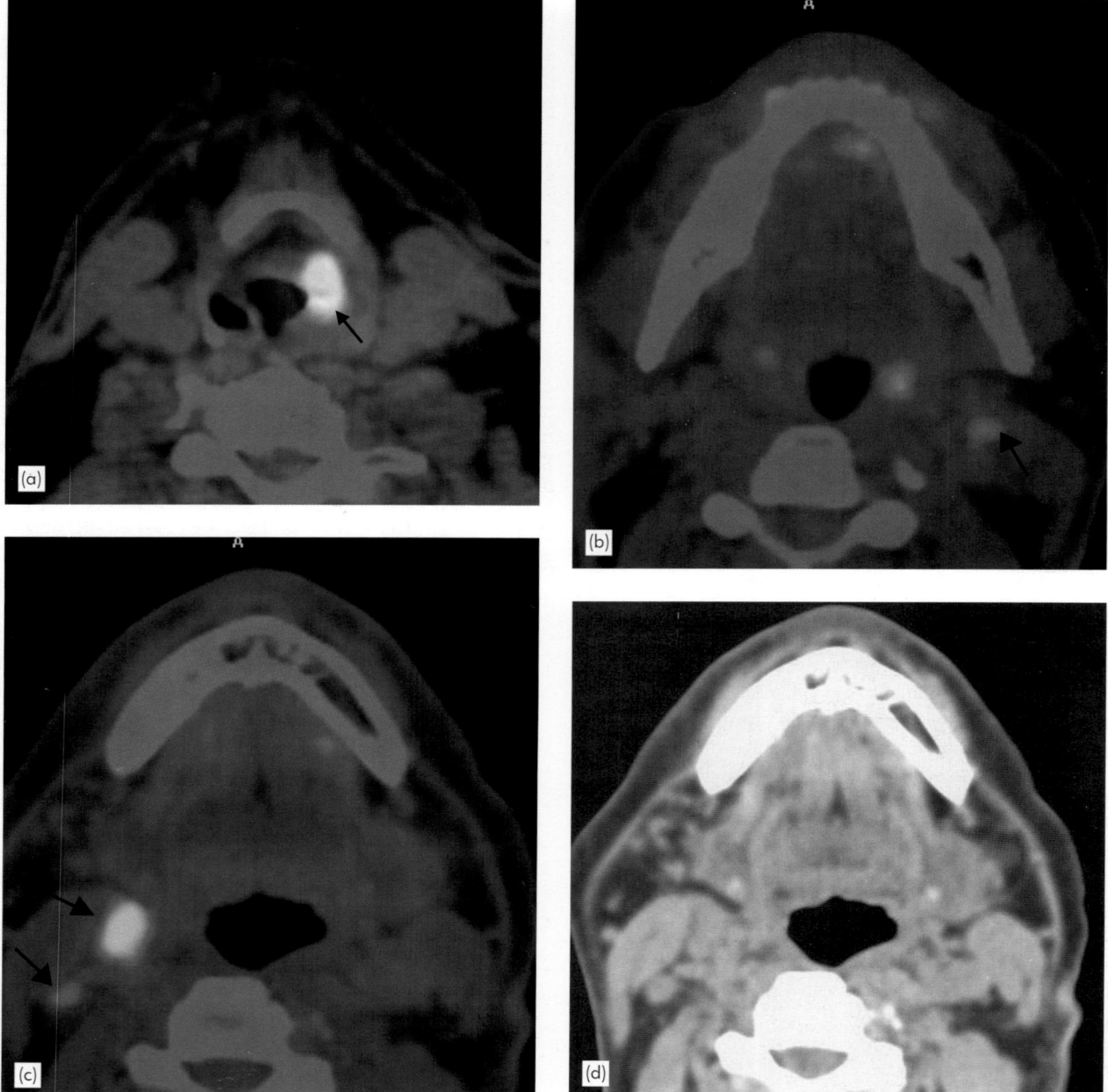

Figure 54.3 A patient referred for assessment of supraglottic laryngeal squamous cell carcinoma with equivocal nodal disease on conventional evaluation. Clinical assessment suggested contralateral nodal disease not confirmed by MR and ultrasound-guided fine needle aspiration cytology examinations. FDG with integrated PET/CT demonstrated **(a)** the primary site (arrow); **(b)** ipsilateral neck nodal disease (arrow); and also **(c)** contralateral neck nodal disease (arrows). **(d)** The contralateral neck nodal disease, which corresponded to a cluster of three subcentimetre nodes on CT, was subsequently confirmed by neck dissection.

Following radiotherapy, the minimum interval that should be allowed before performing FDG-PET for evaluation of recurrent/residual disease has yet to be determined. In a group of 25 radiotherapy (RT) patients who were followed up between 4 and 11 months and where all failures were confirmed by pathological correlation, there were fewer false-negative results when FDG-PET was performed four months after RT compared with one month following RT.[33] In a series of 44 consecutive patients there were no false-negative results, but a significant number of false-positive results when FDG-PET was performed 12 weeks or less following various treatments for recurrent/residual disease.[34] This is in contrast to our own experience of 11 patients with a high risk of recurrence where FDG-PET was performed eight weeks post-RT as part of a surveillance study. Of the nine negative studies, there was one possible false-negative result and no

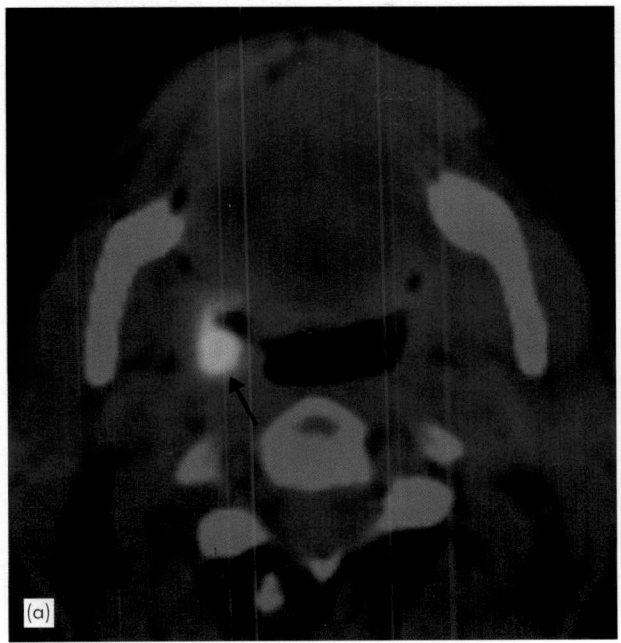

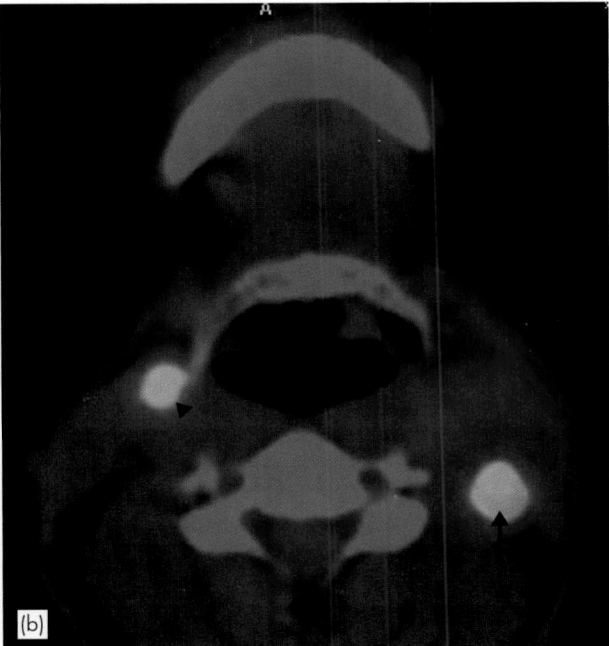

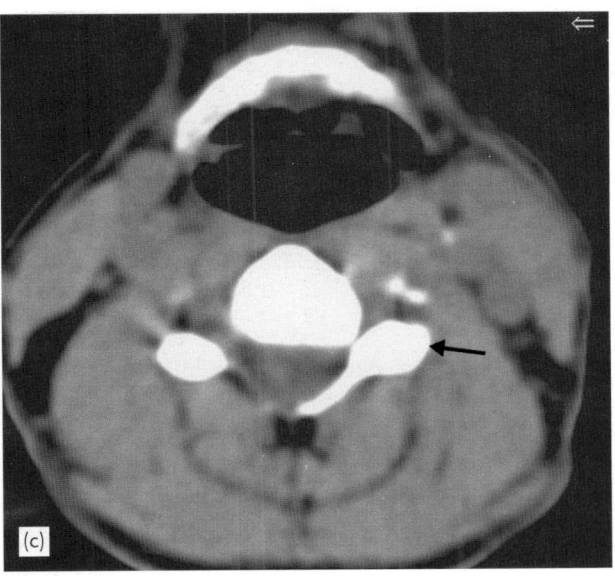

Figure 54.4 A 33-year-old woman presented with a right level II node due to SCC. Conventional assessment including EUA with multiple biopsies and CT/MR did not identify the primary site. FDG with integrated PET/CT **(a)** shows the tonsillar SCC (arrow); **(b)** confirms the level II nodal mass (arrowhead) and also shows contralateral neck nodal disease (arrow); **(c)** corresponds to a node of normal size, short axis diameter of 8 mm, on the CT component of integrated PET/CT (arrow).

false-positive results; both patients with positive FDG-PET scans relapsed.

Recurrent/residual disease as a group show higher FDG uptake compared with sequelae of treatment. Semi-quantitative analysis, however, does not improve discrimination between active disease and post-treatment changes as there is considerable overlap of SUVs between these two groups.[24, 35]

In clinical practice, FDG PET and now FDG with integrated PET/CT is routinely considered eight weeks or more following RT. A definitively positive scan should be taken as highly suspicious of disease as long as there is no infection. A negative scan is highly likely to represent absence of active disease, but still demands careful surveillance as microscopic foci of active disease cannot be excluded. An equivocal scan requires biopsy in areas of FDG activity or an early repeat FDG-PET.

FDG-PET is more accurate than conventional methods for assessment of recurrent/residual disease, but false-positive and false-negative results occur and so must be used in the context of the overall assessment of the patient.[24, 25, 26, 27, 28, 29, 31, 34, 35] A positive scan can influence a more aggressive biopsy approach and a negative scan a more conservative approach. In some instances it can be used to select sites for further biopsies in biopsy-negative patients with suspected recurrent/residual disease, thus increasing the yield of positive biopsies and avoiding unnecessary deep biopsies (**Figure 54.5**).

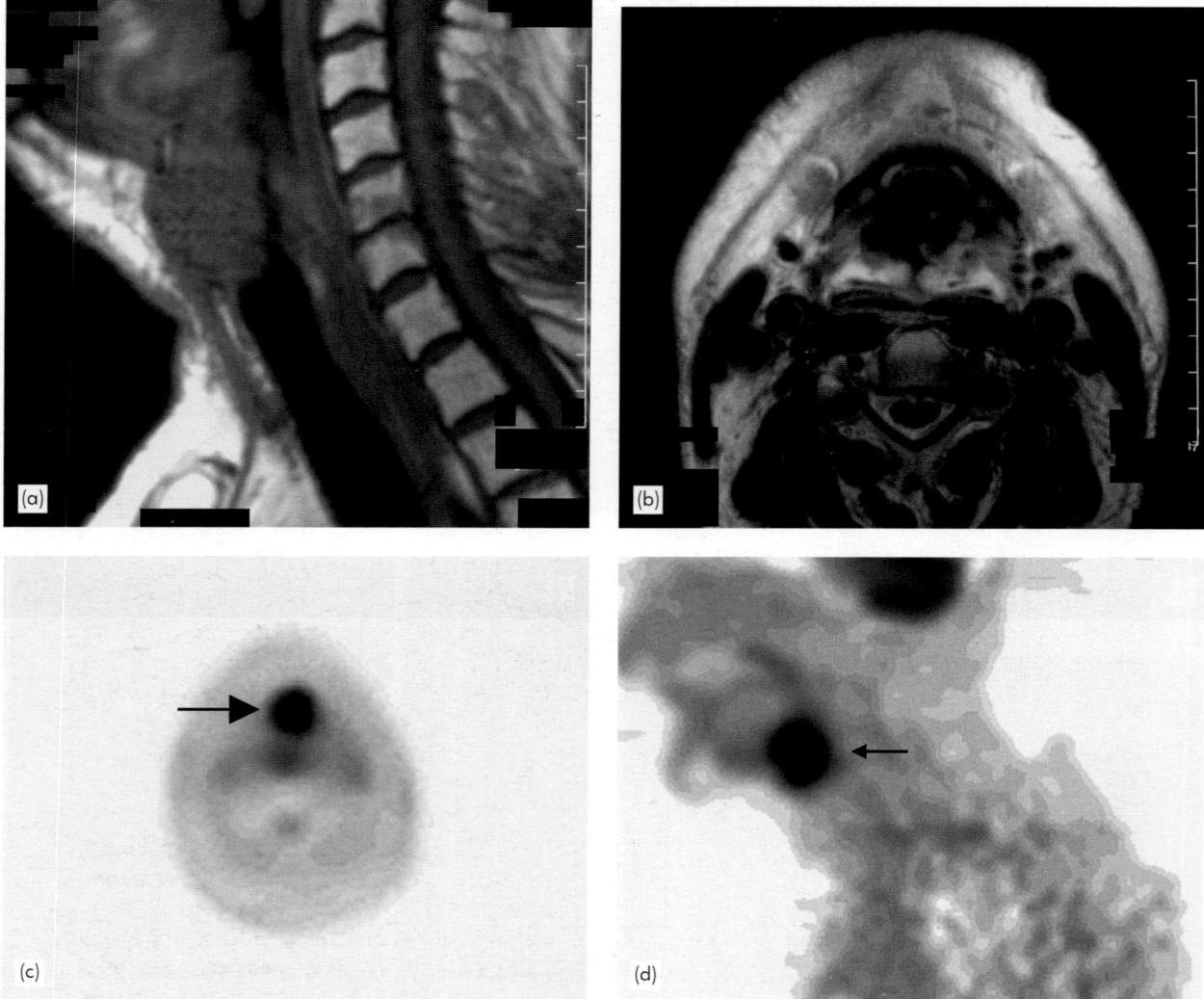

Figure 54.5 A 62-year-old man, nine months after radical RT with curative intent for a T3 N1 laryngeal SCC. EUA, including multiple biopsies, did not show active disease. (a) Sagittal T1-weighted MR scan demonstrating an intermediate signal intensity mass in the supraglottic larynx. (b) Axial T2-weighted MR scan shows the mass to be predominately of low signal. (c) FDG-PET axial and (d) sagittal images shows intensive uptake in the laryngeal oedema consistent with recurrent disease (arrow), confirmed by further biopsies.

Furthermore, as in patients with primary disease, FDG-PET will detect other unexpected cancers in some patients (**Figure 54.6**). [***/**]

Post-treatment neck assessment

Two retrospective reviews, with 34 patients in one study and 36 patients in the other, found FDG-PET had a sensitivity of 100 and 93 percent, specificity of 89 and 77 percent, PPV 70 and 72 percent, NPV 100 and 94 percent, respectively. Both studies suggested FDG-PET to be superior to CT/MR.[26, 27] These results are in agreement with a prospective study where FDG-PET identified recurrent nodal disease in all eight patients seen with suspected nodal recurrence who subsequently had histologically proven disease. In this series, the

sensitivity and specificity of FDG-PET was 100 percent, compared with CT/MR (75 and 80 percent, respectively) and clinical evaluation (100 and 60 percent, respectively).[13] These results suggest that FDG-PET is a potentially useful tool for assessing recurrent disease in the post-treatment neck and is an area that deserves further attention. [***/**]

Preliminary results show that FDG PET is accurate for detection of residual neck disease when performed at least eight weeks after chemoradiotherapy.[36, 37, 38, 39] There is considerable interest in the use of FDG with integrated PET/CT for the detection of residual disease in the neck in patients with advanced (N2 and N3) nodal metastases following chemoradiotherapy. A multicentre UK trial has recently been funded by the department of health to test the hypothesis that FDG with integrated PET/CT guided watch and wait is a valid alternative to the current

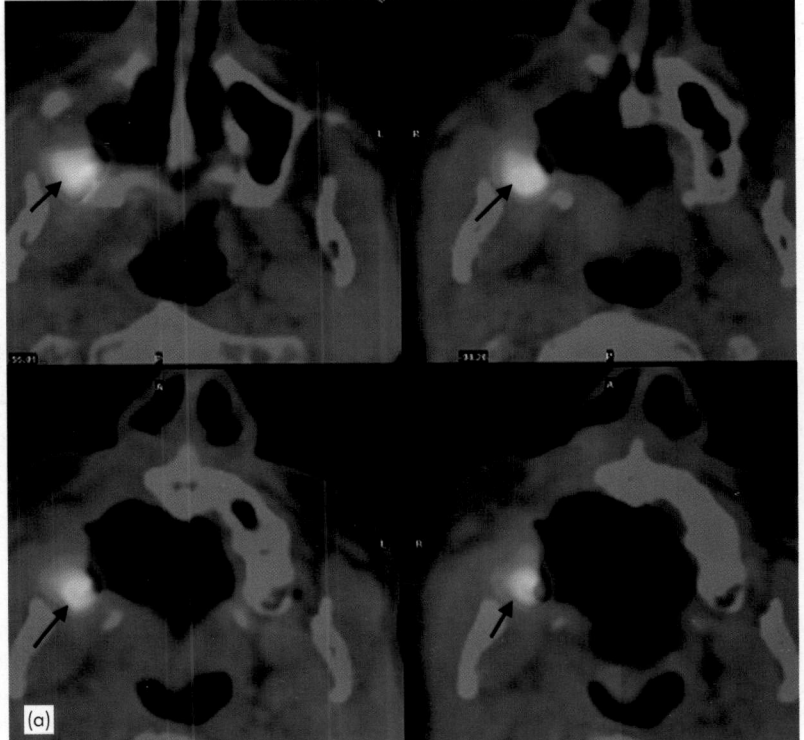

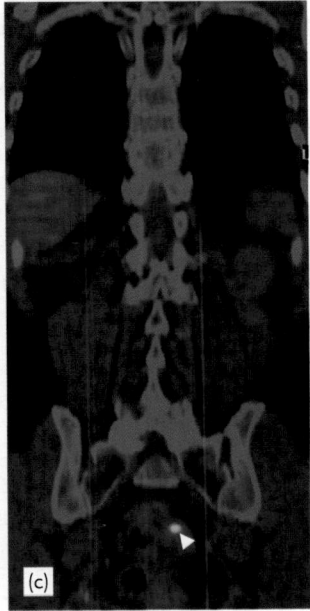

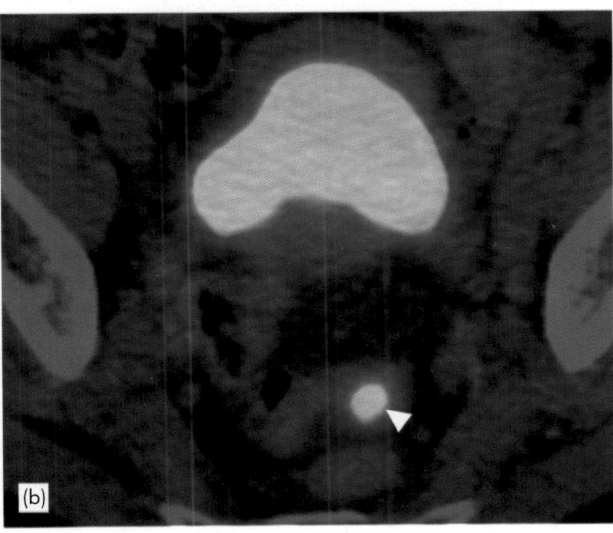

Figure 54.6 A 63-year-old man with clinical suspicion of recurrence at the surgical bed at the primary site. Direct inspection including biopsies, CT and MR did not provide a definitive diagnosis. FDG with integrated PET/CT demonstrated (a) recurrent disease within the surgical bed (arrows); (b) and (c) uptake in the rectum suspicious of rectal carcinoma (arrowheads), confirmed by subsequent colonoscopy and biopsies.

practice of planned neck dissection in this group of patients. Results from this study are awaited with interest.

OCCULT PRIMARY TUMOURS

The cornerstone for investigating this group of patients is with examination under anaesthesia (EUA), including multiple biopsies and CT/MR. As such, FDG-PET can only be justified if it can detect more primary sites following these investigations. The various studies which have investigated FDG-PET in this setting have shown, without exception, that FDG-PET can detect more primary sites compared with conventional assessment.[40, 41, 42, 43, 44, 45, 46] In a study of 27 patients which included 21 squamous cell carcinomas (SCC) and undifferentiated carcinomas, FDG-PET showed 28 percent more histologically proven primary sites.[45] Our own experience is similar with FDG-PET detecting 29 percent more pathologically confirmed primary sites.[46] In four other studies, with 7–14 patients with occult SCC or undifferentiated carcinoma in each study, FDG-PET detected between 8 and 42 percent more histologically verified primary sites compared with conventional work up.[40, 41, 42, 43, 44] Some of the occult primaries detected were lung cancers in patients who did not have chest CT; it is unclear how many of these lung cancers would have been detected by CT. Excluding the lung cancers, FDG-PET detected up to 20 percent more primary sites.[40, 41, 42, 43, 44]

Well-documented false-positive results are unusual in the literature: there were 15 (9 percent) clinically or histologically verified cases from a cumulative total of 173 head and neck sites (nasopharynx, 2; tonsil, 5; tongue base, 3; submandibular gland, 1; oral cavity, 1; thyroid, 2; epiglottis, 1) and a further five (2 percent) in the lungs where no tumour was identified at subsequent broncho-scopy or CT.[27, 40, 41, 42, 43, 44, 45, 46, 47, 48] One study is at variance with a false-positive result of 46 percent (6/13);[43] the authors suggest that it was possible that the biopsy was in error and that the true PPV of the technique was underestimated. In one study, all 17 patients including the three patients where FDG-PET showed a primary site which was not subsequently confirmed, were treated on the basis of the FDG-PET result. No other primary head and neck tumour developed during subsequent follow-up in any of the patients.[46] This result supports the speculation that FDG-PET may be more specific than the current figures indicate. Further clarification may be available with long-term follow-up of larger groups of patients.

Inflammatory pulmonary lesions including granulo-mas and abscesses and recent biopsy can result in false-positive FDG-PET.[40, 42] Dental caries and benign thyroid and salivary gland nodules are recognized causes of intense FDG uptake and so do not usually cause a diagnostic dilemma. We have found that tonsillectomy can cause potential confusion, not on the side of surgery but on the contralateral side, where normal tonsillar uptake in the remaining tonsil can mimic a malignancy.

Considering all the studies with false-negative results reported, there was a cumulative total of over 127 patients and only 10 (8 percent) false-negative results confirmed at histology or subsequent follow-up: tongue carcinoma, 3, including 2 base of tongue carcinomas; tonsillar carcino-ma, 2; nasopharyngeal cancer, 1; lung cancer, 2; mesothe-lioma, 1; and gastric carcinoma, 1.[27, 40, 41, 42, 43, 44, 45, 46] The ability to detect cancers less than 1 cm in diameter with FDG-PET is currently unclear. Using attenuation corrected scanning, FDG-PET showed a 4-mm base of tongue SCC in one study.[40] Even in retrospect, a further study failed to show a 7-mm pharyngeal wall SCC with attenuation correction scanning.[46]

Most studies report that in the majority of patients with an occult primary tumour after staging which includes FDG-PET, no head and neck primary tumour will emerge after treatment during subsequent follow-up.[40, 41, 42, 43, 44, 45, 46, 47, 48]

FDG-PET can influence the therapeutic plan further in up to 59 percent of patients.[41, 42, 44, 45, 46, 47, 48] It can alter management by not only identifying the primary site, but also other occult sites of disease including bony metastases, mediastinal nodal disease and synchronous carcinomas at other sites.[40, 45]

Biopsies carried out after FDG-PET can improve the number of occult primaries detected compared with EUA with speculative biopsies.[40, 41, 42, 45] [***/**]

OTHER MALIGNANT TUMOURS

FDG-PET is of limited value for the preoperative assessment of thyroid nodules as both malignant and benign thyroid lesions can be equally avid for FDG. However, it can have a role in the assessment of the post-treatment patient. In a study of 24 patients with treated differentiated papillary and follicular thyroid cancer, the metastases had an alternating pattern of uptake with 131-iodine and FDG. Either some 131-iodine uptake com-bined with low FDG trapping or no 131-iodine uptake combined with high FDG trapping.[49] The hypothesis was that persistent iodine metabolism is consistent with better cell differentiation, while the loss of this ability together with increased glucose metabolism is consistent with dedifferentiation.[49] Several reports have demonstrated the value of FDG-PET in treated papillary and follicular thyroid cancer patients who have suspected recurrent disease with a high thyroglobulin levels and negative 131-iodine scan.[49, 50, 51, 52, 53] In a retrospective review, FDG-PET was found to be useful in 64 percent (39/61) of patients who had an elevated thyroglobulin and negative 131-iodine scan with a PPV of 83 percent (34/41) and an NPV of 25 percent (5/20). Furthermore, true positive FDG-PET findings correlated positively with increasing thyroglobulin levels.[52] In a study of 18 patients with elevated thyroglobulin levels FDG-PET localized occult disease in 71 percent (12/17) of patients who subse-quently had confirmation of disease, mainly unsuspected neck and chest nodal disease; FDG-PET was of much more limited value in patients with normal thyroglobulin levels.[53]

The overall accuracy of FDG-PET in this setting is unclear. In all published studies, many lesions were not verified histopathologically and in most studies the follow-up period after FDG-PET was unclear. The incremental improvement afforded by FDG-PET over other imaging is also uncertain. Various studies show FDG-PET has an advantage over 131-iodine in its ability to detect more nodal disease in the neck and in the mediastinum.[53, 54, 55, 56] With regard to the neck, however, none of these studies systematically compared neck MR and ultrasound with FDG-PET. In one survey, minimal cervical nodal disease present in three patients not detected by 131-iodine and FDG-PET was shown on ultrasound.[53] In most of the patients where FDG-PET detected mediastinal nodal disease, a comparison with CT (chest) was not made. In the literature, FDG-PET demonstrated lung metastases which were not iodine avid, but these same studies showed that CT was superior to FDG-PET in this area (**Figure 54.7**).[53, 55]

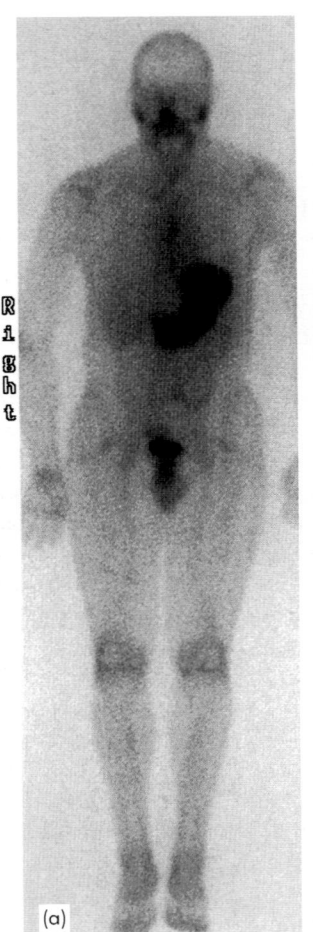 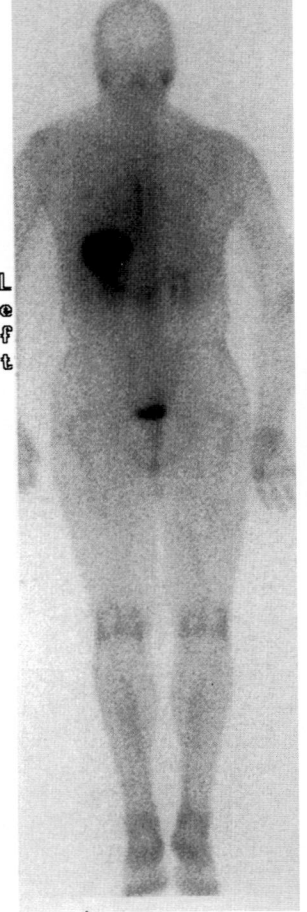

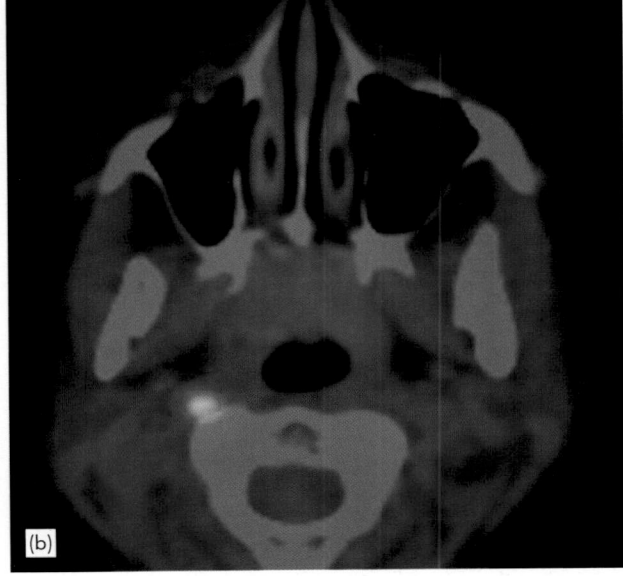

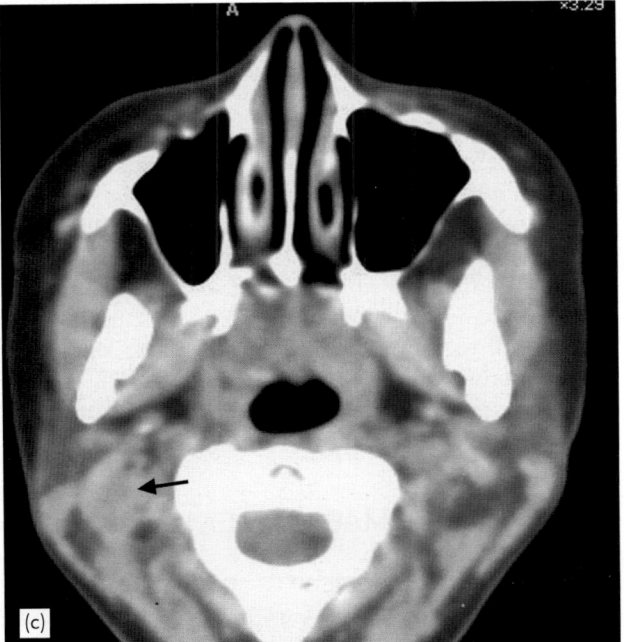

Figure 54.7 A 38-year-old man who presented with elevated thyroglobulin after total thyroidectomy and 131-iodine ablation for papillary thyroid cancer. (a) Whole body 123-iodine scan showed no active disease. (b) FDG with integrated PET/CT shows the nodal recurrence corresponding to (c) normal sized nodes on CT (arrow). Surgery and histological examination confirmed retropharyngeal nodal disease.

Thallium and hexakis (2-methoxyisobutyl-isonitirile) technetium-99m (MIBI) have been proven to be useful radiopharmaceuticals as alternatives to 131-iodine in the follow-up of differentiated thyroid cancer. A retrospective multicentre study evaluated the use of 131-iodine, FDG and MIBI in the follow-up of 222 such patients. FDG was more sensitive than iodine 131 and MIBI, 75, 50 and 53 percent respectively with no compromise in specificity, 90, 99 and 92 percent, respectively.[51]

FDG-PET can detect metastases from Hurthle cell carcinoma and anaplastic carcinoma.[53, 57] Its clinical value in these tumours is currently unclear.

With medullary thyroid cancer, preliminary results suggest FDG-PET to be an accurate technique for detecting metastases and recurrent disease. The largest study in the literature, a German multicentre retrospective survey, reviewed 100 FDG-PET studies performed on 85 patients. The results of the FDG-PET were compared with 46 indium-111 pentetreotide (SMS) studies, 33 pentavalent technetium dimercaptosuccinate acid (DMSA) scans, 8 hexakis (2-methoxyisobutyl-isonitirile) technetium-99m (MIBI) scans, 64 CT and 37 MR. One hundred and eighty-one lesions were identified by at least one technique; FDG-PET detected the majority of lesions with a lesion detection probability of 68 percent compared with 25 percent for SMS, 29 percent for DMSA, 6 percent for MIBI, 53 percent for CT and 58 percent for MR. In the 55 lesions confirmed histologically, FDG-PET had the highest overall accuracy with a sensitivity of 78 percent and specificity of 79 percent; MR had a slightly higher sensitivity of 82 percent, but a specificity of 67 percent and MIBI had a specificity of 100 percent, but a sensitivity of only 25 percent.[58]

In one published report of postoperative parathyroid carcinoma, FDG-PET provided more accurate information compared with other imaging.[59]

FDG-PET cannot reliably distinguish between malignant and benign major salivary gland tumours as both can be equally FDG avid. It can, however, be useful for distinguishing active disease from sequelae of treatment.

FDG-PET is effective for detecting lymphoma except low-grade non-Hodgkin's lymphoma and extranodal marginal zone B-cell lymphoma, which are not consistently FDG avid.[60, 61]

Head and neck malignant melanomas, sarcomas and paraganglionomas have been shown to be FDG avid.[62, 63] FDG-PET can be useful in these rare head and neck tumours for detecting occult sites of disease, especially when more disease is suspected than can be accounted for by conventional assessment, provided the known sites of disease are FDG avid (**Figure 54.8**). [***/**]

INDETERMINATE PULMONARY LESIONS

Cancer patients with indeterminate pulmonary lesions following full clinical and radiological assessment can

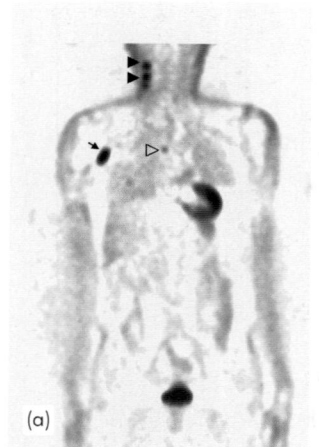
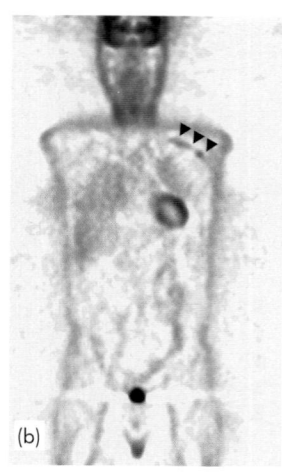

Figure 54.8 A 49-year-old man presented with left neck nodes due to high-grade non-Hodgkin's lymphoma (NHL). He had systemic symptoms but conventional assessment showed disease that was localized to the left neck. **(a)** FDG-PET coronal slice demonstrates disease in the neck (arrowheads) and also in the mediastinum (hollow arrowhead) and axilla (arrow). The patient's management was changed from localized RT to the neck to chemotherapy. **(b)** Following chemotherapy, the FDG abnormalities in the neck, axilla and mediastinum resolved. Increased uptake is seen along an infected Hickmann line (arrowheads).

present a diagnostic dilemma to the surgeon, and head and neck cancer patients are no exception. Accurate characterization of the pulmonary abnormality can alter treatment plan. FDG-PET has been shown to be an accurate noninvasive test for the diagnosis of pulmonary lesions (**Figure 54.9**). A metanalysis of the data from 40 studies showed FDG-PET has a sensitivity of 96.8 percent and specificity of 77.8 percent.[64] Abscesses and granulomas including those due to sarcoid, tuberculosis (TB), anthracite and fungus (asperilloma, blastomycosis, cocidiomycosis, cryptococcis, histolplasmosis) can mimic malignant lesions.[65] False-negative FDG-PET results are very unusual, although bronchoalveolar carcinoma, highly differentiated neuroendocrine carcinoma and adenocarcinoma, especially within a scar, have been reported to cause confusion.[65] Lesions smaller than 1 cm across can be detected by FDG-PET, but false-negative results do occur and so a negative scan must be interpreted with caution.[65] [***/**]

ALTERNATIVE IMAGING METHODS FOR FDG UPTAKE

Owing to the high costs and limited availability of full ring bismuth germinate PET systems, alternative methods of imaging 511 keV photons of positron emitters have been sought. To this end, partial ring bismuth germinate systems, such as the ECAT advanced rotating tomograph (ART), scanners with six positron-sensitive sodium

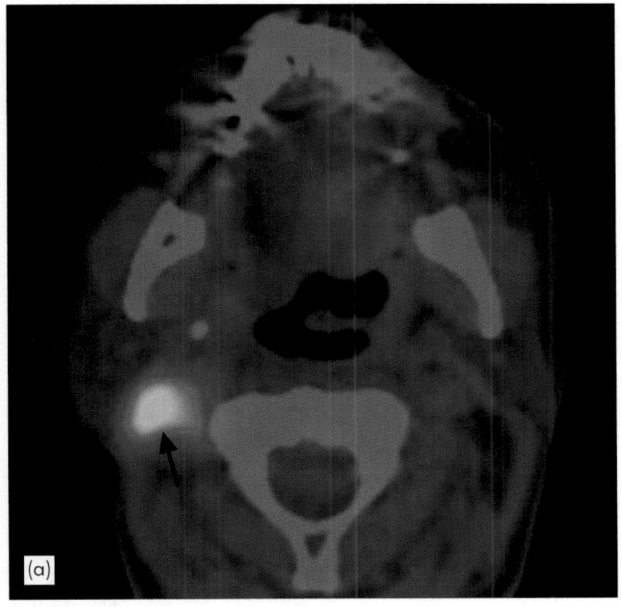

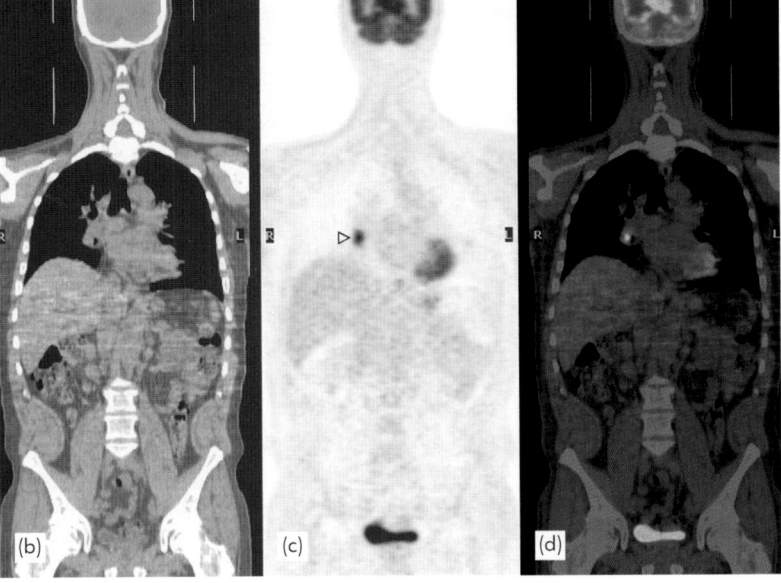

Figure 54.9 A 54-year-old man with clinical suspicion of recurrence of oropharyngeal cancer. CT and MR did not provide a definitive diagnosis. **(a)** FDG with integrated PET/CT demonstrated recurrent disease in the post-treatment neck (arrow); and **(b)**, **(c)** and **(d)** uptake in the right hilum of the lung suspicious of a bronchogenic carcinoma (hollow arrowhead), confirmed by subsequent bronchoscopy and biopsies.

iodide detectors and dual-headed gamma cameras operating in coincidence have been developed. These systems are less sensitive compared with full ring dedicated PET systems. Nevertheless, their performance may be adequate in the specific clinical settings.

Stokkel and colleagues, in a retrospective review of 54 consecutive SCC patients, found FDG dual-head PET a valuable tool for staging the neck.[66] In a prospective study of 48 patients with suspected recurrent laryngeal or hypopharyngeal cancer, the results obtained with FDG dual-headed PET was comparable with those from studies using full ring PET.[67] Similar results were obtained in one study using a sodium iodide detector system and a partial ring PET in another; in both, FDG was superior to CT/MR.[68, 69]

In three studies, non-full ring PET systems detected 28–73 percent more occult head and neck primary tumours compared with conventional imaging. It is unclear how many of the occult malignancies would have been detected by EUA and multiple biopsies, as FDG was performed prior to EUA in all patients studied.[69, 70, 71]

With regards to thyroid cancer, several pilot studies have shown the feasibility of FDG dual-head PET for detecting recurrent disease in patients with elevated thyroglobulin and negative 131-iodine scan.[72, 73]

Despite these encouraging preliminary reports for the use of non-full ring PET for the assessment of head and neck cancer patients, there is now very limited interest in the use of this technology with the advent of combined PET-CT scanners.

RADIOTRACERS OTHER THAN FDG

Carotid artery resection may occasionally offer a chance of cure in patients with advanced head and neck cancer. [15-O] H$_2$O PET has been used a rapid quantitative means of determining cerebral blood flow prior to carotid artery resection in this group of patients.[74]

Beyond clinical studies, PET provides the unique opportunity to assess specific biological characteristics of head and neck cancer with minimal disturbance of tumour physiology. Hypoxic areas in head and neck tumours have been successfully evaluated with PET using radiolabelled nitroimidazole compounds including fluorine-18 fluoromisonidazole (FMISO) and fluorine-18 fluoroerythronitroimidazone (FETNIM).[75, 76] Thymidine labelled with 11-carbon, [methyl-11C] thymidine and L-[methyl-11C] methionine (11-C methionine) have been developed to enable the measurement of the proliferative capacity of head and neck tumours.[77, 78] Chao and others demonstrated the feasibility of using Cu(II)-diacetyl-bis-N4-methylthiosemicarbozone (Cu-ATSM), a hypoxic marker, for planning intensity modulated radiotherapy.[79]

NONONCOLOGICAL APPLICATIONS

FDG-PET is potentially a useful tool in the assessment of cochlea implants and their pattern on stimulation of the central nervous system. A pilot study using FDG-PET and [15-O] H$_2$O demonstrated that the primary auditory cortex does not develop normally in prelingually deaf subjects, but that in post-lingually deaf subjects this is not so and the primary auditory cortex may be reactivated by cochlear implant after many years of deafness.[80]

INTEGRATED PET/CT

Positron emission tomography is limited by the imprecise localization of radiotracer. Software image fusion is labour-intensive and is usually unsuccessful unless data are acquired prospectively. Furthermore, accurate software registration is generally only valid for FDG-PET. The advantages of integrated PET/CT include superior localization of lesions and better distinction between physiological uptake and pathology. With PET/CT, CT is acquired followed by PET. Using CT for attenuation correction also means shorter scanning times; 30 minutes compared with 60 minutes with standard FDG PET. PET/CT should augment the information provided by PET; it will more accurately localize the occult primary in the orophyarnx. In patients with suspected recurrence of thyroid cancer, the CT component will detect pulmonary metastases not identified on FDG and in other patients more precise anatomical localization of active disease within treatment sequelae will influence the treatment plan.[81, 82, 83]

✓ Patients with indeterminate lung lesions which are not accessible to precutaneous biopsy or where a pneumothorax would be particularly hazardous. [Grade C/D]

Deficiencies in current knowledge and areas for future research

➤ Large prospective comparative studies of FDG with integrated PET/CT with state-of-the-art ultrasound (neck) for patients referred for assessment of primary disease and equivocal necks following conventional assessment.

➤ Prospective studies evaluating FDG with integrated PET/CT as an early predictor of response to treatment and as an independent prognostic factor for head and neck SCC.

➤ Large prospective studies evaluating the value of FDG with integrated PET/CT as a surveillance tool in head and neck SCC patients with high risk of recurrence.

➤ Prospective comparative studies including MR and state-of-the-art neck ultrasound, CT (chest) and FDG with integrated PET/CT for the assessment of patients with treated differentiated thyroid cancer, elevated thyroglobulin and negative whole body 131-I scan.

➤ Integrated PET/CT studies with hypoxic and cell proliferation markers for evaluating the biology of malignant head and neck tumours.

ACKNOWLEDGEMENTS

I am very grateful to my clinical oncology and head and neck surgery colleagues with whom I work closely, especially Professor Michele Saunders, Mr Roy Farrell, Dr Katherine Lemon, Dr Kate Goodchild. I also gratefully acknowledge Dr Jane Chambers for her useful critical comments.

REFERENCES

1. Wong WL, Hussain K, Chevretton E, Hawkes DJ, Baddeley H, Maisey M et al. Validation and clinical application of computer-combined computed tomography and positron emission tomography with 2-(18F)fluoro-2-deoxy-d-glucose head and neck images. *American Journal of Surgery*. 1996; **172**: 628–32.

2. Warburg O, Wind F, Negelein G. Uber den stoffwechsel von tumoren im korper. *Klinische Wochenschrift*. 1926; **5**: 829–32.

3. Hustinx R, Benard F, Alavi A. Whole body FDG-PET imaging in the management of patients with cancer. *Seminars in Nuclear Medicine*. 2002; **32**: 35–46.

4. Seifert E, Schadel A, Haberkorn U, Strauss LG. Evaluating the effectiveness of chemotherapy in patients with head and neck tumours using positron emission tomography. *HNO*. 1992; **40**: 90–3.

5. Braams JW, Pruim J, Freling NJM, Nikkels PGJ, Rodenburg JLN, Boering G et al. Detection of lymph node metastases of squamous cell cancer of the head and neck with FDG-PET and MR. *Journal of Nuclear Medicine*. 1995; **36**: 211–6.

6. Adams S, Baum RP, Stuckensen T, Bitter K, Hor G. Prospective comparison of 18-F-FDG with conventional imaging modalities (CT, MRI, US) in lymph node staging of head and neck cancer. *European Journal of Nuclear Medicine*. 1998; **25**: 1255–60.

7. Laubenbacher C, Saumweber D, Wagner-Manslau C, Kau RJ, Herz M, Avril N et al. Comparision of fluorine-18-fluorodeoxyglucose PET, MR and endoscopy for head and neck squamous cell carcinoma. *Journal of Nuclear Medicine*. 1995; **36**: 1747–57.

8. Kau RJ, Alexiou C, Laubenbacher C, Werner M, Schwaiger M, Arnold W. Lymph node detection of head and neck squamous cell carcinomas by positron emission tomography with fluorodeoxyglucose F18 in a routine clinical setting. *Archives of Otoloaryngology – Head and Neck Surgery*. 1999; **125**: 1322–8.

9. McGuirt WF, Williams III DW, Keyes JW, Greven KM, Watson Jr. NE, Geisinger KM et al. A comparative diagnostic study of head and neck metastases using positron emission tomography. *Laryngoscope*. 1995; **105**: 373–5.

10. Myers LL, Wax MK, Nabi H, Simpson GT, Lamonica D. Positron emission tomography in the evaluation of the N0 neck. *Laryngoscope*. 1998; **108**: 232–6.

11. Stoeckli SJ, Steinert H, Pflaltz M, Schmid S. Is there a role for positron emission tomography with 18F-fluorodeoxyglucose in the initial staging of nodal negative oral and oropharyngeal squamous cell carcinoma. *Head and Neck*. 2002; **24**: 345–9.

12. Nowak B, di Martino E, Janicke S, Cremerius U, Adam G, Zimmy M et al. Diagnostik maligner Kopf-Hals-Tumouren durch F-18-FDG PET im vergleich zu CT/MRT. *Nuklearmedizin*. 1999; **38**: 312–8.

13. Wong WL, Chevretton E, McGurk M, Hussain K, Davis J, Beaney R et al. A prospective study of FDG PET imaging for the assessment of head and neck squamous cell carcinoma. *Clinical Otolaryngology*. 1977; **22**: 209–14.

14. di Martino E, Nowak B, Hassan HA, Hausman R, Adam G, Buell U et al. Diagnosis and staging of head and neck cancer – a comparision of modern imaging modalities (positron emission tomography, computed tomography, colour coded duplex sonography) with pan endoscopic and histopathological findings. *Archives of Otolaryngology – Head and Neck Surgery*. 2000; **126**: 1457–61.

15. Brouwer J, de Bree Remco, Comans EFJ, Castelijns JA, Hoekstra OS, Leemans CE. Positron emission tomography using [18F] flurodeoxyglucose (FDG-PET) in the clinically negative neck: is it likely to be superior? *European Archives of Oto-rhino-laryngology.* 2004; **261**: 479–83.

16. Teknos TN, Rosenthal EL, Lee D, Taylor R, Marn CS. Positron emission tomography in the evaluation of stage III and IV head and neck cancer. *Head and Neck.* 2001; **23**: 1056–60.

17. Chang J T-C, Chan S-C, Yen T-C, Liao C-T, Lin C-Y, Lin K-J et al. Nasopharyngeal carcinoma by (18)-F-fluorodeoxyglucose positron emission tomography. *International Journal of Radiation Oncology, Biology, Physics.* 2005; **62**: 501–7.

18. Keyes JW, Chen MYM, Watson Jr. NE, Greven KM, McGuirt WF, Williams III DW. FDG PET evaluation of head and neck cancer: value of imaging the thorax. *Head and Neck.* 2000; **22**: 105–10.

19. Brun E, Ohlsson T, Erlandsson K, Kjellen E, Sandell A, Tennvall J et al. Early prediction of treatment outcome in head and neck cancer with 2-18FDG PET. *Acta Oncologica.* 1997; **36**: 741–7.

20. Halfpenny W, Hain SF, Biassoni L, Maisey MN, Sherman JA, McGurk M. FDG PE. A possible prognostic factor in head and neck cancer. *British Journal of Cancer.* 2002; **86**: 512–6.

21. Minn H, Lapela M, Klemi PJ, Grenman R, Leskinen S, Lindholm P et al. Prediction of survival with fluorine-18-flurodeoxyglucose and PET in head and neck cancer. *Journal of Nuclear Medicine.* 1997; **38**: 1907–11.

22. Rege S, Safa AA, Chaikin L, Hoh C, Juillard G, Withers R. Positron emission tomography: An independent indicator of radiocurability in head and neck carcinomas. *American Journal of Clinical Oncology.* 2000; **23**: 164–9.

23. Allal AS, Dugluerov P, Allaoua M, Haenggeli C-A, El Ghazi EA, Lehmann E et al. Standardized uptake value of 2-[18F] Fluoro-2-Deoxy-D-glucose in predicting outcome in head and neck carcinomas treated with radiotherapy with and without chemotherapy. *Journal of Clinical Oncology.* 2002; **20**: 1398–404.

24. Anzai Y, Carroll WR, Quint DJ, Bradford CR, Minoshima S, Gregory T et al. Recurrence of head and neck cancer after surgery or irradiation: Prospective comparison of 2-deoxy-2-(F-18)fluoro-d-glucose PET and MR imaging diagnoses. *Radiology.* 1996; **200**: 135–41.

25. Bailet JW, Sercarz JA, Abemayor E, Anzai Y, Lufkin RB, Hoh CK. The use of positron emission tomography for early detection of recurrent head and neck squamous cell carcinoma in postradiotherapy patients. *Laryngoscope.* 1995; **105**: 135–9.

26. Fischbein NJ, Aassar OS, Caputo GR, Kaplan MJ, Singer MI, Price DC et al. Clinical utility of positron emission tomography with ^{18}F-fluorodeoxyglucose in detecting residual/recurrent squamous cell carcinoma of the head and neck. *AJNR American Journal of Neuroradiology.* 1998; **19**: 1189–96.

27. Hanasono MM, Kunda LD, Segall GM, Ku GH, Terris DJ. Uses and limitations of FDG positron emission tomography in patients with head and neck cancer. *Laryngoscope.* 1999; **109**: 880–5.

28. Kim HJ, Boyd J, Dunphy F, Lowe AV. F-18 FDG PET scan after radiotherapy for early-stage larynx cancer. *Clinical Nuclear Medicine.* 1998; **23**: 750–2.

29. Lapela M, Grenman R, Kurki T, Joensuu H, Leskinen S, Lindholm P et al. Head and neck cancer: Detection of recurrence with PET and 2-(F-18)Fluoro-2-deoxy-d-glucose. *Radiology.* 1995; **197**: 205–11.

30. McGuirt WF, Greven KM, Keyes JW, Williams III DW, Watson N. Laryngeal radionecrosis versus recurrent cancer: A clinical approach. *Annals of Otology, Rhinology, and Laryngology.* 1998; **107**: 293–6.

31. Li P, Shuang H, Mozley PD, Denittis A, Yeh D, Machtay M et al. Evaluation of recurrent squamous cell carcinoma of the head and neck with FDG positron emission tomography. *Clinical Nuclear Medicine.* 2001; **26**: 131–5.

32. Lowe VJ, Boyd JH, Dunphy FR, Kim H, Dunleavy T, Collins BT et al. Surveillance for recurrent head and neck cancer using positron emission tomography. *Journal of Clinical Oncology.* 2000; **18**: 651–8.

33. Greven KM, Williams III DW, Keyes JW, McGuirt WF, Watson NE, Randall ME et al. Positron emission tomography of patients with head and neck carcinoma before and after high dose irradiation. *Cancer.* 1994; **74**: 1355–9.

34. Lonneux M, Lawson G, Ide C, Bausart R, Remacle M, Pauwels S. Positron emission tomography with fluorodeoxyglucose for suspected head and neck tumor recurrence in the symptomatic patient. *Laryngoscope.* 2000; **110**: 1493–7.

35. Lapela M, Eigtved A, Jyrkkio S, Grenman R, Kurki T, Lindholm P et al. Experience in qualitative and quantitative FDG PET in follow-up of patients with suspected recurrence from head and neck cancer. *European Journal of Cancer.* 2000; **36**: 858–67.

36. Yao M, Smith RB, Graham MM, Hoffman HT, Tan H, Funk GF et al. The role of post-radiation therapy FDG PET in prediction of necessity for post-radiation therapy neck dissection in locally advanced head and neck squamous cell carcinoma. *International Journal of Radiation Oncology, Biology, Physics.* 2005; **63**: 991–9.

37. Porceddu SV, Jarmolowski E, Hicks RJ, Ware R, Weih L, Rischin D et al. Utility of PET for the detection of disease in residual neck nodes after (chemo)radiotherapy in head and neck cancer. *Head and Neck.* 2005; **27**: 175–81.

38. McCullom DA, Burrell SC, Haddad RI, Norris CM, Tishler RB, Case MA et al. PET with 18F-FDG to predict pathological response after induction chemotherapy and definitive chemoradiotherapy in head and neck cancer. *Head and Neck.* 2004; **26**: 890–6.

39. Rogers JW, Greven KM, McGuirt WF, Keyes Jr JW, Williams 3rd DW et al. Can post RT neck dissection be omitted for

patients with head and neck cancer who have a negative
PET scan after definitive radiation therapy? *International
Journal of Radiation Oncology, Biology, Physics*. 2004; **58**:
694–7.

40. Aassar OS, Fischbein NJ, Caputo GR, Kaplan MJ, Price DC,
Singer MJ *et al*. Metastatic head and neck cancer: Role
and usefulness of FDG PET in locating occult primary
tumours. *Radiology*. 1999; **210**: 177–81.

41. Braams JW, Pruim J, Kole AC, Nikkels PJC, Vaalburg W,
Vermey J *et al*. Detection of unknown primary head and
neck tumors by positron emission tomography.
International Journal Oral Maxillofacial Surgery. 1997; **26**:
112–5.

42. Safa AA, Luu MT, Rege S, Brown CV, Mandelkern MA,
Wang MB *et al*. The role of positron emission tomography
in occult primary head and neck cancers. *The Cancer
Journal from Scientific American*. 1999; **5**: 214–8.

43. Greven KM, Keyes JW, Williams III DW, McGuirt WF, Joyce
III WT. Occult primary tumours of the head and neck.
Cancer. 1999; **86**: 114–8.

44. Lassen U, Daugaard G, Eigtved A, Damgaard K, Friberg L.
18F-FDG whole body positron emission tomography (PET)
in patients with unknown primary tumours (UPT).
European Journal of Cancer. 1999; **35**:
1076–82.

45. Jungehulsing M, Scheidhauer K, Damm M, Pietrzyk U,
Eckel H, Schicha H *et al*. 2[^{18}F]-fluoro-2-deoxy-D-glucose
positron emission tomography is a sensitive tool for the
detection of occult primary cancer (cancer of unknown
syndrome) with head and neck lymph node manifestation.
Otolaryngology – Head Neck Surgery. 2000; **123**:
294–301.

46. Wong WL, Saunders M. The impact of FDG PET on the
management of occult primary head and neck tumours.
Clinical Oncology. 2003; **15**: 461–6.

47. Bohuslavizki KH, Klutmann S, Sonnemann U, Thomas J,
Kroger S, Werner JA *et al*. F-18 FDG-PET zur detektion des
okkulten primartumors bei patienten mit
lymphnotedmetastsen der halsregion. *Laryngo-Rhine-
Otologie*. 1999; **78**: 445–9.

48. Schipper JH, Schrader M, Arweiler D, Muller S, Scuik J. Die
positronenemissonstomographie zur primatumoursuche
bei halslyphknotenmetastasen mit unbekanntem
primartumor. *HNO*. 1996; **44**: 254–7.

49. Feine U, Lietzenmayer R, Hanke JP, Wohrle H, Muller-
Schauenburg W. ^{18}FDG-Ganzkorper-PET bei
differenzierten schilddrusenkarzinomen. *Nuclear
Medicine*. 1995; **34**: 127–34.

50. Conti PS, Durski JM, Bacqai F, Grafton ST, Singer PA.
Imaging of locally recurrent and metastatic thyroid cancer
with positron emission tomography. *Thyroid*. 1999; **9**:
797–804.

51. Grunwald F, Kalicke T, Feine U, Lietzenmayer R,
Scheidhauer K, Dietlein M *et al*. Fluorine-18
fluorodeoxyglucose positron emission tomography in
thyroid cancer:results of a multicentre study. *European
Journal of Nuclear Medicine*. 1999; **26**: 1547–52.

52. Schluter B, Bohuslavizki KH, Beyer W, Plotkin M, Buchert
R, Clausen M. Impact of FDG PET on patients with
differentiated thyroid cancer who present with elevated
thyroglobulin and negative ^{131}I scan. *Journal of Nuclear
Medicine*. 2001; **42**: 71–6.

53. Wang W, Macapinlac H, Larson SM, Yeh SDJ, Akhurst T,
Finn RD *et al*. (^{18}F)-2-Fluoro-2-deoxy-D-glucose positron
emission tomography localizes residual thyroid cancer in
patients with negative diagnostic ^{131}I whole body scans
and elevated serum thyroglobulin levels. *The Journal of
Clinical Endocrinology and Metabolism*. 1999; **84**:
2291–302.

54. Chung J-K, So Y, Lee JS, Choi CW, Lim SM, Lee DS *et al*.
Value of FDG PET in papillary thyroid carcinoma with
negative ^{131}I whole-body scan. *Journal of Nuclear
Medicine*. 1999; **40**: 986–92.

55. Dietlein M, Scheidhauer K, Voth E, Theissen P, Schicha H.
Fluorine-18 fluorodeoxyglucose positron emission
tomography and iodine-131 whole-body scintigraphy in
the follow-up of differentiated thyroid cancer. *European
Journal of Nuclear Medicine*. 1997; **24**: 1342–8.

56. Javad H, McDougall IR, Segall GM. Evaluation of suspected
recurrent thyroid carcinoma with [18F]fluorodeoxyglucose
positron emission tomography. *Nuclear Medicine
Communications*. 1998; **19**: 547–54.

57. Lind P, Kumnig G, Matschnig S, Heinisch M, Gallowitsch
HJ, Mikosch P *et al*. The role of F-18FDG PET in thyroid
cancer. *Acta Medica Austriaca*. 2000; **27**: 38–41.

58. Diehl M, Risse JH, Brandt-Mainz K, Dietlein M,
Bohuslavizki KH, Matheja P *et al*. Fluorine-18
fluorodeoxyglucose positron emission tomography in
medullary thyroid cancer: results of a multicentre study.
European Journal of Nuclear Medicine. 2001; **28**: 1671–6.

59. Neumann DR, Esselstyn CB, Kim EY. Recurrent post
operative parathyroid carcinoma: FDG PET and sestamibi
SPECT findings. *Journal of Nuclear Medicine*. 1996; **37**:
2000–1.

60. Walsh RM, Wong WL, Chevretton EB, Beaney RP. The use
of PET-^{18}FDG imaging in the clinical evaluation of head
and neck lymphoma. *Clinical Oncology*. 1996; **8**: 51–4.

61. Hoffman M, Kletter K, Becherer A, Jaeger U, Chott A,
Raderer M. 18F-fluorodeoxyglucose positron emission
tomography (18F FDG PET) for staging and follow-up of
marginal zone B-cell lymphoma. *Oncology*. 2003; **64**:
336–40.

62. Goerres GW, Stoeckli SJ, von Schulthess GK. FDG PET for
mucosal malignant melanoma of the head and neck.
Laryngoscope. 2002; **112**: 381–5.

63. Wittekindt C, Theissen P, Jungehulsing M, Brochhagen HG.
FDG-PET imaging of malignant paraganglioma of the neck.
Annals of Otology, Rhinology, and Laryngology. 1999; **108**:
909–12.

64. Gould MK, Maclean CC, Kushner WG, Ware G, Rydzak CE,
Douglas K. Accuracy of positron emission tomography for
the diagnosis of pulmonary nodules and mass lesions: a
meta-analysis. *Journal of the American Medical
Association*. 2001; **285**: 914–24.

65. Wong WL, Campbell H, Saunders M. Positron emission tomography (PET) - evaluation of indeterminate pulmonary lesions. *Clinical Oncology.* 2002; **14**: 123–8.

66. Stokkel MPM, ten Broek F-W, Hordijk G-J, Koole R, van Rijk PP. Preoperative evaluation of patients with primary head and neck cancer using dual-head [18]fluorodeoxyglucose positron emission tomography. *Annals of Surgery.* 2000; **231**: 229–34.

67. Stokkel MPM, Terhaard CHJ, Hordijk G-J, van Rijk PP. The detection of local recurrent head and neck cancer with fluorine-18 fluorodeoxyglucose dual-head positron emission tomography. *European Journal of Nuclear Medicine.* 1999; **26**: 767–73.

68. Farber LA, Benard F, Machtay N, Smith RJ, Weber RS, Weinstein GS *et al.* Detection of recurrent head and neck squamous cell carcinomas after radiation therapy with 2-^{18}F-fluoro-2-deoxy-D-glucose positron emission tomography. *Laryngoscope.* 1999; **109**: 970–5.

69. Kresnik E, Mikosch P, Gallowitsch HJ, Kogler D, Wieser S, Heinisch M *et al.* Evaluation of head and neck cancer with ^{18}F-FDG PET: a comparison with conventional methods. *European Journal of Nuclear Medicine.* 2001; **28**: 816–21.

70. Mukherji SK, Drane WE, Mancuso AA, Parsons JT, Mendenhall WM, Stringer S. Occult primary tumors of the head and neck: Detection with 2-(F-18)fluoro-2-deoxy-D-glucose SPECT. *Radiology.* 1996; **199**: 761–6.

71. Stokkel MPM, Terhaard CH, Hordijk GJ, van Rijk PP. The detection of unknown primary tumors in patients with cervical metastases by dual-head positron emission tomography. *Oral Oncology.* 1999; **35**: 390–4.

72. Alnafisi NS, Driedger AA, Coates G, Moote DJ, Raphael SJ. FDG PET of recurrent or metastatic ^{131}I-negative papillary thyroid carcinoma. *Journal of Nuclear Medicine.* 2000; **41**: 1010–15.

73. Muros MA, Llamas-Elvira JM, Ramirez-Navarro A, Gomez MJA, Rodriguez-Fernandez A, Muros T *et al.* Utility of fluorine-18-fluorodeoxyglucose positron emission tomography in differentiated thyroid carcinoma with negative radioiodine scans and elevated serum thyroglobulin levels. *American Journal of Surgery.* 2000; **179**: 457–61.

74. Okamoto Y, Inugami A, Matsuzaki Z, Yokomizo M, Konno A, Togawa K *et al.* Carotid artery resection for head and neck cancer. *Surgery.* 1996; **120**: 54–9.

75. Lehtio K, Oikonen V, Gronroos T, Eskola O, Kalliokoski K, Bergman J *et al.* Imaging of blood flow and hypoxia in head and neck cancer: initial evaluation with [15O]H2O and [18F]fluoroerythronitroimidazole. *Nuclear Medicine.* 2001; **42**: 1643–52.

76. Rasey JS, Koh Wui-Jin J, Evans ML, Peterson LM, Lewellen TK, Graham MM *et al.* Quantifying regional hypoxia in human tumours with positron emission tomography of [18F]fluoromisonidazole: a pretherapy study of 37 patients. *International Journal of Radiation Oncology, Biology, Physics.* 1996; **36**: 417–28.

77. Minn H, Clavo AC, Grenman R, Wahl RL. In vitro comparision of cell proliferation kinetic and uptake of tritiated fluorodeoxyglucose and L-Methionine in squamous cell carcinoma of the head and neck. *Journal of Nuclear Medicine.* 1995; **36**: 252–8.

78. Van Eijkeren ME, Thierens H, Seuntjens J, Goethals P, Lemahieu I, Strijckmans K. Kinetics of [methyl-11C]thymidine in patients with squamous cell carcinoma of the head and neck. *Acta Oncologica.* 1996; **35**: 737–41.

79. Chao KSC, Bosch WR, Mutic S, Lewis JS, Dehdashti F, Mintun MA *et al.* A novel approach to overcome hypoxic tumour resistance: Cu-ATSM-guided intensity modulated radiation therapy. *International Journal of Radiation Oncology, Biology, Physics.* 2001; **49**: 1171–82.

80. Okazawa H, Naito Y, Yonekura Y, Sadato N, Hirano S, Nishizawa S *et al.* Cochlear implant efficiency in the pre- and post-lingually deaf subjects. A study with H2(15)O and PET. *Brain.* 1996; **119**: 1297–306.

81. Schoder H, Yeung HWD, Gonen M, Kraus D, Larson SM. Head and neck cancer: Clinical usefulness and accuracy of PET/CT image fusion. *Radiology.* 2004; **231**: 65–72.

82. Branstetter BF, Blodgett TM, Zimmer LA, Snyderman CH, Johnson JT, Raman S *et al.* Head and neck malignancy: is PET/CT more accurate than PET or CT alone? *Radiology.* 2005; **235**: 580–6.

83. Syed R, Bomanji JB, Nagabhushan N, Hughes S, Kayani I, Groves A *et al.* Impact of combined 18F-FDG PET/CT in head and neck tumours. *British Journal of Cancer.* 2005; **92**: 1046–50.

55

Image-guided surgery, 3D planning and reconstruction

GHASSAN ALUSI AND MICHAEL GLEESON

Introduction	701	Image-guided surgery	705
Background and overview	701	Key points	709
Image reconstruction	703	Deficiencies in current knowledge and the areas for	
Visualization of image data	703	future research	709
Surgical planning	704	References	709
Surgical simulation	704		

SEARCH STRATEGY

The data in this chapter are supported by a Medline search using the key words image-guided surgery, endoscopic sinus surgery and skull base surgery.

INTRODUCTION

Image-guided surgery (IGS) has developed as a result of advances in computer science, digital scanning and image processing. It is a relatively new technology that provides surgeons with information before and during an operative intervention. IGS is an important part of modern surgical practice in disciplines that include neurosurgery, otorhinolaryngology, maxillo-facial and orthopaedic surgery. Synonyms for this technology include computer-aided surgery, navigational surgery and computer-guided surgery.

With this technology, magnetic resonance (MR), computed tomography (CT) or combined image data sets are used to create three-dimensional (3D) reconstructions of the operative volume. These 3D reconstructions can be used to plan surgery (surgical planning), practise a certain surgical procedure (surgical simulation) or to navigate during the surgical procedure (image-guided surgery). Computer-aided surgery is the umbrella term that is sometimes used to encompass all these processes.

BACKGROUND AND OVERVIEW

It has been possible to generate 3D models of a specific anatomical region from two-dimensional (2D) CT data sets for some time (**Figure 55.1**).[1] At the outset, these 3D models were used to make measurements, drive numerically controlled milling machines to create physical models and to view a patient's anatomy and disease process from every aspect.[2] The extraction of specific structural detail (segmentation) from the data became possible with the development of sophisticated image-processing software and the advantages of preprocessing data in this way became apparent very quickly. It was then only a matter of time before this technology was used to facilitate live surgery. In the operating theatre, images were presented to the surgeon as 2D slices within the three orthogonal planes of space, or as 3D reconstructions displayed on a 2D computer screen. Surgical tools were developed to enable the localization of anatomical features or to confirm the precise position of a pointer within the operative field.

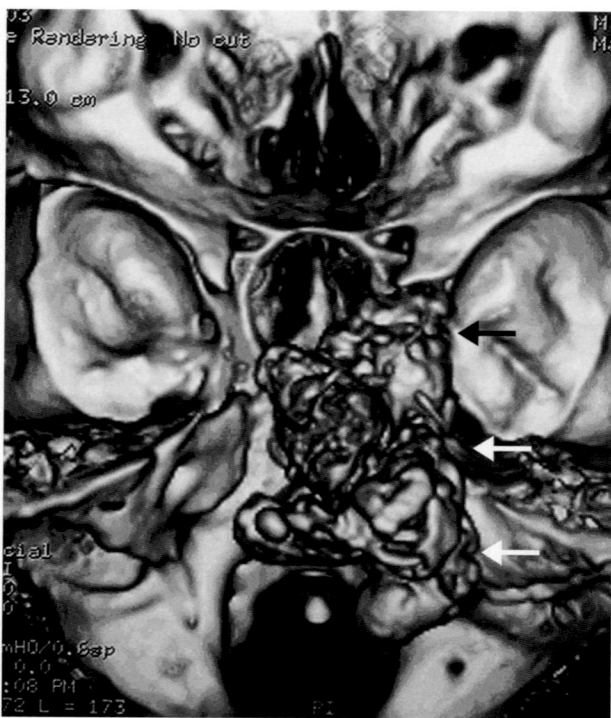

Figure 55.1 3D reconstruction of CT image data showing the involvement of the skull base by an extensive chordoma (arrowed).

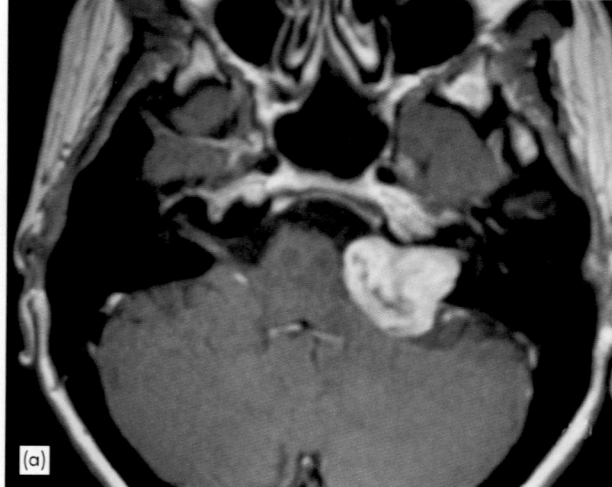

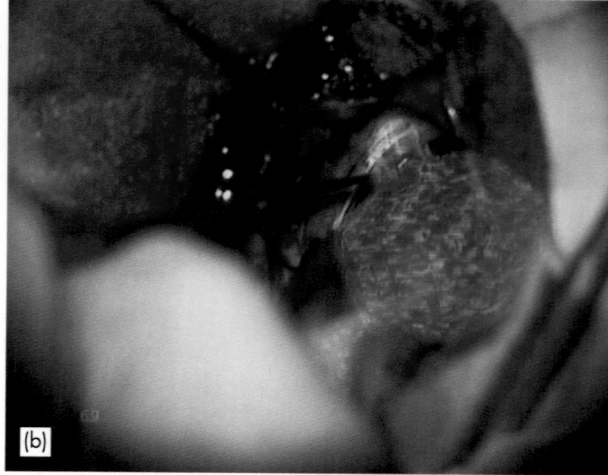

Figure 55.2 Vestibular schwannoma. (a) MR scan; (b) intraoperative view through the microscope with the segmented image data overlain on the operative scene.

Surgeons appreciated that this information was particularly useful in those situations where the disease process or previous surgery has distorted the normal anatomy.[3] Since then, alternative methods of image display have been developed that include image overlays on the surgical field visible through the operating microscope.[4] These computer-generated images may be vector representations of previously segmented and preprocessed data. Alternatively, part of the 3D data set can be superimposed on the patient's anatomy, thus providing the surgeon with an extraordinary 'x-ray' type vision (**Figure 55.2**).[5] Augmented reality is an allied area of research that has yet to fulfil its true potential, but will surely replace conventional IGS in the not too distant future.[4]

Preoperative imaging serves two distinct purposes. First, it is a diagnostic tool. Second, it is used to assess the extent of disease. By careful scrutiny of the images, the surgeon becomes familiar with the anatomy and surgical needs of his patient. The amount of preoperative imaging for complex cases has increased significantly over recent years. Surgeons no longer have to rely so much on their anatomical acumen and intuition in difficult situations. Nowadays, complex and thorough preoperative image processing removes some of the guess work in surgery and utilizes to the full all the information that is acquired. It is hoped that at the least this makes surgery safer and the training of future generations of surgeons better.

Surgeons nowadays plan their approach using data obtained from various imaging modalities. Maxillofacial surgeons were among the first to make use of computers for surgical planning.[6] They used 3D reconstruction of CT scans of the skull to drive a numerically controlled milling machine that produced prostheses for patients, precise replicas of their normal tissues. The outcome was better fitting prostheses and surgery that took a fraction of the time required by more traditional methods where the prostheses were hand-made during the operative process.[6] Orthopaedic surgeons currently use 3D data sets to drive robots designed to perform accurate drilling of the femur or tibia during hip and knee replacements. Robots controlled by computers using patient specific 3D data sets are extremely accurate. The result is better fitting prostheses and fewer failures and morbidity for patients.[7] Image-guided surgery, when used by trainee surgeons in endoscopic sinus surgery, improves surgical accuracy and reduces the risk of major intracranial or intraorbital complications that might be caused by inexperience. It enhances surgical efficiency and accelerates the learning curve by reducing operative time while maintaining greater than 90 percent accuracy in identifying critical anatomical landmarks.[8]

In the sections that follow, we discuss the principles and elements of IGS so that the user can better understand the technology and jargon that accompanies it.

IMAGE RECONSTRUCTION

The creation of a 3D data set from 2D sections is performed by software using highly complex algorithms that are specific to the particular scanner and scanning protocol employed. Powerful computer workstations are required to run these software programs. This process is automated and requires little clinician input. It is important to consider and understand the various aspects of 3D reconstruction as it has a direct effect on accuracy and visualization.

The concept of slices

Conventional CT scan converts one-dimensional x-ray data into a 2D slice. This is referred to as a single image section and may be acquired along axial, coronal or other planes by changing the gantry angle. Tilting the gantry tilt is extremely useful as sections can be acquired that avoid predictable artifacts, for example those caused by dental restorations. Subtle changes to the gantry angle can also help show certain anatomical features better. Each individual section has a width known as a slice thickness, a factor that pertains to the width of the x-ray beam detector window used. Smaller width beams (windows) produce higher resolution 2D images.

Slices are spaced along the area to be scanned with an inter-slice distance that varies depending on the scanning protocol being used and on the size of the anatomical structure that is being imaged. Spiral and multi-slice CT scans are faster and expose the patient to less radiation than their traditional counterparts. They collect x-ray data in a helical fashion that is reconstructed later into 2D sections or indeed 3D volumetric voxel data sets. The resulting data set from a spiral CT scan may be reformatted along the sagital, coronal or axial planes, as well as emulating any gantry tilt.

Pixels and voxels

Two-dimensional slice sections are composed of pixels which are the smallest picture elements. The more pixels in a certain distance, the better the resolution. Currently, the highest resolution available for both CT and MRI is 512×512 pixels per image. In a field that is 30×30 cm, this gives a high definition picture, whereas in a large field this gives a low resolution. By convention, the image resolution is stated by the number of pixels in the x and y axis only and the size of the image field will not be actually defined.

Each pixel has a value ranging, in the case of the CT scan, from −1000 to 3096. This is often referred to as Hounsfield units (HU). CT scans are calibrated such that the value of 0 equates to the density of water. By convention, high pixel values are displayed as white. The lower the value, the lower the density of the tissue and the darker the pixel would appear. Pixels are 2D, but it is possible to convert these picture elements into a 3D block. This 3D block is referred to as a voxel or a volumetric picture element. Voxels can be a cube or cuboid depending on the inter-slice distance.

Volume averaging

If a structure falls partially within a pixel, the true value of that structure will then be assigned a value less than the normal value of the structure. In the case of bone, which has a value of say 1000 HU, the value of a pixel that includes a part of that part of the bone will be much less, perhaps 500. This is referred to as partial volume averaging and is a major problem in delineating where the edge of a structure should lie within a given image. Higher resolution images would overcome that problem to some extent. This is not always possible as higher x-ray dosages would be required and an order of magnitude increase in the complexity of the hardware. Algorithms have been developed to overcome this problem and define the edge of a structure with a greater degree of confidence. Each one has its own unique problems and for clinical use in the area of neurosurgery and otorhinolaryngology the accuracy difference is submillimetric and can be ignored.

VISUALIZATION OF IMAGE DATA

Many factors have to be considered when deciding which visualization technique to use. The clinical purpose for which the data is to be used is the most significant and the image data are rendered for that purpose. Rendering is the process of generating computer images which represent 3D anatomy with some degree of tissue transparency if that is appropriate.

Surface rendering

Optical surface scanners produce structured 3D coordinate point sets that relate to an anatomical surface.[9] Triplets of data points are generally grouped as the vertices of adjacent triangles that interconnect to make up the entire surface. These triangular surface patches are known as facets or polygons.

The rendering of surfaces from volume data requires preprocessing. The properties of voxels containing anatomical surfaces must first be decided and voxels with these properties can then be processed. Usually the voxels are considered to lie on a surface if they are connected and all have the same associated property within a given range of values. The derived surfaces are called isosurfaces and are selected to correspond to the surfaces of anatomical structures or to surfaces of equal functional activity.

Geometric primitives are also derived from volumetric data by processes such as contour tracing, surface extraction or boundary following. Alternatively, voxels belonging to anatomical parts may be isolated from the full data set by applying thresholds to the data values associated with them. This extraction of tissue topology has become known as 'segmentation'. The derived geometric primitives (such as polygon meshes or contours) are rendered for display using conventional computer graphics techniques.

Figure 55.3b shows the rendering of a facial surface that is made up of a large set of triangular facets that are also shown in Figure 55.3a. This type of image can be produced using data from an optical scan of the face.

Volume rendering can be undertaken for notional surfaces between distinct tissue types. The surface normals are derived directly from the voxel values neighbouring the boundary. These derived surface normals are used for calculating the final image using algorithms. A technique of this sort was used to produce the image depicted in Figure 55.3c.

Volume rendering

Volume rendering has become the most commonly used method with which to visualize 3D medical image data. The basic idea is that 3D volumes are composed of voxels and that these are analogues of their 2D counterparts, the pixels. Fine details throughout a volume of interest are displayed, enabling a more direct understanding of visualized data with fewer artifacts.

This visualization technique works by projecting each voxel on to a viewing plane with a value related to the physical property represented in the voxel array. For example, a voxel containing bone with a high x-ray absorption coefficient might be projected with a high value. The most advanced systems allow the operator to construct a look-up table which relates the physical value associated with the voxel to the value it contributes to the image at the chosen viewing plane. A pixel in the viewing plane usually receives contributions from many voxels and the operator may control the manner in which these contributions are composed. For example, the operator may choose to display only the maximum contribution from any voxel along a ray. This produces an image known as the maximum intensity projection (MIP). On

the other hand, any individual voxel-associated value may be assigned a maximum opacity value to produce the same images as would be produced by surface rendering.

Figure 55.4a and b show two volume-rendered images with different look-up tables. These demonstrate how different anatomical structures may be made visible through others which are being rendered transparent. Major blood vessels may, for example, be effectively rendered visible within the anatomical data set.

Generally, a volume-rendered image appears different from that of a surface rendered image in that anatomical structures are presented as having some degree of transparency. For some clinical procedures, such as image-guided biopsy or transcutaneous thermal ablation, transparency may greatly enhance depth perception and thus increase the accuracy of the procedure. It is apparent that surfaces are not explicitly rendered, but human perception reconstructs images that are perceived to be in the correct spatial relationship. The transparency which volume rendering offers also enables the placement of surgical instruments within 3D structures with great accuracy.[10]

SURGICAL PLANNING

Surgical planning is usually carried out in the surgeon's mind, drawing on past experience, knowledge of anatomy and anatomical variation. Some individuals are able to do this very well, others are not. In endoscopic sinus surgery, the surgeon must have the ability to think in 3D, having studied the information available from 2D CT slices. Surgeons may or may not be able to communicate their impressions to other surgeons. Furthermore, their mental image cannot be reviewed, audited or measured by other surgeons or indeed by the surgeon themselves when assessing patients at a later date. Planning using reconstructed 3D data enables the surgeon to assess the patient's anatomy objectively, to communicate this with other surgeons and to review these films at a later date. The data can be segmented and manipulated to familiarize the surgeon with specific features pertinent to that patient and the procedure to be performed.

SURGICAL SIMULATION

The major driving force behind the development of surgical simulators was the morbidity that accompanied the introduction of new techniques such as endoscopic 'key hole' surgery. These techniques were conceptually different from traditional surgery. Surgeons had to operate using a 2D image on a television monitor and had to develop new hand–eye coordination skills not previously required for open surgery. Training surgeons in these new skills and the assessment of their competence was entirely different from the 'apprentice–master' approach that had been the mainstay of traditional surgical teaching.

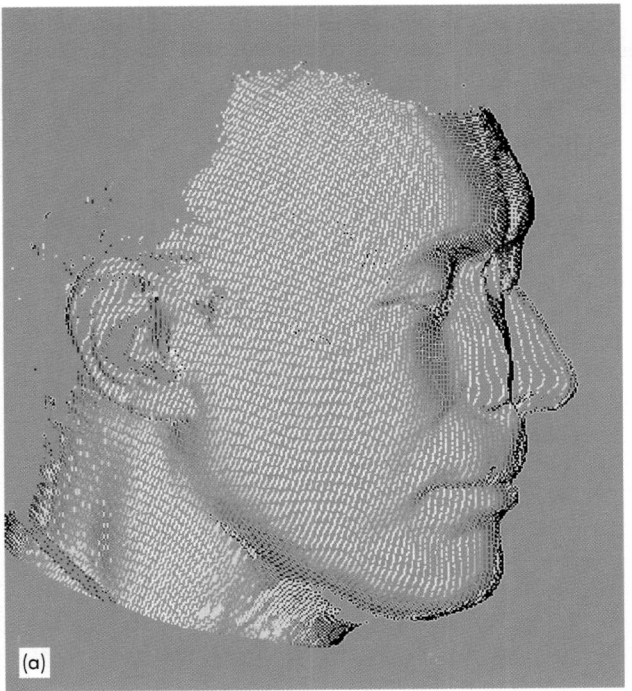

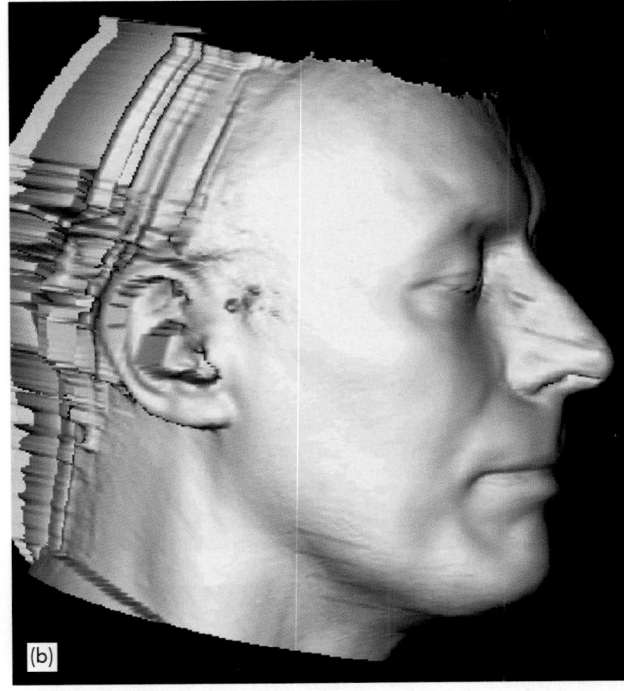

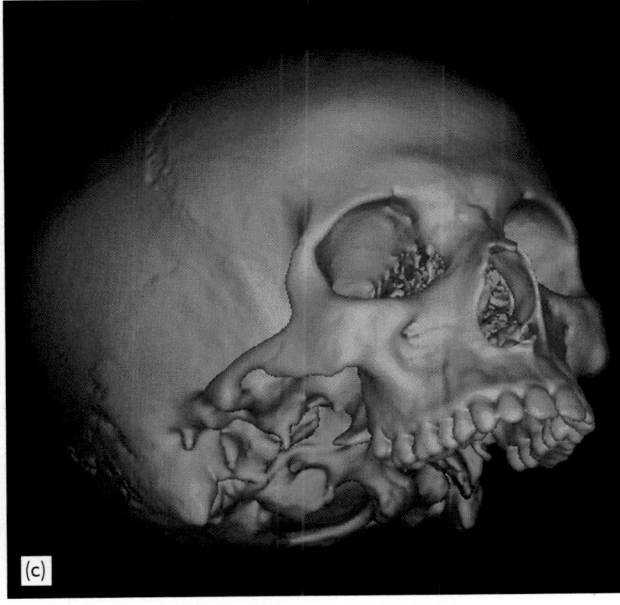

Figure 55.3 (a) Wire mesh; (b) polygon-rendered; and (c) volume surface.

Three-dimensional reconstructions of image data can be used for surgical simulation. Simulators that create a virtual surgical environment or a set of tasks that enhance hand–eye coordination skills seem to be the answer.[11, 12]

Surgical simulators are now being developed and employed in other surgical specialties, for example skull base surgery. They are being used by trainees and experienced surgeons who might find it useful to practise a specific difficult surgical technique before performing the actual operation. Surgeons are able to 'virtually' manipulate, move and drill the mastoid process, to perform laparoscopic or endoscopic sinus procedures. The sensations and resistance encountered during real surgery may be simulated using positive feedback mechanisms in the form of a passive robotic arm.

IMAGE-GUIDED SURGERY

A thorough knowledge of anatomy is essential for all types of surgery, particularly those using microscopes and endoscopes. Preoperative imaging alerts the surgeon to

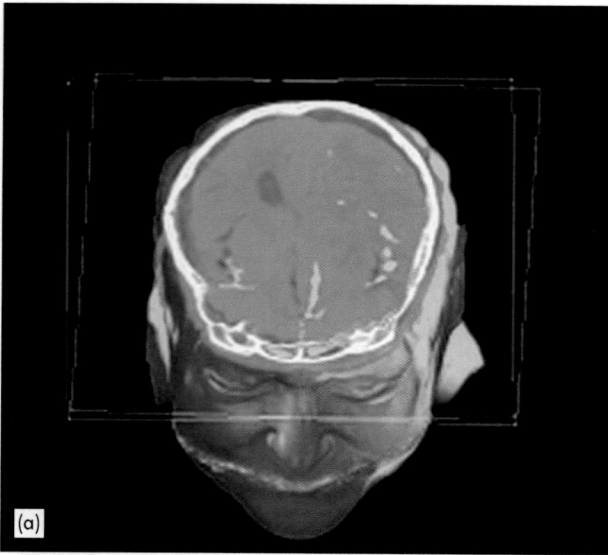

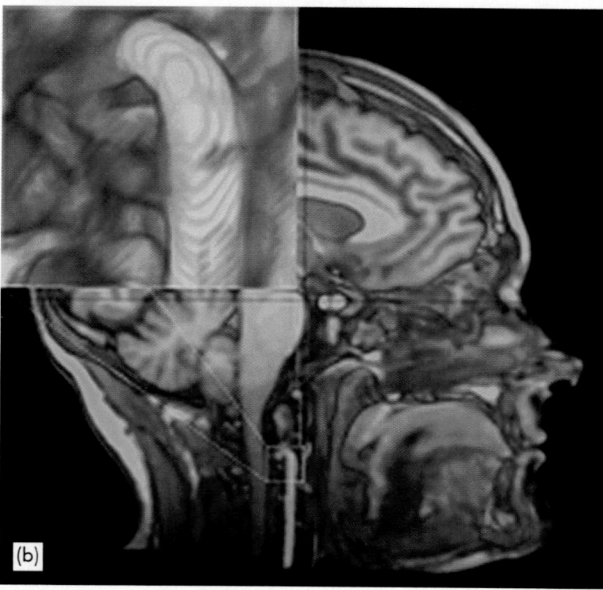

Figure 55.4 Volume-rendered data with different look-up tables

variations of anatomy that are either inherent in the patient or caused by a disease process or previous surgery. As stated before, image guidance offers the surgeon the ability to use the patient's image data intraoperatively to determine position, distance to vital organs and other anatomical features that might be hidden from direct vision. Structures in the vicinity of the skull base are either embedded or closely adherent to bone, making this region ideal for image guidance as CT has great spatial accuracy.

Two fundamental processes are required for intraoperative image guidance, registration and tracking. Registration is the process that relates the patient in the operating theatre to preoperatively acquired image data sets. Tracking is the mechanism of following the position of the patient or an instrument within the operative field.

Both processes are potentially subject to significant mathematical error and it is vital that how this might happen is fully appreciated.

Registration

Once the patient is secured on the operating table, registration of the Cartesian coordinates of the CT scan to that patient in the theatre is achieved by one of two methods. The first is by locating anatomical landmarks visible both on the patient and image data using a probe that is visible to the tracking device. For example, using navigation software, the surgeon would point to pre-specified landmarks, such as the tragus, outer canthus and nasion. This is usually sufficient to achieve a registration accuracy or error of 3–4 mm. This can then be improved by entering a random sample of points from around the operative region (typically 40–100 points) using the probe. The position of the tip of the probe is identified by the tracking device and the coordinates are fed back to the navigation software. In this way, accuracy/errors of 2–3 mm can be achieved.

Other methods of registration use masks[13] and laser scanning tools (**Figure 55.5**).[14] These speed up the acquisition of surface points. With all these methods, calculations made in real time indicate the point accuracy. It is then up to the surgeon to reject or accept that point in order to improve the overall registration accuracy. Some types of IGS systems make use of fiducial markers that are applied to the patient before scanning on the day of surgery. These markers are clearly visible in both MR and CT data sets and, of course, on the patient when in theatre. They help to improve the accuracy of registration.

No matter whether skin fiducials or anatomical landmarks are used for registration, these reference points should describe or be immediately adjacent to the surgical field. Failure to pay attention to this results in navigational inaccuracies. It is important to realize that the registration error is only a measure of the accuracy of correlation between selected points in the virtual data set and the fiducial markers or anatomical landmarks identified on the patient. It is not synonymous with target error, which is the error that could be expected if a probe was placed on a random point of interest within the surgical field. The target error is influenced by the registration error and is unlikely to be much worse if the target is within the volume described by the fiducial markers. However, if the point is outside that volume, the target error will be proportionately greater.

Tracking

Sensors that provide dynamic positional information are known as 'tracking devices'. They are employed in a multitude of everyday situations that range from virtual reality games to missile guidance and electronic tagging of very precise, consistently accurate, fast enough to provide more than 25 readings per second, be insensitive to changes in air temperature, unaffected by metal objects and able to track two objects simultaneously.

Several tracking systems have been employed over the years. Some of the earliest devices were mechanical arms fitted with potentiometers at every joint. These were fast and accurate but were cumbersome, had a restricted range of movement and hindered the movement of the tracked object to which it had to be attached. Systems based on magnetic field distribution are effective and relatively cheap. However, their disadvantage is that tracking accuracy can be both easily and significantly affected by the presence of metal objects.

Infrared light sensors are the most commonly used image-guided surgical systems. They are referred to as either active or passive devices. Active devices sense infrared light from light-emitting diodes (LED) attached to the patient or location probe. Passive tracking devices detect infrared light reflected from metallic balls attached to the patient or probe. In the latter case, the infrared light source is situated on the sensing device itself (**Figures 55.6** and **55.7**). In order to detect changes in the patient's head position, haloes or arches with light-emitting diodes or reflective spheres can be fitted to a Mayfield clamp or the patient's head. Systems based on light-emitting diodes are reliable if the light path is not impeded.[16] Within the operating theatre an accuracy of 2–5 mm can usually be achieved.[4] In general, optical tracking systems are expensive. Cheaper variations do exist, but they lack high degrees of accuracy.

Inertial trackers have also been developed that are small and accurate enough for virtual reality applications. These devices generally provide one rate of change of rotational measurement only; hence, a number would be

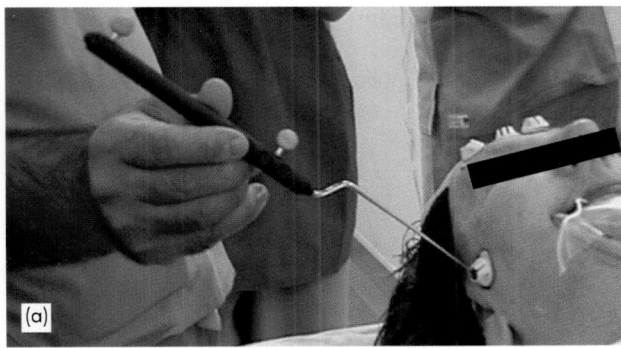
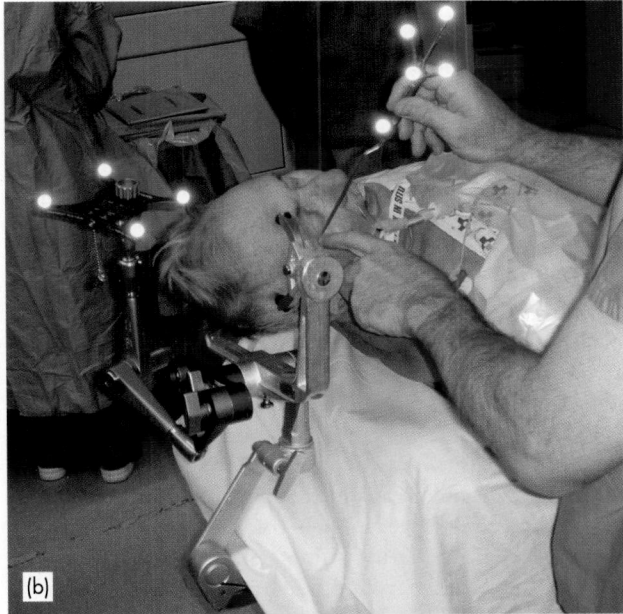
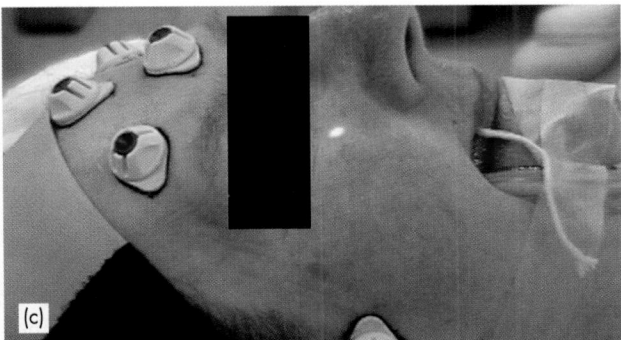

Figure 55.5 (a) A laser registration being undertaken before endoscopic sinus surgery. (b) The laser beam is shone on to the skin around the operative site. (c) A band on to which fiducial balls have been mounted is attached to the patient's head.

prisoners.[15] Although these measurement acquisition systems may be similar, each has different tracking properties that are optimal for a particular application. Without some form of tracking device, it would not be possible to move the patient once they had been registered. In surgical practice, tracking systems must be

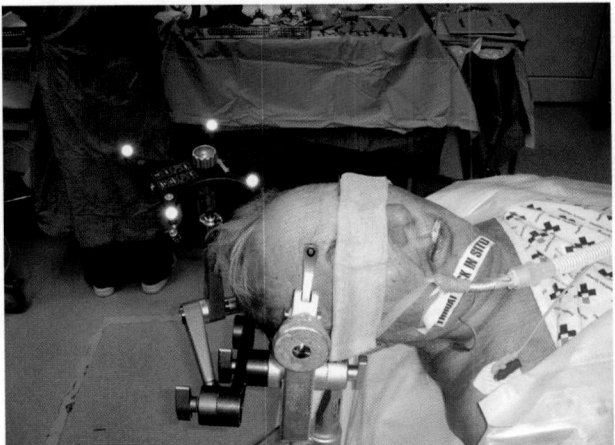

Figure 55.6 A patient with their head held in a Mayfield clamp being prepared for image-guided surgery. An arc with metallic ball fiducials has been attached to the clamp. The arc describes the operative volume. A laser light is being centred on the field to find the optimal position for the tracking device.

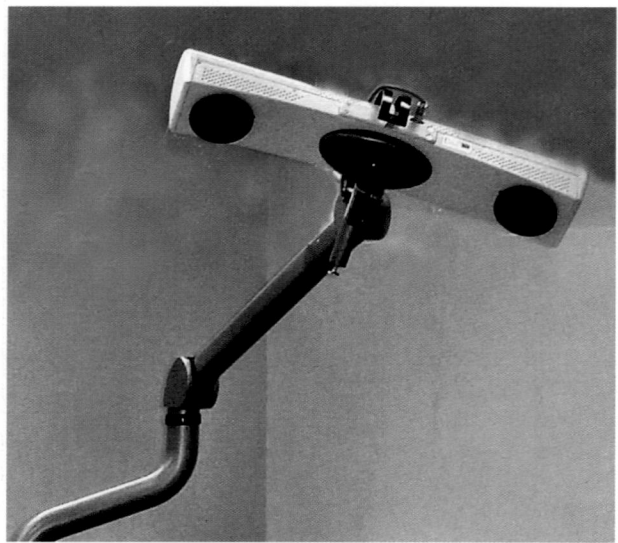

Figure 55.7 An infrared optical tracking system. In the centre of the gantry is a laser light that is used to position the arm during the set-up procedure.

required. They are also not accurate for slow position changes. Systems based on standard ultrasound signals have the potential to achieve much greater accuracy, but are susceptible to changes in temperature and air currents. Other drawbacks include long lag times and interference from echoes and other noises in the environment.

Clinical applications

Image-guided surgery offers most promise in the areas of skull base and endoscopic sinus surgery. Skull base

surgeons have found this technology particularly useful for preoperative surgical planning, design of bone flaps, identification of important structures and for finding small tumours in obscure parts. For example, in **Figure 55.8**, the guidance system had been used to maximize the access for correction of basilar invagination in a patient with osteogenesis imperfecta. The normal anatomical arrangements and landmarks were not present as a result of the disease process.

In rhinology, IGS systems are already in use in difficult revision endoscopic sinus surgery where there are no recognizable anatomical landmarks (**Figure 55.9**).[17] In particular, surgeons have found the guidance systems useful to localize the frontal recess during Draf type 2 and 3 procedures, where the floor of the frontal sinus is to be opened.[18] With the help of these systems, the need to perform open, external procedures will become less. Extended applications of endoscopic sinus surgery include trans-sphenoidal, trans-nasal endoscopic hypophysectomy where conventionally x-ray image intensifiers have been used to localize the sella.[19, 20, 21]

In the field of otology, IGS has been used to aid the surgeon in locating the facial nerve, identifying and localizing lesions of the petrous apex[22] and tumours, particularly in the internal auditory meatus. These include meningiomas and vestibular schwannomas.[23, 24] It is possible that when these systems gain in acceptance, are more accurate and involve shorter set-up times, they may become mainstream intraoperative equipment in all types of mastoid surgery. Their role then would be to aid the surgeon in localizing important atomical structures such as the facial nerve, dura, brain and jugular bulb, as well as diseases, such as cholesteatoma and acoustic schwannoma.

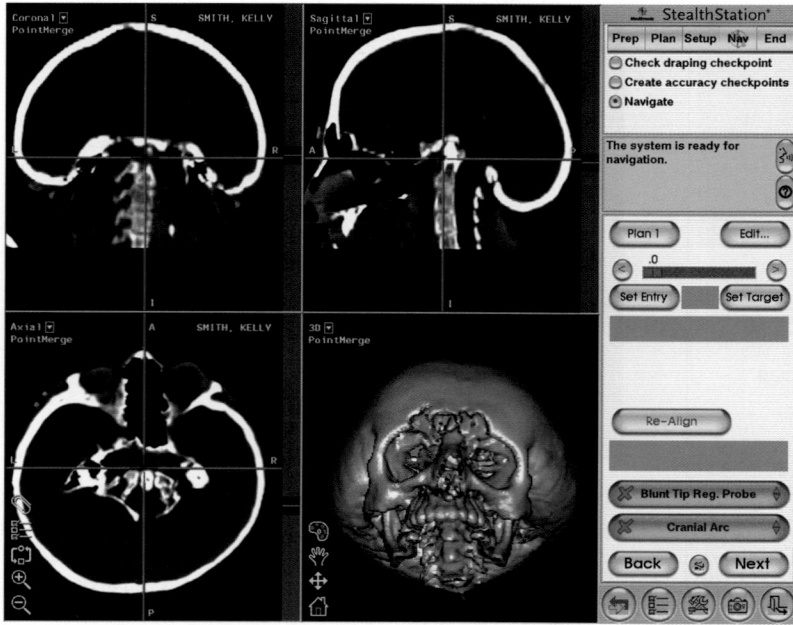

Figure 55.8 Intraoperative screen view during correction of basilar invagination. The cross lines of the cursor are centred over the displaced odontoid peg.

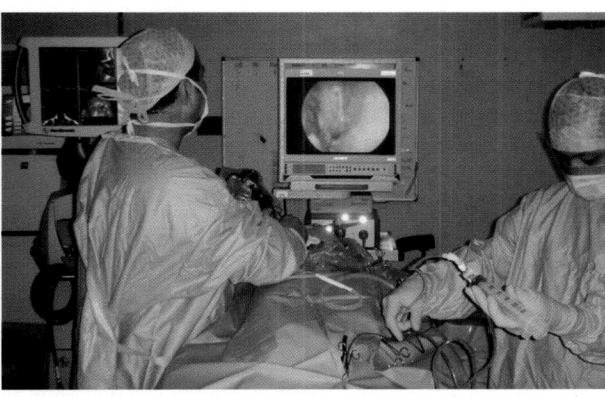

Figure 55.9 Functional endoscopic surgery being undertaken using image guidance.

➤ At present, augmented reality still has to prove its position in surgical practice. Several research groups are producing encouraging results and future reliance on these types of systems is likely to replace traditional IGS systems.

➤ Robots are already being used for drilling in the field of orthopaedics and to manoeuvre and control cameras in laparoscopic surgery. These are far more accurate than humans and are likely to enter other fields of surgery where there is a reliance on power instrumentation, including drills and debriders.

➤ In the future, we are likely to use IGS systems to audit surgical procedures as they already have the inherent capacity to store all information relating to intraoperative navigation. This will be an invaluable and, perhaps, incriminating operative record.

KEY POINTS

- IGS aids the surgeon in diagnosing the extent of disease, planning surgery and providing intraoperative positional information.
- Image-guided surgical techniques may reduce complications in endoscopic sinus surgery.
- IGS techniques offer greater accuracy and confidence in structure and disease localization.
- Major applications are skull base and revision nasal surgery where there is complex or distorted anatomy.

Deficiencies in current knowledge and the areas for future research

➤ Image-guided and augmented reality surgery relies heavily on technology research in the areas of computer hardware (processors, graphics and tracking) and software for segmentation and registration. Developments in these fields are driven by a variety of customer-driven demands. It is vital that clinicians make these demands and provide ideas for the computer scientists.

➤ The most important requirements are for accurate, robust, fail-safe systems that will give clinicians greater confidence. These systems must be user-friendly and ergonomically efficient.

➤ In the future, we are likely to see more developments in the areas of surgical simulation and planning. Surgical training should benefit from simulators that will enable the trainee to develop their hand–eye coordination skills prior to applying them in clinical practice.

REFERENCES

1. Herman GT, Liu HK. Three-dimensional display of human organs from computed tomograms. *Computer Graphics and Image Processing.* 1979; **9**: 1–21.

2. Linney AD, Tan AC, Richards R, Gardner J, Grindrod S, Lees WR. The use of three dimension data on human body for diagnosis and surgical planning. *Revista di Neuroradiologia.* 1992; **5**: 483–8.

3. Olson G, Citardi MJ. Image-guided functional endoscopic sinus surgery. *Otolaryngology – Head and Neck Surgery.* 2000; **123**: 188–94.

∗ 4. Edwards PJ, Hawkes DJ, Hill DL, Jewell D, Spink R, Strong A *et al.* Augmentation of reality using an operating microscope for otolaryngology and neurosurgical guidance. *Journal of Image Guided Surgery.* 1995; **1**: 172–8.

∗ 5. Lapeer RJ, Tan AC, Alusi G, Linney AD. Computer-assisted surgery and planning using augmented reality (CASSPAR): Visualisation and calibration. In: *2003 IEEE/ACM International Symposium on Mixed and Augmented Reality.* Washington: IEEE Computer Society, 2005: 272–3.

6. Vannier MW, Marsh JL, Warren JO. Three-dimensional computer graphics for craniofacial surgical planning and evaluation. *ACM SIGGRAPH Computer Graphics Quarterly.* 1983; **17**: 263–73.

7. Kienzle III TC, Stulberg SD, Peshkin MA, Quaid A, Lea J, Goswami A *et al.* A computer-assisted total knee replacement surgical system using a calibrated robot. In: Taylor RH, Lavallée S, Burdea GS, Mösges R (eds). *Computer integrated surgery.* Cambridge, MA: MIT Press, 1996: 409–16.

8. Casiano RR, Numa Jr. WA. Efficacy of computed tomographic image-guided endoscopic sinus surgery in residency training programs. *Laryngoscope.* 2000; **110**: 1277–82.

9. Cline HE, Dumoulin CL, Hart Jr. HR, Lorensen WE, Ludke S. 3D reconstruction of the brain from magnetic resonance images using a connectivity algorithm. *Magnetic Resonance Imaging.* 1987; **5**: 345–52.

10. Jolesz FA, Kikinis R. Intraoperative imaging revolutionizes therapy. *Diagnostic Imaging.* 1995; **17**: 62–8.

11. Caversaccio M, Eichenberger A, Hausler R. Virtual simulator as a training tool for endonasal surgery. *American Journal of Rhinology.* 2003; **17**: 283–90.

12. Bockholt U, Muller W, Voss G, Ecke U, Klimek L. Real-time simulation of tissue deformation for the nasal endoscopy simulator (NES). *Computer Aided-Surgery.* 1999; **4**: 281–5.

13. Albritton FD, Kingdom TT, DelGaudio JM. Malleable registration mask: application of a novel registration method in image guided sinus surgery. *American Journal of Rhinology.* 2001; **15**: 219–24.

14. Raabe A, Krishnan R, Wolff R, Hermann E, Zimmermann M, Seifert V. Laser surface scanning for patient registration in intracranial image-guided surgery. *Neurosurgery.* 2002; **50**: 797–801; Discussion 802–3.

15. Watanabe K, Kobayashi K, Munekata F. Multiple sensor fusion for navigation systems vehicle navigation and information systems. In: *Vehicle Navigation & Information Systems Conference, 1994 Proceedings.* Washington: IEEE Computer Society, 1994: 575–8.

16. Azuma R, Bishop G. Improving static and dynamic registration in an optical see-through hmd. In: *Proceedings of the 21st Annual Conference on Computer Graphics and Interactive Techniques.* New York: ACM Press, 1994: 197–204.

∗ 17. Metson R. Image-guided sinus surgery: lessons learned from the first 1000 cases. *Otolaryngology – Head and Neck Surgery.* 2003; **128**: 8–13.

∗ 18. Neumann Jr. AM, Pasquale-Niebles K, Bhuta T, Sillers MJ. Image-guided transnasal endoscopic surgery of the paranasal sinuses and anterior skull base. *American Journal of Rhinology.* 1999; **13**: 449–54.

19. Otori N, Haruna S, Yoshiyuki M, Moriyama H. Endoscopic endonasal surgery with image-guidance. *Nippon Jibiinkoka Gakkai Kaiho.* 2000; **103**: 1–6.

20. Kajiwara K, Nishizaki T, Ohmoto Y, Nomura S, Suzuki M. Image-guided transsphenoidal surgery for pituitary lesions using Mehrkoordinaten Manipulator (MKM) navigation system. *Minimally Invasive Neurosurgery.* 2003; **46**: 78–81.

21. Sandeman D, Moufid A. Interactive image-guided pituitary surgery. An experience of 101 procedures. *Neurochirurgie.* 1998; **44**: 331–8.

22. Van-Havenbergh T, Koekelkoren E, De-Ridder D, Van-De-Heyning P, Verlooy J. Image guided surgery for petrous apex lesions. *Acta Neurochirurgica.* 2003; **145**: 737–42; Discussion 742.

23. Sargent EW, Bucholz RD. Middle cranial fossa surgery with image-guided instrumentation. *Otolaryngology – Head and Neck Surgery.* 1997; **117**: 131–4.

24. Klimek L, Mosges R, Schlondorff G, Mann W. Development of computer-aided surgery for otorhinolaryngology. *Computer-Aided Surgery.* 1998; **3**: 194–201.

56

Ultrasound in ear, nose and throat practice

KESHTHRA SATCHITHANANDA AND PAUL S SIDHU

Introduction	711	Reliability of ultrasound examination of thyroid nodules	721
Basic physics and equipment design	711	Cystic lesions	724
Programme software technology advances	713	Soft tissue neoplasms	725
Transducer selection	713	Conclusion	727
Doppler ultrasound	714	Key points	727
Microbubble contrast agents	714	Best clinical practice	727
Advantages of ultrasound	715	Deficiencies in current knowledge and areas for future research	727
Disadvantages of ultrasound	715	References	727
Examination technique	715		
Ultrasound appearances of common abnormalities	715		

SEARCH STRATEGY

The data in this chapter are supported by a Medline search using the key words ultrasound or imaging and neck, head and neck neoplasm, thyroid diseases, parathyroid masses and salivary gland disorders.

INTRODUCTION

Ultrasound has achieved wide clinical use over the past half century. It is a crucial imaging modality in medical practice and now accounts for almost a quarter of all imaging studies carried out in the world. The equipment used has evolved from large expensive B-mode gantry systems with coarse, static, bistable displays, which only demonstrated organ boundaries, to convenient handheld machines with high resolution, real-time imaging with colour Doppler facility making use of digital technology. This chapter will discuss some of the basic physics and principles of both the hardware and software of the ultrasound machine and of real-time B-mode imaging. An overview of the benefits and pitfalls of the more important applications in ear, nose and throat (ENT) practice will be covered, with an emphasis on new advances and future developments.

BASIC PHYSICS AND EQUIPMENT DESIGN

Ultrasound is defined as sound with a frequency above the upper limit of normal hearing (over 20 kHz). In medical practice, much higher ultrasound frequencies are used (2.5–30 MHz) to produce an image based on the detection and display of sound waves reflected from interfaces within the body.

Ultrasound produces tomographic images similar to computed tomography (CT) and magnetic resonance imaging (MRI); however, unlike CT where x-rays are transmitted through the patient to produce an image on the other side of the patient; ultrasound images are formed from reflected sound waves. Sound waves are generated in short bursts by the transducer (or probe) and the sound energy that is reflected back is collected at the point of origin (the transducer) during the relatively long intervals between the sequential generation of sound waves. The ultrasound image is based on the back scattering of sound energy by interfaces of tissues with different physical properties through interactions governed by acoustic physics; the amplitude of the reflected echoes is used to generate the contrast of the different tissues to form the image.

Transducer design

B-mode (brightness mode) real-time imaging is most commonly used in medical practice. The images are formed line by line from the information within the transducer that both transmits and receives ultrasound signals from the body's tissues.

A typical transducer comprises five layers (**Figure 56.1**):

1. a protective layer;
2. mechanical lens ('Hanafy' lens) that allows you to focus the beam in a particular elevation plane;
3. matching layers that overcome the large acoustic impedance mismatch between the ultrasound crystal and the patient's tissues (the acoustic impedance of a material is a measure of how efficiently the sound waves are conducted through the tissue);
4. an active piezoelectric material to produce the sound waves. In practice, this is usually lead zirconate titanate (PZT);
5. a backing block to stop the crystal from freely resonating and thus producing poor echoes that have inadequate axial resolution and are not useful in producing a diagnostic image.

PHYSICS OF ULTRASOUND

Sound is mechanical energy travelling through matter as a wave producing alternating areas of compression and rarefaction.[1] Sound obeys the rules of basic acoustic physics as summarized in the following equation:

$$\text{Velocity } (c) = \text{frequency } (f) \times \text{wavelength } (\lambda)$$

In the clinical setting, the ultrasound transducer generates sound waves in short bursts or pulses of energy that are transmitted into the body where they are propagated through tissues. These acoustic pressure waves may behave either as a transverse wave (travel in a direction perpendicular to the direction of the displaced particle) or as a longitudinal wave (in the same direction as the particle movement). In tissues and fluids, in medical practice, sound behaves in a longitudinal fashion.

Propagation velocity

The speed at which the pressure waves travel through different tissues varies greatly and is affected by the physical properties of the tissues, with this velocity largely

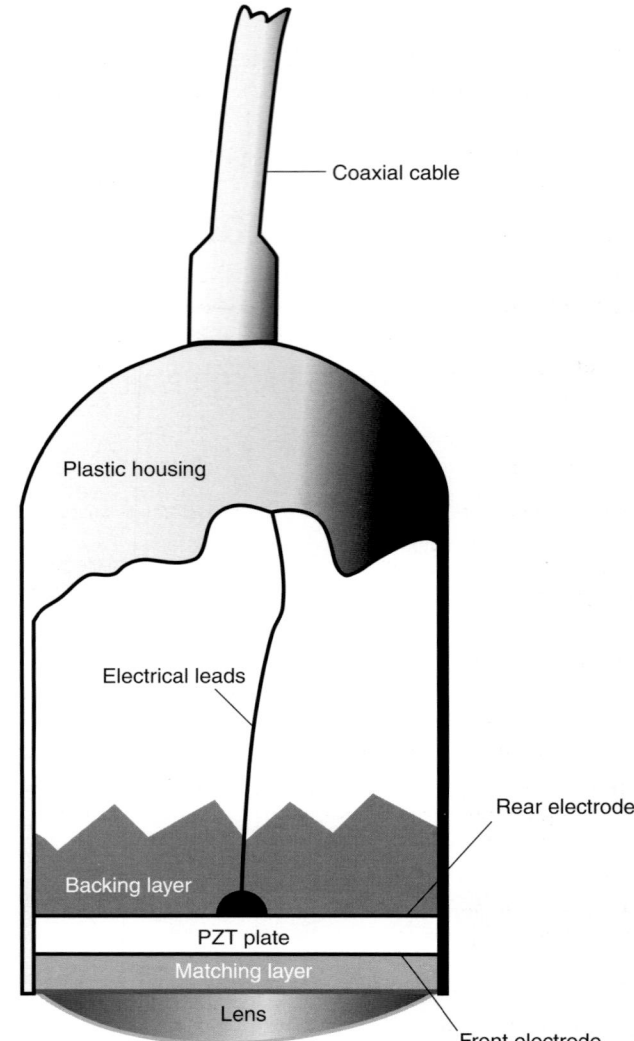

Figure 56.1 Transducer design. Schematic drawing illustrating the design of an ultrasound transducer.

dependent on the resistance of the medium to compression, as well as the tissue stiffness or elasticity. Increasing the stiffness or decreasing the density of the material will increase the propagation velocity.

In the body, the propagation velocity of sound is assumed to be constant, and is quoted at 1540 m/s. This value is the average of measurements for all the tissues and is applicable to most soft tissues of the body. However, it should be noted that some tissues, such as aerated lung and fat, have a much lower velocity than 1540 m/s, whilst others, such as bone, have a much greater velocity. In practice, this property of propagation velocity is critical as it is used to evaluate the distance of a reflecting surface from the transducer. By measuring the time it takes for an echo to return to the probe and knowing the velocity with which the wave travelled, the distance it traversed (which is the depth of the reflecting tissue interface from the probe) can be calculated.

Acoustic impedance

Ultrasound images are formed by detecting and displaying backscattered (reflected) sound waves from a reflecting surface within tissue. Sound travelling in any homogenous medium will not have such a reflecting interface and will consequently appear anechoic (black) as is seen with a simple cyst. At the junction between different tissues with different physical properties, an acoustic interface will be present. In the body, there are many of these interfaces, each of which will produce varying amounts of reflected sound that is detected by the transducer. The strength of the returning sound wave echo is determined by the difference in acoustic impedances of the materials forming the interface. The acoustic impedance is defined by the following formula:

Acoustic impedance (Z) = density (p) × propagation velocity (c)

Interfaces with large differences in acoustic impedances such as soft tissue/air or soft tissue/bone, reflect almost all the incident sound waves, producing returning echoes of higher amplitude, which will form better images. In tissues where there are smaller differences in acoustic impedances, such as muscle and fat, only part of the incident sound wave is reflected and the remainder is allowed to continue on through the material; the returning sound wave echoes will be of smaller strength. It is important to note that both the propagation velocity and acoustic impedance are determined by the physical properties of the tissues and are independent of the frequency of the waves.

Image generation

The foundation of modern ultrasound imaging is with real-time, grey scale, B-mode display where the intensity/brightness of each pixel of the image represents the different amplitudes of the returning sound wave echoes. New digital technology with the consequent improvements in the software of the modern ultrasound machine has allowed improvement of image quality.

To create a two-dimensional (2D) image, multiple ultrasound pulses are sent down a series of successive scan lines, building up a 2D representation of echoes originating from the object being insonnated. The image is normally displayed on a black background, with the greatest amplitude signals appearing as white and no signal as black. Signals of intermediate intensities are displayed as varying shades of grey.

In modern ultrasound machines, a digital memory of 512×512 or 512×640 pixels is used to store values corresponding to the values of the returning echoes, as well as their position in the patient. The digitally stored image can then be displayed on a video monitor by converting the digital signal to an analogue format. The dynamic range of the information stored in the digital memory is much larger than that which can be seen on a video monitor or be appreciated by the human eye. This information needs to be compressed, a technique called 'post-processing', the purpose being to optimally view the information that is likely to be of diagnostic value and selectively eliminate less useful information stored in the memory. One important recent advance is the use of application specific integrated circuits (ASIC), which has led to improving the complexity, speed and reliability of the machines whilst reducing the cost and machine size with lower power consumption. Manufacturers have also developed new techniques to optimize the images by allowing the machine to manipulate the echo signals and therefore reducing the operator-dependent nature of ultrasound.

Real-time ultrasound gives the impression of a moving image by generating a series of 2D images at a rate of 15–60 frames per second, permitting the real-time ultrasound assessment of both anatomy and motion. This innovation has made ultrasound a dynamic examination technique.

PROGRAMME SOFTWARE TECHNOLOGY ADVANCES

Advances in digital technology[2] have allowed electronic and software technology improvement at all stages of the ultrasound imaging systems. Spatial compounding is an example of such a development, improving the quality of the final displayed image. With spatial compounding, the beam is electronically steered so that overlapping scans of an object are acquired at different angles. These entire scan lines are averaged to produce a real-time compound image with better spatial resolution than conventional B-mode imaging. A further example of post-processing to improve imaging is 'coded excitation'. This technique uses the fact that the transmitted pulse is digitally encoded and thus can be modified by changing its frequency or amplitude and the receiver is set to optimally receive this 'code' in the returning echoes, allowing weak signals to be distinguished from background noise. This allows imaging at higher frequency (as used in imaging the superficial structures in the neck) with improved spatial and contrast resolution at greater depth. Other recent advances, less applicable to imaging of neck structures, include 'extended field-of-view' methods that produce a panoramic image to expand diagnostic capabilities particularly in musculoskeletal ultrasound[3] and tissue harmonic imaging, particularly useful in abdominal imaging.[4]

TRANSDUCER SELECTION

When choosing the optimal transducer for a given application, both the requirements for spatial resolution and the distance of a target from the transducer need to be considered. In general, the higher the frequency of the probe, the less the depth of tissue penetration, but the better the spatial resolution. To optimize the imaging, a probe of the highest frequency is chosen that allows penetration to the depth of interest. The imaging of superficial structures requires a higher frequency probe; in the neck, most of the structures of interest are superficial and probes of greater than 7.5 MHz are used. Occasionally, in the larger individual, deeper penetration is required, usually a 5 MHz probe is used. High frequency linear array probes are ideal for imaging superficial structures as the near-field resolution is better; this allows axial resolution of 0.5 mm or less and lateral resolution of 1.0 mm or less and provide a rectangular image format that is well suited to this application.[5] To evaluate the parotid gland area or the floor of the mouth, a curved array or sector transducer may be better suited. Curved array probes make a smaller footprint contact with the skin surface, but give a larger field-of-view at depth as it provides a sector display format.[6]

DOPPLER ULTRASOUND

Doppler ultrasound[7] allows the imaging of blood flow in vessels; an important adjunct to grey scale imaging and has allowed greater diagnostic confidence in image interpretation. The Doppler effect is defined as a change in the apparent frequency of a wave as a result of relative movement between the observer and the source. The observer in this context is the ultrasound transducer and the source is the moving red blood cells within a vessel. The change in frequency (Doppler shift frequency) that is detected can be used to assess movement. The Doppler shift frequency is proportional to the ultrasound frequency, the velocity of the moving target and the angle of insonation of the target. These parameters are summarized in the Doppler equation:

$$\Delta f = 2 \frac{f_t V \cos \phi}{c}$$

where Δf is the Doppler shift frequency; f_t is the frequency of sound emitted from the transducer; V is the velocity of the target towards the transducer; c is the velocity of sound in the medium; and ϕ is the angle of insonation (the angle between the axis of flow and the incident ultrasound beam).

In B-mode imaging, the pulse sound wave echoes are transmitted and the backscattered signal contains information regarding phase and frequency. Precise timing allows the depth from which the echo originates to be measured. However, the additional information contained from these echoes can be used to evaluate moving targets, such as blood flow. The Doppler systems that are in use are of two kinds: continuous wave and pulsed wave Doppler systems.

Continuous-wave Doppler systems use two transducers mounted within the same housing: one transmits sound continuously and one receives the reflected echoes continuously. The traces obtained by this method can be then analysed (spectral analysis). The Doppler shift frequencies are displayed graphically and it is possible to visualize the time-varying waveform of blood flow, measure objective parameters, such as velocity, pulsatility index (PI) and resistance index (RI). The PI is the peak-to-peak value divided by the mean of the peak values throughout the cardiac cycle.

$$\text{Pulsatility index} = \frac{\text{Peak systolic velocity} - \text{End diastolic velocity}}{\text{Mean velocity}}$$

The RI is the peak systole minus the end diastole velocity divided by the peak systole velocity.

$$\text{Resistance index} = \frac{\text{Peak systolic velocity} - \text{End diastolic velocity}}{\text{Peak systolic velocity}}$$

The RI gives an indication of the degree of resistance to blood flow in the distal circulation. The disadvantage of a continuous wave Doppler system is that the range or depth of the moving structure cannot be calculated.

Pulsed-wave Doppler systems overcome this drawback by transmitting short pulses of sound waves and then leaving long intervals between to receive the returning echoes, using a single crystal. The depth of the returning Doppler signal may be calculated by timing the returning signal, with the knowledge of the speed of the sound waves in the tissues.

Duplex scanners combine colour Doppler acquisition equipment with a conventional grey-scale imaging system, allowing visualization of the vessel under interrogation and placing the sample gate over the region of interest to obtain a spectral Doppler signal. In modern machines, the switch from 2D imaging to Doppler mode is instantaneous and many machines allow continued B-mode imaging, whilst acquiring the Doppler information, a practical advantage.

MICROBUBBLE CONTRAST AGENTS

Ultrasound contrast medium[8] is a relatively new technique and is gaining increasing acceptance in improving diagnostic accuracy. Microbubbles are less than 10 μm in diameter, cross capillary membranes and are safe, effective echo enhancers. The agent remains in the vascular compartment and is stable for several minutes after an intravenous bolus. Tissue harmonics is used to image ultrasound contrast agents by tuning the receiver to listen to a band of frequencies that allows the contrast signal to be resolved from the background, allowing visualization of vessels as small as 100 μm, enough to characterize tumour vascularity.[9] Tumour vascularity can be further enhanced using 3D displays to demonstrate the vascular anatomy.

ADVANTAGES OF ULTRASOUND

The benefits of ultrasound imaging are well recognized. The key points to be noted are:

- Ultrasound does not use ionizing radiation making it ideal for paediatric patients, as well as for patients requiring multiple examinations, as in oncology practice.
- Ultrasound is readily available and is relatively cheap.
- Ultrasound allows good spatial resolution and is the 'gold standard' in determining whether a focal lesion is cystic or solid, surpassing even CT or MRI.
- Ultrasound is well tolerated by patients and is a 'patient friendly' technique.
- Ultrasound provides diagnostic information with a high degree of accuracy, allowing for more efficient use of CT and MRI when choosing how, if necessary, to image the patient further.
- An increasingly important role is to guide interventional procedures such as fine needle aspirations, biopsies and drainage catheter insertions accurately and in real time.

DISADVANTAGES OF ULTRASOUND

The disadvantages of ultrasound are few but are very important to consider when making clinical management decisions. The primary disadvantage is that the technique is operator dependent. There should be confidence in your operator and he/she should work in a multi-disciplinary environment to ensure the highest standards. Though the cost of this examination is relatively low, the initial capital costs need to be considered; the equipment has to be high quality. The size and position of the structures and diseases affecting the neck require high-resolution linear array and curvilinear probes with good supporting software to produce images of diagnostic quality. The facility to use colour Doppler is also highly desirable. The images obtained in ultrasound are susceptible to artifact that may cause mistaken diagnoses. The operator has to be aware how to identify, reduce or eliminate such faults from the image.

Despite these disadvantages, ultrasound is a valuable tool in the diagnosis and treatment of diseases of the head and neck and is accepted as the first imaging modality after clinical examination.

EXAMINATION TECHNIQUE

As many conditions that affect the head and neck occur bilaterally and often in an asymmetrical way, it is imperative that both sides of the neck are examined with a systematic and comprehensive approach.

It is best to examine the patient supine and to image the right side of the neck with the patient's head turned to the left and *vice versa*. The areas that should be covered are the thyroid gland, paravascular spaces, cervical triangles, supraclavicular fossae and the major salivary glands. All these areas need to be examined in at least two orthogonal planes. Colour Doppler ultrasound should also be used to assess if there is involvement of the great vessels or if there is increased vascularity in or around abnormalities.

ULTRASOUND APPEARANCES OF COMMON ABNORMALITIES

Lymph nodes

Both surgeons and oncologists use the regional classification of lymph nodes into seven levels adapted by the American Joint Committee on Cancer. Importantly, the retropharyngeal lymph nodes cannot be seen with ultrasound (**Table 56.1**). This group of lymph nodes is important in pharyngeal cancers and in patients who have previously undergone a neck dissection.

Ultrasound is commonly used for the evaluation of patients with enlarged cervical lymph nodes. It has been suggested that, of the numerous lymph nodes in the body, over a third are sited in the cervical region.[10] Although normal lymph nodes may be visualized by ultrasound in healthy subjects, they are often not seen due to both their small size and their similar echo-texture to the surrounding structures.[11] When apparent, lymph nodes are invariably reactive (hyperplastic), inflammatory or neoplastic. Reactive lymph nodes are typically elongated, oval and have smooth margins, predominantly hypoechoic with an eccentric echogenic fatty hilum (**Figure 56.2**). The upper limit of size of a reactive lymph node in the upper jugular chain is 10 mm in the short axis.[12] However, this carries the caveat that in the paediatric population, larger hyperplastic nodes may be encountered.[13]

Table 56.1 Regional classification of lymph nodes into seven levels, adapted by the American Joint Committee on Cancer.

Level	
Level I	Submental and submandibular nodes
Level II	Upper internal jugular chain nodes
Level III	Middle internal jugular chain nodes
Level IV	Lower internal jugular chain nodes
Level V	Spinal accessory chain nodes and transverse cervical chain nodes
Level VI	Anterior cervical nodes
Level VII	Upper mediastinal nodes

See also Chapter 137, Surgical anatomy of the neck, Figure 137.5.

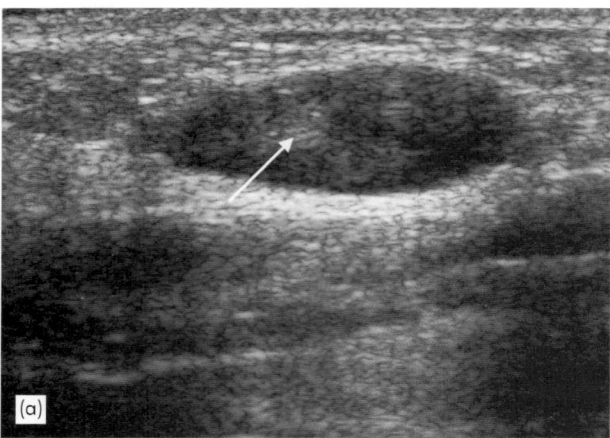

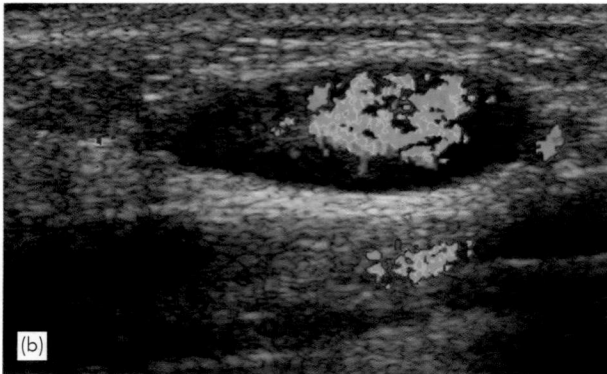

Figure 56.2 Reactive lymph node. (a) An oval-shaped, low-reflective lymph node with an echogenic hilum (arrow), in keeping with a reactive lymph node. (b) Florid colour Doppler flow to the central hilum consistent with a benign reactive lymph node.

Inflammatory nodes are enlarged ($>10\,mm$), round or oval in shape with well-defined borders and in which the hilum is not readily identified. Colour Doppler ultrasound shows hilar vascularization with smooth branching of the intranodal vessels. Ultrasound may assess for the presence of an abscess formation (hypoechoic or anechoic area with no colour Doppler flow) within a mass of inflammatory nodes that may require surgical intervention.[6] Up to 90 percent of cervical lymph node metastases are from squamous cell carcinomas (**Figure 56.3**) and less commonly from a primary tumour in the thyroid, breast, lung, stomach or from a melanoma.[5] Malignant lymph nodes lose the normal ultrasound architecture, have an eccentric hilum, disordered colour Doppler signal and become more rounded (**Figure 56.4**).

Assessment of cervical lymph nodes, the number, level in the neck and the presence of extranodal spread are important prognostic indicators and determine therapeutic options. Most tumours from the upper gastrointestinal tract have a predictable pattern of metastases to the neck depending on the pattern of tumour extent at the primary site. It has been suggested that, if the primary tumour crosses the midline then cervical lymph nodes of both

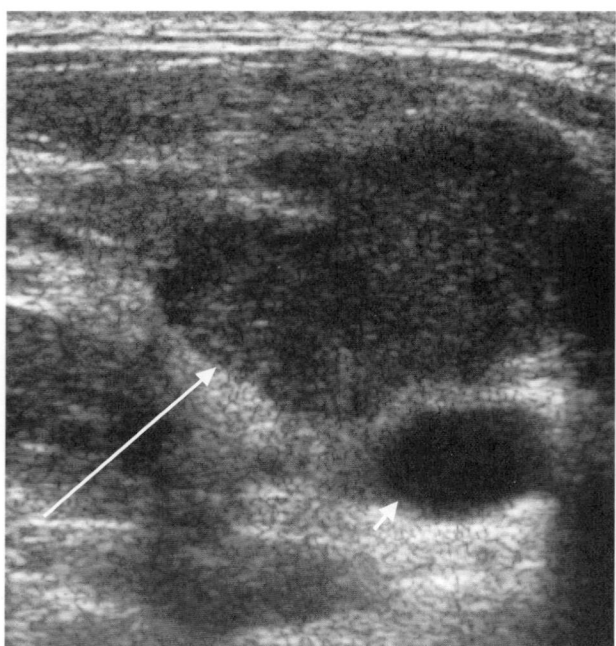

Figure 56.3 Squamous cell carcinoma lymph node metastasis. An enlarged low reflective mass with an irregular border (long arrow), displacing the surrounding soft tissues, anterior to the carotid artery (short arrow), in keeping with a squamous cell metastasis from a primary laryngeal tumour.

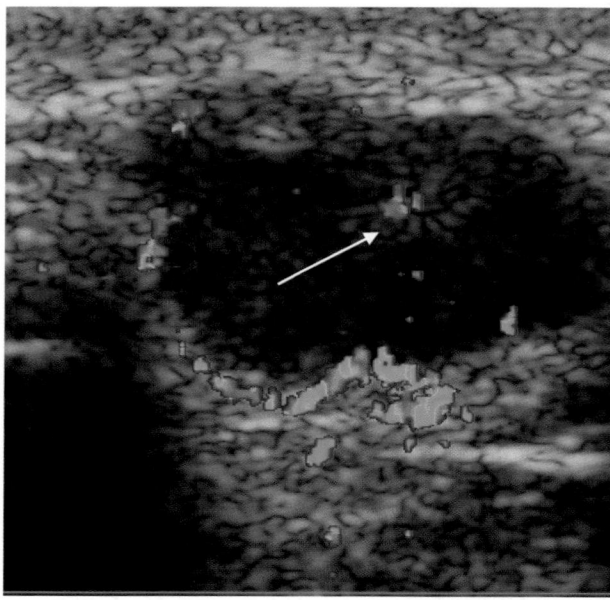

Figure 56.4 Adenocarcinoma lymph node. Colour Doppler images of a low-reflective, irregular, rounded lymph node with an eccentric echogenic hilum (arrow), infiltrated by adenocarcinoma.

sides of the neck are at risk of metastases.[14] [**] The reported prevalence of cervical lymphadenopathy in patients with nasopharyngeal cancer at the time of diagnosis is up to 87 percent.[15] Traditionally, staging was performed by palpation which has a sensitivity and specificity of 60–70 percent, but importantly the rate of occult metastases, undetectable with palpation, with a T1–3 oropharyngeal/supraglottic tumour is 20–50 percent.[16, 17] Ultrasound imaging has a sensitivity of 84 percent, a specificity of 68 percent and an accuracy of 76 percent in detecting abnormal nodes, improved further with the combination of ultrasound-guided fine-needle aspiration cytology (FNAC) to 97 percent sensitivity and 93 percent specificity.[18] [***] The important morphological ultrasound characteristics of lymph nodes to ascertain the presence of malignant change are summarized in **Table 56.2**.[19] [***]

LYMPH NODE SHAPE

The 'roundness index' (longitudinal to transverse diameter ratio) of less than 1.5 indicates metastases in 71 percent of nodes. If the ratio is greater than 2.0, then 84 percent of such nodes are inflammatory or reactive.[20]

LYMPH NODE SIZE

Optimal size is difficult to define as the size of lymph nodes varies with the site in the neck, varying from 5 to 30 mm and the presence of micrometastases does not always cause enlargement.[12, 21] Traditionally, the maximum short axis diameter is quoted in such situations and a cut off of 10 mm is widely accepted. However, when all three lymph node diameters are assessed, the minimal axial diameter is the best criteria for enlargement.[12] The most acceptable size of minimum axial diameter is 7 mm in the upper internal jugular chain and 6 mm for the rest of the neck.[22] It is important to note that the lower the limit criteria for nodal size, the higher the sensitivity in differentiating malignant from benign nodes, but this is at the cost of lower specificity. Conversely, the higher the limit criteria for nodal size, the lower the sensitivity but with increased specificity.

LYMPH NODE ECHOGENICITY

Nodes containing metastases are usually hypoechoic when compared with adjacent muscle.[23] In metastatic papillary

Table 56.2 Ultrasound morphology of malignant infiltrated lymph nodes.

Morphology
Round shape
Short axis diameter of 8 mm or more
Heterogeneous echo-texture
Cystic or necrotic areas
No echogenic (fatty) hilum
Ill-defined margins
Invasion of surrounding tissues

carcinoma of the thyroid, lymph nodes are hyperechoic (87 percent) and homogenous (81 percent). Peripheral echogenic foci are seen in 68 percent of metastatic nodes from papillary carcinoma of the thyroid and have been histologically correlated to psammoma bodies; a characteristic and important feature to recognize.[24] With the newer high-resolution transducers, lymphomatous nodes have a reticular echo pattern, but on the older machines these nodes had a 'pseudocystic' appearance of low reflectivity with posterior enhancement (**Figure 56.5**).[25]

CYSTIC/NECROTIC NODES

The heterogeneous appearance of nodes with cystic spaces, representing areas of necrosis, is seen most commonly with squamous cell carcinoma, but this is a nonspecific finding seen with melanoma, papillary thyroid carcinomas and with tuberculous nodes.[26] Cystic necrosis appears as echo-lucent areas within the lymph nodes (**Figure 56.6**).

CALCIFICATION

Intranodal calcification is unusual in metastatic nodes, except in papillary cell thyroid carcinoma, where calcification is reported in 69 percent.[24] Calcification is also found rarely in irradiated or post-chemotherapy lymph nodes.[26]

ECHOGENIC HILUM

The presence of an echogenic (fatty) hilum is associated with benign disease. Normal lymph nodes have an echogenic hilum in 75–100 percent, whereas it is reported that there is an absent hilum in 96 percent of metastatic lymph nodes,[27] 63 percent of lymphomatous lymph nodes[28] and 83 percent of tuberculous lymph nodes.[23]

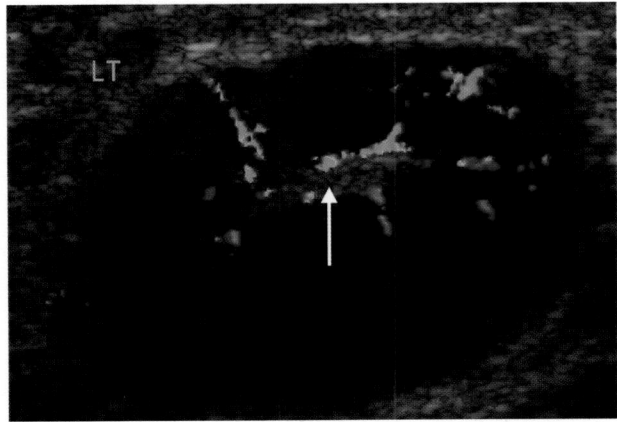

Figure 56.5 Lymphomatous lymph node. An enlarged, rounded, low reflective lymph node that maintains a central echogenic hilum (arrow) infiltrated with lymphoma.

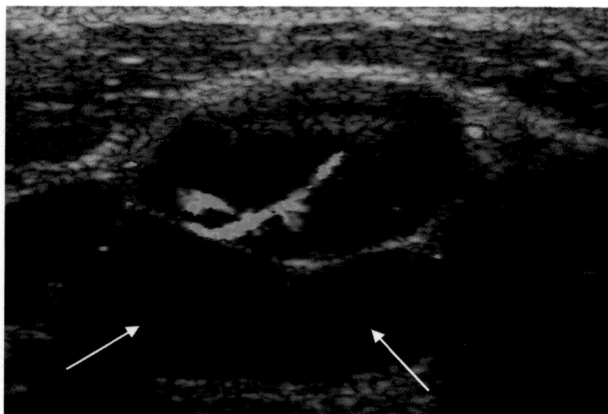

Figure 56.6 Tuberculous lymph nodes. Collection of lymph nodes, with necrosis occurring (arrows) in the posterior lymph nodes, manifest as low reflective fluid. The anteriorly located lymph node has the appearance of a reactive lymph node.

However, as an echogenic hilum is found in both benign and malignant nodes, an echogenic hilum alone should not be used to assess cervical lymph nodes.[29]

VASCULAR PATTERN

Normal and reactive lymph nodes examined with colour Doppler are either avascular or demonstrate hilar vessels with regular branching, whereas metastatic lymph nodes demonstrate tortuous vessels with an aberrant pattern, a peripheral vascular pattern or a mixture of both.[30] The accuracy of differentiating metastases from benign reactive lymph nodes using these criteria is 88 percent (sensitivity 89 percent, specificity 87 percent).[30] Tuberculous lymph nodes may have a variable vascular pattern on colour Doppler imaging and simulate both benign and malignant conditions.[31] Vessels displaced to one side of the lymph node, a relatively common feature in tuberculous lymph nodes (81 percent), is not seen in normal lymph nodes and is uncommon in other pathologies; a useful feature in classifying such lymph nodes.[31]

Using spectral Doppler ultrasound, comparing the highest PI and RI within suspect lymph nodes, malignant nodes showed low resistance flow. Malignant lymph nodes have a PI ≥ 1.1 or an RI ≥ 0.7, with the accuracy of differentiating malignant from benign lymph nodes estimated at 76 and 73 percent, respectively.[30]

Ultrasound microbubble contrast medium has also been used to help evaluate the nature of cervical lymph nodes, where smaller vessels in the lymph nodes are more obvious and the typical pattern of vascular distribution can be ascertained with greater clarity.[32] A high degree of accuracy (99 percent) and a change of diagnosis in 14 percent have been reported with microbubble contrast-enhanced imaging of lymph nodes, with a particularly useful role in smaller or borderline sized lymph nodes.[32] [***]

Thyroid gland

The thyroid gland is a superficial structure and is favourably sited for ultrasound examination. High-frequency B-mode and colour Doppler ultrasound is widely used in both the diagnosis and follow-up of patients with thyroid diseases.

Examination technique consists of obtaining longitudinal and transverse images of the lower half of the neck from the midline. The thyroid gland is made up of two lobes connected medially by the isthmus, which has a transverse course. A third (pyramidal lobe) arises from the isthmus in 10–40 percent of normal individuals. The parenchyma has a homogenous echo texture, which is of higher reflectivity than adjacent muscle.

The thyroid gland is initially assessed for size, which varies with body habitus. Thin subjects have glands that measure 70–80 mm in length and 7–10 mm in depth. Obese patients have glands measuring less than 50 mm in length with an anteroposterior diameter of up to 20 mm.[33] Thyroid volumes have also been used to assess size and are calculated from the right anteroposterior (RAP) diameters and left anteroposterior (LAP) lobes using the following formula:

$$\text{Volume of gland} = (6.91 \times \text{RAP}) + (3.05 \times \text{LAP}) - 3.48$$

Thyroid volume for males is 19.6 ± 4.7 mL and for females is 17.5 ± 3.2 mL.[34] Volumetric studies can be easily performed using 3D ultrasound, but unfortunately this technique is not widely available.

THYROID DISEASE

For ultrasound imaging, thyroid disorders may be broadly considered in two groups: nodular and diffuse. Almost all diffuse thyroid disease and the majority (90 percent) of thyroid nodules are benign, with thyroid malignancy a rare entity accounting for only 1 percent of all cancers.[33]

THYROID NODULES

There are five major roles of ultrasound in the assessment of nodular diseases:

1. detection of focal masses;
2. differentiation of multinodular goiter/hyperplasia from other nodular diseases;
3. to document the extent of a known thyroid malignancy;
4. follow up to look for residual, recurrent or metastatic carcinoma;
5. guidance for FNAC or fine needle aspiration for biopsy (FNAB).

GOITROUS NODULES

Multinodular goiters or hyperplasia is the most common abnormality encountered (80–85 percent).[33] Hyperplasia is recognized as either a diffuse or nodular form. The nodules are separated by normal parenchyma and are mostly isoechoic or hyperechoic with well-defined margins. The adjacent great vessels may be displaced posterior or laterally, but the walls are never involved (**Figure 56.7**). Less than 5 percent of thyroid nodules are hypoechoic, cystic areas are seen in 60–70 percent of cases secondary to haemorrhage or collections of colloid substance.[33] Colloid substance gives a typical 'comet tail' artifact within the nodules.[35] Up to a quarter of goitrous thyroid nodules, particularly in the elderly, have areas of macrocalcification, seen as curvilinear, annular or dystrophic areas of high echoes with posterior acoustic shadowing. Colour Doppler ultrasound shows these thyroid nodules to have less vascularity than the surrounding normal parenchyma.[36]

ADENOMATOUS AND MALIGNANT NODULES

Adenomas and thyroid carcinomas account for most of the nongoitrous nodules, with adenomas accounting for 5–10 percent of all thyroid focal lesions. Thyroid adenomas have a variable appearance on ultrasound, appearing as isoechoic, hypoechoic or hyperechoic masses.[13, 33] Thyroid adenomas have a thick, echo-poor halo, thought to be a fibrous capsule (**Figure 56.8**). The blood supply is often a regular, 'spoke-and-wheel' type of appearance on colour Doppler ultrasound.[33]

Malignant neoplasm of the thyroid are rare (two to three cases per 100,000 individuals) and may be classified as follows:

- papillary cell carcinoma;
- follicular cell carcinoma;
- anaplastic cell carcinoma;
- medullary cell carcinoma;
- lymphoma.

Papillary cell carcinoma

Papillary carcinoma is the most common thyroid neoplasm and makes up 60–70 percent of all thyroid malignancies.[33] On ultrasound, the characteristic appearance is that of a hypoechoic, solid nodule, with up to a third demonstrating cystic changes with detectable blood supply within the intracystic septa (**Figure 56.9**). Punctuate areas of microcalcification are seen in 85–90 percent of lesions; a highly reliable feature in diagnosing papillary carcinoma.[37] Microcalcifications are only seen with the appropriate high frequency imaging, appearing as highly echogenic areas without the posterior acoustic shadowing normally seen with calcification. Colour Doppler studies demonstrate increased vascularity with a chaotic arrangement of blood vessels in 90 percent of lesions, due to arteriovenous shunting, as well as tortuous vessels within the malignant lesion.[38] Regional lymphadenopathy may be present at initial diagnosis in 50 percent of patients.[39] Recurrent lymphadenopathy may develop even after a total thyroidectomy, with the lymph nodes demonstrating microcalcification, cystic change and chaotic hypervascularity, similar in appearance to the primary tumour.[37] [****]

Follicular cell carcinoma

Follicular cell carcinoma accounts for 5–15 percent of all thyroid malignancies, is seen in older patients and often develops in pre-existing thyroid adenomas; approximately 60–70 percent of follicular cell carcinomas are associated with a hyperplastic or adenomatous thyroid nodule.[33] On ultrasound, follicular cell carcinomas are solid,

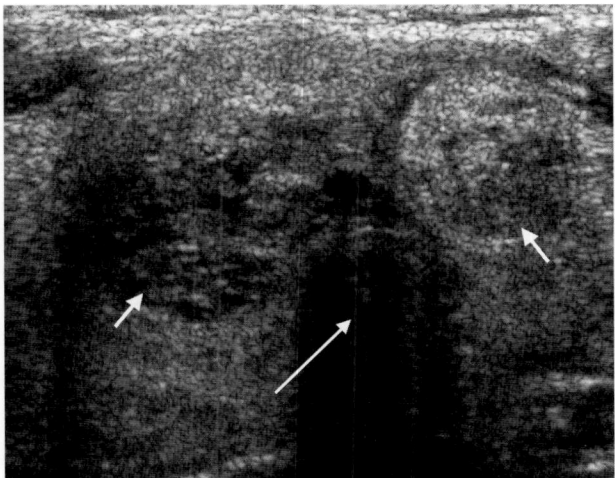

Figure 56.7 Multinodular goitre. A large multinodular goitre, in a transverse view, at the level of the thyroid isthmus and trachea (arrow), demonstrating two large nodules (short arrows).

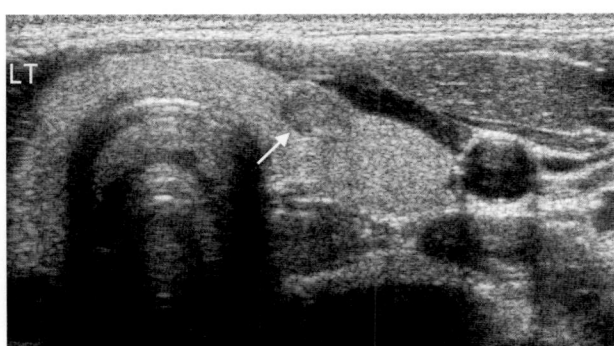

Figure 56.8 Solitary thyroid adenoma. A transverse section through the thyroid gland at the level of the thyroid isthmus, with a left lobe solitary adenoma present as a well-circumscribed isoechoic lesion (arrow).

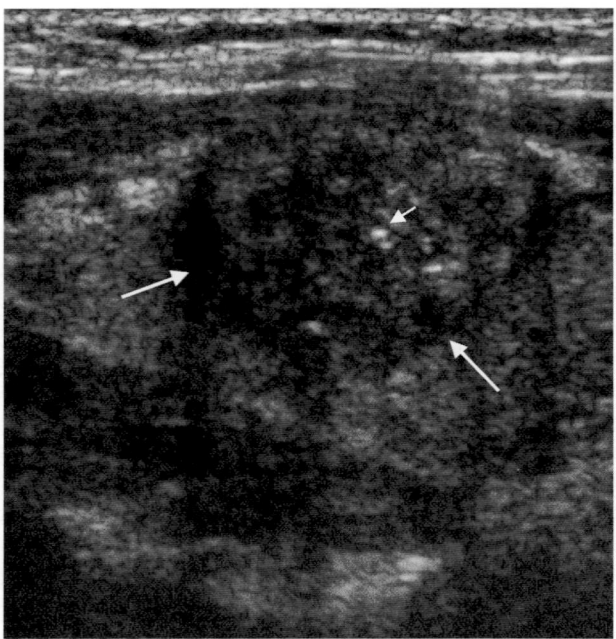

Figure 56.9 Papillary cell carcinoma. A solitary nodule (long arrows) in the right lobe of the thyroid demonstrating an irregular margin and punctate areas of calcification (short arrow).

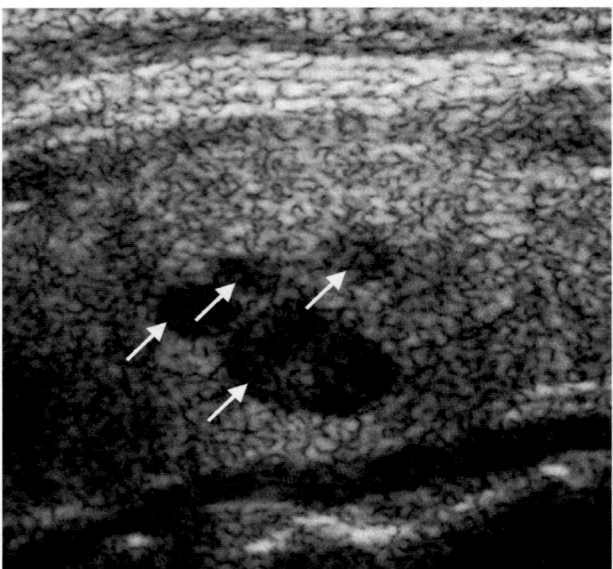

Figure 56.10 Medullary cell carcinoma. Multifocal well-circumscribed, low reflective areas within the left lobe of the thyroid (arrows), with no colour Doppler signal present.

homogenous, hyperechoic or isoechoic nodules with a thick irregular capsule and tortuous perinodular and intranodular vessels often with extracapsular spread. Unfortunately, the presence of extracapsular spread, a crucial feature, may be difficult to demonstrate, the capsular and vascular invasion only being detectable on histology.

Anaplastic carcinoma

Anaplastic carcinomas account for 5–10 percent of all thyroid cancers and, are aggressive tumours seen mostly in the elderly patient. Anaplastic carcinomas are diffusely hypoechoic with areas of necrosis in 78 percent and dense amorphous calcification in 58 percent of lesions.[40] The boundaries of the tumour nodules are irregular due to early invasion of adjacent structures, with nodal or distant metastases seen in 80 percent.[33] [****/*]

Medullary cell carcinoma

Medullary cell carcinoma, an uncommon tumour, is familial in 20 percent with an association with multiple endocrine neoplasia (MEN IIa) syndrome. In MEN IIa, the medullary cell carcinomas are often multicentric, bilateral or both (**Figure 56.10**). On ultrasound, medullary cell carcinoma is similar to papillary cell carcinoma being hypoechoic with irregular margins, demonstrating microcalcifications and irregular vascularity.[41] An important distinguishing feature is the frequent presence of metastatic lymphadenopathy in medullary cell carcinoma.

Primary thyroid lymphoma

Primary thyroid lymphoma is a rare tumour, making up 4 percent of all thyroid tumours, mostly of the non-Hodgkin's type and in 70–80 percent of cases arise from a gland with pre-existing chronic thyroiditis.[33] Primary thyroid lymphoma appears as a hypoechoic, lobulated, vascular mass lesion with large areas of cystic necrosis and encasement of nearby large neck vessels.[42] The adjacent thyroid parenchyma is usually heterogeneous as a consequence of the underlying chronic thyroiditis. [**]

DIFFUSE THYROID DISEASE

Several pathological processes of the thyroid involve the gland in a diffuse manner: acute suppurative thyroiditis, subacute granulomatous (De Quervain's) thyroiditis, chronic lymphocytic thyroiditis (Hashimoto's disease), colloid diffuse goiter and Graves' disease. Colloid diffuse goiter and Graves' disease are the most common cause of thyrotoxicosis. Ultrasound has a limited role in the diagnosis in these disorders, as assessment is based on clinical and biochemical findings.[33]

In Graves' disease, the gland is lobulated and enlarged with a reduction in size used as an indicator of therapeutic success.[43] The parenchyma is more homogenous than a diffuse goiter due to the presence of a large number of intraparenchymal vessels which are seen on colour Doppler ultrasound as turbulent flow within arteriovenous shunts; the 'thyroid inferno' or 'thyroid storm' (**Figure 56.11**).[44] In the normal thyroid gland, Doppler ultrasound of the intrathyroid arteries demonstrates a peak systolic velocity (PSV) of 20–40 cm/s and an end diastolic velocity (EDV) of 10–15 cm/s. However, in thyroid disease, the PSV is

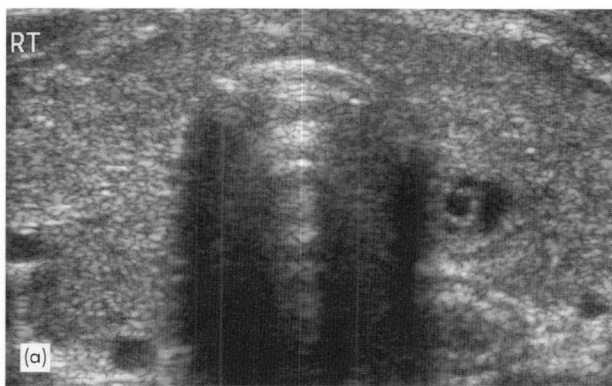

Figure 56.11 Thyrotoxicosis. **(a)** Transverse image through the thyroid gland demonstrating normal parenchymal reflectivity in a patient with thyrotoxicosis. **(b)** The florid colour Doppler signal in the thyroid gland of the same patient is demonstrated, termed a 'thyroid storm'.

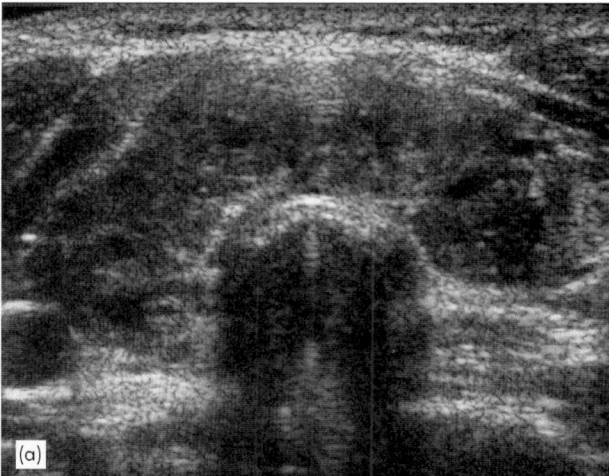

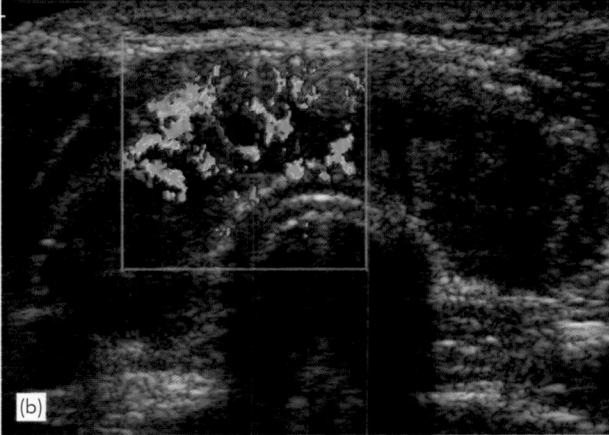

Figure 56.12 Thyroditis. **(a)** An enlarged thyroid gland with scattered 'pockets' of low reflectivity. **(b)** Colour Doppler ultrasound demonstrates a florid increase in vascularity with the inflammatory process.

elevated to 50–120 cm/s due to increased flow rates.[33, 43] There is no correlation between gland hyperfunction and vascularity, measured flow or velocity rates.[33] [***]

In Graves' disease, hypoechoic parenchymal echo-texture with a high flow rate in the thyroid arteries is suggestive of post-treatment relapse.[43] During the course of medical treatment, Doppler studies of the vessels demonstrate a marked fall in flow velocities measured in the superior and inferior thyroid arteries, proportional to the decrease in free circulating thyroid hormone.

Subacute (De Quervain's) thyroiditis is a clinical diagnosis, but on ultrasound the appearances may be characteristic (**Figure 56.12**).[33] Initially, the gland enlarges with ill-defined, irregular margins. Subsequently, the parenchyma becomes hypoechoic and colour Doppler ultrasound demonstrates either normal or decreased flow. As the disease progresses, the gland recovers at different rates and assumes a 'pseudonodular' configuration. Hypoechoic areas may enlarge at follow-up ultrasound, necessitating further medical treatment, where ultrasound assumes an important role.[33]

Chronic autoimmune thyroiditis is visualized as an enlarged gland with lobulated margins, internal fibrous septa and micronodules. The micronodules are seen as

hypoechoic areas measuring 1.0–6.5 mm, dispersed throughout the entire gland.[45] On histology, micronodules represent massive infiltration of plasma cells and lymphocytes. The presence of micronodules is highly suggestive of chronic autoimmune thyroiditis, with a positive predictive value estimated at 94.7 percent.[45] Colour Doppler ultrasound demonstrates increased vascularity similar to the 'thyroid inferno' described in Graves' disease, but the flow velocities are within normal limits both before and during treatment.[33] The end stage of chronic autoimmune thyroiditis is gland atrophy; ultrasounds demonstrating a small gland with ill-defined margins, a heterogeneous echo-texture and absent colour Doppler flow.[33]

RELIABILITY OF ULTRASOUND EXAMINATION OF THYROID NODULES

The finding of a thyroid nodule during an ultrasound examination requires the examiner to try and determine if the nodule is malignant or benign.[36] The reliability of B-mode ultrasound imaging with colour Doppler in differentiating benign from malignant nodules based on morphological and vascular features is reported to have a sensitivity of 63–87 percent, specificity of 61–91 percent with an overall accuracy of 80–94 percent.[33] Early work with ultrasound microbubble agents has been encouraging; in carcinomas, there is a significantly reduced measured arrival time of the contrast agent in comparison to hyperplastic or adenomatous nodules, but no significant difference in arrival time of the contrast agents in benign nodules.[46] FNAC is the most accurate way of distinguishing benign from malignant thyroid nodules with a reported sensitivity of 65–98 percent, specificity of 72–100 percent, false negative rates of 1–11 percent and false positive rates of 1–8 percent.[47] [****] Ultrasound is used to guide such procedures to increase the diagnostic yield of samples.

Parathyroid glands

Normal parathyroid glands are not usually visible due to their small size and similar echo-texture to adjacent thyroid tissue. Occasionally, normal parathyroid glands are seen as either hypoechoic or hyperechoic oval areas adjacent to the lower or upper poles of the thyroid gland.[48] Consequently, the parathyroid glands are usually only imaged when a patient has biochemical evidence of hyperparathyroidism.

Primary hyperparathyroidism may be secondary to either an adenoma (where a single gland is involved), hyperplasia (where all four glands are involved) or rarely a carcinoma. Adenomas are the main cause of primary hyperparathyroidism (80 percent of cases). Secondary hyperparathyroidism is usually a consequence of chronic hypocalcaemia in patients with chronic renal impairment.

Parathyroid adenomas and hyperplastic glands are oval in shape, measuring 7–15 mm in length and are usually hypoechoic in comparison to adjacent thyroid tissue (**Figure 56.13**).[49] Parathyroid adenomas have an echogenic capsule and are usually vascular on colour Doppler ultrasound with prominent diastolic flow demonstrated on spectral Doppler ultrasound. Areas of calcification are rare in parathyroid adenomas, but more common in hyperplasia and carcinoma.[49]

Intrathyroidal parathyroid glands are seen in 1 percent of cases and mimic thyroid nodules as they appear as hypoechoic areas with well-defined margins.[33] Solitary parathyroid cysts are rare, often occurring below the level of the inferior thyroid margin. The cystic fluid in functioning lesions contains high levels of parathyroid hormone.[50]

The sensitivity of ultrasound in localizing parathyroid glands in primary hyperparathyroidism is between 70 and 82 percent.[51, 52] However, in persistent or recurrent hyperparathyroidism, the sensitivity falls and ranges from 36 to 63 percent.[53]

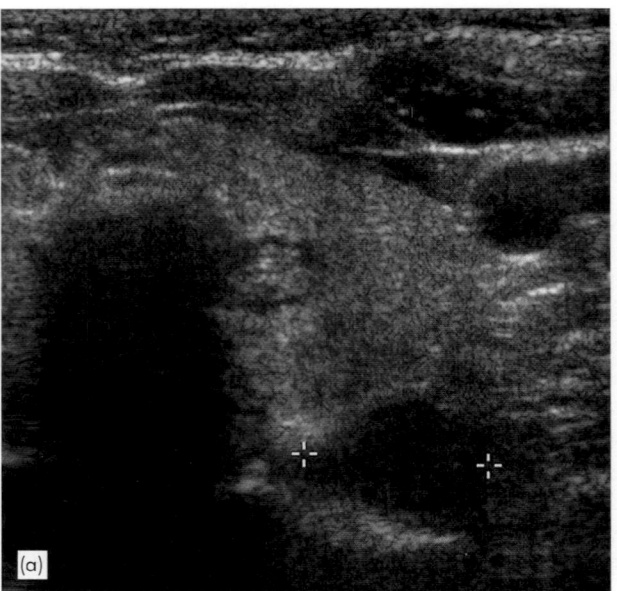

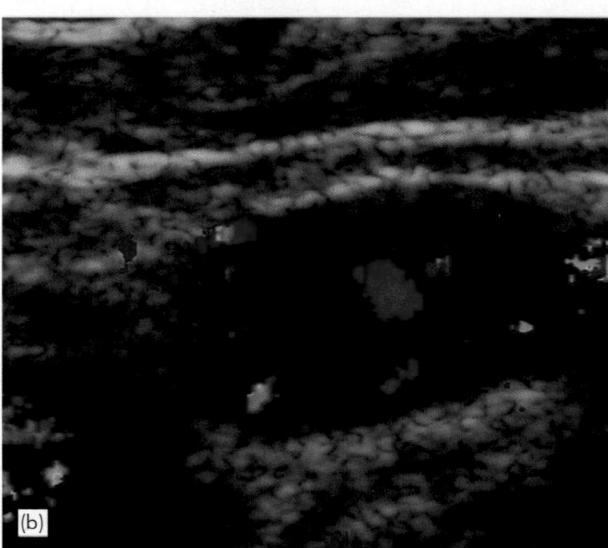

Figure 56.13 Parathyroid adenoma. (a) Low reflective ovoid area at the inferior aspect of the left lobe of the thyroid gland (between cursors). (b) Magnified image of a parathyroid adenoma demonstrating increased vascularity on colour Doppler ultrasound.

Salivary gland disease

Both the parotid and submandibular glands are superficial and well sited for ultrasound examination. The parotid glands are examined, initially in the axial plane in order to identify anatomical landmarks before completing the examination in the coronal plane. The submandibular glands are best seen in the coronal plane with paramandibular images as useful adjuncts. The normal submandibular gland parenchymal echo-texture is of a homogenous, highly reflective nature, well demarcated from surrounding tissues. The parotid gland is generally of higher echogenicity than the submandibular gland. The parotid (Stensen's) and submandibular (Wharton's) ducts are only seen on ultrasound when dilated.[6]

SALIVARY GLAND TUMOURS

Salivary gland tumours account for 3 percent of all head and neck tumours.[54, 55] Ultrasound accurately differentiates salivary gland tumours from other lesions outside the gland in 98 percent of cases.[54, 56] Tumours that arise in the parotid gland are benign pleomorphic adenomas in 80 percent of cases. The accepted treatment for pleomorphic adenomas is parotidectomy, as there is a 40–50 percent recurrence rate if they are only enucleated.[54, 57] Malignant transformation is reported in 3–10 percent of cases, with the risk increasing with time.[55] Pleomorphic adenomas are typically hypoechoic, slightly heterogeneous solid mass lesions with a smooth lobulated outline (**Figure 56.14**). Unusually, unlike other soft tissue masses, pleomorphic adenomas exhibit through transmission of sound in a similar fashion to simple cysts.[56] Ultrasound delineates pleomorphic adenomas in the parotid in 95 percent of cases and further cross-sectional imaging is advised in only in a minority of cases.[55] [**/*]

The second most common tumour in the parotid gland is a Warthin's tumour (adenolymphoma), accounting for 2–24 percent of parotid tumours.[54] Adenolymphomas are markedly hypoechoic due to the increased mucus content of cysts and contain discrete septations, suggested as characteristic of adenolymphomas.[55, 58] Parotid carcinomas are rare and are hypoechoic, heterogeneous lesions with irregular margins.[6] When differentiating malignancy from benign lesions using irregular margins as a marker for malignancy, ultrasound has an accuracy of 94 percent in lesions over 1.0 cm. However, using this as the only criterion is limited, as up to 28 percent of malignant tumours have well-demarcated borders.[56] [*]

SIALOLITHIASIS

The majority of salivary gland calculi (80 percent) occur in the submandibular gland.[56] Calculi larger than 2 mm may be detected on ultrasound, with a typical appearance of an echogenic rim with posterior acoustic shadowing (**Figure 56.15**). Calculi impacted at the ostium are not well seen on ultrasound, but often main salivary duct dilatation as well as intraglandular duct dilatation are present, with gland enlargement and a heterogeneous, hypoechoic appearance (**Figure 56.16**).[59] Both intra- and extraductal calculi may be treated with ultrasound lithotripsy but symptomatic intraparenchymal calculi require surgical removal. Ultrasound is useful in defining the location of calculi in relation to the gland parenchyma, which has important implications for clinical management.[55] [*]

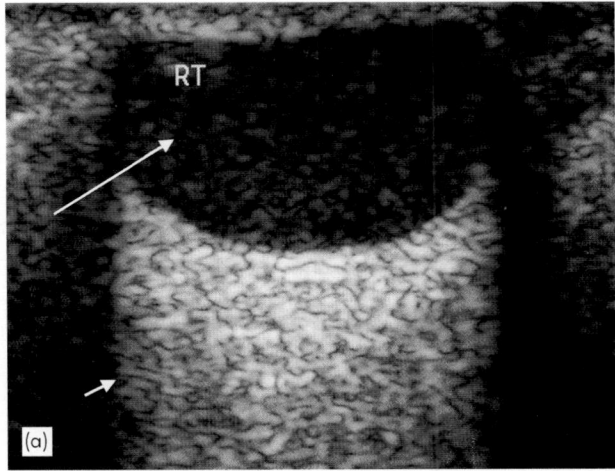

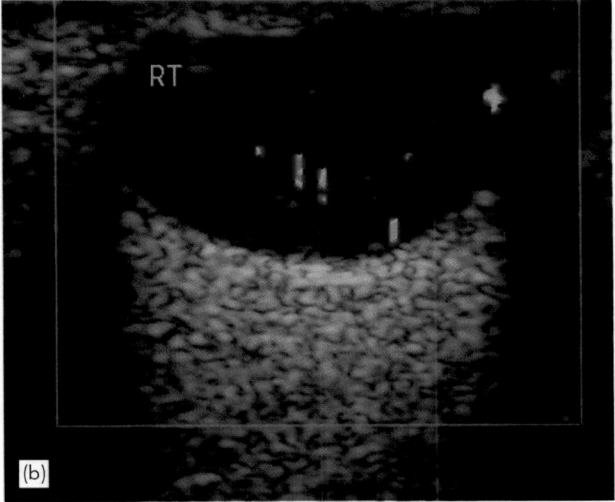

Figure 56.14 Parotid gland pleomorphic adenoma. **(a)** A well-circumscribed low reflective abnormality in the right parotid gland (long arrow) demonstrating through transmission of sound (short arrow), normally a feature of a cystic structure. **(b)** Colour Doppler ultrasound confirms lesion vascularity and the solid nature of the pleomorphic adenoma.

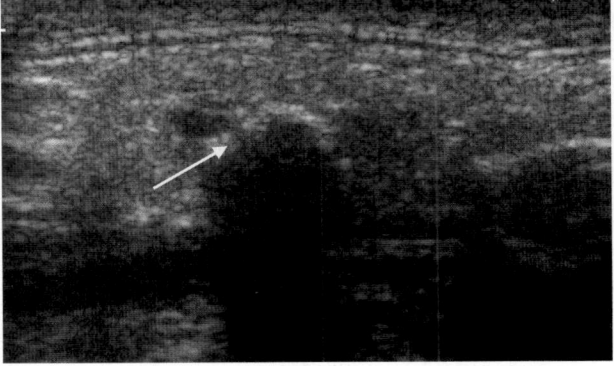

Figure 56.15 Submandibular gland calculus. Linear area of high reflectivity (arrow) and posterior acoustic shadowing present in the submandibular gland, in keeping with a calculus.

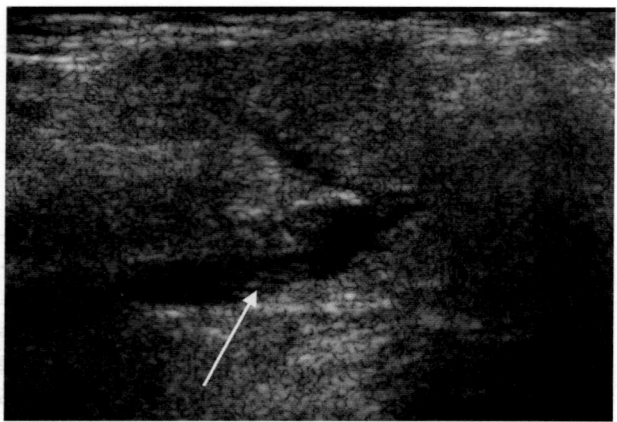

Figure 56.16 Submandibular gland duct dilatation. Dilated main duct in the submandibular gland.

INFLAMMATORY AND AUTOIMMUNE DISORDERS

Acute inflammation causes swollen salivary glands and this enlargement may be documented on ultrasound and compared to the contralateral side if unaffected, or to established normal measurements. Inflammation causes the gland to appear heterogeneous and hypoechoic on ultrasound; the main role of ultrasound is to exclude salivary duct dilatation.[56] Ultrasound may also identify any complications, such as abscess formation, and image guidance could then be used to aspirate fluid for microbiological analysis.

Acute suppurative sialadenitis is a painful condition occurring in postoperative, dehydrated and debilitated patients, seen almost exclusively in the parotid gland. Ultrasound may demonstrate an enlarged, well-defined gland with either a hypoechoic or hyperechoic parenchymal echo-texture. The role of ultrasound in this situation is to detect the presence and extent of any abscess formation.[59]

In chronic inflammation, one or both parotid glands appear heterogeneous with a small number of hypoechoic lesions, measuring up to 10 mm in diameter, often with associated reactive lymph nodes with their characteristic echogenic hilum present.[56] In Sjögren's syndrome, there is bilateral gland enlargement, which on ultrasound may appear of normal or hyperechoic texture with enlargement in the early stages.[59] As the disease progresses, the gland becomes atrophic with multicystic changes and a reticular pattern. The degree of parenchymal damage correlates well with glandular vascularity on colour Doppler ultrasound imaging.[59] As there is an increased risk of developing lymphoma, ultrasound may be used in the follow up of these patients.[60] [**]

CYSTIC LESIONS

Soft tissue cystic lesions occur with a frequency of 1–10 percent in the neck, with ultrasound able to clearly differentiate solid from cystic abnormalities.[61] Necrotic lymph node metastases from squamous cell carcinoma of the head and neck or papillary carcinoma of the thyroid may appear cystic and caution is needed in interpretation. Any lymph node is likely to demonstrate increased vascular flow with colour Doppler ultrasound, which may be used as a discriminator.[5] [*]

Thryoglossal cysts

Thyroglossal cysts occur close to the midline over the anterior aspect of the neck, anywhere between the foramen caecum to the pyramidal lobe of the thyroid gland. Thyroglossal cysts appear as anechoic areas with posterior acoustic enhancement, with the typical appearance of a cyst (**Figure 56.17**).[62, 63] The majority of thyroglossal cysts occur in the region of the hyoid bone and tend to communicate with the bone. This latter finding should be specifically sought on ultrasound, as this will allow the corpus of the hyoid bone to be removed with the cyst at the time of surgery.[56] It is possible on ultrasound imaging to establish if the cyst is multilocular or if a fistula is present.[62]

Branchial cysts

Branchial cysts most commonly arise from the first or second branchial clefts and are found in the region of the parotid glands or anterolateral to the carotid bifurcation. Branchial cysts vary in appearance on ultrasound from anechoic to heterogeneous, depending on the amount of cellular debris or cholesterol crystals in the cysts (**Figure 56.18**).[64] There is no vascularity on colour Doppler ultrasound and if there is colour Doppler signal, the possibility of a branchiogenic carcinoma should be raised.[6]

Dysontogenetic cysts

Epidermoid, dermoid cysts and teratomas are included in the dysontogenetic cyst group, occurring in the midline from the floor of the mouth or tongue.[65] These lesions are usually hypoechoic, but may have high reflective echoes due to the presence of hair, sebum and fluid.[66] The presence of calcification is considered characteristic of teratomas.[6]

Laryngoceles

Laryngoceles are dilatations of the saccule of Morgagni containing mucus, saliva and air, and are classified relative to their position to the larynx. Laryngoceles are seen as anechoic lesions if examined thorough an uncalcified thyroid cartilage.[67]

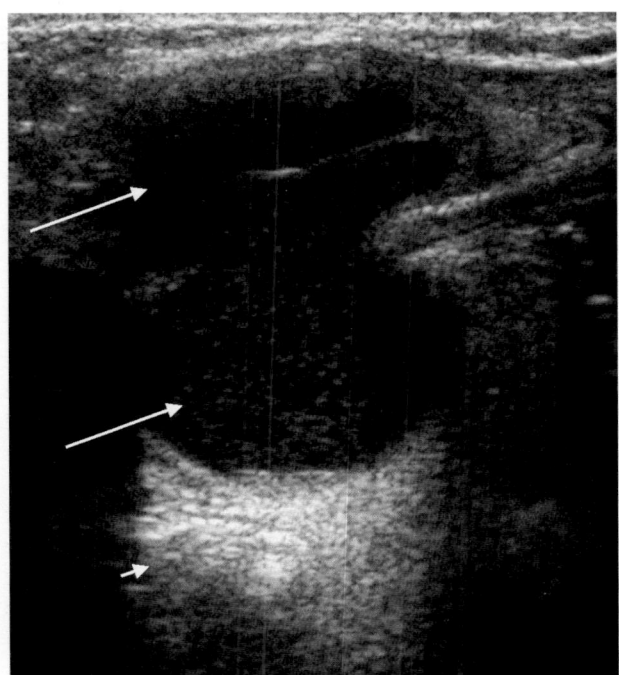

Figure 56.17 Thyroglossal cyst. A thick-walled, bilobulated thyroglossal cyst is present in the soft tissues above the hyoid bone (long arrows). Echogenic debris, manifest as reflective areas, is present within the cyst, which demonstrates characteristic posterior acoustic enhancement (short arrow).

Ranulas

Ranulas are mucous retention cysts of the minor sublingual salivary glands and can extend over the posterolateral aspect of the mylohyoid muscle. Ranulas are recognized as hypoechoic lesions with smooth, well-defined margins with no colour Doppler signal.[6]

SOFT TISSUE NEOPLASMS

Ultrasound is often the only technique used for imaging non-nodal cervical lesions. CT and MRI are used as adjuncts in patients where the lesion is not completely delineated or a specific diagnosis is not made by ultrasound. [*]

Lipomas

Lipomas are common soft tissue masses that are oval, elongated lesions with varying echogenicity depending on the amount of fat and fibrous tissue within the lesion (**Figure 56.19**).[68] The greater the fat content, the more hypoechoic the lesion appears, with the echogenic manifestation due to the presence of multiple fat–water interfaces within the lesion acting as reflectors, thus

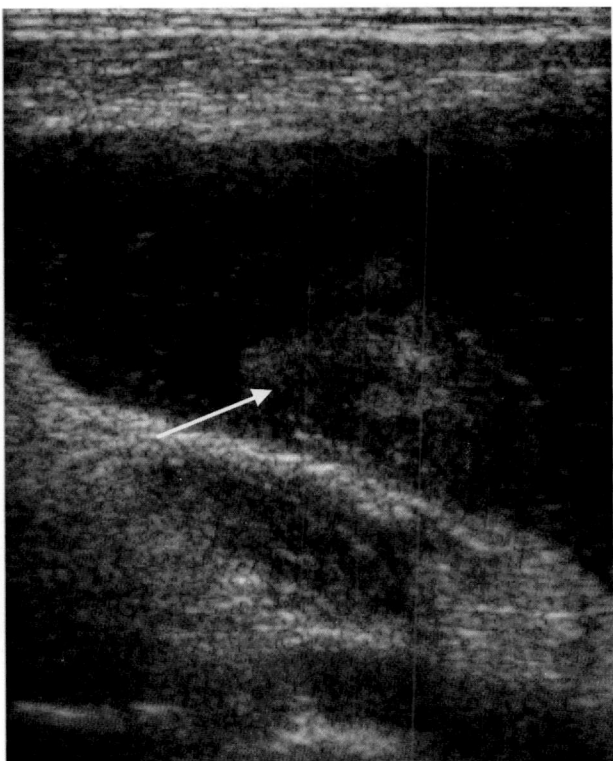

Figure 56.18 Branchial cyst. A cystic abnormality present in the soft tissues of the lateral aspect of the neck, with an area (arrow) of echogenic debris present.

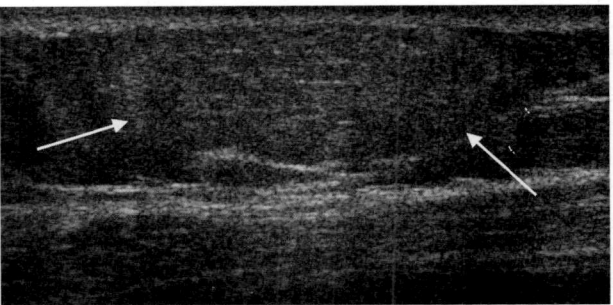

Figure 56.19 Lipoma. A well-circumscribed isoechoic abnormality (arrows) in the soft tissues of the neck causing displacement of the surrounding tissue planes with no increase in colour Doppler signal.

increasing the number and intensity of reflected echoes.[69] In the rare cases where there is doubt, CT or MRI can confirm the presence of fat.

Paragangliomas

Paragangliomas are tumours arising from the autonomic nervous tissue, commonly the carotid body or vagal ganglia (**Figure 56.20**). Paragangliomas appear as hypoechoic solid tumours and lie between the bifurcation

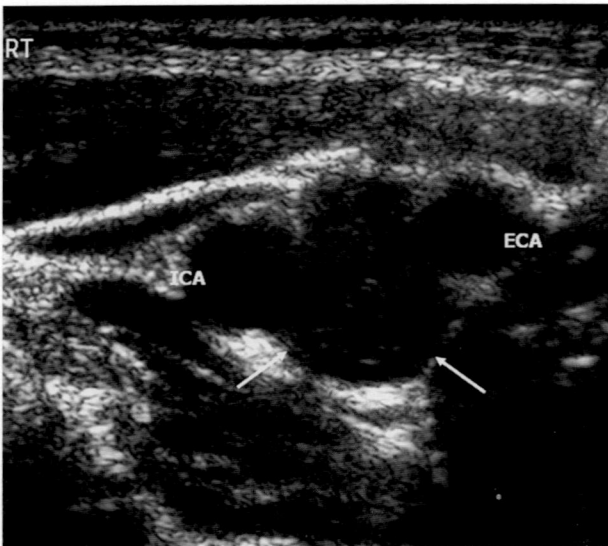

Figure 56.20 Carotid body tumour. A low reflective abnormality (between arrows) with evidence of displacement of the internal carotid artery (ICA) and the external carotid artery (ECA).

of the internal and external carotid arteries. Colour Doppler ultrasound demonstrates a markedly vascular lesion with a low resistance flow, resultant to arteriovenous shunts.[70] Ultrasound is additionally useful in the follow up of these patients to facilitate early detection of recurrence.[6]

Neurogenic tumours

Neurofibromas and schwannomas, when they are present in the neck, are most commonly sited in the posterior triangle. Neurogenic tumours are well-defined, hypoechoic, fusiform lesions with a number of central cystic areas in continuity with a nerve and exhibit posterior acoustic enhancement.[71] With neurofibromas, the nerve enters the centre of the lesion, whereas in schwannomas the mass is eccentric to the nerve and this may be demonstrated on ultrasound. Shwannomas have a variable vascularity but are generally hypervascular, whereas neurofibromas are less vascular which may be an important distinguishing factor between these two entities.[71]

Vascular malformations

Haemangiomas are the most common tumour in infants and up to 60 percent will occur in the head and neck area.[13] Vascular-based lesions may be seen in the prenatal period, are usually evident in the first two years of life and are classified into two broad categories: haemangiomas and other vascular malformations. Vascular malformations are further divided depending on flow characteristics and the presence of anomalous channels.[72] It is important to distinguish between haemangiomas and other vascular malformations as they are treated differentially and have different outcomes. A haemangioma does not regress spontaneously. Haemangiomas are a clinical diagnosis and the role of imaging is to identify deep malformations or if they present as an atypical soft tissue mass. Haemangiomas have a variable ultrasound appearance depending on the number of 'cystic' vascular spaces present. Small lesions are usually echogenic but often the larger lesions are hypoechoic, compressible with increased colour Doppler flow.[73] Lesions in the proliferative phases have increased colour Doppler flow with increased vessel density (>5 vessels/cm^2) and a low resistance pattern on spectral Doppler ultrasound.[72, 74]

Congenital venous malformations occur in the head and neck in 40 percent of cases, but are often not diagnosed at birth.[13, 72] Grey-scale imaging can aid the diagnosis of a venous malformation. The majority of venous malformations are heterogeneous and hypoechoic relative to the subcutaneous tissue and phleboliths are seen in 16 percent.[73] On spectral Doppler ultrasound, venous malformations tend to have a low velocity monophasic flow pattern and mixed vascular lesions tend to have a low velocity, biphasic flow pattern.[73] If the flow velocity is so low to be below the level that can be detected with normal colour Doppler imaging, then the administration of ultrasound microbubble contrast agent may help.[13] Arteriovenous malformations (AVM) have a heterogeneous appearance due to visualization of the feeding vessels; colour and spectral Doppler analysis show high vessel density with high systolic flow from numerous sites of arteriovenous shunting. Distinct from haemangiomas, an AVM always demonstrates pulsatile flow in the veins caused by arterialization of the veins.[72]

Lymphangiomas

Lymphangiomas are thought to originate from sequestered lymphatic sacs that do not communicate with peripheral draining channels. Cystic hygromas, usually diagnosed on antenatal ultrasound examination, are a form of lymphangioma. Seventy-five percent of all lymphangiomas are located in the neck, usually in the posterior triangle, with up to 10 percent extending down to the mediastinum.[75] Four types are classified on histological criteria: cystic hygroma, cavernous lymphangiomas, capillary lymphangiomas and vasculolymphatic malformations. These four types cannot be differentiated by ultrasound as all are multilocular, predominantly cystic masses with both septa and solid components. Ultrasound may also be used to guide therapeutic sclerosing injection in the management of macrocystic lymphangiomas.[76]

Ectopic thymic tissue

Ectopic thymic tissue is seen in the neck in 21–42 percent of infants and resembles a lymphoma, appearing as an echogenic mass with septa that are isoechoic with normal thymus tissue. Increased vascularity on colour Doppler ultrasound allows differentiation of ectopic thymic tissue from a lipoma.[5]

Foreign bodies

Ultrasound is useful in localizing nonradio-opaque foreign bodies, especially in the neck to guide the operator to a suture granuloma with its typical appearance of a hypo-echoic lesion with a central curvilinear echogenic line.[6]

CONCLUSION

Ultrasound is a safe, widely available imaging technique that is patient-friendly and extensively used in most aspects of clinical medicine. In neck imaging, ultrasound use has become more prevalent with the development of real-time, high frequency ultrasound transducers, digital imaging technology coupled with the inherent anatomical advantage of the superficial structures of the head and neck. Ultrasound is currently the imaging modality of choice after clinical examination in ENT practice. Ongoing improvements to ultrasound technology will lead to increased diagnostic accuracy.

KEY POINTS

- High frequency, high resolution ultrasound provides excellent visualization of structures of the neck, allowing guided interventional procedures.
- Ultrasound readily identifies enlarged lymph nodes and may usefully divide the appearances into benign or malignant.
- Ultrasound detects nodular thyroid disease, but is nonspecific in establishing the type of nodule.
- Ultrasound often identifies papillary carcinoma of the thyroid.
- Ultrasound is not sensitive, but specific for the detection of parathyroid adenomas.
- Ultrasound is a reliable method of examination for salivary gland disease.
- Ultrasound should always be the first-line imaging modality in assessing disease of the soft tissues and glandular structures of the neck.

Best clinical practice

✓ A linear high frequency transducer will allow the optimal resolution of the structures of the neck and will guide needle placement in the lesion for tissue sampling.
✓ Ultrasound of lymph nodes using B-mode, colour and spectral Doppler ultrasound allows accurate delineation of lymph nodes into benign and malignant types, but fine needle aspiration is always required.
✓ Ultrasound in the delineation of thyroid nodules is not specific except in papillary cell carcinoma where some ultrasound features are characteristic.
✓ Ultrasound defines an enlarged thyroid and, with the addition of colour Doppler ultrasound, identifies the appearances of thyroiditis and Graves' disease.
✓ Parathyroid adenomas have a characteristic low-reflective ovoid appearance on ultrasound, with colour Doppler flow present in the lesion.
✓ Ultrasound of obstructive salivary gland disease is accurate and will often identify the calculus.

Deficiencies in current knowledge and areas for future research

➤ Ultrasound probe technology and image post-processing will continue to improve, which will allow better visualization of neck structures in difficult patients.
➤ The use of microbubble contrast agents will allow physiological aspects of tumour circulation to be better understood and aid tissue characterization, using transit time and blood vessel distribution.
➤ Better needle visualization will allow better needle guidance for cytological analysis.
➤ An improvement in the identification of benign versus malignant thyroid nodules is desirable.

REFERENCES

1. Merritt CR. Physics of ultrasound. In: Rumack CM, Wilson SR, Charboneau JW (eds). *Diagnostic ultrasound*. St Louis: Mosby, 1998: 3–33.
2. Harvey CJ, Pilcher JM, Eckersley RJ, Blomley MJK, Cosgrove DO. Advances in ultrasound. *Clinical Radiology*. 2002; **57**: 157–177.
3. Weng L, Tirumalai AP, Lowery CM, Nock LF, Gustafson DE, Von Behren PL *et al*. US extended field-of-view imaging technology. *Radiology*. 1997; **203**: 877–80.

4. Whittingham TA. Tissue harmonic imaging. *European Radiology.* 1999; **9**: S323–6.

* 5. Koischwitz D, Gritzmann N. Ultrasound of the neck. *Radiologic Clinics of North America.* 2000; **38**: 1029–45.

* 6. Gritzmann N, Hollerweger A, Macheiner P, Rettenbacher T. Sonography of soft tissue masses of the neck. *Journal of Clinical Ultrasound.* 2002; **30**: 356–73.

7. Merritt CRB. Doppler US: The basics. *Radiographics.* 1991; **11**: 109–19.

8. Harvey CJ, Blomley MJK, Eckersley RJ, Cosgrove DO. Developments in ultrasound contrast media. *European Radiology.* 2001; **11**: 675–89.

9. Ferrara KW, Merritt CR, Burns PN, Foster FS, Mattrey RF, Wickline SA. Evaluation of tumor angiogenesis with US: Imaging, Doppler contrast agents. *Academic Radiology.* 2000; **7**: 824–39.

10. Castelijns JA, van den Brekel MWM. Imaging of lymphadenopathy in the neck. *European Radiology.* 2002; **12**: 727–38.

11. Ying M, Ahuja A. Sonography of neck lymph nodes. Part I. Normal lymph nodes. *Clinical Radiology.* 2003; **58**: 351–8.

12. van den Brekel MWM, Stel HV, Castelijns JA, Nauta JJP, vander Waal I, Valk J *et al.* Cervical lymph node metastasis: assessment of radiologic criteria. *Radiology.* 1990; **177**: 379–84.

13. Toma P, Rossi UG. Paediatric ultrasound. II. Other applications. *European Radiology.* 2001; **11**: 2369–98.

14. Wakisaka M, Mori H, Fuwa N, Matsumoto A. MR analysis of nasopharyngeal carcinoma: Correlation of the pattern of tumor extent at the primary site with the distribution of metastasized cervical lymph nodes. *Preliminary results. European Radiology.* 2000; **10**: 970–7.

15. Khoury GG, Paterson IC. Nasopharyngeal carcinoma: A review of cases treated by radiotherapy and chemotherapy. *Clinical Radiology.* 1987; **38**: 17–20.

16. Shingaki S, Kobyashi T, Suzuki I, Kohno M, Nakajima T. Surgical treatment of stage I and II oral squamous cell carcinomas: analysis of causes of failure. *British Journal of Oral and Maxillofacial Surgery.* 1995; **33**: 304–8.

17. Levendag P, Sessions R, Vikram B, Strong EW, Shah JP, Spiro R *et al.* The problem of neck relapse in early stage supraglottic larynx cancer. *Cancer.* 1989; **63**: 345–8.

18. Stuckensen T, Kovacs AF, Adams S, Baum RP. Staging of the neck in patients with oral cavity squamous cell carcinomas: a prospective comparison of PET, ultrasound, CT and MRI. *Journal of Cranio-Maxillo-Facial surgery.* 2000; **28**: 319–24.

19. Vassallo P, Wernecke K, Roos N, Peters PE. Differentiation of benign from malignant superficial lymphadenopathy: The role of high resolution US. *Radiology.* 1992; **183**: 215–20.

20. Tohnosu N, Onoda S, Isono K. Ultrasonography evaluation of cervical lymph node metastases in esophageal cancer with special reference to the relationship between the short to long axis (S/L) and the cancer content. *Journal of Clinical Ultrasound.* 1989; **17**: 101–6.

* 21. Hajek PC, Salomonowitz E, Turk R, Tscholakoff D, Kumpan W, Czemberik H. Lymph nodes of the neck: Evaluation with US. *Radiology.* 1986; **158**: 739–42.

22. van den Brekel MW, Castelijns JA, Snow GB. The size of lymph nodes in the neck on sonograms as a radiologic criterion for metastasis: how reliable is it? *American Journal of Neuroradiology.* 1998; **19**: 695–700.

23. Ying M, Ahuja AT, Evans R, King W, Metreweli C. Cervical lymphadenopathy: Sonographic differentiation between tuberculous and nodal metastases from non-head and neck carcinomas. *Journal of Clinical Ultrasound.* 1998; **26**: 383–9.

24. Ahuja A, Chow L, Chick W, King W, Metreweli C. Metastatic cervical nodes in papillary carcinoma of the thyroid: Ultrasound and histological correlation. *Clinical Radiology.* 1995; **50**: 229–31.

25. Ahuja AT, Ying M, Yuen HY, Metreweli C. 'Pseudocystic' appearance of non-Hodgkin's lymphomatous nodes: An infrequent finding with high-resolution transducers. *Clinical Radiology.* 2001; **56**: 111–5.

26. Som PM. Lymph nodes of the neck. *Radiology.* 1987; **165**: 593–600.

* 27. Solbiati L, Rizzatto G, Bellotti E, Montali G, Ciotti V, Croce F. High-resolution sonography of cervical lymph nodes in head and neck cancer: Criteria for differentiation of reactive versus malignant nodes. *Radiology.* 1988; **169P**: 113.

28. Ahuja A, Ying M, Yang WT, Evans R, King W, Metreweli C. The use of sonography in differentiating cervical lymphomatous lymph nodes from cervical metastatic lymph nodes. *Clinical Radiology.* 1996; **51**: 186–90.

29. Ahuja AT, Ying M, Evans R, King W, Metreweli C. The application of ultrasound criteria for malignancy in differentiating tuberculous cervical adenitis from metastatic nasopharyngeal carcinoma. *Clinical Radiology.* 1995; **50**: 391–5.

30. Wu CH, Chang YL, Hsu WC, Ko JY, Sheen TS, Hsieh FJ. Usefulness of Doppler spectral analysis and power Doppler sonography in the differentiation of cervical lymphadenopathies. *American Journal of Roentgenology.* 1998; **171**: 503–9.

31. Ahuja A, Ying M, Yuen YH, Metreweli C. Power Doppler sonography to differentiate tuberculous cervical lymphadenopathy from nasopharyngeal carcinoma. *American Journal of Neuroradiology.* 2001; **22**: 735–40.

32. Moritz JD, Ludwig A, Oestmann JW. Contrast-enhanced color Doppler sonography for evaluation of enlarged cervical lymph nodes in head and neck tumors. *American Journal of Roentgenology.* 2000; **174**: 1279–84.

* 33. Solbiati L, Osti V, Cova L, Tonolini M. Ultrasound of thyroid, parathyroid glands and neck lymph nodes. *European Radiology.* 2001; **11**: 2411–24.

34. Hegedus L, Perrild H, Poulsen LR, Andersen JR, Holm B, Schnohr P *et al.* The determination of thyroid volume by ultrasound and its relationship to body weight, age and sex in normal subjects. *Journal of Clinical Endocrinology and Metabolism.* 1983; **56**: 260–3.

35. Ahuja A, Chick W, King W, Metreweli C. Clinical significance of the comet-tail artifact in thyroid ultrasound. *Journal of Clinical Ultrasound*. 1996; **24**: 129–33.

∗ 36. Solbiati L, Osti V, Cova L, Tonolini M. Thyroid nodules: Which sonographic criteria for differentiation between benign and malignant lesions? *British Medical Ultrasound Society Bulletin*. 2001; **9**: 11–8.

37. Ahuja AT, Chow L, Chick W, King W, Metreweli C. Metastatic cervical node in papillary carcinoma of the thyroid: ultrasound and histological correlation. *Clinical Radiology*. 1995; **50**: 229–31.

38. Frates MC, Benson CB, Doubilet PM, Cibas ES, Marqusee E. Can color Doppler sonography aid in the prediction of malignancy of thyroid nodules? *Journal of Ultrasound in Medicien*. 2003; **22**: 127–33.

39. McConahey WM, Hay ID, Woolner LB, van Heerden JA, Taylor WF. Papillary thyroid cancer treated at the Mayo Clinic, 1946 through 1970: Initial manifestations, pathologic findings, therapy, and outcome. *Mayo Clinic Proceedings*. 1986; **61**: 978–96.

40. Takashima S, Morimoyo S, Ikezoe J, Takai S, Kobayashi T, Koyama H *et al*. CT evaluation of anaplastic thyroid carcinoma. *American Journal of Roentgenology*. 1990; **154**: 1079–85.

41. Gorman B, Charboneau JW, James EM, Reading CC, Wold LE, Grant CS *et al*. Medullary thyroid carcinoma: Role of high-resolution US. *Radiology*. 1987; **162**: 147–50.

42. Takashima S, Morimoto S, Ikezoe J, Arisawa J, Hamada S, Ikeda H *et al*. Primary thyroid lymphoma: comparison of CT and US assessment. *Radiology*. 1989; **171**: 439–43.

43. Castagnone D, Rivolta R, Rescalli S, Tozzi R, Cantalamessa L. Color Doppler sonography in Grave's disease: Value in assessing activity of disease and predicting outcome. *American Journal of Roentgenology*. 1996; **166**: 203–7.

44. Ralls PW, Mayekawa DS, Lee KP, Radin DR, Boswell WD, Halls JM. Color-flow Doppler sonography in Graves disease: 'thyroid inferno'. *American Journal of Roentgenology*. 1988; **150**: 781–4.

45. Yeh HC, Futterweit W, Gilbert P. Micronodulation: Ultrasonographic sign of Hashimoto thyroiditis. *Journal of Ultrasound in Medicine*. 1996; **15**: 813–9.

46. Spiezia S, Farina R, Cerbone G, Assanti AP, Iovino V, Siciliani M *et al*. Analysis of color Doppler signal intensity variation after Levovist injection. A new approach to the diagnosis of thyroid nodules. *Journal of Ultrasound in Medicine*. 2001; **20**: 223–31.

47. Gharib H, Goellner JR. Fine-needle aspiration biopsy of the thyroid: An appraisal. *Annals of Internal Medicine*. 1993; **118**: 282–9.

∗ 48. Simeone JF, Mueller PR, Ferrucci JT, vanSonnenberg E, Wang CA, Hall DA *et al*. High-resolution real-time sonography of the parathyroid. *Radiology*. 1981; **141**: 745–51.

49. Reeder SB, Desser TS, Weigel RJ, Jeffrey RB. Sonography in primary hyperparathyroidism. *Journal of Ultrasound in Medicine*. 2002; **21**: 539–52.

50. Forston JK, Patel VG, Henderson VJ. Parathyroid cysts: A case report and review of the literature. *Laryngoscope*. 2001; **111**: 1726–8.

51. Attie JN, Khan A, Rumancik WM, Moskowitz GW, Hirsch MA, Herman PG. Preoperative localization of parathyroid adenomas. *American Journal of Surgery*. 1988; **156**: 323–6.

52. Weinberger MS, Robbins KT. Diagnostic localization studies for primary hyperparathyroidism. A suggested algorithm. *Archives of Otolaryngology – Head and Neck Surgery*. 1994; **120**: 1187–9.

53. Rodriquez JM, Tezelman S, Siperstein AE, Duh QV, Higgins C, Morita E *et al*. Localization procedures in patients with persistent or recurrent hyperparathyroidism. *Archives of Surgery*. 1994; **129**: 870–5.

54. Freling NJM. Imaging of salivary gland disease. *Seminars in Roentgenology*. 2000; **35**: 12–20.

55. Wittich GR, Scheible FW, Hajek PC. Ultrasonography of the salivary glands. *Radiologic Clinics of North America*. 1985; **23**: 29–37.

56. Gritzmann N. Sonography of the salivary glands. *America Journal of Roentgenology*. 1989; **153**: 161–6.

57. Koral K, Seyre J, Bhuta S, Abemayor E, Lufkin R. Recurrent pleomorphic adenoma of the parotid gland in pediatric and adult patients: Value of multiple lesions as a diagnostic indicator. *America Journal of Roentgenology*. 2003; **180**: 1171–4.

58. Howlett DC, Kesse KW, Huges DV, Sallomi DF. The role of imaging in the evaluation of parotid disease. *Clinical Radiology*. 2002; **57**: 692–701.

∗ 59. Ching ASC, Ahuja A. High-resolution sonography of the submandibular space: anatomy and abnormalities. *America Journal of Roentgenology*. 2002; **179**: 703–8.

60. MAkula E, Pokorny G, Kiss M, Voros E, Kovacs L, Kovacs A *et al*. The place of magnetic resonance and ultrasonographic examinations of the parotid gland in the diagnosis and follow-up of primary Sjogrens's syndrome. *Rheumatology*. 2000; **39**: 97–104.

61. Koeller KK, Alamo L, Adair CF, Smirniotopoulos JG. Congenital cystic masses of the neck: radiologic-pathologic correlation. *Radiographics*. 1999; **19**: 121–46.

62. Ahuja AT, King AD, Metreweli C. Sonographic evaluation of thyroglossal duct cysts in children. *Clinical Radiology*. 2000; **55**: 770–4.

63. Ahuja AT, King AD, King W, Metreweli C. Thyroglossal duct cysts: Sonographic appearances in adults. *American Journal of Neuroradiology*. 1999; **20**: 579–82.

64. Badami JP, Athey PA. Sonography in the diagnosis of branchial cysts. *America Journal of Roentgenology*. 1981; **137**: 1245–8.

65. Smirniotopoulos JG, Chiechi MV. Teratomas, dermoids, and epidermoids of the head and neck. *Radiographics*. 1995; **15**: 1437–55.

66. Turetschek K, Hospodka H, Steiner E. Case report: Epidermoid cyst of the floor of the mouth: Diagnostic imaging by sonography, computed tomography and

magnetic resonance imaging. *British Journal of Radiology*. 1995; **68**: 205–97.

67. Baatenburg de Jong RJ, Rongen RJ, Lameris JS, Knegt P, Verwoerd CD. Ultrasound in the diagnosis of laryngoceles. *ORL, Journal for Oto-Rhino-Laryngology and its Related Specialties*. 1993; **55**: 290–3.

68. Fornage BD. Sonographic appearances of superficial soft tissue lipomas. *Journal of Clinical Ultrasound*. 1991; **19**: 215–20.

∗ 69. Behan M, Kazam E. The echographic characteristics of fatty tissues and tumors. *Radiology*. 1978; **129**: 143–51.

70. Derchi L, Serafini G, Rabbia C, De Albertis P, Solbiati L, Candiani F *et al*. Carotid body tumors: US evaluation. *Radiology*. 1992; **182**: 457–9.

71. King AD, Ahuja AT, King W, Metreweli C. Sonography of peripheral nerve tumors of the neck. *America Journal of Roentgenology*. 1997; **169**: 1695–8.

∗ 72. Dubois J, Garel L. Imaging and therapeutic approach of hemangiomas and vascular malformations in the pediatric age group. *Pediatric Radiology*. 1999; **29**: 879–93.

73. Trop I, Dubois J, Guibaud L, Grignon A, Patriquin H, McCuaig C *et al*. Soft-tissue venous malformations in pediatric and young adult patients: Diagnosis with Doppler US. *Radiology*. 1999; **212**: 841–5.

74. Dubois J, Patriquin HB, Garel L, Powell J, Filiatrault D, David M *et al*. Soft-tissue hemangiomas in infants and children: diagnosis using Doppler sonography. *American Journal of Roentgenology*. 1998; **171**: 247–52.

75. Zadvinskis DP, Benson MT, Kerr HH, Mancuso AA, Cacciarelli AA, Madrazo BL *et al*. Congenital malformations of the cervico-thoracic lymphatic system: Embryology and pathogenesis. *Radiographics*. 1992; **12**: 1173–89.

76. Dubois J, Garel L, Abela A, Laberge L, Yazbeck S. Lymphangiomas in children: Percutaneous sclerotherapy with an alcoholic solution of Zein. *Radiology*. 1997; **204**: 651–4.

57

Interventional techniques

JAMES V BYRNE

Introduction	731	Embolization for epistaxis	739
Indications	732	Key points	740
Tools used in interventional neuroradiology techniques	732	Deficiencies in current knowledge and areas for future	
Application of embolization techniques	734	research	740
Embolization for meningiomas and paragangliomas	735	References	740

SEARCH STRATEGY AND EVIDENCE-BASE

The data in this chapter are supported by a Medline search using the key words interventional neuroradiology, endovascular therapy, embolization, meningioma, paraganglioma, epistaxis and tumour embolization.

The evidence base for most INR treatments is lacking. Research has largely involved reports of single institute case audits. Large-scale trials are difficult because relatively small patient numbers are treated at each hospital and multicentre cooperation is needed. This problem is currently being addressed by various specialist interest groups who have organized case registries and a large multicentre trial to study the efficacy of embolization alone for treatment of meningioma is ongoing.

INTRODUCTION

What is interventional neuroradiology and what is its role in the management of patients with pathologies of the head and neck? This chapter is intended to answer these two questions by describing the current (and future) capabilities of the discipline. Interventional radiology originated in surgery, but its complete dependence on accurate *in vivo* corporal imaging places it in radiology. In 1930, Brooks[1] closed an arteriovenous fistula of the cavernous carotid by introducing a muscle embolus via an arteriotomy in the proximal carotid artery. This desperate operation was performed in order to avoid the extensive dissection required to expose and directly repair the fistula. The need of imaging to monitor such embolization was obvious, but the capacity to do so developed slowly after the first description of cerebral angiography by Egas Moniz in 1927,[2] and the technologies needed to navigate catheters through blood vessels and to deposit emboli at specific sites did not become available for another 30 years. In 1964, Lusenhop and Valasquez[3] described an operation to embolize a caroticocavernous fistula using an endovascular catheter under x-ray control and the current form of most procedures was born. Interventions for head and neck pathologies are usually practised within the subspecialty of neuroradiology or, more specifically, interventional neuroradiology (INR).

The term 'most procedures' is used because endovascular embolization is the most common technique. It is used to treat arteriovenous shunts, devascularize tumours and close large arteries prior to surgical resections. However, also included in the INR repertoire are percutaneous techniques for embolization of vascular malformations and tumours, as well as image-guided biopsy and the focussed endovascular delivery of chemotherapy agents. The technologically-driven evolution of the discipline will almost certainly produce new techniques and applications to replace more invasive surgery in the future and it remains to be seen, into which other branch(es) of medicine (or rather surgery) it extends.

INDICATIONS

Detection of head and neck lesions is by magnetic resonance (MR) or computed tomography (CT) scanning and the possible role of INR should be considered before invasive diagnostic x-ray angiography is performed. Combining embolization or functional testing with diagnostic x-ray angiography means that the indications for INR techniques should be considered early in treatment planning.

Preoperative treatment planning of patients with tumours generally involves obtaining biopsy tissue and mapping the lesion's blood supply, as well as its extent and relationship to adjacent normal structures. Information about invasion of large arteries and veins may be vital. Major vessels are at risk, either because of tumour spread or because their sacrifice is a necessary component of the surgical approach. In these situations, preoperative testing of blood supply by temporary vessel occlusion is indicated and endovascular ligation may be appropriate (see Coils and balloons).

Embolization of highly vascular tumours is indicated prior to surgical resection of these tumours in order to reduce intraoperative blood loss and operation times. It may also be indicated to relieve patients of symptoms by inducing tumour shrinkage. Embolization is targeted to occlude the tumour vascular bed, rather than feeding arteries, since occlusion of proximal arteries may fail to reduce blood supply because blood flow from collateral arteries can still be recruited. It is, therefore, most effective in tumours with a rich vascular bed. In most instances, this can be inferred from the degree of contrast enhancement evident on CT or MR scanning, but the uptake of radiographic contrast within a tissue reflects the degree of extravascular leakage of these agents and does not necessarily imply high vascularity, so occasionally tumours showing pronounced enhancement are not suitable for embolization.

The decision to perform embolization therefore depends on clinical and anatomical factors. These should be reviewed in consultation between otolaryngologist and interventional neuroradiologist. The principle guiding the decision to recommend preoperative embolization is that the addition of the INR procedure to the patient's treatment plan should not add to its overall risk. The risk/benefit analysis may require information that can only be obtained at the time of x-ray angiography. For example, embolization via arteries with intracranial territories of supply is obviously more likely to be complicated by stroke than treatments performed entirely in extracranial vessels. Therefore, a team approach is needed to ensure that the risks of complications caused by embolization or preoperative functional testing are acceptable and are likely to improve the results of subsequent surgery. These issues, as they apply to specific tumour types, and the use of embolization in the management of epistaxis, will be discussed below. The purpose and indications for INR techniques are summarized in **Table 57.1**.

TOOLS USED IN INTERVENTIONAL NEURORADIOLOGY TECHNIQUES

Endovascular catheters

Transarterial or transvenous catheterizations are performed for embolization, temporary vessel closures for dynamic testing or intraarterial drug delivery. The catheters used are available in a range of sizes with shaped tips. They are used to select and inject radiographic contrast media in cranial vessels for angiography or as guiding catheters for smaller catheters used for the section of small vessels (i.e. microcatheters). Microcatheters are generally 0.02 inches (0.508 mm) or smaller in diameter and used to inject embolization materials. They are constructed with flexible distal ends for navigation through tortuous vessels and stiffer proximal sections to allow the operator to advance them by pushing.

Two basic types of microcatheters are used: flow-directed and over-the-wire catheters. The former have extremely light and supple distal ends so that they are carried by antegrade blood flow to the target position. The latter are pushed over a guide wire to the objective. Flow-directed catheters work best when blood flow is increased and are therefore used to treat arteriovenous shunts. Their size limits their use to the injection of

Table 57.1 Indications for INR techniques.

Procedure	Technique	Purpose/Benefit
Biopsy	Percutaneous needle	Appropriate treatment selection
Functional testing	Balloon occlusion	Assessment of collateral blood supply prior to surgical or endovascular ligations
Embolization of small vessels	Particles or liquid embolics	Devascularization of tumour to stop haemorrhage
Embolization of large vessels	Balloon or coils	To aid surgical exposure/dissection
Chemotherapy	Superselective injection	To maximize drug delivery

liquids or very small particles. Over-the-wire catheters are used when blood flow is slower. The combination of guide wire and a stiffer catheter makes navigation easier and their larger lumen allows the delivery of both particles and coils. They are usually used in the treatment of head and neck tumours.

Materials used for embolization

PARTICLES

Embolic agents can be categorized on various criteria. Traditionally, they are divided according to whether the resulting devascularization is permanent or temporary. Temporary agents being autologous blood clot, gelfoam powder and microfibrillar collagen, whilst polyvinyl alcohol particles (PVA) are considered permanent agents (see **Table 57.2**). However, embolization using PVA is liable to be temporary because, though the particles are not degraded, their effect may be circumvented by development of new collateral vessels.[4,5] In practice, the development of new vessels is less likely if particles can be deposited in vessels within the tumour, rather than in proximal arteries. To ensure the deep penetration of injected particles, they are engineered to mix well with radiographic contrast so that they can be injected as an even suspension. PVA or Trisacryl gelatin microspheres are currently used in the author's department. These come in a range of sizes varying between 40 and 800 microns in diameter. The choice of particle size is important because, though smaller particles will penetrate to smaller vessels, they are more likely to pass through arteriovenous shunts and reach the lungs. They are also more likely to cause ischaemic damage to normal tissues. On the other hand, larger particles occlude proximal arteries and achieve less reliable tumour devascularization.[6]

The effect of PVA or gelatin particles on tissues is to cause an initial acute inflammatory response, which is followed by a chronic foreign body reaction within weeks.[5,7] Devascularization causes ischaemia and necrosis within hours, which in turn causes tumours to swell and may exacerbate symptoms, particularly pain. Preoperative embolization is therefore best performed the day before or immediately prior to operation.

COILS AND BALLOONS

Coils are made from steel, tungsten or platinium. Because of problems of corrosion, tungsten is generally no longer used and platinium, though expensive, is preferred because it is inert and not liable to magnetization effects during MRI. A new development is to enhance their effect by adding a thrombogenic coating. The materials used to coat coils include collagen, bioabsorbable polymers and dacron fibres.[8]

Balloons are made of latex or silicone. They are either fixed to a catheter tip for temporary test occlusions or can be detached for vessel occlusion. They are inflated by injecting fluid; usually radiographic contrast media. Coils and balloons are used to occlude large vessels. The delivery of coils is easier to control than balloons and they can be positioned very accurately. There are various methods for controlling the detachment of coils from a delivery wire. These include couplings released by mechanical or hydrostatic pressure, electrolysis or thermal heating.[9] Detachable balloons are released mechanically from a delivery microcatheter, but their detachment is less reliable than the newer methods developed for coils. In many centres they have been superseded by coils.

Coils or balloons are used for large artery occlusion (i.e. endovascular ligations) after a satisfactory temporary balloon occlusion test. High blood flow fistulas are occluded with coils or balloons positioned at the point of transition between artery and vein. Coils are also commonly used to embolize large veins or dural sinuses in order to close dural arteriovenous malformations (AVM). They are less often used in tumour embolizations.

LIQUID EMBOLIC AGENTS

Various liquids are used for embolization including sclerosants, adhesives and soluble plastics. They have the advantage over coils and particles of being injectable via small lumen catheters or needles. Most commonly used are quick-setting adhesives and polymers. The latter are used for percutaneous puncture of small vessels within tumours or facial vascular malformations. Examples of liquid agents are the tissue adhesive n-butyl-2-cyano-acrylate (NBCA) and the copolymer ethylene vinyl alcohol. There are various commercial formulations

Table 57.2 Embolic agents.

Agent	Embolization	Target vessels
Autologous blood clot	Temporary	Large arteries
Gelfoam	Temporary	Large arteries
Polyvinyl alcohol particles	Permanent	Tumour vessels
Trisacryl gelatin particles	Permanent	Tumour vessels
Coils	Permanent	Large arteries/veins
Balloons	Permanent	Large arteries
Alcohol (ethanol)	Permanent	Malformations or tumour vessels
Sodium tetradecyl sulphate	Permanent	Malformations or tumour vessels
Cyanoacrylate adhesives	Permanent	Malformations or tumour vessels
Ethylene vinyl alcohol copolymer	Permanent	Malformations or tumour vessels

available. NBCA thickens and sets on exposure to blood and copolymers set after injection because of solvent dispersal. Both agents are liable to stick the delivery catheter to vessels and require considerable expertise to deliver safely, but they are generally regarded as producing the most permanent form of embolization. They are therefore used for definitive or palliative treatments and in situations where immediate surgical resection is not planned. Sclerosants, such as absolute alcohol, are used to treat facial vascular malformations, but replacement agents are being tested because of toxicity problems.

APPLICATION OF EMBOLIZATION TECHNIQUES

Tumour embolization

TRANSARTERIAL

Embolization of tumours of the head and neck is most often performed to reduce blood loss and facilitate surgical resection or for palliation (**Table 57.3**). It is rarely curative. Preoperative embolization is performed for vascular tumours such as meningioma,[7, 9, 10] haemangioblastoma, juvenile nasopharyngeal angiofibroma,[11] schwannoma and paraganglioma.[12] Functional evaluations by temporary balloon occlusion of major arteries at risk during surgery can also be performed. Preoperative embolization is largely reserved for extraaxial intracranial tumours and only rarely are intraaxial central nervous system (CNS) tumours treated.

Preoperative transarterial embolization is usually performed with PVA particles, sized to occlude the pathological circulation. Liquid agents, including alcohol, can be delivered transarterially by catheter, but are more frequently injected percutaneously (see below). Serious procedural complications occur in about 4 percent of patients and these include cranial nerve palsies (including blindness), stroke due to unrecognized spread of emboli and induced bleeding due to vessel perforation or tissue necrosis (see Embolization for epistaxis). Complicating cranial nerve palsies are more common when very small

Table 57.3 Head, neck and skull base tumours treated by embolization.

Commonly treated tumours	Less frequently treated tumours
Meningioma	Schwannoma
Paraganglioma	Carcinoid
Juvenile angiofibroma	Alveolar sarcoma
Haemangiopericytoma	Thyroid carcinoma
	Granular cell myoblastoma
	Capillary haemangioma
	Esthesioneuroblastoma
	Neurinoma

particles or NBCA are used.[13] Though technically relatively straightforward, safe embolization of skull base lesions should only be undertaken after adequate training. Safe embolization demands a sound knowledge of vascular anatomy and the potential sites of spontaneous external to internal carotid artery or vertebral artery anastomoses, if unintended cerebral or spinal migration of emboli is to be avoided.[14]

PERCUTANEOUS EMBOLIZATION

This technique involves the injection of a liquid embolic agent or sclerosant directly into tumour vessels (**Figure 57.1**). The objective is to devascularize tumours before surgical resection or for palliation of symptoms by

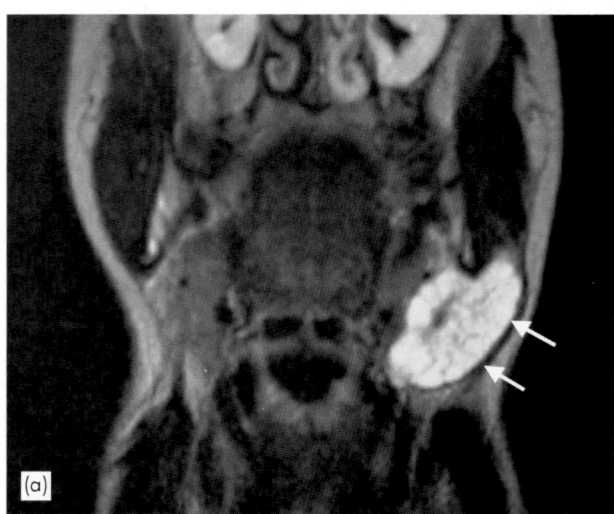

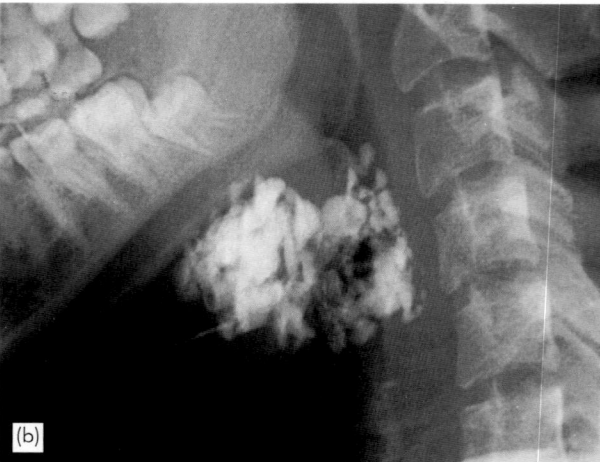

Figure 57.1 Percutaneous embolization of facial venous angioma. (a) A coronal T1W MRI showing the left-sided lesion just below the ramus of the mandible (arrows). In (b), a lateral plain radiograph, a needle has been inserted into the angioma and radiographic contrast injected prior to embolization using ethanol. Because the venous space empties slowly, a sclerosant can be used to obliterate the lesion.

causing tumour involution. Preoperative embolization is usually performed following percutaneous puncture, but perioperative needling can be performed. The technique was first used to devascularize hypervascular juvenile angiofibromas,[15] but has also been used to treat haemangiopericytoma and paraganglioma.[16] The technique is particularly attractive for the management of recurrent lesions and has been reported to achieve total or near-total tumour devascularization.[17]

INTRAARTERIAL CHEMOTHERAPY

Delivery of drugs via selective catheterization of a feeding artery aims to maximize the dose the tumour receives by allowing otherwise systemically toxic dose levels to be administered. The amount of drug delivered to a tumour is proportional to its rate of plasma clearance within the tissue and inversely related to tumour plasma flow.[18] Selective catheterization allows the delivery rate to be fine tuned to the prevailing rate of blood flow. This benefit has been used in various studies of local chemotherapy for head and neck cancers, specifically advanced squamous cell carcinomas.[19] Combination therapies with radio-therapy, for example, RADPLAT, have been effective at inducing remission, and Kumar and Robbins[20] recently reviewed their use. The systemic toxic effects of cisplatin can be mitigated by the simultaneous intravenous administration of its competitive antagonist thiosulphate. Despite logistical problems associated with catheterization and long infusion times, preliminary trials have shown the technique to be highly effective at causing tumour shrinkage.[21]

Temporary and permanent large artery occlusions

Temporary endovascular occlusion of large arteries prior to head and neck surgery allows angiographic and neurological testing of the awake patient to determine the consequences of vessel sacrifice. Rarely is large vessel sacrifice indicated for cancer palliation since the proximal occlusion of arteries is a relatively ineffective method of causing tumour necrosis and/or regression. Large vessel occlusions may be required to manage tumour haemorrhage, as described under Embolization for epistaxis.

There are many described protocols for temporary artery occlusion and dynamic testing. Only two elements are common to all: (1) the procedure is performed under local anaesthesia so that the patient is accessible for neurological examination and (2) anticoagulants are given. Test occlusion involves inflating a balloon in the target artery for 20–30 minutes and assessing the effect on cerebral blood flow. The adequacy of collateral blood flow to the territory of the occluded vessel can be demonstrated by angiography, Doppler ultrasound, xenon CT, SPECT and PET scanning. Additional provocative testing

can be performed by simultaneously lowering the systemic blood pressure or administering a vasodilator drug, such as acetazolamide.[22] All these techniques are designed to improve the reliability of the test but the lack of a consensus protocol testifies to the fact that there remains a risk of the collateral blood flow being inadequate, despite a normal test.

It is generally accepted that preliminary testing reduces the risk of delayed stroke, but the data supporting this conclusion come largely from reports of its use in aneurysm patients.[23] Amongst patients undergoing ligation for skull base tumours, rates for complications range between 5 and 20 percent.[24] The additional risks faced by cancer patients were documented in a single institution report which found their complication rate to be 10 percent, whilst that of aneurysm patients was only 3 percent.[25] Following a satisfactory period of temporary occlusion, the artery is permanently occluded by detaching the balloon used to perform temporary occlusion, or replacing it with embolization coils. Some practitioners prefer the latter because the detachment systems for coils are more reliable. It is obviously important that permanent occlusion is performed at the same arterial level (i.e. at the same place) as the test occlusion.

EMBOLIZATION FOR MENINGIOMAS AND PARAGANGLIOMAS

Two commonly treated tumour types will be described in detail to illustrate the goals of INR in the management of patients with tumour of the skull base and neck.

Meningioma

These typically benign tumours originate from arachnoid cap cells found in arachnoid granulations. They therefore arise in continuity with dura. Though generally intracranial, they are found at extracranial sites by extension from a dural origin or rarely occur entirely extracranially (presumably from ectopic dural rests). Thus tumours may involve the skull base, orbit and cervical spine or the upper neck. They occur in middle age, affect women twice as commonly as men and are linked to a genetic deficit on chromosome 22. Multiple lesions occur in patients with neurofibromatosis II and meningiomatosis.[26, 27] Associations have been reported with exposure to ionizing radiation[28] and hormonal influences due to the presence of androgen and other hormone receptors.[27] They may be locally invasive and the WHO classification of histological findings recognizes three grades (grade 1, benign; grade 2, atypical; grade 3, anaplastic), which are independent of the traditional histopathological descriptions of meningothelial, fibrous, transitional, syncytial and psammomatous subtypes. They are usually highly vascular tumours with the transitional subtype being most vascular and the psammomatous subtype least vascular.

Clinical presentation varies according to location and imaging by CT scan or MRI is usually adequate for diagnosis and preoperative assessment. Tumour calcification and skull hyperostosis is easier to recognize on CT than MRI and suggest a less vascular subtype. Tumour enhancement after intravenous contrast media administration is typical and is more avid in vascular tumours, but such enhancement does not imply that a particular lesion is suitable for embolization. Treatment is by resection and radiotherapy is reserved for more aggressive histological types. Preoperative embolization in indicated for vascular tumours and for the palliation of inoperable newly diagnosed or recurrent tumours.

Intraarterial angiography is required to assess the extent of tumour vascularity and therefore the potential of embolization. In a minority of tumours, dense calcification on CT or lack of enhancement after contrast media administration imply a less vascular tumour and embolization will not contribute to management, but the majority warrant angiography and possible embolization.

The vascular supply to meningioma is typically arranged in a radial pattern of dilated feeding arteries of decreasing size and a delayed venous phase of contrast passage through the tumour bed. Arterial supply may be from external carotid artery branches or from transpial internal carotid artery branches or a mixture of the two (see **Figure 57.2**). The endovascular therapist therefore needs a detailed preembolization angiogram to evaluate the feasibility (and risks) associated with superselective catheterization and injection of particles. In practice, treatment and catheter angiography are usually combined in the same session and scheduled as part of the patient's overall treatment plan.

Embolization is indicated as an adjuvant to tumour resection in order to reduce operative blood loss and facilitate surgery. Since the typical blood supply is by arteries and arterioles of gradually reducing size, small particles (for example, 150 micron) are used first to obstruct intratumour vessels and larger particles injected subsequently to obstruct larger feeding arteries (see **Figure 57.3**). If embolization is performed preoperatively, this technique will cause acute tumour infarction and swelling should be anticipated. Operation is therefore best performed within hours of embolization or if delayed then steps must be taken to ensure that worsening neurological symptoms or signs are quickly detected and treated. Rarely, tumour necrosis causes bleeding and life-threatening expansion of tumours. This complication occurs in about 1–2 percent of instances. Revascularization of tumour after particulate embolization, due to growth of new vessels and collateral routes of blood supply, can also be anticipated within as short a period as two to three weeks.

Another indication for meningioma embolization is to arrest or impede tumour growth when lesions are inoperable and radiotherapy inappropriate. In theory, particles delivered into the tumour bed only will cause tissue ischaemia/necrosis without stimulating growth of collateral blood vessels. In this situation, very small particles (50 microns) are injected slowly and no attempt is made to obstruct larger feeding arteries. Tumour devascularization and shrinkage is monitored by MRI enhanced by intravenous gadolinium administration; induced failure of enhancement implying devascularization.

The efficacy of preoperative embolization is difficult to evaluate objectively. Criteria used in reported studies include comparisons of blood transfusion volumes between tumour resection operations performed with or without preoperative embolization, lengths of hospital stay and clinical outcomes. A reduced need for blood transfusion was reported by Teasdale et al.[29] and Oka et al.,[30] shorter lengths of hospital admission by Dean et al.[31] and Oka et al.,[30] and improved clinical results by Oka et al.[30] when adjuvant embolization was performed. A reduction in neurological complications after surgery was reported by Oka et al.,[30] but this benefit was only evident for patients with large tumours (greater than 6 cm in diameter). The conduct and evaluation of such studies is difficult because of the various sizes and sites of tumours studied.

Several specific complications associated with meningioma embolization have been reported. Intratumoural haemorrhage resulting from devascularization may occur in the 24–36 hours after embolization. In the author's practice, this complication has occurred once in 40 treatments over the last five years. Selective catheterization risks causing vessel damage or rupture. The latter is more likely to occur at sharp bends in vessels. Such bends occur in the course of the middle meningeal artery (a common route for meningioma embolization) and rupture of this artery has been reported to cause bleeding or delayed arteriovenous shunting.[32, 33] The incidence of all procedural complications is about 4 percent, though complications resulting in permanent neurological deficits occur in less than half of affected patients.

Paraganglioma

These benign but locally invasive tumours arise from paraganglionic chemoreceptor cells of neural crest origin. About 50 percent occur in the temporal bone, arising from either the cochlear promontory (i.e. typanicum) or the jugular blub (i.e. jugulare), 35 percent in the carotid body, 12 percent in the region of the high cervical vagus and the rest at various sites of the head and neck.[34]

Though relatively rare tumours, they are usually targets for embolization because of their highly vascular nature. Most occur sporadically though familial cases occur with autosomal dominant inheritancy. In approximately 10 percent of patients, tumours are multifocal and

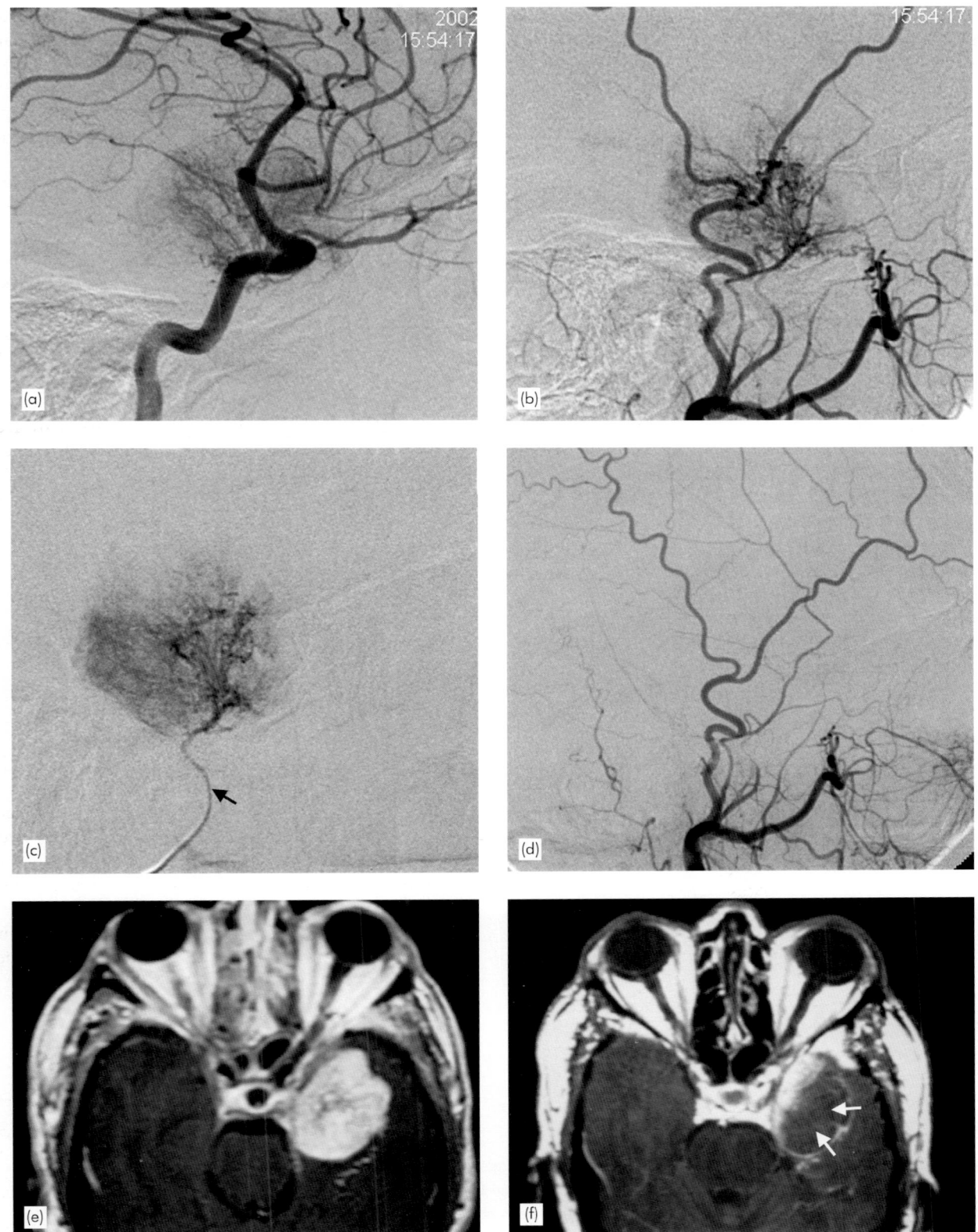

Figure 57.2 Parasellar meningioma. This tumour is supplied by meningeal branches arising from both internal and external carotid arteries. (a) and (b) are lateral views from internal and external carotid injections, respectively. Preoperative embolization of the external carotid supply only was performed. (c) The tumour circulation following selective catheterization of the accessory meningeal artery. The arrow marks the tip of the microcatheter. (d) The effect of embolization on the external carotid angiogram (compare with panel b). (e) and (f) Axial T1W MRI of the tumour before and after embolization of the external carotid blood supply. Note that enhancement occurs in only the medial portion of the tumour on (f) (arrows).

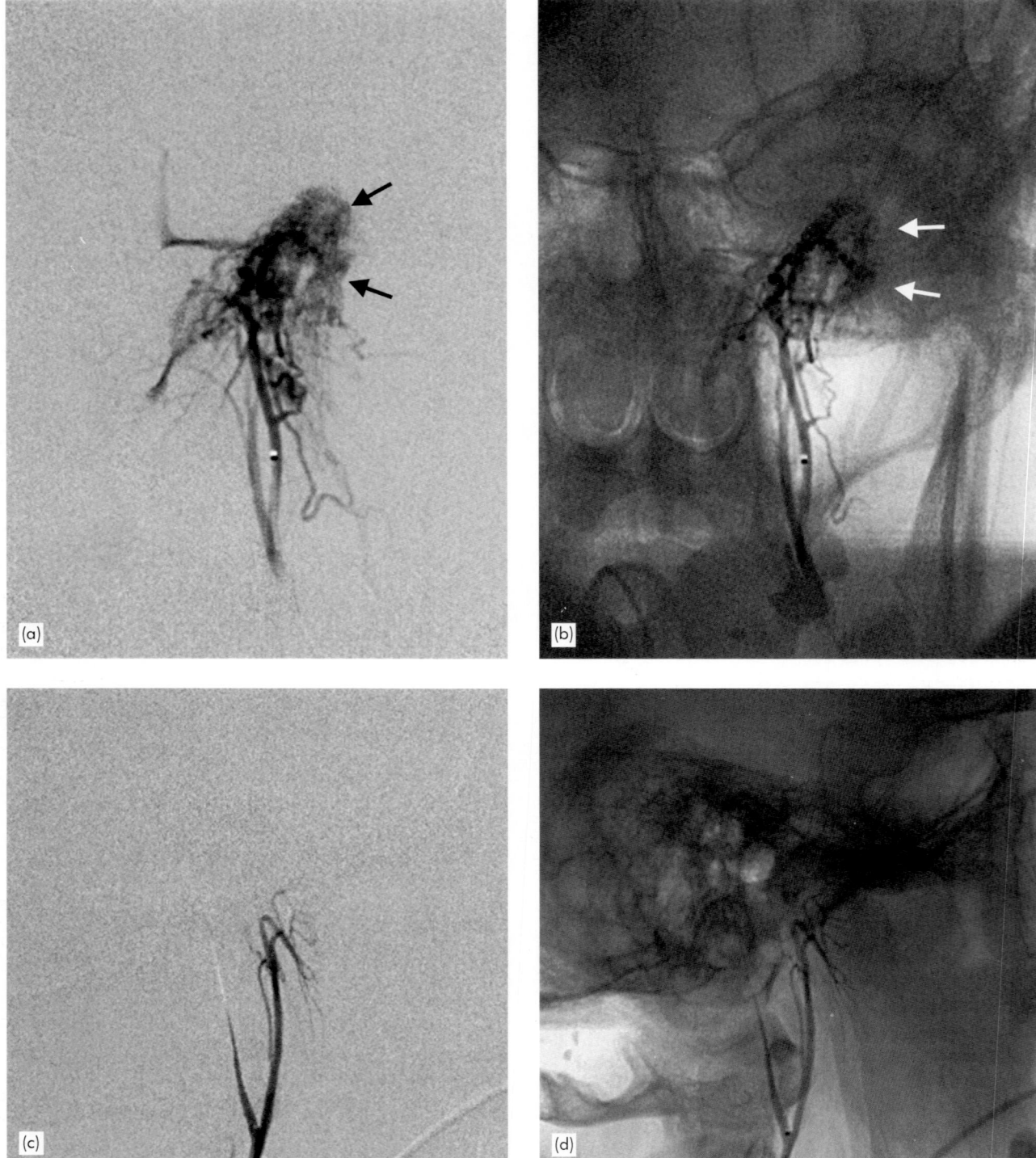

Figure 57.3 Temporal paraganglioma. Lateral angiograms following selective injections into the ascending pharyngeal artery before (a), (b) and after (c), (d) embolization with particles. Images (b) and (d) show the bony details of the digitally subtracted angiograms (a) and (c). The tumour circulation (arrows in (a) and (b)) has been occluded.

up to 5 percent of tumours secrete catacholamines. Symptoms are related to tumour location and typically consist of mass, tinnitus (tympanicum), cranial nerve palsy (jugulare, vagale) and pain. The role of imaging by plannar scanning is to support the clinical diagnosis and

usually includes both CT and MRI. The former (performed with high resolution parameters) will best demonstrate bony involvement and MRI will best demonstrate the soft tissue character of tumours. Tumour vascularity and extent can be assessed from scans performed after intravenous contrast administration and evidence of involvement of the carotid artery or intracranial invasion should be sought. Intraarterial angiography is usually undertaken as part of a preembolization evaluation rather than for surgical planning.[35] The typical angioarchitecture of this tumour type makes angiography a very specific diagnostic test and it should be considered prior to biopsy.

On intraarterial angiography, feeding arteries are found to be enlarged and there is an early and intense blush in the tumour bed. The intratumoural angioarchitecture comprises centripetally orientated arterioles estimated to be 90 mm in diameter at the periphery and 300–600 mm in the centre of the tumour with arteriovenous shunts (see **Figure 57.3**).[36] To further complicate embolization, the majority of tumours show a multicompartment pattern of blood supply with arterial and venous supply confined to a haemodynamic unit so that separate injections of embolic agent have to be made into each feeding artery. The technique for embolization has evolved with the development of embolization particles small enough to penetrate the smaller peripheral arteries (see **Figure 57.4**). The presence of intratumour shunts may justify the use of a percutaneous (or intraoperative) direct puncture technique with injections of a liquid adhesive agent (see Tools used in interventional neuroradiology techniques, above) since spread of emboli to the lungs is less likely. However, arteriovenous (AV) shunting is more rare in paraganglioma than within the vascular bed of some other tumour types (for example, nasopharyngeal angiofibroma).[37]

Embolization is usually performed as an adjuvant to surgical resection. In rare instances, when surgery and/or radiotherapy are considered inappropriate, embolization alone may provide symptomatic relief by stabilizing tumour growth.[38] The benefits of preoperative embolization have been demonstrated in several single institution reports.[39, 40] The efficacy of preoperative embolization has been studied by several groups. Murphy and Brackman compared two groups, totalling 35 patients, and found preoperative embolization reduced the volume of operative blood loss and the lengths of procedure times, but not the length of bed stay.[41] Tikkakoshi *et al.*[42] reported that preoperative embolization improved operating conditions with subjective benefits to surgical results if performed by superselective catheterization and with effective devascularization of the tumour vascular bed.

EMBOLIZATION FOR EPISTAXIS

Transarterial embolization using particles, coils or balloons has been used to control intractable idiopathic epistaxis. For effective embolization, superselective catheterization of the sphenopalatine artery is performed after lateralization of the bleeding site. This goal is frustrated if prior surgical ligation of the internal maxillary artery has been performed or if the site of bleeding cannot be established. In these situations, particles may need to be injected via both internal maxillary and facial arteries.

There is no consensus on the most effective timing of embolization after the onset of spontaneous epistaxis, and different definitions of intractable epistaxis make it difficult to compare published reports. The vast majority of patients admitted to hospital with epistaxis respond to packing, balloon tamponade or local cautery and only a small minority of patients will need embolization.[43] Whether embolization is substantially safer or more effective than internal maxillary artery (IMA) ligation is also debated. In a recent review of the literature comparing embolization with IMA ligation, Cullen and Tami[44] found that embolization was generally reported to be more reliable, but this was not the case in their institution, where outcomes were similar. However, amongst their patients the procedural complication rate was higher after IMA ligation. If the risks are no greater, then it seems logical to employ embolization first, since IMA ligation limits its subsequent use.

For patients with epistaxis secondary to a vascular malformation or nasal tumour, particulate embolization is indicated to stop acute haemorrhage. In patients with Osler–Weber–Rendu disease, multiple sessions may be required to induce remission and embolization is rarely curative.[45] In patients with epistaxis due to the rare internal carotid aneurysm or pseudoaneurysm that erodes the sphenoid bone and bleeds intranasally, emergency embolization using coils or balloons can be life saving. Embolization also has a small but important role in the management of patients bleeding as a result of head and neck cancers elsewhere. Haemorrhage may occur from large or small vessels and may be associated with radiation-induced tissue necrosis. A variety of embolization techniques including particles, coils and balloons may be needed to control such bleeding.[46]

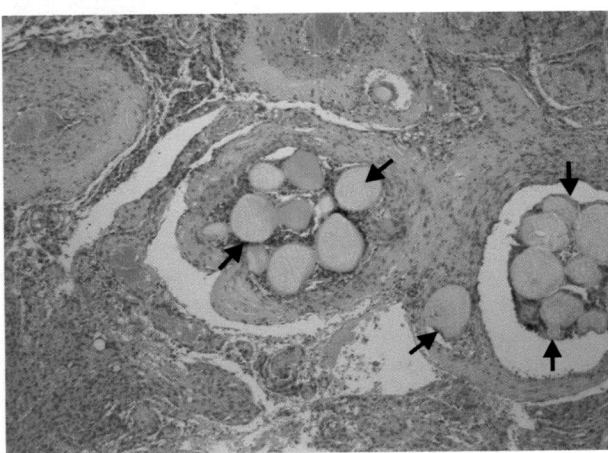

Figure 57.4 Histological section showing embolization particles (arrows) within tumour vessels.

KEY POINTS

- Pre-operative embolization should be considered for all vascular tumours.
- Tumour vascularity can only be inferred from CT and MR scans. Intraarterial angiography is still required to identify tumours suitable for embolization.
- Functional testing of vessels 'at risk' during surgery is performed under local anaesthesia by temporary inflation of an endovascular balloon.
- Most embolizations are performed transarterially, but direct percutaneous injections of tumour or vascular malformation vessels or transvenous injections are also possible.
- Embolization alone is used for palliation and management of inoperable tumours.
- Embolization should be considered early rather than late in the management of intractable epistaxis.

Deficiencies in current knowledge and areas for future research

Technical

➤ Development of non-x-ray imaging. Fluoroscopy using magnetic resonance imaging is now feasible. This avoids the potential hazards of ionizing radiation but requires the development of new catheters and embolic agents. Attempts to develop liquid agents that remain stable in high strength magnetic fields are proving difficult. A great deal of investment is being made to develop ways of monitoring minimally invasive surgical techniques without x-ray fluoroscopy.

➤ Current liquid embolic agents are adhesive and nonadhesive materials that remain coherent during delivery and are permanent need to be developed.

➤ Improvements in reliability of data from functional tests are needed. A great deal of research has been directed at the problem of falsely reassuring temporary vessel occlusion tests. A completely reliable protocol is still needed.

Biological

➤ The evolution of embolized tissue has been studied, but we do not know much about the mechanisms that cause secondary haemorrhage in some tumours.

➤ The potential benefits of local delivery for gene therapy and future chemotherapy agents will

probably open new areas of research. The *in vivo* response of lesions will need further study.

REFERENCES

1. Northfield DWC. Chapter 13. In: *The surgery of the central nervous system*. Oxford: Blackwell Scientific Publication, 1973: 395–6.
2. Miniz E, Lima A, Caldas P. Angiographie en serie de la circulation de la tete. *Revue Neurologique*. 1934; 1: 4.
3. Luessenhop AJ, Velasquez AC. Observations on the tolerance of the intracranial arteries to catheterization. *Journal of Neurosurgery*. 1964; 21: 85–91.
4. Quisling RG, Mickel JP, Ballinger W. Small particle polyvinyl alcohol embolisation of cranial lesions with minimal arteriolar-capillary barriers. *Surgical Neurology*. 1986; 25: 243–52.
5. Hamada J, Kai Y, Nagashiro S, Hashimoto N, Iwata H, Ushio Y. Embolization with porous beads. II: Clinical trial. *American Journal of Neuroradiology*. 1996; 17: 1900–6.
* 6. Latchlow RE. Preoperative intracranial meningioma embolisation: Technical considerations affecting the risk-to-benefit ratio. *American Journal of Neuroradiology*. 1993; 14: 583–6.
7. Kerber CW, Bank WP, Horton JA. Polyvinyl alcohol foam: Prepackaged emboli for therapeutic embolisation. *American Journal of Neuroradiology*. 1978; 130: 1193–4.
8. Sellar R. Endovascular techniques. In: Byrne JV (ed.). *A Textbook of interventional neuroradiology: Theory and practice*. Oxford University Press, 2002: 53–4.
9. Guglielmi G, Vinuela F, Sepetka I, Macellari V. Electrothrombosis of saccular aneurysms via endovascular approach. Part 1: Electrochemical basis, technique and experimental results. *Journal of Neurosurgery*. 1991; 75: 1–7.
10. Manelfe C, Lasjaunias P, Ruscalleda J. Preoperative embolizaton of intracranial meningioma. *American Journal of Neuroradiology*. 1986; 7: 963–72.
11. Davis KR. Debrun. Embolization of juvenile nasopharyngeal angiofibroma. *Seminars in Interventional Radiology*. 1987; 4: 309–20.
12. Lacour P, Doyon D, Manelfe C, Picard L, Salisachs P, Schwaab G. Treatment of chemodectomas by arterial embolization. *Journal of Neuroradiology*. 1975; 2: 275–87.
13. Lasjaunias P, Berenstein A. Chapter 4. In: *Surgical neuroangiography: endovascular treatment of craniofacial lesions*. Berlin: Springer-Verlag, 1987: 90–99.
14. Valavanis A. Preoperative embolization of the head and neck: Indications, patient selection, goals, and precautions. *American Journal of Neuroradiology*. 1986; 7: 943–52.
15. Tranbahuy P, Borsik M, Herman P, Wassel M, Casasco A. Direct intracranial embolisation of juvenile angiofibroma. *American Journal of Otolaryngology*. 1994; 15: 429–35.

16. George B, Casasco A, Deffrennes D, Houdart E. Intratumoral embolisation of intracranial and extracranial tumours: technical note. *Neurosurgery.* 1994; **35**: 771–3.

* 17. Chaloupka JC, Mangla S, Huddle DC, Roth TC, Mitra S, Ross DA *et al.* Evolving experience with direct puncture therapeutic embolization for adjunctive and palliative management of head and neck hypervascular neoplasms. *Laryngoscope.* 1999; **109**: 1864–72.

18. Howell SB. Pharmakokinetic principles of regional chemotherapy. *Contributions to Oncology.* 1988; **29**: 1–8.

19. Lee YY, Dimery IW, Von Tassel P, De Pena C, Blacklock JB, Goepfert H. Superselective intraarterial chemotherapy of advanced paranasal sinus tumours. *Archives of Otolaryngology – Head and Neck Surgery.* 1989; **115**: 503–11.

* 20. Kumar P, Robbins KT. Treatment of advanced head and neck cancer with intra-arterial Cisplatin and concurrent radiation therapy: The RADPLAT protocol. *Current Oncology Reports.* 2001; **3**: 56–65.

21. Kerber CW, Wong WH, Howell SB, Hanchett K, Robbins KT. An organ-preserving selective arterial chemotherapy strategy for head and neck cancer. *American Journal of Neuroradiology.* 1998; **19**: 935–41.

22. Rogg J, Rutigliano H, Yonas H, Johnson DW, Pentheny S, Latchaw RE. The acetazolamide challenge: Imaging techniques designed to evaluate cerebral blood flow reserve. *American Journal of Neuroradiology.* 1989; **10**: 830–910.

23. Byrne JV, Guglielmi G. Chapter 4. In: *Endovascular treatment of intracranial aneurysms.* Berlin Heidelberg, New York: Springer-Verlag, 1998: 120–2.

* 24. Standard SC, Ahuja A, Guterman LR, Chavis TD, Gibbons KJ, Barth AP *et al.* Balloon test occlusion of the internal carotid artery with hypotensive challenge. *American Journal of Neuroradiology.* 1995; **16**: 1453–8.

25. Gonzalez CF, Moret J. Balloon occlusion of the carotid artery prior to surgery for neck tumours. *American Journal of Neuroradiology.* 1990; **11**: 649–52.

26. Langford LA. Pathology of meningiomas. *Journal of Neuro-Oncology.* 1996; **29**: 217–21.

27. Black PMcL. Meningiomas. *Neurosurgery.* 1993; **32**: 643–57.

28. Bondy M, Ligon BL. Epidemiolgy and etiology of intracranial meningiomas: a review. *Journal of Neuro-Oncology.* 1996; **29**: 197–206.

29. Teasdale E, Patterson J, McLellan D, MacPherson P. Subselective preoperative embolisation for meningiomas. A radiological and pathological assessment. *Journal of Neurosurgery.* 1984; **60**: 506–11.

30. Oka H, Kurata A, Kawano N, Seregusa H, Ikuo K, Ohmomo T *et al.* Preoperator superselective embolisation of skull-base meningiomas: indications and limitations. *Journal of Neuro-Oncology.* 1998; **40**: 61–71.

31. Dean BL, Fiom RA, Wallace RC, Khayata MH, Obuchowski NA, Hodak JA *et al.* Efficacy of endovascular treatment of

meningiomas: evaluation with matched sample. *American Journal of Neuroradiology.* 1994; **15**: 1675–80.

32. Terada T, Nakai E, Tsumoto T, Itakura T. Iatrogenic arteriovenous fistula of the middle meningeal artery caused during embolisation for meningioma – case report. *Neurologia Medico-Chirurgica.* 1997; **37**: 677–80.

33. Barr JD, Mathis JM, Horton JA. Iatrogenic carotid-cavernous fistula occurring after embolization of a cavernous sinus meningioma. *American Journal of Neuroradiology.* 1995; **16**: 483–5.

34. Zak FG, Lawson W. *The paraganglionic chemoreceptor system. Physiology, pathology and clinical medicine.* New York: Springer Verlag, 1982.

35. Phelps PD, Cheesman AD. Imaging jugulotympanic glomus tumors. *Archives of Otolaryngology – Head and Neck Surgery.* 1990; **116**: 940–5.

36. Willis AG, Birrel JH. The structure of a carotid body tumour. *Acta Anatomica (Basal).* 1955; **25**: 220–65.

* 37. Schroth G, Haldemann AR, Mariani L, Remonda L, Raveh J. Preoperative embolization of paragangliomas and angiofibromas. *Archives of Otolaryngology – Head and Neck Surgery.* 1996; **122**: 1320–5.

38. Maier W, Marangos N, Laszig R. Paraganglioma as a systemic syndrome: pitfalls and strategies. *Journal of Laryngology and Otology.* 1999; **113**: 978–82.

39. Ogura JH, Spector GJ, Gado M. Glomus jugulare and vagale. *Annals of Otology, Rhinology, and Laryngology.* 1978; **87**: 622–9.

40. Simpson 2nd. GT, Konrad HR, Takahashi M, House J. Immediate postembolization excision of glomus jugulare tumors: advantages of new combined techniques. *Archives of Otolaryngology – Head and Neck Surgery.* 1979; **105**: 639–43.

* 41. Murphy T, Brackmann DE. Effects of preoperative embolization on glomus jugulare tumors. *Laryngoscope.* 1989; **99**: 1244–7.

42. Tikkakoshi T, Luotonen J, Leinonen S, Siniluoto T, Heikkila O, Paivansalo M *et al.* Preoperative embolisation in the management of neck paragangliomas. *Laryngoscope.* 1997; **107**: 821–6.

43. Pollice PA, Yoder MG. Epistaxis: A retrospective review of hospitalised patients. *Otolaryngology and Head and Neck Surgery.* 1997; **117**: 49–53.

44. Cullen MM, Tami T. A Comparison of internal maxillary artery ligation versus embolisation for refractory posterior epistaxis. *Otolaryngology and Head and Neck Surgery.* 1998; **118**: 636–42.

45. Hirsch JA, Choi I-S. Vascular Malformations of the head and neck. In: Byrne JV (ed). *Interventional neuroradiology.* Oxford: Oxford University Press, 2002: 197–212.

46. Morrissey DD, Anderson PE, Nesbit GM, Barnwell SL, Everts EC, Cohen JL. Endovascular management of haemorrhage in patients with head and neck cancer. *Archives of Otolaryngology – Head and Neck Surgery.* 1997; **123**: 15–9.

58

Laser principles in otolaryngology, head and neck surgery

BRIAN JG BINGHAM

Introduction	742	Laser safety	745
History	742	Photodynamic therapy in otorhinolaryngology	745
Principles of laser action	742	Key points	746
Laser light delivery devices	743	Deficiencies in current knowledge and areas for future	
Laser–tissue interaction	745	research	747
Laser applications in otolaryngology	745	References	747

SEARCH STRATEGY

The data in this chapter are supported by a Medline search using the key words head and neck cancer and photodynamic therapy.

INTRODUCTION

Laser is the acronym for light amplification by stimulated emission of radiation. Surgical lasers are devices that amplify light and create coherent light beams ranging from the infrared to the ultraviolet parts of the spectrum.

HISTORY

In 1917, Albert Einstein described the theory of stimulated emission which is the underlying process for laser action. The American physicists, Arthur Schawlow and Charles Townes, described the working principles of lasers in 1958.[1] In 1960 Theodore Maiman demonstrated the first laser action in solid ruby[2] and a year later Ali Javan built the first helium-neon gas laser.[3] C. Kumar N. Patel introduced the carbon dioxide (CO_2) gas laser in 1962. In 1972, in Boston, USA, Jako and Strong were the first to pioneer the use of the CO_2 laser in otolaryngology, head and neck surgery.[4, 5, 6]

PRINCIPLES OF LASER ACTION

A laser empowers atoms to store and emit light in a coherent form. The electrons in the atoms of a laser medium are first pumped or energized to an excited state by an external energy source. These electrons are then stimulated by external photons to emit their stored energy in the form of photons. This process is 'stimulated emission'. The photons emitted have a frequency characteristic to their atoms and travel in step with the stimulating photons. These photons now strike other excited atoms to release even more photons. These photons move back and forth between two parallel mirrors triggering further stimulated emission. This part of the process is known as 'light amplification'. One mirror in the laser tube is partially silvered and it allows the exit or leak of the intense, collimated, monochromatic and coherent laser light.

Nature of laser light

A beam of laser light is:

- **coherent**: the photons or waves travel in step, or in phase with one another.
- **collimated**: the laser light travels in one direction.
- **monochromatic**: one wavelength or colour is in the visible spectrum.

Types of lasers

Depending on the type of laser medium used, lasers can be classified as solid state, gas, semiconductor, liquid or free electron.

A pioneering example of a solid state laser is the ruby laser. The neodymium yttrium aluminium garnate (YAG) laser and the related (frequency doubled) potassium titanyl phosphate (KTP) are examples of solid state lasers in surgical practice.

The carbon dioxide laser (CO_2) is a very efficient gas laser that delivers laser light as an invisible continuous wave beam. The carbon dioxide surgical laser has been the most widely applied laser in oral and laryngological practice. The helium-neon laser is a gas laser with high frequency stability, good colour stability (red) and minimal beam spread. The helium-neon gas laser is often superimposed on an invisible laser beam, such as the CO_2, to facilitate surgical targeting. Activation of chemicals in photodynamic therapy can be achieved with the helium-neon laser.

The gallium arsenide laser is the most commonly used semiconductor laser. This laser is used in CD players and laser printers and has some surgical applications.

The most common medium for a liquid laser is an inorganic dye contained in a glass vessel. This laser is pumped or energized by intense flash lamps or by a gas laser in a continuous wave mode. The frequency of a tuneable dye laser can be altered with the aid of a prism inside the laser cavity. Tuneable dye lasers can be well suited for treating pigmented cutaneous lesions.

Lasers that utilize beams of electrons unattached to atoms and spiralling around magnetic field lines were initially developed in 1977 and are important research instruments. Free-electron lasers are tuneable and, in theory, could cover the electromagnetic spectrum from infrared to x-rays. Free-electron lasers could be capable of producing very high power radiation and may have medical applications in the future.

Patterns of laser output

The configuration of the resonator cavity and the method in which an energy source is applied to the 'active laser medium' will determine the pattern of a laser output. The output may be continuous wave or pulsed. A continuous wave laser operates with a constant intensity. A laser that operates with a continuous output for longer than 0.1 seconds is considered a continuous wave laser. A pulsed laser produces a single or train of pulses with each individual pulse less than 0.1 seconds. A Q-switch is an electro-optical component that facilitates the production of a very short (less than 1 microsecond) but high intensity pulse of laser energy.

Basic laser tissue interaction

The reaction of laser energy with living tissue can be photoablative, photochemical, photomechanical or photothermal. Most lasers react with a combination of all these mechanisms although for a specific wavelength and delivery system one form of tissue reaction may predominate.

- **Photoablative** reactions occur when molecular bonds are divided. The ruby laser, for example, can split the molecular bonds of tattoo ink with minimal local thermal damage. Macrophages remove the tattoo ink after the molecular bonds are broken.
- **Photochemical** reactions occur when infrared, visible or ultraviolet laser light interacts with photosensitizers to produce chemical and physical reactions. This forms the basis for photodynamic therapy that is discussed later in this chapter.
- A **photomechanical** effect occurs when the laser energy is pulsed to disrupt tissue or stones by the mechanism of shock waves. An example of this mechanism would be the use of the Holmium YAG laser to shatter ureteric and renal calculi.
- The conversion of absorbed laser light into heat is a **photothermal** reaction. The tissue effect can be cutting, coagulation or vaporization depending on the laser wavelength and the laser delivery device.

LASER LIGHT DELIVERY DEVICES

Many delivery devices are available to deliver laser energy to tissue in a safe and efficient manner. Some delivery devices are suited ideally for the wavelength that they transmit. Examples of delivery systems would be an articulated arm, a mirror lens system, micromanipulator, fibreoptic fibre, shaped tip fibreoptic fibres and robotized scanners.

An articulated arm uses a system of hollow tubes and mirrors to direct the laser beam to the target area. Most articulated arms have a lens system to focus the emerging beam on the target tissue. The carbon dioxide laser wavelength is absorbed in fibreoptic material and hence this laser energy is delivered with an articulated arm system.

Micromanipulators and other focussing devices can be connected to microscopes. Micromanipulators and focussing devices will create an accurate and reproducible spot on target tissue. This facilitates very accurate multiple laser strikes which is important in otology and laryngology.

Laser energy exits from a micromanipulator or focusing device in a similar style to the 'laser beam weapon' of science fiction. This means that inadvertent strikes beyond the target tissue or misdirection from a reflective surface are a significant operative risk. It also means that a 'laser beam' can be deliberately redirected by a mirror. An example of this would be to use a mirror to redirect CO_2 laser energy on to adenoid tissue or on to lymphoid tissue on the base of the tongue.

The bare fibreoptic fibre is the most common technique for delivering laser energy to tissue. The flexibility and diameter of fibreoptic fibre facilitates their use with both rigid and flexible endoscopes. This means that laser energy can be delivered to almost any tissue that can be seen with an endoscope.

The tissue response to laser energy exiting from the tip of a fibre can be controlled by altering the distance of the fibre from the tissue. Changing the distance between the fibre and the tissue can produce all the tissue photo-thermal effects of coagulation, incision and vaporization. Laser light exits the tip of the fibre in what is called the 'angle of divergence'. The light exiting from the tip of the fibre projects in a similar manner to water projecting from the nozzle of a hosepipe. The smallest light spot and, consequently, the highest concentration of energy are found at the fibre tip. As the distance from the fibre to tissue increases, the projected area of light decreases and the energy intensity reduces.

A fibre 'in contact' with tissue will create an incision. The cut is similar to a saw rather than a knife. This means that some tissue is removed like the kerf of a saw as compared to being split with a scalpel. There is a degree of tactile control with a laser fibre 'in contact' mode. As the fibre is retracted and hovers above the tissue (2–4 mm), it is in the 'near contact' position and vaporizes tissue. As the laser fibre is retracted even further from tissue into the 'noncontact' mode, then the tissue effect is coagulation.

A fibreoptic laser cable can be inserted through the biopsy channel of a fibreoptic endoscope. The end of the laser fibre must protrude beyond the end of the endoscope or heat damage to the endoscope can occur when the laser is fired. To simplify this problem one can perform a preliminary check of the length of fibre required to achieve a satisfactory distal position and then mark the laser fibre with a 'steristrip' at the entry port.

A fibreoptic laser fibre can be inserted through a narrow metal tube to help direct the laser energy. In otology, for example, the laser fibre can be presented through a hollowed out needle. An aspiration channel can be added to the hollow metal fibre carrier to remove smoke from the surgical site. **Figure 58.1** shows a

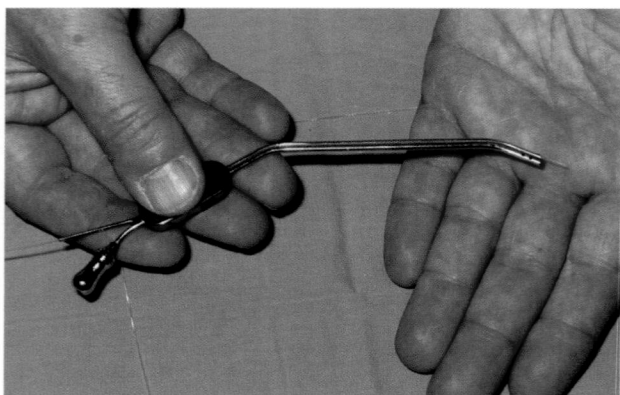

Figure 58.1 A 0.6-micron laser fibre inserted through a modified aural suction tube to create a laser delivery device. The natural torque of the fibre holds the laser fibre in place.

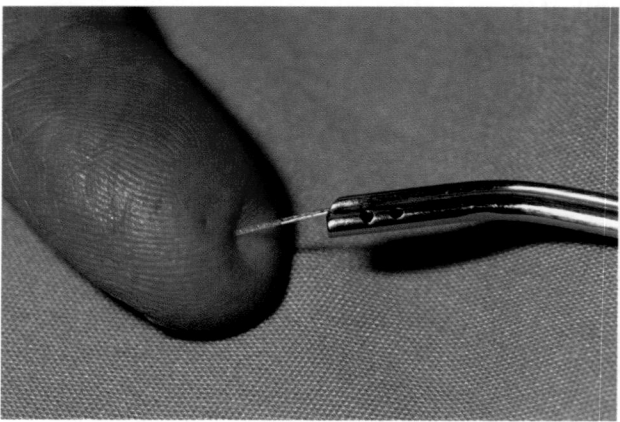

Figure 58.2 The pressure required to move or regress the laser fibre tip into the delivery device.

modified ear suction tube and fibre holder that is used for endoscopic intranasal surgery. In the design of these instruments, the curves of the fibre carrier should create sufficient resistance that when combined with the torque of the laser fibre it results in a fibre that is 'held' in position without any additional mechanism. In **Figure 58.2**, the 0.6-micron laser fibre can be set at the position of choice for the surgeon and will not move unless the surgeon applies additional pressure. The indent of the finger shows the pressure to overcome the self-retaining torque.

A shaped tip laser is a laser fibre with a tip constructed of another material, such as metal or synthetic sapphire. The laser energy heats the tip and it is the conduction of heat from the tip that produces the tissue interaction. Different materials and shapes of tip will create different tissue reactions. Some tips become so hot that a secondary cooling mechanism is required. An example of this type of device in head and neck practice would be a sapphire tipped neodynium YAG fibre used to ablate tracheobronchial tumours.

Robotized scanners can facilitate laser treatment by reproduction of previous instrument settings or by being able to control precisely the distance a laser is placed or 'hovered above' the target tissue. A robotized scanner can 'trace' an area of treatment before delivery of laser energy to ensure accuracy or can apply a pattern to the area of laser treatment. At present, the greatest use for robotized scanners is in the cutaneous treatment of pigmented lesions and for skin resurfacing or recontouring.

LASER–TISSUE INTERACTION

When laser light strikes tissue, it scatters until all the laser energy is either absorbed or reflected. The absorption of laser energy heats tissue. The volume of tissue affected is larger than the area shown by the laser spot size. The depth of penetration by a given wavelength of laser light is determined by the absorption and scattering of the type of tissue and the wavelength of the laser.

The strength of the tissue effect is altered by changing the fluence. Fluence is defined as the laser power in watts, multiplied by the length of exposure in seconds, divided by the area (mm^2) of the target tissue. This implies that when the distance between a fibreoptic tip and the tissue varies, the spot sizes becomes bigger or smaller and the fluence will accordingly increase or decrease.

The heat in the tissue produces a series of changes in the tissue as the temperature rises. The changes are denaturation, coagulation, vaporization, carbonisation and incandescence. Cutting with a laser is narrow controlled vaporization! The heat produced by the absorption of laser light is partly dissipated into air but also produces a secondary thermal effect in surrounding tissue. This lateral thermal effect produces haemostasis by coagulation. The lateral haemostasis effect varies with wavelength of laser, the rate at which the energy is applied, fluence and the nature of the tissue.

LASER APPLICATIONS IN OTOLARYNGOLOGY

The specific clinical applications of lasers are not described in this chapter, but the following list identifies particular lasers for disease-specific regions:

- stapedectomy and tympanomastoid surgery: carbon dioxide laser, KTP laser, argon laser;
- endonasal dacrocystorhinostomy: Holmium YAG laser, KTP laser, 810 nm laser;
- nasal and sinus surgery, including tumour surgery, telangectasia destruction, antrostomy creation and turbinate reduction: Holmium YAG laser, KTP laser, Nd YAG laser, argon laser, 810 nm;
- nasal polyp reduction: CO_2 laser 'swiftlase' (oscillating device).

LASER SAFETY

Each country applies different safety regulations throughout the world. Usually the Medical Devices Agency of a country or state will produce guidance for clinicians and hospitals. In the UK, the local Medical Physics Department will produce local laser rules (based on national guidance) and ensure training of all staff involved in the use of the laser. Training for medical and nursing staff should be mandatory. A laser company will typically provide a safety manual on their particular wavelength of laser. Staff should read the laser safety manual and in many countries produce signed documentation that the manual has been read.

The principles of safety are as follows.

- A laser beam may hit or damage objects outside the target area and cause a fire, tissue damage or eye/visual damage.
- The patient should be shielded by wet gauze or fireproof material from accidental strikes.
- The anaesthetic tube and airway should be protected from accidental strikes that could produce a fire.
- All personnel in the operating room should wear correct eye protection appropriate to the wavelength of the laser.
- A warning sign plus locked doors should prevent unprotected and unprepared individuals from walking into the operating room when the laser is in use.
- The key to switch on the laser should be held by a senior member of the operating team to ensure only properly qualified individuals use the laser.
- The operating room and windows should be laser protected.
- Endoscopic equipment should be blackened to reduce accidental reflective strikes of the laser.

PHOTODYNAMIC THERAPY IN OTORHINOLARYNGOLOGY

Principles of photodynamic therapy

Phototherapy is the use of light in the treatment of disease. An example would be the treatment of neonatal hyperbilirubinaemia with visible light.

Photochemotherapy is a subset of phototherapy where a treatment requires the administration of a drug in addition to the application of light. An example would be treatment of a skin condition such as psoriasis with the combination of a furocoumarin sensitizer drug and UV-A (320–400 nm) light.

Photodynamic therapy (PDT) is a subset of photochemotherapy where, in addition to an administered drug and the application of light, oxygen is required to complete the process. The administered drug is known as a 'photosensitizer'. This type of drug accumulates within a cell and reacts with light and oxygen to form 'singlet' oxygen. The 'singlet' oxygen damages the cell membranes and produces cell death.

One of the attractions of PDT for oncology is that the photosensitizer drug is typically retained in tumour tissue for a longer period than in normal tissue. This improves the therapeutic effect while reducing toxicity to normal tissue. The use of PDT is not affected by prior radiotherapy, chemotherapy or surgery. To date, the principle shortcomings of PDT have been the limited depth of tissue penetration and extensive skin phototoxicity. This skin phototoxicity requires that the patient is not exposed to daylight during treatment or they develop extensive and painful skin reactions.

In photodynamic therapy for head and neck cancer the photosensitizer is usually administered by intravenous infusion. The perfect photosensitizer drug would be absorbed selectively only by tumour tissue in the drug uptake period (also called the drug–light interval). The drug uptake period may last between 3 and 96 hours. The tumour is then irradiated with a measured light dose. Singlet oxygen is released to kill only tumour cells and thus destroy the target tumour.

The tumour targeting arises firstly from the structure of the photosensitizer that leads to the selective uptake by a tumour and secondarily by the accurate application of an appropriate light wave.

The diseases in which trials of photodynamic therapy have taken place include malignant tumours, such as squamous carcinoma of the oral cavity, squamous carcinoma of the nasopharynx, oesophageal carcinoma and metastatic squamous carcinoma of the neck. Non-malignant disease such as inverted papilloma of the sinonasal cavity has also been targeted.

Photodynamic clinical reports in otorhinolaryngology

Both palliative and curative therapy has been reported for oesophageal cancer. The patients receive a photosensitizer followed by light delivered via optical fibres through a flexible endoscope. A phase II trial[7] randomized 218 patients to receive palliative oesophageal PDT (porfimer sodium sensitizer) versus Nd:YAG laser ablative therapy. Each arm gave an equivalent improvement in dysphagia but with fewer perforations in the PDT group (1 versus 7 percent, $p < 0.05$). [***]

Overholt and Panjehpour[8] reported the results of 55 patients with dysplasia or early carcinoma in Barrett's mucosa of the lower end of the oesophagus treated with PDT. The patients received porfimer sensitizer followed at 48 hours with red light therapy. There was a good response at the six-month follow up. Forty-three patients with high-grade dysplasia/adenocarcinoma had endoscopic-proved ablation of their problem. Eleven of the 12

patients with low-grade dysplasia had no dysplasia on endoscopic review. Oesophageal stricture, however, developed in 53 percent of the patients. [***]

There has been hope for PDT in the treatment of head and neck tumours (See Chapter 188, Nasopharyngeal carcinoma; Chapter 192, Oral cavity tumours including the lip; and Chapter 194, Tumours of the larynx). The endoscopic access to squamous tumours of the upper aerodigestive tract combined with the tendency to develop 'field cancerization' make these tumours good candidates for PDT. Gluckman[9] treated a mixture of carcinoma *in situ*, early and advanced squamous cell carcinoma of the head and neck. Dihaematoporphyrin ether and light at 630 nm were used to treat these patients. The best results were obtained in the oral cavity and oropharynx where 11 out of 13 patients had a complete response and two out of 13 a partial response. Four of these tumours had recurrence within one year of treatment. Eight patients with advanced tumours were treated palliatively, but the results were no better that with standard regimes of the time. [**]

Biel[10] treated 25 patients with early squamous cell tumours of the larynx, obtaining a complete response in patients despite the fact that radiation therapy had previously been unsuccessful in 17 of them. [**]

Biel[11] also reported a summary of the results of a collection of studies on the treatment of early squamous cell carcinoma of the head and neck with PDT. There were a total of 217 patients. One hundred and ninety-four (89 percent) showed a complete response to treatment, 23 (10.6 percent) showed a partial response and no patient failed to show any response to the therapy. [**]

Dilkes *et al.*[12] had considerable experience with the use of PDT using the sensitizers m-TPHC, photofrin II and ALA for squamous carcinoma at multiple sites in the head and neck during the mid-1990s. The patients they treated included palliative, primary and adjunctive forms of treatment and, in nearly all cases, the authors identified a visible response to the effects of PDT. Their complications included local pain at the photosensitizer injection site and, in some patients where appropriate precautions had not occurred, post-treatment skin photosensitivity. [**]

Lofgren *et al.*[13] used PDT in five patients with circumscribed nasopharyngeal carcinoma. The drug was activated with laser light under topical anaesthesia and after four years, three of the patients has no evidence of disease. [**]

KEY POINTS

- Light amplification by stimulated emission of radiation.
- Laser light – collimated, coherent and monochromatic.
- Laser tissue action – photoablative, photochemical and photomechanical.

- Laser 'star wars' beam of micromanipulator – hosepipe type jet of fibreoptic laser delivery.
- Read and follow the safety regulations for your laser and operating room.
- PDT requires administered drug, light and oxygen.
- Skin phototoxicity and limited tissue penetration are the current PDT shortcomings.
- PDT has a future place in head and neck cancer management.

Deficiencies in current knowledge and areas for future research

All of the papers on photodynamic therapy for head and neck cancer suggest that photodynamic therapy has a significant place in the future management of this disease. The problem is in determining the exact type of photodynamic therapy associated with which photosensitizer and whether primary therapy, adjunctive therapy or palliation is the optimum course.

REFERENCES

1. Schawlow AL, Townes CH. Infrared and optical lasers. *Physical Review.* 1958; **112**: 1940–9.
2. Maiman TH. Stimulated optical radiation in ruby. *Nature.* 1960; **187**: 493–4.
3. Javan A, Bennett WR, Harriott DR. Population inversion and continuous laser oscillation in a gas discharge containing He-Ne mixtures. *Physical Review Letters.* 1961; **6**: 106.
4. Jako GJ. Laser surgery of the vocal cords. An experimental study with carbon dioxide lasers on dogs. *Laryngoscope.* 1972; **82**: 2204–16.
5. Strong MS, Jako GJ. Laser surgery in the larynx. Early clinical experience with continuous CO2 laser. *Annals of Otology, Rhinology and Laryngology.* 1972; **81**: 791–8.
6. Strong MS, Jako GJ, Vaughan CW, Healy GB, Polanyi T. The use of CO2 laser in otolaryngology: a progress report. *Transactions. Section on Otolaryngology. American Academy of Ophthalmology and Otolaryngology.* 1976; **82**: 595–602.
7. Lightdale CJ, Heier SK, Marcon NE, McCaughan Jr. JS, Gerdes H, Overholt BF *et al.* Photodynamic therapy with porfimer sodium versus thermal ablation therapy with Nd:YAG laser for palliation of esophageal cancer: a multicenter trial. *Gastrointestinal Endoscopy.* 1995; **42**: 507–12.
8. Overholt BF, Panjehpour M. Photodynamic therapy for Barrett's oesophagus. *Gastrointestinal Endoscopy Clinics of North America.* 1997; **2**: 207–20.
9. Gluckman JL. Hematoporphyrin photodynamic therapy: is there truly a future in head and neck oncology? Reflections on a 5 year experience. *Laryngoscope.* 1991; **101**: 36–42.
10. Biel MA. Photodynamic therapy and the treatment of neoplastic diseases of the larynx. *Laryngoscope.* 1994; **104**: 399–403.
11. Biel MA. Photodynamic therapy and the treatment of head and neck neoplasia. *Laryngoscope.* 1998; **108**: 1259–68.
12. Dilkes MG, Alusi G, Djaezeri BJ. Treatment of head and neck cancer with PDT: Clinical experience. *Review of Contemporary Pharmacotherapy.* 1999; **10**: 47–57.
13. Lofgren LA, Hallgren S, Nilsson E, Westerborn A, Nilsson C, Reizenstein J. Photodynamic therapy for recurrent nasopharyngeal cancer. *Archives of Otolaryngology – Head and Neck Surgery.* 1995; **121**: 997–1002.

59

Electrophysiology and monitoring

PATRICK R AXON AND DAVID M BAGULEY

Development of facial nerve monitoring	748	Evidence of the efficacy of monitoring auditory function	751
Technique for continuous facial nerve monitoring	749	Key points	752
Predicting postoperative facial function	749	Best clinical practice	752
Difficulties of monitoring facial function	750	Deficiencies in current knowledge and areas of future	
Monitoring facial function for nonotological procedures	750	research	752
Monitoring auditory function	750	References	752
Techniques	751		

SEARCH STRATEGY

The information presented in this chapter is supported by a Medline search using the key words intraoperative monitoring, facial nerve, cranial nerve and auditory evoked potentials.

DEVELOPMENT OF FACIAL NERVE MONITORING

The first description of intraoperative cranial nerve stimulation was by Fedor Krause in 1898.[1] During cochlear nerve section for tinnitus, he noted '... unipolar faradic stimulation of the (facial) nerve-trunk with the weakest possible current of the induction apparatus resulted in contractions of the right facial region, especially of the orbicularis oculi, as well as the branches supplying the nose and mouth'. Over the next three-quarters of a century, a series of articles refined the technique, all relying on observing movement of the face in order to confirm the functional integrity of the facial nerve.[2, 3, 4, 5, 6, 7] The evoked facial twitch was observed either by the anaesthetist or ancillary staff under the drapes using a flashlight or mirror. These techniques lacked both quantitative control of the stimulus and objective recording of the evoked responses.

In 1979, Delgado and colleagues first described the use of evoked compound muscle action potentials (CMAP) to monitor facial nerve function in response to stimulating the intracranial portion of the facial nerve.[8] The introduction of facial electromyography (EMG) enabled not only facial nerve identification either by electrical stimulation or inadvertent manipulation, but also the possibility of mapping its course through the temporal bone and assessing changes in function during surgical resection of tumour from the nerve's surface.[9] Facial nerve monitoring has proved an invaluable aid during vestibular schwannoma surgery.[10, 11, 12] The introduction of an auditory signal enabled instantaneous real-time auditory feedback to the surgeon during tumour dissection without information passing through an intermediary.[13, 14]

Three trials tested the hypothesis that facial nerve outcome improved when using intraoperative facial nerve monitoring. Harner and colleagues[12] demonstrated the usefulness of facial nerve monitoring in 91 consecutive cases of vestibular Schwannoma resection via the suboccipital route. At one year, 78 percent of those patients who were monitored demonstrated facial function, compared with 65 percent in an unmonitored group, these data were not studied statistically. Niparko and colleagues[15] described the results of 29 patients who underwent translabyrinthine removal of vestibular Schwannoma and compared them with a similar group of 75 unmonitored patients. They demonstrated that monitoring was associated with a significant improvement of facial function at one year for tumours over 2 cm intracranial diameter. Kwartler and colleagues[16] demonstrated that monitored patients with tumours over 2.5 cm had a significant improvement of facial function when compared with a matched unmonitored group. [**]

The benefit of facial nerve monitoring during surgery for chronic middle ear disease is less certain. Facial nerve injury after otological surgery is rare in experienced hands and there are no randomized controlled trials examining its efficacy. Silverstein and others recommend that the facial nerve should be monitored during all general anaesthetic cases where the facial nerve is at risk.[17, 18] This view is in contrast to most American otolaryngologists, although those that trained in the 1990s, those in an academic setting and those who perform more otology than other types of surgery are more likely to use monitoring techniques.[19, 20]

Facial nerve injury often occurs when there is an unexpected change to normal middle ear anatomy, precisely the time when monitoring is so valuable. The senior surgeon must take responsibility to ensure that the equipment is functioning normally. A simple technique for confirming equipment function is described under Technique for continuous facial nerve monitoring. Intraoperative facial nerve monitoring is no substitute for experience in the otological setting and should not replace good surgical practice, but if the operating team adopt the approach that all patients are monitored, the set up technique becomes routine and more reliable.

TECHNIQUE FOR CONTINUOUS FACIAL NERVE MONITORING

The operating theatre is filled with electrical interference generated by the equipment surrounding the anaesthetized patient. Monitoring techniques have developed to minimize this interference and amplify only relevant information. Two sets of subdermal platinum or stainless steel needle recording electrodes are inserted into the upper and lower face. The amplifiers amplify the difference between the potentials recorded at each electrode. This arrangement has the advantage of common mode rejection; electrical interference from other sources is recorded by both electrodes equally and therefore does not create a potential difference between the two closely aligned electrodes. A number of commercial EMG cranial nerve monitoring systems are now available including the NIM-2 (Xomed Treace, Jacksonville, FL, USA) and the Neurosign (Magstim, Whitland, UK). They rely on recording facial muscle activity and delivering the information as a visual and audible representation of the CMAP response. The audible response is either presented as raw EMG activity or a characteristic sound when EMG activity reaches a set threshold.

All systems are isolated and self-contained electrical nerve stimulator and monitoring units. The electrodes are connected to a preamplifier pod, which is attached to the operating table. The recorded electrical signal is filtered through high- and low-pass filters and either rectified and displayed on a logarithmic bar chart or presented as a CMAP waveform. Different systems use different methods of presenting the same information to the surgeon. The logarithmic bar chart has a delayed response decay to enable calculation of rectified CMAP amplitude. Systems that present a CMAP waveform present it as visual and audible real-time information or utilize image capture strategies that also give waveform amplitude information. This allows the surgeon time to examine the waveform and size of the CMAP.

Familiarity with the set up and function of a chosen monitoring system is essential. The senior surgeon must take responsibility and should check that the equipment is functioning normally. Tapping the skin overlying the two sets of subdermal electrodes will generate a recorded response on the monitor. This confirms that electrodes are connected to the preamplifier pod and in turn the preamplifier pod is connected to the monitor, which is switched on. The volume should be checked so that a response is audible over background theatre noise.

Facial nerve stimulation is delivered as a short (0.1 ms) electrical pulse. The stimulating electrode is either monopolar or bipolar. The monopolar electrode is favoured because it is simple to use, but has the disadvantage of stimulating a larger area. The bipolar electrode requires careful positioning of both electrode tips on to the tissue surface; this can prove difficult in the tight confines of the temporal bone. The use of constant voltage stimuli has an advantage over constant current stimuli because it delivers a relatively reliable current to the nerve whatever the medium that surrounds the nerve.

PREDICTING POSTOPERATIVE FACIAL FUNCTION

Recently, a number of studies have described an objective technique that correlates parameters of the evoked CMAP to eventual facial outcome.[15, 21, 22, 23, 24] The test gives non-dichotomous results and therefore a retrospective cut-off point is used to predict those patients who have a good prognosis. Results indicate that a low stimulation threshold, across the site of tumour dissection, is a valuable prognostic indicator of good long-term facial function. The technique, which is simple to perform, assesses the minimum current required to evoke a muscle response after tumour resection. The drawback to the described technique is that the majority of patients have some degree of facial function immediately after surgery. This group will almost certainly have good long-term outcome.[25] It is the small group of patients with poor facial function immediately after surgery that will benefit most from a sensitive and specific predictive test. Axon and Ramsden compared post-dissection minimal stimulation thresholds with immediate postoperative facial function for predicting long-term facial function in 184 patients undergoing vestibular Schwannoma surgery.[25] Post-dissection stimulation thresholds demonstrated only a moderate relation to eventual outcome, which was of limited clinical value. The test criteria were then applied to patients with poor immediate postoperative facial function for predicting long-term outcome, the predictive accuracy fell, further reducing test validity. [**]

Some studies compared the supramaximal CMAP to either facial nerve stimulation proximal and distal to tumour dissection or before and after tumour dissection. These techniques have been advocated as more accurate methods of analysing data, because they remove absolute amplitude comparisons and rely on comparison of ratios.[26, 27] [**]

DIFFICULTIES OF MONITORING FACIAL FUNCTION

All otological procedures rely on a facial muscle response, warning the surgeon that the facial nerve is near. A simple audible noise is all that is required. Recent monitoring systems have increased the amount of information available to the surgeon, stimulating the desire to expand monitoring techniques and so improve patient outcome. This information is superfluous to most procedures and of benefit to only a few. Facial CMAPs represent a complicated interplay between groups of muscle fibres depolarizing in response to facial nerve stimulation. The muscles of the face are very different to those found in the limbs. The facial motor units are small, often having only 25 muscle fibres supplied by each motoneuron compared with many thousands in more peripheral muscles. As a consequence, each muscle has a wide ill-defined motor end-plate zone. The muscles are also arranged in an almost haphazard arrangement, overlying each other and aligned in different directions. This makes meaningful electrophysiological recording difficult. Intra-subject variability (test–retest variability) is high and intersubject comparison almost impossible. The CMAP waveform is usually multiphasic instead of the well-recognized biphasic responses recorded from peripheral muscles, a consequence of phase cancellation. Calculation of maximum amplitude or area under the waveform bears little relation to the number of motoneurons innervating the muscle fibres that create the response.

MONITORING FACIAL FUNCTION FOR NONOTOLOGICAL PROCEDURES

The facial nerve is at risk of iatrogenic injury in the cerebellopontine angle and parotid. Intraoperative facial nerve monitoring has been advocated during microvascular decompression and superficial parotidectomy.[28, 29] Arguments for adopting its use for all surgical procedures are the same as those for otological surgery.

MONITORING AUDITORY FUNCTION

The aim of monitoring the status of the auditory pathway during cerebello-pontine angle (CPA) surgery is the prevention of avoidable postoperative hearing deficit. The achievement of this laudable aim is fraught with difficulty. The cochlear nerve is sensitive to mechanical manipulation and easily damaged, as the intracranial section of the nerve is sheathed in central myelin and has no perineurium.[30] Additionally, the cochlear nerve is intimately involved with pathologies, such as vestibular schwannoma, and hence at very considerable risk during the surgical removal of such lesions, even when every care is taken to preserve the nerve anatomically. The basic principle of intraoperative monitoring is that changes in recordable neuroelectric potentials occur whilst the injury is still reversible and before permanent deficits result.[31] Recent research[32] has demonstrated that this principle holds for changes in auditory brainstem responses (ABR) wave V amplitude (and to a lesser extent latency) in rat auditory nerves manipulated in a fashion analogous to that undergone in humans during vestibular schwannoma removal. It is therefore theoretically feasible that monitoring auditory function may inform the surgeon of reversible injury to the cochlear nerve.

One prerequisite of monitoring auditory function during surgery is that sufficient preoperative hearing must remain such that meaningful recordings may be made in the operating theatre and change observed if and when it occurs. If ABR or electrocochleography (EcochG) are the monitoring techniques of choice, a further prerequisite is for preoperative recordings with that technique. Monitoring with ABR is not possible if waveforms are absent or of grossly abnormal morphology.

Whilst the techniques and equipment utilized for auditory monitoring may seem familiar from the outpatient clinic, their use in monitoring is significantly different. Rather than comparing an individual's data with group data, in monitoring one is comparing a sequence of waveforms over time and evaluating for change. The time allowed for eliciting each recording is limited and this will influence the choice of recording parameters. The decision whether to inform the surgeon of a change in recorded activity is both urgent and crucial. As such, the person undertaking monitoring should be familiar with the operating theatre environment and team, and be able to interpret and communicate observed and measured change to the surgeon confidently and concisely.[33] Such skills are rare and this may prove to be a hindrance to the widespread adoption of these techniques.

TECHNIQUES

Otoacoustic emissions

Cane *et al.*[34] undertook a feasibility study of the use of otoacoustic emissions (OAE) as a technique for monitoring the auditory pathway during surgical removal of a vestibular schwannoma. The experience was that OAE recordings were feasible despite the noise within the surgical environment, but the study did not indicate that OAE would be a useful indicator of early, reversible injury. Theoretically, OAE recording may furnish evidence of cochlear function, but as the site of surgery is the internal auditory canal (IAC), one would not be measuring activity deriving from the point of possible injury. OAE monitoring might therefore give information about ischaemic or noise injury to the cochlea, but it has not yet been demonstrated that this would be at a point where the injury was reversible. At the present time, however, the use of OAE in monitoring auditory function during surgery is rare.

Electrocochleography

Similarly, electrocochleography records activity associated with cochlear function and the distal portion of the cochlear nerve, rather than the intracranial portion of the cochlear nerve, which is acutely at risk during surgery. As such, even strong advocates of EcochG in monitoring have seen it as adjunct to ABR, and not providing the surgeon with the required information when used alone. There is research evidence that responses to auditory stimulation recorded by EcochG persist after complete transection of the VIIth nerve in the rat,[35] and so this technique has the potential to mislead if used in isolation.

One potential advantage of the use of EcochG is the large amplitude of the activity recorded.[36] This allows interpretation of the elicited waveform after fewer averages, so that decision-making may be more rapid.[37] As with ECochG in the outpatient context, there is debate about the optimal site of the recording electrode, with advocates for extratympanic intrameatal placement[36] and transtympanic placement.[38] A further advantage is that EcochG recordings are less compromised by acoustic noise or by electrical artifact as may occur during cautery, and may serve some purpose whilst these are present.[39]

Auditory brainstem responses

Auditory brainstem responses have a theoretical advantage over other techniques in that certain peaks within the waveform derive from anatomical structures at risk of injury during surgery. The generator of wave I is considered to be the distal portion of the cochlear nerve, the site also held to be the generator of the N1 component

of the compound action potential recorded by EcochG.[30] Wave II is associated with the proximal section of the cochlear nerve,[31] wave III with the lower pons (specifically the superior olivary complex)[40] and wave V with the inferior colliculus.[40] The generators of waves III and V are, therefore, unlikely to be directly challenged by surgical manipulation during hearing preservation surgery for space occupying lesions of the CPA, but the latencies of these easily identifiable waves are used during monitoring as change reflects latency change of waves I and II.

Specific methodologies and parameters utilized in intraoperative ABR have been described in detail. The reader who intends to perform this procedure is directed to the comprehensive reviews by Moller[31] and Martin and Mishler.[30] Several points should be noted. There is considerable variability in the methods advocated and clinical trial evidence is not apparent. Second, this variability may account in part for the lack of a strong evidence base for the benefits of auditory monitoring. Further, the reviews cited underline the difference between utilizing ABR in the outpatient clinic and the operating theatre, the need for the technique not to inconvenience surgical techniques and the utility of clear and timely interpretation and communication of change in recordings to the surgeon.

Direct recordings from the cochlear nerve

The need for rapid acquisition of responses may be met by recording directly from the cochlear nerve, the large amplitude of the elicited activity obviating the need for lengthy averaging.[41] This technique was first developed to monitor cochlear nerve function during microvascular decompression surgery, but has been adapted for use during surgical removal of space occupying lesions of the CPA.[37] The site of recording is usually the root entry zone, and both monopolar and bipolar electrodes have their advocates.[42] Click stimuli similar to those used in ABR are used to elicit the response, which comprises a compound action potential. Changes in latency, amplitude and morphology should all be reported to the surgical team.[31]

Combining techniques

Given that each of the techniques described above has technical challenges and shortcomings, many teams choose to utilize more than one, the most common combination being direct cochlear nerve recording and ABR.[43]

EVIDENCE OF THE EFFICACY OF MONITORING AUDITORY FUNCTION

Authors have reported hearing preservation rates following vestibular schwannoma excision, but the heterogeneity of pathological status, surgical technique, surgical experience and criteria for reporting of hearing preservation combine to frustrate analysis of the clinical utility of auditory monitoring. Observational evidence in this area abounds.[44, 45, 46] The need for well-designed, hypothesis-driven clinical trials in this field is paramount.

A similar dearth of evidence is found when determining the relative efficacy of techniques or combinations of techniques. Several studies have reported that direct cochlear nerve recordings are more effective in the maintenance of hearing function than ABR, to an extent that is statistically significant.[47, 48] This effect is said to be due to the immediacy of direct recordings.[49] [**]

Despite the lack of evidence, a consensus is building that monitoring auditory function during CPA surgery is best practice,[42] and that a combination of ABR and direct cochlear nerve recording is optimal,[35] with the adjunctive use of EcochG if desired.[38]

KEY POINTS

- Monitoring facial nerve function is straightforward and neither hampers nor impedes surgery.
- There is a good evidence that monitoring facial nerve function improves outcomes of facial function.
- A consensus has not yet been reached on techniques for monitoring auditory function, but it looks likely that a combination of techniques will be optimal.

Best clinical practice

✓ Regarding monitoring of facial nerve function, there is evidence that these techniques offer benefit in improving facial nerve outcomes in surgery that may challenge the facial nerve. As such it is strongly indicated. [Grade B]
✓ The evidence base for monitoring auditory nerve function is less robust, but it should be regarded as best clinical practice [Grade D/C].

Deficiencies in current knowledge and areas of future research

➤ Further work is required to develop an intraoperative technique that enables accurate assessment of clinical facial nerve function at any point during skull base procedures. Only accurate estimation of motorneuron function will give the surgeon a true representation of immediate facial function and hopefully then enable development of a valid predictive technique.
➤ The speciality as a whole requires a good evidence base to support the use of intraoperative facial nerve monitoring as the standard for all otological procedures that place the facial nerve at risk.

REFERENCES

1. Krause F (ed.). *Surgery of the brain and spinal cord.* New York: Rebman Company, 1912.
2. Frazier CH. Intracranial division of the auditory nerve for persistent aural vertigo. *Surgery, Gynaecology and Obstetrics.* 1912; **15**: 524–9.
3. Olivecrona H. Acoustic tumors. *Journal of Neurology, Neurosurgery, and Psychiatry.* 1940; **3**: 141–6.
4. Hullay J, Tomits GH. Experiences with total removal of tumours of the acoustic nerve. *Journal of Neurosurgery.* 1965; **22**: 127–35.
5. Rand RW, Kurze TL. Facial nerve preservation by posterior fossa transmeatal microdissection in total removal of acoustic tumors. *Journal of Neurology, Neurosurgery, and Psychiatry.* 1965; **28**: 311–6.
6. Poole JL. Suboccipital surgery for acoustic neurinomas: Advantages and disadvantages. *Journal of Neurosurgery.* 1966; **24**: 483–92.
7. Albin MS, Babinski M, Maroon JC. Anesthetic management of posterior fossa surgery in the sitting position. *Acta Anaesthesiologica Scandinavica.* 1976; **20**: 117–28.
8. Delgado TE, Buchheit WA, Rosenholtz HR. Intraoperative monitoring of facial muscle evoked responses obtained by intracranial stimulation of the facial nerve: a more accurate technique for facial nerve dissection. *Neurosurgery.* 1979; **4**: 418–21.
9. Silverstein H, Willcox Jr. TO, Rosenberg SI, Seidman MD. Prediction of facial nerve function following acoustic neuroma resection using intraoperative facial nerve stimulation. *Laryngoscope.* 1994; **104**: 539–44.
10. Moller AR, Janetta PJ. Preservation of facial function during removal of acoustic neuromas. Use of monopolar constant voltage stimulation and EMG. *Journal of Neurosurgery.* 1984; **61**: 757–60.
11. Benecke JE, Calder HB, Chadwick G. Facial nerve monitoring during acoustic neuroma removal. *Laryngoscope.* 1987; **97**: 697–700.
* 12. Harner SG, Daube JR, Beatty CW, Ebersold M. Intraoperative monitoring of the facial nerve. *Laryngoscope.* 1988; **98**: 209–12.
13. Prass RL, Luders H. Acoustic (loudspeaker) facial electromyography (EMG) monitoring: I. Evoked

electromyographic (EMG) activity during acoustic neuroma resection. *Neurosurgery.* 1986; **19**: 392–400.

14. Prass RL, Kenney SE, Hardy RW, Hahn JF, Luders H. Acoustic (loudspeaker) facial EMG monitoring: II. Use of evoked EMG activity during acoustic neuroma resection. *Otolaryngology and Head and Neck Surgery.* 1987; **97**: 541–51.

15. Niparko JK, Kileny PR, Kemink JL. Neurophysiologic intraoperative monitoring: II. Facial nerve function. *American Journal of Otology.* 1989; **10**: 55–61.

16. Kwartler JA, Luxford WM, Atkins J, Shelton C. Facial nerve monitoring in acoustic tumor surgery. *Otolaryngology and Head and Neck Surgery.* 1991; **104**: 814–7.

17. Silverstein H, Smouha EE, Jones R. Routine intraoperative facial nerve monitoring during otologic surgery. *American Journal of Otology.* 1988; **9**: 269–75.

18. Noss RS, Lalwani AK, Yingling CD. Facial nerve monitoring in middle ear surgery. *Laryngoscope.* 2001; **111**: 831–6.

19. Greenberg JS, Manolidis S, Stewart MG, Kahn JB. Facial nerve monitoring in chronic ear surgery: US practice patterns. *Otolaryngology and Head and Neck Surgery.* 2002; **126**: 108–14.

20. Pensak ML, Willging JP, Keith RW. Intraoperative facial nerve monitoring in chronic ear surgery: A resident training program. *American Journal of Otology.* 1994; **15**: 108–10.

21. Selesnick SH, Carew JF, Victor JD, Heise CW, Levine J. Predictive value of facial nerve electrophysiologic stimulation thresholds in cerebellopontine-angle surgery. *Laryngoscope.* 1996; **106**: 633–8.

22. Prasad S, Hirsch BE, Kamerer DB, Durrant J, Sekhar LN. Facial nerve function following cerebellopontine angle surgery: Prognostic value of intraoperative thresholds. *American Journal of Otology.* 1993; **14**: 330–3.

23. Silverstein H, Willcox TO, Rosenberg SI, Seidman MD. Prediction of facial nerve function following acoustic neuroma resection using intraoperative facial nerve stimulation. *Laryngoscope.* 1994; **104**: 539–44.

24. Nissen AJ, Sikand A, Curto FS, Welsh JE, Gardi J. Value of intraoperative threshold stimulus in predicting postoperative facial nerve function after acoustic tumor resection. *American Journal of Otology.* 1997; **18**: 249–51.

∗ 25. Axon PR, Ramsden RT. Intraoperative EMG for predicting facial function in vestibular Schwannoma surgery. *Laryngoscope.* 1999; **109**: 922–6.

26. Axon PR, Ramsden RT. Assessment of real-time clinical facial function during vestibular Schwannoma surgery. *Laryngoscope.* 2000; **110**: 1911–5.

27. Goldbrunner RH, Schlake HP, Milewski C, Tonn JC, Helms J, Roosen K. Quantitative parameters of intraoperative electromyography predict facial nerve outcomes for vestibular schwannoma surgery. *Neurosurgery.* 2000; **46**: 1140–6; discussion 1146–8.

28. Mooj JJ, Mustafa MK, van Weerden TW. Hemifacial spasm: intraoperative electromyographic monitoring as a guide for microvascular decompression. *Neurosurgery.* 2001; **49**: 1365–70; discussion 1370–1.

29. Lopez M, Ouer M, Leon X, Orus C, Recher K, Verges J. Usefulness of facial nerve monitoring during parotidectomy. *Acta Otorrinolaringológica Española.* 2001; **52**: 418–21.

30. Martin WH, Mishler ET. Intraoperative monitoring of auditory evoked potentials and facial nerve electromyography. In: Katz J (ed.). *Handbook of clinical audiology.* Philadelphia: Lippincott Williams and Wilkins, 2001: 323–48.

31. Moller AR. Intraoperative neurophysiological monitoring. In: Roeser RJ, Valente M, Hosford-Dunn H (eds). *Audiology diagnosis.* New York: Thieme, 2000: 545–70.

32. Sekiya T, Shimamura N, Yagihashi A, Suzuki S. Axonal injury in auditory nerve observed in reversible latency changes of brainstem auditory evoked potentials (BAEP) during cerebellopontine angle manipulations in rats. *Hearing Research.* 2002; **173**: 91–9.

33. Fisher RS, Raudzens P, Nunemacher M. Efficacy of intraoperative neurophysiological monitoring. *Journal of Clinical Neurophysiology.* 1995; **12**: 97–109.

34. Cane MA, O'Donoghue GM, Lutman ME. The feasibility of using oto-acoustic emissions to monitor cochlear function during acoustic neuroma surgery. *Scandinavian Audiology.* 1992; **21**: 173–6.

35. Rosahl SK, Tatagiba M, Gharabaghi A, Matthies C, Samii M. Acoustic evoked response following transection of the eighth nerve in the rat. *Acta Neurochirurgica.* 2000; **142**: 1037–45.

36. Mullatti N, Coakham HB, Maw AR, Butler SR, Morgan MH. Intraoperative monitoring during surgery for acoustic neuroma: benefits of an extratympanic intrameatal electrode. *Journal of Neurology, Neurosurgery, and Psychiatry.* 1999; **66**: 591–9.

37. Yingling CD. Intraoperative monitoring of cranial nerves in neurotologic surgery. In: Cummings CW, Fredickson JM, Harker LA, Krause CJ, Schuller DE, Richardson MA (eds). *Otolaryngology head and neck surgery*, 3rd edn. St Louis: Mosby, 1998: 3331–55.

38. Schlake HP, Goldbrunner R, Milewski C, Siebert M, Behr R, Riemann R et al. Technical developments in intra-operative monitoring for the preservation of cranial motor nerves and hearing in skull base surgery. *Neurological Research.* 1999; **21**: 11–24.

39. Schlake HP, Milewski C, Goldbrunner RH, Kindgen A, Riemann R, Helms J et al. Combined intra-operative monitoring of hearing by means of auditory brainstem responses (ABR) and transtympanic electrocochleography (EcochG) during surgery of intra and extrameatal acoustic neurinomas. *Acta Neurochirurgica.* 2001; **143**: 985–95.

40. Legatt AD. Mechanisms of intraoperative brainstem auditory evoked potential changes. *Journal of Clinical Neurophysiology.* 2002; **19**: 396–408.

41. Moller AR. Intraoperative neurophysiologic monitoring. In: Brackmann DE, Shelton C, Arriaga MA (eds). *Otologic surgery.* Philadelphia: WB Saunders, 2001: 645–61.

42. Nguyen BH, Javel E, Levine SC. Physiologic identification of eighth nerve subdivisions: Direct recordings with

bipolar and monopolar electrodes. *American Journal of Otology.* 1999; **20**: 522–34.

∗ 43. Mann WJ, Maurer J, Marangos N. Neural conservation in skull base surgery. *Otolaryngologic Clinics of North America.* 2002; **35**: 411–24.

∗ 44. Radtke RA, Erwin CW, Wilkins RH. Intraoperative brainstem auditory evoked potentials: Significant decrease in postoperative morbidity. *Neurology.* 1989; **39**: 187–91.

45. Harper CM, Harner SG, Slavit DH, Litchy WJ, Daube JR, Beatty CW *et al.* Effect of BAEP monitoring on hearing preservation during acoustic neuroma resection. *Neurology.* 1992; **42**: 1551–3.

46. Fischer G, Fischer C, Remond J. Hearing preservation in acoustic neurinoma surgery. *Journal of Neurosurgery.* 1992; **76**: 910–7.

47. Colletti V, Fiorino FG, Mocella S, Policante Z. EcochG, CNAP and ABR monitoring during vestibular schwannoma surgery. *Audiology.* 1998; **37**: 27–37.

48. Jackson LE, Roberson Jr. JB. Acoustic neuroma surgery: Use of cochlear nerve action potential monitoring for hearing preservation. *American Journal of Otology.* 2000; **21**: 249–59.

∗ 49. Colletti V, Fiorino FG. Advances in monitoring of seventh and eighth cranial nerve function during posterior fossa surgery. *American Journal of Otology.* 1998; **19**: 503–12.

60

Optical coherence tomography

MARIAH HAHN AND BRETT E BOUMA

Introduction	755	Key points	759
Optical coherence tomography: System operation	756	Deficiencies in current knowledge and areas for future	
OCT imaging of the larynx: Preliminary results	757	research	760
Polarization-sensitive optical coherence tomography	757	Acknowledgements	760
Summary	759	References	760

SEARCH STRATEGY AND EVIDENCE-BASE

The data in this chapter are supported by a PubMed search using the key words optical coherence tomography, needle biopsy, surgical guidance, nasal, vocal cord and/or otology. Levels of evidence are not really applicable to this area, but the human studies that underlie the discussion of optical coherence tomography as applied to otorhinolaryngology are observational or at best non-randomized.

INTRODUCTION

Medical imaging technology has advanced rapidly over the past twenty years, providing physicians with essential information on the macroscopic anatomy of patients. Techniques capable of imaging subepithelial structure *in situ*, such as conventional x-ray radiography, magnetic resonance imaging (MRI), computed tomography (CT) and ultrasonography have allowed the noninvasive investigation of relatively large-scale structures in the human body, with resolutions ranging from $100\,\mu m$ to $1\,mm$. Resolution on this scale, however, is insufficient to detect the subtle changes in tissue microstructure characteristic of many ear, nose and throat (ENT) pathologies.

In the field of laryngology, light endoscopy currently forms the cornerstone of clinical imaging and biopsy guidance, yet conventional light endoscopic techniques are unable to reveal information concerning subepithelial tissue. Since many laryngeal pathologies originate near the boundary between the epithelium and the underlying mucosa or within the mucosa itself, the inability to image subepithelial tissue represents a serious limitation of conventional light endoscopy. Even as a method for guiding biopsy, conventional light endoscopy gives only a relatively coarse indication of prospective biopsy locations. Frequently, a large number of biopsies are required to achieve high diagnostic accuracy, a situation that is often undesirable or unfeasible. This is particularly true for the vocal folds, which have a specialized and delicate microstructure that is highly intolerant of trauma. These limitations restrict the effectiveness of light endoscopy for the diagnosis, monitoring and treatment of many laryngeal pathologies. Clinical laryngology would thus greatly benefit from a noninvasive imaging technology capable of resolving subepithelial tissue microstructure in the range of conventional biopsy.

Optical coherence tomography (OCT) is a relatively new optical imaging modality that allows high-resolution, cross-sectional imaging of tissue microstructure. OCT can image with an axial resolution of $1-15\,\mu m$ and has an imaging depth of $2-3\,mm$ in nontransparent tissue. OCT was first applied in 1991 to imaging optically transparent structures, such as the anterior eye and retina.[1,2] Subsequent technological advances have enabled high-resolution imaging of nontransparent tissue in the cardiovascular system[3] and the gastrointestinal,[4] urinary[5] and female reproductive tracts.[6] In addition, the application of OCT to surgical guidance[7] and carcinoma detection[6, 8] has been explored.

The aforementioned imaging studies have demonstrated that OCT is particularly informative in tissues in which nonkeratinized epithelium is separated from underlying stroma by a smooth basement membrane zone, suggesting that OCT may have a strong clinical relevance in laryngology. This indication is further strengthened by several features of the OCT system itself.

- OCT imaging can be performed *in situ* and nondestructively, enabling the imaging of tissue for which biopsy should be avoided or is impossible.
- OCT images are high resolution, 10–100 times that of conventional MRI or ultrasound.
- Imaging can be performed in real time, without the need to process a specimen, as in conventional biopsy, and without the need for a transducing medium, as in ultrasound imaging.
- OCT is fibreoptically based and can thus be interfaced to a wide range of instruments including catheters, endoscopes, laparoscopes and surgical probes.
- OCT systems can be engineered to be compact, portable and low cost, depending on the desired system specifications.

Although this chapter will focus primarily on the potential applications of OCT to laryngeal tissue, OCT has also been applied to imaging of the middle ear[9] and of rat cochlea[10] *ex vivo* with promising results. In addition, OCT has strong potential for improved visualization of nasal tissues.[11] Before presenting and discussing OCT images of larynges *ex vivo*, it is useful to briefly describe the basis by which OCT systems form subepithelial images.

OPTICAL COHERENCE TOMOGRAPHY: SYSTEM OPERATION

Optical coherence tomography performs high-resolution tomographic imaging by measuring light backscattered or backreflected from internal tissue structures. OCT imaging is analogous to ultrasound B-mode imaging, but is based on the detection of infrared light waves, instead of sound. Like acoustic waves, light is characterized by its propagation direction. Light is distinct, however, in that it has an additional vector characteristic known as polarization. The polarization direction is orthogonal to the propagation direction and can be influenced by the medium in which the light propagates. This is known as 'birefringence'. Polarization measurements can be used to provide additional insights into the microscopic structure and integrity of tissues. An adjunct

to conventional OCT, polarization-sensitive OCT (PS-OCT), exploits birefringence as an additional contrast mechanism for imaging tissue. PS-OCT will be discussed in further detail under Polarization-sensitive optical coherence tomography.

The analogy with ultrasound is a useful starting point for understanding the basics of OCT. In ultrasound, a high frequency acoustic pulse travels into the tissue and is reflected or backscattered from internal structures having different acoustic properties. The magnitude and the delay time of the echoes are electronically detected, and the structural properties of the internal tissues are determined from the measured signals. In OCT, imaging is performed by measuring the echo delay time and magnitude of light backreflected or backscattered from internal structures with distinct optical properties. Unlike in ultrasound, though, the speed of light is very high, rendering electronic measurement of the echo delay time of the reflected light impossible. OCT systems circumvent this limitation by using low coherence interferometry, also known as white light interferometry, to characterize optical echoes.

The most common OCT echo detection scheme is based on a Michelson interferometer set up with a scanning reference delay arm, shown in **Figure 60.1**. Within the interferometer, the beam leaving the optical light source is split into two parts, termed the reference and sample beams, at the beam splitter. The reference beam then travels to a mirror, located at a known distance from the detector and subsequently returns to the beam splitter. The sample beam travels to the tissue sample and is reflected back toward the detector by scattering sites within the tissue. Light reflecting from deeper tissue layers has traversed a greater optical pathlength (optical distance) and therefore arrives at the detector at a later time. In addition, the various backreflected parts of the sample beam will have different amplitudes based on the

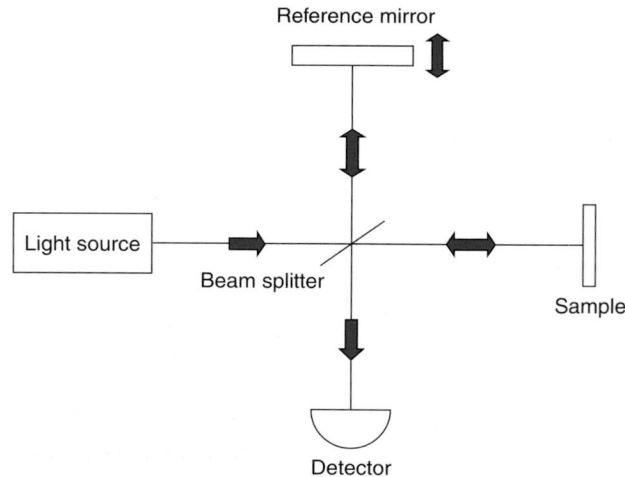

Figure 60.1 Schematic of a optical coherence tomography system using a Michelson interferometer with scanning reference delay arm.

differing strengths of the scattering sites. The reflected portions of the sample beam then return to the beam splitter where they interact with the reflected reference beam and are directed toward the detector.

When two waves from the same source recombine in this manner, an interference pattern will result if the optical pathlength travelled by the two waves is identical. The output detector measures the intensity of this interference pattern and thus only measures information contained in the portion of the sample beam that has travelled the same optical distance as the light in the reference arm. Information about the remaining tissue layers can be extracted by moving the mirror in the reference arm, which changes the optical pathlength travelled by the reference beam. Two- or three-dimensional images are produced by scanning the beam across the sample and recording the optical backscattering versus depth at different transverse positions. The resulting data is a two- or three-dimensional representation of the optical backscattering of the sample on a micron scale.

OCT IMAGING OF THE LARYNX: PRELIMINARY RESULTS

To assess the potential value of OCT imaging technology in improving visualization and pathology, diagnosis and treatment of a given organ system, it is essential to first image normal tissue from that particular organ and then reference the resulting OCT images to parallel histology.

Initial studies of the laryngeal imaging using OCT[12, 13] have focused on the following structures due to clinical relevance:

- the laryngeal surface of the epiglottis;
- the false folds;
- the inferior surface of the true folds.

The images presented are based on a similar focus. It should be mentioned, however, that since OCT can be readily adapted to fibreoptic-based probes, other areas of traditionally poor visibility in light endoscopy, such as the anterior commissure, the subglottis and the laryngeal ventricle, could also be readily imaged using this technology.

In **Figure 60.2**, an OCT image of the laryngeal surface of an ovine (sheep) epiglottis and the associated histological section are shown. Several different layers of the epiglottic tissue are visible, with epithelium, lamina propria and cartilage being clearly demarcated. Glandular structures and vessels are also often visible.

Figure 60.3 presents an OCT image taken along the inferior portion of a porcine true fold, as evidenced by the transition from free-edge nonglandular mucosa to subglottal glandular mucosa observed in the OCT image and corresponding histological section. This image illustrates the ability of OCT to allow visualization of the epithelium, basement membrane and lamina propria of

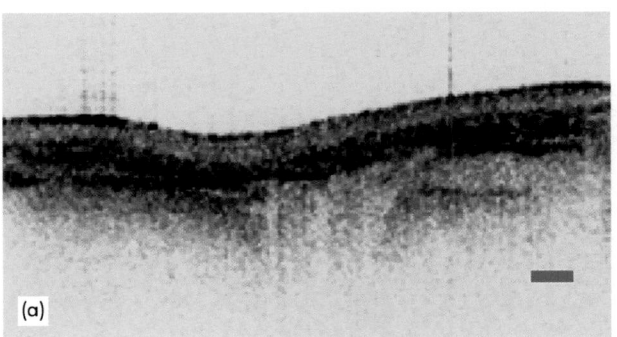

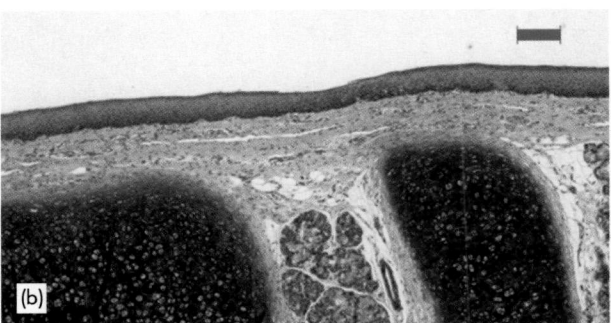

Figure 60.2 (a) OCT image of an ovine epiglottis; (b) corresponding haematoxylin and eosin histology section. Scale bars represent 150 μm.

the true fold, as well as of certain structural features, such as glands and vessels. Note in particular that local epithelial thickness and transparency of the true fold can be readily deduced from these images, implying that OCT may prove useful for the diagnosis of hyperplasia, early-stage keratosis and papillomas, and other pathologies resulting in epithelial abnormalities not normally visible by conventional light endoscopy until an advanced stage. Since many laryngeal pathologies originate at the border between the mucosa and the epithelium, the ability to observe the integrity of the basement membrane via OCT imaging may have important implications for the use of this technology in aiding the diagnosis and monitoring of such laryngeal disorders, possibly including early stage carcinoma.

POLARIZATION–SENSITIVE OPTICAL COHERENCE TOMOGRAPHY

A monochromatic light wave carries three potential sources of information contained in the amplitude, phase and polarization state of its electrical field vector. Conventional OCT, by detecting only the intensity of the interference pattern resulting from interaction of the sample and reference optical beams, fails to quantify the effects of tissue on the polarization state of the sample light beam. An adjunct to conventional OCT, known as polarization-sensitive OCT, therefore has focussed on

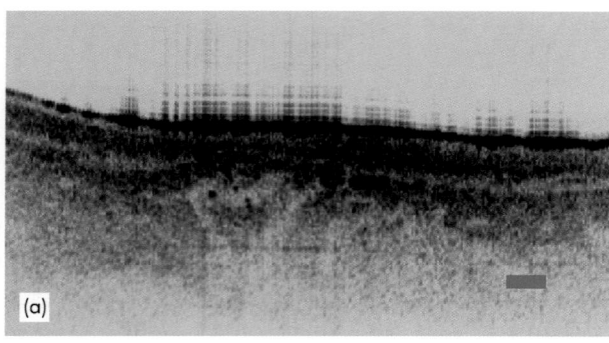

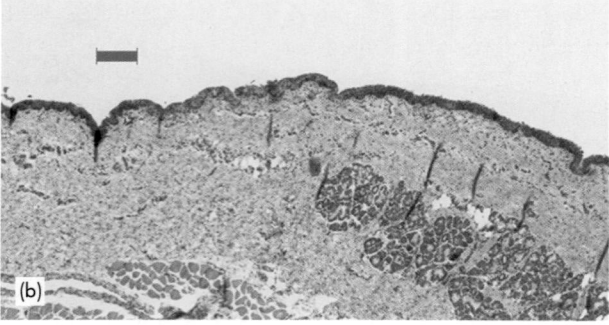

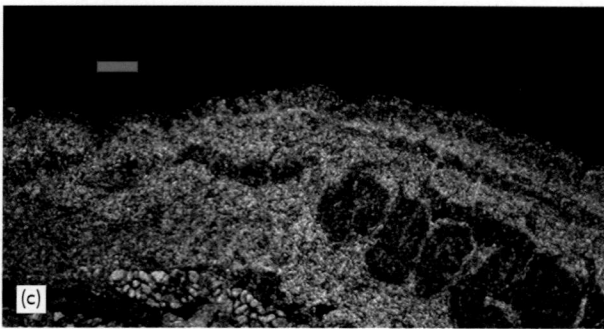

Figure 60.3 (a) OCT image of the inferior surface of a porcine true fold; (b) corresponding haematoxylin and eosin histology section; (c) phase-contrast viewing of the stained histology section. Scale bars represent 150 μm.

exploiting the information contained in the polarization state of the light backreflected or backscattered from the sample relative to that of the reference beam to obtain information about the tissue microstructure.

In order to appreciate the power of PS-OCT and its potential applications, it is helpful to describe briefly the main mechanisms by which tissue alters the polarization state of light. Two mechanisms dominate the changes in the polarization state of light propagating through biological tissue: scattering and birefringence. Scattering changes the polarization of light mainly in a random manner, so it is generally not useful in mapping tissue structure. Organized linear structures, on the other hand, such as collagen fibre bundles with a clear orientation, can exhibit birefringence, resulting in a predictable change in polarization state. Many biological tissues exhibit birefringence, such as tendons, muscle, nerve,

bone, cartilage and teeth.[14] Since changes in birefringence may, for instance, indicate changes in functionality, structure, or viability of tissues, PS-OCT images may contain information which can be used to evaluate tissue microstructure and health beyond the level possible with the use of OCT alone.[15]

The potential implications for clinical laryngology of the sensitivity of PS-OCT to organized linear structures, such as oriented collagen fibre bundles, are numerous. To illustrate, the human vocal fold lamina propria is generally subdivided into the superficial, intermediate and deep layers, with each layer having a characteristic composition and functionality. The relative thickness and integrity of these various layers appear to have a profound impact on voice. This idea is supported by the fact that the average adult will experience marked thinning of the superficial lamina propria relative to the intermediate and deep layers with increasing age,[16] with a concomitant reduction in voice quality.

Histological studies of normal adult human vocal fold tissue have repeatedly noted increased density and longitudinal orientation of collagen fibres as one progresses from more superficial to deeper lamina propria layers.[16] PS-OCT, due to its sensitivity to oriented collagen fibre bundles, may thus allow indirect detection of these lamina propria layers *in situ* and hence monitoring and possibly improving treatment of voice ageing. In the case of vocal fold scarring, the biomechanical integrity of the lamina propria is disrupted, resulting in reduced vocal fold pliability and thus decreased vocal range and quality. Scar tissue has collagen fibre orientation and density that is generally distinct from that of normal tissue and therefore PS-OCT may also prove useful in visualizing, localizing and treating vocal fold scars within the lamina propria. These capabilities could have a profound impact in the area of voice management.

Figure 60.4 compares a PS-OCT image of the inferior surface of a human true fold with the corresponding OCT image and histological section. Note the banding pattern apparent in the PS-OCT image of the vocal fold. A transition from white to black banding indicates a change in the polarization state of light. In particular, observe the marked increase in the thickness of the initial subepithelial white band in the leftmost portion of the PS-OCT image (corresponding to the true fold free edge) relative to that in the more subglottic tissue. The spatial location of this thickened initial band corresponds closely with the increased prominence of the superficial lamina propria in this region. Since collagen in normal superficial lamina propria is sparse and relatively randomly oriented, a net change in the polarization state of light will be slow to occur in this region. Hence, the thickness of the superficial lamina propria can potentially be inferred from the thickness of the initial subepithelial PS-OCT band. The true fold superficial lamina propria features critically in vocal health and disease. Although the presented results are not definitive, the potential of PS-OCT to detect

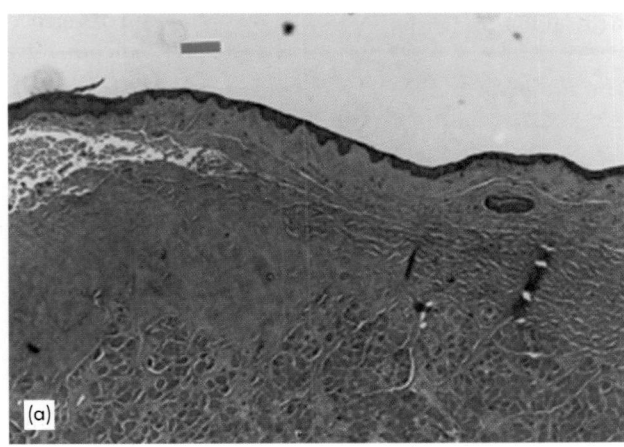

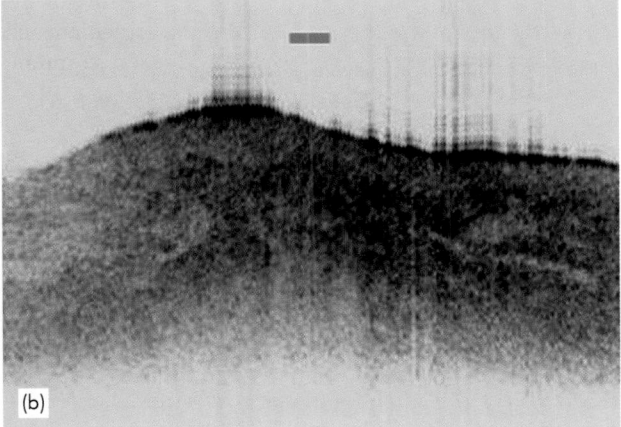

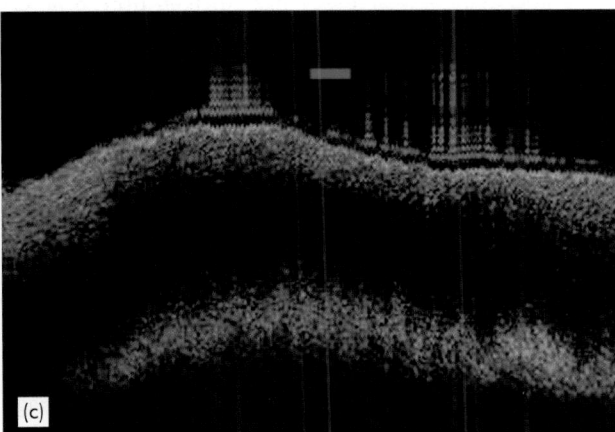

Figure 60.4 (a) Haematoxylin and eosin histology section of the inferior surface of a human true fold; (b) corresponding OCT image; (c) corresponding PS-OCT image. Scale bars represent 150 μm.

changes in the superficial lamina propria thickness and collagen alignment is an exciting area for future study.

Again, it must be stressed that further studies must be carried out to determine what the observed vocal fold polarization patterns truly indicate. In the case that these studies show, that the relative thickness and/or health of the lamina propria layers can indeed be indirectly assessed

by this imaging adjunct, PS-OCT could prove very useful to the study of lamina propria health and in the development of targeted scar treatment strategies.

SUMMARY

OCT and OCT adjuncts have enormous potential for improving the diagnosis, monitoring and both surgical and nonsurgical management of diseased ENT tissues. Conventional OCT provides objective information concerning the structure of tissue elements with distinct optical backscattering and backreflection properties. With regard to the larynx, conventional OCT studies of healthy laryngeal tissues *ex vivo* have demonstrated that OCT can detect spatial changes in the thickness and transparency of the epithelium, the content of the connective tissues in terms of glands and vessels as well as pronounced transitions in connective tissue type and the architecture of the basement membrane.[17] PS-OCT holds promise for permitting indirect visualization of the layers of the true fold lamina propria, as well as of vocal fold scar beds. In addition, a number of other OCT adjuncts, such as spectroscopic OCT[18] and phase dispersion tomography[19] exist or are currently in development, each with distinct imaging advantages and capabilities over conventional OCT imaging. For ENT tissue visualization, the OCT imaging modality represents a rich and vibrant area of future research and discovery.

KEY POINTS

- The diagnosis and treatment of many ENT pathologies would benefit from the ability to image subepithelially and with high resolution *in situ*.
- Optical coherence tomography enables subepithelial imaging of tissue with a resolution ranging from 1 to 15 μm and is fibreoptically based, allowing OCT systems to be interfaced with a wide range of instruments, including catheters and endoscopes.
- With respect to laryngeal tissues, conventional OCT appears to be able to detect spatial changes in the thickness and transparency of the epithelium; the content of the connective tissue, including the presence of glands and vessels; and the integrity of the basement membrane.
- Polarization-sensitive OCT, with its sensitivity to organized linear structures, such as oriented collagen fibre bundles, may prove useful for vocal fold visualization and health assessment.

- OCT and OCT adjuncts hold substantial promise for improved diagnosis and treatment of many ENT disorders, a potential which remains largely untapped and constitutes an exciting avenue for future research, development and discovery.

Deficiencies in current knowledge and areas for future research

Although OCT and OCT adjuncts hold substantial promise for improved visualization of ENT-related tissues, OCT/ OCT-adjunct feasibility studies for most of these tissues are either extremely limited or entirely lacking. For those ENT tissues that have been imaged with OCT, the primary focus of the imaging studies has been the necessary but insufficient first step of assessing the degree to which normal tissue microstructure can be accurately identified from OCT images. Before the OCT imaging modality can be regarded as a diagnostic tool in ENT, rigorous correlation of OCT/OCT-adjunct images of diseased tissue with parallel histology must be carried out to demonstrate that a given disease state can be accurately and reliably identified from OCT image structures. In the case of the larynx, although conventional OCT images of pathological laryngeal structures *in vivo* have been recorded,[12] the corresponding histology necessary to guide OCT image interpretation has most often been lacking. Thus, whether OCT/OCT-adjuncts can reproducibly and accurately identify laryngeal pathology or other ENT pathologies remains to be determined and constitutes an exciting and vital area of future work.

In addition to pathology identification, OCT or certain OCT adjuncts may prove useful in guiding laser and nonlaser-based microsurgery of ENT tissues. In laser microsurgery, PS-OCT may be particularly applicable, since laser damage of collagenous tissue has been shown to alter the tissue's effect on the polarization state of incoming light.[20] This is yet another exciting avenue for future research.

In brief, the following are a few of the many vital areas for current and future investigation:

➤ rigorous correlation of histology with OCT images of pathologic laryngeal specimens;
➤ further investigation of the potential use of PS-OCT in laryngology and correlation of PS-OCT images to laryngeal microstructure;
➤ investigation of other OCT adjuncts, such as spectroscopic OCT, to laryngeal imaging;
➤ further exploration of the possible applications of OCT/OCT adjuncts to ear-related imaging and a feasibility study of OCT applied to nasal tissue;
➤ exploration of the use of OCT or PS-OCT systems to ENT surgical guidance.

ACKNOWLEDGEMENTS

The authors thank Dr Steven Zeitels of the Massachusetts Eye and Ear Infirmary for fruitful discussions. We also thank Joe Seidel, PhD, for cutting and staining the histological sections appearing in this chapter, and Diane Jones of the Massachusetts Eye and Ear Infirmary for helping to procure human laryngeal autopsy specimens.

This work was funded in part by the Advisory Board Foundation, Eugene B Casey Foundation and the National Science Foundation Graduate Fellowships.

REFERENCES

1. Hee MR, Izatt JA, Swanson EA, Huang D, Schuman JS, Lin CP et al. Optical coherence tomography of the human retina. *Archives of Opthalmology – Chicago.* 1995; **113**: 325–32.
2. Swanson EA, Izatt JA, Hee MR, Huang D, Lin CP, Schuman JS et al. *In vivo* retinal imaging by optical coherence tomography. *Optics Letters.* 1993; **18**: 1864–6.
3. Jang IK, Bouma BE, Kang DH, Park SJ, Park SW, Seung HK et al. Visualization of coronary atherosclerotic plaques in patients using optical coherence tomography: comparison with intravascular ultrasound. *Journal of the American College of Cardiology.* 2002; **39**: 604–9.
4. Bouma BE, Tearney GJ, Compton CC, Nishioka NS. Endoscopic optical coherence tomography of the gastrointestinal tract. *Gastrointestinal Endoscopy.* 1999; **49**: 390 Part 2.
5. Tearney GJ, Brezinski ME, Southern JF, Bouma BE, Boppart SA, Fujimoto JG. Optical biopsy in human urologic tissue using optical coherence tomography. *Journal of Urology.* 1997; **157**: 1915–9.
6. Pitris C, Goodman A, Boppart SA, Libus JJ, Fujimoto JG, Brezinski ME. High-resolution imaging of gynecologic neoplasms using optical coherence tomography. *Obstetrics and Gynecology.* 1999; **93**: 135–9.
7. Boppart SA, Bouma BE, Pitris C, Southern JF, Brezinski ME, Fujimoto JG. Intraoperative assessment of microsurgery with three-dimensional optical coherence tomography. *Radiology.* 1998; **208**: 81–6.
8. Jesser CA, Boppart SA, Pitris C, Stamper DL, Nielsen GP, Brezinski ME et al. High resolution imaging of transitional cell carcinoma with optical coherence tomography: Feasibility for the evaluation of bladder pathology. *British Journal of Radiology.* 1999; **72**: 1170–6.
* 9. Pitris C, Saunders KT, Fujimoto JG, Brezinski ME. High-resolution imaging of the middle ear with optical coherence tomography – A feasibility study. *Archives of Otolaryngology – Head and Neck.* 2001; **127**: 637–42. *Recently published study of conventional OCT as applied to ENT-related tissues.*
* 10. Wong BJF, de Boer JF, Park BH, Chen Z, Nelson JS. Optical coherence tomography of the rat cochlea. *Journal of*

Biomedical Optics. 2000; **5**: 367–70. *Recently published study of conventional OCT as applied to ENT-related tissues.*

11. Mahmood U, Ridgway J, Jackson R, Guo SG, Su JP, Armstrong W *et al.* In vivo optical coherence tomography of the nasal mucosa. *American Journal of Rhinology.* 2006; **20**: 155–9.

∗ 12. Gladkova ND, Shakhov AV, Feldschtein F. Capabilities of optical coherence tomography in laryngology. In: Bouma B, Tearney G (eds). *Handbook of optical coherence tomography,* Basel: Marcel Dekkar, 2002: 705–24. *Recently published study of conventional OCT as applied to ENT-related tissues.*

∗ 13. Pitris C, Brezinski ME, Bouma BE, Tearney GJ, Southern JF, Fujimoto JG. High resolution imaging of the upper respiratory tract with optical coherence tomography – A feasibility study. *American Journal of Respiratory and Critical Care Medicine.* 1998; **157**: 1640–4. *Recently published study of conventional OCT as applied to ENT-related tissues.*

14. de Boer JF, Srinivas SM, Nelson JS, Milner TE, Ducros MG. Polarization Sensitive OCT. In: Bouma B, Tearney G (eds). *Handbook of optical coherence tomography.* Basel: Marcel Dekkar, 2002: 237–74.

∗ 15. Drexler W, Stamper D, Jesser C, Li XD, Pitris C, Saunders K *et al.* Correlation of collagen organization with polarization sensitive imaging of *in vitro* cartilage: Implications for osteoarthritis. *Journal of Rheumatology.* 2001; **28**: 1311–8. *Potential uses of PS-OCT are discussed in the context of a clinical example.*

16. Hammond TH, Gray SD, Butler JE. Age- and gender-related collagen distribution in human vocal folds. *Annals of Otology Rhinology and Laryngology.* 2000; **109**: 913–20 Part 1.

17. Burns JA, Zeitels SM, Anderson RR *et al.* Imaging the mucosa of the human vocal fold with optical coherence tomography. *Annals of Otology Rhinology and Laryngology.* 2005; **114**: 671–6.

18. Morgner U, Drexler W, Kartner FX, Li XD, Pitris C, Ippen EP *et al.* Spectroscopic optical coherence tomography. *Optics Letters.* 2000; **25**: 111–3.

19. Yang CH, Wax A, Dasari RR, Feld MS. Phase-dispersion optical tomography. *Optics Letters.* 2001; **26**: 686–8.

20. de Boer JF, Milner TE, vanGemert MJC, Nelson JS. Two-dimensional birefringence imaging in biological tissue by polarization-sensitive optical coherence tomography. *Optics Letters.* 1997; **22**: 934–6.

61

Contact endoscopy

MARIO ANDREA AND OSCAR DIAS

Introduction	762	Summary	767
Technical details	763	Key points	767
Contact endoscopy of the larynx	763	Deficiencies in current knowledge and areas for future	
Contact endoscopy of the nasal cavity	764	research	767
Contact endoscopy of the nasopharynx	766	References	767
Oral cavity and oropharynx	767		

SEARCH STRATEGY AND EVIDENCE-BASE

The data in this chapter are supported by a Medline search using the key words contact endoscopy, *in vivo* diagnosis focusing on the clinical impact of contact endoscopy in the assessment and understanding of diseases of the upper aero digestive tract. The evidence level of contact endoscopic assessment is correlated with its learning curve involving knowledge of cytological, pathological and micro vascular patterns. It is difficult to classify the contact endoscopy findings by levels of evidence because we have direct access to the cell images in its more pure form. In some aspects the level of evidence is 1. However, in general, we would classify it as level 3 and 4 evidence.

INTRODUCTION

Contact endoscopy was first described by Desormeaux in 1865,[1, 2] who managed to obtain a direct view of the bladder mucosa. Interest in this technique then waned for almost a century, until technological advances had been made and Jaupitre[3] began to promote it once more. More recently, Hamou[4, 5] developed and described his technique of microcolpohysteroscopy, in which contact endoscopy played a pivotal role. Its use in research to study the microvasculature of the larynx[6, 7, 8, 9, 10] prompted further clinical applications within the upper airway. Contact endoscopy has now been employed to assess vocal cord pathology, the nasal mucosa, nasopharynx, oral cavity, oropharynx and the trachea.[11, 12, 13, 14, 15, 16, 17, 18, 19, 20, 21, 22]

Contact endoscopy allows *in vivo* and *in situ* observation of the mucosal blood vessels and superficial cells of the epithelium which have been previously stained with methylene blue. The experienced otolaryngologist is able to perform a pathological evaluation during planned endoscopy and in many cases, an immediate diagnosis can be made. The information acquired does not render conventional biopsy and histological evaluation obsolete, rather it gives additional information to complement it. With contact endoscopy it is possible to detect microvascular changes and/or alterations in surface cellular structure that are suggestive of subclinical stages of disease. It is worth noting that because cells migrate towards the surface, most pathological processes can be seen by examining the superficial layers[23, 24, 25] and it is precisely this that contact endoscopy addresses. The surgeon is able to assess the microscopic structure of the entire mucosa, allowing a more complete interpretation of the disease process. In other words, it offers the clinician a global perspective of the disease process with the facility of cellular and vascular mapping at any number of sites in the region. Furthermore, contact endoscopy has the advantage that it can be undertaken with the patient awake in the outpatient setting or while anaesthetized in the theatre.

Contact endoscopy of the upper aerodigestive tract is still in its infancy. More and more centres are using this technique and its principles are being applied in other specialties as well. No doubt further technological advances will be forthcoming and the process will be refined. It is possible that in the future, contact endoscopy will occupy a central role in diagnosis, therapeutic planning and the follow-up of patients with a number of upper aerodigestive tract diseases. This chapter describes the current state of the art of contact endoscopy.

TECHNICAL DETAILS

Contact endoscopy can be undertaken in either the conscious or anaesthetized patient. Topical anaesthesia is all that is required. Several endoscopes have been developed and are commercially available but, for most purposes in the upper airway, only two endoscopes are required (7215 AA and 7215 BA, Karl Storz, Tuttlingen, Germany). With these endoscopes the clinician has direct access to the subsurface microvascular plexus and to the surface epithelium which can be viewed at a magnification of ×60 and ×150.

The mucosal surface to be examined is carefully cleaned by gentle suction or with a swab that has been moistened with saline. The surface is then stained with 1 percent methylene blue applied on a fragment of Spongostan®. The tip of the endoscope is placed gently against the surface of the mucosa allowing examination. Staining lasts for approximately four to five minutes at most sites before gradually disappearing. In the nasal cavity, the stain disappears more quickly as it is moved away towards the nasopharynx along the mucociliary pathway.

CONTACT ENDOSCOPY OF THE LARYNX

Contact endoscopy of the larynx and hypopharynx is performed under general anesthesia with conventional endotracheal intubation and synchronous microlaryngoscopy.

Normal appearance

Squamous cells at the vocal cord edge and in the hypopharynx have a polyhedric shape, being contiguous with each other. Their nuclei are round, darkly stained and the cytoplasm has a light blue tone. The nuclear:cytoplasmic ratio is regular and the overall morphologic pattern is homogeneous. Ciliated epithelium is present in most of the larynx. The nuclei of the cells are round, but the limits of the cytoplasm are difficult to define. Bundles

of cilia appear as filamentous structures that can be displaced by the tip of the contact endoscope. The transition from squamous to ciliated epithelium can be observed. Islands of squamous cells in the middle of ciliated epithelium may be seen and are not abnormal. The duct orifices of glands can also be identified. What is and what is not normal varies between patients and is very much influenced by such factors as age and diet and habits such as voice use and smoking.

Abnormal appearance

Metaplastic substitution of ciliated epithelium by squamous epithelium is most commonly seen in heavy smokers. It also occurs in patients with gastroesophageal reflux where the ciliated epithelium of the posterior commissure is replaced by squamous epithelium. It would seem that this interferes with normal mucus clearance.

When patients with chronic laryngitis are studied by this method, the epithelial pattern is found to be homogeneous, but epithelial cells have larger nuclei than normal and an increased nuclear:cytoplasmic ratio. As cell turnover is accelerated by inflammation, it is possible to visualize immature cells at the surface that are similar to those usually present in the intermediate layers of the normal epithelium. There are more blood vessels within the mucosa, but the vascular network keeps its normal pattern. In some cases of chronic laryngitis, filaments of fungal hyphae are identified and, if seen, should prompt treatment with antifungal agents.

Keratosis is detected very easily. Distinct and different stages of keratinization may be seen in the same patient. In the initial stages of keratinization, isolated cells without nuclei are observed. More advanced stages show groups of cells without nuclei, but with distinct cells still identifiable. With further progression of the disease it is not possible to distinguish the borders of individual cells and only large areas of an amorphous or laminar structure are visible.

In frank leukoplakia, degrees of cellular abnormality are identified that include heterogeneity of cell populations with nuclei of different colour, size and shape. The variation seen is in agreement with the histopathological concept of leukoplakia, in which different pathological alterations such as hyperkeratosis and dysplasia can develop simultaneously.[24]

Contact endoscopy may not detect dysplasia when alterations are confined solely to the deep epithelial layers. However, in most cases, dysplasia is associated with involvement of the superficial layers as well and these are accessible to the endoscope. The most significant dysplastic changes[23, 24, 25] are variations in nuclear size, shape and colour, together with changes of the nuclear:cytoplasmic ratio (dyskaryosis and anysokaryosis). The more pronounced the changes identified by contact endoscopy, the more severe the dysplasia. Vascular changes also develop with dysplasia, where the normal vascular pattern is substituted by vessels of varying size. Unfortunately, when intense keratosis accompanies dysplasia it is not possible to observe the vessels beneath the surface.

In carcinoma, cell morphology is very variable with extreme heterogeneity of nuclear size, shape and staining characteristics. The nuclear:cytoplasmic ratio also changes from cell to cell. Nuclear inclusion bodies, prominent nucleoli and mitoses may be seen. The normal microvascular pattern and architecture is disturbed. Atypical vessels of different sizes and shapes are seen, as are thromboses, ectasias and rupture. In this situation, contact endoscopy enables the assessment of transitional zones between normal and abnormal mucosa and, as a result, a better evaluation of early stage disease. Surgeons also find it useful to guide biopsies and the collection of cytological samples so that safe margins may be identified. Interestingly, adjacent areas with normal squamous and ciliated cells often exhibit vascular changes (vascular loops) that signify an imminent change in status.

Contact endoscopy has also had an impact on the assessment and management of laryngeal papillomata. Typical vascular loops in the core of the papillomata can be seen as long as the associated keratosis is not too severe. In certain phases of the disease it is possible to identify koilocytes (ballooned cells) and inflammatory infiltrate. New lesions and incipient spread can also be detected. It would be hoped that eventually this information would translate into more accurate excision of papillomata and a reduced risk of residual or recurrent disease.

In summary, contact endoscopy helps the surgeon understand the pathophysiology of several common laryngeal conditions, such as metaplasia, caused by smoking, gastroesophageal reflux or vocal abuse, premalignant lesions, the early stages of laryngeal carcinoma, human papilloma virus (HPV) lesions and the association of cancer and HPV infection. In the future, tumour staging may well expand to encompass information on the cellular changes detected by contact endoscopy (**Figure 61.1**).

CONTACT ENDOSCOPY OF THE NASAL CAVITY

The anterior part of the nasal cavity may be examined easily with the patient awake using topical anaesthesia.

Normal appearance

As in the larynx, it is possible to evaluate the distribution and morphological appearance of the squamous and ciliated epithelia, glandular ostia, mucus and submucosal vascular networks. Squamous epithelium is usually present at the anterior tip and inferior border of the inferior turbinate, the septum and nasal vestibule. This epithelium consists of polyhedric cells with dark blue nuclei and a light blue cytoplasm. Ciliated epithelium is present in most of the nasal cavity. The transition between ciliated and squamous epithelium is usually well defined, although in some cases isolated patches of squamous epithelium are seen in the middle of the ciliated epithelium.

The dynamic variation in volume of the turbinates caused by the nasal cycle explains the presence of small folds and papillas that tend to move in front of the endoscope. The duct orifices of glands are most prominent at the anterior end of the turbinates. Characteristically, they appear as concentric accumulations of cells with the innermost cell layers on a deeper plane. Dynamic changes in the glandular ostia are sometimes observed when manipulating the contact endoscope. The orifices of the glands become more noticeable when mucus is expelled. Mucus itself is seen as a moving layer that stains light blue and emanates from distinct papillas. It follows the contours of the papillas and carries away cell debris which either detaches spontaneously or as a result of the movement of the endoscope.

Characteristic features of the microvascular network have also been described. The papillas observed in the turbinates usually contain a small blood vessel. In the anterior part of the septum there are vessels of a very distinct calibre that are linked by anastomoses.

Abnormal appearance

Contact endoscopy in the nasal cavity is probably of most use in the study and management of chronic rhinosinusitis, allergic rhinitis, nasal polyposis and mucocilliary diseases. In these conditions, it can be employed to assess the response to different types of treatment.[26]

In patients with chronic rhinitis, squamous epithelium covers most of the inferior and middle turbinates and anterior septum. The nuclei of these cells look larger than normal. Areas of keratosis predominate in regions exposed to turbulent air flow, such as the anterior end of the inferior surface of the turbinates. Usually in these patients there is overproduction of mucus and the methylene blue stain clears very quickly. The density of mucous glands is increased and consequently more ostia are seen than in normal patients. Inflammatory cell infiltrates can be identified and differentiation of this infiltrate may help define the nature of the inflammatory process.

Mucus production is also increased in patients with allergic rhinitis. The papillae of glands are larger than normal and a U-shaped vascular axis is seen in the papillae. Ciliated epithelium is usually preserved in allergic rhinitis and there are fewer inflammatory changes than in the chronic nonallergic rhinitis group. In chronic nonallergic rhinitis, vascular congestion is diffuse and

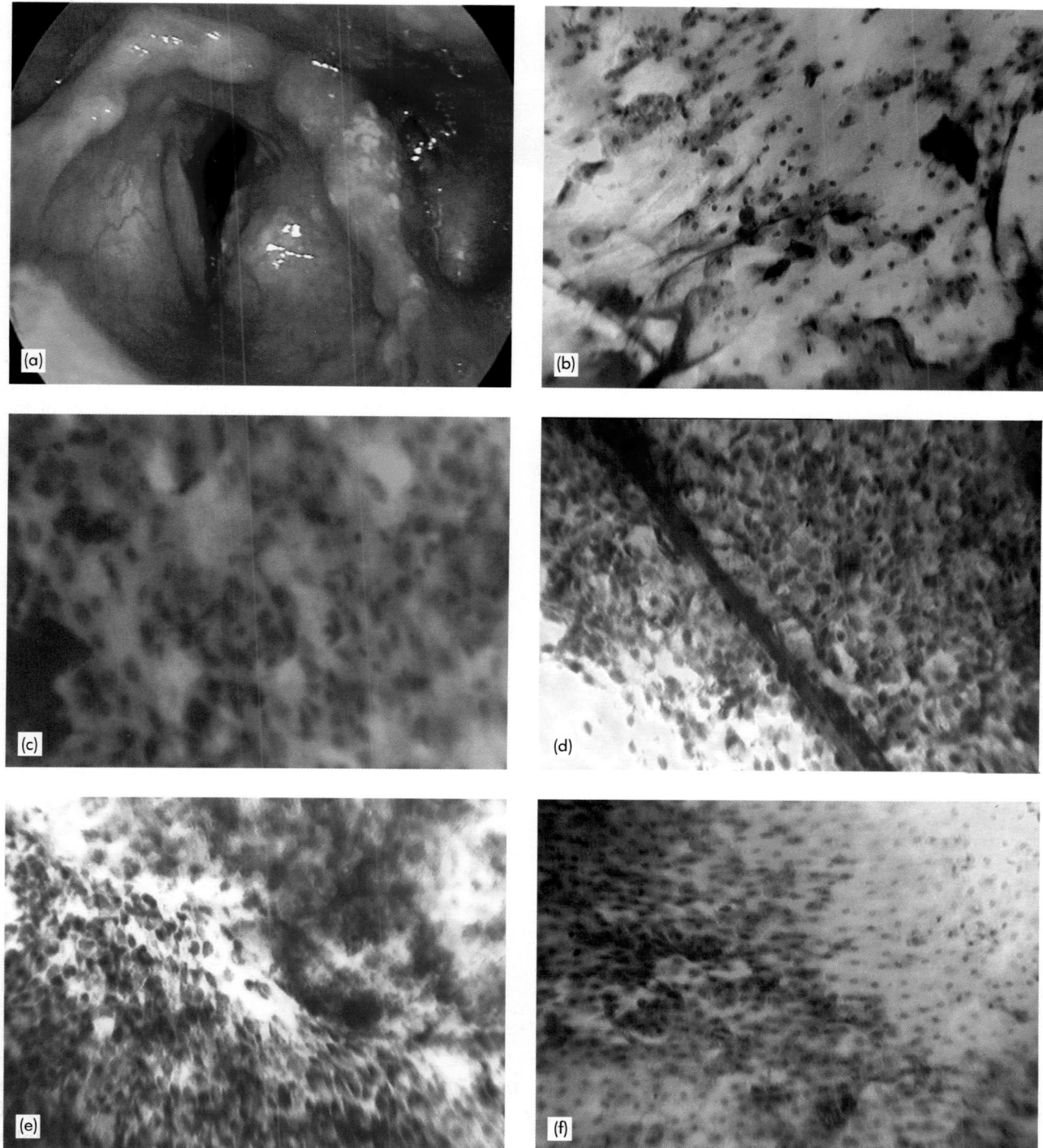

Figure 61.1 Contact endoscopic assessment of a laryngeal tumour. (a) Laryngeal tumour (T_3 N_2 M_x); (b–h) Contact endoscopy ($\times 60$). (b) Right arytenoid region: normal squamous epithelium. Note the regular appearance of the cells and their nuclei. (c) Left arytenoid region: tumour present. The nuclei of the epithelium are irregular in size and shape. Numerous mitoses are visible. (d) Right vocal cord: malignant changes are easily visible, as well as variations in nuclear size and shape. (e) Left vocal cord: tumour pattern. (f) Right false cord: transition from normal epithelium to tumour pattern.

independent of the papillae. Very enlarged vessels are sometimes identified.

Examination of nasal polyps has shown that the anterior face is covered by squamous epithelium while the rest of the polyp is covered with ciliated cells. Metaplastic changes may be present and are related to the duration of exposure to turbulent air flow. Nasal polyposis is usually accompanied by inflammatory cell infiltrates.

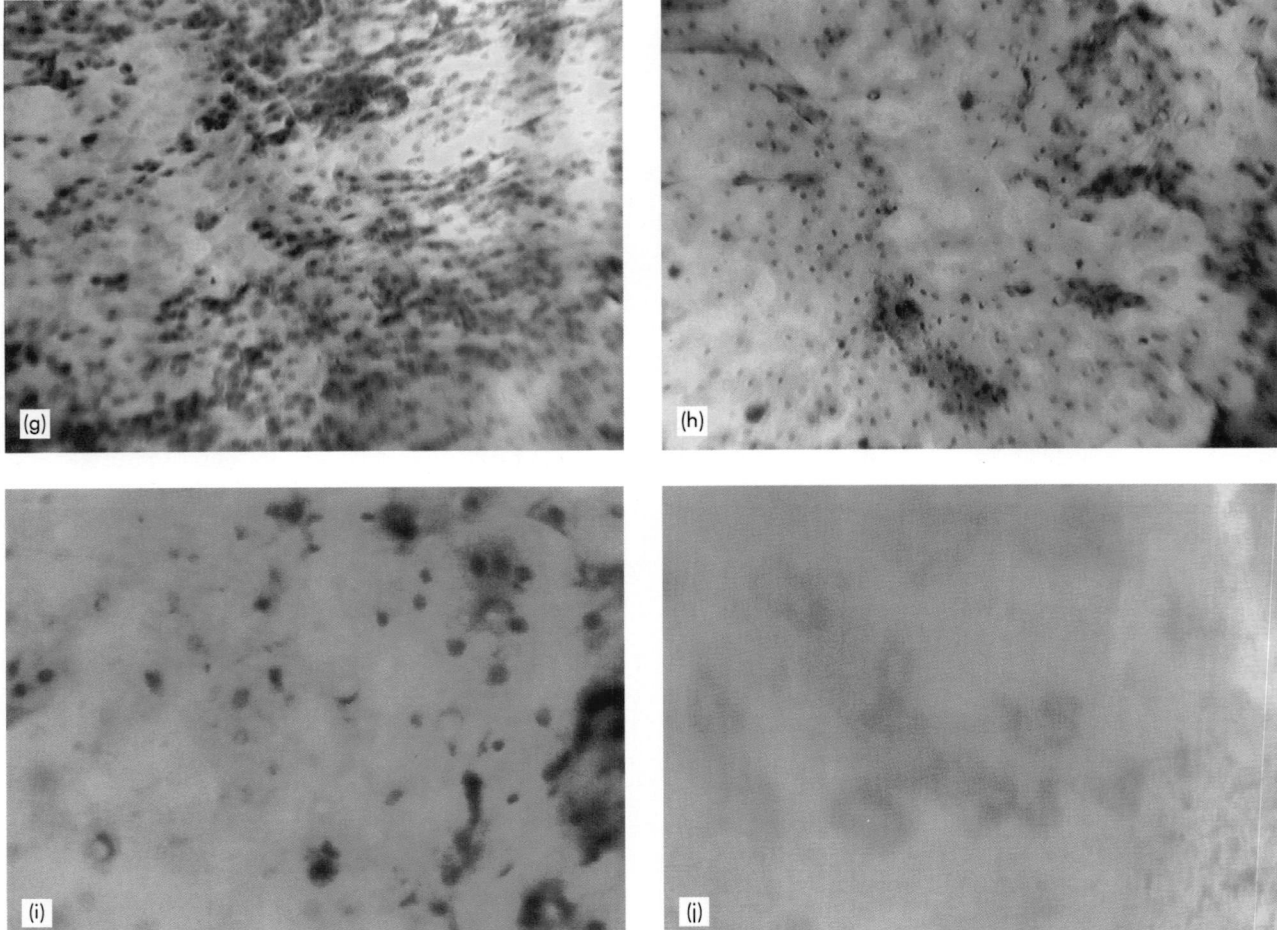

Figure 61.1 Contact endoscopic assessment of a laryngeal tumour. (Continued) (g) Right false cord: islands of atypical cells. (h) Medial aspect of the right arytenoid: tumour pattern associated with presence of koylocytes. (i) Contact endoscopy (×150), koylocytes (ballooned cells), medial aspect of the right arytenoid. (j) Contact endoscopy (60×), vascular loops typical of HPV, right arytenoid region.

Contact endoscopy can, and perhaps should, be used during functional endoscopic sinus surgery to assess the state of the mucosa. The type and degree of abnormalities can help the surgeon decide which areas of mucosa to remove and which to retain.

CONTACT ENDOSCOPY OF THE NASOPHARYNX

Contact endoscopy of the nasopharynx can be performed through the nose under local anaesthesia. Its main use is in the long-term follow-up of patients who have been treated for nasopharyngeal carcinoma.

Normal appearance

Although the majority of the nasopharynx is lined with ciliated epithelium, it is usual to see areas of squamous epithelium, typically in the central and inferior part of the

posterior wall. Orifices of glandular ducts are present throughout the nose.

Abnormal appearance

An irregular vascular pattern is seen in areas with nasopharyngeal carcinoma. Atypical vessels, ectasias, thrombosis, blood cell aggregates and increased vascular fragility are common. The tissue is extremely fragile and will bleed easily if probed too firmly with the endoscope. As with all malignancy, the stained epithelium of the nasopharynx shows anysokaryosis, heterochromasia and hyperchromasia. There are often clusters of malignant cells with hyperchromatic nuclei. Most nuclei are irregular in shape, others fusiform in shape (fibroblast-like) and some are large and oval. Occasionally, it is possible to observe the nucleolus, nuclear inclusions and even mitoses. There is almost always a marked lympho-cytic infiltrate. The transitional zone between the tumour and normal tissues is very important and it is usual to see inflammatory infiltrates and/or keratosis. Small islands of malignant cells are sometimes found in the middle of the apparently normal ciliated epithelium in areas immediately adjacent to the tumour.

It is worth emphasizing that a number of centres regularly use contact endoscopy for both the diagnosis and follow-up of their patients with nasopharyngeal tumours.[27, 28] In particular, this technique is used in areas where nasopharyngeal carcinoma is endemic as an office-based procedure to confirm the diagnosis, identify submucosal disease when malignancy is not detected endoscopically and to identify persistent and recurrent nasopharyngeal carcinoma. Contact endoscopy is also used to select areas for biopsy.

ORAL CAVITY AND OROPHARYNX

Contact endoscopy of the oral cavity and oropharynx is performed either with or without topical local anaesthesia.

Normal appearance

It is important to remember that the morphology of the oral mucosa varies from site to site. In some parts it is keratinized, the so-called masticatory mucosa, while in others it is not, as in the lining of the mucosa or specialized mucosa. These different patterns must be recognized if pathological changes are to be understood and interpreted.

The transition from the keratinized epithelium of the lip to the nonkeratinized epithelium of the vestibule is seen easily. The greater part of the mucosa of the lip, the alveoli, cheek, floor of the mouth, ventral surface of the tongue and soft palate is also nonkeratinized squamous epithelium. Some keratinization is to be expected in the cheek opposite the occlusal plane. The masticatory mucosa covering the hard palate and gingiva is a keratinized epithelium. On the dorsum of the tongue, filiform and fungiform papillae can be seen. Contact endoscopy in the oral cavity and oropharynx has great potential in areas such as the diagnosis of early cancer, the study of tumour margins, the assessment of the response to radiotherapy and chemotherapy and to identify subclinical stages of disease.

SUMMARY

Contact endoscopy allows *in vivo* and *in situ* assessment of the mucosa and underlying microvascular network. With experience, the operator can distinguish between normal and abnormal tissues. It represents a new phase in the development of endoscopy. This technique can

improve the accuracy of diagnosis and give useful information about the extent of disease. It helps identify earlier subclinical stages of disease than was previously possible.

Many centres use this technique and global experience is increasing.[27, 28, 29, 30, 31, 32] The accuracy and clinical applicability of contact endoscopes will continue to be enhanced by improvements in optical systems, new cell dyes, markers, fluorescent products,[22] light sources, image processing and better recording techniques.

KEY POINTS

- Contact endoscopy is a simple, noninvasive technique that offers real-time information about disease processes.
- Contact endoscopy allows the mapping of an entire mucosal surface in the conscious or anaesthetized patient.
- Contact endoscopy may eventually be used to monitor changes that develop in the premalignant stages of the disease.

Deficiencies in current knowledge and areas for future research

➤ Contact endoscopy has great potential for the early diagnosis of nasopharyngeal cancer. However, more experience needs to be gained to define its role as a screening procedure.

➤ More knowledge is needed on the pathogenesis of squamous metaplasia and atypical hyperplasia.

➤ Articulation of contact endoscopy with other technologies such as fluorescence, confocal and narrow band imaging will further enhance the accuracy of *in vivo* and *in situ* diagnosis.

REFERENCES

1. Reuter M, Reuter H, Engel R. *History of endoscopy.* Publication of the Max Nitze Museum, Stuttgart and International Nitze Leiter Research Society of Endoscopy, Vienna, 1999.
2. Desormeaux AJ. De l'endoscope et de ses applications au diagnostique et au traitement des afféctions de l'uréthre et de la vessie. Paris, 1865 (from *History of endoscopy.* Publication of the Max Nitze Museum, Stuttgart and International Nitze Leiter Research Society of Endoscopy, Vienna, 1999).

3. Jaupitre M. La cystocinématographie en couleur. Communications au Congrés Français d'Urologie. October 1955, 128 (from *History of endoscopy*. Publication of the Max Nitze Museum, Stuttgart and International Nitze Leiter Research Society of Endoscopy, Vienna, 1999).

4. Hamou JE. *Microendoscopy and contact endoscopy*. Brevet Français 79,04168, Paris 1979. International patent PCT/FR 80/0024, Paris, 1980. US patent 4,385,810, Washington DC, 1983.

* 5. Hamou JE. *Hysteroscopy and microcolpohysteroscopy*, text and atlas. Appleton & Lange, 1991.

* 6. Andrea M. '*Vascularização arterial da laringe, distribuição macro e microvascular*'. PhD dissertation, University of Lisbon, Portugal, 1975.

7. Andrea M, Guerrier Y. L'Epiglotte et ses amarrages. *Cahiers d'ORL et de Chirurgie Cervico-Facial*. 1979; **14**: 793–803.

8. Andrea M, Guerrier Y. Microvascularization de la muqueuse laryngée et trachéale. Introduction à la physiopathologie des lésions sténosantes. *Annales d'Otolaryngologie et de Chirurgie Cervico Faciale*. 1980; **97**: 409–21.

9. Andrea M, Guerrier Y. The anterior commissure of the larynx. *Clinical Otolaryngology*. 1981; **6**: 259–64.

10. Andrea M. Vasculature of the anterior commissure. *Annals of Otology, Rhinology, and Laryngology*. 1981; **90**: 18–20.

* 11. Andrea M, Dias O, Paço J, Santos A, Fernandes A. Anatomical borders in staging – Rigid endoscopy associated to microlaryngeal surgery. In: Smee R, Bridger G. (eds). *Laryngeal cancer*. Proceedings of the II World Congress of Laryngeal Cancer, Sidney, Australia. Elsevier Science BV, 1994: 233–5.

12. Andrea M, Dias O, Santos A. Contact endoscopy during microlaryngeal surgery. A new technique for endoscopic examination of the larynx. *Annals of Otology, Rhinology, and Laryngology*. 1995; **104**: 333–9.

13. Andrea M, Dias O, Paço J. Endoscopic anatomy of the larynx. In: Fabian R, Gluckman J (eds). *Current review of otolaryngology and head and neck surgery*. London: Churchill Livingstone, 1995: 271–5.

14. Andrea M, Dias O, Santos A. Contact endoscopy of the vocal cord. Normal and pathological patterns. *Acta Otolaryngologica*. 1995; **115**: 314–6.

15. Andrea M, Dias O. Rigid and contact endoscopy associated to microlaryngeal surgery. In: Fried M (ed.). *The larynx: A multidisciplinary approach*, 2nd edn. Mosby Year Book, 1996: 75–9.

16. Andrea M, Dias O. *Atlas of rigid and contact endoscopy in microlaryngeal surgery*. Philadelphia: Lippincott-Raven Publishers, 1995.

17. Andrea M, Dias O. Rigid and Contact endoscopy during microsurgery. In: Yanagisawa E (ed.). *Color atlas of diagnostic endoscopy in otorhinolaryngology*. Tokyo: Igaku Shoin, 1996: 168–73.

18. Andrea M, Dias O. Endoscopic assessment of early vocal cord cancer. Paper presented at the Proceedings of IV International Conference of Head and Neck Tumors, Toronto, 1996.

19. Andrea M, Dias O. Newer techniques of laryngeal assessment. In: Cummings CW, Frederikson JM, Krause CJ, Harker LA, Schuller DE, Richardson MA (eds). *Otolaryngology head and neck surgery*. St Louis: Mosby Year Book, 1998: 1967–78.

20. Andrea M, Dias O. Rigid and contact endoscopy of the larynx. In: Ferlito A (ed.). *Diseases of the Larynx*. London: Arnold, 2000: 1001–111.

21. Andrea M, Dias O. La endoscopia rígida y de contacto en la evaluación de las lesiones premalignas de la laringe. In: Suarez Nieto C (ed.). *Tratado de otolaringologia y cirurgia de cabeza y cuello*. Madrid: Proyectos Médicos, 1999: 3006–9.

* 22. Arens C, Malzahn K, Dias O, Andrea M, Glanz H. Endoskopische bildegebende verfahren in der diagnostik des kehlkopfkarzinoms und seiner vorstufen. *Laryngorhinootologie*. 1999; **78**: 685–91.

23. Crissman J. Pathology of the upper aerodigestive tract mucosa. In: Paparella M, Schumrick D, Gluckman J, Meyerhoff W (eds). *Otolaryngology, head and neck*, 3rd edn. Vol. III, Philadelphia: WB Saunders, 1991.

24. Ferlito A. *Neoplasms of the larynx*. New York: Churchill Livingstone, 1993.

25. Kleinsasser O. *Tumors of the larynx and hypopharynx*. George Thieme Verlag, 1988.

* 26. Andrea M, Dias O, Macor C, Santos A, Varandas J. Contact endoscopy of the nasal mucosa. *Acta Otolaryngologica*. 1997; **117**: 307–11.

27. Xiaoming H, Haiqiang M, Manquan D, Jianyong S, Yong S, Kela L *et al*. Examination of nasopharyngeal epithelium with contact endoscopy. *Acta Otolaryngologica*. 2001; **121**: 98–102.

* 28. Pak MW, To KF, Leung SF, van Hasselt CA. *In vivo* diagnosis of nasopharyngeal carcinoma using contact rhinoscopy. *Laryngoscope*. 2001; **11**: 1453–8.

29. Pau HW, Dommerich S, Just T, Beust M. Cholesteatoma recurrences caused by intraoperative cell seeding? Contact endoscopic and cytologic studies. *Laryngorhinootologie*. 2001; **80**: 499–502.

* 30. Richtsmeier WJ, Huang P, Scher RL. *In situ* identification of normal visceral tissues using contact telescopic microscopy. *Laryngoscope*. 1999; **109**: 216–20.

31. Wardrop PJ, Sim S, Mclaren K. Contact endoscopy of the larynx: a quantitative study. *Journal of Laryngology and Otology*. 2000; **114**: 437–40.

32. Carriero E, Galli J, Fadda G, Di Girolamo S, Ottaviani F, Paludetti G. Preliminary experiences with contact endoscopy of the larynx. *European Archives of Oto-Rhino-Laryngology*. 2000; **257**: 68–71.

PART 12

PAEDIATRIC OTORHINOLARYNGOLOGY

EDITED BY RAY CLARKE

62 Introduction
   Ray Clarke
   771

63 The paediatric consultation
   Ray Clarke and Ken Pearman
   776

64 ENT input for children with special needs
   Francis Lannigan
   783

65 Head and neck embryology
   T Clive Lee
   792

66 Molecular otology, development of the auditory system and recent advances in genetic manipulation
   Henry Pau
   811

67 Hearing loss in preschool children: screening and surveillance
   Kai Uus and John Bamford
   821

68 Hearing tests in children
   Glynnis Parker
   834

69 Investigation and management of the deaf child
   Sujata De, Sue Archbold and Ray Clarke
   844

70 Paediatric cochlear implantation
   Joseph G Toner
   860

71 Congenital middle ear abnormalities in children
   Jonathan P Harcourt
   869

72 Otitis media with effusion
   George Browning
   877

73 Acute otitis media in children
   Peter Rea and John Graham
   912

74 Chronic otitis media in childhood
   John Hamilton
   928

75 Management of congenital deformities of the external and middle ear
   David Gault and Mike Rothera
   965

76 Disorders of speech and language in paediatric otolaryngology
   Ray Clarke and Siobhan McMahon
   990

77 Cleft lip and palate
   Chris Penfold
   996

78 Craniofacial anomalies: genetics and management
   Dean Kissun, David Richardson, Elizabeth Sweeney and Paul May
   1019

79 Vertigo in children   1040
Gavin AJ Morrison

80 Facial paralysis in childhood   1052
SS Musheer Hussain

81 Epistaxis in children   1063
Ray Clarke

82 Nasal obstruction in children   1070
Michelle Wyatt

83 Paediatric rhinosinusitis   1079
Glenis Scadding and Helen Caulfield

84 The adenoid and adenoidectomy   1094
Peter J Robb

85 Obstructive sleep apnoea in childhood   1102
Helen M Caulfield

86 Stridor   1114
David Albert

87 Acute laryngeal infections   1127
Susanna Leighton†

88 Congenital disorders of the larynx, trachea and bronchi   1135
Martin Bailey

89 Laryngeal stenosis   1150
Michael J Rutter and Robin T Cotton

90 Paediatric voice disorders   1167
Ben Hartley

91 Juvenile-onset recurrent respiratory papillomatosis   1174
Michael Kuo and William J Primrose

92 Foreign bodies in the ear and the aerodigestive tract in children   1184
A Simon Carney, Nimesh Patel and Ray Clarke

93 Tracheostomy and home care   1194
Michael Saunders

94 Cervicofacial infections in children   1210
Ben Hartley

95 Diseases of the tonsil   1219
William S McKerrow

96 Tonsillectomy   1229
William S McKerrow and Ray Clarke

97 Salivary gland disorders in childhood   1242
Peter D Bull

98 Tumours of the head and neck in childhood   1251
Fiona B MacGregor

99 Branchial arch fistulae, thyroglossal duct anomalies and lymphangioma   1264
Peter D Bull

100 Gastro-oesophageal reflux and aspiration   1272
Haytham Kubba

101 Diseases of the oesophagus, swallowing disorders and caustic ingestion   1282
Lewis Spitz

102 Imaging in paediatric ENT   1295
Neville Wright

103 Medical negligence in paediatric otolaryngology   1305
Maurice Hawthorne

62

Introduction

RAY CLARKE

Introduction	771	Training the otolaryngologists of the future	775
History	771	Key points	775
Societies	773	Deficiencies in current knowledge and areas for future	
The scope of paediatric practice	773	research	775
Paediatric otolaryngologists	774	Acknowledgements	775
Developing ENT services for children	774	References	775
The general/specialist otolaryngologist	774		

SEARCH STRATEGY

The author has a personal bibliography, which formed the basis for this chapter. The opinions expressed are his own.

INTRODUCTION

Caring for children has been an integral part of otolaryngological practice since the specialty began. Textbooks of paediatric otolaryngology have a shorter history. Although Douglas Guthrie published a small booklet *Diseases of the ear, nose and throat in childhood* in 1921,[1] Wilson's 1955 *Diseases of the ear, nose and throat in children* was the first substantial English-language text devoted to paediatric otorhinolaryngological disorders.[2] This important little book provides early descriptions of aminoglycoside-induced deafness, the technique of tracheobronchoscopy in children and obstructive sleep apnoea, then known as 'aprosexia'. It is a measure of the maturity of paediatric otolaryngology as a discrete subspecialty, and a recognition that the pathophysiology, management and expectations from treatment of diseases in children are often very different from what obtains in adults[2] that this is now the third edition of *Scott-Brown's Otorhinolaryngology, Head and neck surgery* which includes a separate section covering paediatric aspects of our specialty.

HISTORY

Mastoid surgery for the treatment of otological sepsis was popularized by Sir William Wilde (1815–1878) who described what we now know as otitis media with effusion – 'strumous otitis'.[3] Wilde recognized the association between 'strumous otitis' and Eustachian tubal dysfunction, described tympanocentesis as a treatment and popularized the use of a myringotomy knife which is not dissimilar to that used today.[4]

The Victorian and Edwardian laryngologists, notably Morrel McKenzie and Sir Felix Semon in London, had large paediatric practices and dealt with often-fatal upper respiratory tract pathologies, such as diphtheria. McKenzie provides us with the first description of laryngeal papillomatosis. He noted the post-mortem findings in a child who died of airway obstruction in what he poignantly described as a 'home for the friendless'.[5]

In Europe, Gustav Killian pioneered suspension laryngoscopy and tracheobronchoscopy in Freiburg, Bresgau at the beginning of the twentieth century. The principles were soon extended to children. Chevalier

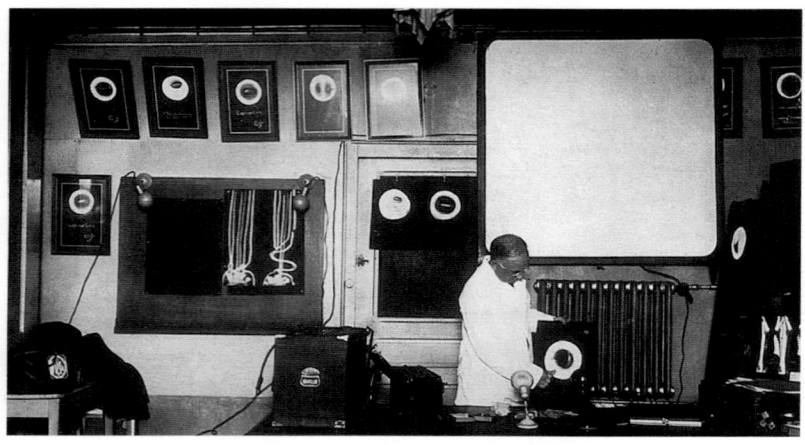

Figure 62.1 *Chevalier Jackson teaching in Paris. Reproduced by kind permission of the John Q Adams Center for the History of Otolaryngology—Head and Neck Surgery, American Academy of Otolaryngology—Head and Neck Surgery Foundation, © 2007. All rights reserved.*

Jackson (**Figure 62.1**) in Philadelphia established a reputation throughout the United States for the skill with which he could extract bronchial foreign bodies. A brilliant teacher, he illustrated his work in his own hand and was probably the single most important figure to popularize airway endoscopy in children on both sides of the Atlantic. The pioneering work of British physicist Harold Hopkins in the design of modern 'rod-lens' telescopes (**Figure 62.2**) moved paediatric airway surgery to new levels.

Modern-day paediatric otolaryngologists are acutely aware of the debt they owe to paediatricians and anaesthesiologists. Sophisticated diagnostic and therapeutic procedures in children are only possible because of the huge advances made in improving the survival and care of small babies.

It is difficult for those of us trained in recent times to appreciate just how harrowing airway disorders in children could become before the equipment and skills which we now take for granted were developed. Joseph O'Dwyer (New York) is credited with the first successful emergency endotracheal intubation in a child. In 1886 he presented 50 cases with a 70 percent mortality. The technique remained controversial but was enthusiastically taken up by a Chicago physician, Dr Frank Waxham, who used it to provide an alternative airway for children with diphtheria.[6] Long-term nasal endotracheal intubation as an alternative to tracheotomy was popularized only from the 1960s onwards. In 1955, Wilson wrote of emergency tracheotomy in children, 'these are desperate cases at best, and it may be a comfort to remember that the worst thing which can happen is that the patient will die. This is unfortunately a likely event in any case.'[2]

The late Sylvan Stool, a pioneer American paediatric otolaryngologist and historian recounts his earliest experiences with the removal of bronchial foreign bodies: 'The telescopes and cameras of today make endoscopy easy. Anybody can remove a foreign body and look like a technical master. You should have been around when we were changing that little bulb on the end of the Jackson bronchoscope three or four times during a case.'[6]

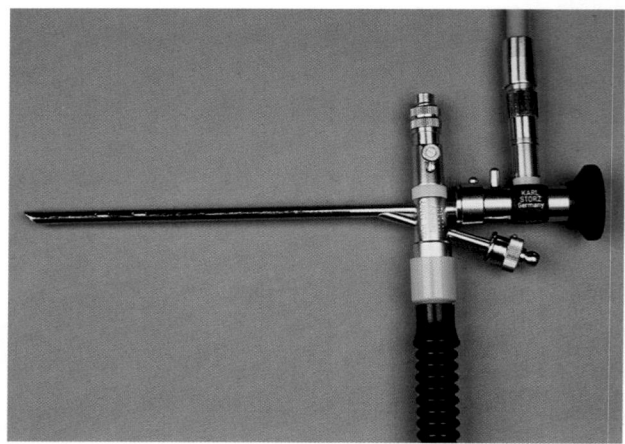

Figure 62.2 *A modern ventilating bronchoscope incorporating a 'Hopkins rod' telescope.*

Airway endoscopy in children is now a highly skilled – and safe – undertaking. This is due to parallel advances in equipment and the training of personnel – otolaryngologists, anaesthesiologists and support staff. The equipment required for this work is now considerable (see Chapter 86, Stridor).

The first paediatric ENT ward was opened in Poland in 1895. This was at the Children's Hospital in Warsaw under the supervision of Dr Jan Gabriel Danielewicz. An independent children's ENT department was established in Budapest immediately after the Second World War. In Italy, Dr Carlo Mancini headed a department in Brezia in 1950. Children's ENT services were quickly established in Czechoslovakia, Slovakia, and Bucharest. In Britain ENT departments were founded in the early part of the twentieth century in the children's hospitals at Great Ormond Street London, Alder Hey Liverpool and in Bristol.

Advances in diagnosis and rehabilitation have greatly improved outcomes and expectations for the deaf child. Although audiological medicine has developed as a separate specialty, and a multiplicity of professionals

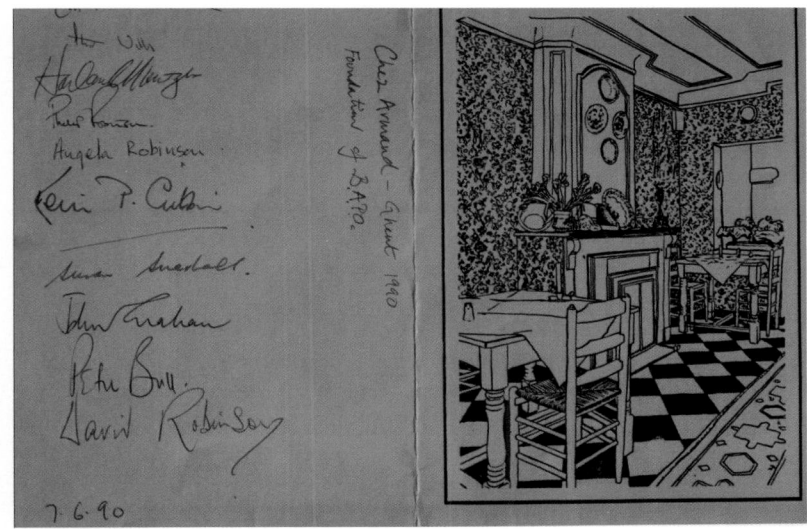

Figure 62.3 Surviving document from the founding of the British Association for Paediatric Otolaryngology (BAPO). Reproduced with kind permission of Mr John Graham FRCS, London, UK.

work in tandem to care for children with hearing loss, this remains a core part of the workload of otolaryngologists who look after children. Hence, much of the foregoing section is devoted to this topic.

SOCIETIES

As new specialties emerge, the societies and associations which promote their aims and allow colleagues to share views, advances and collective wisdom develop. Loose gatherings of otolaryngologists with an interest in children were formed in Eastern Europe from the beginning of the twentieth century. In the United States the Society for Ear Nose and Throat Advances in Children (SENTAC) met in 1977. The American Society for Pediatric Otolaryngology (ASPO) (www.aspo.us) was founded in 1985. The European Working Group in Pediatric ENT was founded in 1977 and later became the European Society for Pediatric Otolaryngology (ESPO) – a forum for discussion and advances in paediatric ORL through international meetings and via its journal the *International Journal of Pediatric Otolaryngology*.

In Britain it was not until 1991 that the British Association for Paediatric Otolaryngology (BAPO) (www.bapo.org/uk) was formed. The idea for a British society came about at a meeting of colleagues attending the international congress at Ghent in 1990. Surviving mementos include a signed menu (**Figures 62.3** and **62.4**) from the Chez Armand restaurant (John Graham FRCS, personal communication).

THE SCOPE OF PAEDIATRIC PRACTICE

Almost all otolaryngologists look after children. For most this represents a vital and rewarding part of their clinical workload. The spectrum of diseases ranges from common problems such as adenotonsillar hypertrophy,

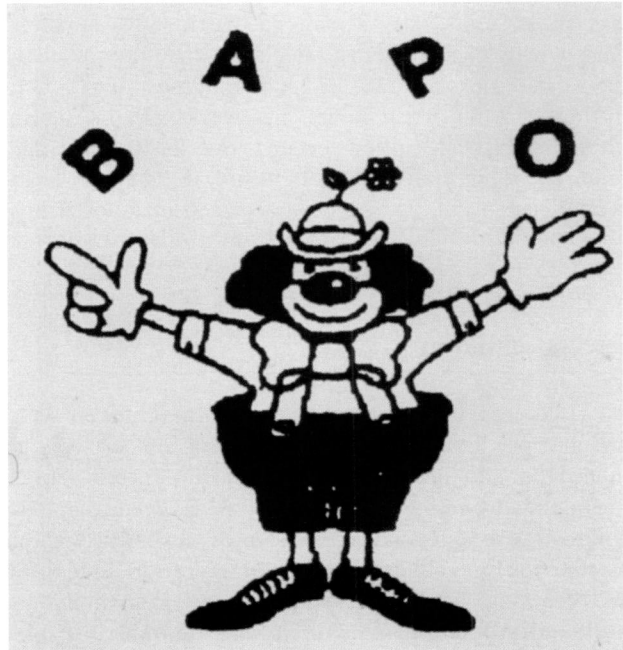

Figure 62.4 The BAPO logo.

rhinosinusitis and otitis media to more esoteric and challenging presentations such as subglottic stenosis, tumours of the salivary glands and congenital deformities of the ear. A general otolaryngologist or an otolaryngologist with a broad-based practice but an interest in children can satisfactorily look after most children. Those with complex or rare conditions, the very young and those with multiple medical pathologies requiring the attention of paediatricians, neonatologists and intensivists are best managed in a designated children's centre in close liaison with other professionals. Hence the skills of 'paediatric otolaryngologists' are increasingly required at these centres.

PAEDIATRIC OTOLARYNGOLOGISTS

Paediatric otolaryngologists look after 'special problems, in special children in a special institution'.[7] Needless to say, they will have had training that reflects this remit.

Special problems

The 'special problems' that paediatric otolaryngologists look after include congenital and acquired airway disease and the otorhinolaryngology (ORL) pathologies which occur in children who require management on a special care baby unit (SCBU) or in the paediatric intensive care unit (PICU). Much of this work is diagnostic and supportive. It lacks the glamour and appeal of laryngotracheal reconstructions, cricotracheal resections, etc., which are procedures now rarely done outside of highly specialized units. Day-to-day paediatric ORL involves liaison with paediatricians, paediatric anaesthesiologists, intensivists, nursing and allied staff and, most of all, often distraught parents and carers. The work is by its nature unpredictable and often occurs 'out of hours'. The required skills are not just technical but relate to the judgement and experience needed to make decisions on small and often very ill babies and to contribute to a multidisciplinary team.

Special children

All children are special but some of the children with whom a paediatric otolaryngologist deals are very special indeed because of their complex medical needs. These include syndromic children, children with genetic diseases, children with often severe locomotor and neurological dysfunction, and children with communication difficulties and learning disabilities, which range from mild to profound. All have parents/carers who are intimately and uniquely involved in the child's health care decisions and who simply cannot be appropriately looked after in a general ENT clinic setting. These children get the range of ORL problems with which we are all familiar, for example adenotonsillar disease, rhinitis, otitis media, often against a background of severe multisystem disease. They need a completely different management approach to that needed for otherwise healthy children. They are best looked after by clinicians with skills that can only be developed by working with such children and parents and who have an appreciation of the natural history of diseases in such settings. If they require surgery it is often wholly inappropriate that this should take place outside of a specialist children's centre where facilities for anaesthesia, recovery and postoperative intensive care are available as required. Special needs children also develop unique problems such as sialorrhoea, obstructive sleep apnoea

and aspiration which are best managed by experienced personnel in a designated setting.

Special hospitals

Children's hospitals or 'centres' are 'special' places not because of their geographic location but because of the availability of skilled personnel in a unique multidisciplinary setting. Support services such as anaesthesia, speech and language therapy, paediatric imaging, children's specialist nurses, feeding clinics, regional facilities such as craniofacial surgery and neonatal surgery are simply not found outside these centres. 'Centres' include not only the specialist children's hospitals but also paediatric facilities in the few large teaching hospitals where supraregional services for children are concentrated. Perhaps the defining features of such a centre are the availability of a dedicated paediatric surgical team and the presence of a designated PICU. A paediatric otolaryngologist will have the major proportion of his/her clinical commitments at such a centre.

DEVELOPING ENT SERVICES FOR CHILDREN

It is essential that otolaryngologists are to the fore in local discussions on service planning that have an impact on children – and that is most discussions in the sphere of health care. Up to 30–50 percent of our workload involves the care of children.[8] Otolaryngologists have, and must maintain, an important role as strong advocates for children.[9, 10]

Otherwise healthy children with common pathologies where anaesthetic risks are minimal are best looked after near their homes in settings that are convenient for parents and carers. Provided support services are adequate there is no merit in relocating all this work to already overstretched children's centres.

Children with airway obstruction who can be cared for locally – for example those with acute infections, croup, the older child with sleep apnoea – are appropriately managed by a designated otolaryngologist with a special paediatric interest.

Increasingly, one or more members of a team of otolaryngologists will assume a lead role in looking after such children and may also lead the development and management of audiology services for children, given the shortage of audiology professionals.

THE GENERAL/SPECIALIST OTOLARYNGOLOGIST

What of the general ENT surgeon or the otolaryngologist with a special interest in, say head and neck disease, skull base surgery or rhinology? Can he/she continue to include children in his/her clinical practice? Emphatically yes. It is essential that the skills of these surgeons are made available as needed for often rare and complex problems in children. Special local arrangements may also be needed for cochlear implantation where otologists with a largely adult practice may be best placed to establish a service with a mixed adult and children base. Rhinologists with an adult base may be best to deal on an ad hoc basis with some of the complex nasal problems that occur in children.

Head and neck problems in children are very different to the range of disease seen in adults. There is much to be said for developing the expertise of a very small number of otolaryngologists who take a particular interest in these challenging cases rather than regarding them as within the ambit of all adult head and neck oncologists.

TRAINING THE OTOLARYNGOLOGISTS OF THE FUTURE

The fortunes of paediatric otolaryngology are very much in the ascendancy. The specialty is particularly popular with trainees, assuring us a bright future. Training programmes in ORL must include sufficient exposure to the diagnosis and management of ENT disease in children to enable otolaryngologists to continue with a broad-based practice that includes the management of children. The specialist paediatric otolaryngologists of the future will need more advanced training. Fellowship programmes are well established in the United States and represent a model that could usefully be adopted elsewhere. Otolaryngologists – paediatric or not – need to act as feisty advocates for children. It is easy for paediatric aspects of services to be marginalized and for children to be disadvantaged, particularly when ENT services or training programmes are reconfigured. Continued vigilance is essential.

KEY POINTS

- Paediatric otolaryngology is as old as the specialty of otolaryngology itself.
- Looking after children is an integral part of the work of an ENT specialist.
- The pathophysiology and natural history of disease may be very different in children.
- Some children will require the specialist knowledge and skill of a paediatric otolaryngologist.
- Training in the generic skills required to care for children is essential to ORL practice.

Deficiencies in current knowledge and areas for future research

➤ There is an increasing trend to centralize children's surgery. Otolaryngologists must ensure they are to the fore in local service planning.
➤ There is a need for careful workforce planning and the establishment of fellowship training programmes to maintain the advances we have made.

ACKNOWLEDGEMENTS

I am grateful to Professor George Browning, Editor, *Clinical Otolaryngology and Allied Sciences* and to Blackwell Publications for permission to use material previously published as an editorial in the journal *Clinical Otolaryngology and Allied Sciences* April 2005.

REFERENCES

1. Guthrie D. *Diseases of the ear nose and throat in childhood.* London: AC Black, 1921.
* 2. Wilson TG. *Diseases of the ear nose and throat in children.* London: William Heinemann, 1955.
3. Wilde WR. *Practical observations on aural surgery and the nature and treatment of diseases of the ear.* London: John Churchill, 1853.
4. Clarke RW. Irish literary otolaryngologists. In: Pirsig W, Willemot J, Weir N (eds). *Ear, nose and throat mirrored in medicine and arts.* Ostend: Wayenborgh Publishing, 2005: 221–36.
5. Mackenzie M. *Diseases of the pharynx, larynx and trachea. A manual of the diseases of the throat and nose.* New York: William Wood and Company, 1880.
* 6. Allen GC, Stool SE. History of paediatric airway management. *Otolaryngologic Clinics of North America.* 2000; **33**: 1–14. *A readable and entertaining account of the developments which have made paediatric airway endoscopy the sophisticated procedure it is today.*
7. Bluestone CD. Paediatric otolaryngology: past, present, and future. *Archives of Otolaryngology – Head and Neck Surgery.* 1995; **121**: 505–8.
8. Osman EZ, Aneeshkumar MK, Clarke RW. Paediatric otolaryngology services in the UK: a postal questionnaire survey of ENT consultants. *Journal of Laryngology and Otology.* 2005; **119**: 259–63.
9. Clarke RW, Osman E. British paediatric otolaryngology – coming of age. *Clinical Otolaryngology and Allied Sciences.* 2005; **30**: 94–7.
10. Bluestone CD. Humans are born too soon: impact on pediatric otolaryngology. *International Journal of Pediatric Otorhinolaryngology.* 2005; **69**: 1–8.

63

The paediatric consultation

RAY CLARKE AND KEN PEARMAN

Introduction	776	Key points	781
Requirements for the clinic	777	Best clinical practice	781
Preparation for the consultation	777	Deficiencies in current knowledge and areas for future	
The consultation	777	research	781
Consent in children	780	References	782

SEARCH STRATEGY

This chapter was complied largely from the authors' personal experience as clinicians and teachers, supplemented by their personal bibliographies. The websites of the Departments of Health (www.doh.gov.uk) and Education and Skills (www.dfes.gov.uk) were consulted for the sections on consent, for information on the National Service Framework for Children and for 'Every Child Matters'.

INTRODUCTION

Major recent developments in UK government policies that relate to children have been informed by the findings of the Kennedy[1] and Laming[2] inquiries. Their recommendations, together with those of subsequent government publications (the *National service framework for children* and *Every child matters*) provide a comprehensive blueprint for best practice in children's services and are universally applicable. While many of their recommendations have been routinely practised for a long time, they are a useful reference source and what follows is in keeping with their spirit.[3, 4]

Children and parents often remember vividly their first encounter with a 'specialist'. For many, it will be the child's first contact with doctors/clinics and hospitals. It is worthwhile investing time and effort into making the experience as pleasant and productive as possible. The principles that make for a satisfactory and productive visit to the otorhinolaryngology (ORL) clinic apply to both adults and children, but some features of the paediatric consultation are unique.

The decision to seek advice will have been made not by the patient but by the child's parent(s) or carer. With infants and young children the history and a discussion concerning diagnosis and management is by proxy, i.e. involving the parent/carer (usually the mother) rather than the child. Often the mother will be anxious, perplexed and 'worried if she is doing the right thing'. While the primary purpose of the visit is for the doctor to make a diagnosis and advise on an investigative/treatment plan, a good consultation is far more than that. It represents an opportunity to establish a rapport with the parent and child that in some cases may last for much of the patient's childhood. It is the forum for explaining, in simple and understandable terms, what the doctor's opinion is on the child's condition and for discussion of treatment options. It provides the chance to familiarize the mother and child with the hospital/clinic, to introduce them to other members of staff who may be involved in the child's care and to reassure them that the child will be well looked after should they need to come into hospital.

Most hospitals demand that a trained children's nurse be available for all paediatric consultations. Specialist nurses who work in paediatric ORL are invaluable. Staff numbers need to be sufficient not only to support the working of the clinic, but also to ensure the safe supervision of patients and their siblings while parents are preoccupied. Thus paediatric clinics need more nurse input than general ENT clinics.

REQUIREMENTS FOR THE CLINIC

The waiting area

A paradox of planning hospitals and clinics for children is that despite children's small size their requirements for space are much greater than those of adults. In an ideal world, children would only be seen in dedicated clinics designed with their unique requirements in mind but this is not always possible. Whatever the setting, seating has to be comfortable and suitable for all ages. Wheelchair access is essential as are facilities for breastfeeding and for changing of babies' clothes. Children become bored and fractious if they wait too long. As well as organizing clinic appointments to minimize waiting, a well-equipped waiting area with toys, paper, coloured pencils and computer games will help to keep children occupied and reduce parental stress. Play therapists greatly enhance the quality of a child's hospital visit. Some progressive hospitals employ clowns and entertainers. Adolescents may feel uncomfortable surrounded by hordes of small children and need to have their particular needs catered for as well. Some hospitals have separate clinics for adolescents scheduled for after school times and they usually appreciate a separate ward or section of a ward if they require inpatient care.

'Special' clinics

There is much to be said for running separate clinics for some categories of patients. These may include 'special needs' clinics and clinics where multidisciplinary input is required, for example audiology, cleft palate, etc. Thought needs to be given to the organization of time and space in such clinics because a balance needs to be struck between making the most efficient use of time by all concerned and the need not to overtire or overwhelm the child by seeing too many adults in one room at one time.

The clinic rooms

An examining room should be able to accommodate not just the patient, doctor and nurse but two parents, one or more siblings, sometimes in 'Moses baskets' or push-chairs, and often a grandparent. In the case of special needs children, there may be a need to accommodate a wheelchair, oxygen cylinders and the various bits and pieces the mother needs for tracheotomy care and gastrostomy management. Ideally, the examining room should have a small play area as well where the child and siblings can occupy themselves while the mother gives the history and the doctor can quietly observe the child. Instruments other than those in frequent use should be discreetly put away. Small children will be frightened at the sight of an array of picks and hooks. Facilities for hand washing are essential. An operating microscope is essential, either in the room or nearby. Endoscopy – both flexible and rigid – is now so frequently performed in an outpatient setting in children that it can be regarded as a mandatory requirement in a paediatric clinic. A suitable range of scopes with facilities for safe storage and ideally a monitor and image capture system should be available, not just for specialized airway or voice clinics but as a routine requirement for any paediatric consultation. The physical environment must be safe for the child, with no spirit lamps, sharp instruments or corners.

PREPARATION FOR THE CONSULTATION

A hospital visit is a routine event in the life of the doctor, but a major event for the mother and child. Arrangements may have been made for sibling childcare, the mother will have had to discuss the visit with the child's teacher and often one or both parents will have taken a day off work. Parents or children must never feel rushed. If you need to hurry them along, the clinic has not been properly planned. It makes for a smoother consultation if the doctor has taken the trouble to read the case notes and learn the child's name before the consultation starts. If the child has a syndrome or an unusual medical condition read up about it in advance. Make sure you have checked any investigations the child may have had, including hearing tests. As far as possible, children and parents appreciate continuity and like to be able to see the same doctor on successive visits. It is not the authors' place to advise on dress code, suffice to say that your best tailored suit and crisp, cotton dress shirt will neither impress the average eight year old or continue to look crisp at the end of a busy morning!

THE CONSULTATION

Welcome the child and carer(s), make eye contact and start by introducing yourself. Introductions should include others in the room and include permission for medical/nursing students to be present and for them to examine the child. Multidisciplinary clinics can be particularly intimidating as by their very nature several specialists are present. It is good practice for all to wear a name badge and many hospitals will demand this. This does not excuse the need to introduce yourself and other members of the team. Learn and use the child's name.

Establish who is with the child and if not the parents note names, for example of foster carers or grandparents. A well-conducted consultation where the mother/carer feels she has been listened to and had the child's symptoms properly and simply explained is an important part of the management of many childhood ailments. Many doctors regard themselves as excellent communicators because of their capacity to talk well. Fewer listen well! Listen, watch the child, look at the mother's facial expressions, pick up as many nuances as you can to help you in your decision making and to improve your rapport with mother and child. Resist the temptation to conduct the entire consultation without involving the child directly in the discussion. Listen and respond to both the child and the family and encourage the child to give her own views. Good consultation skills can be taught, learned and improved upon. Parents may be angry, upset, uncooperative, seeming not to listen, evasive or challenging in a variety of other ways, but it goes without saying that as the child's doctor you must never become short-tempered no matter how difficult the exchange or how great you feel the provocation is.

If interpreters are needed, it is best to make arrangements in advance. Pay attention to the seating plan, especially with signing interpreters. Professional interpreters are preferable to relatives and friends, and using elder siblings to interpret is undesirable. Speak slowly and clearly to the patient's mother at normal volume and use plain English without jargon or colloquial terms.[5]

The history

Doctors are taught to take a history in a structured didactic way. This is not always suited to paediatric work. It is best to start with an open question, such as 'what are your worries about Jennifer?' and let the mother explain in her own words, without interruption until she feels she has got her message across. More direct questions can then be put. Always ask about the impact of symptoms on the child herself and on family life. If parents volunteer to show you the child's 'health book' or growth charts, make sure you look at these even if you feel they are not directly relevant. Parents understandably feel any record of their child's health and progress must be important.

The examination

Most children are happy to be examined (**Figure 63.1**). An astute clinician will have commenced the process as soon as the child enters the room. Stridor, mouth breathing, syndromic features and the child's general alertness may give clues. Smaller children are best examined sitting on the mother's knee. Tell the child in an age-appropriate way what you are going to do at all stages of the examination – do not assume they have been listening and expect it. Children do not need to be

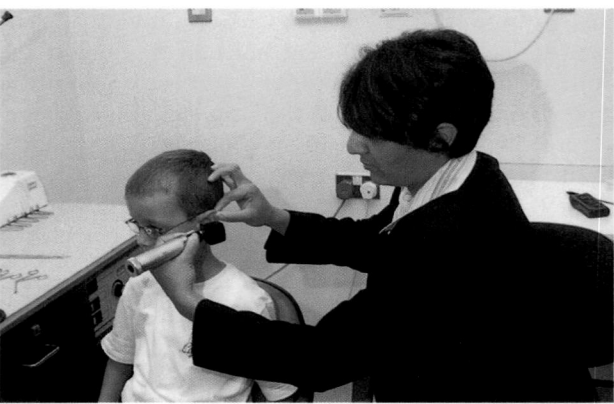

Figure 63.1 Examining a young child.

restrained for clinical examination and if the child is not cooperative it is best not to press or coerce them. When potentially uncomfortable procedures such as the removal of wax or foreign bodies are to be performed, it is important to be truthful and not to tell the child it will not hurt if it may do. If you do hurt the child explain and, where appropriate, apologise.

Otoscopy

Most children will tolerate the gentle introduction of an electric auriscope. Some units use video-otoscopy which has the advantage of enabling the mother and child to see an image of the eardrum on a monitor and also permits pictorial record keeping.

The nose

Children do not like the Thudicum's speculum. A good view of the nasal cavities can be obtained by elevating the tip of the nose or by using an otoscope with a large speculum (**Figures 63.2** and **63.3**). Rigid endoscopy may be tolerated by the very young, where a fine-calibre telescope will be needed, and in older children who will cooperate if the procedure is explained to them. Local anaesthetic sprays often make matters worse and if a child finds the procedure uncomfortable it is best to just abandon it.

The nasal airway can be assessed by gently occluding one nostril at a time and asking the child to breathe gently. The spatula test in which a cold tongue depressor is placed under the nostrils and the condensation pattern inspected to determine whether there is occlusion of the nasal airway is especially helpful in very young children (**Figure 63.4**).

The pharynx and larynx

Try to obtain a view without using a tongue depressor. Many young children will tolerate mirror examination of

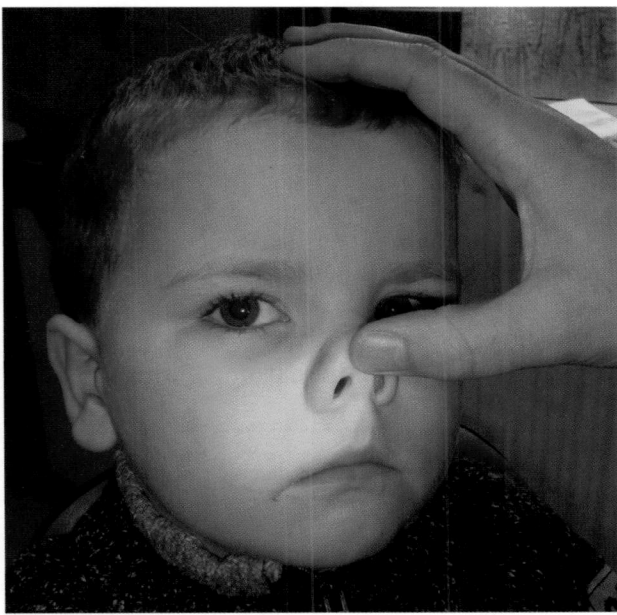

Figure 63.2 Anterior rhinoscopy.

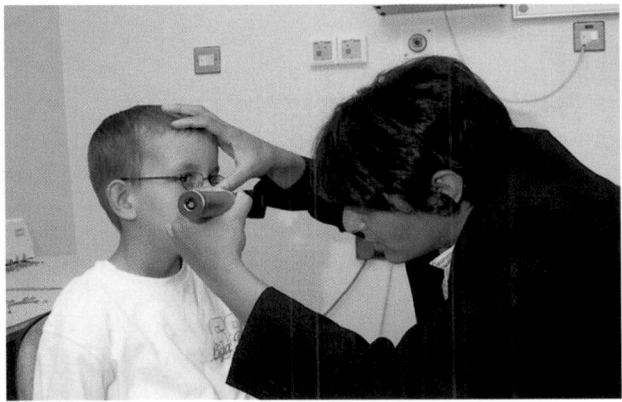

Figure 63.3 Using an aural speculum for nasal examination.

the post-nasal space, but flexible endoscopy is increasingly used and often well tolerated. The adenoids, hypopharynx and larynx can be seen in this way. The function of the velopharyngeal sphincter can also be assessed and recorded.

Some children will tolerate mirror examination but often the view is unsatisfactory and, if the child will permit examination via the mouth a 70° rod lens telescope is very useful as its slim shaft fits easily between large tonsils.

The neck

It is important to inspect and palpate the neck, but remember that enlarged lymph nodes in children are so common as to be normal. Other swellings in the neck include cystic hygroma, thryoglossal cysts and salivary gland swellings. These are dealt with in Chapter 99,

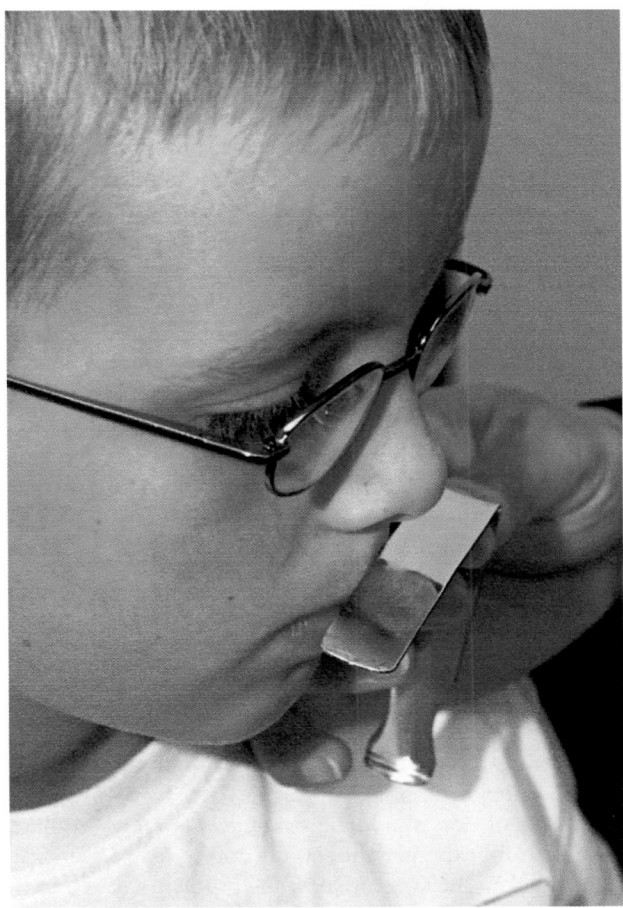

Figure 63.4 The spatula test.

Branchial arch fistulae, thyroglossal duct anomalies and lymphangioma and Chapter 97, Salivary gland disorders in childhood.

Investigations

Other than audiometry and tympanometry, few investigations are needed for the common presentations at a children's ENT clinic. Hearing tests are considered in Chapter 68, Hearing tests in children.

Management plan

The parents have come to see you to hear your opinion on their child's condition and to discuss a management plan with you. This part of the consultation is vital and must never be rushed. Explanations should be straightforward and easy to understand, involving the child where appropriate. Models, diagrams, printed and audiovisual material can aid this process greatly. For many interventions, such as tonsillectomy, adenoidectomy and insertion of tympanostomy tubes, there will be more than one management option and it is important that these are discussed in an open and honest way. This sometimes means doctors have to admit doubts and uncertainties which are best explained without embarrassment so that a way forward can be agreed by consensus. The treatment will be a matter for negotiation between the otolaryngologist and the mother and/or child and questions should be encouraged. Some parents see the ORL consultation as a means to confirm a treatment option they have already decided on with their family doctor, for example tonsillectomy for recurrent sore throats. Others are reluctant to consider any surgery, but all will greatly appreciate an informed discussion and an honest presentation of the evidence for current practice focused on the specific needs of their child. In general, parents appreciate a discussion with the senior clinician, but this needs to be balanced with the need for residents and juniors to see patients and improve their diagnostic and consultation skills.

Functional problems

Problems for which no organic cause can be found are encountered in paediatric ENT practice, particularly in adolescents. They often take the form of unexplained coughs, pains or abnormal hearing tests. It is important to investigate for underlying organic pathology. Where none is found, the patient should not be led to feel that the clinician believes that the problem is entirely imaginary because this breaks down confidence. An approach in which the problem is treated as a disorder of body function rather than mental function is more likely to be helpful.

Breaking bad news

If bad news has to be given, such as a diagnosis of deafness, the need for long-term tracheotomy or suspicion of malignancy, the help of a senior clinician should be sought immediately. Parents and children remember such episodes with chilling clarity – often for a lifetime. Great harm can be done by insensitive or even well-meaning but inexperienced handling of such situations. Many hospitals have policies on the breaking of bad news. In the clinical situation, it is not always possible to follow these blueprints to the letter, but every consideration should be shown to the family. The setting in which the news is to be broken should be considered beforehand and appropriate supporting staff briefed. The consultation must not be rushed. Parents will often be shell-shocked by unexpected bad news and may not remember detailed information. Further discussion should be offered if needed and it is helpful to make a clear management plan beforehand, so that there is no uncertainty about the next steps to be taken or the timing of the next appointment.[6]

Prescribing for children

In general, otolaryngologists do not prescribe a large range of drugs in the outpatient setting. Where drugs are prescribed, it is essential to be aware of the correct dosage and presentation for children and that the child's mother understands how to give the medication. Evidence-based prescribing is not always possible for children, and where unlicensed and off-label medicines are used, local safety standards should be adhered to.

Recording and communication of the outcome of the consultation

Hand-written notes should be legible, signed, dated and clearly identify the writer. Subject to the need for confidentiality, there is often a need to inform more people of the outcome of the consultation in paediatric work than there is with adults (e.g. educators, community paediatricians, geneticists, etc.). Parents should be made aware of this and correspondence should be copied to all appropriate parties including the parents/carers themselves.

Child protection issues

All professionals involved in paediatric work need to be aware of the potential for children to be subject to abuse or neglect. Of those children subject to physical abuse some 75 percent suffer injuries to the head and neck.[7, 8] Examples of presentations that may arouse suspicion include auricular haematomas, traumatic perforations of the eardrum, nasal injuries, pharyngeal lacerations, dental trauma and tears of the lingual frenulum. Children are naturally active and some of these injuries occur in the rough and tumble of normal childhood but if there is a pattern of injury or if the presentation seems inappropriate clinicians have not only an ethical but a legal duty to raise concern. Needless to say, such concerns must be handled with great sensitivity, but prompt action should be taken and comprehensive notes, detailing the injuries and the reasons for suspicion, should be made. All hospitals which look after children should have an agreed mechanism for dealing with such concerns, usually involving the help of a senior and experienced paediatrician.[2] Clinicians who have little direct experience of child protection will need the advice and support of a more experienced colleague.

CONSENT IN CHILDREN

Competence

It is axiomatic that any interventions proposed in children require consent. While the law has primacy this will vary according to the administration or health service that one is working in and it is imperative that doctors who care for children are thoroughly conversant with the law relating to consent and parental responsibility. Whatever the legal requirements it is important to respect the legitimate concerns of parents, be they mothers, fathers, single, married or divorced, to be cognisant of cultural and individual family dynamics and to proceed by consensus wherever possible. What is unique about consent in paediatric practice is that young children will not have the understanding required to give informed consent, although it is good practice at all times to involve the child as much as possible in decision making.

The following is based on English law and on custom and practice in the UK.

Once children have reached the age of 16 years they are deemed to be competent and can therefore give consent themselves. Nevertheless, it is wise to encourage teenagers to involve their families in decision making. 'Competence' implies the capacity to comprehend and retain information material to a decision, and the ability to weigh this information in decision making. Some 16- and 17-year-olds may not be competent by reason of unconsciousness, pain or severe learning disability. In such cases, a person with parental responsibility may take a decision for the child, but over the age of 18 nobody can give consent for another person, and if such a person is not competent clinicians may have to take decisions without consent that are in the best interests of the individual.

Some children under the age of 16 will be able to understand what an intervention involves. The courts have determined that such children are competent if they have 'sufficient understanding and intelligence to enable him or her to understand fully what is proposed'.[9] This is colloquially known as 'Gillick competence'. The determination as to whether the child has Gillick competence rests with the clinician.[10]

Parental responsibility

If a child is not competent, only a person exercising parental responsibility can give valid consent for that child. This is usually one or both of the child's parents. In England and Wales 'parental responsibility' is as defined by the Children's Act 1989 and amended by the Adoption and Children Act 2002. The child's natural mother has parental responsibility as has the father if he is married to the mother or was married to the mother at the time of the child's birth. Unmarried fathers may acquire parental responsibility by order of a court or by a 'parental responsibility agreement'. For births registered after December 2003, a father named on the birth certificate has parental responsibility irrespective of his marital status. Grandparents and others who look after children cannot give consent unless special legal arrangements have been made. Consent is only legally required from one parent, but where applicable it is good practice to

ensure that both parents and the child are involved in the decision-making process.

Consent in children is an issue that causes great sensitivities. The reader is referred to the Department of Health guidelines (www.doh.gov.uk/consent) and trainee surgeons in particular are advised to seek the advice of senior colleagues in the event of any uncertainties.

KEY POINTS

- A clinic visit is a routine event for the doctor. It may be a major episode in the life of the parent and child.
- The organization of children's clinics require more space, more preparation and more attention to detail than is the case for adult clinics.
- Everyone can learn better consultation skills.
- Consent is a sensitive issue in children.
- Clinicians need to be familiar with the law in the jurisdiction in which they work and with best practice.

Best clinical practice

✓ Prepare for the consultation before the child comes into the examining room.
✓ Always introduce yourself to the parent and child.
✓ Explain the current knowledge base for every proposed intervention and listen to the views of the parent/child.
✓ A suitable range of flexible and rigid endoscopes, with facilities for safe storage and ideally a monitor and image capture system should be available, not just for specialized airway or voice clinics, but as a routine requirement for any paediatric consultation.
✓ It is important to know the procedures to be followed in the event of concerns about child protection, and the law on consent for the jurisdiction in which you work.

Deficiencies in current knowledge and areas for future research

➤ Parents are becoming more and more involved in decision making for their children in health care. The old patriarchal model of medical practice is fast disappearing. Doctors will need to discuss the natural history of diseases, treatment options and the uncertainties around evidence for existing practices in much greater detail than before.

REFERENCES

* 1. Kennedy I. Learning from Bristol: the report of the public inquiry into children's heart surgery at the Bristol Royal Infirmary 1984–1995. Command Paper: CM 5207, 2001. Available from: www.bristol-inquiry.org.uk. *A far-reaching set of recommendations to guide clinicians and health care managers regarding the provision of clinical services for children.*

2. Laming H. The Victoria Climbié Inquiry; Report of an Inquiry by Lord Laming. Command Paper CM5730, 2003. Available from: www.victoria-climbie-inquiry.org.uk.

3. British Red Cross, with the advice and funding from the Department of Health. *Emergency multilingual phrasebook.* Rochester, UK: British Red Cross, 2004.

4. National Service Framework for Children, Young People and Maternity Services. Available from: www.doh.gov.uk.

5. Department for Education and Skills. *Every child matters.* London: The Stationery Office, 2003. Available from: www.dfes.gov.uk/everychildmatters.

* 6. Faulkner A. *When the news is bad. A guide for health professionals.* Cheltenham: Nelson Thornes, 1998. *Excellent handbook with guidance applicable to both adults and children.*

7. Crouse CD, Faust A. Child abuse and the otolaryngologist: Part 1. *Otolaryngology Head and Neck Surgery.* 2003; **128**: 305–11.

8. Crouse CD, Faust A. Child abuse and the otolaryngologist: Part 2. *Otolaryngology Head and Neck Surgery.* 2003; **128**: 311–8.

9. *Gillick* v. *Norfolk and Wisbech AHA* [1985] 3 WLR 830, 3 All ER 402.

* 10. DOH website on consent. Available from: www.doh.gov.uk. *Required reading for all UK practitioners.*

64

ENT input for children with special needs

FRANCIS LANNIGAN

Introduction	783	Drooling	788
Clinical environment	783	Key points	789
Communication and rapport	784	Best clinical practice	789
General considerations	785	Deficiencies in current knowledge and areas for future	
The ear and hearing	785	research	790
The upper aerodigestive tract	786	References	790

SEARCH STRATEGY

The opinions in this chapter are supported by a Medline search using the key words cerebral palsy, mental retardation, handicap, special needs, Down syndrome, hearing loss, hearing aids, obstructive sleep apnoea/disorder, adenoidectomy/tonsillectomy, tracheostomy, drooling, sialorrhoea.

INTRODUCTION

Developments in neonatology and improved paediatric intensive care management are such that more infants with extreme prematurity or multiple organ pathologies now survive.[1] Similarly, modern treatments of many genetic and congenital diseases have improved outcomes. A proportion of such infants and children will have multiple medical conditions. These include neuromuscular dysfunction, sensory impairment including deafness, communication disorders and developmental delay. Epilepsy and learning disability are also more common in this group of children.[1]

The prospect of managing a child with special needs may appear daunting, and is often associated with disappointing outcomes. However, in the appropriate clinical setting and with the intent of attaining maximal objective evidence to support a proposed intervention, the disappointment will be minimized. Down syndrome (trisomy 21) raises many of the issues common to managing ENT problems in children with special needs (**Figure 64.1** and **Table 64.1**).

Terminology

The Oxford English dictionary defines a 'handicap' as a condition that markedly restricts a person's ability to function physically, mentally or socially. A 'disability' is a physical or mental condition that limits a person's movements, senses or activities. Some parents and children in the UK in particular dislike the terms handicap and disability as they feel these emphasize negative aspects of the child's needs and potential. The term 'special needs' is now more commonly accepted but much of the literature still relates to children with disabilities or multiple handicaps and these terms are widely accepted internationally.

CLINICAL ENVIRONMENT

An increasing proportion of clinical time is spent by the paediatric otolaryngologist–head and neck surgeon as part of a multidisciplinary team in the provision of treatment to children with special needs, usually in a tertiary setting.

It is neither possible nor desirable to adequately assess a child with multiple pathologies in a general paediatric ENT clinic. These children often have clinical records that extend to several volumes, which require time for meaningful review. It is, therefore, desirable to set aside a specific clinic for evaluating children with special needs. Needless to say this clinic should be conducted by the consultant or senior attending physician. Even with the best clinic administration, some children will 'slip through the net' into a general clinic. It is the author's

practice to explain such an error to the parents/carer and, if appropriate, reschedule the planned consultation. It goes without saying that wheelchair access, facilities for oxygen delivery, and seats for parents/carers and siblings are mandatory.

Clinical examination may be especially challenging; a skilled paediatric nurse is invaluable.

COMMUNICATION AND RAPPORT

The parents/carers of these children are often highly discerning and probe carefully the merits and risks of any proposed medical or surgical intervention. On occasion, more time is required to explain why an accepted surgical intervention may not be appropriate for a child than would be spent obtaining informed consent for that same procedure. The carers and children have multiple interactions with health care staff and will often develop a warm rapport with clinicians. Many will be familiar with the details and expectations of often-rare syndromes and will be affiliated with parent/carer groups that provide information and enable parents to discuss issues common to particular conditions with each other. In Britain, a joint project between parents and carers and the Royal College of Paediatrics and Child Health – 'Contact a Family' – maintains a website (www.cafamily.org.uk) which provides information and support for families of children with a variety of specific conditions.

Planned surgery

It should be remembered that the child with multiple pathologies will usually represent a greater anaesthetic and surgical risk with increased postoperative morbidity. They require the skills of a paediatric anaesthesiologist and may be unsuitable for same-day hospital care – overnight stay or even longer may be required predominantly due to delay in re-establishment of adequate oral intake and increased respiratory complications of

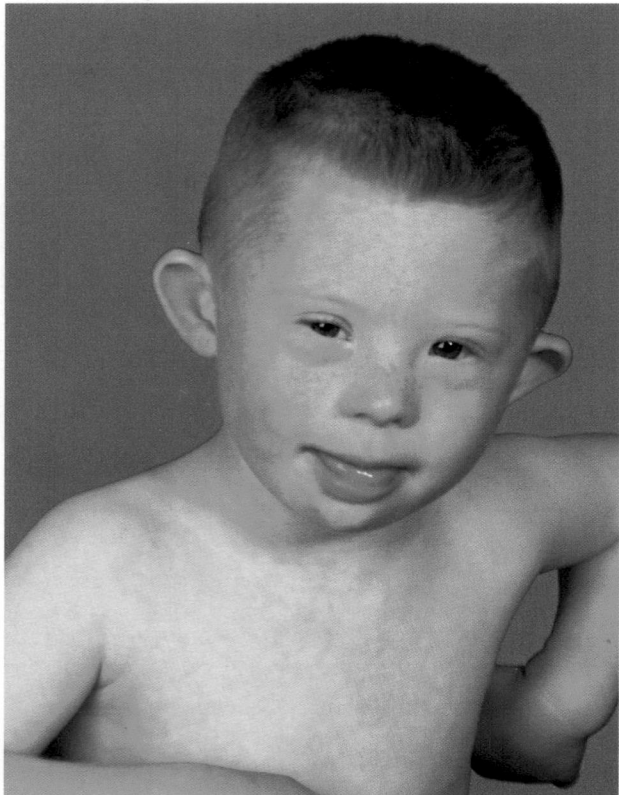

Figure 64.1 Child with Down syndrome.

Table 64.1 ENT problems in Down syndrome.

General	The airway	Ear disorders
Frequent upper respiratory tract infections (URTI)	Airway obstruction	Deafness
Thyroid disease	Narrow subglottis and trachea – may need smaller endotracheal tube during anaesthesia	Frequent acute otitis media and otitis media with effusion
Sialorrhoea		Small pinna and external meatus
Atlantoaxial instability (manipulate the head with extreme care under anaesthesia)	Midfacial hypoplasia – increased incidence of obstructive sleep apnoea syndrome (OSAS)	Premature ossification of the cochlea
		Facial nerve dehiscence common
	Hypotonic pharyngeal airway	Ossicular fixation
	Macroglossia	Mondini malformation more common

anaesthesia.[2] Some will need paediatric intensive care facilities postoperatively and this will need to be planned in advance. Often they require multiple surgical input, e.g. dental treatment, ear surgery and attention to a gastrostomy, and it may be appropriate to coordinate any planned ENT intervention with other treatments/disciplines.

What are routine investigations in the otherwise healthy child may require general anaesthesia in the child with multiple pathologies.

GENERAL CONSIDERATIONS

Common childhood ENT disorders may significantly interfere with the normal development of any child and their impact may be significant. In the child with special needs these common conditions may have a disproportionate impact on development and family life. Conversely, apparently minor clinical gains may have dramatic impacts for the child and their parents/carers, e.g. reduced nocturnal seizures following treatment of obstructive sleep disorder or improved hearing following grommet insertion.

In the child with special needs the maxim remains: maximize input in order to facilitate development to maximum potential. [**/*]

Ethical issues

It is necessary to address some difficult ethical issues when treating children with special needs. These children will naturally make greater demands on the health-care system, irrespective of the quality of care. 'There is no point in treating children like this.' 'The resources spent treating children like this would be better spent elsewhere.' These are common comments that are often heard in relation to the management of such children. It goes without saying that such opinion must never be communicated in any way to the patient or the parent/carer.

A full discussion of the ethical and health economic issues is beyond the scope of this chapter; nevertheless, some practical guidelines are required.

It is probably better if health-care professionals who hold negative opinions regarding intervention, irrespective of their role, excuse themselves from the management of these children; to do otherwise is inviting problems.

Prognosis

The available evidence related to the care of these children is predominantly in the form of retrospective case series. [**/*] Other than for some specific conditions, prognosis

is often uncertain. There are some crude indicators: the necessity for nasogastric tube feeding is a significant adverse prognostic indicator, interestingly unaffected by conversion to gastrostomy feeding. Paradoxically, the addition of a tracheostomy (despite its inherent mortality and morbidity) in the presence of nasogastric/gastrostomy feeding improves outcome, presumably due to improved access for bronchial toilet.[3] These indicators obviously only relate to the most severe end of the spectrum; however, such information may facilitate difficult decisions for parents/carers. Otherwise there is little evidence base to support interventions, other than that available for such interventions in otherwise healthy children.

The prognosis of many childhood medical conditions, for example cystic fibrosis, metabolic diseases, renal failure and congenital cardiac lesions, has been greatly improved by active intervention and the involvement of multidisciplinary teams.[1] [****/**]

It has been demonstrated in other areas that timely intervention may in the long-term reduce expenditure (cf. Chapter 70, Paediatric cochlear implantation). Whilst outcome measures are difficult to assess, there is now evidence that multidisciplinary intervention in children with Down syndrome improves intermediate/long-term hearing outcomes.[4] [**/*]

THE EAR AND HEARING

Assessment

Evaluation of the auditory pathway in the child with multiple pathologies may prove challenging, but is essential in overall management. Many referrals of these children will be from developmental paediatricians who wish to exclude significant hearing loss from a child's spectrum of disability (and also as part of a screening protocol for 'at risk' infants). Where access for audiological assessment is provided without direct assessment by a paediatric otolaryngologist–head and neck surgeon, systems must be in place to initiate appropriate clinical assessment and habilitation/rehabilitation of an identified hearing loss. Conventional age-appropriate audiological evaluation is performed with the understanding that results may not be accurate and that general anaesthesia with objective audiological evaluation is more likely to be required. Under general anaesthesia, any external or middle ear component of the problem should be minimized simultaneously to provide maximal accuracy of obtained thresholds (e.g. ear toilet, myringotomy plus/minus grommet insertion). Little controversy exists when it comes to obtaining accurate hearing thresholds, and apportioning conductive/sensorineural components to hearing loss. The same is not true when it comes to management.

Management

Concern has been raised with respect to the use of ventilation tubes in children with special needs, in particular Down syndrome. Some reports have documented a higher rate of morbidity following ventilation tubes in these children, notably otorrhoea and residual perforation.[5] Overall, however, the majority of children in these reports still benefit from intervention. [**]

The narrow external meatus and the often difficult anatomy of the ear canal associated with Down syndrome make any transcanal middle ear surgery technically difficult (if not impossible); the narrow, and often hairy, meatus also contributes to failure of clearance of skin debris and wax. The proposed alternative is to use amplification for the management of hearing loss; this may prove to be a very acceptable alternative for some children. Often children with Down syndrome develop sensorineural loss in the teenage years and if amplification is anticipated this may be an argument for considering it earlier.

Amplification is not trouble-free. The presence of a hearing aid mould in a congenitally narrow and hairy external meatus may predispose to wax impaction and recurrent otitis externa – ear toilet will often require general anaesthesia in such children. Amplification may not, therefore, have the desired effect of avoiding otorrhoea and/or intervention under general anaesthesia. A rarely mentioned issue with respect to amplification is the small, but potentially disastrous, risk of ingestion of hearing aid batteries by the wearer or a sibling; this should be communicated to parents/carers.[6] The judgement is individual to each child and will involve full discussion of the advantages and disadvantages with the parent/carer and child if he/she is old enough to participate in the decision. [*]

If amplification is the chosen modality for treatment, then regular observation is required for the early detection of the development of retraction changes/atelectasis, which should prompt reconsideration of surgical intervention.[5]

Cholesteatoma

Childhood cholesteatoma is a miserable condition for the patient, the parent/carer and all but the most enthusiastic otologist; this is even worse in the child with special needs. Not least of the expected problems encountered when cholesteatoma occurs is the unusual temporal bone anatomy associated with some syndromes, for example Down syndrome.[7] Computed tomography (CT) scanning is essential to anticipate anatomical anomalies and facilitate planning surgical management – a conventional post-aural approach is ill-advised if there is a sclerotic mastoid, with middle fossa dura at the level of the second genu of the facial nerve. Peroperative facial nerve monitoring is especially valuable in this group. [*] In view of the difficulties associated with cholesteatoma, it is the author's practice to treat retraction pockets/atelectasis aggressively in an incremental manner: from ventilation tubes and management of nasal conditions, to excision and reinforcement grafting. [*]

Otalgia

Recurrent otalgia, particularly at night, is a common feature of otitis media. This symptom may result in sleep deprivation for the child and family. It may also cause daytime behaviour problems, e.g. head-banging. Prolonged conservative management will not alleviate this situation which will often have been present for some time before otherwise asymptomatic middle ear disease is identified. Surgical intervention in the form of tympanostomy tube insertion may have dramatic benefit in such a circumstance. [**/*]

THE UPPER AERODIGESTIVE TRACT

Issues relating to feeding problems, drooling, stridor, nocturnal airway obstruction, dysphonia, aspiration and long-term airway access, may all present either as a single entity or in any combination.

Feeding problems

Most tertiary paediatric institutions have 'feeding teams'. These teams comprise paediatric gastroenterologists, paediatric neurologists, speech and swallowing therapists, dieticians and psychologists. They will manage issues related to feeding from the time of discharge from the neonatal unit through to adolescence. The paediatric otolaryngologist–head and neck surgeon will therefore usually only become involved with purely feeding issues when a surgical problem has already been identified or when feeding problems are associated with aspiration requiring tracheostomy for bronchial toilet. Great care must be taken when explaining to a parent/carer the postoperative management required when tracheostomy is performed for this reason: continued aspiration of oropharyngeal secretions is likely to occur and increase demands for tracheostomy care. Some parents/carers may, on reflection, decline the option of tracheostomy. In this instance, an upper endoscopy should be recommended in order to exclude any other structural or functional abnormality (other than neuromuscular incoordination) contributing to aspiration. If not already performed, a thorough upper endoscopy is mandatory prior to tracheostomy for the same reasons; particular care must be given to the exclusion of an occult laryngeal cleft by the use of an appropriate laryngeal probe for palpation of the posterior glottis and cricoid cartilage (**Figure 64.2**).

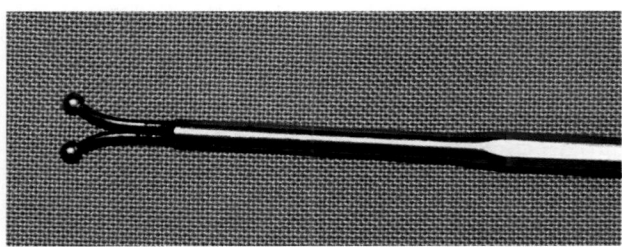

Figure 64.2 Blunt laryngeal probe and measuring device (Lowinger laryngeal probe; Xomed-Medtronic) – useful in older infants and children; not readily manipulated in smaller laryngoscopes where a fine blunt suction probe will suffice.

Often by the time tracheostomy is performed, some degree of reduced respiratory reserve is present; however, once past the anaesthetic and perioperative period, there is often apparent improvement in respiratory function due to reduced dead space and reduced airway resistance. Whilst this apparent improvement remains it may provide considerable respite for the parent/carer.[3]

Laryngotracheal disease

Dysphonia and stridor will often be wrongly attributed to neuromuscular problems intrinsic to the child's overall condition. It is important that the paediatric otolaryngologist–head and neck surgeon should not perpetuate such assumptions; thorough upper endoscopy is required as would be the case for otherwise healthy children. It must be emphasized, however, that any concomitant neuromuscular incoordination will adversely impact upon therapeutic interventions – it is always difficult to be precise about the degree of this adverse impact, and not just because of the varying degree of neuromuscular incoordination. For example, correction of a subglottic stenosis may have a disappointing outcome due to arytenoid prolapse secondary to neuromuscular incoordination; changing the dynamics of the upper airway may have a very unpredictable outcome. Nowhere is this principle better illustrated than in the management of snoring and sleep-related airway obstruction.

Obstructive sleep apnoea

The simplistic notion that snoring equates to adenotonsillar hypertrophy and that each child may be safely treated with adenotonsillectomy will result in disappointment more commonly in the child with multiple pathologies than in the general paediatric population.[8] Adenotonsillectomy alone fails to reduce the Respiratory Disturbance Index below 5 in approximately 15 percent of children undergoing surgery for a presumed obstructive sleep disorder;[9] and it is into this group that the child with multiple pathologies is more likely to fall.[8] Airway noise is

common in these children and is often a respiratory monitor for parents/carers! It is always worth directly enquiring about features of nocturnal airway obstruction, but the usual clinical features (which are notoriously unreliable in the healthy child[9]) may be even more difficult to interpret in the child with a complex medical history. Initial examination should include consideration of dysmorphic features and neuromuscular coordination in addition to the more usual clinical examination. Simple measures to eradicate any bacterial rhinitis or to institute treatment for atopy should be used as appropriate. The myriad of potential causes of sleep disruption, some of which may coexist with an element of an obstructive sleep disorder, makes clinical judgement suspect. Formal polysomnography may prove extremely helpful in the selection of children who are likely to benefit from intervention; it may also identify other causes for sleep disruption.[10] It is common practice for a parent/carer to board with their child for this investigation; the validity of the investigation may be assessed by asking the parent/carer if the night of the sleep study was a typical night for their child. If polysomnography demonstrates significant obstruction, then the next step is to determine the level of that obstruction. Once again it is important to emphasize that whilst adenotonsillar hypertrophy may be significant, and indeed adenotonsillectomy is likely to be the intervention of first choice, other causes of airway obstruction are more likely to coexist.[11] Sleep endoscopy has been suggested to facilitate localization of the level of obstruction, which is more likely to be multiple in this type of patient. This procedure requires experience to be of value, but may demonstrate unexpected levels of airway compromise; and may be of particular importance following failed earlier intervention.[12] Syndromic children are more likely to require tracheostomy in the management of an obstructive sleep disorder, for example, Crouzon syndrome (**Figures 64.3** and **64.4**). However, it may be possible to avoid tracheostomy by management of other levels of obstruction. Modified conservative uvulopalatopharngyoplasty (UPPP),[8, 13] tongue base reduction, hyoid suspension[10] and laser aryepiglottoplasty[14] may have a role depending on the findings at sleep endoscopy. [**/*] Using a stepwise incremental targeted procedure has been reported to avoid tracheostomy in up to 80 percent of children with cerebral palsy.[10] Great caution must be taken with any procedure that has the potential to impact upon velopharyngeal function; there is a much higher risk of postoperative velopharyngeal insufficiency in this group of children.[15] Partial (or superior) adenoidectomy using an endoscopic-powered debrider may minimize this risk.[16, 17] [**/*]

The multidisciplinary sleep clinic

It is the author's practice to coordinate each stepped intervention with the paediatric sleep physician; partial

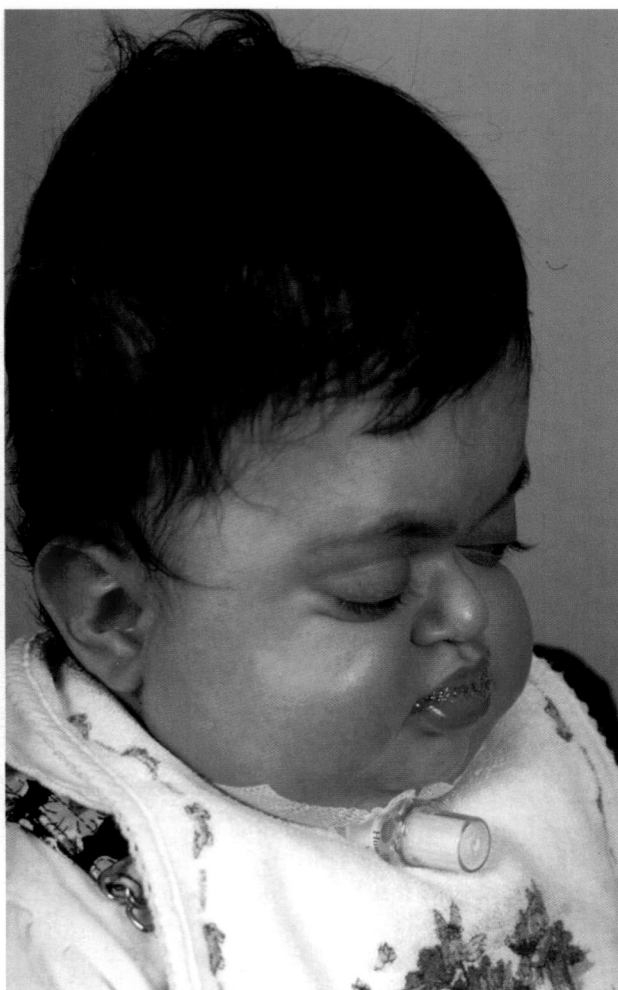

Figure 64.3 Obstructive sleep disorder in a child with Crouzon syndrome treated with tracheostomy.

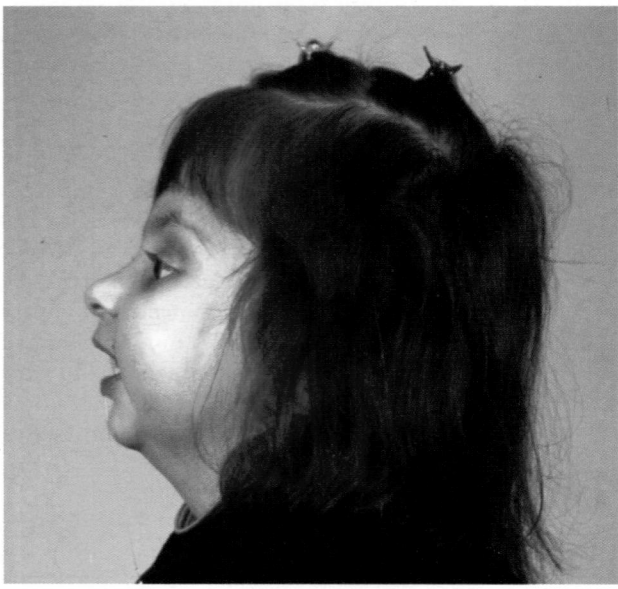

Figure 64.4 Successful decannulation of child in **Figure 64.3** following midfacial advancement.

surgical successes may permit the use of positive airway support devices that had previously been unsuccessful. It is the author's experience that an increasing number of such children require multimodality therapy to adequately control nocturnal airway obstruction without tracheostomy.

Many special needs children have sleep disorders not due to airway obstruction. These may have a profound impact on quality of life for families. Optimum treatment of these disorders involves an interested paediatrician and a multidisciplinary team.[10]

DROOLING

Drooling, or sialorrhoea, is physiological in the early part of life. It will occur in relation to teething, oropharyngeal ulceration and upper respiratory tract infections/upper aerodigestive tract infections. Physiological drooling usually settles around the age of two years when the primary dentition has erupted; however, it may persist on a minor basis in some children up to the age of four. This physiological occurrence is minor by comparison to the sialorrhoea that may occur with cerebral palsy and other forms of severe neurological impairment. Approximately 10 percent of children with cerebral palsy will have problematic drooling.[18] In order to determine this it is necessary to question the parent/carer regarding their management of the drooling – how many times are changes of clothes required per day; are 'quilted' bibs required for management? Some carers will complain that the school-going child soils books and papers and in older children there is the added difficulty of peer acceptance. If the condition has little impact on clothing management, then the drooling is minimal and simple reassurance will usually suffice. The resourcefulness, and tolerance, of parents/carers in dealing with this problem never ceases to amaze the author! Excessive drooling will macerate skin and therefore give rise to dermatological problems around the mouth and along the line that gravity carries it on an individual child. It can be a miserable problem for both parents and the child. General examination should include consideration of posture as well as a full otolaryngology evaluation. Particular consideration should be given to evaluation of nasal obstruction, and the presence of oropharyngeal ulceration (including gingivitis), which may be overlooked or considered noncontributory in the presence of severe neurological impairment.

Treatment

Nonsurgical treatments are often disappointing, and have usually failed by the time a child arrives at the paediatric otolaryngologist–head and neck surgeon. Anticholinergic agents to reduce salivary flow are often poorly tolerated due to nausea, and ocular side effects. Speech and swallowing therapy should also have been tried for a period of six months; occasionally simple posture changes (sometimes using appliances) will improve oral continence.[19]

Surgical treatments utilize the concepts of: the division of parasympathetic neurological supply to major salivary glands; mechanical obstruction of the salivary ducts; and rediversion of salivary flow.

Neurectomy

Division of the anterior branches of the tympanic plexus on the promontory via a relatively simple tympanotomy will reduce, but not eliminate, secretions from the parotid gland. It should be remembered that these branches (usually two) may be covered by a thin layer of bone (more commonly the anterior branch). This necessitates formal identification and division of two nerves in the mucosa overlying the promontory; failing this, a micro-drill is used to find the branch(es) which are always superficial in the bone.[20] It is also possible to reduce the parasympathetic drive to the submandibular salivary gland with simultaneous division of the chorda tympani nerve; however, this necessitates removal of taste from the anterior two-thirds of the tongue. In a child who already has severe limitation of sensory input, it may be difficult to justify the deliberate removal of one route of input. It can be difficult to obtain informed consent, particularly given the usually disappointing results produced by this intervention.[21] In its favour, this technique can be performed bilaterally, with little in the way of post-operative morbidity. The author no longer recommends or performs denervation procedures unless it is the preferred option of the parent/carer. [**/*]

Botulinum toxin

Botox has been used by some authors. Direct injection into the parotid and submandibular glands may reduce salivary flow.[22] Evidence is currently sparse and controlled trials are needed before this can be recommended for routine clinical use.

Mechanical diversion or obstruction of salivary flow

Overall, mechanical diversion or obstruction of salivary flow from the major glands is reported to produce the best outcomes.

Ligation of the submandibular and parotid ducts is reported to be an effective treatment, with surprisingly few sequelae. The procedure is performed intraorally, with postoperative antibiotic prophylaxis. The glands

initially swell and subsequently undergo atrophy.[23] It is interesting to note that a radionucleotide study of submandibular gland function following duct transposition reported 50 percent of the glands are atrophied and nonfunctioning following surgery.[24]

In the past 20 years or so, transposition of the submandibular ducts to the tonsillar fossae has become the most popular and reported procedure for drooling. From its initial description, the procedure has been refined to include intraoral excision of the sublingual salivary glands. The sublingual glands drain via the distal portion of the submandibular salivary duct; therefore leaving the sublingual glands *in situ* may predispose to postoperative ranula formation. Tonsillectomy (if not already performed) is carried out as part of the procedure to facilitate duct transposition. There is often significant postoperative swelling and significant postoperative morbidity may occur. Parental satisfaction is very high with this procedure.[19] Long-term follow-up suggests that improvement in drooling is maintained.[25] There are reports of increased dental caries following submandibular duct transposition; this is presumed to be due to loss of the salivary 'puddle'.[26, 27] It should be mentioned to parents/carers that there will be the need for diligent dental hygiene and increased risk of dental caries following transposition of the submandibular ducts. [**/*]

KEY POINTS

- Children with special needs require extra time for clinical evaluation.
- The maxim remains: maximize sensory input in order to maximize achievement of potential.
- Apparent small clinical gains may have dramatic benefits for the child and family.
- Where possible, maximal information should be obtained to support planned intervention.
- Conventional intervention is less likely to produce the anticipated outcome in a child with special needs.

Best clinical practice

- ✓ Rehabilitation of hearing presents special challenges in this group of children and management must be tailored for a particular child.
- ✓ Airway obstruction is more likely to be complex and multilevel in syndromic children.

✓ Submandibular duct transposition with excision of the sublingual glands is the current procedure of choice for excessive drooling.
✓ Children with Down syndrome present challenges to otolaryngologists and anaesthesiologists and special care is needed when considering surgery in this group.

Deficiencies in current knowledge and areas for future research

➤ There is an increasing trend to centralize the care of special needs children around a tertiary centre where support services including paediatric anaesthesia are available.
➤ Developmental paediatrics is a growing specialty; better classification of developmental disorders and attendant improvements in predicting outcome are already underway.
➤ Multidisciplinary involvement – essential to the optimum management of these children – will improve outcome and hopefully the evidence base for treatment.

REFERENCES

* 1. Colvin M, Maguire W, Fowlie PW. Neurodevelopmental outcomes after pre-term birth. *British Medical Journal*. 2004; **329**: 1390–3. *Excellent review of expected outcomes and improved survival of babies from SCBUs.*

2. Goldstein NA, Armfield DR, Kingsley LA, Borland LM, Allen GC, Post JC. Postoperative complications after tonsillectomy and adenoidectomy in children with Down syndrome. *Archives of Otolaryngology – Head and Neck Surgery*. 1998; **124**: 171–6.

3. Strauss D, Kastner T, Ashwel S, White J. Tube feeding mortality in children with severe disabilities and mental retardation. *Pediatrics*. 1997; **99**: 358–62.

4. Shott SR, Joseph A, Heithaus D. Hearing loss in children with Down syndrome. *International Journal of Pediatric Otorhinolaryngology*. 2001; **61**: 199–205.

5. Iino Y, Imamura Y, Harigai S, Tanaka Y. Efficacy of tympanostomy tube insertion for otitis media with effusion in children with Down syndrome. *International Journal of Pediatric Otorhinolaryngology*. 1999; **49**: 143–9.

6. Litovitz TL. Battery ingestions: product accessibility and clinical course. *Pediatrics*. 1985; **75**: 469–76.

* 7. Kanamori G, Witter M, Brown J, Williams-Smith L. Otolaryngologic manifestations of Down syndrome. *Otolaryngology Clinics of North America*. 2000; **33**: 1285–92. *An excellent overview of this condition.*

* 8. Seid AB, Martin PJ, Pransky SM, Kearns DB. Surgical therapy of obstructive sleep apnea in children with serve mental insufficiency. *Laryngoscope*. 1990; **100**: 507–10. *A good series.*

9. Suen JS, Arnold JE, Brooks LJ. Adenotonsillectomy for treatment of obstructive sleep apnea in children. *Archives of Otolaryngology – Head and Neck Surgery*. 1995; **121**: 525–30.

* 10. Cohen SR, Lefaivre JF, Burstein FD, Simms C, Kattos AV, Scott PH et al. Surgical treatment of obstructive sleep apnea in neurologically compromised patients. *Plastic and Reconstructive Surgery*. 1997; **99**: 638–46. *Comprehensive multi-procedure series, with good work-up.*

11. Magardino TM, Tom LW. Surgical management of obstructive sleep apnea in children with cerebral palsy. *Laryngoscope*. 1999; **109**: 1611–5.

* 12. Myatt HM, Beckenham EJ. The use of diagnostic sleep endoscopy in the management of children with complex upper airway obstruction. *Clinical Otolaryngology*. 2000; **25**: 200–8. *A good series of an emerging technique.*

13. Kosko JR, Derkay CS. Uvulopalatopharyngoplasty: treatment of obstructive sleep apnea in neurologically impaired pediatric patients. *International Journal of Pediatric Otorhinolaryngology*. 1995; **32**: 241–6.

14. Hui Y, Gaffney R, Crysdale WS. Laser aryepiglottoplasty for the treatment of neurasthenic laryngomalacia in cerebral palsy. *Annals of Otology, Rhinology and Laryngology*. 1995; **104**: 432–6.

15. Kavanagh KT, Kahane JC, Kordan B. Risks and benefits of adenotonsillectomy for children with Down syndrome. *American Journal of Mental Deficiency*. 1986; **91**: 22–9.

16. Murray N, Fitzpatrick P, Guarisco JL. Powered partial adenoidectomy. *Archives of Otolaryngology – Head and Neck Surgery*. 2002; **128**: 792–6.

17. Finkelstein Y, Wexler DB, Nachmani A, Ophir D. Endoscopic partial adenoidectomy for children with submucous cleft palate. *Cleft Palate and Craniofacial Journal*. 2002; **39**: 479–86.

18. O'Dwyer TP, Conlon BJ. The surgical management of drooling – a 15 year follow-up. *Clinical Otolaryngology*. 1997; **22**: 284–7.

* 19. Crysdale WS, Raveh E, McCann C, Roske L, Kotler A. Management of drooling in individuals with neurodisability: a surgical experience. *Developmental Medicine and Child Neurology*. 2001; **43**: 379–83. *A large series and clinical experience.*

20. Hollinshead WH. The ear. In: *Anatomy for surgeons: the head and neck*, 3rd edn. Vol 1. London: Harper and Row, 1982: 174–5.

21. Parisier SC, Blitzer A, Binder WJ, Friedman WF, Marovitz WF. Tympanic neurectomy and chorda tympanectomy for the control of drooling. *Archives of Otolaryngology*. 1978; **104**: 273–7.

22. Cordivari C, Misra VP, Catania S, Lee AJ. New therapeutic indications for botulinus toxins. *Movement Disorders*. 2004; **19**: S157–61.

23. Klem C, Mair EA. Four-duct ligation; a simple and effective treatment for chronic aspiration from sialorrhea. *Archives of Otolaryngology – Head and Neck Surgery*. 1999; **125**: 796–800.

24. Hotaling AJ, Madgy DN, Kuhns LR, Filipek L, Belenky WM. Postoperative technetium scanning in patients with submandibular duct diversion. *Archives of Otolaryngology – Head and Neck Surgery*. 1992; **118**: 1331–3.

25. Burton MJ, Leighton SE, Lund WS. Long-term results of submandibular duct transposition for drooling. *Journal of Laryngology and Otology*. 1991; **105**: 101–3.

26. Hallett KB, Lucas JO, Johnston T, Reddihough DS, Hall RK. Dental health of children with cerebral palsy following sialodochoplasty. *Special Care in Dentistry*. 1995; **15**: 234–8.

27. Arnrup K, Crossner CG. Caries prevalence after submandibular duct retroposition in drooling children with neurological disorders. *Pediatric Dentistry*. 1990; **12**: 98–101.

65

Head and neck embryology

T CLIVE LEE

General embryology	792	Larynx	803
Skull	794	Thyroid gland	805
Pharyngeal arches	795	Ear	805
Pharyngeal pouches	796	Key points	809
Pharyngeal clefts	797	Deficiencies in current knowledge and areas for further	
Face	797	research	809
Palate	798	Acknowledgements	809
Mouth	799	References	809
Nose and paranasal sinuses	803		

SEARCH STRATEGY

The data in this chapter are supported by a Medline search using the key words head, skull, ear, nose, palate, tongue, tooth, salivary gland, neck, thyroid, pharynx, oesophagus and larynx and focussing on level 1 evidence on embryology, growth and development. Morphological details are described and their relation to embryological stages, size and age are summarized in **Table 65.1**. References to the underlying genetic and molecular mechanisms governing embryological development are cited.

GENERAL EMBRYOLOGY

Development begins with fertilization when the sperm and oocyte, each haploid with 23 chromosomes, unite to form the diploid zygote containing 46 chromosomes. Chromosomal abnormalities and gene mutations cause major craniofacial defects. Three, rather than two, copies of chromosomes cause trisomy syndromes – trisomy 13, 18 and 21 (Down syndrome). Partial chromosome deletions result in cri-du-chat syndrome (chromosome 5), Angelman syndrome (chromosome 15), Miller–Dieker syndrome (chromosome 17) and Shprintzen syndrome (chromosome 22). Breakage of chromosomes (fragile X syndrome) and gene mutations (MSX2) also cause craniofacial abnormalities.[2]

The zygote divides, producing a morula which cavitates to form a blastocyst that implants in the endometrium during the second week. The inner cell mass of the blastocyst gives rise to the embryo. Initially the inner cell mass forms a bilaminar germ disc which then, by gastrulation, leads to a trilaminar disc comprised of ecto-, meso- and endoderm layers in week 3 (**Figure 65.1**). Weeks 3–8 comprise the embryonic period during which the main organ systems are established and are vulnerable to teratogens such as drugs (thalidomide, alcohol), infectious agents (rubella, HIV) and physical agents (x-rays) which can cause major birth defects.

Ectoderm gives rise to tissues and organs which maintain contact with the outside world – the nervous system, skin, the sensory epithelium of the ear, nose and

Table 65.1 Carnegie embryonic stages in the development of the human head and neck, based on ultrasonic studies.[1]

Stage	Age (days)	Size (mm)	Major features
1	1	0.1–0.15	Fertilization
5	7	0.1–0.2	Implantation
8b	23	1.01–1.5	Neural folds and groove appear
9	25	1.5–2.5	Otic disc, somites appear
10	28	2–3.5	Neural fold fusion; two pharyngeal arches; otic pit
12	30	3–5	3–4 pharyngeal arches
13	32	4–6	Otic vesicle
14	33	5–7	Endolymphatic appendage, cochlear duct begins
15	36	7–9	Nasal pit; auricular hillocks beginning
16	38	8–11	Utricosaccular diverticulum, nasal sacs face ventrally
17	41	11–14	Tubotympanic recess, six auricular hillocks, nasofrontal groove
18	44	13–17	1–3 semicircular ducts, stapes and stapedius, tip of nose; ossification begins oronasal membrane
19	46	16–18	Cartilaginous otic capsule, malleus and incus
20	49	18–22	Tensor tympani
22	53	23–28	External ear developing
23	56	27–31	Cochlear duct with 2.5 turns, head more rounded

Embryonic period: weeks 3–8 (days 8–56); foetal period: weeks 9–38.

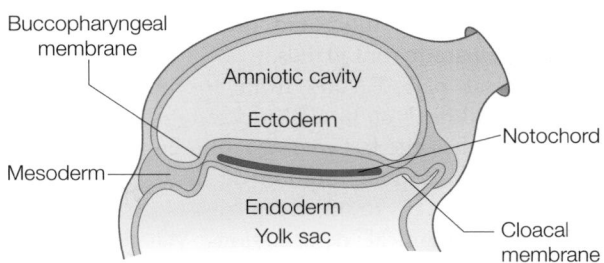

Figure 65.1 Highly diagrammatic representation of a longitudinal section of the developing embryonic disc. The structure never looks like this at any one time since development is progressing at different rates. Nevertheless, mesoderm lies between ectoderm and endoderm, except at the buccopharyngeal and cloacal membranes where the two layers are in contact. The notochord, a derivative of the ectodermal layer, lies within the mass of mesoderm. A connecting stalk attaches the developing disc with its amniotic cavity and yolk sac to the uterine wall, and these structures lie within the extra-embryonic coelom at this stage of development.

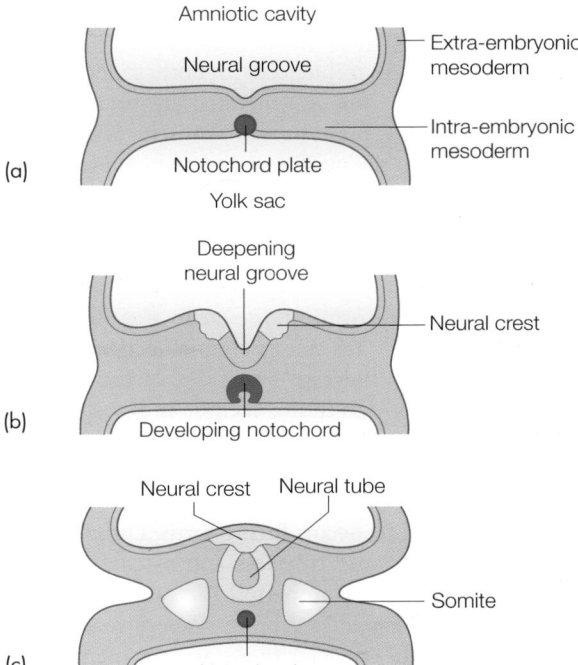

Figure 65.2 Transverse section of the developing embryonic disc at various stages of development. In the early presomite stage (a) a midline neural groove is present above the notochordal plate, which is fused with the endodermal layer. The neural groove deepens (b) and specialized neural crest cells develop on the lips of the groove. The notochord separates from the endodermal layer. By the somite stage (c) the neural tube has formed and the neural crest cells are about to migrate to form cell clusters which, at the head end of the embryo, become the cranial sensory nerve ganglia. Cells from the neural crest also form the posterior root ganglion of the spinal cord and the cells of the sympathetic ganglia.

eye, and tooth enamel. Neurulation is the process by which ectoderm forms a neural plate that folds to form the neural tube, giving rise to the brain and spinal cord, and the neural crest (**Figure 65.2**). Neural crest changes into mesenchyme and contributes to the connective tissue and bones of the face and skull.

Lateral to the neural tube, paraxial mesoderm forms pairs of somites each of which give rise to its own sclerotome (bone and cartilage), myotome (muscle) and dermatome (dermis) component. The occipital bone and cervical vertebrae are derived from sclerotomes, and the related myo- and dermatomes are segmentally innervated. Endoderm provides the epithelial lining of the gastro-intestinal and respiratory tracts, including the tympanic cavity and auditory tube, and the parenchyma of the thyroid and parathyroid glands.

The foetal period runs from the ninth week of gestation until birth at 38 weeks of gestation or 40 weeks after the onset of the last menstruation and is characterized by growth and maturation of tissues and organs. Abnormalities may result from disruption of blood supply or mechanical deformation. Major congenital malformations, due to genetic, environmental or, most commonly, unknown causes, occur in approximately 4 percent of live births, but minor abnormalities are found in a further 15 percent.[3] A *syndrome* is a group of anomalies occurring together with a specific common cause, while in an *association* this cause has yet to be determined. Due to the common germ layer origin of a variety of organs, or the contemporaneous development of different systems, the presence of minor abnormalities may indicate more serious underlying defects. This is particularly true of external ear abnormalities which feature in most common chromosomal syndromes.[2]

SKULL

Skull development is influenced by both genetic factors and the mechanical forces generated by brain growth, development of the pharynx and muscle activity. The skull is divided into the neurocranium, which protects the brain, and the viscerocranium, derived from pharyngeal arches, which forms the face and jaws. Both neurocranium and viscerocranium ossify partly by intramembranous and partly by endochondral ossification.[1] In intramembranous ossification, mesenchyme differentiates directly into bone. This mesenchyme is derived from neural crest cells in the roof and sides of the skull and from paraxial mesoderm in the occiput and posterior otic capsule. Primary ossification centres appear as spicules in the centre of these flat bones and radiate to the periphery. At birth, membranous sutures separate these bony plates, enabling moulding to occur during birth. Osteoblasts lay down new bone on outer surfaces and osteoclasts resorb bone from inner surfaces to permit the vault to grow and accommodate the expanding brain. Where sutures meet at the angles of the parietal bone are six membranous intersections, termed *fontanelles*. The largest is the anterior fontanelle at bregma, between the parietal and frontal bones, which is a useful indicator of raised intracranial pressure or dehydration and provides access to the underlying superior sagittal venous sinus. It is obliterated by two years, while the posterior fontanelle at lambda, between the parietal and occipital bones, closes at about six months after birth.[4]

Premature closure of sutures results in craniosynostosis.[5] Early closure of the coronal suture causes acrocephaly, or tower skull; early closure of the sagittal suture causes a long narrow skull, scaphocephaly (**Figure 65.3**) and unilateral premature closure of the coronal and

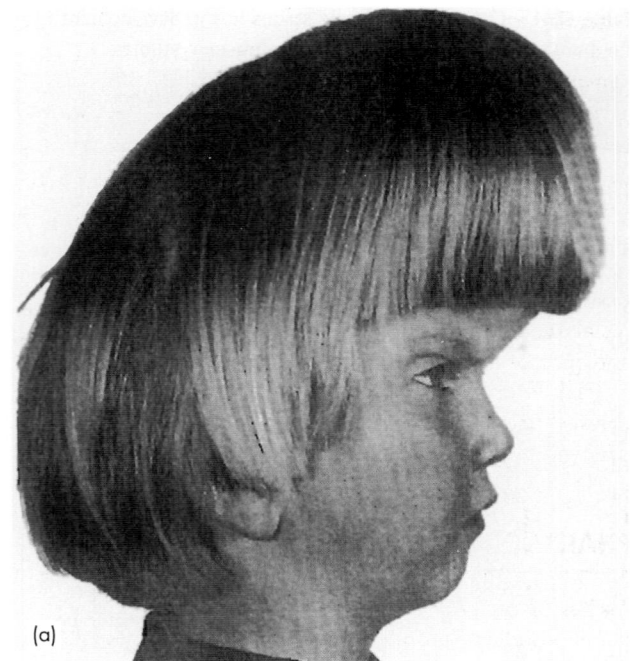

(a)

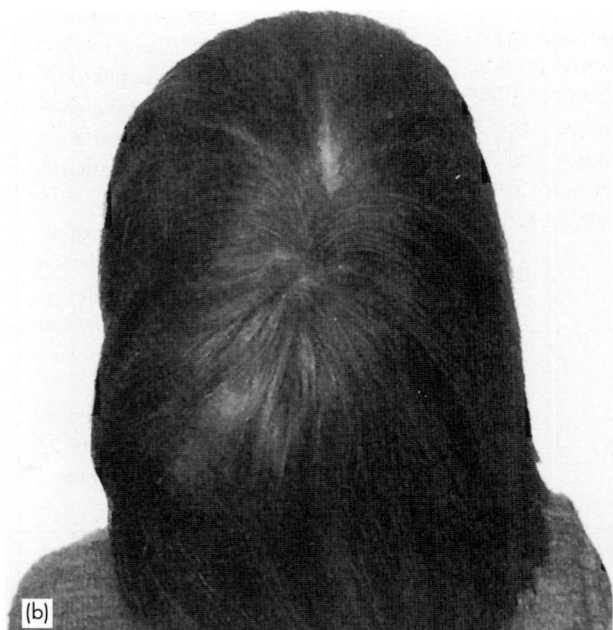

(b)

Figure 65.3 Scaphocephaly. In this child the sagittal suture is completely fused, while the remaining sutures of the cranial vault are normal.

lambdoid sutures results in asymmetry – plagiocephaly (see Chapter 78, Craniofacial anomalies: genetics and management).

In endochondral ossification, mesenchyme forms a cartilaginous model which is then replaced by bone. Anterior to the pituitary gland in the midline, neural crest cells give rise to the ethmoid, inferior nasal concha and body of the sphenoid. Posterior to the pituitary, paraxial mesoderm forms the clivus and base of the occipital bone.

Laterally, the ala orbitalis and ala temporalis form the lesser and greater wings of the sphenoid, while the otic capsule develops around the membranous labyrinth and gives rise to the petrous and mastoid parts of the temporal bone.[2] The sphenooccipital junction remains cartilaginous until puberty, while the cartilage of the foramen lacerum does not undergo ossification. Incomplete ossification may lead to herniation of the meninges, or meningocoele, but larger defects can include neural tissue (meningoencephalocoele) (see Chapter 78, Craniofacial anomalies: genetics and management) or even brain and part of a ventricle (meningohydroencephalocoele).[2]

The viscerocranium, forming the face and jaws, is derived from the first two pharyngeal arches.

PHARYNGEAL ARCHES

Arches of mesenchyme derived from paraxial and lateral plate mesoderm and neural crest cells appear in the fourth and fifth weeks of development. They are covered externally by ectoderm, which forms clefts between successive arches, and internally by endoderm which forms pouches between arches. Morphologically, they resemble gills in fish, but as true gills (branchia) are never formed, the term pharyngeal arches is used in humans. Pharyngeal arches play a role in the formation of the face, ear and neck (**Figure 65.4**) and their derivatives are summarized in **Table 65.2**.[5]

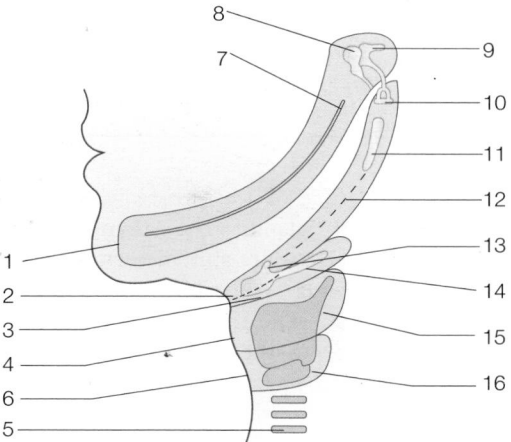

Figure 65.4 A diagram to show the derivatives of the pharyngeal arch cartilages. 1, First arch cartilage; 2, second arch cartilage; 3, third arch cartilage; 4, fourth arch cartilage; 5, tracheal rings; 6, sixth arch cartilage; 7, Meckel's cartilage; 8, malleus; 9, incus; 10, stapes; 11, styloid process; 12, stylohyoid ligament; 13, lesser horn and upper body of hyoid bone; 14, greater horn and lower body of hyoid bone; 15, thyroid cartilage; 16, cricoid cartilage. Modified from Ref. 2, with permission.

First pharyngeal arch

The first arch has a dorsal maxillary process and a ventral mandibular process. The maxillary process gives rise to the premaxilla, maxilla, zygomatic bone, the zygomatic process and squamous part of the temporal bone by intramembranous ossification. The mandibular process contains Meckel's cartilage which persists as the malleus, anterior ligament of malleus, incus and sphenomandibular ligament. The majority of the mandible is formed by membranous ossification of mesenchyme around Meckel's cartilage. This entraps the inferior alveolar branch of the mandibular nerve which enters the bone through the mandibular foramen. Its terminal branch, the mental nerve, exits via the mental foramen. The right and left mandibular processes meet in the midline at the symphysis menti which achieves bony union six months after birth.[4]

The trigeminal (V) nerve supplies sensation to the first arch connective tissues via its ophthalmic, maxillary and mandibular branches. Only the mandibular division has a motor root and supplies eight first arch muscles: four muscles of mastication (temporalis, masseter, medial and lateral pterygoid), two tensors (tympani and palati), mylohyoid and the anterior belly of digastric.

Second pharyngeal arch

The second arch gives rise to the stapes, styloid process of the temporal bone, stylohyoid ligament, lesser cornu and upper body of the hyoid bone. The facial (VII) nerve supplies sensation to second arch connective tissue in the external auditory canal, but is mainly motor supplying: stapedius, stylohyoid, posterior belly of digastric, occipitofrontalis and the muscles of facial expression.

Third pharyngeal arch

The third arch gives rise to the greater cornu and lower body of the hyoid bone. The glossopharyngeal (IX) nerve supplies sensation to third arch connective tissues in the posterior third of the tongue and is motor to glossopharyngeus.

Fourth and sixth pharyngeal arches

The cartilagenous components of the fourth and sixth arches fuse to form the laryngeal cartilages: thyroid, cricoid, arytenoid, corniculate and cuneiform. The superior laryngeal branch of the vagus (X) supplies sensation to fourth arch connective tissue from the valleculae and epiglottis to the true vocal cords and is motor to levator palati, pharyngeal constrictors (partially) and

Table 65.2 Derivatives of the pharyngeal arches and pouches.[1, 2, 5]

Arch	Skeleton	Nerve	Muscles	Artery	Pouch
First	Maxilla, Meckel's cartilage, malleus, anterior ligament of malleus, incus, sphenomandibular ligament, portion of mandible	V. Trigeminal mandibular division	Mastication (temporalis, masseter; medial and lateral pterygoids); mylohyoid; anterior belly of digastric, tensor palati, tensor tympani	Maxillary	Eustacian tube; middle ear cavity; Tubotympanic recess (first cleft forms external auditory meatus)
Second	Staples; styloid process; stylohyoid ligament; lesser horn and upper portion of body of hyoid bone	VII. Facial	Facial expression (buccinator; auricularis; frontalis; platysma; orbicularis oris; orbicularis oculi); posterior belly of diagastric; stylohyoid; stapedius	External carotid	Bed of palatine tonsil
Third	Greater horn and lower portion of body of hyoid bone	IX. Glossopharyngeal	Stylopharyngeus	Common carotid and first part of internal carotid	Thymus; inferior parathyroid
Fourth–sixth	Laryngeal cartilages (thyroid, cricoid, arytenoid, corniculate, cuneiform)	V. Vagus. Superior laryngeal branch (nerve to fourth arch)	Cricothyroid; levator palati; constrictors of pharynx (fourth)	Aortic arch (fourth left)	Superior parathyroid (fourth)
		Recurrent laryngeal branch (nerve to sixth arch)	Intrinsic muscles of larynx (sixth)	First part subclavian (fourth right) Ductus arteriosus (sixth left) Proximal right pulmonary (sixth right)	Ultimobranchial body (fifth)

cricothyroid. The recurrent laryngeal branch of the vagus supplies sensation to sixth arch derivatives, notably the infraglottic larynx, and is motor to the other muscles of the larynx.

PHARYNGEAL POUCHES

On each side, between the six arches, lie five pharyngeal pouches lined by endoderm (**Figure 65.5**). Their derivatives are summarized in **Table 65.2**.

The first pouch extends laterally to form the Eustachian tube, the middle ear cavity and the tubotympanic recess, which extends as far as the tympanic membrane.

The second pouch forms the bed of the palatine tonsil.

The third pouch forms ventral and dorsal wings. The epithelium of the ventral wing differentiates into the thymus, while that of the dorsal wing forms the inferior parathyroid gland. The thymus separates from the pharyngeal wall and descends inferomedially to unite with contralateral thymic tissue behind the sternum. The inferior parathyroid descends to lie posterior to the inferior pole of the ipsilateral thyroid lobe. Thymic tissue may be found embedded in the thyroid, while the inferior parathyroids may lie at sites from the bifurcation of the common carotid artery to the anterior mediastinum behind the sternum.

The dorsal wing of the fourth pouch differentiates into parathyroid tissue which descends to lie posterior to the superior pole of the ipsilateral thyroid lobe.

The fifth pouch (or ventral wing of the fourth) forms the ultimobranchial body, which is incorporated into the thyroid gland and gives rise to parafollicular calcitonin-secreting cells.

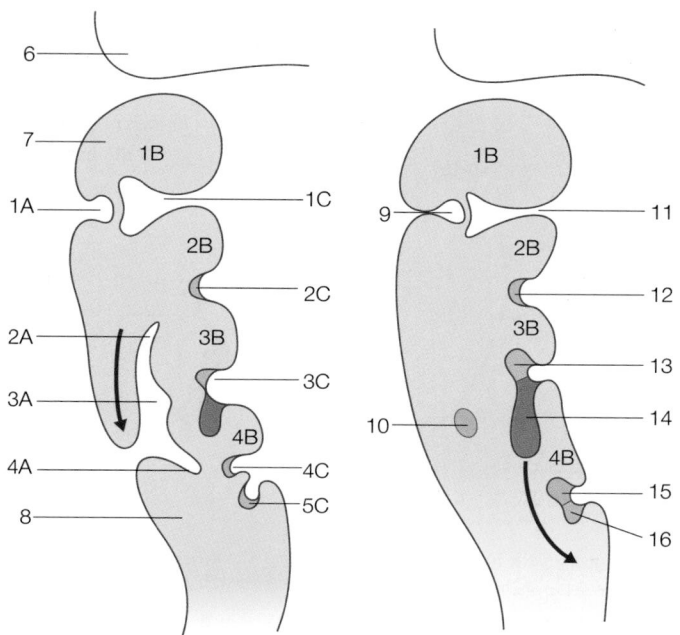

Figure 65.5 A diagram to show the development and derivatives of the pharyngeal pouches and clefts. Note the way in which the second, third and fourth clefts are buried and, if not obliterated, form the cervical sinus. 1A, first cleft; 1B, first arch; 1C, first pouch; 2A, second cleft; 2B, second arch; 2C, second pouch; 3A, third cleft; 3B, third arch; 3C, third pouch; 4A, fourth cleft; 4B, fourth arch; 4C, fourth pouch; 5C, fifth pouch; 6, maxillary process; 7, mandibular process; 8, epicardial ridge; 9, external auditory meatus; 10, cervical sinus; 11, pharyngotympanic tube; 12, palatine tonsil; 13, inferior parathyroid gland; 14, thymus; 15, superior parathyroid gland; 16, ultimobranchial body. Modified from Ref. 2, with permission.

Pharyngeal diverticulum

The structural weakness between thyropharyngeus and cricopharyngeus, Killian's dehiscence, may be the site of an acquired pulsion diverticulum which may be described erroneously as a 'pharyngeal pouch'.[6]

As neural crest cells contribute to both pharyngeal and heart formation, craniofacial and cardiac abnormalites are common to a number of syndromes (see Chapter 78, Craniofacial anomalies: genetics and management). First arch structures are affected in Treacher Collins and Goldenhar syndromes (see Chapter 80, Facial paralysis in childhood), and the Pierre Robin sequence. The DiGeorge sequence affects the third and fourth pouches, as well as the first arch and external ears.[1, 2]

PHARYNGEAL CLEFTS

On each side, between the first five arches, lie four pharyngeal clefts lined by ectoderm. Normally, only the first cleft persists and its dorsal end gives rise to the external auditory meatus, separated from the first pouch by the tympanic membrane. The ventral end is normally obliterated, but may persist as a sinus, cyst or fistula. Such a fistula extends from below the auricle, through the parotid gland and opens into the external auditory meatus. It has a variable relationship with the facial (VII) nerve.[1]

The second arch overgrows the second, third and fourth clefts, forming the cervical sinus which then resorbs. However, if this sinus persists, it gives rise to cervical cysts along the anterior border of sternocleidomastoid (**Figure 65.6**).[7] If the cysts communicate with the

skin, they form external branchial fistulae. The cervical sinus may also communicate with the second pouch in the bed of the palatine tonsil to form an internal branchial fistula. Such fistulae pass over the glossopharyngeal (IX) and hypoglossal (XII) nerves and run between the external and internal carotid arteries (**Figure 65.7**) (see Chapter 99, Branchial arch fistulae, thryoglossal duct anomalies and lymphangioma).[1, 8]

The third cleft may give rise to a fistula extending from the anterior border of sternocleidomastoid, passing superficial to the hypoglossal (XII) nerve, deep to the carotid arteries and piercing the thyrohyoid membrane to open into the piriform fossa.[8] Very rarely a fistula from the fourth cleft may extend from the anterior border of sternocleidomastoid, pass around the arch of the aorta on the left side, or right subclavian artery, ascend in the neck running superficial to the hypoglossal (XII) nerve, deep to the carotid arteries and open into the lower pharynx (see Chapter 99, Branchial arch fistulae, thryoglossal duct anomalies and lymphangioma).[1]

FACE

The face develops from five growth centres or prominences – the frontonasal in the midline and the right and left maxillary and mandibular prominences. The frontonasal prominence forms the forehead and, inferiorly, lies above the primitive mouth or stomodeum with a nasal placode on either side. The nasal placodes invaginate to form nasal pits and their margins form lateral and medial nasal processes. The first arch gives rise to the maxillary prominences lateral to the stomodeum and the mandibular prominences inferiorly.[9]

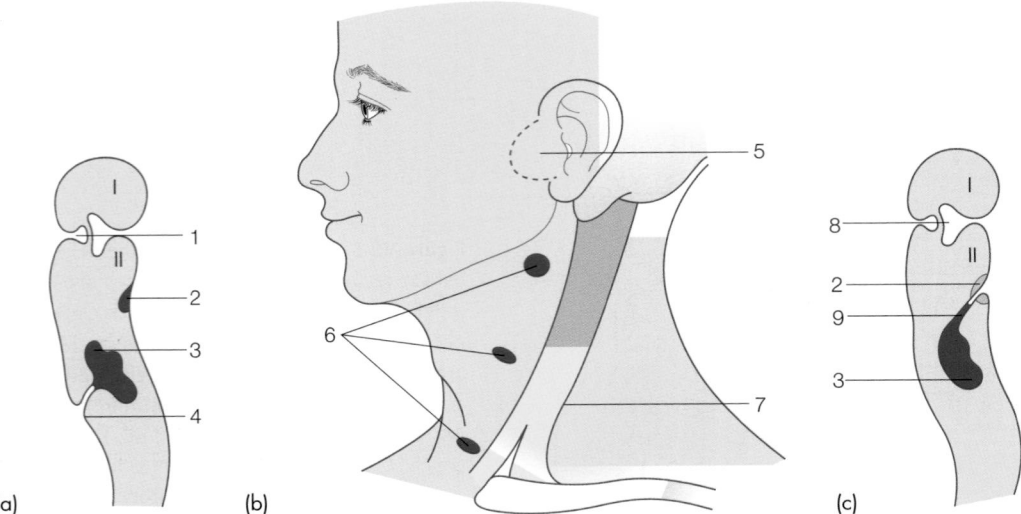

Figure 65.6   A diagram to show a lateral cervical (branchial) cyst opening onto the surface as a fistula (a). (b) Location of cysts and fistulae anterior to the sternocleidomastoid muscle. (c) Internal opening of a fistula by the palatine tonsil. 1, external auditory meatus; 2, palatine tonsil; 3, lateral cervical (branchial) cyst; 4, external branchial fistula; 5, region of preauricular fistulae; 6, region of lateral cervical cysts and fistulae; 7, sternocleidomastoid muscle; 8, tubotympanic recess; 9, internal branchial fistula. Modified from Ref. 2, with permission.

The maxillary prominences grow medially, pushing the medial nasal processes towards the midline and fusing with them to form the upper lip (**Figure 65.8**). The philtrum is derived from the medial nasal process with the maxillary prominence providing the lateral lip and cheek. An alternative theory is that the maxillary prominences fuse in the midline superficial to the frontonasal prominence, thus accounting for the maxillary nerve supplying sensation to all of the upper lip, including the philtrum.[1] The nasolacrimal groove lies between the maxillary prominence and lateral nasal process. This groove separates, forming a duct, and allows the lateral nasal process and maxillary prominence to fuse.

The lower lip and jaw are formed by the fusion of the right and left mandibular prominences. The right and left halves meet anteriorly at the symphysis menti, but fusion, starting at the outer and inferior surfaces, is usually complete by six months after birth.[4] The cheeks develop from the maxillary and mandibular processes which accounts for their sensory innervation. The musculature, however, is derived from mesenchyme of the second pharyngeal arch and so receives its motor supply from the facial (VII) nerve.

PALATE

The palate separates the oral and nasal cavities and is formed in two phases, primary and secondary, under separate genetic and epigenetic controls (see Chapter 77, Cleft lip and palate).[1] The medial nasal processes fuse to form the triangular primary palate which carries the upper medial and lateral incisors and extends posteriorly to the incisive foramen – the premaxilla of the adult. The secondary palate comprises the remainder of the adult hard and soft palates and is formed in three stages where the palatal shelves are, respectively, vertical, horizontal or fused.[10] In stage I, vertical palatal shelves arise from the maxillary prominences and lie lateral to the tongue. The two shelves expand by cell division, hydration and electrostatic forces in the orofacial cavity which is growing in height but not in width.[11] Descent of the tongue as the first arch elongates, combined with shelf expansion, results in the elevation of the shelves to the horizontal position – stage II (**Figures 65.9**). This movement is rapid and occurs in a matter of minutes or hours.[12] In stage III, the palatal shelves fuse separating the nasal and oral cavities.[12] The epithelium on the superior, nasal surface is pseudo-stratified, ciliated columnar, while on the inferior, oral surface are stratified, squamous, nonkeratinizing cells.[10] Bone that forms in the hard palate belongs to the maxillae and palatine bones. The soft palate and uvula probably develop by epithelial displacement due to mesenchymal activity, rather than by midline fusion.[1]

Facial clefts

Cleft palate may result from disturbances at any stage of palatal development.[5, 11] Failure of fusion of the maxillary prominence and medial nasal process gives rise to clefts anterior and posterior to the incisive foramen. Anterior clefts may involve the lip alone or include the palate, may

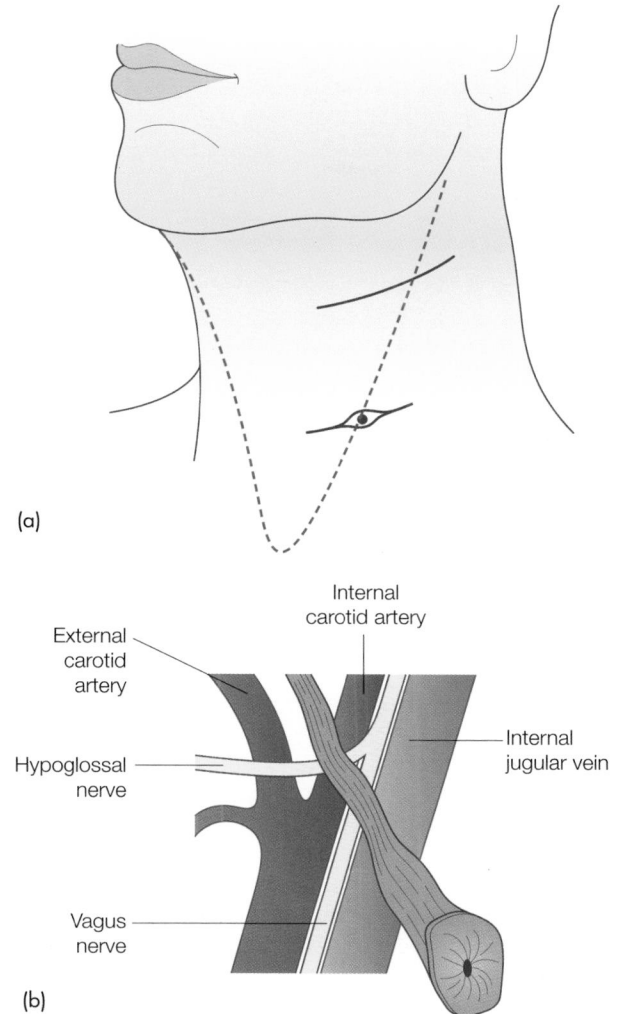

(a)

(b)

Figure 65.7 Operation for second branchial cleft fistula **(a)** showing two horizontal incisions, the lower one to include the fistulous opening; **(b)** the fistula is seen crossing the hypoglossal nerve to pass between the internal and external carotid arteries.

extend into the nose and may be bilateral.[13] Posterior clefts lie in the midline and may involve the uvula alone, or separate both palatine shelves and extend into the nose. Anterior and posterior clefts may be combined. Cleft types are summarized in **Figure 65.10**.[14] A variety of mechanisms have been implicated in clefting, with failure of shelf elevation occurring in the majority of cases.[11]

Failure of fusion of the maxillary prominence and lateral nasal process exposes the nasolacrimal duct to form an oblique facial cleft. However, they may be due to irregular tearing accompanying rupture of the amnion.[1] Craniofacial clefts are summarized in **Figure 65.11**.[15] Rarely, the medial nasal processes may fail to fuse causing a median cleft lip. The entrapment of epithelium along lines of fusion may result in nasolabial, globulomaxillary, median alveolar and median palatal cysts which usually do not present until adulthood (**Figure 65.12**).

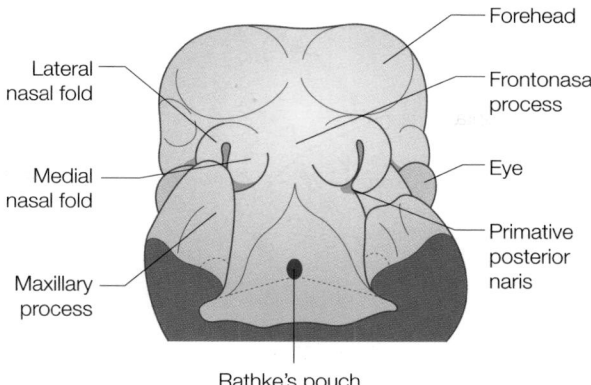

Figure 65.8 The roof of the stomodeum of a 12 mm human embryo illustrating the development of the primitive palate and posterior nares by approximation of the maxillary processes to the lateral and medial nasal folds. The previous site of the attachment of the buccopharyngeal membrane is represented by a dotted line and part of the left maxillary process has been removed. After Hamilton WJ and Mossman HW (eds). *Human embryology*. Cambridge: Heffer, 1972.

MOUTH

The primitive mouth or stomodeum is bounded by the forebrain superiorly and the pericardial cavity inferiorly. The buccopharyngeal membrane separating it from the foregut breaks down and so connects the amniotic cavity and the primitive gut (**Figure 65.13**). The cranial part of the foregut, often termed the pharyngeal gut, thus extends from the buccopharyngeal membrane to the tracheo-bronchial diverticulum.[2] Laterally, pharyngeal mesenchyme segments to form the pharyngeal arches.

Salivary glands

Three pairs of salivary glands arise from the oropharyngeal epithelium and follow similar patterns of development to produce branching ducts and secretory acini.[16] The submandibular gland originates as an epithelial cord in the groove between tongue and mandible which branches into the surrounding mesenchyme. Serous acini appear early, followed by mucous acini postnatally.[1, 17] The sublingual and parotid glands develop in a similar fashion, with the site of opening of the parotid duct dependent upon skeletal development. There is no evidence to suggest that the gland is composed of two lobes, rather the parotid ductules grow around the facial (VII) nerve, making it intimately entwined with the gland.[18]

Teeth

The epithelium of the oral cavity forms the dental lamina on the upper and lower jaws. On each jaw, ten diverticula

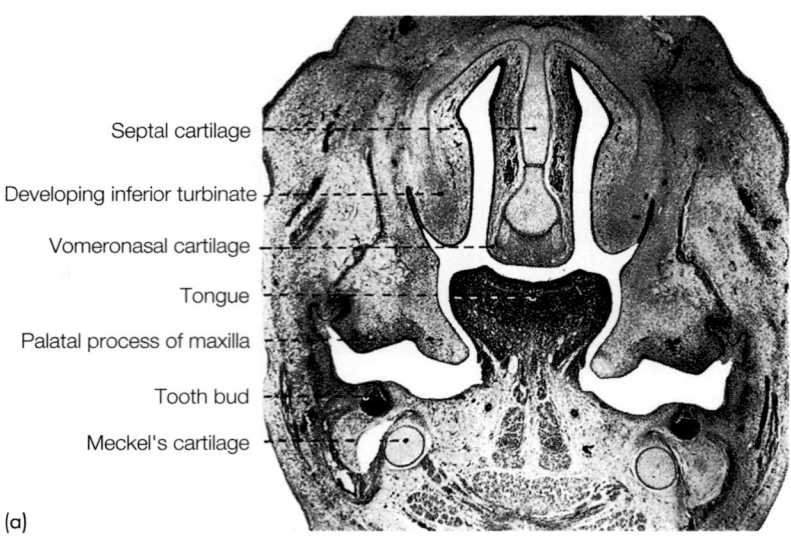

Septal cartilage

Developing inferior turbinate

Vomeronasal cartilage

Tongue

Palatal process of maxilla

Tooth bud

Meckel's cartilage

(a)

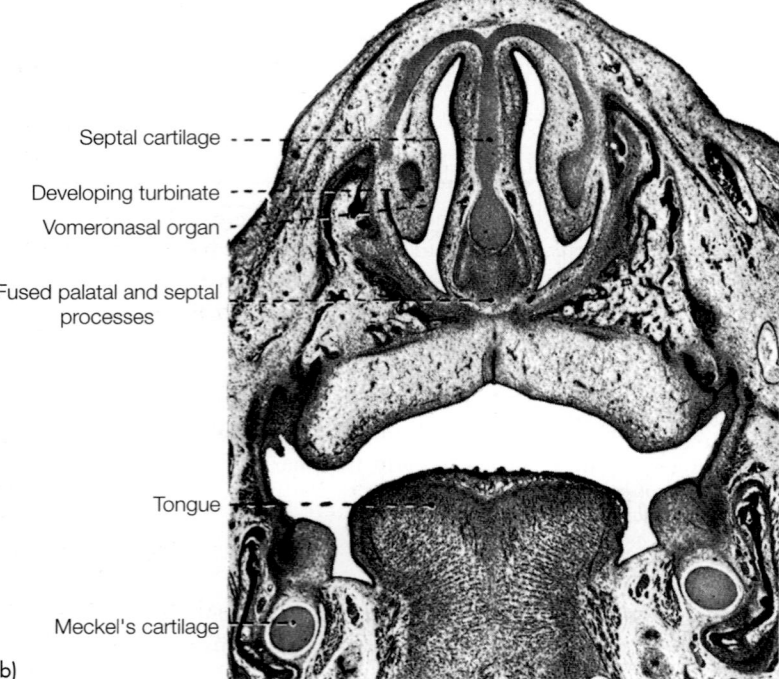

Septal cartilage

Developing turbinate

Vomeronasal organ

Fused palatal and septal processes

Tongue

Meckel's cartilage

(b)

Figure 65.9 Section through the developing palate of (**a**) a 20-mm and (**b**) a 48-mm human foetus. Reprinted from Hamilton WJ and Mossman HW (eds). *Human embryology*. Cambridge: Heffer, 1972.

of the lamina push into the jaw mesenchyme giving rise to a permanent tooth bud and the dental bud from which a deciduous tooth develops in a complex interaction of genetic and epigenetic factors.[19] The deep surface of each bud invaginates to form a dental cap lying on the dental papilla, a neural crest derivative. The cap comprises outer and inner epithelial layers separated by the stellate reticulum. The central part of the dental papilla forms the pulp of the tooth, while cells deep to the inner dental epithelium differentiate into odontoblasts which produce dentine and push themselves inwards into the papilla. The outer dental epithelial cells differentiate into ameloblasts which deposit enamel prisms over the dentine, beginning

at the apex and spreading towards the neck. As the enamel thickens, the ameloblasts are pushed outwards into the stellate reticulum (**Figure 65.14**).

The dental epithelial cells form a root sheath which expands into the jaw mesenchyme. Odontoblasts lay down dentine, continuous with that in the crown, which narrows the pulp chamber to a root canal. In the jaw mesenchyme, cells in contact with dentine differentiate into cementoblasts and secrete cementum. Outside the cementum, the periodontal ligament forms to connect the tooth to the jaw bone. None of the deciduous or primary teeth are impeded by covering bone and lengthening of the root causes the crowns to erupt in sequence from six

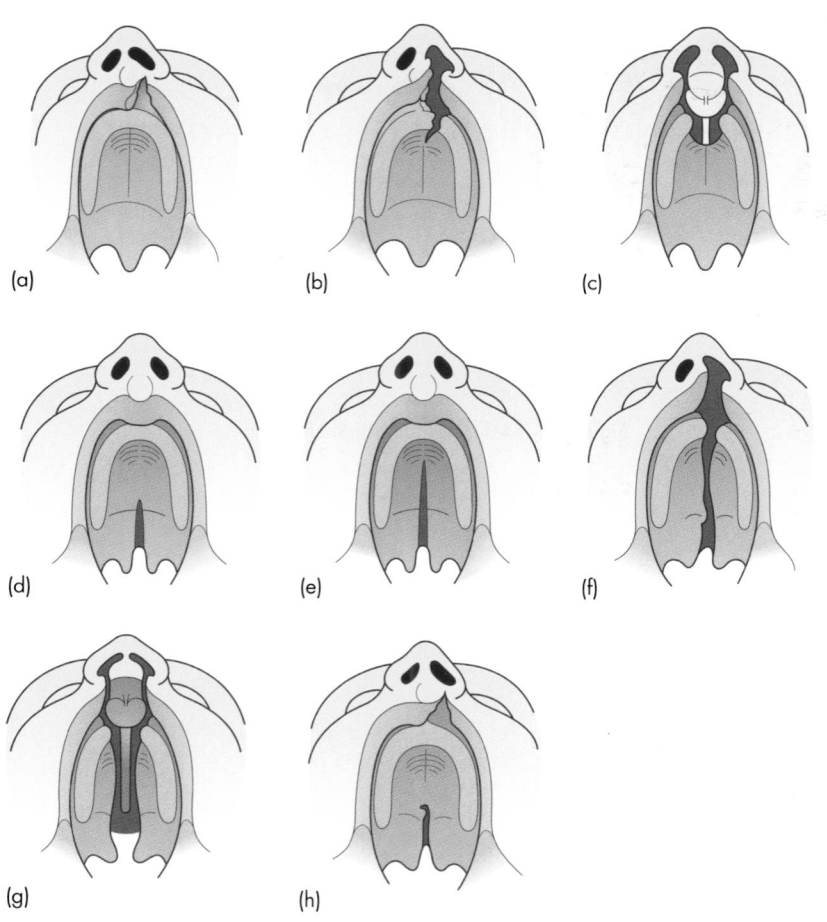

Figure 65.10 Kernahan and Stark classification of cleft lip and palate. **(a)** Group A, incomplete unilateral cleft of primary palate; **(b)** group B, complete unilateral cleft of primary palate; **(c)** group C, complete bilateral cleft of primary palate; **(d)** group D, incomplete midline cleft of secondary palate; **(e)** group E, complete midline cleft of primary and secondary palates; **(f)** group F, complete unilateral cleft of primary and secondary palates; **(g)** group G, complete bilateral clefts of primary and secondary palates; **(h)** group H, cleft of primary palate and incomplete cleft of secondary palate.

to 24 months after birth.[20] The permanent tooth buds remain dormant until the age of six years when they grow, pushing the deciduous teeth up and out.

Tongue

Two lateral lingual swellings from the first pharyngeal arch fuse with the midline tuberculum impar to form the anterior two-thirds of the tongue. In the posterior third, the third branchial arch overgrows the second. The V-shaped sulcus terminalis separates these regions with its apex at the foramen caecum from which the thyroid gland originates. General sensation to the anterior two-thirds of the tongue is from the lingual branch of the mandibular (V) nerve and taste from the chorda tympani branch of the facial (VII) nerve, while both taste and sensation to the posterior third are from the glossopharyngeal (IX) nerve. However, the glossopharyngeal nerve supplies taste and sensation to the vallate papillae anterior to the sulcus (**Figure 65.15**). Behind the posterior third lie the valleculae and epiglottis, fourth arch derivatives innervated by the superior laryngeal nerve from the vagus (X). The musculature is derived from four occipital somites innervated by the hypoglossal (XII) nerve.

Oropharynx and oesophagus

The formation of an oesophagotracheal septum divides the foregut into a respiratory diverticulum anteriorly and the oesophagus posteriorly (**Figure 65.16**). The oesophagus descends with the heart and septum transversum and so is lengthened. It is lined by endoderm which changes from stratified columnar in the embryo, to cuboidal and then to stratified squamous by birth, although ectopic gastric muscosa may also be present. The surrounding mesoderm gives rise to a muscular coat that is striated in its upper two thirds, innervated by the nucleus ambiguus of the vagus (X), and smooth in its lower two thirds and innervated by the dorsal nucleus of the vagus (X), via the oesophageal plexus.[6] Peristalsis is immature at birth along the oesophagus and at the lower oesophageal sphincter, permitting regurgitation of food.

Deviation of the oesophagotracheal septum may give rise to oesophageal atresia and/or tracheooesophageal fistula. Atresia prevents passage of amniotic fluid into the gut resulting in hydramnios, while five types of fistula may result.[2, 21, 22] The most common comprises a blind upper oesophagus with the lower oesophagus joining the trachea near its bifurcation. In the second type, there is a

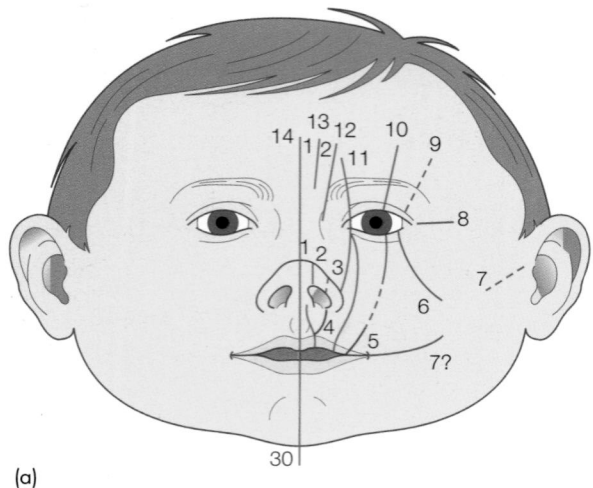

(a)

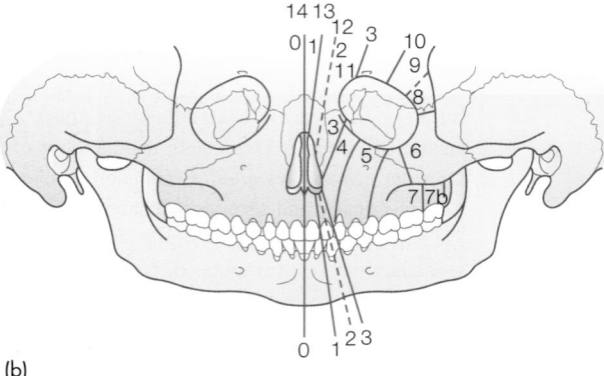

(b)

Figure 65.11 Tessier classification of craniofacial clefts. Localization of (a) soft-tissue clefts; (b) skeletal (bony) clefts. Dotted lines represent either uncertain sites or uncertain clefts.

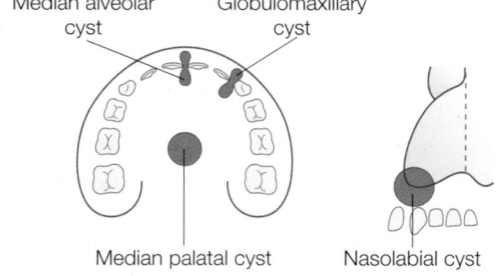

Figure 65.12 Development of cysts of the maxilla.

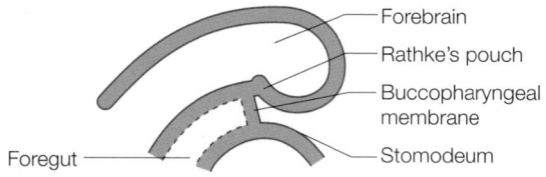

Figure 65.13 Sagittal section of human embryo showing early development of oral cavity.

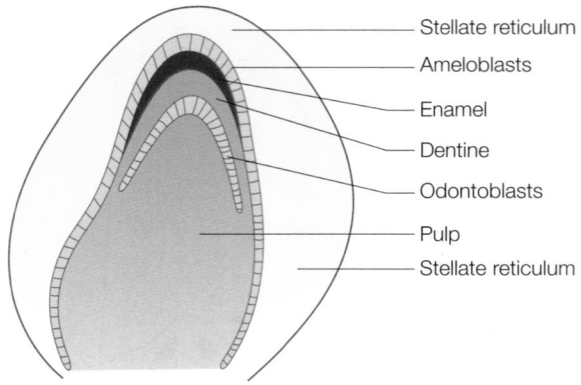

Figure 65.14 Developing human tooth.

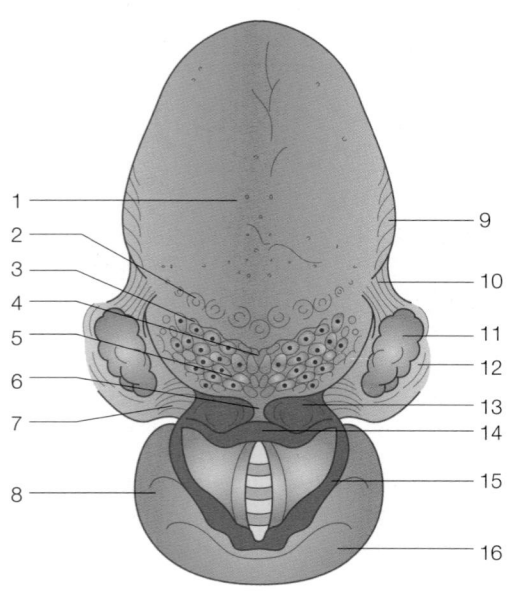

Figure 65.15 The base of tongue and valleculae from above. 1, tongue; 2, vallate papillae; 3, sulcus terminalis; 4, foramen caecum; 5, base of tongue (pharyngeal part); 6, median glossoepiglottic fold; 7, lateral glossoepiglottic fold; 8, pyriform fossa; 9, folia linguae; 10, palatoglossal fold; 11, palatine tonsil; 12, palatopharyngeal fold; 13, vallecula; 14, epiglottis; 15, aryepiglottic fold; 16, posterior pharyngeal wall.

blind upper and lower oesophagus, with no connection (fistula) to the trachea. The third type consists of a proximal tracheooesophageal fistula with a blind lower oesophagus. In the H-type abnormality, there is a proximal and a distal tracheooesophageal fistula. In the fifth type, there is a tracheooesophageal fistula without oesophageal atresia (**Figure 65.17**). Vertebral, anal, tracheooesophageal and radial (VATER) abnormalities are frequently found in the same individual – a VATER association (see Chapter 101, Diseases of oesophagus, swallowing disorders and caustic ingestion).[1]

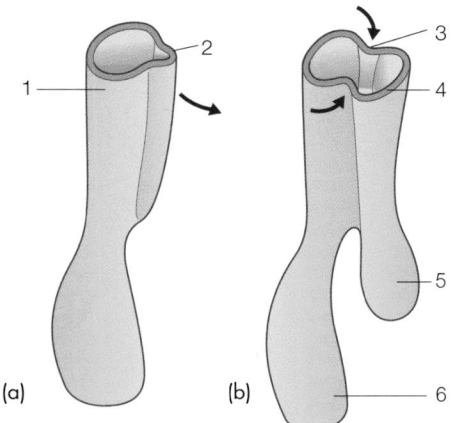

Figure 65.16 The development of the tracheobronchial (respiratory) diverticulum and oesophagus. (a) Laryngotracheal groove appearing in the ventral aspect of the foregut. (b) The lips of the groove closing in to form the oesophagotracheal septum separating the respiratory tract from the alimentary canal. 1, foregut; 2, laryngotracheal groove; 3, oesophagotracheal septum; 4, trachea; 5, lung bud; 6, stomach.

NOSE AND PARANASAL SINUSES

The development of the medial and lateral nasal prominences causes the deepening of the nasal pits which open into the stomodeum between medial and lateral nasal processes (**Figure 65.8**). The nasal pits deepen to form nasal sacs which open at the anterior nares and will form the nasal cavities (see Figure 104.1 in Chapter 104, Anatomy of the nose and paranasal sinuses). Posteriorly, the medial and lateral nasal processes fuse to form a nasal fin of epithelium which then regresses to leave the oronasal membrane caudally.[23] The development of the primary palate (premaxilla) and secondary palate, from the maxillary shelves, separates the oral and nasal cavities. Rupture of the oronasal membrane enables the nasal sac to communicate with the oropharynyngeal cavity via the primary choanae. The definitive posterior choanae will lie further posteriorly due to palatal growth. Unilateral or bilateral choanal atresia may be due to persistence of the oronasal membrane or due to persistence of epithelial cells which normally plug the nasal cavity during the embryonic period (see (see Chapter 82, Nasal obstruction in children).[23, 24]

A midline ridge develops from the posterior edge of the frontonasal prominence in the roof of the nasal cavity and extends posteriorly to the adenohypophyseal (Rathke's) pouch, which ascends from the roof of the oral cavity to form part of the pituitary gland (see Figure 104.4 in Chapter 104 Anatomy of the nose and paranasal sinuses). Anteriorly, the septum is grooved forming the vomeronasal organ, which becomes a blind, tubular pouch 2–6 mm in length, involved in the sensation of pheromones.[1] The primitive septum is initially made

entirely of cartilage. The superior part ossifies to form the perpendicular plate of the ethmoid. Posteroinferiorly, the vomer ossifies from two centres on either side of the cartilage leaving two bony alae. The remaining septal cartilage is quadrilateral and lies anteroinferiorly, surmounted by the two nasal bones.

Conchal cushions appear on the lateral walls of the nasal cavity and fuse to form the conchae or turbinate bones. The superior and middle conchae originate with the ethmoid bone, while a supreme concha is present in up to one-third of cases. The inferior concha may be regarded as a separate bone, but functionally is a detached piece of the ethmoid.[4] A depression or meatus develops beneath each concha and diverticula from these form the paranasal sinuses. The maxillary sinus arises from the middle meatus at the beginning of the foetal period, but most expansion develops after birth with development of the middle third of the face and eruption of the secondary dentition. A few ethmoid cells are present at birth and the frontal sinus, an enlarged anterior ethmoid air cell, invades the frontal bone after birth, while the sphenoid develops during childhood (**Figure 65.18**). The nasolacrimal duct appears along, but independently of, the border of the maxillary and frontonasal prominences to drain into the inferior meatus of the nose.

The frontal prominence gives rise to the bridge and septum of the nose, the fused medial nasal processes form the bridge and tip, while the alae are derived from the lateral nasal processes. Agenesis, clefting, duplication of the nose and supernumerary nostrils are anomalies of embryological development.[25]

LARYNX

The respiratory system develops as a ventral outgrowth of the foregut and grows caudally, on a lengthening stalk.[26] The cephalic end of the stalk develops into the glottis and infraglottis, and the rest becomes the trachea. Above the respiratory diverticulum, pharyngeal mesoderm compresses the foregut lumen ventrodorsally as far cranially as the fourth pharyngeal pouches, forming an epithelial lamina with a narrow pharyngoglottic duct along its dorsal border. This mesoderm also raises an epiglottic and two arytenoid swellings in the pharyngeal floor at the level of the fourth pouches. The triangular laryngeal caecum is bounded by these swellings and grows caudally between the lamina and epiglottis. The epithelial lamina separates cephalocaudally, connecting the laryngeal caecum with the pharyngoglottic duct to form the laryngeal vestibule; when the separation is complete, the vestibule is continuous with the infraglottic cavity.[27] However, incomplete separation gives rise to congenital laryngeal webs (see Chapter 88, Congenital disorders of the larynx, trachea and bronchi).[28] Meanwhile, bilateral pouches arising from the caudal end of the caecum form the

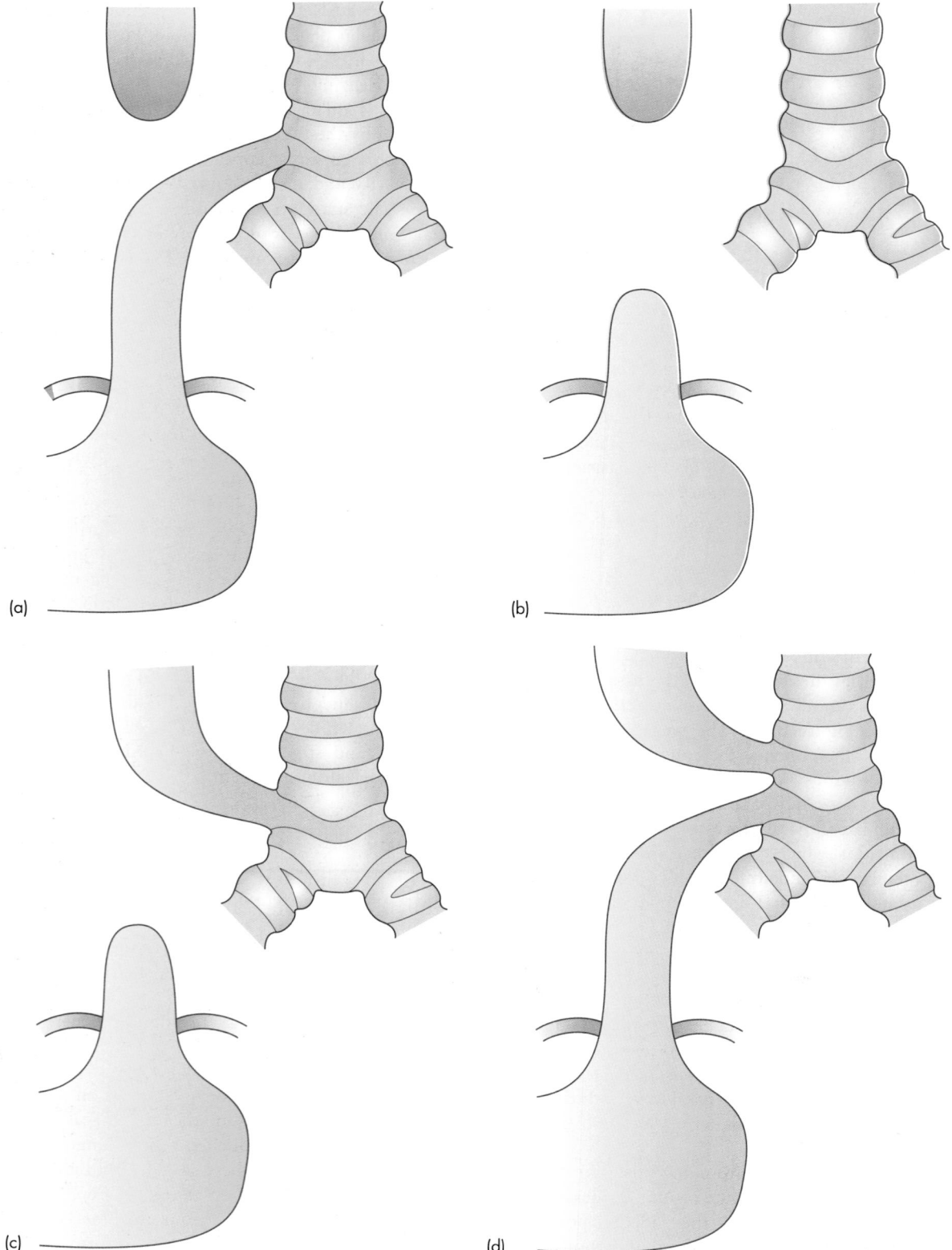

Figure 65.17 Types of oesophageal atresia. **(a)** Oesophageal atresia with distal trachaeooesophageal fistula, 87 percent; **(b)** oesophageal atresia without distal trachaeooesophageal fistula, 6–7 percent; **(c)** oesophageal atresia with proximal trachaeooesophageal fistula, 2 percent; **(d)** oesophageal atresia with proximal and distal trachaeooesophageal fistula, <1 percent (continued over).

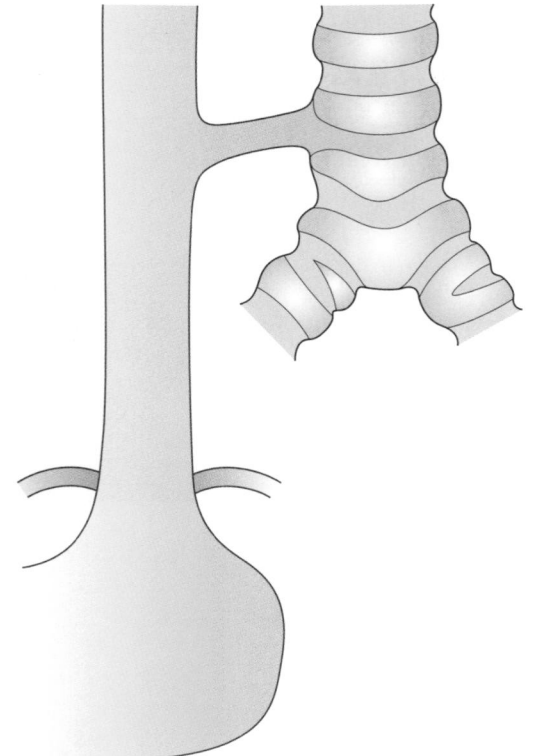

(e)

Figure 65.17 Types of oesophageal atresia (continued). **(e)** trachaeooesophageal fistula without oesophageal atresia, 3–4 percent.

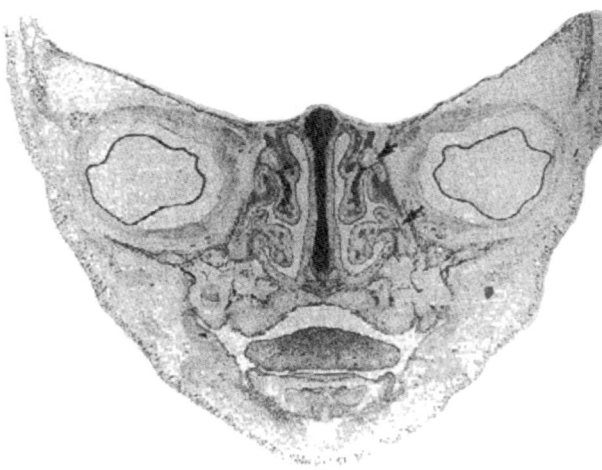

Figure 65.18 Coronal section through the head of a 150-mm human foetus, showing early cavitation of maxillary sinus and ethmoids (arrowed).

ventricles, the lower lips of which become the vocal folds. The vestibule and ventricles receive sensory innervation from the internal branch of the superior laryngeal nerve of the fourth arch, while sensation to the infraglottic larynx is from the recurrent laryngeal nerve of the sixth arch. Motor supply is from the recurrent laryngeal nerve, with the exception of cricothyroid muscle which is supplied by the external branch of the superior laryngeal nerve.

Pharyngeal mesoderm surrounding the laryngeal cavity gives rise to the laryngeal cartilages and intrinsic musculature. The laryngeal cartilages are derived from the fourth and sixth pharyngeal arches. The cricoid chondrifies bilaterally from a single centre in the ventral arch of a precartilaginous template which encircles the infraglottic cavity, and on meeting forms the dorsal lamina. Each arytenoid chondrifies from a single centre and each lamina of the thyroid cartilage chondrifies from two.[27, 28] At birth, the epiglottis is close to the soft palate and apposition of the two structures can close off the oral cavity, so protecting the airway during suckling when breathing and drinking occur simultaneously.[1]

THYROID GLAND

A diverticulum develops behind the tuberculum impar of the tongue and descends anterior to the pharynx and hyoid bone. It then ascends deep to the hyoid and descends again anterior to the thyroid and cricoid cartilages to the level of the upper tracheal rings and expands to form lateral lobes connected by a central isthmus. Epithelial cells develop into thyroid follicles, with hormone synthesis beginning early in the foetal period.[1] The ultimobranchial body from the fourth or fifth pharyngeal pouch provides parafollicular cells which secrete calcitonin.

The descent of the thyroid is marked by the thyroglossal duct which connects the gland to the foramen caecum. It is divided into suprahyoid and infrahyoid portions by the growth of the hyoid bone from the second and third pharyngeal arches. The duct usually atrophies but may persist as a fibrous cord or as a tube.[8] Thyroglossal cysts may develop along its course, usually median in position (**Figures 65.19** and **65.20**), which move on swallowing and protrusion of the tongue.[29]

A small or absent thyroid results in congenital cretinism (see Chapter 99, Branchial arch fistulae, thryoglossal duct anomalies and lymphangioma). Failure of normal descent may result in a lingual thyroid, causing dysphagia or it may be sublingual, prelaryngeal or suprasternal. Between the isthmus and hyoid bone a pyramidal lobe or a fibromuscular band, the levator glandulae thyroidea, may be found.[6] The isthmus, or one lobe, may be absent.[29] More than half of abnormal neck masses are of thyroid origin.[1] Accessory thyroid tissue may be found in the neck, thymus, mediastinum, heart, trachea, oesophagus or liver, due to attachment to an adjacent organ and also, as part of a teratoid tumour, in the ovary.[1]

EAR

The internal, middle and external ear each have a different origin.

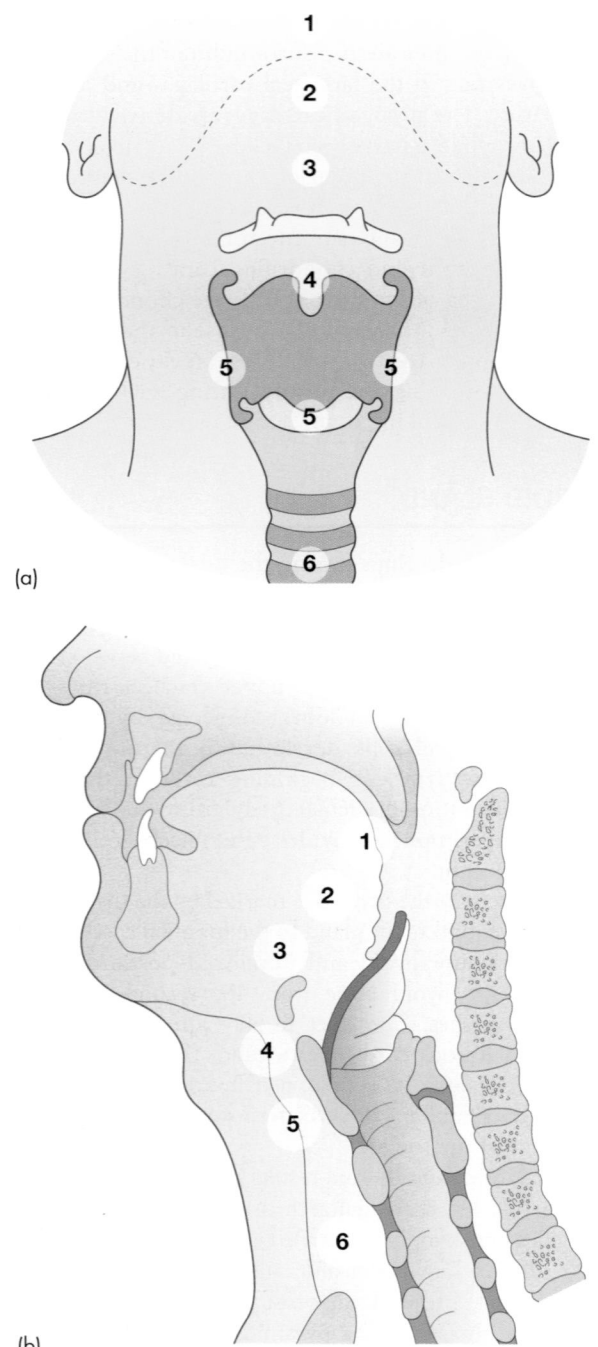

(a)

(b)

Figure 65.19 Possible sites of thyroglossal cysts. 1, Base of tongue; 2, intralingual; 3, suprahyoid; 4, infrahyoid; 5, prethyroid; 6, pretracheal.

Internal ear

Ectoderm over the hindbrain thickens to form otic discs (placodes) which invaginate to form pits and then separate from the surface to form otocysts (**Figure 65.21**).

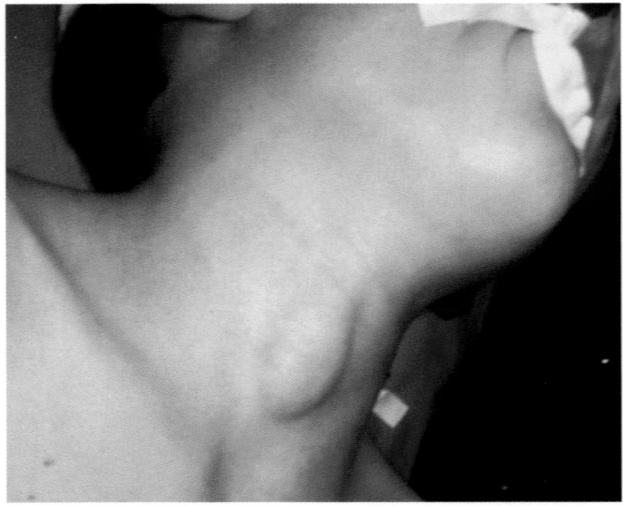

Figure 65.20 Midline thyroglossal cyst.

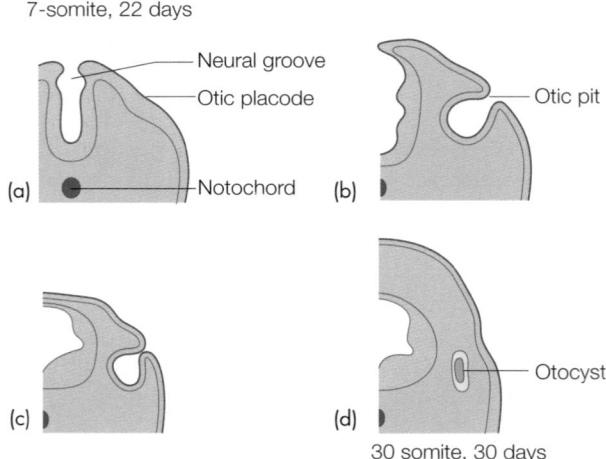

7-somite, 22 days

Neural groove
Otic placode

(a)

Notochord

Otic pit

(b)

(c)

(d)

Otocyst

30 somite, 30 days

Figure 65.21 Diagram to represent the development of the otocyst from the otic placode, which in turn is derived from the ectoderm cranial to the first occipital somite. During the seven days of its development, the neural groove has also become converted into the future brain stem.

Each otocyst subsequently divides into a ventral part, which gives rise to the saccule and cochlear duct, and a dorsal part which forms the utricle, semicircular canals and endolymphatic duct (**Figure 65.22**). These epithelial derivatives are collectively termed the membranous labyrinth. Neural crest cells migrate away from the developing otocyst to form the statoacoustic ganglion from which the vestibulocochlear nerve is derived.[2]

The cochlear duct develops as an outpouching of the saccule and penetrates the surrounding mesenchyme in a spiral fashion forming 2.5 turns. The ductus reuniens connects the saccule and cochlea. This mesenchyme

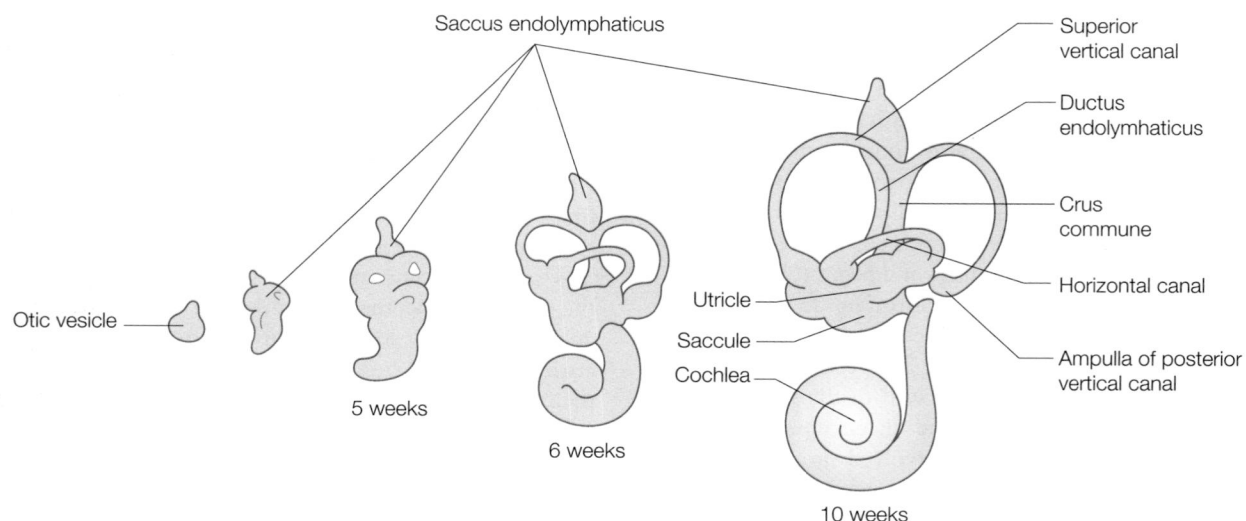

Figure 65.22 Development of the membranous labyrinth from the otocyst. This rapid and complex change occurs over a six-week period.

differentiates into cartilage which then vacuolizes to form two perilymphatic spaces, the scala vestibuli and scala tympani, around the cochlear duct or scala media. The vestibular membrane separates the duct from the scala vestibuli, while the basilar membrane separates the duct from the scala tympani (**Figure 65.23**). An inner sulcus divides the epithelial cells of the cochlear duct into an inner ridge, the future spiral limbus, and an outer ridge. The outer ridge forms one row of inner and three to four rows of outer cells, separated by the tunnel of Corti. On either side of the tunnel, pillar cells give mechanical rigidity, while the sensory cells develop a cluster of

stereocilia and are termed hair cells. These are covered by the tectorial membrane which extends from the spiral limbus. The hair cells and tectorial membrane comprise the organ of Corti which transmits sensory impulses to the spiral ganglion and then, via the cochlear fibres of the vestibulocochlear (VIII) nerve, to the brain. Differentiation proceeds in the basal to apical direction as the duct elongates.

The dorsal part of the otocyst flattens and outpouchings appear to form semicircular canals. The walls between adjacent canals resorb to give rise to three canals – superior, posterior and lateral – emerging from the utricle. One end of each canal dilates to form a crus ampullare in which a fibrogelatinous cupola develops. The crus nonampullare of the lateral canal persists, while those of the superior and posterior canals fuse to form the crus commune nonampullare. In each ampulla, sensory cells form a crest or crista ampullaris. Similar sensory areas, the maculae, develop in areas where vestibular fibres of the vestibulocochlear (VIII) nerve enter the walls of the utricle and saccule. Two cell types differentiate; sensory cells with a single kinocilium and many stereocilia and supporting cells which produce a gelatinous matrix and are responsible for the formation of otoconia.[30]

Congenital malformations of the inner ear ranging from complete cochlear aplasia to incomplete partition of the cochlea, first described by Mondini in 1791, are reviewed by Graham et al.[31]

Middle ear

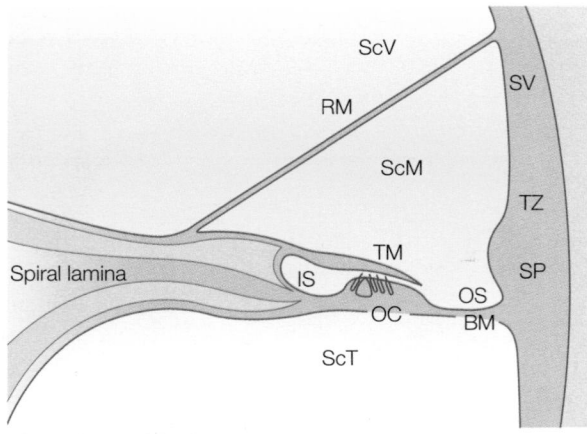

Figure 65.23 Diagram illustrating the structures and relationship of the cochlear duct. BM, basilar membrane; IS, inner sulcus; OC, organ of Corti; OS, outer sulcus; RM, Reissner's membrane; ScM, scala media; ScT, scala tympani; ScV, scala vestibuli; SP, spiral prominence; SV, stria vascularis; TM, tectorial membrane; TZ, transitional zone. Yellow areas show bone.

As the first pharyngeal pouch grows laterally to meet the floor of the first pharyngeal cleft, the ossicles and tympanic branch of the facial (VII) nerve develop in mesenchyme between them. The proximal part of the pouch forms the narrow auditory or Eustachian tube, while its distal part widens to form the tubotympanic recess which gives rise to the primitive tympanic cavity. Cleft ectodem, mesenchyme and pouch endoderm form the three layers of the future tympanic membrane, with the handle of the malleus embedded in it, traversed by the chorda tympani. The malleus and incus are derived from the first pharyngeal arch cartilage and begin to ossify at 16 weeks, reaching adult size and form by 25 weeks. The stapes is derived from the second arch (Reichert's) cartilage and begins to ossify at 18 weeks. The base of the stapes appears in the lateral wall of the otic capsule, surrounding the otocyst, where it occupies the oval window, and hence may be involved in otosclerosis. Rarely the stapedial artery, passing between the crura, may persist. The ossicular ligaments develop within endodermal reflections connecting the ossicles to the walls of the tympanic cavity. The tensor tympani, attached to the malleus, and stapedius, attached to the stapes, are supplied by the mandibular and facial nerves, respectively. The middle ear reaches adult size before birth.[1] Epithelium of the tubotympanic recess invades the mastoid process to form the antrum and, postnatally, the mastoid air cells.

Type 1 malformations of the middle ear are due to abnormal development of the ring surrounding the tympanic membrane. In type 2 malformations, the space between the mandibular fossa and the front of the mastoid process is absent, resulting in an abnormal course of the facial (VII) nerve which may be associated with cochlear malformations.[1, 31] Evolutionary and mechanical influences on middle ear development are discussed by Prendergast.[32]

Temporal bone

The temporal bone is composed of four parts: petromastoid, styloid, squamous and tympanic.[4] The petromastoid originates from the capsule surrounding the otocyst and progresses from mesenchyme to cartilage to bone. It gives rise to the petrous which encloses the bony labyrinth, the tegmen tympani which roofs the tympanic cavity, and forms the mastoid process at one to two years after birth. The styloid process is derived from the second pharyngeal arch cartilage. The squamous part ossifies intramembranously and includes the mandibular fossa and zygomatic process. The tympanic part may be derived from the first pharyngeal arch and develops as an incomplete bony ring which unites with the squamous part before birth at the squamotympanic fissure.[1] The tegmen separates them in part and first arch derivatives pass through the petrotympanic fissure to the spine of the sphenoid and then, as the sphenomandibular ligament, to the lingula of the mandible.

External ear

The external auditory meatus develops from the dorsal portion of the first pharyngeal cleft and canalizes from medial to lateral. Epithelial cells proliferate to form a meatal plug which may persist after birth causing conductive deafness. Auricular hillocks, three from the first and three from the second pharyngeal arch, surround the cleft below the level of the mandible. As they ascend, some mandibular hillocks contribute to the tragus, while the remainder form the bulk of the auricle (**Figure 65.24**), but abnormalities such as auricular appendages and fistulae are common (**Figure 65.25**). Congenital malformations of the ear are often features of common chromosomal syndromes, such as Trisomy 18, Trisomy 21, Fragile X and Treacher Collins syndrome.[2]

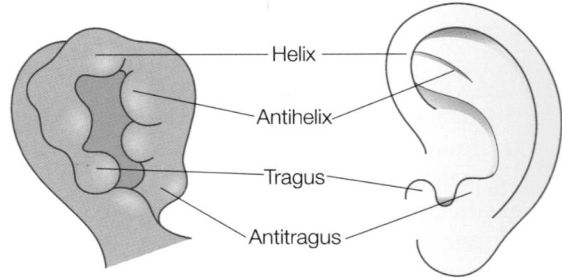

Figure 65.24 Early stages in the development of the auricle. Six cartilaginous hillocks are visible around the first pharyngeal groove. During subsequent development these become the cartilage of the auricle, although the bulk of the auricle appears to be derived from the cartilage of the second arch.

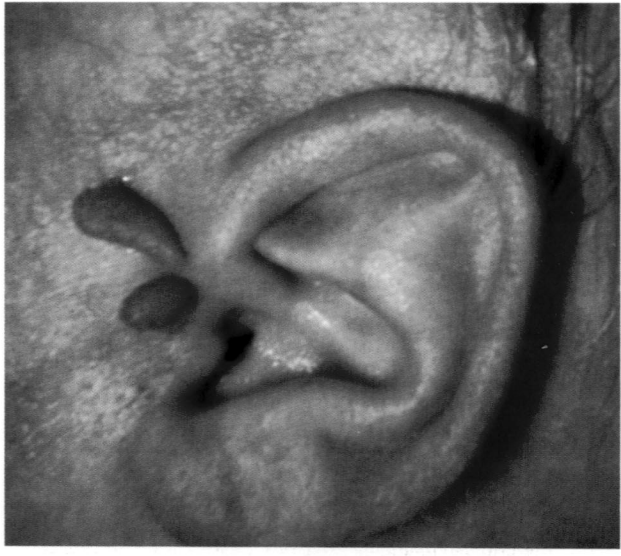

Figure 65.25 Accessory auricle in an infant.

KEY POINTS

- Major organ systems are established during the embryonic period, weeks 3–8.
- Pharyngeal arch, pouch and cleft development explain motor and sensory innervations and common abnormalities.
- Palatogenesis explains most craniofacial clefting.
- Recent advances in laryngeal embryology correlate well with clinical data.
- Thyroglossal duct cysts are the most common congenital cervical abnormality.
- Ear abnormalities are commonly associated with chromosomal syndromes.

Deficiencies in current knowledge and areas for further research

Morphological descriptions of embryological development are well established.[2, 9, 15, 17, 18, 27, 28, 29, 30] The underlying genetic and molecular mechanisms are now beginning to be understood.[5, 10, 12, 19] Detection of molecular markers may lead to earlier and more effective intervention while increased understanding of mesenchymal stem cell and matrix interactions offer the prospect of tissue engineered replacement surgery within the next five years. By clearly understanding the mechanisms by which organs develop, the effects of teratogens may be predicted and birth defects avoided.

ACKNOWLEDGEMENTS

I would like to thank my colleagues, Professor EJ Guiney, Professor MJ Ryan and Professor BE McCartan, for providing illustrations and for their helpful comments on the text.

REFERENCES

1. O'Rahilly R, Muller F. *Human embryology and teratology*, 3rd edn. New York: Wiley-Liss, 2001.
2. Sadler TW. *Langman's medical embryology*, 8th edn. Philadelphia: Lippincott Williams & Wilkins, 2000.
3. Hobbs CA, Cleves MA, Simmons CJ. Genetic epidemiology and congenital malformations: from the chromosome to the crib. *Archives of Pediatrics and Adolescent Medicine*. 2002; **156**: 315–20.
4. Scheuer L, Black S. *Developmental juvenile osteology*. San Diego: Academic Press, 2000.
* 5. Wilkie AO, Morriss-Kay GM. Genetics of craniofacial development and malformation. *Nature Reviews Genetics*. 2001; **2**: 458–68. *This combines embryology, evolution and mouse genetics to describe head development and explain skull vault and pharyngeal arch malformations and clefting.*
6. Standring S (ed.) *Gray's anatomy*, 39th edn. Edinburgh: Churchill Livingstone, 2005.
7. Davenport M. ABC of general surgery in children. Lumps and swellings of the head and neck. *British Medical Journal*. 1996; **312**: 368–71.
8. Ellis PDM. Branchial cleft anomalies, thyroglossal cysts and fistulae. In: Kerr AG (ed.). *Scott-Brown's otolaryngology*, 6th edn. Oxford: Butterworth-Heinemann, 1997: 6.30.1–6.30.13.
9. Hinrichsen K. The early development of morphology and patterns of the face in the human embryo. *Advances in Anatomy, Embryology and Cell Biology*. 1985; **98**: 1–79.
* 10. Kerrigan JJ, Mansell JP, Sengupta A, Brown N, Sandy JR. Palatogenesis and potential mechanisms for clefting. *Journal of the Royal College of Surgeons of Edinburgh*. 2000; **45**: 351–8. *A comprehensive review of the molecular and morphological mechanisms involved in palate formation and the vulnerable points which may lead to clefting.*
11. Ferguson MWJ. Palate development: Mechanisms and malformations. *Irish Journal of Medical Science*. 1987; **156**: 309–15.
12. Sandy JR. Molecular, clinical and political approaches to the problem of cleft lip palate. *The Surgeon, Journal of the Royal Colleges of Surgeons of Edinburgh and Ireland*. 2003; **1**: 9–16.
13. Summerfield Kung T. The anatomy of hare-lip in man. *Journal of Anatomy*. 1954; **88**: 1–12.
14. Kernahan DA, Stark RB. A new classification for cleft lip and palate. *Plastic and Reconstructive Surgery*. 1958; **22**: 435–41.
15. Tessier P. Anatomical classification of facial, cranio-facial and latero-facial clefts. *Journal of Maxillofacial Surgery*. 1976; **4**: 69–92.
16. Denny PC, Ball WD, Redman RS. Salivary glands: A paradigm for diversity of gland development. *Critical Reviews in Oral Biology and Medicine*. 1997; **8**: 51–75.
17. Guizetti B, Radlanski RJ. Development of the submandibular gland and its closer neighboring structures in human embryos and fetuses of 19–67 mm CRL. *Anatomischer Anzeiger*. 1996; **178**: 509–14.
18. Guizetti B, Radlanski RJ. Development of the parotid gland and its closer neighboring structures in human embryos and fetuses of 19–67 mm CRL. *Anatomischer Anzeiger*. 1996; **178**: 503–8.
19. Tucker AS, Sharpe PT. Molecular genetics of tooth morphogenesis and patterning: The right shape in the right place. *Journal of Dental Research*. 1999; **78**: 826–34.

20. Ranly DM. Early orofacial development. *Journal of Clinical Pediatric Dentistry.* 1998; **22**: 267–75.

21. Mansfield LE. Embryonic origins of the relation of gastroesophageal reflux disease and airway disease. *American Journal of Medicine.* 2001; **111**: 3S–7S.

22. Spitz L. Diseases of the oesophagus. In: Kerr AG (ed.). *Scott-Brown's otolaryngology*, 6th edn. Oxford: Butterworth-Heinemann, 1997: 6.29.1–6.29.5.

23. Lund VJ. Anatomy of the nose and paranasal sinuses. In: Kerr AG (ed.). *Scott-Brown's otolaryngology*, 6th edn. Oxford: Butterworth-Heinemann, 1997: 1.5.1–1.5.7.

24. Keller JL, Kacker A. Choanal atresia, CHARGE association and congenital nasal stenosis. *Otolaryngologic Clinics of North America.* 2000; **33**: 1343–51.

25. Williams A, Pizzuto M, Brodsky L, Perry R. Supernumerary nostril: A rare congenital deformity. *International Journal of Pediatric Otorhinolaryngology.* 1998; **44**: 161–7.

26. O'Rahilly R, Muller F. Chevalier Jackson lecture. Respiratory and alimentary relations in staged human embryos. New embryological data and congenital anomalies. *Annals of Otology, Rhinology and Laryngology.* 1984; **93**: 421–9.

27. Zaw-Tun HA, Burdi AR. Reexamination of the origin and early development of the human larynx. *Acta Anatomica.* 1985; **122**: 163–84.

* 28. Milczuk HA, Smith JD, Everts EC. Congenital laryngeal web: Surgical management and clinical embryology. *International Journal of Pediatric Otorhinolaryngology.* 2000; **52**: 1–9. *This illustrates and summarizes recent advances in laryngeal embryology which explain web formation and applies this knowledge to the surgical management of five cases.*

* 29. Organ GM, Organ Jr. CH. Thyroid gland and surgery of the thyroglossal duct: Exercise in applied embryology. *World Journal of Surgery.* 2000; **24**: 886–90. *A review of thyroid and thyroglossal duct embryology, explaining the rationale behind their surgical management in general and the Sistrunk operation in particular.*

30. Wright A. Anatomy and ultrastructure of the human ear. In: Kerr AG (ed.). *Scott-Brown's otolaryngology*, 6th edn. Oxford: Butterworth-Heinemann, 1997: 1.1.1–1.1.11.

* 31. Graham JM, Phelps PD, Michaels L. Congenital malformations of the ear and cochlear implantation in children: Review and temporal bone report of common cavity. *Journal of Laryngology and Otology.* 2000; **114**: 1–14. *A review of the development of the inner, middle and outer ears and the practical aspects of congenital malformations in cochlear implant surgery.*

32. Prendergast PJ. Mechanics applied to skeletal ontogeny and phylogeny. *Meccanica.* 2002; **37**: 317–34.

66

Molecular otology, development of the auditory system and recent advances in genetic manipulation

HENRY PAU

Introduction	811	Key points	818
The development of the ear	813	Deficiencies in current knowledge and areas for future research	819
Recent advances in genetic manipulation in the treatment of congenital deafness	817	References	819

SEARCH STRATEGY

The following databases were consulted: OMIM, PubMed, Web of Science, MedlinePlus, Hereditary Hearing Loss homepage http://webhost.ua.ac.be/hhh/ using the key words congenital deafness, gene therapy and auditory development.

INTRODUCTION

Table 66.1 provides a glossary of terms used in genetics.

Types of deafness

Deafness is a common childhood problem. Serious hearing impairment is found in one in 800 newborns.[1] Abnormal genetic make up accounts for approximately 50 percent of permanent childhood deafness.[2] In addition, several genes have been found that, when mutated, either cause or predispose to progressive hearing loss,[3] suggesting that this type of deafness may also have a significant genetic basis. Genetic deafness, therefore, poses a problem both at birth and later in life. It is therefore important to identify the mutated genes involved and to understand the ear pathology caused by these defective genes.

Deafness can be broadly categorized into **syndromic** (deafness associated with other symptoms) or **nonsyndromic** (deafness associated with no other symptoms). Many more loci have been found for syndromic deafness than nonsyndromic deafness, despite the fact that these make up the minority of all inherited deafness cases (about 30 percent of deafness is thought to be syndromic). This is likely due to the fact that syndromic cases of deafness are more accurately diagnosed due to the additional features of the syndromes.

Nonsyndromic types of deafness are classified on the basis of the mode of inheritance as follows: DFNA (autosomal dominant), DFNB (autosomal recessive) and DFN (X-linked forms). At present, 39 DFNB, 51 DFNA, eight DFN, one modifier DFNM1[4] and two mitochondrial loci (regions on the mitochondrial chromosome) have been identified,[5] and 36 causative genes have been reported (**Table 66.2**).[5, 6]

Clinically, deafness is generally categorized on the basis of which auditory structures are affected. Conductive deafness refers to defects found in the outer or middle ear, whereas sensorineural hearing loss (SNHL) refers to disruptions in the sound transmission from the inner ear to the cortex of the brain. Most SNHL is due to abnormalities at the level of the inner ear. Inner ear pathology is further categorized into three groups: **morphogenetic**, **cochleosaccular** and **neuroepithelial**.[7]

Table 66.1 Glossary of terms used in genetics.

Term	Name	Explanation
Autosomal dominant gene	DFNA	A single, abnormal gene on one of the autosomal chromosomes (one of the first 22 'non-sex' chromosomes) from either parent can cause certain diseases. One of the parents will usually have the disease (since it is dominant) in this mode of inheritance. Only one parent must have an abnormal gene in order for the child to inherit the disease.
Autosomal recessive gene	DFNB	An abnormal gene on one of the autosomal chromosomes (one of the first 22 'non-sex' chromosomes) from each parent is required to cause the disease. People with only one abnormal gene in the gene pair are called carriers, but since the gene is recessive they do not exhibit the disease. The normal gene of the pair can supply the function of the gene so that the abnormal gene is described as acting in a recessive manner. Both parents must be carriers in order for a child to have symptoms of the disease; a child who inherits the gene from one parent will be a carrier.
Genotype		The genetic composition of an organism
Genetic 'mapping'		Technique employed to identify gene by using primers (manufactured genetic markers)
Gene transfer		Transfer of certain genes using vectors, such as viruses
Linkage analysis		Similar technique to genetic mapping in gene identification by using primers
Locus		A region on a chromosome
Modifier genes	DFNM1	Genes that do not cause disease but have the ability to influence the expression of other genes resulting in abnormalities
Mutation		Abnormalities caused by alteration of genome
Phenotype		The physical appearance of an organism
Transfer 'vector'		A carrier employed to enter and introduce genetic materials into a cell, e.g. a virus
Transgenesis		The insertion or deletion of a gene at the embryonic stage of development resulting in different phenotypes
X-linked	DFN	Genes that can only be inherited from the maternal side, e.g. mitochondrial genes

Morphogenetic defects, characterized by abnormal development of the ear leading to a malformation, only occur in 15–20 percent of profoundly deaf humans.[8] This is because important morphogenetic genes are often involved in diverse development processes and mutations in these genes are likely to lead to antenatal death. Cochleosaccular refers to abnormalities in the stria vascularis, which regulates the ionic balance of the endolymph. The third and probably the most common type of inner ear pathology, neuroepithelial, is caused by defects in the organ of Corti, in which the hair cells responsible for the first step of the pathway of transducing sound information to neural code are situated.[8]

Using mouse mutants in understanding human genetic deafness

Identifying the gene that causes a particular type of deafness involves, first of all, localizing the mutation to a specific region of a chromosome (genetic mapping). In human populations, this process is confused by the fact that many types of deafness, particularly nonsyndromic forms, are difficult to diagnose as there are few defining features. To minimize grouping cases of deafness together in which the causative gene may be different, genetic

mapping must be done either in large consanguineous families or in populations that have been isolated from immigration.[9] To a certain degree, this approach has been successful in that researchers have been able to localize over 100 nonsyndromic forms of deafness.[5] However, the step between localizing the gene to a region of the chromosome and actually identifying the mutated gene is a large and difficult one.

The mouse appears to be the best model for understanding genetic hearing and balance defects in humans for several reasons. Firstly, because large numbers of mice which all carry the same mutation can be produced, the region of the chromosome in which the mutation is located can be more specifically pinpointed than in humans, making the mouse a powerful tool for gene identification. Due to genomic conservation between mice and humans, the mutated genes can be positioned and identified in the mouse and the homologous human genes can be identified and sequenced for possible mutations. Secondly, the mouse cochlea is structurally very similar to humans in its organization and specialization. Both species have similar types of inner ear pathology, and in some cases, the orthologous (same gene, but different species) gene is involved in deafness in the two species. Thirdly, there have been recent advances in the manipulation of the mouse genome, such that it is the most appropriate vertebrate in which to perform

Table 66.2 Human syndromes with known causative genes.

Syndromes	Causative genes	Clinical features
Alport syndrome	COL4A5, COL4A3, COL4A4	Nephritis, hearing loss, lenticonus and other eye disorders, immunologic abnormality of skin, disorders of platelets, abnormalities of white blood cells, or smooth muscle tumours
Branchio-oto-renal syndrome	EYA1	Auricular pits/fistulae, blocked/absent nasolacrimal duct, branchial cleft/sinus/cysts, cleft palate, cochlear/saccular abnormalities, deafness, double ureters, facial weakness, hydronephrosis, microphthalmia, atretic auditory canal, renal agenesis/dysplasia or ectopic kidneys
Norrie syndrome	Norrin	Pseudotumour of the retina, retinal hyperplasia, hypoplasia and necrosis of the inner layer of the retina, cataracts, phthisis bulbi, progressive sensorineural hearing loss and mental disturbance
Pendred syndrome	SLC26A4	Goitre, hypothyroidism, deafness
Stickler syndrome	COL2A1, COL11A2, COL11A1	Progressive myopia, vitreoretinal degeneration, premature joint degeneration with abnormal epiphyseal development, midface hypoplasia, irregularities of the vertebral bodies, cleft palate deformity and variable sensorineural hearing loss
Treacher Collins syndrome	TCOF1	Coloboma of the lower eyelid (the upper eyelid is involved in Goldenhar syndrome), micrognathia, microtia, hypoplasia of the zygomatic arches, macrostomia and inferior displacement of the lateral canthi
Usher syndrome	MYO7A, USH1C, CDH23, PCDH15, USH2A, USH3	Hearing impairment and retinitis pigmentosa – there are at least three clinical subtypes
Pfeiffer syndrome, Kallmann syndrome, craniosynostosis	FGFR1	Craniosynostosis, ocular proptosis, mixed deafness, mid-face dysgenesis
Waardenburg syndrome	PAX3, MITF, SLUG, EDNRB, EDN3, SOX10	Dystopia canthorum (lateral displacement of the inner canthus of each eye), pigmentary abnormalities of hair, iris and skin (often white forelock and heterochromia iridis), sensorineural deafness
Jervell and Lange–Nielson	KVLQT1, KCNE1 (IsK)	Long QT syndrome and deafness
Maternally inherited diabetes and deafness (MIDD)	tRNALeu, tRNALys, tRNAGlu	Deafness, diabetes, seizures, migraines, short stature, mental retardation and stroke-like episodes
Mitochondrial encephalopathy, lactic acidosis and stroke-like episodes (MELAS)	tRNALeu	Deafness, mitochondrial myopathy, encephalopathy, lactic acidosis, and stroke-like episodes.
Myoclonic epilepsy and ragged red fibres (MERRF)	tRNALys, tRNALeu	Deafness, myoclonus, ataxia, progressive external ophthalmoplegia and seizures
Kearns–Sayre syndrome (KSS)	Several tRNA genes	Weakness of facial, pharyngeal, trunk and extremity muscles, deafness, small stature, electroencephalographic changes, markedly increased cerebrospinal fluid proteinophthalmoplegia, pigmentary degeneration of the retina and cardiomyopathy
Progressive myoclonic epilepsy, ataxia and deafness	tRNASer	Deafness, ataxia and seizures

Modified from Ref. 5.

transgenesis, a feature which can be useful in both the identification of a mutated gene as well as in the production of potential mouse models. Finally, the mouse is useful in embryological and developmental studies, and invasive physiological tests can also be performed in anaesthetized mice, which provide important clues to the basis of the dysfunction and could not be carried out in humans.

THE DEVELOPMENT OF THE EAR

The branchial apparatus

In the fourth and fifth week of development in the human embryo, five ridges develop in the side walls of the primitive pharynx (**Figure 66.1**). These ridges are known as branchial arches. Initially they consist of a mesodermal

Structurally in mice, the cochlear duct develops from a tubular out-pocketing of the ventral portion of the otocyst on embryonic day 11 (E11) and starts to coil. By embryonic day 17 (E17), it attains its mature shape of one and three-quarters turns. The organ of Corti develops from the thickened epithelial cells of the cochlear duct. This thickened area is formed of tall columnar cell mounds: the lesser and the greater epithelial ridges. It is believed that inner hair cells (IHC) derive from the greater epithelial ridge and the outer hair cells (OHC) derive from the lesser ridge. *Pax2* has been shown to be responsible for the outgrowth of the cochlea.

The main events of semicircular canal formation in a developing mouse occur between 11.5 and 13 days embryonically (E11.5–E13). From the medial aspect of the otocyst, an uncoiled tube grows out and projects dorsally. The first two semicircular canals to form, the superior and the posterior, develop from a shared pocket-shaped rudiment. This out-pocketing begins to develop from the dorsal part of the otocyst by E11.5 and shows the first signs of conversion into a pair of semicircular canals. The canals are formed by fusion of the lateral and medial epithelial surfaces of the out-pocketing and the subsequent disappearance of the fused region of epithelia. The superior canal forms first, followed closely by the posterior; the horizontal canal forms last from a separate rudiment. By E13, all the major changes that

the inner ear undergoes are complete and the inner ear labyrinth resembles a miniature replica of its adult form.[30] The utricle and its macula are derived from the upper middle third of the medial and lateral walls of the otocyst. The saccule and its macula are derived from the lower middle third of the medial wall of the otocyst (**Figure 66.3**).

Origin of the sensory organs

The inner ear houses the receptor cells for two distinct sensory pathways: the auditory and vestibular systems. Patterning of the inner ear into prospective auditory and vestibular sensory areas is associated with restricted gene expression domains during the stages of development from otic placode to otocyst. Ventromedial areas, where the putative auditory epithelium forms, express *Pax2*, *Dlx4*, *Fgf2*, *Fgf3*, *BMP4*, *notch* and *Ncam* genes. Dorsolateral areas which form vestibular epithelium express *Hmx2*, *Hmx3*, *Dlx3*, *MshC*, *MshD*, *Sox9*, *p75*, *Lmx1*, *Gbx3*, *Sek1*, *BMP7* and *Igf1* genes.[31]

Once the sensory hair cells have been specified, their continued differentiation requires transcription factor *Pou4f3*. In the absence of this gene, the hair cell phenotype aborts at an early stage, eventually leading to the death of hair cells and the supporting cells.[32]

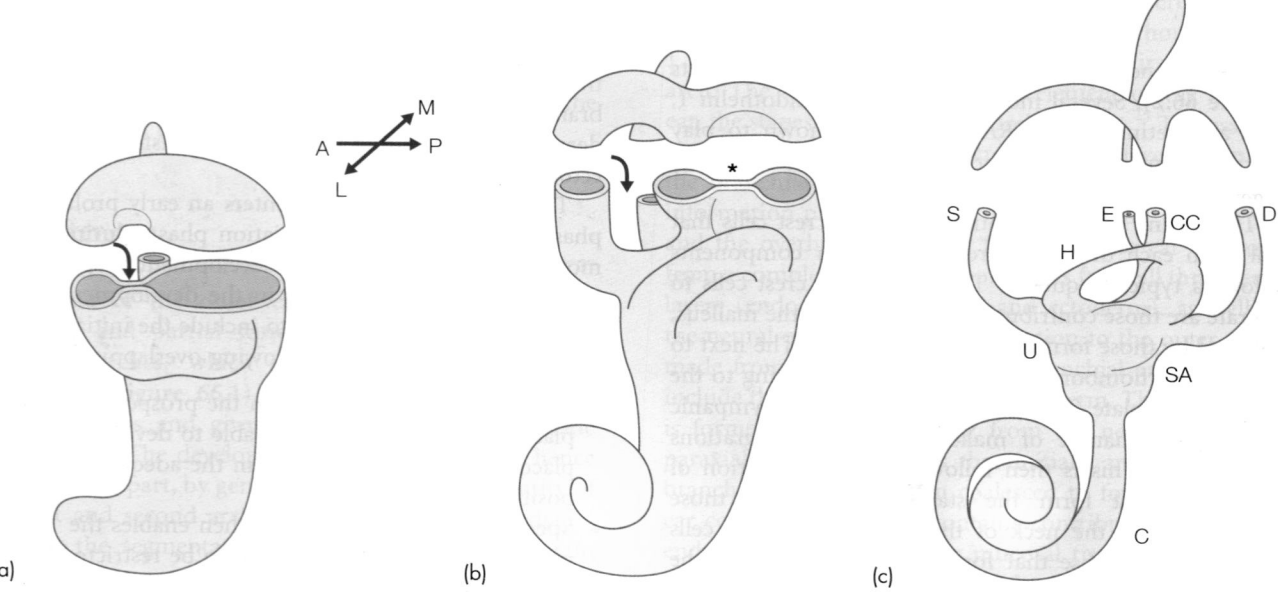

(a)   (b)   (c)

Figure 66.3 Schematic transected diagrams of inner ear morphogenesis during the period of semicircular canal development (left inner ear). (a) The walls of the canal plate have met in the region of the superior semicircular canal (arrow). (b) The fused layer of canal plate epithelium in the region of the superior canal has now disappeared (arrow), during which time the posterior canal walls have come together and are now apposed (asterisk). (c) All fused regions of superior and posterior canal plate have now disappeared leaving two canal tubes that are united centrally by the crus commune. A, anterior; C, cochlea; CC, crus commune; E, endolymphatic duct; H, horizontal; L, lateral; M, medial; P, posterior; SA, saccule; S, superior; U, utricle. Redrawn from Ref. 30, © 1993, with permission from Elsevier.

Modifier genes affecting the development of the auditory system

More often than not, a given genetic disorder may manifest in a variety of ways. Variable phenotypes can result from genetic modifier loci. Modifier genes affect the phenotypic outcome of a given genotype by interacting in the same or parallel biological pathway as a disease gene. The effect can be enhancing, leading to a more severe mutant phenotype, or suppressive, reducing the mutant phenotype even to the extent of completely restoring the normal condition. Modifier genes can also alter the clinical presentations of a given disease, resulting in different combinations of traits. Moreover, multiple modifier genes may act in combination to create a cumulative effect on the expression of a phenotype. Human modifiers of hearing include *DFNM1* locus which suppresses hearing loss among individuals with *DFNB26* mutation[4] and a locus on chromosome 8, which modifies maternally inherited aminoglycoside-induced deafness associated with a mutation (*A1555G*) in the mitochondrial 12S ribosome RNA.[33]

RECENT ADVANCES IN GENETIC MANIPULATION IN THE TREATMENT OF CONGENITAL DEAFNESS

The purpose of any medical research is to apply the findings to clinical use. It may one day be possible to reverse certain types of defect that affect the early development of the auditory and vestibular systems. A prerequisite for treatment will almost certainly be early and accurate diagnosis. Screening programmes can then be established using molecular techniques. Groups with strong family histories of vestibular disorders and/or deafness with any related syndromes and premature newborns should be targeted for screening in the first instance. Molecular techniques can scan for the genetic defect at several levels. They may be used in linkage analysis, where the location of the gene on a particular chromosome is identified; or the techniques may identify the actual gene, the mutation within the gene and the gene product.[34]

Some childhood hearing loss may be progressive during the first few months or years of life. Early diagnosis of hearing impairment in children would be essential if medical or surgical interventions were to stand a good chance of preserving some hearing ability. Intervention would depend on us having a much greater understanding of the likelihood of developing a serious hearing impairment than we presently have, so that a realistic prognosis could be provided to aid a family's decision.[35]

Gene transfer

The prospect of therapeutic insertion of genetic material into the inner ear promises to be an attractive technology for clinical applications. It offers the hope of preventing, arresting, reversing or curing vestibular or hearing disorders caused by hereditary diseases or environmental insults. There are currently very few treatment options for vestibular disorders and sensorineural hearing loss and, therefore, it is important to investigate and develop new technologies for inner ear disease. *In utero* gene transfer may indeed be an option, but this technology will have many technical and ethical issues that remain to be overcome.

A number of different gene transfer vectors have been studied *in vivo* for their efficacy, utility and safety in intracochlear gene transfer. Vectors successfully studied include cationic liposomes, adeno-associated virus, adeno-virus, lentivirus, herpes simplex virus and vaccinia virus, with variable intensities of transgene expression in different parts of the organ of Corti.[36]

For experimental purposes as well as future clinical application, it is important to develop a vector delivery system that preserves hearing and vestibular functions, as well as inner ear architecture. Systemic administration of the vectors has the disadvantage of systemic toxicity including viral hepatitis and encephalitis.[37] Direct instillation, on the other hand, allows high vector concentration to be delivered to the target organ, using a small amount of vector solution, which increases the likelihood of gene delivery to the targeted tissue, while minimizing leakage of the vector to the surrounding organs. Several techniques of intracochlear vector delivery have been developed and their efficacy and safety have been compared and contrasted.[36] They include miniosmotic pump infusion or microinjection into the scala tympani via the round window, infusion or microinjection into the scala tympani through a co-chleostomy, injection into the endolymphatic sac accessed from the posterior fossa and gel foam application to the round window membrane. The first three methods have the advantage of a controlled steady intracochlear perfusion, but have the disadvantage of potentially physically damaging the architecture of the cochlea. Gel-foam soaked with the vector solution applied to the round window is noninvasive and nondestructive, and does not cause disruption to the anatomy of the inner ear.[36] However, the exact mechanism of vector transfer through the round window membrane is poorly understood and hence there is no control over the rate of delivery. It has also been shown that transgene expression in the contralateral, noninjected cochlea occurs, suggesting that systemic dissemination could potentially be associated with direct delivery methods. Three potential routes of spread from the cochlea have been suggested and they include viral spread via the cochlear aqueduct which connects the scala tympani of the basal turn of the cochlea to the cerebrospinal fluid (CSF) space, transmission of vectors through the temporal bone marrow spaces and haemato-genous dissemination.[38] To date, there has been no report of gene transfer being used to successfully treat deafness in an animal model.

Stem cell and gene therapy

In addition to single gene transfer, there has been great interest in the potential of the twin technologies of stem cell and gene therapy for medicine. Hair cells in the cochlea are very vulnerable to disruption of their homeostasis and tend to die if they cannot function normally.[39] Once dead, hair cells are not naturally replaced. One approach to treating deafness could be to trigger regeneration of cochlear hair cells. However, there is no point in stimulating the regeneration of hair cells that are unable to function because of a genetic defect. Accurate diagnosis combined with dual treatment of stem cell insertion and gene transfer would be vital for this approach to succeed. Over recent times, the potential of somatic stem cells for therapeutic applications has become almost infinite, limited only by the ingenuity of investigators in the manipulation of their genomes and culture conditions.[40]

Cochlear gene transfer can offer several potential applications including the study of specific expression and function of certain genes and the delivery of therapeutic agents. However, demonstration of transgene expression in tissues outside the treated cochlea raises concerns about the safety of its application regarding systemic dissemination of the vectors used.[36] Better techniques to improve and enhance specific vector delivery into the cochlea need to be developed and tested.

Timing of intervention

In humans, the otic placode starts to develop when the embryo has reached the seventh somite stage (about 22 days) and by 25 weeks, the development of the organ of Corti and the vestibular system are complete and resemble the adult form. Prenatal tests for congenital abnormalities including Down syndrome, cystic fibrosis and spina bifida are performed by the end of the first trimester and it would be too late if interventions were to be implemented to the developing ear at this stage. The rudimentary pinna has formed by 60 days and in the fourth month convolutions have attained their adult form, although further enlargement continues during the remaining months of gestation and also in the post-natal period.[41] Timing of genetic intervention would therefore be important. Direct gene transfer or stem cell insertion into the inner ear at the embryonic stage would involve some form of intrauterine surgery and surgical intervention on the human foetus has been performed for more than two decades in the United States.[42] In the past, only foetuses with life-threatening defects, for example, giant foetal cervical teratoma[43] have been considered as candidates for prenatal correction. However, more foetal surgical procedures are now being performed for non-lethal conditions, such as congenital diaphagmatic hernia

using fetoscopic repair techniques.[42] Surgical intervention involving inner ear gene transfer on human embryos seems a good idea, but is still rather far-fetched with the technology available to us at present. It may be more feasible to treat post-natal progressive deafness and/or vestibular disorders by using this approach, but the exact pattern of expression and functions of the genes involved must be understood prior to such intervention. In addition, the attitudes of the patients and their families and their views on such intervention must be respected. The deaf community in the United Kingdom is very advanced, with its own culture and there has been anecdotal evidence that deaf couples do not necessarily want their children to be able to hear if it means that they will be excluded from the deaf community to which their parents belong (see Chapter 69, Investigation and management of the deaf child).

Drug therapy

An alternative approach is based on drugs, which, by definition, are small molecules with ready access to the target cells. We may be able to exploit alternative pathways to carry out the task that is affected by a mutation. For example, connexin 26 mutation is thought to the most common cause of nonsyndromic deafness in the Caucasian population. Another connexin may be capable of substituting for connexin 26 in forming gap junctions, but its gene may not normally be expressed in the cochlea. A drug might therefore be developed to activate expression of the alternative connexin gene in the cells needing to form gap junctions. Clues about which alternative pathways might be worth exploiting will come from investigations of interacting genes.[35]

KEY POINTS

- Congenital deafness is a common childhood problem.
- Genetic abnormalities cause not only congenital deafness; several genes have been found that, when mutated, either cause or predispose to progressive hearing loss.
- Mice appear to be the best model for the study of genetic deafness.
- Understanding the molecular biology of the auditory system may be the key to the future development of genetic counselling and treatment for congenital deafness.
- Surgical intervention involving inner ear gene transfer on human embryos seems a good idea, but is still rather far-fetched with the technology currently available.

Deficiencies in current knowledge and areas for future research

Genetic testing for deafness is now a reality and has changed the paradigm for evaluating deaf patients. It will be used by surgeons for diagnostic purposes and as a basis for treatment and management options. Mutation screening is currently available for only a limited number of genes, such as connexin 26. In these cases, diagnosis, carrier detection and reproductive risk counselling can be provided. In the future, there will be an expansion of the role of genetic testing and counselling will not be limited to reproductive planning. Treatment and management decisions will be made based on specific genetic diagnoses. New discoveries and technologies will expand and increase the complexity of genetic testing options. Otolaryngologists will therefore have to familiarize themselves with current discoveries and accepted protocols for genetic testing.

REFERENCES

* 1. Fortnum HM, Summerfield AQ, Marshall DH, Davis AC, Bamford JM. Prevalence of permanent childhood hearing impairment in the United Kingdom and implications for universal neonatal hearing screening: Questionnaire based ascertainment study. *British Medical Journal*. 2001; **323**: 536–40. *A clinically relevant article explaining the incidence of congenital deafness and the need for universal neonatal hearing screening*

2. Marazita ML, Ploughman LM, Rawlings B, Remington E, Arnos KS, Nance WE. Genetic epidemiological studies of early-onset deafness in the U.S. school-age population. *American Journal of Medical Genetics*. 1993; **46**: 486–91.

3. Steel KP. Progress in progressive hearing loss. *Science*. 1998; **279**: 1870–1.

4. Riazuddin S, Castelein CM, Ahmed ZM, Lalwani AK, Mastroianni MA, Naz S *et al*. Dominant modifier DFNM1 suppresses recessive deafness DFNB26. *Nature Genetics*. 2000; **26**: 431–4.

* 5. Van Camp G, Smith R. Hereditary Hearing Loss homepage. 2005. http://webhost.ua.ac.be/hhh/ *The most up-to-date source of information in the genes identified in congenital deafness*.

6. Verpy E, Masmoudi S, Zwaenepoel I, Leibovici M, Hutchin TP, Del Castillo I *et al*. Mutations in a new gene encoding a protein of the hair bundle cause non-syndromic deafness at the DFNB16 locus. *Nature Genetics*. 2001; **29**: 345–9.

7. Steel KP, Bock GR. Hereditary inner-ear abnormalities in animals. Relationships with human abnormalities. *Archives of Otolaryngology*. 1983; **109**: 22–9.

8. Steel KP. Inherited hearing defects in mice. *Annual Review of Genetics*. 1995; **29**: 675–701.

9. Kiernan A, Steel K. Mouse homologues for human deafness. In: Kitamura K, Steel K (eds). *Genetics in otorhinolaryngology. Advances in otorhinolaryngology*. Basel: Karger, 2000; **56**: 233–43.

10. Shanahan D. Cyberanatomy of the branchial arches. Newcastle-upon-Tyne: Newcastle University. Last updated 19th June 2007; cited May 2007. Available from: http://anatome.ncl.ac.uk/tutorials/clinical/arch/text/page1.html

11. Fekete DM, Wu DK. Revisiting cell fate specification in the inner ear. *Current Opinion in Neurobiology*. 2002; **12**: 35–42.

12. Lufkin T, Dierich A, LeMeur M, Mark M, Chambon P. Disruption of the Hox-1.6 homeobox gene results in defects in a region corresponding to its rostral domain of expression. *Cell*. 1991; **66**: 1105–19.

13. Gavalas A, Studer M, Lumsden A, Rijli FM, Krumlauf R, Chambon P. Hoxa1 and Hoxb1 synergize in patterning the hindbrain, cranial nerves and second pharyngeal arch. *Development*. 1998; **125**: 1123–36.

14. Rivera-Perez JA, Wakamiya M, Behringer RR. Goosecoid cell acts autonomously in mesenchyme-derived tissues during craniofacial development. *Development*. 1999; **126**: 3811–21.

15. Yamada G, Mansouri A, Torres M, Stuart ET, Blum M, Schultz M *et al*. Targeted mutation of the murine goosecoid gene results in craniofacial defects and neonatal death. *Development*. 1995; **121**: 2917–22.

16. Kurihara Y, Kurihara H, Suzuki H, Kodama T, Maemura K, Nagai R *et al*. Elevated blood pressure and craniofacial abnormalities in mice deficient in endothelin-1. *Nature*. 1994; **368**: 703–10.

17. Yanagisawa H, Yanagisawa M, Kapur RP, Richardson JA, Williams SC, Clouthier DE *et al*. Dual genetic pathways of endothelin-mediated intercellular signaling revealed by targeted disruption of endothelin converting enzyme-1 gene. *Development*. 1998; **125**: 825–36.

18. Clouthier DE, Williams SC, Yanagisawa H, Wieduwilt M, Richardson JA, Yanagisawa M. Signaling pathways crucial for craniofacial development revealed by endothelin-A receptor-deficient mice. *Developmental Biology*. 2000; **217**: 10–24.

19. Thomas T, Kurihara H, Yamagishi H, Kurihara Y, Yazaki Y, Olson EN *et al*. A signaling cascade involving endothelin-1, dHAND and msx1 regulates development of neural-crest-derived branchial arch mesenchyme. *Development*. 1998; **125**: 3005–14.

20. Qiu M, Bulfone A, Martinez S, Meneses JJ, Shimamura K, Pedersen RA *et al*. Null mutation of Dlx-2 results in abnormal morphogenesis of proximal first and second branchial arch derivatives and abnormal differentiation in the forebrain. *Genes and Development*. 1995; **9**: 2523–38.

21. Lohnes D, Mark M, Mendelsohn C, Dolle P, Dierich A, Gorry P *et al*. Function of the retinoic acid receptors (RARs) during development (I). Craniofacial and skeletal abnormalities in RAR double mutants. *Development*. 1994; **120**: 2723–48.

22. Martin JF, Bradley A, Olson EN. The paired-like homeo box gene MHox is required for early events of skeletogenesis in multiple lineages. *Genes and Development.* 1995; **9**: 1237–49.

23. Matsuo I, Kuratani S, Kimura C, Takeda N, Aizawa S. Mouse Otx2 functions in the formation and patterning of rostral head. *Genes and Development.* 1995; **9**: 2646–58.

24. Mallo M. Formation of the middle ear: Recent progress on the developmental and molecular mechanisms. *Developmental Biology.* 2001; **231**: 410–9.

25. Mallo M. Embryological and genetic aspects of middle ear development. *International Journal of Developmental Biology.* 1998; **42**: 11–22.

26. Francis-West P, Ladher R, Barlow A, Graveson A. Signalling interactions during facial development. *Mechanisms of Development.* 1998; **75**: 3–28.

27. Rijli FM, Mark M, Lakkaraju S, Dierich A, Dolle P, Chambon P. A homeotic transformation is generated in the rostral branchial region of the head by disruption of Hoxa-2, which acts as a selector gene. *Cell.* 1993; **75**: 1333–49.

28. de Kok YJ, van der Maarel SM, Bitner-Glindzicz M, Huber I, Monaco AP, Malcolm S *et al.* Association between X-linked mixed deafness and mutations in the POU domain gene POU3F4. *Science.* 1995; **267**: 685–8.

29. Torres M, Giraldez F. The development of the vertebrate inner ear. *Mechanisms of Development.* 1998; **71**: 5–21.

30. Martin P, Swanson GJ. Descriptive and experimental analysis of the epithelial remodellings that control semicircular canal formation in the developing mouse inner ear. *Developmental Biology.* 1993; **159**: 549–58.

31. Represa J, Frenz DA, Van De Water TR. Genetic patterning of embryonic inner ear development. *Acta Otolaryngologica.* 2000; **120**: 5–10.

32. Xiang M, Gan L, Li D, Zhou L, Chen ZY, Wagner D *et al.* Role of the Brn-3 family of POU-domain genes in the development of the auditory/vestibular, somatosensory, and visual systems. *Cold Spring Harbor Symposia on Quantitative Biology.* 1997; **62**: 325–36.

33. Bykhovskaya Y, Estivill X, Taylor K, Hang T, Hamon M, Casano RA *et al.* Candidate locus for a nuclear modifier gene for maternally inherited deafness. *American Journal of Human Genetics.* 2000; **66**: 1905–10.

34. Smith SD, Kimberling WJ, Schaefer GB, Horton MB, Tinley ST. Medical genetic evaluation for the etiology of hearing loss in children. *Journal of Communication Disorders.* 1998; **31**: 371–88; quiz 388–9.

* 35. Steel KP. Science, medicine, and the future: New interventions in hearing impairment. *British Medical Journal.* 2000; **320**: 622–5. *A beautifully written account of the science behind the various modes of possible gene therapy.*

* 36. Lalwani AK, Jero J, Mhatre AN. Current issues in cochlear gene transfer. *Audiology and Neurootology.* 2002; **7**: 146–51. *A good summary of experiments that have been carried out in cochlear gene transfer in the world literature.*

37. Lalwani AK, Walsh BJ, Carvalho GJ, Muzyczka N, Mhatre AN. Expression of adeno-associated virus integrated transgene within the mammalian vestibular organs. *American Journal of Otology.* 1998; **19**: 390–5.

38. Kho ST, Pettis RM, Mhatre AN, Lalwani AK. Safety of adeno-associated virus as cochlear gene transfer vector: Analysis of distant spread beyond injected cochleae. *Molecular Therapy.* 2000; **2**: 368–73.

39. Steel KP. Perspectives: Biomedicine. The benefits of recycling. *Science.* 1999; **285**: 1363–4.

* 40. Lemoine NR. The power to deliver: stem cells in gene therapy. *Gene Therapy.* 2002; **9**: 603–5. *An interesting and easy to follow article on current issues in stem cell/gene therapy in general.*

41. Wright A. Anatomy and ultrastructure of the human ear. In: Kerr A. (ed.). *Scott-Brown's otolaryngology,* Vol. 1. 1997: pp.1/1/6–8.

42. Farmer D. Fetal surgery. *British Medical Journal.* 2003; **326**: 461–2.

43. Hirose S, Sydorak RM, Tsao K, Cauldwell CB, Newman KD, Mychaliska GB *et al.* Spectrum of intrapartum management strategies for giant fetal cervical teratoma. *Journal of Pediatric Surgery.* 2003; **38**: 446–50.

67

Hearing loss in preschool children: screening and surveillance

KAI UUS AND JOHN BAMFORD

Introduction	821	Surveillance	829
Principles and definitions	821	Surveillance for otitis media with effusion	830
Prevalence and risk factors	823	Key points	830
The rationale for screening	825	Best clinical practice	831
Newborn hearing screening	826	Deficiencies in current knowledge and areas for future	
The eight-month IDT screen	828	research	831
The school-entry screen	829	References	831

SEARCH STRATEGY

The data in this chapter are supported by a Medline and CINAHL search for relevant articles published in English, using key words infant or newborn and hearing screening and hearing loss.

INTRODUCTION

Any discussion of screening must be firmly grounded in an understanding of the principles of screening as a public health exercise, an understanding of some of the key evidence regarding the epidemiology of the condition of interest, in this case childhood hearing loss, and the evidence for or against different approaches to screening and surveillance for that condition. Thus, this chapter starts with an outline of the key definitions and principles of screening, before proceeding to review evidence on the prevalence of different types of childhood hearing loss. The case for newborn screening is summarized and evidence for current performance of newborn screens reviewed. Other approaches to screening and surveillance in the preschool years are also reviewed (the eight-month screen, the school entry screen) and the position with regard to temporary childhood hearing loss discussed.

PRINCIPLES AND DEFINITIONS

Surveillance is a process of ongoing or regular observation of the health of individuals or populations. Traditionally health service professionals have considered surveillance essentially as secondary prevention through early detection. However, the concept that child health depends upon continuous vigilance and supervision by health professionals is fairly narrow and supervisory; child health surveillance is now regarded as just one component of child health promotion programmes which aim to promote partnership between parents, children and health professionals, in which parents are empowered to make use of services and expertise according to their needs.

Screening is a public health activity in which members of a defined population, who do not show any obvious symptoms, are offered a test in order to identify those individuals who are more likely to be helped than harmed by further assessment or treatment to diminish the risk of a disease (or impairment) or its complications (or consequences). Accurate early diagnosis of serious conditions offers the opportunity to initiate treatment before the disease progresses (or to intervene to mitigate the consequences of the impairment). When screening is done well, it can be very beneficial.

Even though screening can potentially help to save lives or improve the quality of life through early diagnosis of serious conditions, it is not an infallible process. Screening can potentially reduce the risk of developing a disease (or impairment) or its complications (or consequences). However, in all screening programmes there are inevitably individuals who are referred as having the condition but do not (**false positives**), and who are not referred but do have the condition (**false negatives**).

From an ethical viewpoint, screening differs from responsive clinical practice, since screening is targeting individuals who appear healthy and is offering to help individuals make an informed choice about their health or the health of their children. It is particularly important for individuals who consent to be screened or have their child screened to be aware of the risks involved and have reasonable expectations of a screening programme.

In the UK, the National Screening Committee 'assesses proposed new screening programmes against a set of internationally recognised criteria covering the condition, the test, the treatment options and the effectiveness and acceptability of the screening programme. Assessing programmes in this way is intended to ensure that they are more beneficial than harmful, and can be implemented at reasonable cost. When research has shown screening to be effective in reducing mortality and morbidity from a particular condition, the National Screening Committee may decide to pilot the proposed screening programme. This provides valuable information on the effectiveness, feasibility and public acceptability of screening when performed in an ordinary health service setting rather than a specialist research site. Pilot studies enable informed decisions to be made about policy priorities; ensuring resources are targeted on services that are proven to work'.[1]

The principles that a screening programme should satisfy have been identified in seminal work by Wilson and Junger.[2] These were extended by Haggard and Hughes[3] in their review of screening for hearing loss in children.

- The condition (hearing impairment) should be an important health problem.
- There should be an accepted treatment, i.e. an acceptable means of habilitation for those identified by the screen.
- Facilities for assessment, diagnosis and treatment should be available.
- The hearing impairment should be recognizable at an early stage.

- There should be a suitable test for use as the screen.
- The test should be acceptable to the parents and to the child.
- The natural history of the condition should be known and understood.
- There should be an agreed policy on who to treat.
- The cost of case finding (including all consequential costs of the screening programme) should not be disproportionate to overall healthcare costs of care for the hearing-impaired child.
- Case finding should be seen as a continuing process.
- The incidental harm should be small compared to the overall benefits.
- There should be guidelines on how to explain results to parents with appropriate support.
- All hearing screening arrangements should be reviewed in the light of changes in demography, epidemiology and other factors.
- Cost and effectiveness of hearing screening should be examined on a case-type basis to maximize the effectiveness and benefit for each type before considering overall costs, effectiveness and benefits.

There are a number of key definitions relevant to screening programmes which should be used in the quality assurance and audit of any screening programme:

Coverage is the proportion of the target population who undergo the screen.

Screen positive result is a screening result that is greater than or equal to a specified cut-off level. In the case of permanent childhood hearing impairment, there is debate about the appropriate cut-off level; at present in the UK the cut-off level is the estimated hearing threshold (averaged across 0.5, 1, 2 and 4 kHz) of 40 dB HL. This level is based upon evidence for the benefits of early intervention in moderate or greater hearing loss. Further research on the effects of and early intervention for mild hearing loss in the 20–40 dB HL range is ongoing. A true-positive is an individual with a screen-positive result who has the condition (impairment). A false-positive is an individual with a screen-positive result who does not have the target condition (impairment).

Screen negative result is a screening result that is less than the specified cut-off level. A true-negative is an individual with a screen-negative result who does not have the condition (impairment). A false-negative is an individual with a screen-negative result who does in fact have the condition (impairment). Effective screening programmes attempt to reduce false-negatives to the irreducible minimum, while keeping false-positives within manageable service levels. The aim of a screen is to refer on a manageable proportion of the population for further (diagnostic) tests, that proportion being likely to contain as many of the true cases in the population as possible.

Sensitivity is the rate of true-positives or the proportion of individuals with the target condition in the population who are correctly identified by the screen. The term can be applied to a screening test, if (as is the case with newborn hearing screening) the screen consists of more than one test, or to the screen as a whole, or indeed to the screening programme. **Test sensitivity** is the proportion of individuals who were given the test, have the condition (impairment) and were detected by the test. **Screen sensitivity** is the proportion of individuals who completed the screen who have the condition (impairment) and who were detected by the screen (which may consist of more than one test with conditional pass/refer rules). **Programme sensitivity** is the proportion of the subjects in the whole population with the specified condition (impairment) who are detected by the screening programme. It is a product of the screen sensitivity and the coverage achieved by the screen programme.

Specificity is the rate of true-negatives or the proportion of individuals free of the target condition in the population who are correctly identified as such by the screen. As with sensitivity, the term specificity may be applied at the level of test, screen or programme. The latter is a product of specificity and coverage. **Positive predictive value** is the proportion of individuals with a positive test result who have the target condition.

Yield is used to indicate the number of cases identified by a screen (e.g. in the first 12 months of the first phase of the Newborn Hearing Screening Programme (NHSP) in England, 40 true cases of bilateral permanent hearing loss were identified via the screen). The yield is sometimes expressed as the number of cases identified via the screen per 1000 individuals screened, thus allowing comparison with published prevalence figures, and acting as a surrogate for sensitivity (since sensitivity can only be established in retrospect, once all false-negative and missed cases have been found). The yield of a screen is affected by coverage and sensitivity, and affects the cost per case identified. Finally, the **incremental yield** is the number of true cases referred by a screen when any true cases that would have been or were identified by preceding screening, surveillance programmes or responsive services are excluded.

Incidence is the number of new instances of the condition (impairment) occurring during a certain period (e.g. a year) in a specified population. Thus, in an average-sized health community with 5000 births per year, an incidence of between five and ten cases of congenital permanent moderate or greater bilateral hearing loss might be expected.

Prevalence is the total number of individuals who have a given disease or condition (impairment) at a given point in time per population figure (e.g. per 1000 live births). Davis et al.[4] have suggested a figure of 1.12 per 1000 for congenital permanent bilateral hearing impairment of moderate or greater degree (see under Prevalence and risk factors below for further discussion of prevalence figures).

The extended Wilson and Junger screening criteria identify costs and effectiveness as important issues for screening programmes (points 9 and 14 above). **Cost-effectiveness analysis** is an economic analysis used to compare effectiveness and cost of health interventions in which either (1) effects of the interventions are known to be equal and so the option to be recommended is that which is least (or less) costly (sometimes known as 'cost-minimization analysis') or (2) effects and costs differ across interventions; hence, the option to be recommended is that with the lowest (or lower) ratio of cost per unit of health gain, as implementation of this option will lead to the most (or more) effective use of a fixed budget.

PREVALENCE AND RISK FACTORS

Congenital permanent bilateral hearing loss

The quality of published studies on the prevalence of congenital permanent hearing loss is variable, with the poorer studies marred by lack of clarity on case definition, uncertain methodology and doubtful case ascertainment. Of the better studies, those reported by Davis et al.[4] and Fortnum et al.[5, 6] are probably the most extensive and reliable. Fortnum et al.[5] report the results of a retrospective ascertainment of all cases of permanent bilateral hearing loss of moderate or greater degree in children born in the UK's Trent health region between 1985 and 1993. Considerable effort was put into the ascertainment process such that the authors believe that over 90 percent of all known cases were found. Based on the birth cohorts for 1985–1990, the prevalence of moderate-to-profound congenital permanent bilateral hearing loss was 1.12 (95 percent CI 1.01–1.23) per 1000 live births (0.64 per 1000 for moderate hearing loss; 0.23 per 1000 for severe hearing loss; 0.24 per 1000 for profound hearing loss). An even more extensive study is reported by Fortnum et al.[6] In this, the authors carried out a full national retrospective ascertainment of all cases of bilateral permanent hearing loss of moderate or greater degree in the UK, born between 1980 and 1997. Data were collected in years 1998–1999 within a strict ethical framework from both health (audiology) and education (support services for hearing impaired children). Once duplicate data had been excluded, there were 17,160 cases, giving an overall prevalence of 1.33 per 1000 births (95 percent CI 1.22–1.45). However, prevalence varied as a function of age, being 0.91 per 1000 (95 percent CI 0.85–0.98) for the three-year-old cohort and rising to 1.65 per 1000 (95 percent CI 1.62–1.68) for the nine-year-old cohort, where it levelled off. The authors argue that the rise in prevalence with age is not because of any change in prevalence with year of birth, nor can it be ascribed only to later acquired losses, and they conclude that there are more late-onset and progressive permanent childhood hearing losses than previously suspected. Furthermore, statistical adjustment of the data indicated the possibility of under-ascertainment, such that the final prevalence figure at age nine years might be as high as 2.0 per thousand. While these data support the use of newborn hearing screening for the identification of the 1.12 (or thereabouts) congenital cases per 1000 births, other processes will be needed for the post-natal onset cases. [**]

Risk factors

Risk factors for permanent congenital hearing loss are well established. The risk factors for permanent hearing loss in neonates as suggested by the US Joint Committee on Infant Hearing position statement 2000 are as follows.[7]

- An illness or condition requiring admission of 48 hours or greater to a NICU.
- Stigmata or other findings associated with a syndrome known to include a sensorineural and/or conductive hearing loss.
- Family history of permanent childhood sensorineural hearing loss.
- Craniofacial anomalies, including those with morphological abnormalities of the pinna and ear canal.
- *In utero* infection such as cytomegalovirus, herpes, toxoplasmosis or rubella.

The three major summary risk factors are:

1. history of treatment in an neonatal intensive care unit (NICU) or special care baby unit (SCBU) for more than 48 hours;
2. family history of early childhood deafness;
3. craniofacial anomaly (e.g. cleft palate) associated with hearing impairment.[4, 8]

About 60 percent of congenital bilateral permanent hearing loss of moderate degree or greater is associated with one or more of these three risk factors, in the proportions 29.3 percent NICU, 26.7 percent family history and 3.9 percent craniofacial anomaly. [**] The high proportion of cases with risk factors led, in the early 1990s, to the widespread introduction of 'at risk' newborn screening in which attempts were made to screen all those babies (perhaps some 10 percent of the birth cohort) with risk factors, in order to identify early this 60 percent of the target true cases of congenital permanent loss. However, in practice, due to the difficulty experienced by maternity services in reliably identifying a family history of permanent childhood hearing loss, the proportion of the target population identified by at risk screening was rarely above 40 percent.[4] [**]

Acquired and late-onset permanent bilateral hearing loss

Acquired hearing loss is a hearing loss acquired postnatally which, on the basis of case history, was not considered to be present and detectable using appropriate tests at or very soon after birth. Post-meningitic hearing loss and hearing loss due to trauma are the most common causes of acquired hearing loss in children. The study by Fortnum *et al*.[6] has indicated that progressive or late-onset hearing losses may be more prevalent than suspected, having an effect through the preschool and early school years (see Prevalence and risk factors). Any newborn hearing screening programme will of course not identify these cases and this therefore points to the importance of addressing other means of finding them.

Unilateral permanent hearing loss

There are few reliable studies on the prevalence of unilateral permanent hearing loss in preschool children. However, there is some reason to suspect that prevalence may be relatively high. In a retrospective study of children up to the age of ten years, Vartiainen and Karjalainen[9] found a prevalence of 1.7 per 1000 live births for permanent unilateral sensorineural or mixed hearing loss (> 25 dB HL at 0.5–4 kHz, including mixed hearing impairments with bone conduction thresholds of ≥ 25 dB HL). [**] The yield for permanent unilateral moderate or greater hearing loss in the Newborn Hearing Screening Programme in England is 0.64 (95 percent CI 0.37–0.91) per 1000 screened. This is new information and has raised a number of issues about the appropriate early management of unilateral permanent hearing loss that have not been faced before.[10] [**]

Auditory neuropathy/dys-synchrony

Auditory neuropathy/auditory dys-synchrony (AN/AD) is caused by damage to inner hair cells, the synaptic juncture between the inner hair cells, auditory neurons in the spiral ganglion, the VIIIth nerve fibres, or any combination. This is observed on clinical audiological tests as normal otoacoustic emissions (OAEs) in the presence of an absent or severely abnormal auditory brainstem response (ABR).

The prevalence of AN/AD is not known. It has been reported that up to 10 percent of all children with confirmed permanent hearing loss have auditory neuropathy.[11, 12]

Infants and children diagnosed with AN/AD typically have a remarkable medical history. It is a condition found predominantly in the NICU population: three in 1000 high-risk babies present with AN/AD[13] and it is considered relatively rare in the well-baby population.[12] [**]

Temporary childhood hearing loss

Temporary childhood hearing loss due to otitis media with effusion (OME) is extremely common, with a point prevalence of some 20 percent and a period prevalence in the under five-year-olds of some 80 percent.[3, 14] [**] The major risk factors are season, passive smoking, bottle-feeding, upper respiratory tract infections, admission to NICU as a newborn, day care and siblings having had OME.[3] [**] The large scale TARGET (Trials of Alternative Regimes in Glue Ear Treatment) studies currently being carried out in the UK are likely to provide much-needed evidence in a number of domains; careful recruitment of over 300 cases aged 3.5 to 7 years has provided more robust data than have been available previously. Refinement of risk factor analyses has indicated season, passive smoking, siblings having had OME and snoring and mouth-breathing as the best indicators for persistence.[15] The TARGET studies indicate material effects of persistent OME on hearing difficulties, speech/language delay, disturbed sleep patterns, behaviour and (consequent on these) parental and child quality of life. [****]

THE RATIONALE FOR SCREENING

In this section, we will consider screening only with respect to permanent childhood hearing loss.

The critical review (1997) of newborn hearing screening carried out as part of the UK's Health Technology Assessment programme[4] identified eight broad reasons for the introduction of newborn hearing screening for all babies.

1. Outcomes for at least some children with congenital permanent hearing loss are the cause of considerable concern.
2. Median identification age in the UK for moderate or greater bilateral congenital permanent hearing loss based on current screening tests was around 22 months.
3. There is evidence that intervention in the first six months of life for children with moderate or greater permanent bilateral hearing loss can improve at least some outcomes.
4. More precise and detailed neural connections depend upon appropriate early stimulation; myelination of auditory pathways by six months of age is delayed by almost any chronic insult.
5. Early identification allows early and more appropriate management decisions, made not from a starting point of developmental deficit.
6. Costs of newborn screening look to be broadly acceptable.
7. Evidence from parents of deaf children strongly suggest that they would have welcomed very early identification.
8. Evidence from parents suggest that they would welcome a newborn hearing screen.

Early deprivation and early plasticity

Studies with animals have shown that deafferentation of the auditory system during early sensitive periods of development results in marked anatomic and physiological changes that occur extensively throughout the central auditory system.[16, 17, 18] [****] The first study to demonstrate that, within the sensitive period, changes wrought by loss of afferent input could be reversed was carried out by Pasic and Rubel.[19] They showed that in neonatal gerbils, changes in cochlear nucleus cell size produced by auditory nerve blocking by tetrodotoxin were completely reversible after seven days. [****] There appears to be considerable plasticity in the whole pathway during early development, but in the adult subject plasticity at lower neural levels (e.g. brainstem, midbrain) is considerably reduced and possibly lost.[20] This indicates that the early post-natal period is crucial for the establishment of auditory pathways that can accurately represent complex sounds at the cortical level. There appears to be a critical period of plasticity at lower pathways of the auditory system. [****]

Outcomes

There is good evidence that outcomes in a number of domains are affected by permanent hearing loss. In most cases this is a severity-dependent effect, with greater effects for more severe hearing losses; there are, however, very great individual differences, with some children performing at levels appropriate to their age and others performing very poorly. These differences are not always a function of degree of hearing loss, but will be a result of a range of intrinsic and extrinsic factors. One such factor is the age at which the hearing loss was identified, as well as habilitative support provided. The evidence of compromised outcomes associated with congenital permanent hearing loss comes from studies looking at communication skills,[21] literacy,[22] behaviour,[23] educational achievement,[24] mental health,[25] family dynamics[26] and quality of life.[23] [**]

Late identification

Since the late 1950s, the UK has had a universal eight-month screen for childhood hearing loss based on the infant distraction test (IDT) (see Chapter 68, Hearing tests in children) and usually carried out by health visitors in community clinic settings. With the introduction of newborn hearing screening this is to be phased out; there is good evidence that it has poor sensitivity, poor specificity and is not cost effective in terms of cost per case found.[5, 27, 28] The retrospective study of permanent childhood hearing impairment greater than or equal to 40 dB HL in children born between 1985 and 1993 and resident in Trent health region, showed that the median ages at referral, confirmation of the impairment, prescription of hearing aids and fitting of hearing aids were, respectively, 10.4, 18.1, 24.4 and 26.3 months.[5] [**] While much of the delay was clearly due to delays in the assessment process after referral, nonetheless the median age of screen referral for children with congenital hearing loss was little short of one year.

Benefits of early identification and intervention

Yoshinaga-Itano et al.[29] compared the receptive and expressive language abilities of 72 children with hearing loss who had been identified by six months of age with 78 children whose hearing losses were identified after six months and showed that early-identified children demonstrated significantly better language scores than the later-identified children. For children with normal cognitive abilities, this language advantage was found across all test ages, communication modes, degrees of hearing loss and socioeconomic backgrounds. It was also independent of gender, ethnicity and the presence or absence of additional disabilities. [***]

This finding is consistent with a number of similar studies of variable quality, all reporting significantly better language scores for children whose hearing losses were identified earlier.[30, 31, 32, 33, 34, 35, 36, 37] [***/**]

Even though evidence from randomized controlled trials is not available to address the question of whether earlier rather than later intervention is better for children with hearing loss, the consistency of findings from a number of quasi-experimental studies provides consistent and convincing evidence about the benefits of earlier intervention.

Assessment and management

Some aspects of audiological assessment are easier in the first few months of life: for example, unsedated electrophysiological tests such as the auditory brainstem response, and habilitative procedures such as real ear measurements for hearing aid fittings, or ear impressions for earmoulds. Perhaps more importantly, the earlier that parents and services know about the child's hearing loss, its degree and the child's progress, the earlier can decisions be made about management (e.g. appropriate hearing aids, first language, extent and type of family support).

Costs

While further cost-effectiveness studies are required, it is clear that the costs of newborn screening are broadly acceptable.[4] Stevens et al.[28] compared the costs of newborn hearing screening of all babies in three areas already implementing such a service, with costs of the IDT screen in seven areas, and found that the mean service costs for the universal newborn hearing screen and the eight-month IDT screen were £13,881 and £24,519, respectively, for a standardized district of 1000 live births; the cost per case found was much lower for newborn screening due to the higher sensitivity of the screen. [**]

Parental wishes

Finally, there is the issue of parental rights to significant information about their child. This has been given expression in a number of surveys, the largest of which is that by Watkin et al.[38] He investigated the attitudes of parents of deaf children to newborn hearing screening. If such a procedure had been available to them when their child was born, 89 percent said they would have wanted it. It is also known that early identification tends to avoid the parental anxiety and anger that may be associated with delayed detection.[38, 39] [**]

NEWBORN HEARING SCREENING

Current screening tests available

The tests used for newborn hearing screening are currently one or more of:

- automated otoacoustic emissions (AOAE);
- transient evoked otoacoustic emissions (TEOAE);
- distortion product otoacoustic emissions (DPOAE);
- automated auditory brainstem response (AABR).

TEOAE reflect the activity in the outer hair cells of the cochlea, while AABR waveforms are affected by cochlear and neural lesions. These methods are described in detail in Chapter 68, Hearing tests in children and Chapter 69, Investigation and management of the deaf child.

It is important to note that a newborn hearing screening programme protocol that regards a clear OAE result as a screen pass will miss neonates with auditory neuropathy, since the latter will manifest with OAE present, but ABR absent. Because auditory neuropathy is predominantly found in the NICU/SCBU population (and according to Sininger[13] as many as three per 1000 neonates enrolled in NICU/SCBU may have auditory neuropathy), AABR is the method of choice in the NICU/SCBU population. [**] In the UK Newborn Hearing Screening Programme (www.hearing.screening.nhs.uk), both AABR and TEOAE is required for NICU babies, while for well babies the two tests are done in series, with only those without clear bilateral responses on OAE going on to AABR. This ordering is driven by the time required and the costs associated with AABR as opposed to OEA.

Cut–off level and case definition

While many North American programmes[40, 41] target all babies with permanent hearing loss, including mild and unilateral hearing losses, the Newborn Hearing Screening Programme in England aims to identify all children with a permanent hearing loss of 40 dB HL or greater averaged over the frequencies 0.5, 1.0, 2.0 and 4.0 kHz for the better hearing ear.[4] As a byproduct, the screen will also identify a number of babies who have unilateral and in some cases mild hearing loss, but the consequences of delay in identification are not well established in these infants, and most are not candidates for hearing aids or other therapies associated with early identification.[42] [**] However, this is lack of evidence for effects rather than evidence of no effects, and research is underway to identify best practice for the early management of congenital permanent mild and unilateral hearing loss.

Models for universal newborn hearing screening

The most commonly used model to date has been a hospital-based screen employing a team of dedicated screeners performing the screening tests on neonates on the maternity unit before discharge. This is backed up by a recall clinic for the babies missed by the initial screen.[27, 42] However, in some European countries, a community-based screening model integrated into an existing framework of preventive health care has been used with considerable success.[43, 44] Owen et al.[45] reported that it was feasible for health visitors to perform neonatal hearing screening in the community and achieve very high coverage and low false-positive rates. The assumption is that community-based screening also results in higher parental satisfaction, but this is yet to be established. [**] Some areas in England are using a community-, rather than hospital-based model and cost-effectiveness comparisons are being undertaken.

'At–risk' screening

Risk factors for permanent congenital hearing loss are well established. Davis and Wood[8] showed that babies admitted to a neonatal intensive care unit for more than 48 hours were 10.2 (95 percent CI 4.4–23.7) times more likely to have a permanent hearing loss (greater than 50 dB HL in this study) than those who did not undergo

intensive care. Fortnum et al.[5] showed that prevalence was increased 14-fold for children with a family history of early permanent childhood deafness. Babies with cranio-facial anomalies associated with hearing impairment (e.g. cleft palate) are also at high risk for hearing loss. The large-scale Wessex study[27] reported that, of 25,000 newborns screened, 8.1 percent fulfilled high-risk criteria for permanent childhood hearing loss.

Thus, targeted newborn hearing screening looks like a desirable option, as only a small proportion of babies would need to be screened. The yield is potentially high: just 86–208 high-risk babies need to be screened to find one baby with hearing loss as opposed to a yield of one per 2041–2794 low-risk babies screened.[27, 46, 47] Thus, it has been argued that targeted newborn hearing screening is a relatively inexpensive way of improving the age of identification for a significant proportion of children with congenital hearing loss.[28]

However, there are a number of disadvantages to targeted newborn hearing screening. Stevens et al.[28] noted that some 'at risk' infants, in particular those with a family history of hearing loss, are not being referred for screening. More importantly, some 40 or 50 percent of babies born with permanent hearing loss demonstrate no risk factors. Numerous studies agree that around half of all affected infants have no risk factors at birth and thus would be missed by a targeted hearing screening.[5, 12, 41, 48]

Performance of universal newborn hearing screening

Davis et al.[4] reported in their critical review of the evidence that high coverage of over 90 percent was possible with hospital-based newborn screening programmes. The current newborn hearing screening programme in England has completed the screening in 96 percent of all target babies,[10] [**] which is well within the set quality standards.

Davis et al.[4] also concluded that screen sensitivity was estimated to range from 80 to nearly 100 percent and that screen specificity was above 90 percent. Specificity has been shown to gradually but significantly improve as advances in technology, use of two-stage screening (i.e. two tests) and training methodology evolve.[41, 49] [****/**] Davis et al.[50] concluded that all methods of neonatal hearing screening appear to have high test and screen sensitivity, which can be extended to programme sensitivity in both universal and targeted neonatal hearing screening programmes given sufficient resources. The authors also concluded that TEOAE screens and TEOAE/AABR combined screens in particular have high screen specificity for full-term babies shown in several different implementations. [**] Screen specificity is influenced by whether the protocol requires a clear response in both ears or in either ear. For example in the Wessex study, to facilitate lower failure rates, more rapid screening and greater coverage, a unilateral clear TEOAE response was accepted as a pass in infants younger than 48 hours.[27] [****]

Programme sensitivity has been shown to be around 80 percent.[4] [***] The yield has been shown to be very high. To find one child with bilateral moderate-to-profound hearing loss 755–1422 newborns have to be screened.[27, 42, 47] Yield is even higher, of course, if unilateral and mild cases are included.[41, 51] [**] The median age of identification for those screened neonatally is of the order of two months.[10, 42, 46, 52] [**]

It is important to note that these data are derived from a rather few, though large, published studies of universal newborn screening.[27, 42, 51] Only the Wessex study[27] is a controlled trial (but not a randomized controlled trial). The extent to which these encouraging results can be translated into a national screen is an issue being addressed by the national evaluation of the first phase of the Newborn Hearing Screening Programme (NHSP) in England.

Cost-effectiveness

Stevens et al.[28] found that in comparison to the IDT screen, universal newborn hearing screening has acceptable costs. They calculated the mean service price for universal hearing screening in three services and, for the IDT test screen, at 1994 prices, these were £13,881 and £24,519, respectively, for a standardized district of 1000 live births. [**]

The cost of universal newborn hearing screening compares favourably with screening for other congenital conditions, e.g. hypothyroidism, phenylketonuria or haemoglobinopathy.[53] It has been argued that universal newborn hearing screening will have paid for itself within ten years in terms of the long-term savings made in special education and social interventions.[53] However, longitudinal data do not yet exist. [**]

'Family-friendliness'

Since screening takes place over the very first days or even hours after the baby's birth, one of the main concerns associated with newborn hearing screening is the risk of causing unnecessary anxiety for the family.

Several studies on parental opinions show that in general parents were very positive about newborn hearing screening and that the risk of disturbing the parent–child relationship by early screening seemed small and could be further minimized by improved information and rapid and effective follow-up.[10, 38, 54, 55, 56, 57] [**] The current implementation of the NHSP in England has developed a number of processes for ensuring high levels of information for mothers/parents, including a national screener-training programme, training and information sessions

for other professionals, plain English information leaflets, written parental consent to the screen and so on. The extent to which these have minimized levels of anxiety in the mothers of babies passing the screen at different stages, and those whose babies are referred by the screen, is being investigated. The effects of early identification on the family are being investigated in true cases by in-depth interviews with parents.

Quality assurance

There is an ethical duty within a screening programme (particularly a national programme) to ensure that good quality services are in place prior to the start of the screening programme and that they continue to meet national guidelines. It is most important to promote an evaluative culture to enable continued service improvement in both technical and family-friendly service delivery.

Quality standards for early identification and management of congenital permanent hearing loss have been developed in the USA[7] and the UK.[58, 59] Consensus statements on newborn hearing screening have been developed in the USA[7] and in Europe.[60]

Some of the quality standards adopted by the current Newborn Hearing Screening Programme in England are shown in **Table 67.1**.

THE EIGHT-MONTH IDT SCREEN

The eight-month IDT screen has been in place as an almost universal screen across the UK since the late 1950s. It is being phased out as the Newborn Hearing Screening Programme is implemented. While protocols and test

Table 67.1 Quality standards for the NHS Newborn Hearing Screening Programme in England.

Quality standards
Initial programme coverage >90% of all live births by discharge
Screen coverage including call back >95% of all births by six months
Coverage of NICU/SCBU 99% of live discharge
Referral rate for non-NICU/SCBU <3%
Referral rate for NICU/SCBU <5%
All screen referrals followed up with audiological assessment by three months of age[a]
True cases confirmed by six months of age for all cases
Hearing aid fitted for all true cases within four weeks of confirmation[b]
Education services informed of all true cases within three working days

[a]Unless deliberately delayed for diagnostic reasons or follow-up refused.
[b]Unless deliberately delayed for management reasons.

details vary from area to area, the most typical format involves a two-person distraction test, using frequency-specific stimuli (low, mid and high frequencies) presented at quiet levels (e.g. 35 dBA) to the side and slightly behind (at 45°) the eight-month-old infant who is seated on the parent's knees. A full localization response to all stimuli on both sides represents an acceptable pass. Failures are usually retested once at a later date, except in the case of obvious concern, and two test failures constitutes a screen referral. This may be made to a secondary or tertiary audiology department, to a general practitioner for onward referral, or to an ear, nose and throat (ENT) department.

The screen cannot be used in the first six months of life and therefore it cannot support the start of intervention before six months of age. Evidence on the performance of this screen is reviewed by Davis et al.[4] The median age of identification through the IDT screen varies from 12 to 20 months; coverage falls in the range of 80–95 percent, although there may be some urban areas where coverage is as low as 60 percent. Sensitivity estimates of the IDT screen vary from 18 to 88 percent according to the service area. Screen sensitivity is greatly influenced by the degree of hearing loss, with higher sensitivity for more severe losses; even so, there have been too many cases of profound hearing losses passing the screen. Low coverage and low sensitivity result in unacceptably low incremental yield, in the range of 25–40 percent. The failure rate is high at 5–10 percent, largely because of poor practice and because of a high number of referrals due to transient OME. The referral rate has considerable resource implications for services. [**]

Because of its low yield, the IDT screen has not proved to be cost-effective. Davis et al.[4] estimate the cost per child detected with permanent bilateral hearing loss to be between £81,700 and £102,100 ($166,366 and $207,906), as opposed to £9900–£19,700 ($20,159 and $40,115) per child detected through a hospital-based newborn hearing screening programme. [****]

There have been consumer concerns about the quality of the IDT screen. Studies have shown that the subjectivity of the test has caused parents not to take the test seriously, which has contributed to low coverage and low interest in attending follow-up appointments.[61, 62] [**]

Because of widespread dissatisfaction with the IDT screen, there have been some attempts to substitute 'vigilance' programmes based on questionnaires to parents. Sutton and Scanlon[63] showed that a vigilance programme was likely to perform as well as the IDT screen (but no better) for severe and profound hearing losses, but less well than the IDT screen in referring moderate hearing losses. [**]

THE SCHOOL-ENTRY SCREEN

The school-entry hearing screen is currently employed universally across the UK. It consists of a modification of standard pure-tone audiometry, with test signals presented at specific frequencies and at fixed levels (the 'sweep' test). The cut-off level is set at 20 or 25 dB HL. One or two tests may be performed, usually during the first year of school entry. The screen is usually carried out by a school nurse, but may be done by a school doctor or audiology technician. Testing is generally done within the school and ambient noise may limit specificity. There is currently very little monitoring or evaluation of the school entry screen. Guidelines for training and testing for non-audiology professionals have been issued.[64]

Apart from referring children with progressive and acquired permanent hearing loss that have not been picked up by parental observation and responsive services, the school-entry screen also has the potential to identify children with mild and unilateral hearing loss, as well as high-frequency hearing loss and other hearing losses with unusual configurations. It may also have a role in identifying children with marked hearing loss due to OME, and is thought to be a reasonably cost-effective way of raising awareness of the importance of good hearing at a crucial stage of the child's education and development. However, these assertions remain to be tested by good quality research.

SURVEILLANCE

As we saw earlier, child health surveillance is regarded as one component of child health promotion programmes which encourage partnership between parents, children and health professionals and in which parents are empowered to make use of services and expertise according to their needs. Surveillance for childhood hearing loss is of considerable importance, since (1) newborn hearing screens will not find all those with preschool permanent hearing loss, because of late onset and progressive hearing loss; (2) any screening programme will miss an irreducible minimum of true cases; and (3) surveillance is a more justifiable approach to identification of children with persistent OME than a screening programme.

At present, there are only rather general guidelines for ongoing surveillance for childhood hearing loss.[65] A UK working group is currently developing more detailed recommendations. These require a hearing assessment by an appropriately trained audiology team at around eight months of age for all babies who did not give clear bilateral responses in the newborn screen, in particular those found to have permanent unilateral or permanent bilateral mild loss. Naturally all babies who missed the newborn screen or audiological follow-up for whatever reason (e.g. declined the newborn hearing screen, moved out of the area, etc.) need a follow-up by an audiologist at eight months of age. They also require that all children who are at risk for late onset or progressive deafness be offered regular hearing assessments by audiologists at appropriate ages, irrespective of the newborn screen outcome. These include infants with family history of childhood hearing loss;[66] a history of severe hyper-bilirubinaemia;[67] evidence or suspicion of congenital infection;[68, 69] presence of neurodegenerative or neuro-developmental disorders; all infants with confirmed or suspected meningitis;[70] those at high risk of persistent middle ear problems as well as sensorineural loss (e.g. children with cleft palate or Down syndrome);[71] and other craniofacial anomalies, including chromosomal or syndromic conditions, including branchial arch and cervical spine anomalies.[72] Surveillance policies should encourage services to be highly responsive to parental or professional concern about a child's hearing or their development of auditory, vocal or communicative behaviour; such infants should be offered a full hearing assessment at any age by an appropriately trained team. The importance of ongoing surveillance by health visitors, family doctors, community health teams, as well as parents (reinforced by appropriate check lists such as those given to parents shortly after the birth of their child), should not be underestimated, since it will help to deal with the increasing prevalence with age found by Fortnum et al.[6] in their extensive prevalence study.

SURVEILLANCE FOR OTITIS MEDIA WITH EFFUSION

Screening for either OME (the pathology) or for the consequent hearing loss (the impairment) fails to meet the criteria for screening programmes outlined under Principles and definitions above. On the other hand, we know that there are material effects upon speech/language, behaviour, physical well-being and quality of life for both parent and child in persistent cases. Some sort of surveillance system needs therefore to be in place for identifying and intervening with those 5 or 10 percent of cases that have OME with a persistence or severity likely to interfere with development. The TARGET group has shown that a screening questionnaire to parents on OME history and hearing loss gives only slightly lower sensitivity but similar specificity to that from school-entry screening. For OME, such questionnaire approaches to surveillance gain over screening, since the fluctuating nature of the condition tends to make a one-off screen misprecise, while parental reports tend usefully to average the observed effects over time.[15] [****]

'Watchful waiting' for three months has been shown to be an effective strategy for confirmed cases picked up by responsive services. Some 50 percent of such cases resolve after three months and do not justify further management unless the condition recurs.[14, 15] The only exception to the advisability of having a watchful-waiting period arises in children with a pure-tone average in the better ear ≥ 30 dB HL at their initial visit, who have a prior audiogram to confirm OME, and who are sent to ENT between August and December. In these children the probability of persistence is greater than 80 percent. [****] If good audiometry is not available in primary care (because of lack of equipment or expertise), tympanometry has been confirmed as sensitive and fairly specific in identifying children with material hearing loss associated with OME.[15] [****] On the other hand, it has been shown that little equipment is available or used to support OME assessment in UK primary care. However, it has also been shown that the use by family doctors of a simple checklist and a training video significantly improves the positive predictive value of their referrals.[15] [****]

The aim for services must be to identify those children who have persistent OME to the extent of being at risk for hearing and speech/language deficits, behaviour problems, quality of life, and, in a few cases, educational deficits.

KEY POINTS

- At least one in 1000 children is born with permanent bilateral hearing loss ≥ 40 dB HL.
- If permanent bilateral congenital hearing loss is identified before six months of age and habilitation started soon thereafter the adverse effects are lessened.
- By the age of nine years, the prevalence of permanent bilateral hearing loss ≥ 40 dB HL is at least 1.65 per 1000 children.
- Newborn hearing screening of all babies is the most cost-effective method of delivering early identification of congenital permanent hearing loss of at least moderate or greater degree.
- More evidence is required on the outcomes for children with permanent mild or unilateral hearing loss, and on alternative approaches to management.
- Screening at eight months using the infant distraction test is not cost-effective.
- School-entry screening may be cost-effective, but there is little evidence to judge as yet.
- Since prevalence continues to rise in the first few years of life, other methods based on surveillance and responsive services need to be in place.
- OME is a very common condition which may lead to hearing loss, delays in speech/language, behaviour problems and reduced quality of life in persistent cases.
- Identification of persistent OME cases depends upon good surveillance systems in primary care and responsive services.

Best clinical practice

✓ Newborn hearing screening of all babies is the most cost-effective way to identify congenital hearing loss.
✓ The eight-month infant distraction test screen is not cost-effective and cannot be justified.
✓ A surveillance programme needs to be in place to help identify late onset and acquired hearing losses, backed up by fast responsive services.
✓ Every effort should be made to minimize family anxiety by good-quality information and rapid and effective follow-up.
✓ Good quality services for true-positive cases based upon informed choices for parents are central to the introduction of a screening programme at any age, but particularly for newborn screening.
✓ Management of true-positive cases will involve close cooperation between health, education and social services.
✓ Parents and professionals in primary care need to be alert to the presence of persistent OME in some children; identification of these children is improved by the use of checklists and a training video by family doctors, and by a standardized 'screening' questionnaire to parents at varying times.

Deficiencies in current knowledge and areas for future research

➤ Even though there is evidence to show that parental anxiety associated with newborn hearing screening is fairly minimal, ways of reducing it further need to be investigated. In addition, more understanding of the experiences of the families whose babies are identified with hearing loss at a very early age is needed, in order to ensure that the service received at this early and sensitive stage is 'family-friendly'.
➤ There are a number of different ways to run a successful newborn hearing screening programme, in terms of equipment, tests and protocols. More work on the modelling of cost-effectiveness under different conditions (e.g. urban versus rural, size of the birthing hospital, the pattern of discharge, etc.) would be helpful.
➤ Auditory neuropathy is a relatively new condition to audiology services. More research is needed concerning the prevalence, aetiology, outcomes, diagnostic and habilitative options for children with this condition.
➤ Currently, children with mild and unilateral hearing loss will be identified as a by-product of newborn hearing screening for permanent bilateral hearing losses of ≥40 dB HL. More research is needed about the prevalence, effects, outcomes and habilitative options for these children.
➤ There is evidence to show that progressive and acquired permanent childhood hearing loss is more prevalent than previously thought. Confirmatory data are needed and evidence on the risk factors for progressive and acquired permanent childhood hearing loss is needed in order to improve surveillance or targeted assessment programmes.
➤ The school entry screen requires a more extensive evidence base.

REFERENCES

1. National Screening Committee. Webpage: http://www.nsc.nhs.uk.
2. Wilson JMG, Junger G. *Principles and practice of screening for disease.* Geneva: World Health Organisation, 1968.
3. Haggard MP, Hughes E. *Screening children's hearing.* London: HMSO, 1991.
* 4. Davis A, Bamford J, Wilson I, Ramkalawan T, Forsaw M, Wright S. A critical review of the role of neonatal hearing screening in the detection of congenital hearing impairment. *Hearing Technology Assessment.* 1997; **1**: 1–105.
* 5. Fortnum H, Davis A. Epidemiology of permanent hearing impairment in Trent region, 1985–1993. *British Journal of Audiology.* 1997; **31**: 409–46.
* 6. Fortnum HM, Summerfield AQ, Marshall DH, Davis AC, Bamford JM. Prevalence of permanent childhood hearing impairment in the United Kingdom and implications for universal neonatal hearing screening: questionnaire based ascertainment study. *British Medical Journal.* 2001; **323**: 536–9.
7. Finitzo T, Sininger Y, Brookhouser P, Epstein S, Erenberg A, Roizen N et al. Year 2000 position statement: Principles and guidelines for early hearing detection and intervention programs. *Pediatrics.* 2000; **106**: 798–817.
8. Davis A, Wood S. The epidemiology of childhood hearing impairment: Factors relevant to planning services. *British Journal of Audiology.* 1992; **26**: 77–90.
9. Vartiainen E, Karjalainen S. Prevalence and etiology of unilateral sensorineural hearing impairment in a Finnish childhood population. *International Journal of Pediatric Otorhinolaryngology.* 1998; **43**: 253–9.
10. Bamford J, Ankjell H, Crockett R, Marteau T, McCracken W, Parker D, et al. Evaluation of the newborn hearing screening programme in England: Studies, results and recommendations. Report to Department of Health and National Screening Committee, May 2005, 242.
11. Rance G, Beer DE, Cone-Wesson B, Shepherd RK, Dowell RC, King AM et al. Clinical findings for a group of infants and young children with auditory neuropathy. *Ear and Hearing.* 1999; **20**: 238–52.

68

Hearing tests in children

GLYNNIS PARKER

Introduction	834	Auditory speech discrimination tests	841
Electrophysiological testing	834	Hearing assessment in children with special needs	841
Behavioural observation audiometry	835	Key points	842
The distraction test	835	Best clinical practice	842
Visual reinforcement audiometry	838	Deficiencies in current knowledge and areas for future	
Performance testing	839	research	842
Pure tone audiometry	840	References	842

SEARCH STRATEGY

The data in this chapter are supported by a Medline search using the key words audiometry/child and hearing test/child.

INTRODUCTION

It is essential that suspected hearing loss in young children is promptly investigated. Accurate assessment of hearing is fundamental to diagnosis, investigation and rehabilitation. The techniques applicable to adults and older children are often inappropriate for the young child and for the older child or adult with special needs, particularly learning disability. Skilled testing by trained personnel in a suitable test environment is essential. Electrophysiological events in response to a sound stimulus may be recorded (electrophysiological testing). This is considered in detail in Chapter 67, Hearing loss in pre-school children: screening and surveillance and Chapter 233, Evoked physiological measurement of auditory sensitivity. The focus of this chapter is on those tests that require skilled observation and recording of the child's response to one or more sound stimuli. Testing is increasingly required to monitor speech perception in children with hearing aids and cochlear implants. These 'functional hearing tests' are also considered.

ELECTROPHYSIOLOGICAL TESTING

Key developmental age: 0–6 months, up to adult if appropriate

Electrophysiological techniques including otoacoustic emission (OAE), auditory brainstem response (ABR) and cortical evoked response audiometry (CERA) are discussed in Chapter 67, Hearing loss in pre-school children: screening and surveillance and Chapter 233, Evoked physiological measurement of auditory sensitivity. These methods are mainly employed in newborn screening (see Chapter 67, Hearing loss in pre-school children: screening and surveillance) and diagnostic testing of infants in the first six months.[1, 2] They can also prove of value in children of any age, when behavioural testing has failed to produce reliable results, in particular, those with severe learning or communication difficulties.[3] They may require general anaesthesia. Electrophysiological techniques are also used to confirm hearing thresholds, for example in children with profound hearing loss, prior to fitting of high power hearing aids or cochlear implantation or where nonorganic factors are suspected. Whilst electrophysiological testing has the advantage of being objective in terms of the child's response, behavioural or speech discrimination testing remain the only functional measures for assessing the complete auditory system.

BEHAVIOURAL OBSERVATION AUDIOMETRY

Key developmental age: 0–6 months

In behavioural observation audiometry (BOA), changes in activity are observed in response to a sound stimulus. Response behaviours in infants up to four months might include eye widening, eye blink (auropalpebral reflex), arousal from sleep, startle or shudder of the body or definite movement of the arms, legs or body. From four to seven months, lateral inclination of the head towards the sound or a listening attitude or stilling may be observed. The test is usually performed with the child cradled in the parent's lap. The child's attention may be lightly engaged in front by a distractor. The sound stimulus is presented for <2 seconds, in a horizontal plane, 15 cm from the child's ear, out of peripheral vision. The distractor observes evidence of a response. A range of sound stimuli may be sometimes employed, including narrow band and warble tones or less frequency-specific examples, such as a small bell, squawky squeeze toy or banging wooden bricks.[4] [***]

Reliability as a diagnostic test is obviously a concern. A wide variability in judgement of response between testers due to misinterpretation of random movements and a tendency to underestimate hearing thresholds has been demonstrated.[5] Attempts have been made to reduce observer bias by use of video recording of the procedure and scoring the playback without knowledge of the sound or no sound trials.[6] [***]

The use of BOA in infants under six months has been largely superseded by the availability of electrophysiological techniques. It does, however, have a continuing role in the assessment of children with severe learning difficulties, who have not reached an appropriate developmental stage for distraction or visual reinforcement audiometry. It may also be of value in cases of auditory neuropathy when ABR is a poor indicator of functional hearing levels.[7]

THE DISTRACTION TEST

Key developmental age: 6–18 months

The test is based on the principle that the normal response observed when sound is presented to a baby is a head turn to locate the source of sound. The test is suitable for babies from 6 to 18 months, corresponding to the stage when the child can sit erect unsupported and perform head turns in a horizontal plane. An appropriate allowance should be made for prematurity. Habituation is increasingly likely to occur after 12 months, although the technique may prove to be useful in older children with learning or communication difficulties where other methods have been unsuccessful.

The credibility of the infant distraction test as a tool for screening for hearing impairment has become questionable. In many areas, it has been discontinued in favour of electrophysiological testing in the newborn period[1] (see Chapter 67, Hearing loss in pre-school children: screening and surveillance). Nevertheless, it remains a valuable diagnostic technique when used by trained, experienced testers in appropriate settings. The infant distraction test was first described by Ewing and Ewing in 1944,[8] but was subsequently modified by McCormick[9] who placed particular emphasis on the use of frequency-specific, calibrated sound stimuli. The test is described with reference to the guidelines outlined by McCormick.[10] [***/**/*]

Test method

The test should be performed in a tidy, uncluttered, suitably sized room (recommended minimum >16 m^2) with ambient noise levels <30 dB(A). Two testers are required, one to present the sound stimuli out of vision and the other to control the baby's attention in the forward direction (the distractor). The latter should be responsible for directing the test. The arrangement is shown in **Figure 68.1**. The child sits on the parent's knee, facing forward and erect, lightly supported around the waist. The distractor directs the attention of the child to a simple activity usually performed on a low table. Suitable examples include spinning a brightly coloured object, using finger puppets or gently pushing a miniature car. In the classic distraction test described by McCormick, the item is covered by the hands which maintain a fine attention control by moving the fingers slightly. The sound stimulus is presented by the second tester, half a second after the item is covered. The distractor observes the child's response.

The second tester should be positioned strictly out of the child's visual field, which can be assumed to extend at least 90° to either side of the child's midline. The sound stimulus should be presented in the horizontal plane to the ears at an angle, set back 45° between 1 m and 15 cm from the child's ear. The shorter distance increases the head shadow effect, thereby increasing the sound stimulus on one side relative to the other. Evidence of asymmetric hearing levels may be indicated by a difference in response thresholds or difficulty in localizing the sound source. Particular care must be taken when presenting the sound close to the ear to avoid visual or tactile clues. The sound

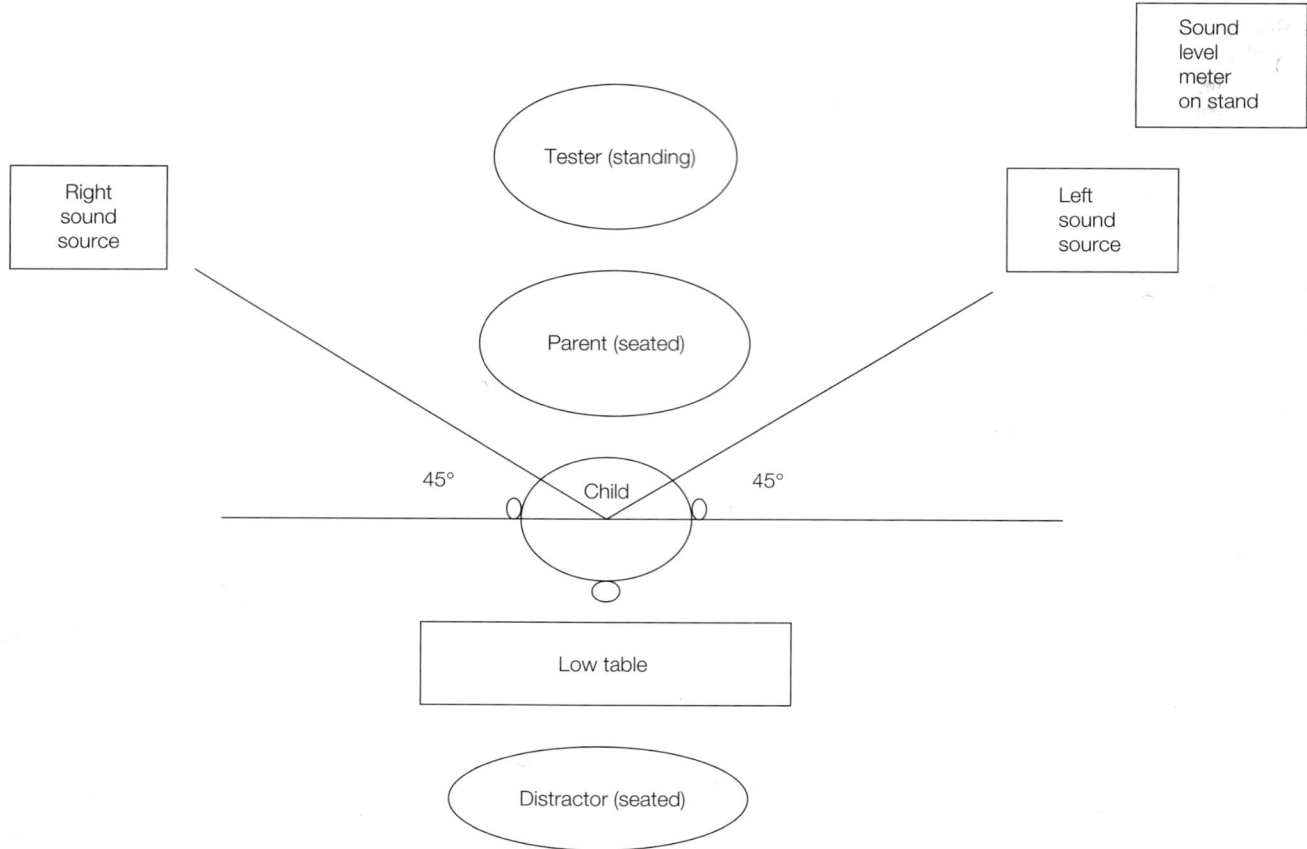

Figure 68.1 Test arrangement for the distraction test.

stimulus should continue up to 10 seconds if there is not an immediate response. During this interval, the distractor should maintain the fine attention control at the front until a response is observed.

The normal response expected is a full head turn in the direction of the sound. This may be rewarded by a smile or vocal praise or gentle tickle from the second tester. Some warble tone generators incorporate a flashing light, which can be activated in response to the turn, providing an incentive to the child and thereby acting as a 'response reinforcer'. The child's attention should then be brought back to the front by the distractor. [**]

The stimulus

A wide range of sound stimuli can be used to elicit a response, including voice, musical toys, 'everyday sounds', narrow band noise and warble tones (see **Figure 68.2**). Pure tones should be avoided due to the potential creation of standing waves, resulting in unpredictable sound levels. Responses to any sound stimulus may be valid, provided the intensity and the frequency spectrum, as delivered at the level of the ear, can be established. A sound level meter should be employed to check the intensity of the stimulus by accurately reproducing the

sound and the distance from the ear. Although it has been demonstrated that babies are more likely to respond to wide band sounds, this will inevitably provide less information regarding frequency-specific hearing as required for diagnosis and possible amplification prescription. Sound generators delivering calibrated narrow band and frequency-modulated warble tones have been demonstrated to be effective at eliciting a response and are therefore generally preferred.[11]

Initially, a sound stimulus is presented which is anticipated to be likely to be suprathreshold, for example at 70 dB(A) in a child with probable normal hearing. A sound is then presented at the anticipated minimal response threshold, for example, 30 dB(A). The intensity for sound field testing is generally measured on the dB(A) scale, but this can be converted to dBSPL (sound pressure level) if required, particularly for hearing aid prescription fitting.[12]

There is no prescribed order for frequency and intensity of sound presentations. The number of reliable responses elicited by distraction testing may be limited, particularly in children over 12 months who may habituate to the test. It is therefore important to prioritize and focus on those thresholds which would be most valuable for each clinical situation, but would normally aim to include high-, medium- and low-frequency information. This, however,

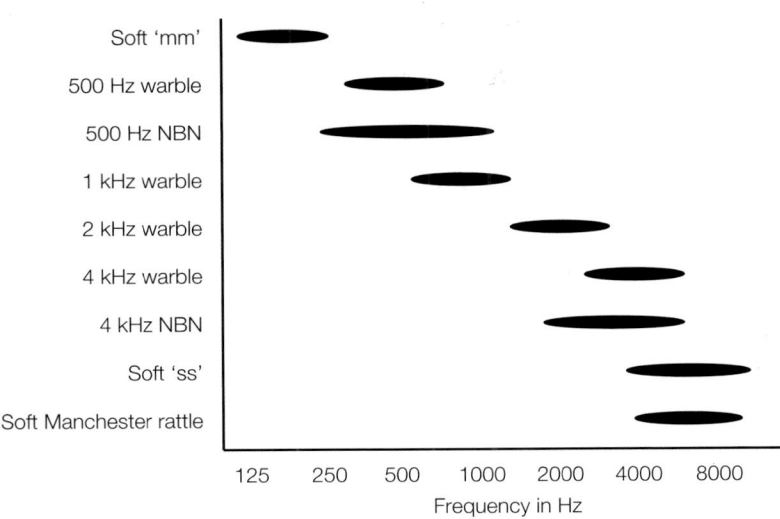

Figure 68.2 The distraction test: examples of frequency spectra for commonly used sound sources. With thanks to JC Stevens, Department of Medical Physics, Royal Hallamshire Hospital, Sheffield, UK.

may need to be balanced against the benefit of varying the order and side of presentation simply to sustain the child's interest. [Grade D]

No sound control trials

No sound trials are essential for the validation of response thresholds in a distraction test. Some children exhibit checking or searching behaviour or simply turn towards their parents for reassurance during the test. This can clearly be misleading if it coincides with a sound presentation. It is therefore appropriate to introduce control trials in which the test is performed in the usual manner by both testers, but no sound is generated. If the child appears to make a response, then it must be assessed how this compares to the responses observed to sound trials. Usually a difference is noted which can be used to confirm a true response. However, if the checking responses are indistinguishable from the sound responses, the results must be interpreted with appropriate caution.

Tactics such as increasing the interest of the distracting activity and/or maintaining that activity whilst the sound/no sound is presented may avoid 'clueing in' the child. This may be particularly helpful in children over one year. Evidence of visual, tactile or even olfactory clues must also be considered and addressed. [*]

Recording the results

The outcome of each valid presentation and no sound trial should be recorded in chart form, specifying the sound source, frequency range if known and intensity. A tick or a cross may be used to indicate whether a response was observed. The response threshold is regarded as the quietest level at which two out of three clear responses were recorded for each particular sound stimulus. Other observations such as the ability to localize the sound source correctly or any concerns about the test reliability should also be recorded. **Table 68.1** lists the most commonly encountered pitfalls in distraction testing and avoidance measures. [**]

Table 68.1 Pitfalls encountered in distraction testing.

Pitfalls	Avoidance measures
Visual, tactile, olfactory clues from parent, distractor or second tester	Critical observation of all parties
	No sound trials
'Checking' responses by child	Critical assessment of responses
	No sound trials, if necessary take a break, or sustain distraction activity
Loss of interest in test, suprathreshold responses	Vary the sound stimulus
	Exchange roles of distractor or second tester
	Use broader band or more interesting sounds
Inaccurate estimation of frequency and intensity of stimulus	Use calibrated sound sources
	Measure accurately with sound level meter, trying to reproduce conditions
Extraneous noise, leading to false responses or only suprathreshold response	Use quiet facilities, ideally a sound-treated room with ambient noise <30 dB(A)
	Observe other auditory clues, e.g. clicking switch on warbler
	No sound trials

VISUAL REINFORCEMENT AUDIOMETRY

Key developmental age: 6–36 months

Visual reinforcement audiometry (VRA) incorporates the principle that young children can be trained by operant conditioning to produce a localizing turn to a visual stimulus in response to a sound stimulus. A technique of conditioned orientation reflex (COR) audiometry was initially described by Suzuki and Ogiba[13] and was further developed by Liden and Kankkunen[14] who introduced the term 'visual reinforcement audiometry'. Further developments and modifications to the technique have been described.[15, 16] VRA is now established as a standard technique within the test battery for hearing assessment in preschool children.[17, 18, 19] A comparison of VRA with the infant distraction test in children aged 12–25 months has demonstrated that VRA generates more auditory-evoked head turns than an unrewarded sound stimulus and delays habituation so that the test was more likely to be completed.[20] The method is described with reference to Widen et al.[21] and Shaw.[22] [***/**/*]

The test arrangement

The test room should be sound-treated to ensure low levels of ambient noise and should ideally be partitioned to provide an observation area with a one-way window, with access to a communication system between the rooms, such as a radio link. If however, this facility is not available, then it is still possible to perform the test within one room, provided the tester operating the audiometer minimizes the distraction to the child and does not provide any additional clues. A suitable arrangement is shown in **Figure 68.3**. The child is seated on the parent's lap or on a low chair in front of a low table, with the parent seated slightly behind. A second tester may sit on the other side of the table or adjacent to the child to provide low level play activity. For sound field testing, the speakers may be placed at 45, 60 or 90° from the child and at the same height as the child's head at a distance of at least 1 m from the ear. Frequency-specific calibration of the sound signal from a test point equivalent to the child's head position is essential. Alternatively, a calibrated signal may be presented via insert earphones using foam tips or the child's own ear moulds, if available. This has the advantage of potentially providing more precise ear-specific response thresholds and even offers an opportunity to introduce masking by appropriate presentation of narrow band noise in the contralateral ear. This is particularly valuable in amplification selection and setting.[23] A standard bone conductor may also be used in conjunction with VRA to differentiate between a conductive and sensorineural hearing loss. [**]

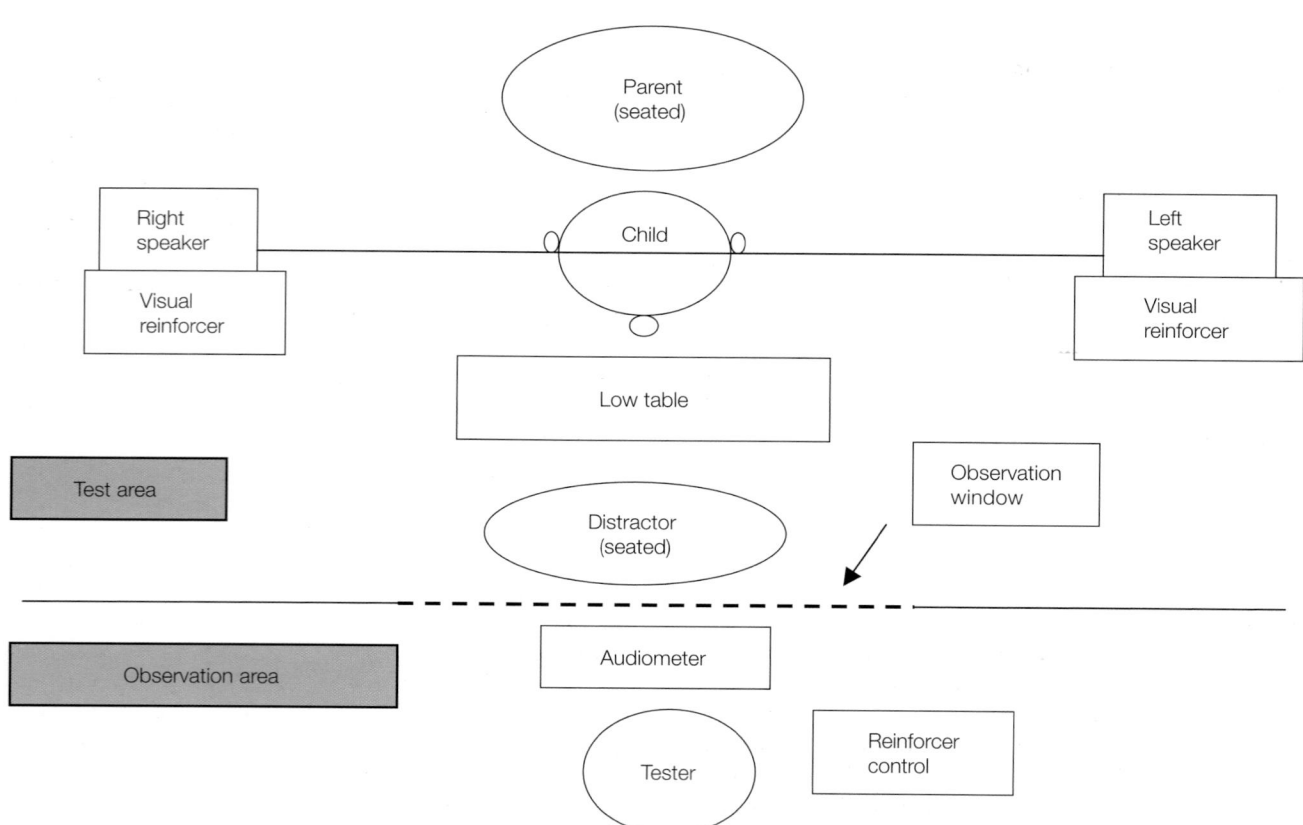

Figure 68.3 The test arrangement for visual reinforcement audiometry.

Thompson and Folsom[24] demonstrated that in VRA, unlike distraction testing, the complexity of the signal, including the bandwidth, had no effect on response rate once the child had been correctly conditioned. Frequency-modulated warble tones are generally employed for sound field testing, but pure tones may be used in conjunction with insert earphones or a bone conductor. The frequency sequence should be prioritized according to the clinical situation, but would most often include 0.5, 1.0, 2.0 and 4.0 kHz and in some cases 0.25 and 3 kHz. The duration of the signal is usually two to three seconds.

Visual reinforcers are generally placed adjacent to or above each speaker. The reinforcer acts as a reward and therefore increasing the attractiveness or appeal to the child and introducing variety is likely to sustain interest and reduce habituation. Commercially available reinforcers, include toys with eyes that light up and puppets in darkened glass cabinets which illuminate and dance. Monitors showing appropriate video displays can also be effective. The reinforcer is generally remotely activated by the tester as required. [**]

Test method

Using the arrangement as described above, the first task must be to establish the conditioned response. Having drawn the child's attention to the front by gentle play activity on the table, a suprathreshold auditory signal should be presented concurrently with the visual reward, for example, for a child with probable near-normal hearing, one might start with a 1 kHz warble tone at 70 dBHL. The child may turn to locate the sound (orientation response) and thereby view the activated reinforcer, but if necessary, the child's attention should be directed towards it. This sequence is repeated several times. The sound stimulus should then be presented alone and the reinforcer only activated after the child has produced an appropriate turning response. Praising the child and making it a game will further help to reinforce the response. If this can be reliably repeated two or three times, then operant conditioning has been established. Children under one year or those with learning difficulties may take longer to successfully condition. If it appears that the initial auditory stimulus may be inadequate, this can be cautiously increased or a different frequency or vibrotactile stimulus used.

Once the child has demonstrated successful conditioning, the aim is to establish minimal response levels (MRL) for each frequency, as prioritized by the clinical situation. One reliably obtained MRL is more valuable than a number of 'maybes'. A flexible descending/ascending technique, similar to that used in play audiometry may be applied. Responses should be charted as described for the distraction test, using the two out of three valid response rule to determine the MRL. No sound control trials should be included to verify a true response and similar measures taken in the event of frequent 'checking behaviour'. MRL less than 20 dBHL can routinely be recorded for frequencies between 0.5 and 4 kHz in normal hearing infants using insert earphone VRA.[25] Primus[26] found test–retest reliability to be good with 50 percent repeatability within 10 dB. Widen[21] demonstrated that MRL for at least four frequencies were successfully recorded in more than 90 percent of over 3000 infants aged 8–12 months, tested using VRA. [***]

PERFORMANCE TESTING

Key developmental age: 2–5 years

The performance test was first described by Ewing and Ewing[8] as a transitional technique suitable for children from 2.5 years and in some cases younger, until co-operation with pure tone audiometry can be achieved. It can be used to assess unaided or aided sound field thresholds. It follows the simple principle that the child is conditioned to wait for a sound and then to respond with a play activity. The test method is described with reference to McCormick.[10] [**]

Test method

The child should be seated on a low chair adjacent to the parent in an uncluttered room with low levels of ambient noise. A toy is placed on a low table in front of the child (**Figure 68.4**). Toys which involve a simple repetitive activity are most suitable, such as the classic 'men in a boat', balls on sticks, knocking down skittles or pegs in a board. The conditioning sequence starts with the tester engaging the child's attention by holding the response item, e.g. the wooden man, poised waiting in front of the child. After a few seconds, a suprathreshold sound stimulus is presented and the tester responds by an appropriate activity, e.g. placing the man in the boat. This sequence is repeated several times often supported by gestures such as a stop sign using the palm of the hand and a cupped hand to the ear to indicate listening. This has the advantage of avoiding dependence on spoken language. The child is then offered the response item and guided to wait and perform the task as shown. Vocal praise should be used to reinforce a correct response. The number of repetitions required to successfully condition the child will depend on their age, developmental status, willingness to co-operate and in particular their ability to inhibit the response until the signal is detected. It may be necessary to increase the intensity of the signal or initiate conditioning using a vibrotactile stimulus.

69

Investigation and management of the deaf child

SUJATA DE, SUE ARCHBOLD AND RAY CLARKE

Introduction	844	Key points	856
Epidemiology	844	Best clinical practice	856
Aetiology	845	Deficiencies in current knowledge and areas for future	
The newly diagnosed deaf child	849	research	857
Support and education	853	References	857

SEARCH STRATEGY

The references for this chapter were compiled from a Medline search using the terms deaf, hearing loss or hearing impairment and child. The World Health Organization (WHO) website (www.who.int), the NHS Newborn Hearing Screening Programme website (www.nhsp.info), the deafness and hereditary hearing loss overview website (www.geneclinics.org/profiles/deafness-overview/details) and the NHS Modernising Childrens' Hearing Aid Service website (www.psych-sci.manchester.ac.uk/mchas) were also consulted.

INTRODUCTION

This chapter focusses on the general principles of management of a moderately to profoundly deaf child. Sensorineural deafness may occur before (prelingual deafness) or after the child has acquired the ability to speak (postlingual deafness). This distinction has important implications for the child's education and management.

Earlier detection with universal neonatal screening is now practised in most developed countries. Advances in detection, genetics, imaging and treatment – including amplification and cochlear implantation – for these children have meant that new guidelines and ways of working are needed for healthcare professionals. There has also been more understanding of the deaf culture, the deaf community and their concerns with these advances. The implication of all levels and types of deafness for education has increasingly been recognized, together with the implications of managing the modern technologies in educational settings. The education of deaf children has

also been challenged with a worldwide move towards the integration of deaf children into mainstream education wherever possible.

EPIDEMIOLOGY

Approximately one child in 1000 (some 900 per year in the UK) is born with a bilateral permanent childhood hearing impairment (PCHI). This is defined as confirmed permanent bilateral hearing impairment exceeding 40 dBHL (hearing level) (average of pure tone thresholds at 0.5, 1, 2 and 4 kHz in the better hearing ear). About 60 percent of these children have a moderate (41–60 dBHL) hearing loss, while the remainder have a severe (61–80 dBHL) or profound (>81 dbHL) loss (www.who.int/pbd/deafness/hearing_impairment_grades/en/index). Hearing loss in a child may be present at birth (congenital) or may develop after birth (acquired). The prevalence of PCHI increases with age, suggesting that a further one in 1000 children develop acquired or progressive hearing impairment.[1] The terms 'deafness' and 'deaf' in this chapter are used to cover both moderate, severe and profound hearing loss.

The WHO estimated in 2005 that there were 278 million people worldwide with bilateral moderate to profound hearing loss, of whom 62 million had deafness that began in childhood. Two-thirds of people with moderate to severe hearing impairment live in developing countries.

In the developing world, the greatest proportion of childhood hearing loss is caused by infection. This includes congenital conditions, such as rubella and cytomegalovirus, and acquired childhood infections such as mumps, measles, meningitis and chronic otitis media. In the developed world, about half of children with PCHI have a genetic cause for their deafness.

AETIOLOGY

Most children with permanent childhood hearing impairment have sensorineural hearing loss. Causes of conductive hearing loss include chronic otitis media and some rare congenital conditions, such as bilateral aural atresia. The causes of PCHI are shown in **Table 69.1**.

Congenital causes

GENETIC

Genetic disease results from aberrations in the coding function or processing of human DNA. In the western world, congenital sensorineural hearing loss is accounted for by genetic factors in approximately half of cases. About 77 percent of these cases of hereditary hearing loss are autosomal recessive, 22 percent are autosomal dominant and 1 percent are X-linked.[2] In addition, a small fraction (less than 1 percent) represents those families with mitochondrial inheritance in which the trait is passed through the maternal lineage. In general, autosomal recessive forms of hearing loss are prelingual. Autosomal dominant forms tend to present later and result in progressive, postlingual hearing loss.[3]

Approximately 30 percent of patients will have a pattern of additional medical anomalies such as to constitute a syndrome – syndromic hearing loss. Nonsyndromic hearing loss constitutes most cases of congenital sensorineural loss. A number of gene mutations thought to be responsible for nonsyndromic hearing loss have recently been identified. The disorder DFNB1, caused by mutations in the GJB2 gene (which encodes the protein connexin 26) and the GJB6 gene (which encodes the protein connexin 30), accounts for 50 percent of autosomal recessive nonsyndromic hearing loss. The carrier rate in the general population for a recessive deafness-causing GJB2 mutation is about one in 33.[4]

Table 69.1 Causes of permanent childhood hearing impairment.

Causes of hearing impairment		
Congenital disorders		
Genetic	Syndromic	Autosomal recessive
		Autosomal dominant
		X-linked
		Mitochondrial
	Nonsyndromic	Autosomal recessive
		Autosomal dominant
		X-linked
		Mitochondrial
Nongenetic	Congenital rubella syndrome	
	Cytomegalovirus	
	Congenital syphilis	
Environmental causes		
Perinatal causes	Hypoxia	
	Hyperbilirubinemia	
	Low birth weight	
Acquired disorders	Infections	Chronic otitis media
		Meningitis
		Mumps
		Measles
		AIDS
	Ototoxic drugs	
	Trauma	
	Neoplastic disease	
Idiopathic		

Syndromic sensorineural hearing loss is found in conditions such as Pendred's syndrome, Branchio-otorenal syndrome, Usher syndrome and Wardenburg syndrome, amongst others. Conductive hearing loss is commonly encountered in Down syndrome and Treacher Collins syndrome.

NONGENETIC

Perinatal factors

In the developed world, approximately half of cases of congenital hearing loss are due to environmental factors. In previous decades, infectious agents such as rubella and cytomegalovirus were common environmental causes of hearing loss. While the frequency of such infections has dropped with the introduction of vaccines, a concomitant improvement in the survival rates of preterm babies has increased the proportion of babies with hearing loss related to perinatal events, including stays in the neonatal intensive care unit (NICU). Thus, the overall incidence of nongenetic deafness has remained approximately unchanged. Preterm and low-birth-weight infants are particularly susceptible to factors, such as hypoxia and hyperbilirubinaemia. Davis and Wood[5] showed that babies admitted to a neonatal intensive care unit for more than 48 hours were 10.2 (95 percent, confidence interval 4.4 – 23.7) times more likely to have a permanent hearing loss (greater than 50 dBHL in this study) than those who did not undergo intensive care. Hypoxia is associated with apnoea, difficult delivery, low Apgar scores and use of ventilation. It is known to be associated with neurodevelopmental deficits, but the exact mechanism of hypoxia-related hearing loss is unclear. Hyperbilirubinemia is an independent risk factor for sensorineural hearing loss in infants. High levels of unconjugated bilirubin cross the immature blood–brain barrier and deposit in the grey matter causing neurotoxicity. This is thought to lead to sensorineural hearing loss, which is usually permanent, although some cases may be reversed once bilirubin levels return to normal.[6] These infants are more often than not nursed on a neonatal intensive care unit, where they may receive ototoxic drugs, such as aminoglycoside antibiotics (e.g. gentamicin, tobramycin and amikacin) and diuretics (e.g. furosemide). There is some evidence of a genetic susceptibility to the damaging effects of these drugs explaining the variability in hearing loss that affects infants treated in neonatal intensive care units.[7]

Maternal infections

Infection is still responsible for a significant proportion of acquired hearing loss, especially in developing countries, although vaccination has greatly reduced the incidence. Congenital cytomegalovirus (CMV) is the most common cause of nonhereditary sensorineural hearing loss in the developed world.[8, 9] Between 22 and 65 percent of symptomatic and 6 and 23 percent of asymptomatic children will have hearing loss following congenital CMV infection.[10] It has been estimated that 12 percent of congenital sensorineural hearing loss is due to CMV infection. The hearing loss can be of delayed onset with threshold fluctuations and/or progressive loss.[3]

Congenital rubella syndrome (CRS) is probably the most important cause of nongenetic congenitally acquired hearing loss in countries with no rubella vaccination programme. CRS occurs when there is maternal infection with the rubella virus in the first trimester of pregnancy. It leads to a number of abnormalities in the child including deafness, ocular defects (cataracts, glaucoma), cardiovascular anomalies (patent ductus arteriosus, pulmonary artery stenosis and ventricular septal defects), central nervous system problems (microcephaly, global retardation) and characteristic skin changes (**Figure 69.1**).[11]

The WHO has recommended vaccination against rubella (www.who.int/immunization/topics/rubella/en/index1). Two approaches have been suggested: (1) prevention of CRS only, through immunization of adolescent girls and/or women of childbearing age; or (b)

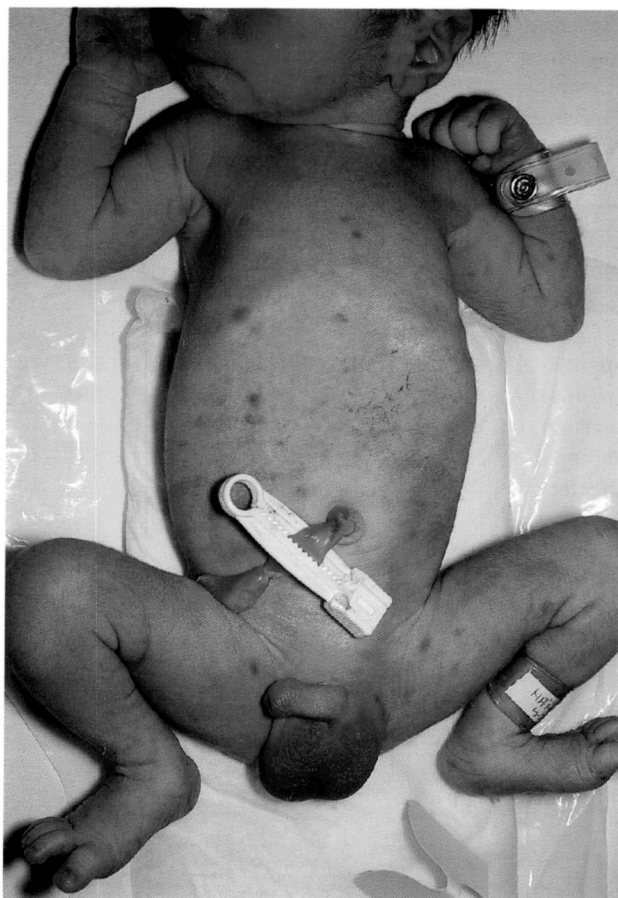

Figure 69.1 Congenital rubella with characteristic skin rash. The child was profoundly deaf. Courtesy of J Verbov, Emeritus Professor of Paediatric Dermatology, Royal Liverpool Children's Hospital, Alder Hey.

elimination of rubella, as well as CRS through universal vaccination of infants and young children (with/without mass campaigns), surveillance and assuring immunity in women of childbearing age.[12] This is the norm in most developed countries where the incidence of CRS deafness is now very rare.[13]

Syphilis is caused by the bacterium *Treponema pallidum*. It is a common infection in most of the developing world and has recently re-emerged in parts of the developed world. The main route of transmission is sexual contact, but syphilis can also be transmitted from an infected mother to her baby (congenital syphilis). Congenital infection can occur at any stage during pregnancy, but the highest likelihood of damage to the foetus is when infection occurs and is untreated during the first or second trimesters. During primary syphilis, the rate of vertical transmission in untreated women is 70–100 percent; this drops to 10–40 percent in the latent stage of the disease. Thus the poorest prognosis is for an infant infected during the first or second trimester by a mother in the primary or secondary stages of disease.

Hearing loss is a late feature of congenital syphilis and often appears as one of a group of signs known as 'Hutchinson's triad'. These signs include inflammation of the cornea giving it an opaque appearance, which leads to loss of vision, peg-shaped upper incisors (Hutchinson's teeth) and eighth cranial nerve deafness. Hearing loss is the least common component of Hutchinson's triad and occurs in around 3 percent of children with late congenital syphilis. It typically appears when the child is eight to ten years of age, although occasionally it may be delayed until adulthood. Onset is sudden and damage to the cranial nerve is thought to result from a persistent and ongoing inflammatory response to the infection. Loss of hearing may be unilateral or bilateral and initially involves higher frequencies, with normal conversational tones affected later.[14]

Congenital syphilis can be treated with high-dose penicillin, but is best prevented by identification and eradication of the infection in the mother. Prenatal screening for syphilis is commonplace in developed countries and is the main priority for prevention of the disease in developing countries.

Acquired causes

Causes of permanent acquired hearing loss include bacterial meningitis, chronic otitis media, mumps, measles, trauma and ototoxic drugs.

MENINGITIS

The most common cause of acquired PCHI is childhood meningitis. The risk of developing significant sensorineural impairment after bacterial meningitis has been estimated at approximately 10 percent.[15, 16, 17, 18] Early assessment of hearing after meningitis is recommended so that appropriate rehabilitation can be initiated. If cochlear implantation is necessary, this should be done with minimal delay as ossification of the cochlear duct can make implantation difficult or even impossible (see Chapter 70, Paediatric cochlear implantation).

MEASLES

Measles is a highly infectious viral illness, which presents acutely with high fever, running nose, characteristic Koplik's spots on the buccal mucosa and a distinctive generalized maculopapular rash (**Figure 69.2**). It occurs worldwide but its incidence has reduced significantly in developed countries since the introduction of an effective vaccine in 1968. It is predominantly a disease of infants and young children and occurs mostly after the age of six months. Globally, measles is the leading cause of vaccine-preventable child deaths.

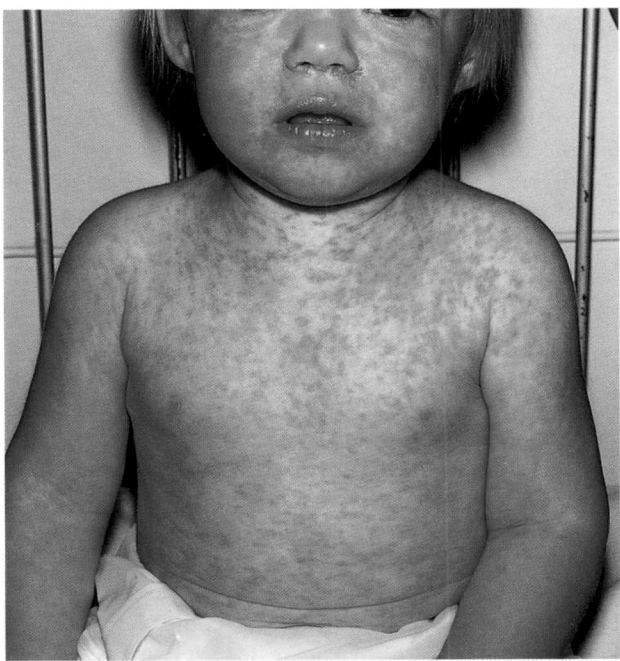

Figure 69.2 Child with maculopapular rash characteristic of measles. Courtesy of J Verbov, Emeritus Professor of Paediatric Dermatology, Royal Liverpool Children's Hospital, Alder Hey.

Measles has been reported as a major aetiological factor for severe to profound bilateral hearing loss in deaf children. As it was known that mucous membranes all over the body were affected, the observed hearing loss was previously thought to be conductive and attributable to suppurative otitis media, chronic perforation and mastoiditis. There are reports of measles virus being found within the cochlea, thus providing the needed evidence in favour of the sensorineural component. This explains the often-reported severe and sometimes progressive/delayed sensorineural hearing loss among affected children.

The WHO and United Nations Children's Fund (UNICEF) have emphasized primary prevention of measles in its global campaign against the prevailing childhood illnesses in the developing world for several decades. Immunization for measles can be administered as a single vaccine or as the triple MMR (measles, mumps and rubella) vaccine (www.who.int/vaccines-documents/DocsPDF01/www573).

MUMPS

Mumps, caused by infection with the mumps virus, is a nonsuppurative enlargement of the salivary glands, particularly the parotids. The infection may be subclinical in up to one-third of the cases and in these the first presentation may be the appearance of complications. Sensorineural hearing loss as a result of mumps is mostly unilateral, although bilateral loss has been described. The incidence of mumps-related sensorineural hearing loss has been documented as 5/100,000.[19]

Mode of presentation

It has been shown that early diagnosis of PCHI has an important bearing on outcome. A landmark study has demonstrated that children whose hearing losses were identified by six months of age demonstrated significantly better receptive and expressive language skills than did children whose hearing losses were identified after the age of six months.[20] [***]

SCREENING

Since the recent introduction of universal neonatal screening in most developed countries, PCHI is identified mainly through this modality. However, some children with PCHI are still missed until a later age. In countries where neonatal screening has not been implemented, diagnosis is still dependent upon parental suspicion, distraction testing and preschool screening. In addition, children with progressive hearing loss may be identified by surveillance and parental/teacher suspicion. Children who develop PCHI as a result of childhood illness are usually identified by a high degree of suspicion by parents and carers and by surveillance.

Prior to the introduction of universal neonatal screening in the UK in 2001/2002, almost a quarter of children born deaf were not identified until they were over 3.5 years of age.[21] As a result of universal neonatal screening in the UK, the median age of detection of PCHI is now ten weeks.[22]

Currently in the UK, all children are screened with automated otoacoustic emissions (AOAE) as close to the time of birth as possible by a trained operator. The result of the test is either a 'pass' or 'refer'. In addition, all infants in neonatal intensive care units have automated auditory brainstem response (AABR) testing. This is because there is a proportion of children with auditory neuropathy (estimated to be up to three in 1000 in the neonatal intensive care unit) whose AOAE test would give a 'pass' result.[23] A child who does not pass the OAE screening test in both ears would go on to have AABR testing. If this too is not passed then the child is referred for further testing.

More information on screening can be found in Chapter 67, Hearing loss in preschool children: screening and surveillance.

SINGLE-SIDED DEAFNESS

Screening has also resulted in early detection of unilateral sensorineural hearing loss. In the past, unilateral hearing loss was considered to be of little consequence because speech and language presumably developed appropriately with one normal-hearing ear. The yield for permanent unilateral moderate or greater hearing loss in the Newborn Hearing Screening Programme in England is 0.64 (95 percent, CI 0.37–0.91) per 1000 screened.[22] Of course, unilateral hearing loss can also be acquired and this occurs as a result of trauma, infection, ototoxicity, metabolic disorders and surgery. Unilateral hearing loss results in an inability to hear from the direction of the deaf side, difficulty in hearing speech in noise and poor localization of sound. A review carried out in 2004 concluded that school children with unilateral hearing loss appear to have increased rates of grade failures, need additional educational assistance and may show behavioural issues in the classroom. Speech and language delays may occur in some children, but it is unclear if children 'catch up' as they grow older.[24]

It would appear that the impact of unilateral hearing loss on the language development and educational performance varies considerably.

Current practice is that unilateral sensorineural hearing loss is investigated to identify progressive pathology or conditions that might affect the other ear, e.g. dilated vestibular aqueducts. At the time of writing, children with single-sided deafness are monitored in the UK, but not treated unless the child complains of a problem with localization or perception of speech in noise.

DELAYED PRESENTATION

The infant distraction test (IDT), which was the screening test used in the UK until recently, had been in place since the 1960s. It involved a health visitor check at the age of nine months within the community. A behavioural test was used which had neither high sensitivity nor specificity. As a result, a large number of children with normal hearing were referred for further investigations. More worryingly, a large number of children with PCHI were not being identified. There are no data available yet on how many children are detected late since the introduction of universal neonatal screening in the UK.

In countries where universal neonatal screening has not yet been established, identification of children with PCHI is still dependent on parental or teacher suspicion, locally arranged behavioural screening programmes and preschool screening. In a questionnaire-based study in Nigeria, only 12 percent of parents of a child with hearing loss suspected hearing difficulty by the age of six months. Parental suspicion occurred mostly at 12–24 months, compared with 8–14 months in developed countries. The most common mode of detection was a child's failure to respond to sound (49 percent).[25]

PROGRESSIVE HEARING LOSS

Some children have normal hearing or only a mild loss at birth, but develop progressive hearing loss with time. A study performed in the UK just before the introduction of universal neonatal screening showed the prevalence of confirmed PCHI to be 1.07 per 1000 (95 percent confidence interval 1.03–1.12) for three-year-olds. Amongst children aged 9–16 years though, the prevalence increased to 2.05 per 1000 (2.02–2.08). This increase in prevalence must be due to either acquired or progressive hearing loss. It is likely that a number of children have progressive hearing loss and would not necessarily be identified by neonatal or early screening.[1]

Progressive hearing loss may be due to genetic or environmental causes. In some syndromes such as Pendred's syndrome, the hearing loss is typically progressive. Nonsyndromic hearing loss related to a variety of known and unknown mutations can also be fluctuant or progressive.[26] Some infectious causes such as congenital CMV and congenital syphilis can cause late-onset or progressive hearing loss.

This group poses a challenge, as neonatal screening will not identify them. Identification of these cases therefore is dependent upon a high degree of suspicion in children with known associated syndromes, surveillance and prompt assessment in response to parent or teacher concern.

HEARING LOSS DUE TO CHILDHOOD ILLNESS

Acquired PCHI can be caused by meningitis, viral infections such as mumps and measles, chronic otitis media, trauma or ototoxicity (streptomycin, cisplatin). Early detection of hearing loss in these groups is based upon surveillance of at-risk groups (e.g. children undergoing chemotherapy) and parent/teacher/medical staff suspicion.

THE NEWLY DIAGNOSED DEAF CHILD

Parents and healthcare professionals are faced with a series of dilemmas and challenges when it is established that a child is deaf. Parents remember with chilling clarity the day they were told their baby was deaf, and cumbersome inexpert handling of this scenario can have profound adverse effects. An experienced empathic team that works in a coordinated way with the family and can present a knowledgeable and nonpartisan approach to the various options and resources available makes for the best outcome for parents and child. Now the diagnosis is likely to take place very early in the child's life before parents have adjusted to being parents and it is even more important that time is made available for them and that they are supported in the early days.

Reactions to the diagnosis

For the majority of parents, having a child with hearing loss is completely unexpected. Parents, when confronted with a diagnosis of hearing loss in their child, go through a grieving process akin to a death experience; they have lost the expectation of the 'perfect' baby. For the parents of a child with a disability, this time frame is less rigid and the grief can be nonfinite and last the lifespan of the child, emerging at critical points. In a survey of parental reactions to the news that their baby had failed a hearing screening test, the feelings elicited were of fear, shock, confusion, depression, frustration, anger, loneliness, sadness, blame and even agression.[27]

Large surveys have shown that the vast majority of parents would like to know whether their child has permanent hearing impairment as close to birth as possible.[28] This is now an expectation, but it places great responsibility on the professionals.

Parents will have questions regarding the development of the child, especially speech and future education needs. Many of these questions cannot be answered straight away. The parents are then bombarded with information regarding intervention and are required to make decisions often without understanding or taking in the information they have been given.

The presence of a child with hearing loss is often linked with psychosocial stress in the parents and other family members.[29] Once a hearing loss has been confirmed, these emotions become even more heightened. The degree of hearing loss does not seem to influence the parents' ability to cope. In fact, stress levels were found to be higher in the parents of children with less severe hearing loss.[30] This might be because the child may at least sometimes respond to sound, which can delay the parents' acceptance of the hearing loss and confuse the diagnosis.

The initial grief may be followed by feelings of anger, despair and helplessness as the diagnosis becomes apparent. Sadness, sorrow, even depression may occur. Parental guilt is also a feature of the reaction to the diagnosis. The expectation of having to make decisions that will hugely impact the future of their child and the amount of information from health professionals that they have to take in within a short span of time leads to confusion and sometimes insecurity.

Stress and quality of life remain factors even after the parents have come to terms with the diagnosis.

The impact on the parents of earlier diagnosis of hearing loss as a result of neonatal screening is a cause for concern. It has been suggested that such an early diagnosis of hearing loss may interfere with parental bonding with a child that is usually otherwise perfectly healthy, and which we know is vital to support the early development of communication skills, the foundations of later language development, whether spoken or signed. This concern is reflected by the experience of some parents. The risk of disturbing the parent–child relationship by early screening could be minimized by improved information and rapid and effective follow up. Young and Tattersall[31] used a narrative approach to parents as evaluators of newborn hearing screening. They reaffirmed the excellence of screening practice but also raised new questions about how to pre-empt the experiences of the minority for whom screening will not be a satisfactory process.

Investigations

In the UK, national guidelines for investigating the aetiology of permanent childhood hearing impairment were developed by the British Association of Audiological Physicians in conjunction with the British Association of Community Doctors in Audiology (BACDA) (www.baap. org.uk/Guidelines/BAAP_guidelines_Jan_2001). It is recommended that core investigations are offered to the parents of all children with newly diagnosed bilateral sensorineural hearing loss and thresholds over 70 dB in the better ear averaged across 500, 1000, 2000 and 4000 Hz, while 'additional' investigations are dictated by individual circumstances and the findings of core investigations (**Tables 69.2** and **69.3**). Parents may not wish to pursue investigations, the results of which in many cases have no immediate impact on the management of the child, but it is essential that healthcare professionals are aware of the baseline investigations and can discuss the rationale behind various tests with parents so they can make an informed choice. There is some evidence, however, that these guidelines are not being fully implemented. This is mainly due to issues of funding and parental choice. In an audit of children diagnosed with severe or profound PCHI between 2002 and 2004, 41 percent were not offered imaging of the inner ears. A total of 47.1 percent accepted and 52.9 percent declined electrocardiograph (ECG) evaluation. A total of 70.6 percent accepted and 29.4 percent declined connexin mutations testing.[32]

The aims of aetiological investigations are as follows:

- to try to answer parents who ask 'why is my child deaf?';
- to identify and treat medical conditions, e.g. 8th nerve aplasia, congenital infection, Jervell and Lange–Nielsen syndrome, Alport's syndrome, neurofibromatosis type 2, Usher syndrome and vestibular hypofunction;
- to assist the family in making decisions about the most appropriate communication mode, educational placement and counselling on cochlear implantation, e.g. in 8th nerve aplasia, Usher syndrome;
- to inform genetic counselling;
- to inform epidemiological research.

The recommendation is that patients should undergo core investigations with additional investigations as dictated by the clinical scenario. [**]

CLINICAL EXAMINATION

All children with hearing loss of unknown cause should be evaluated for features associated with syndromic deafness. Important features include branchial cleft pits, cysts or fistulae, preauricular pits, telecanthus, heterochromia iridis, white forelock, pigmentary anomalies, high myopia, pigmentary retinopathy, goitre and craniofacial anomalies.

Table 69.2 Core investigations for all cases of bilateral severe to profound sensorineural hearing loss.

Investigation	
Paediatric history:	Detailed history of pregnancy delivery and postnatal period. Developmental milestones including speech and language and motor milestones, pre- and postnatal noise exposure, history of ototoxic medications, head injuries, ear disease, meningitis, viral illness and immunization status
Family history:	Deafness or risk factors associated with hearing loss in first- and second-degree relatives
Clinical examination:	Inspection and physical measurement of craniofacial region, assessment of the neck, skin and nails, limbs, chest and abdomen. Developmental examination
Audiology:	Age-appropriate assessment including tympanometry. Audiometry on first-degree relatives
Imaging:	Magnetic resonance imaging of inner ears and/or computed tomography of petrous temporal bones.
Electrocardiograph	
Urine for microscopic haematuria	
Connexin 26 and 30 mutations testing with access to clinical genetics service for counselling	
Ophthalmic assessment	
Referral to clinical geneticist	
Vestibular investigations	

AUDIOLOGY

Skilled audiological testing must be performed to assess the severity of the hearing loss and to determine whether it is conductive, sensorineural or mixed. This is discussed in detail in Chapter 68, Hearing tests in children.

IMAGING

Imaging can detect treatable pathologies such as perilymph fistula, inner ear malformations with an associated

Table 69.3 Additional investigations.[a]

Investigations
Haematological and biochemical tests
Serological test for congenital rubella and cytomegalovirus infections
Thyroid tests
Immunology tests
Metabolic screen blood and urinalysis
Renal ultrasound
Chromosomal analysis

[a]Only used when medical indications are present.

risk of meningitis and the enlarged vestibular aqueduct. Both computed tomography (CT) and magnetic resonance imaging (MRI) can be useful. Imaging modalities and techniques are discussed in Chapter 102, Imaging in paediatric ENT.

Radiological abnormalities either on CT or MRI are found in about one-third of children with PCHI (**Figure 69.3**). On CT scans, a large vestibular aqueduct is the most common isolated finding, while cochlear dysplasia is the most common abnormality in scans showing multiple abnormalities. Other abnormal findings include lateral semicircular canal dysplasia, otic capsular lucency, small internal auditory canals and hypoplastic cochlea. MRI scans are more likely to detect abnormalities primarily involving the central nervous system.[33] There is a slightly higher yield of radiological abnormalities with increasing severity of hearing loss and a significantly higher imaging yield with unilateral sensorineural hearing loss than with bilateral.[34]

At least 40 percent of children with large vestibular aqueduct (LVA) will develop profound sensorineural hearing loss. The identification of LVA should raise the suspicion of Pendred syndrome and thyroid abnormality. Patients with LVA are at risk for progressive deafness after minor head trauma. Identifying this anomaly influences management as it prompts a search for treatable thyroid function anomalies and parents can be counselled with respect to the dangers of incidental head trauma.[35]

SEROLOGY

Universal neonatal screening will detect less than half of all sensorineural hearing loss caused by congenital CMV infection[36] as the hearing loss in a large proportion of children with congenital CMV is progressive. Laboratory testing has to be carried out in neonatal samples within three weeks of life. This presents difficulties as after three weeks of age, virus isolation could be due to acquired infection, which is not usually associated with adverse outcome. Previous studies[9, 37] have shown that dried blood spots on Guthrie cards collected at birth for the screening of metabolic disorders have proved a valuable

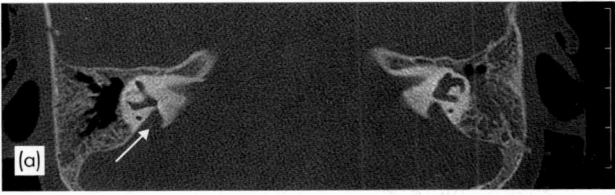

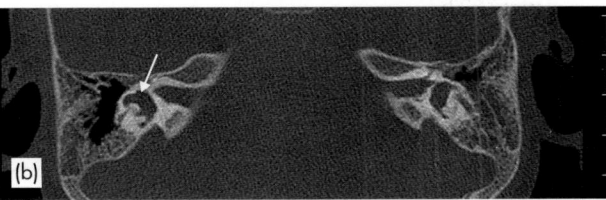

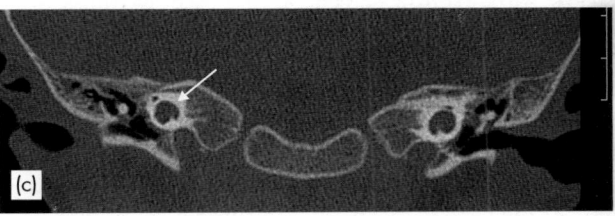

Figure 69.3 Typical appearances of a Mondini deformity in a child with bilateral severe sensorineural deafness. Axial high resolution CT scan through (a) dilated vestibular aqueducts and (b) a more inferior slice that shows bilateral dysplastic vestibules. (c) Coronal image through the abnormal cochlea showing typical Mondini abnormality with incomplete formation of the apical and middle turns of the cochlea. Images kindly supplied by D Saunders, Consultant Neuroradiologist, Great Ormond Street Hospital, London, UK.

tool for demonstrating CMV DNA for diagnosing congenital infection after months or even years of life.

Rubella-specific IgG and IgM synthesized by the foetus are detectable at birth in CRS. However, since maternally derived rubella-specific IgG is also present in infants' sera, laboratory diagnosis of CRS is almost invariably made by detection of rubella-specific IgM responses. This response is detectable in almost 100 percent of CRS cases up to age three months with the most sensitive antibody-capture assays. The response declines progressively to less than 50 percent at 12 months and is rarely detectable after 18 months. It is therefore suggested that there is value in testing for CRS only if the deafness is identified within the first six months of life.[38]

GENETIC SCREENING

The disorder DFNB1, caused by mutations in the GJB2 gene (which encodes the protein connexin 26) and the GJB6 gene (which encodes the protein connexin 30), accounts for 50 percent of autosomal recessive non-syndromic hearing loss. The carrier rate in the general population for a recessive deafness-causing GJB2 mutation is about one in 33. It is current practice that the families of all children with severe/profound hearing loss are offered genetic screening for these two mutations. Establishing a molecular diagnosis of GJB2-related deafness is important clinically since these children can avoid further diagnostic tests and are not at increased risk for medical comorbidity. In general, bony abnormalities of the cochlea are not part of the deafness phenotype and developmental motor milestones and vestibular function are normal.[4] The hearing loss associated with GJB2-related deafness can vary from mild to profound. The diagnostic yield of GJB2 screening is significantly higher in patients with severe to profound sensorineural hearing loss (SNHL) than in all other groups.[34] Preciado *et al.* suggested that a cost-effective approach to screening would be to test children with severe to profound SNHL with a GJB2 screen, as opposed to those with milder SNHL, who should undergo imaging as the initial testing step.[39]

Screening for the mitochondrial aminoglycoside susceptibility gene mutation A1555G is offered to patients who have developed hearing loss following exposure to aminoglycosides, perhaps on the neonatal intensive care unit. If the gene is identified and subsequent administration of aminoglycosides restricted, then the severity of aminoglycoside-induced hearing loss can be limited. Also, as the gene is inherited from the mother, restricting the use of aminoglycosides in maternal relatives will also limit the prevalence of hearing loss caused by these drugs.[40]

Numerous genes have been and continue to be identified relating to hereditary hearing loss. DNA testing can be carried out but at present in the UK, except for the connexins and the aminoglycoside susceptibility genes, routine screening is not performed.

BLOOD TESTS

Although routine blood tests such as full blood count (FBC), thyroid function tests, erythrocyte sedimentation rate (ESR), syphilitic blood tests, cholesterol and triglyceride levels, urea and electrolytes are carried out, abnormalities are rarely related to the cause of the hearing loss.[34]

Genetic counselling

Genetic counselling is the process of providing individuals and families with information on the nature, inheritance and implications of genetic disorders to help them make informed medical and personal decisions. The parents of all children with genetic PCHI should be offered the services of a genetic counsellor; they might not be considering further children themselves, but it is important for their present children and their future plans of families of their own. These discussions are likely to be sensitive and the information needs to be shared sensitively with a counsellor present to follow up issues;

discussion of comparative statistical odds can be very confusing and misunderstandings can lead to repercussions later. When the parents of the child are themselves deaf, then there are other issues that have to be taken into consideration. Many deaf people view deafness as a distinguishing characteristic and not as a handicap, impairment or medical condition requiring a 'treatment' or 'cure', or needing to be 'prevented'. In fact, having a child with deafness may be preferred over having a child with normal hearing.[41] Healthcare professionals need to be sensitive to these feelings and to have a frank discussion with parents to establish their views and aspirations.

Hereditary hearing loss may be inherited in an autosomal dominant, an autosomal recessive or an X-linked manner. Mitochondrial disorders with hearing loss also occur.

The risk to siblings and risk of inheritance can be predicted from the pattern of inheritance. However, clinical severity and disease phenotype may differ between individuals with the same mutation; thus, age of onset and/or disease progression may not be predictable (www.geneclinics.org/profiles/deafness-overview/details).

AUTOSOMAL DOMINANT HEREDITARY HEARING LOSS

Most children diagnosed as having autosomal dominant hereditary hearing loss have a deaf parent; the family history is rarely negative. However, the disorder may be the result of a *de novo* gene mutation. The proportion of cases caused by *de novo* mutations is unknown, but thought to be small.

If one of the parents has the mutant allele, the risk to siblings of inheriting the mutant allele is 50 percent. Individuals with autosomal dominant hereditary hearing loss have a 50 percent chance of transmitting the mutant allele to each child.

When neither parent has the deafness-causing mutation or clinical evidence of the disorder, it is likely that there has been a *de novo* mutation. However, possible nonmedical explanations including alternate paternity or undisclosed adoption could also be explored (www.geneclinics.org/profiles/deafness-overview/details).

AUTOSOMAL RECESSIVE HEREDITARY HEARING LOSS

The parents are obligate heterozygotes and therefore carry a single copy of a deafness-causing mutation. Heterozygotes are asymptomatic.

At conception, each sibling has a 25 percent chance of being deaf, a 50 percent chance of having normal hearing and being a carrier, and a 25 percent chance of having normal hearing and not being a carrier.

For children with GJB2-related (connexin) severe-to-profound deafness, siblings with the identical GJB2 genotype have a 91 percent chance of having severe-to-profound deafness and a 9 percent chance of having mild-to-moderate deafness. For children with GJB2-related deafness and mild-to-moderate deafness, siblings with the identical GJB2 genotype have a 66 percent chance of having mild-to-moderate deafness and a 34 percent chance of having severe-to-profound deafness (www.geneclinics.org/profiles/deafness-overview/details).

X-LINKED HEREDITARY HEARING LOSS

In this pattern of inheritance, the recessive gene is carried on the X chromosome. Therefore, only males are affected.

If pedigree analysis reveals that the deaf male is the only individual in the family with hearing loss, several possibilities regarding his mother's carrier status need to be considered:

- he has a *de novo* deafness-causing mutation and his mother is not a carrier;
- his mother has a *de novo* deafness-causing mutation, as either: a 'germline mutation' (i.e. occurring at the time of her conception and thus present in every cell of her body); or 'germline mosaicism' (i.e. present in some of her germ cells only);
- his maternal grandmother has a *de novo* deafness-causing mutation.

A female who is a carrier has a 50 percent chance of transmitting the deafness-causing mutation with each pregnancy. Sons who inherit the mutation will be deaf; daughters who inherit the mutation are carriers and are likely to have normal hearing.

If the mother is not a carrier, the risk to siblings is low, but greater than that of the general population because of the possibility of germline mosaicism.

Males with X-linked hereditary hearing loss will pass the deafness-causing mutation to all of their daughters and none of their sons (www.geneclinics.org/profiles/deafness-overview/details).

MITOCHONDRIAL DISORDERS WITH HEARING LOSS AS A POSSIBLE FEATURE

Inheritance is via the mother who usually has the mitochondrial mutation and may or may not have symptoms. Alternatively, there may be a *de novo* mitochondrial mutation. If the mother has the mitochondrial mutation, all siblings are at risk of inheriting it. All offspring of females with a mutation are at risk of inheriting the mutation. Offspring of males with a mitochondrial DNA mutation are not at risk.

UNKNOWN DIAGNOSIS/MODE OF INHERITANCE

The subsequent offspring of a hearing couple with one deaf child and an otherwise negative family history of deafness have an 18 percent empiric probability of

deafness in future children. If the deaf child does not have DFNB1 based on molecular genetic testing of GJB2 (which codes for the protein connexin 26), the recurrence risk is 14 percent for deafness unrelated to connexin 26.

If the hearing couple is consanguineous or comes from a highly inbred community, the subsequent offspring have close to a 25 percent probability of deafness because of the high likelihood of autosomal recessive inheritance.

The offspring of a deaf person and a hearing person have a 10 percent empiric risk of deafness.

The child of a nonconsanguineous deaf couple in whom autosomal dominant deafness has been excluded has an approximately 15 percent empiric risk for deafness. However, if both parents have connexin 26-related deafness, the risk to their offspring is 100 percent. Conversely, if the couple has autosomal recessive deafness known to be caused by mutations at two different loci, the chance of deafness in their offspring is lower than that of the general population. (www.geneclinics.org/profiles/deafness-overview/details).

SUPPORT AND EDUCATION

The rationale for intervention

Deafness has a profound effect on both adults and children and can impose a heavy social and economic burden on individuals, families, communities and countries. In normally hearing children, the language of the home is acquired through the channel of hearing. For profoundly deaf children, this normal acquisition is disrupted, leading to the likelihood of communication, speech and language delay, which may result in underachieving educationally and later in employment. Over 90 percent of deaf children are born to hearing families, where the language of the home will be a spoken language; for deaf children of deaf parents who use sign language, language will be acquired naturally through the visual route. For deaf children of deaf parents then language learning may be easier and more effective. As adults, deafness often makes it difficult to obtain, perform and keep employment. Both children and adults may suffer from social isolation as a result of deafness. There is some evidence that access to services for deafness are dependent on social class and income with those in developing countries and in the poorer sectors of society having difficulty in accessing the services they need.

The field of deafness is fraught with controversy for many years and the clinician needs to be sensitive to some contentious issues when working with parents of young deaf children. Deafness can be viewed in differing ways: as a medical condition to be 'cured', as a cultural and linguistic identity to be valued rather than 'cured' and the educational models of deafness and models of intervention often reflect these differences. For parents of newly diagnosed deaf children these issues can be bewildering; although there are differing models of intervention and management, there is little evidence for the efficacy of one over another.[42]

Today's technology of early diagnosis, effective hearing aids and cochlear implants emphasizes the medical model of deafness, in which the technology can be viewed as alleviating the effects of deafness and providing the opportunity for 'normal' development. For those with the traditional view of the deaf community, these developments can be seen as a threat in which sign language with its own grammar and culture will no longer have a place. In fact it may be that our present situation, offering more effective technology than ever before with better and earlier access to hearing and with a better understanding of the importance of early interaction in language development, offers opportunities to move forward from the old arguments and to offer deaf children real potential to develop spoken language, while not denying the value of sign language too. The interested reader is referred to the review by Marshark and Spencer[42] of the historical and theoretical perspectives.

The effects of the rapidly changing technology and of our knowledge of child and language development makes it essential that the clinician keeps up to date with current thinking and practice in these areas, and works as part of a multidisciplinary team to ensure that information and discussions are up to date.

Hearing aids

Amplification in the form of hearing aids is the mainstay for the treatment of PCHI in most cases. Early audiological assessment and provision of hearing aids at the youngest possible age (as young as four weeks in some cases) makes for the best long-term outcome. Supplying, fitting and after-care of young children with hearing aids is a demanding and skilled professional task and an appropriately trained and experienced audiologist is essential.

Behind the ear (BTE) air conduction hearing aids with a soft mould, replaced at regular intervals as the child grows, are most commonly used. The ear mould can be replaced as the child's ear canal grows. The mould may need to be changed as often as monthly in the first year. Older children, where the ear canal volume is greater, may be able to use in the ear (ITE) hearing aids. The principles that govern choice of hearing aid and on-going support are covered in Chapter 239a, Hearing aids.

Children who are unable to use a mould in the ear canal due to conditions such as atresia may be considered for behind the ear hearing aids (Chapter 239a, Hearing aids). As a preliminary measure, while waiting for the skull to mature sufficiently to enable fitting of a bone-anchored hearing aid (BAHA®), a Softband consisting of a microphone mounted on an elastic headband placed around the head may be used (**Figure 69.4**).

The management of conductive or mixed hearing loss is considered in more detail in Chapter 239b, Bone-anchored hearing aids.

Children with bilateral hearing loss should be fitted with bilateral aids unless there is a definite medical contraindication, e.g. infected ears. This gives the child binaural hearing with increased volume, better sound localization, reduction of the head shadow effect, improved speech recognition in noise, improvements in spacial balance and listening ease (www.psych-sci.manchester.ac.uk/mchas/).

In the UK, the median age at hearing aid fitting is now 16 weeks. The median delay from detection of hearing loss to provision of hearing aids is five weeks.[22] The situation in the developing world is far less satisfactory; current annual production of hearing aids is estimated to meet less than 10 percent of global need (whqlibdoc.who.int/publications/2004/9241592435_eng).

Cochlear implantation has transformed the rehabilitation of severe and profoundly deaf children in healthcare systems where it is available, and is considered in detail in Chapter 70, Paediatric cochlear implantation.

The education of deaf children

The education of deaf children has long been the subject of controversy with the questions of where and how deaf children should be taught being hotly debated throughout the world. Often the debate has not been fuelled with evidence but rather by rhetoric, and decisions about the education of deaf children have often been dependent on

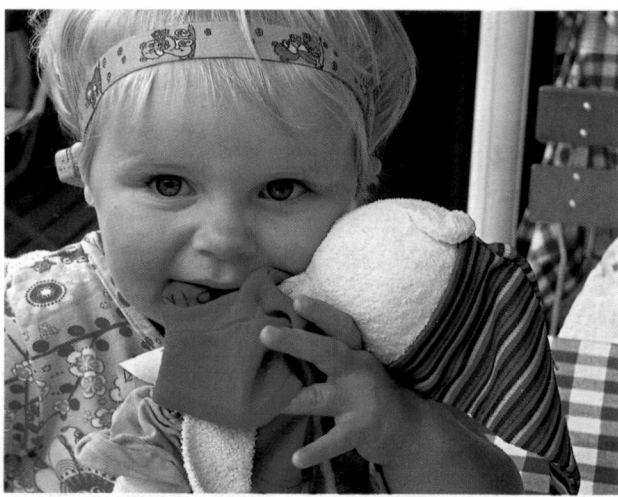

Figure 69.4 Child wearing a BAHA® Softband. Photograph by courtesy of Cochlear Europe Ltd.

where the child lived rather than upon their needs or their parents' wishes. Interestingly, the arguments, choices and debates have taken place throughout the world, and today the advent of modern technologies for deaf children are influencing these decisions.

Traditionally, deaf children were educated in special schools, usually residential and often in isolated areas. Large schools for deaf children were established in many countries in the latter half of the nineteenth century and children were taught according to the prevailing philosophy in the school. During the second half of the twentieth century more deaf children were educated in integrated settings, i.e. with their hearing peers, supported by improved technology, such as the fitting of FM systems which enabled teachers to use a microphone to aid communication with the deaf child (**Figure 69.5**) (Chapter 239a, Hearing aids) coupled with the political will to include more children with disabilities in mainstream education. Now the terms 'inclusive education' and 'least restrictive environment' are used internationally and supported by the legal requirement in many developed countries for deaf children to have an individual education programme with their needs identified. The options for educational placement can be described as:

- mainstream education with varying levels of specialist support: this may be a teacher of the deaf visiting on a regular basis and/or in-class support from a nonspecialist assistant. This may support the development of spoken or sign language, and the in-class support will vary according to the needs of the child; it may be in the form of a note-taker, or an interpreter;
- a unit, resource base, or special class in a mainstream school, with specialist teaching always available; this can be a very flexible way of providing access to specialist teacher of the deaf support and the child's time in mainstream or resource class can be varied according to changing needs over time;

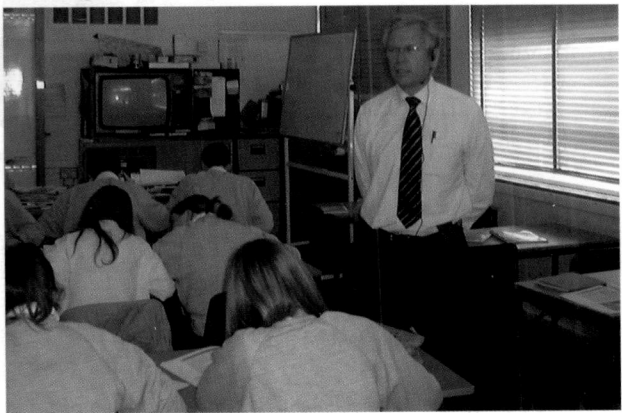

Figure 69.5 A teacher of the deaf using an FM microphone.

- a school for the deaf, which may be a day school or a residential school. The school for the deaf may have a specialist philosophy, using a sign bilingual approach or an oral approach, for example. It allows deaf children to have a peer group and to access specialist teaching, but can provide limited access to the broader world and, with small numbers, it can be difficult to provide specialist teaching in specialist subjects and to overcome these difficulties.

Whatever the educational placement of the child, it is important to ensure that the child's educational and social needs are met: medical and audiological services have the goal of improving hearing – for the educator there may be differing goals: those of literacy and numeracy and of social and emotional well-being. However, it is also vital that the technology supporting the child's access to the curriculum is used effectively; the acoustics in schools are often poor, the technology can be difficult to manage, particularly in a mainstream setting, and there may be considerable discrepancy between the child's functioning in the clinic and in school. A clinician involved in the fitting of hearing aids or implants should ensure that the child's teacher of the deaf understands the technology, can carry out simple trouble-shooting and has access to spares to ensure that the child is not without their amplification during the day. Accessories such as radio hearing aid systems (or FM) or sound field systems are increasingly common, but need to be managed in the classroom rather than in the clinic. Children and young people are unlikely to use their equipment if it is not functioning properly, and the growing complexity of the technology demands increasing competence from teachers and increasing liaison with the audiology clinic.

The other major decision that needs to be made on behalf of deaf children is that of communication mode, and whether to use a signed or oral approach. The Milan conference of 1860 concluded that the deaf were to be taught by oral means with the 'uncontestable superiority of speech over sign' and thus began a hundred years of the dominance of oral education over sign. The oral view was challenged strongly by the reports of poor linguistic and educational outcomes, for example,[43] and by the increasing voice of the deaf community, promoting its own culture and language.[44] Initially, this took the form of total or simultaneous communication with the use of spoken language and signed support. However, sign language has a grammar of its own and cannot be used with spoken language, and an interest in sign bilingual programmes where sign language is used independently of spoken language grew. In the UK, sign bilingualism began in the 1980s, interestingly at the same time as cochlear implantation, with its focus on spoken language. To summarize, communication choices used

interventions and profile of cases. *Pediatrics*. 2006; **117**: e887–93.

23. Rance G, Beer DE, Cone-Wesson B, Shepherd RK, Dowell RC, King AM *et al*. Clinical findings for a group of infants and young children with auditory neuropathy. *Ear and Hearing*. 1999; **20**: 238–52.

∗ 24. Lieu JEC. Speech-language and educational consequences of unilateral hearing loss in children. *Archives of Otolaryngology, Head and Neck Surgery*. 2004; **130**: 524–30.

25. Olusanya BO, Luxon LM, Wirz SL. Childhood deafness poses problems in developing countries. *British Medical Journal*. 2005; **330**: 480c.

26. Smith SD, Taggart RT. Genetic hearing loss with no associated abnormalities. In: Toriello HV, Reardon W, Gorlin RJ (eds). *Hereditary hearing loss and its syndromes*. New York: Oxford University Press, 2004: 37–82.

27. Kurtzer-White E, Luterman D. Families and children with hearing loss: grief and coping. *Mental Retardation and Developmental Disabilities Research Reviews*. 2003; **9**: 232–5.

28. Watkin PM, Beckman A, Baldwin M. The views of parents of hearing impaired children on the need for neonatal hearing screening. *British Journal of Audiology*. 1995; **29**: 259–62.

29. Feher-Prout T. Stress and coping in families with deaf children. *Journal of Deaf Studies and Deaf Education*. 1996; **1**: 155–65.

30. Burger T, Spahn C, Richter B, Eissele S, Lohle E, Bengel J. Parental distress: the initial phase of hearing aid and cochlear implant fitting. *American Annals of the Deaf*. 2005; **150**: 5–10.

31. Young A, Tattersall H. Parents' of deaf children evaluative accounts of the process and practice of universal newborn hearing screening. *Journal of Deaf Studies and Deaf Education*. 2005; **10**: 134–45.

32. Yoong S, Spencer N. Audit of local performance compared with standards recommended by the national guidelines for aetiologic investigation of permanent childhood hearing impairment. *Child: Care, Health and Development*. 2005; **31**: 649–57.

33. Mafong DD, Shin EJ, Lalwani AK. Use of laboratory evaluation and radiologic imaging in the diagnostic evaluation of children with sensorineural hearing loss. *Laryngoscope*. 2002; **112**: 1–7.

∗ 34. Preciado DA, Lim LHY, Cohen AP, Madden C, Myer D, Ngo C *et al*. A diagnostic paradigm for childhood idiopathic sensorineural hearing loss. *Otolaryngology – Head and Neck Surgery*. 2004; **131**: 804–9.

35. Walsh RM, Ayshford CA, Chavda SV, Proops DW. Large vestibular aqueduct syndrome. ORL. *Journal for Otorhinolaryngology and its Related Specialties*. 1999; **61**: 41–4.

36. Fowler KB, Dahle AJ, Boppana SB, Pass RF. Newborn hearing screening: will children with hearing loss caused by congenital cytomegalovirus infection be missed? *Journal of Pediatrics*. 1999; **135**: 60–4.

37. Barbi M, Binda S, Primache V, Caroppo S, Dido P, Guidotti P *et al*. Cytomegalovirus DNA detection in Guthrie cards: a powerful tool for diagnosing congenital infection. *Journal of Clinical Virology*. 2000; **17**: 159–65.

38. Reardon W. Syndrome diagnosis and investigation. In: Toriello HV, Reardon W, Gorlin RJ (eds). *Hereditary hearing loss and its syndromes*. New York: Oxford University Press, 2004: 3–7.

39. Preciado DA, Lawson L, Madden C, Myer D, Ngo C, Bradshaw JK *et al*. Improved diagnostic effectiveness with a sequential diagnostic paradigm in idiopathic pediatric sensorineural hearing loss. *Otology and Neurotology*. 2005; **26**: 610–5.

40. Fischel-Ghodsian N, Prezant TR, Chaltraw WE, Wendt KA, Nelson RA, Arnos KS *et al*. Mitochondrial gene mutation is a significant predisposing factor in aminoglycoside ototoxicity. *American Journal of Otolaryngology*. 1997; **18**: 173–8.

41. Arnos KS, Israel J, Cunningham M. Genetic counseling of the deaf. Medical and cultural considerations. *Annals of the New York Academy of Sciences*. 1991; **630**: 212–22.

∗ 42. Marschark M, Spencer PE. Spoken language development of deaf and hard-of-hearing children: Historical and theoretical perspectives. In: Spencer PE, Marschark M (eds). *Advances in the spoken language development of deaf and hard-of-hearing children*. New York: Oxford University Press, 2006: 3–21.

43. Conrad R. *The deaf school child*. London: Harper & Row, 1979.

44. Nevins N, Chute P. *Children with cochlear implants in educational settings*. San Diego: Singular Publishing Group, 1996.

45. Lynas W. Communication options. In: Stokes J (ed.). *Hearing impaired infants: Support in the first eighteen months*. London: Whurr Publishers, 1999: 98–128.

46. Archbold SM, Nikolopoulos TP, Lutman ME, O'Donoghue GM. The educational settings of profoundly deaf children with cochlear implants compared with age-matched peers with hearing aids: implications for management. *International Journal of Audiology*. 2002; **41**: 157–61.

∗ 47. Stacey PC, Fortnum HM, Barton GR, Summerfield AQ. Hearing-impaired children in the United Kingdom, I: Auditory performance, communication skills, educational achievements, quality of life, and cochlear implantation. *Ear and Hearing*. 2006; **27**: 161–86.

48. Tait M, Lutman ME, Robinson K. Preimplant measures of preverbal communicative behavior as predictors of cochlear implant outcomes in children. *Ear and Hearing*. 2000; **21**: 18–24.

49. Thoutenhoofd E. Cochlear implanted pupils in scottish schools: 4-year school attainment data (2000–2004). *Journal of Deaf Studies and Deaf Education*. 2006; **11**: 171–88.

50. Vermeulen AM, van Bon W, Schreuder R. Reading comprehension of deaf children with cochlear implants.

Journal of Deaf Studies and Deaf Education. 2007; **12**: 283–302.

51. Damen GW, van den Oever-Goltstein MH, Langereis MC, Chute PM, Mylanus EA. Classroom performance of children with cochlear implants in mainstream education. *Annals of Otology, Rhinology and Laryngology.* 2006; **115**: 542–52.

52. Yoshinaga-Itano C. Benefits of early intervention for children with hearing loss. *Otolaryngologic Clinics of North America.* 1999; **32**: 1089–102.

53. Dauman R, Daubech Q, Gavilan I, Colmet L, Delaroche M, Michas N *et al.* Long-term outcome of childhood hearing deficiency. *Acta Otolaryngologica.* 2000; **120**: 205–8.

70

Paediatric cochlear implantation

JOSEPH G TONER

Introduction	860	Controversies in management	866
Timing of implantation	861	Quality of life measures	866
Assessment	863	Key points	867
Preoperative counselling	864	Best clinical practice	867
Surgery	864	Deficiencies in current knowledge and areas for future	
Special surgical circumstances	865	research	867
Postoperative habilitation	865	References	867

SEARCH STRATEGY

The data in this chapter are supported by a PubMed search using the key words cochlear implantation and cochlear implants, limited to randomized controlled trials, human, children 0–18 years. The Cochrane and TRIP databases were also consulted.

INTRODUCTION

Hair cell loss is the principal cause of senorineural deafness. Sufficient neural elements usually survive and are available for electrical stimulation enabling meaningful activation of the auditory cortex. A cochlear implant is a prosthetic device which replaces the transducer function of damaged hair cells and provide this electrical stimulation.

History

Electrical stimulation of the ear was attempted as early as the eighteenth century.[1] The modern era of cochlear implantation began with Djourno and Eyries[2] who inserted a device that produced awareness of sound, but no speech discrimination. Animal models were developed in the 1960s.[3, 4] Prototype implants were introduced in the early 1970s and rapid development took place over the next decade.

In 1969, William House recommended clinical use of electrical stimulation in profoundly deaf patients.[3] Several were implanted and outcomes evaluated in detail. In the 1980s, commercially available devices were used in routine clinical practice. The Food and Drug Administration (FDA) approved their use in adults in 1984. Increased confidence in results obtained in adults led to more widespread paediatric implantation in the late 1980s. In 1990, the FDA approved the use of cochlear implants in children.

Current status

Almost all children with severe to profound sensorineural hearing loss may now be considered for implantation subject to the provisos outlined below. The potential candidate population of children in the UK is thus some 600 per annum. Most have congenital loss (1 in 1000 births), but a small number have acquired loss mainly due to meningitis.

The aetiology of severe congenital hearing loss is considered in Chapter 66, Molecular otology, development of the auditory system and recent advances in genetic manipulation. Genetic disorders account for more than 50 percent of all cases.

Devices

Implantation involves insertion of a receiver/stimulator into a bony recess in the squamous temporal bone. The cochlea is opened (cochleostomy) and an electrode array connected to the receiver is inserted. These constitute the internal device. The internal receiver/stimulator package has an embedded magnet to secure the transmitting coil. A microphone, microprocessor and transmitter coil (external device) is positioned by magnetic coupling over the internal device and delivers the encoded signal (**Figure 70.1**).

The microphone is connected to a speech processor, which digitally processes and then encodes the auditory signal. The signal is then transmitted transcutaneously to the implanted receiver/stimulator, which stimulates the surviving neural elements in the modiolus. This enables selective stimulation of the relevant segments of the surviving ganglion cell population with the tonotopically determined frequency information.

All the current cochlear implant devices used in the UK enable good auditory habilitation in most patients. There is still a significant variability in individual results. Although there are many technical differences between the implant devices in relation to speech processing and device specifications, there is no conclusive evidence that any one implant device has performance benefits over the others.

TIMING OF IMPLANTATION

Prelingual deafness

Depending on the time of onset, deafness can be prelingual or post-lingual, i.e. occurring before or after the development of normal speech and language. The critical period for speech and language development lasts for a significant portion of the first decade of life, but is a continuum rather than a discrete event. Hence there is a transitional category that is referred to as perilingual deafness, i.e. deafness arising during acquisition of key speech and language skills. In outcome, these children are equivalent to those in the prelingual category.

Neuroplasticity (the ability of the brain to respond adaptively to behaviorally relevant stimuli) is a feature of both motor and sensory functions. If a congenitally blind child has vision restored after the first few years of life then, although the child is able to 'see' objects and different colours, they are unable to recognize them. This is referred to as cortical blindness. The same phenomenon is observed in relation to hearing and speech and language development. Where auditory input is restored to patients only after the first decade of life, they are unable to acquire normal speech and language. The existence of a critical period for language development during the first five years of life is well established.[5] Providing auditory stimulation during this period is critical.[6] Deafness significantly reduces language development. A normally hearing child

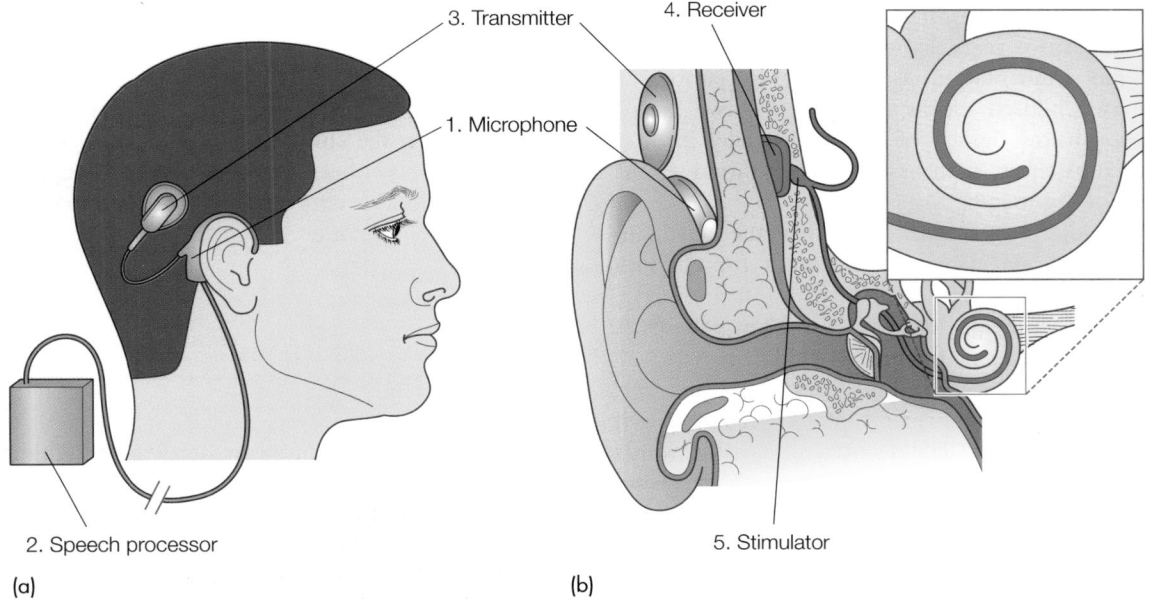

Figure 70.1 Implantation of a device. **(a)** Side view; **(b)** front view.

may have a vocabulary of between five and 26 thousand words by the age of five years. A profoundly deaf child of the same age typically has only 200 spoken or signed words.[7] Developmental studies support the potential benefits of early implantation. Ryals and colleagues[8] have demonstrated that the auditory system requires early stimulation to develop normally and that auditory deprivation may prevent development of normal frequency and place coding. Studies of animal models have shown that electrical stimulation commenced shortly after inducement of deafness enhances neural survival and may prevent changes in the central auditory system.

Animal experiments indicate that changes take place both in the brain stem and auditory cortex that produce a neurophysiological barrier to successful implantation after the 'critical period'.[9, 10]

There is increasing evidence from functional brain imaging studies with positron emission tomography (PET) to confirm this auditory critical period. In effect, unused brain capacity is reassigned to other tasks if not hard-wired for its primary designated purpose within the first few years of life. This confirms the judgement of experienced clinicians that early implantation, probably before the age of two and possibly significantly earlier, is required to maximize the potential for normal language development in prelingually deaf children. Conversely, if a congenitally deaf child presents late, e.g. after the age of seven, it is likely that the benefit of implantation in relation to speech and language acquisition and recognition will be very limited. Many centres would therefore counsel parents against implantation.

Early implantation

The National Institutes of Health (NIH) consensus statement in 1995[11] advocated implantation in children after the age of two years. However, clinical practice has evolved and implantation is now being performed regularly in children below the age of two years. Implantation below the age of one year usually requires special circumstances, such as rapid obliteration of the cochlea following meningitis.

Several studies have begun to confirm the benefit in terms of speech and language outcomes for children implanted at an earlier age.[6, 12, 13, 14, 15, 16]

Kileny et al.[6] studied a group of 48 implant patients at the age of seven years and a further study involving 53 patients who were assessed three years following implantation. The study confirmed that in terms of speech recognition with monosyllables and multisyllabic words and sentences, children perform better with increased duration of use of cochlear implantation and reduced age at implantation. Children implanted at a younger age performed better than children implanted at an older age.

Harrison et al.[13] reported a retrospective analysis of 70 profoundly deaf children, 78 percent of whom were congenital. The age range of this group was 2–15 years and they achieved a five-year follow up. Several standard speech perception tasks were administered (phonetically balanced kindergarten (PBK), Glendonald auditory screening procedure (GASP), test of auditory comprehension (TAC), word intelligibility by picture identification (WIPI)). A binary partitioning algorithm was used to divide the dataset on the basis of age and implantation. This allowed the data to be divided into two age categories, those above and those below the age of 4.4 years. Analysis of speech perception performance indicated that there was a statistically significant improvement in scores in those implanted at a younger age compared with those implanted later.[13]

Govaerts et al.[15] analyzed a retrospective longitudinal cross-sectional study of 70 paediatric cochlear implant patients and demonstrated that for children implanted after the age of four years categories of auditory performance (CAP) scores rarely reached normal. However, for patients implanted between two and four years, normal CAP scores were usually reached and two-thirds were integrated into mainstream primary schools. Implantation below the age of two years always resulted in a normal CAP score with 90 percent being integrated into mainstream preschooling. A possible bias in this study related to the fact that children implanted at a young age have normally been identified as having a significant hearing loss at a younger age and therefore received hearing aids at an earlier age. Although the numbers are not sufficiently large to avoid this source of bias, some of the children implanted at an older age had received hearing aids at an early age, but still had outcomes related to their age at implantation.[15] All of these studies are cohort studies with no controls. It is extremely unlikely that a study which randomized subjects to either a prolonged hearing aid use group or cochlear implant group would be accepted by parents. So, although Yoshinaga-Itano et al.[17] have reported early intervention of whatever kind as being beneficial to the ultimate outcome in terms of language development, a view supported by the study by Moeller,[18] the precise reason for this has never been proved. The hypothesis that it may be the habilitative effort that is important in determining the positive outcomes in cochlear implant children is unlikely to be tested.

Post-lingual candidates

Post-lingual deafness in children is most frequently a consequence of meningitis or head injury. Although the duration of deafness is a factor in speech perception outcome after cochlear implantation, it is not an overriding issue. In adults with cochlear implants, the trend in most reported series indicates that the longer the duration of deafness, the poorer will be the outcome in relation to speech perception. However, most children who become profoundly deaf after a significant period of normal language development (five to ten years) and who receive a cochlear implant will regain excellent open-set auditory-only speech discrimination skills.

ASSESSMENT

Assessment is a multiprofessional evaluation of hearing, communication ability, cochlear morphology, middle ear/mastoid status and other relevant general developmental issues.

Audiological tests

Many infants will have already undergone electrophysiological tests as part of their diagnostic assessment, usually either auditory brainstem responses (ABR) or electrocochleography (ECochG). While these tests provide some indication of the severity of the hearing loss, behavioural testing when available is preferred as it is a test of the entire auditory pathway (not just the peripheral system and brain stem connections). Behavioural aided and unaided responses are obtained using visual reinforcement audiometry (VRA). In very young children, the level of language competency means that speech discrimination tests are not available. Therefore, audiological candidacy is informed mostly by the aided responses. The criterion adopted now by most UK centres is that if aided thresholds at frequencies above 2 kHz are greater than 50 dBA, then benefit from a cochlear implant is likely.

In older children (post-lingual deafness), standard pure tone and aided free field tests are performed, but speech discrimination tests are more critical. Assessment is similar to adults though the test material will need to be 'language-age' appropriate. An aided audiogram is a reasonable surrogate predictor of speech discrimination ability. Speech discrimination scores are performed both in the auditory-only and auditory with lip-reading modes. An auditory-only open-set sentence score of below 30 percent is generally regarded as being an indicator of likely benefit from cochlear implantation; however, some centres may implant candidates with 50 percent discrimination scores. Vestibular testing is not routinely performed on children.

Imaging

High-resolution computed tomography (CT) scanning shows the bony morphology of the cochlea and labyrinth. Congenital abnormalities include the Mondini dysplasia, common cavity deformity or a large vestibular aqueduct. The internal auditory meatus may be narrow and raise the possibility of auditory nerve aplasia. Meningitis can cause significant obliteration of the cochlea. Ossification is usually found in the basal turn of the cochlea near the round window, but sometimes ossification is complete.

The accuracy of high-resolution CT scanning to predict patency of the cochlea is extremely variable; high-resolution magnetic resonance imaging (MRI) is regarded as being superior to CT in this respect, but it can still underestimate the degree of cochlea ossification.[12, 19, 20, 21]

Imaging is particularly important in post-meningitic patients in confirming the presence of a fluid-filled basal turn. High resolution three-dimensional (3D) reconstructions may provide information on patency of the individual scalae. In cases where there is no auditory response, high-resolution MRI scans may demonstrate the presence of an auditory nerve. This is particularly important if a CT has demonstrated an abnormally narrow internal auditory canal (IAC).

Infants may require sedation or anaesthesia to undergo imaging and therefore it is advantageous to be able to perform MRI and CT together.

PET or functional magnetic resonance imaging (fMRI) will increasingly provide functional information in relation to persistent plasticity and in the future may provide valuable information in relation to candidacy.

Medical assessment

The trend towards decreasing implantation at a younger age means that anaesthetic and perioperative risk must be evaluated, particularly for children with complex medical conditions. Young[22] found that in implanting infants less than 12 months of age there are physiological issues that require the anaesthetic risks to be considered seriously. The benefits of early surgery must be weighed against these risks. He acknowledges that there may be factors such as rapidly progressing obliteration in post-meningitis cases which may alter the risk/benefit balance, but the anaesthetic risks need to be carefully discussed as part of the informed consent process.

Neurodevelopmental issues

This is a complex area for implant teams. Candidacy has recently been extended to children with learning disabilities and other developmental problems. Outcomes are more difficult to demonstrate, but benefit in communication is achieved by some. Careful consideration is needed to assess likely benefit to hearing and to quality of life. Problems with lack of reliable reporting of auditory sensations may make devising optimum stimulation parameters difficult, and there is the risk of causing distress due to overstimulation. Some of these issues may be overcome with electrically evoked ABR response testing, now possible on the newest generation of implant devices.

PREOPERATIVE COUNSELLING

The potential implant candidate must not be looked at in isolation. Consideration should be given to the assessment of parental or care-givers attitudes, particularly the ability to assist in the delivery of an intense postoperative programme to enable the child to develop receptive and expressive oral language skills. This will include commitment to an appropriate educational environment to maximize potential. Social workers and/or psychologists may help to ensure the importance of these issues is recognized.

Following the assessment process and determination of likely benefit, the parents are counselled regarding the surgery and the habilitative management process. This will include explanation of the benefits and risks of surgery, variability of outcome and the requirement for intensive and prolonged input from the implant centre team and local professionals.

SURGERY

A low complication rate is now reported from most established centres, with a 'learning curve' in new centres.

Technique

The surgery involves several steps.

- **Incision and flap design**. Implant surgery was initially performed via a large incision. Gibson *et al.*[23] were the first to advocate a much smaller post-aural incision and by the late 1990s most surgeons had begun to adopt some version of what resembles a standard post-aural mastoidectomy incision. This reduces flap-related problems and is more acceptable to children and their parents since a large head shave is not required.[24] A recent survey of UK implant centres reported a flap-related complication rate of 2.4 percent in children, but that included earlier cases preformed with larger incisions.[25]
- **Bony approach to cochlea**. A standard mastoidectomy is followed by a posterior tympanotomy preserving the chorda tympani. The round window region is visualized through a posterior tympanotomy. The scala tympani is entered via a cochleostomy anterior to the round window niche. Following electrode insertion, any space between the electrode and the cochleostomy can be sealed with soft tissue, usually fascia or muscle. There is an increasing trend in the UK towards use of a facial nerve monitor.[25]
- **Bony recess for and fixation of receiver/stimulator**. A device-specific contoured bony recess is fashioned for the receiver/stimulator package. In children this

almost always involves exposure of the dura. Most surgeons prefer to preserve a bony island over the dura if possible. Fixation of the device can be with either absorbable or nonabsorbable sutures. Bone cement is also used for electrode fixation at the mastoid rim or posterior tympanotomy.

- **Closure and postoperative care**. Drains are rarely required. Most patients receive some form of antibiotic cover, though there is no generally accepted regime. Many patients have some form of imaging of the electrode array (most frequently via a modified Stenvers view) to confirm satisfactory position prior to discharge.

Complications

THE FACIAL NERVE

The incidence of facial nerve damage is very low. Hoffman and Cohen[26] reported 0.58 percent in children ($n = 1905$); in a UK series, 0.2 percent had permanent facial nerve injury.[25]

Non-auditory stimulation, usually of the facial nerve, is relatively common following cochlear implantation, particularly in post-meningitic patients. It is thought that bony channels develop, allowing electrical stimulation of the horizontal segment of the facial nerve. Often these problems can be overcome by programming out the relevant electrodes. Care must be taken in these cases as this aberrant effect of stimulation may upset the child and lead to an aversion to device use.

Bigelow *et al.*[27] reported an incidence of 14 percent of some form of non-auditory or facial nerve stimulation. In a very small number of cases, if a significant number of electrodes have to be switched off, implant performance may be degraded.

MENINGITIS

There are concerns about a possible increased risk of meningitis – particularly pneumococcal – in children who have had cochlear implantation. Epidemiological studies are complicated by the fact that the cochlear implant population has a higher incidence of meningitis before cochlear implantation than the general population. A survey in the United States showed that of roughly 5000 children under the age of five who had been implanted, 300–400 had had an episode of meningitis prior to the implantation; 17 had had meningitis after implantation. This increased risk of meningitis in deaf individuals may be due to structural abnormalities such as common cavity deformity or enlarged vestibular aqueduct.[28]

The advice from the Department of Health in the UK is that all patients who have been implanted should be offered pneumococcal vaccination. Prospective patients should be advised regarding immunization prior to implantation. Patients who have implantation and develop otitis media or signs of other febrile illnesses should be urgently assessed by either their general practitioner or the implant centre.

DEVICE EXTRUSIONS

This is one of the most serious complications following implant surgery. Hoffman and Cohen[26] reported an incidence in children of 0.16 percent ($n = 1905$). Gibbin et al.[25] reported the experience of UK centres with a similar incidence of 0.25 percent.

DEVICE FAILURES

Earlier implants had various design faults, which provided some device reliability problems. Cumulative survival rates for all the devices in use in the UK are in the range of 97–99 percent.

SPECIAL SURGICAL CIRCUMSTANCES

Cochlear anatomical abnormalities

Implantation of the malformed cochlea is technically feasible.[29] Patients with an enlarged vestibular aqueduct or enlarged vestibule may have 'gushers' intraoperatively. Several authors have concluded that outcomes in terms of speech discrimination in these patients are similar to those with no structural abnormalities.

Obliterated cochlea

Ossification develops as a consequence of meningitis, temporal bone trauma and some autoimmune disorders. The basal turn of the scala tympani is most frequently affected due to the connection between the subarachnoid space with the scala tympani via the cochlear aqueduct. Scala vestibuli ossification is less common and may take place later in the ossification process.[30, 31]

Ossification was initially thought to be a contra-indication to cochlear implantation, but various surgical procedures have been developed to allow at least partial implantation in those cochleas with significant degrees of ossification. Gantz et al.[32] described a drill-out procedure by creating a trough around the modiolus, drilling out the entire basal turn. Balkany et al.[33, 34] modified this technique using an intact canal wall procedure. Steenerson et al.[31] described scali vestibuli electrode insertion in which the scali vestibuli is opened anterior to the round window by drilling above the spiral ligament. The outcome in patients whose implant was inserted into the scala vestibuli was compared to matched controls who

had standard scala tympani insertion. The outcome measures including sentence recognition scores and vowel and consonant speech scores were similar in both groups. He concluded therefore that scala vestibuli insertion was an acceptable alternative to scala tympani insertion in partially obliterated cases.

Cohen and Waltzman[35] described partial insertion through a short inferior tunnel drilled along the basal turn. In some cases, this partial drill out will reach a patent segment of the basal turn and a full insertion is then possible.

More recently, the implant manufacturers have produced different electrode configurations to deal with the problem of the ossified cochlea.[36, 37] A dual/split array is available; one electrode is inserted into an inferior tunnel drilled along the basal turn and the other electrode is inserted into a separate cochleostomy drilled into the superior limb of the basal turn. A compressed electrode array with an increased number of electrodes along a shorter distance is an alternative in a basal turn drill-out procedure.

Chronic suppurative otitis media and open mastoid cavities

Patients with mastoid cavities were initially considered unsuitable for implantation. However, increasing experience has led most centres to offer surgery to these patients. Various techniques are described.[38] Surgery is performed as a one- or two-stage procedure. In the two-stage procedure, all squamous epithelium is removed from the cavity, which is then obliterated behind a blind sac closure of the external canal. After an interval, the cochlear implant device is inserted at a second-stage operation. In the one-stage technique, the device is inserted following removal of disease and the cavity obliterated and closed.

POSTOPERATIVE HABILITATION

This is a multidisciplinary effort involving audiologists, speech and language therapist and specialist educators; it begins with programming the device with stimulation parameters for the electrode array which will provide auditory perception across the speech range. In the very young, this can be assisted by electrophysiological measures which can predict the threshold and comfort levels for electrical stimulation. In older children, behavioural responses can be used to refine the implant stimulation parameters. These parameters can change over time and therefore need to be regularly confirmed at 'programming' sessions. The role of the speech and language therapist and specialist educators is to maximize the potential provided by the auditory input to develop speech perception and intelligibility, and thereby to permit access to the educational curriculum as fully as possible.

CONTROVERSIES IN MANAGEMENT

Implantation in older children and adolescents

The ideal age for implantation in congenitally deaf children has been discussed. The current recommendation is around or just before the age of two years. Several studies have examined the benefits of implantation in older children and adults. Waltzman et al.[39] examined the outcomes in 35 congenitally deaf children who received implants after the age of eight years and 14 congenitally deaf adults. The results indicated that there was improvement in open-set speech perception in children. Adults demonstrated improvement in mean scores for word and sentence recognition, although the improvement was not as significant as in children implanted at a younger age. Results were adversely influenced by increasing duration of deafness and older age at time of implantation.

Bilateral cochlear implantation

In the last few years, experience has grown with bilateral implantation and studies in adults report the benefits binaural hearing should provide, including sound localization and enhanced speech recognition in background noise.

Muller et al.[40] reported a study of nine bilaterally implanted adult patients tested for speech understanding in quiet and in noise. They were tested in three situations, left implant only, right implant only and both implants activated. The speech discrimination tests included monosyllables in quiet and sentences in noise. Results indicated higher speech scores for all subjects with bilateral stimulation. This has encouraged bilateral implantation in children and preliminary results indicate that outcomes measured by auditory perception and speech intelligibility are improved.[41] Bilateral implantation will require further longitudinal evaluation of significant numbers of children in order to confirm these early reports indicating that additional benefits accrue from the second implant.

MRI following cochlear implantation

The presence of a magnet in the current implant systems has led to MRI being contraindicated in implanted patients. The devices have a removable magnet; a small incision over the posterior half of the receiver/stimulator package will allow the implanted magnet to be removed to enable MRI to be performed. This requires a small surgical procedure with the risk of introducing infection.

A recent study[42] shows that it is possible to perform an MRI scan provided the scanner is equipped with a 1-Tesla magnet.

QUALITY OF LIFE MEASURES

Cheng et al.[43] have reported that cochlear implants in profoundly deaf children have a positive effect on quality of life at reasonable direct costs and appear to result in net savings to society.

The cost–utility of paediatric cochlear implantation was analyzed by O'Neill et al.[44] They concluded that it was an effective intervention with a quality adjusted life year (QALY) gain of £10.341 ($21.00), and recommended the intervention as effective for profoundly hearing-impaired children. QALYs are a measure of the benefit of a medical intervention. The measure takes into account both quantity and quality of life generated by a healthcare intervention and is based on the number of years of life that would be added by the intervention. Each year in perfect health is assigned the value of 1.0 down to a value of 0 for death. If the extra years would not be lived in full health, for example if the patient were to lose a limb, become blind, or be confined to a wheelchair, then the extra life-years are given a value between 0 and 1 to account for this.[45]

Francis et al.[46] reported that cochlear implantation accompanied by aural rehabilitation increases access to acoustic information of spoken language, leading to higher rates of mainstream placement in schools and lower dependence on special education support services. The cost savings that result from a decrease in the use of support services indicates an educational cost benefit of cochlear implant rehabilitation for many children. However, larger more methodologically robust studies will be required to strengthen evidence and deal with confounding variables such as socioeconomic status, cognitive function, age of diagnosis of deafness and language intervention, and the mode of communication.

Although now a decade old, the NIH consensus statement[11] is still the outcome of the most extensive systematic review, it concluded that:

Cochlear implantation improves communication ability in most adults with severe to profound deafness and frequently leads to positive psychological and social benefits as well. Currently, children at least two years old and adults with profound deafness are candidates for implantation. Cochlear implant candidacy should be extended to adults with severe hearing impairment and open-set sentence discrimination that is less than or equal to 30 percent in the best aided condition. Access to optimal education and (re)habilitation services is important for adults and is critical for children to maximize the benefits available from cochlear implantation.

KEY POINTS

- Cochlear implantation is a proven effective treatment for the management of severe to profound sensorineural hearing loss in children.
- All infants and children who are diagnosed as having a severe to profound congenital hearing loss should be referred urgently for assessment.
- Increasingly, implantation is undertaken between the ages of one and two years.
- The results in older children are less good, but assessment by an implant centre is still worthwhile.
- Patients in the UK are managed within a multidisciplinary team in a small number of specialized centres.
- Complication rates are low.
- Studies have confirmed the cost effectiveness of paediatric implantation.

Best clinical practice

- ✓ Any child with a hearing loss >70 dB (unaided), acquired or congenital, should be referred for assessment.
- ✓ Children with aided levels >50 dB at frequencies of 2 Hz and above should be referred to a specialist centre.
- ✓ Children with significant deafness post-meningitis should be referred urgently because of the risk of progressive obliteration of the cochlea.
- ✓ Age at implantation in the pre- or perilingual deaf has an inverse relationship to outcomes of enhanced oral communication.
- ✓ Implantation should take place in a designated centre, with experienced staff working in a multiprofessional team.

Deficiencies in current knowledge and areas for future research

- ➤ The implementation of universal neonatal hearing loss screening with resultant early intervention should lead to improved outcomes for all children with hearing loss, particularly those requiring cochlear implantation.
- ➤ Lack of RCT based evidence is a deficiency but is unlikely to be resolved due to the perceived effectiveness of implantation and therefore difficulty in recruiting to a hearing aid arm of such a trial.

REFERENCES

1. Loeb GB. Cochlear prosthetics. *Annual Review of Neurosciences.* 1990; **13**: 357–71.
2. Djourno A, Eyries C. Prothese auditive par excitation electrique a distance du nerf sensoriel a l'aide d'un bobinage inclus a demeure. *Presse Médicale.* 1957; **36**: 14–17.
3. Simmons FB. History of cochlear implants in the United States: A personal perspective In: Schindler RA and Merzenich MM (eds). *Cochlear Implants.* New York: Raven Press, 1985: 1–7.
4. Clarke GM. Responses of cells in the superior olivary complex of the cat to electrical stimulation of the auditory nerve. *Experimental Neurology.* 1969; **24**: 124–36.
5. Cairns H. *The acquisition of language.* Austin, TX: Pro-ed, 1986.
6. Kileny PR, Zwolan TA, Ashbaugh C. The influence of age at implantation on performance with a cochlear implant in children. *Otology and Neurotology.* 2001; **22**: 42–6.
7. Schabb WA. Effects of hearing loss on education. In Jaffe BF (ed.). *Hearing loss in children: A comprehensive text.* Baltimore: University Park Press, 1977: 650–4.
8. Ryals BM, Rubel EW, Lippe W. Issues in neural plasticity as related to cochlear implants in children. *American Journal of Otology.* 1991; **12**: 22–7.
9. Harrison RV, Nagasawa A, Smith DW, Stanton S, Mount RJ. Reorganisation of the auditory cortex after neo-natal high frequency cochlear hearing loss. *Hearing Research.* 1991; **54**: 11–9.
10. Larsen SA, Kirchhoff TM. Anatomical evidence of synaptic plasticity in the cochlear nucleii of deaf white cats. *Experimental Neurology.* 1992; **115**: 151–7.
11. NIH Consensus Statement. Cochlear implants in adults and children. 1995; **13**: 1–30.
12. Nikolopoulos TP, O'Donoghue GM, Robinson KL, Holland IM, Ludman C, Gibbin KP. Preoperative radiologic evaluation in cochlear implantation. *American Journal of Otology.* 1997; **18**: S73–4.
13. Harrison RV, Panesar J, El-Hakim H, Abdolell M, Mount RJ, Papsin B. The effects of age of cochlear implantation on speech perception outcomes in prelingually deaf children. *Scandinavian Audiology Supplement.* 2001; **53**: 73–8.
14. Illg A, von der Haar-Heise S, Goldring JE, Lesinski-Schiedat A, Battmer RD, Lenarz T. Speech perception results for children implanted with the CLARION cochlear implant at the Medical University of Hannover. *Annals of Otology, Rhinology and Laryngology.* 1999; **177**: 93–8.
15. Govaerts PJ, De Beukelaer C, Daemers K, De Ceulaer G, Yperman M, Somers T *et al.* Outcome of cochlear implantation at different ages from 0 to 6 years. *Otology and Neurotology.* 2002; **23**: 885–90.
16. Miyamoto RT, Kirk KI, Svirsky M, Sehgal ST. Communication skills in pediatric cochlear implant recipients. *Acta Otolaryngologica.* 1999; **119**: 219–24.

17. Yoshinaga-Itano C, Sedey AL, Coulter DK, Mehl AL. Language of early- and later-identified children with hearing loss. *Pediatrics.* 1998; **102**: 1161–71.

18. Moeller MP. Early intervention and language development in children who are deaf and hard of hearing. *Pediatrics.* 2000; **106**: E43.

19. Jackler RK, Luxford WM, Schindler RA, McKerrow WS. Cochlear patency problems in cochlear implantation. *Laryngoscope.* 1987; **97**: 801–5.

20. Nair SB, Abou-Elhamd KA, Hawthorne M. A retrospective analysis of high resolution computed tomography in the assessment of cochlear implant patients. *Clinical Otolaryngology.* 2000; **25**: 55–61.

21. Seidman DA, Chute PM, Parisier S. Temporal bone imaging for cochlear implantation. *Laryngoscope.* 1994; **104**: 562–5.

22. Young NM. Infant cochlear implantation and anaesthetic risk. *Annals of Otology, Rhinology and Laryngology.* 2002; **111**: 49–51.

23. Gibson WPR, Harrison HC, Prowse C. A new incision for placement of the cochlear multi-channel cochlear implant. *Journal of Laryngology and Otology.* 1995; **109**: 821–5.

24. Gibson WPR, Harrison HC. Further experience with a straight, vertical incision for placement of cochlear implants. *Journal of Laryngology and Otology.* 1997; **111**: 924–7.

25. Gibbin KP, Raine CH, Summerfield AQ. Cochlear implantation – UK and Ireland surgical survey. *Cochlear Implants International.* 2003; **4**: 10–21.

26. Hoffman RA, Cohen NL. Complications of cochlear implant surgery. *Annals of Otology, Rhinology and Laryngology.* 1995; **166**: 420–2.

27. Bigelow DC, Kay DJ, Rafter KO, Montes M, Knox TW, Yousem DM. Facial nerve stimulation from cochlear implants. *American Journal of Otology.* 1998; **19**: 163–9.

28. O'Donaghue G, Balkany T, Cohen N, Lenarz T, Lustig L, Niparko J Editorial. Meningitis and cochlear implantation. *Otology and Neurotology.* 2003; **23**: 823–4.

29. Eisenman DJ, Ashbaugh C, Zwolan TA, Zwolan H, Alexander T, Telian SA. Implantation of the malformed cochlea. *Otology and Neurotology.* 2001; **22**: 834–43.

30. Telian SA, Zinnerman-Philips S, Kileny PR. Successful revision of failed cochlear implants in severe labyrinthitis ossificans. *American Journal of Otology.* 1996; **17**: 53–60.

31. Steenerson RL, Gary LB, Wynes MS. Scali vestbuli cochlear implantation for labyrinthine ossification. *American Journal of Otology.* 1990; **11**: 360–3.

32. Gantz BJ, McCabe BF, Tyler RS. Use of multichannel implants in obstructed and obliterated cochleas. *Otolaryngology – Head and Neck Surgery.* 1988; **98**: 72–81.

33. Balkany T, Hodges AV, Luntz M. Update on cochlear implantation. *Otolaryngologic Clinics of North America.* 1996; **29**: 277–88.

34. Balkany T, Luntz M, Telischi FF, Hodges AV. Intact canal wall drill-out procedure for implantation of a totally ossified cochlea. *American Journal of Otology.* 1997; **18**: 558–9.

35. Cohen NL, Waltzman SB. Partial insertion of the Nucleus multichannel cochlear implant: Technique and results. *American Journal of Otology.* 1993; **14**: 357–61.

36. Bredberg G, Lindström B, Löppönen H, Skarzynski H, Hyodo M, Sato H. Electrodes for ossified cochleas. *American Journal of Otology.* 1997; **18**: S42–3.

37. Lenarz T, Lesinski-Schiedat A, Weber BP, Issing PR, Frohne C, Buchner A *et al.* The Nucleus double array cochlear implant: A new concept for the obliterated cochlea. *Otology and Neurotology.* 2001; **22**: 24–32.

38. Babighian G. Problems in cochlear implant surgery. *Advances in Otorhinolaryngology.* 1993; **48**: 65–9.

39. Waltzman SB, Roland JT, Cohen NL. Delayed implantation in congenitally deaf children and adults. *Otology and Neurotology.* 2003; **23**: 333–40.

40. Muller J, Schon F, Helms J. Speech understanding in quiet and noise in bilateral users of the MED-EL COMBI 40/ 40 + cochlear implant system. *Ear and Hearing.* 2002; **23**: 198–206.

41. Kuhn-Inacker H, Shehata-Dieler W, Muller J, Helms J. Bilateral cochlear implants: A way to optimize auditory perception abilities in deaf children? *International Journal of Pediatric Otorhinolaryngology.* 2004; **68**: 1257–66.

42. Baumgartner WD, Youssefzadeh S, Hamzavi J, Czerny C, Gstoettner W. Clinical applications of MRI imaging in early implant patients. *Otology and Neurotology.* 2001; **22**: 818–22.

43. Cheng AK, Rubin HR, Powe NR, Mellon NK, Francis HW, Niparko JK. Cost–utility analysis of the cochlear implant in children. *Journal of the American Medical Association.* 2000; **284**: 850–6.

44. O'Neill C, O'Donoghue GM, Archbold SM, Normand C. A cost–utility analysis of paediatric cochlear implantation. *Laryngoscope.* 2000; **110**: 156–60.

45. Phillips C, Thompson G. What is a QALY? London: Hayward Medical Communications. Last updated 2003; cited May 2007. Available from: www.evidence-based-medicine.co.uk/ebmfiles/WhatisaQALY.pdf

46. Francis HW, Koch ME, Wyatt JR, Niparko JK. Trends in educational placement and cost–benefit considerations in children with cochlear implants. *Archives of Otolaryngology – Head and Neck Surgery.* 1999; **125**: 499–505.

Congenital middle ear abnormalities in children

JONATHAN P HARCOURT

Introduction	869	Nonossicular congenital middle ear abnormalities	873
Classification of congenital ossicular abnormalities	869	Key points	874
Incidence of congenital ossicular abnormalities	870	Best clinical practice	875
Clinical presentation of congenital ossicular abnormalities	871	Deficiencies in current knowledge and areas for future research	875
Investigation of congenital ossicular abnormalities	871	References	875
Principles of management	871		
Management of specific congenital ossicular abnormalities	871		

SEARCH STRATEGY

The data in this chapter are supported by a search of the Guidelines databases on www.nelh.nhs.uk, the Cochrane library and TRIP databases using the key words congenital, middle ear and ossicle. This was supplemented by a PubMed search using the key words congenital and middle ear or ear, ossicle.

INTRODUCTION

Conductive hearing loss in children is usually acquired. The most common aetiology is otitis media with effusion (OME) but it may be the result of chronic otitis media (mucosal or squamous). In the presence of severe congenital deformity of the external ear, associated abnormalities of the ossicular chain are common but in isolation they are rare and often have a delayed diagnosis, particularly if unilateral.

A variety of nonossicular congenital middle ear abnormalities may also be associated with ossicular deformities. They may be symptomatic in themselves or be important aspects of other middle ear conditions and surgery. They include:

- persistent stapedial artery;
- anomalous course of the facial nerve;
- congenital perilymphatic fistula;
- high jugular bulb;
- aberrant internal carotid artery.

Definition of congenital ossicular abnormalities

Congenital ossicular fixation and defect is defined as a malformation affecting the ossicular chain, present at birth, which leads to a dysfunction of the ossicular mechanism due to immobility or discontinuity of the ossicular chain.

Major malformations involve both the tympanic cavity and the external ear (ear canal and pinna) and are described as congenital aural atresia or microtia. In association with these conditions, in either sporadic cases or as part of a syndrome such as Treacher Collins or Goldenhar, there may be a variable degree of ossicular abnormality and there may also be associated inner ear dysplasia.

Minor malformations affect the ossicular chain alone and the tympanic membrane and ear canal are normal.

CLASSIFICATION OF CONGENITAL OSSICULAR ABNORMALITIES

There have been many published classifications based on individual surgeons' series.[1] Cremers' classification describes the largest published series of operated minor congenital ear anomalies (104 cases).[2] It has been modified by Tos[3] and seems to be the most inclusive and descriptive of all the published schemes (**Table 71.1**).

Minor malformations are divided into four main groups, each of which may be subdivided: isolated stapes ankylosis, ankylosis with other ossicular anomaly, isolated ossicular anomaly and aplasia or severe dysplasia of the oval or round windows. [*]

INCIDENCE OF CONGENITAL OSSICULAR ABNORMALITIES

Bergstrøm[4] reported that out of a group of 687 children with congenital hearing loss, only eight (1.2 percent) were found to have isolated middle ear anomalies. There is no systematic report of absolute incidence though Thringer et al.[5] reported the incidence of conductive hearing loss, severe enough to require amplification, to be 0.6:1000. These cases were all bilateral. The incidence of unilateral cases is unclear.

Cremers and Teunissen's series[2] does provide a relative incidence with stapes ankylosis with another associated ossicular chain anomaly being the most common finding (38 percent) with isolated stapes ankylosis being the other largest group (30 percent). Isolated anomaly of the ossicular chain was found in 22 percent and aplasia or severe dysplasia of the oval or round windows in 10 percent.

In a Japanese surgical series, Hashimoto et al.[6] reported a much higher rate of incudostapedial joint

Table 71.1 Cremers' classification of minor congenital anomalies of the ossicular chain in 144 operated ears (modified by Tos).

Class	Main anomaly	Subclassification	% 144 ears

1	Isolated congenital stapes ankylosis (or fixation)	a. **Footplate fixation**
		  1. Normal stapedial arch
		  2. Monopodial stapedial arch
		  3. Monocrural stapedial arch
		b. **Stapes suprastructure fixation**
		  1. Elongation of the pyramidal eminence
		  2. Stapes-pyramidal process bony bar
		  3. Stapes facial canal bony bar
		  4. Stapes-promontory wall bony bar
		  5. More than one bony bar
			30.6

2	Stapes ankylosis associated with another congenital ossicular chain anomaly	a. **Incus and/or malleus deformation or aplasia of the long process of the incus** b. **Bony fixations of the malleus and/or incus**	38.2
3	Congenital anomaly of the ossicular chain but mobile stapes footplate	**Discontinuity of the ossicular chain** Aplasia of the long process of the incus Dysplasia of the long process of the incus	15.3

		Epitympanic fixation
		Malleus
		  Anterior
		  Superior
		  Lateral
		Incus body
		  Superior
		  Lateral
		  Medial
		Short process of the incus
		  In incudal fossa
		Tympanic fixation
		  Of the malleus handle
		  Of the long process of the incus
			6.3

4	Congenital aplasia or severe dysplasia of the oval or round window	**Aplasia**	6.9
		Dysplasia	
		Crossing (prolapsed) facial nerve	2.1
		Persistent stapedial artery	0.7

defects, either in isolation or with stapes fixation, making up nearly 50 percent of cases.

The majority of Cremers' cases were sporadic though in 25 percent they were part of a recognizable congenital syndrome including branchio-oto-renal, hemifacial microsomia, Klippel-Feil, Crouzon and Pfeiffer syndromes. [**]

CLINICAL PRESENTATION OF CONGENITAL OSSICULAR ABNORMALITIES

Children with bilateral ossicular abnormalities will often present at a similar age to children with OME because of poor hearing performance and speech delay. It is not unusual that the children are managed with one or more sets of ventilation tubes before the diagnosis is made. The observation of a conductive hearing loss, normal tympanic membrane and normal middle ear pressures should lead to the general diagnosis.

INVESTIGATION OF CONGENITAL OSSICULAR ABNORMALITIES

Audiometry

There is an average threshold of approximately 50 dB, producing a flat air conduction line, with no low frequency bias as with otitis media. There is an average air–bone gap of 35 dB between 0.5 and 2 kHz, either due to Carhart's effect or because of the presence of an underlying sensorineural hearing loss. Tympanometry usually demonstrates a normal middle ear pressure with reduced compliance due to fixation of the ossicular chain.

Imaging

High resolution computed tomography (CT) scanning remains the primary imaging modality though complementary magnetic resonance imaging (MRI) studies may demonstrate associated labyrinthine and internal auditory meatal abnormalities. CT virtual endoscopy may offer a further mode of presenting the images for preoperative surgical planning though as yet it fails to image satisfactorily the stapes suprastructure.[7]

Exploratory surgery

The diagnosis may only be made during a tympanotomy, though an interesting alternative to lifting the tympanic membrane is to attempt to visualize the ossicles via Eustachian tube and middle ear endoscopy.[8] The innate risk of damage to the ossicles and extent of view with this technique is as yet not well defined.

PRINCIPLES OF MANAGEMENT

As with all cases of hearing loss, children and adults with congenital ossicular abnormalities need to be managed with thought to their overall hearing performance and requirements.

In the presence of a bilateral moderate hearing loss due to a maximal or near maximal conductive hearing loss, some form of auditory rehabilitation should be recommended. For the majority, this will mean a conventional unilateral or bilateral air conduction hearing aid. With minor malformations there should be a stable external ear canal as a platform for amplification. If the patient develops local complications in the external ear canal, such as recurrent or chronic otitis externa, a bone-anchored hearing aid (BAHA) would be a suitable alternative. [*]

Unilateral cases are less well defined in terms of best management. In the presence of ipsilateral tinnitus, amplification may act as a tinnitus masker. A hearing aid may improve the patient's hearing performance in background noise and optimize sound localization. The positive benefits need to be weighed against the potential morbidity of a conventional hearing aid, which includes the occlusion effect, otitis externa and the body image issues involved in wearing hearing aids, particularly amongst children and adolescents.

Surgery for congenital ossicular abnormalities should only be undertaken by dedicated otologists with experience of complex middle ear reconstruction. When the diagnosis has been made in childhood, consideration for surgery should be preceded by an adequate trial of amplification. Whatever middle ear surgery is contemplated, but particularly with stapedotomy, there is a significantly higher risk of delayed sensorineural hearing loss due to sporadic episodes of acute otitis media in children under ten years of age. By this time it may be appropriate to involve the child in the decision-making process or to wait until adolescence or adulthood to allow the patient to come to their own decision regarding surgical treatment.

A preoperative CT scan would be a mandatory investigation to attempt to identify the ossicular abnormality, but also to visualize any other middle or inner ear abnormality such as an anomalous facial nerve, congenital cholesteatoma, aberrant vascular structures or labyrinthine dysplasia.

MANAGEMENT OF SPECIFIC CONGENITAL OSSICULAR ABNORMALITIES

Isolated stapes ankylosis

Tos[3] subdivided Cremers' basic classification to separate stapes ankylosis into two main groups, depending on

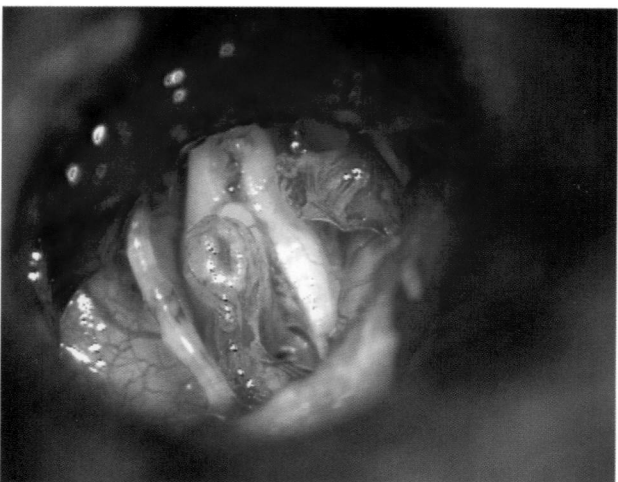

Figure 71.2 Stapes may be normal and mobile, even in the presence of a bifurcated facial nerve.

Congenital perilymphatic fistula

Congenital perilymphatic fistula (PLF) is an abnormal communication between the middle and inner ear. It may be associated with:

- microfissures around the oval and round windows;
- labyrinthine or IAM dysplasia.

The diagnosis is controversial as there is no reliable preoperative test which identifies the condition and management is based on the suggestive diagnosis of a child presenting with progressive or fluctuating sensorineural hearing loss, possibly associated with vertigo. Weber et al.[21] define the intraoperative diagnosis as being based on the identification of clear fluid which reaccumulates with anaesthetic Valsalva or Trendelenburg manoeuvre. Beta-transferrin positive samples are consistent with CSF being a constituent of the leak and this will be a feature of some but not all cases of PLF, usually associated with labyrinthine or IAM dysplasia. This is not a real-time test during the surgical procedure and is very specific but not very sensitive for PLF, which may not contain CSF.[22]

In view of the difficulties of diagnosis, Weber et al.[21] suggest the policy of packing temporalis muscle around the oval and round windows in all suspected cases. This is based on the observation that packing does not seem to cause any significant complications (such as a subsequent conductive hearing loss) and he argues that it may be beneficial despite no confirmation of a PLF. In his series of 160 ears with suspected PLF there was a greater than 90 percent rate of stabilization or improvement in hearing in both PLF positive and negative cases, though he acknowledges that in other series there is a similar outcome in nearly half of cases without packing. [**]

High jugular bulb

A high jugular bulb (HJB) is usually asymptomatic and discovered as an incidental finding on otoscopy or during middle ear surgery. It can cause heavy bleeding from accidental puncture while lifting a tympanomeatal flap or even inserting a ventilation tube.

The jugular bulb can be defined as 'high' if it reaches the level of the inferior bony annulus and is often covered by thin bone or is dehiscent. In the presence of a plethoric mass within the tympanic cavity, the differential diagnosis will include HJB, aberrant ICA, a PSA and a glomus tympanicum tumour.

An HJB can be associated with hearing loss. If it includes a medial portion impinging on the cochlear or vestibular aqueduct, a connection with vestibular symptoms and a sensorineural hearing loss has been suggested. There may be a more direct association with a conductive hearing[23] loss due to interference with the ossicles, contact with the tympanic membrane and obstruction of the round window niche.

Major surgery to occlude or re-route an HJB is unlikely to be justified by symptoms alone, though there are occasional reports of intrusive pulsatile tinnitus associated with an HJB. It is possible to consider endovascular occlusion in the rare case of persistent haemorrhage, when tympanic cavity surgery is contraindicated.[24]

Aberrant internal carotid artery

This may be associated with other vascular abnormalities such as a PSA and likewise present as a vascular middle ear mass. Associated symptoms include pulsatile tinnitus, which may be objective, and hearing loss. In approximately 20 percent of cases it is bilateral.[25]

An aberrant ICA is an important differential diagnosis of a glomus tympanicum tumour, which can be resolved by CT scanning. Brisk bleeding, hemiparesis, aphasia, deafness, Horner syndrome and intractable vertigo may result if the vessel is unintentionally injured.[25]

KEY POINTS

- Congenital abnormalities of the middle ear may occur in association with major malformations such as microtia.
- Isolated malformations are rare but include anomalies of the ossicular chain and the middle ear vasculature.
- Diagnostic delay is common. Deafness due to ossicular pathology is often misdiagnosed as otitis media with effusion. It is not unusual for children to have repeated ventilation tubes before the correct diagnosis is made.

Best clinical practice

✓ Unless deafness is bilateral management can be conservative. [Grade D]

✓ If there is bilateral hearing loss, auditory rehabilitation will be required. [Grade D]

✓ Surgery is difficult with uncertain outcomes and best considered only by those with specific training and experience. [Grade D]

✓ Surgery may be best deferred until children can participate in the process of informed consent. [Grade D]

Deficiencies in current knowledge and areas for future research

➤ The incidence, aetiology and pathogenesis of congenital ossicular abnormalities is poorly understood.

➤ The role of otoendoscopy in the diagnosis and management of these conditions needs to be better defined.

➤ Developments in middle-ear implantation may render corrective surgery almost redundant.

REFERENCES

* 1. Nandapalan V, Tos M. Isolated congenital stapes suprastructure fixation. *Journal of Laryngology and Otology*. 1999; **113**: 798–802.

2. Cremers CWRJ, Teunissen E. A classification of minor congenital ear anomalies and short- and long-term results of surgery in 104 ears. In: Charachon R, Garcia-Ibanes E (eds). *Long-term results and indications in otology and otoneurosurgery*. Amsterdam/New York: Kugler Publications, 1991: 11–2.

3. Tos M. Congenital ossicular fixations and defects. In *Surgical solutions for conductive hearing loss*. New York: Thieme, 2000: 212–39.

4. Bergstrøm L. Assessment and consequence of malformations of the middle ear. *Birth Defects*. 1980; **16**: 217–41.

5. Thringer K, Kankkunen A, Liden G, Nikalson A. Prenatal risk factors in the aetiology of hearing loss in pre-school children. *Developmental Medicine and Child Neurology*. 1984; **26**: 799–807.

6. Hashimoto S, Yamamoto Y, Satoh H, Takahashi S. Surgical treatment of 52 cases of auditory ossicular malformations. *Auris, Nasus, Larynx*. 2002; **29**: 15–8.

7. Nakasato T, Sasaki M, Ehara S, Tamakawa Y, Muranaka K, Yamaoto T et al. Virtual CT endoscopy of ossicles in the middle ear. *Clinical Imaging*. 2001; **25**: 171–7.

8. Karhuketo TS, Ilomaki JH, Dastidar PS, Laasonen EM, Puhakka HJ. Comparison of CT and fiberoptic video-endoscopy findings in congenital dysplasia of the external and middle ear. *European Archives of Otorhinolaryngology*. 2001; **258**: 345–8.

9. Ombredanne M. Chirurgie des surdites congenitales par malformations ossiculaires de 10 nouveaux cas. *Annales d'Oto-laryngologie et de Chirurgie Cervico Faciale*. 1960; **77**: 423–49.

10. Shambaugh GE. Developmental anomalies of the sound conducting apparatus and their surgical correction. *Annals of Otology, Rhinology and Laryngology*. 1952; **61**: 873–87.

11. Lindsay JR, Sanders SH, Nager GT. Histopathologic observation in so-called congenital fixation of the stapedial footplate. *Laryngoscope*. 1960; **70**: 1587–602.

12. Nandapalan V, Tos M. Isolated congenital stapes ankylosis: an embryologic survey and literature review. *Otology and Neurotology*. 2000; **21**: 71–80.

13. Cremers CWRJ, Hombergen GCHJ, Scaf JJ, Huygen PLM, Volkers WS, Pinckers AJLG. X-linked progressive mixed hearing deafness with perilymphatic gusher during stapes surgery. *Archives of Otolaryngology*. 1985; **111**: 249–54.

14. Jackler RK, Hwang PH. Enlargement of the cochlear aqueduct: fact or fiction? *Otolaryngology – Head and Neck Surgery*. 1993; **109**: 14–25.

15. Nishizaki K, Kariya S, Fukushima K, Orita Y, Okano M, Maeta M. A novel laser-assisted stapedotomy technique for congenital stapes fixation. *International Journal of Pediatric Otorhinolaryngology*. 2004; **68**: 341–5.

16. Welling DB, Merrell JA, Merz M, Dodson EE. Predictive factors in pediatric stapedectomy. *Laryngoscope*. 2003; **113**: 1515–9.

17. De La Cruz A, Angell S, Slattery W. Stapedectomy in children. *Otolaryngology – Head and Neck Surgery*. 1999; **120**: 487–92.

18. Silbergleit R, Quint DJ, Mehta BA, Patel SC, Metes JJ, Noujaim SE. The persistent stapedial artery. *American Journal of Neuroradiology*. 2000; **21**: 572–7.

19. Govaerts PJ, Cremers CWRJ, Marquet TF, Offeciers FE. The persistent stapedial artery: does it prevent successful surgery? *Annals of Otology, Rhinology and Laryngology*. 1993; **102**: 724–8.

20. Rohrt T, Lorentzen P. Facial nerve displacement within the middle ear (report of 3 cases). *Journal of Laryngology and Otology*. 1976; **90**: 1093–8.

21. Weber PC, Bluestone CD, Perez B. Outcome of hearing and vertigo after surgery for congenital perilymphatic fistula in children. *American Journal of Otolaryngology*. 2003; **24**: 138–42.

22. Bluestone C. Implications of beta-2 transferrin assay as a marker for perilymphatic versus cerebrospinal fluid labyrinthine fistula. *American Journal of Otology*. 1999; **20**: 701.

Contact with other children at home and at playgroups

Table 72.3[29] [***] shows the risk factors in addition to AOM in a multivariate analysis for the occurrence of OME. This confirms the increasing effect of age up to two years of age, but also the effect of having siblings and a family history of them having OME. In another study that otoscopically examined family members of children with OME, rather than rely on historical reports, 32 percent of siblings and 19 percent of parents were also classified as otoscopically affected.[38] [**]

Other multivariate studies have suggested that in addition to the number of siblings, attendance for daycare with four or more other children up to 3.5 years of age can double the risk (CI 1, 3).[30] [***] This risk has been confirmed by others.[12] [**]

Some have advocated that the number of children in daycare settings could be reduced to lessen this risk, but for most parents availability, convenience and cost are limiting determinants.

Hereditability

In a same sex twin/triplet prospective cohort study, Casselbrandt et al.[39] [***] looked at sets where the zygosity was known. In children who had OME during the first two years of life, there was greater concordance in monozygotic sets in the number and duration of OME episodes than in dizygotic sets. The magnitude of the effect of heredity in comparison to other risk factors for OME was not investigated.

Race

Whether the prevalence of OME is different in different races requires control for many other factors. When factors including socioeconomic group and child contacts are controlled for in a multivariate analysis, the prevalence in black children is no different from white children.[40] [***] Chinese children may have a lower prevalence, but a multifactorial analysis has not been reported.[35] [**]

Table 72.3 Risk factors significant in a multivariate model for OME under two years of age.

Risk factor	Category	OR	95% CI
AOM	Yes/No	1.6	1.2, 2.1
Previous AOM	Yes/No	1.7	1.2, 2.4
Age	Increase per month	1.0	1.0, 1.0
No. of siblings	Increase per sibling	1.6	1.3, 2.0
OME family history	Yes/No	1.4	1.1, 1.7

Reprinted from Ref. 29, with permission.

It must be concluded that at present there is insufficient evidence to examine any effect of race, apart from black and white where no difference has been shown.

Gender

Some multivariate studies report the risk of developing OME to be no different in boys and girls.[30, 31, 41] Some report a higher risk in boys[11, 38] and others a higher risk in girls.[29]

It must be concluded that there is likely to be little difference, if any, in the risk for boys compared to girls.

Smoking

For public health reasons, parental smoking has frequently been reported as a risk factor for the occurrence of OME. However, in multivariate analysis when other factors have been controlled for, no effect of parental smoking is detected[31] [***] or it is present for smokers of up to 20 cigarettes per day, but the risk reduces if it is more than 20 cigarettes per day.[30] [***]

The conclusion must be that, in comparison to the other material risk factors for the occurrence of OME in children under the age of two years, the effect of parental smoking must be negligible. [***]

Risk factors for occurrence in children older than three years

No literature has been identified that reports a multifactorial analysis of risk factors in children older that three years of age. However, episodes of acute otitis media are likely to be less important because of its lower prevalence in this age group.

Duration and recurrence of episodes in children under the age of three years

The natural history of the duration, recovery and recurrence of OME in 1328 children from one to two years of age is shown by ear in Figure 72.5.[42] [***] The distribution of the duration of episodes is very skewed; the median duration of OME was three months or less, but the 95th percentile was at 12 months. Fifty percent of affected ears had resolved after three months. However, around 50 percent of the ears that resolved had a further episode.

What happens in individual infants rather than in ears has been documented by Paradise et al.[40] [***] In a large cohort (n = 2253) followed up from 2 months of age to 6, 12, 24 months of age, 49, 79 and 91 percent respectively had at least one episode of OME.

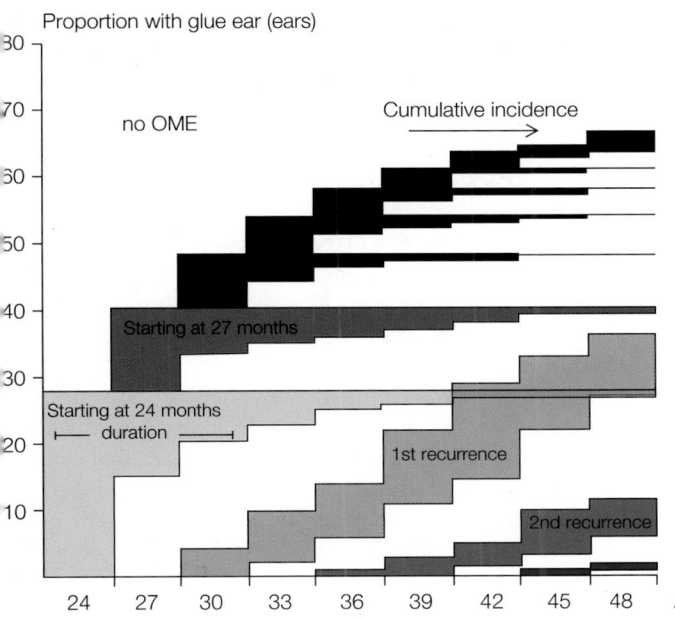

Proportion with glue ear (ears)

Figure 72.5 Natural history of OME (*n* = 1217 ears). Shaded areas indicate the presence of OME by episode of occurrence. The breadth of the hatched areas indicates the duration of the episode in various proportions of the total sample of ears. Redrawn from Ref. 42, with permission.

Hogan *et al.*[43] [***] followed up 95 full-term infants monthly for three years. The infants fell into three groups. The majority (65 percent) had OME at less than a third of monthly visits. Of the other 35 percent with OME at more than one visit, half of them had OME in one or both ears for more than 18 (50 percent) of their first 36 months of life. Though the mean duration of OME was longer in those with a propensity for developing OME (unilateral six weeks; bilateral ten weeks), the main difference was time between episodes. On average this was longer in children who had less OME (every 31 weeks compared with every 11 weeks).

Overall, infants were twice as likely to develop unilateral as opposed to bilateral OME. One month later, in infants with a unilateral effusion, the majority (50 percent) had resolved, a minority (20 percent) had become bilateral and the other 30 percent remained unilateral. In those with bilateral effusions at the start, one month later the majority (60 percent) remained bilateral. In the others (40 percent), bilateral resolution was more frequent than unilateral resolution (in a ratio of 3:1).

Duration and recurrence of episodes in children older than three years

A cohort of 856 British children, aged five to eight years was screened three times a year (approximately every four months) for three successive years to study the prevalence and natural history of OME defined by a type B tympanogram.[24] [***] **Table 72.2** confirms the already reported age and season effect. There was no gender effect. The proportion of unilateral to bilateral OME was equal.

In a subsample of 67 ears with OME, the resolution rates at 4, 8 and 12 months were 52, 78 and 91 percent, respectively. The overall recurrence rate was low (7 percent).

A more detailed monthly study of seven-year-old Danish pupils (*n* = 387) reported the mean overall duration of an ear episode to be 1.8 months with 12 percent lasting more than 6 months.[44] [***] Ears first diagnosed to have OME between September and February persisted longer than those first diagnosed between March and August.

Risk factors for persistence

Three studies have been identified that have followed up children to identify risk factors that might be used to predict those that are more likely to have persistent bilateral OME. One study was carried out in primary care and followed up children who were six months or older for three months.[13] [***] Another study was of children aged between three and seven years referred from primary care with suspected OME and seen at secondary care on average 13 weeks later.[15] [***] The third study was of children of the same age identified at secondary care to have bilateral OME with an associated hearing impairment in both ears of at least 20 dB hearing loss (HL). These children were followed up for three months to identify those in whom the OME persisted bilaterally with the same degree of impairment.[14, 16, 17] [***]

In these three studies, which all followed up the children for three months, the persistence rates of bilateral OME were 56, 35 and 51 percent, respectively. All studies identified the second half of the year (July–December) as a major risk factor with odds ratios of between 2 and 3. In primary care, whether a child has frequent or upper respiratory symptoms at the time of assessment is also an important determinant of persistence. In secondary care, the degree of associated hearing impairment predicted persistence. The only factor that might have an influence and has the potential to be modified was whether or not the mother smoked and this was a significant multivariate factor in the secondary care study.[15] [***]

In all three studies, the magnitude of the effect of any factor singly or in combination was insufficient to predict with certainty those likely to persist or resolve.

Clinical applicability of best epidemiological evidence

The prevalence of OME in childhood is age dependent, with two peaks in the distribution; one centred around one to two years of age and the other around three to seven years of age. [***]

In temperate countries, twice as many children have OME in the winter as opposed to the summer. The increased frequency of upper respiratory infections and close contact with other children during the winter months contribute to this association. [***]

Under three years of age, episodes of acute otitis media, contact with other children and heredity are factors that increase the risk of occurrence. No easily modifiable factors in the age group have been identified. [***]

Under three years of age, unilateral OME is twice as common as bilateral OME. Those with a propensity to develop OME have more frequent episodes rather than longer episodes. Bilateral OME is more likely to persist than unilateral OME. Therefore, most effort should be expended on children with bilateral OME. [***]

In primary care, children with bilateral OME and a history of upper respiratory infections are more likely to persist. In secondary care, children with bilateral OME seen in the second half of the year (July–December) with a hearing impairment of 30 dB HL in both ears are more likely to persist. [***]

None of the factors for persistence singly or in combination are sufficient to negate a requirement for watchful waiting before considering surgery. [***]

DIAGNOSIS

The initial diagnosis in most cases of childhood OME will be by otoscopy, the examiner having been alerted to the possibility by ear or hearing problems. The otoscopic appearances of OME are extremely variable and take experience to reliably detect, but can be aided by the use of a pneumatic otoscope. Hence, in many children a confirmatory method would be helpful. In some ears it will not be possible to see the tympanic membrane because of wax and again an alternative way of diagnosing OME without needing to remove the wax is helpful. The investigations available will be those that are used. In primary care this may be tympanometry and occasionally audiometry. In secondary care, both these investigations should be readily available.

Reference gold standard

In most diagnostic situations, the reference gold standard as to whether OME is present or not has to be by some other investigation. In addition, the ears that are being used as the controls are important to define. Ears that have recently had an episode of OME are likely to be different from ears that have never had OME.

Because of its availability and semi-objective nature, tympanometry is perhaps the most common reference standard used. In children who are being operated on for OME, the surgical finding of middle ear fluid can be the reference standard. Unfortunately, the surgical series has to have an undesirable 'dry tap' rate in order to calculate the ability of the investigation to detect ears that do not have fluid. Even the surgical findings are prone to error as the absence of OME may be due to the anaesthetic gases aerating the middle ear before the myringotomy is performed.

History

Though this will often initiate the assessment and be an indicator of previous problems, it is not a reliable indicator of the current presence of OME or the degree of hearing impairment. Several level 1 evidence papers support this statement. In particular, in a cohort study of 216 children followed from birth to 27 months of age at three-monthly intervals, the sensitivity of parental report of current OME and hearing impairment was poor.[45] The lack of correlation between parent report of hearing and the current pure-tone thresholds has been further illustrated by Stewart et al.[46] (**Figure 72.6**) [****] In this figure there is no correlation whatsoever between parental reports of their child's hearing and the child's hearing thresholds.

As might be expected if an infant's parents give a history of ear problems, recurrent upper respiratory infections, mouth breathing and snoring, such a child is more likely to

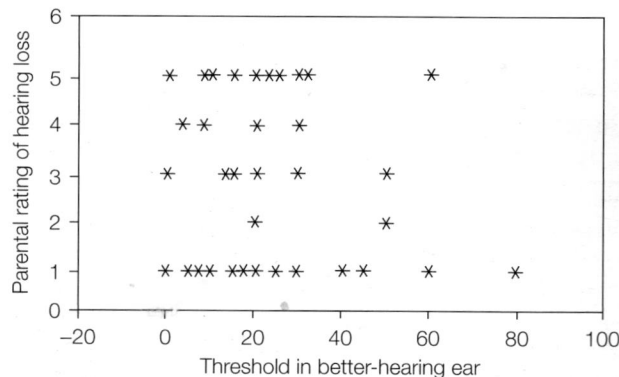

Figure 72.6 Parental perception of hearing loss (from 1 = definitely no to 5 = definitely yes) versus the actual hearing thresholds in the better ear, n = 84 children. Redrawn from Ref. 46, with permission.

have recurrent OME in the future than if there is no such history.[23] [**] It remains to be investigated whether children with such a history merit monitoring.

Diagnostic tools

OTOSCOPY

Unfortunately the otoscopic appearances of OME are extremely varied. **Figures 72.7, 72.8, 72.9, 72.10, 72.11, 72.12** and **72.13** are some examples of what can be seen. Not included are ears with residual fluid following acute otitis media which would add additional variety, particularly in abnormalities of thickness and inflammation of the pars tensa. In such ears, the tympanic membrane may also be bulging rather than retracted.

The otoscopic findings in OME are mainly different combinations of retraction of the pars tensa and variations in its colour. Retractions may be evident by indrawing of the handle of the malleus (**Figures 72.8, 72.9, 72.10, 72.11, 72.12** and **72.13**) or the presence of a neo-annular fold (particularly evident in **Figure 72.10**, but also in **Figures 72.7, 72.8, 72.9, 72.11, 72.14, 72.15**).

In some ears the retractions may be more localized than others (in **Figures 72.8** and **72.12** there is a Sade grade 3 retraction to the promontory). In **Figure 72.10**, the pars tensa retraction is particularly evident inferiorly.

Colour changes can be more yellow (**Figure 72.11**), more blue (**Figure 72.15**) or just clear (**Figure 72.7**).

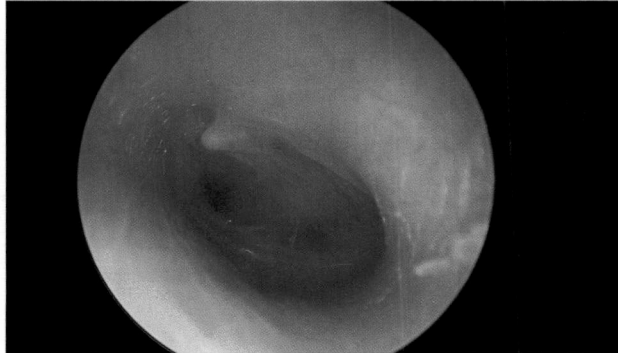

Figure 72.9   Otitis media with effusion (left). Malleus handle markedly retracted.

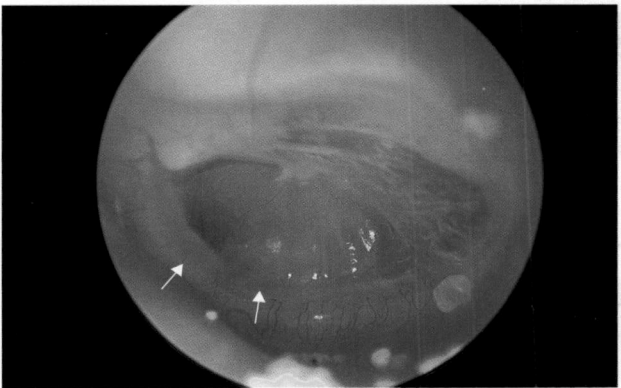

Figure 72.10   Severely retracted position of malleus handle in otitis media with effusion (left). As the retraction develops a neoannular fold may develop (arrow).

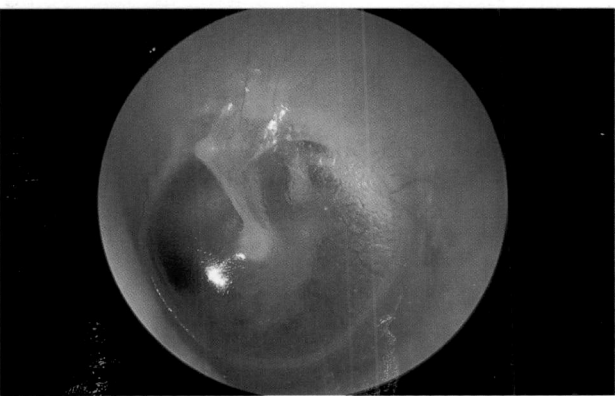

Figure 72.7   Otitis media with effusion (left). Malleus handle in normal position.

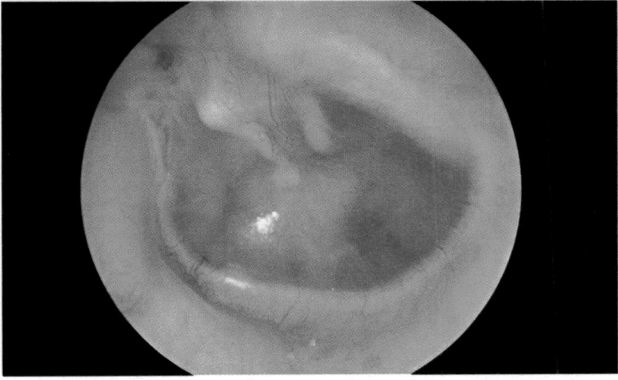

Figure 72.11   Left tympanic membrane in otitis media with effusion showing yellowish colour.

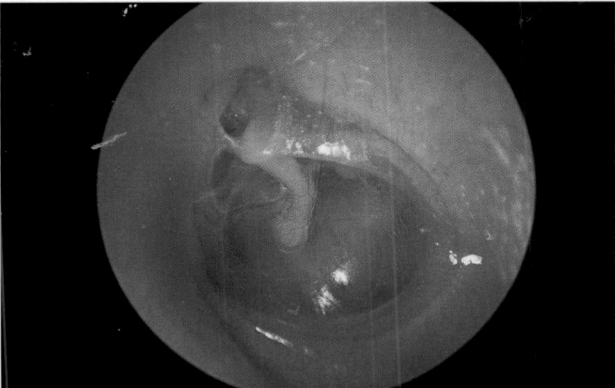

Figure 72.8   Otitis media with effusion (left). Malleus handle slightly retracted.

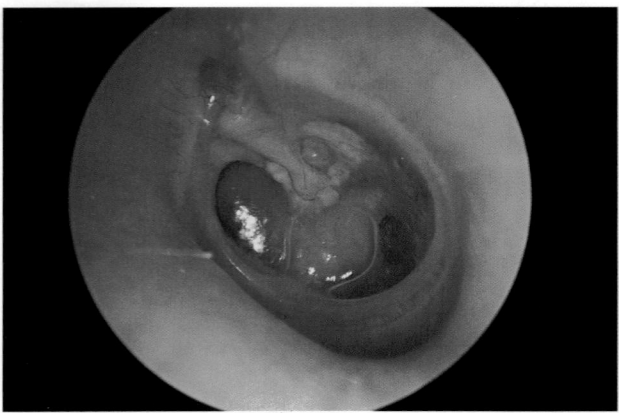

Figure 72.12   Fluid level in otitis media with effusion (left).

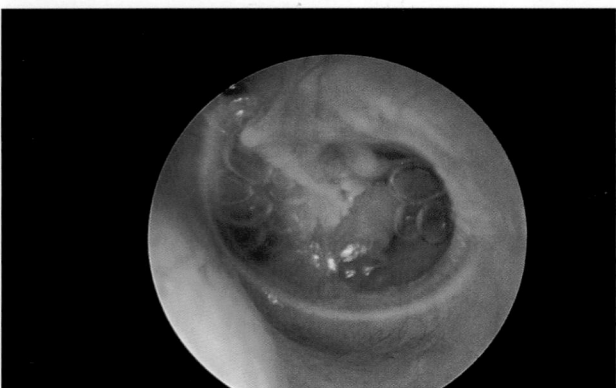

Figure 72.13   Air bubbles in otitis media with effusion (left).

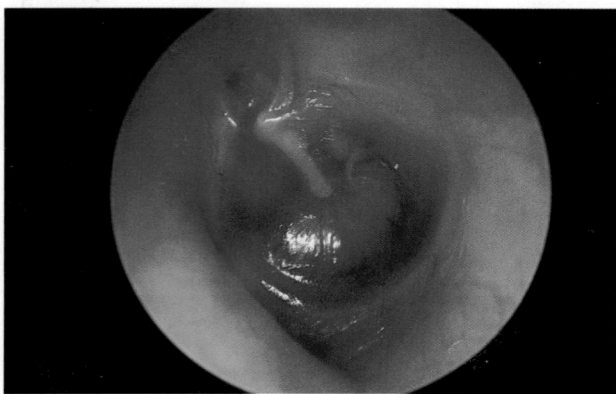

Figure 72.14   Left tympanic membrane in otitis media with effusion showing clear colour.

Fluid levels (**Figure 72.12**) or air bubbles (**Figure 72.13**) are relatively uncommon.

In some children, otoscopy may not be practicable because the view is obscured by wax. This occurs in approximately 10 percent of ears (Trial of Alternative Regimens of Glue Ear Treatment: TARGET, unpublished data). Whether it is necessary to remove the wax is

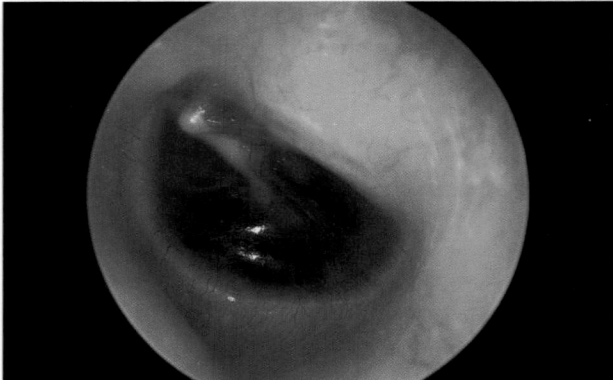

Figure 72.15   Left tympanic membrane in otitis media with effusion showing bluish colour.

doubtful. In secondary care, tympanometry and audiometry will usually be practicable and provide sufficient information to allow decisions to be made.

Pneumatic otoscopy

This can be carried out with a closed system in a hand-held otoscope or with a Siegle's pneumatic speculum, viewed with headlight illumination or microscope. Though acceptable to most children, the inability to gain a seal with the available speculum can occur in up to 20 percent of children aged over 18 months.[47] [***] If the tympanic membrane is seen to move, the lack of a seal is irrelevant as the middle ear is obviously aerated. The problem arises when no movement is seen and air escape is evident. Most reports of the sensitivity and specificity of pneumatic otoscopy do no include such children, nor do they include children in whom the tympanic membrane could not be visualized.

Simulated otoscopy using static videos has been compared with simulated pneumatic otoscopy using dynamic videos to compare their accuracy.[48] [****] The 'true' middle ear status was determined in 'most ears by tympanometry and myringotomy data'. Overall, there was a relative improvement of 26 percent in the overall score of trainees and consultants with the addition of pneumatic otoscopy. This improvement was greater for the consultants than for the trainees. Whether the results of this simulated study can be generalized to the clinical situation remains to be reported. In practice, many clinicians use pneumatic otoscopy when they have doubts as to whether there is OME rather than routinely.

Studies that compare pneumatic otoscopy with tympanometry are available, but studies that compare pneumatic otoscopy with the findings at surgery are chosen as the type of study to report because they are a better reference standard (**Table 72.4**). The sensitivity of pneumatic otoscopy caried out by trained specialists ranges from 85 to 93 percent and its specificity from 71 to 89 percent. These calculations omit children in whom pneumatic otoscopy was not possible (up to 20 percent of

Table 72.4 Sensitivity (Sens), specificity (Spec), positive predictive (PPV) and negative predictive values (NPV) of otoscopy in the detection of OME with surgical findings as the reference standard.

Author	OME (%)	Pneumatic otoscopy			
		Sens	PPV	Spec	NPV
Toner and Main[49]	56	87	84	89	84
Finitzo et al.[50]	70	93	84	58	78
Vaughan-Jones and Mills[51]	68	90	88	75	78
Nozza et al.[52]	55	85	78	71	79

Ears in which the tympanic membrane could not be visualized or a seal obtained are not included.

children). If they were to be included, the sensitivities and specificities would alter dramatically. The sensitivity and specificity of pneumatic otoscopy, even where practicable, would be markedly poorer in practitioners whose skills have not been validated.[53]

Over the years, American clinical practice guidelines have strongly advocated the use of pneumatic otoscopy as the primary diagnostic method for OME.[54, 55, 56] It is certainly to be recommended to those in primary care where the examiners are perhaps less experienced than specialists who also will have access to additional methods of assessment, including tympanometry and audiometry.

Video otoscopy

Video recordings of otoscopy, including pneumatic otoscopy, can be documented and used to monitor changes with time. It can also be used for teaching and research purposes.

FREE-FIELD VOICE TESTING

In primary care, audiometry is seldom available, particularly for younger children. Under these circumstances, the practitioner could perform free-field voice testing of hearing. Though not reported in a primary care setting, in those over the age of three years the sensitivity of modifications of the voice test (e.g. use of pictures to point at or two-syllable words) is 80–96 percent and the specificity is 90–98 percent.[57] [****] Unfortunately, these satisfactory levels are unlikely to be achieved when carried out by less experienced examiners in a primary-care setting.

TYMPANOMETRY

Tympanometry with an impedance meter (see Chapter 232, Psychoacoustic audiometry) has been advocated since the 1970s as a reliable method of detecting OME. Since then, there have been many publications on its use as a screening instrument using otoscopy as the reference standard. Its role as a confirmatory test has also been assessed in secondary care using otoscopy, pure-tone audiometry or surgical findings as the reference standard.

Though an acoustic seal is sometimes difficult to achieve, bilateral tympanograms should be obtainable in the majority (98 percent) of children between the ages of 3.5 and 7 years,[58] in a slightly lower percentage (90–94 percent) of infants 2–11 months of age[59, 60] and 78–88 percent of infants 12–24 months of age are included.[60]

Tympanograms can be classified in multiple ways, the simplest being peaked/no-peaked, usually with the additional subclassification of peaked tympanograms depending on the pressure at which the peak is recorded. Numerical evaluation of various parameters[61, 62] has also been advocated. These have the scientific advantages of being able to be analyzed in multiple different ways to produce ROC (receiver operating characteristic) curves. They have the disadvantage of being more difficult to apply in comparison to visually scanning the tympanogram for a peak and noting the pressure at that peak.

Peaked versus flat (non-peaked) tympanograms

The classification most commonly used is that of Jerger[63] modified by Zielhaus et al.[21] which uses compliance and pressure as the numerical parameters. The classification can be presented in many ways; visually as examples (e.g. Orchik et al.[64]), in a summary figure as in **Figure 72.16** or in **Table 72.5**. Analyzing papers with the findings at myringotomy (soon after tympanometry) as the reference 'gold' standard, suggest that a type B tympanogram is frequently associated with OME, a type A is infrequently associated with OME and a type C falls in between (**Table 72.6**). This study[64] is particularly informative because

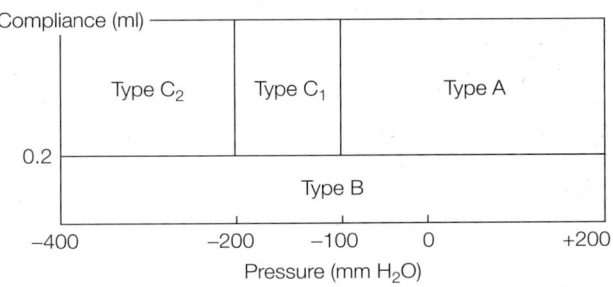

Figure 72.16 Classification of tympanogram types according to Jerger. Modified from Ref. 63, with permission.

Table 72.5 Classification of tympanograms.

	Type	Description
Peaked	A	Between + 200 and −99 daPa
	C₁	Between −100 and −199 daPa
	C₂	Between −200 and −399 daPa
Non-peaked	B	No observable peak between + 200 and −600 daPa

Reprinted from Ref. 63, with permission.

Table 72.6 Relationship between tympanogram type and effusion at myringotomy.

Tympanogram type	% Effusion			
	None	Minimal	Moderate	Impacted
A	27	36	15	22
B	0	12	13	75
C	18	35	24	23

Reprinted from Ref. 64, with permission.

the amount of middle ear fluid is quantified. Unfortunately, in this study type C tympanograms were not subcategorized as type C_1 and C_2.

Taking a variety of level 1 evidence studies (**Table 72.7**), a type B tympanogram compared with all other types of tympanogram has a sensitivity of between 56 and 73 percent and a specificity of between 50 and 98 percent in detecting OME confirmed surgically. Compared with all other types, a type B plus C_2 has a sensitivity of between 73 and 99 percent and a specificity of between 40 and 74 percent (**Table 72.8**). [****] Why there is such a range of values can only be partly explained by the differing proportion of ears with OME and the fact that the anaesthetic can itself aerate the middle ear giving a 'false' dry tap.

Pittsburgh algorithm

Table 72.9[62] [****] shows the sensitivity and specificity of various tympanometric measures, including the gradient, which is taken alongside acoustic reflexes (see Acoustic reflexes) appears to give good positive and negative predictive values. Unfortunately, no comparison of this algorithm is made with the easier to apply peak/no-peak distinction.

Tympanoscopes

Tympanometry can also be performed with a hand-held otoscope that automatically prints out the results. Compared with the more complicated, scientific impedance bridge, these have the advantage of portability and lower cost. Hence, they are commonly advocated for use in primary care. In such a setting and with training,[66, 67] if a type B tympanogram is classified with a type C_2 tympanogram, the sensitivity and specificity (100 and 75 percent) are comparable to conventional methods.[68, 69] Using a type B tympanogram alone to diagnose OME gave poor sensitivity and specificity and is not recommended.

TYMPANOMETRY IN COMBINATION WITH OTOSCOPY

The results of otoscopy can either be in agreement or disagreement with tympanometry. If in agreement, their diagnostic value can be assessed against the findings at myringotomy.[50] [****] Thus, when otoscopy suggests OME and is associated with a type B tympanogram, the

Table 72.7 Sensitivity (Sens), specificity (Spec), positive (PPV) and negative predictive values (NPV) of a Type B tympanogram versus Type A and C in the detection of OME with surgical findings as the reference standard.

Author	OME (%)	Type B alone			
		Sens	PPV	Spec	NPV
Orchik et al.[64]	59	55	88	90	58
Toner and Mains 1990[49]	56	86	94	93	84
Finitzo et al. 1992[50]	70	57	95	94	47
Vaughan–Jones and Mills[51]	68	67	96	94	58
Nozza et al.[52]	55	85	78	71	79
Sassen et al.[65]	73	90	83	50	66
Palmu et al.[59]	74	70	93	98	94

Table 72.8 Sensitivity (Sens), specificity (Spec), positive (PPV) and negative predictive values (NPV) of a Type B + C_2 tympanogram versus Type A + C in the detection of OME with surgical findings as the reference standard.

Author	OME (%)	Type B and C_2			
		Sens	PPV	Spec	NPV
Finitzo et al. 1992[50]	70	73	87	73	53
Vaughan–Jones and Mills[51]	68	89	75	40	67
Sassen et al.[65]	73	99	91	74	97

combined sensitivity is 98 percent. When otoscopy suggests no OME and is combined with a type A tympanogram, the specificity is 98 percent. However, in this study the findings were in agreement in only 44 percent of ears. In the other 66 percent, where the results are not in agreement, another indicator of OME such as audiometry would be required.

ACOUSTIC REFLEXES

Two papers[70, 71] [****] showed that the results of measuring the acoustic reflexes in association with classification of tympanometry as peaked/non-peaked substantially lowered its specificity whilst adding little to the sensitivity. Such testing is therefore not advocated if this classification is used. On the other hand, if the Pittsburgh algorithm is used it would appear to add value.[70] [****]

EUSTACHIAN TUBE FUNCTION TESTS

Reliably assessing Eustachian tube function requires a method that does not depend on a child's ability to perform a task. It also has to be applicable when the

Table 72.9 Sensitivity, specificity and predictive values of various criteria using acoustic emittance measures for the diagnosis of MEE, as determined at myringotomy, in ears with a history of chronic or recurrent otitis media ($n = 111$).

Variables	Criterion	Sens (%)	Spec (%)	PPV (%)	NPV (%)
Gr + AR	Gr < 0.1, or Gr = 0.2, or 0.3 with AR absent	90	86	95	75
	Gr ≤ 0.1, or Gr = 0.2 with AR absent	88	86	95	71
Y_{tm} + AR	Y_{tm} ≤ 0.2, or Y_{tm} = 0.3, 0.4, or 0.5 with AR absent	83	86	94	65
	Y_{tm} < 0.3, or Y_{tm} = 0.4 or 0.5 with AR absent	85	76	90	65
AR alone	AR absent	88	85	94	72
GR alone	Gr ≤ 0.1	78	90	96	60
	Gr ≤ 0.2	91	70	89	75
Y_{tm} alone	Y_{tm} ≤ 0.1	31	97	96	34
	Y_{tm} ≤ 0.2	56	93	96	44
	Y_{tm} ≤ 0.3	73	80	91	52
	Y_{tm} ≤ 0.4	82	63	86	56
Gr and Y_{tm}	Gr ≤ 0.1 or Y_{tm} ≤ 0.2	83	87	94	65

Gr, gradient; AR, Acoustic reflex; Y_{tm}, peak compensated admittance; NPV, negative predictive value; PPV, positive predictive value. Sens, sensitivity; Spec. specificity. Reprinted from Ref. 52, with permission.

tympanic membrane is intact rather than just when a ventilating tube is in place. Sonotubometry is such a method, but needs to be improved further for it to be clinically applicable.[72]

ACOUSTIC REFLECTOMETRY

This is performed with a hand-held acoustic otoscope that does not require a seal. It is moved around whilst emitting a sound of 80 dB A over a frequency range. The amount of sound reflected back is recorded and analyzed in various ways. Unfortunately, the sensitivity and specificity of the test is poorer than tympanometry when pneumatic otoscopy or the surgical findings are used as the reference standards.[73, 74, 75] [****]

AUDIOMETRY

In secondary care, audiometric assessment of the hearing is mandatory in all children referred with a suspected persistent hearing impairment, irrespective as to whether OME is diagnosed at the time. If OME is diagnosed then the laterality and severity of the impairment will dictate management. If there is no OME and if the air-conduction thresholds are elevated, bone-conduction thresholds will detect the 1 percent of children with previously undiagnosed congenital, sensorineural impairments.[76] [**]

The method used to assess the hearing thresholds depends on the equipment available, the age of the child and the assessor's preference.[77] In essence, it can be performed binaurally free-field or monaurally with headphones. Tones or speech can be presented and the method of response can be by turning to the sound source or by performing a task, which can range from doing something with a toy, to raising a hand or pointing at an object or picture. Conventional air- and bone-conduction

testing is the preferred method as it tests each ear separately and can quantify any conductive component present. In children over 3.5 years of age, air- and bone-conduction thresholds are obtainable in the majority of children (95 and 92 percent, respectively) on the first occasion.[78] [**] Age is the main determinant of whether thresholds are obtainable, rather than the method of audiometry. Even if the child's concentration is poor, the results on average are only 5 dB poorer and can still be used to guide management.[78] [**]

Air–bone gap

The presence of an air–bone gap of at least 10 dB is a poor predictor of concurrent OME. Of children referred with a history of OME, 80 percent (1234 of 1551 children) will have an air–bone gap of > 10 dB, but only 32 percent will have otoscopic evidence of OME associated with a type B or C_2 tympanogram (MRC (Medical Research Council) Multicentre Otitis Media Study Group, unpublished data). Using findings at myringotomy as the reference standard, 37 percent (28 of 75) of ears with an air–bone gap of greater than 10 dB had a dry tap. It was only when the air–bone gap was greater than 30 dB was the dry tap rate reduced to 4 percent (1 of 27).[79] [***] The most likely reason for the air–bone gap being such a poor predictor is that children studied prospectively with OME will have a small residual conductive impairment after otoscopic and tympanometric resolution of their OME (personal communication). [***]

Carhart notch in the bone-conduction thresholds

As with any pure conductive impairment, one would expect OME to be associated with a Carhart notch in the bone-conduction thresholds around 2 kHz. By definition, the notch has to be 10 dB or greater between 0.5 and 4 kHz as any lesser dips could be due to test/retest error.

As such, accurate bone-conduction thresholds are required and this may be problematic in younger children. Notches are reported to be present in 48 percent of children with OME whose mean age was nine years.[80] [**] In those able to perform the audiometry, the positive predictive value of a Carhart notch in diagnosing fluid at myringotomy was 97 percent and the negative predictive value was 87 percent.[79] [**]

Ideal diagnostic strategy for OME

The ideal strategy for the diagnosis of childhood OME should be applicable to the majority of children being assessed. This rules out myringotomy and means that it has to be based on any combination of otoscopy, tympanometry and audiometry.

The first thing to consider is the percentage of children in whom one of these investigations is not possible. In the TARGET study (unpublished data), at the first visit to a specialist clinic of children with suspected OME aged between 3.25 and 7 years, it was not possible in both ears to obtain tympanometry in 1.6 percent, air-conduction thresholds in 3 percent, bone-conduction thresholds in 6 percent and otoscopy in 9 percent of children. The ability to assess the hearing thresholds was age related, ranging from 12 percent in three year olds to 11 percent in seven year olds. The inability to perform otoscopy in such a high proportion of children is partly because aural toilet to visualize the tympanic membrane was not enforced, but this is probably the usual practice of most clinicians for children in this age group.

Otoscopy should be attempted in all children not just to diagnose OME, but also acute and chronic otitis media. Pneumatic otoscopy can be of added value where there is uncertainty. In those with OME on otoscopy, audiometry is required to help determine management. Thus, in such children, tympanometry is probably only a confirmatory investigation. In those in whom the tympanic membrane cannot be visualized or the findings are uncertain, then tympanometry is essential. In those with a type B or C_2 tympanogram, audiometry will detect those with a bilateral hearing impairment of 20 dB or greater that merit follow up. [Grade D] Unfortunately, a review article of the methods of diagnosing OME[81] does not address the question of whether the diagnostic method was practicable and what difference that would make to the comparisons they make. If they were to have done so, they might have proposed the above strategy rather than the use of pneumatic otoscopy.

Assessment of hearing

This is important to assess not just for the diagnostic reasons stated above, but in secondary care the current hearing thresholds are the main determinant as to management.

HISTORY

Unfortunately, reliance cannot be placed on parental report of the current hearing, though it may reflect the hearing in the past (see under Diagnosis; and History above).

AUDIOMETRY

Routine audiometric testing of the hearing of every child with OME seen at secondary care is recommended, as the associated hearing impairment can vary enormously from negligible to moderately severe (see Outcomes of childhood OME below).

TYMPANOMETRY AS A SCREEN FOR AUDIOMETRY

Having excluded a sensorineural impairment by audiometry at a child's first visit, at subsequent visits tympanometry can be used as a screen to identify those most likely to have a material hearing impairment associated with their OME. This was first proposed by Dempster and McKenzie.[82] [****] Since then, others have examined this possibility in more detail using different audiometric cut-offs.[58, 71] [****] The results are not materially different between papers, but the later publication[58] has analyzed a greater variety of outcomes and cut-offs (**Table 72.10**). Thus, for example, taking 25 dB HL in the better ear as the level requiring detection, limiting audiometry to those with a bilateral type B reduces the workload by 50 percent, but will detect 90 percent of such impaired children. Limiting audiometry to those with bilateral type B or C_2 tympanograms reduces the workload to 69 percent of the sample, yet 95 percent of the impaired children will be detected.

Tympanometry can be particularly helpful if resources are limited in choosing children for more time-consuming audiometry. This should only be done once a coexisting sensorineural impairment has been excluded. [****]

OTHER CLINICAL EXAMINATIONS

What other examination is undertaken depends on whether there are any other nonotological symptoms, such as recurrent sore throats, blocked nose and snoring.

POPULATION SCREENING FOR OME

As OME is highly prevalent in the childhood population and is frequently asymptomatic, some have suggested that universal screening so that early treatment could be implemented. A Cochrane review[83] identified three trials where a population was screened and those with OME were then randomized to ventilation tubes or watchful waiting. No benefit was identified on language development or behaviour, the outcomes that one might hope would benefit from early intervention. Population screening is thus not considered to be efficacious at present. [Grade A]

OUTCOMES OF CHILDHOOD OME

Natural history

As discussed earlier (see above under Epidemiology), the majority of epidemiological studies are point prevalence studies of a cohort of children at different times rather than longitudinal studies of specific children over time. There are considerably fewer data on the natural history in individual children available, this being the information most relevant to clinical practice.

As children with bilateral OME are more likely to have more severe outcomes, studies that report such children are those that are concentrated upon. Hogan et al.[43] [***] found that in children under three years of age with a propensity to have bilateral OME, the effusions lasted on average ten weeks, albeit the children were likely to have a further episode within 11 weeks.

Older children between the ages of 3.25 and seven years have been studied extensively in the UK MRC-funded

TARGET study. A total of 3831 children of this age were referred from primary care because of suspected OME. When screened at the trial clinic, only 34 percent (**Table 72.11**) satisfied the criterion for further study of having bilateral OME associated with a hearing impairment of at least 20 dB HL in both ears.[14, 16, 17] [***] This cohort underwent a 12-week watchful waiting period, following which 49 percent of children no longer met the bilateral OME hearing criterion. That is, only 51 percent persisted. At that stage, children with persistent OME were randomized and in those who had nonspecific medical management, three months later only 49 percent were persistent.[84] [****] It was only three months later that a group of children was identified that could be truly considered to have persistent bilateral OME with a hearing.

To summarize the above data, of the children aged 3.25–7 years referred to secondary care with bilateral OME, if they waited 13 weeks to be seen, underwent a watchful waiting period of three months and then waited a further three months for surgery, by then in 92 percent of them the hearing impairment associated with their OME will have resolved (**Table 72.11**). Thus, even in secondary care, the vast majority of children with bilateral OME resolve spontaneously over a nine-month period, albeit the OME might recur.

Table 72.10 Sensitivity, specificity and positive predictive value (PPV) as percentages for tympanometry in all children in seven centres.

	% of sample	Type B + B tymp versus others			Type B + B or B + C$_2$ tymp versus others			Type B + B or B + C$_2$ or C$_2$ + C$_2$ tymp versus others		
		Sensitivity	Specificity	PPV	Sensitivity	Specificity	PPV	Sensitivity	Specificity	PPV
Better ear HL ≥ 15	76	65	91	96	80	80	93	84	75	92
Better ear HL ≥ 20	53	81	81	82	90	62	72	92	54	69
Better ear HL ≥ 25	34	90	69	60	94	49	49	95	43	46
Better ear HL ≥ 30	23	92	60	41	94	43	33	94	37	31
ABG ≥ 10	88	58	92	98	72	84	97	77	79	96
ABG ≥ 15	75	65	87	94	80	77	90	84	72	90
ABG ≥ 20	59	75	80	84	86	64	77	89	57	75
ABG ≥ 25	44	83	72	70	91	54	61	93	48	58
ABG ≥ 30	32	89	66	55	94	48	46	93	42	43

n = 1153. ABG, air–bone gap. Reprinted from Ref. 58, with permission.

Table 72.11 Natural resolution of OME in children (n = 3831) referred to otolaryngology from primary care (GP). Persistence is defined as bilateral OME associated with hearing ≥ 20 dB HL in both ears.

Wait	Wait time (months)	Total wait	% persistence	% persistence of original cohort
GP to otorhinolaryngologist	3	3	34	34
Otorhinolaryngologist watchful wait	3	6	51	17
Nonsurgical cases	3	9	49	8
Nonsurgical cases	3	12	89	7

Reprinted from Ref. 14, with permission.

As might be expected if a less strict definition of what constitutes persistence is taken, such as not having an associated requirement for the degree of hearing impairment, the resolution rates by ear of chronic OME are materially lower; 19, 25, 31 and 33 percent at 3, 6, 12 and 24 months, respectively.[85] [****]

Outcomes

OTOPATHOLOGY

To answer the question, 'does OME cause pars flaccida and tensa retractions that can progress to a cholesteatoma?' would require a cohort of children with documented OME to be followed up and compared with a cohort that do not have OME. Ideally the OME cohort would have no effective therapy for their OME, including the insertion of ventilation tubes as these themselves might cause pathology.

The best alternative evidence is from a large cohort ($n = 964$) of children who were screened for OME every three months between the ages of two and four years and were otoscopically reassessed when they were seven or eight years of age.[86] [***] The children were classified as:

- never OME (never a type B tympanogram);
- persistent OME/no surgery (type B tympanogram on at least two consecutive visits);
- transient OME/no surgery (type B tympanograms that were not consecutive);
- OME surgery (those with OME that had ventilation tubes inserted; 60 percent had only one tube inserted).

Table 72.12 shows the otoscopic sequel in these four groups of children. What one is primarily looking for is a dose–response effect, albeit the OME surgery group would be the most severe group and include any additive effect of ventilation tubes. There is a clear dose–response effect for attic retractions. This is, therefore, a disease effect. There is also a dose–response effect for tympanosclerosis and atrophy of the pars tensa, but with a particularly large increase in the ventilation tube group.

Hence, these are most likely to be disease effects, but with an increased risk following the insertion of ventilation tubes. No dose–response effect is apparent for retractions of the pars tensa. The high incidence (14 percent) of this in the OME surgery group can therefore be mainly attributed to the ventilation tubes.

It is concluded [***] that attic retractions are an OME disease effect with an incidence of approximately 14 percent in the most severe children. What proportion of these retractions progress to cholesteatoma is not known. There is no evidence that the risk of attic retraction is altered by the insertion of ventilation tubes.

Tympanosclerosis and atrophy of the pars tensa are OME disease effects, the risk of which is increased by the insertion of ventilation tubes to >45 percent and around 70 percent, respectively.

Long-term pars tensa retractions are more likely caused by the insertion of ventilation tubes than by the disease process itself with an incidence of 15 percent.

CONDUCTIVE HEARING IMPAIRMENT

The hearing impairment associated with OME varies greatly. Table 72.13 shows the percentage of OME children aged between 2 and 12 years with confirmed, bilateral OME who have various pure-tone air-conduction averages in their better hearing ear. Overall, the mean threshold in the better ear was 21 dB HL (s.d. 10), but in 54 percent of those with bilateral OME the pure-tone average in the better ear was better than 20 dB HL.[87] [***] The mean threshold in the poorer hearing ears was 31 dB HL (s.d. 13). The speech reception or speech awareness thresholds in infants in this study were of a similar distribution. This suggests that the majority of children with bilateral OME have an insufficient hearing impairment to be materially disabling. This paper also reports a group of children with unilateral OME. In them the mean threshold in the better ear was 11 dB HL (s.d. 7) and 23 dB HL (s.d. 10) in the poorer ear.

Coincidentally, 'normal' children in this age group on average do not have 'normal' thresholds, the mean

Table 72.12 Otopathologic sequelae at seven to eight years of age in four groups of right ears.

OME persistence groups	Tympanosclerosis %	Atrophy %	Retractions pars tensa % stage ≥2	Attic retraction % stage ≥2
No OME (reference group) ($n = 264$)	0	3.4	1.9	0.4
Transient OME ($n = 251$)	2.4[a]	4.4	2.0	4.4
Persistent OME ($n = 219$)	3.7[c]	8.8[b]	1.9	7.4
Ventilation tube ($n = 64$)	47.6[d]	68.2[d]	14.3[b]	14.3[b]

Ears classified according to the persistence of OME at preschool age and surgical treatment (96 ears with signs of active middle ear disease, perforation or ventilation tube still present excluded).

p-value associated with chi-square test or Fisher's exact test for the transient OME, persistent OME and ventilation tube groups as related to the no-OME group (i.e. reference group).

[a] <0.05; [b] <0.01; [c] <0.005; [d] <0.001.

Reprinted from Ref. 86, with permission.

Table 72.13 Pure-tone average air-conduction thresholds in the better hearing ear in 385 children aged 2–11 years with bilateral OME confirmed by a diagnostic algorithm, including pneumatic otoscopy, tympanometry and reflexes.

PTA dB HL	Percentage
0–4	4
5–9	10
10–14	20
15–19	20
20–24	14
25–29	13
30–34	6
35–39	4
40–44	1
45–49	2
50–54	1

Reprinted from Ref. 87, with permission.

air-conduction thresholds in three- to six-year-old children being 3 dB HL.[88, 89] [***]

Though it might be expected that the viscosity of the middle ear fluid would be a determinant of the hearing, it would not appear to be so. In particular, there is no difference in the hearing levels in ears with serous fluid compared with those with mucoid fluid.[90] [***]

HEARING DISABILITY SECONDARY TO CONDUCTIVE IMPAIRMENT

The main method of assessing a child's hearing disability is by questioning the parents. Four of the nine questions in the MRC Reported Hearing Disability (RHD) questionnaire are sufficient to predict the overall disability (**Table 72.14**) (personal communication). [***]

Many hold that audiometric measures such as speech-in-noise would be a superior way to measure disability rather than using the pure-tone thresholds. If this were to be the case, such a measure in a specific child might more likely reflect the detrimental effect of OME and predict their likely benefit of management. Research in this area is ongoing.

Sensorineural hearing impairment

There is no evidence to suggest that OME is associated with a sensorineural hearing impairment in the short term.[78] [***]

Long-term hearing impairment

There is now considerable evidence that following the otoscopic and tympanometric resolution of fluid, ears that have had OME still have a small residual conductive impairment in the order of 10 dB HL (personal communication). [****] The reason for this is not known, but is likely to be due to ossicular chain immobility caused by some residual fluid or mucosal oedema around them.

Table 72.14 Four questions that predict a child's hearing disability associated with OME.

Question	Response	Weighting
How would you describe your child's hearing?	Normal	0
	Slightly below normal	0.4
	Poor	0.6
	Very poor	0.6
	Not sure	0
	Missing	0
Has he/she misheard words when not looking at you?	No	0
	Rarely	0.1
	Often	0.6
	Always	0.6
	Not sure	0
	Missing	0
Has he/she had difficulty hearing when with a group of people?	No	0
	Rarely	0.1
	Often	0.5
	Always	0.6
	Not sure	0.1
	Missing	0
Has he asked for things to be repeated?	No	0
	Rarely	0.1
	Often	0.5
	Always	0.6
	Not sure	0
	Missing	0

Unpublished data.

In a cohort followed from birth to 18 years of age, those who had had otitis media (acute and with effusion) had air-conduction thresholds that were 4 dB on average poorer that those that had not had otitis media.[91] [***] Their bone-conduction thresholds were also 2 dB poorer. Whether these poorer thresholds are a disease effect or the result of surgery has yet to be elucidated.

High frequency sensorineural damage above 8 kHz has also been reported in a case series of children with OME who had been operated on and followed up for between three and five years.[92] [**]

SPEECH AND LANGUAGE

The development of normal speech and language in a child depends on many interrelated factors, the age of the child being the major factor, but the ethnic background and the degree of interfamily communication, particularly by the mother, are important. Any hearing impairment a child might have due to their OME obviously interplays with these factors.

Assessment of speech and language is complicated by it having many components, including speech reception, speech and sound production, expressive language and cognitive understanding. When a parent expresses concern regarding their child's speech and language, this can be partly investigated by comparing the child's performance with standard milestones. Thus, at 18 months they would be expected to have a vocabulary of ten words with meaning. More formal objective assessments can be undertaken for each of the components of speech and language and related to the results in normal age-matched controls.

Total bilateral loss of hearing during the first few years of life will obviously have a profound effect on speech and development. Whether the usually intermittent, mild to moderate conductive impairment that can be associated with otitis media with effusion in the first two to three years of life makes an impact has been extensively studied.[93] [****] Prospective cohort studies do indeed suggest that there is an impact of otitis media that is related to the number of days with bilateral fluid during the first two to three years of life. However, follow up of these children when they are seven to eight years of age suggests that by then the children have caught up with their nonaffected peers.[94] [***] Thus, overall, the data would suggest at most a mild effect on speech production and reception in early childhood,[93, 95] that is not modified by surgical intervention (see Surgery) and spontaneously resolves with age.

COGNITION

The factors that interplay and influence a child's intellectual development are even more complex than those that affect speech and language development. Many objective measures are available with age-related 'normal' values, but whether these are affected by a child having had OME is difficult to determine. Cohorts of children can be grouped as to how much OME they have had and this is correlated to a particular outcome, having controlled for demographic and environmental factors. Any effect of OME that has been identified occurs early in a child's academic development, around the ages of three to four years, and has been minor compared with the demographic and environmental ones. Any effect corrects itself with time and is no longer detectable once the child is seven or eight years of age.[96, 97, 98] [***]

BEHAVIOUR

Abnormalities of behaviour can be reported in questionnaires by the parents or by the teachers. These can be analyzed to give a global behaviour score or be broken down into various components of behaviour. These vary between questionnaires. Thus, the Rutter score[99] can be broken down into antisocial, neurotic, hyperactive and inattentive behaviour. The MRC Behaviour Questionnaire can be broken down into anxiety, aggressive, context-related and social immaturity components. Many factors influence a child's behaviour which have to be controlled for before calculating the effect of the hearing impairment associated with OME.

Whether this is the case has been best reported in OME children being randomized in randomized controlled trials (RCT). Fifty-five percent of three-year-old children with bilateral, three-month persistent OME have abnormal overall Rutter scores. This compares with 10–15 percent of unselected three year olds.[100] [***] The overall behaviour scores in children aged between three and seven years with three-month persistent bilateral OME, associated with a hearing impairment of at least 20 dB HL in both ears, is 0.6 s.d. poorer (i.e. moderately) than the population scores (MRC Otitis Media Study Group, unpublished data). There is some evidence that even when a child has reached the age of 15 years, they have still poorer behaviour than non-OME children, particularly in the inattentive and hyperactive aspects.[101] [***]

BALANCE

Around 30 percent of parents of children with OME report that they are clumsy, often imbalanced and can fall. These symptoms would appear to be more common than in non-OME children.[102] [***] The pathophysiology as to why OME might cause such symptoms is difficult to understand. However, laboratory assessments of balance suggest that these are abnormal in children with a history of OME,[103] [***] but the clinical significance and relation to symptoms is unclear. It is highly likely that if they are due to vestibular dysfunction they will compensate naturally with time. There are reports that laboratory assessments improve after surgery, but these observations are uncontrolled.[104] [**] Improvement in such tests is also likely to occur with practice and is an alternative reason for the improvements reported.

It must be concluded that at present there is insufficient knowledge and understanding to guide the assessment and management of balance symptoms in childhood OME.

QUALITY OF LIFE

Because there are so many potential outcomes that might be attributed to a child having a mild to moderate hearing impairment due to OME, it would be helpful if an overall OME disease score could be calculated. Two such disease-specific 'otitis media' quality of life questionnaires are available. The OME-6 covers physical suffering, hearing loss, speech impairment, emotional distress, activity limitations and caregiver concern and is applicable to two-month to 12-year-old children with OME or recurrent AOM. This has been shown to improve in children who have had ventilation tubes inserted, but because of the lack of a control group it is not possible to conclude that surgery was beneficial.[105, 106] [**] There is also some concern that the OME-6 does not relate to the severity of the hearing impairment that might limit its usefulness.[107]

A longer questionnaire, the OM7-27, was developed to summarize the outcomes in the MRC TARGET study.[108]

The 27 questions cover the seven domains of hearing difficulty, upper respiratory symptoms, sleep patterns, behaviour problems, ENT-related parental quality of life, global physical health and speech/language impairment. It is applicable to children between the ages of three and seven years with OME. The effect of surgery in comparison to nonsurgical management awaits reporting.

Both these questionnaires are potentially useful for research studies, but cannot be described as true quality-of-life instruments. This requires a generic questionnaire that can be used to compare outcomes for different conditions. Many such instruments are available for adults (e.g. the SF-36), but those for children are still in the development stage. A generic Dutch quality-of-life instrument for preschool children (TAPQOL) has been used in a surgical RCT (see Quality of life, under Surgery below) and the communication, positive mood, sleep and aggression domains in this questionnaire relate well to the OME-6 and the Health Utilities Index mark 111.[109]

To assess the benefit from interventions, the Glasgow Children's Benefit Inventory has been shown to reflect the parental satisfaction of ventilation tube insertion and allows a comparison to be made between different interventions for different paediatric otolaryngological conditions.[110]

MANAGEMENT

Counselling and hearing tactics

Parents of children with OME are often misinformed about many aspects of the condition. In particular, they can have overpessimistic views about its severity and be overoptimistic about the merits of surgery. At their first visit to their general practitioner or to a specialist, time has to be spent explaining that, in general, OME is a benign condition with a high spontaneous recovery rate and no long-term sequelae. In most children, the main concern will be the hearing. It should be explained to the parents that the impairment associated with OME is very variable in degree and mild or moderate at most.

It is important that all parents of children with OME receive appropriate general counselling about the natural history and relative benign nature of the condition. Those in contact with the child, including any minder or teacher, should be made aware that the disability can be minimized by hearing tactics, including those shown below:

- getting the child's attention before starting to talk;
- reducing the background noise as much as possible by turning off the television, etc.;
- facing the child so that they can see you talk;
- speaking in a normal voice both in volume, speed and emphasis, as close as possible to the child;
- leaflets such as *Glue ear explained*[111] given to the parents can reinforce the above messages.

Medical

Medical management would potentially be of greatest benefit if it could speed the resolution of an episode of OME. Hence, randomized controlled trials carried out in primary care settings would be those most appropriate to consider using resolution of OME as the outcome. Such studies are uncommon and often include heterogeneous groups of children with otitis media rather than OME. The effect of most medications has been systematically reviewed, but the advisability of performing a metanalysis on the data must be questioned because of the heterogeneity of the studies.

Most trials follow up children for one to two weeks after therapy. If at this point the therapy is ineffective, there is no reason for further follow up as it is unlikely to be of benefit thereafter. However, if it is effective after one to two weeks, then follow up for the recommended watchful waiting period of 12 weeks is necessary to see if it is of benefit in the longer term and might be used to reduce the proportion of children being considered for surgery.

NASAL TOPICAL STEROIDS

Systematic reviews[112] [****] of the randomized controlled trials in August 2002 identified one study of topical nasal steroids versus placebo ($n = 44$) that found no difference in resolution of the OME at three weeks.[113] [****] Another study which gave antibiotics in addition to nasal steroids also found no difference.[114] [****] Both studies randomized small numbers and no subsequent trials have been identified. It must be concluded that there is insufficient evidence to support the use of topical nasal steroids at present for childhood OME.

SYSTEMIC STEROIDS

Considerable concern has been expressed about the use of oral steroids being given to children for a nonlife-threatening and spontaneously resolving condition. Consequently, it would have to be highly effective in the long term before it could be recommended. There is no evidence to suggest that oral steroids are effective for longer than in the short term (two weeks) even when combined with antibiotics.[112, 115, 116, 117] [****] Systemic steroids cannot be recommended at present for childhood OME.

ANTIBIOTICS

Multiple randomized controlled trials of antibiotics have been published in heterogeneous groups of patients. Two metanalyses,[118, 119] [****] covering the years 1966–1991 and 1993 respectively, reported that though there might be initial benefit in the first two weeks, there was no evidence of benefit in the longer term (> 6 weeks). Later literature reviews up to 1999[120] [****] and 2006[115] [****]

confirmed that antibiotics had no significant effect on longer-term outcomes. Hence, it is not recommended that antibiotics be used for the longer term (>6 weeks) management of childhood OME.

NASAL DECONGESTANTS

A meta-analysis of four trials (n = 1202) found that antihistamine/decongestants had no significant effect on the resolution rate of OME.[115, 121] [****] Nasal decongestants are not recommended for use in childhood OME. [Grade B]

MUCOLYTICS

A systematic review of six randomized controlled trials of S-carboxymethylcysteine (Mucodyne) published before 1993 could not demonstrate that they had an effect.[122] [****] A later trial also showed no significant effect.[123] [****] Because of a nonsignificant trend for increased benefit in these small, biased trials, a larger well-designed study is merited.

Other approaches

AUTOINFLATION

A systematic review of autoinflation for the treatment of glue ear in children[124] identified five randomized controlled trials and considered them to be of variable and low quality. Though a metanalysis of the three studies that investigated Otovent balloons indicated that children allocated to autoinflation were 3.5 times more likely to improve than controls (CI 2.0, 6.1), the authors could not recommend autoinflation for clinical practice. [****] The ability to autoinflate with the balloon is a particular problem in younger children.

If some form of nonsurgical management is required during a period of watchful waiting, autoinflation is the therapy with the strongest evidence of efficacy for older children.[115] [****]

HOMEOPATHY

No randomized controlled trials have been identified. A small, nonblinded study did not show homeopathy to be of benefit.[125] [**]

Surgery

MYRINGOTOMY AND ASPIRATION

From three trials, myringotomy with aspiration has not been shown to be effective in restoring the hearing levels in children with OME.[126] [****]

VENTILATION TUBES

Ventilation tubes can be of different materials (teflon, silicone, titanium, gold, etc.) and be coated with materials such as silver oxide. Their shapes vary but can be categorized as grommets or T-tubes. In general, the larger and stiffer the flange that goes in the middle ear, the longer it stays *in situ*. The longer a tube stays *in situ* the longer it can be potentially of benefit. On the other hand, the longer a tube is *in situ* the greater the chance of complications, including infection, granulation tissue, permanent perforation and thinning of the tympanic membrane with possible retraction.[127] [****] The object is then to try and estimate the likely duration of the OME and choose the appropriate tube. Unfortunately, prediction in children of the likely duration of the OME is difficult if not impossible. However, in adults T-tubes are justified routinely, as in them OME is likely to be persistent over years rather than months.

Though some classify ventilation tubes as short, medium or long term, data are lacking on 'duration of tube function' as opposed to the more commonly reported and less relevant 'duration till extrusion'. An additional problem is that in studies, follow-up intervals are never less than every three months and often every six months. In general, the time of extrusion is taken as the midpoint between visits. This means that duration times are fairly crude estimates. Therefore, most authors prefer to report at set time periods postoperatively. Thus, if one of the most commonly reported tubes is taken, at six months post-operation 55 percent of Shepard teflon ventilation tubes are functioning[15] [****] and between 30 and 55 percent are extruded.[127, 128, 129] [****] Armstrong tubes have similar extrusion rates, but only 10 percent of T-tubes will have been extruded at six months.[127] [****] One potential reason for the range between studies in extrusion times of the same tube is likely to be the varying incidence of recurrent acute otitis media in the children being studied, acute otitis media being more frequent in younger children. Another problem is that even though a tube might have a lower extrusion rate at 24 months (66 percent for Reuter Bobbin compared with 94 percent for Shepard for example), the difference is hardly relevant if 74 percent of the Reuter Bobbins are obstructed.[127] [****] Thus, at present there is only sufficient evidence to classify ventilation tubes as short or long term.

SURGICAL TECHNIQUE

Site

Insertion of the ventilation tube posterosuperiorly is not recommended because of the potential for damaging the ossicular chain. It makes no difference to the extrusion rate as to whether the tube is inserted through a radial or circumferential incision[130] and whether sited anterosuperiorly rather than antero-inferiorly.[131, 132, 133] [****] Placement antero-inferiorly compared with placement postero-inferiorly lengthens the time a ventilation tube is *in situ* (for a Shepard tube 80 versus 45 percent at 6 months and 30 versus 15 percent at 12 months are *in situ*).[131] [****]

To maximize the duration of potential tube function, the preferred insertion site is antero-inferior through a circumferential or radial incision. [****]

Associated aspiration

Though it is accepted practice to aspirate as much of the middle ear fluid as possible through the myringotomy before inserting a ventilation tube, there is no evidence that this is required. The hearing levels three months following insertion of a ventilation tube was no different in ears that were aspirated compared with those that were not aspirated.[134, 135] [****] However, no data are given immediately post-operation when the ears that were aspirated may have had better hearing.

There is no necessity to go to great lengths to remove all middle ear fluid when inserting a ventilation tube. [***]

Topical preparations

These can be used after insertion of the tube to prevent tube blockage with blood and infection in the postoperative period. Their efficacy is discussed under Complications of ventilation tubes.

OUTCOMES OF VENTILATION TUBES

The most up-to-date Cochrane systematic review of 'grommets (ventilation tubes) for hearing loss associated with otitis media with effusion in children'[136] [****] is based on a systematic literature search to March 2003 with some subsequent papers to August 2004 included. The RCTs of satisfactory quality identified could be divided into those that randomized within a child, one ear to have ventilation tubes and the other ear not to have ventilation tubes ($n = 7$) and those where children were randomized to have bilateral ventilation tubes or to watchful waiting ($n = 6$). Within the first by-ear category, in three trials all children had adenoidectomy and the other four the children were randomized to have adenoidectomy or no adenoidectomy. In the second category, in five trials none of the children had adenoidectomy and in the other trial children were also randomized to have adenoidectomy or no adenoidectomy.

Time with effusion

In the three studies that provided such data, children who had ventilation tubes without adenoidectomy spent 32 percent (CI 17, 48) less time with effusion during the first year after insertion. After that time most ventilation tubes had become nonfunctioning or had been extruded. In another study[137] at nine months post-insertion, those that had had ventilation tubes had 46 percent (CI 32, 61) less OME on otoscopy.

Hearing

Ventilation tubes alone will improve the hearing level by 9 dB (CI 4, 14) at six months, 6 dB (CI 3, 9) at 12 months and 4 dB (CI 2, 6) at 24 months. Adenoidectomy has an additional effect of 3–4 dB (CI 2, 5) at six months and 1 dB (CI 0.1, 2.8) at 12 months (**Figure 72.17**).

A subsequent individual patient data metanalysis of three by-ear trials confirmed that the effect of a ventilation tube in those with an impairment of 25 dB HL or greater when randomized was 10 dB at six months and 3 dB at 12 months.[141] [****]

How this magnitude of improvement translates to reduction in hearing disability is not possible to assess in the 'by-ear' studies. Since 1992, the majority of studies have randomized ventilation tubes 'by child' so that hearing disability and other child-centred outcomes can be studied in addition to the hearing levels.

TARGET is a UK multicentre study that looked at the effect of ventilation tubes alone or with adjuvant adenoidectomy on child-centred outcomes. To be eligible, children had to be aged between 3.5 and 7 years and have bilateral OME, persistent over a 12-week 'watchful waiting' period and associated with a hearing impairment in both ears of 20 dB HL or poorer. Children were randomized to one of three arms: no-surgical management, bilateral ventilation tubes (Shepard) or bilateral ventilation tubes with adjuvant adenoidectomy. **Figure 72.18** shows the binaural hearing average in the two surgical groups in comparison with the nonsurgical group. The hearing in the nonsurgical group improves with time, mainly due to the natural resolution of the OME. Children randomized to have ventilation tubes had a marked improvement three months following surgery of 12 dB compared with the nonsurgical group.

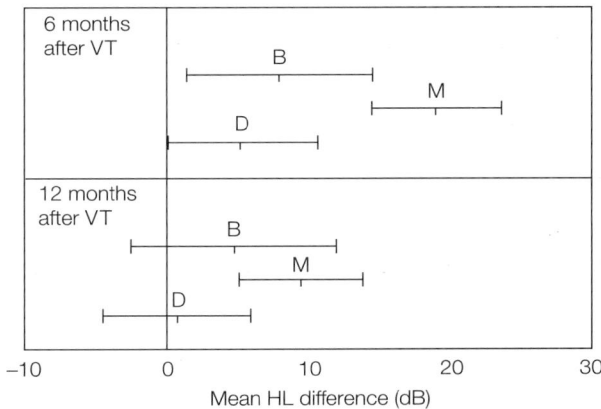

Figure 72.17 Mean improvement in hearing level and 95 percent confidence intervals after ventilation tube (VT) insertion compared to no surgery (NS). B, Black *et al.*;[138] D, Dempster *et al.*;[139] M, Maw and Herod.[140] Redrawn from Ref. 126, with permission.

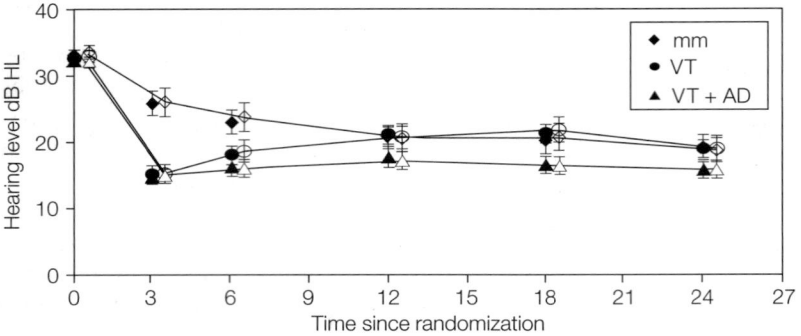

Figure 72.18 Means and 95 percent confidence intervals of the binaural hearing over the two-year follow up in the ventilation tube (VT), ventilation tube with adenoidectomy (VT + AD) and nonsurgical/medical management (mm) arms of TARGET. Redrawn from Ref. 142, with permission.

It should be noted that in both ventilation tube groups the hearing at three months does not become 'normal'; that is 0 dB HL. If one excludes the small number of ears in which the ventilation tube is nonfunctioning, there is still a material air–bone gap of 13 dB SD 7.[142] [****] At all other postoperative visits, when a tube is functioning, the air–bone gap is of a similar magnitude and, as the middle ear space is well ventilated, is considered due to effusion and oedema around the ossicular chain.

The difference in hearing between the two surgical groups and the nonsurgical group becomes almost negligible at 12 months. The reason for the deterioration in the hearing levels over time in those with a ventilation tube is due to a combination of two factors. The proportion of tubes that become nonfunctioning increases with time, though children were eligible to have them reinserted if the hearing entry criteria were resatisfied. The other reason is that in ears where the ventilation tube has extruded and the OME has resolved, there is still a small but material conduction deficit of approximately 14 dB.[142] [****] The reason why those in the nonsurgical arm improves over that period is mainly due to the natural spontaneous resolution rate of the OME combined with a much smaller contribution from those that switched management arms to surgery.

To summarize from this trial, the improvement in hearing effected by ventilation tubes averaged over the first year was 5.7 dB (CI 3.6, 7.7). In the second year, the difference between the two groups became negligible. Hence, when averaged over two years the benefit of ventilation tubes is reduced to 3.1 dB (CI 1.3, 4.8). These data are not dissimilar to the 'by-ear' studies reported earlier.

A more recent individual data metanalysis of four trials that randomized children to ventilation tubes or watchful waiting confirmed the benefit of short-term ventilation tube at six months, but not at 12 months, with a magnitude of difference of 4.5 dB (CI 2.5, 6.5).[141] [****]

It is concluded that short-term ventilation tubes give a benefit to the hearing of 4–5 dB at six months following insertion in those with documented persistent bilateral OME over a three-month period and a hearing impairment of at least 20 dB HL in both ears. This short-term benefit has to be balanced against the 5–10 dB poorer hearing in late teenage years in ears that have had OME ventilation tubes inserted having controlled for OME severity (see under Long-term hearing impairment above).

Predictive factors for benefit to hearing

To date, no individual study has identified factors that predict which children are likely to benefit most from ventilation tubes. To do this requires a larger study than any performed to date. Alternatively, a metanalysis could attempt to do this, albeit the predictive factors that one might wish to investigate might not have been recorded in all studies. Individual child data have been made available for metanalysis from seven trials that randomized children ($n = 1232$) with 12-week persistent bilateral OME to ventilation tubes or nonsurgical management.[141] [****] The only factor predictive of a better hearing outcome at six months was attendance at daycare with an impairment of 20/25 dB in both ears. Those without daycare had no benefit (>1 dB) at six months. No effect of age, sex or socioeconomic group was evident. In three trials which randomized children 'by-ear', those with a binaural hearing level of >25 dB HL benefited by 10 dB at six months compared with the 4 dB of those with lesser hearing thresholds.

These data suggest that when the aim is improvement in the hearing, then younger children at daycare and those with binaural hearing thresholds poorer than 25 dB HL and persistent over at least 12 weeks will benefit most.

Hearing disability

In TARGET, the childrens' hearing disability was assessed by a Reported Hearing Difficulty questionnaire. Using standard deviations as a unit of measurement, the difference between ventilation tubes and no surgery over the first year is 'large' even when adjusted for the expectation effect of surgery.[142] [****] Over the two-year time period, the reduction in hearing disability with ventilation tubes was 'modest'.

Speech and language

Three randomized controlled trials have specifically looked at whether ventilation tubes affect speech and language development. The study of Paradise et al.[143] [****] randomized children when they were on average 18 months of age, that of Rovers et al.[144] [****] when they were on average 20 months of age and that of Maw et al.[137] [****] when they were 36 months of age. All obtained objective measures of speech and language, including receptive and expressive aspects. All assessed the hearing audiometrically. The design of all three studies was to randomize children to 'early' or 'late' surgery. As with this form of randomization, there is always the potential for those randomized to 'late' surgery to have surgery earlier.

Paradise et al.[143] identified eligible children from a birth cohort of 6350 children. Nine percent were eligible because of the duration of their unilateral or bilateral OME. There was no difference between the early and late surgery groups when followed 18 months after randomization up to when the children were on average three years of age. By then, 34 percent of the early surgery group had had surgery. The children in this trial have now been reported twice subsequently, the last when they were six years of age, which confirmed the lack of benefit of ventilation tubes.[145] [****] The negative outcome of this study may in part be due to the inclusion of children with unilateral OME (63 percent of the sample). Unfortunately, the authors did not report the results of the children with bilateral OME separately.

Rovers et al.[144] identified their eligible children from a Dutch birth cohort of 30,099 children. Those who failed a hearing screen at nine months of age three times ($n = 1081$) were followed up over four to six months. Those who had persistent bilateral OME ($n = 386$; 1 percent of total cohort) were eligible for randomization to 'early' or 'late' surgery. Children were followed up for 12 months at which time, once adjusted for the effects of the mother's education and the child's intelligence, there was no effect of early surgery. In this study, only 9 percent of the late surgery group had early surgery. This study would suggest that children aged 20 months with bilateral persistent OME do not benefit, regarding their speech and language development, from ventilation tubes. This does not mean that children with more severe problems do not benefit; it is just that they have not been studied.

Maw et al.[137] considered children from a birth cohort to be eligible for randomization if they had documented bilateral OME associated with a hearing impairment of more than 25 dB HL persistent over a three-month watchful waiting period. Children also had disruptions to 'speech, language, learning or behaviour', though how this was defined was not stated. The mean age of the children at randomization was three years. At nine months following randomization, those that had not had surgery were 3.2 months behind in their speech and language, but this difference had disappeared at 18 months. Unfortunately by then 85 percent in the late surgery group had had surgery. Their conclusions were that there is no difference between early and late surgery, but they could not comment upon whether surgery had an effect on speech and language in this age group.

A subsequent metanalysis of two of these studies[141] [****] and a systematic review of all trials[83, 136] [****] confirmed the null effect of ventilation tubes on children in the first four years of life with OME.

It must be concluded that, in general, ventilation tubes are not indicated to aid speech and language development in children three years and younger.

Randomized controlled trials on severely affected children are merited, but might be difficult to achieve because of their relative rarity.

Behaviour

The UK randomized controlled trial of surgery, described under Speech and language above, of three-year-old children[137] included serial behaviour questionnaires (Richman) and these were reported in a separate publication.[100] [****] The mean change in the Richman behaviour score nine months following randomization was no different in the children receiving early ventilation tubes as opposed to the watchful waiting group. However at that time, the proportion of children with extremely poor scores was fewer in the surgery group (30 percent compared with 47 percent). The authors chose to highlight the latter finding, but it could be argued that using the mean scores rather than taking an arbitrary cut off is a more relevant and sensitive analysis.

It must be concluded that the effect of bilateral persistent OME associated with a hearing impairment on a child's behaviour is likely to be small and correct spontaneously with time, irrespective of whether they have surgery.

Quality of life

The Dutch study described under Speech and language included a generic quality-of-life questionnaire that covers 13 domains, nine of which would be applicable to children with OME (vitality, appetite, communication, motor problems, social, anxiety, aggression, eating and sleeping). No effect of surgery on this measure of quality of life was identified in the 18-month-old (on average) children with persistent bilateral OME.[144] [****]

Cost–benefit analysis

Such an analyis requires the cost of an intervention to be calculated in terms of a change in a generic quality of life outcome. So, though the cost of surgery was obtained in the Dutch study, as there was no change in the quality of life such an analysis was not relevant.[146] The TARGET study has yet to report a cost–benefit analysis.

COMPLICATIONS OF VENTILATION TUBES

At surgery

The most common immediate complication at the time of surgery is displacement of the ventilation tube into the middle ear (0.5 percent, CI 0.3, 0.7).[147] [****] Efforts should be made to retrieve the tube at the time, but failure to remove it seldom causes problems. Ossicular chain damage will only occur if the myringotomy is placed incorrectly, i.e. posterosuperiorly. Very rarely, a high jugular bulb may be pierced by an inferiorly placed myringotomy.

Immediately post-operation

Blockage of the tube with blood can be prevented to some extent by aspiration at the time of surgery. Syringing has been suggested but is only likely to be effective before the blood dries. [****]

Early infection around the tube occurs in 9 percent of ears (CI 8.5, 9.7).[147] [****] Topical antibiotic steroid drops at the time of surgery can reduce the incidence to 1 percent (CI of difference 3, 12).[148] [****] Some clinicians prolong topical therapy for three to five days after surgery with similar results.[149] [****] The same short-term effect can be achieved with two weeks of prednisolone and trimethoprim,[150] [****] but whether this reduction of infection has any effect on longer-term tube function is doubtful.[151] [****]

Otorrhoea

When a ventilation tube is *in situ*, it can be associated with otoscopic evidence of infection with the production of pus that may be clinically evident as otorrhoea. The reason for the infection could be the presence of the tube acting as a foreign body, an episode of acute otitis media with the middle ear pus coming through the ventilation tube, or a combination of both. Making a distinction is difficult, but the younger the child the higher the chances are that the infection is due to an episode of acute otitis media. In addition, the pus can dry and block the tube, increasing the chances of it being extruded.

In a literature review of case-controlled studies and randomized controlled trials of the complications of ventilation tubes inserted in children of all ages and for all indications, approximately 9 percent of parents report early postoperative otorrhoea (**Table 72.15**).[147] [***] Thereafter, approximately 7 percent report recurrent acute episodes and 3 percent chronic discharge. However, in children aged between 3.5 and 7 years, where the indication for ventilation tubes is persistent OME, parental report of otorrhoea is of the same magnitude but the otoscopic incidence of infection at any time is <1 percent during the two-year follow-up period (personal communication). [****]

Management of infection is mainly aural toilet with topical antibiotic steroid drops. [*] Secondary granulation tissue occurs in approximately 1 percent of all cases (CI 0.7, 1.3).[147] [***] Granulation tissue is similarly treated with topical preparations. The tube, especially long-term ones, occasionally has to be removed (approximately 4 percent of ears).[147] [***]

Permanent perforation

When a ventilation tube extrudes, an initial pars tensa perforation is inevitable. In the majority, this will heal spontaneously (personal communication). [****] A perforation may then subsequently reoccur at the same site due to a subsequent episode of acute otitis media. Again, in the majority this will heal spontaneously. Thus at any one time following tube extrusion, a proportion of ears will have a perforation which may or may not heal spontaneously. What the proportion is depends on the age of the child and the type of tube inserted. Overall, short-term tubes are associated with a 2 percent incidence of perforations and longer-term tubes an incidence of 17 percent (**Table 72.15**) an increased relative risk of 3.5 (CI 1.5, 7.1) (**Table 72.16**).

Once a perforation has been documented as chronic, myringoplasty is the management of choice. This is not usually performed until the child has outgrown having recurrent acute otitis media.

Tympanosclerosis

Hyaline degeneration of the collagen tissue in the fibrous layer of the pars tensa becomes evident otoscopically as localized white patches or plaques of tympanosclerosis. These do not occur in the absence of a history of otitis media. The frequency of tympanosclerosis increases with the frequency of OME (**Table 72.12**). However, there is a dramatic increased risk difference of 0.33 (CI 21, 45) if a

Table 72.15 Incidence of otorrhoea with indwelling tympanostomy tubes.

Type of otorrhoea	Unit of analysis	Incidence		
		Rate %	95% CI	Range
Early postoperative	Patients	16.0	14.2–17.9	8.8–19.6
Recurrent acute	Patients	7.4	6.0–9.1	0.7–19.6
Chronic	Patients	3.8	2.2–6.0	1.4–9.9
Requiring tube removal	Ears	4.0	3.5–4.5	0–34.3

Reprinted from Ref. 147, with permission.

Table 72.16 Incidence of tympanic membrane sequelae after tympanostomy tube extrusion.

Tympanic membrane sequelae	No of ears	Incidence %	95% CI
Tympanosclerosis	7197	31.7	30.6–32.8
Atrophy or retraction at short-term tube site	1467	25.5	24.2–26.8
Atrophy or retraction at long-term tube site	460	23.3	22.0–24.6
Retraction pocket of pars tensa	543	3.1	1.8–5.0
Chronic perforation, short-term tube	8107	2.2	1.8–2.5
Chronic perforation, long-term tube	3356	16.6	15.3–17.8
Cholesteatoma, short-term tube	8231	0.8	0.6–1.0
Cholesteatoma, long-term tube	1899	1.4	0.9–2.0

Reprinted from Ref. 147, with permission.

ventilation tube has been inserted;[136] [****] in this instance there being no difference between short- and long-term tubes (**Tables 72.15** and **72.16**).

In a small proportion of ears, tympanosclerosis is a dynamic process with resolution and occurrence occurring with time.[152] [**] What effect, if any, tympanosclerosis has on the hearing is debated, but has been reported to be up to 3 dB in the short term.[153] [****] In the longer term at the age of 18 years, there is an impairment of 5–10 dB with a 3–4 dB sensorineural component in those who have had ventilation tubes, having controlled for the OME disease load in childhood.[154] [***] The more tubes that had been inserted, the greater the impairment.

Pars tensa atrophy and retraction

Thinning and retraction of the tympanic membrane is itself considered to be a complication of persistent OME. In children initially referred with bilateral OME, pars tensa retraction to the incus or promintory (Sade grade 3/4) occurs in 8 percent of the better and 10 percent of the poorer hearing ears.[14, 16, 17] [***] Such retractions were not associated with a history of longer ear problems. Such retractions followed up over a 12-week watchful waiting period resolved in 69 percent of the better and 65 percent of the poorer ears. The OME had also resolved in 14 percent of the better and 10 percent of the poorer ears with a pars tensa retraction, respectively.

Pars tensa atrophy also occurs in approximately 3 percent and retraction to the incus or promintory in 2 percent of ears in seven- to eight-year-old children in whom there is no history of OME (**Table 72.12**). This incidence is similar to that in children with transient episodes of OME. However, the incidence of atrophy, but not of retraction, increases to approximately 9 percent in those with persistent OME. In those who still have a ventilation tube *in situ* for their OME, the incidence of atrophy increases to approximately 68 percent and retraction to approximately 14 percent. It could be argued that this increase in ears with a ventilation tube still *in situ* is because these are more persistent cases, rather than because of the ventilation tube itself. This is in part supported by the fact that the incidence is the same with short- and long-term tubes (**Table 72.16** and **72.17**).

What can be conclusively inferred is that ventilation tubes do not prevent the occurrence of atrophy or retraction and should not be inserted for that reason alone. [Grade B]

Effect of swimming

A review of the literature in 1993[155] and a Scottish Intercollegiate Guidelines Network review[120] both come to the conclusion that swimming has no effect on the incidence of reported otorrhoea in children with ventilation tubes. This is supported by the one randomized controlled trial of 212 consecutive children. Of the 50

Table 72.17 Meta-analysis of tympanostomy tube sequelae.

Outcome assessed	Rate difference (%) (95% CI)[a]	Relative risk (95% CI)[b]
Increase in otorrhoea (long- versus short-term tube)	13.7 (−0.7–28.0)	2.1 (1.0–4.1)
Increase in chronic perforation (long- versus short-term tube)	7.3 (1.3–13.3)	3.5 (1.5–7.1)
Increase in cholesteatoma (long- versus short-term tube)	1.3 (0.4–2.2)	2.6 (1.5–4.4)
Increase in atrophy/retraction (tube versus no surgery or myringotomy)	11.0 (2.6–10.3)	1.7 (1.1–2.7)
Increase in tympanosclerosis (tube versus no surgery or myringotomy)	29.9 (21.9–38.0)	3.5 (2.6–4.9)

[a]Absolute difference in outcomes between groups; $p < 0.05$ when the 95% CI does not include zero.
[b]Ratio of sequelae incidence between groups; $p < 0.05$ when the 95% CI does not include one.
Reprinted from Ref. 147, with permission.

percent followed up for one year, 68 percent in the swimming compared with 60 percent in the no-swimming group reported otorrhoea. The mean number of episodes was one per year in both groups.[156] [****] It is also unlikely that getting shower or bath water in the ears increases the incidence of otorrhoea. However, there is no substantive literature addressing this question, except laboratory studies that suggest that the pressure would be insufficient for bath water to be forced into the middle ear.

There is therefore no reason to advise against getting water in the ear in children who are fitted with ventilation tubes.

ADENOIDECTOMY

Surgical techniques

Conventionally, adenoidectomy has been performed by blind curettage. This has the advantage of speed, but the disadvantage of relying on the haemorrhage ceasing spontaneously. Temporary nasal packs can be used to encourage haemostasis. Unfortunately, in the immediate postoperative period, bleeding occurs in approximately four percent of children.[157] [**] Suction diathermy ablation, where the tissue is first diathermied then removed by suction, may be associated with less intraoperative blood loss, but haemorrhage in the immediate postoperative period is no less.[157] [**]

Some do not perform the procedure blindly but inspect the adenoids at intervals with a mirror. This has the potential of allowing more selective removal of adenoid tissue and avoiding palatopharyngeal incompetence by leaving an inferior pad of tissue. Microdebriders have also been advocated as allowing more selective removal of tissue. Though visualization is better with this because the tissue and blood are removed by suction, the intraoperative blood loss is no less than by curettage.[158] [***]

Outcomes of adenoidectomy

The mechanism whereby adenoidectomy resolves the OME in some children is unclear, the most popular unproven hypothesis being that it removes a chronic source of infection in the nasopharynx rather than because it removes tissue that physically obstructs the Eustachian tube.

Hearing

Adenoidectomy alone was the conventional surgical management for many years. Since the introduction of ventilation tubes its use has gradually declined because of its lesser overall effect on the persistence of OME and hearing. In the three UK trials, the overall effect at six months on the hearing of adenoidectomy was 8 dB compared with 12 dB for ventilation tubes. Current practice is to perform adenoidectomy as an adjunct to the insertion of ventilation tubes.

Figure 72.19 shows the effect of ventilation tubes along with adenoidectomy in the three UK trials and is presented in a similar manner to the results for ventilation tubes alone (**Figure 72.17**). The additional benefit of adenoidectomy was approximately 2 dB at 6 and at 12 months. In addition, adenoidectomy reduced the necessity for the reinsertion of short-term ventilation tubes where reinsertion is determined by recurrence of a hearing impairment due to OME (see Revision surgery). Follow up of the children in the Maw and Herod study[140] for a further 12 years[159] [****] showed that the difference of 1–2 dB continues long term. Rather surprisingly, in this study the hearing in all the 12-year-old children who had previous OME was still not normal (approximately 15 dB HL).

The TARGET study confirms the additional benefit of adenoidectomy during the second year of that study (**Figure 72.18**). Over the first year, the magnitude of the adjuvant effect of adenoidectomy was 2.3 dB (CI 0.6, 4.0) and over two years was 3.3 dB (CI 1.7, 4.8).

Hearing disability

In TARGET, over the two-year follow-up period, the adjuvant benefit of adenoidectomy on the reported hearing difficulty was 'modest' (personal communication). [****]

Revision surgery

The proportion of children meriting reinsertion of the ventilation tubes after extrusion because there was still bilateral OME with a material hearing impairment is significantly reduced by adenoidectomy from 47 to 28 percent ($p = 0.01$) of children (personal communication). [****]

Detailed data regarding revision after two years of follow up are currently unavailable in any RCT. However,

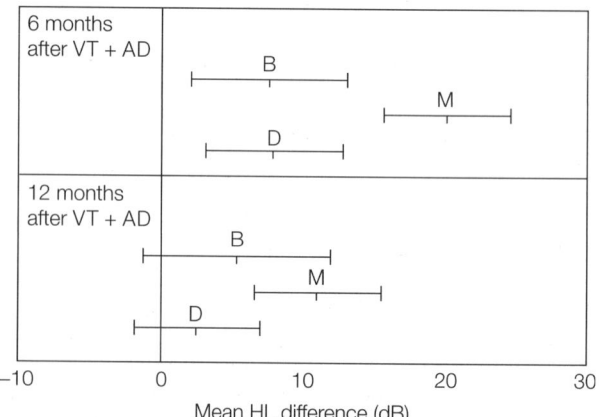

Figure 72.19 Mean improvement in hearing level and 95 percent confidence intervals after ventilation tube with adenoidectomy (VT + AD) compared to no surgery (NS). B, Black et al.;[138] D, Dempster et al.;[139] M, Maw and Herod.[140] Redrawn from Ref. 126, with permission.

hospital activity data suggest that the children who have had an adenoidectomy are less likely to be admitted to hospital and have further surgery for OME extending for a longer period.[160] [***]

Upper respiratory tract symptoms

Adjuvant adenoidectomy improved the reported upper respiratory tract symptoms, as well as the hearing to a 'modest' extent in the TARGET study. The extra benefit is variable and has yet to be shown to be predictable so that adenoidectomy can be offered to children selectively. Interestingly, the mechanism of any benefit is unclear, but it is unlikely to be due to an improvement in Eustachian tube function.[161] [****]

Indicators of benefit

Many authors have attempted to analyze which children in their studies are most likely to benefit from adjuvant adenoidectomy. A metanalysis has yet to be reported.

Complications of adenoidectomy

Haemorrhage in the postoperative period is the most feared complication, the incidence depending on how haemorrhage is defined. This can be any blood however small (0.5–8 percent) or the numbers requiring intervention such as blood transfusion or return to theatre (0.5 percent).[157, 162, 163] [***] Transient velopharyngeal insufficiency can occur in up to 5 percent, but more permanent insufficiency is uncommon (<0.1 percent).[164] [****]

Hearing aids

While hearing aids have been used in children with persistent OME, to avoid repeated surgery their use as the preferred initial management has not been extensively reported. In case series,[165] aids were acceptable to the majority of parents and gave aided thresholds with a mean of 17 dB. [**] The unaided thresholds were not reported, but this improvement is at least in the same range as expected of ventilation tubes. The main concern is potential noise trauma if the aid continues to be worn after the OME has resolved.

BONE-CONDUCTION HEARING AIDS

These have not been considered a viable option until the production of a Softband bone-conduction aid which incorporates a BAHA® (bone anchored hearing aid) in a head-band. This method of amplification has the potential advantage over an air-conduction aid in that should the hearing impairment improve during the period of aid issue due to resolution of the OME, then potentially damaging noise trauma would not occur. No report has been identified that has looked at the benefit from the Soft-band aid.

MANAGEMENT OF OME IN CHILDREN WITH CRANIOFACIAL ABNORMALITIES

Children with a cleft palate even subsequent to its surgical repair have a high incidence of OME which in some is a constant condition. As such, how to alleviate their hearing impairment without increasing the risk of developing chronic otitis media has increasingly been achieved with the use of hearing aids rather than ventilation tubes.[166, 167] [***] The same attitudes apply to the management of OME in children with Down syndrome.[168] [**]

KEY POINTS

- Otitis media with effusion (OME) is the chronic accumulation of mucus within the middle ear and sometimes the mastoid air cell system.
- In children, the prevalence is bimodal with the first and largest peak of ~20 percent at two years of age and a second peak of ~16 percent at around five years of age. [***]
- Natural resolution of the OME is the most likely outcome, albeit there may be further episodes. [***]
- In the majority of children their OME causes only a mild hearing impairment that is unlikely to be disabling. [***]
- Any effect of this hearing impairment on speech and language and cognition is small, of minor significance and likely to spontaneously correct with age. [***]
- The effect of persistent OME on behaviour, though evident, is small. [***]
- Follow-up studies suggest that children who have had OME will still have a small conductive impairment (~10 dB) once the OME has resolved. [***]
- A small conductive impairment is even evident when in their late teens, albeit whether this is a disease effect or the effect of surgery at this age has yet to be clarified. [***]
- Attic retractions are an OME disease effect with an incidence of ~14 percent in the most severely affected children. [***] What proportion of these retractions progress to cholesteatoma is not known.
- There is no evidence that the risk of developing an attic retraction and the potential to develop a cholesteatoma is altered by the insertion of ventilation tubes. [***]
- Tympanosclerosis and atrophy of the pars tensa are OME disease effects, the risk of which is increased by the insertion of ventilation tubes to ~30 and ~25 percent respectively. [***]

- Long-term pars tensa retractions are more likely caused by the insertion of ventilation tubes than by the disease process itself, with an incidence of ~3 percent. [***]
- The benefit of ventilation tubes on children under three years of age with significant language, development or behaviour problems requires investigation.
- In children over the age of three years, the binaural hearing average can be taken as a surrogate of hearing disability, behaviour and impact upon quality of life. In children of this age, OME is unlikely to have a major effect on language or cognition. [***]
- The arbitrary cut-off in hearing thresholds that is taken to indicate a potentially disabling effect that could be improved by ventilation tubes is now taken as 25 dB HL or poorer in both ears. [****]
- All children with hearing thresholds at these levels or poorer should have their hearing documented over at least a 12 week watchful waiting period before any decisions regarding surgery are made. [***]
- Children whose hearing thresholds do not satisfy the hearing criterion of 25 dB HL bilaterally may or may not be followed up 12 weeks later with repeat audiometry.
- Children who persist with OME and a bilateral 25 dB HL over a 12-week-period can benefit from the beneficial effects of ventilation tubes on the hearing over the next nine months. However, the effect is small and is maximal at three months of a magnitude of 12 dB. [****]
- Even when a ventilation tube is functioning, there is still a residual conductive impairment of around 13 dB. [****]
- This relatively small benefit to the hearing has to be balanced against the longer term deleterious effects of ventilation tubes on the tympanic membrane which are associated with poorer hearing. This balance of benefit against harm has to be fully discussed with and appreciated by the parents or carers.
- There is no evidence that a pars tensa retraction in association with OME is an indicator of chronicity or greater benefit from ventilation tubes. [***]
- If ventilation tubes are to be inserted there is a strong argument that adenoidectomy should be performed at the same time, particularly if there is concern regarding the general health of the upper respiratory tract. [***]
- Adenoidectomy extends the period of benefit to the hearing of short-term ventilation tubes up to two years by a magnitude of around 2 to 3 dB. [****] It also reduces the proportion

of children eligible for reinsertion of short-term tubes from around 50 to 25 percent. [****]
- No predictors of benefit from adenoidectomy have been identified. Whether adjuvant adenoidectomy is merited for this small gain in hearing, given the risk of postoperative bleeding in 4 percent of children, is unresolved.

Best clinical practice

In primary care

✓ OME should be suspected in children who have recently recovered from an episode of acute otitis media and in those presenting because of parental concern regarding their hearing. [Grade B]
✓ Attention should be paid to parental concern regarding their child's hearing, particularly if there is a history of recurrent acute otitis media. [Grade B]
✓ All children should have otoscopy to confirm OME and exclude AOM or COM. [Grade C]
✓ Unless specifically trained in otoscopy, this is likely to be insufficiently sensitive or specific even if performed with a pneumatic otoscope to reliably make the diagnosis of OME. [Grade B] Tympanometry should perhaps be more available in primary care.
✓ In primary care the unreliability of otoscopy and non-availability of tympanometry should not cause concern as it is the disability of a bilateral hearing impairment persistent for longer than 12 weeks that is the indicator for referral for audiometric assessment, rather than suspicion of OME.
✓ Free-field voice testing is therefore a more meaningful assessment to perform. [Grade B]
✓ No medical therapy has been shown to be effective longer term (more than six weeks) including antibiotics [Grade A], topical nasal steroids, systemic steroids, nasal decongestants and mucolytics. [Grade B]
✓ In the older child, auto-inflation with the help of 'Otovent' balloons may be beneficial. [Grade B]
✓ It is important that all parents of children with OME receive appropriate general counselling about the natural history and relative benign nature of the condition. [Grade D] This includes advice regarding hearing tactics (see above under Counselling and hearing tactics).
✓ If there is persistent concern regarding the hearing in any child, then referral for hearing assessment is indicated. This will detect previously unsuspected sensorineural impairments as well as quantify any hearing impairment associated with OME. [Grade D]

✓ In most cases, such referral should be for hearing assessment and a further period of audiometric monitoring, rather than for consideration of ventilation tubes. [Grade B]

In secondary care

✓ Pure-tone air-conduction thresholds should be assessed in all children referred with suspected OME and a hearing impairment at their first visit. Not masked bone-conduction thresholds should be obtainable in the majority of 3.5 years or older children. This will aid management of those with OME and detect the ~1 percent with previously undiagnosed sensorineural hearing impairments. [Grade B]

✓ Otoscopy and parental reports of hearing are insufficient to predict current hearing thresholds. [Grade B]

✓ Otoscopy, supplemented by tympanometry if there is any doubt as to whether there is OME, should be performed in all children. This, along with the hearing thresholds, should enable the children with OME to be categorized as having unilateral or bilateral disease, and if bilateral whether the impairment in both ears is > = 25 dB HL. This distinction is relevant to future management in secondary care. [Grade B]

✓ Thereafter, all parents of children with OME should receive appropriate general counselling about the natural history and relative benign nature of OME. [Grade D]

✓ The hearing levels associated with the child's OME should be discussed with the parents and advice about hearing tactics given to help the parents mitigate any disability (see above under Counselling and hearing tactics). [Grade D]

✓ There is insufficient evidence to support the use of topical nasal steroids at present for childhood OME. [Grade B]

✓ Systemic steroids cannot be recommended at present for childhood OME. [Grade B]

✓ It is not recommended that antibiotics be used for the longer term (more than six weeks) in the management of childhood OME. [Grade A]

✓ If some form of nonsurgical management is required, auto-inflation is the therapy with the strongest evidence of efficacy for older children. [Grade B]

✓ As there is no evidence that medical therapy is beneficial, clinicians in secondary care have the task of identifying those that might benefit from surgery after a period of watchful waiting.

✓ Children with unilateral OME are unlikely to develop bilateral OME. [***] In general, children with unilateral OME do not merit follow-up at secondary care and should not have ventilation tubes inserted. [Grade A]

✓ Myringotomy with aspiration has not been shown to be effective in restoring the hearing levels in children with OME and is not recommended without the insertion of ventilation tubes. [Grade A]

✓ In children under the age of three years, ventilation tubes are not indicated even in cases with persistent bilateral OME if there are no language, development or behaviour problems. [Grade A] They therefore do not merit routine follow-up at secondary care.

✓ In general, ventilation tubes are not indicated to aid speech and language development in children aged three years and younger. [Grade A]

✓ The effect of bilateral persistent OME associated with a hearing impairment on a child's behaviour is likely to be small and correct spontaneously with time. Correspondingly, a child's behaviour is not an indication for surgery. [Grade B]

✓ Ventilation tubes do not prevent the occurrence of atrophy or retraction and should not be inserted for that reason alone. [Grade B]

✓ Short-term ventilation tubes are of proven benefit to the hearing up to nine months following insertion in children with bilateral OME documented to have been persistent for at least 12 weeks. The magnitude of the effect is around 4 to 5 dB. It is recommended that such ventilation tubes be limited to those most likely to benefit; children with a hearing impairment of at least 25 dB HL in both ears audiometrically documented to have persisted for at least three months. [Grade A]

✓ To maximize the duration of potential tube function, the preferred insertion site is antero-inferior through a circumferential or radial incision. [Grade A]

✓ In arriving at a decision regarding surgery, the deleterious effects of ventilation tubes in the longer term on tympanic membrane scarring (RR 0.33), thinning and poorer hearing (5 to 10 dB) must be discussed with the parents to enable any consent to be fully informed. [Grade D]

✓ There is no reason to give advice against getting water in the ears in children who have ventilation tubes. [Grade D]

Deficiencies in current knowledge and areas for future research

➤ Otitis media with effusion and acute otitis media in children is the most researched area in otology.

➤ As such, a high proportion of the important clinical questions on otitis media with effusion have already been satisfactorily addressed for the mild to moderately affected child.

➤ What requires investigation are children with the extremes of persistence of OME, such as occurs in children with craniofacial abnormalities.

➤ The ideal therapy would be a preventative one, such as immunization to reduce the frequency of upper respiratory viral and bacterial infections.

> For those who develop OME, medical therapy which manages the mucosal aspects of the condition are more likely to be beneficial than surgical therapy.

> It is important to have confirmation by better controlled studies of the more serious otological damage, such as retraction that occurs to the tympanic membrane following ventilation tube insertion.

> How to best change the attitudes to ventilation tubes of surgeons and parents given their paucity of benefit for any length of time and their permanent damaging effect is perhaps the aspect most requiring research in OME.

ACKNOWLEDGEMENTS

Figures 72.7 to **72.15** are reprinted from Wormald PJ and Browning GG. *Otoscopy: a structured approach*. London: Hodder Arnold, 1996.

REFERENCES

1. Bluestone CD. State of the art: definitions and classifications. In: Liu DJ, Bluestone CD, Klien JO, Nelson JD. (eds). *Recent advances in otitis media with effusion.* Proceedings of the 3rd International Conference. Ontario: Decker and Mosby; 1984

2. Shimada T, Lim DJ. Distribution of ciliated cells in the human middle ear. Electron and light microscopic observations. *The Annals of Otology, Rhinology, and Laryngology.* 1972; **81**: 203–11.

3. Lim D. Normal and pathological mucosa of the middle ear and Eustachian tube. *Clinical Otolaryngology.* 1979; **4**: 213–34.

4. Tos M. Pathogenisis and pathology of chronic secretory otitis media. *Annals of Otology, Rhinology and Laryngology.* 1980; **89**: 91–7.

5. Ishii T, Toriyama M, Suzuki JI. Histopathological study of otitis media with effusion. *Annals of Otology and Laryngology.* 1980; **89**: 83–6.

6. Takkeuchi K, Majima Y, Hirata K, Hattori M, Sakakura Y. Quantitation of tubotympanal mucociliary clearance of otitis media with effusion. *Annals of Otology, Rhinology, and Laryngology.* 1990; **99**: 211–4.

7. Kubba H, Pearson JP, Birchall JP. The aetiology of otitis media with effusion: a review. *Clinical Otolaryngology.* 2000; **25**: 181–94.

8. Jero J, Karma P. Bacteriological findings and persistence of middle ear effusion in otitis media with effusion. *Acta Otolaryngologica.* 1997; **529**: 22–6.

9. Sheanan P, Blaney AW, Sheanan JN, Earley MJ. Sequelae of otitis media with effusion among children with cleft lip and/or palate. *Clinical Otolaryngology.* 2002; **27**: 494–500.

10. Rivron RP. Bifid uvula: prevalence and association in otitis media with effusion in children admitted for routine otolaryngological operations. *Journal of Laryngology and Otology.* 1989; **103**: 249–52.

11. Alho OP, Oja H, Koivu M, Sorri M. Risk factors for chronic otitis media with effusion in infancy. *Archives of Otolaryngology – Head and Neck Surgery.* 1995; **121**: 839–43.

12. Marx J, Osguthorpe JD, Parsons G. Day care and the incidence of otitis media in young children. *Otolaryngology – Head and Neck Surgery.* 1995; **112**: 695–9.

13. van Balen FAM, de Melker RA. Persistent otits media with effusion; can it be predicted? A family practice follow-up study in children aged 6 months to 6 years. *Journal of Family Practice.* 2000; **49**: 605–11.

14. Medical Research Council Multicentre Otitis Media Study Group. Risk factors for persistence of bilateral otitis media with effusion. *Clinical Otolaryngology.* 2001; **27**: 147–56.

15. Medical Research Council Multicentre Otitis Media Study Group. Selecting persistent glue ear for referral in general practice; a risk factor approach. *British Journal of General Practice.* 2002; **52**: 549–53.

16. Medical Research Council Multicentre Otitis Media Study Group. Pars tensa and pars flaccida retraction in persistent otitis media with effusion. *Otology and Neurotology.* 2001; **22**: 291–8.

17. Medical Research Council Multicentre Otitis Media Study Group. Surgery for persistent otitis media with effusion: generalizability of results from the UK trial (TARGET). *Clinical Otolaryngology.* 2001; **26**: 417–24.

18. Tasker A, Dettmar PW, Panetti M, Koufman JA, Birchall JP, Pearson JP. Reflux of gastric juice and glue ear in children. *Lancet.* 2002; **359**: 493.

19. Lieu JEC, Nuthappan BS, Uppaluri R. Association of reflux with otitis media in children. *Otolaryngology – Head and Neck Surgery.* 2005; **133**: 357–61.

20. Daly KA. Epidemiology of otitis media. *Otolaryngologic Clinics of North America.* 1991; **24**: 775–86.

21. Zielhuis GA, Rach GH, van den Basch A, van den Broek P. The prevalence of otitis media with effusion: a critical review of the literature. *Clinical Otolaryngology.* 1990; **15**: 283–8.

22. Engel J, Anteunis L, Volovics A, Hendriks J, Marres E. Prevalence rates of otitis media with effusion from 0 to 2 years of age: healthy-born versus high-risk born infants. *International Journal of Pediatric Otolaryngology.* 1999a; **47**: 243–51.

23. Engel JAM, Anteunis LJC, Volvics A, Hendricks JJT, Manni JJ. Chronic otitis media with effusion during infancy, have parent-reported symptoms prognostic value? A prospective longitudinal study from 0 to 2 years of age. *Clinical Otology.* 1999; **24**: 417–23.

24. Williamson IG, Dunleavey J, Bain J, Robinson D. The natural history of otitis media with effusion – a three-year

study of the incidence and prevalence of abnormal tympanograms in four South West Hampshire infant and first schools. *Journal of Laryngology and Otology.* 1994; **108**: 930-4.

25. Tos M, Holm-Jensen S, Sorensen CH, Mogensen C. Spontaneous course and frequency of secretory otitis in 4-year-old children. *Archives of Otolaryngology.* 1982; **108**: 4-10.

26. Rovers MM, Straatman H, Zielhuis GA, Ingels K, van der Wilt GJ. Seasonal variation in the prevalence of persistent otitis media with effusion in one-year-old infants. *Paediatric and Perinatal Epidemiology.* 2000; **14**: 268-74.

27. Rovers MM, Straatman H, Ingels K, van der Wilt GJ, van den Broek P, Zielhuis GA. The effect of ventilation tubes on language development in infants with otitis media with effusion: A randomized trial. *Pediatrics.* 2000; **106**: E42.

28. Midgley EJ, Dewey C, Pryce K, Maw AR. ALSPAC study team. The frequency of otitis media with effusion in British pre-school children: a guide for treatment. *Clinical Otology.* 2000; **25**: 485-91.

29. Sassen ML, Brand R, Grote JJ. Risk factors for otitis media with effusion in children 0 to 2 years of age. *American Journal of Otolaryngology.* 1997; **18**: 324-30.

∗ 30. Dewey C, Midgeley E, Maw R. The ALSPAC study team. The relationship between otitis media with effusion and contact with other children in a British cohort studied from 8 months to 3.5 years of age. *International Journal of Pediatric Otorhinolaryngology.* 2000; **55**: 33-45. *Good multivariate analysis.*

∗ 31. Engel J, Anteunis L, Volovics A, Hendriks J, Marres E. Risk factors of otitis media with effusion during infancy. *International Journal of Pediatric Otolaryngology.* 1999b; **48**: 239-49. *Good multivariate analysis including 19 pertinent risk factors.*

32. Apostolopoulos K, Xenelis J, Tzagaroulakis A, Kandiloros D, Yiotakis J, Papafragou K. The point prevalence of otitis media with effusion among school children in Greece. *International Journal of Pediatric Otorhinolaryngology.* 1998; **44**: 207-14.

33. Marchisio P, Principi N, Passali D, Salpietro DC, Boschi G, Chetri G *et al.* Epidemiology and treatment of otitis media with effusion in children in the first year of life. *Acta Otolaryngologica.* 1998; **118**: 557-62.

34. Saim A, Siam L, Siam S, Ruszymah BHI, Sani A. Prevalence of otitis media with effusion amongst pre-school children in Malaysia. *International Journal of Pediatric Otorhinolaryngology.* 1997; **41**: 21-8.

35. Rushton HC, Tong CF, Yue V, Wormald PJ, van Hasselt CA. Prevalence of otitis media with effusion in multicultural schools in Hong Kong. *Journal of Laryngology and Otology.* 1997; **111**: 804-6.

36. Son DH, Son NT, Tri L, Phuong TK, Mai TTT, Tien VM *et al.* Point prevalence of secretory otitis media in children in Southern Vietnam. *Annals of Otology and Laryngology.* 1998; **1107**: 406-10.

37. Del Mar C, Glasziou P, Hayem M. Are antibiotics indicated as initial treatment for children with acute otitis media? A

meta-analysis. *British Medical Journal.* 1997; **314**: 1526-9.

38. Daly KA, Rich SS, Levine S, Margolis RH, Le CT, Lindgren L *et al.* The family study of otitis media: design and disease and risk factor profiles. *Genetic Epidemiology.* 1996; **13**: 451-68.

39. Casselbrant ML, Mandel EM, Fall PA, Rockette HE, Kurs-Lasky M, Bluestone CD *et al.* The heritability if otitis media; a twin and triplet study. *Journal of the American Medical Association.* 1999; **282**: 2125-30.

40. Paradise JL, Rockette HE, Colburn DK, Bernard BS, Smith CG, Kurs-Lasky M *et al.* Otitis media in 2253 Pittsburgh-area infants prevalence and risk factors during the first two years of life. *Pediatrics.* 1997; **99**: 318-33.

41. Rovers MM, Hofstad EA, vann den Brand KI, Ingels K, van den Wilt GJ, Zielhius GA. Prognostic factors for otitis media with effusion. *Clinical Otolaryngology.* 1998; **23**: 543-6.

42. Zielhius GA, Rach GH, van den Broek P. Screening for otitis media with effusion in preschool children. *Lancet.* 1989; **1**: 311-3.

43. Hogan SC, Stratford KJ, Moore DR. Duration and recurrence of otitis media with effusion in children from birth to 3 years: prospective study using monthly otoscopy and tympanometry. *British Medical Journal.* 1997; **314**: 350-3.

44. Lous J, Fiellau-Nikolajsen M. Epidemiology of middle ear effusion and tubal dysfunction. A one-year prospective study comprising monthly tympanometry in 387 non-selected 7-year-old children. *International Journal of Pediatric Otorhinolaryngology.* 1981; **3**: 303-17.

45. Anteunis LJC, Engel JAM, Hendriks JJT, Manni JJ. A longitudinal study of the validity of parental reporting in the detection of otitis media and related hearing impairment in infancy. *Audiology.* 1999; **38**: 75-82.

46. Stewart MG, Friedman EM, Sulek M, Duncan NO, Fernandez AD, Bautista MH. Is parental perception an accurate predictor of childhood hearing loss? A prospective study. *Otolaryngology and Head and Neck Surgery.* 1999; **120**: 340-4.

47. Cavanaugh RM. Obtaining a seal with otic specula: Must we rely on an air of uncertainty? *Pediatrics.* 1991; **87**: 114-6.

48. Jones WS, Kaleida PH. How helpful is pneumatic otoscopy in improving diagnostic accuracy? *Pediatrics.* 2003; **112**: 510-3.

49. Toner JG, Mains B. Pneumatic otoscopy and tympanometry in the detection of middle ear effusion. *Clinical Otolaryngology.* 1990; **15**: 121-3.

50. Finitzo T, Freil-Patti S, Chinn K, Brown O. Tympanometry and otoscopy prior to myringotomy; issues in diagnosis or otitis media. *International Journal of Pediatric Otorhinolaryngology.* 1992; **24**: 101-10.

51. Vaughan-Jones R, Mills RP. The Welch Allyn audioscope and microtymp: their accuracy and that of pneumatic otoscopy, tympanometry and pure tone audiometry as

predictors of otitis media with effusion. *Journal of Laryngology and Otology.* 1992; **106**: 600–2.

52. Nozza RJ, Bluestone CD, Kardatzke D, Bachman R. Identification of middle ear effusion by aural acoustic admittance and otoscopy. *Ear and Hearing.* 1994; **15**: 310–23.

53. Steinbach WJ, Sectish TC, Benjamin DK, Chang KW, Messner AH. Pediatric residents' clinical diagnositic accuracy of otitis media. *Pediatrics.* 2002; **109**: 993–9.

* 54. American Academy of Pediatrics. Otitis media with effusion; clinical practice guideline. *Pediatrics.* 2004; **113**: 1412–29. *OME guidelines.*

55. Rosenfeld RM, Culpepper L, Doyle KJ, Grundfast KM, Hoberman A, Kenna MA *et al.* American Academy of Pediatrics Subcommittee on Otitis Media with Effusion, American Academy of Family Physicians, American Academy of Otolaryngology – Head and Neck Surgery. Clinical practice guideline: Otitis media with effusion. *Otolaryngology and Head and Neck Surgery.* 2004; **130**: S95–118.

* 56. Preston K. Pneumatic otoscopy: a review of the literature. *Issues in Comprehensive Pediatric Nursing.* 1998; **21**: 117–28. *Good literature review.*

57. Pirozzo S, Papinczak T, Glasziou P. Whispered voice test for screening for hearing impairment in adults and children: systematic review. *British Medical Journal.* 2003; **327**: 967–70.

58. Medical Research Council Multicentre Otitis Media Study Group. Sensitivity, specificity and predictive value of tympanometry in predicting a hearing impairment in otitis media with effusion. *Clinical Otolaryngology.* 1999; **24**: 294–300.

59. Palmu A, Puhakka H, Rahko T, Takala AK. Diagnostic value of tympanometry in infants in clinical practice. *International Journal of Pediatric Otorhinolaryngology.* 1999; **49**: 207–13.

60. Engel J, Anteunis L, Chenault M. Otoscopic findings in relation to tympanometry during infancy. *European Archives of Otorhinolaryngology.* 2000; **257**: 366–71.

61. American Speech-Language-Hearing Association. Guidelines for screening for hearing impairments and middle ear disorders. *ASHA.* 1989; **31**: 71–7.

62. Nozza RJ, Bluestone CD, Kardatzke D, Bachman R. Towards the validation of aural acoustic immittance measures for diagnosis of middle ear effusion in children. *Ear and Hearing.* 1992; **13**: 442–53.

63. Jerger J. Clinical experience with impedance audiometry. *Archives of Otolaryngology.* 1970; **92**: 311–24.

64. Orchik DJ, Dunn JW, McNutt L. Tympanometry as a predictor of middle ear effusion. *Archives of Otolaryngology.* 1978; **104**: 4–6.

65. Sassen ML, Van Aarem A, Grote JJ. Validity of tympanometry in the diagnosis of middle ear effusion. *Clinical Otolaryngology.* 1994; **19**: 185–9.

66. De Melker RA. Diagnositic value of microtympanometry in primary care. *British Medical Journal.* 1992; **304**: 96–8.

67. Van Balen FAM, Aarts AM, de Melker RA. Tympanometry by general practitioners: reliable? *International Journal of Pediatric Otorhinolaryngology.* 1999; **48**: 117–23.

68. Mooler H, Tos M. Daily impedance audiometric screening of children. *Scandinavian Audiology.* 1992; **21**: 9–14.

69. Fields MJ, Corwin P, White PS, Doherty J. Microtympanometry, microscopy and tympanometry in evaluating middle ear effusion prior to myringotomy. *New Zealand Medical Journal.* 1993; **106**: 386–7.

70. Roush J, Drake A, Sexton JE. Identification of middle ear dysfunction in young children: a comparison of tympanometric screening procedures. *Ear and Hearing.* 1992; **13**: 63–9.

71. Kazanas SG, Maw R. Tympanometry, stapedius reflex and hearing impairment in children with otitis media with effusion. *Acta Otolaryngologica.* 1994; **114**: 410–4.

72. Van der Avoort SJC, van Heerbeek N, Zeilhuis GA, Cremers CWRJ. Sonotubometry: Eustachian tube ventilatory function test; A state-of-the art review. *Otology and Neurotology.* 2005; **26**: 538–43.

73. Pellett FS, Cox LC, MacDonald CB. Use of acoustic reflectometry in the detection of middle ear effusion. *Journal of the American Academy of Audiology.* 1997; **8**: 181–7.

74. Kemaloglu YK, Sener T, Beder L, Bayazit Y, Goksu N. Predictive value of acoustic reflectometry and tympanometry. *Interantional Journal of Pediatric Otorhinolaryngology.* 1999; **48**: 137–42.

75. Oyiborhoro JMA, Olaniyan SO, Newman CW, Balakrishnan SL. Efficacy of acoustic otoscope in detecting middle ear effusion in children. *Laryngoscope.* 1987; **97**: 495–8.

76. Vartiainen E. Otitis media with effusion in children with congenital or early-onset hearing impairment. *Journal of Otolaryngology.* 2000; **29**: 221–3.

77. McCormick B. Behavioural hearing tests 6 months to 5 years. In: McCormack B (ed.). *Paediatric audiology: 0–5 years.* London: Whurr Publisher, 1989: 97–116.

78. Medical Research Council Multicentre Otitis Media Study Group. Influence of age, type of audiometry and child's concentration on hearing thresholds. *British Journal of Audiology.* 2000; **34**: 231–40.

79. Kumar M, Meheshwar A, Mahendran S, Oluwasamni A, Clayton MI. Could the presence of a Carhart notch predict the presence of glue at myringotomy? *Clinical Otolaryngology.* 2003; **28**: 183–6.

80. Ahmad I, Pahor AL. Carhart's notch: a finding in otitis media with effusion. *International Journal of Pediatric Otorhinolaryngology.* 2002; **64**: 165–70.

81. Takata GS, Chan LS, Morphew T, Mangione-Smith R, Morton SC, Shekelle P. Evidence assessment of the accuracy of methods of diagnosing middle ear fluid in children with otitis media with effusion. *Paediatrics.* 2003; **112**: 1379–87.

82. Dempster JH, MacKenzie K. Tympanometry in the detection of hearing impairments associated with otitis media with effusion. *Clinical Otolaryngology and Allied Sciences.* 1991; **16**: 157–9.

83. Butler CC, van der Linden MK, MacMillan H, van der Wouden JC. Screening in the first four years of life to undergo early treatment for otitis media with effusion. *Cochrane Database of Systematic Reviews.* 2003: CD004163.

84. Browning GG. Watchful waiting in childhood otitis media with effusion. *Clinical Otolaryngology.* 2001; **26**: 1–2.

85. Rosenfeld AR, Kay D. Natural history of untreated otitis media. *Laryngoscope.* 2003; **113**: 1645–57.

86. Schilder AGM, Zielhuis GA, Haggard MP, van den Brook P. Long-term effect on otitis media with effusion: otomicroscopic findings. *American Journal of Otology.* 1995; **16**: 365–72.

87. Fria TJ, Cantekin EI, Eichler JA. Hearing acuity of children with otitis media with effusion. *Archives of Otolaryngology.* 1985; **111**: 10–6.

88. Rakho T, Karma P. Pure-tone hearing thresholds in otologically healthy 5-year-old children in Finland. *Archives of Otorhinolaryngology.* 1989; **246**: 137–41.

89. Hunter LL, Margolis RH, Giebink GS. Identification of hearing loss in children with otitis media. *Annals of Otology, Rhinology, and Laryngology.* 1994; **163**: 59–61.

90. Bluestone CD, Beery QC, Paradise JL. Audiometry and tympanometry in relation to middle era effusions in children. *Laryngoscope.* 1973; **83**: 594–604.

91. Brechtje A de Beer, Graamans K, Snik AFM, Ingels K, Zeilhuis GA. Hearing deficits in young adults who had a history of otitis media in childhood: Use of personal stereos had no effect on hearing. *Pediatrics.* 2003; **111**: e304–8.

92. Hunter LL, Margolis RH, Rykken JR, Le CT, Daly KA, Geibink GS. High frequency hearing loss associated with otitis media. *Ear and Hearing.* 1996; **17**: 1–11.

93. Roberts JE, Rosenfeld RM, Zeisel SA. Otitis media and speech and language: a meta-analysis of prospective studies. *Pediatrics.* 2004; **113**: e238–48.

94. Butler CC, MacMillan H. Does early detection of otitis media with effusion prevent delayed language development? *Archives of Disease in Childhood.* 2001; **85**: 96–103.

95. Roberts J, Hunter L, Gravel J, Rosenfeld AR, Berman S, Haggard M et al. Otitis media; hearing loss, and language learning: controversies and current research. *Journal of Developmental and Behavioral Pediatrics.* 2004; **25**: 110–22.

96. Lous J. Otitis media and reading achievement: a review. *International Journal of Pediatric Otorhinolaryngology.* 1995; **32**: 105–21.

97. Johnson DL, Swank PR, Owen MJ, Baldwin CD, Howie VM, McCormick DP. Effect of early middle ear effusion on child intelligence at three, five, and seven years of age. *Journal of Pediatric Psychology.* 2000; **25**: 5–13.

98. Augustsoon I, Engstand I. Otitis media and academic achievements. *International Journal of Pediatric Otorhinolaryngology.* 2001; **57**: 31–40.

99. Rutter M. A children's behaviour questionnaire for completion by teachers: preliminary findings. *Journal of Child Psychology and Psychiatry, and Allied Disciplines.* 1967; **8**: 1–11.

100. Wilks J, Maw R, Peters TJ, Harvey I, Golding J. Randomised controlled trial of early surgery versus watchful waiting for glue ear: the effect on behavioural problems in pre-school children. *Clinical Otolaryngology.* 2000; **25**: 209–14.

101. Bennett KE, Haggard MP, Silva PA, Stewart IA. Behaviour and developmental effect of otitis media with effusion in the teens. *Archives of Disease in Childhood.* 2001; **85**: 91–5.

102. Golz A, Angel-Yeger B, Parush S. Evaluation of balance disturbances in children with middle ear effusion. *International Journal of Pediatric Otorhinolaryngology.* 1998; **43**: 21–6.

103. Casselbrant ML, Furman JM, Mandel EM, Fall PA, Kurs-Lasky M, Rockette HE. Past history of otitis media and balance in four-year-old children. *Laryngoscope.* 2000; **110**: 773–8.

104. Waldron MNH, Matthews JNS, Johnson IJM. The effect of otitis media with effusions on balance in children. *Clinical Otolaryngology.* 2004; **29**: 318–20.

105. Rosenfeld RM, Baya MH, Bower CM, Brookhouser PE, Casselbrant ML, Chan KH et al. Impact of tympanostomy tubes on child quality of life. *Archives of Otolaryngology – Head and Neck Surgery.* 2000; **126**: 585–92.

106. Richards M, Giannoni C. Quality-of-life outcomes after surgical intervention for otitis media. *Archives of Otolaryngology – Head and Neck Surgery.* 2002; **128**: 776–82.

107. Kubba H, Swan IRC, Gatehouse S. How appropriate is the OM6 as a discriminative instrument in children with otitis media. *Archives of Otolaryngology – Head and Neck Surgery.* 2004; **130**: 705–9.

108. Haggard MP, Smith SC, Nicholls EE. Measurement of quality of life outcomes in otitis media. In: Rosenfeld RM, Bluestone CD (eds). *Evidence-based otitis media*, 2nd edn. Hamilton, Ontario: BC Decker, 2003: 401–29.

109. Kubba H, Swan IRC, Gatehouse S. Measuring quality of life in preschool children with sore throats and otitis media using the TAPQOL questionnaire. *Otolaryngology and Head and Neck Surgery.* 2005; **132**: 647–52.

110. Kubba H, Swan IRC, Gatehouse S. The Glasgow children's benefit inventory: a new instrument for assessing health-related benefit after an intervention. *Annals of Otology and Laryngology.* 2004; **113**: 980–6.

111. Deafness Research UK. *Glue ear: A guide for parents.* London: Deafness Research UK, 2003.

112. Butler CC, van der Voort JH, Oral or topical nasal steroids for hearing loss associated with otitis media with effusion. *Cochrane Database of Systematic Reviews.* 2002: CD001935.

113. Shapiro GG, Bierman CW, Furukuwa CT. Treatment of persistent Eustachian tube dysfunction with aerosolized nasal dexamethasone phosphate versus placebo. *Annals of Allergy.* 1982; **49**: 81–5.

114. Tracy JM, Demain JG, Hoffman KM, Goetz DW. Intranasal beclomethasone as an adjunct to treatment of chronic

middle ear effusion. *Annals of Allergy, Asthma and Immunology.* 1998; **80**: 198–206.

115. Williamson I. Otitis media with effusion. *Clinical Evidence Concise.* 2006; **16**: 245–7.

116. Mandel EM, Casselbrant ML, Rockette HE, Fireman P, Kurs-Lasky M, Bluestone CD. Sytemic steroid for chronic otitis media with effusion in children. *Pediatrics.* 2002; **110**: 1071–80.

117. Thomas CL, Simpson S, Butler CC, van der Voort JH. Oral or topical nasal steroids for hearing loss associated with otitis media with effusion in children. *Cochrane Database of Systematic Reviews.* 2006; **3**: CD001935.

118. Rosenfeld RM, Post JC. Meta-analysis of antibiotics for the treatment of otitis media with effusion. *Otolaryngology and Head and Neck Surgery.* 1992; **106**: 378–86.

119. Williams RL, Chalmers TC, Stange KC, Chalmers FT, Bowlin SJ. Use of antibiotics in preventing recurrent acute otitis media and treating otitis media with effusion. *Journal of the American Medical Association.* 1993; **270**: 1344–51.

120. Scottish Intercollegiate Guidelines Network. Diagnosis and management of childhood otitis media in primary care. A national clinical guideline. No 6, February 2003.

121. Griffin GH, Flynn C, Bailey RE, Schultz JK. Antihistamines and/or decongestants for otitis media with effusion (OME) in children. *Cochrane Database of Systematic Reviews.* 2006; **4**: CD003423.

122. Pignataro O, Pignataro LD, Gallus G, Calori G, Cordaro CI. Otitis media with effusion and S-carboxymethylcysteine and/or its lysine salt: a critical overview. *International Journal of Pediatric Otorhinolaryngology.* 1996; **35**: 231–41.

123. Commins DJ, Koay BC, Bates GJ, Moore RA, Sleeman K, Mitchell B *et al.* The role of Mucodyne in reducing the need for surgery in patients with persistent otitis media with effusion. *Clinical Otology.* 2000; **25**: 274–9.

124. Reidpath DD, Glasziou PP, Del Mar C. Systematic review of autoinflation for treatment of glue ear in children. *British Medical Journal.* 1999; **318**: 1177–8.

125. Harrison H, Fixsen A, Vickers A. A randomised comparison of homeopathy and standard care for treatment of glue ear in children. *Complementary Therapies in Medicine.* 1999; **7**: 132–5.

126. Freemantle N, Sheldon TA, Song F, Long A. *The treatment of persistent glue ear in children.* Effective Health Care Bulletin No. 4. York: University of York, NHS Centre for Reviews and Dissemination, 1992.

127. Weigel MT, Parker MY, Goldsmith MM, Postma DS, Pilsbury HC. A prospective randomised study of four commonly used tympanostomy tubes. *Laryngoscope.* 1989; **99**: 252–6.

128. Richards SH, Kilby D, Shaw JD, Campbell H. Grommets and glue ears: A clinical trial. *Journal of Laryngology and Otology.* 1971; **85**: 17–22.

129. Shone GR, Griffith IP. Titanium grommets: a trial to assess function and extrusion rates. *Journal of Laryngology and Otology.* 1990; **104**: 197–9.

130. Guttenplan MD, Tom WC, DeVito MA, Handler SD, Wetmore RF, Potsic WP. Radial versus circumferential incision in myringotomy and tube placement. *International Journal of Pediatric Otorhinolaryngology.* 1991; **21**: 211–5.

131. Heaton JM, Bingham BJG, Osbourne J. A comparison of performance of Shepard and Sheehy collar button ventilation tubes. *Journal of Laryngology and Otology.* 1991; **105**: 896–8.

132. Walker P. Ventilation tube duration versus site of placement. *Australian and New Zealand Journal of Surgery.* 1997; **67**: 571–2.

133. Hern JD, Jonathan DA. Insertion of ventilation tubes: does the site matter? *Clinical Otology.* 1999; **24**: 424–5.

134. Youngs RP, Gatland DJ. Is aspiration of middle ear effusions prior to ventilation tube insertion really neccesary? *Journal of Otolaryngology.* 1988; **17**: 204–6.

135. Egeli E, Muzaffer K. Is aspiration necessary before tympanostomy tube insertion? *Laryngoscope.* 1998; **108**: 443–4.

136. Lous J, Burton MJ, Felding JU, Ovesen T, Rovers MM, Williamson I. Grommets (ventilation tubes) for hearing loss associated with otitis media in children. *Cochrane Database of Systematic Reviews.* 2005: CD001801.

137. Maw R, Wilks J, Harvey I, Golding J. Early surgery compared with watchful waiting for glue ear and effect on language development in preschool children: a randomised trial. *Lancet.* 1999; **353**: 960–3.

138. Black NA, Sanderson CF, Freeland AP, Vessey MP. A randomised controlled trial of surgery for glue ear. *British Medical Journal.* 1990; **300**: 1551–6.

139. Dempster JH, Browning GG, Gatehouse S. A randomised study of the surgical management of children with persistent otitis media with effusion associated with a hearing impairment. *Journal of Laryngology and Otology.* 1993; **107**: 284–9.

140. Maw R, Herod F. Otoscopic, impedance and audiometric findings in glue ear treated by adenoidectomy and tonsillectomy; a prospective randomised trial. *Lancet.* 1986; **1**: 1399–402.

141. Rovers MM, Black N, Browning GG, Maw R, Zielhius GA, Haggard MP. Grommets in otitis media with effusion: an individual patient data meta-analysis. *Archives of Disease in Childhood.* 2005; **90**: 480–5.

142. Medical Research Council Multicentre Otitis Media Study Group. The role of ventilation tube status in the hearing levels in children managed for bilateral persistent otitis media with effusion. *Clinical Otolaryngology.* 2003; **28**: 146–53.

143. Paradise JL, Feldman HM, Campbell TF, Dollaghan CA, Colburn DK, Bernard BS *et al.* Effect of early or delayed insertion of tympanostomy tubes for persistent otitis media on developmental outcomes at the age of three years. *New England Journal of Medicine.* 2001; **344**: 1179–87.

144. Rovers MM, Krabbe PFM, Straatman H, Ingels K, van der Wilt G-J, Zielhuis GA. Randomised controlled trial of the

effect of ventilation tubes (grommets) on quality of life at age 1–2 years. *Archives of Disease in Childhood.* 2001; **84**: 45–9.

145. Paradise JL, Campbell TF, Dollaghan CA, Feldman HM, Bernard BS, Colburn DK *et al.* Developmental outcomes after early or delayed insertion of tympanostomy tubes. *New England Journal of Medicine.* 2005; **353**: 576–86.

146. Hartman M, Rovers MM, Ingels K, Zeilhius GA, Severns JL, van der Wilt GJ. Economic evaluation of ventilation tubes in otitis media with effusion. *Archives of Otolaryngology – Head and Neck Surgery.* 2001; **127**: 1471–6.

147. Kay DJ, Nelson M, Rosenfeld RM. Meta-analysis of tympanostomy tube sequelae. *Otolaryngology and Head and Neck Surgery.* 2001; **124**: 374–80.

148. Shinkwin CA, Murty GE, Simo R, Jones NS. Per-operative antibiotic/steroid prophylaxis of tympanostomy tube otorrhoea; Chemical or mechanical effect? *Journal of Laryngology and Otology.* 1996; **110**: 531–3.

149. Garcia P, Gates GA, Schechtman KB. Does topical antibiotic prophylaxis reduce post-tympanostomy tube otorrhoea? *Annals of Otology, Rhinology, and Laryngology.* 1994; **103**: 54–8.

150. Daly KA, Giebink GS, Lindgren B, Margolis RH, Westover D, Hunter LL *et al.* Randomized trial of the efficacy of trimethoprim-sulfamethoxazole and prednisolone in preventing post-tympanostomy tube morbidity. *Pediatric Infectious Disease Journal.* 1995; **14**: 1068–74.

151. Pearson CR, Thomas MR, Cox HJ, Garth JN. A cost–benefit analysis of the post-operative use of antibiotic ear drops following grommet insertion. *Journal of Laryngology and Otology.* 1996; **110**: 527–30.

152. Tos M, Stangerup S-E, Larsen P. Dynamics of eardrum changes following secretory otitis media. *Archives of Otolaryngology – Head and Neck Surgery.* 1987; **113**: 380–5.

153. Johnston LC, Feldman HM, Paradise JL, Bernard BS, Colburn K, Casselbrant ML *et al.* Tympanic membrane abnormalities and hearing levels at the ages of 5 and 6 years in relation to persistent otitis media and tympanostomy tube insertion in the first 3 years of life: A prospective study incorporating a randomised controlled trial. *Pediatrics.* 2004; **114**: e58–67.

154. De Beer BA, Schilder AGM, Ingels KI, Snik AF, Zielhuis GA, Graamans K. Hearing loss in young adults who had ventilation tube insertion in childhood. *Annals of Otology, Rhinology, and Laryngology.* 2004; **113**: 438–44.

155. Pringle MB. Grommets, swimming and otorrhoea – a review. *Journal of Laryngology and Otology.* 1993; **107**: 190–4.

156. Parker GS, Tami TA, Madox MR, Wilson JF. The effect of water exposure after tympanostomy tube insertion. *American Journal of Otolaryngology.* 1994; **15**: 193–6.

157. Walker P. Pediatric adenoidectomy under vision using suction-diathermy ablation. *Laryngoscope.* 2001; **111**: 2173–7.

158. Murray N, Fitzpatrick P, Guarisco JL. Powered partial adenoidectomy. *Archives of Otolaryngology – Head and Neck Surgery.* 2002; **128**: 792–6.

159. Maw R, Bawden R. Spontaneous resolution of severe chronic glue ear in children and the effect of adenoidectomy, tonsillectomy and insertion of ventilation tubes (grommets). *British Medical Journal.* 1993; **306**: 756–60.

160. Coyte PC, Croxford R, McIsaac W, Feldman W, Friedberg J. The role of adjuvant adenoidectomy and tonsillectomy in the outcome of the insertion of tympanostomy tubes. *New England Journal of Medicine.* 2001; **344**: 1188–95.

161. Dempster JH, Browning GG. Eustachian tube function following adenoidectomy: an evaluation by sniffing. *Clinical Otology.* 1989; **14**: 411–4.

162. Leighton SEJ, Rowe-Jones JM, Knight JR, Moore-Gillon VL. Day case adenoidectomy. *Clinical Otology.* 1993; **18**: 215–9.

163. Ahmed K, McCormick MS, Baruah AK. Day-case adenoidectomy – is it safe? *Clinical Otolaryngology and Allied Sciences.* 1993; **18**: 406–9.

164. Paradise JL, Bluestone CD, Colburn DK, Bernard BS, Smith CG, Rockette HE *et al.* Adenoidectomy and adenotonsillectomy for recurrent acute otitis media: parallel randomised clinical trials in children not previously treated with tympanostomy tubes. *Journal of the American Medical Association.* 1999; **282**: 945–53.

165. Jardine AH, Griffiths MV, Midgley E. The acceptance of hearing aids for children with otitis media with effusion. *Journal of Laryngology and Otology.* 1999; **113**: 314–7.

166. Maheshwar AA, Milling MAP, Kumar M, Clayton AT. Use of hearing aids in the management of children with cleft palate. *International Journal of Pediatric Otorhinolaryngology.* 2002; **66**: 55–62.

167. Sheahan P, Blayney AW. Cleft palate and otitis media with effusion. *Revue de Laryngologie Otologie Rhinologie.* 2003; **124**: 171–7.

168. Iino Y, Imamura Y, Harigai S, Tanaka Y. Efficacy of tympanostomy tube insertion for otitis media with effusion in children with Down syndrome. *International Journal of Pediatric Otorhinolaryngology.* 1999; **49**: 143–9.

73

Acute otitis media in children

PETER REA AND JOHN GRAHAM

Introduction	912	Conclusion	925
Definition	912	Key points	925
Diagnosis	913	Best clinical practice	925
Aetiology	914	Deficiencies in current knowledge and areas for future	
Epidemiology	917	research	926
Management options	917	Acknowledgements	926
Outcomes	921	References	926
Complications	921		

SEARCH STRATEGY

The data in this chapter are supported by searches of Medline and the Cochrane Controlled Trials Register, using the term acute otitis media. Reference lists were reviewed for further articles, and authors of recent presentations contacted personally for their reference lists.

INTRODUCTION

For such a common childhood infection, acute otitis media (AOM) remains something of an enigma. It is hard to diagnose accurately and on existing evidence, as opposed to custom and tradition, there is still a high level of uncertainty over how it should best be treated. This is against a background of increasing bacterial resistance to antibiotics. There is plenty of evidence in the literature of the relative frequencies of viral and bacterial pathogens in AOM, but this is often of little help to the clinician on the spot in an individual case. Some of the epidemiological evidence is also relatively 'soft', since it is based on the flawed premise that AOM can accurately be diagnosed from the history and otoscopy alone, unsupported by tympanometry or tympanocentesis. In this chapter, the authors have tried to thread their way through the often conflicting evidence about the practical management of AOM at the same time as covering what is known of the pathology, epidemiology and complications of this commonest of childhood illnesses.

We have found ourselves uncomfortably often using expressions such as 'uncertainty,' 'insufficient evidence,' or 'limited information,' and quoting [****] and [***] levels of evidence. Even a metanalysis, the supposed gold standard of evidence, is only as good as the studies it covers. It must be remembered that the prevalence of otitis media with effusion (OME), 'glue ear,' only began to be widely appreciated after the development of the twin tools of universal hearing screening and the tympanometer in the 1960s and early 1970s, respectively. The accuracy of correct reporting of cases of AOM lags behind that of OME mainly because in the majority of large population studies of AOM the essential presence of fluid in the middle ear is not confirmed by tympanometry and audiometry.

DEFINITION

AOM may be defined clinicopathologically as inflammation of the middle ear cleft of rapid onset and infective origin, associated with a middle ear effusion and a varied collection of clinical symptoms and signs. It is synonymous with acute suppurative otitis media. It normally develops behind an intact tympanic membrane, but may include acute infections arising in the presence of ventilation tubes or existing tympanic membrane perforations. The requirement to confirm a middle ear effusion, and the nature of the symptoms and signs, vary between authors.[1, 2]

The literature supports four broadly defined subgroups of AOM.

1. **Sporadic** episodes occurring as infrequent isolated events, typically occurring with upper respiratory tract infections.
2. **Resistant** AOM: persistence of symptoms and signs of middle ear infection beyond three to five days of antibiotic treatment.
3. **Persistent** AOM: persistence or recurrence of symptoms and signs of AOM within six days of finishing a course of antibiotics.
4. **Recurrent** AOM: either three or more episodes of AOM occurring within a six-month period, or at least four or six episodes within a 12 month period (no consensus has been reached on the latter).

Groups two and three appear similar at first glance and this distinction may be questioned. It is included to maintain some consistency with the wider literature.

Grading of the severity of an episode has been attempted and has merit both clinically and for research. Pyrexia from 37.5–39°C, vomiting and severity of otalgia have been used.[3, 4] [*]

DIAGNOSIS

Diagnosis is based on the combination of often nonspecific symptoms, evidence of inflammation of the middle ear cleft and, by some authors, by the additional confirmation of a middle ear effusion. Diagnostic difficulty has affected the quality of research into AOM. There may well not be a clear history of a crescendo of otalgia in a coryzal child, followed by rapid symptomatic relief associated with tympanic membrane perforation and associated blood-stained otorrhoea. The difficulty in establishing clear diagnostic guidelines has been highlighted in an analysis of 80 studies of AOM.[5] In diagnosing AOM, only 52.5 percent of the studies cited middle ear effusions, 32.5 percent included symptoms and signs of inflammation and 2.5 percent considered the rapidity of onset. Clinicians recognize this difficulty. A large multinational study rated clinicians diagnostic certainty in children under one year of age at only 58 percent, rising to 73 percent in those over 31 months.[6]

Symptoms

Diagnosis by symptomatology alone is inaccurate because of the young age of most patients, and the nonspecific nature of the symptoms. One-third of children may have no ear-related symptoms. Two-thirds may be apyrexial.[7] Symptoms suggestive of AOM include rapid onset of otalgia, hearing loss, otorrhoea, fever, excessive crying, irritability, coryzal symptoms, vomiting, poor feeding, ear-pulling and clumsiness (**Table 73.1**). AOM most commonly develops three to four days after the onset of coryzal symptoms. The otalgia will settle within 24 hours in two-thirds of children without treatment.[9] The otorrhoea, if present, is mucopurulent and may be blood-stained. Symptomatic relief is obtained without treatment in 88 percent by day four to seven. The hearing loss, caused by the middle-ear effusion, occurs early in the illness and may persist at greater than 20 dB for one month in over 30 percent, and two months in 20 percent of children. [**/*]

Signs

The child may appear unwell, and may rub his or her ear. The diagnosis is often confirmed, rightly or wrongly, by an attempt at otoscopic assessment of the tympanic membrane. However, a poorly functioning otoscope, the moving target of a child's head, the narrow ear canal of an infant, the natural redness of the tympanic membrane of a screaming child, wax and, above all, the inaccuracy of an untrained (or even trained) eye, straining to interpret a two-dimensional image, all combine to make otoscopy an imprecise art. Since trained observers have been shown to have only an 85 percent accuracy in otoscopic diagnosis,[10] it would not be surprising for a sensible primary care physician to rely more on history and the general aspect of a child than on otoscopic findings. With these reservations, diagnosis may be supported by otoscopic assessment of tympanic membrane colour, position and mobility (**Figure 73.1**). In AOM the tympanic membrane is usually opaque. It is most commonly yellow, or

Table 73.1 Relation of reported symptoms to presence of AOM in 302 children under four years of age.

Symptom	Sensitivity	Specificity	Positive predictive value	Negative predictive value
Earache	60	92	83	78
Restlessness	64	51	46	68
Rhinitis	96	8	41	74
Cough	83	17	40	61
Fever	69	23	38	53

Reprinted from Ref. 8, with permission.

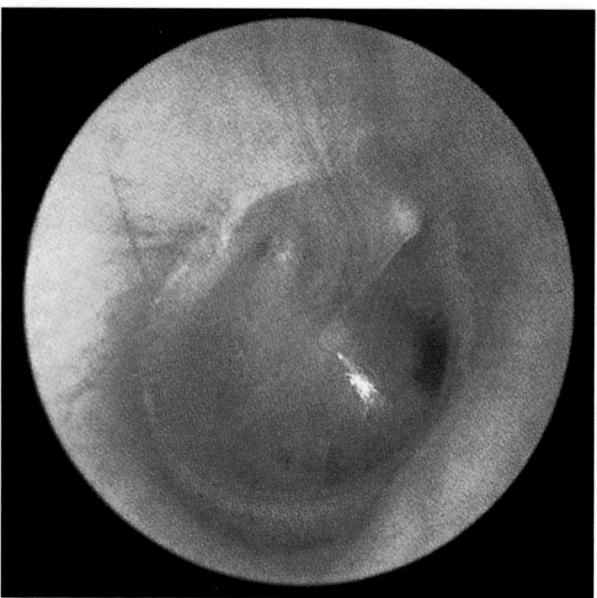

Figure 73.1 Otoscopic findings in early AOM.

yellowish pink in colour, being red in only 18–19 percent.[7, 10] The position of the tympanic membrane reliably predicts AOM only when it is bulging. Hypomobility of the drum demonstrated by pneumatic otoscopy has been shown to aid diagnosis[10] and is felt essential in some countries,[1] although others including the Dutch[2] take a more pragmatic view and do not include this in their diagnostic criteria. Should the drum have perforated, or a ventilation tube be *in situ*, mucopurulent otorrhoea will be seen. [**/*]

Investigations

Tympanometry may be used to establish the presence of a middle ear effusion, but is not usually available. Tympanocentesis and culture of middle ear effusion have been used in a number of studies assessing diagnostic accuracy of clinical signs, and establishing the organisms prevalent in a community. It is rarely required to make the diagnosis, though may be considered in high risk children such as the immunocompromised, an unwell neonate, those that fail to respond to conventional treatment and children who are seriously ill or have complications of AOM. Taking a bacterial swab of persistent otorrhoea following perforation is recommended. Nasopharyngeal swabbing for bacterial culture has been assessed but the correlation with middle ear organisms has been too weak to recommend it clinically.[11]

Specific investigation may be prompted by recurrent AOM not responsive to conventional treatment. Both iron deficiency anaemia and white blood cell disorders have been associated with AOM, so a full blood count is indicated. Immunoglobulin assay may be appropriate: Ig A, G (with subclasses) and M are typically assessed. Children

with recurrent infection of ventilation tubes may also merit investigation for primary ciliary dyskinesia, particularly if nasal and pulmonary symptoms coexist. [**/*]

Differential diagnosis

Pain may be referred from tonsillitis, teething, temporomandibular joint disorders or simply be the result of an uncomplicated upper respiratory tract infection. In a screaming child, the tympanic membrane may well appear red. Diagnostic confusion may occur with acute mastoiditis, otitis media with effusion, otitis externa, trauma, Ramsey Hunt syndrome and bullous myringitis. Very rarely, AOM may be the first indication of serious underlying disease, such as Wegener's granulomatosis or leukaemia.

AETIOLOGY

Microbiological, anatomical and environmental factors combine with altered host defence mechanisms to predispose to infection. Genetic predisposition to recurrent AOM is being increasingly cited in the literature.

Infective agents

AOM results from infection of the middle ear cleft. Both bacterial and viral infections are implicated. These infections may occur in isolation or combination.

VIRUSES

Clinically it is apparent that AOM is commonly associated with viral upper respiratory tract infections. As our ability to identify these improves, the role of viruses in the aetiology of AOM is becoming clearer. Increasing use of polymerase chain reaction assays for respiratory viruses suggests 60–90 percent of cases of AOM may be associated with viral infection.[12] In one study, a specific viral cause of upper respiratory tract infection was shown in 41 percent of children with AOM.[13] The viruses most commonly associated with AOM vary between studies, but in decreasing frequency include:

- respiratory syncytial virus (RSV);
- influenza A virus;
- parainfluenza viruses;
- human rhinovirus;
- adenoviruses.

This heterogeneity is important when considering vaccination against viruses as a prophylactic measure.

The mechanism by which they give rise to AOM is likely to vary between viruses. Viral material has been demonstrated in the middle ear aspirates of children with

AOM in 48–71 percent of cases.[12] The viral material may arrive either passively along the Eustachian tube along with other nasopharyngeal secretions or may actively invade the middle ear cleft possibly by haematogenous spread. These alternative routes of entry are suggested by the wide variation in rates of isolation of specific viral strains in the middle ear during systemic infection, ranging from 4 to 74 percent of cases dependent upon the specific virus. If all arrived passively, similar rates of isolation would be expected. This implies some viruses may be actively invading the middle ear cleft, and may be contributing directly to mucosal inflammation. RSV invaded the middle ear most frequently.[13] In contrast, those arriving passively appear to cause AOM by virtue of their action on the Eustachian tube, on bacterial adherence, and on host immunity.

There is good clinical and animal evidence that viral infection affects Eustachian tube function.[12] At a cellular level there is release of multiple inflammatory mediators from cells within the nasopharynx. Ciliated epithelial cells numbers decline, mucus production increases in the Eustachian tube and negative middle ear pressure results. This is likely to predispose to AOM.

Alteration of host immunity has been documented after viral infections, increasing susceptibility to bacterial infections. Cell-mediated immunity has been shown to be affected by RSV infection, and neutrophil function altered by influenza viruses. In a study of children with bronchiolitis caused by RSV, 62 percent developed AOM. Bacteria were isolated from the middle ear in all these children.

The ability of bacteria to colonize and adhere to the nasopharyngeal epithelium appears to be increased by certain viral infections. Increased colonization by pathogenic bacteria may predispose to AOM.

Viral and bacterial infection coexist in the middle ear cleft in AOM in as many as two-thirds of cases where viruses have been identified. This is important as clinical studies show that children who have both viruses and bacteria in their middle ear are very much more likely to have a poor response to antibiotics when compared to those with bacteria only (33 versus 3 percent failure respectively, in one study[14]). Why this should be is unclear, but may be related to the greater concentrations of inflammatory mediators in ears in which both bacteria and viruses are present. [**/*]

BACTERIA

The bacteria isolated from the middle ear in AOM are shown in **Table 73.2**.[15, 16]

In persistent or recurrent bacterial AOM, repeat culture of middle ear aspirates has failed to grow pathogenic bacteria in 30–50 percent of patients, implying that inflammation may persist despite the eradication of the infecting organism. The spectrum of organisms is similar to that in isolated episodes. In the 1980s *H. influenzae* was the most common organism identified

Table 73.2 Bacteria associated with AOM.

Bacteria	Incidence (%)
Haemophilus influenzae	16–37[a]
Moraxella catarrhalis	11–23
Streptococcus pyogenes	Up to 13
Staphylococcus aureus	Up to 5

[a]There are some 90 serotypes.

in persistent or recurrent AOM, but this has been replaced by drug-resistant *Pneumococcus*. After antibiotic treatment for recurrent AOM it is now estimated that 50 percent of *H. influenzae* are beta-lactamase producing. A similar proportion of pneumococci are penicillin resistant.[16] Penicillin resistance in pneumococci results from decreased penicillin binding protein on the bacterial cell walls, so reducing the affinity for penicillin-related drugs, but means that resistance may often be overcome by increasing drug dosage. This is not the case with beta-lactamase producing organisms. Most *Moraxella catarrhalis* are now beta-lactamase producing.

Studies on HIV-positive children suggest a similar spectrum and prevalence of infecting organisms as occurs in immunocompetent children, except where the child is severely immunosuppressed, when a higher percentage of *Staphylococcus aureus* has been reported. [**]

Routes of spread of infection

Three potential routes are described: the Eustachian tube, tympanic membrane perforations or grommets, and haematogenous.

The Eustachian tube is traditionally assumed to be the main route by which organisms reach the middle ear, though there are relatively few studies to confirm this. It is speculated that negative middle ear pressure may facilitate the movement of bacteria up the Eustachian tube.[17] Circumstantial evidence is also gained from similarities in organisms cultured from the post-nasal space and the middle ear cleft in AOM. Whether anatomical or physiological differences predispose to AOM is unclear. Studies of Native Americans, who are prone to otitis media, suggest their Eustachian tubes are shorter, straighter and more patulous than in whites, but also that they have a low passive tubal resistance.[18] Research has found no difference in tubal dimensions in otitis prone and non-prone children. However, altered tubal function may play a role. Specifically, otitis-prone children have been shown to have significantly poorer active tubal function (muscular opening function).

Pathogen entry through tympanic membrane perforations or ventilation tubes is most commonly associated with water exposure.

Haematogenous spread is inferred from the evidence provided by studies of viral identification in the blood and middle ear as described previously. It was shown that the wide variation in rates of identification of specific viral strains from the middle ear could not be explained by passive Eustachian tube transport alone.[12] [**/*]

Risk factors

GENETIC FACTORS

There is growing evidence that recurrent AOM is largely genetically determined. It is likely many genes are involved. There are numerous studies suggesting a familial association. A metanalysis of risk factors has shown that when one family member had AOM the risk increased for other family members (relative risk 2.63).[19] Racial differences are well described with increases in American Indians, Eskimos and Australian Aboriginals. However, environmental factors, such as poor economic status, may contribute to the increased risks in these groups. The most powerful evidence comes from twin studies, in particular comparison of monozygotic and dizygotic twins in whom the occurrence of AOM was compared.[18] Many immune related mechanisms, which are likely to have a genetic basis, have been proposed. Certain human leukocyte antigen (HLA) classes have been shown to be significantly associated with increased risk of AOM. Maternal blood group A is reported to an independent risk factor (relative risk 2.82). Atopy has also been associated with increased risk of developing AOM. [****/***/**]

IMMUNE FACTORS

Our understanding of the immune response to AOM remains incomplete. However, a number of specific associations have been identified which suggest that certain defective or immature pathways may predispose to infection. Low levels of IgG2 subclasses have been reported in several studies to be more common in otitis-prone children. Those with IgG2 deficiency were shown to be three times more likely to develop post-ventilation tube insertion otorrhoea for example. Delayed maturation of anti-pneumococcal antibodies (IgG1 and IgG2 were studied) does appear to predispose to AOM. This may explain in part why children grow out of AOM as immunity matures.

Defective complement-dependent opsonization has been associated with recurrent AOM and diarrhoea in infancy.[18] This is caused in some examples by low concentrations of mannose-binding protein which acts as an opsonin. This appears to be a common defect with over 20 percent of children with recurrent AOM affected in some studies. This may be particularly important in infancy when the antibody repertoire is limited.

Aberrant expression of critical cytokines, such as tumour necrosis factor and interleukins, resulting in suboptimal host defence, has been postulated as a cause for persistent infection. Expression of mucin genes, at least nine of which have been identified, may differ in those predisposed to AOM. Middle ear mucosa expresses specifically the MUC5B gene. Mucin genes regulate the production of mucin. Limited evidence is beginning to emerge that over-expression may alter the mucociliary transport system.[18]

A number of studies on children with HIV infection have yielded conflicting results. Advanced disease associated with low CD4 counts does seem to be associated with an increased incidence of AOM. [**/*]

ENVIRONMENTAL FACTORS

There are many reports on the relative contribution of environmental factors. These are important as it may be possible to modify them. The most important is almost invariably stated to be day-care attendance outside the home. The larger the number of children in the group, the greater the risk. Day care outside the home carries a relative risk (rr) for AOM of 2.45, compared to a risk of 1.59 for children cared for in their own home. The incidence of AOM appears to follow that of seasonal upper respiratory tract infections (URTI) in the winter months. Breastfeeding for three months is protective (rr, 0.87). Use of a pacifier (dummy) carries a relative risk of 1.45.[19] Poor socioeconomic status associated with poor housing and overcrowding has been reported to be associated with AOM (overcrowding: rr, 5.55 in a Greenlandic population, for example). Passive smoke exposure from parental smoking is weakly associated (rr, 1.0–1.6). There is more limited evidence to support the role of dietary factors, in particular cow's milk allergy, in predisposing to AOM. [****]

SYNDROMIC ASSOCIATIONS

Syndromes associated with abnormalities of skull base anatomy are well recognized as being associated with chronic middle ear disease, but less is published on associations with AOM. Children with Turner's syndrome do suffer more frequent episodes of AOM. Down syndrome predisposes to middle ear disease, including AOM. In cleft palate there is only a minor increase reported. Certainly Eustachian tube dysfunction in these groups predisposes to middle ear effusion, but it is not clear whether it is this dysfunction or an increase in risk secondary to subtle immunological factors that predisposed to infection. No increase is found in children with primary ciliary dyskinesia if grommets are not inserted, or cystic fibrosis.

A direct association between iron deficiency anaemia, and the degree of anaemia and frequency of AOM has been reported. [**]

EPIDEMIOLOGY

AOM is one of the commonest illnesses of childhood. It accounts for approximately 25 percent of all prescriptions for children under ten years of age in the USA, for example. Its incidence appears highest in the first year of life, more specifically the second six months of life in most studies, and gradually reduces with increasing age. This progression was shown by Strangerup and Tos[20] who reported an incidence of a first episode of AOM in 22 percent in the first year of life, 15 percent in year two and 10 percent in year three, falling to 2 percent by year eight (**Figure 73.2**). Epidemiological studies have been compromised by difficulty in achieving accuracy in diagnosis when large numbers of children are being assessed, hence there are wide variations in reported numbers. Incidences of over 60 percent are stated in some reports of infants up to age one year. By age three years, some 50–70 percent of all children will have had at least one episode of AOM, and at least 75 percent by the age of nine years.

The incidence of AOM certainly varies with the seasonal incidence of viral upper respiratory infections. There are reports that it is increasing over a period of years. Possible reasons include increased day nursery attendance and changes in diagnostic awareness.

Recurrent AOM has been reported in 5 percent of children under two years of age. Others have reported that by age three, half of children will have had at least three episodes. An important indicator of future problems is a first episode before nine months of age: these children have a one in four risk of developing recurrent AOM.

In the first two years of life, AOM occurs bilaterally in 80 percent of cases. After six years of age, it is unilateral in 86 percent.[20]

MANAGEMENT OPTIONS

Most children with AOM will get better quickly and without treatment. Some will not. A very small number

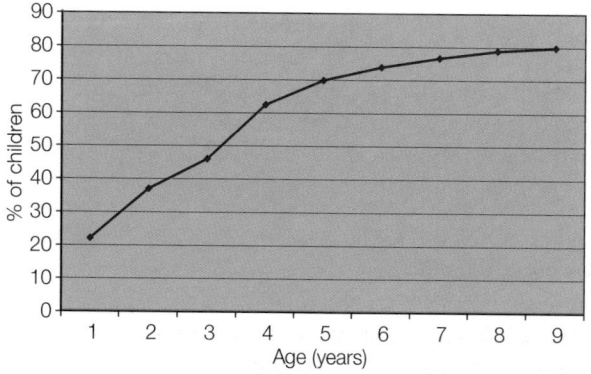

Figure 73.2 Cumulative incidence of acute otitis media (i.e. how many children have had at least one episode in their life). Redrawn from Ref. 20, with permission.

may develop potentially serious complications. Current debate questions whether and for whom treatment is required, and the role of prophylactic strategies. As serious complications are rare it can be difficult to obtain high quality evidence of how effective are prophylaxis and the treatment of episodes of AOM in preventing such complications.

Management of acute episodes

CONSERVATIVE TREATMENT

Most children will benefit from simple analgesics and anti-pyrexials, in a quiet supportive environment. Paracetamol and ibuprofen are most commonly used in the UK. There is limited experimental animal evidence showing that ibuprofen provides additional benefit by reducing mucosal inflammation when taken in combination with amoxicillin.

MEDICAL TREATMENT

Antibiotics

Uncertainty over the use of antibiotics is reflected in wide variations in usage between countries, ranging from 31 percent in the Netherlands to 98 percent in the USA.[9] There is, however, an increasingly good evidence-base for the most appropriate management in children over two years of age. In children under two, the evidence-base is weaker.

Antibiotics, if not prescribed initially, should be given to a child who fails to improve after two to three days of 'watchful waiting', and to all children with an 'irregular' illness course. They should also be given to 'high risk' children, defined by the Dutch as children with craniofacial abnormalities, Down syndrome, immuno-deficiencies and those under the age of two years suffering a recurrent episode of AOM.[2] Guidelines must be adapted to suit local experience, for example in regions of the world with a high incidence of complications of AOM where all patients may be regarded as high risk.

A recent metanalysis[9] has addressed the question of whether antibiotics should be given at initial consultation. Two-thirds of children recovered within 24 hours of the start of treatment, and 80 percent by days two to seven, with or without antibiotics. This, of course, raises the question as to whether the children did indeed have AOM in the first place. Antibiotics did lead to 5 percent fewer children overall having pain between days two and seven. That equates to 17 children needing to be treated to prevent one child experiencing pain during days two to seven. Relatively few data were available on hearing loss at one and two months post-infection, but no differences were found between those who received antibiotics and those who did not. No significant differences were found on progression of disease or relapse of symptoms. Similarly, no differences were found in complications of AOM. However, those taking antibiotics suffer nearly double the side effects, such as diarrhoea, than those who do not, and run a greater risk of developing antibiotic resistant bacteria.

The length of treatment was addressed in a separate metanalysis.[21] Short (five day) and long (ten day) courses of treatment were compared. At 8–19 days the weighted mean failure rate in the short course was 19 percent and 13.7 percent in the long course. By days 20–30, this had converged to 15.7 versus 12.5 percent, which was nonsignificant. It implied that 17 children would need to receive the long course to avoid one treatment failure. The authors concluded that five days of treatment was appropriate in uncomplicated infections in low risk children over two years of age without recurrent AOM or tympanic membrane perforation. Under two years of age evidence is weaker that short course treatment is adequate.

Attempts have been made to identify a subgroup of children who may benefit from antibiotics. Younger age may be an important determinant, but good evidence is lacking because of diagnostic difficulties in this group. However, while published data show only modest benefit from antibiotic treatment between six and 24 months of age[22] (number needed to treat (NNT) = seven for one symptomatic improvement at day four), most would recommend treatment below two years of age. Using short-term symptomatic outcome markers at day three, it has been shown that immediate antibiotics may benefit those children presenting with higher temperatures (>37.5°C) or vomiting (NNT = 3–6).[4]

AOM occurring in the presence of a tympanic membrane perforation or ventilation tubes may be treated equally successfully with oral or topical antibiotics. The potential ototoxicity of topical aminoglycoside ear drops in these cases is well recognized and dose dependent, therefore prolonged topical treatment should be avoided. [****]

Which antibiotic?

This should be determined by national recommendations. Amoxicillin remains the first choice in most centres, but at higher than previously recommended doses (80 mg/kg/day) if drug-resistant pneumococci are common in a particular country or region, or macrolides for penicillin-sensitive patients. For persistent or resistant episodes, national policies should be sought depending on the prevalence of beta-lactamase-producing organisms and culture results if available. Options include amoxicillin-clavulonate or cefuroxime axetil orally, or intra-muscular ceftriaxone (US Centre for Disease Control and Prevention).

Antihistamines and decongestants

A metanalysis of the use of oral or intranasal antihistamines and/or decongestants concluded that their use could not be supported, and that medication side effects were higher when they were used together. While combining the two treatments was shown to slightly reduce persistent AOM at two weeks (NNT = 10.5) the result may have been biased by the design of the studies.[23] [****]

SURGICAL TREATMENT

Surgery has a limited role in the treatment of an uncomplicated episode of AOM. Myringotomy was practised in the pre-antibiotic era, and indeed was continued until the late 1980s in some countries as a first-line treatment for AOM. However, there are now a number of good studies showing that myringotomy plus antibiotics offers no advantage over antibiotics alone. Myringotomy alone has a worse outcome than either of the antibiotic groups.[24] Myringotomy is reserved for severe cases where complication is present or suspected, to relieve severe pain or when microbiology is strongly required. [****]

Management of recurrent acute otitis media

ALTERATION OF RISK FACTORS

It may be possible to alter many of the environmental risk factors discussed previously. Parents should be reassured of the benign natural history of AOM, as these children have been shown to be more demanding than those without recurrent disease, and their mothers more anxious about their care. The most readily modifiable risk factor is exposure to other children. AOM increases with the number of children in day care, the length of time a child spends in day care each week, how young a child is when introduced into day care, the presence of children under two years of age in the day-care setting and having a sibling in day care. Advice should include sitting a child semi-upright if bottle-fed and avoiding passive smoke inhalation. Restricting the use of pacifiers, particularly after infancy, should be recommended for otitis-prone children. The mother may be advised to continue breastfeeding for at least six months after future pregnancies and increasing vitamin C intake and avoiding alcohol in the third trimester, both of which have been weakly associated with AOM. The role of food allergies, in particular cow's milk, is still unclear. No effective role has as yet been shown for homeopathic remedies. [**]

MEDICAL PROPHYLAXIS

Antibiotics

Antibiotic prophylaxis has the potential to cause problems, but should be considered for recurrent AOM. Many organisms need to be covered so a broad-spectrum drug is required. Risks for the development of resistant organisms increase, adverse drug reactions may occur and active disease may be masked. Studies of prophylaxis of recurrent AOM invariably treat each individual recurrence with additional antibiotics. Trials therefore compare antibiotic prophylaxis versus placebo between acute episodes. The natural history of recurrent AOM is reassuring. Over 50 percent of children having no treatment between attacks will not suffer a further episode in the following six months. Indeed, only one in eight continues to suffer recurrent AOM (i.e. three or more episodes) during the trials, if treated only for acute episodes. However, metanalysis does show a benefit of antibiotic prophylaxis equating to a reduction of approximately 1.5 episodes per 12 months of antibiotic treatment given, above that expected from the natural history. So one child would need eight months of treatment to avoid one episode of AOM. There was a trend for those treated with sulfisoxazole to do better than those treated with amoxicillin, both being used at half the therapeutic dosage.[25] Recommendations are for six months of treatment through the winter months in children who do not have background OME.

Those studies that assessed the length of time a child has OME in association with AOM showed that while antibiotic prophylaxis may reduce the incidence of AOM, it does not reduce the length of time with OME. This is important as antibiotic prophylaxis may therefore be most appropriate for children not prone to OME, while ventilation tubes may be indicated for those prone to OME.

Most trials exclude 'high risk' children, who are often most in need of treatment. On the basis of the metanalysis described above, which shows a modest benefit with the use of antibiotic prophylaxis, there may also be a place for its use in the management of high-risk children with recurrent AOM, despite the absence of specifically targeted studies. [****]

Xylitol

Xylitol is a commonly used sweetener that inhibits pneumococcal growth and the attachment of pneumococci and Haemophilus to nasopharyngeal cells. Studies in daycare nurseries using chewing gum or syrup have suggested reductions of 30–40 percent in the occurrence of AOM. However, this translates to 1–1.5 episodes per year.[26] It is ineffective if used in acute upper respiratory infections. Given the very large quantities that must be consumed, and potential concerns over the safety of such consumption, its use cannot yet be recommended. [***]

Vaccination

Vaccines have been used effectively against most common childhood infections caused by single specific organisms such as mumps, measles and rubella. The concept of vaccinating against AOM therefore is an attractive one that is being actively explored. Potential obstacles include the wide range of causative organisms, both bacterial and viral, the varied serotypes, technical difficulties in producing an effective immune response, obtaining an immune response before six months of age, parental resistance to multiple vaccination and the possibility that the successfully targeted pathogens will simply be replaced by others.

Vaccination against viruses

Since 60–90 percent of episodes are initially associated with viral infections (see above under Viruses) viral vaccination seems the most logical first step. AOM secondary to infection by the measles virus is now relatively uncommon in industrialized countries, for example.

Influenza A vaccination is currently the only commercially available preparation for the prophylaxis of viral upper respiratory infections. Three trials of children in daycare have shown its efficacy in preventing AOM, resulting in 30–36 percent fewer episodes during a subsequent influenza epidemic, and reducing influenza-associated AOM by 83–93 percent.[27] This is not an absolute reduction in episodes, and this indication is not yet within the UK Department of Health guidelines.[28] This does show, however, that preventing viral URTI can be an effective method of reducing AOM. [***]

RSV vaccines are undergoing clinical trials for lower respiratory tract infection, but as yet do not seem to be providing significant protection. No studies are under way assessing a role in AOM.

Parainfluenza virus vaccines have been evaluated in animals and need to target types 1, 2 and 3 viruses. Limited human studies demonstrate relative safety and immunogenicity, but efficacy studies are not available.[29]

Vaccination against bacteria

Vaccination against *Streptococcus pneumoniae*, nontypeable *Haemophilus influenzae* and *Moraxella catarrhalis* is made difficult by the low immunogenicity of the polysaccharide capsule of these bacteria in young children and infants. Success against *Haemophilus influenzae* type B (which causes epiglottitis and meningitis) using a polysaccharide-protein conjugated vaccine provides one potential solution.

Streptococcus pneumoniae vaccination is particularly challenging because of the 90 serotypes of the bacteria. However, as only a small number of these cause most pneumococcal AOM, and it has been shown that anti-capsular antibodies can prevent pneumococcal AOM, progress has been made. Early attempts with unconjugated pneumococcal polysaccharide vaccines proved unsuccessful in children under two years of age. However, a heptavalent conjugated vaccine (Prevenar, Wyeth-Lederle Vaccines) has been shown to be highly effective in preventing invasive pneumococcal disease and modestly successful in reducing AOM in two major studies. Immunization occurs at two, four, six and 12, and in one study also 15 months of age. Episodes of AOM from any cause were reduced by 6 and 7 percent, respectively, and pneumococcal AOM by 34 percent.[29] To improve cover during the critical first six months of life, trials are under way to see if immunizing the mother in the third trimester of pregnancy is effective. Immunization after two years of age is with 23-valent pneumococcal polysaccharide vaccine. Whilst vaccination is recommended in certain 'at risk' children,[28] its place in the management of AOM is not yet clear. It may be, for example, that vaccinating a child presenting with recurrent AOM will be ineffective because colonization of the upper respiratory tract has already occurred. Publications on this are pending. Debate on the quality of systematic reviews on this topic continues and clear guidance cannot yet be given.[30] [***]

Non-typeable *Haemophilus influenzae* vaccines are being developed by several techniques.[27] Phase I clinical trials using a conjugated vaccine are under way. Animal experiments using a chinchilla model have shown some reduction in AOM with this type of vaccine.

Moraxella catarrhalis vaccine research is at a preclinical stage, but products are under development.

Experts in the field hope vaccination against all three of these bacteria may be possible within a decade.[29]

Special attention should be drawn to children with, or awaiting, cochlear implants. Concern has been raised about a number of cases of meningitis. Whether it is implant related or reflects inner ear abnormalities in many of these children is unclear. All such children are recommended to have the heptavalent pneumococcal vaccine before the age of two years and the 23-valent pneumococcal polysaccharide vaccine at the age of two or over (see Chapter 70, Paediatric cochlear implantation). Hib conjugate vaccine is recommended for all children up to four years of age.

Immunoglobulins

The importance of immunological immaturity in the occurrence of recurrent AOM has been emphasized. Intramuscular pooled gamma-globulin in otitis-prone children has been shown not to reduce the incidence of AOM. However, in a Japanese study, intravenous immunoglobulin (GB-0998) in IgG2-deficient infants has been shown to be an effective prophylaxis for AOM, as well as pneumonia in this specific group of children. [**]

Benign commensals

A recent paper considered whether spraying benign commensals (alpha streptococci) into the nose to recolonize the nasopharynx following antibiotics might reduce AOM by inhibiting the growth of pathogenic bacteria. A significant reduction was reported.[31] A separate smaller study, which did not pretreat with antibiotics, showed no difference. [***]

SURGICAL PROPHYLAXIS

In contrast to the large number of trials comparing antibiotic treatments, there are relatively few addressing

surgical prophylaxis. Surgery is potentially attractive, however, in that it may reduce problems of antibiotic resistance and also treat subsequent OME.

Ventilation tubes

A recent metanalysis of five trials concluded that the presence of ventilation tubes versus no tubes yielded a relative decrease in episodes of AOM of 56 percent, equivalent to an absolute reduction of 1.0 episode per child per year.[32] The effect occurred mostly in the first year of follow up, presumably as this covered the period when the tubes were in place. Of equal importance is the reduction in the prevalence of OME by 115 days per child-year. Seventy-nine percent were reported to have an improved quality of life. Side effects included recurrent otorrhoea in 7 percent and chronic otorrhoea in 4 percent. Other studies have shown a higher incidence of tympanosclerosis and focal areas of tympanic membrane atrophy of questionable significance in the ventilation tube groups.

These findings need careful interpretation. One of the studies compares antibiotic prophylaxis with amoxicillin to tubes to placebo.[33] The amoxicillin group had a significant reduction in episodes of AOM. The tube and placebo group did not. However, when AOM occurred in the placebo group, it was more distressing than when otorrhoea occurred with AOM in the group with tubes in place. Also, over a two-year period, the surgical group had 26 and 61 days fewer with OME than the antibiotic and placebo groups, respectively.

It is difficult to draw conclusions about the role of ventilation tubes. On the evidence available they may be considered for children with recurrent AOM, but no persistent effusion, in whom medical strategies have failed. There may be a greater role for them in preference to, or following failure of, medical prophylaxis in the child with recurrent AOM and persistent OME. [****]

Adenoidectomy and adenotonsillectomy

The limited evidence-base for best practice is most striking when considering adenoidectomy. Two papers are particularly worth discussing, both with a cohort of children from Pittsburgh. Randomization methods have been questioned in these studies, as has follow up. The first concluded that adenoidectomy may be beneficial in children who had previously had ventilation tube insertion and suffered subsequent AOM. AOM was reduced by 31 percent relative to the control group in a two-year follow up (or 0.32 episodes per child-year), and subjects spent 42 percent less time with OME. Additionally, the need for further tubes was reduced by 50 percent.[34]

Their second trial was of children who had not previously had ventilation tube insertion. Considering children without overt adenotonsillar disease, a modest reduction in the number of episodes of AOM was recorded in the first year after surgery from 2.1 to 1.4

following adenotonsillectomy, but not adenoidectomy. Similarly, OME was reduced from 30 to 19 days in year one in the adenotonsillectomy group, and to 22 days in the adenoidectomy group. The effect was not apparent after the first year. Drop out from the trial was particularly high in the adenoidectomy group, and the results should be viewed cautiously. For children with adenotonsillar symptoms, no AOM benefit was reported from adenotonsillectomy. The authors concluded the risks of surgery were not warranted in children who had not previously had ventilation tube insertion.

In summary, there is little evidence to support adenotonsillectomy. Adenoidectomy may be considered in those children who have failed medical therapy and had further AOM following ventilation tube insertion. The presence of OME increases the benefit of adenoidectomy. [***]

OUTCOMES

An episode of acute otitis media may resolve rapidly with or without antibiotics; it may prove resistant to first-line antibiotics; it may persist or recur shortly after a course of antibiotics has finished; it may subsequently recur; or it may progress to tympanic membrane perforation or other complication of infection. Here we consider the medium- and long-term consequences of infection: the natural history of AOM, middle ear effusions, auditory functioning and speech and language development.

Natural history

Data come from the control arms of randomized controlled trials, and hence usually exclude high-risk children, complicated cases, and those under two years old. Without antibiotic treatment, symptomatic relief from pain and fever occurs in approximately 60 percent of children within 24 hours of diagnosis, in over 80 percent by day two to three, and 88 percent by days four to seven.[9, 25] These data do not equate with complete resolution, for example otorrhoea may still be present without pain or fever, and only 73 percent reach the stage of complete resolution by day seven to fourteen. In all studies, those with resistant or persistent disease will have received antibiotic treatment.

For recurrent AOM the prognosis is also generally favourable. Following study entry, and with only acute episodes treated, recurrence rates fell to 0.13 episodes per child per month in the subsequent 6–24 months – approximately 1.6 episodes per year. Indeed, over half had no further attack in the following six months, and only one in eight continued to satisfy the diagnostic criteria for recurrent AOM.[25] Other work has shown that even in early recurrences of infection three to four weeks after a previous episode, a new organism is usually involved.

Caution should be attached to these findings. Though pooled numbers are large, high risk children and those with baseline OME were generally excluded.

MIDDLE EAR EFFUSIONS

Middle ear effusions are an important outcome of AOM. Looking again at those children randomized to placebo, pooled data show rates of OME of 63 percent two weeks after AOM, 40 percent at one month and 26 percent at three months. Antibiotics did not appear to have any effect.[9, 25]

AUDITORY FUNCTIONING

What little work has been carried out on short-term audiometric outcomes suggests that approximately one in three children will have an air–bone gap greater than 20 dB at one month after infection, and one in five at three months. There is limited evidence to suggest that AOM may reduce long-term audiometric thresholds. Several studies following cohorts of children have reported small but significant loss of very high frequency hearing (11–16 kHz) in those with many episodes of AOM. There is a suggestion that this may be more a consequence of disturbed middle ear mechanics than cochlear damage. The significance for auditory functioning as the child grows older is not established.

SPEECH AND LANGUAGE DEVELOPMENT

It is difficult to separate the literature on AOM and OME outcomes. Little is written on speech production or reception. In children with OME, a significant effect seems to occur in the early years of life on expressive language development, but not receptive language. A small number of studies point to persisting effects on expressive language in school-age children. There is little evidence showing different cognitive development in school-age children with a history of otitis media in the first three years of life. There are suggestions that poor behavioural traits may be more common by school age, but more work is required before conclusions are drawn.

COMPLICATIONS

Extracranial

TYMPANIC MEMBRANE

Tympanic membrane perforation is considered a complication of AOM. It is the commonest complication of infection and is reported in 0–10 percent of episodes. Perforation is associated with a purulent or bloody otorrhoea and immediate relief of pain. It typically occurs in the posterior half of the pars tensa, and is associated with loss of the fibrous middle layer of the drum. This may predispose to future posterior retraction pockets. Four outcomes of perforation may result. In most cases the perforation heals spontaneously and the infection resolves. Second, the infection may resolve, but the perforation persists. This may predispose the ear to future AOM or chronic suppurative otitis media. Third, the perforation and otorrhoea may persist, manifesting as chronic suppurative otitis media. 'Chronicity' is generally deemed to have occurred by three months. Fourth, a further complication may arise.

The long-term outcomes were assessed in a cohort of otitis-prone children followed up from 3 to 14 years of age. By the end of the study 7 percent had collapse of the posterior superior tympanic membrane, chronic suppurative otitis media, or central perforation.[35] Scarring or tympanosclerosis was present in 27 percent, although several studies report that ventilation tubes increase this risk.

ACUTE MASTOIDITIS

Four classes of mastoiditis are defined. During episodes of acute otitis media, infection and inflammation may naturally extend into the mastoid cavity, and be visualized radiologically. This is not associated with the typical signs of acute mastoiditis and is not considered a complication of AOM.

Infection may spread to the mastoid periosteum by emissary veins: acute mastoiditis with periosteitis. At this stage no abscess is present but the post-auricular crease may be full, the pinna may be pushed forward and there may be mild swelling, erythema and tenderness of the post-aural region.

When acute mastoid osteitis develops, the infection has begun to destroy the bone of the mastoid air cells and a subperiosteal abscess may develop. Signs may be similar to those when periosteitis is present. A subperiosteal abscess develops most commonly in the post-auricular region. A zygomatic abscess may develop above and in front of the pinna. A Bezold's abscess may result from perforation of the medial mastoid cortex, tracking down the sternomastoid to the posterior triangle. Pus tracking down peritubal cells may result in a retropharyngeal or parapharyngeal abscess (**Figure 73.3**).

A fourth stage may be reached, subacute ('masked') mastoiditis, in incompletely treated AOM after 10–14 days of infection. Signs may be absent, but otalgia and fever persist. This stage can also progress to serious complications.[3]

In the pre-antibiotic era, mastoiditis was a common and serious complication of AOM. In a study in 1954 the control group was reported to have developed mastoiditis in 17 percent of cases.[9] In some developing countries rates of 5 percent are still quoted. In the 1970s it was estimated that 0.004 percent of cases of AOM resulted in surgery for

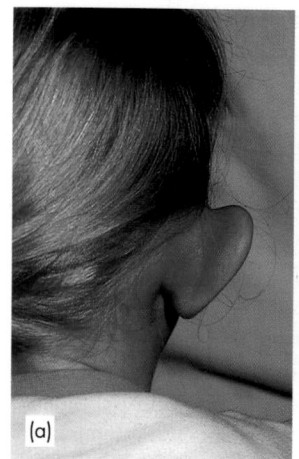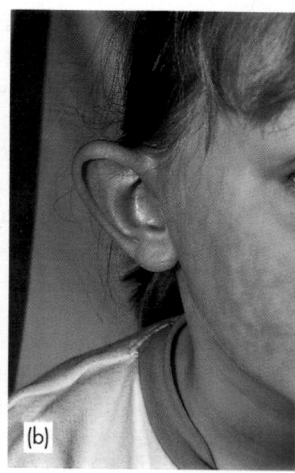

Figure 73.3 (a) and (b) Acute mastoiditis.

mastoiditis. The incidence is reported by several authors to be increasing gradually again. The incidence varies between countries. In the UK, Canada, Australia and the United States, where antibiotic prescription rates are over 96 percent, the incidence ranges from 1.2 to 2.0 per 100,000 population per year. In Norway, Denmark and The Netherlands (prescription rates 67, 76 and 31 percent, respectively) rates are higher at 3.5, 4.2 and 3.8 respectively.[36]

Acute mastoiditis is a disease of childhood. A large multicentre study found 28 percent to be in children less than one year of age, 38 percent in one to four year olds, 21 percent in four to eight year olds, 8 percent in 8–18 year olds and 4 percent in those over 18 years of age.[37] This higher incidence in younger children reflects the peak ages for AOM.

Traditional teaching was that acute mastoiditis is preceded by 10–14 days of middle ear symptoms. However, in many papers the short length of middle ear symptoms prior to presentation is noteworthy. For example, in one large study approximately 32 percent had one to two days symptoms, 34 percent had three to six days, 26 percent seven to fourteen days and 8 percent over 14 days.[37] Prior antibiotic treatment of the infection is common, reported in 22–55 percent of children. Clearly antibiotics do not fully protect against mastoiditis.

Symptoms are of otalgia and irritability in most children. Pyrexia is less common in those treated with antibiotics. Otorrhoea is present in only approximately 30 percent. Clinically, a red or bulging tympanic membrane will often be seen. A normal drum is reported in a very variable proportion of cases, but certainly does not exclude the diagnosis and is believed to result from resolution of the mesotympanic infection following antibiotic treatment, while the osteitis in the mastoid progresses. Retro-auricular swelling is seen in approximately 80 percent and retro-auricular erythema in 50–84 percent (less in previously treated children). Tenderness is typically sited over MacEwen's triangle (on palpation through the conchal bowl). Pinna protrusion is present in two-thirds of cases. Sagging of the posterior wall of the external auditory canal, resulting from subperiosteal abscess formation, should be looked for, but is quoted as an uncommon finding. Few patients will have a 'full house' of the classic signs.

A somewhat different incidence of organisms has been identified from those gained from culture in AOM. Around 20 percent of samples do not grow bacteria. *Streptococcus pneumoniae*, *Streptococcus pyogenes*, *Pseudomonas aeruginosa* and *Staphylococcus aureus* are the most commonly reported. *Haemophilus influenzae* is less commonly reported, and *Moraxella catarrhalis*, *Proteus mirabilis* and Gram-negative anaerobes rarely.

Recommended investigations vary between institutions. A full blood count, C-reactive protein (CRP), and blood cultures are often obtained. A CT scan of the mastoid is recommended when intracranial complications are present or suspected (though MRI may be more helpful in identifying specific intracranial pathology), when mastoidectomy is to be performed and in those not improving on antibiotic treatment. A CT may show evidence of osteitis, abscesses and intracranial complications.

Differential diagnosis includes AOM, otitis externa, furunculosis and reactive lymphadenopathy. Rarely, undiagnosed cholesteatoma, Wegener's granulomatosis, leukaemia and histiocytosis may first present with AOM, hence tissue should be sent for histology if mastoidectomy is performed.

Myringotomy with or without ventilation tube placement, culture of the aspirate and high-dose intravenous antibiotics is the most commonly recommended initial treatment in acute mastoiditis. This is adequate in 75 percent of cases. Failure to improve, subperiosteal abscess formation (occurring in 10–30 percent) or development of complications merits at least abscess drainage with or without cortical mastoidectomy. This can be challenging surgery for the less experienced as the mastoid is often full of granulations and the facial nerve superficial in the young child.

A most important message is that intracranial complications from acute mastoiditis develop in 6–17 percent of cases, and many of these may develop during hospitalization. Although acute mastoiditis may be less common than in the past, its severe complications still occur. [**]

PETROSITIS

Infection may extend to the petrous apex. The classic features of Gradenigo's triad (VI nerve palsy, severe pain in the trigeminal nerve distribution and middle ear infection) are not always present. Patients commonly present with other intracranial complications. Recent papers recommend high-dose broad spectrum antibiotics and a variety of mastoidectomy, from cortical to radical, though drainage of the petrous apex is no longer felt necessary. [*]

FACIAL NERVE PALSY

In the pre-antibiotic era, it was estimated that acute lower motor neurone facial palsy complicated 0.5 percent of episodes of AOM (see Chapter 80, Facial paralysis in childhood). It is now quoted at 0.005 percent.[38] Most are related to bacterial infection but case reports with viral AOM exist. Approximately four out of five children present with a partial paralysis. The case series in the literature report that approximately 80 percent of palsies respond well to ventilation tube insertion and intravenous antibiotics. The remainder undergo cortical mastoidectomy. Advice is conflicting about when and in whom mastoidectomy is required and the role of facial nerve decompression. As recovery is generally so good, a more conservative approach without facial nerve decompression seems appropriate. Most children achieve rapid restoration of normal facial function, with a mean time to complete recovery of four months. Those with a total paralysis at presentation have a recovery stretching over many months.

Sixth nerve palsy in the absence of petrositis has also been reported. It is speculated this may stem from phlebitis spreading along the inferior petrosal sinus from the lateral sinus. [*]

LABYRINTHITIS

Round window permeability changes during acute infection are important as these may allow entry of bacterial toxins. There is some experimental evidence that permeability can be increased by streptococcal toxins. Preformed channels for bacterial entry may also exist, such as surgical or congenital perilymph fistulae. These may allow infection to spread directly to the subarachnoid space causing meningitis. Particular concern arises in children with congenital inner ear abnormalities and those with cochlear implants. Three types of labyrinthitis are recognized. *Perilabyrinthitis* is not associated with AOM. *Serous labyrinthitis* is inflammation of the labyrinth without pus formation, and is characterized by recovery of auditory and vestibular function. *Suppurative labyrinthitis* may result from spread of infection from the mastoid or middle ear. Severe vertigo, nausea, vomiting, nystagmus and permanent hearing loss result. Suppurative labyrinthitis is rare, and the treatment of cases presented in the literature ranges from ventilation tube insertion and aggressive antibiotic use, to tympanomastoidectomy and cochleotomy. [*]

Intracranial

In the pre-antibiotic era, intracranial complications of AOM were more common and mortality rates of over 75 percent are presented. Published mortality rates from intracranial complications now average approximately 5 percent in industrialized countries.

Persistent headache and fever are the most common early symptoms of an intracranial complication. In half of cases there may be signs only of AOM and not mastoiditis. Frequently two or more complications coexist. Early diagnosis is important for improving outcomes.

Seven classical intracranial suppurative complications of AOM are described.[3]

1. **Meningitis** is usually cited as the commonest intracranial complication of AOM, accounting for 54–91 percent of cases. In contrast, studies assessing the aetiology of meningitis are conflicting. One of the largest recent studies found no association between bacterial meningitis and AOM, while another found an antecedent history of AOM in 29 percent,[39] though this does not equate to a causal relationship. Special mention has already been made of possible associations between congenital inner ear malformations such as cochlear dysplasia, cochlear implants and meningitis. Younger children, average age two years, are most commonly infected. Studies focus almost exclusively on bacterial aetiologies. The rate of *Haemophilus influenzae* type B meningitis has dropped dramatically since vaccination was introduced. *Streptococcus pneumoniae* is the causal agent in a greater proportion because of this reduction.[39] A second intracranial complication should be looked for in any infant with meningitis with MR scanning. Myringotomy may help to establish the infective agent if evidence has not been obtained from lumbar puncture. Treatment is medical. If mastoid surgery is required, it is usual to try and wait for an improvement in the medical condition of the child first if possible. [*]

2. **Extradural abscess** is the next commonest intracranial complication. It is more commonly associated with chronic disease. Pus collects between dura and bone, usually after bone erosion. If lying in the posterior fossa medial to the sigmoid sinus, it is termed an extradural (epidural) abscess, if within the split of dura enclosing the sigmoid sinus it is called a peri-sinus abscess. It may be discovered only at mastoidectomy, but may be suspected in the patient with persistent headache and fever or severe otalgia. Treatment is surgical drainage. [*]

3. **Subdural empyema** is a collection of pus between the dura and arachnoid membranes and is termed a subdural empyema. It is rare. It develops by direct extension of infection or thrombophlebitis. In addition to headaches and pyrexia, focal neurological signs, seizures and signs of meningeal irritation may be present. Paranasal sinusitis is reported to be a much commoner cause than AOM. Surgical drainage of the abscess through burr holes or craniectomy may be indicated. Mastoidectomy may sometimes be required, though many cases cited in the literature were treated medically. [*]

4. **Sigmoid sinus thrombosis** most commonly results from erosion of the bone over the sinus from mastoiditis and may also be associated with other complications. However, it occurs in association with otitis media alone in 43 percent of cases. Infected thrombus develops within the sinus and may then extend proximally and distally to the internal jugular vein and superior vena cava, entering the systemic circulation and causing septicaemia. In addition to headache and otorrhoea, a spiking pyrexia may develop. Griesinger's sign is mastoid tenderness and oedema secondary to thrombophlebitis of the mastoid emissary vein. MRI is the imaging of choice showing high signal intensity in the sigmoid sinus on both T_1-and T_2-weighted images and absent flow. If caused only by otitis media, myringotomy and antibiotics may suffice. However, in the presence of mastoid infection, it is more usual to perform a canal wall up mastoidectomy, needle the sinus to assess blood flow and occasionally to remove infected thrombus. As persistent sepsis and distant thrombosis are uncommon, the role of anticoagulation is unclear in the literature.[40] Serial imaging to look for propagation of thrombus has been recommended. [**/*]

5. **Focal otitic encephalitis (cerebritis).** Focal inflammation and oedema of brain tissue may occur independent of, or in association with, any suppurative complication of AOM. Intensive antibiotic treatment is required. [*]

6. **Brain abscess** is more commonly associated with chronic ear disease but may occur in association with AOM and its complications (**Figure 73.4**). Brain abscess forms a larger proportion of complications in developing countries. It may develop in both the temporal lobe and cerebellum. Persistent headaches are the commonest symptom. Initial symptoms may be of encephalitis, but these often settle as the abscess organizes over days or weeks. Eventually, signs of raised intracranial pressure, focal neurology and infection develop. Invstigations include CT imaging followed by lumbar puncture, if safe. In the early stages of cerebritis, neurosurgical drainage may be avoided but will be required if the abscesses are expanding. Brain abscesses carry a potentially high mortality rate, although in industrialized countries the few large

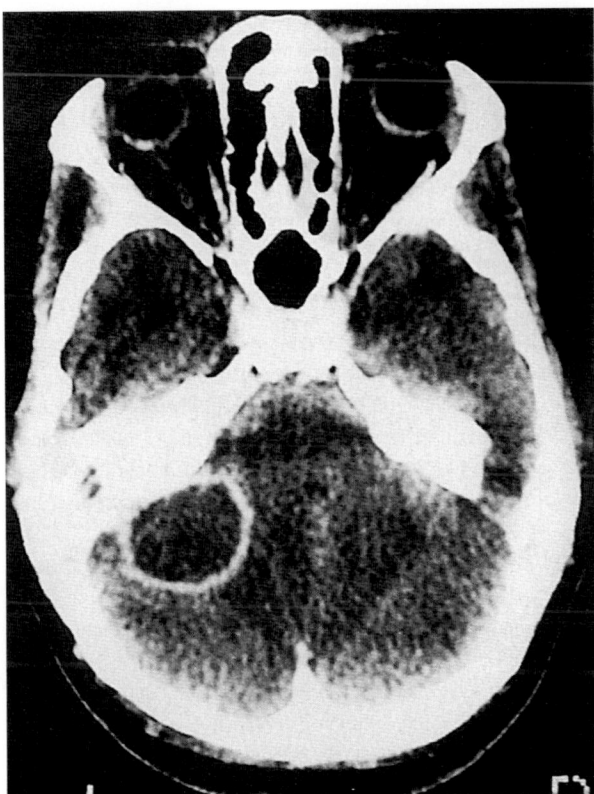

Figure 73.4 Brain abscess secondary to AOM.

series now quote rates of below 10 percent. One large review found the mortality from otogenic causes, at 3.8 percent, was much lower than from other causes. [*].

7. **Otitic hydrocephalus** is a complication of AOM manifesting as raised intracranial pressure in the absence of any space-occupying lesion, and without obstruction to the flow of cerebrospinal fluid (CSF). Benign intracranial hypertension is a synonym. The aetiology is obscure. Headache is the predominant symptom. It is commonly associated with sigmoid or transverse sinus thrombosis and so MRI is an important investigation. Lumbar puncture will show raised CSF pressure, but normal CSF composition. A number of medical treatments may be tried and liaison with a paediatric neurologist is recommended. [*].

CONCLUSION

It can be seen from this chapter that there are deficiencies in our current knowledge of both the diagnosis and aetiology of AOM, and uncertainties in management strategies. However, we have been able to describe a number of potentially exciting developments that have occurred in the past few years.

KEY POINTS

- Acute otitis media is one of the commonest illnesses of childhood.
- Diagnosis can be difficult particularly in very young children.
- Management recommendations vary widely between countries.
- A range of modifiable risk factors should be addressed.
- Evidence is emerging to support new prophylactic strategies.
- Intracranial complications are still seen despite prior antibiotic treatment.

Best clinical practice

✓ AOM is one of the commonest illnesses of childhood. Accurate diagnosis is notoriously difficult. A high index of suspicion is required in the unwell child. [Grade B]

✓ The clinician should distinguish between sporadic, resistant, persistent or recurrent AOM as management strategies differ. [Grade A]

✓ Two-thirds of children recover within 24 hours with or without treatment, so a period of watchful waiting may be reasonable in uncomplicated AOM. [Grade A]

✓ Antibiotics should not be withheld in severe or irregular infections, should be given if a child fails to improve within two to three days of the onset of AOM and should be given in sufficiently high doses. [Grade A]

✓ Pyrexia (>37.5°C), severe otalgia, vomiting, age under two years and 'high risk' children have all been used as indicators to use antibiotics sooner rather than later. [Grade B/C]

✓ Practitioners should be aware of local bacterial antibiotic resistance patterns and prescribing policies. Broad spectrum antibiotics are not generally required as first-line therapy. [Grade A]

✓ In otherwise healthy children over two years of age, five days of antibiotics is usually adequate. [Grade A]

✓ For persistent or resistant AOMs it should be noted that whilst pneumococcal drug resistance can usually be overcome by increased antibiotic doses, *Haemophilus* may be beta-lactam producing, so broader spectrum antibiotics may be required. [Grade B]

✓ Modifiable risk factors should be discussed with parents. These include nursery attendance, parental smoking, breastfeeding and the use of pacifiers. [Grade C]

✓ In the management of recurrent AOM, on average eight months of antibiotic prophylaxis would be needed to prevent one episode of AOM. This strategy may be preferred in the absence of effusions between episodes of AOM. [Grade A]

✓ Ventilation tube insertion reduces the number of episodes of AOM by over 50 percent. This option may be preferred when effusions persist between episodes of AOM. [Grade A]

✓ Additional adenoidectomy may further reduce the number of episodes of AOM. [Grade A]

✓ The benefits of tonsillectomy on episodes of AOM are not sufficient to warrant its use in the management of recurrent AOM. [Grade A]

✓ Vigilance should be maintained for complications of AOM, the most common symptoms being persistent pyrexia and headache. [Grade C].

Deficiencies in current knowledge and areas for future research

The following list summarizes what we feel this chapter should be able to report on when the next edition is being prepared.

➤ Greater standardization and reproducibility of diagnostic criteria is required to compare trials.

➤ As most children appear to recover without treatment, better characterization of those who may have initial antibiotic treatment withheld is needed.

➤ Trials should be set up to study high risk groups of children who are currently excluded from most studies: those with conditions predisposing them to acute otitis media and children under 18 months of age. These are the children likely to benefit the most from our intervention.

➤ We know many important risk factors, but trials are needed to show whether attempts to modify them actually help.

➤ The potential benefit of vaccination to older children with recurrent infection needs exploring. As more vaccines are developed, we must know to whom we should be recommending them.

➤ The number and quality of trials of surgical intervention does not allow confident guidance to be given as to the long-term benefits or consequences of ventilation tube insertion.

➤ More data are required on the long-term consequences of recurrent infection in terms of altered audiometric thresholds, quality of life and language and cognitive development.

ACKNOWLEDGEMENTS

We would like to thank Dr Anne Schilder from the University Medical Center, Utrecht, for her data on management practices in the Netherlands.

REFERENCES

1. Diagnosis and Treatment of Otitis Media in Children. Bloomington (MN): Institute for Clinical Systems Improvement (ICSI); 2001 July. http://www.guideline.gov

2. Appleman CLM, van Balen FAM, van de Lisdonk EH, van Weert HCLM, Eizinga WH. NGH-standaard Otitis Media Acuta (eerste herziening). *Huisarts en Wetenschap.* 1999; **42**: 362–6, and www.artsennet.nl/nhg

* 3. Bluestone CD, Gates GA, Klein JO, Lim DJ, Mogi G, Ogra PL *et al.* Definitions, terminology, and classification of otitis media. *Annals of Otology, Rhinology and Laryngology.* 2002; **188**: 8–18. *Up-to-date and succinct account of terminology in otitis media.*

4. Little P, Gould C, Moore M, Warner G, Dunleavey J, Williamson I. Predictors of poor outcome and benefits from antibiotics in children with acute otitis media: pragmatic randomised trial. *British Medical Journal.* 2002; **325**: 22–5.

5. Chan LS, Takata GS, Shekelee P, Morton SC, Mason W, Marcy SM. Evidence assessment of management of acute otitis media: II. Research gaps and priorities for future research. *Pediatrics.* 2001; **108**: 248–54.

6. Froom J, Culpepper L, Grob P, Bartelds A, Bowers P, Bridges-Webb C *et al.* Diagnosis and antibiotic treatment of acute otitis media: report from International Primary Care Network. *British Medical Journal.* 1990; **300**: 582–6.

7. Schwartz RH, Stool SE, Rodriguez WJ, Grundfast KM. Acute otitis media: towards a more precise definition. *Clinical Pediatrics.* 1981; **20**: 549–54.

* 8. Heikkinen T, Ruuskanen O. Signs and symptoms predicting acute otitis media. *Archives of Pediatrics and Adolescent Medicine.* 1995; **149**: 26–9. *Well-researched systematic review on the role of antibiotics.*

9. Glasziou PP, Del Mar CB, Sanders SL, Hayem M. Antibiotics for acute otitis media in children (Cochrane Review). *The Cochrane Library.* Oxford: Update Software Ltd, 2002.

10. Karma PH, Pentilla MA, Sipila MM, Kataja MJ. Otoscopic diagnosis of middle ear effusion in acute and non-acute otitis media. I. The value of different otoscopic findings. *International Journal of Pediatric Otorhinolaryngology.* 1989; **17**: 37–49.

11. Gehano P, Lenoir G, Barry B, Bons J, Boucot I, Berche P. Evaluation of nasopharyngeal cultures for bacteriologic assessment of acute otitis media in children. *Pediatric Infectious Disease Journal.* 1996; **15**: 329–32.

12. Heikkinen T. The role of respiratory viruses in otitis media. *Vaccine.* 2001; **19**: S51–5.

13. Heikkinen T, Thint M, Chonmaitree T. Prevalence of various respiratory viruses in the middle ear during acute otitis media. *New England Journal of Medicine*. 1999; **340**: 260–4.

14. Chonmaitree T, Owen MJ, Howie VM. Respiratory viruses interfere with bacteriologic response to antibiotic in children with acute otitis media. *Journal of Infectious Diseases*. 1990; **162**: 546–9.

15. Eskola J. Polysaccharide-based pneumococcal vaccines in the prevention of acute otitis media. *Vaccine*. 2000; **19**: S78–82.

16. Pichichero ME, Reiner SA, Brook I, Gooch 3rd WM, Yamauchi T, Jenkins SG et al. Controversies in the medical management of persistent and recurrent acute otitis media. *Annals of Otology, Rhinology and Laryngology*. 2000; **183**: 1–12.

17. Buchman CA, Doyle WJ, Skoner DP, Post JC, Alper CM, Seroky JT et al. Influenza A virus induces acute otitis media. *Journal of Infectious Diseases*. 1995; **172**: 1348–51.

18. Casselbrant ML, Mandel EM. The genetics of otitis media. *Current Allergy and Asthma Reports*. 2001; **1**: 353–7.

19. Uhari M, Mantysarri K, Niemela M. A meta-analysis of the risk factors for acute otitis media. *Clinical Infectious Diseases*. 1996; **22**: 1079–83.

20. Strangerup SE, Tos M. Epidemiology of acute suppurative otitis media. *American Journal of Otolaryngology*. 1986; **7**: 47–54.

21. Kozyrskyi AL, Hildes-Ripstein GE, Longstaff SEA, Wincott JL, Sitar DS, Klassen TP et al. Short course antibiotics for acute otitis media (Cochrane review). In: *The Cochrane Library*. Oxford: Update Software Ltd, 2002.

22. Damoiseaux RA, van Balen FA, Hoes AW, Verheij TJ, de Melker RA. Primary care based randomised, double blind trial of amoxicillin versus placebo for acute otitis media in children under 2 years. *British Medical Journal*. 2000; **320**: 350–4.

23. Flynn CA, Griffin T, Tudiver F. Decongestants and antihistamines for acute otitis media in children (Cochrane Review). In: *The Cochrane Library*. Oxford: Update Software Ltd, 2002.

24. Kaleida PH, Casselbrant ML, Rockette HE, Paradise JL, Bluestone CD, Blatter MM et al. Amoxicillin or myringotomy or both for acute otitis media: results of a randomised clinical trial. *Pediatrics*. 1991; **87**: 466–74.

25. Rosenfeld RM. Natural history of untreated otitis media and what to expect from medical therapy. In: Rosenfeld RM, Bluestone CD (eds). *Evidence-based otitis media*. New York: Decker Inc, 1999: 157–221.

26. Uhari M, Kontiokari T, Niemela M. A novel use of xylitol sugar in preventing acute otitis media. *Pediatrics*. 1998; **102**: 879–84.

27. Giebink GS, Bakaletz LO, Barenkamp SJ, Eskola J, Green B, Gu X-X et al. Recent advances in otitis media: vaccine.

Annals of Otology, Rhinology and Laryngology. 2002; **111**: 82–94.

28. Donaldson L, Mullally S, Smith J. Update on immunisations. Department of Health. August 2002: 1–8. http://www.doh.uk/cmo/index.htm

* 29. Snow JB. Progress in the prevention of otitis media through immunization. *Otology and Neurotology*. 2002; **23**: 1–2. *Account of current evidence on the possible preventive role of vaccination.*

30. Jefferson T, Demicheli V. Polysaccharide pneumococcal vaccines. Existing guidance is at variance with the evidence. *British Medical Journal*. 2002; **325**: 292–3.

31. Roos K, Hakansson EG, Holm S. Effect of recolonisation with 'interfering' alpha streptococci on recurrences of acute and secretory otitis media in children: randomised placebo controlled trial. *British Medical Journal*. 2001; **322**: 210–2.

32. Rosenfeld RM. Surgical prevention of otitis media. *Vaccine*. 2000; **19**: S134–9.

33. Casselbrant ML, Kaleida PH, Rockette HE, Paradise JL, Bluestone CD, Kurs-Lasky M et al. Efficacy of antimicrobial prophylaxis and of tympanostomy tube insertion for prevention of recurrent acute otitis media: results of a randomised clinical trial. *Pediatric Infectious Disease Journal*. 1992; **11**: 278–86.

34. Paradise JL, Bluestone CD, Rogers KD, Taylor FH, Colborn DK, Bachman RZ et al. Efficacy of adenoidectomy for recurrent otitis media in children previously treated with tympanostomy-tube placement. *Journal of the American Medical Association*. 1990; **263**: 2066–73.

* 35. Stenstrom C, Invarsson L. Late effects on ear disease in otitis-prone children: a long-term follow-up study. *Acta-Otolaryngology*. 1995; **115**: 658–63. *Highlights national variations in prescribing patterns for acute otitis media.*

36. Van-Zuijlen DA, Schilder AG, Van-Balen FA, Hoes AW. National differences in incidence of acute mastoiditis: relationship to prescribing patterns of antibiotics for acute otitis media? *Pediatric Infectious Diseases Journal*. 2001; **20**: 140–4.

37. Luntz M, Brodsky A, Nusem S, Kronenberg J, Keren G, Migirov L et al. Acute mastoiditis: a multicentre study. *International Journal of Pediatric Otorhinolaryngology*. 2001; **57**: 1–9.

38. Ellefsen B, Bonding P. Facial palsy in acute otitis media. *Clinical Otolaryngology and Allied Sciences*. 1996; **21**: 393–5.

39. Ryan MW, Antonelli PJ. Pneumococcal antibiotic resistance and rates of meningitis in children. *Laryngoscope*. 2000; **110**: 961–4.

40. Bradley DT, Hashisaki GT, Mason JC. Otogenic sigmoid sinus thrombosis: what is the role of anticoagulation? *Laryngoscope*. 2002; **112**: 1726–9.

74

Chronic otitis media in childhood

JOHN HAMILTON

Introduction and definitions 928
Histology and pathogenesis of chronic otitis media 930
What may prevent resolution of otitis media? 931
Chronic perforation of the tympanic membrane 932
Atrophy of the pars tensa of the tympanic membrane
(including retraction pockets) 941
Cholesteatoma 947
Ossicular erosion in chronic otitis media 954

Conclusions 956
Key points 957
Best clinical practice 958
Deficiencies in current knowledge and areas for future
research 958
Acknowledgements 959
References 959

SEARCH STRATEGY

The data in this chapter are supported by Medline searches through the PubMed online database using medical subject headings (*inter alia* otitis media; otitis media, suppurative; tympanic membrane perforation; tympanoplasty; myringoplasty; cholesteatoma, ossicular prosthesis, etc.). Searches were curtailed by using the 'child (0–18)' limiter and by focusing on appropriate subheadings in the medical subject headings database. Free text searches using terms not included in the medical subject headings database such as 'tympanic membrane atrophy' and 'tympanic membrane retraction' were expanded and refined using Boolean operators. Results were stored using reference manager software (Endnote), which also allowed searches to be combined without duplication of results. The Cochrane database was also consulted. These electronic searches were extended by reference to proceedings of major international symposia, particularly the series of international otitis media conferences, the international cholesteatoma meetings and the middle ear mechanics series.

INTRODUCTION AND DEFINITIONS

In any specialized field new terminology is introduced to facilitate dialogue between interested parties. These specialized terms require precise definition in order that communication and comparison between centres can have any value at all. However, in any developing area of human endeavour a rudimentary subject may be found to harbour several new aspects of interest. This development not only leads to the introduction of new terms in the field of study but also the reclassification of the parent subject. In this way, the progressive change caused by increasing understanding of a subject paradoxically may complicate its teaching. The following problems may arise.

- Older classifications and definitions may become obsolete.
- Some terms may become repeatedly defined and therefore ambiguous.
- Increasing complexity of classifications, whilst of value to those developing the subject, may hinder their widespread use. The balance between precision and utility may have no perfect solution.

The study of chronic otitis media has resulted in all these problems.

WHO definition of chronic otitis media, 1996

A WHO/CIBA Foundation Workshop[1] in 1996 produced the following definitions:

- **Chronic suppurative otitis media**: 'a stage of ear disease in which there is chronic infection of the middle ear cleft, i.e. Eustachian tube, middle ear and mastoid, and in which a non-intact tympanic membrane (e.g. perforation or tympanostomy tube) and discharge (otorrhoea) are present'. The same report qualifies this definition by stating that the otorrhoea should be present for two weeks or longer.
- **Chronic otitis media**: 'includes both chronic suppurative otitis media and chronic perforation of the tympanic membrane'.

International Symposium on Recent Advances in Otitis Media, 1978

A task force was appointed on behalf of this symposium[2] to provide definitions of terms relevant to otitis media, as well as a classification of the subject. It proposed *inter alia*:

- **chronic otitis media**: 'a chronic discharge from the middle ear through a perforation of the tympanic membrane'.
- **chronic otitis media** and **ronic suppurative otitis media** were defined as synonymous.

However, the definitions continued that 'suppurative refers to active clinical infection'. Furthermore, 'a perforation without discharge can be an inactive stage of the infection'.

As the term 'chronic suppurative otitis media' appears here to be considered equal to 'active chronic otitis media' there is not only some inconsistency within this set of definitions but a clear path for this evolution of these terms. As a result, the terms 'active chronic otitis media' and 'inactive chronic otitis media' have also enjoyed widespread use.

The unambiguous part of the original definition was the perforation. Unfortunately, this elevated the presence of a perforation as sufficient to establish the existence of chronic otitis media. Given that tympanic membrane perforations need not be caused by chronic otitis media, this was manifestly wrong. This is particularly true in the paediatric population in which a common cause for tympanic membrane perforation is acute otitis media. In most such cases, the perforation heals with resolution of the acute infection without a phase of chronic infection.

International Symposium on Recent Advances in Otitis Media, 1999

A panel reporting to the Post-Symposium Research Conference of this Symposium has issued a revised classification of otitis media.[3] The panel produced an exhaustive and hierarchical classification of otitis media (see **Table 74.1**). Nonetheless, the new classification continues to have difficulty with 'chronic otitis media', not only denying the term its significance as an immediate subclassification of otitis media but also refuting the validity of the term. The panel report states that: 'the term chronic otitis media is confusing and potentially mis-leading and should not be used, since some consider it to mean chronic otitis media with effusion, others think it means chronic suppurative otitis media, and still others include cholesteatoma under this term'.

The panel prefers the term 'chronic suppurative otitis media' and define this to mean 'a chronic perforation with chronic otitis media'.

Resolution: new classification

Hitherto, the definition of chronic otitis media has been either that of a clinical syndrome, or as a mixture of pathological entity and clinical syndrome. The tension seems most easily resolved by considering chronic otitis media to be a purely pathological entity.

- 'Chronic otitis media' is a pathological term only, indicating chronic inflammation affecting the middle ear cleft.
- Chronic otitis media may be attended by various pathological complications affecting the structures of the middle ear cleft, including perforated tympanic membrane, tympanic membrane retraction pockets, cholesteatoma, ossicular defects, tympanosclerosis and myringitis.
- The patient may be troubled by symptoms and signs caused by a mixture of these pathologies.

This framework (see **Figure 74.1**) provides the basis for the organization of this chapter, since this model predicts:

- multiple complications of chronic otitis media may present simultaneously (see **Figure 74.1** and **74.2**);
- treatment of an ear affected by chronic otitis media may require attention to each of many complications;
- treatment of complications of chronic otitis media does not necessarily influence the severity of the underlying chronic otitis media;
- the treated ear remains at risk of further complications of chronic otitis media.

The last of these points is of particular importance when considering chronic otitis media in children. If otitis media in children is more vigorous than in adults, it is possible to predict further that the complications of chronic otitis media are more prevalent in children than in adults; and the outcomes of the treatment of ears affected by chronic otitis media in children, particularly in the long term, are worse than in adults. These two assertions clearly justify a greater understanding of this condition in children and are examined throughout this chapter.

Table 74.1 Recent advances in classification of otitis media.

Classification			
Otitis media	Acute otitis media		
	Otitis media with effusion		
Eustachian tube dysfunction			
Intratemporal (extracranial) complications	Perforation of tympanic membrane	Acute perforation	
		Chronic perforation	Acute otitis media
			Chronic otitis media (and mastoiditis; chronic suppurative otitis media)
	Mastoiditis		
	Apical petrositis	Acute	
		Chronic	
	Facial paralysis	Acute	
		Chronic	
	Labyrinthitis	Acute	
		Serous	
		Suppurative	
		Chronic	
	Atelectasis of middle ear	Localized	
		Generalized	
	Aural acquired cholesteatoma	Without infection	
		With infection	
	Cholesterol granuloma		
	Ossicular discontinuity		
	Adhesive otitis media		
	Tympanosclerosis		
	Ossicular fixation		
Intracranial complications	Meningitis		
	Extradural abscess		
	Subdural ernpyema		
	Encephalitis		
	Brain abscess		
	Dural sinus thrombosis		
	Hydrocephalus		

Modified from Ref. 3, with permission. This classification is widely recognized, but the concepts which underpin it are not used in this chapter. Please refer to Resolution: new classification and **Figure 74.1**.

HISTOLOGY AND PATHOGENESIS OF CHRONIC OTITIS MEDIA

Histological analysis of human temporal bones with various types of otitis media has revealed that although the clinical subgroups of otitis media may be considered to be distinct, the histology of these groups overlaps considerably.[4, 5]

- All forms of otitis media display submucosal inflammatory infiltrates and mucosal metaplasia with the development of glandular structures, mucus-producing cells and ciliated cells on histological examination.
- Chronic inflammation is characterized by tissue destruction, as well as attempts at healing.

- The general histological features include mononuclear cell infiltrates, submucosal fibrosis, the formation of highly vascular granulation tissue and osteitis.
- Mucosal complications such as cholesterol granuloma and tympanosclerosis may be seen.
- Changes in special structures associated with the middle ear cleft, such as the tympanic membrane, are also seen.
- It is of particular importance that histologically discernible chronic otitis media occurs quite frequently in the absence of tympanic membrane perforation.[4]
- Animal experiments indicate that features of chronic inflammation appear within 14 days if acute otitis media fails to resolve.[6]

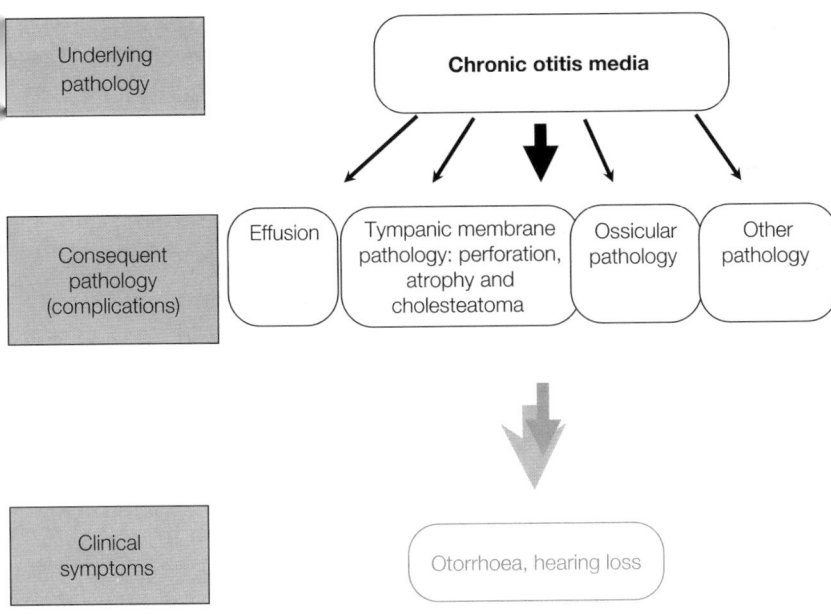

Figure 74.1 Model for the classification of chronic otitis media. In this model, chronic otitis media is regarded as a pathological entity only. The arrows indicate a one-way relationship. Thus, chronic otitis media may be complicated by a wide variety of largely independent pathological complications and the clinical presentation is governed by which complications are present. This model predicts that treatment of a complicating pathology will not influence the nature of the underlying chronic otitis media, a problem of considerable significance in the management of this disease in children.

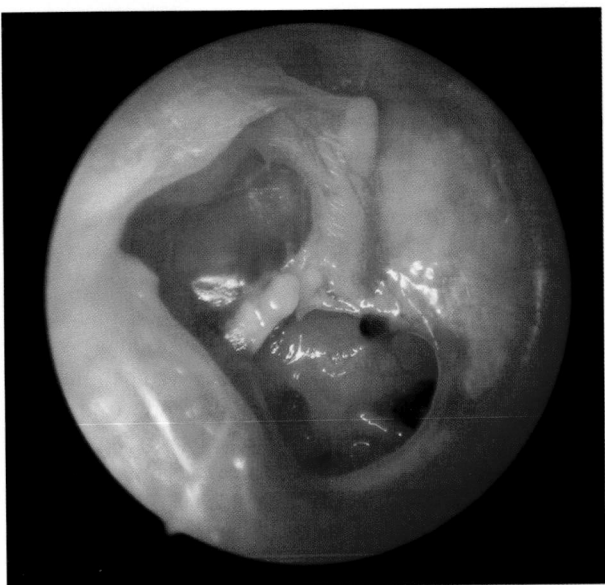

Figure 74.2 Chronic otitis media and its complications. In this ear chronic otitis media has been complicated by tympanic membrane perforation, tympanic membrane sclerosis, tympanic membrane atrophy, ossicular erosion and erosion of the posterior annulus. Although gross inspection suggests the middle ear mucosa to be healthy, published histological survey has established that microscopic analysis will confirm the presence of chronic inflammation.

WHAT MAY PREVENT RESOLUTION OF OTITIS MEDIA?

Repeated infection from the nasophaynx

Acute upper respiratory tract infections may spread to the middle ear cleft from the nasopharynx via the Eustachian tube. The following mechanisms are suggested to enhance transfer between the nasopharynx and middle ear.

- In the presence of an intact tympanic membrane, inflammation of the pharyngeal end of the Eustachian tube may prevent gas exchange along the Eustachian tube. Isolation of the middle ear allows diffusion effects with the middle ear mucosa to dominate the physiology of the middle ear cleft gas pocket. Over long periods this results in lowering of the middle ear pressure. In turn, this may predispose to aspiration of nasopharyngeal microbes into the middle ear cleft on the rare occasion when the Eustachian tube does manage to open.
- In the presence of a perforated tympanic membrane, the middle ear air cushion no longer impedes the movement of gas from the nasopharynx into a closed box, predisposing to reflux from the nasopharynx to the middle ear cleft.[7]

Repeated infection from the external ear canal

In the presence of a perforated tympanic membrane, microbes can be transported in fluid media from the ear canal into the middle ear. In particular, water that gains access to the external ear canal can flow without impediment into the middle ear through the perforation. In addition, mucus from the middle ear may straddle the tympanic membrane and provide a vehicle for the transfer of microbes from the external ear into the mesotympanum.

Persistent colonization by bacterial biofilms

There is evidence that many chronic infections are caused by the ability of bacteria to alter their form to create nonmotile communities adherent to mucosa and protected by polysaccharide matrix. Such biofilms are able to resist most forms of host resistance as well as antibiotics and are not detected by conventional microbiological assays. The biofilms often consist of many microbial strains and are capable of converting back to more conventional planktonic bacterial populations. Biofilms have long been recognized in chronic infections.[8] Recent microscopic evidence of biofilms in otitis media has indicated that this mechanism may be important in maintaining chronic ear infections.[9]

CHRONIC PERFORATION OF THE TYMPANIC MEMBRANE

Definitions

According to the panel reporting to the Seventh Post-Symposium Research Conference of the International Symposium on Recent Advances in Otitis Media a perforation of the tympanic membrane is deemed to be chronic if present for three months.[3] Chronic suppurative otitis media is defined by otorrhoea of at least six weeks duration in the presence of a chronic tympanic membrane perforation.[3]

By contrast, the WHO defines chronic suppurative otitis media as 'a stage of ear disease in which there is chronic infection of the middle ear cleft, i.e. Eustachian tube, middle ear and mastoid, and in which a non-intact tympanic membrane (e.g. perforation or tympanostomy tube) and discharge (otorrhoea) are present'.[1] The same report qualifies this definition by stating that the otorrhoea should be present for two weeks or longer.[1]

Chronic otitis media and the pathology of tympanic membrane perforation

Tympanic membrane perforation usually occurs secondary to acute otitis media. The process by which acute traumatic tympanic membrane perforations heal has been studied in animals. These investigations indicate that healing is mediated by hyperplasia, proliferation and migration of the outer keratinizing squamous epithelium.[10] This advances ahead of connective tissue rich in fibroblasts. Failure of this process has been attributed primarily to persistent infection.

One study examined 30 entire perforated tympanic membranes taken from patients receiving tympanic allografts for the treatment of their perforations. All showed evidence of inflammation, epithelial hyperplasia and fibrosis as if still trying to heal.[11] A second study of the margins of surgically treated chronic perforations indicated that the connective tissue was inadequately vascularized and extracellular matrix substances and growth factors were deficient. In 5 of the 30 cases in the former study, squamous epithelium extended medially more than 0.7 mm from the perforation edge.[11]

A tympanic membrane perforation associated with chronic otitis media is not just a defect in an otherwise normal structure. Not only is the tympanic membrane participating in the chronic inflammation, but the endoepithelial junction need not be located at the perforation edge.

Chronic otitis media need not be associated with tympanic membrane changes.[12] By contrast, inflammatory changes in the tympanic membrane are almost universally associated with chronic otitis media.[12]

Classification

Older textbooks distinguish between tubotympanic disease, which is a defect of the anterior and inferior tympanic membrane and atticoantral disease, which is a defect of the posterior and superior tympanic membrane. The former group is also termed safe and the latter unsafe.

Older textbooks also distinguish between central and marginal perforations.

These classifications do not clearly distinguish tympanic membrane perforation from other tympanic membrane pathology, such as retraction pockets or cholesteatoma. By grouping a number of complications of chronic otitis media, these classifications draw conclusions about their combined behaviour instead of informing us about perforations alone.

There is no evidence that true perforations (perforations with no retraction) in the epitympanum and posterior mesotympanum behave differently from other tympanic membrane perforations. However, tympanic membrane disease affecting the epitympanum and posterior mesotympanum is more likely to be cholesteatoma or a retraction pocket. These do behave differently to perforations.

There is no evidence that true marginal perforations behave differently from other tympanic membrane perforations. However, marginal tympanic membrane disease is more likely to be cholesteatoma or a retraction pocket. These do behave differently to perforations.

As both perforations and retractions can affect any part of the tympanic membrane, a classification based on tympanic membrane locations is not an accurate means of distinguishing between them.

These classifications attempt on an anatomical basis to distinguish tympanic membrane pathologies which behave differently from one another. It is more germane to distinguish between tympanic membrane perforation and tympanic membrane retraction pockets (including cholesteatoma). This distinction is not difficult to make with the help of the otological microscope.

There is evidence that granulation tissue, which is a feature of all forms of chronic otitis media, can also give rise to acute intracranial infections. Thus even the distinction between cholesteatoma and perforations is not a valid means of identifying safe and unsafe disease.[13]

Epidemiology

The epidemiology of chronic ear discharge associated with chronic ear perforations (chronic suppurative otitis media) has been widely studied in children. The WHO recognize a prevalence of chronic suppurative otitis media of more than 1 percent of children as presenting an 'avoidable burden' which can be managed in the 'general health care context'[1] and more than 4 percent as representing a 'massive' public health problem requiring urgent attention.[1]

The populations with the highest prevalence of childhood chronic suppurative otitis media are found among the Inuit and Australian Aboriginals. The most extreme rates of tympanic membrane perforation in a series have been recorded at 67 percent in Australian Aboriginals and 46 percent in the Inuit.[14, 15] Apache and Navaho Indians, rural Maori and Solomon Islanders as well as some rural Indian and African populations have been found to have a point prevalence of chronic suppurative otitis media of over 5 percent. Other Native American, Indian and African populations have prevalence rates of 1–2 percent.[1]

Prospective studies of large populations of urban children in Saudi Arabia and Brazil found point prevalence of chronic suppurative otitis media of 1.3 and 0.9 percent, respectively.[16, 17] A well-planned national study in South Korea found a rate of less than 1 percent in the paediatric population.[18]

No such thorough or representative population screening of paediatric populations has been performed recently in Europe or the USA. Audiometric screening studies of small populations suggests a point prevalence of less than 1 percent in these countries. By contrast, the UK National Study of Hearing found a somewhat higher rate (4.1 percent) of tympanic membrane perforation in the British adult population.[19]

Risk factors

A firm understanding of the causes of the exceptionally high prevalence of chronic suppurative otitis media in Inuit and Australian Aboriginals remains elusive. In the past focus has been directed at the biological antecedents of disease. For instance, the racial variations in Eustachian tube anatomy at one time attracted attention as a possible cause for the early onset and persistence of otitis media. Subsequently, nasopharyngeal colonization by a wide variety of otological pathogens became recognized as a more pivotal risk factor.[20] Early nasopharyngeal colonization is associated with early acute otitis media,[21] which in turn is associated with the early onset of tympanic

membrane perforation. More recently, the social factors underlying the biological parameters have been determined. It has been established that these populations acquire pathogens early because of high rates of cross-infection from infected siblings in overcrowded conditions.[22, 23] This problem also helps to perpetuate the carriage of pathogens, a process assisted by factors that reduce the child's ability to clear the disease (see **Table 74.2**).

AGE

Data from aboriginal populations indicate a high prevalence of tympanic membrane perforation in very young children with a somewhat lower prevalence in adulthood. The highest rate of perforation is seen in the two- to four-year-old age group, at which stage the rate of perforation is roughly three times the rate seen in adulthood (see **Figure 74.3**).[24, 29] By contrast, in South Korea, a rising prevalence with age is found (see **Figure 74.4**).[18] No information was presented regarding whether these perforations were symptomatic or not, so these data may reflect a steady reduction in perforation rates in childhood over the last 50 years.

TYMPANOSTOMY TUBES

Tympanostomy tube insertion is a recognized cause of subsequent tympanic membrane perforation. A recent review of 62 studies revealed that chronic perforation of the tympanic membrane occurred in 964 of 20,222 ears (4.8 percent).[30] Short-term tubes caused chronic perforations in 175 of 8107 ears (2.2 percent). Long-term tubes resulted in chronic perforation in 556 of 3356 ears (16.6 percent). More detailed metaanalysis from eight studies providing separate outcomes for both long-term and short-term tubes indicated that long-term tubes increased the relative risk of chronic perforation by 3.5 (CI: 1.5–7.1)[30] compared with short-term tubes.

Table 74.2 Risk factors proposed for high rates of chronic suppurative otitis media in indigenous children.

Risk factor
Early nasopharyngeal acquisition of otological pathogens due to high rates of cross-infection[20, 22, 23]
More siblings under the age of five[24]
More crowded accommodation[23]
Higher number of siblings with a history of ear inflammation[23]
Prolonged carriage rates of nasopharyngeal pathogens[21, 25]
Age at first episode of acute otitis media[26]
Poorer nutritional status[27]
Reduced exposure to medical services and supportive therapies

Other biological factors
Eustachian tube anatomy
Differences in immune genes[28]

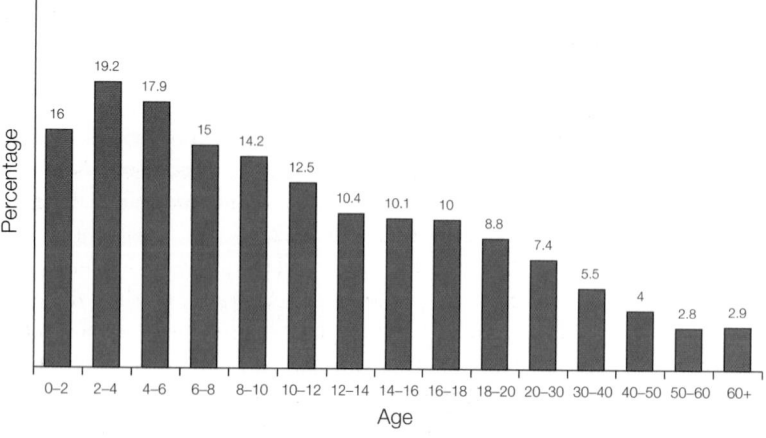

Figure 74.3 Point prevalence of ear infection in Australian Aboriginals.[29]

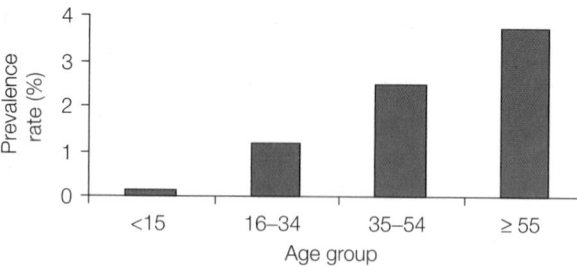

Figure 74.4 Prevalence rate of tympanic membrane perforation by age in Korea (1991 survey estimates).[18]

CLINICAL SYNDROMES

Syndromes that involve skull base, midfacial and Eustachian tube disorders are well known to be associated with an increased prevalence and persistence of otitis media with effusion. The commonest of these disorders are Down syndrome and cleft palate. There is little evidence concerning the prevalence of tympanic membrane disorders in these groups in the literature. One prospective survey of 50 patients has confirmed that those with cleft palate also have a significantly raised prevalence of tympanic membrane perforation (11 percent).[31] A survey of 201 adults with Down syndrome did not find an increased rate of of tympanic membrane perforation (1 percent).[32] This study relied on history, however, and did not include tympanic membrane inspection.

Microbiology

Animal studies reveal that a histological picture of chronic inflammation can be found as early as two weeks after inoculation.[33]

A review of studies of microorganisms implicated in chronic suppurative otitis media of at least two weeks duration found that in children, as in adults, the most commonly isolated organism is *Pseudomonas aeruginosa*.[34] *P. aeruginosa* is an extracellular opportunistic pathogen that is frequently encountered in chronic infections. It utilizes two major mechanisms to evade

the host defence system. One of these mechanisms is the production of a large number of extracellular products, such as proteases, toxins and lipases. Inhibition of the local immune response by bacterial proteases provides an environment for the colonization and establishment of chronic infection. The other mechanism by which *P. aeruginosa* evades the host defence system is through the production of a biofilm. The biofilm induces a low phagocyte response, and provides a barrier for the bacteria against antibodies, complement and the cells of the immune system.[35] Mixed infection is common and other aerobes commonly isolated include *Staphylococcus aureus*, diphtheroids, streptococci and Gram-negative bacilli including *Proteus mirabilis*. Anaerobes and fungi are also reported, although less frequently evaluated. When assessed, Bacteroides and Fusobacterium species, as well as *Peptococci* and *Peptostreptococci* are found to be common.[34] Synergism between anaerobes and aerobes is a widely recognized mechanism for increased virulence in mixed infections and it is notable that intracranial complications of otogenic infection usually have mixed flora including anaerobes.

Clinical presentation

Children with tympanic membrane perforations that are not inflamed may have minimal or no symptoms. Children with tympanic membrane perforations usually have minimal hearing loss except when their ears are discharging or when there is associated ossicular disease. Ear discharge in the presence of a tympanic membrane perforation is usually profuse. The discharge is usually pale and opaque, but not offensive. If the child has received no information on aural health care, the ears may discharge continuously. If the patient knows to keep the ears dry, the ears usually discharge only when water is accidentally admitted into the ear canals or during an upper respiratory tract infection. If the chronic otitis media is associated with profuse granulation or polyp formation, the ear discharge may become bloodstained. Otalgia is unusual in the presence of a tympanic membrane perforation. Itching is unusual and occurs only when a secondary otitis externa complicates the presentation. Tinnitus and dizziness are very unusual. When they are reported in the presence of tympanic membrane perforation that is actively discharging, examination and investigation to exclude labyrinthine involvement is urgent and essential.

Clinical examination

A child presenting with profuse chronic ear discharge and hearing loss has chronic otitis media in almost all cases. The precise complication of chronic otitis media associated with the symptoms is determined by examination of the tympanic membrane (see **Figure 74.5**), which can only be performed once adequate access to the tympanic membrane has been obtained.

Initial inspection of the ear may reveal mucopus filling the lumen of the ear canal. This can be removed either by suction with microscopic control or by mopping the ear. Most children are frightened by the loud sound caused by aural suction. By contrast, even tiny infants will tolerate mopping very well (see **Figure 74.6**).

Once the ear canal has been cleared, the tympanic membrane should be inspected carefully and systematically. It is a minimum requirement that the entire tympanic membrane be inspected. It should first be determined whether the entire tympanic membrane can be seen. Some ear canals are narrow or tortuous and only part of the tympanic membrane can be seen. If the attic area cannot be seen then a further examination with the otoendoscope may improve the view. If this is not possible in the outpatient department, the child's ear should be inspected under general anaesthesia. If the pars flaccida is normal, the pars tensa should be fully inspected.

The general condition of the tympanic membrane should be noted. A healthy tympanic membrane is only a few cells thick and is translucent. The incus and features on the medial wall of the mesotympanum are just discernible. The chronically inflamed tympanic membrane is thicker and opaque. The appearance of the tympanic membrane is more homogenous. The blood vessels on the tympanic membrane surface may be more prominent, standing out in contrast to the rest of the drum.

Defects in the pars tensa should be noted, along with their location and size. Whether the defect is a perforation or a retraction pocket should be noted. This cannot always be reliably determined using a hand-held otoscope so inspection using the otological microscope is essential. If this is not possible in the outpatient department, the child's ear should be inspected under general anaesthesia.

Tympanic membrane inflammation associated with the defect should be recorded.

Other tympanic membrane pathology, such as tympanosclerosis or myringitis, should also be documented. An endoscopic photographic image provides a useful alternative view of the tympanic membrane and improves the identification of these extra pathological details.

Features visible through the perforation should be recorded. These include the degree of inflammation of the middle ear mucosa and the integrity of the ossicular chain. Anatomical features on the medial wall of the middle ear space may be visible, particularly if the mucosa is not inflamed.

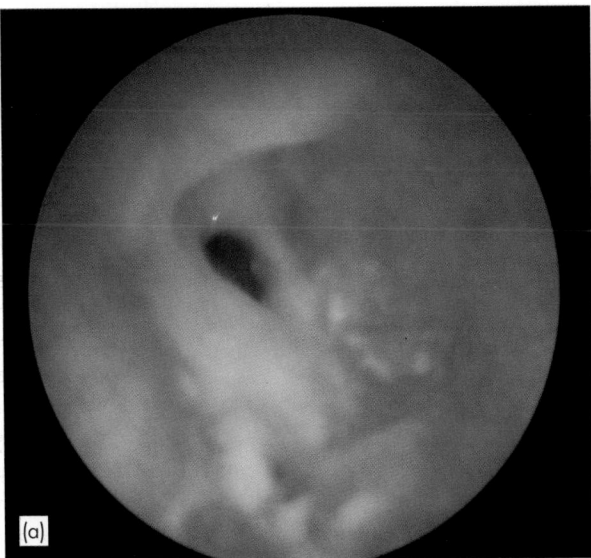 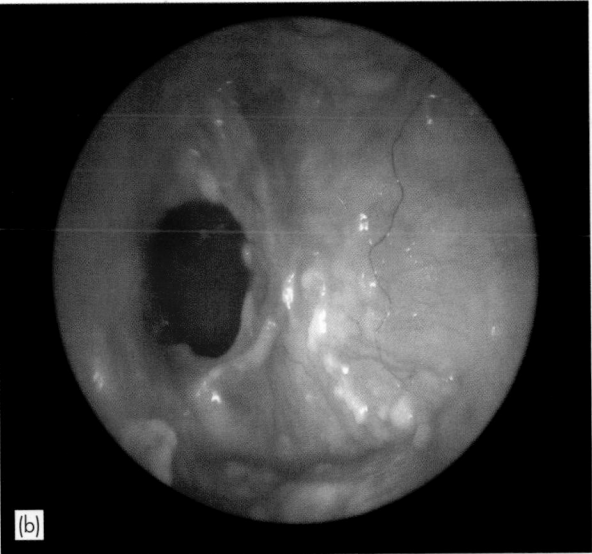

Figure 74.5 Chronic suppurative otitis media. **(a)** In a child with chronic ear discharge, very little information will be gained by inspection of the ear if the physician is unable to clear the ear canal. The child with chronic ear discharge should be considered to have a cholesteatoma until otherwise proven. **(b)** After cleaning the child's ear by mopping with cotton wool until the entire tympanic membrane is visible, the ear discharge in this case is confirmed to be associated with a tympanic membrane perforation with no evidence of cholesteatoma.

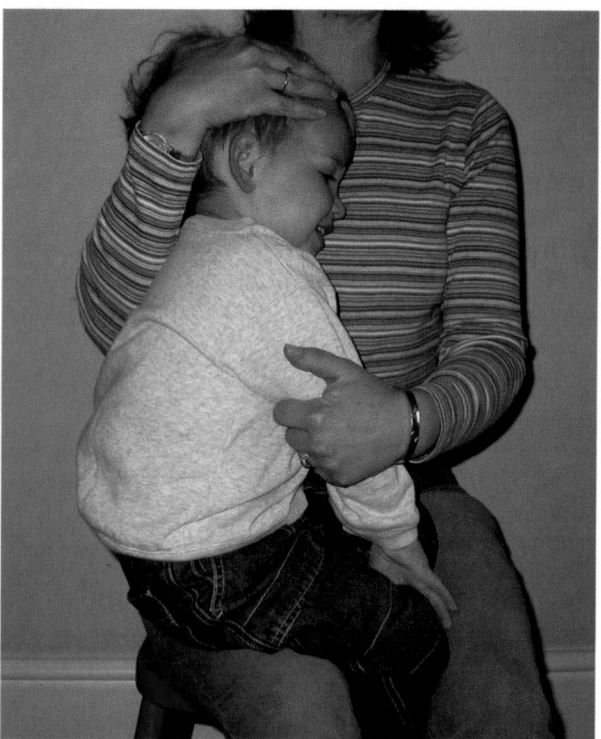

Figure 74.6 Aural toilet in small children. Mopping the ear canal with cotton wool is well tolerated in small children. Nonetheless, it is important to keep the head still during the procedure. The child's parent can assist by gently securing the head and limbs as shown. The child can also be visually distracted with an attractive toy.

Investigation

EAR SWAB

A prospective study to evaluate the value of performing microbiological culture of all discharging ears did not show any statistically discernible benefit over empirically treated ears.[36]

EXAMINATION UNDER ANAESTHETIC

This is rarely necessary as the tympanic membrane perforation can usually be readily identified in the outpatient department after aural mopping. If the child will not tolerate inspection or mopping in the clinic, examination under anaesthetic is necessary to exclude tympanic membrane retraction disease or cholesteatoma.

AUDIOLOGY

Children from the age of four can usually cooperate so that an accurate pure tone audiogram can be obtained. The audiogram will estimate the cochlear and middle ear hearing loss in each ear. Tympanic membrane perforations rarely cause more than 15 dB hearing loss. Larger conductive losses are caused by associated ossicular

pathology. The audiogram may alert the surgeon to this additional problem. Occasionally, associated tympanic membrane pathology, namely tympanic membrane sclerosis, can fix the malleus and cause a greater conductive loss. Significant ipsilateral sensorineural hearing loss may ensure that the patient will not gain any discernible hearing benefit from surgery. Significant contralateral hearing loss may render the patient and surgeon wary of undertaking ear surgery on the ipsilateral ear.

Treatment of ear discharge in the presence of a tympanic membrane perforation

COMMUNITY INTERVENTION

Early uncontrolled reports from Maori and Inuit communities demonstrated a reduction of the prevalence of chronic suppurative otitis media since the introduction of improved housing and better access to healthcare.[37, 38] These reports have not been replicated in other communities in the past 15 years. The ideal treatment of otorrhoea through a chronic tympanic membrane perforation in high-risk communities should include improvements in nutritional status, in living environment and education about the disease, as well as more overtly medical strategies.[39] Despite the identification of risk factors and the introduction of guidelines for the community management of otitis media in severely affected autochthonous populations, there has been no change in prevalence of the disease in the most affected Australian Aboriginal and Inuit communities over the past 20 years.[40, 41]

There exists only one published controlled community intervention trial of the effectiveness of improving public health or primary care services to a community with a high prevalence of paediatric tympanic membrane perforation. This intervention study assessed the impact of introducing well-managed salt water swimming pools to remote Aboriginal communities where children were swimming in stagnant water holes. A significant reduction in tympanic membrane perforation rates ensued.[42] [***]

MEDICAL TREATMENT

Most clinicians regard keeping the ears scrupulously dry as the fundamental step in the prevention of chronic ear discharge in the presence of a perforated tympanic membrane. There is no high quality evidence to support this treatment. It may be that belief in the pathological model presented under Repeated infection from the external ear canal is so firmly held that no one has sought to test the treatment based upon it. Possibly, the futility of any treatment plan which does not include this component may be so obvious to clinicians treating chronic suppurative otitis media that failure to advise patients to keep their ears dry may be considered unethical, and a trial impossible to sanction.[43]

Nonetheless, the salt-water swimming pool trial in Western Australia (see under Community intervention) raises some questions about this conviction. Whilst the trial principally confirms that swimming in dirty water is worse than swimming in clean water, it does also demonstrate that it is possible for some children to allow water into their perforated ears without the development of chronic ear discharge.

Medical treatment includes aural toilet and the provision of topical or systemic antibiotics, topical steroids and topical antiseptics. A systematic review of these interventions was published in 1998[44] and has since been updated.[45] [****] Twenty-four randomized trials were identified. Ten of these trials contained no children and only four trials dealt mainly or exclusively with children.[46, 47, 48, 49] It should be noted in advance that most randomized trials on this topic are of low quality with few offering near complete follow-up records. Details confirming blinding of investigators, randomization and concealment of treatment allocation, as well as data concerning inclusion and exclusion criteria, measures of compliance as well as recording of drop-outs is often lacking. The metaanalysis of randomized trials of nonsurgical treatment of ear discharge in the presence of a perforated tympanic membrane revealed the following in children.[44] Aural toilet alone by mopping with cotton wool wisps was no better in alleviating ear discharge than no treatment at all. Two trials were of markedly different design and came to significantly different conclusions on this point.[46, 47] Topical antibiotics and antiseptics after aural toilet were more effective than no treatment and also more effective than aural toilet alone.[46, 47] There was no difference in effectiveness between topical antiseptics and topical antibiotics in one study involving children.[46]

In adults (but not specifically studied in children), five studies have found that topical antibiotics and antiseptics were generally more effective than systemic antibiotics. The addition of a systemic antibiotic to a topical antibiotic did not improve the effectiveness of treatment.[46] Topical quinolones were significantly more effective than other topical or systemic antibiotics in resolving otorrhoea.[44]

None of the papers assessing fluroquinolones studied in the systematic review included children. More recently, however, a randomized controlled trial in children only has demonstrated a significantly higher cessation of ear discharge with topical ciprofloxacin than a combined antibiotics, steroid and antiseptic preparation.[49] [****] Eleven studies monitored ototoxicity and these found negligible or no changes in hearing levels after topical treatment.[44] The treatments were not effective in promoting the healing of the tympanic membrane perforations.[44]

The following recommendations summarize the findings:

- topical antibiotics with aural toilet is the most effective method of treatment; [****]
- quinolones appear to be more effective than other types of antibiotics in resolving otorrhoea; [****]
- antiseptics may be just as effective as antibiotics. [**]

These conclusions are based on short-term outcome measures and, at best, offer guidance to the temporary management of chronic suppurative otitis media.

Aminoglycosides and ototoxicity

Although clinical studies have not identified hearing impairment as an adverse outcome in the medical treatment of ear discharge associated with chronic tympanic membrane perforation,[45] a review paper in 1993 identified animal studies which associated the use of topical aminoglycosides with ototoxicity.[50] In accordance with this, the Committee on Safety in Medicines published a guideline in 1997 updating doctors of their 1981 warning that topical aminoglycosides were not indicated in patients with perforated ears. A further committee meeting in 1998 did not consider that a submission from the British Association of Otolaryngologists/Head and Neck Surgeons provided any grounds to reverse this warning. At the time of writing, no topical aminoglycoside is officially recognized for use in patients with perforated ears.

The Clinical Audit and Practice Advisory Group, British Association of Otolaryngologists – Head and Neck Surgeons (ENT-UK) have published a consensus statement on the use of aminoglycoside ear drops in the presence of a tympanic membrane perforation.[51] The advisory group recommend that the following be adopted as guidance.

When treating a patient with a discharging ear in whom there is a perforation or patent grommet:

- if a topical aminoglycoside is used, this should only be in the presence of obvious infection;
- topical aminoglycosides should be used for no longer than two weeks;
- the justification for using topical aminoglycosides should be explained to the patient;
- baseline audiometry should be performed, if possible or practical, before treatment with topical aminoglycosides.

Topical otic fluoroquinolones in children

A randomized controlled trial of 0.3 percent ciprofloxacin drops against framycetin, gramicidin and dexamethasone drops for chronic suppurative otitis media in a paediatric Australian Aboriginal population found a significantly higher rate of elimination of ear discharge in the the ciprofloxacin group.[49] [****] The study was double-blinded, the method of allocation was stated, inclusion and exclusion criteria were defined. Almost one-quarter of the original 147 study patients was lost to follow-up. The cure rates were: ciprofloxacin 42 of 55 children (74.6 percent) and framycetin 29 of 56 (51.8 percent). The type of treatment was significantly associated with the outcome ($p = 0.009$). The absolute rate difference is 24.6 percent (CI: 15.8 percent, 33.4 percent). There were no confounding factors. There were minor adverse reactions only, with no rate difference between the treatment arms.

A randomized controlled trial of topical ofloxacin against co-amoxiclav in an entirely paediatric population with acute otitis media noted that the topical fluoroquinolone was well tolerated by the paediatric patients. Treatment-related adverse event rates were 31 percent for augmentin and 6 percent for ofloxacin ($p < 0.001$). Neither treatment significantly altered hearing acuity.[52]

A study of the systemic availability of fluoroquinolones after topical application found minimal systemic uptake and side effects from this class of medicines remains low.[53]

In keeping with their efficacy and lack of side effects in otitis media, the Food and Drug Administration in the USA approved the use of a combined ciprofloxacin and hydrocortisone preparation in 1998. Despite a call for similar approval in the UK,[54] the Committee of Safety in Medicines has still not recognized this preparation.

Antiseptics

The Cochrane Review[44] concluded that topical antiseptics may be just as effective as antibiotics. The reviewers recommended that the effectiveness of cheap topical antiseptics should be studied further. Since then only one randomized controlled trial investigating the efficacy of a topical antiseptic in chronic suppurative otitis media has been published. This work investigated the efficacy of three concentrations of aluminium acetate solution. No difference in the cure rate of the 13 and 3.25 percent solutions was found, but a 1.3 percent solution was less effective.[55] [****] Further work in this area would be of considerable interest as topical antiseptics are cheap.

SURGICAL CLOSURE OF THE TYMPANIC MEMBRANE PERFORATION IN CHILDREN

Spontaneous healing of chronic tympanic membrane perforations is uncommon, and medical interventions are not effective in promoting perforation closure. Surgical intervention is the treatment of choice to effect closure of the perforation. The medical literature provides ample evidence that when this is performed in an adept manner, a high rate of closure is possible in adults, in the short to medium term at least. However, there remains controversy concerning the reperforation rate in children.

Age of the patient

The most important and controversial issue regarding the surgical closure of tympanic membrane perforations in

children is that of the age of the patient at the time of the procedure. Although earlier reports indicated an increased failure rate in small children, studies concluding that age makes no difference now outnumber those that find a difference by five to one. However, in most papers a small sample size leading to insufficient power compromises the accuracy of these conclusions. Because of this limitation, a metaanalysis of paediatric tympanoplasty provides the most authoritative analysis of parameters that correlate with closure of the tympanic membrane. One such study, based on a Medline search of the English language literature, has been published.[56]

Nineteen articles provided sufficient age-related data of surgical outcomes for a linear regression of success rate against age to be performed. Success was defined as an intact tympanic membrane following surgery. The success rate was defined as the number of intact tympanic membranes following surgery divided by the total number undergoing surgery. These data are shown in **Figure 74.7**.

A more thorough statistical analysis was performed. The mean weighted differences of success rate were calculated by age for each age from 6 to 13 years in one-year increments. Linear regression of this statistic against age in years indicated a significant association of greater success with advancing age ($p < 0.005$).

Exclusion of the youngest patients does not eliminate the relationship between success rate and age, for when the analysis is repeated in the age group 9 to 13 years an association persists ($p < 0.03$).

Other potential risk factors

In the belief that something that is more prevalent in the younger age groups must account for this result, the same authors sought to identify the cause of this relationship. A metaanalysis of supposed risk factors for surgical failure of tympanic membrane repair was performed using data from 30 studies. None of the following had any discernible influence on the outcome of surgery in comparative studies: perforation size (less versus greater than 50 percent), prior or concurrent adenoidectomy

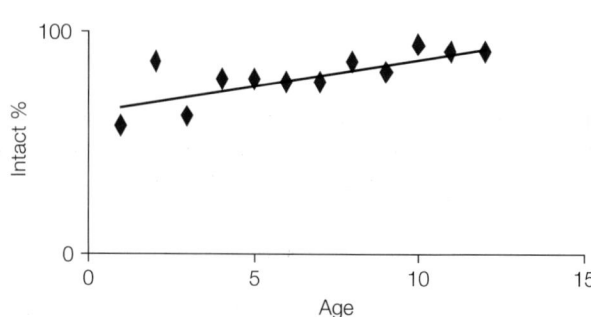

Figure 74.7 Results of tympanoplasty from 19 published articles according to patient age. Unweighted data (previously unpublished) and regression line are shown. Courtesy of Jeffrey T Vrabec.

(yes/no), status of the contralateral ear (normal/not normal) or Eustachian tube test result (good/poor) (see **Table 74.3**). They also compared variables between studies which had not been quantitatively assessed within any existing paper: infection at the time of surgery (yes/no) and surgical technique (overlay/underlay) and, again, found no significantly discernible influence on outcome.

Subsequent papers

Since the tympanoplasty metaanalysis, there have been a number of papers describing tympanoplasty with cartilage repair of the tympanic membrane.[57] The authors suggest that there is no increased rate of tympanic membrane repair failure in small children with this technique. It should be remembered that the same claims were made about fascia repair of the tympanic membrane in small children. Until such time as rigorous analysis of sufficient numbers with age-related data is performed then such can claims cannot be regarded as proven.

OTHER AIMS OF SURGICAL CLOSURE OF THE TYMPANIC MEMBRANE

Hearing impairment

It is well established that the hearing impairment caused by tympanic membrane perforations is dependent on the size of the perforation and many tiny perforations cause minimal hearing impairment. In general, the hearing gain from tympanic membrane closure alone is small.

Detailed analysis of hearing outcomes in paediatric tympanoplasty is restricted because of the lack of raw data from existing studies. Pooled data indicate that: 85 percent of 567 children had postoperative speech reception thresholds of less than 30 dB HL; 70 percent had postoperative speech reception thresholds of less than 20 dB HL; 87 percent had a postoperative air-bone gap of less than 20 dB HL.[56] No correlation of these data with preoperative factors was performed.

Elimination of middle ear pathology

Sheehy and Shelton have suggested that tympanoplasty should eradicate pathological conditions from the middle

ear.[58] In children, the surgeon may not be able to achieve this aim. Indeed, histological analysis of temporal bones not infrequently identifies the presence of middle ear inflammation behind an intact tympanic membrane.[4]

The following sequelae suggesting the persistence of middle ear inflammation despite closure of the perforation were tabulated in the metaanalysis of paediatric tympanoplasty[56] – otitis media with effusion: 75/708 (10.6 percent); atelectasis: 31/478 (6.7 percent).

Cases of postoperative cholesteatoma were also seen. These may be iatrogenic or due to progression of disease.

LONG-TERM RESULTS

Long-term follow-up of patients inevitably results in some loss of data as patients move away, are unable to attend or even die from other causes. There are statistical techniques to compensate for this loss of information. Long-term follow-up data which do not use such probabilistic techniques are often meaningless and possibly misleading. The only paper using life-table analysis to study tympanoplasty in children has shown a deterioration over time of the repaired tympanic membrane due to increasing perforation and myringitis. Even at one year following surgery, untreated middle ear inflammation has caused, through effusion, perforation and myringitis, the disease free rate to drop to 0.63 (CI 0.42, 0.81).[59]

TIMING OF TYMPANOPLASTY IN CHILDREN

While the factors causing an increased failure rate in young children have not been unequivocally identified, there appears to be some merit in delaying the operation until such time that the likelihood of surgical failure is minimized (has fallen to or near adult levels). The decision to offer surgical treatment in a child with a tympanic membrane perforation should therefore not be a reflex initiated by sighting the perforation.

A planned delay in surgical treatment prolongs the period during which infection may enter from the ear canal so diligent use of prophylactic manoeuvres must be employed to maintain a dry ear.

Table 74.3 Factors that do not influence the outcome of tympanoplasty in children.

Parameter	Perforation size (less versus greater than 50%)	Prior or concurrent adenoidectomy (Y/N)	Status of the contralateral ear (normal/not)	Eustachian tube test result (good/poor)	Infection at the time of surgery (Y/N)	Surgical technique (underlay/overlay)
Number	388/484 versus 102/147	115/146 versus 187/235	401/495 versus 182/254	83/95 versus 41/53	44/60 versus 408/514	872/1069 versus 692/830
WMD	1.46 (CI −25.2, 28.1)	3.10 (CI −23.6, 29.8)	6.48 (CI −15.0, 27.9)	14.69 (CI −20.8, 50.1)	73.31 versus 81.18	88.16 versus 90.40
P	0.91	0.82	0.55	0.42	0.26	0.86

WMD, weighed mean difference. Reprinted from Ref. 56, with permission.

Preventing the ingress of water is the most important of these in the industrial world. For the patient with no interest in swimming the extra care required to control infections may be very small. The child should be taught how to keep water away from the ear when washing. When washing the hair or face, a water-resistant barrier should also be used to exclude any stray drops.

Maintaining a dry ear requires extra care when the child takes an interest in swimming. The options for care include banning swimming or permitting limited surface swimming with the use of a barrier in the ear canal. Since most children greatly enjoy swimming, provision of swim plugs and advice about avoiding diving below the surface of the water should be routinely provided while awaiting surgical closure of the perforation.

It will rarely be possible for the surgeon to confidently offer a discernible improvement in hearing. The most tangible benefit will arise if there exists some compromise of the patient's health or activity by the risk of infection. Some patients with no ear discharge, minimal hearing loss and no compromise of daily activity may justifiably prefer to decline an offer of surgical intervention.

SURGICAL TECHNIQUE

The tympanic membrane perforation may be only one of several complications of chronic otitis media present in the affected ear. These other complications may also affect the tympanic membrane. Tympanosclerosis, atelectasis and myringitis may all be found accompanying a perforation on the same eardrum. The complications may also affect the remainder of the middle ear. Mucosal hyperplasia due to chronic suppurative otitis media may still be present. Ossicular fixation or defects may be evident. The aim of tympanoplasty is to restore the middle ear including the sound transformer.[58] In keeping with this approach, adequate repair of a tympanic membrane perforation requires adequate repair of the middle ear not just closure of the defect. Thus, the extent of surgery deemed to be adequate varies according to the severity of the disease. Very mild disease may require no more than attention to the perforation alone. More severe disease may require attention to the middle ear space and tympanic membrane, as well as the perforation.

The tympanic membrane may be entirely healthy apart from the presence of a small perforation. In this circumstance the intervention required to close the hole may be no more than excision of the rim of the perforation with the placement of a small graft to close the defect.[60] The procedure may be performed as a day case and healing occurs within weeks. There is no requirement to pack the ear postoperatively. There are series reported using this technique that have excellent results.[61] [*] A key point for achievement of these results appears to be careful selection of patients.[61]

If there is ancillary tympanic membrane disease, treatment of the tympanic membrane as well as the perforation may be necessary.[62] [*] Excision of the rim of the perforation remains important. This procedure also requires secure reinforcement of the entire tympanic membrane around the defect so that the graft obturates the perforation and is in contact with the entire rim of the perforation. Although reabsorbable materials are sometimes inserted into the middle ear to support this tissue, it is possible to support the graft on the annulus and manubrium. Because of extensive coexisting tympanic membrane disease, reinforcement of the entire tympanic membrane with temporalis fascia, tragal perichondrium or cartilage is frequently necessary.[63] [*]

Grossly inflamed mucosa has been identified as an independent risk factor for later abnormality of the repaired tympanic membrane.[64] [**] It has been suggested that under this circumstance repair be performed with cartilage rather than temporalis fascia. It is also possible to reduce thickened mucosa that physically impedes placement of a graft. This is most effectively performed with a KTP laser which acts as a haemostat as it vaporizes the excess tissue.

Injury to the mucosa of the medial surface of the middle ear may cause adhesions to the tympanic membrane graft during healing. Division of pre-existing adhesions may promote this. In addition, factors that narrow the slender middle ear cleft, such as thickened middle ear mucosa or retraction of the umbo increase this risk. Under any of the preceding circumstances, it is prudent to insert a barrier to prevent contact between the medial and lateral surfaces during healing. Thin (0.25 mm) silastic or ophthalmic gelfilm are suitable.

Umbo retraction is particularly common in perforations with extensive loss of the inferior part of the tympanic membrane. If the umbo retraction is particularly marked, it may be necessary to disarticulate the ossicular chain to lateralize the manubrium satisfactorily. The malleus head is excised and a malleus to stapes assembly is performed in addition to the tympanic membrane repair. Amputation of the umbo should not be performed as this greatly diminishes acoustic transmission through the middle ear.

Anterior perforations present a great problem to many surgeons (see below). Good access to these perforations can be obtained with an anterior canalplasty.[62] All suggestions concerning surgical technique are grade D recommendations.

OUTCOMES OF SURGERY FOR TYMPANIC MEMBRANE PERFORATION

The metaanalysis of the surgical repair of tympanic membrane perforations suggests that perforation closure can be expected in 90 percent of cases. It should be that this figure is gleaned from case series proffered by motivated individuals with a special interest in otology in children. More typical figures for success rate by British surgeons seems to be between 74 percent (small perforation) and 56 percent (large perforation).[65, 66] This raises a number of important points.

- The surgical repair of the tympanic membrane is a difficult procedure requiring considerable skill.
- There is considerable variation in outcomes from surgeon to surgeon.
- Patients cannot be informed as part of the consent process if no audit of the operating surgeon's results is performed.
- It is debatable whether any surgeon should continue to offer this treatment if his/her success rate for the procedure is as low as 56 percent.
- An appropriate response to audit is essential.
- Training of tympanic membrane repair should include techniques to improve access.

ATROPHY OF THE PARS TENSA OF THE TYMPANIC MEMBRANE (INCLUDING RETRACTION POCKETS)

Introduction

The study of the treatment of pars tensa atrophy and its sequelae is particularly short of high-quality evidence. Consequently this topic is intensely controversial.

Chronic otitis media and the pathology of atrophy of the pars tensa of the tympanic membrane

Atrophy of the pars tensa of the tympanic membrane occurs through loss of the collagenous fibrous layer.[67] The cause of this pathology is not fully understood; however, pars tensa atrophy is associated with chronic middle ear inflammatory changes in histological studies in human temporal bones.[68, 69] Animal model studies have demonstrated that pars tensa atrophy can result from middle ear inflammation.[70, 71]

There is also evidence that some cases of tympanic membrane atrophy are associated with sniffing. In the presence of an open Eustachian tube, sniffing results in a sharp reduction in Eustachian tube and middle ear pressure. An unwanted consequence of the sharp drop in middle ear pressure is retraction of the tympanic membrane.[72] The stimulus for this behaviour appears to be the sensation of pressure and range of abnormal sounds perceived by the patient during the period that the Eustachian tube is open. The benefit resulting from sniffing is closure of the tube and cessation of the unpleasant symptoms.[73] That this behaviour is learnt has been suggested by studies which have identified that the Eustachian tube need not be a passive bystander but is sometimes actively opened in preparation for the sniff.

Following the loss of this stiff structural element, the thinned area of tympanic membrane can be more easily displaced by the pressure difference across the tympanic membrane. The relative negative middle ear pressure found in association with chronic otitis media results in a visible medial displacement ('retraction') of the weakened area.[69] Reduced middle ear pressures are usually attributed to increased rates of gas exchange across the middle ear mucosa during periods of inflammation, but may be consequent upon gas extraction caused by sniffing.

Should the middle ear pressure be raised, as after sleep, the tympanic membrane may bulge laterally.[74, 75]

Pars tensa atrophy with retraction may focally affect any segment of the tympanic membrane and may affect the entire tympanic membrane.[76]

The tendency of retraction pockets caused by chronic otitis media to form in the posterosuperior part of the tympanic membrane may be due to a combination of the following factors. The posterosuperior pars tensa is more vascular than other areas of the tympanic membrane and may be subject to more marked inflammatory reactions.[77] The fibrous layer in this region is less complete and can be devoid of circular fibres.[78]

Atrophy of the pars tensa ranges from mild through to more severe retraction with fixation of the atrophic segment to the bony walls of the middle ear (see **Figure 74.8**). Some cases of tympanic membrane collapse are

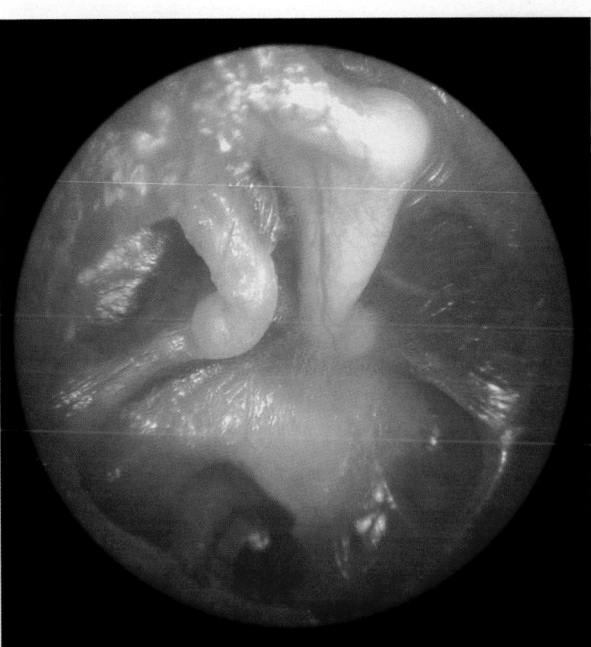

Figure 74.8 Retraction of the pars tensa. The tympanic membrane of this seven-year-old girl's ear is atrophic and retracted. The fundus of the retraction pocket is not wholly visible and there is some accumulation of skin in the retracted area. Although there is a fluid level visible behind the anterior part of the tympanic membrane, the ossicular chain is intact and the child's hearing remained normal. Two years after this photograph was taken the girl's ear remains unchanged.

progressive. They may become associated with erosion of the ossicles (see **Figure 74.9**).[79] A small proportion of advanced pars tensa retraction pockets progress to become cholesteatoma (see **Figure 74.10**).[80]

Definitions and classification

Thus, pars tensa retraction includes not only a range of appearances, but also a clinically important minority which will insidiously deteriorate. Terminology and classifications were specifically designed to attempt to distinguish the high-risk subgroup, which progresses to cholesteatoma.

Sade's classifications of retraction of the pars tensa of the tympanic membrane defined two types of retraction and classified each on an ordinal scale.

1. Atelectasis, defined as diffuse 'retraction of the tympanic membrane towards the promontorium' (see **Table 74.4**).[69]
2. Retraction pocket, defined as focal 'retraction of the pars tensa towards or into the attic'.[79]

The distinction between Sade's two types of retraction has faded, with the terms defined for retraction towards the promontorium now freely used for all pars tensa retractions.

Further classifications of atelectasis have been defined. These have largely followed the original, using an ordinal scale largely based on anatomical features of the retraction pocket. For the most advanced stage of most of these classifications, the definition reflects the role of retraction pockets in the genesis of cholesteatoma by including a nonanatomical feature such as adherence of the pocket or keratin accumulation within the pocket. A recent, innovative classification has also reflected the tendency of retraction pockets to damage the ossicular chain by including an audiometric parameter.[81] No evidence has been presented to date that any of these provides a more precise prediction of disease progression than the Sade classification.

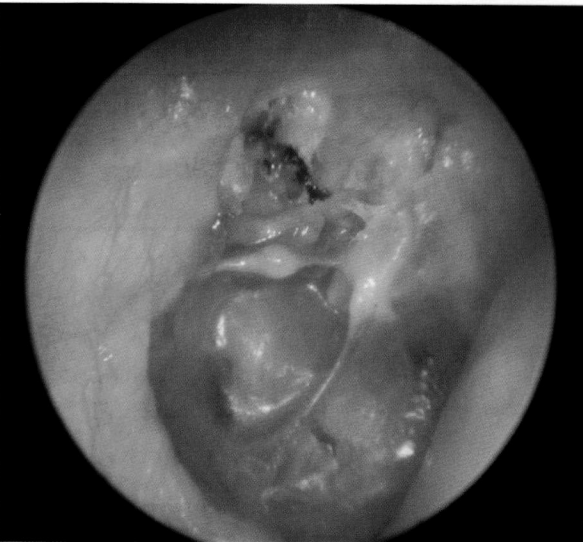

Figure 74.10 Retraction of the pars tensa with cholesteatoma. A small proportion of retraction pockets progress to form cholesteatoma. In this ear there is erosion of the manubrium, the incus, the scutum and the posterior annulus as well as the development of a cholesteatoma. Note that the anterior mesotympanum/protympanum remains ventilated.

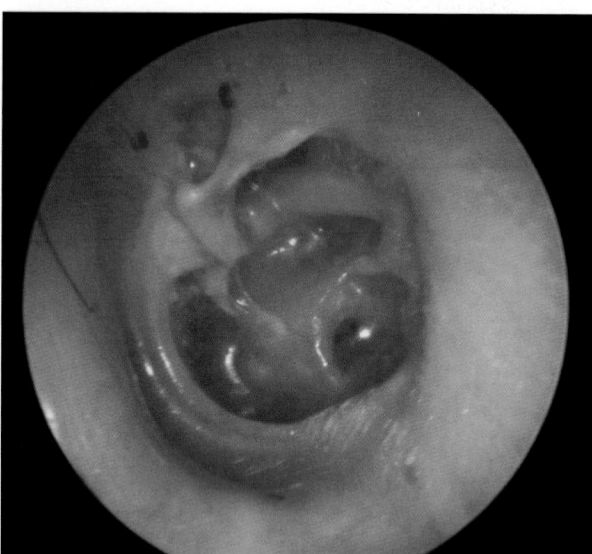

Figure 74.9 Retraction of the pars tensa with ossicular erosion. The tympanic membrane of this young man is almost entirely atrophic and retracted. The fundus of the retraction pocket is not entirely visible but the pocket remains self-cleaning. The manubrium, the long process of the incus and the stapes superstructure have all been eroded. Although there is air in the protympanum, the atrophic tympanic membrane is draped over the facial nerve and the stapes footplate. The last feature has resulted in elevation of the hearing threshold being restricted to 30 dB hearing loss. This is his better hearing ear and the hospital notes indicate his ear has remained unchanged for over a decade.

Table 74.4 Sade classification of atelectasis.

Grade	Title	Description
1	Retracted ear	Slight retraction of the tympanic membrane
2	Severe retraction	Retraction of the tympanic membrane, touching the incus or the stapes
3[a]	Atelectasis	Tympanic membrane touching the promontorium
4	Adhesive otitis	Tympanic membrane adherent to the promontorium

[a]Of these, stage III was, itself, called 'tympanic membrane touching the promontorium' or 'atelectasis'. The ambiguous nature of the term 'atelectasis' has been compounded as the distinction between retraction 'towards the promontorium' and 'towards the attic' has been neglected. For many surgeons, 'atelectasis' has metamorphosed into a term describing any retraction pocket of the pars tensa. Reprinted from Ref. 79, with permission.

Epidemiology of retraction of the tympanic membrane

POPULATION-BASED STUDIES

A population-based survey of 15,890 Navajo children determined the point prevalence of tympanic membrane retraction in this population at 1.9 percent.[82] Another such survey of 794 children followed up in the Dunedin area of New Zealand identified a point prevalence of 1.3 percent retracted tympanic membranes in this cohort at the age of 15.[83]

PREVALENCE IN THE POPULATION OF CHILDREN WITH PERSISTENT OTITIS MEDIA WITH EFFUSION

Prospective follow-up of children with persistent otitis media with effusion has confirmed an increase in the prevalence of pars tensa retraction with increasing duration of follow-up. Fifteen percent developed some degree of retraction.[84, 85] Only 2 percent of patients were found to have advanced (Sade grade III/IV) pars tensa retraction. The age distribution of patients whose retracted tympanic membranes cause sufficient concern to prompt surgery is not necessarily the same as the prevalence of retracted tympanic membranes in the community. The former distribution is shown in (**Figure 74.11**). This strikingly confirms that intervention for tympanic membrane retraction is predominantly a paediatric problem.

Natural history of progression of retraction of the tympanic membrane

Follow-up of patients with tympanic membrane retraction over a mean of three to five years using the Sade classifications has established the following.

- Retraction without atrophy (grade I atelectasis) is usually a transitory condition. It rarely progresses to more advanced stages and frequently reverts to a normal tympanic membrane. This behaviour is discernibly different to more advanced stages of this disease (see **Table 74.5**).[86]
- Grades II and III of the disease are quite dynamic, having the ability to improve, deteriorate or remain the same. Over three to five years, 16 percent may be expected to deteriorate.[79]
- Grade IV atelectasis, on the other hand, does not spontaneously revert back to earlier stages of the disease. This is significantly different to the behaviour of the other stages of the disease (see **Table 74.5**).[79]
- Sixteen percent of grade IV retraction towards the promontory will progress to perforation.[79]
- Ten percent of clean pockets retracting towards the attic will progress to the accumulation of keratin debris.[79]
- A large number of retraction pockets which progress towards the attic present at a late stage.[79]

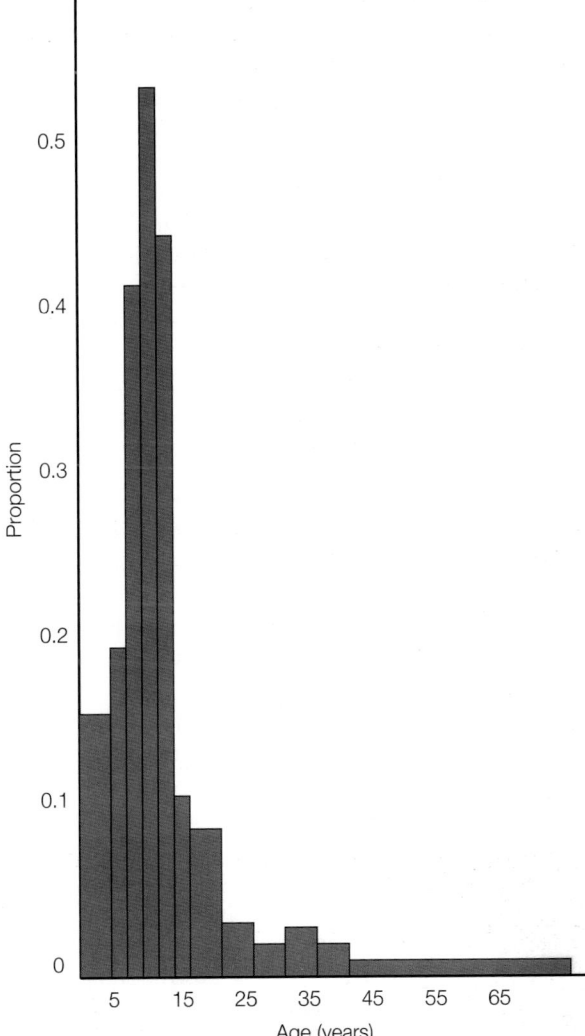

Figure 74.11 Histogram of age of patient at time of surgical excision of pars tensa retraction pocket.

Table 74.5 Natural history of pars tensa retraction towards the promontory.

Investigator	Sade grade assessed	Change	Probability of change
Tay (1995)[86]	I	Improve	0.85
	II, III, IV	Improve	0.29
Sade (1981)[79]	I, II, III	Improve	0.42
	IV	Improve	0
	I, II, III	Worsen	0.17
	IV	Worsen	0.20

It should be noted that the distinction between Sade's two types of pars tensa retraction has not been widely followed. As a result, the results of the quantitative analysis of the behaviour of retraction towards the promontory has been freely interchanged with that of retraction towards the attic.

The only factor associated with the progression of pars tensa retraction is progression of disease beyond Sade grade I.[86] In fact, this evidence might more clearly be interpreted as showing that grade I retractions do not progress. Once atrophy has occurred progression is a possibility.

Although the Sade grade remains the most widely accepted adopted means of monitoring disease progression, the risk of deterioration from one grade to the next is low and the classification provides a low predictive value for disease progression.

Symptoms

Retraction of the pars tensa of the tympanic membrane may be associated with a complex and highly variable set of symptoms and signs. These result not just from the atrophy of the tympanic membrane itself, but also from the underlying chronic otitis media, as well as Eustachian tube phenomena. Furthermore, complications of the retraction such as erosion of the ossicles or infection of keratin accumulating within the retraction pocket also contribute to the melange of symptoms.

Frequently there may be no symptoms at all. Variable hearing loss due to chronic inflammation with accumulation of a middle ear effusion may occur. Persistent hearing loss may result if the tip of the long process of the incus has been eroded. In general, hearing loss is mild when there is a contact between the retracted tympanic membrane and an intact stapes. Erosion of the stapes superstructure results in a larger and more clinically significant conductive hearing loss. Episodic or recurrent otalgia or otorrhoea may occur. These may be due to episodes of acute otitis media or infection of debris within the pocket. Some patients with retraction of the pars tensa experience pain on performing Valsalva's manoeuvre. Variable sound perception due to variable Eustachian tube patency also occurs.[73] For a similar reason, some patients experience a feeling of fullness or pressure in their ears. They find that sniffing, which reduces the middle ear pressure and locks the Eustachian tube, eases this sensation.[72]

Signs

Examination of the retracted tympanic membrane requires the following steps:

- provision of an adequate view of the tympanic membrane;
- establishing the diagnosis;
- staging the disease.

OBTAINING AN ADEQUATE VIEW OF THE TYMPANIC MEMBRANE

Please refer to Clinical examination in the section on Chronic perforation of the tympanic membrane above.

ESTABLISHING THE DIAGNOSIS

Careful microscopic examination of the retracted pars tensa is required to determine the fine details necessary to diagnose and stage the disease.

Care is required to differentiate a retraction pocket from a perforated tympanic membrane and the two-dimensional view provided by a hand-held otoscope may not be sufficient. The otological microscope will help determine if the retracted area is perforated, if other tympanic membrane disease is present and whether there is any evidence for acute or chronic middle ear inflammation.

If keratin is accumulating within the retraction pocket, some authorities would consider that the pathology is better considered a cholesteatoma. However, a minor accumulation of dry keratin, associated with streaming of the keratin out of the retraction pocket, usually remains asymptomatic and is not always associated with disease progression.

STAGING THE RETRACTION POCKET

It is important to attempt to identify the margins and entire fundus of the retraction pocket. It may disappear behind the posterior annulus, the manubrium or the chorda tympani.

The structures under the floor of the retracted tympanic membrane should be carefully inspected. The promontory and round window and ossicles are readily identifiable when the inferior pars tensa is retracted. If there is retraction of the posterior tympanic membrane, the abnormality is readily recognized because the long process of the incus will be clearly visible.

The state of the incus and stapes should be carefully inspected. The retraction may be in contact with the long process of the incus only or may envelop the incus and stapes like clingfilm. The lenticular process of the incus may be eroded so that the capitulum is partly visible. The long process may be eroded so that it no longer makes contact with the stapes. There may be erosion of the posterior annulus so that the stapedius tendon and pyramid are clearly visible. The stapes superstructure may be absent so that the oval window is visible.

There may be keratin accumulating within the pocket. An early sign of this accumulation is a stream of wax emanating from the pocket around the posterior annulus and along the posterior canal wall. In more advanced cases, keratin may accumulate within the retracted area. This may be a generalized feature of the pocket. Keratin accumulation may be focal and associated with areas where the fundus of the pocket is no longer visible.

There may be granulation tissue associated with the retraction if this accumulating keratin becomes infected. There may be granulation tissue within the pocket itself. It may extend onto the adjoining canal wall, in which case the underlying bony annulus may become devitalized (see **Figures 74.8, 74.9** and **74.10**).

Investigations

PURE TONE AUDIOMETRY

Pars tensa retraction pockets cause morbidity not just through progression to cholesteatoma, but also by eroding the ossicular chain resulting in hearing loss. Although ignored in the Sade classification, quantitative assessment of hearing status is an important parameter in the complex process of deciding whether to offer intervention for a retraction pocket. To this end, some classifications require hearing evaluation as part of retraction pocket staging.[81]

EXAMINATION UNDER ANAESTHETIC

If the child cannot tolerate aural cleaning in the clinic and inspection of the entire tympanic membrane cannot be performed, examination of the ear under anaesthetic should be arranged.

Management of retraction of the pars tensa of the tympanic membrane

The management of the variable and uncertain behaviour of retracted tympanic membranes is highly controversial. The data presented above under Natural history of progression of retraction of the tympanic membrane indicate that most cases do not progress. Nonetheless, some retracted tympanic membranes progress to form cholesteatoma. At present we cannot predict with certainty which cases will progress. As a result, there are two possible management strategies. The simpler is to wait until cholesteatoma has developed, at which stage intervention is clearly justifiable. The more controversial is to intervene before cholesteatoma develops, using the best available risk factors.

The argument for early intervention asserts that a minor procedure can prevent progression of the disease and the development of complications prior to the development of cholesteatoma. One refinement of this strategy argues that fixation of the tympanic membrane to the promontory is an indication for surgical intervention, since grade IV retractions do not spontaneously improve.

A second scheme proposes that grade III retractions which are progressing are the ideal indication for surgical intervention, since fixation of the tympanic membrane is, itself, associated with a higher incidence of postoperative residual cholesteatoma.[87, 88] [**] Given that a diagnosis of late stage retraction provides a low positive predictive value for the subsequent emergence of cholesteatoma, this strategy will necessarily result in some patients undergoing an intervention which could be considered unnecessary.

The specific risks associated with surgery for tympanic membrane retraction include the following.

- Surgical elevation of the collapsed tympanic membrane from the ossicles carries some risk of cochlear injury.
- Failure of the tympanic membrane to heal after surgery may result in an iatrogenic perforation.
- There is also a risk of spawning an iatrogenic cholesteatoma by leaving epithelium capable of generating keratin in the mesotympanum in those cases with adherence of the tympanic membrane to the walls of the middle ear.
- Even if the tympanic membrane heals, the tympanic membrane may retract again.

Offering surgery which could be considered unnecessary and which carries some risk of morbidity requires some justification. The justification is that allowing the disease to progress to cholesteatoma exposes the patient to the complications of this disease and condemns the affected patient to extensive surgery as the only treatment option. This, in turn, exposes the patient to a high risk of associated morbidity.

It follows that the debate about intervention pivots on the balance of the risks of surgical intervention at various stages of this progression, as well as the risks associated with the complications of the natural course of the disease. At present, there are no controlled trials of interventions for retraction of the pars tensa. The comparative data required to quantify the above arguments are, therefore, unavailable. Even if such data were already published, the information is unlikely to be generalizable, given the highly operator-dependent nature of the outcome of otological surgery. Since many surgeons performing otological surgery do not keep detailed data about the morbidity associated with their surgery, there is little consensus on the indications for surgical intervention for pars tensa retraction pockets.

Surgical intervention for retraction pockets

GROMMET INSERTION

Treatment of tympanic membrane atelectasis with insertion of a ventilation tube into the remaining healthy tympanic membrane is widely practised. However the best available evidence at present suggests that this treatment does not influence the development of tympanic membrane retraction.[84, 89] Insertion of multiple ventilation tubes results in more tympanic membrane scarring and no benefit in limiting the progression of tympanic membrane retraction.[30]

REINFORCEMENT TYMPANOPLASTY

Excision of the retraction pocket with grafting of the tympanic membrane is also widely performed. The graft material is usually temporalis fascia, perichondrium or cartilage. If the pocket is removed intact there need be no concern about residual disease. If the pocket is adherent to the middle ear walls and tears during removal a second-look procedure may be necessary since the risk of residual disease is as high as with cholesteatoma surgery.[87] If the retraction pocket is firmly adherent to the ossicles, particularly the stapes, there is a risk of sensorineural hearing loss while removing the disease. Using a KTP laser to remove the disease on the ossicles can lessen this. The laser vaporizes the epithelium and, in contrast to mechanical techniques, does not require movement to remove disease.[90]

RETRACTION POCKET EXCISION

The realization that simple excision of the retraction is usually associated with spontaneous healing of the tympanic membrane has introduced a less invasive procedure for the management of pars tensa retraction pockets (see **Figure 74.12**).[91, 92] As this simple operation does not require insertion of a graft, it is simpler than other techniques for tympanic membrane repair, can usually be performed permeatally, does not require packing of the ear and can be performed as a day case procedure. By virtue of its simplicity, excision of the retraction pocket can be genuinely offered as prophylaxis

against the development of cholesteatoma. The introduction of this procedure has heightened the intensity of the debate concerning the indications for intervention. The results of excision of series of pars tensa retractions are shown in **Table 74.6**.

Long term results after surgery for retraction pockets

As yet there are no published long-term studies using life table methods of the outcome of surgery on pars tensa retraction pockets. An unpublished, long-term follow-up study of patients in Gloucestershire using life table analysis indicates that many procedures are followed by further retraction of the tympanic membrane (see **Figure 74.13**). As such, surgery for pars tensa retraction might best be viewed as a temporizing procedure, much in the manner of the insertion of grommets for symptomatic persistent glue ear, rather than a definitive cure.

Table 74.6 Outcomes of tympanic membrane retraction pocket excision.

Author	Number	Normal	Recurrence	Follow-up (months)
Stewart[91]	31	12	12	60
Wayloff[93]	21	9	6	n/a
Ars[94]	149	126	23	60
Robinson[88]	66	43	18	14
Bowdler[95]	46	21	13	
O'Sullivan[96]	31	23	7	16

n/a, not available.

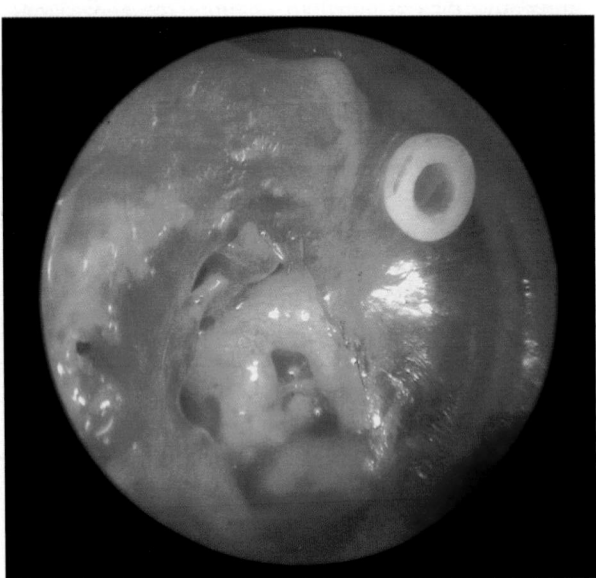

Figure 74.12 Excision of a tympanic membrane retraction pocket. This child has undergone an Ars-Marquet procedure, in which the tympanic membrane retraction pocket is excised and a minigrommet is inserted through the healthy tympanic membrane remnant. No repair of the defect is undertaken as in the majority of cases the tympanic membrane repairs itself, much as after a traumatic perforation. This 11-year-old girl's tympanic membrane healed normally even though she had an acute otitis media five days after surgery.

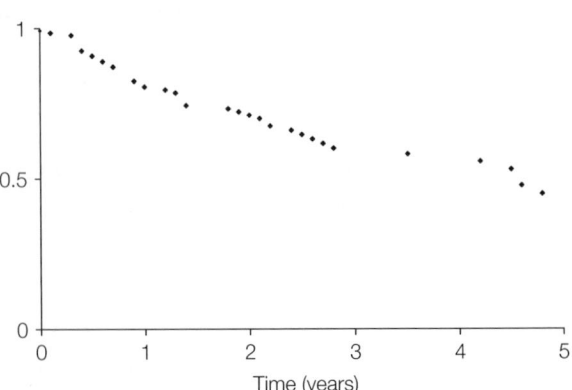

Figure 74.13 Life table analysis of long-term follow up after excision of pars tensa retraction pocket. The outcome measure was the development of further atrophy and retraction (at least Sade grade II). The outcome does not indicate the need for reoperation. The data are gleaned predominantly from children operated at Gloucestershire Royal Hospital between 1990 and 1995 (unpublished data).

Ossicular chain defects associated with retraction pockets

The commonest ossicular defect associated with pars tensa tympanic membrane atrophy is erosion of the tip of the long process of the incus.[97] This can be directly repaired by interposing a graft or prosthesis between the residual long process and the capitulum.[98, 99, 100] Larger defects of the long process can be repaired by removal of the incus and repositioning it as a malleus-stapes assembly.[99]

CHOLESTEATOMA

Definition

The stratified squamous epithelium of the tympanic membrane and external ear canal can migrate prior to being shed at the entrance to the external meatus. In this way, the ear canal protects itself from filling with shed keratinocytes.

Under some circumstances, squamous epithelium accumulates within the temporal bone. If the squamous epithelium and accumulating keratinocytes are within the middle ear space, this condition is termed 'cholesteatoma'.[101]

Failure of epithelial migration and accumulation of keratin within the ear canal (or surgically modified ear canal) is not generally termed cholesteatoma. However, if there is also focal erosion of external ear canal bone in association with keratin accumulation some authorities term this 'external canal cholesteatoma'.

Pathogenesis and classification

Following the ascendancy of histological examination for pathological diagnosis in the mid-nineteenth century, early theories that cholesteatoma was a tumour were superseded by hypotheses that the condition was due either to a vestigial structure or a metaplastic process. This distinction between congenital and acquired forms of cholesteatoma remains important to this day, particularly in children.

Congenital cholesteatoma

Keratin cysts may accumulate because the epithelium from which they arise is closed. In general, such cysts may arise as a result of developmental abnormality or may be iatrogenic. Epidermal cysts which are found medial to an intact tympanic membrane (see **Figure 74.14**) are considered to be 'congenital' if they fulfil the criteria of Derlaki and Clemis:

- white mass medial to an intact tympanic membrane;
- normal pars tensa and flaccida;

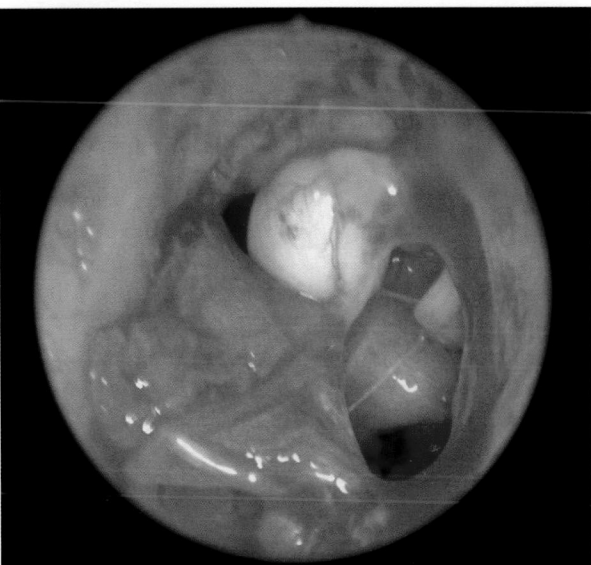

Figure 74.14 Congenital cholesteatoma. This three-year-old boy presented with hearing loss and in addition to glue ear was noted to have a white mass behind the anterosuperior part of the intact tympanic membrane. He had no previous history of surgical intervention and satisfied the criteria for congenital cholesteatoma. The epidermoid cyst was removed intact and the ossicular chain was preserved. His hearing remains normal.

- no previous history of ear discharge, perforation or previous otological procedures;[102]
- it has been proposed that prior bouts of acute otitis media are not grounds for excluding the possibility of congenital cholesteatoma since it is very rare for a child to have no episodes of otitis media in its first five years.[103]

A vestigial structure, the epidermoid formation, from which congenital cholesteatoma may originate has been identified in the anterior epitympanum.[104] However, not all congenital cholesteatomas are located anterosuperiorly[105] and not all are found to be epithelial cysts.[106] It therefore remains possible that other processes, such as the invagination of squamous epithelium from the developing ear canal[107] or the ingestion of squamous elements in amniotic fluid,[108] may be involved.

Some epithelial cysts that satisfy the definition of a congenital cholesteatoma do not present until the fourth or fifth decade. It has been suggested that the origins of these may in fact be metaplastic[109] or acquired from the aberrant resolution of a pars tensa retraction pocket.[110]

Surgical causes of middle ear epithelial cysts include failure to completely remove a previous cholesteatoma or implantation of squamous epithelium as a consequence of careless handling of normal tympanic membrane.

Acquired cholesteatoma

More commonly, keratin accumulates within a diverticulum of tympanic membrane squamous epithelium which extends into the middle ear. Even though this structure communicates with the external ear, keratin accumulates as a result of inadequate epithelial migration.

Recognized mechanisms leading to such acquired cholesteatoma include the following.

- **Immigration**: migration of squamous epithelium into the middle ear through a defect in the tympanic membrane.[111] While this mechanism continues to be recognized, it is responsible for only a very small proportion of cholesteatomas.
- **Retraction**: progressive retraction of the tympanic membrane, either in the pars flaccida or associated with atrophy of the pars tensa.[112]
- **Basal cell hyperplasia**: proliferation of the basal layers of the keratinizing epithelium of pars flaccida.[113]

Animal models have confirmed that squamous epithelial proliferation is promoted by chronic middle ear inflammation.[113]

The distinction between congenital and acquired cholesteatoma may be blurred by the following mechanisms.

- Metaplasia: epithelial transformation from the columnar endothelium of the middle ear cleft into keratinizing epithelium in response to chronic middle ear inflammation.[109] This acquired cholesteatoma gives rise to epithelial cysts.
- Some apparently acquired cholesteatoma may be due to late perforation of congenital epithelial cysts through the tympanic membrane.
- A mechanism whereby a retraction cholesteatoma might present behind an intact tympanic membrane has recently been proposed.[110]

Iatrogenic cholesteatoma

Implantation of squamous epithelium as a result of blunt or sharp trauma to the tympanic membrane may result in a cholesteatoma. The otologist must always be aware of this possibility when operating on the tympanic membrane. Failure to remove all squamous epithelium from the middle ear during cholesteatoma allows the disease to persist and return. This iatrogenic form is known as 'residual' cholesteatoma. Cholesteatoma that returns *de novo* after surgery is termed 'recurrent' (see **Table 74.7**).

Epidemiology

INCIDENCE

Estimates based on retrospective analysis of hospital operation data and the population served have demonstrated an incidence of 0.3/10,000 per year in Denmark,[114] 0.7/10,000 per year in children in Iowa,[115] 0.9/10,000 per

Table 74.7 Classification of cholesteatoma by aetiology.

Congenital	Acquired
Vestigial	Invagination
Hamartoma	Invasion
Metaplasia	Basal cell hyperplasia
Invagination	Metaplasia
Amniotic migration	Trauma
	Iatrogenic (residual)

year in Finland,[116] 1.3/10,000 per year in Scotland[117] and 0.1–1.6/10,000 per year in Northern Ireland.[118] Extremes of 0.04/10,000 per year in Gothenburg[119] and 6.6/10,000 per year in Israel[120] have also been reported.

PREVALENCE

It is possible to estimate the prevalence of cholesteatoma from epidemiological studies of tympanic membrane disorders. These population-based studies generally observe a population of less than 10,000 patients and may not be accurate if the prevalence of cholesteatoma is very low. A survey in Jerusalem has suggested a prevalence of cholesteatoma as high as 7/10,000 children,[121] with a survey in Vietnam suggesting a similar prevalence of 6/10,000 children.[122] The Inuit population, which has a high incidence of chronic suppurative otitis media, has a somewhat lower prevalence of cholesteatoma – 0.5/10,000 in a population-based survey of children.[123] In Aboriginal children, the prevalence of cholesteatoma was 5/10,000 in a study of 7326 ears.[124]

CHANGE IN PREVALENCE

The change in the incidence of cholesteatoma over recent decades varies from report to report. In Northern Ireland[118] and Scotland,[117] no change in the incidence of cholesteatoma has been demonstrated. Over the same period in Finland,[116] Israel[120] and Merseyside,[125] by contrast, a drop in the prevalence of cholesteatoma has been noted.

AGE DISTRIBUTION

The age and sex distribution of the patients undergoing cholesteatoma surgery in a population-based study from Iowa a quarter of a century ago[115] is shown in **Figure 74.15**. The peak incidence in the second decade of life corresponds well with information collected from a database of patients undergoing cholesteatoma surgery in Gloucestershire from 1980 to 2002 (see **Figure 74.16**).

SEX

Cholesteatoma affects approximately three males for every two females. The proportion of males to females

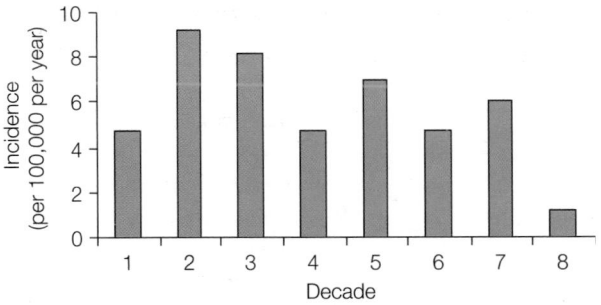

Figure 74.15 Incidence of cholesteatoma by age in Iowa in 1975/6. Redrawn from Ref. 115, with permission.

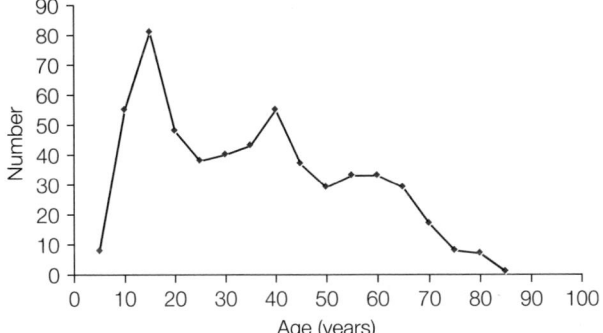

Figure 74.16 Cumulative prevalence of cholesteatoma by age in Gloucestershire 1980–2002. Previously unpublished data.

in childhood in the population aged less than 16 years is not statistically different to the ratio in adulthood (see **Table 74.8**).

ANATOMICAL FEATURES OF CHOLESTEATOMA

The distribution of tympanic membrane pathology in cholesteatoma in children is different to that of adults. In children there is a significantly higher rate of cholesteatoma associated with pars tensa pathology than in adults (see **Figure 74.17**). In adults attic cholesteatoma is more frequent (see **Table 74.9**).

EXTENT OF CHOLESTEATOMA

The spread of middle ear cholesteatoma through the temporal bone is also different in children compared with adults. Paediatric cholesteatoma more frequently involves the extremes of the middle ear space (the Eustachian tube, the anterior mesotympanum, the retrolabyrinthine area and the mastoid tip) than cholesteatoma in adults. Adult cholesteatoma, however, more frequently involves the anterior epitympanum (see **Table 74.10**).

Symptoms

Children with cholesteatoma are nearly always affected by either ear discharge or hearing loss, or both, in the

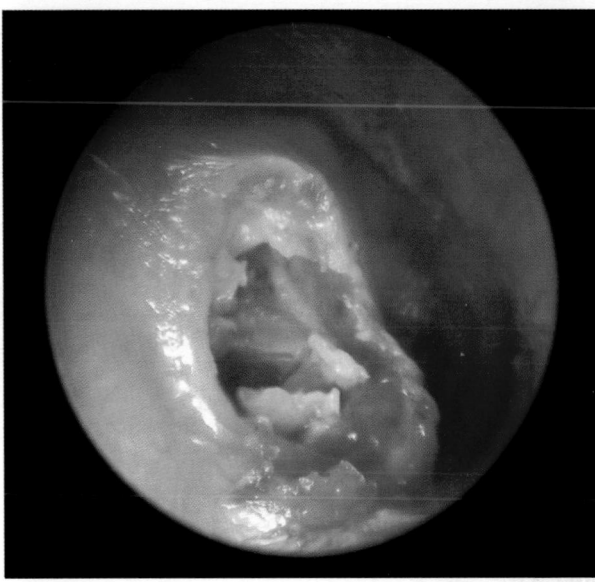

Figure 74.17 Posterior mesotympanic cholesteatoma. Cholesteatoma extending from this part of the tympanic membrane is more frequent in children than in adults. Involvement of the posterior mesotympanum commonly results in erosion of the long process of the incus and less frequently the stapes superstructure. Involvement of posterior mesotympanum and sinus tympani is a recognized risk factor for residual cholesteatoma after surgery. This six-year-old boy had loss of the stapes superstructure and although a malleus to footplate prosthesis was inserted he does not have useful hearing in this ear.

Table 74.8 Sex incidence of cholesteatoma.

	Number (age <16)	Number (age ≥16)
Male	124	345
Female	81	249

$\chi^2 = 0.52$. Previously unpublished data from personal database.

Table 74.9 Anatomical features of cholesteatoma.

	Age <16	Age ≥16
Attic	23	65
Pars tensa	48	51

$p < 0.005$ (χ^2, df = 1). Previously unpublished data from personal database.

diseased ear. Only 2 percent of children with cholesteatoma have neither of these symptoms. Only one in eight children with cholesteatoma has pain and other symptoms are rare. The pattern of symptoms is similar to that seen in adults except that dizziness is rarely seen in the paediatric population (see **Table 74.11**).

Table 74.10   Extent of cholesteatoma.

	Age <16	Age ≥16
Eustachian tube	46	25
Anterior mesotympanum	51	64
Anterior epitympanum	15	13
Retrolabyrinthine area	10	4
Mastoid tip	15	1
Patient total	67	156

$p < 0.0007$ ($\chi^2 = 19.25$, $v = 4$). Previously unpublished data from personal database.

Table 74.11   Comparison of prevalence of presenting symptom of cholesteatoma in adults and children.

Symptoms	Adult (%)	Child (%)	Significance (χ^2)
Otorrhoea	85.1	88.9	
Hearing loss	68.8	66.3	
Pain	14.4	12.6	
Dizziness	8.2	0	$p < 0.001$
Facial palsy	1.2	0.5	
Tinnitus	6.5	2.0	
Abscess	1.3	0	
Neither deaf nor discharge	1.7	2.1	

Previously unpublished data from personal database.

Signs

A child presenting with profuse ear discharge and hearing loss has symptoms caused by chronic otitis media until proven otherwise. The precise complication of chronic otitis media associated with the symptoms is determined by examination of the tympanic membrane. Thus the diagnosis of cholesteatoma is not made and, more importantly, cholesteatoma cannot be excluded until the entire tympanic membrane has been examined. Inspection of the ear often requires two stages: obtaining a view of the tympanic membrane and systematic examination of the tympanic membrane.

OBTAINING A VIEW OF THE TYMPANIC MEMBRANE

Mucus, keratin, polyps or even wax may prevent a clear view of the eardrum. The reader is referred to Clinical examination under Chronic perforation of the tympanic membrane above for the general approach to cleaning children's ears (see **Figure 74.6**). Once the debris has been removed from the child's ear, further inspection may reveal the presence of a polyp filling the lumen. Aural polyps associated with mucopus are almost always due to exuberant granulation tissue. The collagen content of polyps is very low so that most can be avulsed painlessly using microsuction. Once the polyp has been removed its base can be cauterized with silver nitrate to obtain haemostasis.

INSPECTION OF THE TYMPANIC MEMBRANE

Once the tympanic membrane can be clearly seen, it should be systematically inspected for areas of retraction.

It should first be determined whether the entire tympanic membrane can be seen. Some ear canals are narrow or tortuous and only part of the tympanic membrane can be seen. It is a minimum requirement that the entire tympanic membrane be inspected. If this is not possible in the outpatient department the child's ear should be inspected under general anaesthesia.

Defects in the pars tensa should be noted, along with their location and size. Most important of all to note is whether the defect is a perforation or a retraction pocket. This cannot always be reliably determined using a handheld otoscope, so inspection using the otological microscope is essential. If this is not possible in the outpatient department, the child's ear should be inspected under general anaesthesia.

If the pars tensa is normal, the pars flaccida should be fully inspected. Considerable care may be required to exclude an attic cholesteatoma. In most cases, retraction of the pars flaccida can be readily identified. Some attic retractions, however, can barely be seen even on prolonged and careful examination. They may have a very narrow opening. The anatomy of the ear canal may limit the view of the area. If the attic area cannot be seen then a further examination with the otoendoscope may improve the view. If this is not possible in the outpatient department, the child's ear should be inspected under general anaesthesia. The attic area may be obscured by polyps, keratin or even apparently innocuous mucus or wax. Wax and mucus covering the attic area should be removed. Granulation tissue and moist keratin within this area confirms the diagnosis.

On occasion, a cholesteatoma sac can be seen through an otherwise normal tympanic membrane as a vague white mass with a convex border. A myringotomy to remove any middle ear mucus may help to clarify this sign. Occasionally, a limited tympanotomy may be required to confirm the diagnosis. Rarely such mesotympanic disease may have an attic origin so a further inspection of the attic should be performed.

Investigation of cholesteatoma

AUDIOLOGY

The patient's ipsilateral middle ear hearing function may change as a result of cholesteatoma surgery. It may be unaffected, impaired or improved. The impact this will have on the patient depends on not just the operation but also the preoperative hearing in each of the patient's ears. It is therefore essential to obtain a measure of the hearing in both ears prior to surgery.

With the information provided by a preoperative audiogram, the surgeon can plan for the possible outcomes of surgery and advise the patient on these possibilities.

- In all cases the patient should be advised that the hearing in the operated ear may deteriorate.
- If the preoperative ipsilateral air conduction is normal, loss of hearing in the operated ear will have more impact if the contralateral hearing is impaired. It is therefore essential that the opposite air conduction threshold be determined so that any appropriate mitigating action, such as the provision of a hearing aid, can be planned.
- If the preoperative ipsilateral air conduction is impaired, the possibility of improving the hearing through surgery should be determined. The ipsilateral bone conduction threshold is essential under these circumstances. If it is also impaired the patient should be advised that improvement in hearing effected by surgery alone is unlikely. If the bone conduction threshold is normal, there remains a chance that the hearing can be improved by surgery, but the likelihood of this happening will depend on the cause of the hearing loss.

EXAMINATION UNDER ANAESTHETIC

This procedure may be essential in small children in order to inspect the tympanic membrane closely. Since acquired cholesteatomas arise from the tympanic membrane, the majority can be diagnosed with this evaluation. Nonetheless, it is important to realize that even acquired cholesteatomas, particularly in the attic, may be difficult to identify and a systematic and careful exploration of the tympanic membrane, including the attic area, is essential. A fine sucker is a useful multipurpose probe, retractor and elevator, as well as microsucker in this venture.

COMPUTED TOMOGRAPHY OF TEMPORAL BONE

In most cases, cholesteatoma is diagnosed by direct inspection of the tympanic membrane. Computed tomography (CT) may be of value in establishing a diagnosis of cholesteatoma under the following circumstances:[126]

- indeterminate examination under anaesthesia;
- suspected epidermal cyst;
- symptomatic ear with apparently clear attic retraction pocket.

CT scan also may be of value in planning the operation when the following particulars pertain:

- revision cholesteatoma surgery;
- suspected inner ear complication;
- suspected intracranial complication.

This information can improve the planning of the case and inform the patient and family of risks specific to the operation.

CT scanning is not valuable in every case. However, the benefit the surgeon gains from the scan parallels his/her ability to interpret it. Accordingly, there exists a body of opinion which feels that expertise in interpreting temporal bone CT scans can only come by regular assessment of scans. Furthermore, scan definition continues to improve, hence all opportunities to view new scans should be taken and therefore all cholesteatoma cases should include CT investigation.

MAGNETIC RESONANCE SCAN OF TEMPORAL BONE

Magnetic resonance (MR) scans are currently of less general use in the assessment of cholesteatoma than CT scans because they lack any information about the bony anatomy of the temporal bone.

Although cholesteatoma has specific signal characteristics (see **Table 74.12**), MR scan does not yet adequately discriminate between other chronic middle ear inflammation and cholesteatoma, especially when the cholesteatoma is less than 0.5 cm in diameter. This limits the role of MR scan as a diagnostic test and, in particular, means that it cannot be used yet as a screening tool to diagnose residual cholesteatoma after first stage intact canal wall surgery.[127]

Improvements with diffusion scanning and delayed contrast-enhanced multiplanar imaging may encourage the use of MR as a tool for diagnosing residual cholesteatoma.[128] MR scanning is of particular value in determining the presence of suspected inner ear and intracranial complications of cholesteatoma.

Treatment

MEDICAL

Cholesteatoma is a relentless disease. Once the diagnosis of cholesteatoma has been established in a child who can tolerate a general anaesthetic, there is no justification for withholding the surgical removal of the keratin matrix.

SURGICAL

The definitive treatment of cholesteatoma is surgical.

Table 74.12 MR characteristics of cholesteatoma.

Image character	Signal character
T1 (unenhanced)	Low
T1 (with gadolinium)	Low
T2	High
b-800 diffusion weighted	High

Reprinted from Ref. 127, with permission.

Aims

The aims of cholesteatoma surgery are:

- removal of all cholesteatoma;
- prevention of the development of further cholesteatoma;
- to obtain a 'robust' ear, which remains dry, self-cleaning and free of infection after exposure to water;
- restoration of hearing.

Removal of cholesteatoma encourages radical resection of the mastoid air cells and removal of the posterior and superior ear canal wall to obtain good exposure of the disease. By contrast, maintaining a dry, hearing ear, requires a conservative technique with the preservation or reconstruction of important functional elements. The treatment of cholesteatoma therefore requires the resolution of aims that are antagonistic. This ensures that the successful treatment of cholesteatoma is one of the most challenging endeavours in the entire spectrum of surgical intervention.

REMOVAL OF ALL CHOLESTEATOMA

It is well established that there is a high rate of disease left within the temporal bone ('residual' disease) after primary surgery, whatever the surgical technique. This has been emphasized in many retrospective reviews,[129] as well as in one prospective, controlled trial.[130]

Three retrospective analyses of risk factors for residual cholesteatoma, two specifically in children, using multivariate analysis have been published.[87, 131, 132] The presence of the factors listed in **Table 74.13** independently heightened the risk of residual disease. These results emphasize not only that the temporal bone is a highly complex and heterogeneous anatomical structure but also that the disease is capable of insinuating its way into the interstices of this configuration. The results also confirm that it is particularly difficult to remove disease from the posterior mesotympanum/sinus tympani and from around the ossicular chain.

Improvements in the complete clearance of cholesteatoma have come partly through technological advances that appropriately confront the difficulties presented by the disease and the terrain. Significant advances have been in visual access to the disease and instruments for removal of the disease from around the ossicles. Thus angled endoscopes or mirrors must be available in order that cholesteatoma lurking in the sinus tympani or behind the ossicles can be clearly seen.

The most significant improvement has come from the introduction of the fibre-guided laser as a tool for removing cholesteatoma from around the ossicles (see **Figure 74.18**). Adjacent to the ossicles, removal of disease is improved by using an instrument which does not cause movement of the ossicular chain and which can be passed into the recesses of the posterior mesotympanum, as well as those spaces behind the ossicular chain. The fibre-guided laser fulfils the requirements for removal of cholesteatoma in these areas.

A prospective trial of cholesteatoma surgery with and without a KTP laser has confirmed that the rate of residual disease is lower by a whole order of magnitude when the laser is used.[132] [***] The results are shown in **Table 74.14**.

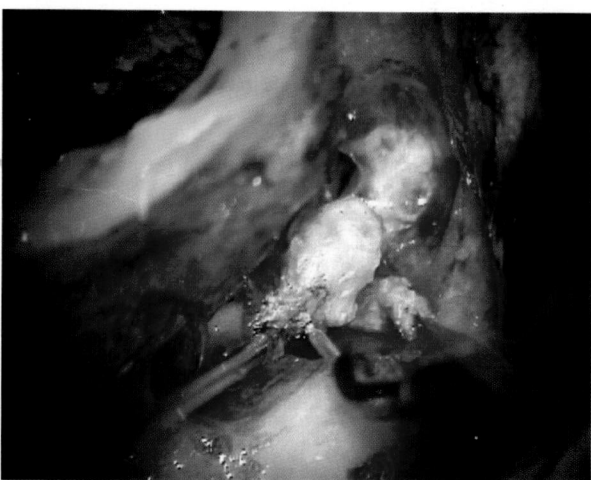

Figure 74.18 Removal of firmly adherent cholesteatoma from the intact ossicular chain. Until recently the surgeon could not avulse firmly adherent cholesteatoma from the intact ossicular chain for fear of causing cochlear damage. The most prudent course of action was to dismantle the chain. The fibre-guided laser can vaporize this cholesteatoma without ossicular movement, thereby achieving the conflicting aims of disease removal and hearing preservation.

Table 74.13 Risk factors for residual cholesteatoma in children.[87, 131, 133]

Risk factor
Erosion of the ossicular chain
Presence of posterior mesotympanic cholesteatoma, especially if adherent
Presence of inflamed middle ear mucosa
Operator ability

Table 74.14 Effect of ancillary use of KTP laser on residual disease rate in intact canal wall cholesteatoma surgery.

	KTP+	KTP−	p (Fisher's exact test)
Number treated	35	33	<0.003
Number residual	1	10	

Reprinted from Ref. 132, with permission.

OBTAIN A ROBUST, DRY EAR

The presence of an unstable ear after surgery is an ongoing burden to the affected child. The ear may feel uncomfortable and may be associated with otitis externa or excoriation of the pinna. The child may be unable to escape a cycle of regular visits to the ENT department for aural toilet. The discharging ear may exacerbate hearing loss by preventing the use of a hearing aid. A child with an ear that will not tolerate exposure to water may, at the least, need to learn protective measures to prevent the ingress of water to the ear and may be excluded from swimming. Sometimes the ear may continually smell offensive. In this sad circumstance the child may become isolated by his or her peers.

The stability of the external element of the ear is dependent upon the self-cleaning mechanism. This mechanism can continue to act when the ear canal is surgically enlarged, up to a point. There is thus some latitude within which the resolution of the conflicting aims stated above can be achieved. This has allowed the development of a variety of procedures for the removal of cholesteatoma. A dry ear after cholesteatoma surgery can be achieved by:

- working around the intact ear canal wall, gaining access to disease using a combined approach through the mastoid air cells and ear canal;
- lowering the canal wall and incorporating the mastoid space into the canal only in temporal bones with a small mastoid air cell system;
- partially obliterating the mastoid bowl after its exposure by removing the canal wall.

The greatest advantage of intact canal wall surgery is that the resultant ear is almost always dry. [**]

Removal of the canal wall and dissection through the mastoid air cells to facilitate the removal of disease less reliably results in a dry ear. If heed is paid only to the 'disease removal' aim of cholesteatoma surgery, then the ear canal wall may be removed without care, making the mastoid bowl part of the subsequent ear canal. If the surgically created canal is irregular, the self-cleaning mechanism fails and the canal either collects keratin or fails to maintain a keratinizing epithelium or both. Only if this bowl is smooth and free of recesses will the new canal tolerate exposure to the external environment. [*]

Multivariate analysis of factors influencing the stability of the mastoid cavity has indicated that adequate lowering of the facial ridge is the most important factor influencing the outcome of a dry ear in canal wall down surgery.[134] [**]

PREVENTION OF RECURRENT CHOLESTEATOMA

Cholesteatoma also has a tendency to return *de novo*. This is particularly the case if there exists the combination of a large space behind the plane of the keratinizing epithelium, as well as a small opening through which the keratinizing epithelium can retract. This will allow the formation of a new narrow-necked sac with subsequent accumulation of keratin ('recurrent' cholesteatoma). Clearly, these circumstances are most likely after intact canal wall surgery although they can also occur after partial obliteration of a large cavity or when a small cavity is attempted in a well-pneumatized temporal bone.

The return of cholesteatoma is partly dependent on the time elapsed since surgery.[135] It is therefore inadequate to baldly state a simple figure as a percentage of patients in whom cholesteatoma has recurred. At the very least the figure should be qualified by the duration of follow-up.

Provided that temporal information about the thoroughness of follow-up, as well as disease recurrence is available, it is possible to calculate the conditional probability of disease recurring in a particular time interval given that it has not recurred by the beginning of that interval. The technique is called life table analysis and provides useful long-term follow-up data. Two studies using life table analysis have confirmed the higher rate of recurrent disease in canal wall up surgery (see **Figure 74.19**).[135, 136] [***]

However, improved surgical technique has corrected this deficiency in the intact canal wall technique. Long-term recurrence rates have been reduced to levels seen in good canal wall down surgery by taking great care to reconstruct any defect through which the disease may return and by staging the surgery. The materials most commonly used for this reconstruction are cartilage and bone pate. One prospective trial of cartilage against bone pate for the repair of such defects has shown no significant difference between the treatment groups in the rate of return of cholesteatoma up to five years after surgery.[137] [***]

Staging of intact canal wall surgery, originally introduced to permit a check for the presence of residual cholesteatoma, allows an opportunity to inspect the scutum repair. This offers an opportunity to repair any persisting

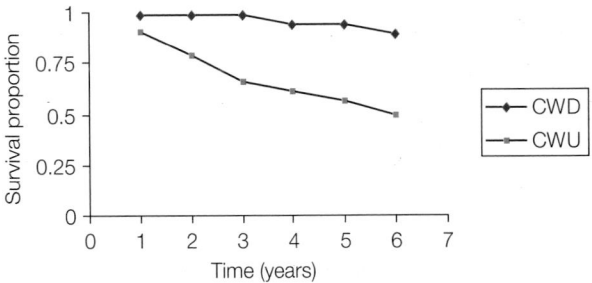

Figure 74.19 Longstanding concerns exist about the rate of recurrent disease with canal wall up surgery. Comparison of recurrence rates of cholesteatoma after single-stage canal wall up (CWU) and canal wall down (CWD) surgery published in 1989. These data encapsulate the widely perceived disadvantage of canal wall preservation in cholesteatoma surgery. Advances in canal wall reconstruction with bone pate or cartilage have now reduced the recurrence rate (see **Figure 74.21**).[135]

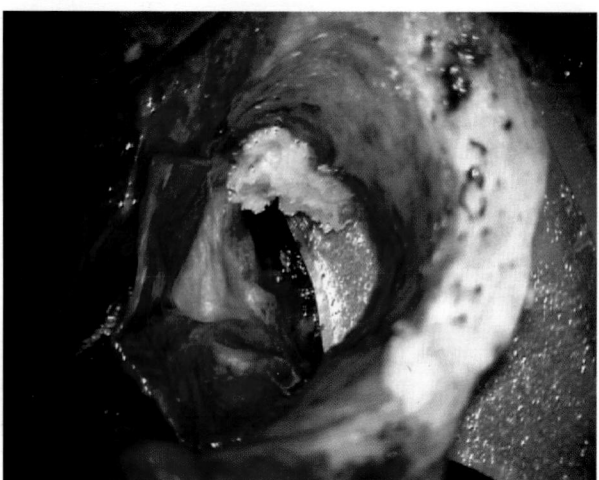

Figure 74.20 Prevention of recurrent cholesteatoma when the canal wall is preserved. Preservation of the intact canal wall was formerly associated with high rates of recurrent cholesteatoma. Reconstruction of the lateral attic wall with bone pate stabilized on a rigid support, such as the silastic strut seen in the plate, has resulted in recurrence rates after intact canal wall surgery being reduced to the levels associated with canal wall down surgery. Nonetheless, recurrence in children remains higher than in adults.

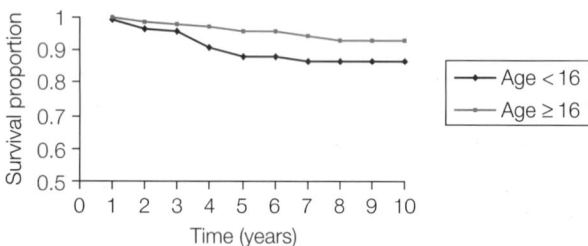

Figure 74.21 Actuarial recurrence rates of cholesteatoma in children and adults after staged intact canal wall surgery with bone pate repair of the lateral attic wall. Previously unpublished data.

defect. Rates of residual cholesteatoma after staged bone pate repair of the scutum are comparable to those seen in canal wall down surgery (see **Figure 74.20**).[138]

The rate of cholesteatoma recurrence in children is compared with the rate in adults in **Figure 74.21**. Both groups underwent staged intact canal wall surgery with repair of the lateral attic wall using bone pate. Children have a slightly higher risk of developing recurrent cholesteatoma. [**]

OSSICULAR EROSION IN CHRONIC OTITIS MEDIA

Epidemiology

Chronic otitis media is associated with erosion of the ossicles. Pars tensa retraction pockets and cholesteatoma are often associated with ossicular erosion.[139] The commonest defect is erosion of the long process of the incus.[97] Erosion of any of the ossicles can occur, but erosion of the entire chain is uncommon.

Pathology

Loss of ossicular integrity secondary to chronic otitis media has been termed resorptive osteitis.[140] The cause of this erosion appears to involve inflammatory cells secreting collagenases. Other pathological processes that contribute to hearing loss include tympanosclerosis, fibrocystic sclerosis, sclerosing osteitis and fibrosis of the tympanic membrane, as well as tympanic membrane perforation.[141]

Classification

Reconstruction of the ossicular chain by interposing rigid prostheses, including the patient's own ossicular remnants, is possible. The geometry of the ossicular defect does not always lend itself to stability of the prosthesis so some reconstructions are more favoured than others. Reconstruction is usually performed between the tympanic membrane, manubrium or long process of incus on the one hand and the capitulum, stapes footplate or vestibule on the other.

There are many surgical techniques for restoring contact between the tympanic membrane and the oval window by bridging the defects in the ossicular chain. Various classifications of this work have arisen.

- Wullstein's original classification of middle ear repair preceded the development of ossicular surgery and is simply based on a topographical sequence of places on the ossicular chain onto which the tympanic membrane could be placed.[142] Although based on procedures which in some cases soon became obsolete, the influence of this classification has been considerable. A number of subsequent classifications of tympanoplasty have adapted the Wullstein system to incorporate ossicular reconstruction.[143]
- Some classifications of ossiculoplasty alone are also based on the nature of the preoperative defect.[144]
- Further classifications of ossiculoplasty also incorporate information about the manner of reconstruction.[145]

Outcome measures

The success of middle ear reconstruction is often measured by the magnitude of the conductive hearing loss in the operated ear. This measure of middle ear function is of technical value to surgeons comparing surgical techniques, but is not of itself of much relevance to the patient, as the operated ear may also be afflicted by sensorineural hearing loss. The value of the end result to the patient is more reliably indicated by the overall hearing loss.[146]

The contribution of the hearing in the operated ear needs also to be evaluated in the context of the hearing in the opposite ear.[146] These effects are concisely summarized by the 'Belfast rules of thumb',[147] which state that the postoperative hearing in the operated ear will be useful to the patient if:

1. the air conduction threshold is less than 30 db HL (regardless of the hearing in the opposite ear);
2. the air conduction threshold is within 15 db HL of the air conduction threshold in a better contralateral ear.

These effects are also summarized in the 'Glasgow benefit plot'.[148]

Risk factors

Three studies have performed multivariate analysis of the factors which influence the audiological outcome of ossicular reconstruction.[149, 150, 151] The outcome measure in each of these was the difference between the air-bone gap, considered to be a reasonable guide to the magnitude of the conductive hearing loss. In one of these studies,[149] detailed analysis was limited by a small sample size: the only independent risk factor for good audiological outcome was the presence of the stapes superstructure. A larger sample size permitted the assessment of more baseline variates and determined that the presence of the manubrium and stapes superstructure together was the most important predictor of good hearing outcome after surgery.[151] By contrast, the absence of the stapes superstructure predicted strongly against a good outcome (see Table 74.15).

This type of study is limited by the quality of the entry data. There are many types of ossiculoplasty and if a type of ossiculoplasty is not included in the entry data, no conclusions can be formulated concerning the relative efficacy of that procedure. For instance, no multivariate assessment of newer procedures, such as malleostapedotomy or malleus dislocation, is available.

Table 74.15 Parameters found to be independently and statistically significant predictors of outcome in ossicular surgery.

	P (multivariate analysis)[a]
Manubrium +, stapes arch +	<0.0001
Stapes only	<0.001
Preop air-bone gap >50 dB (negative indicator)	<0.01

[a]Multivariate analysis using a logistic regression model on the outcome of 600 cases of ossicular surgery.[150]

Three scoring systems have been formulated which are intended to indicate the outcome of ossicular reconstruction. Only the most recent system is based on multivariate analysis of risk factors. It has not been applied to other surgeons' data.[152] The earlier systems did not provide any useful predictive value when applied to other surgeons' data.[151]

Results

Two prospective controlled studies of ossicular reconstruction have been performed. Mangham and Lindemann compared two materials in the reconstruction of ossicular defects.[153] They found no difference between the two materials; however, they did discern a difference between the two surgeons' results. [****] Maassen and Zenner reported a study comparing two different techniques for the reconstruction of the eroded long process of the incus. They found that reconnecting the long process to the stapes head provided significantly better closure of the air-bone gap than malleus to stapes reconstruction.[154] However, no account of the surgeons performing the procedures was provided. [****]

LONG-TERM RESULTS

One actuarial study on long-term hearing, using an outcome similar to the Belfast rules, after surgery for cholesteatoma has been presented (see **Figure 74.22**).[155] [**] This confirmed the following:

- Hearing outcome was dependent on the state of the ossicular chain prior to surgery. In general, the more intact the chain prior to surgery, the more effective the reconstruction.
- There is nearly always good hearing in the presence of an intact ossicular chain.
- The success of surgery ranged from 40 percent when the stapes superstructure was absent to 89 percent for restoration of an intact chain through reconstruction of the long process of the incus.
- Most differences in success rates for the different types of reconstruction were due to failure before the first evaluation.
- Late failure was uncommon.
- The presence of even mild sensorineural hearing loss limited the usefulness of any ossicular reconstruction. This subgroup contributed heavily to the early failures.
- A higher rate of useful hearing in children is largely due to their better cochlear function (**Table 74.16**).
- It is worth reflecting on whether any ossicular reconstruction should be performed in an ear with sensorineural hearing loss, particularly if there is little of the remaining chain. Under these circumstances, a hearing aid may offer some benefit provided that the external ear canal is stable.

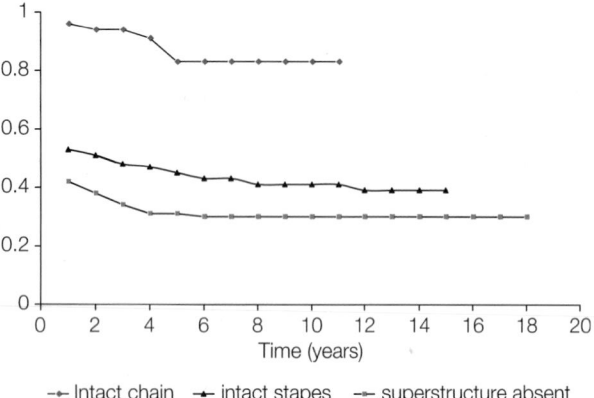

-•- Intact chain   -▲- intact stapes   -■- superstructure absent

Figure 74.22 Long-term results of ossiculoplasty. These data show that although there is some deterioration in useful hearing with time, the value of the intervention is mainly determined at the time of surgery. Hearing is measured here as 'useful' if the air conduction threshold in the operated ear is less than 30 dB ISO. This outcome is slightly more stringent than the more widely used Belfast rules of thumb. The data were gleaned from surgery on both children and adults.

Table 74.16 Hearing results (dB HL) after ossiculoplasty (performed as part of cholesteatoma surgery) in 77 children and 217 adults.

Age (years)	Bone conduction threshold	Air conduction threshold	Air-bone gap
<16	5.8	29.5	24.7
>16	19.1	43.2	24.6

The figures shown are averages for the sample groups. Although the average conductive loss does not differ between the two groups, the overall hearing is better in children because they have a much smaller sensorineural loss.

Technical aspects of ossiculoplasty

There is greater variance in the results of ossicular surgery than the results of other forms of otological surgery. In the last decade, laboratory work using laser Doppler vibrometry and mathematical modelling using finite element analysis has provided insights into the mechanism of the ossicular chain and the optimum techniques for its reconstruction.[156, 157, 158, 159] **Table 74.17** summarizes some of these findings.

Timing of intervention in children

In all patients, whether adult or child, the decision to offer surgical reconstruction of the eroded ossicular chain should be guided by:

- the likelihood of benefit according to the Belfast rules of thumb or the Glasgow benefit plot;
- the surgeon's own audit of outcomes.

Table 74.17 Guidelines for surgical technique from laboratory results.

Factor	
Adhesions	Adhesions to the promontory have a profoundly adverse effect
Displacement	To prevent displacement and rotation of the prosthesis, ensure secure attachment to stapes head or footplate
Tension	Low tension is best; do not stretch the tympanic membrane
Malleus	Using the malleus handle gives better results
Prosthesis mass	High mass has an adverse effect on high frequencies
Prosthesis stiffness	Low stiffness (e.g. cartilage, polyethylene) has an adverse effect at all frequencies

There are some special considerations about ossicular reconstruction in children. The younger the child, the greater the risk that other features of chronic middle ear inflammation, such as middle ear effusion, may still be present. The adverse effect this may have on surgical repair of the tympanic membrane has been presented above in Elimination of middle ear pathology under Chronic perforation of the tympanic membrane. Clearly such problems may both mask any benefit from surgical reconstruction.

In children some concern has been raised about the use of middle ear implants because data on their long-term effects are not available. If only the patient's own ossicles are to be used then it is important that these should not become involved in the underlying disease. For example, ossicular reconstruction in children with cholesteatoma should not be undertaken until it has been demonstrated that there is no residual disease.

CONCLUSIONS

The term 'chronic otitis media' has become ambiguous through confusion with similar terms and through multiple different classifications but is best considered a pathological term. Chronic otitis media can affect all structures within and adjacent to the temporal bone. Its presence can be confirmed by histological assessment and be inferred from its complications. The causes of chronic otitis media are poorly understood; there is no proven prophylaxis against it.

'Chronic suppurative otitis media' is an historic but useful term. It is defined as the presence of chronic ear discharge in the presence of a chronic tympanic membrane perforation. The duration required to satisfy the term 'chronic' varies from definition to definition.

The prevalence of chronic suppurative otitis media is highest in children in Aboriginal communities in otherwise developed countries and represents a massive public health problem. In nonindigenous communities in developed countries, the prevalence of tympanic membrane perforation is higher in adults than in children. Medical treatment of the symptom of ear discharge in chronic suppurative otitis media is best treated with aural toilet and topical fluoroquinolones.

Below the age of 13 years, the rate of successful tympanic membrane repair diminishes with younger age. The nature of the surgical repair of the tympanic membrane depends on the size of the perforation and the state of the remainder of the tympanic membrane and middle ear cleft. The rate of surgical closure of the tympanic membrane can be over 90 percent in the short to medium term in subspecialist hands. The national average rate in Britain is nearer 65 percent. Personal audit of surgical results is essential to provide the patient with the accurate information on which the decision to proceed or reject surgery will be based.

Pars tensa retraction starts in childhood. Tympanic membrane retraction is associated with progression of disease in one case in six once atrophy occurs. The progression of disease following atrophy of the tympanic membrane is slow, but may result in ossicular erosion or cholesteatoma. Tympanic membrane retraction without atrophy does not progress. Risk factors that accurately identify those cases that will progress to cholesteatoma have not been identified.

Tympanic membrane retraction pocket excision is a surgical procedure which acts as prophylaxis against the development of cholesteatoma. Selection of suitable cases for this procedure remains controversial. Personal audit of surgical results is necessary to inform decision making in the management of tympanic membrane retraction pockets.

Cholesteatoma reaches peak prevalence in the second decade. It is more extensive in children than in adults, but less commonly erodes into important temporal bone structures. In general, surgical treatment of cholesteatoma in children is associated with higher rates of residual and recurrent disease. There are many different surgical techniques that aim to satisfy the conflicting requirements of cholesteatoma surgery. Personal audit of surgical results using multiple long-term outcome measures is necessary to inform decision making in the management of cholesteatoma.

The results of ossicular surgery are influenced by the nature of the ossicular defect, but are also operator dependent, being highly sensitive to tiny variations in position and tension. These results, when measured according to a scale that correlates well with patient satisfaction, are better in children than in adults. This is mainly because the contribution of sensorineural hearing loss in children is less than in adults.

KEY POINTS

- The study and teaching of chronic otitis media has been hindered by multiple, ambiguous definitions of the term.
- In this chapter, chronic otitis media is considered to be a pathological term referring to persistent inflammation of the mucosa and submucosa of the middle ear. It is considered to be complicated by chronic inflammatory changes in the structures comprising and adjacent to the middle ear. According to this model surgical treatment is viewed as correcting these complications, but not materially affecting the underlying chronic otitis media. The model predicts that surgery may be compromised by the ongoing effects of middle ear inflammation and this appears to be particularly true after the treatment of children. Nontheless, modern management strategies and surgical techniques have progressed a long way in the past two decades and it is now possible to offer treatment outcomes for the complications of chronic otitis media in children which approach those obtained for adults.
- Recent microscopic evidence of biofilms in otitis media has indicated that this mechanism may be important in maintaining chronic ear infections.
- The social basis of the very high rates of chronic suppurative otitis media in some indigenous communities, particularly in children, has been recognized and forms the basis of new health policies, following the failure of medical treatment strategies to impact on this problem.
- Success rates in surgical closure of the tympanic membrane are, in general, low. The British national average successful closure rate is 65 percent. Surgeons with a specialist interest report higher rates of closure.
- Atrophy and retraction of the tympanic membrane is most prevalent in the second decade of life.
- Atrophy of the tympanic membrane ranges from mild through to more severe retraction with fixation of the atrophic segment to the bony walls of the middle ear. Approximately one case in six of tympanic membrane collapse is progressive. In these cases tympanic membrane retraction may become associated with erosion of the ossicles. A small proportion of advanced tympanic membrane retraction pockets progress to become cholesteatoma.

- The only actuarial data concerning long-term results after pars tensa retraction pocket excision in children suggest that the deleterious effects of the underlying pathology remain vigorous; in half of cases, the retraction pocket returns.
- We have only a limited understanding of which collapsed tympanic membranes will progress, so the management of this condition is extremely controversial.
- Cholesteatoma is most prevalent in the second decade of life.
- Children have a higher rate of recurrent cholesteatoma after surgery than adults.
- As a general rule, the more erosion of the ossicular chain the more difficult it is to surgically reconstruct useful hearing.
- Surgery for ossicular erosion, cholesteatoma and tympanic membrane perforation are all difficult and therefore highly operator dependent.
- A highly operator-dependent environment weakens the generalizabilty of individual prospective randomized studies on surgical treatment.
- Surgeons should be encouraged to carefully audit their own practice to inform themselves (and their patients) about likely outcomes for planned procedures.

Best clinical practice

✓ In purulent otorrhoea, topical antibiotics with aural toilet is the most effective method of treatment and quinolones appear to be more effective than other types of antibiotics in resolving otorrhoea. [Grade C]
✓ No topical aminoglycoside is officially recognized for use in patients with perforated ears. Any doctor who wishes to offer a medicine containing an aminoglycoside for topical application in a child with a perforated tympanic membrane should inform the patient and the patient's carer, prior to offering the treatment, of a potential risk of imbalance or permanent sensorineural hearing loss. [Grade C]
✓ Short-term success rates in surgical closure of the tympanic membrane are lower in very young children. In the longer term, the situation is aggravated by persistence of the effects of chronic otitis media, including middle ear effusion, reperforation and myringitis. The surgeon faced with a young child with a chronic perforated tympanic membrane should consider whether surgical repair would be better delayed. [Grade C]

✓ The management of cholesteatoma in children is surgical. The two main principles that underpin good surgery for this condition, thorough extenteration of disease and the preservation of a robust dry ear are difficult to balance, hence tympanomastoid surgery for cholesteatoma in children is particularly challenging. [Grade C]
✓ Cholesteatoma in children differs from that in adults in that it more often arises from the pars tensa and it is more commonly extensive. It is more difficult to remove in children and has a greater tendency to recur. [Grade C]
✓ Surgeons should be encouraged to carefully audit their own practice to inform themselves (and their patients) about likely outcomes for planned procedures. [Grade D]

Deficiencies in current knowledge and areas for future research

➤ Real understanding of the aetiology of chronic otitis media is lacking. At present there is considerable interest in the relationship between biofilms and chronic middle ear inflammatory disease. Future developments in this area of research are keenly awaited.
➤ Further results from the research into management of the social factors that result in high rates of chronic suppurative otitis media in indigenous communities are expected. The long-term outcome of this treatment, as well as how effectively it can be implemented elsewhere, will be of considerable interest.
➤ Results from studies investigating the role of topical antiseptics in chronic suppurative otitis media should be received soon. Prospective, randomized controlled trials of topical antiseptics against topical quinolones should clarify the treatment of choice for reducing otorrhoea in this disease.
➤ Steps to improve the national rate of successful tympanoplasty are needed. Improved access through canalplasty seems likely to be rewarding and further research into the benefits of this technique is needed.
➤ Improved understanding of the factors driving the deterioration of the tympanic membrane from atrophy through retraction to cholesteatoma may improve decision making in this disease.
➤ The role of the fibre-guided laser in cholesteatoma surgery should be further investigated. The laser offers a new means of accommodating the conflict between disease removal and functional integrity of the ear. There remains the exciting possibility of increased preservation of the ossicular chain with this technique.

- Surgical outcomes for the complications of chronic otitis media are highly dependent on the operator so efforts to promote a wholly evidence-based approach will continue to be bedevilled by lack of generalizability. Nonetheless, there are many aspects of surgery of the tympanic membrane, cholesteatoma and ossicles that could be evaluated with prospective and randomized studies.
- In the absence of high-level evidence, the most effective means of improving decision making for most surgeons will be through recording personal outcomes of surgery. A database of such outcomes will provide the surgeon about his/her success with different strategies for given surgical problems.
- It seems increasingly unlikely that patients will accept advice about the merits of surgical intervention without quantitative information from their prospective surgeon's own practice. Improvements in the collection and awareness of outcome data will be the first step in this direction.

ACKNOWLEDGEMENTS

Thanks to James Robinson for sharing his painstakingly kept database; Francis Lannigan for details concerning the swimming pool trial in Western Australia; Jeffrey Vrabec for sharing the unpublished raw data from his metaanalysis of paediatric tympanoplasty; Manohar Bance for sharing the results of his ossiculoplasty research, not all of which has been published at the time of writing.

REFERENCES

1. WHO/CIBA Foundation Workshop. Prevention of hearing impairment from chronic otitis media. WHO/PDH/98.4. London: CIBA Foundation, 1996.
2. Senturia BH, Paparella MM, Lowery HW. Definition and classification. *Annals of Otology, Rhinology, and Laryngology.* 1980; **89**: 4–8.
3. Bluestone CD, Gates GA, Klein JO, Lim DJ, Mogi G, Ogra PL et al. Definitions, terminology and classification of otitis media. *Annals of Otology, Rhinology and Laryngology.* 2002; **111**: 8–18.
4. da Costa SS, Paparella MM, Schachern PA, Yoon TH, Kimberley BP. Temporal bone histopathology in chronically infected ears with intact and perforated tympanic membranes. *Laryngoscope.* 1992; **102**: 1229–36.
5. Meyerhoff WL, Kim CS, Paparella MM. Pathology of chronic otitis media. *Annals of Otology, Rhinology and Laryngology.* 1978; **87**: 749–60.
6. Meyerhoff WL, Shea DA, Giebink GS. Experimental pneumococcal otitis media: a histolopathological study. *Otolaryngology and Head and Neck Surgery.* 1980; **88**: 606–12.
7. Bluestone CD, Paradise JL, Beery QC. Physiology of the eustachian tube in the pathogenesis and management of middle ear effusions. *Laryngoscope.* 1972; **82**: 1654–70.
8. Gristina AG, Oga M, Webb LX, Hobgood CD. Adherent bacterial colonization in the pathogenesis of osteomyelitis. *Science.* 1985; **228**: 990–3.
9. Ehrlich GD, Veeh R, Wang X, Costerton JW, Hayes JD, Hu FZ et al. Mucosal biofilm formation on middle-ear mucosa in the chinchilla model of otitis media. *Journal of the American Medical Association.* 2002; **287**: 1710–5.
10. Spandow O, Hellstrom S, Dahlstrom M. Structural characterization of persistent tympanic membrane perforations in man. *Laryngoscope.* 1996; **106**: 346–52.
11. Somers T, Houben V, Goovaerts G, Govaerts P, Offeciers E. Histology of the perforated tympanic membrane and its muco-epithelial junction. *Clinical Otolaryngology and Allied Sciences.* 1997; **22**: 162–6.
12. Jaisinghani VJ, Paparella MM, Schachern PA, Le CT. Tympanic membrane/middle ear pathologic correlates in chronic otitis media. *Laryngoscope.* 1999; **109**: 712–6.
13. Browning GG. The unsafeness of 'safe' ears. *Journal of Laryngology and Otology.* 1984; **98**: 23–6.
14. Morris PS. A systematic review of clinical research addressing the prevalence, aetiology, diagnosis, prognosis and therapy of otitis media in Australian Aboriginal children. *Journal of Paediatric and Child Health.* 1998; **34**: 487–97.
15. Baxter JD. Otitis media in Inuit children in the Eastern Canadian Arctic – an overview – 1968 to date. *International Journal of Pediatric Otorhinolaryngology.* 1999; **49**: S165–8.
16. Zazouk SM, Hajjaj MF. Epidemiology of chronic suppurative otitis media among Saudi children – a comparative study of two decades. *International Journal of Pediatric Otorhinolaryngology.* 2002; **62**: 215–8.
17. Godinho RN, Goncalves TM, Nunes FB, Becker CG. Prevalence and impact of chronic otitis media in school age children in Brazil. First epidemiologic study concerning chronic otitis media in Latin America. *International Journal of Pediatric Otorhinolaryngology.* 2001; **61**: 223–32.
18. Kim CS, Jung HW, Yoo KY. Prevalence and risk factors of chronic otitis media in Korea: results of a nation-wide survey. *Acta Oto-Laryngologica.* 1993; **113**: 369–75.
19. Browning GG, Gatehouse S. The prevalence of middle ear disease in the adult British population. *Clinical Otolaryngology and Allied Sciences.* 1992; **17**: 317–21.
20. Leach AJ, Boswell J, Asche V. Bacterial colonisation of the nasopharynx predicts very early onset and persistence of otitis media in Australian Aboriginal infants. *Pediatric Infectious Disease Journal.* 1994; **13**: 983–9.
21. Boswell JB, Niehuys TG, Rickards FW. Onset of otitis media in Australian Aboriginal infants in a longitudinal study from birth. *Australian Journal of Otolaryngology.* 1993; **1**: 232–7.
22. Faden H, Duffy L, Williams A, Krystofik D, Wolf J. Epidemiology of nasopharyngeal colonization with

nontypeable *Haemophilus influenzae* in the first two years of life. *Journal of Infectious Diseases.* 1995; **172**: 132–5.

23. Bruneau S, Ayukawa H, Proulx JF, Baxter JD, Kost K. Longitudinal observations (1987–1997) on the prevalence of middle ear disease and associated risk factors among Inuit children of Inukjuak, Nunavik, Quebec, Canada. *International Journal of Circumpolar Health.* 2001; **60**: 632–9.

24. Rebgetz P, Trennery P, Powers J, Mathews J. Incidence of otitis media in the first year of life. Menzies School of Health Annual Report 1988–89. 1989; 67.

25. Boswell JB, Niehuys TG. Patterns of persistent otitis media in the first year of life in Aboriginal and non-Aboriginal infants. *Annals of Otology, Rhinology, and Laryngology.* 1996; **105**: 893–900.

26. Boswell JB, Nienhuis TG. Onset of otitis media in the first eight weeks of life in Aboriginal and non-Aboriginal Australian. *Annals of Otology, Rhinology, and Laryngology.* 1995; **104**: 542–9.

27. Eason RJ, Harding E, Nicholson R, Nicholson D, Pada J, Gathercole J. Chronic suppurative otitis media in the Solomon Islands: a prospective, microbiological, audiometric and therapeutic survey. *New Zealand Medical Journal.* 1986; **99**: 812–5.

28. Young E. Genes may be key to poor health in Aborigines. *New Scientist.* 2003; **2416**: 10.

29. McGilchrist CA, Hills LJ. A semi-Markov model for ear infection. *Australian Journal of Statisitics.* 1991; **33**: 5–16.

30. Kay DJ, Nelson M, Rosenfeld RM. Meta-analysis of tympanostomy tube sequelae. *Otolaryngology and Head and Neck Surgery.* 2001; **124**: 374–80.

31. Koempel JA, Kumar A. Long-term otologic status of older cleft palate patients. *Indian Journal of Pediatrics.* 1997; **64**: 793–800.

32. Prasher VP. Screening of medical problems in adults with Down Syndrome. Available from: http://down-syndrome.info/library/periodicals/dsrp/02/2/059/DSRP-02-2-059-EN-GB.htm.

33. Fulghum RS, Hoogmoed RP, Brinn JE, Smith AM. Experimental pneumococcal otitis media: longitudinal studies in the gerbil model. *International Journal of Pediatric Otorhinolaryngology.* 1985; **10**: 9–20.

34. Wintermeyer SM, Nahata MC. Chronic suppurative otitis media. *Annals of Pharmacotherapy.* 1994; **28**: 1089–99.

35. Stewart PS, Costerton JW. Antibiotic resistance of bacteria in biofilms. *Lancet.* 2001; **358**: 135–8.

36. Khanna V, Chander J, Nagarkar NM, Dass A. Clinicomicrobiologic evaluation of active tubotympanic type chronic suppurative otitis media. *Journal of Otolaryngology.* 2000; **29**: 148–53.

37. Giles M, Asher I. Prevalence and natural history of otitis media with perforation in Maori school children. *Journal of Laryngology and Otology.* 1991; **105**: 257–60.

38. Baxter JD, Stubbing P, Goodbody L, Terraza O. The light at the end of the tunnel associated with the high prevalence

of chronic otitis media among Inuit elementary school children in the Eastern Canadian Arctic is now visible. *Arctic Medical Research.* 1992; **51**: 29–31.

39. Leach AJ. Otitis media in Australian Aboriginal children: an overview. *International Journal of Pediatric Otorhinolaryngology.* 1999; **49**: S173–8.

40. Bruneau S, Ayukawa H, Proulx JF, Baxter JD, Kost K. Longitudinal observations (1987–1997) on the prevalence of middle ear disease and associated risk factors among Inuit children of Inukjuak, Nunavik, Quebec, Canada. *International Journal of Circumpolar Health.* 2001; **60**: 632–9.

41. Coates HL, Morris PS, Leach AJ, Couzos S. Otitis media in Aboriginal children: tackling a major health problem. *Medical Journal of Australia.* 2002; **177**: 177–8.

42. Lehmann D, Tennant MT, Silva DT, McAullay D, Lannigan F, Coates H *et al.* Benefits of swimming pools in two remote Aboriginal communities in Western Australia: an intervention study. *BMJ.* 2003; **327**: 415–9.

43. Browning GG. Editorial summary: Time to re-evaluate Cochrane reviews? *Clinical Otolaryngology.* 2006; **31**: 487.

44. Acuin J, Smith A, Mackenzie I. Interventions for chronic suppurative otitis media (Cochrane Review). The Cochrane Library, 2003, CD000473.

∗ 45. Acuin J. Chronic suppurative otitis media. Clinical Evidence 2003 http://www.clinicalevidence.com/ceweb/conditions/ent/0507 visited on 20 July 2004.

46. Smith A, Hatcher J, Mackenzie I, Thompson S, Bai I, Macharia I *et al.* Randomised controlled trial of treatment of chronic suppurative otitis media in Kenyan schoolchildren. *Lancet.* 1996; **348**: 1128–33.

47. Fliss D, Dagan R, Houri Z, Leibermann A. Medical management of chronic suppurative otitis media without cholesteatoma in children. *Journal of Pediatrics.* 1990; **116**: 991–6.

48. Rotimi V, Olabiyi D, Banjo T, Okeowo P. Randomised comparitive efficacy of clindamycin, metronidazole and lincomycin, plus gentamicin in chronic suppurative otitis media. *West African Journal of Medicine.* 1990; **9**: 89–97.

49. Couzos S, Lea T, Mueller R, Murray R, Culbong M. Effectiveness of ototopical antibiotics for chronic otitis media in Aboriginal children: a community-based, multicentre, double-blind randomised controlled trial. *Medical Journal of Australia.* 2003; **179**: 185–90.

50. Rohn GN, Meyerhoff WL, Wright CG. Ototoxicity of topical agents. *Otolaryngologic Clinics of North America.* 1993; **26**: 747–58.

51. Phillips JS, Yung MW, Burton M, Swan I. Use of aminoglycoside-containing ear drops in the presence of a perforation: evidence review. ENT-UK Consensus Statement, 2007.

52. Goldblatt EL, Dohar J, Nozza RJ, Nielsen RW, Goldberg T, Sidman JD *et al.* Topical ofloxacin versus systemic amoxicillin/clavulanate in purulent otorrhea in children with tympanostomy tubes. *International Journal of Pediatric Otorhinolaryngology.* 1998; **46**: 91–101.

53. Gates GA. Safety of ofloxacin otic and other ototopical treatments in animal models and in humans. *Pediatric Infectious Disease Journal*. 2001; **20**: 104–7.

54. Ghosh S, Panarese A, Parker AJ, Bull PD. Quinolone drops for chronic otitis media. *BMJ*. 2000; **321**: 126–7.

55. Thorp MA, Gardiner IB, Prescott CA. Burow's solution in the treatment of active mucosal chronic suppurative otitis media: determining an effective dilution. *Journal of Laryngology and Otology*. 2000; **114**: 432–6.

∗ 56. Vrabec JT, Deskin RW, Grady JJ. Meta-analysis of pediatric tympanoplasty. *Archives of Otolaryngology – Head and Neck Surgery*. 1999; **125**: 530–4.

57. Duckert LG, Muller J, Makielski K, Helms J. Composite autograft "shield" reconstruction of remnant tympanic membranes. *American Journal of Otology*. 1995; **16**: 21–6.

58. Sheehy JL, Shelton C. Tympanoplasty: to stage or not to stage. *Otolaryngology and Head and Neck Surgery*. 1991; **104**: 399–407.

59. Yung M, Neumann C, Vowler S. A longitudinal study on pediatric myringoplasty. *Otology and Neurotology*. 2007; **28**: 353–5.

60. Eavey RD. Inlay tympanoplasty: cartilage butterfly technique. *Laryngoscope*. 1998; **108**: 657–61.

61. Mitchell RB, Pereira KD, Lazar RH. Fat graft myringoplasty in children – a safe and successful day-stay procedure. *Journal of Laryngology and Otology*. 1997; **111**: 106–8.

62. Fisch U. Myringoplasty. In: Fisch U, May J (eds). *Tympanoplasty, mastoidectomy, and stapes surgery*. Stuttgart: Georg Thieme Verlag, 1994: 9–41.

63. El-Hennawi DM. Cartilage perichondrium composite graft (CPCG) in pediatric tympanoplasty. *International Journal of Pediatric Otorhinolaryngology*. 2001; **59**: 1–5.

64. Denoyelle F, Roger G, Chauvin P, Garabedian EN. Myringoplasty in children: predictive factors of outcome. *Laryngoscope*. 1999; **109**: 47–51.

65. Lee P, Kelly G, Mills RP. Myringoplasty: does the size of the perforation matter? *Clinical Otolaryngology and Allied Sciences*. 2002; **27**: 331–4.

66. Ryan RM, Brown PM, Cameron JM, Fowler SM, Grant HR, Topham JH. Royal College of Surgeons comparative ENT audit 1990. *Clinical Otolaryngology and Allied Sciences*. 1993; **18**: 541–6.

67. Sade J. Atelectatic tympanic membrane: histologic study. *Annals of Otology, Rhinology, and Laryngology*. 1993; **102**: 712–6.

68. Yoon TH, Schachern PA, Paparella MM, Aeppli DM. Pathology and pathogenesis of tympanic membrane retraction. *American Journal of Otolaryngology*. 1990; **11**: 10–17.

69. Sade J, Berco E. Atelectasis and secretory otitis media. *Annals of Otology, Rhinology, and Laryngology*. 1976; **85**: 66–72.

70. Wolfman DE, Chole RA. Experimental retraction pocket cholesteatoma. *Annals of Otology, Rhinology, and Laryngology*. 1986; **95**: 639–44.

71. Imamura S, Nozawa I, Imamura M, Murakami Y. Pathogenesis of experimental aural cholesteatoma in the chinchilla. *Journal for Oto-Rhino-Laryngology and its Related Specialties*. 1999; **61**: 84–91.

72. Magnuson B. The atelectatic ear. *International Journal of Pediatric Otorhinolaryngology*. 1981; **3**: 25–35.

73. Bunne M, Falk B, Hellstrom S, Magnuson B. The character and consequences of disturbing sound sensations in retraction type middle ear disease. *International Journal of Pediatric Otorhinolaryngology*. 1999; **51**: 11–21.

74. Hergils L, Magnuson B. Morning pressure in the middle ear. *Archives of Otolaryngology*. 1985; **111**: 86–9.

75. Tideholm B, Brattmo M, Carlborg B. Middle ear pressure: effect of body position and sleep. *Acta Oto-Laryngologica*. 1999; **119**: 880–5.

76. Ars B, de Craemer W. Tympanic membrane lamina propria and middle ear cholesteatoma. In: Tos M, Thomsen J, Pietersen E (eds). *Cholesteatoma and middle ear surgery*. Amstelveen: Kugler Publications, 1988: 429–31.

77. Ruah CB, Schachern PA, Paparella MM, Zelterman D. Mechanisms of retraction pocket formation in the pediatric tympanic membrane. *Archives of Otolaryngology – Head and Neck Surgery*. 1992; **118**: 1298–305.

78. Ars B. Tympanic membrane retraction pocket. *Acta Oto-Rhino-Laryngologica Belgica*. 1995; **49**: 163–71.

∗ 79. Sade J, Avraham S, Brown M. Atelectasis, retraction pockets and cholesteatoma. *Acta Oto-Laryngologica*. 1981; **92**: 501–12.

80. Buckingham RA, Valvassori GE. Middle ear cholesteatoma – etiology, relation to chronic adhesive otitis media, and treatment: an otophotographic study. *Transactions – American Academy of Ophthalmology and Otolaryngology*. 1969; **73**: 873–85.

81. Black B. The collapsed pars tensa: surgical classification and management. In: Magnan J, Chays A (eds). *Proceedings of the Sixth International Conference on Cholesteatoma and Ear Surgery*. Marseille: Label Publications, 2001: 267–9.

82. Nelson SM, Berry RI. Ear disease and hearing loss among Navajo children – a mass survey. *Laryngoscope*. 1984; **94**: 316–23.

83. Stewart IA, Silva PA, Said S, Takazawa A, Webster G. Attic and posterior marginal retractions in a random sample of 794 children. In: Tos M, Thomsen J, Pietersen E (eds). *Cholesteatoma and middle ear surgery*. Amstelveen: Kugler Publications, 1988: 419–20.

84. Maw AR, Bawden R. Tympanic membrane atrophy, scarring, atelectasis and attic retraction in persistent, untreated otitis media with effusion and following ventilation tube insertion. *International Journal of Pediatric Otorhinolaryngology*. 1994; **30**: 189–204.

85. Kay DJ, Nelson M, Rosenfeld RM. Meta-analysis of tympanostomy tube sequelae. *Otolaryngology and Head and Neck Surgery*. 2001; **124**: 374–80.

86. Tay HL, Mills RP. Tympanic membrane atelectasis in childhood otitis media with effusion. *Journal of Laryngology and Otology*. 1995; **109**: 495–8.

87. Roger G, Denoyelle F, Chauvin P, Schlegel-Stuhl N, Garabedian EN. Predictive risk factors of residual

cholesteatoma in children: a study of 256 cases. *American Journal of Otology.* 1997; **18**: 550–8.

88. Sharp JF, Robinson JM. Treatment of tympanic membrane retraction pockets by excision. A prospective study. *Journal of Laryngology and Otology.* 1992; **106**: 882–6.

89. Schilder AG. Assessment of complications of the condition and of the treatment of otitis media with effusion. *International Journal of Pediatric Otorhinolaryngology.* 1999; **49**: S247–51.

90. Hamilton JW. The role of the KTP Laser in cholesteatoma surgery. *Acta Oto-Rhino-Laryngologica Belgica.* 2004; **58**: 101–2.

91. Stewart IA. Surgical treatment of retraction pockets. In: Tos M, Thomsen J, Pietersen E (eds). *Cholesteatoma and mastoid surgery.* Amstelveen: Kugler Publications, 1989: 443–8.

92. Marquet J. My current cholesteatoma techniques. *American Journal of Otology.* 1989; **10**: 124–30.

93. Wayloff MR. Excision of typanic membrane retraction pockets. In: Sade J (ed.). *Acute and secretory otitis media.* Amsterdam: Kugler Publications, 1986: 55–6.

94. Ars B. Middle ear cleft atelectasis. In: Magnan J, Chays A (eds). *Proceedings of the Sixth International Conference on Cholesteatoma and Ear Surgery.* Marseille: Label Production, 2001: 279–93.

95. Blaney SP, Tierney P, Bowdler DA. The surgical management of the pars tensa retraction pocket in the child – results following simple excision and ventilation tube. *International Journal of Pediatric Otorhinolaryngology.* 1999; **50**: 133–7.

96. Srinivasan V, Banhegyi G, O'Sullivan G, Sherman IW. Pars tensa retraction pockets in children: treatment by excision and ventilation tube insertion. *Clinical Otolaryngology.* 2000; **25**: 253–6.

97. Tos M. Pathology of the ossicular chain in various chronic middle ear diseases. *Journal of Laryngology and Otology.* 1979; **93**: 769–80.

98. Solomons NB, Robinson JM. Bone pate repair of the eroded incus. *Journal of Laryngology and Otology.* 1989; **103**: 41–2.

99. Mills RP. Physiological reconstruction of defects of the incus long process. *Clinical Otolaryngology and Allied Sciences.* 1996; **21**: 499–503.

100. Maassen MM, Zenner HP. Tympanoplasty type II with ionomeric cement and titanium–gold-angle prostheses. *American Journal of Otology.* 1998; **19**: 693–9.

101. Bluestone CD, Klein JO. Intratemporal complications and sequelae of otitis media. In: Bluestone CD, Stool SE, Alper CM, Casselbrant ML, Dohar JE, Yellon RF (eds). *Pediatric otolaryngology.* Philadelphia: Saunders, 2003: 687–783.

102. Derlacki EL, Clemis JD. Congenital cholesteatoma of the middle ear and mastoid. *Annals of Otology, Rhinology and Laryngology.* 1965; **74**: 706–27.

103. Levenson MJ, Parisier SC, Chute P, Wenig S, Juarbe C. A review of twenty congenital cholesteatomas of the middle ear in children. *Otolaryngology and Head and Neck Surgery.* 1986; **94**: 560–7.

104. Michaels L. An epidermoid formation in the developing middle ear. Possible source of cholesteatoma. *Journal of Otolaryngology.* 1986; **15**: 169–74.

105. Kamarkar S, Bhatia S, Khashaba A, Saleh E, Russo A, Sanna M. Congenital cholesteatomas of the middle ear: a different experience. *American Journal of Otology.* 1996; **17**: 288–92.

106. McGill TJ, Merchant S, Healy GB, Friedman EM. Congenital cholesteatoma of the middle ear in children: a clinical and histopathological report. *Laryngoscope.* 1991; **101**: 606–13.

107. Aimi K. Role of the tympanic ring in the pathogenesis of congenital cholesteatoma. *Laryngoscope.* 1983; **93**: 1140–6.

108. Northrop C. Histological observations of amniotic fluid cellular content in the ear of neonates and infants. *International Journal of Pediatric Otorhinolaryngology.* 1986; **11**: 113–27.

109. Sade J. The pathogenesis of attic cholesteatoma: the metaplasia theory. In: *Cholesteatoma First International Conference.* Birmingham, AL: Aesculapius Publishing Company, 1977: 212–32.

110. Sudhoff H, Linthicum Jr. FH. Cholesteatoma behind an intact tympanic membrane: histopathologic evidence for a tympanic membrane origin. *Otology and Neurotology.* 2001; **22**: 444–6.

111. Habermann J. Zur Entstehung des Cholesteatoms des Mittelohrs. *Archiv für Ohrenheilkunde.* 1888; **27**: 43–51.

112. Bezold F. Perforation der Membrana flaccida und Tubenverscluss. *Zeitschrift Hals Nasen Ohrenheilkunde.* 1890; **20**: 5–29.

113. Rueedi L. Cholesteatoma formation in the middle ear in animal experiments. *Acta Oto-Laryngologica.* 1959; **50**: 233–42.

114. Tos M. Incidence, etiology and pathogenesis of cholesteatoma in children. *Advances in Oto-Rhino-Laryngology.* 1988; **40**: 110–7.

115. Harker LA. Cholesteatoma: An incidence study. In: *Cholesteatoma First International Conference.* Birmingham, AL: Aesculapius Publishing Company, 1977: 308–9.

116. Kemppainen HO, Puhakka HJ, Laippala PJ, Sipila MM, Manninen MP, Karma PH. Epidemiology and aetiology of middle ear cholesteatoma. *Acta Oto-Laryngologica.* 1999; **119**: 568–72.

117. Padgham N, Mills R, Christmas H. Has the increasing use of grommets influenced the frequency of surgery for cholesteatoma? *Journal of Laryngology and Otology.* 1989; **103**: 1034–5.

118. Kinsella JB. Ventilation tubes and cholesteatoma. *Irish Medical Journal.* 1996; **89**: 223.

119. Rigner P, Renvall U, Tjellstrom A. Late results after cholesteatoma surgery in early childhood. *International Journal of Pediatric Otorhinolaryngology.* 1991; **22**: 213–8.

120. Rakover Y, Keywan K, Rosen G. Comparison of the incidence of cholesteatoma surgery before and after using

ventilation tubes for secretory otitis media. *International Journal of Pediatric Otorhinolaryngology.* 2000; **56**: 41–4.

121. Cohen D, Tamir D. The prevalence of middle ear pathologies in Jerusalem school children. *American Journal of Otology.* 1989; **10**: 456–9.

122. Balle VH, Tos M, Dang HS, Nhan TS, Le T, Tran KP et al. Prevalence of chronic otitis media in a randomly selected population from two communes in southern Vietnam. *Acta Oto-Laryngologica Supplementum.* 2000; **543**: 51–3.

123. Homoe P, Bretlau P. Cholesteatomas in Greenlandic Inuit. A retrospective study and follow-up of treated cases from 1976-91. *Arctic Medical Research.* 1994; **53**: 86–90.

124. McCafferty GJ, Coman WB, Shaw E, Lewis N. In: *Cholesteatoma in Australian aboriginal children. Cholesteatoma First International Conference.* Birmingham, AL: Aesculapius Publishing Company, 1975: 293–301.

125. Roland NJ, Phillips DE, Rogers JH, Singh SD. The use of ventilation tubes and the incidence of cholesteatoma surgery in the paediatric population of Liverpool. *Clinical Otolaryngology and Allied Sciences.* 1992; **17**: 437–9.

126. Falcioni M, Taibah A, De Donato G, Piccirillo E, Caruso A, Russo A et al. Preoperative imaging in chronic otitis surgery. *Acta Otorhinolaryngologica Italica.* 2002; **22**: 19–27.

127. Williams MT, Ayache D, Alberti C, Heran F, Lafitte F, Elmaleh-Berges M et al. Detection of postoperative residual cholesteatomas with delayed contrast-enhanced MR imaging: initial findings. *European Radiology.* 2003; **13**: 169–74.

128. Casselman JW, Kuhweide R, Dehaene I, Ampe W, Devlies F. Magnetic resonance examination of the inner ear and cerebellopontine angle in patients with vertigo and/or abnormal findings at vestibular testing. *Acta Oto-Laryngologica Supplementum.* 1994; **513**: 15–27.

129. Gersdorff M, Vilain J. Long-term results of various surgical treatments for cholesteatoma. *Acta Oto-Rhino-Laryngologica Belgica.* 1990; **44**: 393–8.

130. Smyth GD, Singh R, Hassard TH. Postoperative cholesteatoma: are claims for the canal wall down technique justified? *Otolaryngology and Head and Neck Surgery.* 1980; **88**: 473–6.

131. Rosenfeld RM, Moura RL, Bluestone CD. Predictors of residual-recurrent cholesteatoma in children. *Archives of Otolaryngology – Head and Neck Surgery.* 1992; **118**: 384–91.

*132. Hamilton JW. The efficacy of the KTP laser in cholesteatoma surgery. *Otology and Neurotology.* 2005; **26**: 135–9.

133. Gristwood RE, Venables WN. Factors influencing the probability of residual cholesteatoma. *Annals of Otology, Rhinology, and Laryngology.* 1990; **99**: 120–3.

134. Wormald PJ, Nilssen EL. The facial ridge and the discharging mastoid cavity. *Laryngoscope.* 1998; **108**: 92–6.

135. Austin DF. Single-stage surgery for cholesteatoma: an actuarial analysis. *American Journal of Otology.* 1989; **10**: 419–25.

136. Edelstein DR, Parisier SC. Surgical techniques and recidivism in cholesteatoma. *Otolaryngologic Clinics of North America.* 1989; **22**: 1029–40.

137. Bacciu S, Pasanisi E, Perez Raffo G, Avendano Arambula J, Piazza F, Bacciu A et al. Scutumplasty: costal cartilage versus bone pate. *Auris Nasis Larynx.* 1998; **25**: 155–9.

138. Hamilton JW. Recurrence after staged cholesteatoma surgery with bone pate repair of the lateral attic wall. Paper presented at Seventh International Cholesteatoma Conference, The Hague, 2004.

139. Sade J, Berco E, Buyanover D, Brown M. Ossicular damage in chronic middle ear inflammation. *Acta Oto-Laryngologica.* 1981; **92**: 273–83.

140. Schuknecht HF. *Pathology of the ear,* 2nd edn. Philadelphia, PA: Lea & Febiger, 1993.

141. Nadol JB. Histopathological correlates of residual and recurrent conductive hearing loss following tympanoplasty and stapedectomy. In: Rosowski JJ, Merchant SN (eds). *The function and mechanics of normal, diseased and reconstructed middle ears.* The Hague: Kugler Publications, 2000: 189–203.

142. Wullstein H. Theory and practice of tympanoplasty. *Laryngoscope.* 1956; **66**: 1076–93.

143. Farrior JB. Classification of tympanoplasty. *Archives of Otolaryngology.* 1971; **93**: 548–50.

144. Austin DF. Ossicular reconstruction. *Archives of Otolaryngology.* 1971; **94**: 525–35.

145. Fisch U. Basic situations in ossiculoplasty. In: Fisch U, May J (eds). *Tympanoplasty, mastoidectomy, and stapes surgery.* Stuttgart: Georg Thieme Verlag, 1994: 44.

*146. Smyth GD, Patterson CC. Results of middle ear reconstruction: do patients and surgeons agree? *American Journal of Otology.* 1985; **6**: 276–9.

147. Toner JC, Smyth GD, Kerr AG. Realities in ossiculoplasty. *Journal of Laryngology and Otology.* 1991; **105**: 529–33.

148. Browning GG, Gatehouse S, Swan IR. The Glasgow Benefit Plot: a new method for reporting benefits from middle ear surgery. *Laryngoscope.* 1991; **101**: 180–5.

149. Mills RP. The influence of pathological and technical variables on hearing results in ossiculoplasty. *Clinical Otolaryngology and Allied Sciences.* 1993; **18**: 202–5.

150. Albu S, Babighian G, Trabalzini F. Prognostic factors in tympanoplasty. *American Journal of Otology.* 1998; **19**: 136–40.

151. Modugno GC, Pirodda A, Saggese D, Magnani F, Soprani F. Multivariate analysis in predicting functional results in tympanoplasty. In: Magnan J, Chays A (eds). *Proceedings of the sixth international conference on cholesteatoma and ear surgery.* Marseille: Label Production, 2001: 973–6.

152. Dornhoffer JL, Gardner E. Prognostic factors in ossiculoplasty: a statistical staging system. *Otology and Neurotology.* 2001; **22**: 299–304.

153. Mangham CA, Lindeman RC. Ceravital versus plastipore in tympanoplasty: a randomized prospective trial. *Annals of Otology, Rhinology, and Laryngology.* 1990; **99**: 112–6.

154. Maassen MM, Zenner HP. Tympanoplasty type II with ionomeric cement and titanium-gold-angle prostheses. *American Journal of Otology.* 1998; **19**: 693–9.

155. Hamilton JW, Robinson JM. Short- and long-term hearing results after middle ear surgery. In: Rosowski JJ, Merchant SN (eds). *The function and mechanics of normal, diseased and reconstructed middle ears.* The Hague: Kugler Publications, 2000: 205–14.

156. Koike T, Wada H, Kobayashi T. Analysis of the finite-element method of tranfer function of reconstructed middle ears and their postoperative changes. In: Rosowski JJ, Merchant SN (eds). *The function and mechanics of normal, diseased and reconstructed middle ears.* The Hague: Kugler Publications, 2000: 309–20.

157. Morris DP, Bance M, van Wijhe RG, Kiefte M, Smith R. Optimum tension for partial ossicular replacement prosthesis reconstruction in the human middle ear. *Laryngoscope.* 2004; **114**: 305–8.

158. Bance M, Morris DP, van Wijhe RG, Kiefte M, Funnell WR. Comparison of the mechanical performance of ossiculoplasty using prosthetic malleus-to-stapes head with a tympanic membrane-to-stapes head assembly in a cadaveri middle ear model. *Otology and Neurotology.* 2004; **25**: 903–9.

159. Zahnert T, Huettenbrink KB. Pitfalls in ossicular chain reconstruction. *HNO.* 2005; **53**: 89–102 (in German).

75

Management of congenital deformities of the external and middle ear

DAVID GAULT AND MIKE ROTHERA

Introduction	965	Reconstructive middle ear surgery	982
Embryology	965	The bone-anchored hearing aid	985
Epidemiology and aetiology of ear deformity	967	Key points	986
The range and treatment of external ear deformities	968	Best clinical practice	986
Major congential malformations – microtia and atresia	975	Deficiencies in current knowledge and areas for future	
Assessment and management of the child with aural		research	987
atresia	980	References	987

SEARCH STRATEGY

The references for this chapter were compiled from a Medline search using the search terms congenital, ear and child. The opinions expressed are largely based on the personal experience of the authors.

INTRODUCTION

The embryology of the ear is complex and congenital anomalies are common. This chapter presents a résumé of the common anomalies and a discussion of the treatment options. Both hearing problems and deformity of the pinna can cause a great deal of distress. High quality surgery can lead to major improvements.

EMBRYOLOGY

A detailed knowledge of the normal embryology of the ear is a prerequisite to understanding the spectrum of congenital deformities that can occur and helps the surgeon predict the probable association between anomalies of the pinna, ear canal, middle and inner ear and facial nerve based on the time of embryological interruption.

Pinna

By the end of the fifth week, five branchial arches are discernable. In a 38-day-old embryo, six hillocks have developed in the mesenchymal tissue of the first (mandibular) and second (hyoid) arch and a process of fusion produces a primitive ear in the 50-day-old embryo. Hillocks 1–3 come from the mandibular arch and 4–6 from the hyoid. [****] The process of accretion is complicated and there is controversy over which hillock produces each part of the ear but Park,[1] after analysis of clinical cases makes a strong case for the theory that hillock 1 produces the anterior portion of the ear lobe, hillock 2 the tragus and hillock 3 the ascending helix. Of the second arch hillocks, 4 and 5 produce the anti-helix and the helix, with 6 contributing to the posterior lobule. This is supported by the arterial supply of the ear where hillocks 1, 2 and 3 correspond to the territory of the superficial temporal artery and hillocks 4, 5 and 6 to the distribution of the posterior auricular artery.[1] [****]

The conchal bowl originates from the first branchial groove. Incomplete fusion of the hillocks may cause clefts and hypergenesis may cause tubercles, tags and polyotia. The normal size of the auricle at birth is 66 percent of the length and 76 percent of the width of an adult ear.[2] By the age of six, the auricle has attained 90 percent of adult proportions. The pinna develops around the external meatus, which begins to canalize at week 28. The ear initially forms in the neck region and moves upward onto the head by week ten. In many anomalies, this migration is disturbed and the ear remains low set.

Malformation, such as anotia and microtia, are likely to be caused by the disturbance of development at seven to eight weeks gestational age, whereas deformations (lop, cup and prominent ears) are caused by a problem later in the development or by external compression.

External ear canal

The external ear canal arises from the ectoderm of the first branchial cleft, which appears at four weeks and extends medially towards the mesoderm of the first groove (developing tympanic ring) and first branchial pouch (the embryonic middle ear) during the eighth week. The ectoderm of the ear canal is separated from the endoderm of the first branchial pouch by a layer of mesoderm which becomes the middle fibrous layer of the ear drum. The tympanic ring begins ossification at 12 weeks and forms the bony portion of the external auditory canal. At 28 weeks, a core of ectoderm canalizes from medial to lateral and eventually breaks through to communicate with the conchal depression. [****] Failure of canalization or more rarely lack of ectodermal migration can lead to atresia of the external auditory meatus (EAM),[3] and partial canalization leads to meatal stenosis (an EAM with a diameter of less than 4 mm). Disruption of normal canalization or ectodermal migration can lead to arrested development of the tympanic ring mesoderm with the formation of a dense atretic bony plate in place of the tympanic membrane, an almost universal finding in canal atresia.

Middle ear and ossicles

The first branchial pouch starts to expand to form the Eustachian tube, middle ear and mastoid between the fourth and sixth weeks, but remains filled with mesenchyme until resorption, ossicular development and expansion of the pharyngeal pouch replaces this tissue.[3]

The ossicles are developed from the mesoderm of the first and second branchial arches with the exception of the stapes foot plate which also derives tissue from the otic capsule. The first arch derivatives form the head of the malleus and body and short process of the incus, whereas the more caudal structures, the manubrium of the malleus, long process of the incus and stapes suprastructure arise from the second arch. They start to develop during the fifth week of life. The incudostapedial joint forms during the seventh week. The endoderm of the middle ear cleft develops into the mucosal lining as supporting mesenchymal tissue resorbs, freeing the ossicular chain. [****] Failure of this process leads to a fused incudomalleolar mass which is often attached to the atretic bony plate.

The stapes has two developmental origins. The second arch cartilage forms the suprastructure and tympanic part of the foot plate. The vestibular portion of the foot plate and annular ligament are derived from the otic capsule. The process starts at five weeks and is not completed until 26 weeks. The developing stapedial anlage folds around the stapedial artery and meets the depression (lamina stapedialis) which form independently from the otic capsule. Any structure that interposes (such as a facial nerve or aberrant artery) can adversely effect the development of the oval window.

Ossicular abnormalities are frequently encountered in atresia surgery. They range from near normal development to ossicular fusion and a rudimentary monoblock ossicular mass. If an atretic plate is present, the malleus is always fused to it.[4] Other abnormalities include absence of the manubrium of the malleus, a shortened long process of the incus, failure of the incus to connect with the stapes and fusion of the incudostapedial joint (ISJ). Stapedial abnormalities are fortunately not as common as other ossicular anomalies[5] and although stapedial mobility can be hard to assess due to incudomalleolar fixation, in the presence of a reasonably well-developed suprastructure, a mobile foot plate can be expected.

Inner ear

Although the inner ear and labyrinthine windows have a different embryological origin from the middle and outer ear, abnormalities such as failure of the oval or round window to develop or congenital abnormalities of the cochlea, particularly a Mondini malformation can occur. Based on audiometric and polytomographic studies,[6] 10 percent of patients with atresia will have an inner ear abnormality, usually in the affected ear, but occasionally in the contralateral 'normal' ear. More recent studies using high resolution computed tomography (HRCT) suggest a higher rate of inner ear congenital anomalies affecting between 10 and 47 percent of patients with atresia.[3, 7]

Facial nerve

For the otologist, the ability to predict the course of an aberrant facial nerve in atresia is one of the most important aspects of surgical planning. Satoloff[8] and

Gulya[3] provide a comprehensive review of facial nerve embryology and its practical application, and it is usually possible to deduce the course of the facial nerve by careful analysis of the arrested development[9] supplemented by HRCT scanning.

The facial nerve first appears as the facio-acoustic primordium, the nerve of the second branchial arch at three weeks. At four to five weeks, the sprouting facial nerve and chorda tympani divide the primitive mesenchyme of the second arch into the stapes, stapedius muscle and posterior middle ear wall precursor. At seven weeks, five branches appear in the parotid bud and by 16 weeks the neural communications with the facial muscles are complete (see also Chapter 80, Facial paralysis in childhood). At this stage the course of the facial nerve is much more anterosuperior than in adults.

At eight weeks, a sulcus develops on the posterior otic capsule (the primitive Fallopian canal) and this first genu is remarkably constant. Dehiscence of the horizontal portion and second genu occurs in 25–55 percent of postmortem temporal bones,[8, 10] but displacement is much less common. At ten weeks, the vertical (mastoid) segment of the facial nerve is anterolateral to the middle ear (ME) and external auditory canal (EAC). Failure of the tympanic ring and mastoid to develop over the next 16 weeks places the nerve in a more primitive position. The angle at the second genu at ten weeks is 60°, only reaching the more normal angle of 120° by 26 weeks. Failure of the normal separation between the mastoid and temporomandibular joint (TMJ) leads to a more acute angle at the second genu, increasing the risk of dehiscence and inferior displacement over the oval window. In early developmental arrest, the nerve can pass between the oval and round window, passing through the postero-inferior portion of the atretic plate and exiting through the glenoid fossa. In severe cases the nerve or branches may exit just below a rudimentary tragus.[11] Other abnormalities include a bifurcating facial nerve and a large chorda tympani containing motor fibres.[12]

EPIDEMIOLOGY AND AETIOLOGY OF EAR DEFORMITY

Epidemiology

Microtia occurs once in every 6000 births. The occurrence is estimated at one in 4000 in the Japanese and as high as one in 1:1200 births in Navajo Indians. In 10 percent of cases, the problem is bilateral. The right side is more commonly affected than the left and males are more often affected than females. The overall frequency of prominent ears in North America is 4.5 percent.[13, 14] Skin tags occur in 0.2 percent of the population. Congenital atresia/microtia can occur sporadically as an isolated congenital anomaly, associated with other anomalies or as part of a

recognized syndrome. In most cases the cause is unknown, but in a minority (15 percent) a genetic or environmental cause (foetal alcohol syndrome, maternal diabetic embryopathy, thalidomide and isotretinoin exposure) can be identified. A small number of familial cases of isolated atresia have been reported with autosomal dominant, recessive and x-linked inheritance. Several pairs of identical twins are identified where only one twin has microtia. This lends support to the theory that an intrauterine event rather that a genetic trigger suppresses ear development. At present, haemorrhage in the region of the stapedial artery at a critical phase is the most likely local cause.[15] Thalidomide was thought to induce this.

Syndromic associations

A syndrome does not infer a genetic cause. Whilst the gene mutation causing mandibular facial dystostosis has been identified[16] and brachio-otorenal syndrome is known to be genetic, hemifacial microsomia is just a constellation of abnormalities that are clinically recognizable but at present regarded as idiopathic with no inherited tendency. The causes are probably pathologically heterogeneous with defective genes, teratogens or vascular anomalies acting singly or collectively to disrupt normal development.[17, 18] Syndromic conditions associated with congenital aural atresia include:

- hemifacial microsomia (HM);
- Treacher Collins;
- brachio-otorenal;
- Sticklers;
- Crouzons;
- Noonan syndrome;
- foetal alcohol syndrome;
- coloboma, heart defects, choanal atresia, developmental and growth retardation, genito-urinary malformations and ear anomalies (CHARGE) (see also Chapter 82, Nasal obstruction in children).

See also Chapter 78, Craniofacial anomalies: genetics and management.

HEMIFACIAL MICROSOMIA

Hemifacial microsomia (HM) is a spectrum of malformations involving the orbit, mandible, ears, facial nerve and soft tissues of the face occurring in 1 in 5600 births.[17] Most cases are sporadic, but in rare cases there are familial patterns consistent with autosomal dominant or autosomal recessive inheritance. The presence of a twin is thought to make the causal event more likely to occur.[19] It is generally unilateral but bilateral cases occur in 17 percent. There is a prediction for the right ear (58 percent) and males (63 percent).[20] Isolated microtia has been considered a minor form of HM. Facial weakness and hearing loss are the most common functional defects with 86 percent having a conductive hearing loss and 10–16 percent having a sensorineural hearing loss, a feature that is underappreciated (incidence in the general population is 0.001 percent and in other craniofacial syndromes, 3–4 percent). There is little correlation between the severity of the dysmorphic features and hearing loss. Patients with mildly dysmorphic features can have a moderately severe degree of deafness. The five major features (orbital, mandibular, ear, nerve and soft tissue) form the basis for the most comprehensive and clinically useful classification system, the OMENS score.[17] See also Chapter 80, Facial paralysis in childhood and Chapter 78, Craniofacial anomalies: genetics and management.

Mandibular facial dystostosis or Treacher Collins syndrome is a more specific condition caused by an abnormality on chromosome 5 (5q32-33.2).[16] This is an autosomal dominant condition causing a first and second arch malformation. Six percent occur as a sporadic mutation.[21] The condition is characterized by downsloping palpebral fissures, coloboma of the eyes, hypoplasia of the mandible and maxilla, cleft palate and microtia with atresia. The incidence is 1 in 50,000 live births. Most have bilateral malformed pinna and aural atresia. It is common for the mastoids and middle ears to be poorly developed and in many patients the middle cranial fossa descends to the level of the superior semicircular canal[22] and the jugular bulb protrudes into the small tympanic cavity, making most of these patients unsuitable for middle ear surgery. Most patients have normal inner ear function.

Brachio-oto-renal (BOR) syndrome occurs in 1 in 40,000 children as an autosomal dominant condition. Branchial clefts, fistulae and cysts occur with a malformed pinna and preauricular pits. The syndrome is associated with various renal anomalies. Seventy-five percent of patients with BOR syndrome have a significant hearing loss. Of these, 30 percent are conductive, 20 percent sensorineural and 50 percent mixed.[23] Recent mutational studies in *Drosophila* have shown that gene EYA1 causes the syndrome. The encoded protein or transcriptional activator has been located to chromosome 8 in humans.[24] See also Chapter 66, Molecular otology, development of the auditory system and recent advances in genetic manipulation.

Stickler syndrome is another autosomal dominant condition presenting with cleft palate, micrognathia, severe myopia and retinal detachment. Most of the conductive hearing loss is due to Eustachian tube dysfunction secondary to the cleft palate, but ossicular abnormalities may be present. Some cases have a progressive high frequency sensorineural hearing loss. Mutation of the COL2A1 gene on chromosome 12 has been implicated.[23] See also Chapter 66, Molecular otology, development of the auditory system and recent

advances in genetic manipulation and Chapter 78, Craniofacial anomalies: genetics and management.

Crouzon syndrome (craniofacial dystostosis) is an autosomal dominant craniofacial anomaly with a prevalence of 1 in 50,000, but with marked variability of phenotypic expression characterized by craniosynostosis, maxillary hypoplasia and shallow orbits causing proptosis. A conductive hearing loss is present in 50 percent of cases with 13 percent having aural atresia. See also Chapter 78, Craniofacial anomalies: genetics and management.

Noonan syndrome is a craniofacial abnormality associated with short stature, webbed neck and cardiac abnormalities. The incidence is 1 in 25,000 births[25] and otological problems consist of low set and posteriorly rotated ears, infolding of the helix and a 10–15 percent incidence of sensorineural hearing loss.

Foetal alcohol syndrome is the leading cause of mental retardation in the western world[26] with an incidence of 2 in 1000 live births. Midfacial hypoplasia is common and the condition accounts for 10 percent of children with Pierre Robin sequence. Otological features are posteriorly rotated ears with a poorly formed concha and mixed hearing loss.

The acronym 'CHARGE' describes a nonrandom clustering of malformations and includes coloboma, heart defects, choanal atresia, developmental and growth retardation, genito-urinary malformations and ear anomalies. The head and neck anomalies, in addition to choanal atresia, include external ear abnormalities in 68 percent of cases, congenital middle ear ossicular anomalies in 10 percent and sensorineural hearing loss in 8 percent. Facial nerve dysfunction occurs in 38 percent and was found to be a statistically significant predictor of profound hearing loss which was not true of the severity of the external ear deformity.[27]

THE RANGE AND TREATMENT OF EXTERNAL EAR DEFORMITIES

What is normal?

It is important to have a sense of the normal ear in order to fully appreciate the concerns of patients with abnormalities of ear size, position and slope (**Figure 75.1**). The average adult female ear is 59 mm tall and the average male ear 63 mm tall. In boys, the ear length is 48 mm at six months increasing to 55 mm at five years and 59 mm at ten years. The values are a little reduced for girls. The ear is thus almost fully grown at ten years. Thereafter, it seems to remain much the same size until the age of 60 when it gradually enlarges, particularly the lobe (**Figure 75.2**). The average adult ear protrudes 19 mm from the mastoid skin. The long axis of the ear slopes backwards in line with the slope of the nose. The

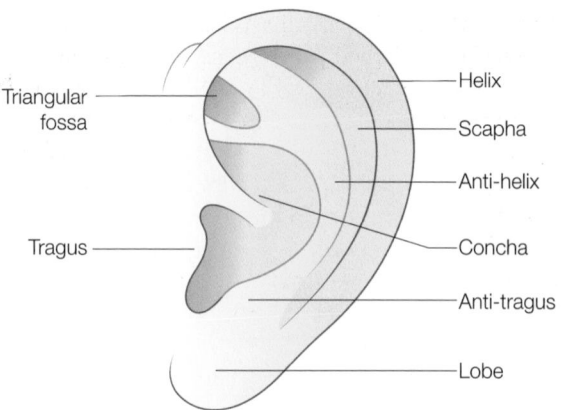

Figure 75.1 The external ear.

Triangular fossa
Tragus
Helix
Scapha
Anti-helix
Concha
Anti-tragus
Lobe

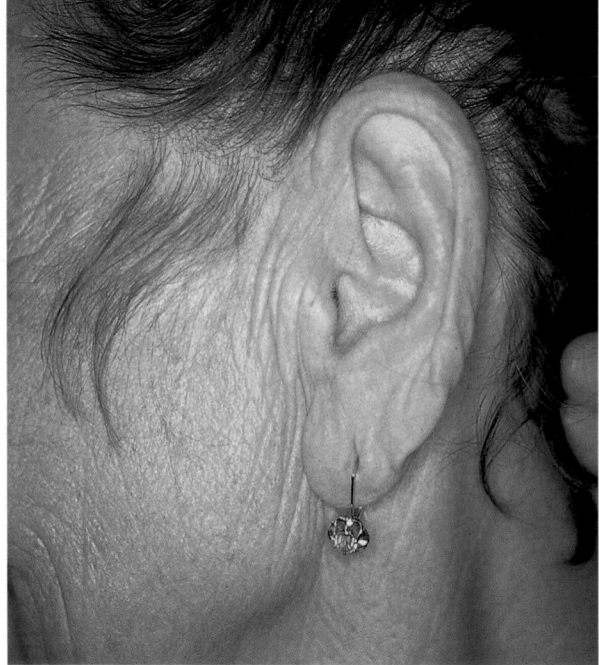

Figure 75.2 The ear often enlarges with age.

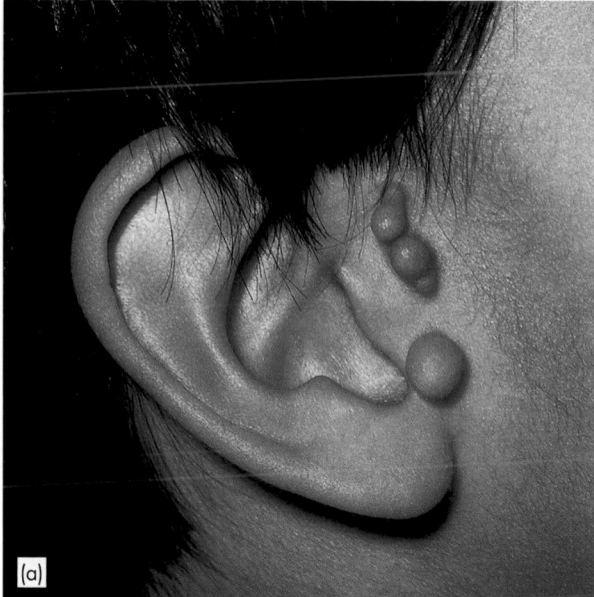

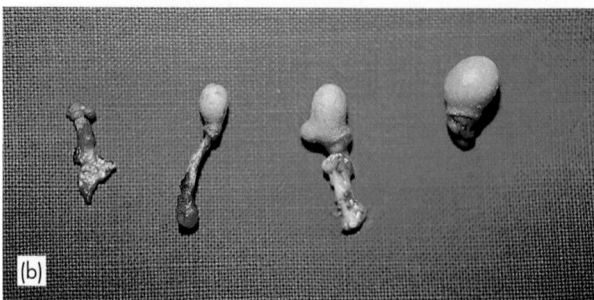

Figure 75.3 (a) A patient presents with preauricular skin tags. (b) When removed, they are often seen to have long cartilage stalks.

ear lies between the level of the eyebrow and a line a few millimetres beneath the nasal columella. The distance from the lateral canthus of the eye to the front of the ear is just over the length of the ear.

A number of patients are extremely sensitive about ears that are excessively large, protruding or which slope forwards. The variety of ear deformity is wide.

Tags

Preauricular skin tags are very common (**Figure 75.3a**). Sometimes the lesion involves only skin but usually the tag contains a long tail of cartilage extending into the cheek (**Figure 75.3b**). It is commonplace to ligate preauricular skin tags in the neonatal period. A new technique is to apply a Liga clip – this is quick and easy to do and a few days later the tag drops off.

Tags with a substantial cartilage core are best treated by elective excision of the skin tag and cartilage spindle under general anaesthetic. A vertical ellipse is recommended.

Mirror ear or polyotia

Rarely, persistent preauricular tissues are so large that they resemble an extra ear and the term 'polyotia' is used. The 'second' ear can appear as a mirror image folded forward and lying on the posterior cheek, and the term mirror ear is also applied (**Figure 75.4a**). It is recommended that skin is peeled off the extra-auricular tissue and protruding cartilage remnants are trimmed. The trimmed cartilage fragments are packed into the anterior conchal hollow and then the skin of the extra ear is redraped to give the cheek a flatter shape (**Figure 75.4b**).[28]

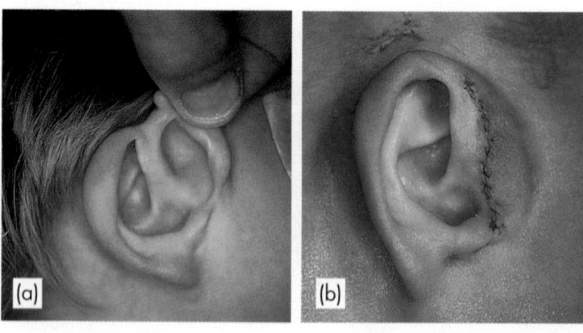

Figure 75.4 (a) Polyotia or mirror ear; (b) postoperative view.

Pits and sinuses

Preauricular sinuses can be difficult to excise and may recur after treatment (**Figure 75.5**). Very occasionally, the sinuses track deeply near to the facial nerve. They are often bilateral and frequently asymptomatic. However, if recurrent infections occur which fail to settle with anti-staphlococcal antibiotics, surgical excision is appropriate. Although most are simple branching sinuses they can pass close to the facial nerve and the use of a microscope or loupes is a great help. It is advisable to use active facial nerve monitoring and avoid local anaesthetic infiltration.

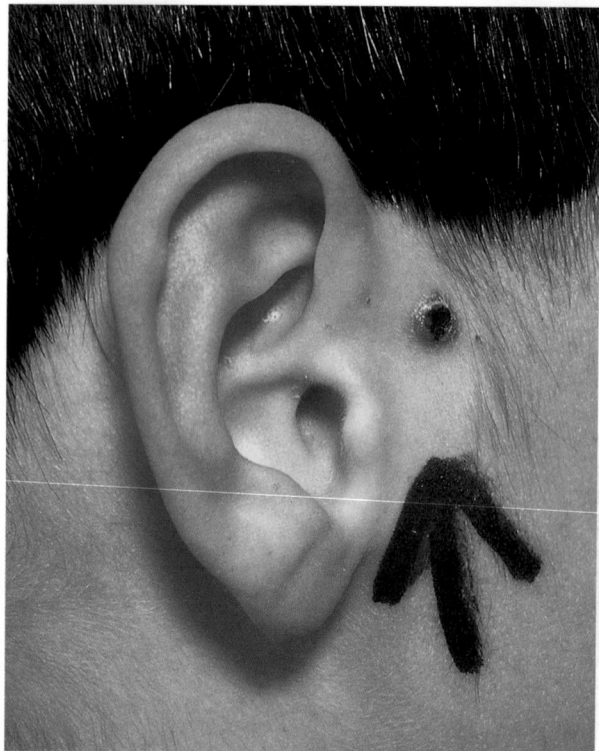

Figure 75.5 An infected preauricular sinus.

Abnormal folds (Stahl's bar)

Abnormal folding of the ear is common (**Figure 75.6a**). A Stahl's bar or third crus is a frequent finding (**Figure 75.6b**). In a small number of cases, the upper pole of the ear flops over and here the term 'lop ear' is used. In some ears, a kink of the helical rim or abnormal fusion of the helical rim to the antihelical fold is observed. In some patients the whole ear appears collapsed vertically to give an ear of reduced height. Stahl's bar is easily and temporarily corrected by finger pressure, but surgical correction often turns out to be difficult to execute.

Attempts to reshape the cartilage by either scoring or tie-bar type tethering sutures are rarely successful and a splint (**Figure 75.6c**) gives a better result. The technique in which the offending cartilage kink is excised as a disc, turned over and through 90° so that the trough is in line with the scaphal hollow, is attractive but not usually wholly successful. A direct wedge excision of the Stahl's bar (skin and cartilage) is a more reliable technique. As the cut edges of the helical rim are sutured together it tends to gain a more normal curl, and although the ear is made smaller it is usually much more attractive.[29]

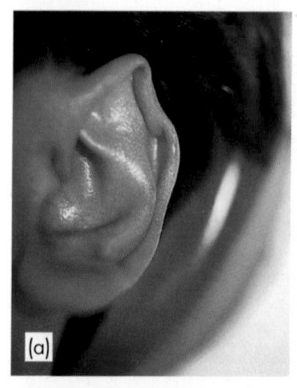
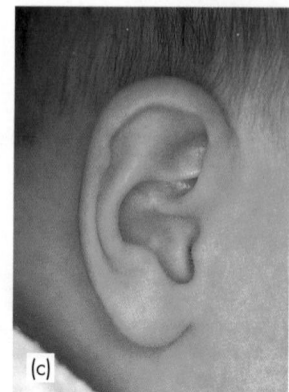
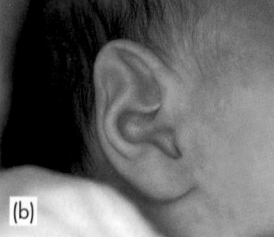

Figure 75.6 (a) Abnormal folds; (b and c) Stahl's bar pre- and post correction with a splint.

Prominent ('bat') ears

Prominent ears are sometimes present at birth (61 percent), while other cases become obvious as the infant head shape changes (**Figure 75.7a**).[30] The condition is not viewed as a deformity in all cultures. The prominence is usually due to an absent antihelical fold but, in some cases, the conchal bowl is excessively deep. A prominent lobe or antitragus is less common. A grading scale for

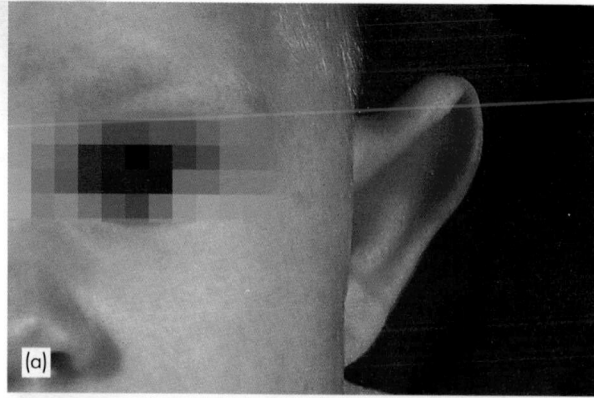

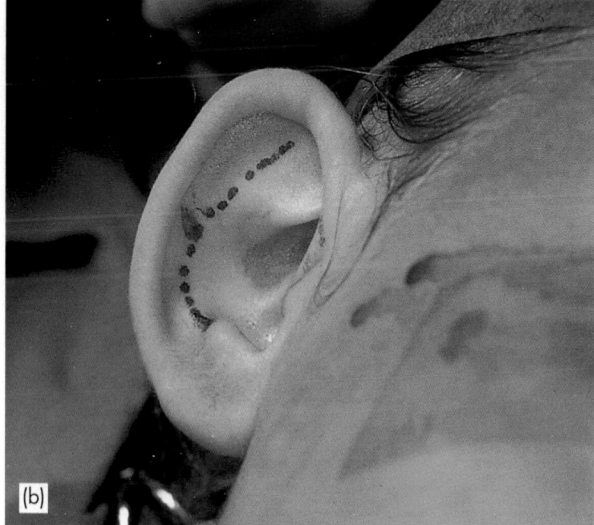

Figure 75.7 (a) Prominent (bat) ear; (b) a prominent ear which lacks an antehelical fold.

prominent ears has been put forward by Graham and Gault,[31] which, in addition to the above features, factors in elasticity and memory of the cartilage. Digital pressure on the relevant part of the ear determines the cause for prominence and gauges the strength of the cartilage. It is recommended that surgery to set back ears be delayed until after the age of five years. Prior to this, the cartilage is especially soft and efforts to reshape it may instead cause irregularity.

Sometimes parents (quite understandably) want prominent ears corrected when the child (equally understandably) is reluctant to have the operation. It is safest in such a situation to put the wishes of the child first. Children who are teased are usually willing to have surgery. Sometimes the need to wear hair up in a ballet class, for example, will prompt a request for surgery.

It is essential to discuss preoperatively the desired position of the ears. Some patients want only a gentle change whilst, for others, only ears which are flat to the side of the head are acceptable.

No two prominent ears are the same. The most common problem is an inadequate antehelical fold (**Figure 75.7b**). This can cause the ear to protrude at

right angles to the mastoid skin. In other ears the conchal bowl is excessively deep, but the antihelical fold is normal. During correction, some ears will need additional attention to a protruding lobe or isolated protrusion of the upper pole alone. In some ears, the reshaping is specifically intended to improve hearing aid retention, and in these, space must be left for the device.

Surgical techniques to remould the cartilage include anterior scoring (**Figure 75.8**),[32] reshaping of the curves by the use of posterior sutures (to emphasize the antihelical fold or to setback the concha)[33] and excision techniques to set back the concha. It is not conventional to rely on skin excision alone to hold back the ear, since this may increase the risk of hypertrophic scarring. Correction of bat ears is challenging surgery and unsatisfactory results can give rise to litigation. It is essential that surgeons who undertake this sort of work are adequately trained and carefully audit their outcomes. Inadequate set back, abnormal shape or folding, keloid scars and significant tissue destruction can cause patients to seek legal redress (**Figure 75.9**). It is important to record that adequate warning of potential problems has been given. Vigilance and prompt treatment of any problems is advised.

Collapsed ears

In a number of patients, the helical rim is adequate but the scaphal hollow is folded backwards to rest on the conchal hollow. The height and shape of the ear is readily improved by undoing soft tissue tethering between the scaphal and conchal cartilages and splinting these structures apart with a cartilage graft. The conchal hollow is a suitable donor site for such grafts.

Folded-over helical rim

When the helical rim cartilage is sharply folded over to provide a double layer covered in a single skin envelope, the ear looks pinched. To correct this, the folded-over

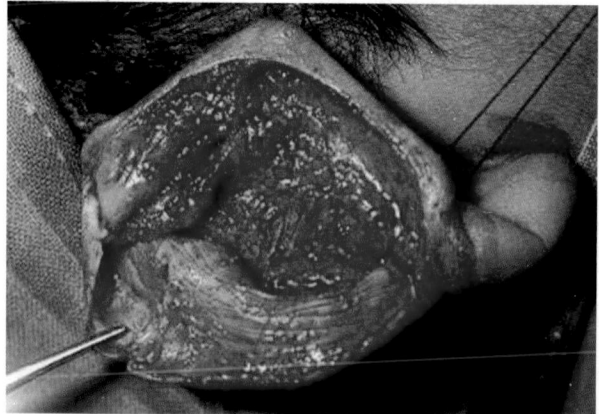

Figure 75.8 The use of anterior scoring to reshape the antehelical fold of a prominent ear.

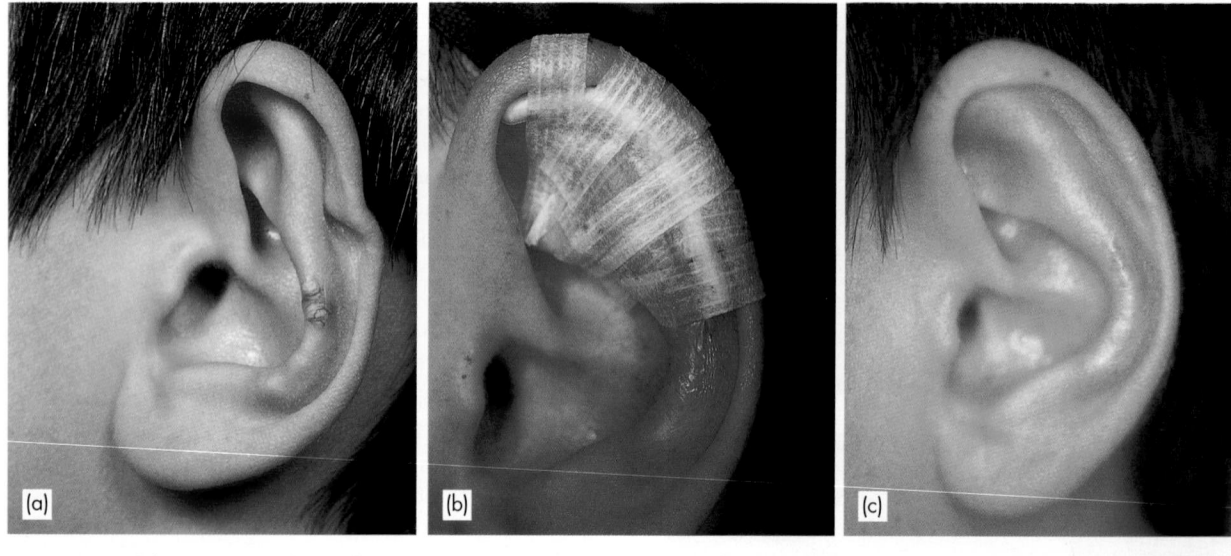

Figure 75.9 (a) An ear kink after prominent ear surgery; (b) the thin indented rim cartilage is reinforced with a cartilage graft and the rim is splinted; (c) the final result.

cartilage (Noonan syndrome, described under Hemifacial microsomia) is excised and then repositioned behind the scaphal hollow to open up the upper pole.

Lop ears

To support a lop ear, 'Mustarde'-type sutures can be used to create a U-shaped cartilage prop at the site of the missing upper antihelical fold.[33] As reinforcement, it is recommended that the ear be hitched to the mastoid fascia (**Figure 75.10**).[34]

'Bumps' and clefts

A bump on the helical rim is a common finding, often referred to as a 'Darwin's tubercle'. This swelling lies at the point at which hillocks 3 and 4 normally fuse.

A cleft of the ear lobe is not a common finding (**Figure 75.11**). In some patients, it is a groove or notch due to poor fusion of hillocks 6 and 1. In others, a significant portion of the lobe is missing due to absence of hillock 6.

The standard cleft of the ear lobe leaves a notch. The anterior fragment is often more medial than the posterior fragment, such that the lobe components lie in different planes. It is possible to raise interposing skin flaps from the notch and to realign the deep tissues with a fine suture. Skin flaps are then redraped and trimmed over the new lobe to resurface it.

In some cases a lobe may be underdeveloped or absent. Such lobes must be rebuilt around a cartilage framework; a disc of conchal cartilage usually suffices.

A partial cleft may interrupt the smooth helical rim as an oblique notch. After peeling the skin off, the

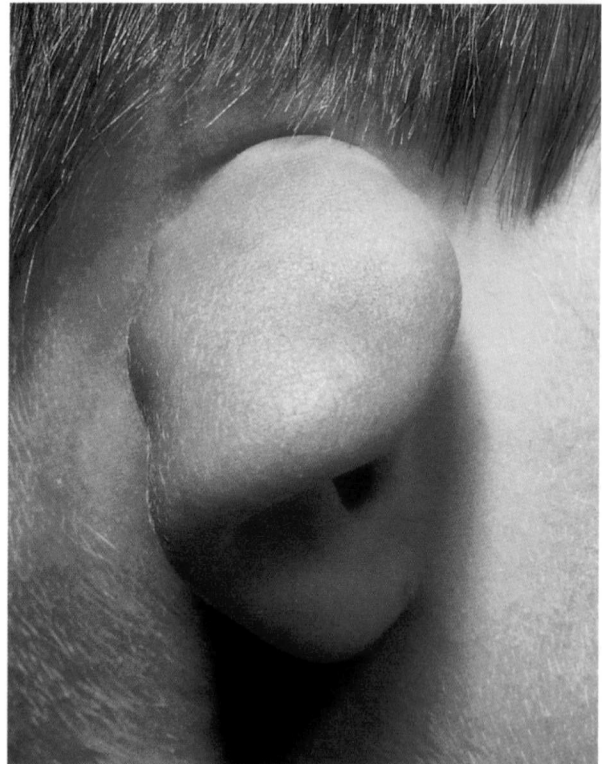

Figure 75.10 Lop ear.

cartilage can be divided in a zig-zag fashion and the leaves resutured to expand the arch of the ear.

Another variation is the absent helical rim.

Macrotia

Excessively large ears are a common cause of teasing. Various components of the ear may be overlarge. In a

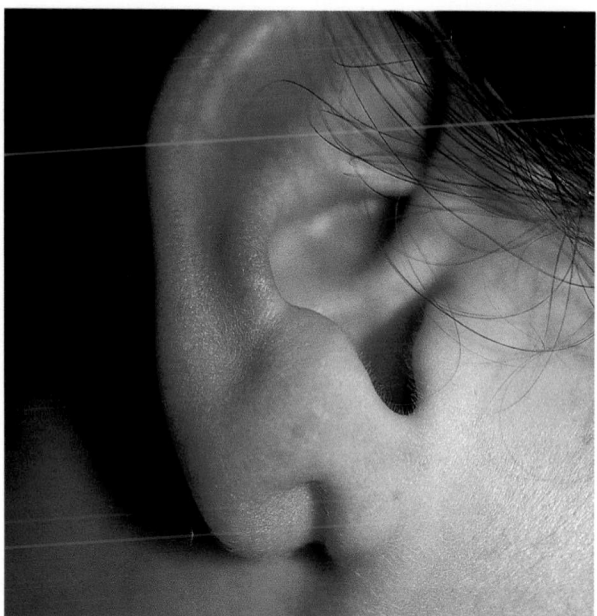

Figure 75.11 A congenital cleft of the ear lobe.

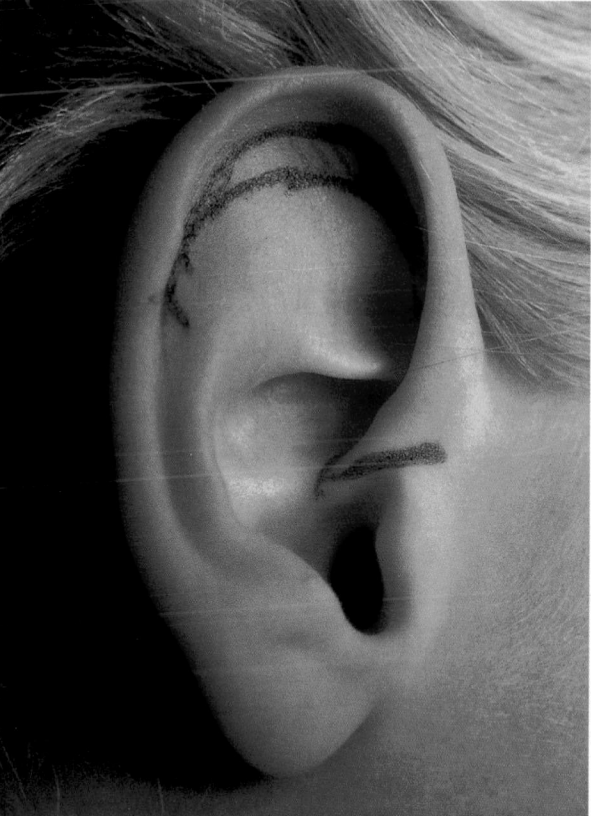

Figure 75.12 Macrotia – the scaphal hollow is overlarge.

normal ear, the upper pole, conchal hollow and lobe take up an equal amount of the height of the ear, splitting it into thirds. In many cases of macrotia, the scaphal hollow is too big, causing the ear to appear top-heavy (**Figure 75.12**). In others, the lobe is too big, so that the ear appears bottom-heavy.

To reduce an excessively large upper ear, it is recommended that an anterior crescent of skin and cartilage be removed from the scaphal hollow of the ear.[35] The helical rim is then advanced around the now smaller ear, preserving the posterior skin to ensure blood supply to the rim. As the root of the helix is approached, spare rim skin and cartilage is trimmed. The cartilage is sutured with fine absorbable sutures. The scars are hidden in the curve of the helical rim and are usually inconspicuous. To reduce an oversized lobe, a wedge of tissue is removed.

Cup ears

In these ears the helical rim is constricted to give a prominent, cone-shaped ear. This is particularly difficult to correct. The constricted rim of a cup ear must be expanded in order to allow it to flatten. A number of techniques have been described. The cartilage can be incised in a zig-zag fashion to expand it once the skin has been peeled off the rim. An alternative is to make a series of radial incisions and to splint them open with a cartilage graft. Another technique is the use of a V–Y plasty at the root of the helix combined with undermining of adjacent skin. Where the ear is severely constricted (conchal-type microtia) a formal reconstruction using a carved costal cartilage framework is advised.

Cryptotia ('the hidden ear')

Sometimes, only the lower two-thirds of an ear is visible and the upper auricular sulcus seems lost (**Figure 75.13**). When the ear is gently pulled away from the side of the head, the upper pole cartilage becomes evident, having been hidden beneath scalp skin. The upper pole is excessively tethered and the lower pole is prominent. To attempt an early, nonsurgical correction, a small Ear Buddies™ splint should be applied as soon as possible after birth to create the upper sulcus. Later, surgical treatment requires the insertion of a skin graft or local flap to release the tethered portion of the ear. The upper auricular sulcus must be recreated with flaps or skin grafts. A simple technique is to widely release the ear by dividing all the fascia and muscles responsible for the tethering and to rotate a superiorly hinged pedicled flap of post-auricular skin from the lower pole into the resulting defect. Occasionally, a revision procedure is required.

Positional problems

An ear which slopes in line with the nose gives a harmonious appearance to the head. Some ears may be too low set. They can often be hitched upwards

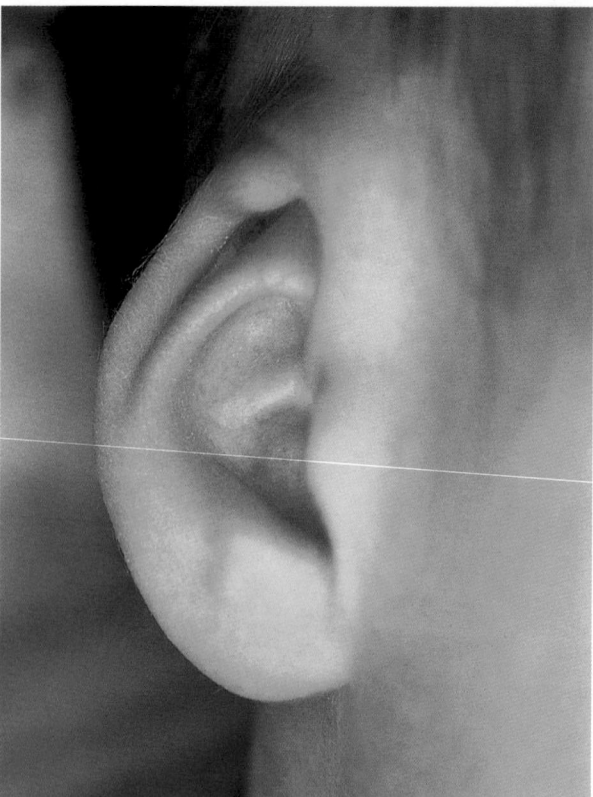

Figure 75.13 In cryptotia, the upper ear cartilage is buried beneath the scalp.

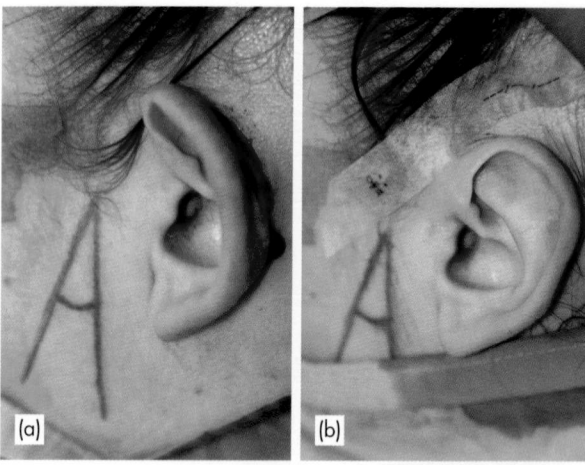

Figure 75.14 (a) An ear with a very vertical axis; (b) after correction.

(auropexy). Sometimes the axis of the ear may be abnormal, such that patients complain about their ears, but are unsure of what is wrong. These ears are usually excessively vertical and it is possible with conchomastoid sutures to adjust the slope (**Figure 75.14**).

Unusual malformations

Vascular malformations including capillary haemangiomata and port wine stain can involve the ear. Hypertrophy of the lobe is common in patients in whom a giant naevus involves the ear. In patients with neurofibromatosis, the ear is often enlarged and malpositioned. Lymphangiomata can present on the ear and sometimes occlude the meatus (**Figure 75.15**).

Splintage

The cartilage of the newborn ear is extremely soft and pliable, possibly due to the influence of circulating maternal oestrogen. In a number of ear deformities in which there is a normal amount of skin and cartilage but the ear is abnormally shaped or prominent, splintage can be curative if performed soon after birth.[36] This technique is applicable to prominent ears, Stahl's bars, lop ears,

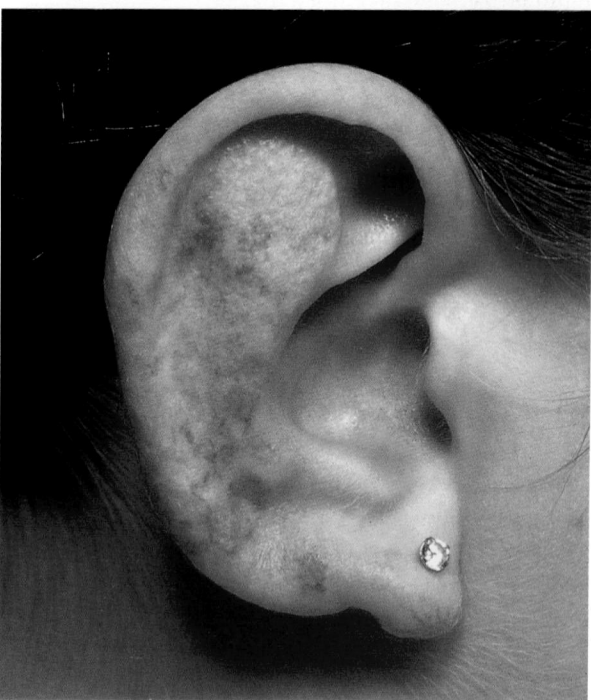

Figure 75.15 Macrotia due to a resolving haemangioma.

cryptotia and kinks of the rim (**Figure 75.16**). It has no role in treating microtia.

It is several weeks before the ear cartilage begins to harden and ideally splintage should be started in the first few days of life. At this stage the cartilage is easily remoulded, the sweat glands are poorly developed so that the tapes which hold the splint in place stick well, and the child moves its head little, and does not reach up to the ears to dislodge or pick at the splints.

Flexible wire splints totally encased in silicone are now commercially available for parents themselves to apply to their child (Ear Buddies). For prominence, rim kinks, Stahl's bar and other abnormal folds, the splints are taped into the scaphal hollow of the ear and then the ear is taped back to the side of the head. The splint exerts

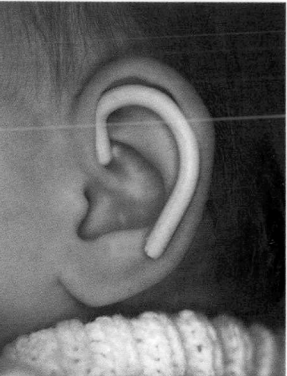

Figure 75.16 A splint *in situ*.

pressure on the scaphal hollow of the ear and emphasizes the antihelical fold and the helical rim. Simply taping the ear back without the splint *in situ* does little to effect an improvement and risks distortion of the rim of the ear. The splint is used in the upper auricular sulcus to correct cryptotia.

In the newborn, splintage for one to two weeks is all that is necessary, whereas in older children (up to six months of age) the splints should be used for several months. If the parents are not diligent in applying the splint then a good correction is less likely. By contrast, some persistent parents achieve a worthwhile correction in children as old as one year. Compliance is increased by the simple expedient of an attractive, though purely cosmetic headband, which hides the tapes and splint on the affected ear or ears from prying eyes.

Early splintage may improve ear shape without the need for later surgery or anaesthetic. Splintage has the additional advantage of preventing presurgery teasing. It is not yet a widespread practice, despite a number of reports which show neonatal splintage of misshapen ears to be of benefit, cheap and safe.[37] Nevertheless, it is clear that the future treatment of such deformities lies in this direction.[38]

MAJOR CONGENTITAL MALFORMATIONS – MICROTIA AND ATRESIA

Classification of microtia

There is great variety in the shape of underdeveloped ears. Total anotia is rare; there is no ear structure and a very low hairline (**Figure 75.17**). The standard microtia patient has a small dependent lobe hanging beneath a cartilage nubbin (**Figure 75.18a**). In a small number of patients, a narrow strip of normal skin separates two small ear remnants (**Figure 75.18b**). It is probable that one of these remnants comes from the first and the other from the second branchial arch, which have failed to fuse. Patients in this group usually have facial nerve weakness on the affected side. The facial nerve is prone to damage

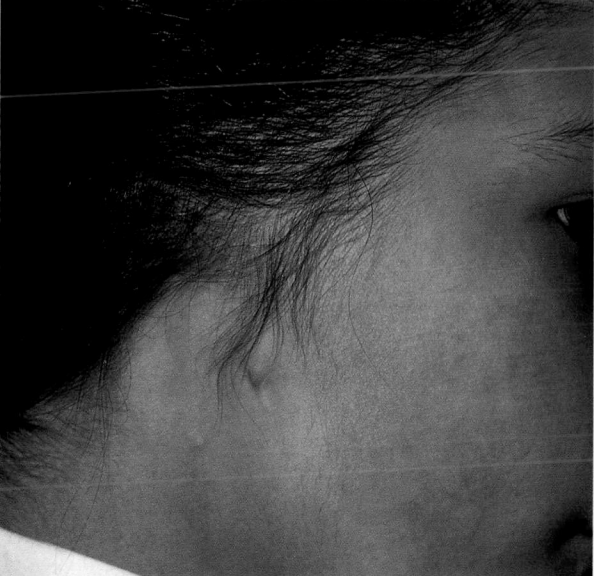

Figure 75.17 Anotia.

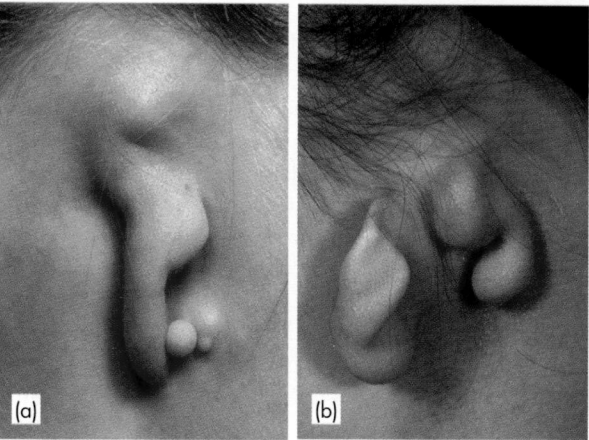

Figure 75.18 (a) Standard microtia; (b) two remnant microtia.

during reconstructive surgery, probably because it runs a very superficial course.

Other variations of microtia include the conchal type (**Figure 75.19**) in which the tragus and a primitive external auditory meatus are present. The term 'constricted ear' or 'cup ear' is used for those cases in which a considerable amount of ear tissue is present. In many of these, when the ear is unfolded, there is a considerable structural defect in the upper pole.

Various classification systems for grades of microtia and atresia have been proposed over the years. All have their merits, but those that reflect the degree of surgical complexity and potential success are clinically more useful. Although there is a recognizable correlation between the degree of microtia and severity of atresia and facial nerve anomalies, this can only be partially predicted from the type of atresia, and trying to impose a unified classification system underestimates the

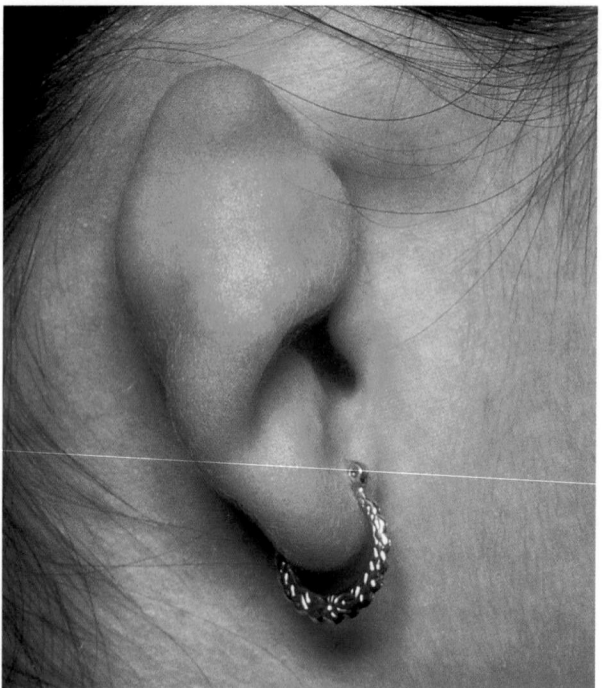

Figure 75.19   A conchal-type microtia.

embryological complexity and diversity of this group. Careful analysis in each case of clinical, audiological and radiological criteria is essential if the patient is to receive the best advice and treatment. Marx's classification of the external ear in 1926[39] proposed four descriptive groups (**Table 75.1**) and has formed the basis of most subsequent systems.

A very detailed classification was suggested by Weerda,[40] that incorporated a surgical plan for each type of defect, but there are valid differences of opinion regarding which type of procedures are appropriate for a particular degree of microtia and a broader classification has generally been accepted. Aguilar and Jahrsdoerfer[41] amended the Marx grading system (**Table 75.2**), which enabled a surgeon to categorize the auricular deformity easily. Grade I, i.e. a smaller but essentially normal ear, needs no correction. Grade II and III deformities can be treated by a variety of surgical techniques described below.

Classification of atresia

Congenital aural atresia also represents a failure of embryological development but over a longer potential time-frame than auricular deformities. Although the severity of microtia has been shown to correlate with the degree of hearing loss[42] and middle ear development[43] up to 10 percent of atresias occur in isolation and minor auricular abnormalities carry a risk factor for middle ear anomalies. There is also an increased risk (10–25 percent) of contralateral congenital conductive hearing loss in unilateral microtia/atresia.[9]

Table 75.1   Descriptive classification of auricular detects proposed by Marx.

Group	Description
Grade I	The auricle is abnormal; different structures of each part of the ear may be recognizable
Grade II	The auricle is abnormal, parts of the ear are not recognizable
Grade III	Very small auricular tag is present
Grade IV	Anotia

Reprinted from Ref. 39, with permission.

Table 75.2   Classification of congenital deformities.

Group	Description
Grade I	Any normal ear that is simply smaller in size in any given dimension
Grade II	An ear with structural deficiencies, such as absent scapha, absent lobule, broadened helical rim, missing helix, missing conchal bowl or missing anti-helical fold
Grade III	An ear exhibiting the classic 'peanut' deformity with no recognizable structures present, anotia

Adapted from Ref. 41, with permission.

A detailed review of the major classifications of congenital atresia is presented by Declan *et al.*[44] From a surgical point of view, the anatomical classification of Altman[45] and its later modification by Marquet[46] and Cremers *et al.*[47] is comprehensive, user-friendly and useful for predicting those patients who might benefit from reconstructive surgery (**Table 75.3**).

Marquet subdivided moderate type II depending on the course of the facial nerve in its third segment, the morphology of the atretic plate, the presence of a tympanic bone and the distance between the glenoid cavity and the anterior surface of the mastoid tip. Surgical outcome was highly related to the proposed classification.[46]

In type IIa, the course of the facial nerve is normal in the third segment. The tympanic bone is hypoplastic, but present with an upper part formed by the squamosal bone and an inferior part from the tympanic bone and extending laterally to the scutum. The distance between the temporomandibular joint and mastoid tip is normal.

In type IIb, the facial nerve is more anteriorly placed in the third segment. The tympanic bone is almost absent and the atretic plate, formed by the squamous bone superiorly and by a length of bone inferiorly extending from the otic capsule but never lateral to the scutum. In between these is often a fibrous ridge containing the facial nerve. A hypoplastic Reichart's cartilage may be present and the distance between the glenoid cavity and mastoid is significantly reduced.

Table 75.3 Classification of aural atresia.

Group	Description
Grade I	The tympanic membrane is still present but hypoplastic. The tympanic bone is normal or hypoplastic. Various types of ossicular malformation have been described, but the stapes is usually mobile
Grade II	An atretic plate is present. The tympanic bone is hypoplastic or absent. The course of the facial nerve may be abnormal. The tympanic cavity is within normal limits
Grade III	The above abnormalities may be found with a severely hypoplastic tympanic cavity

After Marquet[46] and Cremers et al.[47]

Table 75.4 Scoring systems for candidacy for surgery for congenital aural atresia.

	Score
Stapes present	2
Oval window open	1
Middle ear space	1
Facial nerve	1
Malleus incus complex	1
Mastoid pneumatization	1
Incus stapes connection	1
Round window	1
Appearance of external ear	1
Total available points	10

Rating: Type of candidate for surgery. $n = 10$; 10, excellent; 9, very good; 8, good; 7, fair; 6, marginal; 5 or less, poor.
Reprinted from Ref. 48, with permission.

Cremers et al.[47] introduced a further subclassification of type II, again related to surgical outcome. In type IIa they place patients who had only partial bony atresia where a fistulous track could be found that connected with the rudimentary tympanic membrane. In type IIb, there is total bony atresia over the full length of the canal.

Attempts have been made to correlate the degree of auricular malformation and atresia into a single unified classification system, but some clarity and clinical usefulness is lost in the amalgamation. There is an interdependence between the two conditions embryologically, audiologically and when planning treatment, but the factors that influence cosmetic intervention are very different from those that determine the most appropriate treatment for the hearing loss.

Many of the parameters of atresia that determine the potential for surgical success or suggest caution can be defined with HRCT scanning. In 1992, Jahrsdoefer et al.[48] proposed a scoring system for the selection of patients with congenital aural atresia using a ten-point scale based on CT scan elements and the appearances of the external ear (**Table 75.4**). They reported that 82 percent of patients graded 8–10 achieved a postoperative speech reception threshold (SRT) of 15–25 dB. This system has been validated by several investigators.[48]

A subsequent report[43] found that the grade of microtia correlated with the Jahrsdoefer CT grade for aural atresia. Grade I averages 8.5, grade II 7.2 and grade III 5.9. Patients with syndromes involving craniofacial malformations, including Treacher Collins, Goldenhar syndrome, Crouzon and Pierre Robin are considered poor surgical candidates for atresia repair.[21, 49]

Principles of treatment, discussing the options and the role of the congenital ear team

The realization that their child has a congenital deformity of the ear is inevitably traumatic for parents. They need high quality information and reassurance as early as possible to reduce apprehension and a commonly felt sense of guilt. There is often a sense of frantic urgency for corrective surgery. This requires thoughtful and realistic parental counselling from all members of the team. Reassurance if appropriate that this is not an inherited condition nor related to any specific event during pregnancy always helps, as does a comprehensible explanation of the condition in terms that the parents can fully understand.

A positive approach will help the child develop a more self-confident attitude to the 'deformity'. One has to be careful before recommending an irreversible course of action. The two principal surgical approaches – autogenous reconstruction of the residual structures and the use of a prosthetic implant or a bone-anchored hearing aid (BAHA) are complementary rather than competing modalities. If the patient and parents are fully informed, the individual decision becomes much more straightforward. Anyone who has worked in this field will have seen adults who strongly resent having been put through multiple operations as a young child with only limited or no long-term benefit.

Audiologists, geneticists, otologists and plastic surgeons are essential members of the congenital ear team. Psychologists and social workers help the family come to terms with the condition. One of the main functions of the team is to act as an information centre so that the family understand all of the options and have an appreciation of the timescale involved.

Whilst there are psychological reasons to intervene early, particularly in more severe cases of microtia, a more conservative approach allows the child time to make a more mature informed decision. This process of education is at the centre of any congenital ear programme. True informed consent means discussing both the advantages and disadvantages of each treatment option. We insist that each family meets children who have completed treatment, both with reconstructive surgery and with implant-retained prostheses and BAHAs if appropriate. Half an hour with such a family is worth more than any number of consultations with the surgeon.

To achieve consistently good results, patients need to be referred to a specialist unit. There is no room for the occasional operator and very powerful arguments for establishing a number of regional treatment centres.

If ever there was a need for a partnership between patient/family and a surgical team, this is it. Decisions taken with or on behalf of the child will have lifelong implications. No single treatment is ideal, all involve compromise and choice and there is always a third option to do nothing. Parents need to understand that even if there is an associated atresia, the underlying cochlea function will usually be normal. If unilateral then the hearing in the unaffected ear is very likely to be normal and their child's speech and educational development will not be affected.

In bilateral atresia, the principles of bone conduction hearing aids need to be carefully explained, again emphasizing that 'normal' hearing and development are to be expected. The audiologists are involved from the first consultation and reinforce all this information with appropriate testing and hearing aid provision.

The parents' main concern with microtia is inevitably cosmetic. They need to know that there have been significant advances over the last 15 years and that these will continue in the future. The essential principles of autogenous reconstruction and of an implant-retained prosthesis are explained together with the very definite third option of doing nothing. Although many children do want surgical correction, a significant minority are happy to defer treatment or make a conscious decision not to correct their microtia, particularly if they have a well-developed lobule in the correct position which gives a good impression of symmetry when the patient is first seen. This is especially true for girls and for boys when fashion dictates that they should have longer hair.

The key factor in these early consultations is to inform the family as fully as possible about the condition, the potential for hearing and the options for cosmetic correction in the future. Most children and parents are reassured to know that something can be done, even although this may be many years in the future, and then relax into a more open bonding relationship with their child which helps to develop his or her self-confidence. There are inevitably difficult times when starting or changing schools. Some children yearn for ear reconstruction and the benefits in terms of self-esteem are well established.[50] In a number of children, bedwetting, truancy and poor concentration at school have resolved when an ear deformity is corrected.

We spend a great deal of time talking to children, and arrange meetings with families whose children have completed autogenous reconstruction and implantation surgery, preferably without a doctor being present. If they wish to consider osseointegration, we use computer-generated images (Adobe® Photoshop®)[51] to show precisely what they would look like with the remnant ear removed and with the abutments and gold bar in place and with a prosthetic ear attached. Only when we are sure that they are fully informed do we proceed and a significant number of patients elect to have no treatment at this time in the knowledge that they can change their mind at any stage in the future. The results of autogenous reconstruction have improved due to the dedicated work of a few highly skilled surgeons who have modified and refined the technique. Brent, Nagata, Park, Aguilia, Firmin, Weerda and Gault all achieve remarkable results, but it must be recognized that they are superspecialists performing complex multi-stage operations and there will be relatively few centres in any country where work of this high standard can be routinely achieved.[20, 52, 53, 54, 55]

Ear reconstruction for a standard microtia case is carried out in two stages. At the first operation, an ear-shaped framework is carved from costal cartilage and is placed beneath the non-hair-bearing mastoid skin. Suction drains are used to coapt the skin and thus the framework detail shows through. Tissue from the microtia remnant is repositioned to form a lobe (**Figure 75.20a** and **b**).

At the second operation six months later, the reconstructed ear is released and held in normal projection with a small cartilage wedge (**Figure 75.20c**). It is very important that the ear is in the ideal position and, in low hair cases, the framework is covered with a temporoparietal fascial flap and skin graft (**Figure 75.21**).

In the past, many operations did not achieve the desired results and left the patient feeling resentful that they had been put through multiple operations at a young age without their consent. Many have subsequently had an implant-retained prosthesis and felt it has been a marked improvement. However, although an implant-retained artificial ear does provide a visually normal ear, virtually identical to the other side with secure attachment to a stable percutaneous implant site in the majority of cases, there are disadvantages. Percutaneous implantation requires subcutaneous tissue reduction that effectively excludes any future autogenous reconstruction. The remnant pinna, particularly the lobule, has to be removed if an ideal result is to be achieved. The percutaneous site has to last for the rest of the child's life, with a replacement prosthesis every 18 months. Life-long commitment to cleaning the percutaneous site (similar to looking after teeth) is also a prerequisite.

The advantages are a very realistic ear with all the three-dimensional intricacies of a normal pinna and a consequent increase in the patient's self-confidence. Despite 15 years of experience of this technique, in over 40 patients, we still regard autogenous reconstruction as the treatment of first choice, reserving implant surgery for

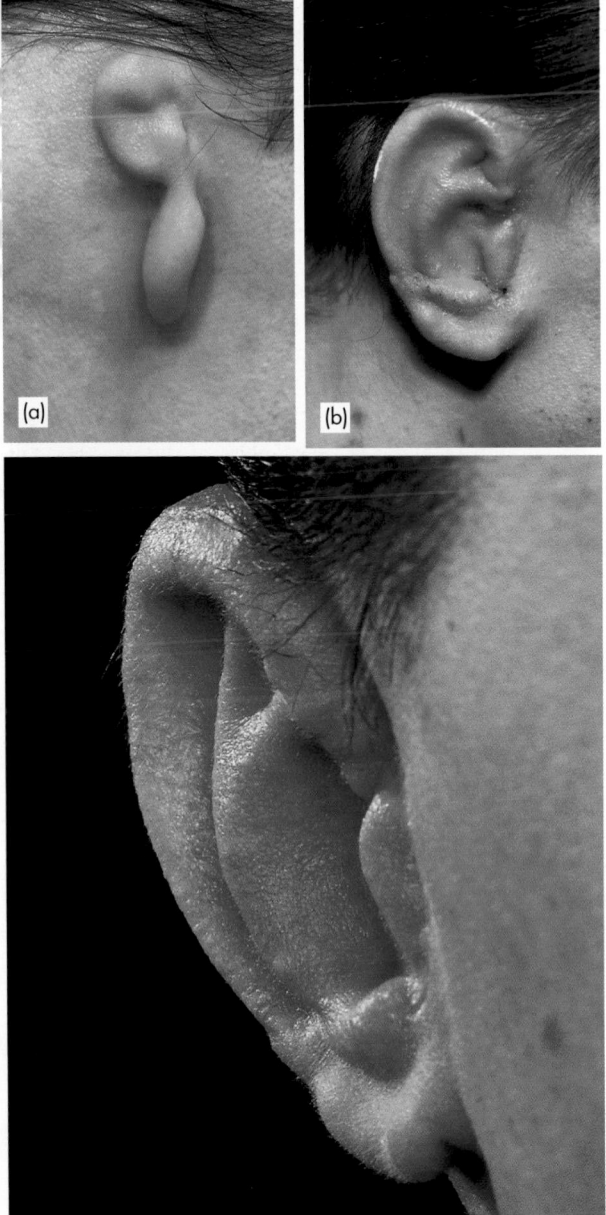

Figure 75.20 (a) A standard microtia deformity; (b) the framework inserted, suction applied. (c) The final result.

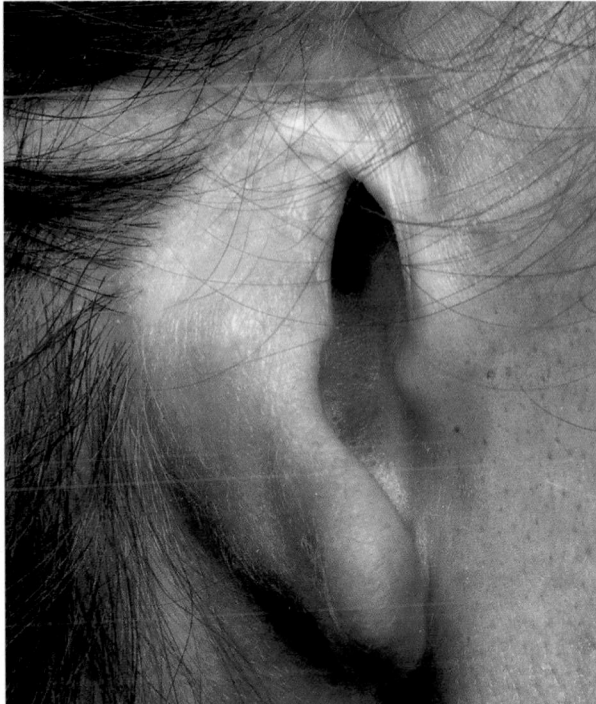

Figure 75.21 In this microtia case, the hair line is very low.

children who make a very conscious decision not to have reconstruction or those referred to us following unsatisfactory plastic surgery.

MICROTIA AND ANOTIA

Treatment for microtia is not essential and some patients will not seek treatment. The surgical options are autogenous reconstruction or a bone-anchored prosthesis. Patients with anotia usually have a low hairline and also require lobe reconstruction.

The gold standard of ear reconstruction is an ear of carved autogenous costal cartilage. Results have improved enormously in recent years.[56] The cartilage framework is placed beneath the mastoid skin and suction drains are used to coapt the skin onto it. Local skin can also be draped over other frameworks, such as porous polyethylene and silastic ear shapes. Although their use saves a donor site scar, these nonautogenous materials are currently more prone to infection in the long term.[57]

It is important to stress that autogenous reconstruction is best carried out on previously unoperated sites, as previous surgery can remove valuable skin and causes scars that tend to interfere with blood supply to the skin envelope. It is not uncommon for well-meaning surgeons to perform interim procedures, such as lobe or lop setback, to make the ear look a little better until the child is old enough for a formal reconstruction without realizing that they are compromising the final result.

Autogenous tissue reconstruction is best delayed until the child is ten years of age. By this time, an adequate amount of chest cartilage is available to create a good three-dimensional framework and the risk of chest deformity after harvest is minimal. Prior to this, the ear shape is sometimes difficult to construct because the floating rib is too short to make a complete helical rim or because the pieces that form the base plate are of inadequate thickness to bear the carved detail.

There is in theory no upper age limit to autogenous ear reconstruction and some children who are fearful of surgery at an early age can wait until they feel able to cope. Other children who are the victims of teasing may wish to have the surgery carried out as early as possible, but surgery prior to the age of seven years may compromise the shape of the framework. If a bone-anchored prosthesis is to be used, then the mastoid bone needs to be of adequate thickness to accept the fixtures. Again, the chance of successful surgery increases with age.

Reconstruction of the microtic ear is technically exacting and only with experience and great attention to detail are realistic results achieved. A framework of costal cartilage is carved and then draped with non-hair-bearing skin. The primitive lobe is repositioned to blend with the framework, a tragus is created and then the reconstructed ear is released from the side of the head to create a post-auricular sulcus. In unilateral cases, a map of the opposite normal ear is made using blank x-ray film (the template). In bilateral cases, it is helpful to ask a relative to act as a model for a template. The design is sketched on to this clear material with a felt tip pen, and the outline is cut out, together with holes for the scaphal hollow and triangular fossa.

With the template positioned on to the side of the head to give a symmetrical appearance, it can be seen whether the lobe will need to be lowered, raised or set back during the reconstruction. In some patients the length of the head (from front to back) on the side of the microtia is reduced and some adjustment of the distances from lateral canthus to ear will be required to give an optimal result. Various techniques are described,[20, 52] but it must be emphasized that this is exacting surgery and few centres can offer consistently good results.

Implant-retained prosthesis

Surgery for establishing percutaneous fixtures for a prosthetic ear is considerably more complex than for a BAHA. Ideally there should be 3 mm of cortical bone in the optimal position for two abutments. Bone thickness can be measured by HRCT. It is usually possible to find adequate bone in the region of the suprameatal crest where there is a triangle of dense bone between the middle cranial fossa and middle ear cleft, but the mastoid is often poorly developed, which makes it difficult to place the inferior implant at least 2 cm from the superior fixture. If the mastoid has developed, the position of the air cells is unpredictable and the lower fixture may have to be placed anteriorly where the mastoid is shelving medially or posterior towards the lateral sinus.

The cortical bone in children is 'softer' than adults and a lower torque setting is used (20–30 Ncm). If the bone is very thin, the implant can be inserted using the hand-held torque wrench. We always try to use a 4-mm fixture, but if there is less than 2 mm of cortical bone, the flange is left 1 mm above the bone surface and covered with bone dust under a periosteal graft or a Gore-Tex® cover, which is known to stimulate new bone formation.[58]

A two-stage procedure is used in children with an interval of four months in an ideal case (4 mm of bone) or six months if one of the above techniques has been used. The main reason is to ensure that the implants are osseointegrated before making the irreversible decision to remove the remnant pinna or reduce the soft tissue.

The importance of subcutaneous tissue reduction so that the epidermis lies on the periosteum for at least 1 cm around the implant cannot be overemphasized. Children show a remarkable capacity for subcutaneous tissue regeneration and inadequate removal leads to mobile skin around the implant with subsequent infection and an unstable percutaneous site.

It is also important to ensure that the abutments are long enough to allow the base plate of the prosthesis to clip on to the gold bar and still maintain an adequate air space around the abutment, which also facilitates easier cleaning. The family must understand that a long-term commitment to the care of the abutments and prosthesis is essential.

With careful patient selection and meticulous attention to surgical detail, this technique offers a remarkably life-like, secure prosthesis and many patients' lives have been transformed. Compared to autogenous reconstruction, the surgery is relatively simple, predictable and carries a high rate of success (94 percent).[59] There are no donor site scars and the patient only stays in hospital for two days. The downside is that this is still an artificial ear and precludes future autogenous reconstruction. The patient is committed to the care of the implant for life and requires a new prosthesis every 18 months. Whilst the skill of the surgeon is important, the technique is useless without a talented prosthetic expert.

We are cautious about recommending a percutaneous implant in children with congenital heart disease because of the risk of endocarditis.[60, 61, 62]

ASSESSMENT AND MANAGEMENT OF THE CHILD WITH AURAL ATRESIA

History and examination

Most patients who attend our congenital ear clinic have microtia as well as atresia, but 15 percent present with isolated atresia. Fortunately, unilateral cases are far more common than bilateral which only account for 20 percent. As noted, the condition is more common in males (63 percent) and on the right side (58 percent).[20] It is important to understand that 10 percent of children with a unilateral atresia will have a congenital conductive hearing loss in the contralateral 'normal' ear and 5 percent may have an associated sensorineural hearing loss. Microtia/atresia may occur as an isolated anomaly or associated with other malformations. A detailed general paediatric history and examination are required to establish a syndromic diagnosis, not just of the craniofacial region but of other organ systems particularly the spine and genitourinary system. Exposure to medicines[63, 64] or infection during pregnancy, amniocentesis or chorionic villous biopsy-threatened abortions or trauma may be relevant together with any family history of similar anomalies or deafness. A general assessment of the physical and mental milestones is made.

The grade of microtia is recorded with particular attention to anterior-inferior displacement of the ears, development of the mastoid tip and the distance between this structure and the TMJ. Evidence of hemifacial microsomia is recorded. The eyes and orbits are examined and the facial nerve function assessed. The external canal is graded as narrow, stenotic (i.e. less then 4 mm), blind ending or atretic. The majority of patients with atresia/microtia have an ipsilateral palatal weakness. The degree of atresia, failure of the tympanic ring to develop as determined by the distance between the TMJ and the mastoid, mastoid size and antero-inferior displacement of the ear, are all clinical features that help predict a potentially aberrant facial nerve.

Audiological investigations

This condition should automatically place the child on a high-risk register for sensorineural hearing loss even if unilateral. Although the majority of children have normal cochlea function even minor congenital anomalies of the middle ear can cause a 40–60 dB hearing loss. Age-appropriate audiological investigations determine the presence or absence of normal cochlea function. If normal hearing can be demonstrated in unilateral cases, no further treatment is necessary at this stage. In bilateral cases or where doubt remains, an appropriate hearing aid is fitted.

The BAHA® Softband has been particularly useful, but we use a variety of techniques including a transducer held in a sweatband, a standard paediatric bone conductor hearing aid (BCHA) on a headspring and a BAHA on a headband. Children with cranial synostosis have proved difficult to fit with a conventional BCHA after the age of 18 months and we now routinely use the BAHA® Softband. Air conduction (AC) aids are also used whenever possible. All children with atresia have problems localizing sound and we emphasize how important it is to instil the practice of stopping and looking carefully in both directions before crossing roads, as there is an increased risk of road traffic accidents in these children.

Imaging

High resolution computed tomography scanning, which forms the foundation of classification of patient selection for reconstructive surgery, is rarely necessary before the age of five as it will not influence management. It may help establish a diagnosis in some syndromic cases and is essential if a child presents with any symptoms or signs suggestive of an underlying ear infection. Cases of meatal stenosis (less than 2 mm) should be scanned between five and ten years of age to exclude cholesteatoma (see under Cholesteatoma in atretic ears). In younger children, a HRCT scan can predict bone thickness at the preferred site of implantation.

Otological surveillance

The child should be kept under otological surveillance to exclude conductive deafness due to otitis media with effusion (OME), particularly in unilateral cases and treatment started as appropriate. Conservative treatment with or without amplification is our standard approach, but if there are signs of retraction or structural changes to the drum, ventilation may be necessary.

Acute otitis media is fortunately rare in atretic ears, but parents and health professionals looking after such children should initiate immediate referral to an otologist if an infection is suspected. Prompt antibiotic treatment usually aborts the infection before mastoiditis or a subdural abscess develop. Failure to improve or signs of intracranial complications necessitate exploration after a HRCT scan. The safest method is to use a transmastoid approach.

Cholesteatoma in atretic ears

Congenital aural stenosis as compared to congenital aural atresia, carries a much greater risk of cholesteatoma. Jahrsdoerfer and Cole[65] reviewed 600 cases of major congenital ear malformations. Fifty patients (54 ears) were found to have aural stenosis. No cholesteatoma were found in children under three years of age regardless of the stenosis size. No bony erosion or middle ear involvement was encountered in children under the age of 12, but in patients over the age of 20, 60 percent had destructive changes. The most significant finding was that in children of 12 years or older with a meatus narrower than 2 mm, 91 percent develop cholesteatoma. Surgery is therefore recommended for these cases between the age of 6 and 12 years before any irreversible damage occurs. Surgery is similar to that for atresia.

Surgical treatment

Reconstruction of an atretic ear is possibly one of the most complex forms of otological surgery. Establishing and maintaining a canal, removing the atretic plate, identifying and mobilizing the ossicular complex and establishing a stable vibratory and medialized tympanic membrane, which will provide hearing thresholds better than 25 dB, is an elusive goal achieved only by the most talented and experienced otologists. While the surgery for autogenous reconstruction of the pinna has progressed in recent years, improved outcomes in reconstructive middle ear surgery have generally been achieved by refining the criteria for selection. Conversely, Tjellstrom's pioneering work,[66] which led to the widespread introduction of the BAHA in Europe and more recently in the USA, has revolutionized the treatment of congenital conductive hearing loss.

Patients with congenital atresia have a number of options, which must be presented honestly to the family. Information about the likely success, potential complications and any alternative devices must be given in an unbiased fashion. Although there are problems with the steel band BCHA, the Softband or hard band BAHA adapter provides very good hearing, albeit with reduced speech discrimination in background noise and the recognized aesthetic and pressure problems.

The surgery for a BAHA is now well established[66] (see Chapter 239b, Bone-anchored hearing aids) and has proved to be a simple, safe and highly effective procedure. There is still some debate about the most appropriate age for implantation. We prefer to have 3 mm of cortical bone and a co-operative child who understands how to look after the aid and abutment, but in unusual circumstances children as young as two have been successfully implanted. Bone in children is softer and the potential for subcutaneous tissue regeneration greater, but if performed as a two-stage procedure with meticulous attention to detail, good osseointegration and a stable percutaneous implant site can be achieved.[67]

RECONSTRUCTIVE MIDDLE EAR SURGERY

Preoperative considerations

Even the most experienced surgeons have problems providing useful hearing improvement, except in mild/moderate cases if evaluated against the Glasgow Benefit Scale. Surgical complications include damage to the facial nerve, a low but ever present risk and the possibility of a high frequency sensory neural hearing loss from transmitted acoustic trauma and postoperatively there is a significant risk of lateralization of the reconstructed drum and restenosis of the canal or meatus which contribute to concerns about long-term stability of any hearing improvement. In contrast, the BAHA offers a technically simple solution with a high success rate (greater than 94 percent) and no risk to the facial nerve or cochlea. It is an electronically processed sound, but studies suggest it provides a high quality of auditory rehabilitation.[68] Both techniques require periodic supervision from an otologist.

In the UK, Scandinavian and other EU countries, the BAHA has gained wide acceptance in the treatment of complex conductive hearing losses caused by chronic suppurative otitis media (CSOM), stenosing otitis externa and complicated otosclerosis and is the preferred method of treatment for congenital aural atresia.[44] The commonly sited reason for avoiding a BAHA in patients with microtia and atresia (that it might adversely affect microtia repair) can be avoided by placing the implant site more posteriorly, away from any area of skin used in auricular reconstruction (**Figure 75.22**).[69]

There are still patients who either need or could benefit from reconstructive middle ear surgery, particularly with grade I or grade IIa atresia or those patients with canal stenosis at risk of developing a cholesteatoma[70] and each case needs to be carefully assessed.

Despite the fact that BAHA implants have transformed the treatment of children with atresia, reconstructive surgery should still have a place in the surgical armamentarium of any unit treating such children. Jahsdoerfer has been responsible for much of the work over the last 25 years on correcting atresia and his contribution stems partly from his pursuit of surgical excellence and in part due to careful analysis of factors in patient selection that directly influence outcomes. His grading system (**Table 75.4**) is widely accepted as definitive for selecting patients for this type of surgery. In his hands, 80 percent of patients who score 8 or more will have thresholds better than 20 dB over 1, 2 and 4 kH. A score of 7 indicates that approximately 70 percent of patients will achieve the same results.[71]

In Schucknecht's series[49] of 69 patients with varying degrees of atresia, only 30 percent of his patients who underwent canaloplasty and ossicular replacement had postoperative hearing better than 20 dB. De la Cruz et al.[72] reported short-term success in closing the air-bone gap to less than 30 dB hearing loss (HL) in 58 percent of 116 cases undergoing atresia surgery, but this dropped to 50 percent with long-term follow-up. All these cases were categorized as moderate/severe atresia.

Important complications that might influence the decision to proceed with reconstruction are damage to the facial nerve, sensory neural hearing loss, restenosis of the canal and meatus, chronic infection and the stability of the improved hearing over time.

The course of the facial nerve can be reasonably accurately predicted by careful analysis of the stage of embryological arrest (see below under Embryology). HRCT may confirm these clinical impressions, but active facial monitoring and meticulous surgical technique are essential if damage is to be avoided. The danger areas are the acutely angled second genu, with the nerve passing anterolaterally in the lower portion of the atretic plate or even in the fibrous tissue lateral to a poorly formed plate (Cremers type IIb) with passage of the nerve through the glenoid fossa, rather than the stylomastoid foramen. It is also at risk when exiting from the lateral aspect of a micromastoid in patients with a low set microtia and, in some cases, the superficial portion of the facial nerve

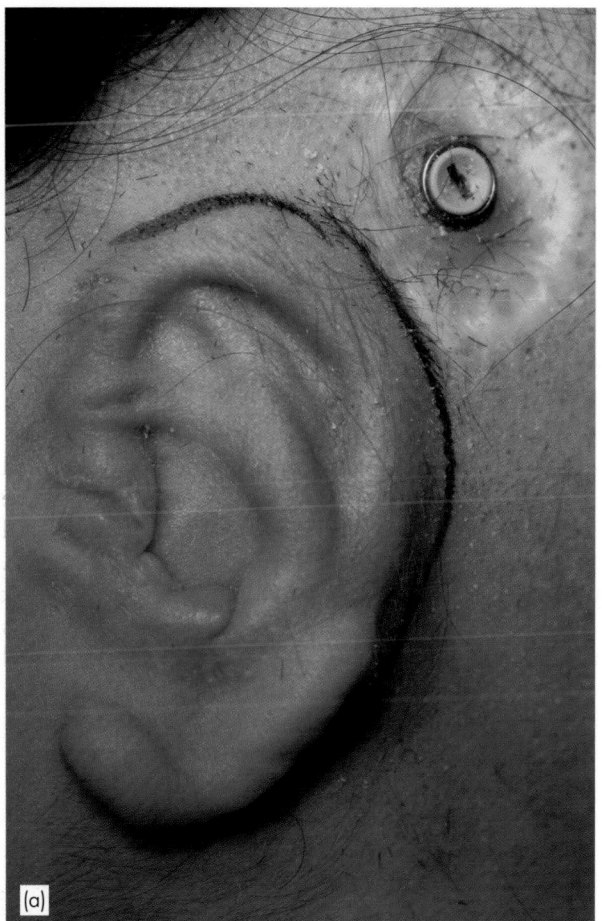

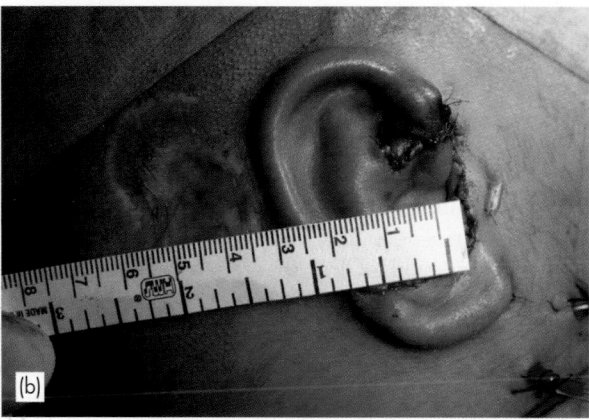

Figure 75.22 (a) The abutment for a bone-anchored hearing aid in a patient with bilateral microtia; (b) It is very important to insert the abutments posterior enough to allow ear reconstruction.

courses anterior to the tragus placing it at risk from soft tissue work over the anterior meatus and damage can occur even with flap elevation in autogenous or inplant reconstruction. The reported incidence of temporary facial nerve palsy is 9 percent and of permanent weakness, 1.5 percent, all from extremely experienced surgeons.[49, 73]

A high frequency sensorineural hearing loss caused by acoustic trauma occurs in up to 12 percent of cases.

Lateralization of the tympanic membrane (TM) from a foreshortened malleus handle or ossicular monoblock occurs in 9–15 percent, canal stenosis due to bony regrowth in 12 percent and soft tissue meatal stenosis in a further 10 percent. There is a significant rate of persistent or intermittent discharge from the neomeatus, particularly if a hearing aid is still required.

The anterior approach

This is the most popular of the three main surgical approaches, popularized by Jahrsdoerfer,[9] de la Cruz[72] and Lambert.[5] Surgery is performed after microtia repair, via a post-auricular incision. Care is taken to avoid exposure of the autogenous cartilage of the reconstructed pinna. A temporalis fascia graft (TFG) is harvested and the periosteum incised at the posterior margin of the temporomandibular fossa and horizontally along the inferior margin of the temporal line. The posterior aspect of the glenoid fossa is identified, but deep dissection should be avoided as the facial nerve can occasionally exit the temporal bone into the TMJ. The tegmen tympani and glenoid fossa form the superior and anterior limits of dissection. If a remnant tympanic bone can be identified, drilling starts at this site, as it will lead to the atretic plate and middle ear (ME). If not, drilling starts over the cribriform area and the atretic plate is usually found at a depth of 1.5 cm. By drilling anterosuperiorly along the tegmen towards the epitympanum, the surgeon remains in a safe area away from the facial nerve. The mastoid is not opened as this creates a larger cavity with all the attendant postoperative problems. The dense atretic plate is 'egg shelled' with diamond burrs and partly removed with curettes. The fused incus and malleus may be seen superiorly on entering the middle ear cleft and produce the 'buttock sign', with a similar configuration to that noted at breach presentation. The atretic plate is commonly fused to the neck of the malleus whose handle may be absent and this is not disturbed until the ear canal has been widened, centred on the ossicular mass. The constraints of the new canal are the TMJ, middle cranial fossa, mastoid air cells and, inferiorly, the facial nerve. Finally, the bony attachment to the ossicular chain is removed by a slowly rotating burr or laser to minimize the risk of sensorineural hearing loss.

The mobility and continuity of the ossicles must be carefully assessed. Ideally, the chain will be mobile but if fixed or not in contact with the stapes the monoblock should be removed and replaced with a sculptured bony columellar or partial ossicular replacement prosthesis (PORP). Fixation of the stapes foot plate is fortunately rare and a contraindication to further surgery. The TFG is placed laterally, draped over the ossicular mass/columellar and extending 2–3 mm into the bony meatus. A 0.01-inch thick split skin graft measuring 5 × 7 cm is taken from the medial aspect of the upper arm, preferably with a mechanical dermatome. After careful measurement, it is cut to form the exact lining of the new ear canal. If there is a thinner edge, it is placed medially with four notches but to create flaps which will cover the fascial graft. A silastic disc is placed over the new TM and the canal filled with a Merocel® ear wick hydrated with antibiotic and steroid eardrops. The lateral graft is folded over the wick, while the new meatus is created.

The reconstructed ear may not be in the correct anatomical position for the meatus. Generally it needs to be elevated in a posterosuperior direction. This is achieved by freeing the ear anteriorly and excising an elipse of skin from the superior aspect of the post-auricular incision. With the ear held in this new position the meatus is marked and an oval of skin and cartilage removed. If conchal cartilage is present, less contraction occurs and a diameter of 1.5 times normal will suffice. The cartilage framework is sutured into its new position with 3/0 Vicryl and the skin graft stitched to the meatal skin with 5/0 Vicryl Rapide. A further Merocel wick is inserted and hydrated and the lateral aspect covered with Bactroban® ointment. The post-aural wound is closed and a mastoid pressure dressing applied.

All of the packs and post-auricular sutures are removed at one week and the new ear canal is filled with antibiotic steroid drops, which are removed with micro-suction after five minutes. The drops are used at home for a further week and the patient is seen two weeks later when the desquamated layer of the skin graft can be removed and the new canal and TM inspected. Granulation tissues are treated with silver nitrate cautery and most resolve with careful microsuction and Triadcortyl® ointment, but it can take several weeks for the ear to stabilize.

Transmastoid approach

This employs a more posterior route to the middle ear cleft using the dura of the middle cranial fossa, the sigmoid sinus and sinodural angles as landmarks to the antrum with subsequent identification of the lateral semicircular canal (LSCC), atretic plate and, if possible, the facial nerve. The atretic plate is removed in a similar fashion, trying to centre the cavity on the stapes. The aim is to create a stable, small, cavity lined with squamous epithelium. A split skin graft (SSG) of 0.01 inch is used to line the cavity after a temporalis fascia tympanoplasty. Obliteration of the cavity with soft tissue flaps and bone pâte have had mixed results.[74] The soft surgery and postoperative management are similar to the anterior approach.

Modified approach

In patients with thick non-pneumatized atretic plates, a modified anterior approach has been proposed.[75] The sinodural angle is opened with limited dissection anteriorly to expose the posterior antrum identifying the lateral semicircular canal and ossicular mass. An anterior approach can then be performed with much more certainty. Image-guided surgery may provide a similar degree of reassurance.

Complications

The major operative concerns for the patient and surgeon are potential damage to the facial nerve and the risk of sensorineural hearing loss from transmitted energy from the drill. Three-dimensional HRCT scanning helps provide an accurate spacial template for the surgeon and image-guided surgery is becoming simpler to configure and more accurate. Some systems, such as BrainLAB (Cambridge, UK), offer accuracy to within 1 mm and as these systems come online they may become as indispensable as active facial nerve monitoring.

There has been considerable debate about the hearing results and long-term stability of atresia surgery. Unless the hearing is better than 25 dB HL, a patient is likely to require a hearing aid which increases the incidence of infection in the neomeatus and begs the question – why not use a BAHA which has none of the attendant risks and a very high success rate both in terms of osseointegration, implant site stability and patient satisfaction? In unilateral cases, the arguments in favour of nonintervention, at least until the patient is old enough to sign their own consent form is even greater. The Glasgow Benefit Scale merely confirms what many otologists have known for years that unless the hearing is within 20 dB of the normal ear, the patient is unlikely to perceive any benefit. Realistically, this limits selection for surgical reconstruction to types I and Ia, with a score of 8+ on the Jahrsdoerfer scale. The long-term stability of hearing improvement has been questioned. Lambert[5] reported a series of 55 patients on whom an initial speech reception threshold of less than 25 dB was achieved in 60 percent of patients in the early postoperative period, but in the longer term (mean 2.8 years) this was maintained in only 46 percent of patients and revision surgery was necessary in one-third of those patients. Chandrasekhar et al.[75] reported closure of the air-bone gap to less than 30 dB in 60 percent of patients with a mean follow-up time of 2.6 years and in only 54 percent in cases of revision surgery.

Lateralization of the TM and ear canal stenosis is common. Schucknecht[49] reported that 26 percent of 69 ears developed stenosis requiring revision surgery and Jahrsdoerfer and Hall[76] found that 50 percent of patients with grade III microtia developed the same complication. Chandrasekhar et al.[75] found that 22 percent of his cases developed restenosis and 9 percent developed lateralization of the TM. Linstrom et al.[77] found some degree of postoperative blunting and cicatrization of the neomeatus in 75 percent of children in his series of 69 ears.

THE BONE-ANCHORED HEARING AID

Patient selection and age at implantation

Even in the very best hands the success rates for aural atresia surgery are less than ideal, both in terms of hearing improvement, restenosis and long-term stability. With very careful selection, more predictable results can be obtained, but in the majority of cases the BAHA offers a low risk, highly acceptable and predictable method of auditory rehabilitation.

Many factors influence the age of implantation. After the age of five, there is usually sufficient bone and a co-operative child. In cases where it is difficult to use a bone conduction hearing aid or BAHA® Softband, for example, craniosynostosis, implants have been successfully inserted at two years of age. Use in adults has been widely reported and a study on 100 children under the age of 16 years[59] confirmed that 95 percent achieved a successful percutaneous implant over an average eight-year period. Skin reactions were noted in 9 percent of patients over a 21-year follow-up period, soft tissue regeneration and appositional bone growth are recognized problems and revision surgery in some form is required in 22 percent of children.[59] Parents and children need to have realistic expectations, helped by the introduction of the trial headband for the BAHA. Family support and commitment to cleaning the skin around the abutment is vital.

Otological and audiological criteria

Patients with congenital atresia are good candidates for implantation, particularly if they have good cochlea function and are not suitable for reconstructive surgery of the ear canal and middle ear. Patients who have had an unsuccessful reconstruction or particularly if the ear discharges with the air conduction hearing aid are suitable, as are patients with unilateral atresia if they find the 'blind area' a handicap.

Average bone conduction thresholds (0.5–4 kHz) should be better than 45 dB for the Baha Divino™, better than 55 dB for the Baha Intenso™, or up to 60 dB average for the more powerful body-worn Baha® Cordelle II aid. Speech discrimination should be better than 60 percent, but in the rare case of a congenital atresia with sensorineural loss, implantation may be the only way of introducing sound to the cochlea. Directional microphones and radio-aid links are available.

Surgery for BAHA

The technique for implantation is discussed in Chapter 239b, Bone-anchored hearing aids and the BAHA operating theatre manual produced by Entific Medical Systems

(now part of Cochlear) is available online at www.cochlearamericas.com/Professional/login.asp. We use a two-stage procedure in children under 12 years to protect the site of osseointegration, but would use single-stage surgery if 4 mm of bone were present. The local skin graft is thinned to 0.2–0.5 mm to remove all the hair follicles. Particular attention is given to subcutaneous tissue reduction, as the potential for regeneration is greater in children and the most common cause for skin reactions. A 4-mm flange fixture is used whenever possible. The bone tends to be softer in children and only gentle pressure is needed on the countersink drill and the torque settings are kept low (20–30 Ncm). If the bone is thin, the flange is left 1 mm proud of the surface and the space augmented with bone dust under a periosteal flap or an expanded polytetrafluoroethylene membrane.[66] In both cases, the interval between the stages is extended to six months. The site of implantation and subcutaneous tissue reduction must be kept away from any skin that might be needed for autogenous reconstruction of the pinna.[78] The BAHA should be 65 mm behind the site of the anticipated external auditory meatus which is often further posterior than expected to take into account any possible future ear reconstruction (**Figure 75.22**).[69]

Parents must be taught how to clean the percutaneous site to minimize the risk of infection. Skin reactions are slightly more common in children during the first year, but are managed by cleaning with Bactroban ointment or occasionally the use of an anti-staphylococcal antibiotic. Thereafter, rates of inflammation at the percutaneous site are similar to adults. Eighteen percent of our children have required revision surgery, mainly for soft tissue reduction, but increasingly for appositional bone growth, which buries the fixture. An elongated snap coupling (8.5 mm) is available, but removal of bone or reimplantation is occasionally needed. Loss of the implant over a prolonged period of 15 years has occurred in 6 percent of our children, consistent with reports from other centres.[66]

Audiological evaluation of BAHA

BAHA provide a reliable and predictable adjunct for auditory rehabilitation in patients with a conductive or mixed hearing loss who are unable to benefit from conventional hearing aids.[79] Many studies report that audiometric benefit from the BAHA is greater than from conventional bone conduction hearing aids both with regard to warble tone thresholds and speech discrimination in a noisy environment.[80] It is suggested that patients with congenital atresia achieve marginally the best freefield thresholds and speech discrimination compared to other BAHA cases.[44] Improved sound quality, appearance and practicality were also noted. Ninety percent of more than 300 patients in the Birmingham study used their implants for more than eight hours every day.[81]

In a study of 19 children implanted with a BAHA for congenital aural atresia, Powell found all of the children who had previously used air conduction aids achieved better freefield warble tones and 71 percent had improved speech discrimination. Of the children who had used conventional conductive hearing aids, 50 percent were found to have improved speech discrimination with the BAHA. Most of the children felt the BAHA was more effective in a noisy environment.[82] Bosman et al.[83] evaluated the audiometric results of fitting bilateral BAHAs in 25 patients (with congenital bilateral atresia) and found improved speech reception thresholds in quiet environments and with noise, symmetrical localization resulting in binaural hearing. These results are supported by the Birmingham group.[84] Wazen et al.[85] studied the effect of fitting a BAHA in unilateral conductive and mixed losses and found significant improvement in the hearing handicap score with the BAHA.

Complications

Inadvertent penetration of the lateral venous sinus due to thin bone can occur. The implant seals the hole. Skin reactions are not uncommon in the first year and loss of the fixture due to late failure of osseointegration or direct trauma occurs in 6 percent of cases. The practice of fitting a 'sleeper' fixture at the time of the first operation remains open to debate. In cases of resistant percutaneous inflammation, the abutment can be removed and reattached when the skin has healed. If this fails, revision subcutaneous tissue reduction is probably needed.

KEY POINTS

- Minor congenital anomalies of the ear are common.
- Major congenital anomalies of the outer or middle ear demand coordinated care from a highly skilled multidisciplinary team able to offer the full spectrum of otological, cosmetic and psychological support.
- One of the main functions of the team is to act as an information centre so that the family understand all of the options and have an appreciation of the timescale involved.
- The major options for microtia are autogenous reconstruction and an implant-retained prosthesis with the very definite third option of doing nothing.
- Good results with autogenous reconstruction are only available in a few centres.
- The authors regard autogenous reconstruction as the treatment of first choice for microtia, reserving implant surgery for

children who make a very conscious decision not to have reconstruction or for those referred following unsatisfactory plastic surgery.
- Despite the fact that BAHA implants have transformed the treatment of children with aural atresia, middle ear reconstructive surgery should still have a place in the surgical armamentarium of any unit treating such children.
- Reconstructive surgery for atresia is some of the most demanding surgery in otology.

Best clinical practice

✓ Flexible wire splints (Ear Buddies) totally encased in silicone are now commercially available for parents themselves to apply to their child's ears. For prominence, rim kinks, Stahl's bar and other abnormal folds, the splints used carefully in infancy may avoid the need for later surgery. [Grade C/D]

✓ Surgeons who engage in the correction of 'bat ears' need to be adequately trained for this work and should audit their results. [Grade D]

✓ Autogenous reconstruction for microtia is best delayed until the child is ten years old. [Grade C]

✓ All children with atresia have problems localizing sound and we emphasize how important it is to instil the practice of stopping and looking carefully in both directions before crossing roads, as there is an increased risk of road traffic accidents in these children. [Grade C]

✓ Microtia and atresia should automatically place the child on a high-risk register for sensorineural hearing loss even if unilateral. [Grade A]

✓ Patients with syndromes involving craniofacial malformations, including Treacher Collins, Goldenhar syndrome, Crouzons and Pierre Robin sequence are considered poor surgical candidates for atresia repair. [Grade C/D]

✓ Cases of meatal stenosis (less than 2 mm) should be scanned between five and ten years of age to exclude cholesteatoma. [Grade C/D]

✓ In unilateral atresia, unless the hearing is within 20 dB of the normal ear, the patient is unlikely to perceive any benefit from reconstructive surgery. Realistically, this limits selection for surgical reconstruction to types I and Ia, with a score of 8+ on the Jahrsdoerfer scale. [Grade C/D]

✓ With very careful selection, more predictable results can be obtained in reconstructive middle ear surgery, but in the majority of cases the BAHA offers a low risk, highly acceptable and predictable method of auditory rehabilitation. [Grade B]

Deficiencies in current knowledge and areas for future research

➤ 'Splints' applied by parents are assuming an ever more important role in the management of minor cartilaginous deformities.

➤ The establishment of specialist centres for BAHA and for the management of congenital ear deformity is enabling more focused, controlled trials and better comparison of results.

➤ The technology that underpins osseointegration is improving rapidly. As experience with these techniques develops more reliable results and lower complication rates are possible.

REFERENCES

1. Park C. Lower auricular malformations: their representation, correction, and embryologic correlation. *Plastic and Reconstructive Surgery*. 1999; **104**: 29–40.

2. Brent B. Auricular repair with autogenous rib cartilage grafts: two decades of experience with 600 cases. *Plastic and Reconstructive Surgery*. 1992; **90**: 355–74; discussion 375–6.

3. Gulya AJ, Schucknecht HF. Phylogeny and embryology. In: Gulya AJ, Schuknecht HF (eds). *Anatomy of the temporal bone with surgical implications*, 2nd edn. New York: Parthenon, 1993: 235–88.

4. Jahrsdoerfer RA, Hall 3rd JW. Congenital malformations of the ear. *American Journal of Otology*. 1986; **7**: 267–9.

5. Lambert PR. Major congenital ear malformations: surgical management and results. *Annals of Otology, Rhinology and Laryngology*. 1988; **97**: 641–9.

6. Naunton RF, Valvassori GE. Inner ear anomalies: their association with atresia. *Laryngoscope*. 1968; **78**: 1041–9.

7. Swartz JD, Faerber EN. Congenital malformations of the external and middle ear: high-resolution CT findings of surgical import. *AJR American Journal of Roentgenology*. 1985; **144**: 501–6.

8. Sataloff RT. Embryology of the facial nerve and its clinical applications. *Laryngoscope*. 1990; **100**: 969–84.

9. Jahrsdoerfer RA. Congenital atresia of the ear. *Laryngoscope*. 1978; **88**: 1–48 (review).

10. Baxter A. Dehiscence of the Fallopian canal. An anatomical study. *Journal of Laryngology and Otology*. 1971; **85**: 587–94.

11. Krowiak EJ, Gurndfast KM. Congenital malformations in the ear. In: Wetmore RF, Muntz HR, McGill TJ (eds). *Pediatric otolaryngology*. New York: Thieme Medical, 2000: 235–52.

12. Cressman WR, Pensak ML. Surgical aspects of congenital aural atresia. *Otolaryngologic Clinics of North America*. 1994; **27**: 621–33 (review).

13. Farkas LG, Cheung G. Facial asymmetry in healthy North American Caucasians. An anthropometrical study. *The Angle Orthodontist*. 1981; **51**: 70–7.

14. Farkas LG. *Anthropometry of the head and face in medicine*. New York: Elsevier, 1981.

15. Poswillo D. The pathogenesis of the first and second branchial arch syndrome. *Journal of Oral Surgery*. 1973; **35**: 302–27.

16. The Treacher Collins Syndrome Collaborative Group. Dixon positional cloning of a gene involved in the pathogenesis of Treacher Collins syndrome. *Nature Genetics*. 1996; **12**: 130–6.

17. Vento AR, LaBrie RA, Mulliken JB. The O.M.E.N.S. classification of hemifacial microsomia. *Cleft Palate – Craniofacial Journal*. 1991; **28**: 68–76; discussion 77.

18. Kelberman D, Tyson J, Chandler DC, McInerney AM, Slee J, Albert D et al. Hemifacial microsomia: progress in understanding the genetic basis of a complex malformation syndrome. *Human Genetics*. 2001; **109**: 638–45.

19. Lawson K, Waterhouse N, Gault DT, Calvert ML, Botma M, Ng R. Is hemifacial microsomia linked to multiple maternities? *British Journal of Plastic Surgery*. 2002; **55**: 474–8.

20. Brent B. Microtia repair with rib cartilage grafts: a review of personal experience with 1000 cases. *Clinics in Plastic Surgery*. 2002; **29**: 257–71 vii.

21. Jahrsdoerfer RA, Jacobson JT. Treacher Collins syndrome: otologic and auditory management. *Journal of the American Academy of Audiology*. 1995; **6**: 93–102.

22. Takegoshi H, Kaga K, Kikuchi S, Ito K. Mandibulofacial dysostosis: CT evaluation of the temporal bones for surgical risk assessment in patients of bilateral aural atresia. *International Journal of Pediatric Otorhinolaryngology*. 2000; **54**: 33–40.

23. Grundfast KM, Siparsky N, Chuong D, Genetics and molecular biology of deafness. Update. *Otolaryngologic Clinics of North America*. 2000; **33**: 1367–94 (review).

24. Abdelhak S, Kalatzis V, Heilig R, Compain S, Samson D, Vincent C et al. Clustering of mutations responsible for branchio-oto-renal (BOR) syndrome in the eyes absent homologous region (eyaHR) of EYA1. *Human Molecular Genetics*. 1997; **6**: 2247–55.

25. Naficy S, Shepard NT, Telian SA. Multiple temporal bone anomalies associated with Noonan syndrome. *Otolaryngology and Head and Neck Surgery*. 1997; **116**: 265–7.

26. Gorlin RJ, Pindborg JJ, Cohen Jr. MM. *Syndromes of the head and neck*, 2nd edn. New York: McGraw-Hill, 1976.

27. Shah UK, Ohlms LA, Neault MW, Willson KD, McGuirt Jr. WF, Hobbs N et al. Otologic management in children with the CHARGE association. *International Journal of Pediatric Otorhinolaryngology*. 1998; **44**: 139–47.

28. Gore SM, Myers SR, Gault D. Mirror ear: a reconstructive technique for substantial tragal anomalies or polyotia. *Journal of Plastic, Reconstructive and Aesthetic Surgery*. 2006; **59**: 499–504.

29. Kaplan HA, Hudson DA. A novel surgical method of repair of Stahl's ear: A case report and review of current treatment modalities. *Plastic and Reconstructive Surgery.* 1999; **103**: 566–9.

30. Tan ST, Gault DT. When do ears become prominent? *British Journal of Plastic Surgery.* 1994; **47**: 573–4.

31. Graham KE, Gault DT. Endoscopic assisted otoplasty: a preliminary report. *British Journal of Plastic Surgery.* 1997; **50**: 47–57.

32. Chongchet V. A method of antihelix reconstruction. *British Journal of Plastic Surgery.* 1963; **16**: 268–72.

33. Mustarde JC. The correction of prominent ears using simple mattress sutures. *British Journal of Plastic Surgery.* 1963; **16**: 170–8.

34. Horlock N, Grobbelaar AO, Gault DT. 5 year series of constricted (lop and cup) ear corrections; Development of the mastoid hitch as an adjunctive technique. *Plastic and Reconstructive Surgery.* 1998; **102**: 2325–32.

35. Gault DT, Grippaudo FR, Tyler M. Ear reduction. *British Journal of Plastic Surgery.* 1995; **48**: 53–4.

36. Tan ST, Abramson DL, MacDonald DM, Mulliken JB. Molding therapy for infants with deformational auricular anomalies. *Annals of Plastic Surgery.* 1997; **38**: 263–8.

37. Ullmann Y, Blazer S, Ramon Y, Blumenfeld I, Peled IJ. Early nonsurgical correction of congenital auricular deformities. *Plastic and Reconstructive Surgery.* 2002; **109**: 907–13; discussion 914–5.

* 38. Lindford AJ, Hettiaratchy S, Schonauer F. Postpartum splinting of ear deformities. *British Medical Journal.* 2007; **334**: 366–8. *This is the latest in a series of papers on ear splintage in newborn infants. The opportunity to reshape an ear without surgery has enormous appeal, and the technique is gaining ground. The reduction in the rate of prominent ear surgery in the UK (down 20 percent in 2006) coincides with the introduction of splintage eight to nine years ago.*

39. Marx H. Die Missbildungen des Ohres. In: Denker A, Kahler O (ed.). *Handbuch der Hals-, Nasen- und Ohrenheilkunde, Bd. VI.* Berlin: Springer, 1926: 620–5.

40. Weerda H. Classification of congenital deformities of the auricle. *Facial Plastic Surgery.* 1988; **5**: 385–8.

41. Aguilar 3rd EA, Jahrsdoerfer RA. The surgical repair of congenital microtia and atresia. *Otolaryngology and Head and Neck Surgery.* 1988; **98**: 600–6.

42. Jafek BW, Nager GT, Strife J, Gayler RW. Congenital aural atresia: an analysis of 311 cases. *Transactions of the American Academy of Ophthalmology and Otolaryngology.* 1975; **80**: 588–95.

43. Kountakis SE, Helidonis E, Jahrsdoerfer RA. Microtia grade as an indicator of middle ear development in aural atresia. *Archives of Otolaryngology and Head and Neck Surgery.* 1995; **121**: 885–6.

44. Declan F, Cremers C, Van de Heyning P. Diagnosis and management strategies in congenital atresia of the external auditory canal. Study Group on Otological Malformations and Hearing Impairment. *British Journal of Audiology.* 1999; **33**: 313–27; (review).

45. Altman F. Congenital atresia of the ear in man and animals. *Annals of Otology, Rhinology and Laryngology.* 1955; **64**: 824–58.

46. Marquet J. [Tympano-ossicular homografts in the surgical treatment of agenesis of the ear. Preliminary report] *Acta Oto-rhino-laryngologica Belgica.* 1971; **25**: 885–97 (in French).

47. Cremers CW, Oudenhoven JM, Marres EH. Congenital aural atresia. A new subclassification and surgical management. *Clinical Otolaryngology.* 1984; **9**: 119–27.

48. Jahrsdoerfer RA, Yeakley JW, Aguilar EA, Cole RR, Gray LC. Grading system for the selection of patients with congenital aural atresia. *American Journal of Otology.* 1992; **13**: 6–12.

49. Schucknecht HF. Congenital aural atresia. *Laryngoscope.* 1989; **99**: 908–17.

50. Horlock N, Vogelin E, Bradbury ET, Grobbelaar AO, Gault DT. Psychosocial outcome of patients after ear reconstruction – a retrospective study of 62 patients. *Annals of Plastic Surgery.* 2005; **54**: 517–24.

51. Morris DP, Rothera MP. The application of computer-enhanced imaging to improve preoperative counselling and informed consent in children considering bone anchored auricular prosthesis surgery. *International Journal of Pediatric Otorhinolaryngology.* 2000; **55**: 181–6.

52. Aguilar EF. Auricular reconstruction in congenital anomalies of the ear. *Facial Plastic Surgery Clinics of North America.* 2001; **9**: 159–69 (review).

53. Firmin F. Auricular reconstruction in cases of microtia. Principles, methods and classification. *Annales de Chirurgie Plastique et Esthétique.* 2001; **46**: 447–66 (in French).

54. Firmin T. Ear reconstruction in cases of typical microtia. Personal experience based on 352 microtic ear corrections. *Scandinavian Journal of Plastic and Reconstructive Surgery and Hand Surgery.* 1998; **32**: 35–47.

* 55. Nagata S. Modification of the stages in total reconstruction of the auricle: Part I–IV. *Plastic and Reconstructive Surgery.* 1994; **93**: 221–66; discussion 267–8. *This paper presents a reliable two-stage technique of ear reconstruction, modifying the previous four-stage procedure introduced by Brent. It has become the standard operation for microtia in recent times.*

56. Botma M, Aymat A, Gault D, Albert D. Ribgraft reconstruction vs osseointegration prosthesis for microtia; A significant change in patient preference. *Clinical Otolaryngology.* 2001; **26**: 274–7.

57. Romo 3rd. T, Fozo MS, Sclafani AP. Microtia reconstruction using a porous polyethylene framework. *Facial Plastic Surgery.* 2000; **16**: 15–22.

58. Granstrom G, Tjellstrom A. Guided tissue generation in the temporal bone. *Annals of Otology, Rhinology and Laryngology.* 1999; **108**: 349–54.

59. Granstrom G, Bergstrom K, Odersjo M, Tjellstrom A. Osseointegrated implants in children: experience from our first 100 patients. *Otolaryngology and Head and Neck Surgery.* 2001; **125**: 85–92.

60. Somers T, De Cubber J, Govaerts P, Offeciers FE. Total auricular repair: bone anchored prosthesis or plastic reconstruction? *Acta Otorhinolaryngologica Belgica.* 1998; **52**: 317–27.

61. Wilkes GH, Wolfaardt JF. Osseointegrated alloplastic versus autogenous ear reconstruction: criteria for treatment selection. *Plastic and Reconstructive Surgery.* 1994; **93**: 967–79.

62. Thorne CH, Brecht LE, Bradley JP, Levine JP, Hammerschlag P, Longaker MT. Auricular reconstruction: indications for autogenous and prosthetic techniques. *Plastic and Reconstructive Surgery.* 2001; **107**: 1241–52.

63. Smithells RW, Newman CG. Recognition of thalidomide defects. *Journal of Medical Genetics.* 1999; **29**: 716–23.

64. Melnick M, Myrianthopoulos NC, Paul NW. External ear malformations: epidemiology, genetics, and natural history. *Birth Defects Original Article Series.* 1979; **15**: I–ix, 1–40.

65. Cole RR, Jahrsdoerfer RA. The risk of cholesteatoma in congenital aural stenosis. *Laryngoscope.* 1990; **100**: 576–8.

∗ 66. Tjellstrom A, Hakansson B, Granstrom G. Bone-anchored hearing aids: current status in adults and children. *Otolaryngologic Clinics of North America.* 2001; **34**: 337–64 (review). *The introduction of the bone-anchored hearing aid has changed the outlook for children with bilateral microtia.*

67. Granstrom G. Osseointegrated implants in children. *Acta Otolaryngologica Supplementum.* 2000; **543**: 118–21.

68. Dutt SN, McDermott AL, Burrell SP, Cooper HR, Reid AP, Proops DW. Patient satisfaction with bilateral bone-anchored hearing aids: the Birmingham experience. *Journal of Laryngology and Otology.* 2002; **28**: 37–46.

69. Bajaj Y, Wyatt ME, Gault D, Bailey CM, Albert DM. How we do it: Baha® positioning in patients with microtia requiring auricular reconstruction. *Clinical Otolaryngology.* 2005; **30**: 468–71.

70. Cole RR, Jahrsdoerfer RA. The risk of cholesteatoma in congenital aural stenosis. *Laryngoscope.* 1990; **100**: 576–8.

71. McKinnon BJ, Jahrsdoerfer RA. Congenital auricular atresia: update on options for intervention and timing of repair. *Otolaryngologic Clinics of North America.* 2002; **35**: 877–90 (review).

72. de la Cruz A, Teufert KB. Congenital aural atresia surgery: long-term results. *Otolaryngology and Head and Neck Surgery.* 2003; **129**: 121–7.

73. Jahrsdoerfer RA, Lambert PR. Facial nerve injury in congenital aural atresia surgery. *American Journal of Otology.* 1998; **19**: 283–7.

74. Shih L, Crabtree JA. Long-term surgical results for congenital aural atresia. *Laryngoscope.* 1993; **103**: 1097–102 (review).

75. Chandrasekhar SS, De la Cruz A, Garrido E. Surgery of congenital aural atresia. *American Journal of Otology.* 1995; **16**: 713–7.

76. Jahrsdoerfer RA, Hall Jr. JW. Congenital malformations of the ear. *American Journal of Otology.* 1986; **7**: 267–9.

77. Linstrom CJ, Aziz MH, Romo T. Unilateral aural atresia in childhood: case selection and rehabilitation. *Journal of Otolaryngology.* 1995; **24**: 168–79.

78. Sabbagh W, Gault DT. Location, location, location. *Journal of Laryngology and Otology.* 2004; **118**: 738–40.

79. Lustig LR, Arts HA, Brackmann DE, Francis HF, Molony T, Megerian CA *et al.* Hearing rehabilitation using the Baha® bone-anchored hearing aid: results in 40 patients. *Otology and Neurotology.* 2001; **22**: 328–34.

80. van der Pouw CT, Snik AF, Cremers CW. The BAHA HC200/300 in comparison with conventional bone conduction hearing aids. *Clinical Otolaryngology and Allied Sciences.* 1999; **24**: 171–6.

81. Dutt SN, McDermott AL, Jelbert A, Reid AP, Proops DW. Day to day use and service-related issues with the bone-anchored hearing aid: the Entific Medical Systems questionnaire. *Journal of Laryngology and Otology.* 2002; **28**: 20–28.

82. Powell RH, Burrell SP, Cooper HR, Proops DW. The Birmingham bone anchored hearing aid programme: paediatric experience and results. *Journal of Laryngology and Otology.* 1996; **21**: 21–29.

83. Bosman AJ, Snik AF, van der Pouw CT, Mylanus EA, Cremers CW. Audiometric evaluation of bilaterally fitted bone-anchored hearing aids. *Audiology.* 2001; **40**: 158–67.

84. Proops DW *et al.* It works – the patients say so: the evidence base for aural rehabilitation with bone-anchored hearing aids. *Journal of Laryngology and Otology.* 2002; **28**: 1–51.

85. Wazen JJ, Spitzer J, Ghossaini SN, Kacker A, Zschommler A. Results of the bone-anchored hearing aid in unilateral hearing loss. *Laryngoscope.* 2001; **111**: 955–8.

76

Disorders of speech and language in paediatric otolaryngology

RAY CLARKE AND SIOBHAN McMAHON

Introduction	990	Key points	994
Normal development of speech and language	990	Best clinical practice	994
Classification and presentation of disorders	991	Deficiencies in current knowledge and areas for future	
Speech and language delay	992	research	994
Sound and speech production and disorders	992	References	994

SEARCH STRATEGY

The references for this chapter were complied from a Medline search using the terms 'speech and language disorders' and 'child'. The Cochrane database was also consulted.

INTRODUCTION

Communication is a fundamental part of the development and maturation of the child. Otolaryngologists are often directly involved in the investigation and management of disorders of communication, be they receptive disorders such as hearing loss, or expressive disorders, for example dysphonia and dysarthria.[1] Speech and language therapists (SLT) have particular expertise in the assessment and treatment of children with such disorders and optimum care of these children is brought about by close cooperation between SLTs, otorhinolaryngology (ORL) paediatricians and other health care professionals.

Speech and language therapists are independent professionals with a large body of scientific knowledge, diagnostic and therapeutic skills. In a short chapter such as this, it is possible only to make ORL clinicians aware of the commoner clinical presentations and to highlight the main principles that underpin SLT as it applies to children who may attend an ORL clinic.

NORMAL DEVELOPMENT OF SPEECH AND LANGUAGE

The development of speech and language starts at birth. Sensory stimulation is essential. Children learn by imitation, experimentation and feedback. Although there is considerable variation, progress is through a series of defined stages.[2] Some of the key stages are shown in **Figure 76.1**. In the first few weeks, some degree of differentiation of cry, for example 'hunger' and 'pain', becomes apparent. The **phonation stage** describes the period in the first two to three months of life when the infant produces predominantly vowel-like sounds, commonly known as 'cooing'. The infant then begins to articulate sounds while vocalizing. This **primitive articulation stage** is frequently referred to as 'gooing'. The normally developing infant continues to produce a wider repertoire of sounds and in the **expansion phase** begins to combine vowels and consonants. The process for the infant culminates in the **canonical babbling phase** with

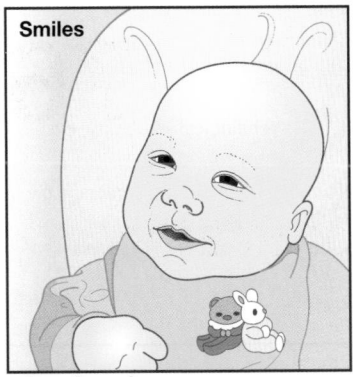

Smiles
Age: 6 weeks

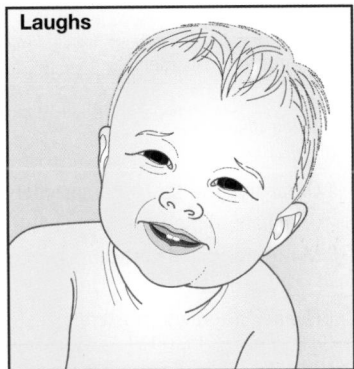

Laughs
Age: 3-4 months

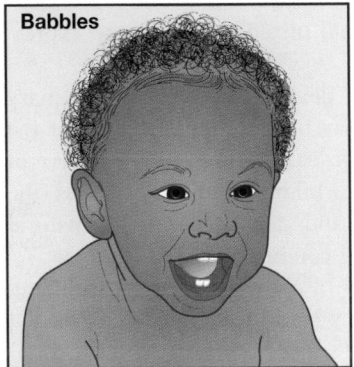

Babbles
Age: 4-6 months

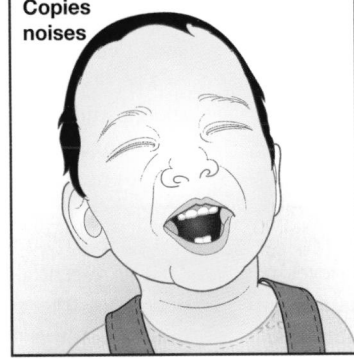

Copies noises
Age: 6-9 months

Figure 76.1 Stages in the development of speech and language.

the infant producing strings of syllable-like sounds, for example 'baba', 'mama' or 'dada'. This phase typically begins to emerge at around six months of age. Multiple studies report that normally developing babies rarely begin canonical babbling later than ten months of age.[3, 4, 5, 6] Thus the absence of the canonical babbling phase at this age has been proposed as an early indication of developmental speech and language problems.

Vocabulary, verbal and linguistic skills develop rapidly in the next two years. Throughout the second year of life normally developing children acquire an increasing vocabulary of single words. By two years, most infants will use at least 50 single words and will be beginning to produce two-word phrases. However, language development is not restricted to the knowledge and use of an increasing number of words.

Receptive language skills emerge as the child begins to understand simple instructions accompanied by gestures, for example 'give it to me', and progresses through following simple instructions in a familiar, predictable situation, for example 'wave bye-bye' while walking away. By two years of age typically developing children can identify familiar items from a small range without gestures or other cues. Receptive language skills develop prior to expressive skills.

A child who has no words by 20–24 months, no phrases at 28 months or who is not speaking intelligibly at three years is a cause for concern and should be investigated. It is axiomatic that parental concern about a child's development should always be acknowledged and warrants investigation. While parental concern may be a lack of expressive language, potential deficits in comprehension should also be explored.

CLASSIFICATION AND PRESENTATION OF DISORDERS

There are several systems for the classification of speech and language disorders but for practical purposes it is useful to consider **receptive**, **expressive** and **mixed** disorders (**Table 76.1**).[7] Children in whom the pattern of speech and language development is atypical and who do not appear to have other developmental disorders are often referred to as having a **specific language impairment** (SLI), although this distinction is not always clear and its validity as a precise diagnostic label has been questioned.[8] Clinical presentations range from complete inability to speak in children with severe developmental disorders to minor errors of fluency or pronunciation. In practice, otolaryngologists are asked to deal with children in one of two categories, i.e. those who are 'slow to speak' (speech or language delay) or those in whom there is concern regarding pronunciation or intelligibility (sound and speech production disorders or disorders of articulation or fluency).

Delay in either speech or language is reported in 6 percent of otherwise healthy preschool children.[9] The proportion is much higher in children with global developmental delay, cerebral palsy or neurological

Table 76.1 Classification of speech and language disorders in children.

Receptive disorders	Expressive disorders[a]	Combined disorders
Neurological: secondary to cognitive impairment (language comprehension)	Voice disorders	Psychological morbidity, e.g. autism, ADHD
Sensory: secondary to hearing or visual impairment	Oropharyngeal structural disorders, e.g. cleft palate, rhinolalia	Developmental disorders, e.g. cerebral palsy
Environmental: poor sensory stimulation	Motor nerve and cortical disorders, e.g. dysarthria	
	Fluency disorders (stuttering)	

[a]Sound and speech production.

disorders, in children on the autistic spectrum, and in children with attention deficit hyperactivity disorder (ADHD).[10] Co-morbidity is common and it is important for clinicians to have a high index of suspicion as the presentation of any one of the above conditions may be with a speech and language disorder. Screening programmes and vigilance among primary care health workers in western countries have ensured that congenital deafness is usually diagnosed before the child develops speech. In developing countries, speech delay is still an important mode of presentation of congenital deafness.

SPEECH AND LANGUAGE DELAY

Delay in speech and language development is the most common developmental disorder affecting children between 3 and 16 years.[7] Children who are slower than their peers to speak cause significant anxiety to their parents and other caregivers. Although delayed speech is 'a delay in speech and/or language development compared with controls matched for age, sex, cultural background and intelligence',[7] there is no universal definition of 'late talkers' that focuses on particular developmental milestones. Using the criteria of Rescorla,[11] children who at 24 months use fewer than 50 single words and/or use no two-word combinations, the prevalence of 'late talking' is between 10 and 15 percent of the population. Law *et al.*[9] in a Cochrane review quote a prevalence rate of 6 percent.

While some late talkers spontaneously improve, more than half of children who are late to talk have continuing language delay at three years and those who have little or no speech at 30 months are at increased risk of persistent problems. Children with persisting difficulties are at risk of ongoing problems with literacy, behaviour, socialization and educational performance. Rescorla[11] reports persistent weaknesses in language-related skills in a group of adolescents who were identified as late talkers between 24 and 30 months. Brownlie *et al.*[12] report adolescents with a history of language impairment had higher rates of arrests and convictions than those with isolated speech impairment or their normally developing peers. Risk factors for poorer outcomes for late talkers include hearing impairment, a positive family history of speech

and/or language delay and mixed (receptive and expressive) delay.

Most children with delayed speech have primary speech and language delay but in almost 50 percent the speech and language disorder is part of a global pattern of developmental delay. In children with global delay the prognosis is less good and dependent on the natural history of the underlying condition.[9]

It is essential to take a thorough history including details of the pregnancy and delivery, developmental milestones and the child's feeding history. A full clinical developmental assessment including age-appropriate testing of cognitive function may be needed. The otolaryngologist must arrange for age-appropriate assessment of the child's hearing and check the status of the middle ears, as otitis media may be a factor in reducing sensory input.

The challenge is to identify those children whose problems will not spontaneously resolve and to identify appropriate interventions for them.

In a systematic review of the effectiveness of speech and language interventions for children with primary speech and language delay/disorder, the authors report that overall there is a positive effect of SLT interventions with best results for children with expressive disorders. The effect of intervention for children with receptive disorders is less predictable.[9] [****]

SOUND AND SPEECH PRODUCTION AND DISORDERS

Normal speech production

Speech production is dependent on three components: respiration, phonation and articulation. Respiration is the current of air from the lungs, which forms the medium for the production of sound. This is modified by the vibration of the vocal folds (**phonation**) to produce 'voice' and then by alteration of the size, shape and position of the structures in the mouth and pharynx notably the tongue, lips and palate (**articulation**). Subtle changes in the quality or 'timbre' of the spoken word (**resonance**) are also brought about by the air-containing cavities of the pharynx, the nose and the paranasal sinuses.

The velopharyngeal sphincter is important in the production of speech. The sphincter marks the junction between the nasopharynx and the oropharynx and closes during swallowing to prevent reflux of food and fluids into the nasal cavity. It is open during nasal inspiration and closes for the most part during speech except for the sounds 'm', 'n' and 'ng'. Disorders of voice where the pathology is in the larynx are dealt with in Chapter 90, Paediatric voice disorders.

Disorders of articulation

Articulation disorders may be idiopathic but neurological dysfunction, developmental delay, lack of coordination of movements in the mouth or pharynx, dental anomalies, malocclusion, or tongue problems, such as microglossia and macroglossia, must be considered. A thorough otolaryngological asessment will include age-appropriate assessment of hearing and examination of all of the structures of the head and neck involved in the production of speech.

Nasal speech (rhinolalia)

Otolaryngologists may be asked to see children with abnormalities of pronunciation described as 'nasal' speech. Excessive nasal air escape during speech gives rise to **hypernasal speech** or **rhinolalia aperta**. In **rhinolalia clausa** the normal pattern of nasal escape when speaking 'nasal' sounds, for example nn, mm and ng, is obstructed. There may be a mixed hypo- and hypernasal pattern.

The distinction between these varieties of nasal speech can be difficult for the untrained ear; hence thorough assessment by a speech and language therapist is essential before commencing treatment.

HYPERNASAL SPEECH

In hypernasal speech (rhinolalia aperta) the velopharyngeal sphincter remains open or partly open during speech and air escapes into the nasal cavity. Causes include palatal paralysis, for example diptheria, cerebral palsy, cleft palate, submucous cleft, adenoidectomy, and craniofacial surgery such as midfacial osteotomy. Placing a cold steel spatula under the nostrils and observing the misting pattern as the child speaks is a useful clinical test for the condition. Some nasal escape is normal during 'nasal' sounds such as mm, nn and ng, but misting when the child speaks a phrase with no nasal sounds, for example 'Katie's sister was six yesterday', is suggestive of

palatal dysfunction. In established cases, there may be compensatory nasal grimacing as the child attempts to correct the nasal escape. Velopharyngeal insufficiency and submucous palatal clefts are dealt with in Chapter 77, Cleft lip and palate.

HYPONASAL SPEECH

Hyponasal speech (rhinolalia clausa) can be caused by septal deviation, polyps, gross turbinate hypertrophy, adenoids or a space-ccupying nasopharyngeal lesion. The spatula test shows no escape when the child is asked to speak words with 'nasal' sounds, for example 'Mummy and nanny are mending' will be pronounced 'Bubby and daddy are bedding'.

Tonsils, adenoids and speech

Tonsillectomy may affect the 'timbre' or resonance of the singing voice and in the case of children who sing it is wise to inform them and their parents of this. Adenoidectomy causes transient velopharyngeal sphincter dysfunction in about 5 percent of cases. This can cause troublesome rhinolalia aperta. In a small minority (0.01 percent) this may be longstanding.[13, 14]

Children with submucous palatal clefting – where the only external sign may be a bifid uvula – should have adenoidectomy with extreme caution if at all. Partial adenoidectomy, under direct or endoscopic vision and preserving a buttress of tissue around the lateral margins may preserve the velopharyngeal closure mechanism.[15]

Hyponasal speech due to large adenoids rarely constitutes an indication for adenoidectomy on its own. Usually there will be an independent indication for surgery, for example airway obstruction. Adenoids regress and parents should be made aware of this when giving informed consent if adenoidectomy is offered to improve the child's speech.

Fluency disorders (stuttering)

'Fluency' refers to the organization, structure and sequence of speech patterns. Some degree of dysfluency is developmental but persistent stuttering – characterized by abnormal prolongations interruptions and syllable repetitions – can cause significant difficulties which persist into adult life.

Stuttering typically starts in the third and fourth years of life, typically in children whose speech and language development is otherwise normal. The aetiology is unknown, but there is a familial association and boys are more commonly affected than girls. There is no association with tongue tie or with adenotonsillar disorders and no evidence to justify surgery of any sort for stuttering.

The available evidence supports early intervention – in the preschool years – under the supervision of a speech and language therapist.[16] [****]

Tongue tie

Tongue tie (ankyloglossia) is characterized by tethering of the anterior part of the tongue to the floor of the mouth by a short lingual frenulum. It is usually asymptomatic but may restrict tongue mobility in the newborn and give rise to difficulties with breastfeeding. Many parents present for treatment as they are concerned about the appearance of the tongue or about the potential for the condition to interfere with activities such as licking the lips and kissing. The condition tends to improve as the child gets older.[17]

There is no evidence to link tongue tie with speech and language disorders. Nevertheless, parents often request treatment. If treatment is required, a simple division of the frenulum is adequate. In the newborn, this can be undertaken without anaesthesia but older children require a general anaesthetic.

KEY POINTS

- Speech and language disorders – particularly delayed speech – are common in children.
- In very young children most cases of speech and language delay resolve spontaneously.
- Persistent speech and language difficulties in young children are predictive of long-term problems affecting behaviour, learning and school achievement.
- Adequate stimulation is essential for normal development of speech and language.
- Deafness may be a key factor in the aetiology of speech and language disorders. Delayed speech is still a common mode of presentation of deafness.

Best clinical practice

✓ Normally developing babies rarely begin 'canonical babbling' later than ten months of age. Absence of the canonical babbling phase at this age is an early indication of developmental speech and language problems. [Grade B]

✓ A child who has no words by 20–24 months, no phrases at 28 months or who is not speaking intelligibly at three years is a cause for concern and should be investigated. [Grade B/C]

✓ Global developmental delay, cerebral palsy, neurological disorders, children on the autistic spectrum and children with ADHD may present with a speech and language disorder. [Grade B]

✓ The distinction between the different varieties of nasal speech (rhinolalia) can be difficult for the untrained ear; hence thorough assessment by a speech and language therapist is essential before commencing treatment. [Grade C/D]

✓ Stuttering is best managed by early intervention – in the preschool years – under the supervision of a speech and language therapist. [Grade A]

✓ There is no good evidence of an association between tongue tie and disorders of speech and language. [Grade A]

Deficiencies in current knowledge and areas for future research

➤ The evidence base that underpins current practice in speech and language therapy is improving steadily. Many treatments are now the subject of randomized controlled trials and systematic reviews.

➤ Developmental paediatrics is a well-established subspecialty. Children with developmental disorders often have speech and language disorders and are increasingly being seen in multidisciplinary clinics where access to speech and language therapy is improving.

REFERENCES

1. Ruben RJ. Valedictory – why paediatric otorhinolaryngology is important. *International Journal of Pediatric Otolaryngology.* 2003; 67: S53–61.
2. Oller DK, Eilers RE, Neal AR, Schwartz HK. Precursors to speech in infancy; the prediction of speech and language disorders. *Journal of Communication Disorders.* 1999; 32: 223–5.
3. Rescorla L, Mirak J. Normal language acquisition. *Seminars in Pediatric Neurology.* 1997; 4: 70–6.
4. Dodd B, Holm A, Hua Z, Crosbie S. Phonological development: a normative study of British-English speaking children. *Clinical Linguistics and Phonetics.* 2003; 17: 617–43.
5. Brady NC, Marquis J, Fleming K, McLean L. Prelinguistic predictors of language growth in children with developmental disabilities. *Journal of Speech, Language and Hearing Research.* 2004; 47: 663–77.

6. Ingram D. *First language acquisition: method, description and explanation.* Cambridge, UK: Cambridge University Press, 1989.

∗ 7. Busari JO, Weggelaar NM. How to investigate and manage the child who is slow to speak. *British Medical Journal.* 2004; **328**: 272–6. *A valuable practical guide for clinicians.*

8. Dollaghan CA. Taxometric analyses of specific language impairment in 3- and 4-year old children. *Journal of Speech, Language and Hearing Research.* 2004; **47**: 464–75.

∗ 9. Law J, Garrett Z, Nye C. Speech and language therapy interventions for children with primary speech and language delay or disorder (Cochrane Review). In: *The Cochrane Library.* Oxford: Update Software, 2003. *A meta-analysis of current evidence for speech and language therapy in the management of children with delayed speech.*

10. Bruinsma Y, Koegel RL, Koegel LK. Joint attention and children with autism: a review of the literature. *Mental Retardation and Developmental Disabilities Research Reviews.* 2004; **10**: 169–75.

11. Rescorla L. Age 13 language and reading outcomes in late talking toddlers. *Journal of Speech, Language and Hearing Research.* 2005; **48**: 459–72.

12. Brownlie EB, Beitchman JH, Escobar M, Young A, Atkinson L, Johnson C *et al.* Early language impairment and young adult delinquent and aggressive behaviour. *Journal of Abnormal Child Psychology.* 2004; **32**: 453–67.

13. Maryn Y, Van Lierde K, DeBodt M, Van Cauwenberge P. The effects of adenoidectomy and tonsillectomy on speech and nasal resonance. *Folio Phoniatrica et Logopedica.* 2004; **56**: 182–91.

14. Andreassen ML, Leeper HA, MacRae DL. Changes in vocal resonance and nasalization following adenoidectomy in normal children: preliminary findings. *Journal of Otolaryngology.* 1991; **20**: 237–42.

15. Finkelstein Y, Wexler DB, Nachmani A, Ophir D. Endoscopic partial adenoidectomy for children with submucous cleft palate. *Cleft Palate-Craniofacial Journal.* 2002; **39**: 479–86.

∗ 16. Jones M, Onslow M, Packham A, Williams S, Ormond T, Schwartz I *et al.* Randomised controlled trial of the Lidcombe programme of early stuttering intervention. *British Medical Journal.* 2005; **331**: 659–61. *A review of stuttering with an account of an intervention programme with a sound evidence-base.*

∗ 17. Lalakea ML, Messner AH. Ankyloglossia: does it matter? *Pediatric Clinics of North America.* 2003; **50**: 381–97. *Well-written review of a common and poorly understood paediatric presentation.*

77

Cleft lip and palate

CHRIS PENFOLD

Introduction	996	Robin sequence and Robin complexes	1000
Classification	996	Management of cleft lip and palate	1001
Epidemiology	997	Otitis media in cleft palate	1010
Normal embryogenesis	998	Key points	1013
Embryopathy of facial clefting	999	Best clinical practice	1013
Genetic factors	999	Deficiencies in current knowledge and areas for future	
Environmental factors and gene/environment interactions		research	1013
– the 'Greenspan' model	1000	Acknowledgements	1013
Clefts as part of a syndrome	1000	References	1014

SEARCH STRATEGY

The data in this chapter are supported by a Medline search using the search terms cleft palate, cleft lip, clinical trials and focusing on aetiology and treatment. The Cochrane database was also consulted.

INTRODUCTION

Clefts of the lip and palate are the among the most common congenital birth anomalies. The reported incidence varies between 0.4/1000 and 3.7/1000 live births.[1] The condition usually presents as an isolated anomaly (nonsyndromic cleft lip and/or palate) but may be associated with other congenital defects (syndromic cleft lip and/or palate). This chapter describes the epidemiology, embryogenesis and aetiology of cleft lip and palate and then focusses on the principles of treatment.

CLASSIFICATION

Many different classification systems of varying complexity have been proposed for cleft lip and palate. The simple ones are easy to use, but fail to distinguish between phenotypic characteristics that may be significant with regard to aetiology and treatment outcome.

Veau's 1931 classification, which has four categories, is an example of a simple system.[2] It is incomplete since it makes no provision for isolated cleft lip or alveolus. The earliest symbolic representation appears to have been developed by Pfeifer in 1966 (**Figure 77.1**).[3] Kernahan and Stark's classification was developed and represented symbolically as a 'striped Y' by Kernahan in 1971 (**Figure 77.2**).[4]

Kriens introduced a simple coding system for paraphrasing cleft lip and palate in 1987.[5] This system represents the anatomic site, and the side and type of cleft (complete, partial, microform) in a simple alphabetical code – LAHSHAL. Complete clefts are recorded in upper case, partial clefts in lower case and microform clefts are denoted by an asterisk (**Figure 77.3**). This system has been widely used and has the advantage of being easy to record in medical records and electronically.

Two systems of contrasting complexity in use today are the American Cleft Palate Association's detailed classification designed in 1962 and a much simpler variation of the symbolic 'Y' system currently used in the UK.

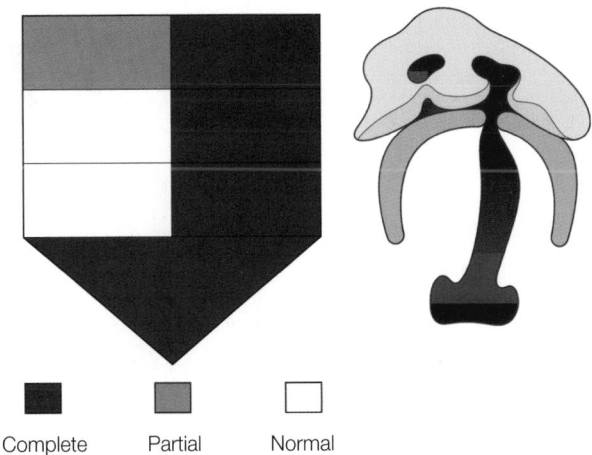

Figure 77.1 Pfeifer's symbolic classification.

Complete   Partial   Normal

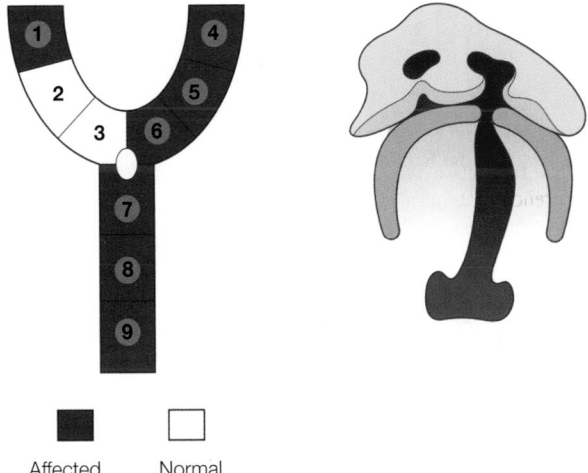

Affected   Normal

Figure 77.2 Kernahan's striped 'Y' classification. 1, 4, lip; 2, 5, alveolus; 3, 6, hard palate anterior to incisive foramen; 7, 8, hard palate; 9, soft palate; 0, incisive foramen.

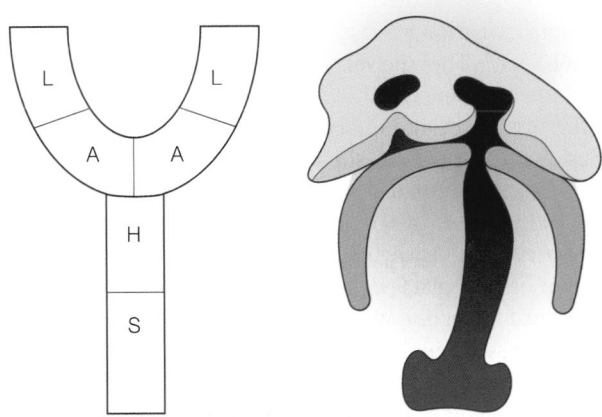

Figure 77.3 LAHSHAL - anatomic paraphrase of cleft lip, alveolus and palate. A, alveolus; H, hard palate; L, lip; S, soft palate.

True median clefts fall into a category outside the classification systems for clefts of the lip and palate described. They can occur as an isolated malformation or may occur with holoprosencephaly (failure of the prosencephalon to sufficiently divide into the double lobes of the cerebral hemispheres). The result is a single-lobed brain structure and severe skull and facial defects.[6]

Tessier[7] described an anatomical system of classification for craniofacial clefts, which depended on the site and the relationship of the cleft to the midline sagittal plane. The classification describes 14 different types of clefts according to whether they are cranial or facial and their relation to the midsagittal line. The system facilitates description of both the site and severity of clefting. Clefts of the lip and alveolus are numbered 1, 2 and 3. The causes of most clefts are unknown; some are malformations and some represent disruptions caused for example, by amniotic bands. The vast majority are sporadic with a few exceptions including the autosomal dominant inherited Treacher Collins syndrome.

EPIDEMIOLOGY

There are racial differences in incidence with the highest incidence of cleft lip and palate reported in Native Americans (3.7/1000 live births) and the lowest in children of Afro-Carribean descent (0.3/1000 births).[1] In Europe, there appears to be a clear difference between north and south with the lowest rate of 6.3 per 10,000 in El Valles, Spain and the highest (2.62/1000) in Finland.[8] [**]

Cleft lip with or without cleft palate (CL/P) is more common in boys. The more severe the defect, the greater the proportion of males affected. The male:female ratio is 2:1 for cleft lip and palate reducing to 1.5:1 for isolated cleft lip (CL). This contrasts with the incidence of isolated cleft palate (cleft palate only, CPO) which is lower at around 0.62/1000, shows less variation in different racial groups and is more common in girls (sex ratio = 0.83).[8] Associated malformations occur more frequently in infants who have CPO than in those with CL/P.[9, 10, 11, 12] [**]

Clefts of the lip may be incomplete or complete, unilateral or bilateral. Unilateral cleft lip occurs twice as commonly on the left side. Approximately 10–30 percent are associated with skin bridges that connect the medial and lateral cleft elements known as Simonart's bands. Cleft palate (CP) may involve just the soft palate or extend into the hard palate. Submucous cleft of the soft palate where the mucosa is intact but the underlying tissues are 'cleft' has been reported in approximately 1 in 1200 to 1 in 2000 births,[9] similar to the incidence of overt CPO. [**]

There is evidence from epidemiological studies that infants with cleft lip and palate have an increased risk of mortality in the first years of life.[13] This increased mortality is greater than that accounted for by the presence of other associated anomalies. [**]

NORMAL EMBRYOGENESIS

In the embryo, the face appears to develop at the end of the fourth week and is complete by the eighth week of pregnancy. The palate is completely formed by the end of the tenth week. The process of facial development starts with the migration of neural crest cells into the facial region to form the facial mesenchyme. This migration starts just before the neural folds fuse to form the neural tube at the end of the third week.

A series of swellings appear around the stomodeum at the end of the fourth week (**Figure 77.4**). These correspond to the frontonasal process, the bilateral maxillary process and the mandibular process. The developing nasal placodes arise as thickenings on either side of the frontonasal process. During the fifth week, the nasal placode becomes surrounded by a horseshoe-shaped ridge consisting of lateral and medial nasal processes creating a nasal pit in the middle. The nasal pits continue to deepen and eventually rupture, forming communications between the nasal and oral cavities, called primary choanae.

By the seventh week, the maxillary processes have advanced medially underneath the lateral nasal swellings and fused with the medial nasal swellings which themselves have merged with each other. This complex comprising the fused medial nasal swellings and maxillary swellings forms the primary palate and is complete by the end of the seventh week (**Figure 77.5**).

During the sixth week, two shelf-like swellings project medially from the maxillary process behind the primary palate (**Figure 77.6a**). Their medial edges hang vertically downwards either side of the tongue surrounded by a layer of undifferentiated epithelial cells, two to three layers

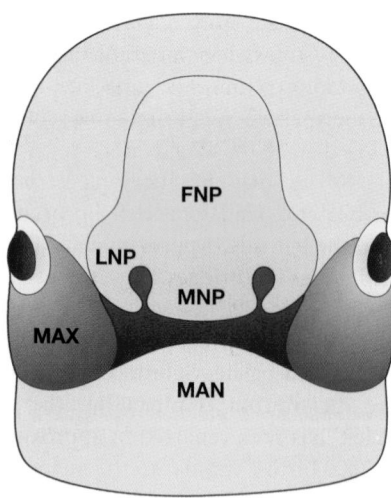

Figure 77.4 Development and fate of the facial processes. Representation of a 30–32-day-old human embryo showing the development of the facial processes. FNP, frontonasal process; MAX, maxillary process; MAN, mandibular process; MNP, medial nasal process; LNP, lateral nasal process.

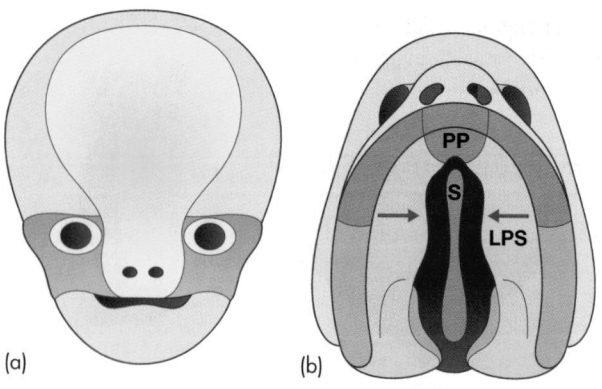

Figure 77.5 Representation of seven-week-old embryo showing the fate of the facial processes (a) frontal view; (b) ventral view of primary and secondary palate. LPS, lateral palatal shelf; PP, primary palate; S, nasal septum.

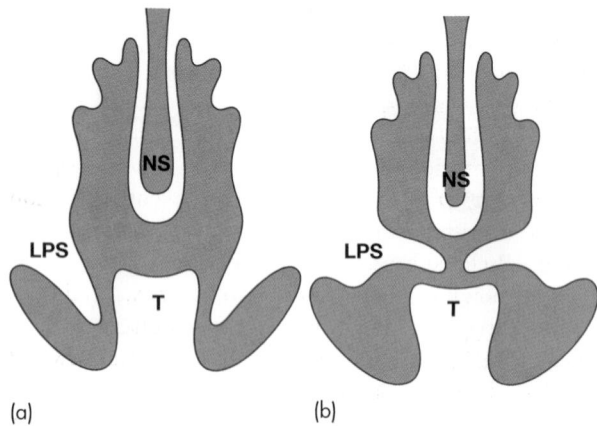

Figure 77.6 Elevation of the palatal shelves. Coronal section of (a) seven-week-old embryo; (b) eight-week-old embryo after elevation of the palatal shelves. LPP, lateral palatal process; S, nasal septum.

thick and referred to as medial edge epithelium (MEE). At a precise moment during the seventh week (about seven days later in female compared to male embryos), the drooping palatal shelves rapidly elevate during a matter of minutes or hours to a horizontal position (**Figure 77.6b**).[14, 15] The shelves make contact in the midline and the opposing layers of MEE adhere to each other. The MEE disappears and mesenchyme flows across the palate. Fusion of the palatal shelves is complete by the tenth week. Although there is some controversy as to the fate of the MEE there is no doubt that its role in exposing underlying mesenchymal tissue is crucial to successful fusion of the palatal shelves.

Bone formation in the palatal processes of the maxillary and palatine bones is dependent on the differentiation of osteogenic blastomas from the mesenchyme of the hard palate. The muscles of the soft palate are formed by the migration of mesoderm from the pharyngeal walls. Formation of the nose is completed by the development of the secondary nasal septum from mesenchyme which extends down from the roof of the primitive nasal cavity to fuse with the palatal shelves in the midline.

EMBRYOPATHY OF FACIAL CLEFTING

Facial clefts can occur as part of a syndrome or as isolated clefts. Nonsyndromic cleft lip with or without cleft palate is considered as aetiologically distinct from cleft palate only. Nonsyndromic cleft lip and palate is the result of an embryopathy culminating in a failure of fusion between maxillary mesenchymal processes. It is composed of two separate entities: cleft lip with or without cleft palate and cleft palate only. This distinction is supported by embryological considerations, as well as genetic studies.

Evidence on the aetiology of facial clefting is derived from a combination of epidemiological studies, animal model studies (mainly murine models) and human genetic and in vitro studies. A positive family history can be identified in 20 percent of patients in different populations, which supports the view that genetic factors have an important role in the aetiology of facial clefting. A picture has emerged which supports a genetic predisposition to disruption of the normal development and fusion of the mesenchymal processes resulting in malformations that are disclosed by environmental factors.

Essentially a cleft is caused by one or a combination of the following: hypoplasia, abnormal directional growth of mesenchymal processes, failure of fusion or breakdown of fusion of mesenchymal processes.

Failure of palatal shelf elevation may be responsible for 90 percent of palatal clefting.[9] In some cases obstruction of palatal shelf elevation by the tongue secondary to micrognathia may be a contributory factor in palatal clefting as may occur in Pierre Robin sequence.

GENETIC FACTORS

The development of detailed structures of the head and face is mainly determined genetically.[16] Nonsyndromic clefting occurs in the absence of other physical problems or any evidence of delay in motor or cognitive development. Both nonsyndromic CPO and CL/P have a genetic background that is probably disclosed by environmental factors. About 70 percent of cases of CL/P and 50 percent of CPO are nonsyndromic.[17, 18] Evidence that genetic factors play an important role in the aetiology of CPO and CL/P is forthcoming from population studies, most notably the study by Fogh-Anderson in 1942.[19] A recent study that compared CL/P and CPO showed concordance values in CL/P for monozygotic twins and dizygotic twins of 40 percent and 4.2 percent compared with values in CPO of 35 and 7.8 percent, respectively.[20] [**]

Most of the genetic studies are based on segregation, allelic association and linkage analyses.[21, 22] Proposed aetiologies include single gene causes, chromosomal disorders and polygenic interactions. The proposition of divergent models for orofacial clefting has implications for genetic counselling which continues to be informed by empirically derived risk data (Table 77.1).[23]

Association and linkage analysis attempt to map a disease gene on a chromosome using genetic markers. One of the first cleft lip and palate candidate gene association studies using a case–control approach provided evidence for the role of transforming growth factor alpha (TGFα) in CL/P.[24] [**]

Linkage analysis examines the cosegregation of a disease and a genetic marker in a family unit in order to determine if they segregate independently or together. Genetic linkage studies using from 1 to 40 families[20, 21, 25] have suggested loci for clefts on chromosomes 4, 6, 17 and 19, but results have been inconsistent[18] with only loci on 6p consistently showing linkage to CL/P in studies from Denmark,[26] Italy[27] and the UK.[28] The UK study, which involved a genome-wide screen carried out on 100 sibling pairs, confirmed nine regions of interest. One of these regions at 1p36 is of particular interest because its deletion is associated with an increased frequency of clefting[29] and contains the genes SKI, P73 and MTHFR which are candidate genes for CL/P.[18] There is an expanding list of

Table 77.1 Genetic risks of cleft lip and or palate in the absence of a defined syndrome or Mendelian pattern.

Relationship to index case	Cleft lip with or without palate (%)	Cleft palate alone (%)
Siblings (overall risk)	4	1.8
Sibling (no other affected members)	2.2	
Sibling (two affected siblings)	10	8
Sibling and affected parent	10	
Children	4.3	3
Second-degree relatives	0.6	
Third-degree relatives	0.3	
General population	0.1	0.04

Reprinted from Ref. 23, with permission.

genes that have already been shown to play an important role in facial development that includes genes identified as growth factors, cytokines, self-signalling molecules and structural proteins. Gene linkage and association studies have confirmed a possible role for a number of these (**Table 77.2**).[24, 30, 31, 32, 33, 34, 35, 36, 37, 38, 39, 40]

ENVIRONMENTAL FACTORS AND GENE/ENVIRONMENT INTERACTIONS – THE 'GREENSPAN' MODEL

A relation between some environmental factors – notably smoking, alcohol, anticonvulsants, steroids taken during pregnancy and the risk of having a baby with an orofacial cleft is well established. The model for complex diseases presented by Greenspan[41] can be applied to CL/P and CPO both of which have a multifactorial aetiology. According to Greenspan's model, the same output or phenotype can be produced in different ways with a network of interactions, including the type of gene mutation, the effect of other genes and environmental factors. Complex pathways through this network of gene–gene interaction and gene–environment interaction may provide alternative routes through which CL/P and CPO can be developed and avoided. An example of a possible gene–environment interaction important for the development of orofacial clefts is that between folate and the methylenetetrahydrofolate reductase (MTHFR) gene.

The role of folic acid metabolism in the aetiology of orofacial clefting is less clear than that demonstrated for neural tube defects (NTD).[42] There is conflicting evidence about the beneficial role of dietary folate supplement in preventing orofacial clefts, although the weight of evidence does support the view that there is some benefit if folate is taken periconceptually in high doses.[43] Recent studies have indicated a role for folic acid and the MTHFR gene in the aetiology of CL/P, but the strength and direction of this genetic–environment interaction has not been clarified.[44, 35, 38] The study of gene–environment interactions in orofacial clefting has achieved some remarkable successes and developments in genetic technology promise that such successes are only the beginning.[45, 46] [**]

CLEFTS AS PART OF A SYNDROME

Most orofacial clefts are nonsyndromic and occur as an isolated anomaly. Additional malformations are more frequently associated with CPO than with CL/P and least of all with isolated cleft lip, but reported rates of associated malformations vary considerably. Recent studies have reported rates of associated anomalies varying between 22 and 47 percent for CPO and 28 and 37 percent for CL/P, similar to previous estimates of 50 percent for CPO and 30 percent for CLP.[11, 47, 48, 49] Malformations of the upper or lower limbs or the vertebral column are the most common associated anomalies, accounting for 33 percent of all associated defects followed by cardiovascular anomalies which make up 24 percent.[50] [**]

An increasing number of syndromes with orofacial clefting as part of the spectrum of anomalies has been reported since 1970.[51] There are now over 400 syndromes associated with CPO and CL/P in the London Dysmorphology Database.[52] Cleft lip and palate and cleft palate only are the most common syndromic cleft subtypes; cleft lip on its own is only rarely syndromic. Syndromic clefts have a variety of causes, including single gene disorders that exhibit Mendelian inheritance, chromosome abnormalities and teratogens. In over 50 craniofacial syndromes a gene has been either mapped to a chromosomal location or actually isolated and its structure identified. In most cases different genes have been responsible for different syndromes but occasionally there are cases where identical mutations produce different syndromes suggesting the influence of other genes or environmental factors. **Table 77.3** shows some of the common syndromes associated with clefting.

ROBIN SEQUENCE AND ROBIN COMPLEXES

Pierre Robin sequence is a common condition that includes a combination of micrognathia or retrognathia, cleft palate, glossoptosis (backward prolapse of the tongue) and upper airway obstruction. What is now recognized as Pierre Robin sequence was first described in

Table 77.2 Some of the candidate genes suggested by allelic association and/or linkage analysis for orofacial clefting.

Candidate gene	Gene map locus	Name of gene	Reference
TGF alpha	2P13	Transforming growth factor alpha	21, 30, 31
MSX1	4p16.1	Homeobox gene (HOX7)	31, 32, 33
MTHFR	1p36	Methylenetetrahydrofolate reductase	34, 35, 36, 37, 38
TGF beta 3	14q24	Transforming growth factor beta 3	31, 33

Reproduced from Penfold CN. Etiology, growth, audit and trends in cleft lip, alveolus and palate. In: Ward-Booth P, Schendel S (eds). *Maxillofacial surgery*, 2nd edn, by permission of Elsevier.

Table 77.3 Some common syndromes associated with cleft palate.

Syndrome	Detail
Chromosomal	
Velocardiofacial syndrome	Deletion chromosome 22q11
Non-Mendelian	
Goldenhar	
Mendelian disorders	
Orofacial digital syndrome	X-linked
Stickler syndrome	Autosomal dominant
Treacher Collins syndrome	Autosomal dominant (treacle gene mapped to 5q32-q33.1)
Van der Woude syndrome	Autosomal dominant (gene maps to 1q32-q41)

Reproduced from Penfold CN. Etiology, growth, audit and trends in cleft lip, alveolus and palate. In: Ward-Booth P, Schendel S (eds). *Maxillofacial surgery*, 2nd edn, by permission of Elsevier.

1923 as a 'syndrome consisting of micrognathia and upper airway obstruction'.[53] The term 'sequence' denotes a series of anomalies caused by a cascade of events initiated by a single malformation. This is in contrast to the term 'syndrome', which is reserved for those errors of morphogenesis where the simultaneous presence of multiple anomalies can be attributed to a single cause. Robin sequence denotes a cascade of events starting with retrognathia or micrognathia (**Figure 77.7**). The consequent posterior position of the tongue prevents normal elevation of the palatal shelves resulting in a 'U'-shaped cleft palate. Respiratory compromise is produced by true glossoptosis. Because of causal, pathogenetic and phenotypic differences Robin sequences of various types can occur alone or as part of a syndrome, which may be genetically determined.[54, 55] In many cases of apparent Robin sequence, the manifestations are causally but not sequentially related. For example, the clinical

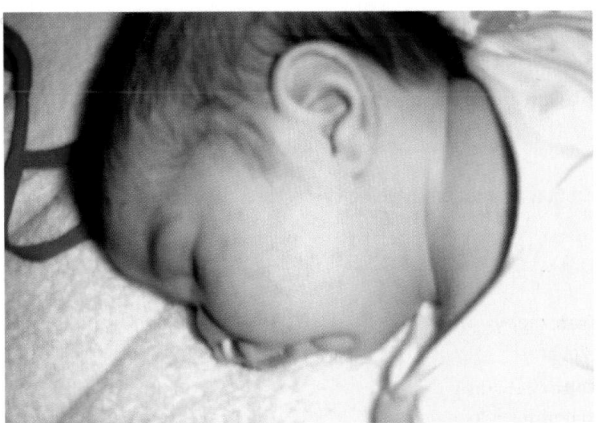

Figure 77.7 Baby with retrognathia, part of Pierre Robin sequence.

manifestations of del(22q11.2) or velocardiofacial syndrome include retrognathia (caused by an obtuse cranial base angle), cleft palate (submucous or true) and airway obstruction. In this syndrome the mechanism of airway obstruction, when present, is not caused by retrognathia, but by hypotonia. The term 'Robin complex' has been suggested to describe those cases where the manifestations are causally but not sequentially related.[56]

MANAGEMENT OF CLEFT LIP AND PALATE

Diagnosis

In the past, clefts of the lip and palate were diagnosed at birth. This is still largely true today. One exception is the diagnosis of submucous cleft palate which usually only becomes manifest if and when speech problems, in the form of velopharyngeal insufficiency (VPI), are identified. Diagnosis is often delayed until after the age of three years and sometimes much later. Early identification of submucous cleft palate would allow early treatment before speech problems develop, but this is complicated by the fact that not all cases of submucous cleft cause such problems. The mere presence of a submucous cleft is not in itself an indication for treatment. Careful monitoring of speech development is essential. Identification of feeding difficulties in the neonatal period may be a marker for the subsequent development of VPI.

During the last decade, technological advances in obstetric ultrasound have facilitated prenatal diagnosis of cleft lip and palate. Cleft lip can now be accurately detected by transvaginal sonography as early as 13–16 weeks gestation.[57] The size and severity of the cleft cannot as yet be accurately assessed. Isolated cleft palate cannot be detected or ruled out prenatally.

Prenatal diagnosis in cleft lip and palate has inevitably raised difficult ethical issues. There is evidence from a study in Israel that the adoption of widespread prenatal screening for cleft lip and palate at 14–16 weeks gestation is associated with a high incidence of termination in cases where a cleft lip has been diagnosed, even in the absence of other major congenital anomalies.[58] This is in contrast to a study in California where the reported incidence of termination in prenatally diagnosed cleft lip was much smaller at around 10 percent.[59] Factors that may influence the uptake of termination include the timing of prenatal screening, the perception of the 'burden of clefting', which is influenced by cultural, religious and socioeconomic factors, and the provision of genetic counselling at the time of prenatal diagnosis. It is likely that prenatal diagnosis will have an impact on the incidence of cleft lip and palate in live-born infants in certain countries. This in turn will have an impact on the demand for provision of treatment.

General principles

Management of patients with cleft lip and palate requires a multidisciplinary approach delivered by a team. This will ideally include a nurse specialist, paediatrician, feeding specialist, speech and language therapist, cleft surgeon, orthodontist, audiologist, otolaryngologist and psychologist.

CP/CLP can cause impairment of feeding, hearing, nasal breathing, speech, dentofacial growth and development, facial appearance and psychosocial well-being.[60, 61] **Table 77.4** lists examples of outcomes associated with facial appearance, growth and function, psychosocial state and patient satisfaction that have been measured by investigators in the field of cleft lip and palate research.

The goal of cleft care is to correct all the problems attributable either directly or indirectly to the original malformation. The burden of prolonged treatment – which often extends over many years and involves multiple surgical procedures – can cause significant disruption to family life.[63] [**/*]

Most clinical evidence supporting contemporary treatment regimes for cleft lip and palate is based on case reports and observational studies. This is the case in most if not all surgical disciplines where until recently, studies of operations were retrospective case series with randomized controlled trials accounting for less than 10 percent of the total.[64, 65] There is little objective evidence to help choose between various treatments. A recent survey of European cleft services revealed that 194 different surgical protocols were performed by 201 teams for unilateral cleft lip and palate alone.[66]

We still do not know for certain what are the best operations, when to do them and what ancillary treatments should be employed.

Early management – airway and feeding

Parents of a child born with cleft lip and palate need psychological support and access to early specialist feeding advice. Babies with cleft lip or cleft lip and palate can experience feeding problems that usually resolve in the early neonatal period. Babies with an isolated cleft palate may continue to experience problems for many months and require careful management.[67] Palatal obturator plates have enjoyed widespread use, but their popularity has declined in the absence of evidence to show any real benefit.[68, 69] [****/***] Babies with additional anomalies are at increased risk of feeding problems and may also have difficulty maintaining a satisfactory airway. Pierre Robin sequence is a well-recognized set of anomalies that presents with retrognathia, cleft palate, glossoptosis and varying degrees of upper airway obstruction. Mild cases can be managed conservatively by careful postural management during feeding and sleep. More severe cases may require airway support during the early months of life with a nasopharyngeal tube and nasogastric or gastrostomy feeding.[70] [**]

Presurgical orthopaedics

Preoperative preparation using presurgical orthopaedics has been used for centuries to try to realign the bony

Table 77.4 Examples of outcome measures used in cleft lip and or palate research.

Variable category	Outcome measure	Method	Data form
Facial appearance	Lip and nose form	Standardized subjective analysis using reference examples, anthropometric analysis, rating specific features or pairwise matching[62]	Photographs
Facial growth and development	Facial profile	Cephalometric analysis Soft tissue profile analysis	X-rays
Facial growth and development	Dental arch relationship	GOSLON yardstick	Dental model casts
Speech	Nasal resonance Nasal emission Articulation Intelligibility	Perceptual evaluation, nasometry	Standardized speech sample
Hearing	Tympanic membrane compliance Frequency thresholds	Tympanometry Audiometry	Direct measurement
Nasal breathing	Nasal airflow	Nasometry	Direct measurement
Quality of life	Psychosocial well-being	Validated questionnaire	Direct measurement

Reproduced from Penfold CN. Etiology, growth, audit and trends in cleft lip, alveolus and palate. In: Ward-Booth P, Schendel S (eds). *Maxillofacial surgery*, 2nd edn, by permission of Elsevier.

elements of the cleft and facilitate surgical repair.[71] More recently, appliances have been directed at moulding the alar cartilages of the nose to facilitate primary nasolabial reconstruction.[72] Active appliances are designed to transfer forces produced by springs, elastic strapping or screws to the bone elements. Passive appliances align segments by channelling growth into prepared spaces underneath an acrylic plate which has to be continuously adjusted, keeping the tongue out of the cleft. Treatment is usually prolonged, requires a high degree of co-operation and can be demanding for parents. There is no doubt that these techniques can in many cases facilitate operative closure of cleft lip and palate, but paradoxically there is no evidence that creating a more normal bone alignment prior to surgery results in an improved surgical outcome. Extravagant claims that presurgical orthopaedics promotes growth have not been substantiated. Current evidence does not support its use as a cost-effective treatment.[73] [****]

Expectations from surgery

Improved understanding of the mechanisms of facial growth together with a detailed appreciation of the complex arrangement and function of muscles involved in the cleft lip and palate deformity have contributed to recent advances in surgical care of cleft lip and palate. Enthusiasm for radical surgery has been tempered by an ever-increasing awareness that surgery itself can have a detrimental effect on facial growth. Cleft lip and palate surgery should aim to achieve the following:

- isolation of the nasal cavity from the mouth;
- bone continuity throughout the maxillary alveolus to facilitate the eruption of the permanent dentition;
- a functional velum that will permit normal speech;
- an aesthetic and functional lip and nose.

In order to achieve these aims, it is best to restore nasolabial form and function at the earliest opportunity – usually before age six months – and to complete repair of the secondary palate by the time 'babbling' has become established – usually before 9–12 months. Bony restoration of the alveolar cleft in order to facilitate eruption of the permanent teeth is usually completed by age 11 years.

In the past, attempts at restoration of nasal form and function were delayed often until age 12 years in order to reduce the risk of growth impairment. Recognition of the importance of nasal breathing and the intimate relationship between form and function of the nose and lip has encouraged an earlier radical approach to nasal repair which is now often attempted at the time of primary lip repair. There is still controversy about the best way to repair a cleft lip and palate. This is largely due to the wide degree of variability in the deformity itself and debate about the relative contribution of inherent tissue hypoplasia and secondary functional hypoplasia.

Traditional methods of lip repair focused on achieving balanced length and proportion of lip skin and vermillion and the production of a symmetrical 'Cupid's bow' by the transposition of skin flaps. A detailed analysis of the skin around the cleft lip deformity shows that it is both retracted and displaced secondary to the initial hypoplasia and a lack of normal muscle function. The skin of the nasal floor, which is quite different from lip skin being thinner and hairless is pulled down into the upper part of the lip.[74, 75, 76] Respect for these boundaries in the design of skin incisions avoids transposition of nasal skin on to the lip. Incisions should ideally not cross aesthetic boundaries such as the alar and columellar bases. The length of the repaired cleft lip is influenced to a large degree by underlying muscle function. It is now recognized that optimum results can only be consistently achieved if a detailed nasolabial muscle repair is performed.[77, 78, 79, 80] [**/*] The nasolabial muscle rings are disrupted in complete cleft lip deformity and their abnormal insertions result in unbalanced muscle function, which further worsens the degree of deformity (**Figure 77.8**).

Timing of surgery

Operative procedures for cleft lip and palate can be categorized into primary and secondary procedures depending on the timing of intervention. Primary procedures include repair of the cleft lip/nose and palate deformity and repair of the alveolar bone defect with or without alveolar bone grafting. Secondary or revision procedures are often directed at improving speech. They include fistula repair, soft palate revision surgery,

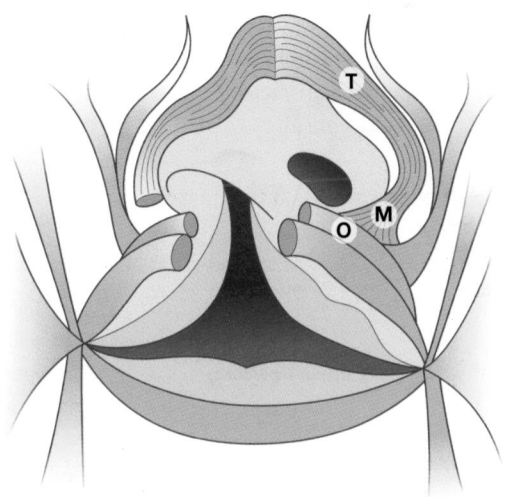

Figure 77.8 Nasolabial muscle ring in unilateral cleft lip. M, myrtiform head of nasalis muscle; O, oblique head of orbicularis oris; T, transverse head of nasalis muscle.

pharyngoplasty, posterior pharyngeal wall implant, secondary or revision surgery to the lip/nose complex and orthognathic surgery.

Timing of lip repair varies from a few days to six months according to the surgeon's preference. Some surgeons carry out neonatal repair, but as yet there is no clear evidence to justify the increased risk of surgery at this age. It is difficult to carry out detailed muscle reconstruction before three months of age. Some surgeons perform preliminary 'lip adhesion' (which essentially involves joining the skin and leaving the muscle alone at the margins of the cleft) on wide clefts to try to reduce the size of the cleft prior to a definitive repair.[81] There is no evidence to show that this contributes to improved outcomes, but some surgeons still use it as an alternative to preoperative orthopaedics.

Table 77.5 outlines the timing of surgical procedures performed in the treatment of cleft lip and palate.

Unilateral cleft lip

Various flaps involving rotation, advancement and triangular designs have been and are used in the repair of unilateral cleft lip (**Figure 77.9**).[82, 83] The most popular is the rotation advancement technique first described by Millard in 1976 (**Figure 77.10**).[82] Numerous modifications of Millard's original design have since been proposed, including measures to lengthen the columella and reduce scarring across the columella base.[84] Delaire has described a design that respects the anatomical boundaries between lip and nasal skin and avoids crossing aesthetically sensitive areas, such as the columella base and alar rim (**Figure 77.11**). Although this incision in itself has little facility to lengthen the lip, the incorporation of wavy lines and small triangular flaps above the vermillion allow some degree of lengthening. Delaire emphasizes the important contribution that the restoration of labiomaxillary muscle function makes towards achieving satisfactory lip length and aesthetics.[74, 75, 76] and considers this to be as important as

geometric arrangement of skin flaps (**Figure 77.12**). [**/*] Some postoperative support is required to maintain the nasal correction. This can take the form of nasal splinting[79] or internal support sutures.[85]

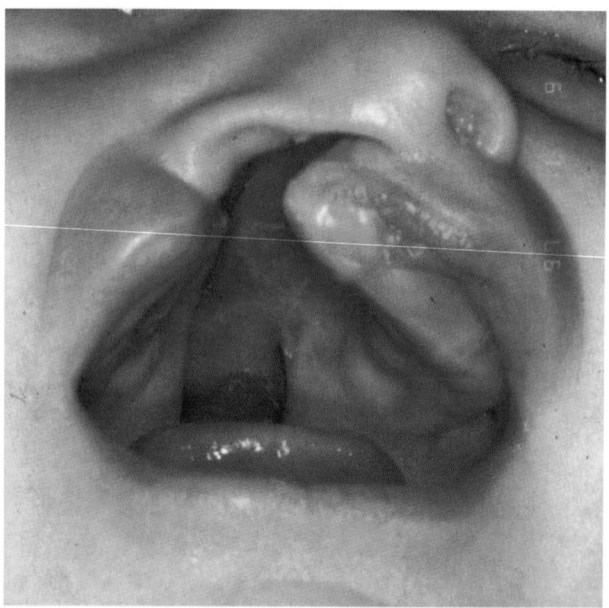

Figure 77.9 Unilateral cleft lip.

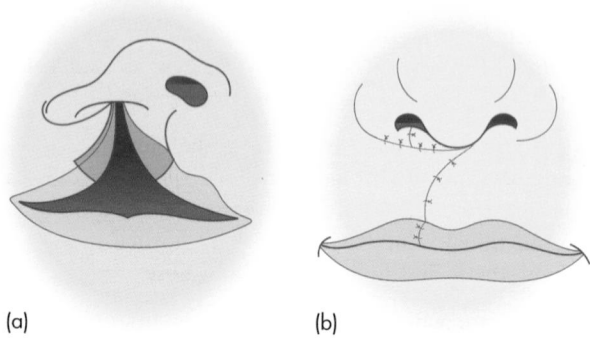

(a)   (b)

Figure 77.10 (a,b) Incision design for Millard rotation – advancement repair of complete unilateral cleft lip.

Table 77.5 Timing of surgery.

Surgery		Timing
Primary repair	Cleft lip/nose	<6 months
	Cleft palate	<12 months
Repair of bone defect in cleft alveolus	Gingivoperiosteoplasty	12 months–3 years
	Primary alveolar bone grafting	12 months–3 years
	Secondary alveolar bone grafting	9–11 years
Secondary/revision surgery to improve speech	Palatal fistula repair	Variable
	Soft palate revision	<3 years
	Pharyngoplasty	Variable
Secondary/revision surgery to lip/nose		Variable
Orthognathic surgery		>17 years

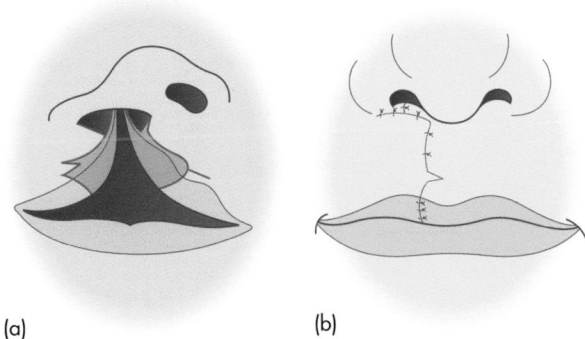

Figure 77.11 (a,b) Incision design for modified Delaire-type repair of complete unilateral cleft lip.

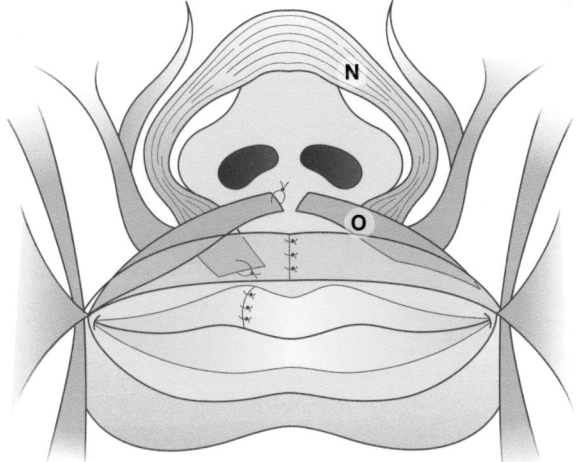

Figure 77.12 Repair of the nasolabial muscle ring in complete unilateral cleft lip.

Bilateral cleft lip

Bilateral cleft lip (**Figure 77.13**) is a more severe deformity than unilateral. There is often a significant degree of hypoplasia in the midline prolabium, which is bereft of muscle and normal vermillion. The short columella, which characterizes bilateral clefts is seldom fully corrected by functional surgery alone. A characteristic feature of complete bilateral clefts is the marked projection of the prolabium and premaxilla, which further compounds the surgical problem. Lip adhesions and presurgical orthopaedics in the form of lip strapping are often employed to lessen the degree of projection and facilitate primary lip repair.

Restoration of labiomaxillary muscle function helps achieve satisfactory lip length and aesthetics, but achieving muscle continuity across the prolabium can be difficult. Lip adhesion has been advocated as a primary procedure in order to facilitate the muscle repair at a second operation. Alternatively, a two-stage procedure repairing one side at a time can be carried out, although it has the disadvantage of introducing a degree of asymmetry into what was otherwise a symmetrical deformity. There is little evidence to support the use of

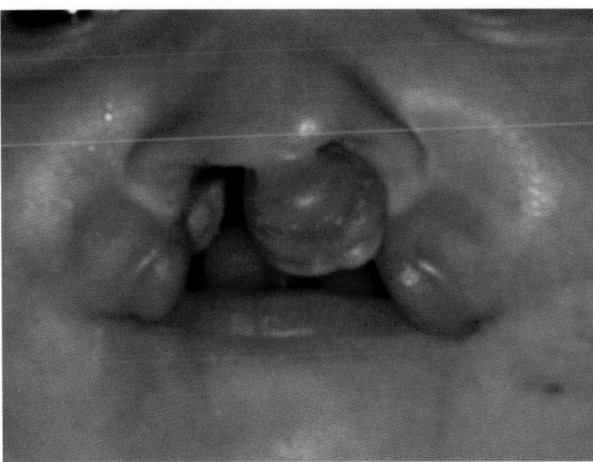

Figure 77.13 Complete bilateral cleft lip.

either of these approaches. An example of a single-stage surgical approach which facilitates labiomaxillary muscle reconstruction and nasal dome reshaping is shown in **Figure 77.14**.

The management of the short columella is controversial. Techniques have been devised which import skin from the prolabium or nasal sill into the columella to provide length. An example of this approach is the elevation of forked flaps from the sides of the prolabium, which are initially stored in the nasal sill and then elevated into the columella at a second-stage operation.[86, 87] The disadvantage of this technique is that it produces unsightly scars under the columella and an unnatural appearance to the external nares, which often appears overtly large. The latter problem is a consequence of ignoring the real nature of the alar cartilage deformity. The domes of the alar cartilages are grossly flattened, but the cartilage itself is seldom hypoplastic. The shortened medial element is compensated by increased length of the lateral element – the effect of which is to drag the columella 'into the nose'. Importing tissue into the columella magnifies this aspect of the deformity. A better approach is to retrieve the columella from where it has been hidden in the nose and correct the imbalance between the medial and lateral elements of the alar cartilage. This requires careful dissection under and between the domes of the lower alar cartilage (**Figure 77.14c**). The lower alar cartilage is released from the mucosa and overlying skin, repositioned and supported by direct suturing or long-term nasal splints.[88] Nasolabial moulding is a form of presurgical orthopaedics that expands the columella preoperatively. This facilitates correction of the nasal tip cartilages through a retrograde approach under the prolabium and columella.[89] [**/*]

Alveolar cleft

It is important to repair the alveolar cleft and to achieve bone continuity in order to create an intact alveolar arch

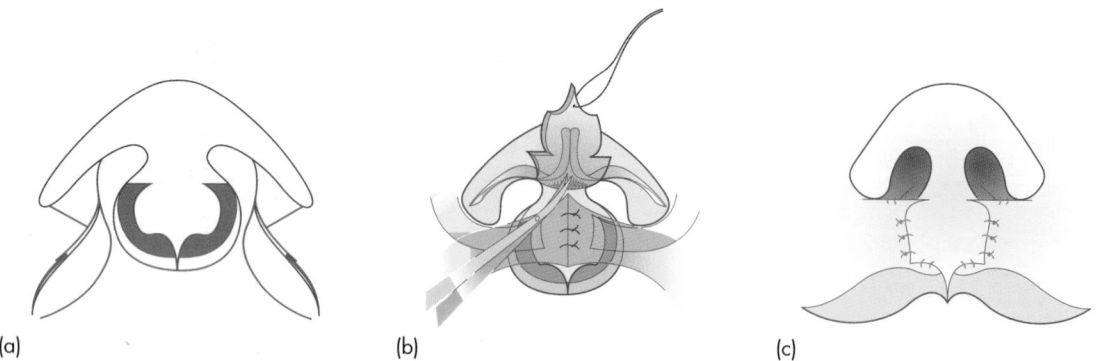

(a)   (b)   (c)

Figure 77.14   Repair of complete bilateral cleft lip. (a) Incision design for single-stage repair of bilateral cleft lip (shaded area excised); (b) prolabial flap elevated and dissection underneath and between domes of lower alar cartilages; (c) wound closure.

and to allow eruption of the lateral incisor and canine. There are two main ways in which this can be achieved.

1. Secondary alveolar bone grafting at age 9–11 years (**Figure 77.15**). This is often preceded by primary soft-tissue closure with a vomer flap at the time of primary lip repair, although the alveolar cleft may be left unrepaired at the time of primary surgery.
2. Primary gingivo-periosteoplasty (GPP) at either the time of palate closure or delayed until the age of three to five years.

There is good evidence that secondary alveolar bone grafting produces consistently good results.[90, 91] [**/*] Timing of the bone graft is usually determined by the development of the canine tooth, although earlier bone grafting may be indicated to support the eruption of the lateral incisor. There is no evidence that secondary bone grafting has a detrimental effect on facial growth when performed between 9 and 11 years of age. This is in contrast with primary bone grafting carried out before two to three years of age where evidence from retrospective case series suggests that these early bone grafts were associated with significant growth impairment.[92, 93] [**/*]

The concept of stimulating bone growth in the alveolar cleft underneath transposed mucoperiosteal flaps (gingivo-periosteoplasty) has been around for many years. It has the obvious advantage of removing the need for a later bone graft and has the potential for establishing an intact alveolus at a much earlier age than secondary bone grafting. GPP is carried out before three years of age and often at the time of primary palate repair. Success depends on achieving approximation of the alveolar segments, which usually requires some form of presurgical orthopaedics. There is concern that early surgery on the alveolus may impair maxillary growth,[94] but preliminary results have been encouraging.[95, 96, 97] [**] The results of treatment after completion of facial growth are awaited before the efficacy of this technique can be confirmed.

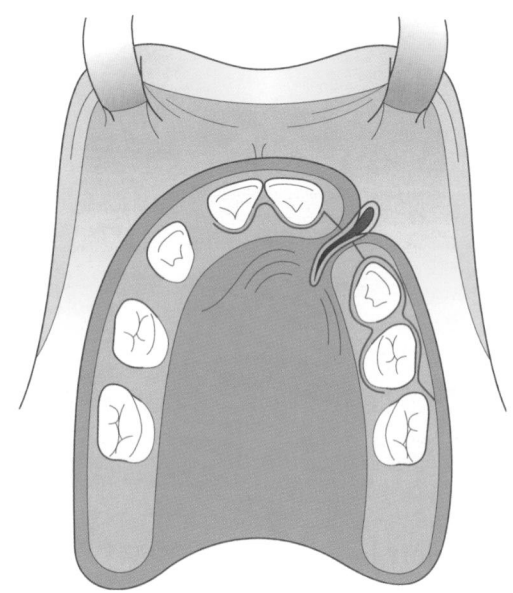

Figure 77.15   Incision design for secondary alveolar bone graft.

Hard palate repair

Palate repair has invoked much controversy over the years mainly because of the detrimental effect that palatal surgery has on maxillary growth. Traditional methods of closure involve transposition of either bipedicled flaps (Langenbeck flap) or axial flaps based on the greater palatine vessels (Veau flap, Veau–Wardill–Kilner). These methods can be used to repair the hard and soft palate (secondary palate) cleft in one stage (**Figure 77.16**). It is now recognized that scars formed by leaving areas of exposed bone in the hard palate, especially the anterior and lateral margins of the palate produced by 'push back procedures', have the potential to inhibit both anterior and transverse growth of the maxilla.[98] [**/*] Modifications of the Langenbeck flap have been introduced whereby the flap is designed inside the greater palatine pedicle in order to move the area of denuded palatal bone

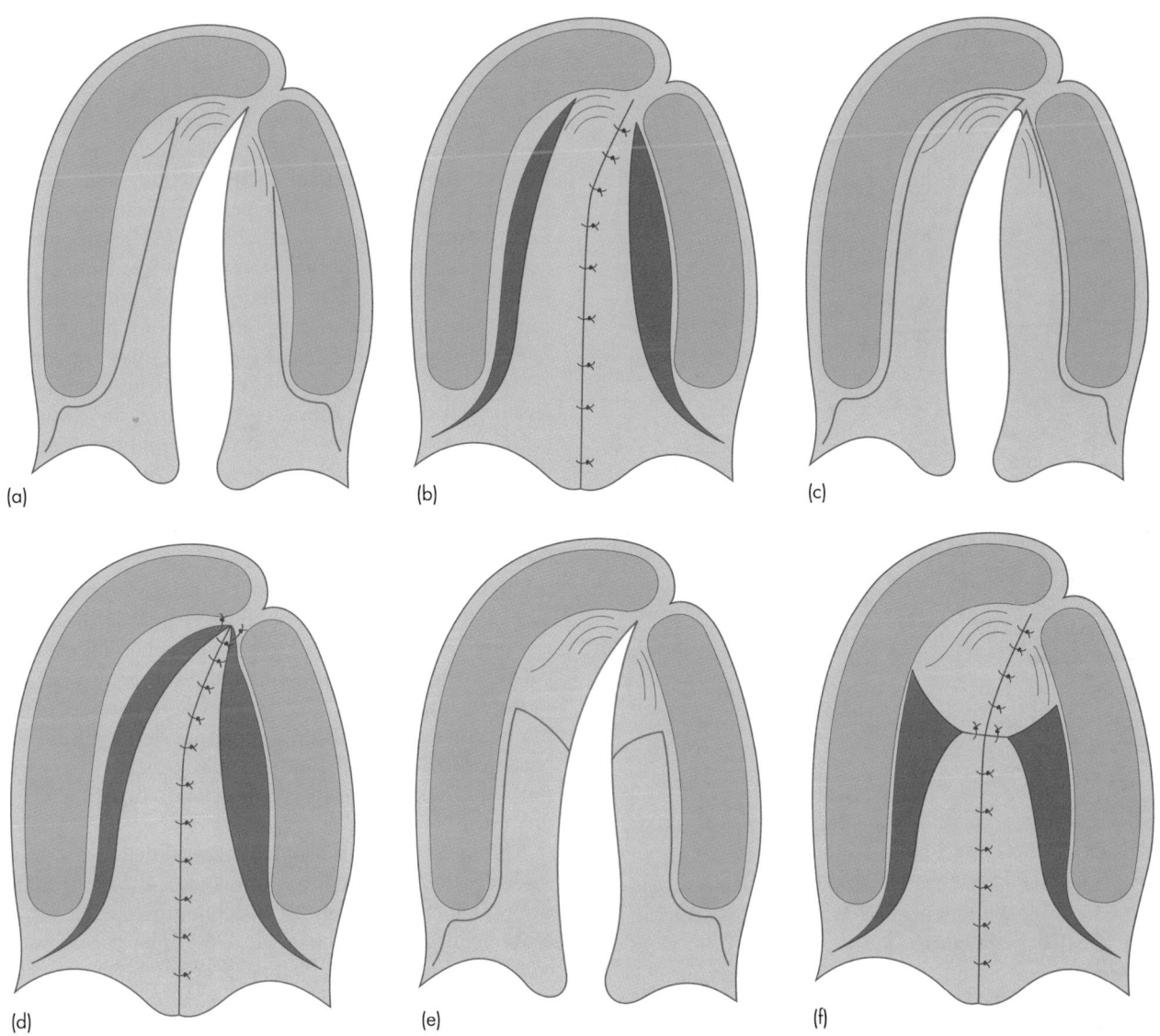

Figure 77.16 Methods of cleft palate repair: (a,b) Langenbeck; (c,d) Veau; (e,f) Veau–Wardill–Kilner.

more medially. There is, however, no evidence other than occasional case series using historical controls to suggest that this approach has any benefit.[99] [**/*] Two other strategies designed to lessen the impact of palatal surgery on facial growth include delayed closure of the hard palate and the vomer flap. In delayed closure, the soft palate is repaired at the usual time around six to nine months of age, but no attempt is made to repair the hard palate. Delaying hard palate closure for a number of years results in a reduction in the width of the cleft and facilitates repair without the need for transposed palatal flaps. (**Figure 77.17**).[76] The main objection to this approach is the detrimental effect that delay in hard palate closure beyond 12–18 months may have on speech development, in addition to the problems associated with a persistent hard palate fistula.

The use of a vomer flap to repair the hard palate cleft was first described by Pichler in 1926.[100] Used as a single layer closure, the periosteal surface of the flap is transposed to the palatal side where it becomes epithelialized leaving a large part of the vomer exposed to heal by secondary intention (**Figure 77.18**). Alternatively, it can be used as part of a two-layer closure. The main objection to this method is that like traditional palatal flap repairs, the transposed vomer flap may have a negative impact on maxillary growth.[101] [*] This would seem to be a logical expectation, but evidence from analysis of case series from the Oslo group in particular show that it has only a minimal effect, if any, on anterior maxillary growth.[91] [**] The effect on vertical maxillary growth is less clear and needs to be confirmed by further research.

Anatomy and function of the soft palate

An understanding of normal soft palate anatomy is fundamental to achieving a satisfactory muscle

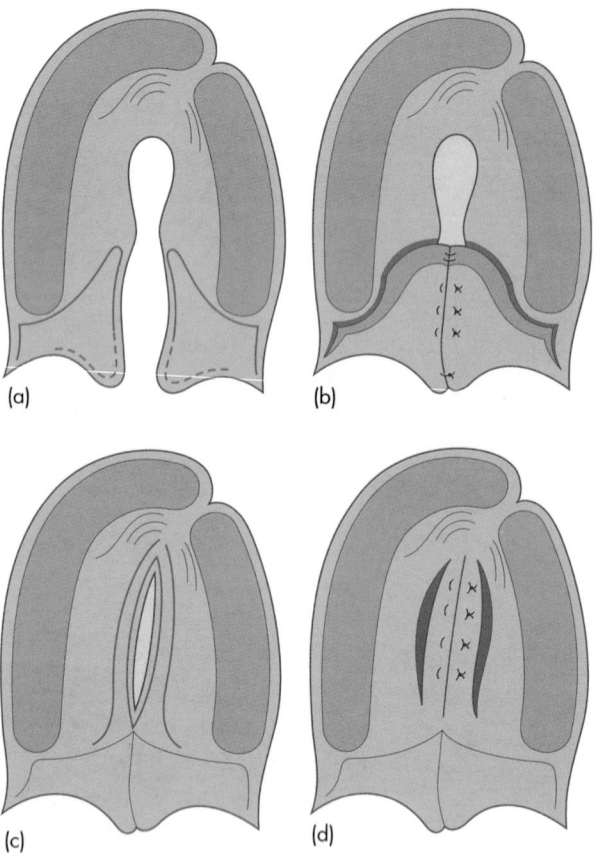

Figure 77.17 Two-stage method of cleft palate repair: (a) incision design for soft palate repair; (b) wound closure of soft palate repair; (c) medial Langenbeck incision design for second-stage hard palate repair; (d) wound closure of hard palate repair. After Delaire.[76]

winds around the hamulus to which it is partly attached and ascends to its origin in the scaphoid fossa, spine of the sphenoid bone and membranous portion of the tympanic tube. It is this latter attachment which suggests that the tensor's primary function is related to Eustachian tube function rather than velar function. The primary velar muscles are the levator palatini, palatopharyngeus and palatoglossus. The palatoglossus and palatopharyngeus arise from the back of the palatal aponeurosis and maxillary tuberosity. The palatoglossus is a thin sheet of muscle that extends to form the anterior pillar of the fauces. The palatopharyngeus is a much more substantial muscle that is spilt into two heads by the insertion of the levator palatini and runs down to form the posterior pillar of fauces and inserts into the thyroid cartilage and pharyngeal aponeurosis. The levator palatini muscle originates from the medial part of the Eustachian tube and from the petrous temporal bone. It runs down forwards and medially to enter the middle third of the velum between the two heads of palatopharyngeus to join with its partner from the opposite side. It is the prime elevator of the velum. The palatopharyngeus and palatoglossus act as depressors and all three muscles act to lengthen the velum. The last muscle to consider is the muscularis uvulae, which runs anteroposteriorly from the posterior nasal spine to the uvula beneath the nasal mucosa. The function of the muscularis uvulae remains unknown.

The mechanism of velopharyngeal function has been studied qualitatively by nasendoscopy and both qualitatively and quantitatively by videofluoroscopy.[102, 103, 104] Movement of both the velum and pharyngeal walls contribute to normal velopharyngeal function. The pattern of closure differs between individuals and between different speech sounds. Closure during swallowing is much slower and occurs at a lower level in the pharynx than that which occurs during speech.

reconstruction (**Figure 77.19**). A fibrous aponeurosis occupies the anterior third of the velum. It is attached to the posterior edge of the hard palate and is continuous with the tendon of tensor veli palatini. The tensor tendon

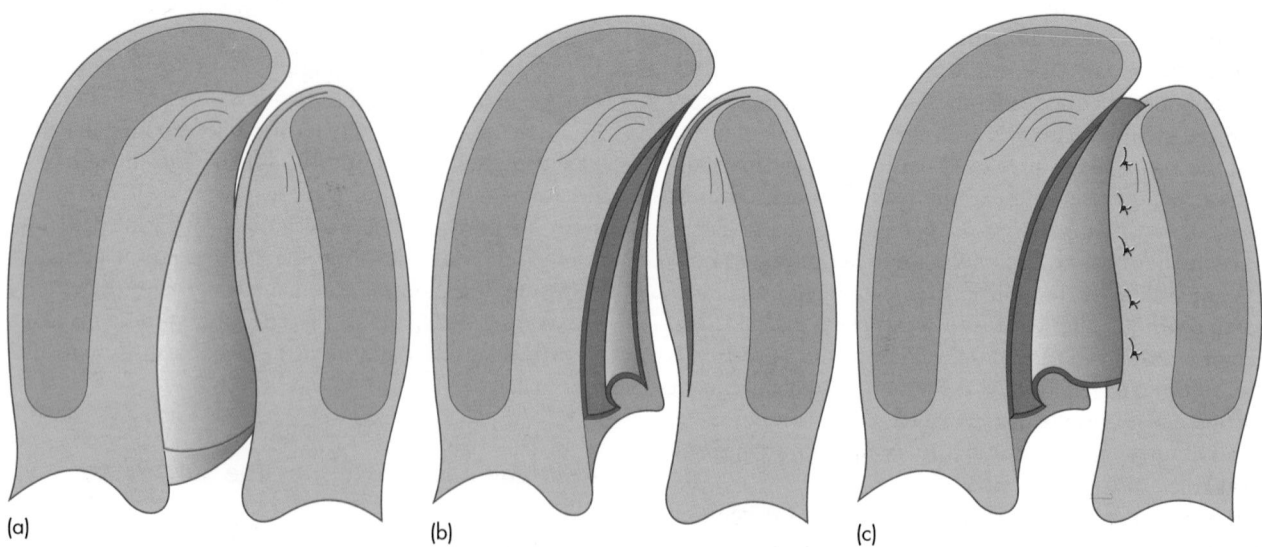

Figure 77.18 (a,b,c) Vomer flap repair of unilateral cleft palate.

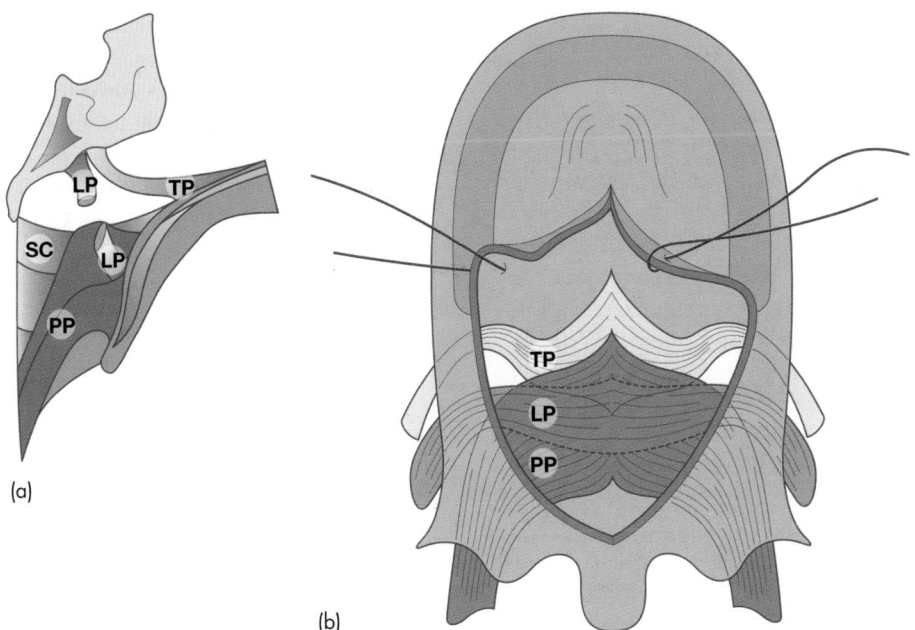

Figure 77.19 Velum muscles: (a) sagittal view from midline; (b) inferior view. LP, levator palatini; PP, palatopharyngeus; SP, superior constrictor; TP, tensor palatini.

Anatomical variables which affect velopharyngeal closure include:

- the size of the velum in relation to the depth and width of the oropharynx and the slope of the posterior pharyngeal wall. The area of contact between the velum and posterior pharyngeal wall includes adenoid tissue, which can make an important contribution to velopharyngeal closure.[105] [***]
- the extensibility of the velum;
- the degree of lift of the velum.

Soft palate repair

The goal of soft palate repair is to achieve velopharyngeal competence. Early attempts at repairing the soft palate were limited to achieving surgical closure of the cleft by joining the muscle and mucosa at the margin of the cleft. Later attempts at lengthening the soft palate with 'push back' procedures not only failed to achieve extra length, but also left large areas of denuded bone in the anterior hard palate, which had a detrimental effect on growth.[98] [**] More recently, surgeons have attempted to address the underlying muscle abnormality in an attempt to create a levator sling imparting improved function to the velum. The cleft muscle deformity was first described by Veau[2] and has since been elaborated on by several authors.[106] In cleft palate, the tensor aponeurosis is thickened into a fan shape that inserts into the lateral part of the posterior edge of the hard palate. The levator palatini and palatopharyngeus being unable to meet in the midline run forward to insert into the medial part of

the posterior edge of the hard palate, as well as into the edge of the contracted aponeurosis (**Figure 77.20**).

Various methods of surgical repair that attempt to posteriorly reposition and repair the abnormal velar muscles have been described. Furlow[107] described a novel approach to soft palate repair which incorporated a double opposing 'Z plasty'. This method results in posterior repositioning of the velar muscles, albeit with a degree of asymmetry, and results in some degree of

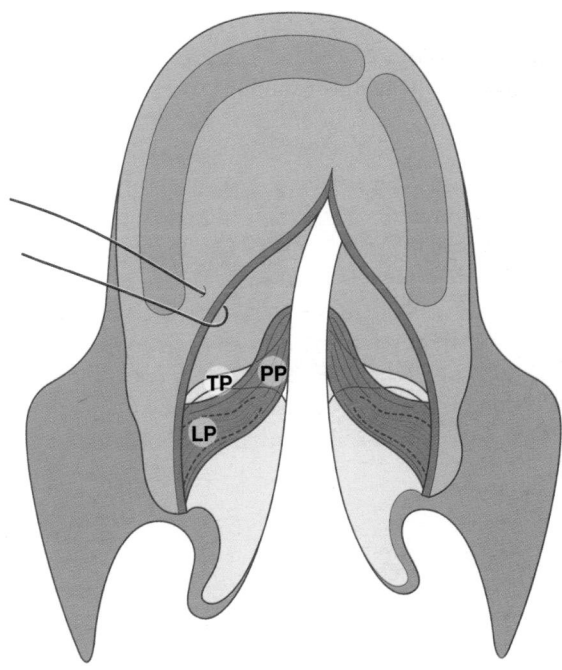

Figure 77.20 Cleft palate muscles. LP, levator palatini; PP, palatopharyngeus; TP, tensor palatini.

palatal lengthening. Good speech results have been reported using this technique[108] and it has become a popular method of soft palate repair. [**]

Other authors have primarily focused on muscle repair as a way of lengthening the velum.[109, 110, 111, 112] The first step in muscle repair of the cleft velum is to separate the abnormal attachment of the aponeurosis and muscles from the posterior edge of the hard palate. The muscles are then dissected from their attachment to the nasal and oral mucosa and reorientated to a varying degree. Despite initial enthusiasm, significant improvement in velopharyngeal function following muscle repair has not been unequivocally demonstrated by prospective studies.[109] [**] There is some confusion, however, as to what constitutes an anatomical muscle repair and the degree to which the levator muscle, rather than the palatopharyngeus muscle, is dissected and reorientated. The efficacy of a radical approach to velar repair, which includes dissection and repair of both the levator and palatopharyngeus muscle aided by the operating microscope, has been recently demonstrated by Sommerlad in a prospective case series.[111] [**]

Secondary surgery – lip, nose and alveolus

Although the benefits of secondary surgery may seem obvious to clinicians, the views of the patient should ultimately determine whether such procedures are carried out. Secondary surgery is often required to correct those problems that were not managed adequately by primary operations. Secondary procedures may be indicated for functional and aesthetic correction of the lip and nose, to close palatal fistulas and to correct velopharyngeal incompetence.

Lip and nose procedures may vary from simple procedures to align the vermillion or lengthen the lip scar to complete revision of the lip and nose encompassing muscle reconstruction and nasal correction. The secondary unilateral cleft nose deformity is characterized by an asymmetric nasal tip, deviated septum and asymmetry of the nasal bones. The secondary bilateral cleft nose deformity is usually characterized by a short columella and wide alar base. Complete correction of these deformities is facilitated by an open approach to the nasal tip. This technique allows direct visualization and correction of the alar cartilage deformity. Attention to the bone deformity is usually delayed until after ten years of age. [**/*]

Palatal fistula

Palatal fistulas can occur as a result of wound breakdown at the time of hard palate repair. They usually occur just behind the alveolus or at the junction between the hard and soft palate. Palatal fistulas that are causing problems with

speech or nasal regurgitation can be repaired at any age, but the success of the secondary repair is adversely affected by scarring from the primary procedure. Those fistulas near an alveolar cleft can usually be left until bone grafting is carried out at nine to ten years of age. Most fistulas can be closed by local flaps. Large fistulas may require tissue to be imported from elsewhere, such as a tongue flap.

OTITIS MEDIA IN CLEFT PALATE

Eustachian tube dysfunction is almost universal in children with cleft palate.[113] The majority will demonstrate some evidence of otopathology, most frequently otitis media with effusion (OME) (see Chapter 72, Otitis media with effusion). Sensorineural hearing loss is also more common in this group of children.[114] Cholesteatoma and conductive hearing loss persisting into adult life are more prevalent than in age-matched controls.[115, 116] [**] This tendency to develop OME is not reversed by early palatal surgery and children should have careful ENT and audiological surveillance even after the palate has been repaired.

Management strategies for otitis media in cleft palate children vary among different teams. Most clinicians agree on the need for a concerted multidisciplinary approach.[117] Some teams feel that the frequency of OME in cleft palate is such as to warrant early tympanostomy tubes and report good audiological outcomes.[118] [**] The alternative approach is to offer tympanostomy tubes only when there is overt evidence of OME.[119] The provision of hearing aids is increasingly considered, avoiding the morbidity associated with often-multiple grommets.[120] Long-stay tympanostomy tubes are associated with even higher complication rates, notably persistent perforation of the tympanic membrane (see Chapter 72, Otitis media with effusion).

The optimum approach is unknown. Current advice is that cleft palate teams should ensure careful otological and audiological surveillance of all cleft palate children with intervention as appropriate for each child.

Velopharyngeal insufficiency

PATHOPHYSIOLOGY AND ASSESSMENT

Velopharyngeal insufficiency (VPI) is an inability to completely close the velopharyngeal port during speech. This results in leakage of air into the nasal cavity and produces hypernasal vocal resonance and nasal air emission. Patients with VPI may develop compensatory misarticulations, which can be difficult to resolve even if the VPI is corrected. Causes include:

- cleft palate;
- submucous cleft palate;
- congenital or acquired neuromuscular abnormalities;

- iatrogenic;
- adenoidectomy;
- palatopharyngoplasty for sleep apnoea;
- maxillary advancement procedures;
- unknown.

Cleft palate is the most common cause, but any congenital or acquired condition that interferes with velopharyngeal closure can result in VPI.

The incidence of post-adenoidectomy VPI is about 1/1200 and often occurs because underlying pathology such as submucous cleft palate becomes unmasked.[121] [**] It is important to examine patients for stigmata of submucous cleft palate, i.e. bifid uvula, before adenoidectomy is performed. Occasionally a remnant of adenoid tissue forms an irregularity in the posterior pharyngeal wall. Large tonsils occasionally obstruct velopharyngeal closure. VPI occurring after adenoidectomy will spontaneously resolve in about 50 percent of cases.[121] [**] Therapeutic measures used to treat VPI include speech and language therapy, surgery, a prosthetic obturator or palatal lift appliances. The choice of therapy will depend on a number of factors including aetiology of the VPI, age of the patient, length of time VPI has been present and the presence of articulatory compensations.

A specialist speech and language therapy assessment is an essential first step in diagnosis. This can be supported by airflow/pressure studies and acoustic analysis. Videofluoroscopy and nasendoscopy provide useful information about the structure and dynamics of the velopharyngeal mechanism. Videofluoroscopy involves a significant radiation dose and co-operation may be a problem with nasendoscopy especially in young children. Magnetic resonance imaging (MRI) may offer a solution in the future, but image acquisition is too slow for real-time studies at present.

PALATE REPAIR

Surgery to improve velar length and function may be indicated especially where there is evidence of anterior insertion of the levator muscles, or in the case of a submucous cleft. Palate rerepair in the form of a radical intravelar veloplasty or Furlow double opposing 'Z' plasty has been shown to be effective in treating VPI following cleft palate repair in selected cases where the velopharyngeal gap is small.[122, 123] [**] These procedures have a lower morbidity than a pharyngoplasty.[124] [***]

Pharyngoplasty

In those patients where palate rerepair is not appropriate or is unsuccessful, surgery to alter the form and function of the pharyngeal wall may be considered. Augmenting the posterior wall with an implant is perhaps the simplest method, but the outcomes are often unsatisfactory and extrusion of the implant is common.[125] [**] The alternative is a pharyngoplasty. There are two main types

of pharyngoplasty: those employing medial transposition of flaps from the lateral pharyngeal wall and those that employ flaps from the midline of the pharyngeal wall. In lateral flap pharyngoplasty (**Figure 77.21**), muscle flaps derived from the posterior pillar of the fauces can be used to augment the posterior and lateral walls of the pharynx and decrease the velopharyngeal gap. If the nerve supply to these flaps is preserved they may also remain contractile, providing a sphincteric closure. In the Hynes type of pharyngoplasty, flaps from the posterior pillar of the fauces containing palatopharyngeus and salpingopharyngeus are inserted as high as possible in the posterior pharyngeal wall at the projected level of contact with the velum.[126] This usually necessitates division of the posterior part of the velum to provide access. In another type of lateral flap pharyngoplasty, described by Orticochoea,[127] the flaps are inserted lower down below the projected point of contact with the velum. Insertion of the flaps into the posterior pharyngeal wall is assisted by the elevation of a small posterior pharyngeal flap. The success of this procedure is dependent on active contraction of the transposed palatopharyngeus muscle. A number of reports have found a correlation between the level of flap insertion and improvement in nasalance scores during speech. Several authors have concluded that the flaps should be placed as high as possible in the nasopharynx at the point of velopharyngeal contact,[128, 129] similar to the procedure originally described by Hynes. [**/*]

Midline flap pharyngoplasty involves inserting an inferiorly or more commonly a superiorly based flap (**Figure 77.22**) from the posterior pharyngeal wall into the posterior edge of the velum.[130, 131] The flap forms a static bridge with lateral ports on either side that are closed by medial movement of the lateral pharyngeal walls. Shrinkage of the flap occurs to a variable degree. Lining the flap as much as possible with nasal mucosa can minimize this. Midline flaps are entirely static and rely on lateral wall movement to effect closure. If there is no lateral wall movement, velopharyngeal competence can only be achieved by making the flaps so wide that they obstruct the nasopharynx. In contrast, the effectiveness of lateral flap pharyngoplasty is dependent on sphincteric contraction of the flaps themselves, as well as movement of the velum.

It would seem logical that the choice of operation should be guided by the preoperative pattern of closure. This approach has been supported by some prospective studies which show that it is possible to achieve normal resonance in up to 85 percent of cases.[132, 133, 134] [***/**] However, a recent randomized controlled trial comparing sphincter pharyngoplasty to a pharyngeal flap has failed to show a difference in speech outcome between the two types of procedure.[135] [****]

Complications of pharyngoplasty

Common side effects of pharyngoplasty include snoring, mouth breathing, catarrh and nasal obstruction. A less

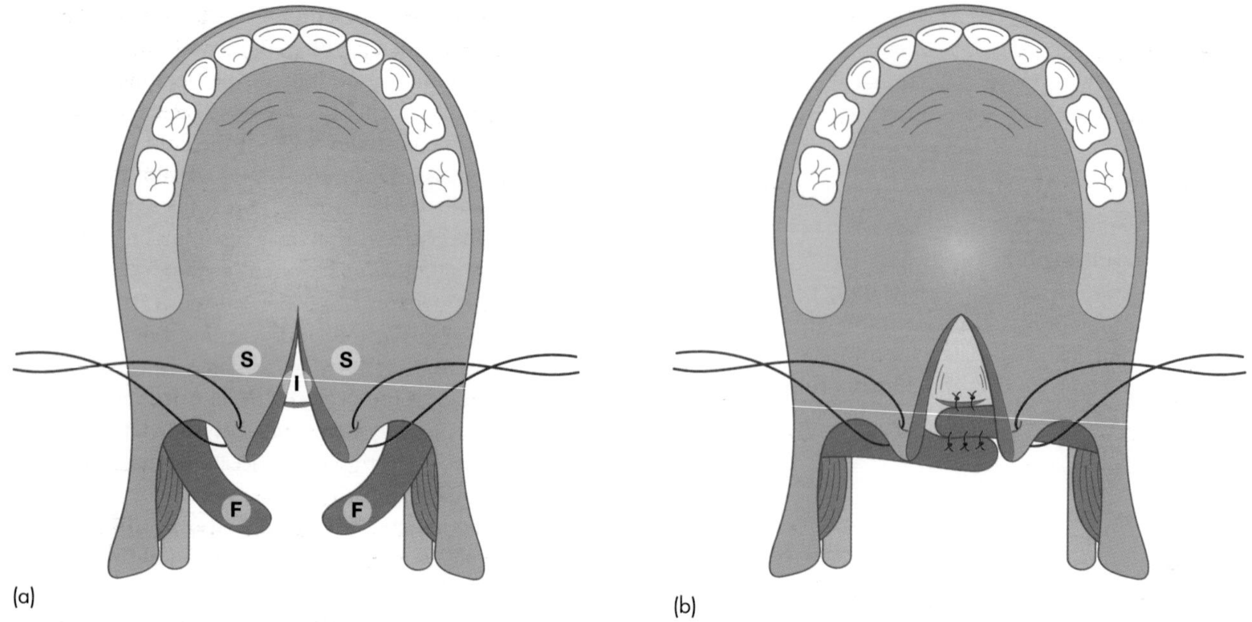

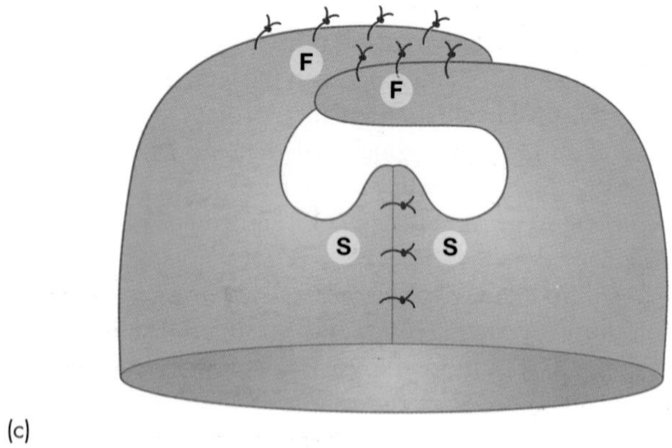

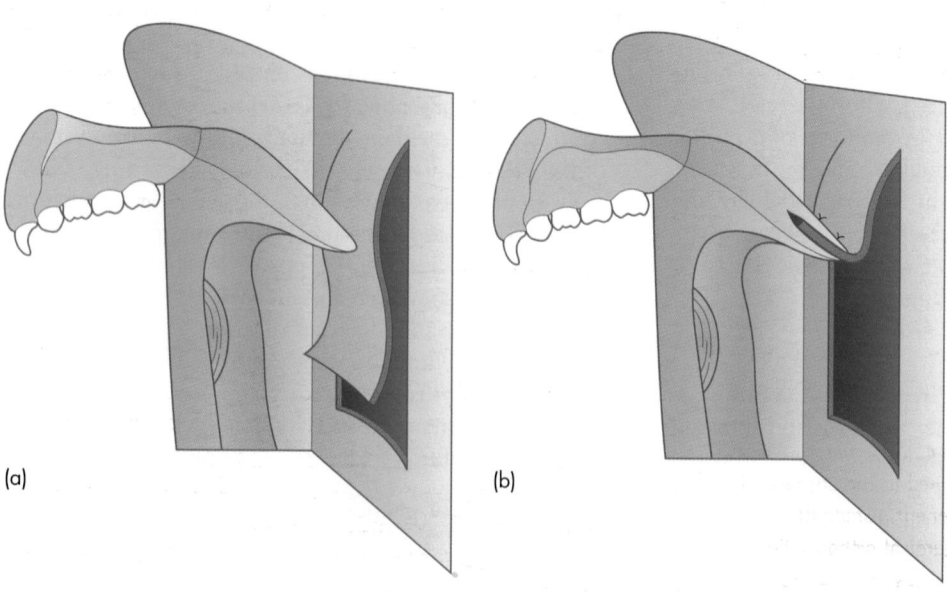

Figure 77.21 Lateral flap pharyngoplasty. Oral view with soft palate divided in midline for access. (a) F, posterior tonsillar pillar flaps containing palatopharyngeus elevated; I, horizontal incision high up in posterior pharyngeal wall – at level of contact with posterior edge of elevated velum; (b) flaps rotated posteromedially, overlapped and sutured to fascia in posterior pharyngeal wall; (c) anterosuperior view of lateral flaps overlapped and sutured to fascia in posterior pharyngeal wall. F, flaps; S, soft palate.

Figure 77.22 Superior flap pharyngoplasty – sagittal view from midline. (a) Midline flap elevated from posterior pharyngeal wall; (b) flap sutured into pocket in posterior border of soft palate.

common but more serious side effect is obstructive sleep apnoea (OSA) which has a reported incidence ranging between 4 and 90 percent and can occur in all types of pharyngoplasty.[135, 136] [****/***/**] The large range in the reported incidence of OSA probably reflects the different measurement protocols used to diagnose OSA, as well as patient and operative variables. There is evidence from the VPI surgical trial group that severity of OSA tends to decrease with time so that by 12 months post-operation significant OSA is rare irrespective of the type of pharyngoplasty.[135] [****]

Our incomplete understanding of the side effects represents a significant limitation when advising patients on the risks and benefits of surgery for VPI, especially in patients with mild symptoms.

KEY POINTS

- Clefts of the lip and palate are common congenital birth anomalies.
- Aetiology is complex. Known associations are with antenatal anticonvulsants, steroids, maternal smoking and alcohol. Some of the genes associated with orofacial clefting have now been identified.
- Prenatal screening for cleft lip is now routinely available in many centres.
- Management of patients with cleft lip and palate requires a multidisciplinary approach delivered by a team which includes an otolaryngologist.
- Otitis media is a significant problem in cleft palate children and requires careful surveillance and management.
- Eustachian tubal dysfunction and otitis media with effusion are almost universal in cleft palate children.
- Minor abnormalities of palatal function may cause velopharyngeal insufficiency with an adverse effect on the child's speech.

Best clinical practice

- ✓ In Pierre Robin sequence, severe cases may require airway support during the early months of life with a nasopharyngeal tube. A tracheostomy is nowadays very rarely required. [Grade C/D]
- ✓ Palatal obturator plates have enjoyed widespread use, but their popularity has declined in the absence of evidence to show any real benefit. [Grade B]
- ✓ Extravagant claims that presurgical orthopaedics promotes growth have not been substantiated.

Current evidence does not support its use as a cost-effective treatment. [Grade A]
- ✓ Optimum management of otitis media should be customized to the individual child. Ventilating tubes are not always appropriate. [Grade B]
- ✓ Otolaryngologists need to be particularly vigilant in recognizing submucous cleft palate. [Grade C/D]
- ✓ The mere presence of a submucous cleft is not in itself an indication for treatment. [Grade B]
- ✓ Careful monitoring of speech development is essential in submucous cleft. [Grade C/D]
- ✓ Otological and audiological surveillance is an essential part of the management of cleft palate. Children with hearing loss require active intervention and support with a management strategy and treatment plan established for each child. [Grade C/D]
- ✓ Many cases of velopharyngeal insufficiency occurring after adenoidectomy can be treated expectantly. [Grade C/D]

Deficiencies in current knowledge and areas for future research

- ➤ Advances in genetics are helping to unravel the aetiology of orofacial clefting. Many candidate genes are now being sequenced.
- ➤ Reorganization of cleft palate services and the concentration of expertise in centres where a multidisciplinary team is available has the potential to improve data collection, clinical audit and research, as well as outcomes for cleft palate children in the UK.
- ➤ Dedicated training in cleft palate surgery is likely to improve outcomes further.
- ➤ The optimum management of OME in cleft palate is unknown. Centralized collection and analysis of data from the many teams looking after these children with careful monitoring of otological and audiological outcomes would greatly help rationalize treatment planning.

ACKNOWLEDGEMENTS

Figures 77.1 to 77.6 are redrawn from Penfold CN. Cleft lip and palate and evidence-based care. In: Ward-Booth P, Schendel S (eds). *Maxillofacial surgery*, Volume 2, 2nd edn. 2007; 1001–25, by permission of Elsevier.

REFERENCES

* 1. Vanderas AP. Incidence of cleft lip, cleft palate, and cleft lip and palate among races: a review. *Cleft Palate Journal.* 1987; **24**: 216–25.

2. Veau V. *Division palatine.* Paris: Masson, 1931.

3. Pfeifer G. *Classification of Northwestern German Jaw Clinic in treatment of patients with cleft of lip, alveolus and palate.* Presented at the Second Hamburg International Symposium. Stuttgart: Thieme, 1966.

4. Kernahan DA. The striped Y – a symbolic classification for cleft lip and palate. *Plastic and Reconstructive Surgery.* 1971; **47**: 469–70.

5. Kriens O. LAHSHAL: An easy clinical system of cleft lip, alveolus and palate documentation. In: Kriens O (ed.). *Proceedings of the Advanced Workshop: 'What is a cleft?'* Stuttgart: Thieme, 1989.

6. Cohen Jr MM. *The child with multiple birth defects.* New York: Oxford University Press, 1997.

* 7. Tessier P. Anatomical classification of facial, cranio-facial and latero-facial clefts. *Journal of Maxillofacial Surgery.* 1976; **4**: 69–92.

* 8. Special report: EUROCAT and orofacial clefts: the epidemiology of orofacial clefts in 30 European regions. Online. Available from: http://www.eurocat.ulster.ac.uk/pubdata.

9. Gorlin RJ, Cohen Jr MM, Hennekam RCM. *Syndromes of the head and neck*, 4th edn. New York: Oxford University Press, 2003.

10. Hagberg C, Larson O, Milerad J. Incidence of cleft lip and palate and risks of additional malformations. *Cleft Palate – Craniofacial Journal.* 1997; **35**: 40–5.

11. Kallen B, Harris J, Robert E. The epidemiology orofacial clefts: 2. Associated malformations. *Journal of Craniofacial Genetics and Developmental Biology.* 1996; **26**: 242–8.

12. Shprintzen RJ, Siegel-Sadewitz VL, Amato J, Goldberg RB. Anomalies associated with cleft lip, cleft palate or both. *American Journal of Medical Genetics.* 1985; **20**: 585–95.

13. Christensen K, Juel K, Herskind M, Murray JC. Long term follow up study of survival associated with cleft lip and palate at birth. *British Medical Journal.* 2004; **328**: 1405–6.

* 14. Ferguson MWJ. Palate development. *Development.* 1988; **103**: 41–60.

15. Ferguson MWJ. Developmental mechanisms in normal and abnormal palate formation with particular reference to the aetiology, pathogenesis and prevention of cleft palate. *British Journal of Orthodontics.* 1981; **8**: 115–37.

16. Wilkie AO, Morriss-Kay GM. Genetics of craniofacial development and malformation. *Nature Reviews Genetics.* 2001; **2**: 458–68.

17. Jones MC. Etiology of facial clefts. Prospective evaluation of 428 patients. *Cleft Palate Journal.* 1988; **25**: 16–20.

* 18. Murray JC. Gene/environment causes of cleft lip and/or palate. *Clinical Genetics.* 2002; **61**: 248–56.

* 19. Fogh-Anderson P. *Inheritance of harelip and cleft palate.* Copenhagen: Munksgaard, 1942.

20. Wyszynski DF, Beaty TH, Maestri NE. Genetics of nonsyndromic oral clefts revisited. *Cleft Palate – Craniofacial Journal.* 1996; **33**: 406–17.

* 21. Gorlin RJ, Cohen Jr. MM. The orofacial region. In: Wigglesworth JS, Singer DB (eds). *Textbook of fetal and perinatal pathology*, 2nd edn. Malden, MA: Blackwell Science, 1998: 732–78 (Chapter 22).

22. Carinci F, Pezzetti F, Scapoli L, Martinelli M, Avantaggiato A, Carinci P et al. Recent developments in orofacial cleft genetics. *Journal of Craniofacial Surgery.* 2003; **14**: 131–43.

23. Harper P. Oral and craniofacial disorders. In: *Practical genetic counselling*, 5th edn. Oxford: Butterworth-Heinemann, 1998: 211.

24. Ardinger HH, Buetow KH, Bell GI, Bardach J, Van Demark DR, Murray JC. Association of genetic variation of the transforming growth factor-alpha gene with cleft lip and palate. *American Journal of Human Genetics.* 1989; **54**: 348–53.

25. Schutte BC, Murray JC. The many faces and factors of orofacial clefts. *Human Molecular Genetics.* 1999; **8**: 1853–9.

26. Eiberg H, Bixler D, Nielsen LS et al. Suggestion of linkage of a major locus of nonsyndromic orofacial cleft with F13A and tentative assignment to chromosome 6. *Clinical Genetics.* 1987; **32**: 129–32.

27. Carinci F, Pezzetti F, Scapoli L, Padula E, Baciliero O, Curioni C et al. Nonsyndromic cleft lip and palate: evidence of linkage to a microsatellite marker on 6p23. *American Journal of Human Genetics.* 1995; **56**: 337–9.

28. Scapoli L, Pezzetti F, Carinci F, Martinelli M, Carinci P, Tognon M. Evidence of linkage to 6p23 and genetic heterogeneity in nonsyndromic cleft lip with or without cleft palate. *Genomics.* 1997; **43**: 216–20.

29. Shapira SK, McCaskill C, Northrup H, Spikes AS, Elder FF, Sutton VR et al. Chromosome 1P36 deletions: the clinical phenotype and molecular characterization of a common newly delineated syndrome. *American Journal of Human Genetics.* 1997; **61**: 642–50.

30. Mitchell LE. Transforming growth factor alpha locus and non syndromic cleft lip with or without cleft palate: a reappraisal. *Genetic Epidemiology.* 1997; **14**: 231–40.

31. Lidral AC, Murray JC, Buetow KH, Basart AM, Schearer H, Shiang R et al. Studies of the candidate genes TGB2, MSX1, TGFA and TGFB3 in the aetiology of cleft lip and palate in the Philippines. *Cleft Palate – Craniofacial Journal.* 1997; **34**: 1–6.

32. van den Boogaard MJH, Dorland M, Beemer FA, van Amstel HK. MSX1 mutation is associated with orofacial clefting and tooth agenesis in humans. *Nature Genetics.* 2000; **24**: 342–3.

33. Lidral AC, Romitti PA, Basart AM, Doetschman T, Leysens NJ, Daack-Hirsch S et al. Association of MSX1 and TGFB3

with nonsyndromic clefting in humans. *American Journal of Human Genetics.* 1998; **63**: 557–68.

34. Gaspar DA, Pavanello RC, Zatz M, Passos-Bueno MR, Andre M, Steman S *et al.* Role of the C677T polymorphism at the MTHFR gene on risk to nonsyndromic cleft lip with/ without cleft palate: results from a case-control study in Brasil. *American Journal of Medical Genetics.* 1999; **87**: 197–9.

35. Martinelli M, Scapoli L, Pezzetti F, Carinci P, Stabellini G, Bisceglia L *et al.* C677T variant form at the MTHFR gene and CL/P: a risk factor for mothers? *American Journal of Medical Genetics.* 2001; **98**: 357–60.

36. Wysinski DF, Diel SR. Infant C677T mutation in MTHFR, maternal preconception vitamin use, and risk of nonsyndromic cleft lip. *American Journal of Medical Genetics.* 2000; **92**: 79–80.

37. Mills JL, Kirke PN, Molloy AM, Burke H, Conley MR, Lee YJ *et al.* Methylenetetrahydrofolate reductase thermolabile variant and oral clefts. *American Journal of Medical Genetics.* 1999; **86**: 71–4.

38. Shaw GM, Todroff K, Finnell RH, Rozen R, Lammer EJ. Maternal vitamin use, infant C677T mutation in MTHFR, and isolated cleft palate risk. *American Journal of Medical Genetics.* 1999; **85**: 84–5.

39. Beaty TH, Hetmanski JB, Zeiger JS, Fan YT, Liang KY, VanderKolk CA *et al.* Testing candidate genes for nonsyndromic oral clefts using a case-parent trio design. *Genetic Epidemiology.* 2002; **22**: 1–11.

40. Tanabe A, Taketani S, Endo-Ichikawa Y, Tokunaga R, Ogawa Y, Hiramoto M. Analysis of the candidate genes responsible for nonsyndromic cleft lip and palate in Japanese people. *Clinical Science (London).* 2000; **99**: 105–11.

* 41. Greenspan RJ. The flexible genome. *Nature Reviews. Genetics.* 2001; **2**: 383–7.

42. Czeizal AE, Dudas I. Prevention of the first occurrence of neural-tube defects by periconceptional vitamin supplementation. *New England Journal of Medicine.* 1992; **327**: 1832–5.

43. Ceizal A, Timar L, Sarkozi A. Dose-dependent effect of folic acid on the prevention of orofacial clefts. *Pediatrics.* 1999; **104**: e66.

44. Jugessur A, Wilcox AJ, Lie RT, Murray JC, Taylor JA, Ulvik A *et al.* Exploring the effects of methylenetetrahydrofolate reductase gene variants C677T and A1298C on the risk of orofacial clefts in 261 Norwegian case-parent triads. *American Journal of Epidemiology.* 2003; **157**: 1083–91.

45. Calzolari E, Bianchi F, Rubini M, Ritvanen A, Neville AJ, EUROCAT Working Group. Epidemiology of cleft palate in Europe: implications for genetic research. *Cleft Palate – Craniofacial Journal* 2004; **41**: 244–9.

* 46. World Health Organisation. *Global strategies to reduce the health-care burden of craniofacial anomalies.* Report of WHO Meetings on International Collaborative Research on Craniofacial Anomalies. Geneva: World Health Organization, 2002.

47. Tolarova MM, Cervenka J. Classification and birth prevalence of orofacial clefts. *American*

Journal of Medical Genetics. 1998; **75**: 126–37.

48. Stoll C, Alembik Y, Dott B, Roth MP. Associated malformations in cases with oral clefts. *Cleft Palate – Craniofacial Journal.* 2000; **37**: 41–7.

49. Milerad J, Larson O, Hagberg C, Ideberg M. Associated malformations in infants with cleft lip and palate: a prospective, population based study. *Pediatrics.* 1997; **100**: 180–6.

50. Lees M. Genetics of cleft lip and palate. In: Watson ACH, Sell DA, Grunwell P (eds). *Management of cleft lip and palate.* London and Philadelphia: Whurr Publishers, 2001.

51. Cohen Jr. MM, Bankier A. Syndrome delineation involving orofacial clefting. *Cleft Palate – Craniofacial Journal.* 1991; **28**: 119–20.

* 52. Winter R, Baraitser M. *London dysmorphology database.* Oxford: Oxford University Press, 1998.

53. Robin P. La chute de la base de la langue considéreé comme une nouvelle cause de gene dans la respiration naso-pharyngienne. *Bulletin de l'Académie Nationale de Médecine.* 1923; **89**: 37–41.

54. Pruzansky S. Not all dwarfed mandibles are alike. *Birth Defects.* 1969; **5**: 120–9.

* 55. Cohen Jr MM. Etiology and pathogenesis of orofacial clefting. *Oral and Maxillofacial Clinics of North America.* 2000; **12**: 379–97.

56. Cohen Jr MM. Robin sequences and complexes: causal heterogeneity and pathogenetic/phenotypic variability. *American Journal of Medical Genetics.* 1999; **84**: 311–5.

57. Bronstein M, Yoffe N, Zimmer E, Blumenfeld Z. Early detection of fetal anomalies by transvaginal sonography. *Fetal and Maternal Medicine Review.* 1993; **5**: 137–46.

* 58. Blumenfeld Z, Blumenfeld I, Bronstein M. The early prenatal diagnosis of cleft lip and the decision making process. *Cleft Palate – Craniofacial Journal.* 1999; **36**: 105–7.

59. Jones MC. Prenatal diagnosis of cleft lip and palate: experiences in Southern California. *Cleft Palate – Craniofacial Journal.* 1999; **36**: 107–9.

60. American Cleft Palate, Craniofacial Association. Parameters for the evaluation of patients with cleft lip/ palate or other craniofacial anomalies. *Cleft Palate – Craniofacial Journal.* 1993; **30**: S1–12.

61. Turner SR, Rumsey N, Sandy JR. Psychological aspects of cleft lip and palate. *European Journal of Orthodontics.* 1998; **20**: 407–15.

62. Tobiasen JM. Scaling facial impairment. *Cleft Palate Journal.* 1989; **26**: 249–54.

63. Endriga MC, Kapp-Simon KA. Psychological issues in craniofacial care: state of the art. *Cleft Palate – Craniofacial Journal.* 1999; **36**: 3–11.

64. McCulloch P, Taylor I, Sasako M, Lovett B, Griffin D. Randomised trials in surgery: problems and possible solutions. *British Medical Journal.* 2002; **324**: 1448–51.

65. Pollock AV. Surgical evaluation at the crossroads. *British Journal of Surgery*. 1993; **80**: 964-6.

∗ 66. Shaw WC, Semb G, Nelson PA, Brattstrom V, Molsted K, Prahl-Andersen B et al. The Eurocleft project 1996-2000: overview. *Journal of Craniomaxillofacial Surgery*. 2001; **29**: 131-40.

67. Bannister P. Early feeding management. In: Watson ACH, Sell DA, Grunwell P (eds). *Management of cleft lip and palate*. London and Philadephia: Whurr Publishers, 2001.

68. Shaw WC, Bannister P, Roberts CT. Assisted feeding is more reliable for infants with clefts – a randomised trial. *Cleft Palate – Craniofacial Journal*. 1999; **36**: 262-8.

∗ 69. Prahl C, Kuijpers-Jagtman AM, Van't Hof MA, Prahl-Andersen B. Infant orthopedics in UCLP: effect on feeding, weight, and length: a randomized clinical trial (Dutchcleft). *Cleft Palate – Craniofacial Journal*. 2005; **42**: 171-7.

∗ 70. Wagener S, Rayatt S, Tatman A, Gornall P, Slator R. Management of infants with Pierre Robin sequence. *Cleft Palate – Craniofacial Journal*. 2003; **40**: 180-5.

71. Winters JC, Hurwitz DJ. Presurgical orthopedics in the surgical management of unilateral cleft lip palate. *Plastic and Reconstructive Surgery*. 1995; **95**: 755-64.

72. Santiago PE, Grayson BH, Cutting CB, Gianoutsos MP, Brecht LE, Kwon SM. Reduced need for alveolar bone grafting by presurgical orthopedics and primary gingivoperiosteoplasty. *Cleft Palate – Craniofacial Journal*. 1998; **35**: 77-80.

73. Bongaarts CAM, Kuijpers-Jagtman AM, Van 't Hof MA, Prahl-Andersen B. The effect of infant orthopedics on the occlusion of the deciduous dentition in children with complete unilateral cleft lip and palate (Dutchcleft). *Cleft Palate – Craniofacial Journal*. 2004; **41**: 633-41.

74. Delaire J. [Primary cheilorhinoplasty for congenital unilateral labiomaxillary fissure. Trial schematization of a technic]. *Revue de Stomatologie et de Chirurgie Maxillo-Faciale*. 1975; **76**: 193-215 (in French).

∗ 75. Delaire J. Theoretical principles and technique of functional closure of the lip and nasal aperture. *Journal of Maxillofacial Surgery*. 1978; **6**: 109-16.

∗ 76. Delaire J. General considerations regarding primary physiological surgical treatment of labiomaxillopalatine clefts. *Oral and Maxillofacial Surgery Clinics of North America*. 2000; **12**: 361-78.

77. Randall P. The importance of muscle. In: Bardach J, Morris UL (eds). *Multidisciplinary management of cleft lip and palate*. Philadelphia: WB Saunders, 1990: 1133-71.

78. Schendel S. Cleft lip repair: an alternative approach. In: Vistnes L (ed.). *How they do it*. Boston: Little Brown, 1991: 338-50.

79. Talmant JC. Correction de la narine du bec de lièvre unilateral: ses grands principes. *Annales de Chirurgie Plastique*. 1984; **29**: 123-32.

80. Markus AF, Delaire J, Smith WP. Facial balance in cleft lip and palate II. Cleft lip and palate and secondary deformities. *British Journal of Oral and Maxillofacial Surgery*. 1992; **30**: 296-304.

81. Randall P. A lip adhesion operation in cleft surgery. *Plastic and Reconstructive Surgery*. 1965; **35**: 371-6.

∗ 82. Millard DR. *Cleft craft – The evolution of its surgery. 1. The unilateral deformity*, 1st edn. Boston: Little Brown, 1976.

83. Tennison CW. The repair of the unilateral cleft lip by the stensil method. *Plastic and Reconstructive Surgery*. 1952; **9**: 115.

84. Mohler L. Unilateral cleft lip repair. *Plastic and Reconstructive Surgery*. 1987; **80**: 511.

85. McComb H. Treatment of the unilateral cleft lip nose. *Plastic and Reconstructive Surgery*. 1975; **55**: 596-601.

86. McComb H. Primary repair of the bilateral cleft lip nose. *British Journal of Plastic Surgery*. 1975; **28**: 262.

87. Millard DR. Closure of bilateral cleft lip and elongation of columella by two operations in infancy. *Plastic and Reconstructive Surgery*. 1971; **47**: 324.

88. Mulliken JB. Principles and techniques of of bilateral complete cleft lip repair. *Plastic and Reconstructive Surgery*. 1985; **75**: 477-86.

89. Randall P, Whitaker L, LaRossa D. Cleft lip repair: the importance of muscle repositioning. *Plastic and Reconstructive Surgery*. 1974; **54**: 316-23.

∗ 90. Bergland O, Semb G, Abyholm FE. Elimination of the residual alveolar cleft by secondary bone grafting and subsequent orthodontic treatment. *Cleft Palate Journal*. 1986; **23**: 175-205.

91. Semb G, Borchgrevink H, Saelher IL, Ramsted T. Multidisciplinary management of cleft lip and palate in Oslo, Norway. In: Bardach J, Morris HL (eds). *Multidisciplinary management of cleft palate*. Philadelphia: WB Saunders, 1990: 27-37.

92. Jolleys A, Robertson NRE. A study of the effects of early bone grafting in complete clefts of the lip and palate – five year study. *British Journal of Plastic Surgery*. 1972; **25**: 229-37.

93. Rehrmann AH, Koberg WR, Koch H. Long term post-operative results of primary and secondary bone grafting in complete clefts of the lip and palate. *Cleft Palate Journal*. 1970; **7**: 206-21.

94. Henkel KO, Gundlach KK. Analysis of primary gingivoperiosteoplasty in alveolar cleft repair. Part I: Facial growth. *Journal of Craniomaxillofacial Surgery*. 1977; **25**: 266-9.

95. Lee CT, Grayson BH, Cutting CB, Brecht LE, Lin WY. Prepubertal midface growth in unilateral cleft lip and palate following alveolar molding and gingivoperiosteoplasty. *Cleft Palate – Craniofacial Journal*. 2004; **41**: 375-80.

96. Smith WP, Markus AF, Delaire J. Primary closure of the cleft alveolus: a functional approach. *British Journal of Oral and Maxillofacial Surgery*. 1995; **33**: 156-65.

97. Brusati R, Mannucci N. The early gingivoalveoloplasty. Preliminary results. *Scandinavian Journal of Plastic and Reconstructive Surgery*. 1992; **26**: 65-70.

* 98. Ross B. Treatment variables affecting facial growth in complete unilateral cleft lip and palate. Part 7: an overview of treatment and facial growth. *Cleft Palate Journal.* 1987; **24**: 71–7.

99. Pigott RW, Albery EH, Hathorn IS, Atack NE, Williams A, Harland K et al. A comparison of three methods of repairing the hard palate. *Cleft Palate – Craniofacial Journal.* 2002; **39**: 383–91.

100. Pichler H. Zur operation der doppelten lippen-gaumenspalten. *Deutsche Zeitschrift für Chirurgie.* 1926; **195**: 104.

101. Delaire J, Precious D. Avoidance of the use of vomerine mucosa in primary surgical management of velopalatine clefts. *Oral Surgery, Oral Medicine, Oral Pathology.* 1985; **60**: 589–97.

102. Birch M, Sommerlad BC, Bhatt A. Image analysis of lateral velopharyngeal closure in repaired cleft palates and normal palates. *British Journal of Plastic Surgery.* 1994; **47**: 400–5 [erratum appears in *British Journal of Plastic Surgery.* 1995; **48**: 178].

*103. Pigott RW, Bensen JF, White FD. Nasendoscopy in the diagnosis of velopharyngeal incompetence. *Plastic and Reconstructive Surgery.* 1969; **43**: 141–7.

104. Ramamurthy L, Wyatt RA, Whitby D, Martin D, Davenport P. The evaluation of velopharyngeal function using flexible nasendoscopy. *Journal of Laryngology and Otology.* 1997; **111**: 739–45.

105. Finkelstein Y, Berger G, Nachmani A, Ophir D. The functional role of the adenoids in speech. *International Journal of Pediatric Otorhinolaryngology.* 1996; **34**: 61–74.

106. Boorman JG, Freelander E (eds). Surgical anatomy of the velum and pharynx. In: *Recent advances in plastic surgery 4.* Edinburgh: Churchill Livingstone 1992: 17–28 (Chapter 2).

107. Furlow Jr LT. Cleft palate repair by double opposing Z-plasty. *Plastic and Reconstructive Surgery.* 1986; **78**: 724–38.

108. Randall P, LaRossa D, Solomon M, Cohen M. Experience with the Furlow double-reversing Z-plasty for cleft palate repair. *Plastic and Reconstructive Surgery.* 1986; **77**: 569–76.

109. Kriens O. Anatomical approach to veloplasty. *Plastic and Reconstructive Surgery.* 1969; **43**: 29.

110. Marsh JL, Grames LM, Holtman B. Intravelar-veloplasty: a prospective study. *Cleft Palate Journal.* 1989; **26**: 46–50.

*111. Sommerlad BC. A technique for cleft palate repair. *Plastic and Reconstructive Surgery.* 2003; **112**: 1542–8.

112. Malek R, Psaume J. Nouvelle conception de la chronologie et de la technique du traitement des fentes labio-palatines. *Annales de Chirurgie Plastique.* 1983; **28**: 237.

113. Hocevar-Boltezar I, Jarc J, Kozelj V. Ear, nose and voice problems in children with orofacial clefts. *Journal of Laryngology and Otology.* 2006; **120**: 276–81.

114. Schonweiler R, Schonweiler B, Schmelzeisen R. [Hearing capacity and speech production in 417 children with facial cleft abnormalities]. *HNO.* 1994; **42**: 691–6.

*115. Goudy S, Lott D, Canady J, Smith RJ. Conductive hearing loss and otopathology in cleft palate patients. *Otolaryngology – Head and Neck Surgery.* 2006; **134**: 946–8.

116. Gudziol V, Mann WJ. Chronic eustachian tube dysfunction and its sequelae in adult patients with cleft lip and palate. *HNO.* 2006; **54**: 684–8.

117. Moss AL, Fonseca S. Audiological issues in children with cleft lip and palate in one area of the U.K. *Cleft Palate – Craniofacial Journal.* 2006; **43**: 420–8.

118. Valtonen H, Dietz A, Qvarnberg Y. Long-term clinical, audiologic, and radiologic outcomes in palate cleft children treated with early tympanostomy for otitis media with effusion: a controlled prospective study. *Laryngoscope.* 2005; **115**: 15112–6.

119. Shaw R, Richardson D, McMahon S. Conservative management of otitis media in cleft palate. *Journal of Craniomaxillofacial Surgery.* 2003; **31**: 316–20.

120. Sheahan P, Blayney AW. Cleft palate and otitis media with effusion: a review. *Revue de Laryngologie, Otologie, Rhinologie.* 2003; **124**: 171–7.

*121. Stewart KJ, Ahmad T, Razzell RE, Watson AC. Altered speech following adenoidectomy: a 20 year experience. *British Journal of Plastic Surgery.* 2002; **55**: 469–73.

122. Sie KC, Tampakopoulou DA, Sorom J, Gruss JS, Eblen LE. Results with Furlow palatoplasty in management of velopharyngeal insufficiency. *Plastic and Reconstructive Surgery.* 2001; **108**: 17–25; discussion 26–9.

123. Sommerlad BC, Mehendale FV, Birch MJ, Sell D, Hattee C, Harland K. Palate re-repair revisited. *Cleft Palate – Craniofacial Journal.* 2002; **39**: 295–307.

124. Liao YF, Noordhoff MS, Huang CS, Chen PK, Chen NH, Yun C et al. Comparison of obstructive sleep apnea syndrome in children with cleft palate following Furlow palatoplasty or pharyngeal flap for velopharyngeal insufficiency. *Cleft Palate – Craniofacial Journal.* 2004; **41**: 152–6.

125. Witt PD, O'Daniel TG, Marsh JL, Grames LM, Muntz HR, Pilgram TK. Surgical management of velopharyngeal dysfunction: outcome analysis of autogenous posterior pharyngeal wall augmentation. *Plastic and Reconstructive Surgery.* 1997; **99**: 1287–96; discussion 1297–300.

*126. Hynes W. Observations on pharyngoplasty. *British Journal of Plastic Surgery.* 1967; **20**: 244–56.

*127. Orticochea M. Construction of a dynamic muscle sphincter in cleft palates. *Plastic and Reconstructive Surgery.* 1968; **41**: 323–7.

128. Riski JE, Serafin D, Riefkohl R, Georgiade GS, Georgiade NG. A rationale for modifying the site of insertion of the orticochea pharyngoplasty. *Plastic and Reconstructive Surgery.* 1984; **73**: 882–94.

*129. Jackson IT, Silverton JS. The sphincter pharyngoplasty as a secondary procedure in cleft palates. *Plastic and Reconstructive Surgery.* 1977; **59**: 518–24.

130. Schoenborn K. Ueber eine neue methode der staphylorrapie. *Archiv fur Klinische Chirurgie.* 1876; **19**:

527–31. (Stellmach RK. *Plastic and reconstructive surgery* 1972; **49**: 558–62, trans.)

131. Rosenthal W. Pathologie und therapie der gaumendefecte. *Fortschritte Zahnheilkunde.* 1932; **8**: 890.

132. Argamaso RV, Shprintzen RJ, Strauch B, Lewin ML, Ship AG, Croft CB. The role of lateral pharyngeal movement in pharyngeal flap surgery. *Plastic and Reconstructive Surgery.* 1980; **66**: 214–9.

133. Peat B, Albery EH, Jones K, Pigott RW. Tailoring velopharyngeal surgery. The influence of aetiology and type of operation. *Plastic and Reconstructive Surgery.* 1980; **66**: 214–9.

134. Armour A, Fischbach S, Klaiman P, Fisher DM. Does velopharyngeal closure pattern affect the success of pharyngeal flap pharyngoplasty? *Plastic and Reconstructive Surgery.* 2005; **115**: 45–52; discussion 53.

135. VPI Surgical Trial Group. Pharyngeal flap and sphincterplasty for velopharyngeal insufficiency have equal outcome at 1 year postoperatively: results of a randomised trial. *Cleft Palate – Craniofacial Journal.* 2005; **42**: 501–11.

136. Yu-Fang Liao DDS, Noordhoff MS, Chiung-Shing H, Philip KT, Chen MD, Ning-Hung C. Comparison of obstructive sleep apnea syndrome in children with cleft palate following furlow palatoplasty or pharyngeal flap for velopharyngeal insufficiency. *Cleft Palate – Craniofacial Journal.* 2004; **41**: 152–6.

Craniofacial anomalies: genetics and management

DEAN KISSUN, DAVID RICHARDSON, ELIZABETH SWEENEY AND PAUL MAY

Introduction	1019	Encephalomeningocoele	1034
General principles of management	1019	Craniofacial clefts	1035
Classification	1019	Key points	1036
Craniosynostosis	1020	Best clinical practice	1036
Syndromic craniosynostosis	1027	Deficiencies in current knowledge and areas for future	
Hemifacial microsomia	1032	research	1037
Treacher Collins syndrome (mandibulofacial dysostosis)	1033	References	1037

SEARCH STRATEGY

The data in this chapter are supported by a Medline search using the key words craniofacial anomalies, craniosynostosis, hemifacial microsomia, Treacher Collins syndrome, encephalocoele and craniofacial clefts.

INTRODUCTION

The term 'craniofacial anomalies' encompasses a large number of different conditions, usually present at birth, and variable in their aetiology, extent, severity and clinical presentation. Different terminologies, classification systems and treatment protocols can add difficulties for those trying to gain an understanding of the subject. Management usually requires multidisciplinary input and coordination, often from a large number of different specialists working as part of a dedicated craniofacial team. For many conditions, monitoring and intervention is required from birth to maturity and often beyond, well into adult life. The aim of this chapter is to describe some of the more commonly encountered groups of craniofacial anomalies, to outline the principles of their management, and review the contribution of genetics to the understanding of these conditions.

GENERAL PRINCIPLES OF MANAGEMENT

The craniofacial region is particularly complex in its anatomy and function, evidenced by the large number of medical and surgical specialities, and professions allied to medicine, that are devoted to this anatomical area. All of these specialists have key roles to play in the management of patients with craniofacial anomalies. The systemic consequences of localized functional impairment in craniofacial anomalies, as well as the frequent presence of associated (noncraniofacial) anomalies, require the expertise of a wide variety of other specialists. Management of paediatric craniofacial anomalies requires all the facilities and expertise available in a modern dedicated paediatric setting.

All patients require screening/assessment by the core members of the team, followed by further in-depth assessment (if necessary by other specialists) and treatment if indicated (see **Table 78.1**). [*]

CLASSIFICATION

Owing to the complexity and heterogeneity of craniofacial anomalies there is no universal classification system. Many classification systems have been proposed, based on embryology, aetiology, anatomical location, morphology and genetics. In England, the National Specialist

Table 78.1 Multidisciplinary team: the roles of each discipline.

Discipline	Role
Genetics	Diagnosis, associated conditions, risk of future siblings having the condition, risk of patient passing on the condition to his/her children
SALT	Speech and language, feeding, general developmental milestones
Psychologist	Parental anxiety, preparation for operations, intervention for older patients, coping strategies, cognitive assessment
Paediatrician	General development, associated abnormalities
Ophthalmology	ICP, acuity and motility
ENT	Airway problems, hearing and middle ear disease
Neurosurgery	ICP, hydrocephalus, associated abnormalities, surgical treatment of the condition
Maxillofacial	Surgical correction of deformity
Plastic surgery	Surgical correction of deformity
Orthodontist	Craniofacial growth and development, dental condition and occlusion
Anaesthetist	Experience of paediatric craniofacial and neurosurgical anaesthesia. Access to paediatric intensive care unit (PICU)

SALT, Speech and language therapist.

Commissioning Advisory Group (NSCAG) recognize six categories of patients:[1]

1. craniofacial clefts;
2. craniofacial dysostosis;
3. craniosynostosis;
4. encephalocoele;
5. overgrowth, undergrowth or dysraphia associated with unilateral or bilateral orbital dystopia or displacement;
6. any other complex anomaly where referring specialists feel that the expertise present within the service would substantially benefit the treatment of the condition.

For the purposes of this chapter we present the most common conditions that present to the craniofacial surgeon.

CRANIOSYNOSTOSIS

Craniosynostosis is the term applied to the premature fusion of one or more of the sutures of the growing cranium, and manifests as abnormal cranial growth. In order to understand the pathophysiology of craniosynostosis, normal skull growth must be considered.

Normal skull growth

The stimulus for growth of the cranium comes from the expanding brain, which grows rapidly in the first two years of life, doubling in weight in the first year and achieving 90 percent of its adult size by the age of two years. This rapid brain growth has to be accommodated by a concomitant expansion in volume of the skull. The cranial vault consists of the frontal, parietal, temporal and occipital bones, which are separated from each other by the cranial sutures (metopic, sagittal, coronal and lambdoid). These sutures allow gradual displacement of the individual bones, allowing the brain to expand. In order to avoid large gaps developing between the bones as the expansion proceeds, new bone is deposited at the free margins of the bones adjacent to the sutures. Bone resorbtion and deposition also takes place on the inner and outer surfaces of the calvarial bones to produce changes in their curvature and thickness.

The patent cranial sutures therefore allow for growth to take place in response to the stimulus of the growing brain and, unlike the epiphyseal plates of the long bones, cranial bones do not have intrinsic growth potential. The sutures only remain patent while brain growth is taking place. If brain growth ceases, cranial growth ceases, and the cranial sutures will be replaced by bone, resulting in fusion – a normal phenomenon once growth is complete.

Classification

Premature fusion of calvarial sutures has a variety of underlying causes, broadly divided into **primary** and **secondary** craniosynostosis.[2]

Secondary craniosynostosis is uncommon, but may be seen in microcephaly, where there is a lack of underlying brain growth, in some haematologic (polycythaemia, thalassaemia) and metabolic abnormalities (rickets, hyperthyroidism), and may be drug induced (retinoic acid).

Primary craniosynostosis is much commoner than secondary craniosynostosis. It can be classified on the basis of the number of sutures involved (single suture, multiple or total), the site of the involved suture(s) (metopic, coronal, sagittal, lambdoid) and whether it is an isolated condition (nonsyndromic) or associated with other malformations (syndromic). Primary craniosynostosis constitutes a significant workload in craniofacial units.

Incidence

Primary nonsyndromic craniosynostosis occurs in approximately 1:2000 live births. Of the nonsyndromic craniosynostoses, sagittal synostosis is the most common accounting for 60 percent of cases. In cases of nonsyndromic craniosynostosis there is a male predominance with male to female ratios of 4:1 in sagittal synostosis and 3:1 in metopic synostosis. Of the syndromic craniosynostoses, Crouzon syndrome has the highest incidence with 1:25,000 live births[3] and Apert syndrome is 1:60,000 live births.[4]

Aetiology

Craniosynostosis is aetiologically heterogeneous.[4] Both nonsyndromic and syndromic craniosynostoses result from an interaction between genetic factors, molecular and cellular events, mechanical and deformational forces and secondary effects of each of these on normal growth and development. Premature fusion of the sutures may take place alone or, in syndromic craniosynostosis, with other anomalies. Most cases of isolated craniosynostosis are sporadic. However, familial cases do happen and a positive family history can be found in 14.4 percent of coronal, 6 percent of sagittal and 5.6 percent of metopic synostosis cases, but very rarely in lambdoid synostosis.[5, 6, 7, 8, 9] For isolated, single suture synostosis with unaffected parents, the recurrence risks range from 1 percent in sagittal synostosis to 5 percent in coronal and metopic synostosis.[10]

Chromosomal abnormalities may also cause craniosynostosis, particularly in patients with other anomalies or problems with growth or development. Teratogens may also be causative, as in the case of sodium valproate and trigonocephaly. The syndromic craniosynostoses are usually genetically determined, often occurring as new mutations. There is an increasing recognition that some of the so-called isolated nonsyndromic synostoses also have a genetic basis.

Genetics of craniofacial anomalies

The vast array of genetic conditions causing craniofacial anomalies precludes an exhaustive discussion of their genetics in this text. However, it is appropriate to discuss the more common conditions and encourage a low threshold for the involvement of the clinical genetics team in the management of patients with craniofacial anomalies. Clinical geneticists can contribute to both diagnosis and counselling of affected individuals and also their families. Interested readers are encouraged to consult the texts of Gorlin et al.[11] and Cohen and MacLean[4] for more extensive details on craniofacial anomaly syndromes.

When considering the aetiology of craniofacial anomalies it is helpful to consider their aetiology in terms of **malformations** (e.g. genetic syndromes, teratogens), **deformations** (e.g. positional plagiocephaly) and **disruptions** (e.g. amniotic bands). Some craniofacial anomalies are multifactorial.

Genetic testing is not indicated in patients with isolated sagittal or metopic synostosis in whom there are no associated abnormalities or concerns about growth or development, and no significant family history. However, coronal synostosis, even when isolated, warrants analysis of at least FGFR3 for the Pro250Arg mutation (see below under FGFR3-associated coronal synostosis syndrome – Muenke craniosynostosis) and possibly analysis of the TWIST gene (see below under Saethre-Chotzen syndrome).

Genetic testing by DNA analysis of specific genes is available only for syndromes where the causative gene has been identified. This facilitates diagnosis and also counselling of family members, particularly when a parent may be a gene carrier with a very mild phenotype. Chromosomal analysis should be considered in any patient with complex or multiple abnormalities, or in whom there are concerns regarding a child's growth or development. Informed consent should be obtained prior to any genetic testing, especially as abnormal results may have implications for other family members as well as the child. Failure to identify a genetic abnormality in a syndromic patient does not, however, rule out a genetic cause for their condition, and involvement of a clinical geneticist is essential.

Prenatal diagnosis by genetic analysis of chorionic villus sample or amniotic fluid may be available for conditions in which the causative genetic abnormality is known. Prenatal ultrasound scanning later in pregnancy may reveal abnormal craniofacial contour or associated skeletal or systemic abnormalities in syndromic conditions; however, the premature sutural fusion of isolated craniosynostosis is much more difficult to detect.

Pathogenesis and consequences

Premature suture fusion results in inhibition of skull growth in a direction perpendicular to the affected suture. Despite this localized failure of skull growth, the brain continues to grow, and expands in different directions, where expansion can be accommodated by normal (patent) sutures, producing compensatory changes at a distance from the abnormal suture and usually parallel to it.[12] In the latter half of the last century, Moss[13] postulated that the cranial base was the site of abnormal physical stresses, and that these could be transmitted to the dura of the cranial vault, resulting in suture fusion. [***/**/*] Whatever the underlying mechanism, the restriction of growth perpendicular to the fused suture, and the compensatory changes elsewhere in the cranium,

Table 78.2   The craniosynostoses. Affected sutures and resultant head shapes. The anterior aspect of the skull (the forehead) is towards the top of the table.

Shape of skull	Suture affected	Name
	Saggital	Scaphocephaly
	Metopic	Trigonocephaly
	Unilateral coronal	Frontal plagiocephaly
	Bilateral coronal	Brachycephaly
	Unilateral lambdoid	True posterior synostotic plagiocephaly

may result in a reduction in cranial volume (and hence raised intracranial pressure (ICP)) and a change in shape (resulting in characteristic changes dependent on the suture or sutures involved) (see **Table 78.2**).

Clinical assessment

The history may be of a baby with an abnormal head shape, present at birth, gradually becoming worse. Examination reveals the characteristic head shape (see **Table 78.2**) with ridging of the affected suture.

Imaging

Plain films allow assessment of sutural patency and the overall morphology of the skull. All sutures are easily visible in the normal growing skull, with the exception of the metopic suture which normally fuses early. A prematurely fused suture may be sclerotic (**Figure 78.1**) or may not be visible at all. The abnormal shape of the head will be apparent, and skull base abnormalities not apparent on clinical examination may be seen (e.g. the 'harlequin eye' appearance of the sphenoid ridge in coronal synostosis). Computed tomography (CT), especially when reconstituted via a three-dimensional format, provides even more detail of the morphology of the skull (**Figure 78.2**). In addition, a CT scan allows evaluation of the intracranial contents. [**]

Raised intracranial pressure

It is logical to think of raised ICP developing as a result of failure of cranial expansion in the presence of continuing

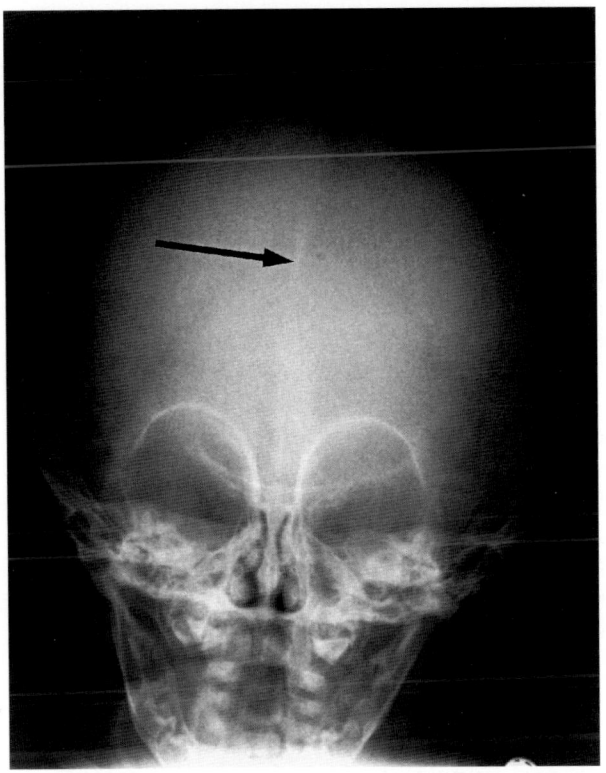

Figure 78.1 Skull x-ray showing sclerosed suture. Arrow points to sclerosed metopic suture.

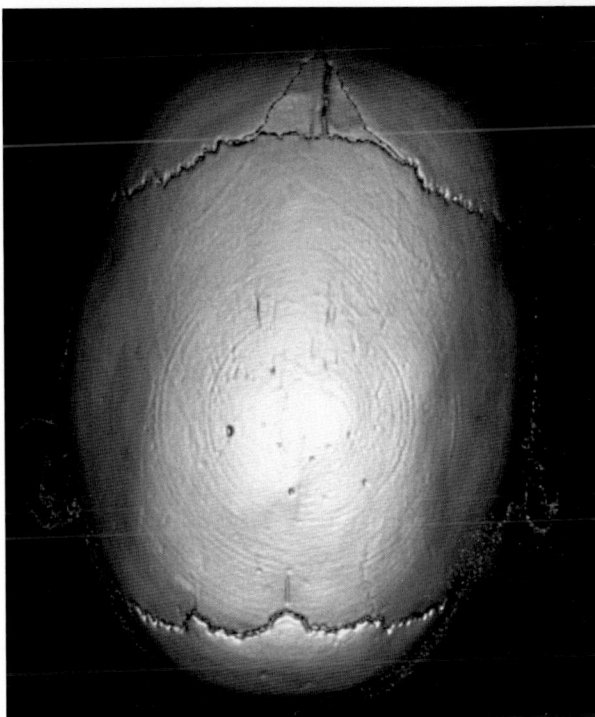

Figure 78.2 CT scan of patient with scaphocephaly. Note the absence of sagittal suture.

pressure from the growing brain. However, the relationship is complex, and other factors have been implicated. Raised ICP is not directly related to a decrease in intracranial volume,[14] and venous hypertension has been identified as a result of a significantly narrower jugular foramen (6.5 mm versus 11.5 mm) in complex and syndromic patients with raised ICP.[15]

The reported incidence of raised ICP in patients with craniosynosotosis shows wide variation, and there is variability in the threshold for diagnosis in reported studies, with values of 15 or 20 mm Hg chosen.[16] Reported incidence in mixed cohorts of nonsyndromic and syndromic patients vary from 17 to 92 percent.[14, 17, 18, 19] Studies that have compared the incidence of raised ICP in nonsyndromic and syndromic patients have shown a higher incidence in syndromic patients (approximately 50 percent) compared with nonsyndromic patients (approximately 25 percent).[20, 21]

Diagnosis may be difficult because the classic clinical features of raised ICP are often absent. Thus, the child's development, in particular the acquisition of normal developmental milestones, vision, reading and language comprehension, motor skills, and general behaviour are important, and may require detailed specialist investigation, including ophthalmological assessment. Changes in visual-evoked potentials have been shown to be early indicators of raised ICP.[22, 23]

Plain skull films may show the classic 'copper-beaten' appearance of chronically raised ICP (**Figure 78.3**) but

the absence of changes does not exclude raised ICP.[24] CT/ magnetic resonance (MR) scan may be helpful but in cases where clinical assessment is equivocal, invasive ICP monitoring may be indicated, using either a traditional ICP bolt or, more recently, parenchymal fibre-optic transducers which have been shown to be reliable as recorders of ICP and are associated with a low rate of complications.[20]

Transcranial Doppler ultrasonography has been proposed as an alternative noninvasive, inexpensive and safe alternative.[25] [*]

Hydrocephalus

Hydrocephalus is characterized by enlargement of the cerebral ventricles due to obstructed outflow of cerebrospinal fluid (CSF) somewhere along its path from the lateral ventricles, through the interventricular foramina, third ventricle, cerebral aqueduct, fourth ventricle and subarachnoid space to the sites of absorption. Hydrocephalus can occur in up to 20 percent of patients with craniosynostosis. It may be associated with chronic venous hypertension and hindbrain herniation, particularly in multisutural synostosis. The neurosurgical treatment of clinically significant hydrocephalus should be undertaken before more major craniofacial corrective surgery. [**/*]

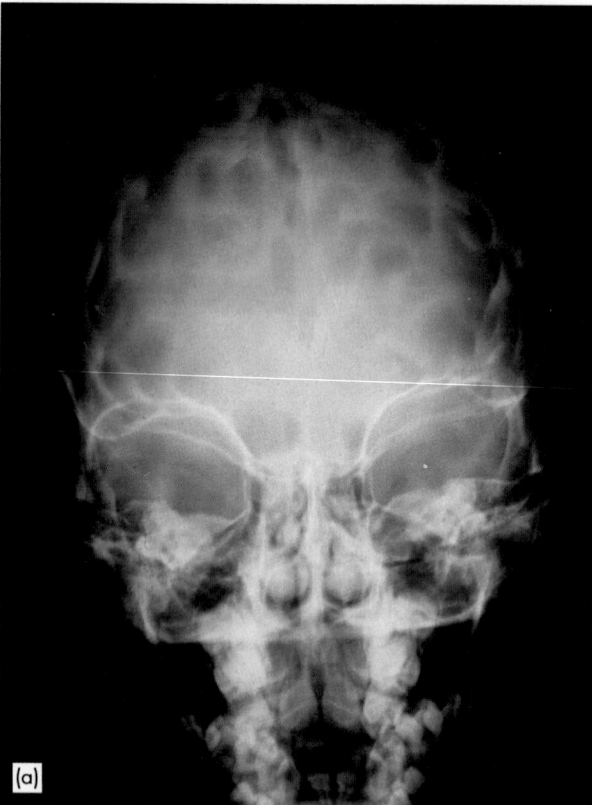

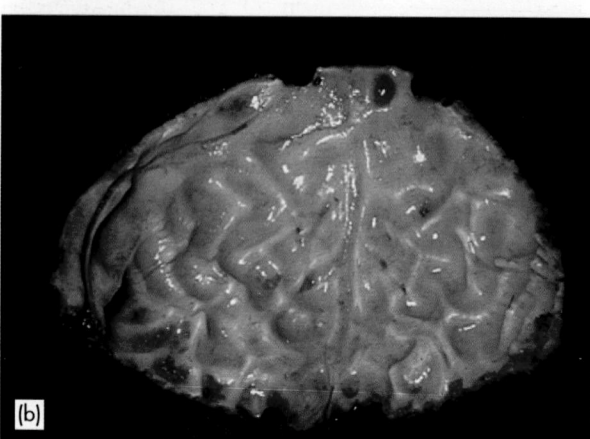

Figure 78.3 Skull x-ray of patient with raised ICP showing 'copper beating'. Removed frontal bone shows indentation of underlying brain tissue.

Differential diagnosis

Not all abnormal head shapes are due to craniosynostosis, and accurate diagnosis is essential since the management of nonsynostotic head shape abnormalities is nonsurgical. The bones of the skull in early life are relatively soft and deformable, rendering the head susceptible to alteration in shape for a variety of reasons. Nonsynostotic causes of abnormal head shape include intrauterine and birth canal moulding, assisted delivery, e.g. Ventouse, intracranial abnormalities and post-natal deformational forces on the growing skull due to external pressure on the head or to uneven muscle tension in the muscles attached to the skull base.

Intrauterine, birth canal and assisted delivery moulding will be present at birth but improve fairly quickly. Intracranial abnormalities will present at birth but persist. Post-natal deformational changes are not present at birth, develop gradually, and if the cause is removed, will improve. This is in contrast to craniosynostosis, which is usually apparent at birth and progresses with growth. Diagnosis is usually possible based on the history and examination alone, but confirmation of the patency of sutures can be confirmed by plain radiographs or CT scan if needed.

The most common presentation of nonsynostotic abnormalities of head shape is occipital plagiocephaly (for more detail see under Posterior skull deformity (including lambdoid synostosis)) due to habitual sleep position (the 'Back to sleep' campaign, encouraging parents to ensure babies sleep as far as possible on their backs, has contributed to this in recent years) or torticollis. Other causes include abnormal head posture due to vertebral abnormalities or ocular squint.

General principles of surgical management

The indications for surgery are treatment of raised ICP, correction of significant cosmetic deformity and prevention of future deformity by allowing normal growth to take place.

The general principles of surgery for the craniosynostoses are to remove the cause by excising the affected suture, correct the existing deformity by reshaping the affected area of the cranium and moving it into the position it would have been in had it grown normally. This leaves an expanded intracranial volume, with a space between the dura and the repositioned bone, into which the brain can expand, thus relieving raised ICP if present. It also corrects the cosmetic deformity. Leaving a gap in the region of the excised suture, which will mimic a normal suture, will allow future growth to take place by movement of the bone in response to continued brain growth.

Timing of surgery is important. Early surgery has the advantage that ICP is normalized without delay, and the deformity may be less severe since it has had less time to develop. However, early surgery may be followed by reossification at the site of the excised suture (restenosis), with a re-emergence of the condition requiring further surgery. The timing of surgery is, therefore, a balance between operating too early with the risk of restenosis and operating too late when there may be prolonged raised ICP, the deformity is greater and its correction may require more extensive surgery because of lack of future brain growth and, thus, capacity for skull remodelling in response to brain growth. Optimum timing is different for different sutures, and is discussed below under Timing of surgery.

Major craniofacial surgery carries significant risks and complications, and a dedicated team familiar with all aspects of the management of these patients is a prerequisite for surgery to be performed. This will include a dedicated ward and theatre with appropriately trained staff, a paediatric anaesthetist and HDU/PICU facilities. [**/*]

Single suture nonsyndromic craniosynostosis

SAGITTAL SYNOSTOSIS (SCAPHOCEPHALY)

This is the commonest isolated craniosynostosis, accounting for approximately 60 percent of nonsyndromic cases. It is far more common in males than females (4:1 ratio). The characteristic head shape is narrow transversely (due to lack of widening of the cranium perpendicular to the fused sagittal suture) and long anteroposteriorly (due to compensatory growth at the patent coronal and lambdoid sutures). The whole suture may be affected, with compensatory changes at the front and back, or the fusion may be predominantly anterior (with anterior compensatory growth resulting in frontal bossing) or posterior (with compensatory occipital bulging) (**Figure 78.4**).

The optimum age for operation is six to nine months, when suturectomy (midline linear strip craniectomy) with lateral osteotomies to permit brain growth ('lateral barrel staving') are performed. At this age, there is sufficient future brain growth to effect a continued gradual improvement, giving good results without the need for more extensive surgery, although some centres prefer a more complete operative correction when operating at an early age. In older patients in whom the diagnosis may have been delayed, more extensive procedures are necessary, and total calvarial remodelling may be needed.

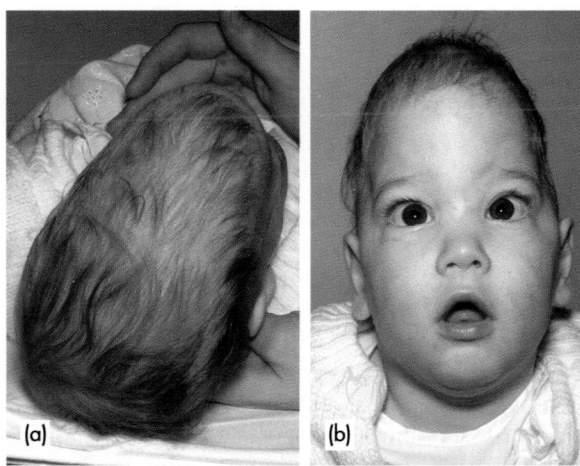

(a) (b)

Figure 78.4 Patient with scaphocephaly. The skull is long from front to back and narrow from side to side ('boat shaped').

ANTERIOR SYNOSTOSES

Coronal and metopic synostosis predominantly affect the forehead and supraorbital region, and surgical management is similar, irrespective of the involved suture.

CORONAL SYNOSTOSIS (FRONTAL PLAGIOCEPHALY AND BRACHYCEPHALY)

This is the second commonest simple craniosynostosis, accounting for approximately 30 percent of all cases. Coronal synostosis may be either unilateral or bilateral and can be associated with significant deformity of the facial skeleton, particularly in unilateral cases.

Unilateral (frontal plagiocephaly)

In unilateral cases there is flattening of the forehead on the ipsilateral side with a decrease in the anteroposterior dimension of the anterior cranial fossa and a resultant decrease in its volume. There are compensatory changes on the contralateral side with frontal bossing. Changes may affect the facial skeleton and result in significant complex facial asymmetry in more severe cases.

Bilateral (brachycephaly)

In bilateral cases there is a (usually) symmetrical reduction in anterior growth of the forehead, with compensatory widening of the skull, particularly in the temporal region. The forehead is recessed, there is poor brow projection and frontotemporal bossing may be present. The upper face is usually broad and there may be telecanthus or hypertelorism.

METOPIC SYNOSTOSIS (TRIGONOCEPHALY)

This represents approximately 10 percent of the total number of patients presenting with single suture craniosynostosis, although there is some early evidence from the experience of craniofacial centres that incidence of trigonocephaly may be on the increase. There is a deficiency of lateral growth of the frontal bones, with compensatory growth in the parietal and occipital regions, resulting in a widening of the back of the head. This, along with the narrow forehead, produces the characteristic triangularly shaped head (trigonocephaly) The fused metopic suture is often markedly elevated (ridged), further emphasizing the triangular shape. Owing to the reduction in lateral growth of the skull anteriorly, there is a decrease in the interorbital and intercanthal distances.

SURGERY

Fronto-orbital advancement and remodelling

Surgical correction of coronal and metopic synostosis is usually carried out between the ages of 12 and 15 months.

Earlier than this risks the need to repeat surgery because of restenosis, particularly if surgery is carried out before six months of age.[26]

Surgery involves fronto-orbital advancement and remodelling (FOAR) described by Paul Tessier.[27] It is now the standard technique for expansion of the anterior fossa and correction of deformities involving the forehead and orbital rims. This involves removal of the frontal bone and supra orbital bone (supra orbital bar), remodelling and replacement in a forward position (**Figure 78.5**). This is usually carried out as a bilateral procedure, even in cases of unilateral coronal synostosis, since the deformity is never confined totally to the side of the fused suture, and results of bilateral surgery tend to be better than unilateral surgery in many cases.

Posterior skull deformity (including lambdoid synostosis)

Flattening of the occipital region is seen frequently and can happen for a variety of reasons, the most common of which is due to prolonged pressure on the occipital region during sleep, where the child is put to sleep on its back. The pressure causes deformation of the relatively soft occipital bones, resulting in deformational posterior plagiocephaly. The deformity is not present at birth, but develops gradually over the first few months of life. As the child gets older, gains head control and becomes more mobile, spending less time on its back, the cause is removed or lessened, and the condition often improves spontaneously. However, the deformity may be rather marked, and in moderate or severe cases, may remain noticeable despite the tendency for improvement. Similarly, torticollis with an imbalance in the action of the sternocleidomastoid muscles on each side may result in similar changes. Physiotherapy will usually correct limitations in neck movement, removing the underlying cause and allowing some spontaneous improvement. Other conditions affecting head posture (e.g. ocular squint and hemivertebral abnormalities) may have similar effects.

True lambdoid synostosis may cause occipital flattening, but is the rarest of all the isolated craniosynostoses (approximately 1 percent). It is usually unilateral, but in 15 percent of cases is bilateral. There is still controversy regarding the true relationship of lambdoid synostosis and posterior plagiocephaly.

Diagnosis is dependent on the history (present at birth), examination (ridged suture and specific indicators, e.g. ear position) (**Figure 78.6**) and radiological investigations (plain film or CT) demonstrating a fused suture.

Surgery is rarely indicated for posterior skull deformity, even when synostosis is suspected. The deformity is rarely very noticeable once it is covered by hair and the risk of raised intracranial pressure is very low. Surgery may be undertaken in very severe deformity but full correction is not possible because the skull base deformity, which manifests as change in ear position, is not correctable, and the presence of the dural venous sinuses (torcula) limits the extent of safe bone removal for remodelling.

Recently, there has been increasing interest in the use of moulding helmets to treat posterior plagiocephaly, but there is a lack of good evidence with regard to efficacy,

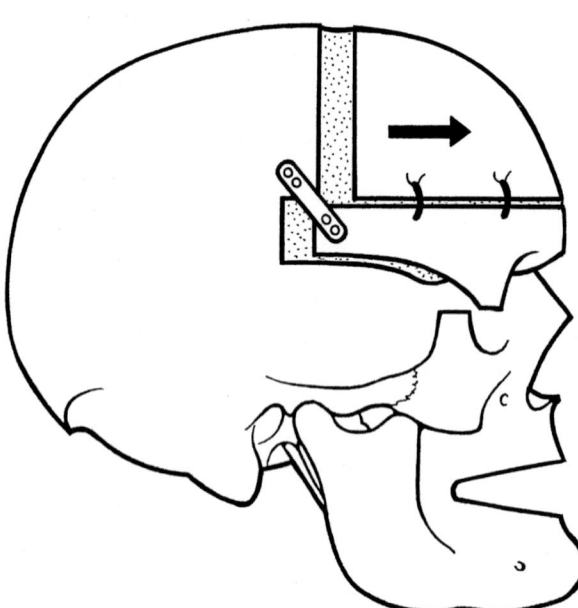

Figure 78.5 Diagram of FOAR. The frontal bone and supraorbital bar are removed, reshaped and replaced in an anterior position (see Fronto-orbital advancement and remodelling).

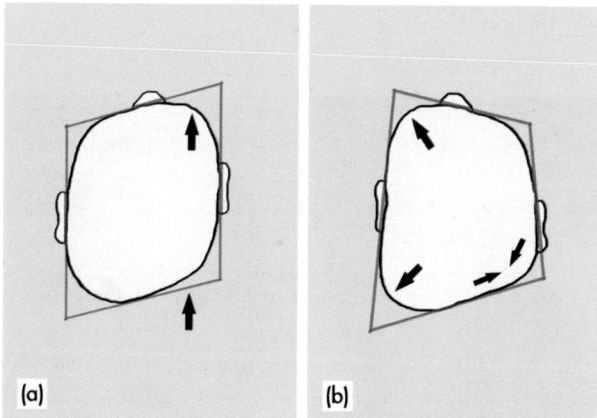

Figure 78.6 Differences between positional and true lambdoid synostosis. Positional moulding produces a parallelogram-shaped head and the ear moves anteriorly on the affected side. Unilambdoid synostosis produces a trapezoid-shaped head and the ear moves posteriorly towards the affected suture.

and properly designed scientific study is required to establish their place in the management of craniofacial patients.

Endoscopic treatment of craniosynostosis

Over the last few years, surgeons in America have been using endoscopic techniques to treat stenosed calvarial sutures. Purpose-built systems utilizing 4 mm 0° and 30° rigid endoscopes allow visualization of the subgaleal space and the undersurface of the skull when dissecting the dura. Such techniques allow strip craniectomies (but not remodelling) to be performed, with a significant reduction in blood loss and blood transfusion rates. To date, successful treatment of sagittal, metopic, lambdoid and coronal suture synostosis has been performed when such methods have been allied to the use of custom-made cranial orthotic moulding helmets. Further studies are required to establish the efficacy of this method of treatment. Successful treatment of isolated suture synostosis for 70 patients treated over a four-year period has been reported.[28]

SYNDROMIC CRANIOSYNOSTOSIS

A syndrome is defined as a constellation of symptoms and signs that collectively characterize an abnormal condition or disease state. Syndromic craniosynostoses result from an interaction between genetic factors, molecular and cellular events, mechanical and deformational forces, and secondary effects of each of these on normal growth and development.

The clinical manifestation of some syndromes may vary from mild (unnoticeable) to severe.

Crouzon syndrome

Described in 1912 by a French neurosurgeon, this syndrome affects the face and cranium and occurs in 1:25,000 live births. Crouzon syndrome is characterized by craniosynostosis and maxillary hypoplasia with shallow orbits causing ocular proptosis. There is often bicoronal synostosis (brachycephaly) but occasionally the sagittal suture may also be affected. The main abnormality is an underdeveloped midface which results in prolapse of the globes ('exorbitism'), hypoplasia of the malar bones, retromaxillism and a resultant malocclusion. Anomalies of the middle ear and atresia of the external auditory canal may give rise to a conductive hearing loss. Abnormalities are usually confined to the craniofacial region although there may be systemic anomalies.[4] Intelligence is usually normal. Crouzon syndrome is caused by mutations in FGFR2 and is autosomal dominant, although new mutations frequently arise.[29] The severity of this condition is extremely variable, even within the same family, and

therefore a mildly affected parent may only be diagnosed after the birth of a more severely affected child. Severity may vary from a barely noticeable degree of proptosis and midfacial hypoplasia to, more rarely, cloverleaf skull.

Apert syndrome

Described in 1906 by Apert, this syndrome has an incidence of 1:60,000 live births. There is an autosomal dominant pattern of inheritance although most cases of Apert syndrome occur without a family history as a result of new mutations and there is a link with advanced paternal age.[30] The main features of this condition include craniosynostosis, abnormal midfacial development and fusion of the digits of the hands and feet (syndactyly). Abnormalities of the midface and cranium are evident at birth with brachycephaly and midface retrusion causing an anterior open bite (malocclusion). Cleft soft palate or bifid uvula is present in 30 percent of cases. Fixation of the stapes footplate may cause a conductive hearing loss. There may be other associated malformations and intellectual ability may vary from normal to significantly impaired.[31] Apert syndrome is caused by mutations in FGFR2; in two-thirds of cases the mutation is Ser252Trp, and is Pro253Arg in the remaining one-third.[32]

Pfeiffer syndrome

First described in 1964, Pfeiffer syndrome is similar to Crouzon syndrome, and is characterized by craniosynostosis and midfacial hypoplasia with shallow orbits. However, additional features of Pfeiffer syndrome are broad thumbs and broad great toes. Severity of craniofacial anomalies can vary from mild midfacial hypoplasia to cloverleaf skull. Coronal sutures are most commonly affected with resultant brachycephaly. Other features may include skeletal anomalies such as fusion of the elbow joint, solid cartilaginous trachea and choanal stenosis. Three clinical subtypes have been suggested depending on the extent of associated features.[4] Pfeiffer syndrome is caused by mutations in FRFR1 and FGFR2, in some cases the same mutations that can cause Crouzon syndrome. Inheritance is autosomal dominant although many cases arise as a result of new mutations. Intelligence varies from normal to mild learning difficulties, although central nervous system abnormalities may occur in severe cases.[11]

FGFR3-associated coronal synostosis syndrome (Muenke craniosynostosis)

This increasingly recognized autosomal dominant condition is associated with unilateral or bilateral coronal synostosis and a variety of minor anomalies. The cause is a specific mutation of FGFR3, the Pro250Arg mutation.[33]

The phenotype this causes is extremely variable, even within the same family, and includes coronal synostosis, macrocephaly without synostosis, ptosis and minor anomalies of the hands and feet. Intelligence is usually within normal limits although learning difficulties, usually mild, may be present. The effect of the mutation may be so mild in some family members that they are unaware of any craniofacial problems and could be offered gene testing to clarify their carrier status.

Saethre–Chotzen syndrome

This was first described in 1931. This is an extremely variable autosomal dominant condition, although abnormalities may be milder than in other syndromic craniosynostosis conditions. Owing to this, a mildly affected parent may not be aware that they also have the condition until after their more obviously affected child is diagnosed. The most commonly affected suture is the coronal suture and the craniofacial abnormalities are frequently asymmetric. Associated features may include ptosis, a low anterior hairline, small ears with a prominent horizontal crus, mild cutaneous syndactyly and broad thumbs and great toes. Mutations in the gene TWIST cause Saethre-Chotzen syndrome but the phenotype has also been seen in association with Pro250Arg mutations in FGFR3.[34]

Craniofrontonasal syndrome

This condition is characterized by craniosynostosis which is usually coronal, frontonasal dysplasia, curly or frizzy hair, sloping shoulders and ridged nails. As part of the frontonasal dysplasia there is hypertelorism, a broad nasal bridge and, occasionally, a bifid nasal tip. There may also be skeletal anomalies such as joint hyperextensibilty, scoliosis and broad toes. The inheritance is X-linked and, unusually for this form of inheritance, females are more severely affected than males. The gene EFBN1 has recently been identified as causative.[35]

Carpenter syndrome

This very rare autosomal recessive condition is characterized by craniosynostosis which may affect all sutures causing a cloverleaf skull, and also polysyndactyly (accessory digits with fusion of the digits) and brachydactyly (shortened digits). Mixed hearing loss may also occur. Patients may have obesity and may show learning difficulties.[36] The causative gene has been identified as RAB23.[37]

Kleeblattschädel anomaly (clover leaf skull)

This describes a trilobar skull and is usually caused by pansynostosis involving the coronal, lambdoid and metopic sutures, with bulging of the brain through open sagittal and sometimes squamosal sutures. The prognosis is often, but not universally, poor. Cloverleaf skull is a nonspecific anomaly and may be an isolated defect or part of wider syndromes. As such, the aetiology of cloverleaf skull is varied. It may be seen in patients with certain chromosomal abnormalities or be a feature of syndromes such as Pfeiffer, Apert, Crouzon and Carpenter.

Management

The aim of treatment in the craniofacial dysostosis group of patients is the same as for nonsyndromic craniosynostosis patients, which is to provide surgical correction for the abnormal shape (cosmetic) and restore volume (function).

Before treatment of the craniofacial anomaly, associated factors may need to be addressed. These include the compromised airway, globe protrusion, feeding and other medical abnormalities (heart, lung, etc.). Correction of craniosynostosis in infancy and midface retrusion in childhood are the mainstays of surgical treatment and require coordination with dentists, orthodontists, speech and language therapists and psychologists.

Airway

Respiratory problems may arise due to maxillary hypoplasia and, in some instances, tracheomalacia and choanal stenosis. Measures that may be useful include specific positioning of the patient, nasal stents, insertion of a nasopharyngeal airway and more complex strategies such as continuous positive airway pressure, endotracheal intubation or even tracheostomy. In the older child it may be necessary to perform adenoidectomy and/or tonsillectomy if indicated. This should be approached with caution where a cleft palate – often a submucous cleft – is present owing to potential creation or exacerbation of velopharyngeal insufficiency. Compromise of the airway may only be apparent when the child is asleep. Sleep studies may be required in some patients. Obstructive sleep apnoea is dealt with in more detail in Chapter 85, Obstructive sleep apnoea in childhood.

Visual complications

Owing to midfacial hypoplasia allied with temporal bulging, the orbits may be shallow and globe protrusion may happen. Most patients do not develop complications. Papilloedema, optic atrophy and progressive optic nerve dysfunction may accompany increased ICP even without evidence of hydrocephalus and even with open fontanelles. Uncorrected refractive error, strabismus, ptosis and corneal abrasion can lead to amblyopia, which if not reversed can lead to permanent visual disability. Proptosis due to the inability to close the eyelids can lead to corneal abrasion. Craniosynostosis syndromes can be associated with missing extraocular muscles or muscles with abnormal insertions, resulting in ocular motility disorders.[38, 39]

Emergency treatment is usually conservative with the use of protective eye chambers or tarsorraphy. Rarely, early forehead/midface advancement may be indicated where corneal protection is impossible. In the older child the cosmetic aspects of ocular problems will be addressed with fronto-orbital advancement and midface surgery.

Papilloedema, optic atrophy and progressive optic nerve dysfunction may accompany increased ICP.

Uncorrected refractive error, strabismus, ptosis and corneal abrasion can lead to amblyopia.

Feeding

In cases of midface hypoplasia there is the potential for maldevelopment of oropharyngeal function. Difficulties may include problems achieving lip seal (sucking may be impaired), airway reduction and the presence of cleft palate. This, in the short-term, will have an impact on swallowing and thus feeding and in the long-term, an influence on the development of speech and language. Assessment by speech and language therapists and nutritionists is thus very important. It may be necessary to insert a naso-gastric tube or, in some cases, provide a feeding gastrostomy.

Intracranial pressure

The incidence of raised ICP in the syndromic patient is approximately twice that of the nonsyndromic patient. Assessment and manifestations have already been covered in a previous section (see Single suture nonsyndromic craniosynostosis above). In cases where there is evidence of raised ICP in a patient who is less than the ideal age for fronto-orbital advancement (particularly in the presence of a posterior constriction), early posterior skull release should be considered as an initial procedure.[26] Posterior skull release involves a posterior craniotomy allowing a free segment or a segment fixed in new position allowing increased intracranial volume.

Definitive correction of syndromic craniosynostis

This usually involves correcting the skull base and vault abnormality with FOAR early, in order to restore appearance and reduce the risk of development of raised ICP. Surgery to the midface is performed later; this restores appearance, enlarges the airway and improves the dental occlusion.

Timing of surgery

There is a balance between the risk of developing raised ICP if surgery is performed late and the risk of restenosis if surgery is performed early. Taking into account this balance, FOAR is usually performed at approximately 12–14 months age, as it is in nonsyndromic patients.

Timing of surgery to the midface is a matter of debate. Within the UK, surgery is usually delayed until the age of five to six years, or older, prior to the child starting secondary education. This delay is intended to allow growth of the child so that the weight increases, as does the circulating blood volume. Midface surgery often results in significant loss of blood volume with much of the haemorrhage not directly amenable to local control.

There are instances when surgery is performed early if there is risk to the eyes or there is an ongoing airway problem.

Surgical procedures

The type of surgery is dictated by the pattern of the deformity. There are three basic operations available.

1. The **Le Fort III** osteotomy involves advancement of all midfacial structures inferior to the frontal bone, i.e. nose, zygomas and maxilla en bloc. This requires a bicoronal flap for access to the nasal root, orbits and zygomatic bones and osteotomies of the nasal root, medial orbital walls, orbital floor, lateral orbital wall, frontozygomatic suture and pterygomaxillary complex. This allows mobilization of the midface. Internal fixation and bone grafts ensure satisfactory healing and stability.
2. Where midface hypoplasia is associated with hypertelorism, a **facial bipartition** may be carried out. It essentially involves a Le Fort III osteotomy to advance the midface and excision of a V-shaped segment of bone from the midline, creating two independent hemifacial segments, which can then be brought together to reduce the interorbital distance.
3. **Monobloc** procedure involves advancement of the forehead and midface at the same time by combining a Le Fort III procedure with FOAR.

Distraction osteogenesis

Conventional surgery involves osteotomy, mobilization and bone movement at one operation. Bone grafting and internal fixation are required to ensure healing and stability. It has the advantage of completing treatment at one operation. However, where the required bone movement is large (greater than 10 mm in the midface) or there is significant scarring of surrounding soft tissues, the desired movement may be difficult or impossible to achieve. The alternative of distraction osteogenesis can overcome these difficulties. Distraction osteogenesis involves initial osteotomy without mobilization and application of an internal or external distraction device, which is activated after a one-week latent period and produces a movement of 1 mm per day. This allows gradual adaptation of a surrounding soft tissue envelope, as well as osteogenesis within the osteotomy gap, allowing for greater movements without the need for bone grafting or internal fixation. Once the desired movement has been achieved, the distractors are left *in situ* for a further eight weeks to allow consolidation of the newly formed bone. Distraction therefore has the advantage of being able to produce larger movements without the requirement for bone grafts or internal fixation. The disadvantages are that the treatment is prolonged, the patient has to tolerate the distraction devices and a second operation is often required for distractor removal. In most craniofacial patients, the advantages of distraction outweigh the disadvantages compared with conventional surgery and, therefore, the majority of midface advancements are now carried out using distraction (see **Figure 78.7**). [***/**/*]

Complications of surgery

Craniofacial surgery carries significant risks. Intubation may be difficult because of abnormal anatomy, there may be coincident systemic abnormalities and the operation may be prolonged.

Complications vary with the extent of the surgery. In the literature, death is reported in 1.5–2 percent of cases as a result of uncontrolled haemorrhage, meningitis, respiratory obstruction or cerebral oedema. The major complications of surgery will be addressed in turn.

BLOOD LOSS

The patient has a small absolute blood volume and there may be appreciable sudden haemorrhage, in particular from the cerebral sinuses. Blood loss varies with the timing and extent of the surgery. In a simple suture release, blood loss is in the region of 100 mL. Blood transfusion is commonplace for infants undergoing this surgery and for older children having more extensive procedures. Risk of viral transmission is low but the consequences are potentially devastating. Avoiding

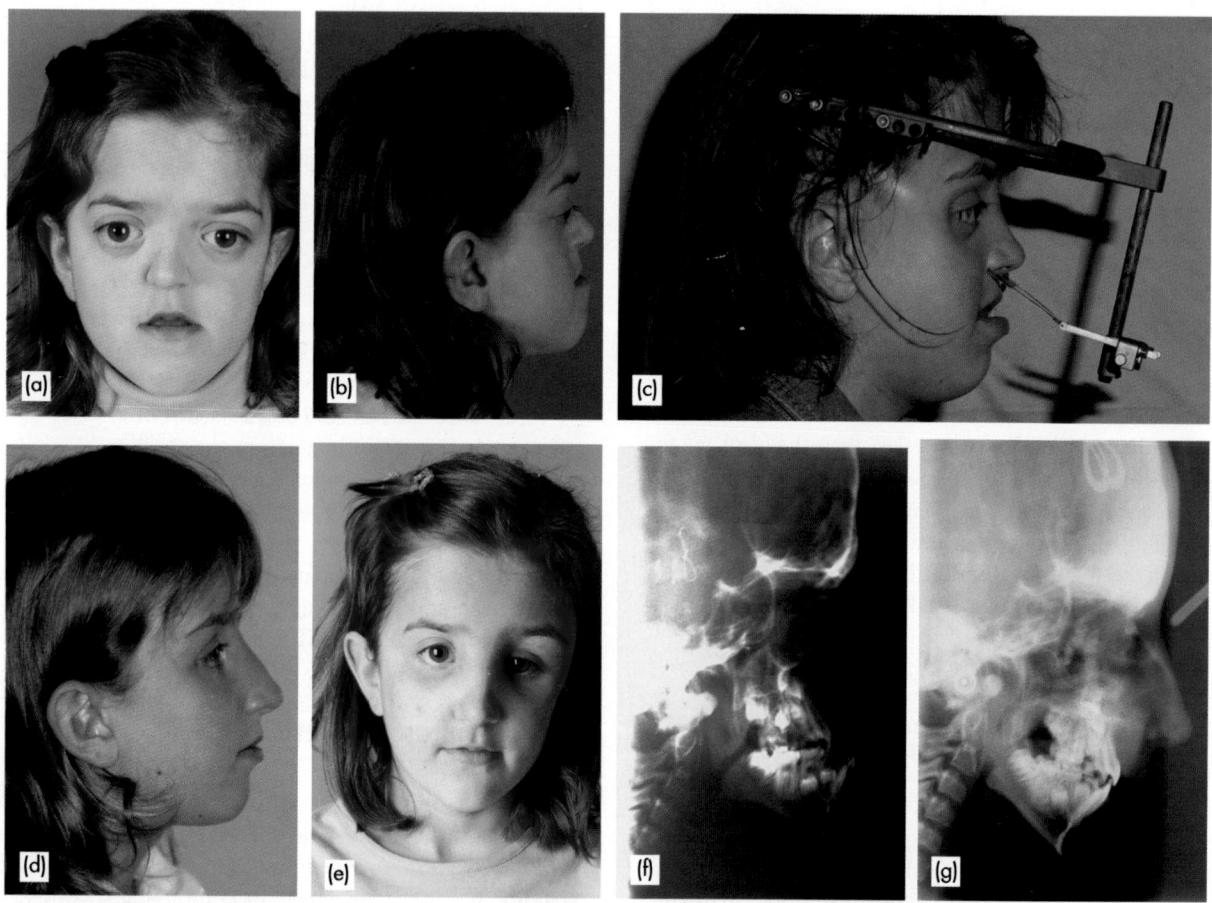

Figure 78.7 Patient with Crouzon syndrome treated with midface distraction. Previously having undergone FOAR at 15 months, now undergoing midface distraction (Le Fort III) at the age of nine years with rigid external distractor (RED frame). The end position is a midface that has been advanced and brought inferiorly.

transfusion is not always possible but providing the intravascular volume is maintained then patients can tolerate low haemoglobin levels.[40, 41]

AIR EMBOLISM

A major danger in craniofacial surgery is ingress and embolization of air through the circulation. This can occur at any stage during surgery, from inserting large-calibre central lines, raising a scalp flap or opening into the major sinuses. In anticipation of blood loss and air embolization, an arterial and central venous line are routinely used along with a number of peripheral lines. A significant air embolism will result in hypotension, bradycardia and cardiac arrest.

CEREBRAL OEDEMA

All measures should be taken to avoid cerebral oedema. Positioning the patient correctly, ensuring correct endotracheal tube positioning and maintaining the correct intravascular fluid replacement are all vital. There should be minimal brain retraction and handling, particularly in cases of pre-existing raised intracranial pressure as this predisposes the patient to a developing cerebral oedema. In many cases the use of systemic steroids (e.g. dexamethasone) may be useful in minimizing cerebral oedema.

DURAL TEAR

Craniofacial surgery such as suturectomy and vault expansion are essentially extra dural procedures. In certain circumstances, for example repeat surgery or when 'copper beating' of the inner table of the skull is present, it may be impossible to avoid tears of the dura mater.

CEREBROSPINAL FLUID FISTULA

Cerebrospinal fluid leak is uncommon but will take place if a dural tear is not either recognized or adequately repaired. CSF can then leak through the scalp wound or, perhaps more commonly, leak into the nose and present as CSF rhinorrhoea. Often this is transient, lasting a few days and sealing spontaneously. Obvious fistulae that fail to resolve must be treated. Of more concern are those that persist unnoticed and lead to infection at some later date.

INFECTION

Infection can occur, particularly in cases involving communication with the paranasal sinuses, and result in meningitis, intracerebral abscess or subdural empyema. Chronic infection can also manifest as lost bone graft or

implants. Treatment of postoperative infection is aggressive but conservative, systemic antibiotics and local debridement but with preservation of bone flaps at all costs.

INTRACEREBRAL/SUBDURAL HAEMATOMA

Haematoma can present in the early postoperative phase with unexpected signs of raised intracranial pressure or 'lateralizing' signs.

BLINDNESS

Surgery around the optic apex and skull base has the potential to damage the optic nerves or tracts. In particular, hypertelorism procedures and monobloc midfacial advancement carry a risk to these structures.

RESTENOSIS

The aim of much cranial vault surgery is to release the prematurely fused sutures, thereby allowing unimpeded brain growth. The gaps created gradually reossify. Occasionally, restenosis takes place, and with continued brain growth there is a rise in intracranial pressure. This tends to happen more commonly in syndromic craniosynostosis than in nonsyndromic cases.

The potential for reossification declines with increasing age of the child. In children over one year of age large bony defects of the skull vault may not close entirely. In some cases it is necessary to repair these defects using a split calvarial bone switch procedure.

Outcome of surgery for craniosynostosis

Measurement of the outcome of craniofacial surgery is difficult and multifaceted. Assessment of the aesthetic result is subjective and surgeons, parents, families and patients may have different perspectives. The various forms of craniosynostosis are heterogenous and even within a single diagnostic category severity is variable. This includes both the skull and facial components of the deformity.[26] A generally accepted, simple and limited outcome measure is the reoperation rate; Whittaker et al.[42] have devised a four-point scale to describe this (see **Table 78.3**). Most of the published follow-up studies, not surprisingly, report a better outcome for single suture compared with multisuture involvement and for nonsyndromic compared with syndromic patients. Major secondary procedures were required in 37 percent of syndromic[43] compared with 13 percent of nonsyndromic patients,[44] while other authors reported reoperation rates of 17 percent for syndromic and 5 percent for nonsyndromic patients.[26]

Aetiology

Unlike hemifacial microsomia, this is an autosomal dominant condition, although approximately 50 percent of cases have no family history and therefore represent new mutations. Its incidence is approximately 1:50,000 live births.[51] Severity is very variable and other family members may be very mildly affected. Intelligence is usually normal. Treacher Collins syndrome is caused by mutations in the gene TCOF1.[52]

Clinical manifestations

The palpebral fissures may be down-slanting, with colobomas of the lower eyelid and eyelash/follicle malformations being common. A hypoplastic midface with poorly developed or absent zygomas, associated with mandibular hypoplasia results in a very characteristic facial appearance (**Figure 78.9**). Features are bilateral and often symmetrical. Bilateral ear abnormalities including hypoplasia, microtia or anotia, hypoplasia or atresia of the external auditory meatus, middle ear anomalies and associated hearing defects are common. There is cleft palate in 35 percent of cases.

Management

Management of the airway in the neonate is required to overcome respiratory obstruction associated with mandibular hypoplasia or choanal atresia. Early feeding difficulties may also need to be addressed. Further management may include repair of cleft palate, provision of bone conducting hearing aid followed by a bone anchored hearing aid, and close monitoring and intervention for speech and language development. Eyelid abnormalities may need surgical correction, hypoplastic or absent zygomas may be reconstructed, usually using calvarial bone grafts, and mandibular deficiency can be corrected with conventional osteotomy or distraction osteogenesis. [**/*]

ENCEPHALOMENINGOCOELE

Encephalomeningocoele represents a herniation of meninges with or without associated brain tissue, through a bony defect of the calvarium. They are a congenital anomaly representing one end of the spectrum of neural tube defects. Its diagnosis is based on the finding of either meninges and CSF (meningocoele) or nervous tissue (encephalocoele) beyond the confines of the calvarium.

The incidence of encephalocoele is reported to be as high as 1:3000 live births in South-East Asia and as low as 1:10,000 live births in North America.[53]

Aetiology

Encephalocoeles may be isolated or associated with other anomalies. When other problems coexist, causes include chromosomal abnormalities, single gene disorders, teratogens and disruptions such as amniotic bands. The primary abnormality in the development of an encephalocoele is a mesodermal defect that develops when the surface ectoderm fails to separate from the neuroectoderm. This results in a defect in the calvarium and dura. Within the calvarium itself there may be failure of bone formation or pressure erosion from expanding intracranial contents. The aetiology of isolated cases is thought to be multifactorial, with both genetic and environmental

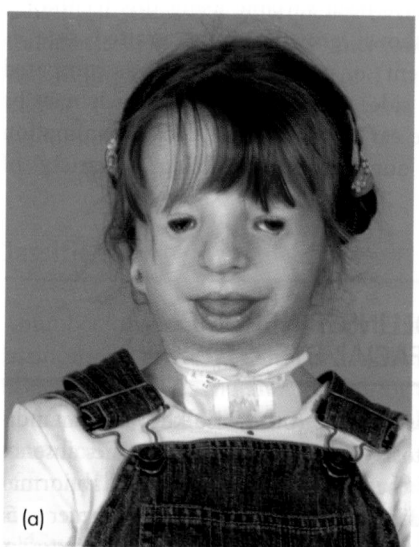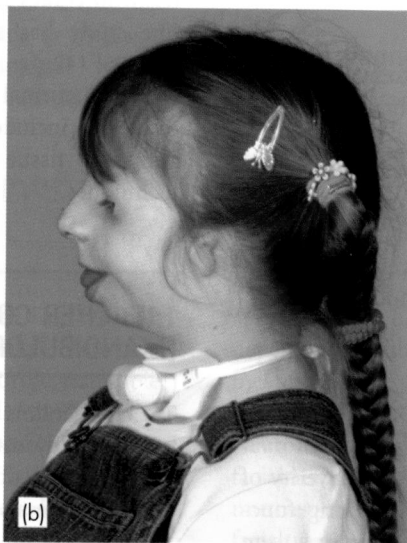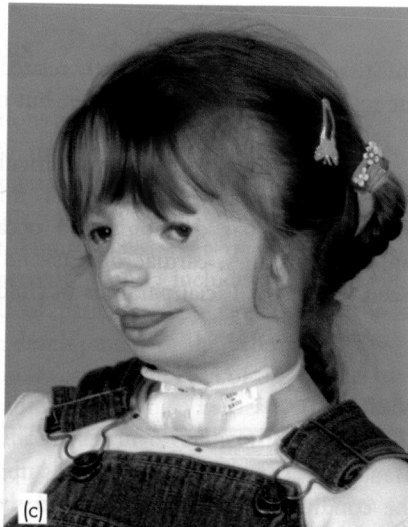

Figure 78.9   Treacher Collins. Abnormalities of zygomatic bones, ears, eyelids and mandible. Note tracheostomy.

factors playing a part. The widespread use of folic acid prior to conception and during pregnancy aims to reduce the frequency of neural tube defects in the general population. After the birth of an affected child, the use of high-dose folic acid prior to and after conception is recommended for subsequent pregnancies.[54]

Diagnosis

Detailed imaging is required for any nasal mass in the neonate prior to biopsy since anterior encephalocoeles may be confused with dermoids, neurofibromas and teratomas. Investigations may include an MR scan demonstrating a mass with intracranial connection and a CT scan demonstrating a bony defect in the calvarium (see **Figure 78.10** and Chapter 82, Nasal obstruction in children).

Classification

There are various classification systems for encephalocoele, based on the contents of the sac, site of the swelling, location of the skull defect and whether the swelling is overt or occult. The most commonly applied system is that relating to the location of the cranial defect. Encephalocoele may be **occipital**, **frontoethmoidal**, **parietal** or **sphenoidal**. Whereas occipital sites are most common in Europe, frontoethmoidal encephalocoeles are most common in Asia.

Management

Indications for treatment are the presence of a CSF leak or high probability of a CSF leak. Functional issues include patency of airway, allowance of normal feeding and

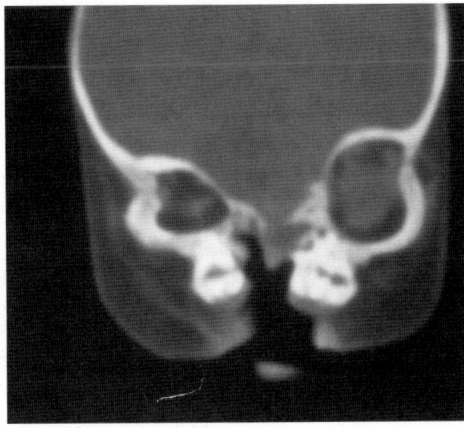

Figure 78.10 CT scan of encephalocoele. Note deficiencies of cranium.

unobstructed vision. In cases where the encephalocoele is large and visible there may be cosmetic issues.

There is an indication for early treatment when a CSF leak is present, otherwise surgery may be deferred until the child is older. This extra time allows the child to grow and further investigations, i.e. imaging, to be performed.

Technique

Principles of treatment involve excision of the hernial sac/reduction of contents, dural repair, bony repair and correction of any associated secondary deformity. Secondary deformity may include hypertelorism, orbital dystopia and destruction of the nasal bridge (in cases of anterior encephalocoeles).

Outcome

The prognosis is dependent upon the contents, site and size of the defect. Some encephalocoeles are incompatible with survival. Approximately three-quarters of the patients with encephalomeningocoele who survive will have a long-term mental deficit, and the best overall prognostic factor is the absence of brain tissue within the herniated sac. Outcome for treated anterior encephalocoeles tends to be better than occipital encephalocoeles, with figures as low as four of 65 with long-term intellectual impairment.[53] [**/*]

CRANIOFACIAL CLEFTS

A craniofacial cleft happens as a result of a failure of fusion of the various embryonic processes from which the craniofacial complex is formed. The exact incidence of craniofacial clefts is not known but can be estimated to be approximately 2:100,000 live births.[55]

Aetiology

The interplay of hereditary and environmental factors is complex and with few total cases is yet to be elucidated in detail. The majority of craniofacial clefts occur sporadically. Many factors have been implicated in the formation of craniofacial clefts, including drugs, e.g. anticonvulsants, corticosteroids and chemotherapeutic agents, radiation, infection, amniotic bands and metabolic disturbances during pregnancy. Craniofacial clefts may also be seen as part of wider syndromes such as Goldenhar syndrome.

Classification

Tessier[56] classified facial clefts according to their relationship with the orbit, nose and mouth. Numbering the clefts from 0 to 14 allowed the lower numbers to relate to the facial clefts and the higher numbers the cranial extensions (See Chapter 77, Cleft lip and palate).

Clinical features

The clinical features are variable depending on the type of cleft. Clefts affecting the interorbital area result in hypertelorism and orbital dystopia (see **Figure 78.11**).

Management

Surgical treatment will depend upon the site, size and severity of the cleft. The extent of the cleft can be variable, ranging from a notch in the soft tissues or soft tissue deficiency, or may be severe affecting skin, bone and brain.

Treatment will usually involve reconstitution of the layers, replacement of missing anatomical structures and normalization of secondary distortions. [**/*]

Frontonasal dysplasia

Frontonasal malformation, or frontonasal dysplasia, is characterized by wide spacing of the eyes (hypertelorism), a characteristic hairline ('widow's peak'), a broad nasal bridge and bifid nasal tip. Occasionally, there may be midline clefting of the skull or palate. Most cases are sporadic and aetiology is unclear.

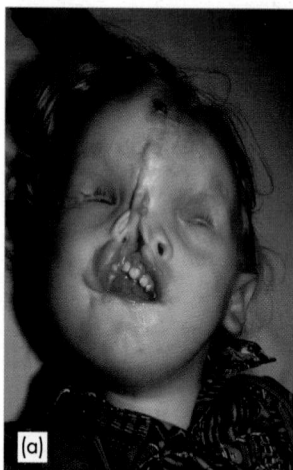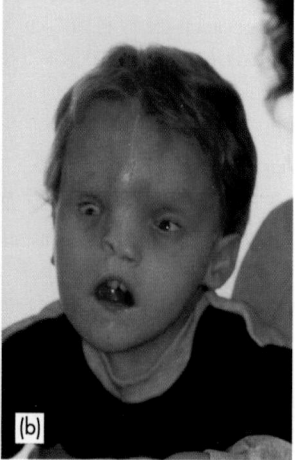

Figure 78.11 Facial cleft. Preoperative and postoperative views (see under Craniofacial clefts above).

Deficiencies in current knowledge and areas for future research

➤ The aetiology of craniosynostosis is still not understood. The complex interactions between the environment, genetic factors and other unknown stimuli are yet to be elicited.

➤ The role of moulding helmets and the possibility of more widespread use of endoscopic techniques for the treatment of craniosynostosis is yet to be confirmed.

➤ The best timing for many of the surgical procedures performed for many of the craniofacial anomalies is still uncertain and is a matter for debate and future research.

REFERENCES

1. National Specialist Commissioning Advisory Group. Annual report 2001–2002. Department of Health. 21–22.
2. Thompson DNP, Hayward RD. Craniosynostosis-pathophysiology, clinical presentation and investigation. In: Choux M, Di Rocco C, Hockley A, Walker M (eds). *Paediatric neurosurgery.* London: Churchill Livingstone, 1999: 275–90.
3. Cohen MM. The aetiology of craniosynostosis. In: Persing JA, Jane JA, Edgerton MI (eds). *Scientific foundations and surgical treatment of craniosynostosis.* Baltimore: Williams and Wilkins, 1989.
4. Cohen Jr MM, MacLean RE. *Craniosynostosis: Diagnosis, evaluation, and management,* 2nd edn. New York: Oxford University Press, 2000.
5. Fryburg J, Hwang V, Lin KY. Recurrent lambdoid synostosis within two families. *American Journal of Medical Genetics.* 1995; **58**: 262–6.
6. Hennekam RCM, Van der Boogaard M. Autosomal dominant craniosynostosis of the sutura metopica. *Clinical Genetics.* 1990; **38**: 374–7.
7. Lajeunie E, Le Merrer M, Bonaiti-Pellie C, Marchac D, Renier D. Genetic study of nonsyndromic coronal craniosynostosis. *American Journal of Medical Genetics.* 1995; **55**: 500–4.
8. Lajeunie E, Le Merrer M, Marchac D, Renier D. Genetic study of scaphocephaly. *American Journal of Medical Genetics.* 1996; **62**: 282–5.
9. Lajeunie E, Le Merrer M, Marchac D, Renier D. Primary trigonocephaly: Isolated, associated and syndromic forms. Analysis of a series of 237 patients. *American Journal of Medical Genetics.* 1998; **75**: 211–5.
10. Harper PS. *Practical genetic counseling,* 6th edn. London: Hodder Arnold, 2004.
* 11. Gorlin RJ, Cohen MM, Hennekam RCM. *Syndromes of the head and neck.* Oxford Monographs on Medical Genetics No. 42, 4th edn. New York: Oxford University Press, 2001.
12. Virchow R. Uber den Cretinismus, namentlich in Franken, and uber pathologische Schadelformen. *Verhandlungen der Physische-Medizinische Gesellschaft Wurzburg.* 1851; **2**: 230–70.
13. Moss ML. The pathogenesis of premature cranial synostosis in man. *Acta Anatomica (Basel).* 1959; **37**: 351–70.
14. Fok H, Jones BM, Gault DG, Andar U, Hayward R. Relationship between intracranial pressure and intracranial volume in craniosynostosis. *British Journal of Plastic Surgery.* 1992; **45**: 394–7.
15. Rich PM, Cox TC, Hayward RD. The jugular foramen in complex and syndromic craniosynostosis and its relationship to raised intracranial pressure. *American Journal of Neuroradiology.* 2003; **24**: 45–51.
16. Eide PK, Helseth E, Due-Tonnesen B, Lundar T. Assessment of intracranial pressure. *Pediatric Neurosurgery.* 2002; **37**: 310–20.
17. Thompson DN, Harkness W, Jones B, Gonsalez S, Andar U, Hayward R. Subdural intracranial pressure monitoring in craniosynostosis: its role in surgical management. *Child's Nervous System.* 1995; **11**: 269–75.
18. Gault DT, Renier D, Marchac D, Jones BM. Intracranial pressure and intracranial volume in children with craniosynostosis. *Plastic and Reconstructive Surgery.* 1992; **90**: 377–81.
19. Whittle IR, Johnston IH, Besser M. Intracranial pressure changes in craniostenosis. *Surgical Neurology.* 1984; **21**: 367–72.
20. Tamburrini G, Di Rocco C, Velardi F, Santini P. Prolonged intracranial pressure monitoring in non-traumatic paediatric neurosurgical diseases. *Medical Science Monitor.* 2004; **10**: 53–63.
21. Thompson DN, Harkness W, Jones BM, Hayward RD. Aetiology of herniation of the hindbrain in craniosynostosis. An investigation incorporating intracranial pressure monitoring and magnetic resonance imaging. *Pediatric Neurosurgery.* 1997; **26**: 288–95.
22. Tuite GF, Chong WK, Evanson J, Narita A, Taylor D, Harkness WF et al. The effectiveness of papilloedema as an indicator of raised intracranial pressure in children with craniosynostosis. *Neurosurgery.* 1996; **38**: 272–8.
23. Mursch K, Brockmann K, Lang JK, Markakis E, Benke-Mursch J. Visual evoked potentials in 52 children requiring operative repair of craniosynsostosis. *Pediatric Neurosurgery.* 1998; **29**: 320–3.
24. Tuite GF, Evanson J, Chong WK, Thompson DN, Harkness WF, Jones BM et al. The beaten copper cranium: a correlation between intracranial pressure, cranial radiographs, and computed tomographic scans in children with craniosynostosis. *Neurosurgery.* 1996; **39**: 691–9.
25. Govender PV, Nadvi SS, Madaree A. The value of transcranial Doppler ultrasonography in craniosynostosis. *Journal of Craniofacial Surgery.* 1999; **10**: 260–3.
26. Wall SA, Goldin JH, Hockley AD, Wake MJC, Poole MD, Briggs M. Fronto-orbital re-operation in

craniosynostosis. *British Journal of Plastic Surgery*. 1994; **47**: 180–4.

27. Tessier P. Osteotomies totales de la face. Syndrome de Crouzon, syndrome d'Apert:oxycephalies, scaphocephalies, turricephalies. [Total facial osteotomy. Crouzon's syndrome, Apert's syndrome: oxycephaly, scaphocephaly, turricephaly.] *Annales de Chirurgie Plastique*. 1967; **12**: 273–86.

28. Jimenez DF, Barone CM. Role of endoscopy in craniofacial surgery. In: Lin KY, Ogle RC, Jane JA (eds). *Craniofacial surgery: science and surgical technique*. Philadelphia: WB Saunders, 2002: 173–87.

29. Kreiborg S. Crouzon syndrome. *Scandinavian Journal of Plastic and Reconstructive Surgery. Supplementum*. 1981; **18**: 1–198.

30. Tolarová MM, Harris JA, Ordway DE, Vargervik K. Birth prevalence, mutation rate, sex ratio, parents' age, and ethnicity in Apert syndrome. *American Journal of Medical Genetics*. 1997; **72**: 394–8.

31. Cohen Jr MM, Kreiborg S. An updated pediatric perspective on the Apert syndrome. *American Journal of Diseases of Children*. 1993; **147**: 989–93.

32. Wilkie AO, Slaney SF, Oldridge M, Poole MD, Ashworth GJ, Hayward RD *et al*. Apert syndrome results from localized mutations of FGFR2 and is allelic with Crouzon syndrome. *Nature Genetics*. 1995; **9**: 165–72.

33. Muenke AM, Gripp KW, McDonald-McGinn DM, Gaudenz K, Whitaker LA, Bartlett SP *et al*. A unique point mutation in the fibroblast growth factor receptor 3 gene (FGFR3) defines a new craniosynostosis syndrome. *American Journal of Human Genetics*. 1997; **60**: 555–64.

34. Howard TD, Paznekas WA, Green ED, Chiang LC, Ma N, Ortiz De Luna RI *et al*. Mutations in TWIST, a basic helix–loop–helix transcription factor, in Saethre-Chotzen syndrome. *Nature Genetics*. 1997; **15**: 36–41.

35. Wieland I, Jakubiczka S, Muschke P, Cohen M, Thiele H, Gerlach KL *et al*. Mutations of the ephrin-B1 gene cause craniofrontonasal syndrome. *American Journal of Human Genetics*. 2004; **74**: 1209–15.

* 36. Panchal J, Uttchin V. Management of craniosynostosis. *Plastic and Reconstructive Surgery*. 2003; **111**: 2032–48.

37. Jenkins D, Seelow D, Jehee FS, Perlyn CA, Alonso LG, Donnai D *et al*. RAB23 mutations in Carpenter syndrome imply an unexpected role for Hedgehog signaling in cranial suture development and obesity. *American Journal of Human Genetics*. 2007; **80**: 1162–70.

38. Clement R, Nischal K. Simulation of oculomotility in craniosynostosis patients. *Strabismus*. 2003; **11**: 239–42.

39. Somani S, Mackeen LD, Morad Y, Buncic JR, Armstrong DC, Phillips JH *et al*. Assessment of extra-ocular muscles position and anatomy by 3-dimensional ultrasongraphy: a trial in craniosynostosis patients. *Journal of AAPOS*. 2003; **7**: 54–9.

40. Harrop CW, Avery BS, Marks SM, Putnam GD. Craniosynostosis in babies: complications and management of 40 cases. *British Journal of Oral and Maxillofacial Surgery*. 1996; **34**: 158–61.

41. Meyer P, Renier D, Arnard E. Blood loss during repair of craniosynostosis. *British Journal of Anaesthesia*. 1993; **71**: 854–7.

42. Whitaker LA, Bartlett SP, Schut L, Bruce D. Craniosynostosis: an analysis of the timing, treatment and complications in 164 consecutive patients. *Plastic and Reconstructive Surgery*. 1987; **80**: 195–212.

43. McCarthy JG, Glasberg SB, Cutting CB, Epstein FJ, Grayson BH, Ruff G *et al*. Twenty year experience with early surgery for craniosynostosis: II. The craniofacial synostosis syndromes and pansynostosis–results and unsolved problems. *Plastic and Reconstructive Surgery*. 1995; **96**: 284–95.

44. McCarthy JG, Glasberg SB, Cutting CB, Epstein FJ, Grayson BH, Ruff G *et al*. Twenty year experience with early surgery for craniosynostosis: I. Isolated craniofacial synostosis–results and unsolved problems. *Plastic and Reconstructive Surgery*. 1995; **96**: 272–83.

* 45. Kearns GJ, Padwa BL, Kaban LB. Hemifacial microsomia: the disorder and its surgical management. In: Ward Booth P, Schendel SA, Hausamen JE (eds). *Maxillofacial surgery*. Philadelphia: Churchill Livingstone, 1999: 917–42.

46. Vento AR, La Brie RA, Mulliken JB. The OMENS classification of hemifacial microsomia. *Cleft Palate-craniofacial Journal*. 1991; **28**: 68–77.

47. Pruzansky S. Not all dwarfed mandibles are alike. *Birth Defects*. 1969; **1**: 120–9.

48. Kaban LB, Moses ML, Mulliken JB. Surgical correction of hemifacial microsomia in the growing child. *Plastic and Reconstructive Surgery*. 1988; **82**: 9–19.

49. Rahbar R, Robson CD, Mulliken JB, Schwartz L, Dicanzio J, Kenna MA *et al*. Craniofacial, temporal bone, and audiologic abnormalities in the spectrum of hemifacial microsomia. *Archives of Otolaryngology – Head and Neck Surgery*. 2001; **127**: 265–71.

50. Molina F. Hemifacial microsomia and Goldenhar syndrome. In: Lin KY, Ogle RC, Jane JA (eds). *Craniofacial surgery: science and surgical technique*. Philadelphia: WB Saunders, 2002.

51. Koppel DA, Moos KF. Treacher Collins Syndrome. In: Ward Booth P, Schendel SA, Hausamen JE (eds). *Maxillofacial surgery*. Philadelphia: Churchill Livingstone, 1999: 943–52.

52. Wise CA, Chiang LC, Paznekas WA, Sharma M, Musy MM, Ashley JA *et al*. TCOF1 gene encodes a putative nucleolar phosphoprotein that exhibits mutations in Treacher Collins syndrome throughout its coding region. *Proceedings of the National Academy of Sciences of the United States of America*. 1997; **94**: 3110–5.

53. Bhagwati SN, Mahapatra AK. Encephalocoele and anomalies of the scalp. In: Choux M, Di Rocco C, Hockley

A, Walker M (eds). *Paediatric Neurosurgery.* London: Churchill Livingstone, 1999: 101–20.

54. [No authors listed]. Prevention of neural tube defects: results of the Medical Research Council Vitamin Study. MRC Vitamin Study Research Group. *Lancet.* 1991; **338**: 131–7.

55. Kawamoto HK. The kaleidoscopic world of rare craniofacial clefts: Order out of chaos. *Clinics in Plastic Surgery.* 1976; **3**: 529–72.

56. Tessier P. Anatomical classification of facial, craniofacial and latero-facial clefts. *Journal of Maxillofacial Surgery.* 1976; **4**: 69–92.

79

Vertigo in children

GAVIN AJ MORRISON

Introduction	1040	Ataxia	1048
Maturation of the vestibular system	1040	Treatments for vertigo	1049
Assessment of the dizzy child	1041	Key points	1049
Causes of childhood vestibular symptoms	1042	Best clinical practice	1050
Vestibular conditions with normal hearing	1042	Deficiencies in current knowledge and areas for future	
Vestibular conditions with associated hearing loss	1045	research	1050
Persistent imbalance and ataxia: central disorders	1048	References	1050

SEARCH STRATEGY

A number of search strategies were employed for this chapter. Using dizziness, vertigo, paediatric/pediatric/child and the major conditions as key words the following databases were consulted: Embase, Ovid Medline (R) and Journals @ Ovid full text subset.

INTRODUCTION

Children do not usually complain of vertigo; history and diagnosis can be elusive. Owing to this, the pattern of symptoms in the very young has a wide differential diagnosis. Once middle ear disease and congenital or hereditary sensorineural conditions have been excluded, a large percentage will have dizziness associated with migraine. Posterior fossa neurological disease should be considered; in older children, adult causes of vertigo may be seen. Reassurance that the prognosis is favourable, and antihistamines such as cinnarizine or, if appropriate, antimigraine treatments are usually effective.

MATURATION OF THE VESTIBULAR SYSTEM

The otic capsule develops early in gestation between the 4th and 12th weeks of intrauterine life. As the vestibular system is phylogenetically older than its auditory counterpart, each stage in development is in advance of the auditory system, and therefore less vulnerable to environmental insult. The semicircular canals have formed from the utricular portion of the otic vesicle by the 30-mm stage, while the cochlear duct has two and a half coils by the 50-mm stage.[1] The vestibular nerve myelinates by 16 weeks in utero. By 24 weeks there is even a primitive vestibulo-ocular reflex present. After birth, at four months of age, the baby can tilt its head to keep it vertical. Bithermal caloric responses can be made in nine-month-old babies if necessary, to measure the vestibulo-ocular reflex. Vestibular nystagmus in children, however, tends to be of a lower frequency and greater amplitude. Maximum slow phase velocity readings are often similar to those in adults, but the normal range for the canal paresis and directional preponderance calculations are wider than that seen in adults. Congenital nystagmus resultant from macular visual loss differs however. [***]

Infantile reflex responses and motor milestones

The Moro response comprises a sudden bilateral extension of the upper limbs evoked by sudden jarring of the cot or dropping the head backwards by a few centimetres. This response is present in normal children at birth, and disappears by the sixth month. The secondary inherent responses are righting responses and protective reactions. From four months, the infant will tilt the head to maintain it vertical if the trunk is tilted through 30°. The ages of sitting unsupported, crawling and walking, bear some relation to vestibular function but also depend upon neurodevelopment. Vision also plays an important part in postural control.

ASSESSMENT OF THE DIZZY CHILD

Symptoms of vertigo in children

Childhood vertigo results from a mismatch of information from the three different sensory systems: vestibular, visual and proprioceptive. Vertigo, however, is much more difficult to recognize in babies and children than in adults; children are not able to describe what they are experiencing and may present with other somatic symptoms such as cowering in the corner of the cot, falling to the ground crying, burying their head in their hands and vomiting. Interestingly, children born with a congenital lack of normal vestibular function often have no balance disturbance at all. Vision remains by far the most important sense for locomotor and balance acquisition.

It is helpful to direct the history taking with a number of principal and most likely diagnoses in mind. In the paediatric age group the principal conditions to consider are:

- benign paroxysmal vertigo of childhood;
- basilar migraine;
- epilepsy;
- central causes of ataxia and loss of balance;
- vestibular neuronitis;
- BPPV;
- adult causes, e.g. Menière's disease.

A more complete list appears in **Table 79.1**.

The presentation of vertigo varies quite dramatically according to the age of the child. While it is possible for two year olds to experience acute vertigo, young children cannot describe this, and may even present with torticollis. If there is a delay in motor milestones, children may present with poor balance or falling; this can also be associated with simple conditions such as 'glue ear'. By five years of age, short-lived dizzy episodes can be described, the common cause being benign paroxysmal vertigo (BPV) of childhood. By the teenage years, migrainous vertigo, psychogenic vertigo and the adult vertiginous conditions are much more common.

History taking

It is helpful to establish the nature of the dizziness, whether it is true vertigo, loss of balance or a light-headed faint feeling. The duration and periodicity can be useful guides as may precipitating factors such as head or neck injury.

Table 79.1 Causes of childhood vestibular symptoms.

Conditions with hearing loss	Conditions with normal hearing
OME	Motion sickness
Suppurative ear disease	BPV of childhood
Cholesteatoma with fistula	Basilar migraine
Temporal bone trauma	Seizure disorders
Barotraumatic perilymph fistula	BPPV
Menière's disease	Post-traumatic vertigo
Post-traumatic vertigo	Viral labyrinthitis or neuronitis
Enlarged vestibular aqueduct syndrome	Posterior fossa tumours
Other congenital temporal bone anomalies, e.g. CHARGE association	Cardiac causes: syncope and arrhythmias
	Acute poisoning
Dehiscent superior semicircular canal syndrome	Multiple sclerosis and Lyme disease
Drug-induced ototoxicity	CNS infections: Coxsackie A and B, echovirus encephalitis or HIV infection
Congenital syphilis	
Herpes zoster oticus	Meningitis: viral or bacterial
Congenital CMV infection	Chiari malformations
Metabolic conditions: Hurler's syndrome, hypothyroidism	Hereditary cerebellar ataxias
	Acute cerebellar ataxia
Usher's syndrome	

The presence of frequent headaches and whether they occur with vertigo or at other times is important. Associated vomiting may be an indication of an acute true vertigo, a migraine phenomenon or the presence of raised intracranial pressure. Associated hearing loss, otalgia or otorrhoea are important. It can be helpful to categorize childhood dizziness into conditions with normal hearing and those with associated deafness (**Table 79.1**).

A neurological history is helpful, specifically if there is anything to suggest temporal lobe seizures, visual or olfactory hallucinations. The developmental history, in terms of the motor milestones, or any regression should be ascertained. The presence of a recent pyrexial illness, the drug history both current, past and, indeed, *in utero* can be important, and various sorts of poisoning should be borne in mind in the child who becomes acutely ill with vertigo and may have ingested something while playing. In the ill febrile child a range of serious infectious diseases should be considered. In a slightly older child, it may be more apparent that the problem is one of fainting or hyperventilation, or that there are cyanotic attacks or palpitations in association with the dizziness.

The family history is relevant, especially one of maternal migraine, familial sensorineural deafness or neurofibromatosis type 2 (NF2).

Examination of the dizzy child

The routine paediatric examination will include otoscopy. Facial nerve function, tongue movements and the gag reflex should be checked. It is important to look at eye movements and, in particular, to search for nystagmus, which can be unmasked with the use of Frenzel glasses. The standard clinical balance assessments can be undertaken, for example Romberg's test, Untenberger's stepping test and the tandem heel-toe gait. It is helpful to make this fun for the child by introducing games, such as hopping and kicking a football, to assess balance function better. Optokinetic nystagmus may be viewed by watching a rotating drum, and a marked directional preponderance may be diagnosed. Dix-Hallpike positional testing should also be undertaken (see Chapter 240b, Evaluation of balance).

Cerebellar ataxia is seen on heel-toe tandem gait with dysmetria, but with normal ranges of lower limb motion and unchanged gait velocity and stride length. Characteristically, gait is wide based with dyssynergia and dysrhythmia, and balance is poor.[2]

Investigations

Audiometry is mandatory. This should comprise a pure tone audiogram or alternative threshold assessment, such as visual reinforcement audiometry, if the child's age or development demands it. Objective testing with brainstem auditory-evoked responses may be indicated. Tympanometry should also be undertaken.

Routine blood tests to exclude anaemia or other blood dyscrasias are worthwhile. The white cell count and inflammatory markers (erythrocyte sedimentation rate or C-reactive protein) may give a clue to an infective condition which could have led, for example, to cerebellar encephalitis. Serology should exclude congenital syphilis, and human immunodeficiency virus (HIV) disease might be considered.

Depending on the history and the level of concern, other investigations might include formal bithermal caloric testing with video-nystagmography or electronystagmography recordings.

Imaging the head and inner ears with magnetic resonance (MR) scanning and/or a high resolution computed tomography (CT) scan for the bony labyrinth and temporal bones will be indicated in selected children. For example, reassurance that there is no space-occupying lesion in a child with headaches and vertebrobasilar migraine or defining an enlarged vestibular aqueduct in association with sensorineural hearing loss could be important. If the diagnosis is clinically obvious however, then it is unnecessary to undertake brain scanning.

Where the history indicates it, referral for an electroencephalogram (EEG) and neurological opinion or for an electrocardiogram and cardiac review may have to be considered. [*]

CAUSES OF CHILDHOOD VESTIBULAR SYMPTOMS

The diagnostic flow chart (**Figure 79.1**) summarizes the diagnostic process in managing the child with vestibular symptoms. The conditions are discussed in more detail below.

VESTIBULAR CONDITIONS WITH NORMAL HEARING

Table 79.1 lists most of the conditions that can present with childhood vertigo, dizziness or balance problems. Although the differential diagnosis is extensive, in over half the children who present to the paediatric otolaryngologist with dizziness or disequilibrium, the cause will be otitis media with effusion (OME or 'glue ear'), BPV of childhood or dizziness as a migraine phenomenon.[3] A further study indicates the most common causes for vertigo in children to be migraine in 31 percent and BPV of childhood in 25 percent.[4] Other less frequent causes include trauma with deafness, delayed endolymphatic hydrops, benign positional vertigo and, more rarely, cerebellopontine angle tumour, seizures, acute vestibular neuritis or juvenile rheumatoid arthritis. In this study,

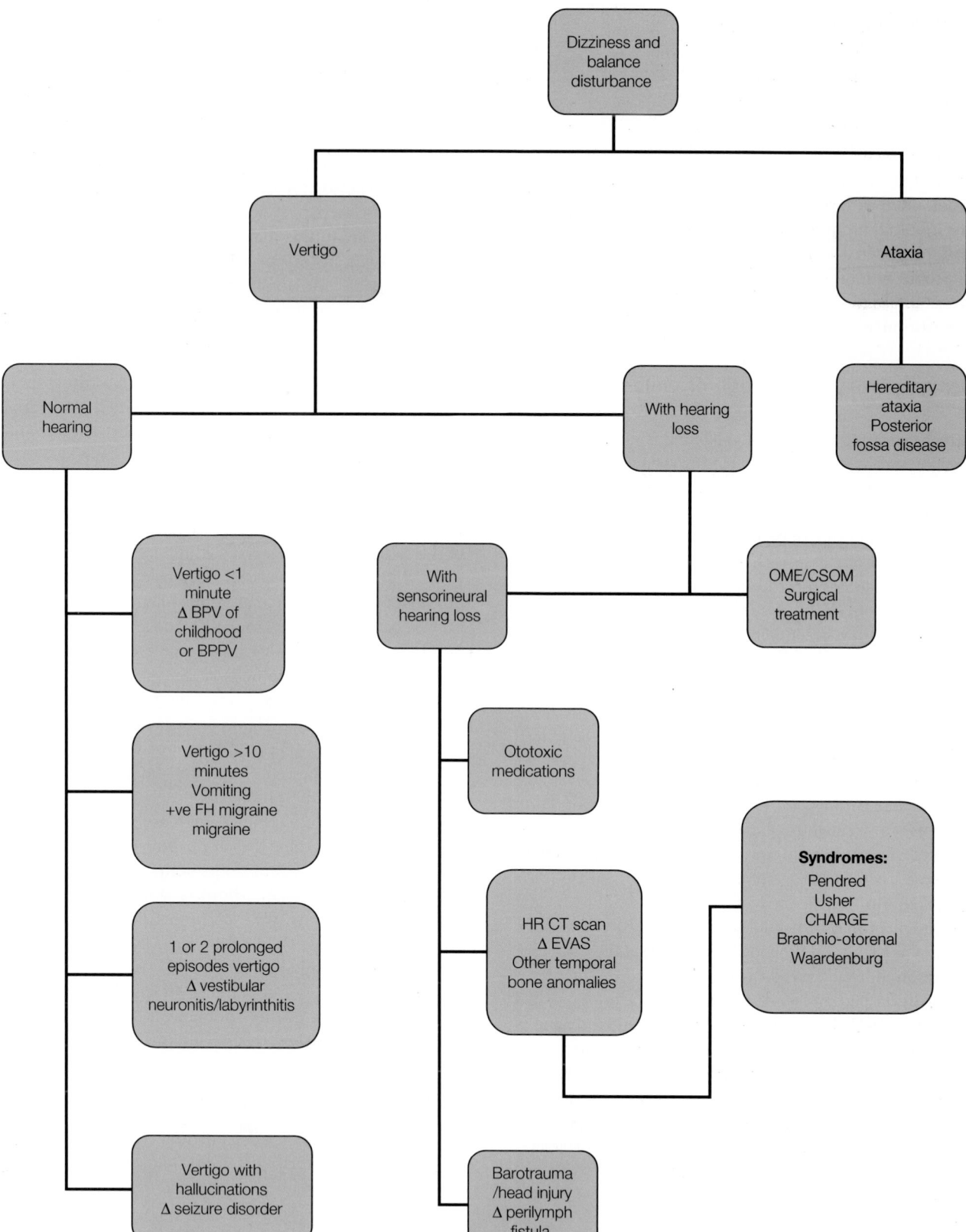

Figure 79.1   Diagnostic flow chart for balance disturbances in children.

abnormalities were found in hearing in 24 percent, in positional testing in 5 percent, in 11 percent of bithermal caloric tests, and in 65 percent on rotational chair testing.[4]

Motion sickness

Motion sickness is caused by a conflict in the kinetic input, often with an excessive vestibular stimulation. Girls are more commonly affected than boys and it tends to settle at puberty. Interestingly, motion sickness can occur in people with blindness, but can also be caused by purely visual stimulation. There is an association with migraine and vestibular dysfunction.[5]

Benign paroxysmal vertigo of childhood

Benign paroxysmal vertigo of childhood is not a positional vertigo and is quite different from benign paroxysmal positional vertigo (BPPV). It occurs in children who are aged four or over, with no obvious precipitating factors. It is a very frequent cause of paediatric dizziness, being found in 35 percent of children with dizziness in one series.[6] The child experiences short-lived acute vertigo for 30–60 seconds. He or she may fall or hold onto something suddenly and cry, becoming pale and sweaty. There is then a rapid return to complete normality a few minutes later. Nystagmus is present during attacks which are recurrent and variable in frequency. They can continue in older children but usually subside. Half of these children go on to develop migraine in adolescence. Most have a family history of migraine. Caloric abnormalities are quite likely to be present if recordings are made. A very similar condition presents in a slightly younger age group as benign paroxysmal torticollis. All torticollis is not related to vertigo however. There is a suggestion that creatinine kinase levels are likely to be elevated in BPV of childhood, and measurement may be helpful in diagnosis.[7] BPV has a very favourable long-term prognosis. In one study the condition had resolved by about eight years of age, and on long-term follow-up 21 percent had developed migraine but none had any vertigo or balance disorder.[8] The differential diagnosis of a child or baby presenting with marked torticollis is large and varied and should include congenital torticollis, paroxysmal torticollis with vertigo, mastoiditis or neck abscess, skull base tumour and neurological extrapyramidal spasmodic torticollis or psychogenic spasmodic torticollis.

Basilar migraine

Migraine is a common multifactorial neurovascular disorder. Several genes have been discovered for migraine; the CACNA1A gene on chromosome 19p13, encoding for part of a neuronal calcium channel is one. Other loci and genes associated with migraine have also been described. Familial hemiplegic migraine has been similarly linked.

Migraine, in general, affects 5 percent of schoolchildren and can occur at any age. Half of children with basilar artery migraine do not have headaches, but when present, the headaches are synchronous with the dizzy attacks in only one-third. Vomiting with attacks is common. The child is likely to be unwell for a few days at a time. If there is no headache the history of some transient neurological disturbance such as hemiparesis, ataxia or facial paresis will indicate the diagnosis. An important clue to this diagnosis is the family history; 85 percent have a history of a first-degree relative suffering from migraine. In one study into migraine-related vestibulopathy, common vestibular test abnormalities included a directional preponderance on rotational testing, unilateral reduced caloric responsiveness and vestibular system dysfunction patterns on posturography. Treatment was usually directed at the underlying migraine condition by identifying and avoiding dietary triggers and prescribing prophylactic antimigraine medications. Symptomatic relief was also provided using anti-motion sickness medications, vestibular rehabilitation and pharmacotherapy directed at any associated anxiety.[9] Review of the symptoms of aura revealed the following: migraine with typical aura in 63.1 percent; migraine with prolonged aura in 4 percent; familial hemiplegic migraine in 6.5 percent, basilar migraine in 15.9 percent; and ophthalmoplegic migraine in 4 percent. The average age at the onset of migraine was 8.8 years and of the appearance of aura 10.9 years. The most frequent aura symptoms were visual. Hemiparaesthesia was seen in 34 percent, vertigo in 14.5 percent, hemiparesis in 13 percent and ataxia in 6.6 percent. Vaproate and flunarizine were effective for migraine prophylaxis.[10]

Electroencephalographic changes are seen during and shortly after a migraine attack but fully resolve in time. EEG, carried out within four hours of the onset of symptoms (initial stage), shows a diffuse polymorphic subdelta-delta activity. EEG, performed 16 hours after the onset of symptoms, shows delta-theta activity predominant over the occipital regions.[11]

Video-nystagmography studies in children with migraine, undertaken during spontaneous nystagmus, gaze nystagmus, eye tracking test, optokinetic and positional nystagmus and caloric testing, showed that all patients with migraine had abnormalities in vestibular testing. Analysis of the results suggested a mainly central localization of vestibular dysfunction.[12]

There is an overlap between children with chronic tension type headache and migraine headache, usually without aura. Nausea, noise and light intolerance are common in these patients but vertigo is unusual.

Vestibular neuronitis

This presents as it does in adults, with acute severe vertigo, nausea and often vomiting but normal hearing.

Children recover more quickly from this disorder than do adults. Half of patients can have repeated episodes, although within a few years attacks become progressively less severe and are likely to cease.

Benign paroxysmal positional vertigo

While in adults BPPV most commonly occurs spontaneously or follows vestibular neuronitis sometime previously, in children it is rare and BPPV is more likely to occur following a head injury or marked whiplash injury. It has a good prognosis. In one study on children's temporal bones in Boston, 12.7 percent of paediatric temporal bones examined had basophilic deposits, many of them with otoconial crystals in the semicircular canals. That is much higher than the incidence in children who had any vertigo symptoms, a temporal bone finding mirrored for this condition in adults.[13] The exact pathogenesis of BPPV is not yet fully explained.

Post-traumatic vertigo

The complaint of dizziness and headaches quite commonly follows head injury in children. The relatively high incidence of these persistent post-traumatic symptoms in children and adolescents presents a diagnostic challenge. It is often difficult to differentiate between functional complaints generated by psychological trauma or compensation seeking and an organic aetiology.[14]

Seizure disorders

Recurrent unprovoked seizures due to epilepsy are either generalized or localized (focal). Seizure disorders can give rise to vertigo in two ways: first, in the aura of a generalized (grand mal) fit; second, as vertiginous epilepsy or vestibulogenic epilepsy. In temporal lobe or occipital lobe focal epilepsy there may be transient loss of consciousness or amnesia; the child may describe the sensation of movement and may have visual or auditory hallucinations. There may be motor or emotional components. Convulsive epilepsies are generally unmistakable. Absence epilepsies may be recognized by the provocation of an episode during hyperventilation. Complex partial seizures in children can be difficult to distinguish from behavioural problems, shuddering attacks, paroxysmal vertigo, breath-holding spells, cardiogenic syncope, night terrors and movement disorders, such as paroxysmal kinesigenic choreoathetosis.[15]

A comparison of the elementary visual hallucinations of 50 patients with migraine and 20 patients with occipital epileptic seizures showed that in epileptic seizures they are predominantly multicoloured with circular or spherical patterns as opposed to the predominantly black and white linear patterns of migraine.

This simple clinical symptom of elementary visual hallucinations may be helpful in distinguishing between classic or basilar migraine and visual partial epileptic seizures, particularly in children.[16] Referral to paediatric neurology is required if vertiginous epilepsy is suspected.

Psychogenic (conversion reaction) vertigo

Psychogenic dizziness should be diagnosed after excluding organic pathology. Sometimes seen in adolescents, more commonly girls, it is said to occur in children who are put under parental pressure to achieve. Recurrent fainting episodes can be seen in adolescence, when the possibility of a cardiac cause should be considered. In surdocardiac syndrome, for example, there is a prolonged QT interval, fainting and a risk of sudden death.

Psychogenic vertigo as a conversion reaction can be seen alone or in association with psychogenic hearing loss. The discrepancy between symptoms and findings in audiometric or vestibular tests is the essential clue for reaching a diagnosis of a conversion disorder. Referral to a psychiatrist may be necessary because many patients have problems in school or at home, and recovery may take a long time.[17] [**/*]

Miscellaneous conditions with normal hearing

There are a number of other conditions which can mimic vertigo that are worth considering in the infant or child with unusual symptoms. These include toddler breath-holding attacks.

POISONING

In a child with dizziness, nausea and vertigo, among other symptoms, acute poisoning from plants, chemicals or drugs should be considered.

ATAXIA

Ataxia and other primarily neurological, hereditary or degenerative conditions are rare. They are discussed in a separate section (see later under Persistent imbalance and ataxia: central disorders).

VESTIBULAR CONDITIONS WITH ASSOCIATED HEARING LOSS

Otitis media with effusion and chronic suppurative ear disease

Glue ear may be detected in the clumsy child with poor balance who is more prone to falls than his siblings or peers. Chronic suppurative otitis media (CSOM) with perforation and infections can influence general balance and CSOM with cholesteatoma carries the possibility of a fistula to the lateral semicircular canal or oval window accounting for dizziness or leading to suppurative labyrinthitis.

Menière's disease

Childhood or adolescent onset of Menière's disease, although uncommon, is well documented. In one series, sporadic Menière's disease began in childhood in less than 3 percent, although, in the less common familial Menière's disease in more than 9 percent, no doubt due to the phenomenon of anticipation. The clinical features are indistinguishable from those in adults; however, early onset tends to be associated with more aggressive disease and a likelihood of relatively early bilateral involvement.[18]

Associated temporal bone abnormalities and hearing loss

In numerous conditions and syndromes there is sensorineural hearing loss with temporal bone anomalies. In only a small number of these conditions are children likely to present with vestibular symptoms. Vision remains the most important special sense in acquiring balance. Children with bilateral vestibular impairment may be delayed somewhat in motor development but rarely present with vertigo. Not surprisingly, in conditions where there is abnormal or absent vestibular development and visual loss, children are more likely to present with balance disturbances. Children with Usher's syndrome have vestibular hypofunction and may therefore have balance difficulties when vision is also impaired.

In CHARGE association (see Chapter 82, Nasal obstruction in children), there are frequently abnormalities, for example a primitive otocyst, and such children may have absent semicircular canals and an aberrant facial nerve. A study from Ann Arbor researched patients with severe sensorineural hearing loss and agenesis of the semicircular canals. Most had CHARGE syndrome, some were nonsyndromic, and one had Noonan's syndrome. They did not present with vertigo.[19] X-linked hereditary deafness is another example in which vestibular symptoms are uncommon despite vestibular hypofunction. Vestibular hypofunction may be present in Down's syndrome.

Enlarged vestibular aqueduct syndrome

Enlarged vestibular aqueduct syndrome is a rare congenital anomaly; vestibular disturbance is uncommon but is seen in 4 percent of children. Fluctuant and progressive

sensorineural hearing loss is the norm and is bilateral in 87 percent of cases. A vestibular aqueduct radiologically wider than 1.5 mm at its midpoint or wider than 2 mm at the operculum is defined as enlarged.[20] Most patients maintain stable hearing in at least one ear over a four-year period. It can occur in nonsyndromic conditions but is also found in 50 percent of patients with Waardenburg's syndrome (types 1 and 2), in which there may be significant widening of the vestibular aqueduct at its midpoint together with other temporal bone anomalies.[21] These children tend to have profound or severe hearing loss. Up to 30 percent of children with Waardenburg's syndrome have vestibular impairment and some experience episodic vertigo. Enlarged vestibular aqueduct syndrome is also seen in Pendred and the branchio-otorenal syndromes, often with an associated Mondini deformity in the former. Patients with enlarged vestibular aqueduct syndrome may show an autosomal recessive inheritance (see Chapter 66, Molecular otology, development of the auditory system and recent advances in genetic manipulation).[22] Avoidance of head injuries is recommended, but may not influence the progression of deafness. The pathogenesis is ill-understood. Surgery to occlude the vestibular aqueduct remains controversial. Conservative management is advised.

The patent cochlear aqueduct

The cochlear aqueduct at its narrowest portion is 0.14 mm wide. It widens as it opens into the posterior fossa with a very variable size at this point. The late Peter Phelps, who had extensive experience in the histopathology of temporal bones, stated that after study of 1400 normal temporal bones and 29 with dysmorphic labyrinths he had failed to show a dilated cochlear aqueduct, and believed that sensorineural deafness attributed to this, in fact, related to defects at the fundus of the internal auditory canal (Phelps P, personal communication).

Dehiscent superior semicircular canal syndrome

Dehiscent superior semicircular canal syndrome has been described but is quite rare. It can be demonstrated on high resolution CT scanning. Typically, vertigo or oscillopsia is evoked by loud noises or by stimuli that result in changes in middle ear or intracranial pressure. The Tullio phenomenon (vertigo in response to sound) and Hennebert's sign (a positive fistula test with a normal middle ear) may therefore be found. Three-quarters of patients also experience chronic dysequilibrium – often the most debilitating symptom.[23] The condition may also present with an apparent conductive hearing loss. Evoked eye movements, by Valsalva manoeuvre against pinched nostrils, tragal compression or sounds over 100 dB at 500–2000 Hz, produce vertical and torsional components. Surgical repair via the middle fossa approach is successful.

Perilymph fistulae

Perilymph fistulae in children are usually seen in association with temporal bone anomalies and pre-existing severe or total hearing loss in the affected ear. They may present with recurrent meningitis or with cerebrospinal fluid (CSF) behind the tympanic membrane. Perilymph fistulae can arise directly from blunt trauma to the middle ear or from temporal bone fractures and, iatrogenically, after ear surgery for CSOM or poststapedotomy. More rarely, marked barotrauma may lead to a fistula from the round or oval windows. In all these situations surgical exploration to seal the fistula is indicated. Spontaneous perilymph fistula in the normal temporal bone however is probably almost never seen.

In the late 1980s there was a vogue for clinically diagnosing a spontaneous perilymph fistula in children and adults who presented with symptoms of hearing loss, vertigo and sometimes tinnitus. These patients were subjected to surgical exploration of the middle ear with sealing of the apparent fistula. In general, the hearing outcomes from surgery did not seem to correlate with the finding of a fistula and, indeed, it can be very difficult at surgery to be sure if there is any real perilymph leak. To address some of the problems inherent in the diagnosis and treatment of perilymph fistulae, records of patients operated on at the House Ear Clinic over 12 years were reviewed retrospectively. Eighty-six patients were surgically explored for fistulae during this period. Thirty-five (40.7 percent) fistulae were found and 51 ears were patched whether fistulae were found or not. Of the 80 patients who were seen for follow-up, 35 (43.8 percent) were subjectively better and 45 (56.2 percent) were the same. Although the number of fistulae found and the number of patients improved were similar, the composition of the two groups was different. On the basis of audiometric results, improvement in hearing happened in only 18.7 percent of patients. None of the demographic factors or diagnostic tests was predictive of either the presence of a fistula or the therapeutic outcome.[24]

Another retrospective study by Bluestone et al. on patients undergoing perilymph fistula repair compared pre- and postoperative hearing levels, vertiginous complaints and recurrences. In 92 percent of ears there was either stabilized or improved hearing and in 3 percent a decrease was noticed, but this was much later and believed not to be related. The results were similar however in the nonperilymph fistula ears, of which 95 percent had stabilized or improved hearing and, again, 3 percent had a much delayed decrease. Of the children with vertiginous complaints before surgery, 91 percent were improved or stable. Only one child felt somewhat

worse, but, as with hearing loss, this was later than six months after the surgery.[25]

In yet another series of cases operated on for suspected perilymph fistula, ears with a surgically demonstrated fistula and sensorineural hearing loss had either flat or downward-sloping audiograms. At follow-up, vestibular symptoms were found to be eliminated or improved in 96 percent of cases with surgically demonstrated fistulae and in 68 percent of cases in which no fistula was detected at tympanotomy, but hearing improved significantly in only one ear (4 percent) of the former group and in five ears (20 percent) of the latter group.[26]

To conclude, perilymph fistulae can be a cause of hearing loss, vertigo or tinnitus and these symptoms may be fluctuant and possibly progressive. There is currently no good diagnostic test for a small fistula. In the paediatric population the most frequent cause is a congenital fistula. Severe or profound hearing loss is, in this instance, always associated with temporal bone anomalies when a peripymph/CSF leak may be present with fluid behind the tympanic membrane. A defect in the stapes and continuity with the fundus of the internal auditory meatus is one such example. This can be found with a true Mondini deformity in which case some hearing from the basal turn of the cochlea is possible. These cases will require surgical exploration and closure of the leak, not to improve or restore hearing but in an attempt to prevent subsequent meningitis.

Traumatic perilymph fistulae with normal temporal bone anatomy are rare. They are described following head injury and penetrating injury to the middle ear with or without temporal bone fracture, but diagnosis is difficult.[27] A persistent perilymph fistula following ear surgery requires re-exploration. Severe barotrauma can also produce a fistula from the round window or oval window. Clinical suspicion will lead to the decision to explore the ear surgically. More obvious bony erosion with fistula is not infrequently encountered in the presence of cholesteatoma. Exploration and closure of the fistula is indicated. Spontaneous perilymph fistula, in the absence of head injury, direct injury or barotrauma can be virtually discounted. [***/**]

Drug-induced vertigo or imbalance

Ototoxic medications, in particular aminoglycosides, can cause marked vestibular dysfunction with acute vertigo at the time of administration or poor balance, ataxia and motor delay. These drugs might have been administered systemically prenatally to the mother or in post-natal life, but occasionally topically in the presence of a chronic perforation or grommets. Fortunately, however, hearing loss from systemic aminoglycosides given to an infant is unusual. Some degree of vestibular loss may be more common and underdiagnosed. Streptomycin and gentamicin are more selectively vestibulotoxic. In one study, children who had previously been treated with streptomycin commonly showed delay in walking.[28]

Antimalarials such as mefloquine, which is only slowly cleared from the body, can cause dizziness or hearing loss. Platinum-based cytotoxic agents can cause ototoxicity, usually high tone hearing loss and tinnitus rather than dizziness.

Miscellaneous conditions with hearing loss

Infectious aetiologies such as congenital cytomegalovirus (CMV) infection can include sensorineural hearing loss with vestibular symptoms and metabolic diseases such as Hurler's syndrome can be seen with a retrocochlear type of hearing loss and vestibular impairment. Herpes zoster oticus can occur in children.

PERSISTENT IMBALANCE AND ATAXIA: CENTRAL DISORDERS

Toddlers may present with imbalance and a delay in motor development, or with a subsequent deterioration in vestibular function. They can have falls, fear of the dark, abnormal gait and vomiting. Primary developmental delay with motor delay and poor balance suggests a congenital or early acquired neurodevelopmental disorder, while regression of balance and locomotor function that was previously acquired indicates the need to exclude a space-occupying lesion such as meningioma or medulloblastoma. A family history of NF2 would raise suspicion. Any severe illness or even major surgery in a baby or smaller child will not infrequently lead to temporary loss of previously acquired skills such as the ability to walk.

ATAXIA

Ataxia is a common mode of presentation of cerebellar, posterior column and vestibular disease in children. The aetiology of ataxia covers a broad range, from infections to rare hereditary metabolic diseases. The importance of recognizing potentially reversible conditions such as vitamin E deficiency and Refsum's disease has been stressed.[29]

Hereditary cerebellar ataxia

Hereditary cerebellar ataxia present with a slowly progressive ataxia although a posterior fossa tumour must be excluded by imaging. Cerebellar disorders display a variety of inherited and sporadic causes. Advances in genetics have led to the successful classification of over 20 forms of autosomal dominant and recessive cerebellar ataxia with variable phenotypes and have shed light on the underlying pathophysiology of many of these

disorders. Successful disease-modifying or symptomatic treatments for these conditions, thus far, have remained limited.[30]

Refsum's disease

Refsum's disease is a disorder of lipid metabolism with pigmentary retinopathy, demyelinating neuropathy, ataxia and hearing loss. There is progressive difficulty in walking which develops between the ages of four and seven years. In some cases the site of the hearing abnormality in Refsum's disease may be 'post-outer hair cells'.[31]

Charcot-Marie-Tooth disease

The most common hereditary degenerative condition is Charcot-Marie-Tooth disease. Inheritance is autosomal dominant. Perineal muscle atrophy is usual, congenital sensorineural deafness is present in some cases and there can be vestibular weakness. These children develop spinal scolioses and pes cavus.[32]

Acute cerebellar ataxia

Acute cerebellar ataxia occurs, usually in the first three years of life, in a child who was previously normal. It follows a viral febrile illness a few weeks beforehand. There is sudden ataxia, and the condition may take a number of months to resolve or leave some permanent sequelae.

Chiari malformations

Type 1 Chiari malformation is characterized by cerebellar tonsil herniation through the foramen magnum. Children most commonly present with bilateral vocal cord paralysis and associated upper airway obstruction but they can also present with positional vertigo and a central type of nystagmus. The condition can be more severe and associated with syringomyelia, in which case there can be neurological improvement after foramen magnum surgical decompression. Type 1 may present to otolaryngologists.

Type 2 Chiari malformation is the same as type 1, except that in addition there is a noncommunicating hydrocephalus and lumbosacral spina bifida. Type 3 can have any of these features but with cervical or occipital bifida. Children with types 2 and 3 have widespread neurological abnormalities and are unlikely to attend ENT clinics.

Miscellaneous conditions

Demyelination can present in post-pubertal children, in which case vertigo is quite commonly seen. NF2 with posterior fossa meningiomas or vestibular schwannoma are occasionally seen in children, and other intracranial posterior fossa lesions such as medulloblastoma may present with ataxia and vomiting.

Infectious causes

Infectious causes include Lyme disease. Viral infections include meningitis, Coxsackie A and B and echovirus; they can involve the central nervous system with vertigo, nystagmus and cerebellar signs. HIV infection is another possible cause. Bacterial infections include primary meningitis, labyrinthitis as a complication of meningitis or CSOM and tertiary or congenital syphilis. [**/*]

TREATMENTS FOR VERTIGO

Medical treatments

The causative condition should be treated directly if possible. The mainstay of treatment, however, is usually an explanation to the parents and the child and reassurance.

Symptomatically, vestibular sedatives can be helpful. Antihistamines such as cyclizine or cinnarizine can be taken for more prolonged attacks. Hyoscine patches have been advocated and domperidone is helpful for associated sickness.

Dopamine antagonists including phenothiazines such as prochlorperazine are effective vestibular suppressants. However, there is a greater risk of extrapyramidal side effects when using phenothiazines, especially in children. They should be avoided in babies under 10 kg. Should these medications lead to extrapyramidal effects such as oculogyric crisis, it can be treated acutely with the antagonist, procyclidine, by injection.

HT3 antagonists such as ondansetron are powerful antiemetics which block serotonin binding at vagal afferents in the gut and in the regions of the central nervous system (CNS) involved in emesis, including the chemoreceptor trigger zone and the nucleus tractus solitarii. Although principally used in postoperative nausea and vomiting or with cytotoxic drug therapy, they may have a role in the vertiginous child, especially if vomiting.

Migrainous vertigo can be treated with metaclopramide, or serotonin 5-HT1 receptor agonists such as sumatriptan. Rizatriptan is reported to be more effective than other drugs of this class and other simple analgesics.[33] Dietary exclusions can be helpful. Preventative measures, if necessary, would be those currently recognized – pizotifen or propanolol – and if those fail, a neurologist might prescribe anticonvulsants.

Menière's disease may be treated with betahistine, a low salt diet and possibly diuretics or intermittently by dehydration therapy such as Glycerol taken orally. Surgery may occasionally be indicated in severe variants of the disease.

The seizure disorders are usually well controlled with anticonvulsants under the paediatric neurologist's guidance.

Physical treatments for vertigo

If there is benign positional vertigo, the Epley manoeuvre (see Chapter 240d, Vertigo: clinical management and rehabilitation) or the Brandt-Daroff exercises can be employed successfully. Other vestibular rehabilitation exercises for children who have suffered unilateral labyrinthine damage might be helpful in achieving full central compensation and in speeding recovery.

Surgery for vertigo

Surgery relates to that indicated for specific underlying conditions. Unilateral glue ear with poor balance can be corrected by insertion of grommets (preferably bilaterally, the contralateral ear as a prophylactic measure).

If there is a perilymph fistula from barotrauma, middle ear or mastoid disease, or following surgery, that should be explored and closed. Likewise, suppurative ear disease and congenital or acquired cholesteatoma will require tympanomastoid surgery.

A perilymph/CSF fistula from congenital temporal bone anomalies should be closed surgically in an attempt to prevent future meningitis.

Childhood-onset Menière's disease tends to run an aggressive course with debilitating bilateral disease later in life. Destructive surgery is not advised at an early stage although endolymphatic sac decompression and drainage may have a role. [**/*]

KEY POINTS

- Vertigo results from a mismatch of three different sensory inputs, i.e. vision, proprioception and the vestibular system.
- Presentation of balance disorders in children differs from that in adults; very young children cannot complain of vertigo.
- Fifty percent of cases of childhood dizziness and imbalance are caused by one of the three most common causes: BPV of childhood, migraine or OME.
- Adult causes of vertigo are seen in older children/adolescents.
- The mainstay of treatment is reassurance; symptomatic control with medication such as cinnarizine or antimigraine treatments is usually effective.

Best clinical practice

✓ A full history, neurotologic examination and audiometry are required in assessing any child with vertigo. [Grade C/D]

✓ Middle ear disease and congenital sensorineural conditions with vestibular deficits should be excluded. [Grade C/D]

✓ Posterior fossa disease must be excluded where there is ataxia. [Grade C/D]

✓ In some cases, a full blood count, inflammatory markers, glucose, creatinine kinase, thyroid function and special serological tests are helpful. [Grade C]

✓ High resolution CT scanning of the temporal bones and an MR brain scan are often indicated for dizziness with hearing loss. [Grade C]

✓ An MR brain scan is indicated for ataxic conditions. [Grade C]

✓ Special vestibular tests including bithermal caloric stimulation and rotational chair testing can be helpful in reaching a diagnosis and planning treatment. [Grade B]

✓ Referral to a paediatric neurologist is recommended if the diagnosis of a seizure disorder or basilar migraine is considered probable. [Grade D]

✓ Treatment should comprise explanation and reassurance about the condition and symptomatic medical treatment for the vertigo. [Grade D]

✓ Surgical treatment is recommended for significant balance disturbance with OME and for CSOM with cholesteatoma as well as for a persistent perilymph fistula from other causes. [Grade D]

Deficiencies in current knowledge and areas for future research

➤ The value of bithermal caloric tests, video-nystagmography and rotational chair tests has not been demonstrated in the varied paediatric population with vertigo.

➤ The benefit of vestibular rehabilitation exercises over encouraging straightforward everyday activities has not been studied in childrens' treatment regimens.

➤ Motion sickness has been subject to observational studies and effects of drug treatments but further research into aetiology and other treatments could be profitable.

➤ The role and efficacy (if any) of HT3 antagonists such as ondansetron in the management of childhood vertigo has not been studied.

REFERENCES

1. Anniko M. Embryonic development of the vestibular sense organs and their innovation. In: Romand R (ed.). *Development of auditory and vestibular symptoms.* London: Academic Press, 1983: 378–423.

2. Stolze H, Klebe S, Petersen G, Raethjen J, Wenzelburger R, Witt K et al. Typical features of cerebellar ataxic gait. *Journal of Neurology, Neurosurgery, and Psychiatry.* 2002; **73**: 310–2.

* 3. Bower CM, Cotton RT. The spectrum of vertigo in children. *Archives of Otolaryngology – Head and Neck Surgery.* 1995; **121**: 911–5.

* 4. Choung YH, Park K, Moon SK, Kim CH, Ryu SJ. Various causes and clinical characteristics in vertigo in children with normal eardrum. *International Journal of Pediatric Otorhinolaryngology.* 2003; **67**: 889–94.

5. Dobie T, McBride D, Dobie Jr. T, May J. The effects of age and sex on susceptibility to motion sickness. *Aviation, Space, and Environmental Medicine.* 2001; **72**: 13–20.

6. Herraiz C, Calvin FJ, Tapia MC, De Lucas P, Arroyo R. The migraine: Benign paroxysmal vertigo of childhood complex. *International Tinnitus Journal.* 1999; **5**: 50–2.

7. Rodoo P, Hellberg D. Creatine kinase MB (CK-MB) in benign paroxysmal vertigo of childhood: A new diagnostic marker. *Journal of Pediatrics.* 2005; **146**: 548–51.

* 8. Lindskog U, Odkvist L, Noaksson L, Wallquist J. Benign paroxysmal vertigo in childhood: A long-term follow-up. *Headache.* 1999; **39**: 33–7.

9. Cass SP, Furman JM, Ankerstjerne JKP, Balaban C, Yetiser S, Aydogan B. Migraine-related vestibulopathy. *Annals of Otology, Rhinology, and Laryngology.* 1997; **106**: 182–9.

10. Bojinova B, Dimova P, Belopitova L. Clinical characteristics, diagnostic and therapeutic approach of migraine with aura in childhood. *Pediatriya.* 2004; **44**: 14–21.

11. Ramelli GP, Sturzenegger M, Donati F, Karbowski K. EEG findings during basilar migraine attacks in children. *Electroencephalography and Clinical Neurophysiology.* 1998; **107**: 374–8.

12. Mierzwinski J, Pawlak-Osinska K, Kazmierczak H, Korbal P, Muller M, Piziewicz A et al. [The vestibular system and migraine in children.] [Polish] Original Title Uklad przedsionkowy a migrena u dzieci. *Otolaryngologia Polska.* 2000; **54**: 537–40.

13. Bachor E, Wright CG, Karmody CS. The incidence and distribution of cupular deposits in the paediatric vestibular labyrinth. *Laryngoscope.* 2002; **112**: 147–51.

14. Eviatar L, Bergtraum M, Randel RM. Post-traumatic vertigo in children: A diagnostic approach. *Pediatric Neurology.* 1986; **2**: 61–6.

* 15. Murphy JV, Dehkharghani F. Diagnosis of childhood seizure disorders. *Epilepsia.* 1994; **35**: S7–17.

16. Panayiotopoulos CP. Elementary visual hallucinations in migraine and epilepsy. *Journal of Neurology, Neurosurgery, and Psychiatry.* 1994; **57**: 1371–4.

17. Seki S, Inukai K, Watanabe K, Takahashi S, Takahashi S. Three child cases of conversion disorders presented with

psychogenic vertigo and gait disturbance. *Equilibrium Research*. 2004; **63**: 346-52.

18. Morrison AW, Johnson KJ. Genetics (molecular biology) and Menière's disease. *Otolaryngologic Clinics of North America*. 2002; **35**: 497-516.

19. Satar B, Mukherji S, Telian SA. Congenital aplasia of the semicircular canals. *Otology and Neurotology*. 2003; **24**: 437-44.

20. Madden C, Halstead M, Benton M, Greinwald J, Choo D. Enlarged vestibular aqueduct syndrome in the paediatric population. *Otology and Neurotology*. 2003; **24**: 625-32.

21. Madden C, Halstead MJ, Hopkin RJ, Choo DI, Benton C, Greinwald JH. Temporal bone abnormalities associated with hearing loss in Waardenburg syndrome. *Laryngoscope*. 2003; **113**: 2035-41.

22. Lasak JM, Welling DB. The enlarged vestibular aqueduct syndrome: Current opinion. *Otolaryngology and Head and Neck Surgery*. 2000; **8**: 380-3.

23. Minor LB. Superior canal dehiscence syndrome. *American Journal of Otology*. 2000; **21**: 9-19.

∗ 24. Rizer FM, House JW. Perilymph fistulas: The House Ear Clinic experience. *Otolaryngology and Head and Neck Surgery*. 1991; **104**: 239-43.

25. Weber PC, Bluestone CD, Perez B. Outcome of hearing and vertigo after surgery for congenital perilymphatic fistula in children. *American Journal of Otolaryngology*. 2003; **24**: 138-42.

26. Vartiainen E, Nuutinen J, Karjalainen S, Nykanen K. Perilymph fistula – A diagnostic dilemma. *Journal of Laryngology and Otology*. 1991; **105**: 270-3.

27. Kazahaya K, Handler SD. Traumatic perilymphatic fistulas in children: Etiology, diagnosis and management. *International Journal of Pediatric Otorhinolaryngology*. 2001; **60**: 147-53.

∗ 28. Camarda V, Moreno AM, Boschi V. Vestibular ototoxicity in children: A retrospective study of 52 cases. *International Journal of Pediatric Otorhinolaryngology*. 1981; **3**: 195-8.

∗ 29. Gosalakkal JA. Ataxias of childhood. *Neurologist*. 2001; **7**: 300-6.

∗ 30. Blindauer KA. Cerebellar disorders and spinocerebellar ataxia. *Continuum: Lifelong Learning in Neurology. Movement Disorders*. 2004; **10**: 154-73.

31. Oysu C, Aslan I, Basaran B, Baserer N. The site of the hearing loss in Refsum's disease. *International Journal of Pediatric Otorhinolaryngology*. 2001; **61**: 129-34.

32. Sabir M, Lyttle D. Pathogenesis of Charcot-Marie-Tooth disease. Gait analysis and electrophysiologic, genetic, histopathologic, and enzyme studies in a kinship. *Clinical Orthopaedics and Related Research*. 1984; **184**: 223-35.

33. Wellington K, Plosker GL. Rizatriptan: an update of its use and management in migraine. *Drugs*. 2002; **62**: 1539-74.

80

Facial paralysis in childhood

SS MUSHEER HUSSAIN

Introduction	1052	Key points	1059
Embryology and applied anatomy of the facial nerve	1052	Best clinical practice	1059
Diagnosis	1054	Deficiencies in current knowledge and areas for future	
Congenital facial paralysis	1055	research	1060
Acquired facial paralysis	1056	References	1060
Idiopathic	1059		

SEARCH STRATEGY

The data in this chapter are supported by a PubMed search using the key words facial paralysis, otitis media, congenital facial paralysis, ear trauma, facial nerve injury, Wegener's, Bell's palsy and parotid surgery. The focus was restricted to neonates and children.

INTRODUCTION

Bell's palsy remains the most common aetiology for facial paralysis in children[1] although it is much less common than in adults. May et al.,[2] in their study of 170 patients aged from birth to 18 years, found the following aetiology for facial paralysis: Bell's palsy (42 percent), trauma (21 percent), infections (13 percent), congenital (8 percent) and neoplasm (2 percent).

Bell's palsy in children is considered to have a better prognosis than in adults, regardless of treatment.

EMBRYOLOGY AND APPLIED ANATOMY OF THE FACIAL NERVE

Knowledge of the embryology and developmental anatomy of the facial nerve allows for a clear understanding of the various anomalies and clinical presentations of disorders of the facial nerve. The reader is referred to Chapter 65, Head and neck embryology.

By the third week of embryonic development the facioacoustic crest is visible on the dorsolateral aspect of the hindbrain just cranial to the otic placode. The otic placode forms the otocyst giving rise to the membranous labyrinth in the fourth week and the facial nerve becomes distinct. The geniculate ganglion has formed by the fifth week (**Figure 80.1**). The facial nerve divides into its main trunk descending into the second branchial arch and the chorda tympani, which being the pretrematic branch curves cranially into the first branchial arch. A pretrematic branch of a cranial nerve is one that supplies the arch preceding the arch to which the cranial nerve belongs. The chorda tympani and the main trunk of the facial nerve are equal in size at this stage. Malformations of the branchial arches are associated with anomalies of the chorda tympani, such as elongation of the posterior canaliculus, reduplication and low position of the nerve.[3, 4]

The facial nucleus is formed by neuroblasts in the pons, with the sixth nerve nucleus in close proximity. As the brain develops and the pons expands, the sixth nucleus ascends so that the facial nerve fibres have to whirl round the sixth nucleus thus forming an internal genu. Clinically, therefore, an inflammatory or vascular event in this part of the brain will necessarily involve both these nerves. In developmental anomalies such as Mobius syndrome there is agenesis of the facial nucleus and, among other defects, there is also agenesis of the sixth nucleus.[5]

The geniculate ganglion has a separate origin from the facial nerve.[6] It is well defined by the seventh week and gives rise to the sensory roots that form the nervus intermedius. As the main facial trunk descends down the second branchial arch there is caudal movement of the first arch due to rapid expansion, producing the horizontal segment and the first and second genu of the nerve, with the greater superficial petrosal nerve acting as an anchor. Proctor and Nager's seminal papers[7, 8] describe the many variations encountered in the vertical segment of the facial nerve including a bipartite nerve, an anteriorly displaced nerve or one with a posterior hump. Failure to appreciate an anomaly of the facial nerve during surgery can have serious consequences.[9, 10, 11, 12]

Conditions related to malformations of the first or second arch, such as Treacher Collins and Goldenhar

syndromes, will usually mean that the facial nerve is abnormal too. At birth, the normal temporal bone has no mastoid process and an incomplete tympanic ring. The 'u-shaped' tympanic ring has nodular prominences on each arm, which separate the annulus from the future external canal and the foramen of Huschke (**Figure 80.2**). By the end of the first post-natal year these processes fuse, lengthening the canal (**Figure 80.3**). The foramen usually closes some time later. In the newborn the chorda tympani and the facial nerve may exit through the stylomastoid foramen. The mastoid process and external auditory canal are undeveloped so the nerve is very superficial.

The mastoid process develops and reaches adult proportions by the age of 12 years. In neonates and small children the second genu of the facial nerve is more acute and courses more laterally. The most common variation in the course of the facial nerve canal involves the tympanic segment; the bony wall may be dehiscent in 35–55 percent of the population, particularly above the oval window.[7, 8, 13, 14] Acute suppurative otitis media in neonates and children may therefore present with facial paralysis from neuropraxia or bacterial infiltration of the

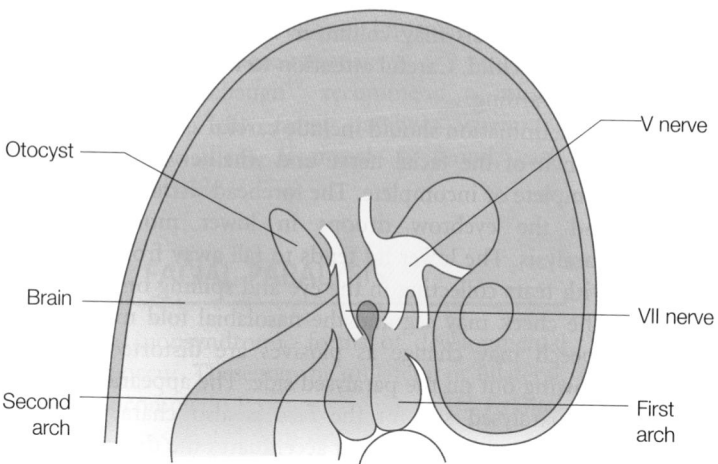

Figure 80.1 The foetal head aged five weeks.

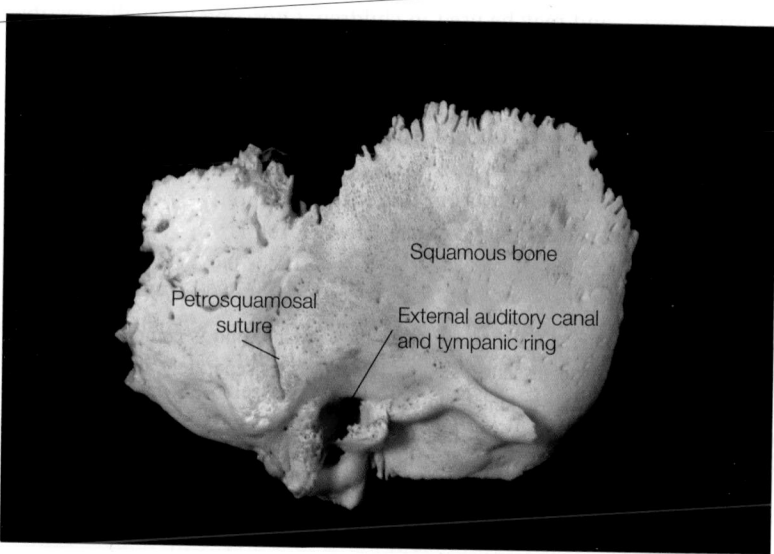

Figure 80.2 The neonatal temporal bone.

ACQUIRED FACIAL PARALYSIS

Infections

ACUTE OTITIS MEDIA

Acute otitis media in neonates and children can present with facial paralysis. This is usually incomplete but the paralysis may progress in the first two to three days of onset. There is suppuration in the middle ear behind an intact tympanic membrane. This may appear red and bulging. The child may be toxic but is typically not unwell. In some cases, where antibiotic have been given, the signs of acute inflammation may not be pronounced. The underlying pathology may be an erosion of the bony Fallopian canal or congenital dehiscence and nerve inflammation. Spread along structures such as the stapedial tendon, chorda tympani or the posterior tympanic artery have been suggested. Moreano et al.[14] studied 1000 temporal bones and noted at least one facial canal dehiscence in 56 percent of temporal bones with the most common site of dehiscence being the oval window area. They introduced the concept of microdehiscence of the facial canal and found this in one-third of the temporal bones. The most common pathogen in middle ear cleft infections in children is pneumococci (80 percent).[32] A wide myringotomy and systemic antibiotics are the initial treatment (**Figure 80.4**). [Grade D] If mastoiditis is suspected, a CT scan and a cortical mastoidectomy may be needed. There is usually full recovery of facial nerve function.

CHRONIC OTITIS MEDIA

Facial paralysis in chronic otitis media is very uncommon. Sheehy et al.[33] report 11 cases of facial paralysis out of 1024 patients with chronic middle ear disease and cholesteatoma. Complications of chronic middle ear disease including facial paralysis are more common in the developing world.[34]

LYME DISEASE

This multisystem disease is caused by the tick-borne spirochaete *Borrelia burgdorferi*.[35] A skin lesion appears after an incubation period of one to four weeks. Ipsilateral or bilateral facial paralysis may appear weeks or months later in 11 percent of cases.[36] A report from Connecticut, an endemic area, describes Lyme disease as the cause of more than 50 percent of facial paralysis in children.[37] Serological tests with enzyme-linked immunosorbent assay to detect immunoglobulin G and M antibodies are used for diagnosis. Doxycycline is the oral antibacterial of choice, while amoxicillin and cefuroxime are alternatives that may be preferred in young children. Tick avoidance has long been the mainstay for preventing Lyme disease.[38]

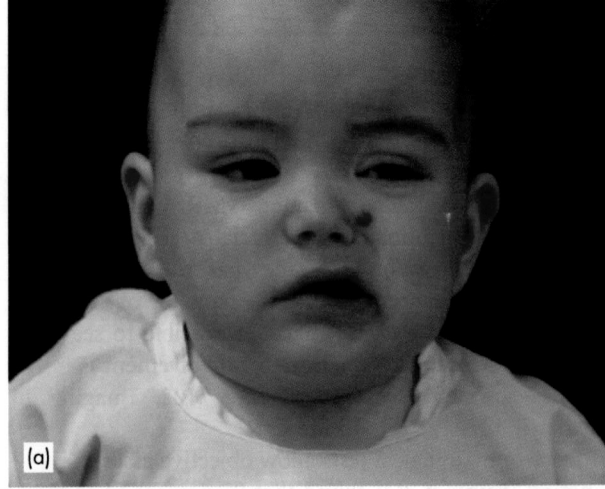

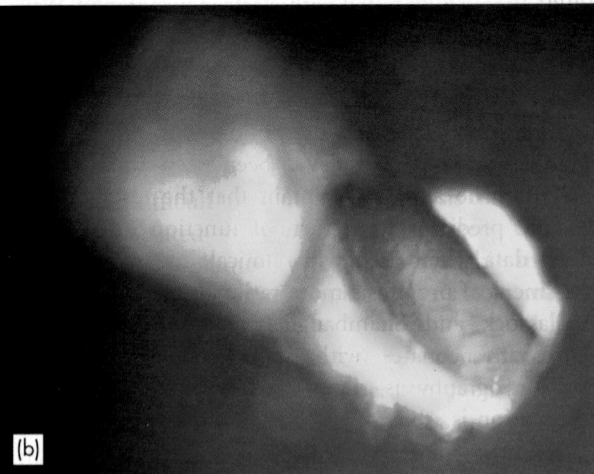

Figure 80.4 (a) Facial paralysis in a neonate from acute otitis media; (b) the state of the eardrum.

VIRAL INFECTIONS

Recrudescence of herpes zoster virus in the geniculate ganglion leads to the classical syndrome of Ramsay Hunt. The disease is uncommon in children. Hato et al.,[39] in a retrospective study of 52 children with Ramsay Hunt syndrome, found that facial paralysis was milder, complete recovery of the function more likely (79 percent) and associated cranial neuropathies less common in children than in adults. The timing of vesicle appearance tended to be delayed in children. The disease was rare in preschool children but relatively more common in older children. Treatment with oral or intravenous acyclovir and prednisolone has been recommended.[40, 41] Facial paralysis has been noted in Epstein–Barr virus infection and this may be bilateral in 40 percent of cases.[42] Facial palsy is an early ENT manifestation of human immunodeficiency virus infection and is seen in 11 percent of cases.[43]

TUBERCULOSIS

The presence of facial paralysis with purulent otorrhoea that does not respond to conventional antibiotics should alert the physician to the possibility of tuberculosis. Antituberculous chemotherapy early in the disease may reduce the need for radical surgery.[44, 45] CT scan is reported to be of value in the diagnosis of facial paralysis due to tuberculosis.[46]

Traumatic

BLUNT TRAUMA

Perinatal trauma

Birth-related trauma is a known cause of facial paralysis. The incidence of facial palsy in the newborn is 1.8 in 1000, the majority associated with forceps delivery.[47] In their report on neonatal facial paralysis, Smith et al.[48] found 74 of 95 cases to be secondary to trauma associated with pregnancy and delivery. The diploic bone of the infant mastoid process, the paper-thin bone covering the facial nerve and the very superficial position of the marginal mandibular branch over the mandible all add to the problem. The pressure of the mother's sacrum on the infant facial nerve may also contribute.

In differentiating between congenital and perinatally acquired facial paralysis the history and physical examination usually suffice. A history of forceps delivery, a baby weighing over 3.5 kg, a primipara mother, prolonged labour and the absence of associated craniofacial anomalies point to perinatal trauma as the cause. The presence of bruising on the side of the face and the mastoid region are suggestive of birth trauma as are other complications associated with birth.

Electrophysiological tests may be used to aid diagnosis; voluntary action potentials on electromyography indicate muscle innervation. Electromyography performed after ten days of paralysis will show fibrillation or polyphasic potential in traumatic cases and absent electrical activity in congenital facial paralysis.[49] A CT scan may show a concealed fracture of the temporal bone.

Temporal bone fracture

An injury to the skull may cause temporal bone fracture. The fracture may be longitudinal, transverse or a combination of both. Classically, longitudinal fractures cause conductive hearing loss whereas transverse fractures usually cause irreversible sensorineural deafness. One-third of fractures are transverse and these have associated facial paralysis in 50 percent of cases. Longitudinal fractures are more common and although the incidence of facial paralysis is less (20 percent), longitudinal fractures cause more facial paralysis than transverse fractures. As discussed previously (see Embryology and applied anatomy of the facial nerve) the greater superficial petrosal nerve in the region of the geniculate ganglion tethers the facial nerve. In head injury the sudden deceleration creates a shearing force on the facial nerve leading to damage. Lee et al.[50] reviewed 72 children with

temporal bone fractures ranging from 6 months to 14 years of age, with a bimodal distribution with peaks at 3 and 12 years of age. The most common causes of fractures were motor vehicle accidents (47 percent), falls (40 percent), biking accidents (8 percent) and blows to the head (7 percent). Common presenting signs and symptoms[51] include hearing loss (82 percent), haemotympanum (81 percent), loss of consciousness (63 percent), intracranial injuries (58 percent), bloody otorrhea (58 percent), extremity fractures (8 percent) and facial nerve weakness (3 percent). The diagnosis of temporal bone fractures is best made clinically and radiographically. The early care of temporal bone fractures is directed toward the treatment of cerebrospinal fluid otorrhoea and immediate-onset facial paralysis. The delayed care is primarily concerned with hearing rehabilitation.[52] Surgical exploration as an option remains controversial, with no randomized controlled study available. It does seem reasonable, however, to explore when nerve entrapment is suspected or where the integrity of the nerve is compromised.

PENETRATING TRAUMA

Injury to the face may damage the facial nerve or one or more of its branches. This may be the result of falling on to a sharp object or a dog bite. The wound needs to be explored and the degree of damage established. This will allow repair with the functioning distal branches in a clean wound. Local control of infection should precede repair in a contaminated wound. [**/*] [Grade C/D]

IATROGENIC TRAUMA

Ear surgery

Mastoid surgery carries a higher risk of injury to the facial nerve in children, even in experienced hands. This is because of the absence of the mastoid process in small children and the superficial position of the facial nerve, which is at risk from a low incision. The operating space within the mastoid cleft is small and if, in addition, an anomaly is encountered, the problems multiply. The injury may not be identified at the time of surgery and may become obvious when the patient is awake.[53] The most common site of injury is the tympanic segment and the second genu of the nerve.[53, 54] Anomalies of the facial nerve encountered in patients with congenital malformation of the middle ear include displacement of the nerve and lack of bony cover.[10] A low-lying tegmen in a sclerotic mastoid is particularly serious and requires skill to protect the nerve at the second genu when drilling in this restricted area. The presence of granulating disease in revision surgery may obscure the usual landmarks and put the nerve at risk. Erosion of the bone by cholesteatoma and its spread to the supra tubal recess[55] puts the geniculate ganglion and the first genu of the facial nerve at risk of injury during disease clearance in the anterior attic. In patients with atresia or stenosis of the external canal, the facial nerve may be damaged in its vertical segment owing to the vertical segment being relatively lateral to the tympanic annulus. Intraoperative monitoring is advisable. [Grade D] Injury to the facial nerve and the chorda tympani are recognized complications of cochlear implantation surgery.[56, 57, 58]

Parotid surgery

The superficial course of the facial nerve in infants and the underdevelopment of surrounding structures mean that the standard techniques for identification of the facial nerve trunk in adults could jeopardize the nerve in children. An alternative technique for identifying the facial nerve has been proposed by Farrior and Santini.[17] Anatomic dissection demonstrates that the facial nerve trunk can be consistently found in a triangle formed by the sternocleidomastoid muscle, posterior belly of the digastric muscle and the cartilaginous ear canal. As in adults, the nerve canal can be identified in the mastoid cavity and followed into the neck. Unlike in adults it is inadvisable to use retrograde dissection of the marginal mandibular branch to find the trunk. [Grade D] Surgery for nontuberculous mycobacteria of the parotid gland and adjacent lymph nodes requires very careful dissection to preserve the facial skin and the nerve (**Figure 80.5**).

Branchial cleft sinus and fistula excision

The variable relationship of the branchial cleft sinus and fistula with the facial nerve makes the nerve vulnerable to injury during surgery. Very careful dissection with intraoperative monitoring is required. D'Souza et al.[59] reviewed the available English, French and German literature between 1923 and 2000 and found 158 cases with fistulae and sinuses. The fistulous tracts were more likely to lie deep to the facial nerve compared with sinus tracts. Lesions with openings in the external auditory meati were associated with a tract superficial to the facial nerve. Younger children were more likely to have a deep tract with consequent increased risk of facial nerve damage. The fistula may be found anywhere along the anterior border of the sternocleidomastoid muscle.[60] Solares et al.,[61] in their report on ten patients with a mean age of nine years, found seven lesions medial to the facial nerve, two lateral and one between branches of the facial nerve. [**/*]

Neoplasms

In children, the two most common causes of facial paralysis from malignancy are leukaemic infiltration of the temporal bone[62, 63] and rhabdomyosarcoma of the head and neck.[64, 65, 66] Levy et al.[67] describe a case of acute mastoiditis and facial paralysis in a five-year-old girl; the diagnosis of leukaemic infiltration of the middle ear cleft

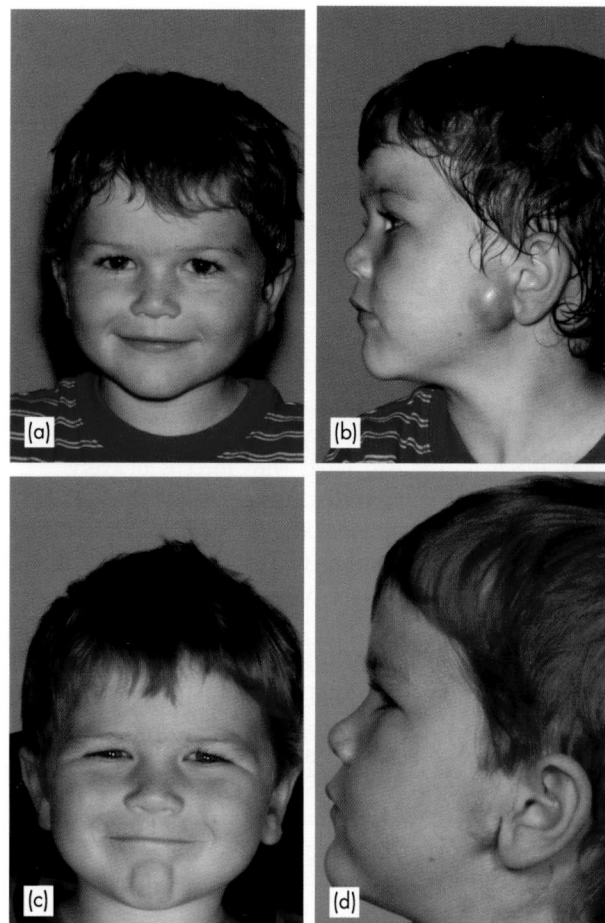

Figure 80.5 Surgery for non-tuberculous mycobacteria (NTM) of the parotid with preservation of the facial nerve. (a, b) Presurgery; (c, d) one week postsurgery.

was made only after surgery and histological examination. Chemotherapy or combined chemo- and radiotherapy are the treatment of choice in known leukaemic patients without symptoms of superimposed infection of the ear or the mastoid process. Surgical management is restricted to cases in which tissue for histological diagnosis is required or drainage of acute infection is needed.

In the Durve et al.[64] series of 14 patients the median age at presentation of rhabdomyosarcoma was 4.5 years with a mean time of onset of symptoms to diagnosis of 21 weeks. Symptoms mimicked those of chronic otitis media, delaying diagnosis. Histological subtype was embryonal in 13 patients and alveolar in 1. All patients underwent multimodality treatment; the five-year disease-free survival rate was 81 percent. Facial paralysis was the most common regional post-treatment morbidity (8 of 14).

The presence of facial paralysis and lymphadenopathy or a mass with aural discharge, hearing loss and aural polyp should prompt urgent investigation and biopsy.

Benign neoplasm of the facial nerve is very rare in children. Facial paralysis from an intracranial neoplasm is uncommon. [**/*]

IDIOPATHIC

Bell's palsy

This is the most common cause of facial paralysis during childhood (42 percent).[2] It is an acute, unilateral, lower motor neurone facial paralysis diagnosed by exclusion. It is essential that otoscopy is normal, that there is no middle ear infection and the hearing is not impaired. There is a body of opinion that attributes Bell's palsy to infection by herpes virus although the evidence for this is inconclusive. The hypothesis is a reactivation of latent herpes simplex virus within the geniculate ganglion. There is a family history of Bell's palsy in a small number of patients and occasionally a viral prodrome. Steroids are sometimes advocated in the acute stage but the evidence supporting their use is equivocal. The Medical Research Council All Scotland Bell's Palsy randomized double-blind trial (in progress) may answer some of the questions related to the use of steroid and antiviral medication. However, this study is restricted to adult patients with Bell's palsy. Facial paralysis in children is considered to have a good prognosis (90 percent recovery) regardless of treatment. Steroid administration is not recommended.[68] [**] [Grade C]

Melkersson–Rosenthal syndrome

Episodes of facial paralysis begin in early childhood or adolescence, predominately in the second decade of life. There is swelling of the lips, palatal mucosa and face, and the tongue is fissured. The facial weakness usually takes a recurring course and is seen in 20 percent of cases. A conservative approach is usually recommended.[69] A preliminary report on the benefit of facial nerve decompression for recurrent facial paralysis in Melkersson-Rosenthal syndrome has recently been further substantiated.[70, 71, 72]

Wegener's granulomatosis

This is a systemic disease characterized by the classical triad of vasculitis, necrosis and granulomatous inflammation, usually of the upper and lower respiratory tract and the kidneys. Primary otological presentation occurs in 20–25 percent of patients[73] and this includes facial paralysis.[74] A high index of suspicion, erythrocyte sedimentation rate, circulating antineutrophil cytoplasmic antibody and histopathology help diagnose this condition. Combination therapy with corticosteroids and cyclophosphamide is given and co-trimoxazole may be used in the long term to reduce remissions.[75]

Hypertension

Hypertension is a rare cause of facial paralysis in children. Misdiagnosis may lead to serious consequences, as reported by Aynaci and Sen.[76] in a case of a hypertensive child with facial paralysis. Bell's palsy was suspected and steroids were given resulting in hypertensive pontine haemorrhage. Recurrent alternating facial paralyses have been reported in a child with hypertension. Antihypertensive treatment and control lead to cessation of further relapse.[77] [**/*][Grade C]

KEY POINTS

- The most common cause of facial paralysis in children is Bell's palsy.
- Knowledge of the embryology and developmental anatomy of the facial nerve allows for a clear understanding of the various anomalies and clinical presentations of disorders of the facial nerve.
- There are important anatomical differences between the topography of the facial nerve in adults and children.
- These anatomical differences and the confined surgical space can make tympanomastoid surgery and surgery of the parotid region in children particularly challenging. Surgeons must be extra vigilant to avoid iatrogenic facial palsy.

Best clinical practice

- ✓ MRI is the only imaging modality that demonstrates the facial nerve comprehensively from the pons to the parotid gland; with gadolinium enhancement it is capable of showing inflammatory changes. [Grade C/D]
- ✓ Electroneurography is a useful adjunct to clinical findings in predicting recovery from facial nerve palsy. [Grade C/D]
- ✓ In facial palsy secondary to acute otitis media, optimum management is wide myringotomy and systemic antibiotics. [Grade C/D]
- ✓ Congenital and acquired facial paralysis in the neonate can be differentiated on the basis of examination, supplemented as required, by electrophysiologic investigations. [Grade C/D]
- ✓ Consider facial nerve monitoring during parotid and tympanomastoid surgery, particularly in children with a high incidence of anatomical abnormalities of the facial nerve, e.g. Down syndrome, craniofacial anomalies. [Grade D]
- ✓ Retrograde dissection of the marginal mandibular branch of the facial nerve to find the trunk is particularly unreliable in children. [Grade D]

Deficiencies in current knowledge and areas for future research

➤ The treatment for facial paralysis remains largely empirical; randomized controlled trials may help answer some of the questions. In view of the small number of cases and the generally good prognosis, a multicentred trial with a sufficiently large number of cases is required.

➤ The currently available monitoring systems for facial nerve function during surgery lack total reliability and are limited in scope. More sophisticated systems including stealth technology offer the prospect of reduced iatrogenic damage and more precise surgery in areas where the facial nerve is at risk.

REFERENCES

1. Lin JC, Ho KY, Kuo WR, Wang LF, Chai CY, Tsai SM. Incidence of dehiscence of the facial nerve at surgery for middle ear cholesteatoma. *Otolaryngology and Head and Neck Surgery.* 2004; **131**: 452–6.
* 2. May M, Fria TJ, Blumenthal F, Curtin H. Facial paralysis in children: differential diagnosis. *Otolaryngology and Head and Neck Surgery.* 1981; **89**: 841–8.
3. Leng TJ. Malformations of chorda tympani nerve. *Lin Chuang Er Bi Yan Hou Ke Za Zhi.* 2000; **14**: 308–10.
4. Kraus P, Ziv M. Incus fixation due to congenital anomaly of chorda tympani. *Acta Oto-laryngologica.* 1971; **72**: 358–60.
5. Stromland K, Sjogreen L, Miller M, Gillberg C, Wentz E, Johansson M et al. Mobius syndrome. *European Journal of Paediatric Neurology.* 2002; **6**: 35–45.
6. D'Amico-Martel A, Noden DM. Contributions of placodal and neural crest cells to avain cranial peripheral ganglia. *American Journal of Anatomy.* 1983; **166**: 445–68.
* 7. Nager GT, Procter B. The facial canal: normal anatomy, variations and anomalies. II. Anatomical variations and anomalies involving the facial canal. *Annals of Otology, Rhinology, and Laryngology.* 1982; **97**: 45–61.
8. Procter B, Nager GT. The facial canal: normal anatomy, variations and anomalies. I. Normal anatomy of the facial canal. *Annals of Otology, Rhinology, and Laryngology. Supplement.* 1982; **97**: 33–44.
9. Raine CH, Hussain SSM, Khan S, Setia RN. Anomaly of the facial nerve and cochlear implantation. *Annals of Otology, Rhinology, and Laryngology. Supplement.* 1995; **166**: 430–1.
10. Jahrsdoerfer RA. The facial nerve in congenital middle ear malformations. *Laryngoscope.* 1981; **91**: 1217–25.
11. Glastonbury CM, Fischbein NJ, Harnsberger HR, Dillon WP, Kertesz TR. Congenital bifurcation of the intratemporal facial nerve. *AJNR. American Journal of Neuroradiology.* 2003; **24**: 1334–7.
12. Al-Mazrou KA, Alorainy IA, Al-Dousary SH, Richardson MA. Facial nerve anomalies in association with congenital hearing loss. *International Journal of Pediatric Otorhinolaryngology.* 2003; **67**: 1347–53.
13. Baxter A. Dehiscence of the Fallopian canal: an anatomical study. *Journal of Laryngology and Otology.* 1971; **85**: 587–94.
14. Moreano EH, Paparella MM, Zelterman D, Goycoolea MV. Prevalence of facial canal dehiscence and of persistent stapedial artery in the human middle ear: a report of 1000 temporal bones. *Laryngoscope.* 1994; **104**: 309–20.
15. Guinto FC, Garrabrant EC, Radcliff WB. Radiology of the persistent stapedial artery. *Radiology.* 1972; **105**: 365–9.
16. Pahor AL, Hussain SSM. Persistent stapedial artery. *Journal of Laryngology and Otology.* 1992; **106**: 254–7.
17. Farrior JB, Santini H. Facial nerve identification in children. *Otolaryngology and Head and Neck Surgery.* 1985; **93**: 173–6.
18. Eavey RD, Herrmann BS, Joseph JM, Thornton AR. Clinical experience with electroneurography in the pediatric patient. *Archives of Otolaryngology – Head and Neck Surgery.* 1989; **115**: 600–7.
19. Glassock ME, Shambaugh GE. *Surgery of the ear.* Philadelphia: W.B. Saunders & Co., 1990: 441–2.
20. Harris JP, Davidson TM, May M, Fria T. Evaluation and treatment of congenital facial paralysis. *Archives of Otolaryngology – Head and Neck Surgery.* 1983; **109**: 145–51.
21. Toelle SP, Boltshauser E. Long-term outcome in children with congenital unilateral facial nerve palsy. *Neuropediatrics.* 2001; **32**: 130–5.
22. Jervis PN, Bull PD. Congenital facial nerve agenesis. *Journal of Laryngology and Otology.* 2001; **115**: 53–4.
23. Carr MM, Ross DA, Zuker RM. Cranial nerve defects in congenital facial palsy. *Journal of Otolaryngology.* 1997; **26**: 80–7.
24. Berker N, Acaroglu G, Soykan E. Goldenhar's Syndrome (oculo-auriculo-vertebral dysplasia) with congenital facial nerve palsy. *Yonsei Medical Journal.* 2004; **45**: 157–60.
25. Yanagihara N, Yanagihara H, Kabasawa I. Goldenhar's syndrome associated with anomalous internal auditory meatus. *Journal of Laryngology and Otology.* 1979; **93**: 1217–22.
26. Parving A. Progressive hearing loss in Goldenhar's syndrome. *Scandinavian Audiology.* 1978; **7**: 101–3.
27. Caksen H, Odabas D, Tuncer O, Kirimi E, Tombul T, Ikbal M et al. Review of 35 cases of asymmetric crying facies. *Genetic Counseling.* 2004; **15**: 159–65.
28. Shah UK, Ohlms LA, Neault MW, Willson KD, McGuirt Jr. WF, Hobbs N et al. Otologic management in children with the CHARGE association. *International Journal of Pediatric Otorhinolaryngology.* 1998; **44**: 139–47.
29. Bauer PW, Wippold 2nd FJ, Goldin J, Lusk RP. Cochlear implantation in children with CHARGE association. *Archives of Otolaryngology – Head and Neck Surgery.* 2002; **128**: 1013–7.

30. Byerly KA, Pauli RM. Cranial nerve abnormalities in CHARGE association. *American Journal of Medical Genetics.* 1993; **45**: 751–7.

31. Kondev L, Bhadelia RA, Douglass LM. Familial congenital facial palsy. *Pediatric Neurology.* 2004; **30**: 367–70.

32. Moriniere S, Lanotte P, Celebi Z, Ployet MJ, Robier A, Lescanne E. [Acute mastoiditis in children: clinical and bacteriological study of 17 cases.] *La Presse Médicale.* 2003; **32**: 1445–9.

33. Sheehy JL, Brackmann DE, Graham MD. Cholesteatoma surgery: residual and recurrent disease. A review of 1024 cases. *Annals of Otology, Rhinology, and Laryngology.* 1977; **86**: 451–4.

34. Mathews TJ. Acute and acute-on-chronic mastoiditis: a five-year experience at Groote Schuur Hospital. *Journal of Laryngology and Otology.* 1988; **102**: 115–7.

35. Burgdorfer W, Barbour AG, Hayes SF, Benach JL, Grunwaldt E, Davis JP. Lyme disease – a tick borne spirochetosis? *Science.* 1982; **216**: 1317–9.

36. Clark JR, Carlson RD, Sasaki CT, Pachner AR, Steere AC. Facial paralysis in Lyme disease. *Laryngoscope.* 1985; **95**: 1341–5.

37. Siwula JM, Mathieu G. Acute onset of facial nerve palsy associated with Lyme disease in a 6 year-old child. *Pediatric Dentistry.* 2002; **24**: 572–4.

38. Eppes SC. Diagnosis, treatment, and prevention of Lyme disease in children. *Paediatric Drugs.* 2003; **5**: 363–72.

39. Hato N, Kisaki H, Honda N, Gyo K, Murakami S, Yanagihara N. Ramsay Hunt syndrome in children. *Herpes zoster syndrome. Annals of Neurology.* 2000; **48**: 254–6.

40. Dickins JR, Smith JT, Graham SS. Herpes zoster oticus: treatment with intravenous acyclovir. *Laryngoscope.* 1988; **98**: 776–9.

41. Stafford FW, Welch AR. The use of acyclovir in Ramsay Hunt syndrome. *Journal of Laryngology and Otology.* 1986; **100**: 337–40.

42. Terada K, Niizuma T, Kosaka Y, Inoue M, Ogita S, Kataoka N. Bilateral facial nerve palsy associated with Epstein–Barr virus infection with a review of the literature. *Scandinavian Journal of Infectious Diseases.* 2004; **36**: 75–7.

43. Ndjolo A, Njock R, Ngowe NM, Ebogo MM, Toukam M, Nko'o S et al. Early ENT manifestations of HIV infection/ AIDS. An analysis of 76 cases observed in Africa. *Revue de Laryngologie – Otologie – Rhinologie.* 2004; **125**: 39–43.

44. Saunders NC, Albert DM. Tuberculous mastoiditis: when is surgery indicated? *International Journal of Pediatric Otorhinolaryngology.* 2002; **65**: 59–63.

45. Weiner GM, O'Connell JE, Pahor AL. The role of surgery in tuberculous mastoiditis: appropriate chemotherapy is not always enough. *Journal of Laryngology and Otology.* 1997; **111**: 752–3.

46. Hadfield PJ, Shah BK, Glover GW. Facial palsy due to tuberculosis: the value of CT. *Journal of Laryngology and Otology.* 1995; **109**: 1010–2.

47. Falco NA, Eriksson E. Facial nerve palsy in the newborn: incidence and outcome. *Plastic and Reconstructive Surgery.* 1990; **85**: 1–4.

48. Smith JD, Crumley RL, Harker LA. Facial paralysis in the newborn. *Otolaryngology and Head and Neck Surgery.* 1981; **89**: 1021–4.

49. Frances HW. Facial nerve emergencies. In: Eisele DW, McQuone SJ (eds). *Emergencies of the head and neck.* St. Louis USA: Mosby, 2000: 337–66.

50. Lee D, Honrado C, Har-El G, Goldsmith A. Pediatric temporal bone fractures. *Laryngoscope.* 1998; **108**: 816–21.

51. Liu-Shindo M, Hawkins DB. Basilar skull fractures in children. *International Journal of Pediatric Otolaryngology.* 1989; **17**: 109–17.

52. Cannon CR, Jahrsdoefer RA. Temporal bone fractures: review of 90 cases. *Archives of Otolaryngology – Head and Neck Surgery.* 1983; **109**: 285–8.

* 53. Green Jr JD, Shelton C, Brackmann DE. Iatrogenic facial nerve injury during otologic surgery. *Laryngoscope.* 1994; **104**: 922–6.

54. Graham MD. Prevention and management of iatrogenic facial palsy. *American Journal of Otology.* 1984; **5**: 513.

55. Horn KL, Brackmann DE, Luxford WM, Shea 3rd JJ. The supratubal recess in cholesteatoma surgery. *Annals of Otology, Rhinology, and Laryngology.* 1986; **95**: 12–5.

56. House 3rd JR, Luxford WM. Facial nerve injury in cochlear implantation. *Otolaryngology and Head and Neck Surgery.* 1993; **109**: 1078–82.

57. Miyamoto RT, Young M, Myres WA, Kessler K, Wolfert K, Kirk KI. Complications of pediatric cochlear implantation. *European Archives of Oto-rhino-laryngology.* 1996; **253**: 1–4.

58. Luetje CM, Jackson K. Cochlear implants in children: what constitutes a complication? *Otolaryngology and Head and Neck Surgery.* 1997; **117**: 243–7.

59. D'Souza AR, Uppal HS, De R, Zeitoun H. Updating concepts of first branchial cleft defects: a literature review. *International Journal of Pediatric Otorhinolaryngology.* 2002; **62**: 103–9.

60. Hussain SSM, Mclay KA. Otolaryngology, head and neck surgery. In: Eremin O (ed.). *The scientific and clinical basis of surgical practice.* Oxford: Oxford University Press, 2001: 620–1.

61. Solares CA, Chan J, Koltai PJ. Anatomical variations of the facial nerve in first branchial cleft anomalies. *Archives of Otolaryngology – Head and Neck Surgery.* 2003; **129**: 351–5.

62. Lilleyman JS, Antoniou AG, Sugden PJ. Facial nerve palsy in acute leukaemia. *Scandinavian Journal of Haematology.* 1979; **22**: 87–90.

63. Zappia JJ, Bunge FA, Koopmann Jr CF, McClatchey KD. Facial nerve paresis as the presenting symptom of leukemia. *International Journal of Pediatric Otorhinolaryngology.* 1990; **19**: 259–64.

64. Durve DV, Kanegaonkar RG, Albert D, Levitt G. Paediatric rhabdomyosarcoma of the ear and temporal bone. *Clinical Otolaryngology and Allied Sciences.* 2004; **29**: 32–7.

the nose and paranasal sinuses), often the source in children is the mucosa over a prominent retrocolumellar vein or varix.

Common aetiological associations include infection, digital trauma from repeated nose picking and upper respiratory tract allergy, a nasal foreign body or a deviated nasal septum. Most cases are idiopathic. The mechanism is thought to be drying of the nasal mucosa due to passing air currents such that an area of excoriation or crusting develops and the friable vessels in the nasal lining break down (**Figure 81.1**). This may explain why the anterior nares is so much more often implicated as inspired air is more thoroughly humidified by the time it reaches the posterior nares.

There are some rare documented causes of nosebleeds in children and it is important to bear these in mind, particularly in recurrent cases with severe recalcitrant bleeds or in an unusual clinical presentation. These are detailed in **Table 81.1**.

ASSESSMENT AND MANAGEMENT

The acute bleed

Simple measures, such as pinching the nares and ensuring that the child keeps her head forward, are usually sufficient to deal with an acute bleed. If the bleeding is persistent, it is important to reassure the child and the

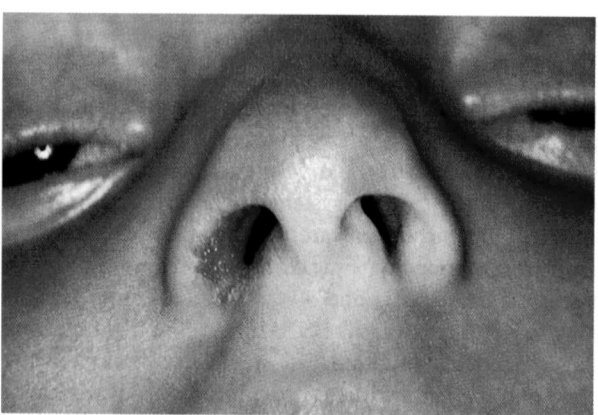

Figure 81.1 Nasal vestibulitis.

parent that the condition is benign. Sit the child up in an examining chair and use a good light source or in the case of a very young or frightened child the nose can be examined while the child is sitting on the parent's knee. A good view of the nasal cavities can be obtained by elevating the tip of the nose using the examiner's thumb and using a conventional head mirror before considering a nasal speculum or an endoscope. Primary care clinicians and accident and emergency doctors should be encouraged to develop the skill of examining the nares in a child using an auriscope with a good-sized speculum introduced into the nose as an excellent view can be obtained in this way with minimum distress to the child (see Chapter 63, The paediatric consultation). If there are clots, the child can be asked to blow his/her nose to remove them and in a cooperative child gentle low pressure suction can be used to further clear the nose. If the bleeding site is apparent and the bleeding is not too profuse, it may be possible to cauterize the source using a silver nitrate stick. If using an anaesthetic/decongestant agent, cophenalcaine™ can be applied directly using a cotton wool bud as the child will find this less distressing than a spray. In the fractious child, local anaesthesia can often compound the child's anxiety and for a simple cautery it is best to explain to the child that it may sting a little, (s)he can tell you if (s)he finds it uncomfortable and you will then stop.

If the bleeding is profuse and uncontrollable, resuscitation may be required and it may be necessary to insert a nasal pack or balloon. Children rarely tolerate nasal packing – or balloon tamponade – well. If anterior packing is unsuccessful a post-nasal pack may be considered but this is a major undertaking in a child and will usually require general anaesthesia for insertion – and often for removal – ideally in a high-dependency or intensive care unit with sedation when the pack is *in situ*.

Recurrent epistaxis

ASSESSMENT

It is important to take a careful history. Enquire if there are any precipitating features, if the child has a background of allergy, if the child is using any medication and

Table 81.1 Causes of epistaxis

Common	Less common
Idiopathic: septal arteries, i.e. Little's area; prominent septal veins Infection Trauma: nose picking; surgery; septal perforation Vestibulitis: Includes foreign body Nasal allergy	Local: septal deformity; tumours; vascular abnormalities Systemic: Coagulopathies, primary or secondary; hereditary haemorrhagic telangiectasia

enquire which side the bleeding commonly arises from. It is important to thoroughly examine the nasal cavity as detailed above. If the history is of recurrent self-limiting epistaxis in an otherwise healthy child in whom clinical examination is normal or the only findings are of prominent vessels in the typical 'bleeding sites', i.e. Little's area or a retrocolumellar vein, investigations are not routinely required.

Although epistaxis is usually idiopathic, it is prudent to be alert to some of the unusual pathologies which can present this way. Investigations, if needed, must be tailored to the clinical findings.

If there is clinical evidence of allergic rhinitis, such as nasal obstruction, rhinorhoea, sneezing or the appearance of hyperaemic oedematous nasal mucosa, this may require investigation and management in its own right (see Chapter 83, Paediatric rhinosinusitis).

Enquire about the use of nasal sprays as intranasal steroid sprays can cause localized nasal mucosal trauma often in the region of the anterior end of the inferior turbinate which can give rise to epistaxis.[5]

A concomitant vestibulitis should raise the suspicion of a retained nasal foreign body (**Figure 81.1**).

Epistaxis alone does not require coagulation screening but if there is evidence of bleeding from other sites, easy bruising or a family history of bleeding, investigations should include full blood count and coagulation screen. Idiopathic thrombocytopoenic purpura (ITPP) may present as epistaxis. If a coagulopathy, primary or secondary, is to be excluded it is wise to seek advice from a paediatric haematology colleague as many conditions – such as Von Willebrand's disease – are not easily tested for using conventional coagulation screening.[6]

Nosebleeds in infants and the newborn are especially uncommon. As meningocoeles and encephalocoeles may present in this way, careful examination including thorough endoscopy and imaging may be required (see Chapter 82, Nasal obstruction in children).

Examination under anaesthesia may be needed in a very young or fractious child in whom clinical examination is difficult and will certainly be needed for biopsy if a tumour is suspected. Intranasal biopsies in children should only be undertaken with extreme care and having excluded conditions, such as meningocoele, vascular abnormalities and angiofibroma by careful imaging in consultation with a paediatric radiologist and under the supervision of a paediatric otolaryngologist.

Although angiofibroma is uncommon, epistaxis is the most frequent mode of presentation and vigilance is especially important in adolescent boys in whom thorough examination of the nasopharynx is mandatory. This is now best carried out using a nasendoscope. Urgent imaging including MR scanning must be arranged in consultation with a radiologist (see Chapter 102, Imaging in paediatric ENT).

Nasal parasitosis is uncommon in the UK, but in areas where parasites are endemic they may be implicated in childhood epistaxis (see Chapter 115, Specific chronic infections).

Nasal mycoses may need to be considered, particularly in immunocompromised children, such as those receiving chemotherapy (see Chapter 114, Fungal rhinosinusitis).

Rhabdomyosarcoma can also present with epistaxis (**Figure 81.2**), although there are usually other signs of an expanding intranasal mass such as craniopathies or Eustachian tubal dysfunction (see Chapter 98, Tumours of the head and neck in childhood).

Vascular abnormalities such as arteriovenous malformations and haemangiomata are rare causes of childhood epistaxis but may, if suspected, dictate the need for careful imaging, ideally in consultation with a paediatric radiologist.[7]

CONTROVERSIES IN MANAGEMENT

Commonly used methods for the management of recurrent epistaxis in children are the prophylactic application of petroleum jelly to the nasal vestibule and septum, the use of topical antiseptic creams, and cautery of Little's area or the retrocolumellar veins. If the bleeding is persistently from one side, often you will find either a leash of vessels around Little's area on the affected side or a prominent retrocolumellar vein. Both of these are easy to deal with by cautery. Cautery nowadays is most often undertaken using a silver nitrate impregnated stick (**Figure 81.3**). The use of strong caustic agents,

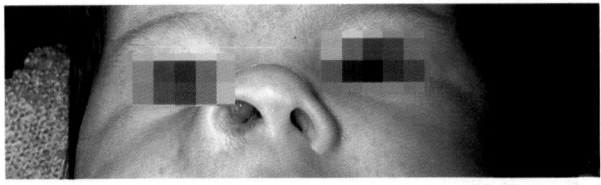

Figure 81.2 A nasal mass (for example, rhabdomyosarcoma) may present with epistaxis.

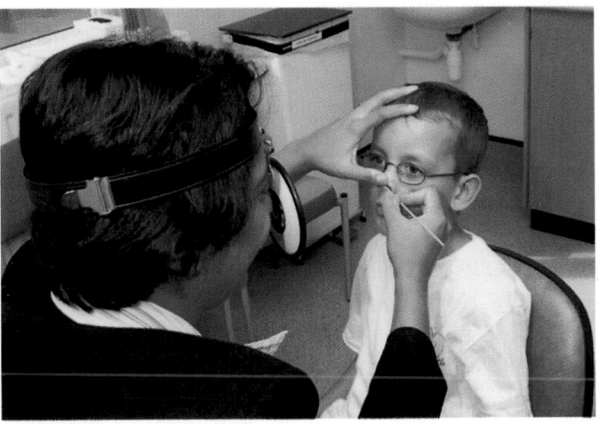

Figure 81.3 Silver nitrate cautery.

such as trichloroacetic acid, which can burn skin and adjacent structures, is to be deprecated.

Petroleum jelly is thought to be effective because it forms a water-resistant film over the affected area of mucosa. In addition, antiseptic creams are thought to sterilize localized infection in the region of the vestibule and the nasal septum.

The evidential base for management of recurrent nosebleeds in children is poor.[8, 9] Commonly used therapeutic options which have been evaluated are:

- expectant treatment, i.e. first aid management of acute bleeds as they arise;
- use of an oil-based antiseptic cream;
- application of petroleum jelly;
- nasal cautery using silver nitrate;
- electrocautery ('hot wire') to the suspected bleeding point.

Less common inverventions include laser therapy, limited septoplasty, local application of tranexamic acid gel[10] and fibrin glue,[11] endoscopic treatment of offending vessels by diathermy or ligation and in recalcitrant cases embolization under the supervision of a radiologist[12] (see Chapter 126, Epistaxis, for a full discussion on treatment options for epistaxis in adults).

As the majority of children with recurrent nosebleeds do not come to the attention of an otolaryngologist, 'expectant' treatment is the most frequently used option. Outcomes following treatment are difficult to standardize and evaluate.

There are few data on the long-term history of children with recurrent epistaxis, but anecdotal evidence suggests that most children spontaneously improve.

Creams and petroleum jelly are widely recommended by primary care clinicians and otolaryngologists. Ruddy et al.[13] conducted a prospective randomized controlled trial (PRCT) comparing antiseptic cream alone with nasal cautery using recurrence as an outcome measure and found no difference. Murthy et al.,[14] in a PCRT, compared the use of silver nitrate cautery alone with silver nitrate cautery and adjunctive treatment with an antiseptic cream. Using self-reported recurrent epistaxis rate as an outcome measure, he found no difference between the groups. Kubba et al.[15] compared chlorhexidine cream with no treatment and found a significant reduction in bleeding in the treatment group. In a small PCRT of children referred to an otolaryngology service and using as an outcome measure the frequency of reported bleeds in the four weeks prior to consultation with an otolaryngologist, Loughran et al.[16] compared the efficacy of vaseline jelly applied twice daily by the parent to the nasal mucosa with no treatment. He found no difference in the groups.

All of the above studies were dogged by low study power, incomplete follow up and variable outcome measures.

Furthermore, nasal carrier cream delivery is difficult to standardize and depends on parental cooperation and compliance. Nasal cautery is a surgical procedure requiring some training and skill (**Figure 81.3**), but it is often delegated to surgeons in training and to nursing personnel with varying degrees of supervision. Follow-up arrangements vary greatly and 'blind' cautery of the nasal septum is often advised even if there is no visible source for bleeding. It seems reasonable to regard the success or otherwise of nasal cautery as operator-dependent. The anecdotal experience of otolaryngologists is that judicious cautery of an obvious offending vessel is worthwhile and is associated with reduced recurrence.

Extensive cautery may be complicated by the development of a nasal septal perforation (**Figure 81.4**). Traditional advice has been that this is more likely if adjacent areas on both sides of the nasal septum are cauterized at one sitting. Although there is no direct evidence for this, it seems prudent to defer cautery of the second side if needed, until the result of cautery on one side can be evaluated over a period of four to six weeks.

Tradition once dictated that children who did not tolerate silver nitrate cautery, or who had recurrent bleeding following outpatient cautery, were offered electrocautery. This usually requires general anaesthesia. The evidence that this is in any way better than silver nitrate is weak. Toner and Walby,[17] in a PRCT, compared electrocautery with cautery with silver nitrate and adjunctive use of an antiseptic cream and found no difference in the two groups using the number with recurrent bleeding in each group as an outcome measure.

Makura et al. conducted a prospective audit and looked at tolerance to outpatient cautery, which he found was as high as 98 percent, but the application of silver nitrate to the mucosa is painful.[9, 18]

Based on the evidence presented, there is no certainty that nasal cautery is better than no active treatment, but if the child has been referred to a paediatric ENT clinic and has had treatment under the supervision of a primary care team, usually consisting of application of creams or jelly,

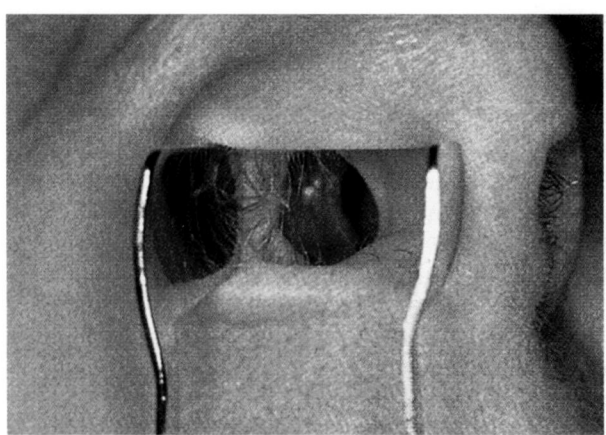

Figure 81.4 Nasal septal perforation.

it seems reasonable if there is a visible prominent nasal vessel to cauterize it. The morbidity is low and anecdotal evidence suggests that it is worthwhile. The evidence from randomized controlled trials comparing petroleum jelly with antiseptic creams suggest that there is little to choose between them on clinical grounds and as the jelly is cheaper and more widely available it should be considered first. [**] The most widely used antiseptic cream is Naseptin^{TM} – a combination of chlorhexidine and neomycin. As it contains peanut oil it must not be used in suspected peanut allergy.

Less commonly considered interventions, such as laser treatment, fibrin glue, septoplasty and endoscopic diathermy, are only applicable on an individual case basis and do not currently have a strong evidential base. [**/*]

MANAGEMENT OF EPISTAXIS IN THE CHILD WITH AN ASSOCIATED MEDICAL CONDITION

Children with upper respiratory tract allergy should be managed in the first instance with treatment appropriate to the primary allergy, i.e. intranasal steroids and antihistamines. Paradoxically, one of the troublesome side effects of intranasal steroid treatment is nosebleeds, thought to be due to the effect of the propellant in nasal steroid delivery systems on the mucosa. This is usually mild and self-limiting (see Chapter 83, Paediatric rhinosinusitis).

Septal deviation can cause epistaxis particularly if there is a prominent septal spur. This can subject an area of nasal mucosa to dry cold air currents which can cause mucosal excoriation. A limited septoplasty may be curative but with the usual caveats that apply to nasal septal surgery in children (see Chapter 123, The septum).

Although the condition is congenital, hereditary haemorrhagic telangiectasia (HHT) is rarely diagnosed in children. Most adult patients will recollect episodes of troublesome bleeding in adolescence (see Chapter 126, Epistaxis). If there is a family history, or if there are telangiectasia on the nasal or buccal mucosa, genetic testing should be considered. Treatment is directed at managing acute bleeds and the gamut of treatment options available in adults may be considered, but the condition is rarely florid in childhood or adolescence. Nasal cautery in these children should be considered with extreme care as nasal septal perforation, and indeed collapse, may complicate multiple cauteries.

Children with advanced malignant disease may have profuse and uncontrollable nosebleeds. As treatment strategies and survival in paediatric oncology improves, otolaryngologists are increasingly asked to help in the management of these children. Thrombocytopenia is a common factor. Severe bleeding can cause great distress and may be life threatening. These children are managed in liaison with a paediatric oncology team or a palliative care clinician. They may require nasal packing, repeated transfusion and platelet therapy. Exceptionally, balloon tamponade or a postnasal pack can be considered. Management of the child's nosebleeds can be an important element of palliative care. Nasal tampons are gentler and easier to insert than BIPP^{TM} packs.

CLINICAL GUIDELINES

Based on the above, the following clinical guidelines seem appropriate for recurrent epistaxis in childhood where there is no systemic disease and no anatomical aetiology other than a plexus in Little's area or a varix in the retrocollumellar area.

- Expectant treatment may be recommended in mild cases. [Grade C/D]
- Petroleum jelly is associated with little or no morbidity and is a reasonable primary care treatment. [Grade C]
- A nasal barrier cream offers limited benefit but morbidity is low and the treatment can be prescribed in primary care. [Grade C]
- If cautery is considered, silver nitrate is the optimum method. [Grade B]
- Nasal cautery is a procedure requiring skill, training and the evaluation of outcome. Haphazard application of caustic agents to the child's nasal mucosa is unwise. [Grade D]
- Electrocautery should rarely be considered. [Grade C/D]
- Very few children require general anaesthesia. [Grade C/D]
- There are no studies comparing antiseptic cream with petroleum jelly, but it seems reasonable to recommend antiseptic preparations in the presence of a concomitant vestibulitis, otherwise cost and ease of application should dictate the choice. [Grade C]
- Laser therapy, fibrin glue and septoplasty have essentially not been evaluated and can only be considered on an individual basis. [Grade D]
- Neither systemic nor local tranexamic acid has any place in the treatment of childhood epistaxis. [Grade C]
- The innovative techniques for epistaxis which have been pioneered by adult rhinologists, such as endoscopic ligation of the sphenopalatine artery, have not yet been widely applied in children but may have a limited role (see Chapter 126, Epistaxis).

KEY POINTS

- Epistaxis in children is extremely common and usually innocuous.

- Most acute bleeds settle with simple therapeutic interventions that parents and carers can administer at home.
- Investigations are rarely required.
- Spontaneous resolution is common for children with recurrent epistaxis.

Best clinical practice

✓ Other than careful rhinoscopy, no formal investigations are required for children with recurrent epistaxis who are otherwise in good health and where clinical history and findings on examination are unremarkable.

✓ Indications for referral to an otolaryngologist include:
  - troublesome recurrent epistaxis where treatment with nasal barrier creams has been unsuccessful;
  - associated nasal discharge;
  - children with a known or suspected haematological disorder;
  - a short history of severe bleeds;
  - persistent unilateral symptoms;
  - associated vestibulitis;
  - parental concern;
  - systemic disease or upset.

✓ Adolescent boys with unexplained epistaxis need urgent referral.

✓ Nasal cautery using silver nitrate in the hands of an appropriately trained clinician is an innocuous well-tolerated procedure with little morbidity and should be undertaken where there is an evident blood vessel.

✓ Naseptin cream™ contains peanut oil and must not be used in children with suspected peanut allergy.

Deficiencies in current knowledge and areas for future research

➤ The role of silver nitrate seems unlikely to be validated by randomized controlled trials as the technique is operator dependent.

➤ There are no good studies looking at the effect of epistaxis on quality of life and at the effect of intervention on quality of life indices.

➤ If we are to conduct large population studies on the natural history of epistaxis and the effect of intervention, these will need to be primary-care centred as most children with epistaxis do not come to the attention of an otolaryngologist.

➤ Optimum treatment of nosebleeds in systemic malignant diseases needs to be streamlined and improved.

REFERENCES

1. Petruson B. Epistaxis in childhood. *Rhinology.* 1979; **17**: 83–90.
2. Murray AB, Milner RA. Allergic rhinitis; A common cause of recurrent epistaxis in children. *Annals of Allergy, Asthma and Immunology.* 1995; **74**: 30–3.
3. Juselius H. Epistaxis: A clinical study of 1724 patients. *Journal of Laryngology and Otology.* 1974; **88**: 317–27.
4. Jackson K, Jackson R. Factors associated with active refractory epistaxis. *Archives of Otolaryngology – Head and Neck Surgery.* 1988; **114**: 862–5.
5. Transgrud AJ, Whitaker A, Small-Ralph E. Intranasal corticosteroids for allergic rhinitis. *Pharmacotherapy.* 2002; **22**: 1458–67.
* 6. Katsanis E, Luke K, Hsu E. Prevalence and significance of mild bleeding disorders in children with recurrent epistaxis. *Journal of Pediatrics.* 1988; **113**: 73–6. *Good overview of relationship between coagulopathy and nosebleeds and summary of laboratory tests.*
7. Giridharan W, Belloso A, Pau H, McEwan J, Clarke RW. Epistaxis in children with vascular malformations – commentary of two cases and literature review. *International Journal of pediatric otorhinolaryngology.* 2002; **65**: 137–41.
* 8. McGarry G. Nosebleeds in children. *Clinical Evidence.* 2005: 399–402. *Summary of current evidence.*
* 9. Burton M, Doree C. Interventions for recurrent idiopathic epistaxis (nosebleeds) in children. *Cochrane Database Systematic Review.* 2004; **1**: CD 004461. *A systematic review of treatment strategies.*
10. Tibbelin A, Aust R, Bende M, Holgersson M, Petruson B, Rundcrantz H *et al.* Effect of local tranexamic acid gel in the treatment of epistaxis. *Journal of Oto-Rhino-Laryngology and its Related Specialties.* 1995; **57**: 207–9.
11. Vaiman M, Segal S, Eviatar E. Fibrin glue treatment for epistaxis. *Rhinology.* 2002; **40**: 88–91.
12. Elden L, Montanera W, Terbrugge K, Willinsky R, Lasjaunias P, Charles D. Angiographic embolization for the treatment of epistaxis: a review of 108 cases. *Otolaryngology – Head and Neck Surgery.* 1994; **111**: 44–50.
13. Ruddy J, Proops DW, Pearman K, Ruddy H. Management of epistaxis in children. *International Journal of Pediatric Otorhinolaryngology.* 1991; **21**: 139–42.
14. Murthy P, Nilssen EL, Rao S, McClymont LG. A randomised clinical trial of antiseptic nasal carrier cream and silver nitrate. *Clinical Otolaryngology and Allied Sciences.* 1999; **24**: 228–31.
15. Kubba H, MacAndie C, Botma M, Robison J, O'Donnell M, Robertson G *et al.* A prospective, single-blind, randomised controlled trial of antiseptic cream for recurrent epistaxis in childhood. *Clinical Otolaryngology.* 2001; **26**: 465–8.
16. Loughran S, Spinou E, Clement WA, Cathcart R, Kubba H, Geddes NK. A prospective, single-blind, randomized

controlled trial of petroleum jelly/vaseline for recurrent paediatric epistaxis.. *Clinical Otolaryngology and Allied Sciences*. 2004; **29**: 266–9.

17. Toner JG, Walby AP. Comparison of electro and chemical cautery in the treatment of anterior epistaxis. *Journal of Laryngology and Otology*. 1990; **104**: 617–8.

18. Makura ZG, Porter GC, McCormick MS. Paediatric epistaxis: Alder Hey experience. *Journal of Laryngology and Otology*. 2002; **116**: 903–6.

82

Nasal obstruction in children

MICHELLE WYATT

Introduction	1070	Best clinical practice	1078
Congenital disorders	1070	Deficiencies in current knowledge and areas for future	
Acquired abnormalities	1076	research	1078
Key points	1077	References	1078

SEARCH STRATEGY

The evidence-base for this chapter is supported by a Medline search using the key words nasal obstruction and children and focusing on a variety of key words appropriate to the individual topics. These include all the subheadings listed below (e.g. choanal atresia, pyriform aperture stenosis, etc.). The Cochrane database and the National Electronic Library for Health for ENT were also consulted.

INTRODUCTION

The causes of nasal obstruction in children are numerous and diverse, but the symptoms are essentially similar. Stertor, mouth breathing, feeding problems, sleep disturbance and rhinorrhoea are all frequently reported. Concern should be heightened if there is failure to thrive, significant nocturnal obstruction, intermittent cyanosis or apnoea.

The severity of the problem will depend on the degree of the blockage and the size of the child. A clinical history will ascertain whether the problem is uni- or bilateral, complete or partial, intermittent or constant, acute or chronic. It is useful to know whether the symptoms were with the child from birth or have developed subsequently and whether the onset has been gradual or sudden. Newborns are generally obligate nasal breathers for the first few months of life and so nasal obstruction in this group can present as an acute respiratory emergency. The extent of the problem will alter related to the child's ability to breathe orally, which corresponds to their level of maturity and neurological development. An oral airway is often enough to relieve distress until definitive treatment can be undertaken.

Examination is essential. It can be particularly helpful if the child will permit the use of flexible or rigid endoscopy. Imaging via computed tomography (CT) and magnetic resonance imaging (MRI) has been shown to be of great value in delineating both nasal and post-nasal lesions.

Tables 82.1, 82.2 and **82.3** outline the variety of causes of nasal obstruction in children. This chapter aims to review those conditions not covered elsewhere in this book.

CONGENITAL DISORDERS

Skeletal anomalies

CHOANAL ATRESIA

In this rare condition (incidence 1 in 7000 live births), there is complete obstruction of the posterior nasal openings on one or both sides (**Figure 82.1**). The blockage has been thought to be either bony or membranous in origin. In reality, a mixed picture is usually seen (70 percent of cases) with the remainder

Table 82.1   Congenital causes of nasal obstruction in children.

Anatomical/skeletal abnormalities	Nasal cysts	Nasal masses
Choanal atresia	Dermoid	Meningo-/encephalocoele
Pyriform aperture stenosis	Nasoalveolar	Glioma
Nasal agenesis	Nasolacrimal	Hamartoma
Craniosynostosis syndromes	Dentigenerous	Chordoma
'Cleft palate' nose	Mucous	Teratoma
	Pharyngeal bursa (Thornwaldt cyst)	

Table 82.2   Acquired causes of nasal obstruction in children.

Structural	Inflammatory	Tumours
Osseocartilagenous nasal deformity	Infective	Angiofibroma
Foreign body	Allergic	Olfactory neuroblastoma
	Rhinosinusitis/polyposis	Rhabdomyosarcoma
	Physiological	Nasopharyngeal carcinoma
	Neonatal rhinitis	(Haemangioma (vasoformative disorder))
	Pubertal rhinitis	(Fibro-osseous disease)

Table 82.3   Systemic diseases causing nasal obstruction in children.

Diseases
Cystic fibrosis
Ciliary dyskinesia
Immune deficiency
Sarcoidosis
Wegener's granulomatosis

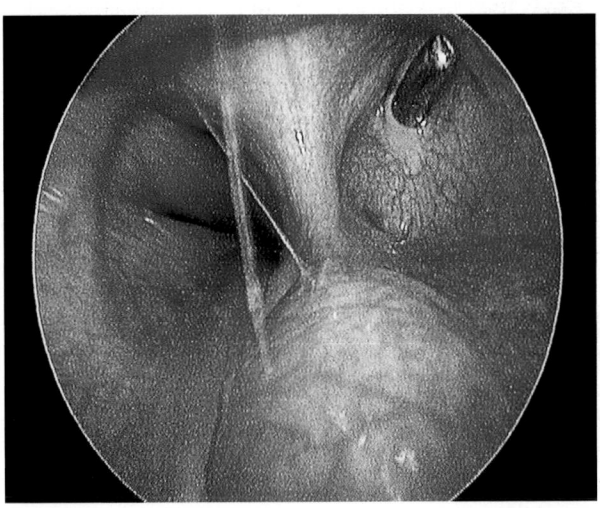

Figure 82.1   Unilateral choanal atresia as viewed from the nasopharynx with a 120° endoscope. A sound is perforating the membrane.

being purely bony. It is believed to be secondary to persistence of the nasobuccal membrane (see Chapter 65, Head and neck embryology).

Bilateral choanal atresia will present as an acute respiratory emergency at birth as newborns are obligate nasal breathers. The classical picture of cyclical cyanosis (blue spells relieved by crying) is seen. Placement of an appropriately sized oral airway usually resolves the distress. It may be helpful to place a metal spatula just below the child's external nasal aperture; misting excludes a diagnosis of choanal atresia. The inability to pass nasal catheters suggests the diagnosis which can be confirmed by flexible endoscopy or CT scanning (with suction clearance of the nose and the application of 0.5 percent ephedrine drops 30 minutes previously) (**Figure 82.2**). If an oral airway is well tolerated, transfer is often possible without endotracheal intubation, though this may be required in certain cases.

Choanal atresia may be an isolated anomaly or one feature of a number of associated congenital anomalies, e.g. CHARGE association (coloboma, heart defects, atresia choanae, retardation of growth, genital

anomalies and ear abnormalities). These associated anomalies should be excluded in a baby with choanal atresia. Minimum investigations in addition to the nasal CT scan are cardiac echo, renal ultrasound scan and an ophthalmology and audiology review.

Unilateral problems often come to light in an older child with a persistent profuse one-sided nasal discharge in whom there is no history of foreign body insertion.

Numerous techniques have been described for the correction of choanal atresia with little direct comparisons made. Outcomes are themselves hard to define objectively. Most studies rely on clinical judgements made by the surgeon as to the size of the nasal airway and

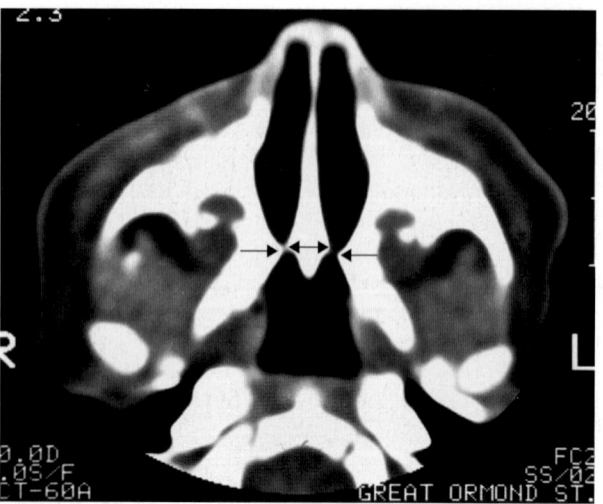

Figure 82.2 CT scan (axial view) to illustrate the expansion of the posterior vomer and medial maxillary walls of the nasopharynx in choanal atresia (arrowed).

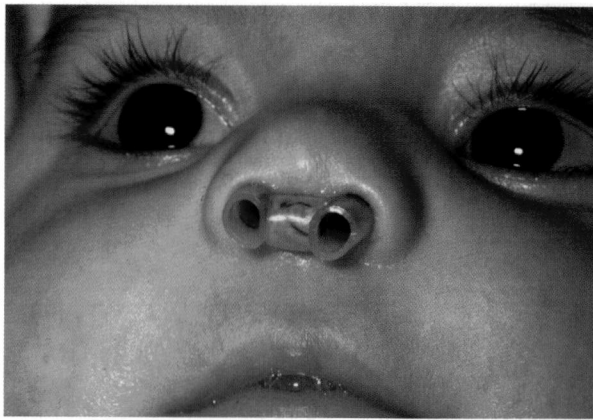

Figure 82.3 Bilateral nasal stents with an endotracheal tube bridging piece.

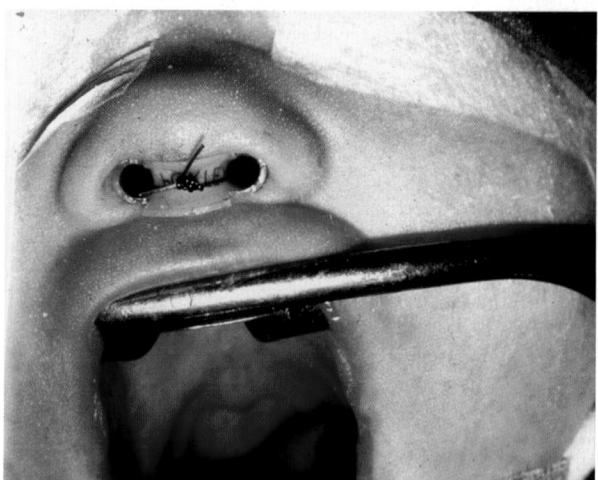

Figure 82.4 Bilateral nasal stents without a bridging piece.

opinion from the patient and their family as to whether they are 'asymptomatic'. The number of surgeries required and time taken to obtain a satisfactory outcome are also used to make comparison.

Transpalatal and transnasal surgery have been shown to have similar outcomes.[1] [**] Endoscopic transnasal approaches have also been successfully reported.[2] [**] The technique described in three papers from Great Ormond Street Hospital, London[3, 4, 5] [**] represents the largest reported experience at 161 patients and involves a transnasal repair under direct vision. A 120° endoscope is placed in the mouth and positioned in the nasopharynx behind the soft palate. The atretic plate is perforated initially with a sound and currently is removed with the specifically designed microdebrider attachment (previously a diamond paste burr was used). Bilateral nasal stents are fashioned from two Ivory Portex[TM] endotracheal tubes cut to length, with the bevelled end of each sitting in the nasopharynx orientated towards the septum. The philtrum is protected by either a small length of size 12 suction catheter cut to act as a bridging piece or a further small piece of endotracheal tube (**Figure 82.3**). The stents are secured by a circumseptal '0' prolene suture and are left *in situ* for six weeks. Others use a single tube as a stent which has a window cut in the middle to allow access for the securing suture and avoids the need for a bridging piece (**Figure 82.4**). Scrupulous stent care is vital to prevent obstruction or damage to the nasal soft tissues. Some authors do not favour stenting in unilateral or even bilateral cases. It is suggested that removal of the posterior aspect of the vomer along with the atretic plate and the use of powered instruments have made stents unnecessary. Authors who support this view do stress the need for early repeat examination for removal of granulations and dilatation as required.[2, 6] [**]

Given the limitations in the definition of outcome as described above, success rates have been shown to be similar over the past 20 years with the three Great Ormond Street Hospital (GOSH) papers showing rates of between 68 and 80 percent for bilateral and 82–93 percent for unilateral atresia. The length of time for follow-up has been variable, but is only quoted in months in the GOSH papers. A group of 78 children from the Philadelphia Children's Hospital were followed up for 35 months on average with similar results.[7] [**]

The role of mitomycin C (MMC) in the treatment of choanal atresia is still being clarified. MMC is an antineoplastic agent which acts to inhibit fibroblasts and angioneogenesis and so reduces granulation tissue and fibrosis. It is suggested that its use at the time of stent removal and at subsequent dilatations improves outcome. A variety of doses and protocols have been described and some benefit has been reported.[8] [**] The KTP laser has also been shown to be helpful in the treatment of granulation tissue which develops postoperatively.[1] [**]

PYRIFORM APERTURE STENOSIS

This abnormality, first described in 1988, arises due to bony overgrowth of the nasal process of the maxilla

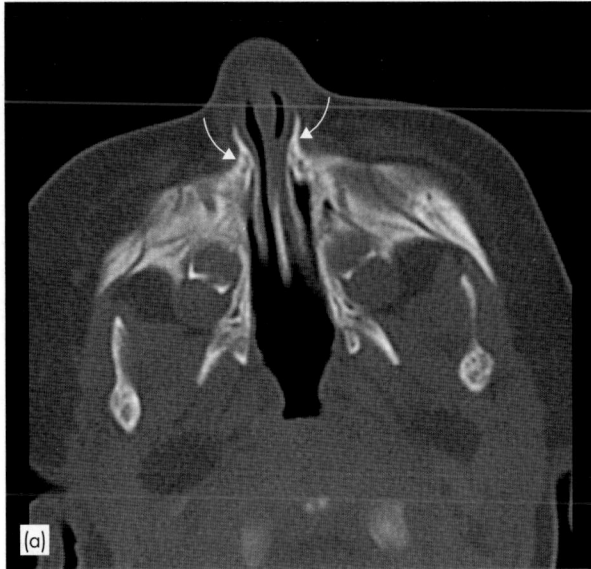
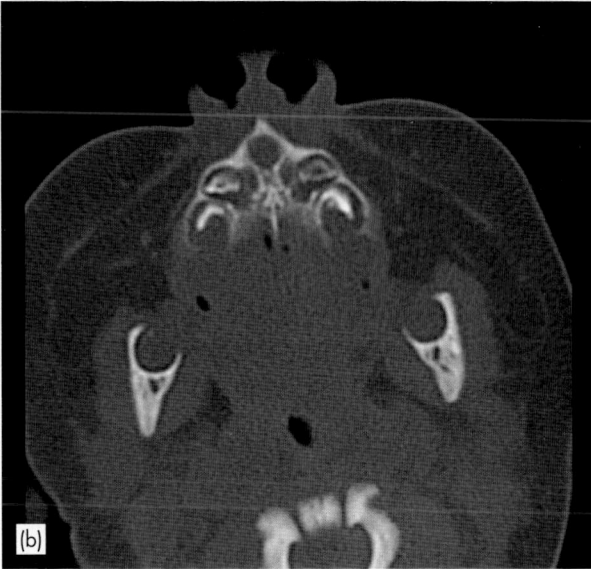

Figure 82.5 CT scan (axial view) of bilateral pyriform aperture stenosis. Note the single central incisor.

(**Figure 82.5**).[9] The pyriform aperture is the narrowest part of the nasal airway and so even minimal reduction in diameter here can cause significant problems. Symptoms similar to bilateral choanal atresia occur and epiphora is also often seen secondary to bony involvement of the nasolacrimal ducts. Endoscopy is prevented by the bony obstruction at the vestibule. CT scan confirms the diagnosis and shows the single central incisor which exists in some affected individuals. In this subgroup with a 'mega-incisor', there is a suggested association with holoprosencephaly, a rare congenital condition in which the developing forebrain fails to divide appropriately to form the cerebral hemispheres, diencephalon and optic and olfactory bulbs. These patients should undergo further evaluation for central nervous system (CNS) defects and particularly the hypothalamic–pituitary–thyroid axis.

Conservative treatment in the form of nasal topical medication is often sufficient, but if there is severe obstruction, respiratory distress or failure to thrive, surgical intervention is necessary. The approach can be transnasal with an alar-releasing incision or sublabial. The mucosa is lifted and the abnormal bone drilled away. Nasal stents are then placed for several weeks.

NASAL AGENESIS

Complete arhinia is very rare but can occur either in isolation or as part of a syndrome. It originates at the fifth week *in utero* when the nasal placode fails to canalize to form the nasal passages. Presentation at birth with acute respiratory distress is usual (neonates are obligate nasal breathers), though problems sometimes do not arise until feeding is attempted. Management is with an oral airway and tube feeding prior to definitive treatment.

Congenital nasal cysts

Congenital cysts, as described in **Table 82.1**, can either obstruct the nose or cause discharge from an associated sinus tract.

DERMOID CYST

Dermoid cysts (**Figure 82.6**) derive from ectoderm and mesoderm and can contain all the structures of normal skin. Nasal lesions account for between 1 and 3 percent of all dermoids and are the most common midline nasal mass. There is debate as to their origin. One theory is that they originate from an embryological aberration resulting in inadequate closure of the fonticulus frontalis, which then allows dermal tissue to extend between the nasal bones and cartilage. Dura can also extend down through this area. Another suggestion is that there is a persistence of residual dura in the prenasal space. The prenasal space runs in the midline between the developing nasal bone and underlying cartilage from the brain to the nasal tip. The misplaced dura is believed to form a contact with the skin and then it retracts to result in a sinus, in which a cyst can then develop.

Dermoids usually present as a slowly growing cystic midline mass over the nasal dorsum. An associated pit can often be seen in any position from the nasal tip to the glabella, hair may be present at its opening. Infection of a dermoid can result in abscess formation requiring drainage. Early surgical excision is recommended to prevent either this complication or further expansion of the cyst with associated destruction of local tissue.

Preoperative assessment for intracranial extension is essential. CT is helpful for bony anatomy, while MRI delineates a CNS connection.

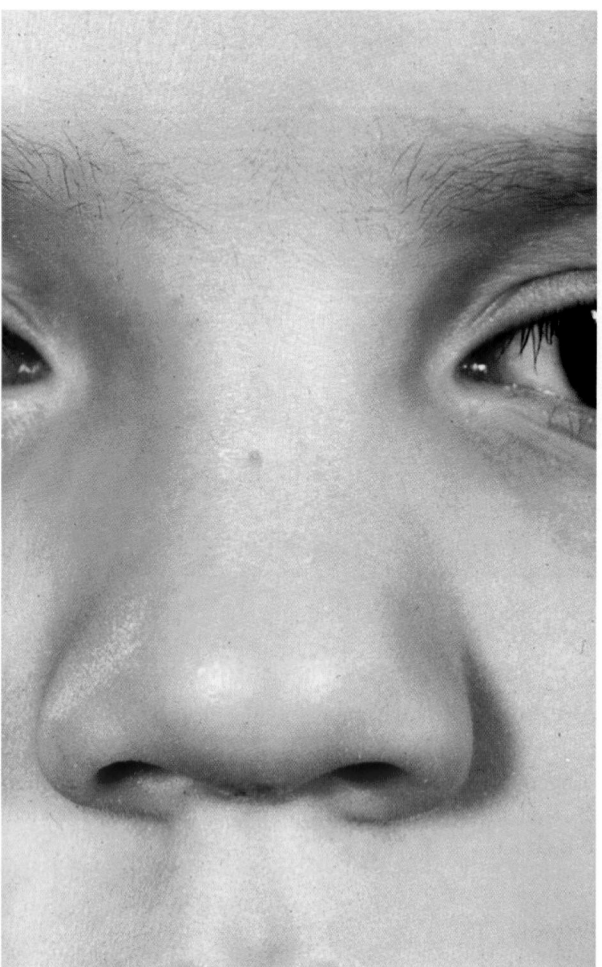

Figure 82.6 Midline nasal sinus associated with an underlying dermoid cyst.

Surgical approaches depend on the position of the cyst. If it is in the lower half of the nose, an open rhinoplasty procedure is an excellent way of removing pathology and obtaining a good cosmetic result. Cysts higher up the nose may need direct excision via an elliptical incision. Extension of the sinus tract deep to the nasal bones usually necessitates a medial osteotomy to permit adequate exposure for removal. Some find a lateral rhinotomy a useful approach to expose the septum and so allow complete removal of the cyst and associated tract. Any punctum in the skin will require local excision.

Careful consideration is required for intracranial extension. If this occurs, a combined intracranial/extracranial procedure is recommended. If it is only suspected, it is appropriate to approach the lesion via the nose first and only proceed with the craniotomy if absolutely required.[10] [**]

NASOLACRIMAL DUCT CYSTS

The nasolacrimal duct system should canalize *in utero* from a superior to inferior direction, but at birth the lower end not infrequently can remain closed. Thirty percent of babies are born with nasolacrimal duct blockage. If there is no lumen at both ends of the system, fluid builds up resulting in a cyst. These lesions cause epiphora and nasal obstruction sometimes leading to feeding difficulties and respiratory distress. They can be unilateral or bilateral. Eighty-five percent of cases resolve spontaneously by nine months of age.

Diagnosis is made by clinical examination and CT. On the latter, a dilated nasolacrimal duct, an intranasal cyst and cystic dilation of the lacrimal sac are seen. If surgical removal is required, endonasal marsupialization under endoscopic guidance is recommended, though endonasal ablation with a carbon dioxide laser has been described.[11] [**] Ophthalmology input is helpful as intraoperative nasolacrimal probing and stenting may be needed.

THORNWALDT'S CYST

The pharyngeal recess or bursa sits in the midline of the posterior wall of the nasopharynx. It ends next to the adenoids and is lined by the pharyngeal mucous membrane. Cystic transformation of this recess was first described by Thornwaldt in 1885 and so bears his name. Inflammation of this lesion causes nasal obstruction, occipital pain, fullness in the ears and discharge. Endoscopic examination will confirm the diagnosis. Imaging by CT and MRI will show any adhesion to the cervical vertebrae. Incision or excision of the cyst have been described, while total clearance would involve a transpalatal approach.

NASOALVEOLAR CYSTS

These are rare, nonodontogenic, soft tissue lesions arising from the incisive canal during the development of the maxilla. They present lateral to the midline at the alar base and can cause asymmetrical alar flare. Excision is usually via a sublabial approach.

DENTIGEROUS CYSTS

These present in the floor of the nose or maxillary sinus and have a dental origin. Endoscopic marsupialization or removal via the nose is usually satisfactory.

MUCOUS CYSTS

Mucous cysts have been described anywhere in the nose, but appear to be more common in the floor. They may be congenital, but are more usually seen as a complication of rhinoplasty. Endoscopic and open approaches are used, depending on the position of the lesion.

Congenital nasal masses

A congenital nasal mass can consist of ectopic intracranial tissue. The structures may have prolapsed into the nasal cavity and become disconnected, but in many cases an intracranial connection is maintained.

ENCEPHALOCOELE, MENINGOCOELE AND GLIOMA

A nasal encephalomenigocoele represents a herniation of meninges with or without associated brain through bony defects of the calvarium. A meningocoele consists of either meninges alone or with cerebrospinal fluid (CSF) and an encephalocoele contains nervous tissue. Gliomas (**Figure 82.7**) are benign midline masses containing glial cells, fibrous and vascular tissue. Gliomas are similar to encephalocoeles, but have become separated from the intracranial structures. However, 15 percent do remain attached to the brain via a fibrous stalk. Presentation is usually early on as a firm, noncompressible, reddish swelling. If the diagnosis is not obvious, differentiation between these lesions and encephalocoeles can be made in a number of ways. A probe will pass laterally but not medially to an intranasal encephalocoele, while an intranasal glioma can arise from the lateral nasal wall. Furstenberg's test (compression of the internal jugular vein) usually causes an encephalocoele to enlarge, but not a glioma. Imaging (CT/MRI) confirms the nature of the lesion.

If the obstruction is causing significant problems, surgical removal of a glioma is recommended. The approach depends on the size and position of the lesion and can be performed intranasally or via a lateral rhinotomy or external rhinoplasty procedure.[12] Encephalocoeles and meningocoeles that need surgery usually require a combined transnasal and neurosurgical approach.

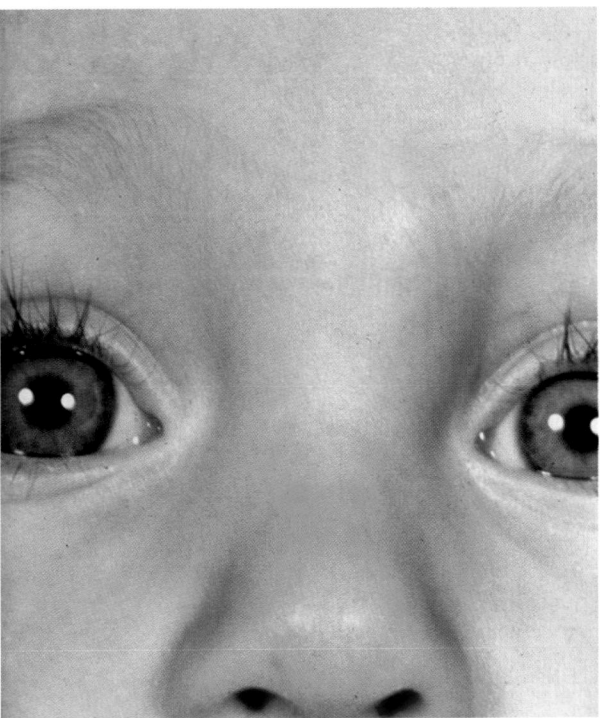

Figure 82.7 Broadened nasal dorsum in a child with a glioma.

NASAL HAEMANGIOMA

These are benign lesions which come under the general classification of vascular malformations (**Figure 82.8**). They can occur in the nose either externally or internally, the latter often arising from the turbinates.

Classically, a haemangioma is either absent or flat at birth and then undergoes a period of rapid growth to present as a mass at around six weeks of age. Growth then continues for the first six months of life before gradual involution occurs and the lesion generally disappears by around the age of six years. This natural history supports conservative management if possible. MRI is the recommended mode of imaging if required and it is particularly useful to exclude an intracranial connection. Liaison with a paediatric dermatology team is vital in patient management as their experience with haemangiomas elsewhere gives invaluable expertise. The first-line intervention would be the use of oral steroids, which are of greatest

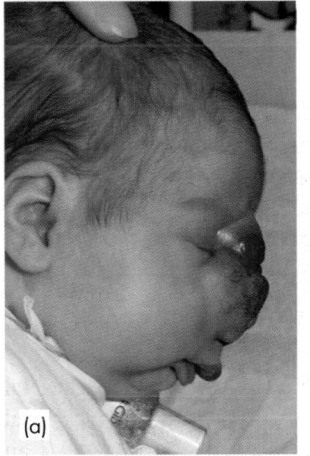
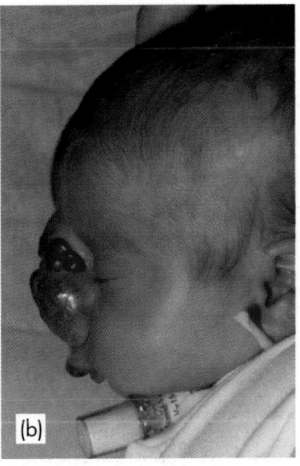
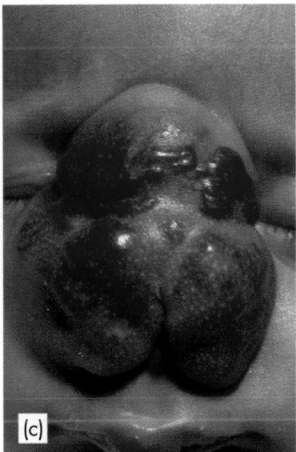
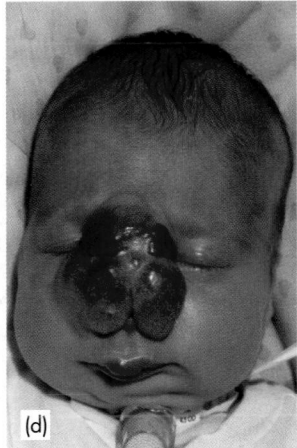

(a) (b) (c) (d)

Figure 82.8 External nasal haemangioma in a 10-week-old girl.

benefit in the rapid growth phase. If rapidly enlarging and encroaching on surrounding structures, e.g. the orbit, a short course of treatment with an anti-proliferative agent, such as methotrexate or vincristine, may be considered under the supervision of a paediatric oncologist.

Surgical treatment may be required, particularly if there are airway or feeding issues. Rarely there can be bleeding, ulceration, platelet consumption, cardiovascular compromise or infection.

MISCELLANEOUS NASAL MASSES

Hamartomas, chordomas, teratomas and craniopharyngiomas are extremely rare causes of nasal obstruction in the child.

ACQUIRED ABNORMALITIES

Osseocartilagenous septal deformity

A number of babies are born with a septal deviation either in isolation or in association with an abnormality of the bony pyramid. It is felt that this problem is either due to intrauterine positioning or to birth trauma (moulding). Closed reduction of the septal deformity with topical anaesthetic in each nostril in the first few days of life has been described by a number of authors and a recent review of long-term follow-up has stressed its importance.[13] It may be appropriate, however, only when there is a significant problem with airway compromise as others have shown complete resolution of the problem without any intervention.[14]

Deformity in older children is usually felt to be due to some form of injury that may have been subtle and unnoticed by either parent or child. There is much debate as to whether septal surgery is appropriate in the growing nose. The main growth centre of the nose is at the septovomerine angle and there is concern that even minor disruption here can lead to significant problems with the final midfacial contour.

Animal studies have shown the development of further septal deviations and poor cartilage regeneration following cartilage resection, crushing and reimplantation.[15] However, a study of anthropometric measurements before and after external septoplasty in 26 children (mean age 9.5 years, with mean follow-up of 3.1 years) showed no deleterious effect of surgery on the development of the nose and midface.[16] Corrective surgery for nasal cartilaginous abnormality in children with cleft lip and palate has been carried out at around seven to eight years of age without affecting midfacial growth.

Generally, if the symptoms are significant, a limited septoplasty with the minimal removal of cartilage is acceptable. Care should be taken not to disrupt the upper lateral cartilages.

Similar concerns have been raised regarding surgery to the bony septum and nasal pyramid. Waiting until at least the early teenage years is felt to be appropriate. Interestingly, though the external rhinoplasty approach has been used for other reasons in very young children no detrimental effects on nasal growth have been reported.

Septal haematoma/abscess

Persistent nasal obstruction following injury should raise concern regarding the possibility of a septal haematoma. These are more common in children than adults, as the former have a thicker and more elastic mucoperichondrium, which often remains intact while the septal vessels below rupture. Pain and fever occur if a septal abscess develops. Both these conditions require drainage to prevent septal perforation.

Foreign bodies

In a small child with unilateral foul discharge, a nasal foreign body must be excluded. If the object has been present for some time, calcareous deposits can form around it resulting in a rhinolith. Care must be taken to act quickly if a battery has been placed in the nose as septal erosion can rapidly occur (see Chapter 92, Foreign bodies in the ear and the aerodigestive tract in children, for further details).

Physiological rhinitis

NEONATAL RHINITIS

Swelling of the nasal mucosa in newborn infants can cause significant airway problems, particularly when feeding, as babies are obligate nasal breathers.

Idiopathic neonatal rhinitis is characterized by mucoid rhinorrhoea with nasal mucosal oedema in the afebrile newborn. This results in stertor, poor feeding and respiratory distress.[17] Structural abnormality, such as choanal atresia or pyriform aperture stenosis, must be excluded before making the diagnosis. Treatment of neonatal rhinitis depends on the severity of symptoms. Nasal bulb suction with saline drops in the first instance is recommended. A short-term course of steroid nose drops would be the next step. This should be closely monitored to avoid the potential side effects from systemic absorption.

Children with infective rhinitis have purulent rhinorrhoea and sometimes associated fever, while allergic rhinitis with sneezing and lacrimation is very unusual in the neonatal period.

It is important to consider chlamydia infection acquired in the birth canal. This usually results in conjunctivitis, but involvement of the nose is seen in around 25 percent of affected individuals. Presentation is with obstruction, rhinorrhoea and a markedly erythematous nasal mucosa on examination. Swabs are diagnostic and the appropriate antibiotic should be prescribed.

Rarely congenital syphilis (*Treponema pallidum*) can cause nasal symptoms in the newborn. Thin, clear secretions are seen between the second week and third month of life. This progresses to a mucopurulent discharge with significant obstruction and crusting of the nostrils. Antibiotic treatment is required both for symptomatic relief and to prevent chronic infection of the cartilage resulting in a saddle deformity.

PUBERTAL RHINITIS

The symptoms of rhinitis are reported as coinciding with the onset of puberty, often in girls and less so in boys. The aetiology is felt mainly to be due to the rise in blood oestrogen levels that occur at this time with some effect also from increased testosterone levels. Oestrogen is known to increase acetylcholine levels by inhibiting acetylcholinesterase. Acetylcholine is a potent vasodilator produced by parasympathetic nerve endings which pass to the nasal mucosa in the vidian nerve. The net result is swelling of the nasal mucosa with increased nasal secretions.[18]

Fibro–osseous disease

This term is used to describe a group of rare disorders, which can affect any bone in the body, including those of the nasal skeleton. They are characterized by the replacement of normal bony architecture with fibroblasts, collagen fibres and a variable amount of mineralized material. Nasal problems are caused by a lesion developing from the upper jaw and spreading out to block the paranasal sinuses and nostrils (**Figure 82.9**). There may also be significant aesthetic concerns, interruption to the development of the dentition and orbital involvement.

Fibro-osseous disease encompasses fibrous dysplasia (FD), benign fibro-osseous neoplasms (including ossifying fibroma) and reactive dysplastic lesions. However, a precise classification of this group of lesions is still a matter of debate. Fibrous dysplasia and ossifying fibroma can present a nasal obstruction in a young child and differentiating between the two conditions may not always be possible. Fibrous dysplasia has three subtypes: monostotic, which involves one site and accounts for 70 percent of cases; polyostotic, which involves multiple bony sites and a polyostotic form with extraskeletal abnormalities (McCune–Albright syndrome) in which there are café-au-lait spots and multiple endocrinopathies due to autonomous secretion of hormones. A mutation in a stimulatory G protein subunit (Gsα) has been found in all three subtypes of fibrous dysplasia.

Imaging is helpful in diagnosis. Fibrous dysplasia has diffusely blending margins, unlike the clearly defined ossifying fibroma. Areas within FD will show an opaque appearance (ground-glass effect), be cystic or multiloculated. The thinned overlying bone has reactive periosteal new bone formation.

Fibrous dysplasia will stop growing at skeletal maturity, whereas the progression of ossifying fibroma is uncertain. Complete surgical excision of ossifying fibroma is ideal, but may not always be possible. In fibrous dysplasia, surgery is performed if significant compression of adjacent structures is occurring. Treatment is surgical, but total excision is often not possible. The aim is to preserve function and limit disability. Endoscopic techniques have been described to excise small lesions limited to the nose or paranasal sinuses, but with extensive disease, the midface degloving approach is recommended. Postoperative baseline imaging is required as recurrence rates are high and repeated procedures may be necessary. Radiotherapy is not used because of the risk of sarcomatous change. Spontaneous malignant change has been reported and is more common in the polyostotic form.

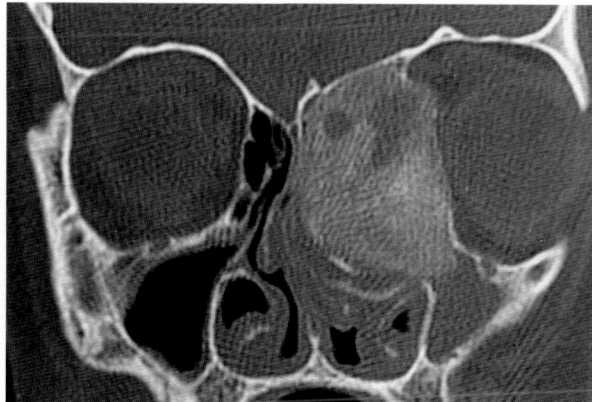

Figure 82.9 CT scan of fibrous dysplasia.

KEY POINTS

- Newborn infants are obligate nasal breathers; nasal obstruction can cause significant respiratory compromise.
- Affected infants may develop stertor, mouth breathing, feeding problems, sleep disturbance and rhinorrhoea.
- Immediate relief can be brought about by placement of an oral airway.
- Choanal atresia may occur in isolation, but is often one of a number of associated anomalies.
- A congenital nasal mass can consist of ectopic intracranial tissue.

Best clinical practice

✓ Use of an oral airway in neonates with nasal obstruction can facilitate transfer for definitive treatment. [Grade C/D]

✓ Minimum additional investigations required in a child with choanal atresia to look for CHARGE association are echocardiography, renal ultrasound and ophthalmology/audiology review. [Grade C/D]

✓ Early surgical excision of dermoid cysts is recommended before infection or further expansion occurs. [Grade C/D]

✓ Nasal masses may not be as innocuous as they seem; always consider intracranial extension and arrange appropriate imaging. CT is helpful for bony anatomy. MRI may identify a CNS connection. [Grade C/D]

✓ Compression of the internal jugular vein (Furstenberg's test) usually causes an encephalocoele, but not a glioma, to enlarge. [Grade C/D]

✓ Idiopathic neonatal rhinitis is underdiagnosed and improves with intranasal steroids. [Grade C/D]

✓ The external rhinoplasty approach causes minimal cosmetic deformity and is extremely useful in the surgical management of nasal masses. [Grade C/D]

✓ Despite the uncertainty about long-term outcomes, septoplasty in children can be undertaken with caution, but only when there are significant symptoms. Cartilage excision should be minimized. [Grade C/D]

Deficiencies in current knowledge and areas for future research

➤ Multi-centre studies are required to clarify the role of mitomycin C in the treatment of choanal atresia.

➤ The long-term outcomes of nasal septal surgery in children are still uncertain.

REFERENCES

∗ 1. Triglia JM, Nicollas R, Roman S, Paris J. Choanal atresia: therapeutic management and results in a series of 58 children. *Revue de Laryngologie-Otologie-Rhinologie.* 2003; **124**: 139–43. *Up-to-date account of the main principles of management of choanal atresia with good follow-up.*

2. Van Den Abbeele T, Francois M, Narcy P. Transnasal endoscopic treatment of choanal atresia without prolonged stenting. *Archives of Otolaryngology – Head and Neck Surgery.* 2002; **128**: 936–40.

3. Morgan DW, Bailey CM. Current management of choanal atresia. *International Journal of Pediatric Otorhinolaryngology.* 1990; **19**: 1–13.

4. Friedman NR, Mitchell RB, Bailey CM, Albert DM, Leighton SE. Management and outcome of choanal atresia correction. *International Journal of Pediatric Otorhinolaryngology.* 2000; **52**: 45–51.

∗ 5. Kubba H, Bennett A, Bailey CM. An update on choanal atresia surgery at Great Ormond Street Hospital for Children: preliminary results with mitomycin C and the KTP laser. *International Journal of Pediatric Otorhinolaryngology.* 2004; **68**: 939–45.

6. Schoem SR. Transnasal endoscopic repair of choanal atresia: why stent? *Otolaryngology – Head and Neck Surgery.* 2004; **131**: 362–6.

∗ 7. Samadi D, Shah U, Handler D. Choanal atresia: a twenty year review of medical comorbidities and surgical outcomes. *Laryngoscope.* 2003; **113**: 254–8. *A good review focussing on outcomes.*

8. Prasad M, Ward R, April MM, Bent J, Froehlich P. Topical mitomycin as an adjunct to choanal atresia repair. *Archives of Otolaryngology – Head and Neck Surgery.* 2002; **128**: 398–400.

9. Ey EH, Han RB, Juon WK. Bony inlet stenosis as a cause of nasal airway obstruction. *Radiology.* 1988; **168**: 477.

∗ 10. Rahbar R, Shah P, Mulliken J, Robson C, Perez-Atayde A, Proctor M *et al.* The presentation and management of nasal dermoid. *Archives of Otolaryngology – Head and Neck Surgery.* 2003; **129**: 464–71.

11. Helper KM. Respiratory distress in the neonate. *Archives of Otolaryngology – Head and Neck Surgery.* 1995; **121**: 1423–5.

12. Koltai PJ, Hoehn J, Bailey CM. The external rhinoplasty approach for rhinologic surgery in children. *Archives of Otolaryngology – Head and Neck Surgery.* 1992; **118**: 401–5.

13. Tasca I, Compadretti GC. Immediate correction of nasal septum dislocation in newborns: long term results. *American Journal of Rhinology.* 2004; **18**: 47–51.

14. Sorri M, Laitakari K, Vainio-Mattila J, Hartikainen-Sorri AL. Immediate correction of congenital nasal deformities; follow up of 8 years. *International Journal of Pediatric Otorhinolaryngology.* 1990; **19**: 277–83.

15. Boenisch M, Tamas H, Nolst-Trenite GJ. Influence of polydioxanone foil on growing septal cartilage after surgery in an animal model: new aspects of cartilage healing and regeneration (preliminary results). *Archives of Facial Plastic Surgery.* 2003; **5**: 316–9.

16. El-Hakim H, Crysdale WS, Abdollel M, Farkas LG. A study of anthropometric measures before and after external sepoplasty in children: a preliminary study. *Archives of Otolaryngology – Head and Neck Surgery.* 2001; **127**: 1362–6.

∗ 17. Nathan CA, Seid AB. Neonatal rhinitis. *International Journal of Pediatric Otorhinolaryngology.* 1997; **39**: 59–65. *A good review of a common condition.*

18. Lekas MD. Rhinitis during pregnancy and rhinitis medicamentosa. *Otolaryngology – Head and Neck Surgery.* 1992; **107**: 845–8.

83

Paediatric rhinosinusitis

GLENIS SCADDING AND HELEN CAULFIELD

Introduction and definition	1079	Treatment	1083
Epidemiology	1080	Surgery for paediatric rhinosinusitis	1084
Allergic rhinitis	1080	Complications of sinusitis in children	1085
Viral rhinitis	1080	Key points	1089
Acute sinusitis and rhinosinusitis	1080	Best clinical practice	1089
Chronic rhinosinusitis	1080	Deficiencies in current knowledge and areas for future	
Diagnosis	1082	research	1089
Examination	1082	References	1089
Investigations	1082		

SEARCH STRATEGY

The data in this chapter are supported by a Medline search using the key words paediatric rhinosinusitis, complications, sinusitis, upper respiratory tract infections, immune deficiency, reflux, primary ciliary dyskinesia, cystic fibrosis, orbital cellulitis, endoscopic sinus surgery, adenoidectomy and by reference to the Oxford textbook of paediatrics, plus articles already in the authors' bibliographies.

INTRODUCTION AND DEFINITION

'Rhinosinusitis' implies inflammation of the mucus membrane lining the nose and sinuses resulting in two or more of the following symptoms. One to be:

- blockage/congestion or
- nasal discharge (anterior/posterior);
- facial pain/ pressure;
- decrease or loss of smell;

with one or more of the following:

- endoscopic signs of polyps;
- mucopurulent discharge from the middle meatus;
- oedema and mucosal obstruction, primarily in the middle meatus;
- CT mucosal changes in the ostiomeatal complex and/ or sinuses.[1]

The nature and pattern of inflammation varies between patients from allergic (with eosinophil predominance) to infectious with neutrophil predominance. The pattern may also vary with time and treatment within an individual. Rhinitis may exist alone, but is frequently accompanied by sinus mucosal changes – rhinosinusitis. The condition may be acute or chronic.

Acute sinusitis lasts under 12 weeks or occurs under six times per year. Bacterial sinusitis complicates 0.2 to 2 percent of viral upper respiratory tract infections.[2] Five to 13 percent of the general population may have experienced sinusitis during childhood,[3] but less than 0.5 percent of those affected are likely to require hospital care.[4]

Recognized factors predisposing to paediatric rhinosinusitis include the following:[5, 6, 7, 8, 9, 10, 11, 12,13, 14, 15, 16, 17, 18, 19, 20, 21]

- allergy: intermittent and/or persistent;
- innate immune deficiency: primary ciliary dyskinesia, cystic fibrosis;
- acquired immune deficiency: IgA deficiency, IgG subclass deficiency, variable immune deficiency;
- gastroesophageal reflux disorder;
- environmental pollution: malnutrition, hyposplenism, diabetes mellitus, immune suppression, biochemical abnormalities.

Diabetes mellitus, if poorly controlled, can be associated with acute sinusitis or with a chronic form, sometimes with fungi present. Chronic diseases such as renal failure are associated with an increased prevalence of upper respiratory tract infections.

Lack of splenic function, either due to previous surgical removal or compromise by diseases such as sickle cell anaemia and malaria, is associated with impaired resistance to infection, particularly with Pneumococci. Polyvalent pneumococcal vaccine should be given prior to splenectomy and patients followed for their ability to make anti-pneumococcal responses.

Protein–calorie malnutrition is common in poorer countries, but milder forms exist in affluent western societies where children frequently have poor diets due to excess consumption of junk foods. Iron deficiency anaemia was thought to be associated with susceptibility to infection, but a recent paper disputes this.[60]

DIAGNOSIS

Diagnosis rests on a detailed history, supported by examination findings. A standard proforma may be helpful. Particularly relevant points are: past evidence of allergic disease (atopic dermatitis, asthma), purulence of nasal discharge, whether this ever remits, and the length of the history.

Associated conditions are common and enquiries should be made about otitis media with effusion, tonsillitis, sleep disorders, asthma and chest infections.

Environmental influences such as allergens present in the home, parental smoking and day care are relevant.[61, 62] In small children a feeding history, particularly of colic or other food reactions, or drinking a bottle whilst lying down, may point to reflux as a possible cause.

A differential diagnosis includes obstructive disorders such as choanal atresia and foreign body, particularly if the problem is unilateral. Adenoid hypertrophy with post-nasal space bacterial colonization also presents with similar symptoms to those of chronic rhinosinusitis.

EXAMINATION

External examination should include a check for an allergic nasal crease or Denny's lines (extra creases under the eyes) plus other evidence of allergy such as atopic dermatitis. Ability to nose-breathe should be tested together with some estimation of the nasal airway which can be as simple as spatula testing.

Internal examination of the nose can be carried out gently with an otoscope. Nasendoscopy will provide more detail, but is difficult in small children without anaesthetic.

The state of the mucus membranes, nature of any discharge and any structural abnormalities should be noted.

Examination of the throat, ears and lower respiratory tract should also be undertaken, together with some functional lower respiratory tract measurement such as peak flow, in all children with upper respiratory tract disease.[26]

INVESTIGATIONS

Skin prick testing

This can be undertaken even in small children, in whom the back is a useful site whilst they are being cuddled by a parent or carer. As with adults it is wise to exclude patients with anaphylaxis, severe atopic dermatitis, recent antihistamines and dermagraphism. Blood RAST (see Chapter 109, Allergic rhinitis) tests be can be substituted looking for allergens suggested by the history.

As with adults, a positive and negative control should be included. A wheal 2 mm greater than the negative control is regarded as positive. However, false positive results occur and observations must be interpreted in the light of the patient's history (**Figure 83.1**).

Blood tests

In refractory rhinitis and rhinosinusitis, some if not all of the following investigations may prove helpful:

- full blood count and differential, including eosinophil count;
- iron studies;
- immunoglobulins;
- IgG subclasses, MBL;
- total IgE and IgE to specific allergens which are either unavailable for skin prick testing or when skin prick testing is contraindicated.

Radiology

Sinus x-rays correlate poorly with computed tomograhy (CT) scans[63] and are very rarely necessary. One possible

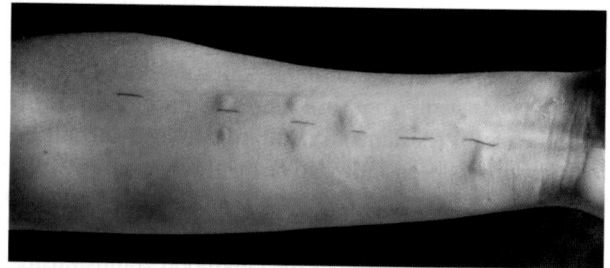

Figure 83.1 Skin prick testing.

exception is acute rhinosinusitis not resolving with therapy after 48 hours, when a plain x-ray may show an empyema of the maxillary antrum. A chest x-ray can be helpful if primary ciliary dyskinesia is suspected since it may show dextrocardia in Kartagener's syndrome.

CT scans of the paranasal sinuses are abnormal in over one-third of children for six weeks after a viral cold, demonstrating sinus inflammation. They are rarely helpful as a diagnostic procedure unless abnormalities such as choanal atresia or encephalocoele are suspected in a child with predominately obstructive symptoms or if extension of acute sinusitis to the orbit or the brain is suspected. Otherwise they provide a useful road map in rare cases where surgical intervention is necessary.[64]

Other specialist tests include:[65]

- nasal mucosal ciliary clearance as assessed by saccharin clearance time;
- ciliary beat frequency as assessed by phase contrast electron microscopy;
- ciliary ultrastructure using the electron microscope;
- nitric oxide measured by chemiluminescence on expired air and intranasally;
- sweat tests and/or genetic analysis for cystic fibrosis;
- pH or impedance monitoring in suspected gastro-oesophageal reflux disease;
- audiometry and tympanometry where there is a suspicion of hearing impairment or speech and language disorder.

TREATMENT

Treatment of allergic rhinitis detailed in the ARIA guidelines[26] is based upon the frequency and severity of disease (see Figures 109.1 and 109.4 in Chapter 109, Allergic rhinitis).

Allergen avoidance

Since hayfever sufferers do not experience hayfever symptoms outside the grass pollen season, it seems that allergen avoidance is effective. However, evidence for the effectiveness of allergen avoidance measures in the treatment of rhinosinusitis is lacking.

Pharmacotherapy

The same preparations are used in paediatric as in adult rhinitis. Special paediatric considerations are as follows:

- **antihistamines**: sedating antihistamines impair academic performance and should be completely avoided;[66]
- **sodium cromoglicate**: this is weakly effective and needs to be used several times a day, but is the only nasal spray licensed for children under four years in the UK;

- **topical corticosteroids**: the metanalysis demonstrates that these are the most effective form of treatment for allergic rhinitis[67, 68] [****] and this is also true in children under four years of age where fluticasone propionate was shown to be superior to ketotifen syrup.[69] They are licensed either for four, six or twelve years upwards and it is important that those which have a systemic bioavailability (betamethasone, dexamethasone, second generation topical corticosteroids) are used only briefly. For long-term use, fluticasone or mometasone appear to be least absorbed.[70] Care should be taken to monitor growth since this is a very sensitive measure of systemic effect, particularly in children receiving corticosteroids at more than one site;
- **leukotriene receptor antagonists** (LTRAs): although these drugs have efficacy in allergic rhinitis, they are no more effective than antihistamines and are similarly expensive. As with adults, some individuals obtain more benefit than others from this form of therapy. Even if combined with an antihistamine the efficacy is not greater than that of an inhaled corticosteroid.[71] Consideration should be given to the use of LTRAs in order to try and reduce steroid dose in children with multiple problems (such as rhinitis, asthma and eczema) who are receiving corticosteroids at more than one site;[72]
- **Decongestants**: oral decongestants are ineffective and have significant side effects such as hyperactivity and insomnia. [****] Topical decongestants can cause rebound with a blocked unresponsive nasal mucosa (rhinitis medicamentosa) if used for more than a few days at a time.[73] They are best used during the thick phase of a cold, on flying or at the start of therapy when the nose is considerably blocked.

There are very few trials of therapy for chronic rhinosinusitis, especially in children. Removal of possible underlying contributing factors (allergens, pollution, infection), would seem sensible. Nasal douching in adults reduces symptoms and improves quality of life. The literature on antibiotics and antifungal agents topical or oral remains confused,[64] but there is evidence of benefit from tobramycin topically in cystic fibrosis.[74]

Immunotherapy

IMMUNE REPLACEMENT THERAPY

Some individuals with severe immunoglobulin defects respond to immunoglobulin replacement therapy.[56] However, this is not usually employed for rhinosinusitis in isolation. Very severe immune deficiency such as T-cell problems may necessitate bone marrow replacement therapy.

BACTERIAL VACCINES

Once widely used, mixed vaccines containing several bacterial antigens were abandoned in the UK after double-blind, placebo-controlled studies showed no efficacy. Some are some available in Europe, with small trials suggesting reduction of reinfection in children.[75]

PNEUMOVAX® (ANTI-PNEUMOCOCCAL VACCINE)

This is effective presplenectomy.

Sublingual immunotherapy

Immunotherapy using preparations of the rhinitis-producing allergen to induce tolerance (densensitization) has been in vogue for many years, usually relying on subcutaneous injection. Sublingual immunotherapy (SLIT) has recently been proposed as an alternative to the subcutaneous route and has been shown in both rhinitis and asthmatic patients to have a good safety profile with no severe systemic reactions reported.[76, 77] A recent Cochrane metanalysis[78] concluded 'SLIT is a safe treatment which significantly reduces symptoms and medication requirements in allergic rhinitis. The size of the benefit compared to that of other available therapies, particularly injection immunotherapy, is not clear, having been assessed directly in very few studies. Further research is required concentrating on optimising allergen dosage and patient selection'.

Recent studies performed in large samples of patients have shown a clear dose-effect of tablet-based SLIT in patients with grass-pollen induced rhinoconjunctivitis.[79, 80, 81] In one study in which subcutaneous and sublingual immunotherapy for seasonal rhinitis were compared, both were effective compared to placebo, although the study was underpowered to detect differences between the treatments.[82] A further recent trial of grass allergen tablets for sublingual use demonstrated a 30–40 percent improvement in symptom and medication scores and an approximate 50 percent increase in the responder rate, compared to placebo.[83] A further follow-up for five years is planned in order to assess possible beneficial long-term effects.

SURGERY FOR PAEDIATRIC RHINOSINUSITIS

Adenoidectomy

There is growing evidence in the literature for adenoidectomy as a first line surgical intervention for chronic rhinosinusitis in children who have failed maximal medical treatment.[84] Hypertrophic adenoids block the posterior choanae, interfering with nasal airflow and the drainage of secretions. They harbour pathogenic bacteria which proliferate rapidly after viral infection. In a recent prospective study, children with large obstructive adenoids showed a significant reduction in the number of episodes of infective rhinosinusitis per year following adenoidectomy.[85] However, a recent metanalysis of (adeno-) tonsillectomy involving six randomized and seven nonrandomized trials with 1596 person years data on upper respiratory tract infections demonstrated a pooled risk difference of only -0.5 episodes per year postoperatively (95 percent CI -0.7 to -0.3).[86] [****] The advent of suction diathermy adenoidectomy has greatly reduced the risks of primary and secondary haemorrhage and, due to the greatly reduced perioperative blood loss, has made adenoidectomy safe in young children.[87] [***]

Maxillary antral washout

Maxillary antral washout used to be the most commonly performed sinus procedure performed in children. The rationale behind it is that it irrigates infective material out of the sinus through the natural ostium, thereby restoring its patency. Infected secretions were washed out and mucosal blood flow improved. However, since the advent of CT scanning it is has been found that over 70 percent of children have involvement of their ethmoid sinuses in chronic rhinosinusisitis and that one irrigation of the maxillary antrum rarely clears the symptoms.[88]

Inferior meatal antrostomy

Creation of an inferior meatal antrostomy does not improve the movement of secretions towards the natural ostium. Despite the creation of an inferior meatal antrostomy, continued obstruction of the osteomeatal complex results in retained secretions and persistent disease. A high failure rate has been reported for this procedure in children with chronic rhinosinusitis and most surgeons have abandoned this procedure, except in children with cystic fibrosis and primary ciliary dyskinesia where gravity is needed to drain sinus secretions as normal mucociliary function is absent. [***]

Turbinate reduction surgery

Surgery to reduce the bulk of the inferior turbinates is sometimes advocated to improve symptomatic nasal obstruction. A multitude of techniques – linear cautery, diathermy, cryosurgery, laser reduction partial excision and submucous resection – have been described. Benefits are short lived and there is significant morbidity with risk of bleeding, postoperative pain and discomfort, troublesome crusting of the nasal secretions and intranasal adhesions. The evidence base for these techniques is weak but best results seem to be with formal submucous resection and a turbinate lateralization procedure.[89] [***/**] Many otolaryngologists empirically offer turbinate reduction surgery where the predominant symptom is nasal obstruction. Turbinectomy is considered in Chapter 125, The management of enlarged turbinates.

Endoscopic sinus surgery

In 1996 a group of otolaryngologists with a specific interest in paediatric rhinosinusitis met in Brussels and created a consensus document in which they described absolute and possible indications for paediatric endoscopic sinus surgery (ESS).[90] These are shown in **Table 83.1**.

A coronal CT scan of the paranasal sinuses with coronal 4 mm cuts using bony windows should be obtained in all patients in whom endoscopic sinus surgery is being considered. This will both define the extent of the disease and provide a road map of the anatomy so that damage to vital structures may be avoided.

The most commonly used technique is an anterior to posterior dissection, as described by Messerklinger in 1978,[91] which is well suited to limited disease affecting the anterior ethmoids, maxillary sinus and frontal sinus. Fashioning of a middle meatal antrostomy can be difficult in the child due to the narrow infundibulum. Paediatric endoscopes (2.7 mm) and instruments are now available, which together with the microdebrider have greatly improved surgical precision. In an attempt to reduce adhesions, some surgeons leave stents in the middle meatus. These are usually removed under general anaesthetic at seven to ten days.[92]

Metanalysis of all the current evidence suggests that paediatric ESS for chronic sinusitis achieves treatment goals in 88 percent.[93] Unfortunately, the results in children with cystic fibrosis are not so encouraging with a recurrence rate of 50 percent within 12 months.[94]

In the early 1990s, two studies involving piglets demonstrated significant changes in facial growth following sinus surgery.[95, 96] Subsequently, two papers involving humans suggest that the risk is less substantial and no discernable change in facial anthropometric measurements were seen ten years after ESS.[97, 98]

The role of endoscopic sinus surgery in paediatric sinusitis is still evolving but the technique appears safe without long-term side effects; however adenoidectomy should be the first step in young children with adenoidal hypertrophy and nasal symptoms unresponsive to medical treatment. [****]

COMPLICATIONS OF SINUSITIS IN CHILDREN

Complications of paranasal sinus disease are more common in children than adults. The spread of infection from the nose and paranasal cavities to the surrounding brain and orbit is facilitated in children by dehiscences in the common bony walls at the suture lines, the thinness of the cranial bones and the relative immunosuppression of the child under the age of five.

The incidence of serious complications of sinusitis has steadily declined since the advent of antibiotics, but orbital and intracranial complications still occur (**Table 83.2**). Intracranial spread occurs through septic venous phlebitis in the venous system which drains the brain and paranasal sinuses. This whole venous system is devoid of valves and there are no lymphatic vessels or lymph nodes in the orbit to trap infection. [****/**]

Local complications

ORO ANTRAL FISTULA

An oro antral fistula is an abnormal communication between the floor of the maxillary sinus and the roof of the oral cavity. It is usually caused by extraction of a molar tooth in the older child. If identified early, simple gingival closure can be successful. Once the fistula is established it discharges foul smelling green pus which requires systemic antibiotics and maxillary antral lavage. Large oro antral fistulae require surgical repair using local mucosal flaps with or without buccal fat grafts.[99]

Table 83.1 Indications for paediatric endoscopic sinus surgery.

Indications	Relative indications
Complications of sinusitis	Persistent signs and symptoms with CT findings consistent with clinical disease
Symptomatic mucocoeles	Symptomatic concha bullosa
Systemic disease complicating sinusitis	Chronic headache with abnormal CT
Recurrent or chronic sinusitis persisting for six months despite medical therapy	Chronic nasal discharge
	Recurrent sinusitis with normal CT

Table 83.2 Complications of paediatric rhinosinusitis.

Local complications	Orbital complications	Intracranial complications
Oro antral fistula	Periorbital cellulitis	Meningitis
Mucocoele	Subperiosteal abscess	Intracranial abscess
Osteomyelitis	Orbital abscess	
	Cavernous sinus thrombosis	

MUCOCOELES

Mucocoeles are epithelial-lined mucous containing cysts which can completely fill a paranasal sinus. They can be classified as primary or secondary. Primary mucocoeles are mucous retention cysts which are common and usually asymptomatic, situated in the floor of the maxillary sinus. Secondary mucocoeles are due to obstruction of a sinus osteum due to inflammation, which causes the retention of secretions under pressure. Secondary mucocoeles are very rare in children but when they do occur the most common site is the frontoethmoids. In children with cystic fibrosis, however, the maxillary sinus is most commonly affected. The wall of the cyst releases osteolytic substances and can cause expansion of bone, presenting as a space-occupying lesion and acting as a benign tumour.[100]

Frontoethmoid mucocoeles cause displacement of the orbit leading to progressive diplopia, proptosis and limitation of ocular movement. It is not uncommon for children to initially present to an ophthalmologist because of this. Bulging of the medial nasal wall causes nasal obstruction. Vertex headache is frequent and may be the only symptom in the cases of isolated sphenoid mucocoeles although pressure on the optic nerve will cause visual disturbance.[101]

Plain x-rays of the paranasal sinuses are of little use in evaluating mucocoeles. The investigation of choice is CT scanning. Mucocoeles are seen as round or oval homogenous masses involving one or more paranasal sinuses and causing compression of the surrounding structures due to expansion of the bony walls of the affected sinus.

Mucocoeles require surgical intervention. Frontoethmoid mucocoeles have traditionally been marsupialized using an external frontoethmoidectomy approach and extensive surgery using osteoplastic flaps and cranialization of the frontal sinus has also been described. Within the last decade, however, there is increasing evidence of the suitability of endoscopic sinus surgery in the treatment of paediatric mucocoeles and thus avoiding external scars.[102, 103]

OSTEOMYELITIS

Osteomyelitis of the frontal bone is a rare complication of frontal sinusitis. Less than 20 cases have been reported in the literature within the last decade. Teenagers are most commonly affected and initial presentation is with local headache and tenderness. Infection in the frontal sinus can cause an osteomyelitis of the frontal bone. Suppurative material may then breach the cortex of the frontal bone causing subperiosteal abscess formation in the tissues of the forehead. This creates a boggy swelling which was first described by Sir Percival Pott in 1760 and consequently is named 'Pott's puffy tumour'.

Frontal bone osteomyelitis can also cause subdural, epidural and periorbital abscesses as well as secondary septic thrombosis of the dural sinuses and is associated with severe neurological sequelae in 20 percent of patients.[104]

The causative organisms are Gram-positive cocci including *Streptococcus*, *Staphylococcus* and oral anaerobes. Initial treatment consists of the administration of intravenous antibiotics such as penicillin, flucloxacillin and metronidazole.

CT scanning of the brain and paranasal sinuses is the most appropriate investigation as it will show which sinuses are involved and can detect intracranial or soft tissue spread of infection. Chronic or early osteomyelitis can be detected using a technetium 99 bone scan.

Surgical intervention is needed if the CT scan shows a complication of frontal sinusitis such as abscess formation. Frontal sinus trephine through an external eyebrow incision and maxillary antral washout under anaesthetic are usually sufficient to clear the pus in the sinuses. The osteoplastic flap procedure removing sequestrated frontal bone with secondary acrylic plate reconstruction is very rarely needed. [**]

Orbital complications

Infection may spread through the thin party wall (lamina papyracea) separating the ethmoidal sinuses from the orbit. If confined to the anterior part of the orbit in front of the fibrous septum, which protects the more posterior contents of the globe, 'periorbital' or 'pre-septal' cellulitis ensues. Spread behind the septum and into the globe proper is the far more dangerous 'orbital cellulitis' (**Figure 83.2**). Periorbital cellulitis is the most frequently occurring complication in children. Children with orbital complications of sinusitis commonly present to ophthalmologists and paediatricians, as well as otolaryngologists, and their successful management depends on cooperation between these specialities.[105] The reason for this is the importance of the assessment of the child's eye and general clinical condition. The difficulty for the clinician lies in distinguishing periorbital cellulitis, which will usually resolve with antibiotics, from subperiosteal or orbital abscess which requires surgical drainage.

In one series, 70 percent of children presenting with periorbital cellulitis were under nine years old and 70 percent of these had medically treatable periorbital

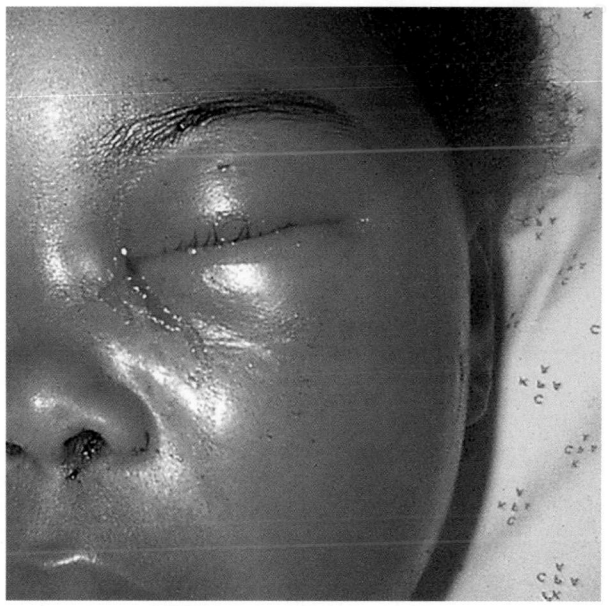

Figure 83.2 Orbital cellulitis.

cellulitis. Despite modern surgical techniques and appropriate antibiotics, blindness is still a real risk in children as a result of orbital infection. The older the child at presentation the greater the risk of subperiosteal abscess, orbital abscess or cavernous sinus thrombosis.[106]

In 1970, James Chandler published an excellent paper in which he describes both the pathogenesis and management of the orbital complications of sinusitis and his classification system, as shown in **Table 83.3**, is still used today.[107]

PERIORBITAL CELLULITIS/SUBPERIOSTEAL ABSCESS/ ORBITAL ABSCESS

Unfortunately, when a child presents with periorbital cellulitis it is not easy to define which stage the disease has reached on clinical signs alone and it must be remembered that half of cases with intracranial complications present with periorbital cellulitis.[108] On the other hand, the great majority (75–80 percent) of periorbital cellulitis in children resolves with antibiotic treatment alone.[109] For these reasons protocols are needed to ensure that each patient is appropriately treated and to reduce the incidence of complications.[110] In the UK, all children with periorbital cellulitis are admitted for the administration of

Table 83.3 Chandler's classification of orbital infection.

Stage	
1	Inflammatory oedema
2	Orbital cellulitis
3	Subperiosteal abscess
4	Orbital abscess
5	Cavernous sinus thrombosis

intravenous antibiotics. Traditionally, penicillin, flucloxacillin and metronidazole have been used as the commonest pathogens isolated were *Streptococcus*, *Staphylococcus* and *Haemophilus influenza* type b. Since the advent of the Hib vaccine, haemophilus infections are much rarer and only occur in unimmunized children.[111] Anaerobes such as bacteroides are part of the natural nasal flora and rarely cultured except in chronic rhinosinusitis and some brain abscesses. However, it is prudent to include anaerobic cover from the outset. In areas where beta lactamase-producing bacteria are common, the antibiotic combination should be changed to either cefuroxime and metronidazole or co-amoxyclavulanic acid. Intranasal decongestants and irrigation with saline are routinely used but their benefit has not been scientifically evaluated. Regular and adequate analgesia is required.

The patient should be closely monitored by documenting neurological state, the temperature and white-cell count. Colour vision, visual acuity, eye movements and papillary reflexes should be checked once or twice per day by an ophthalmologist.[111] Worrying features include worsening proptosis, visual disturbance, reduced or painful eye movement and high fever. If there is no improvement in clinical signs after 24 hours of appropriate intravenous antibiotics, a CT scan of the paranasal sinuses and brain with contrast should be ordered urgently. Other indications for CT scanning are as follows:[110]

- central neurological signs;
- inability to perform adequate opthalmological examination;
- no improvement in orbital signs or general clinical condition after 24 hours of appropriate intravenous antibiotics;
- deterioration of orbital signs (proptosis, opthalmoplegia, altered colour vision, or visual acuity).

Surgical intervention is required if there is evidence of a collection of pus, either subperiosteally, within the orbit or intracranially. The aim of surgery is to drain the pus, release the pressure on the orbit and to provide material for microbiological culture. Extensive sinus surgery is unjustified as orbital complications are usually the result of acute sinus infections. The location of the abscess will dictate if an endoscopic approach is feasible.[112] Endoscopic drainage avoids external scars and results in rapid resolution of periorbital inflammation. The anatomical limits of the paediatric nose and the vascular mucosa make it technically difficult but excellent results have been reported in expert hands.[113] An external ethmoidectomy with bilateral maxillary antral washout has stood the test of time. If a subperiosteal abscess is encountered, it can be drained into the nose through a subtotal ethmoidectomy. In the presence of pus trapped in the frontal sinus, a trephination of the frontal sinus floor can be performed at the same time. If an orbital abscess is present, it can be drained via a linear incision around the orbit through the tarsal plate of the upper eyelid. Intravenous antibiotics should be continued for a further 48 hours and then oral antibiotics for a further 10–14 days.[114]

CAVERNOUS SINUS THROMBOSIS

Cavernous sinus thrombosis results from septic phlebitis of the ophthalmic veins and involvement of the cavernous sinus. Initially, the orbital signs are unilateral but these become progressively bilateral causing proptosis with third, fourth and sixth cranial nerve palsies. Signs of meningitis are frequently present and there is dilation of the episcleral veins, which is a distinctive feature. It can prove to be fatal with quoted mortality rates of 30 percent.[115] CT scanning of the head with contrast will confirm the diagnosis. Intravenous broad-spectrum antibiotics should be started immediately, together with heparin anticoagulation. *Staphylococcus aureus*, *Streptococcus* and *Pneumococcus* are the most likely organisms. High-dose systemic steroids will reduce oedema around the orbital apex and should be given. Orbital exploration and drainage of involved paranasal sinuses is urgently needed so as to drain an orbital abscess and decompress the orbit. Intravenous antibiotics will be needed for several weeks for an optimal outcome.[116] [**]

Intracranial complications

MENINGITIS

Meningitis is regarded as the most common intracranial sinogenic complication.[117] The clinical presentation is headache, neck stiffness and a high fever in the presence of purulent rhinorrhea. Febrile convulsions and vomiting may occur. However, it must be remembered that, in one-third of children, neck stiffness will not be demonstrable.[114] In young children it can be difficult to distinguish meningitis from intracranial abscess or encephalitis. CT scan of the brain with contrast should be undertaken before lumbar pucture to exclude intracranial lesions that could cause raised intracranial pressure.[118]

First-line treatment is with intravenous antibiotics. *Streptococcus pneumoniae*, *Haemophilus influenza* type b (Hib) and *Neisseria meningitidis* are the most common pathogens, although vaccination has virtually eradicated Hib meningitis in some countries. Drainage of the involved sinus is needed if either there is no improvement in clinical condition or intracranial involvement on CT scanning. Unfortunately, neurological sequelae such as sensorineural deafness and global delay are common after meningitis. The use of adjuvant corticosteroids is controversial but is beneficial in reducing the incidence of neurological sequelae in children.[119] [**/*]

INTRACRANIAL ABSCESS

All intracranial complications of sinusitis are more common in male adolescents.[120] The management of intracranial abscess requires close cooperation between the otolaryngologist, neurosurgeon and paediatrician as it is life-threatening and requires immediate treatment. Intravenous broad-spectrum antibiotics with good cerebrospinal (CSF) penetration are needed, together with drainage of the involved sinus and its intracranial focus of infection.

Intracranial abscesses can be classified as extradural, subdural and intracerebral, depending on their anatomical location. Intracranial extradural abscess is due to infection in the space between the dura and bone and is almost exclusively a complication of frontal sinusitis with secondary osteomyelitis. It presents with local tenderness, fever and headache, but focal neurological signs and changes in conscious level are rarely seen. Both the affected sinus and the extradural abscess require surgical drainage, either endoscopically or externally.

Subdural infection (**Figure 83.3**) is very rare but is a serious complication of frontal sinusitis. It carries a 25–35 percent mortality rate and, of those who survive, 30 percent will have permanent neurological impairment.[117] It tracks over the frontal lobes in the subdural space and can spread into the interhemispheric region leading to a parafalcine abscess. The presenting features are of worsening headache, vomiting, seizures and rapid loss

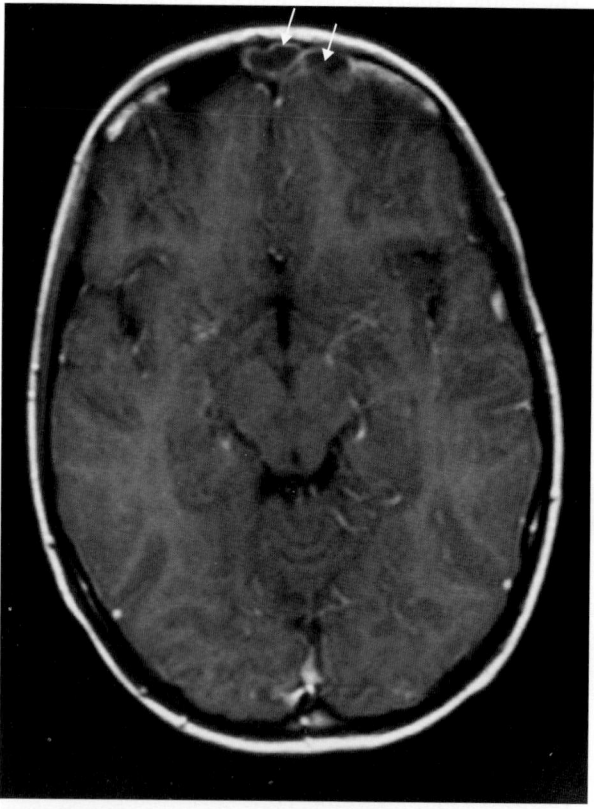

Figure 83.3 Subdural empyema due to frontal sinusitis (arrowed).

of consciousness with specific neurological signs depending on the site of the abscess. CT or MRI are used to make the diagnosis. Treatment consists of intravenous broad-spectrum antibiotics and a combined neurosurgical and otolaryngological procedure to achieve drainage of the affected sinus and subdural abscess. Perioperative steroids and anticonvulsants are used to reduce the effects of raised intracranial pressure.

Ten percent of intracerebral abscesses in children are secondary to sinusitis or mastoiditis. This is significantly less frequent when compared to data collected prior to the 1980s.[121] Unfortunately, the mortality rate of those affected remains unchanged at about 25 percent. The frontal and parietal lobes are most commonly affected. The symptoms are those of raised intracranial pressure, fever, seizures and loss of consciousness. Diagnosis is by imaging with CT or MRI. Lumbar puncture is contra-indicated as there is a distinct likelihood that it will cause coning of the brainstem. As a result of scarring of cerebral tissue, postoperative epilepsy occurs in approximately one-third of children who undergo excision of their intracerebral abscess and therefore CT guided aspiration and intravenous antibiotic treatment is advocated to reduce this risk.[122] [**]

KEY POINTS

- Paediatric rhinitis/rhinosinusitis is very common.
- Paediatric rhinosinusitis is usually treatable with medication and surgery is rarely needed.
- Imaging is rarely needed to make the diagnosis.
- In allergic rhinitis, skin prick tests may be negative for the first year or two of symptoms in children.
- IgA/IgG subclass deficiency is common in the population and should be considered as a cause of recurrent rhinosinusitis.
- Complications of infective sinusitis are rare but potentially fatal. Early recognition and treatment help to reduce morbidity.

Best clinical practice

- ✓ Indications for prescribing antibiotics in rhinosinusitis are: moderately severe maxillary pain with tenderness in the face and purulent rhinorrhea lasting more than seven days following a cold. [Grade B]
- ✓ The antibiotic chosen should be the most narrow spectrum agent available against the likely pathogens. [Grade B]

- ✓ Additional use of topical nasal corticosteroids or antihistamine plus antibiotics is associated with a more rapid resolution of symptoms in acute sinusitis. [Grade B]
- ✓ Intranasal steroids are the most effective form of treatment for allergic rhinitis. [Grade A]
- ✓ Oral decongestants are ineffective in rhinitis. [Grade A]
- ✓ There is growing evidence in the literature for adenoidectomy as a first line surgical intervention for chronic rhinosinusitis in children who have failed maximal medical treatment. [Grade C]
- ✓ In orbital cellulitis, if there is no improvement in clinical signs after 24 hours of appropriate intravenous antibiotics, a CT scan of the paranasal sinuses and brain with contrast should be ordered urgently. Surgical drainage of a subperiosteal or orbital abscess may be required. [Grade C]
- ✓ Lumbar puncture is contraindicated in sinogenic meningitis as there is a risk that it will cause coning of the brainstem. [Grade C/D]

Deficiencies in current knowledge and areas for future research

- ➤ There is much ongoing work on the epidemiology of upper respiratory tract allergy in children. The respective roles of hereditary factors, viral infections in early infancy and early exposure to antigens are still unclear.
- ➤ Knowledge of the pathophysiology of allergic rhinitis – including the role of nitric oxide – continues to be refined.
- ➤ The evidence base for surgical interventions in paediatric rhinosinusitis needs to be improved.

REFERENCES

1. Fokkens W, Lund VJ, Mullol J *et al.* On behalf of the European Rhinosinusitis and Nasal Polyps Group. European position paper on rhinosinusitis and nasal polyps. *Rhinology EPOS.* 2007; **Suppl 20**: 1–136.
2. Scadding GK. Paediatric chronic rhinosinusitis. In: Sih T, Clement P (eds). Published in *Paediatric ENT*, Brazil (2001), published in UK 2002.
3. Wald ER, Guerva N, Byers C. Upper respiratory tract infections in young children: Duration and frequency of complications. *Paediatrics.* 1991; **87**: 129–33.
4. Henriksson G, Westrin KM, Kumlien J, Pontus. A 13-year report on childhood sinusitis: Clinical presentations

predisposing factors and possible means of prevention. *Rhinology*. 1996; **34**: 171–5.

5. Kogutt MS, Shwachman H. Diagnosis of sinusitis in infants and children. *Paediatrics*. 1973; **52**: 121–4.

6. Crockett DM, McGill TJ, Friedman EM, Healy GB, Salkeld LJ. Nasal and paranasal sinus surgery in children with cystic fibrosis. *Annals of Otology, Rhinology and Laryngology*. 1987; **96**: 367–72.

7. Aberg N, Engstrom I, Lindberg U. Allergic disease in Swedish school children. *Acta Paediatrica Scandinavica*. 1989; **78**: 246–52.

8. Rachelefsky GS, Katz RM, Siegel SC. Chronic sinusitis in the allergic child. *Pediatric Clinics of North America*. 1988; **35**: 1091–101.

9. Savolainen S. Allergy in patients with acute maxillary sinusitis. *Allergy*. 1989; **44**: 116–22.

10. Fireman P. Diagnosis of sinusitis in children: Emphasis on the history and physical examination. *Journal of Allergy and Clinical Immunology*. 1992; **90**: 433–6.

11. Furukawa CT, Sharpe M, Bierman CW, Pierson WE, Shapiro GC, Altman LC et al. Allergic patients have more frequent sinus infections than non-allergic patients. *Journal of Allergy and Clinical Immunology*. 1992; **89**: 332.

12. Rachelefsky GS, Katz RM, Siegel SC, Spector MD, Rohr AS. Chronic sinusitis in children. *Journal of Allergy and Clinical Immunology*. 1992; **87**: 219.

13. Shapiro GC, Virant FS, Furakawa CT, Pierson WE, Bierman CW. Immunologic defects in patients with refractory sinusitis. *Paediatrics*. 1991; **87**: 311–6.

14. Orobello RW, Park RI, Belcher LJ, Eggleston P, Lederman HM, Banks JR et al. Microbiology of chronic sinusitis in children. *Archives of Otolaryngology – Head and Neck Surgery*. 1991; **117**: 980–3.

15. Sapiro ED, Milmoe GJ, Wald ER, Rodman JB, Bowen AD. Bacteriology of the maxillary sinuses in patients with cystic fibrosis. *Journal of Infectious Diseases*. 1982; **146**: 589–93.

16. Stern RC, Boat TF, Wood RE, Matthews LW, Doerahuk CF. Treatment and prognosis of nasal polyps in cystic fibrosis. *American Journal of Otolaryngology*. 1982; **136**: 1067.

17. Reilly JS, Kenna MA, Stool SE, Bluestone CD. Nasal surgery in children with cystic fibrosis: Complications and risk management. *Laryngoscope*. 1985; **95**: 1491.

18. Ceporor R, Smith RJH, Catlin FI, Bressler KL, Furuta GT, Shandera KC. Cystic fibriosis: An otolaryngologic perspective. *Otolaryngology – Head and Neck Surgery*. 1987; **97**: 356.

19. Cuyler JP, Monaghan AJ. Cystic fibrosis and sinusitis. *Journal of Otolaryngology*. 1989; **18**: 173–5.

20. Drake Lee AB, Morgan DW. Nasal polyps and sinusitis in children with cystic fibrosis. *Journal of Laryngology and Otology*. 1989; **103**: 753–5.

21. Rudolph CD. Supraesophageal complications of gastroesophageal reflux in children: challenges in diagnosis and treatment. *American Journal of Medicine*. 2003; **115**: 150S–156S.

22. Ellwood P, Asher MI, Bjorksten B, Burr M, Pearce N, Robertson CF. Diet and asthma, allergic rhinoconjunctivitis and atopic eczema symptom prevalence: an ecological analysis of the Internation Study of asthma Allergies in Childhood (ISAAC) data. ISAAC Phase One Study Group. *European Respiratory Journal*. 2001; **17**: 436–43.

23. Otten FW, Van Aarem A, Grote JJ. Long term follow up of chronic therapy resistant purulent rhinitis in children. *Clinical Otolaryngology*. 1992; **17**: 32–2.

24. Clement PA, Bijloos J, Kaufman L, Lauwers L, Maes JJ, Van der Vaken P et al. Incidence and aetiology of rhinosinusitis in children. *Acta Otorhinologolgy*. 1989; **43**: 523–43.

25. Manning SC, Biavati MJ, Phillips DL. Correlation of clinical sinusitis signs and symptoms to imaging findings in pediatric patients. *International Journal of Pediatric Otorhinolaryngology*. 1996; **37**: 65–74.

* 26. Bousquet J, van Cauwenberge P, Khaltaev N. Allergic rhinitis and its impact on asthma (ARIA). *Journal of Allergy and Clinical Immunology*. 2001; **108**: S147–334. *An account of current thinking re the association between asthma and allergic rhinitis.*

27. Kulig M, Bergmann R, Klettke U, Wahn V, Tacke U, Wahn U. Natural course of sensitization to food and inhalant allergens during the first 6 years of life. *Journal of Allergy and Clinical Immunology*. 1999; **103**: 1173–9.

28. Gwaltney Jr. JM. Acute community acquired bacterial sinusitis: To treat or not to treat. *Canadian Respiratory Journal*. 1999; **6**: 46A–50A. Review.

29. Johnston NW, Sears MR. Asthma exacerbations. 1: epidemiology. *Thorax*. 2006; **61**: 722–728S.

30. Murray CS, Poletti G, Kebadze T, Morris J, Woodcock A, Johnston SL et al. Study of modifiable risk factors for asthma exacerbations: virus infection and allergen exposure increase the risk of asthma hospital admissions in children. *Thorax*. 2006; **61**: 376–82.

* 31. Hickner JM, Bartlett JG, Besser RE, Gonzales R, Hoffman JR, Sande MA et al. Principles of appropriate antibiotic use for acute rhinosinusitis in adults – a background. *Annals of Internal Medicine*. 2001; **134**: 498–505. *Recommendations on the management of acute sinusitis particularly relevant in primary care.*

32. Turner BW, Cail WS, Hendley JO, Hayden FG, Doyle WJ, Sorrentino JV et al. Physiologic abnormalities in the paranasal sinuses during experimental rhinovirus colds. *Journal of Allergy and Clinical Immunology*. 1992; **90**: 474–8.

* 33. Arroll B. Antibiotics for upper respiratory tract infections: an overview of Cochrane reviews. *Respiratory Medicine*. 2005; **99**: 255–61. *A systematic review of this controversial topic.*

34. Nayak AS, Settipane GA, Pedinoff A, Charous BL, Meltzer EO, Busse WW et al. Effective dose range of mometasone furoate nasal spray in the treatment of acute rhinosinusitis. *Annals of Allergy, Asthma and Immunology*. 2002; **89**: 271–8.

35. Meltzer EO, Charous BL, Busse WW, Zinreich SJ, Lorber RR, Danzig MR. Added relief in the treatment of acute

recurrent sinusitis with adjunctive mometasone furoate nasal spray. The Nasonex Sinusitis Group. *Journal of Allergy and Clinical Immunology.* 2000; **106**: 630–7.

36. Braun JJ, Alabert JP, Michel FB, Quiniou M, Rat C, Cougnard J *et al.* Adjunct effect of loratadine in the treatment of acute sinusitis in patients with allergic rhinitis. *Allergy.* 1997; **52**: 650–5.

37. Meltzer EO, Bachert C, Staudinger H. Treating acute rhinosinusitis: comparing efficacy and safety of memetasone furoate nasal spray, amoxicillin, and placebo. *Journal of Allergy and Clinical Immunology.* 2005; **116**: 1289–95.

38. Gordts F, Clement PA, Destryker A, Desprechins B, Kaufman L. Prevalence of sinusitis signs on MRI in a non-ENT paediatric population. *Rhinology.* 1997; **35**: 154–7.

39. Rachelefsky GS, Spector SL. Sinusitis and asthma. *Journal of Asthma.* 1990; **27**: 1–3.

40. Bush A, O'Callaghan C, Boon A. Primary ciliary dyskinesia. *Archives of Disease in Childhood.* 2002; **87**: 363–5.

41. Wodehouse T, Kharitonov SA, Mackay IS, Barnes PJ, Wilson R, Cole PJ. Nasal nitric oxide measurements for the screening of primary ciliary dyskinesia. *European Respiratory Journal.* 2003; **21**: 43–7.

42. Kerem B, Rommons JM, Buchanan JA, Markiewicz D, Cox TK, Chakravarti A *et al.* Identification of the cystic fibrosis gene: genetic analysis. *Science.* 1989; **245**: 1073–80.

43. Shwachman H, Kulczycki L, Mueller H, Flake C. Nasal polyps in patiens with cystic fibrosis. *Paediatrics.* 1962; **30**: 389–401.

44. Bak-Pedersen K, Larsen PK. Inflammatory middle ear diseases in patients with cystic fibrosis. *Acta Oto-laryngologica.* Supplementum 1979; **360**: 138–40.

45. Stern RC, Boat TF, Wood RE, Matthews LW, Doershuk CF. Treatment and prognosis of nasal polyps in cystic fibrosis. *American Journal of Diseases of Children.* 1982; **136**: 1067–70.

46. Henderson Jr. WR, Chi EY. Degranulation of cystic fibrosis nasal polyp mast cells. *Journal of Pathology.* 1992; **166**: 395–404.

47. Henriksson G, Westrin KM, Karpati F, Wikstrom AC, Stierna P, Hjelte L. Nasal polyps in cystic fibrosis: clinical endoscopic study with nasal lavage fluid analysis. *Chest.* 2002; **121**: 40–7.

48. Klossek JM, Neukirch F, Pribil C, Jankowski R, Serrano E, Chanal I *et al.* Prevalence of nasal polyposis in France: a cross-sectional, case-control study. *Allergy.* 2005; **60**: 233–7.

49. Davidson TM, Murphy C, Mitchell M, Smith C. Management of chronic sinusitis in cystic fibrosis. *Laryngoscope.* 1995; **105**: 354–8.

50. Raman V, Clary R, Siegreist KL, Zehnbauer B, Chatila TA. Increased prevalence of mutations in the cystic fibrosis transmembrane conductance regulator in children with chronic rhinosinusitis. *Paediatrics.* 2001; **109**: E13.

51. Harris JP, South MA. Immunodeficiency diseases: head and neck manifestations. *Head and Neck Surgery.* 1982; **5**: 114–24.

52. Kowalcyk D, Mytar B, Zembala M. Cytokine production in transient hypogammaglobulinemia and isolated 1 deficiency. *Journal of Allergy and Clinical Immunology.* 1997; **100**: 556–62.

53. Buckley RH. Clinical and immunologic features of selective IgA deficiency. *Birth Defects Original Article Series.* 1975; **11**: 134–42.

54. Hanson LA, Soderstrom R, Avanzini A, Bengtsson U, Bjorkander J, Soderstrom T. Immunoglobulin subclass deficiency. *Pediatric Infectious Diseases Journal.* 1988; **7**: S17–21.

55. Epstein MM, Gruskay F. Selective deficiency in pneumococcal antibody response in children with recurrent infections. *Annals of Allergy, Asthma and Immunology.* 1995; **75**: 125–31.

56. Silk H, Ambrosino D, Geha RS. Effect of intravenous gammaglobulin therapy in igG2 deficient and IgG2 sufficient children with recurrent infections and poor response to immunization with Hemophilus influenzae type b capsular polysaccharide antigen. *Annals of Allergy.* 1990; **64**: 21–5.

57. Turner MW. The role of mannose-binding lectin in health and disease. *Molecular Immunology.* 2003; **40**: 423–9.

58. Cedzynsk M, Szemraj J, Swierzko AS, Bak-Romaniszyn L, Banasik Seman K, Kilpatrick DC. *Mannan-binding lectin insufficiency in children with recurrent infections of the respiratory system.* Lodz Poland: Laboratory of Immunobiology of Infections, Centre of Medical Biology, Polish Academy of Sciences, 2004.

59. Baughmann RP, Dohn MN. Respiratory tract infections in the immunocompromised (non-HIV) patient. *Current Opinion in Infectious Diseases.* 1995; **8**: 110–5.

60. Ali NS, Zuberi RW. Association of iron deficiency anaemia in children of 1-2 years of age with low birth weight, recurrent diarrhoea or recurrent respiratory tract infections: myth or fact. *Journal of the Pakistan Medical Association.* 2003; **53**: 133–6.

61. Couriel JM. Passive smoking and the health of children. *Thorax.* 1994; **49**: 731–4.

62. Colley JR, Douglas JW, Reid DD. Respiratory disease in young adults: influence of early childhood lower respiratory tract illness, social class, air pollution and smoking. *British Medical Journal.* 1973; **3**: 195–8.

63. McAlister WH, Lusk R, Muntz HR. Comparison of plain radiographs and coronal CT scans in children with recurrent sinusitis. *AJR. American Journal of Roentgenology.* 1990; **155**: 425.

64. Jones NS. Current concepts in the management of paediatric rhinosinusitis. *Journal of Laryngology and Otology.* 1999; **113**: 1–9.

65. Moss RB, King VV. Management of sinusitis in cystic fibrosis by endoscopic surgery and serial antimicrobial lavage. Reduction in recurrence requiring surgery. *Archives of Otolaryngology – Head/Neck Surgery.* 1995; **121**: 566–72.

66. Vuurman EF, van Veggel LM, Uiterwijk MM, Leutner D, O'Hanlon JF. Seasonal allergic rhinitis and antihistamine

84

The adenoid and adenoidectomy

PETER J ROBB

Introduction	1094	Complications of adenoidectomy	1097
Development of the adenoid	1094	Key points	1098
Immune function of the adenoid	1094	Best clinical practice	1099
Pathological effects of the adenoid	1095	Deficiencies in current knowledge and areas for future	
Assessment and management	1096	research	1099
Adenoidectomy	1097	References	1099

SEARCH STRATEGY

The data in this chapter are supported by searches from the Guidelines database at the National Electronic Library for Health, The Cochrane Library, Medline and PubMed using the key words adenoid, adenoidectomy and children.

INTRODUCTION

Santorini described the nasopharyngeal lymphoid aggregate or 'Lushka's tonsil' in 1724. Wilhelm Meyer coined the term 'adenoid' to apply to what he described as 'nasopharyngeal vegetations' in 1870. The adenoid forms part of Waldeyer's ring of lymphoid tissue at the portal of the upper respiratory tract. In early childhood this is the first site of immunological contact for inhaled antigens.

Historically, the adenoid has been associated with upper airway obstruction, as a focus of sepsis, and more recently with the persistence of otitis media with effusion.

DEVELOPMENT OF THE ADENOID

Lymphoid tissue can be identified at four to six weeks gestation, lying within the mucous membrane of the roof and posterior wall of the nasopharynx. Lymphoid tissue of the adenoid may extend to the fossa of Rosenmüller and to the Eustachian tube orifice as Gerlach's tonsil. The membrane is covered with stratified squamous epithelium. The adenoid receives a rich arterial supply from branches of the facial and maxillary arteries and the thyrocervical trunk. Venous drainage is to the internal jugular and facial veins. Lymphatic drainage is to the retropharyngeal lymph nodes and upper deep cervical nodes, particularly the posterior triangle of the neck. Nerve supply is from sensory branches of the glossopharyngeal and vagus nerves.[1]

The adenoid can be identified by magnetic resonance imaging (MRI) from the age of four months in 18 percent of children.[2] By five months of age, the adenoid could be identified in all of 290 children studied. Growth continues rapidly during infancy and plateaus between 2 and 14 years of age. Regression of the adenoid occurs rapidly after 15 years of age in most children. The adenoid appears to be at its largest in the seven-year-old age group.[3] However, clinical symptoms are more common in a younger age group, due to the relative small volume of the nasopharynx and the increased frequency of upper respiratory tract infections. [****/***/**]

IMMUNE FUNCTION OF THE ADENOID

The function of the lymphoid tissue of Waldeyer's ring is to produce antibodies. The adenoid produces B cells, which give rise to IgG and IgA plasma cells. Exposure to antigens via the nasal route is an important part of natural acquired immunity in early childhood. The adenoid appears to have an important role in the development of an 'immunological memory' in younger children.[4] The removal of this tissue at a young age may be immunologically undesirable.[5]

In children aged four to ten years, adenotonsillectomy does not appear to cause significant immune deficiency, although a slight decrease in IgG, IgA and IgM levels was found in the postoperative period four to six weeks after surgery.[6] The authors concluded that this represents a compensatory response of the developing immune system following a reduction of chronic antigen stimulation. Specific reduction in IgG may represent a reduction in antigenic stimulation. There appears to be no decrease in IgE after adenoidectomy.[7, 8]

The evidence that immune status is compromised by removal of the adenoid alone is inconclusive, as studies generally include children also having tonsillectomy.[9] [***/**]

PATHOLOGICAL EFFECTS OF THE ADENOID

The adenoid may be implicated in upper respiratory tract disease due to partial or complete obstruction of the nasal choanae or as a result of sepsis.

Pathological manifestations include rhinitis, rhinosinusitis, otitis media and otitis media with effusion. Adenoiditis, acute or chronic, is considered by some to be a related but distinct infective entity.[10]

Otitis media with effusion

The benefit of adenoidectomy in the management of otitis media with effusion (OME) has traditionally been ascribed to the relief of anatomical obstruction of the Eustachian tube.[11] While this may be a contributory factor, it is clear that adenoid size and physical obstruction alone cannot account for the benefit following adenoidectomy where the adenoid is small.[12] Adenoid size in children with and without OME is not significantly different. It is likely that recurrent acute or chronic inflammation of the adenoid and increased bacterial load, particularly of *Haemophilus influenzae*,[13, 14] results in squamous cell metaplasia, reticular epithelium extension, fibrosis of the interfollicular interconnective tissue and reduced mucociliary clearance in children with OME compared to those without OME.[15] These changes increase bacterial adherence. This is likely to contribute to the development of a 'biofilm' infection resulting in middle ear effusion (a biofilm infection may be defined as 'a structured community of bacterial cells enclosed in a self-produced polymeric matrix and adherent to an inert or living surface').[16] There is now good evidence,

particularly from the TARGET study, to support consideration of 'adjuvant' adenoidectomy in children over the age of three who are undergoing insertion of tympanostomy tubes (see Chapter 72, Otitis media with effusion).

Chronic gastro-oesophageal reflux has also been implicated in the development of OME, as a result of inflammation of the nasopharynx and the adenoid.[17] [***/**]

Recurrent acute otitis media

Randomized controlled trials of the management of recurrent acute otitis media have shown that adenoidectomy was not effective in reducing episodes of infection in children younger than two years during the follow-up periods of 7–24 months after surgery.[18, 19] It is likely that a partial maturational selective IgA deficiency is a causative factor in these 'otitis-prone' children.[20] Low-dose prophylactic antibiotic treatment is preferred to adenoidectomy in this group as a means of preventing recurrent otitis media and the sequelae of infection until maturation of the immune system occurs naturally.[21] [****/***/**]

Upper airway obstruction and obstructive sleep apnoea

Obstructive sleep apnoea in childhood is considered in detail in Chapter 85, Obstructive sleep apnoea in childhood. The prevalence of severe sleep disturbance in children due to upper airway obstruction is estimated to be approximately 1 percent, with a peak incidence between three and six years of age, and an equal sex incidence.[22, 23]

Airway obstruction due to adenoidal hypertrophy may produce depressed arterial PaO_2 and elevated $PaCO_2$ levels, which return to normal after adenoidectomy.[24] The respiratory improvement following adenotonsillectomy also results in a significant increase in serum insulin-like growth factor-I (IGF-I),[25] accounting in part for the clinically observed growth spurt following surgery. Despite the widespread acceptance of the benefits of adenotonsillar surgery in these children, a Cochrane review of adenotonsillectomy for obstructive sleep apnoea found no randomized trials addressing the efficacy of surgery in managing obstructive sleep apnoea syndrome (OSAS) in children.[26]

In a prospective study of 40 children undergoing adenoidectomy, with or without tonsillectomy, for upper airway obstruction, the radiographic estimate of the adenoid size correlated highly with the improvement in polysomnographic scores following surgery. No correlation between tonsil size and grade of obstructive sleep apnoea was found.[27] [**/*]

Rhinosinusitis

The reader is referred to Chapter 83, Paediatric rhinosinusitis. In a retrospective study of 48 children with chronic sinusitis undergoing adenoidectomy or adenotonsillectomy, improvement was reported in the majority following surgery, and only three children subsequently required functional endoscopic sinus surgery.[28]

A prospective study of children with recurrent rhinosinusitis showed that adenoidectomy was effective in abolishing infective episodes of infection, and that few children went on to require functional endoscopic sinus surgery.[29] [**]

Olfaction

Olfactory sensitivity is reduced in relation to adenoid size, and this improves after adenoidectomy.[30] This may, in part, account for the poor appetite reported in children with adenoidal hypertrophy. [**]

Neoplasia

Unsuspected neoplasia of the adenoid (and tonsils) in childhood is rare. Non-Hodgkin's lymphoma is reported in a series of six children.[31] Atypical lymphadenopathy, and persistent and asymmetric enlargement of the tonsils and adenoid, in the absence of infection are suspicious and should prompt early imaging and biopsy. Presentation is often assumed to be due to the more common infective and obstructive manifestations of adenotonsillar disease so the diagnosis is often delayed. [**]

ASSESSMENT AND MANAGEMENT

Clinical history

The history should form part of a full paediatric ENT history with special attention to symptoms of middle ear disease and nasal obstruction. Specific questions regarding sleep disturbance, eating and atopic symptoms are important. A family history of atopy may be relevant. A full history of medication, prescribed, over the counter and alternative or complementary, is important. In children in whom adenoidectomy is being considered, it is essential to positively exclude a history or family tendency of unusual bleeding or bruising, as a routine clotting screen may not confirm mild von Willebrand's disease.

Clinical examination

Assessment of the external nose should be made before rhinoscopy. In particular, look for a skin crease in the supra-tip region that may indicate frequent nose rubbing from symptoms of rhinitis.

Simple anterior rhinoscopy in children may be carried out using a halogen light otoscope with a large speculum. This is generally tolerated better in children than examination with a Thudicum's speculum.

Assessment of the nasal airway may be made with a cold Lack's tongue depressor or large laryngeal mirror. Posterior mirror rhinoscopy is not usually possible in children, but many will tolerate nasendoscopy with topical intranasal local anaesthetic spray, such as co-phenylcaine. Topical cocaine should not be used in children.

Nasendoscopy is increasingly used to assess adenoidal status in an outpatient setting. It may be well tolerated by children and is recommended prior to a decision to undertake surgery where adenoidectomy is the only procedure being considered (**Figure 84.1**).[32]

A grading system has been proposed to assist in the decision to recommend surgery.[33] In another study of 817 children, endoscopic assessment of adenoid size was highly correlated ($p < 0.001$) with nasal obstruction, snoring and the results of tympanometry, but not with purulent rhinorrhoea.[32]

In children undergoing another surgical procedure, peroperative assessment of the adenoid with a rigid endoscope or mirror is recommended to confirm the need for adenoidectomy.[34] [**]

The correlation of adenoid size with lateral soft tissue radiograph of the nasopharynx is poor, but plain radiography may be helpful if adenoidectomy is the only surgical procedure indicated and the child is unable to tolerate nasendoscopy in the clinic.[35] A classification of adenoid size has been described by Clemens et al. (**Table 84.1**).[36]

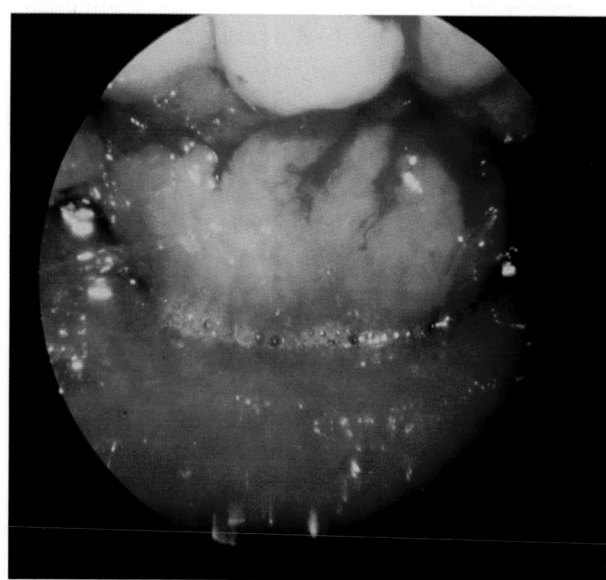

Figure 84.1 Endoscopic view of the adenoids.

Table 84.1 Clinical grading of adenoid size.

Grade	Description
Grade I	Adenoid tissue filling one-third of the vertical portion of the choanae
Grade II	Adenoid tissue filling from one-third to two-thirds of the choanae
Grade III	From two-thirds to nearly complete obstruction of the choanae
Grade IV	Complete choanal obstruction

Reprinted from Ref. 36, with permission from Elsevier.

While acoustic rhinomanometry is a useful research tool, and MRI provides extremely accurate volumetric estimation of the adenoid, these investigations are not applicable in clinical practice.[3, 37]

Nasendoscopy of the nasopharynx to assess adenoid size at the time of surgery is probably the gold standard, while mirror examination underestimates choanal occlusion, and palpation is a poor measure of adenoid hypertrophy.[38] [***/**/*]

Preoperative investigations

Routine preoperative investigations are not indicated prior to adenoidectomy for children who are ASA grade 1 (a normal healthy patient, without any clinically important co-morbidity and without a clinically significant past/present medical history).[39]

Guidance for children who are ASA grade 2 (a patient with mild systemic disease) is not given in the National Institute for Health and Clinical Excellence (NICE) guideline on preoperative tests. Specific investigations for sickle-cell disease, thalassaemia, Down syndrome and congenital heart disease are indicated as appropriate. Management of type 2 diabetes mellitus should follow local paediatric guidelines for diabetic children undergoing elective surgery.

ADENOIDECTOMY

Adenoidectomy with or without tonsillectomy and/or insertion of ventilation tubes is one of the most frequently performed surgical procedures in children. Traditional adenoidectomy is carried out under general anaesthesia with the child in the tonsillectomy position using the blind technique of curettage. Assessment of the adenoid is made digitally prior to curetting the adenoid from the nasopharynx, and haemostasis achieved with gauze swab tamponade. Techniques employing direct vision have the advantage of reduced blood loss (<4 mL versus >50 mL),[36] and the ability to remove adenoid tissue from the choanae, while avoiding trauma to the Eustachian cushions.[40] Of these techniques, those with the largest clinical experience are the suction coagulator and the microdebrider. In a randomized controlled trial, the microdebrider was 20 percent faster than the curettage technique,[41] but the suction coagulator is significantly cheaper than the microdebrider.[42] Single use instruments such as these abolish any potential risk of infection transmission.[43] The Coblator® plasma field device may prove suitable for adenoidectomy, but as yet no published data are available. The KTP laser is associated with a high incidence of postoperative nasopharyngeal stenosis and is not recommended for adenoidectomy.[44]

Where social and geographical factors allow,[45] and with appropriate surgical and anaesthetic techniques, pre-emptive fluid replacement, antiemetics and analgesia, the majority of children may be safely discharged home within six hours of adenoidectomy.[46, 47, 48] [***/**]

COMPLICATIONS OF ADENOIDECTOMY

The complications of adenoidectomy include:

- bleeding;
- dental trauma;
- airway obstruction, due to:
  - retained swab;
  - nasopharyngeal blood clot;
- infection;
- cervical spine injury (particularly in Down syndrome);
- velopharyngeal dysfunction;
- regrowth of the adenoid.

Death

No data assessing the risk of death following adenoidectomy independent of tonsillectomy or general anaesthesia were found.

Bleeding

The reactionary haemorrhage rate, that is, bleeding following adenoidectomy, within 6–20 hours of operation is less than 0.7 percent, and if severe enough to require a return to theatre, postnasal packing is the preferred management in the UK for haemostasis.[49] This study suggests that postnasal packing left *in situ* for four hours post-haemorrhage is as effective as packs left for 24 hours. A small number of consultants in this questionnaire study (3/285) electively admitted children to an intensive care facility following postnasal packing and 4/285 routinely prescribed antibiotics. The increase in the use of direct-vision techniques and controlled haemostasis at the time of operation may lead to a fall in the reactionary haemorrhage rate.

Secondary haemorrhage after adenoidectomy is rare. It may be due to bleeding from an aberrant ascending pharyngeal artery.[50] Unusual reactionary or secondary bleeding should raise the possibility of a clotting or coagulation defect. This will require specialist haematological advice to confirm or exclude.

Dental trauma

Damage to the teeth during adenoidectomy may be accidental due to slippage of the gag or supports. Great care is needed, particularly if the secondary incisors have erupted: the teeth are large, but the mandible immature, and it is safer to use an adult gag, which will rest lateral to the incisors. It is customary to warn parents about damage to teeth, but damage to the teeth will usually be considered negligent. Where there are loose deciduous teeth, consent should be taken preoperatively to remove these under anaesthetic to avoid the possibility of inhalation by the child during the operation or while recovering from anaesthesia.

Retained swab

It is mandatory to confirm that if swabs are used, the count is correct at the end of the operation before the gag is removed and the anaesthesia reversed. A swab may be retained either in the nasopharynx or in the laryngopharynx, hidden from the operator's view.

Nasopharyngeal blood clot

Blood may pool and clot in the nasopharynx during the procedure. The nasopharynx should be gently suctioned to clear any clot before removing the gag. Failure to do so may lead to the clot falling onto the larynx during recovery and causing potentially fatal acute airway obstruction (the 'coroner's clot').

Infection

Infection in the nasopharynx following adenoidectomy is clinically uncommon, although many parents report fetor from the child in the week following surgery. Rarely, retropharyngeal and mediastinal abscess may occur as a result of trauma and secondary infection of the adenoid bed.[51]

Cervical spine

Nontraumatic atlantoaxial subluxation (Grisel syndrome) is rare, but associated with overuse of diathermy either for removal of the adenoid or following curettage when used for haemostasis.[52] Minimum power settings for diathermy should always be used.

Children with Down syndrome may have atlantoaxial instability. Traditionally, such children have plain imaging of the cervical spine prior to surgery. Vigilant attention to the child's peroperative neck position is essential.

Velopharyngeal dysfunction

Severe velopharyngeal incompetence is rare following adenoidectomy, estimated to occur in between 1:1500 and 1:10,000 procedures. It may lead to significant problems with hypernasal speech and swallowing, severe enough to cause nasal regurgitation of fluids. It is mandatory to assess the palate and uvula for submucous cleft of the palate prior to surgery as surgery often unmasks pre-existing palatal dysfunction.[53] Opinion is divided, and no evidence exists as to the management of a child with a bifid uvula with or without a submucous cleft about to undergo adenoidectomy. Using a direct-vision technique, it is possible to perform a partial adenoidectomy, clearing the choanal airway, but leaving the adenoid intact at the velopharyngeal junction.

Long-term velopharyngeal insufficiency is rare. In a retrospective review this occurred after 1 in 1200 adenoidectomies. Reconstructive surgery to correct hypernasal speech may be required if speech and swallowing are severely affected.[54]

Regrowth of the adenoid

A cross-sectional follow-up study of children after adenoidectomy two to five years after surgery concluded that 71 percent had no residual obstructing adenoid. However, the criterion for adenoid sufficient to cause nasal obstruction was tissue occupying more than 40 percent of the nasopharynx.[55] Empirically, many surgeons may consider this significant enough to warrant further surgery.

KEY POINTS

- Adenoidal hyperplasia in childhood is common and self-limiting; mild symptoms of obstruction are not an indication for surgery.
- Significant obstructive symptoms, short of obstructive sleep apnoea, may have effects on daytime behaviour and cognitive function.
- Adenoidectomy is effective in the surgical management of children with upper airway obstruction.
- Adenoidectomy may not be effective in the management of recurrent acute otitis media.

Best clinical practice

✓ It is no longer appropriate to combine adenoidectomy with tonsillectomy, unless there is a specific indication for adenoidectomy [Grade C]

✓ Adjuvant adenoidectomy may be considered as part of the surgical management of children over the age of three years with otitis media with effusion. [Grade B]

✓ Routine preoperative investigations are not indicated prior to adenoidectomy for children who are ASA grade 1. [Grade C]

✓ Adenoidectomy under direct vision using single use instrumentation – excepting the KTP laser – is now a preferred alternative to curettage. [Grade B]

Deficiencies in current knowledge and areas for future research

For each of the following topics there is no currently available evidence at level 1, and further studies are recommended:

➤ Efficacy and morbidity of different techniques of adenoidectomy.

➤ Efficacy of adenoidectomy in the management of obstructive sleep apnoea in children.

➤ Efficacy of adenoidectomy in the management of chronic and recurrent acute sinusitis in children.

➤ The effects of adenoidectomy on the development of childhood immunity.

➤ The relationship between adenoidal hypertrophy and childhood rhinitis.

➤ The role of the adenoid in facilitating a biofilm infection in the upper respiratory tract.

REFERENCES

1. Pachigolla R. 1996. University of Texas Medical Section Grand Rounds. http://www.utmb.edu/otoref/grnds/tnaprobs.htm Accessed 17th July 2004.

2. Jaw TS, Sheu RS, Liu GC, Lin WC. Development of adenoids: a study by measurement with MRI images. *Kaohsiung Journal of Medical Sciences.* 1999; 15: 12–8.

3. Vogler RC, Ii FJ, Pilgram TK. Age-specific size of the normal adenoid pad on magnetic resonance imaging. *Clinical Otolaryngology and Allied Sciences.* 2000; 25: 392–5.

4. Wysocka J, Hassmann E, Lipska A, Musiatowicz M. Naïve and memory T cells in hypertrophied adenoids in children according to age. *International Journal of Pediatric Otorhinolaryngology.* 2003; 67: 237–41.

* 5. Brandtzaeg P. Immunology of the tonsils and adenoids: everything the ENT surgeon needs to know. *International Journal of Pediatric Otorhinolaryngology.* 2003; 67: 69–76.

6. Ikinciogullari A, Dogu F, Ikinciogullari A, Egin Y, Babacan E. Is the immune system influenced by adenotonsillectomy in children? *International Journal of Pediatric Otorhinolaryngology.* 2002; 66: 251–7.

7. Modrzynski M, Zawisza E, Rapiejko P. Serum immunoglobulin E levels in relation to Waldeyer's ring surgery. *Przegi-Lekarski.* 2003; 60: 325–8.

8. Prados M, Sanchez F, Olivencia M, Paulino A, Aragon R. Serum immunoglobulin E levels in relation to adenoid surgery. *Allergologia et Immunopathologia (Madr).* 1998; 26: 52–4.

9. Friday Jr. GA, Paradise JL, Rabin BS, Colborn DK, Taylor FH. Serum immunoglobulin changes in relation to tonsil and adenoid surgery. *Annals of Allergy.* 1992; 69: 225–320.

10. Richardson MA. Sore throat, tonsillitis and adenoiditis. *Medical Clinics of North America.* 1999; 83: 75–83.

11. Nguyen LHP, Manoukian JJ, Yoskovitch A, Al-Sebeih KH. Adenoidectomy: selection criteria for surgical cases of otitis media. *Laryngoscope.* 2004; 114: 863–6.

12. Gates GA. Adenoidectomy for otitis media with effusion. *Annals of Otology, Rhinology and Laryngology.* 1994; 163: 54–8.

13. Suzuki M, Watanabe T, Mogi G. Clinical, bacteriological and histological study of adenoids in children. *American Journal of Otolaryngology.* 1999; 20: 85–90.

14. Brook I, Shah K, Jackson W. Microbiology of healthy and diseased adenoids. *Laryngoscope.* 2000; 110: 994–9.

* 15. Yasan H, Dogru H, Tuz M, Candir O, Uygur K, Yariktas M. Otitis media with effusion and histopathologic properties of adenoid tissue. *International Journal of Pediatric Otorhinolaryngology.* 2003; 67: 1179–83.

16. Fergie N, Bayston R, Pearson JP, Birchall JP. Is otitis media with effusion a biofilm infection? *Clinical Otolaryngology and Allied Sciences.* 2004; 29: 38–46.

17. Tasker A, Dettmar PW, Panetti M, Koufman JA, Birchall JP, Pearson JP. Reflux of gastric juice and glue ear in children. *Lancet.* 2002; 359: 493.

18. Mattila P-S, Joki EVP, Kilpi T, Jokinen J, Herva E, Puhakka H. Prevention of otitis media by adenoidectomy in children younger than 2 years. *Archives of Otolaryngology – Head and Neck Surgery.* 2003; 129: 163–8.

* 19. Koivunen P, Uhari M, Luotonen J, Kristo A, Raski R, Pokka T et al. Adenoidectomy versus chemoprophylaxis and placebo for recurrent acute otits media in children. *British Medical Journal.* 2004; 328: 487–90.

20. Robb RJ, Gowrinath K. Selective IgA maturational deficiency and the "otitis-prone" child. In: McCafferty G, Cauman W, Carroll R (eds). *XVI Proceedings of the World Congress of Otorhinolaryngology,* Bologna: Monduzi Editore, 1997: 981–5.

21. Rovers MM, Schilder AGM, Zeilhuis GA, Rosenfeld RM. Otitis media. *Lancet.* 2004; **363**: 465–73.

22. Ali NJ, Pitson DJ, Stradling JR. Snoring, sleep disturbance and behaviour in 4–5 year olds. *Archives of Disease in Childhood.* 1993; **68**: 360–6.

23. Brouillete RT, Fernbach SK, Hunt CE. Obstructive sleep apnoea in infants and children. *Journal of Pediatrics.* 1982; **100**: 31–40.

24. Khalifa MS, Kamei RH, Zikry MA, Kandil TM. Effects of enlarged adenoids on arterial blood gases in children. *Journal of Laryngology and Otology.* 1991; **105**: 436–8.

25. Bar A, Tarasuik A, Segev Y, Phillip M, Tal A. The effect of adenotonsillectomy on serum insulin-like growth factor-I and growth in children with obstructive sleep apnea syndrome. *Journal of Pediatrics.* 1999; **135**: 76–80.

26. Lim J, McKean M. Adenotonsillectomy for obstructive sleep apnoea in children (Cochrane Review). In: *The Cochrane Library,* Issue 2, 2004, Chichester, UK: John Wiley and Sons Ltd, 2004.

27. Jain A, Sahni JK. Polysomnographic studies of children undergoing adenoidectomy and/or tonsillectomy. *Journal of Laryology and Otology.* 2002; **116**: 711–5.

* 28. Vandenberg SJ, Heatley DG. Efficacy of adenoidectomy in relieving symptoms of chronic sinusitis in children. *Archives of Otolaryngology – Head and Neck Surgery.* 1997; **123**: 675–8.

29. Ungkanont K, Damrongsak S. Effect of adenoidectomy in children with complex problems of rhinosinusitis and associated diseases. *International Journal of Pediatric Otorhinolaryngology.* 2004; **68**: 447–51.

30. Delank KW. Olfactory sensitivity in adenoid hyperplasia. *Laryngorhinootolgie.* 1992; **71**: 293–7.

31. Ridgway D, Wolff LJ, Neerhout RC, Tilford DL. Unsuspected non-Hodgkins lymphoma of the tonsils and adenoids in children. *Pediatrics.* 1987; **79**: 399–402.

32. Wang DY, Bernheim N, Kaufman L, Clement P. Assessment of adenoid size in children by fiberoptic examination. *Clinical Otolaryngology and Allied Sciences.* 1997; **22**: 172–7.

33. Cassano P, Matteo G, Cassano M, Fiorella M-L, Fiorella R. Adenoid tissue rhinopharyngeal obstruction grading based on fibrendoscopic findings: a novel approach to therapeutic management. *International Journal of Pediatric Otorhinolaryngology.* 2003; **67**: 1303–09.

34. Phillips DE, Bates GJ, Parker AJ, Griffiths MV, Green J. Digital and mirror assessment of the adenoids at operation. *Clinical Otolaryngology and Allied Sciences.* 1989; **14**: 131–3.

35. Cohen LM, Koltai PJ, Scott JR. Lateral cervical radiographs and adenoid size: do they correlate? *Ear Nose and Throat Journal.* 1992; **71**: 638–42.

36. Clemens J, McMurray JS, Willging JP. Electrocautery versus curette adenoidectomy: comparison of postoperative results. *Interhational Journal of Pediatric Otorhinolaryngology.* 1998; **43**: 115–22.

37. Cho JH, Lee DH, Lee NS, Won YS, Yoon HR, Suh BD. Size assessment of adenoid and nasopharyngeal airway by acoustic rhinomanometry in children. *Journal of Larynology and Otology.* 1999; **113**: 899–905.

38. Chisholm EJ, Lew-Gor S, Hajioff D, Caulfield H. Adenoid size: a comparison of palapation, nasendoscopy and mirror examination. *Clinical Otolaryngology.* 2005; **30**: 39–41.

39. National Institute for Clinical Excellence. *The use of routine preoperative tests for elective surgery.* London: NICE, 2003.

40. Havas T, Lowinger D. Obstructive adenoid tissue: an indication for powered-shaver adenoidectomy. *Archives of Otolaryngology – Head and Neck Surgery.* 2002; **128**: 789–91.

41. Stanislaw Jr. P, Koltai PJ, Feustel PJ. Comparison of power-assisted adenoidectomy vs adenoid curette adenoidectomy. *Archives of Otolaryngology – Head and Neck Surgery.* 2000; **126**: 845–9.

* 42. Elluru RG, Johnson L, Myers 3rd. CM. Electrocautery adenoidectomy compared with curettage and power-assisted methods. *Laryngoscope.* 2002; **112**: 23–5.

43. Walker P. Pediatric adenoidectomy under vision using suction diathermy ablation. *Laryngoscope.* 2001; **111**: 2173–7.

44. Giannoni C, Sulek M, Friedman EM, Duncan III M. Acquired nasopharyngeal stenosis. *A warning and review. Archives of Otolaryngology – Head and Neck Surgery.* 1998; **124**: 163–6.

45. Kishore A, Haider AAM, Geddes NK. Patient eligibility for day case paediatric adenotonsillectomy. *Clinical Otolaryngology and Allied Sciences.* 2001; **26**: 47–9.

46. Yardley MP, Fairley JW, Durham LH, Parker AJ. Day case tonsil and adenoid surgery: how many are eligible? *Journal of Royal College of Surgeons of Edinburgh.* 1994; **39**: 162–3.

47. Callanan V, Capper R, Gurr P, Baldwin DL. Day-case adenoidectomy, parental opinions and concerns. *Journal of Larynology and Otology.* 1994; **108**: 470–3.

48. Sheppard IJ, Moir AA, Thomas RS, Narula AA. Organisation of day case adenoidectomy in the management of chronic otitis media with effusion – preliminary results. *Journal of the Royal Society of Medicine.* 1993; **86**: 76–8.

49. Tzifa KT, Skinner DW. A survey on the management of reactionary haemorrhage following adenoidectomy in the UK and our practice. *Clinical Otolaryngology and Allied Sciences.* 2004; **29**: 153–6.

50. Windfuhr JP. An aberrant artery as a cause of massive bleeding following adenoidectomy. *Journal of Laryngology and Otology.* 2002; **116**: 299–300.

51. Tuerlinckx D, Bodart E, Lawson G, De Wispelaere JF, De-Bilderling G. Retropharyngeal and mediastinal abscess following adenoidectomy. *Pediatric Pulmonology.* 2003; **36**: 257–8.

52. Tschopp K. Monopolar cautery in adenoidectomy as a possible risk for Grisel's syndrome. *Laryngoscope.* 2002; **112**: 1445–9.

53. Saunders NC, Hartley BEJ, Sell D, Sommerlad B. Velopharyngeal insufficiency following adenoidectomy. *Clinical Otolaryngology and Allied Sciences.* 2004; **29**: 686–8.

54. Stewart KJ, Ahmad T, Raxxell RE, Watson ACH. Altered speech following adenoidectomy: a 20 year experience. *British Journal of Plastic Surgery.* 2002; **55**: 469–73.

55. Buchinsky FJ, Lowry MA, Isaacson G. Do adenoids grow after excision? *Otolaryngology – Head and Neck Surgery.* 2000; **123**: 576–81.

85

Obstructive sleep apnoea in childhood

HELEN M CAULFIELD

Definitions and epidemiology	1102	Postoperative complications and reduction of perioperative risk	1110
Mechanism of sleep-disordered breathing and physiological affects	1103	Long-term postoperative follow-up	1110
Clinical symptoms	1104	Conclusion	1111
Clinical examination	1104	Key points	1111
Investigations	1105	Best clinical practice	1111
Recommendations for investigations	1108	Deficiencies in current knowledge and areas for future research	1111
Treatment	1108	References	1111

SEARCH STRATEGY

The data in this chapter are supported by a Medline search using the key words obstructive sleep apnoea, sleep-disordered breathing, child, paediatric, snoring, sleep disorders, heart failure, pulmonary hypertension, polysomnography and focussing on definitions, symptoms, sleep studies and outcomes of intervention.

DEFINITIONS AND EPIDEMIOLOGY

Obstructive sleep apnoea (OSA) is characterized by episodic partial or complete obstruction of the upper airway during sleep. This causes apnoea or cessation of breathing. Intermittent episodes of brief cessation of breathing may be physiological. An 'apnoea' is defined in adults as cessation of breathing for ten seconds or more. Six seconds or less may be pathological in children. The differences in sleep physiology between adults and children have bedevilled attempts to define OSA in children with the same precision as in adult medicine.[1, 2] Upper airway obstructions during sleep affect pulmonary ventilation and can lead to a drop in peripheral oxygen saturation (hypoxaemia) and retention of carbon dioxide (hypercarbia). Upper airway obstruction disrupts normal sleeping patterns by causing arousals, presumably induced by the effect of hypoxaemia and hypercarbia on the respiratory centre. It is now recognized that sleep-disordered breathing is a spectrum of airway obstruction, and the term encompasses simple snoring, upper airway resistance syndrome (UARS) and the more severe OSA.

Simple snoring

Simple snoring is defined as snoring without obstructive apnoeas, frequent arousals or gas exchange abnormalities. It is generally considered benign although there is growing evidence that it may not be as innocuous a condition as has been believed. In addition to evidence that the secretion of growth hormone is reduced in children with simple snoring,[3] cohort studies of children with habitual snoring suggest they have a higher incidence of neurocognitive disorders, with demonstrable adverse effects on quality of life. Furthermore, these effects are reversible by adenotonsillectomy, and it may be that we need to revise our criteria for intervention in this group of children.[4]

Upper airways resistance syndrome

Upper airways resistance syndrome is a more subtle form of sleep-disordered breathing than OSA. It is characterized by partial upper airway obstruction. The frequency and severity of apnoeas is insufficient to warrant a diagnosis of OSA. UARS can lead to significant clinical symptoms as a result of night-time arousals and pulmonary hypoventilation.[5] This disorder is more common than OSA but is often underdiagnosed.[6] [****/***]

Obstructive sleep apnoea

OSA causes loud persistent snoring interrupted by gasping or choking episodes and silent periods which are apnoeas. It causes significant sleep disruption. This can lead to daytime neurobehavioural problems such as an increase in total sleep time, hyperactivity, irritability, bed-wetting and morning headaches.[7] OSA may significantly affect a child and their family's quality of life.[8] [***]

Untreated OSA can result in significant morbidity such as failure to thrive, pulmonary hypertension and right heart failure.[9] Failure to thrive is not common in these times but children with OSA tend to have a growth spurt following adenotonsillectomy.[3] Although overt right heart failure occurs less frequently, asymptomatic degrees of pulmonary hypertension may be common.[10]

Difficulties concerning definition mean that the exact prevalence of sleep-disordered breathing in children is unknown but may be as high as 11 percent,[11] and it affects between 26 and 65 percent of all children attending otolaryngology clinics in the UK.[12] OSA has a prevalence of approximately 2 percent in the paediatric population and is more common in African children.[13, 14] Sleep-disordered breathing can affect children of all ages but its peak incidence is between the ages of three and seven, when the adenoid and tonsillar lymphoid tissue is disproportionately large relative to the pharyngeal airway.[15] There is an equal incidence in boys and girls but it presents earlier in boys.[13]

Factors that increase the risk of OSA in otherwise healthy children include adenotonsillar hypertrophy, family predisposition, obesity and mild craniofacial disproportion.[11, 14] OSA is also associated with a number of craniofacial syndromes and systemic diseases, in which it has a much higher incidence than in otherwise healthy children (**Table 85.1**). This is a result of craniofacial disproportion and the presence of coexisting upper airway hypotonia. The site of upper airway obstruction is not confined to the adenotonsillar area in these children, and requires investigation.[16] [***/**]

Table 85.1 Children with increased risk of OSA.

Craniofacial syndromes	Systemic illness
Pierre Robin sequence	Cerebral palsy
Crouzon syndrome	Myotonic dystrophies
Goldenhar syndrome	Obesity
Treacher Collins syndrome	Sickle cell disease
Apert syndrome	Glycogen storage disorder
Down syndrome	Achondroplasia
Hunter syndrome	
Velocardiofacial syndrome	
Beckwith–Wiedemann syndrome	

MECHANISM OF SLEEP-DISORDERED BREATHING AND PHYSIOLOGICAL AFFECTS

Breathing against a partially or completely obstructed upper airway causes the clinical signs of sleep-disordered breathing, which include loud snoring, increased respiratory effort with flaring of the nostrils, suprasternal and intercostal recession. Complete obstruction of the pharyngeal airway, as in OSA, leads to silent periods followed by choking or gasping as the child rouses from sleep to re-establish their airway.

Partial (hypopnoea) or complete upper airway obstruction (apnoea) during sleep can lead to hypoxia and hypercarbia. The degree of hypoxia is influenced by the duration of the apnoeic event, the condition of the cardiopulmonary system and whether a coexisting neuromuscular disorder is present. Hypoxia leads to a rise in sympathetic output causing peripheral vasoconstriction, which results in tachycardia and a rise in blood pressure. Changes in the pulse and blood pressure reflect increased sympathetic activity and are markers of subcortical arousal. They correlate directly with the severity of the sleep-disordered breathing and can be used to quantify it. The diastolic blood pressure during rapid eye movement (REM) sleep shows a significant correlation with the number of apnoeas and hypopnoeas.[17] The pulse transit time is a noninvasive marker of blood pressure. It is the interval between the R wave on an electrocardiogram (ECG) and the arrival of the pulse at the finger. The pulse transit time is increased in the presence of increased respiratory effort and decreased in the presence of tachycardia associated with arousal. It is a more sensitive measure of obstructive events than visible electroencephalogram (EEG) arousals found on full polysomnography recording.[18]

Upper airway obstructive events are terminated by these subcortical arousals. The child is unaware of these but they may occur several hundred times a night. Repeated arousals greatly disturb a child's sleep pattern which can lead to changes in behaviour and concentration ability as well as having general effects on a child's quality of life.[4, 5] The rise in pulmonary blood pressure as a result of increased sympathetic activity leads to transient pulmonary hypertension. Long-standing sleep apnoea can result in irreversible pulmonary hypertension and if sustained this will lead to right heart failure and cor pulmonale.[9]

A gradual, improved understanding of these physiological changes that occur during sleep has helped clinicians identify the parameters that need to be measured to ascertain the severity of the sleep-disordered breathing. Full polysomnography is the 'gold standard' investigation for sleep disorders. It can differentiate sleep-disordered breathing from other types of sleep disorder, such as periodic leg movement and narcolepsy. However, if sleep-disordered breathing is suspected, full polysomnography can be substituted by less elaborate sleep studies which measure and analyze pulse rate and oxygen saturation complemented with video and sound recordings of the sleeping child, for example the Visi-Lab[TM] analysis. [***]

CLINICAL SYMPTOMS

The cardinal symptom of sleep-disordered breathing in children is snoring. Severe sleep apnoea with loud, persistent snoring is more likely in younger children. Children with significant obstruction sweat during sleep, particularly in the nuchal area, and have a tracheal tug and intercostal recession with loud stertorous breathing. Children who have repeated apnoeas leading to arousals are very restless at night, often adopting unusual sleeping positions in an attempt to relieve their upper airway obstruction. They may also complain of very dry mouth and morning headaches. The high intrathoracic pressures generated in a child with OSA may cause oesophageal reflux leading to unexplained regurgitation or vomiting during sleep.

A further commonly witnessed symptom is choking episodes. This is best enquired about by imitating a guttural noise, as parents are often not aware of why the noise is being created. Parents often describe witnessed apnoeas as momentary breath holding. Most parents, if asked directly, will deny that their child stops breathing at night. This can lead to an underestimation of the presence of sleep apnoea if the clinical history is not taken with enough attention to detail.

True daytime somnolence as described in adults is unusual in children. Hyperactivity is more common and affected children are often irritable on waking.[7]

It is also important to identify whether the affected child has associated rhinosinusitis as this can exacerbate their sleep-disordered breathing. Rhinosinusitis may be allergic, infective or structural in origin. Medical treatment of this will improve the child's sleep-disordered breathing. Similarly, pulmonary disease may also exacerbate sleep apnoea by causing increased work in breathing requiring higher intrathoracic pressures. The child with severe OSA has chronic hypoventilation at night, which

may lead to pulmonary atelectasia. These children develop a cough with most viral upper respiratory tract infections. A history of previous hospital admission with acute airway compromise heralds an increased risk of complications following surgical intervention.

CLINICAL EXAMINATION

Clinical examination should include a full ENT examination, height and weight measurements and cardiopulmonary examination. Sleep-disordered breathing is more common in the obese child. Conversely, sleep-disordered breathing in a child can cause failure to thrive or a decrease in growth rate.

Subtle craniofacial disproportion should be looked for. Children with a triangular chin, steep mandibular angle, retrognathia, narrow high-arched palate and long soft palate are likely to have sleep-disordered breathing. Mouth breathing indicates nasal obstruction, and examination within the nose should look at the structure of the septum and the quality of the nasal lining for the presence of rhinosinusitis. Many children with sleep-disordered breathing are daytime mouth breathers and therefore the presence of chronic mouth breathing should raise the index of clinical suspicion.

Hyporesonant voice points to enlarged adenoids. In some children it may be possible to perform nasendoscopy with a fibreoptic endoscope to ascertain the size of the adenoid pad and extent of choanal obstruction (**Figure 85.1**). Examination within the oral cavity should exclude a submucous cleft and be used to document the size of the tonsils (**Figure 85.2**). Although most children with OSA have large tonsils, studies show that there is little correlation between the size of the tonsils and the severity of sleep-disordered breathing.[19] Small tonsils can cause upper airway obstruction if there is excessive medialization of the lateral pharyngeal walls during sleep. This can be the result of poor neuromuscular control of the pharyngeal airway, as in cerebral palsy, and previous cleft palate repair. Alternatively, a very large adenoid pad can cause a marked reduction in the calibre of the airway even in the presence of relatively small tonsils. Also, the site of upper airway obstruction is not necessarily adenotonsillar, particularly in syndromic children.[16]

Daytime stertorous breathing is indicative of severe sleep apnoea, as is growth retardation, which has been shown to be due to a reduction in growth hormone secretion.[3, 20] The presence of broken veins on the face indicates raised venous pressure in the face due to upper airway obstruction. Pectus excavatum can result from long-standing intercostal recession during sleep. The presence of noisy breathing, other than stertor, should alert the clinician to the presence of possible distal airway pathology.

Clinical history and examination will confirm the presence of sleep-disordered breathing but cannot reliably

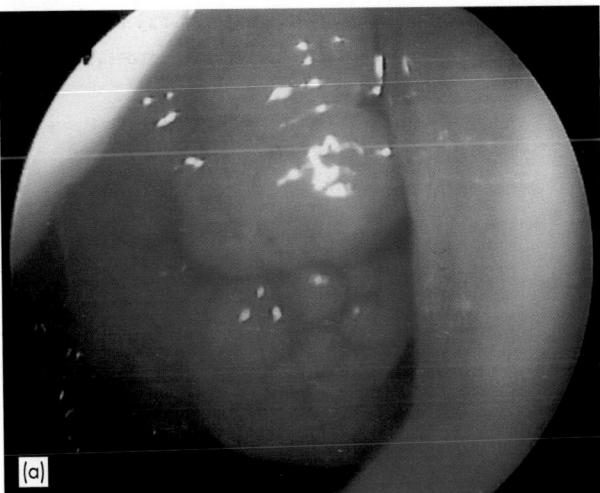

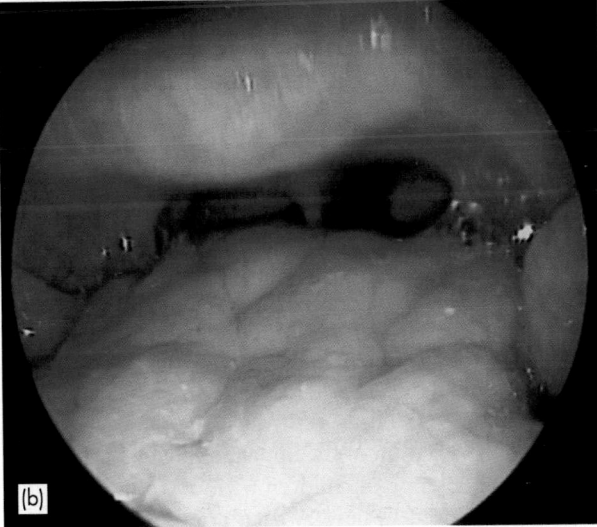

Figure 85.1 (a) A nasendoscopic view of the adenoids in a child showing >50 percent choanal obstruction. (b) An endoscopic view of the same adenoids using a 90° rigid fibreoptic telescope introduced through the mouth.

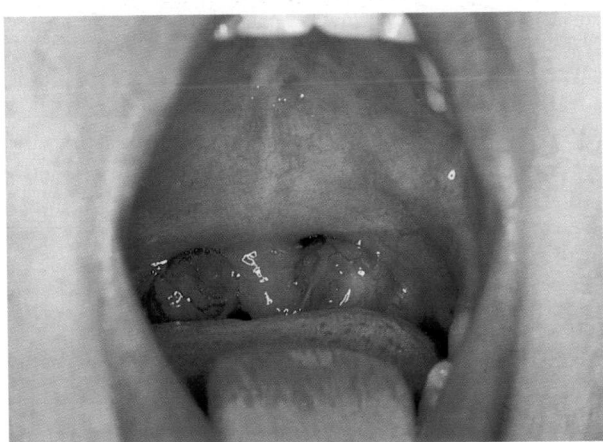

Figure 85.2 An intraoral photograph of a seven-year-old child showing large obstructive tonsils.

distinguish between children with simple snoring and OSA. The clinical history will overdiagnose mild sleep apnoea and under diagnose severe OSA. There are a number of reasons why the history can be misleading. Children with OSA experience most of their obstruction during rapid eye movement sleep (REM sleep), which occurs primarily in the early hours of the morning when parents are not observing them.[21] Children with UARS have a pattern of partial upper airway obstruction which leads to gas exchange abnormalities rather than true apnoeas and may be underreported.[6]

The history and clinical examination will enable the clinician to decide which child needs further investigation but it cannot always determine the need for intervention. An accurate diagnosis is, therefore, needed to ensure appropriate treatment, avoid unnecessary treatment and identify children at risk of developing complications of treatment. [***/**]

INVESTIGATIONS

Investigations are needed in paediatric sleep-disordered breathing to:

- identify children who are at increased risk of the complications associated with sleep-disordered breathing;
- avoid unnecessary intervention in children with simple snoring;
- identify children who are at increased risk of complications following surgical intervention;
- identify the site of upper airway obstruction in a child with sleep-disordered breathing.

Sleep studies

The clinical history and examination will identify most children with sleep-disordered breathing but are not sensitive enough to define severity or differentiate between simple snoring and more severe forms of sleep-disordered breathing. Symptom questionnaires designed to complement the clinical history are good at identifying more severe cases.[22] However, more objective evidence of the severity of sleep-disordered breathing may be sought.

Pulse oxymetry is a screening tool. It relies on indirect measurement of the arterial oxygen saturation using a probe, usually applied to the finger.[23] It is minimally invasive, and can be undertaken in a child's home if a recording device is available. Readings above 97 percent exclude serious hypoxia or hypercarbia.[24] Readings below 87 percent may suggest coexistent cardiac or broncho-pulmonary disease. Between these two extremes it gives little information as to the severity of the sleep apnoea and will miss apnoeic episodes not associated with oxygen desaturation.[25] However, despite these shortcomings, pulse oxymetry does provide some information regarding the severity of OSA, as it will identify severe cases with significant desaturations. It has a high positive predictive value of approximately 97 percent. It is not so helpful in assessing mild-to-moderate OSA, with a low negative predictive value of approximately 47 percent.[26]

One step up from simple pulse oxymetry is a 'mini-sleep' study system. These systems combine pulse oxymetry with video footage and sound recording. Computer software measures movement from the movement detector, snoring from the microphone and analyzes the pulse oxymeter output. The best known is the Visi-Lab. Increased work of breathing (hypopnoeas) and apnoeic episodes without significant oxygen desaturation can be detected using this form of sleep study. A rise in pulse rate associated with a desaturation signifies an arousal and corresponds to the number of apnoeas and hypopnoeas. This data is more useful in adult sleep medicine as age-appropriate criteria for children are not yet standardized.[2]

The American Sleep Apnoea Association currently grades sleep apnoea in the form of the apnoea/hypopnoea index. This is the total number of apnoeas and hypopnoeas divided by the total sleep time, which gives an index per hour (**Table 85.2**).

The gold standard investigation for sleep disorders is full polysomnography. This monitors EEG activity, chest and abdominal movement, oxygen saturation, nasal or oral airflow, end tidal carbon dioxide and continuous ECG recordings. Video monitoring during polysomnography is also helpful but is not standard. Full polysomnography identifies EEG arousal and provides an apnoea/hypopnoea index. It also differentiates between different types of sleep disorder and identifies central apnoeas.

Although ideal, full polysomnography is detailed and expensive and cannot be provided for every child suspected of suffering with sleep-disordered breathing. There is, therefore, the need for rationalization of sleep study investigations depending on the clinical needs of the child (**Table 85.3**). [Grade B]

Sleep nasendoscopy

Although polysomnography is invaluable and essential in documenting the severity of OSA it provides no information concerning the site of upper airway obstruction.

Table 85.2 The apnoea/hypopnoea index.

Apnoea/Hypopnoea index (per hour)	Level of OSA
5–20	Mild
20–40	Moderate
>40	Severe

Table 85.3 Recommendations for investigation.

Which child?	Type of investigation
Healthy child >3 years	No investigations necessary
Healthy child >3 years with increased risk of postoperative respiratory complications	Chest x-ray and ECG Visi-Lab study
Healthy child <3 years	Chest x-ray and ECG Overnight pulse oxymetry Visi-Lab study
Healthy children with: obesity; small tonsils; mild cranofacial disproportion	Sleep nasendoscopy Microlaryngobronchoscopy Post-intervention sleep study
Neuromuscular disease	Full polysomonography Sleep nasendoscopy Post-intervention sleep study

Ascertaining the site of upper airway obstruction is essential in children with obesity, small tonsils or craniofacial disproportion and in those with syndromes and neuromuscular disease. The reason for this is that the site of upper airway obstruction is not necessarily adenotonsillar and may be anywhere from the palate to the supraglottis.[16] The site of upper airway obstruction varies not only between children with different syndromes but also between children with the same syndrome.

Direct visualization of the upper airway using a flexible fibreoptic endoscope in children with obstructive 'awake' apnoea has proved to be very accurate in diagnosing the site of airway obstruction which occur during sleep.[27] It has also become the first-line investigation in the management of children with stridor.

Sleep endoscopy using a flexible fibreoptic endoscope (sleep nasendoscopy) was first described by Croft and Pringle,[28] and is routinely used to assess the site of snoring and airway obstruction in adults. In children, sleep nasendoscopy can be performed with the child breathing spontaneously a mixture of halothane and oxygen. This is thought to provide a relaxation of the upper airway musculature that mimics natural sleep.[16]

Sleep nasendoscopy should be performed in the operating theatre with a skilled paediatric anaesthetist and full cardiopulmonary monitoring. The sites of upper airway obstruction can be documented using a four-level classification system (**Figure 85.3**). The site or level at which the upper airway obstruction is occurring will define the intervention that is needed to correct it. To classify the site of obstruction the upper aerodigestive tract can be divided into the following four functional levels:

1. level 1 or adenoid pad and velopharyngeal obstruction;

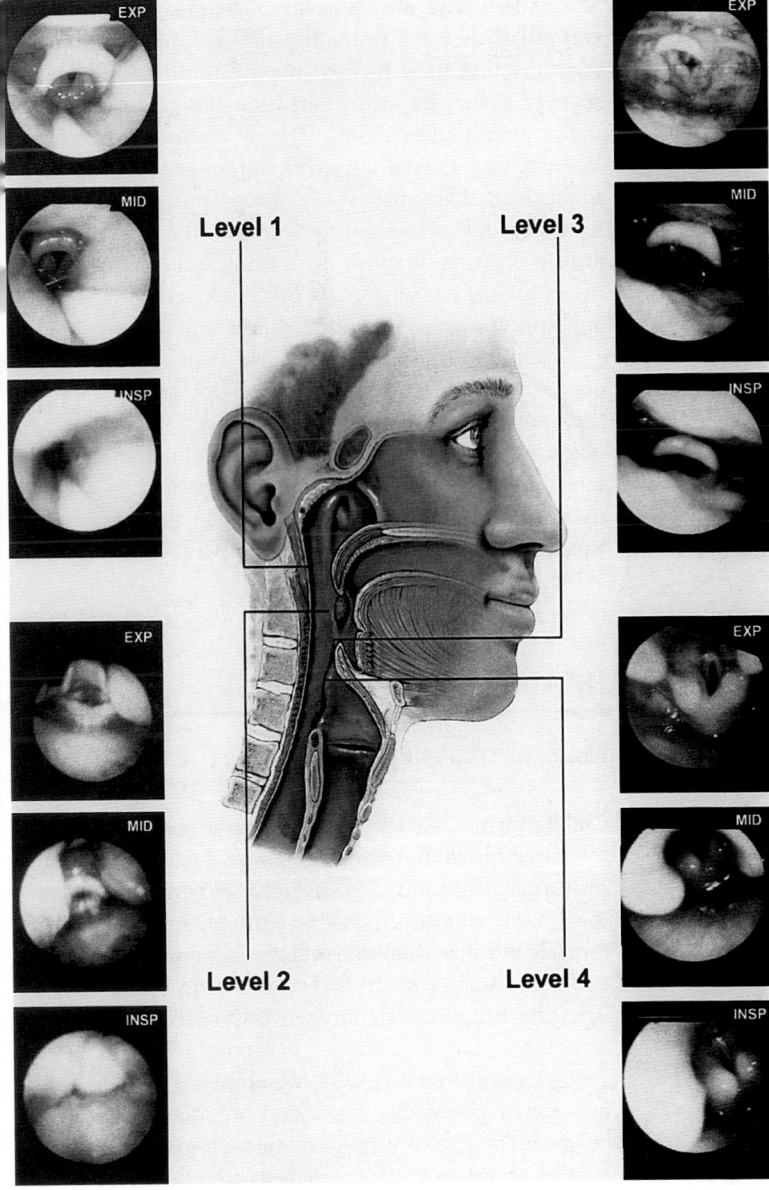

Level 1

Level 3

Level 2

Level 4

Figure 85.3 A classification system for documenting the findings at sleep nasendoscopy. The photographs show the endoscopic view of the obstruction at each level from 1 to 4.

2. level 2 or tonsillar obstruction;
3. level 3 or tongue base obstruction;
4. level 4 or supraglottic obstruction. [Grade B]

Rigid laryngobronchoscopy

Formal rigid laryngobronchoscopy should be performed in the assessment of syndromic children with complex obstructive breathing and in children who have a history of prematurity and prolonged inhalation on a neonatal intensive care unit.[16] It is important to exclude the presence of pathology distal to the glottis that may be exacerbating the upper airway symptoms, for example subglottic stenosis, tracheomalacia, innominate artery compression, bronchomalacia or vascular rings. The incidence of distal airway pathology is higher in Down syndrome patients than in the general population. In one

study, approximately 28 percent of children with Down syndrome and sleep-disordered breathing were found to have laryngeal or tracheal abnormalities on rigid laryngobronchoscopy.[29] The incidence of distal airway pathology in other syndromes is unknown but laryngeal abnormalities have been described in Goldenhar syndrome,[30] and major aortic arch abnormalities in velocardiofacial syndrome can cause tracheal compression.[31] [Grade C]

Imaging

A chest x-ray is mandatory in all children with moderate-to-severe OSA. It will identify pulmonary hypertension and right ventricular hypertrophy causing cardiomegaly. A chest x-ray also detects atelectasia caused by chronic hyperventilation. A lateral x-ray of the post-nasal space is useful in ascertaining adenoid size in children in whom flexible nasendoscopy has not been possible (**Figure 85.4**). Cardiac echocardiography is needed to exclude pulmonary hypertension or right-sided heart failure if EEG or chest x-ray are suggestive. Cardiac catheterization may then be necessary to measure pulmonary venous pressures in severe cases. Cephalometry, fluoroscopy and dynamic magnetic resonance imaging have been used in the assessment of OSA in children but have a limited role.[32] [Grade B]

RECOMMENDATIONS FOR INVESTIGATIONS

In otherwise healthy children over three years old with a history compatible with OSA and large tonsils and adenoids on examination, further investigation of their sleep-disordered breathing is not essential prior to adenotonsillectomy unless they are suspected of having severe OSA. In such cases, pulse oxymetry or a Visi-Lab study should be undertaken. A chest x-ray should be performed to look for atelectasia and an ECG to look for signs of right ventricular hypertrophy or pulmonary hypertension.

Otherwise healthy children under three years of age and other 'at risk' children (listed in **Table 85.1**) are likely to have severe OSA and should have a chest x-ray, ECG and a Visi-Lab study.

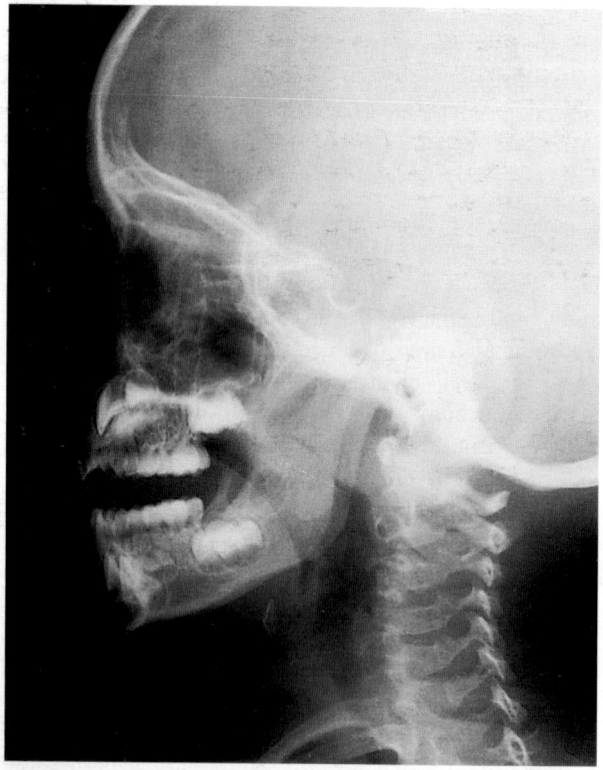

Figure 85.4 A lateral soft tissue x-ray of the head and neck of a three-year-old child with significant obstruction of the nasopharyngeal airway by enlarged adenoids.

Children who are clinically obese, have small tonsils and adenoids on examination or have mild craniofacial disproportion need further investigation to ascertain the severity of the sleep-disordered breathing and the site of upper airway obstruction. This is because adenotonsillectomy may not be curative, and an outcome measure is needed. A Visi-Lab study would provide this. Sleep nasendoscopy is needed to confirm the site of upper airway obstruction prior to adenotonsillectomy so that upper airway obstruction at other sites can be identified and appropriate intervention can be planned.

Syndromic children and those with neuromuscular disease need investigation with full polysomnography as they are likely to have associated central apnoeas and ongoing problems throughout their childhood despite intervention. Sleep nasendoscopy is needed to confirm the site of upper airway obstruction in these children if site-specific treatment is planned. [Grade B] (See also **Table 85.3**.)

TREATMENT

Medical treatment

Children with OSA who present with mucopurulent nasal discharge should have this treated, as it will improve their nocturnal symptoms. Treatment should consist of a four- to six-week course of systemic antibiotics combined with topical intranasal steroids. These children should be tested for sensitivity to airborne allergens that may be irritating the mucosal lining of the nose and paranasal sinuses.

Children with severe OSA, who have a persistent cough or signs of pulmonary atelectasia on chest x-ray, should be given systemic antibiotics and steroids prior to a general anaesthetic. This will help clear bronchial secretions and improve pulmonary function, thereby reducing the risk of postoperative respiratory failure. [Grade D]

CONTINUOUS POSITIVE AIRWAY PRESSURE

Continuous positive airway pressure (CPAP) provides continuous insufflation of the nasopharyngeal airway during sleep, thereby splinting the airway and maintaining its patency. It is usually delivered via a nasal mask and has to be used every night on an indefinite basis. It is a long-term therapy and requires frequent assessment of compliance and efficacy by a paediatric sleep physician. The CPAP pressures are titrated using polysomnography in the sleep laboratory and are periodically adjusted thereafter. Recent work with autotitrated CPAP in children has shown promise.[1] Patients such as the obese child, syndromic children and children with cerebral palsy may not be considered surgical candidates and may benefit from long-term CPAP.[33] CPAP can be started from birth and is well tolerated in older children. CPAP can also be used prior to planned surgical intervention in cases of severe OSA to minimize postoperative risk by improving pulmonary ventilation. [Grade B]

NASOPHARYNGEAL AIRWAY

Pharyngeal airway obstruction may be dramatically relieved with the use of a nasopharyngeal airway. This is of particular use in the newborn and in the first few months of life. It has been traditionally used in children with Pierre Robin sequence but also has a role in children with Apert and Crouzon syndrome. The length of the nasopharyngeal airway can be tailored according to the site of airway obstruction. In Pierre Robin sequence the tip of the nasopharyngeal airway needs to lie just above the epiglottis and in Apert's syndrome to the free edge of the soft palate. Many children with Pierre Robin sequence improve in the first few months of life, and the nasopharyngeal airway may be sufficient treatment of their upper airway obstruction. A sleep study can be performed with the tube *in situ* to assess its effectiveness, and another study performed on planned removal of the airway a few months later to assess progress. [Grade C]

MANDIBULAR ADVANCEMENT SPLINTS

Mandibular advancement splints have been used in some paediatric patients with OSA who cannot tolerate CPAP and are not suitable for surgical intervention. However, a recent study in adults has shown that the symptom relief and improvement in sleep parameters was better with CPAP than with splints.[34] [Grade B]

Surgical treatment

Adenotonsillectomy is the treatment of choice for otherwise healthy children suffering with sleep-disordered breathing. The results of surgery are an improvement in nocturnal hypoxia, behaviour, quality of life and growth rate.[1, 2, 3, 4, 5, 7] [***/***] Polysomnography performed before and after adenotonsillectomy in children with sleep-disordered breathing has demonstrated a universal improvement in their apnoea/hypopnoea index and an abolition of OSA in approximately 90 percent of cases.[35] However, this means that 10 percent of apparently healthy children continue to have OSA after adenotonsillectomy. This group consists of the clinically obese, those with mild craniofacial disproportion, deviated nasal septum, and those with small tonsils on examination. Adenotonsillectomy should still be considered in these children as it can have a satisfactory outcome in some cases.[36] Performing sleep nasendoscopy at the induction of anesthesia will identify the site of the upper airway obstruction, which may be at more than one level and thus help with the long term management.[16]

The results of adenotonsillectomy in children with Down syndrome, cerebral palsy and craniofacial abnormalities are not so encouraging. Recent studies show that between 54 and 100 percent of children with Down syndrome have OSA on polysomnography and the results of adenotonsillectomy are disappointing.[37] Other surgical treatments for OSA in Down syndrome include tonsillar pillar plication after tonsillectomy, midface advancement, uvulopalatopharyngoplasty (UVPP), anterior tongue reduction and hyoid suspension. Even with these forms of surgery an improvement in the child's symptoms is seen in only approximately 70 percent of cases, and deaths from upper airway obstruction are still not uncommon.[38]

Children with cerebral palsy also have much a higher incidence of OSA and sleep-disrupted breathing than age-matched controls when investigated with polysomnography.[39] Adenotonsillectomy in this group is rarely curative and UVPP has been advocated as an alternative to tracheostomy.[40] The difficulty with predicting outcome with UVPP is the multifactorial nature of the airway obstruction, notably the presence of central apnoeas, the general hypotonia of the pharynx, the poor gag reflex, salivary pooling and the multisegment collapse of the upper airway. These factors contribute to a progression from OSA to obstructive awake apnoea and noisy daytime breathing. Laser supraglottoplasty has been used to treat selected cases, with resolution of the noisy breathing (**Figure 85.5**). Other treatments tried as an alternative to tracheostomy include hyoid suspension, mandibular advancement and tongue reduction.

Children with craniofacial syndromes can be treated with a nasopharyngeal airway or tracheostomy until formal midface advancement is performed at about five years of age. Distraction osteogenesis has shown some early promising results and can be performed at a much earlier age (see Chapter 78, Craniofacial anomalies: genetics and management).[41] [Grade B/C]

TREATMENT OPTIONS ACCORDING TO THE LEVEL OF OBSTRUCTION SEEN AT SLEEP NASENDOSCOPY

Depending on the level of obstruction seen at sleep nasendoscopy, the following are treatment options.

- Level 1 obstruction (velopharyngeal obstruction) is relieved by adenoidectomy or UVPP.
- Level 2 obstruction (tonsillar) is relieved by tonsillectomy.
- Level 3 obstruction (tongue base) can be relieved with the use of nasopharyngeal airways, glossopexy, mandibular advancement splints or CPAP.
- Level 4 obstruction (supraglottic) is due to collapse of the supraglottic tissues and manifests in its commonest form as laryngomalacia. It is a common finding in children with cerebral palsy who have upper airway obstruction. The treatment of

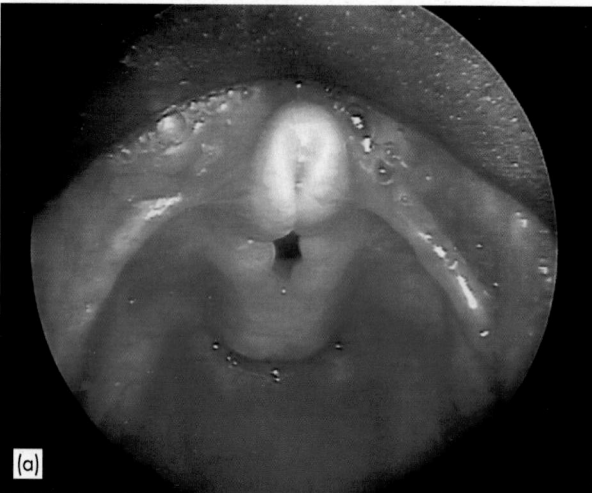

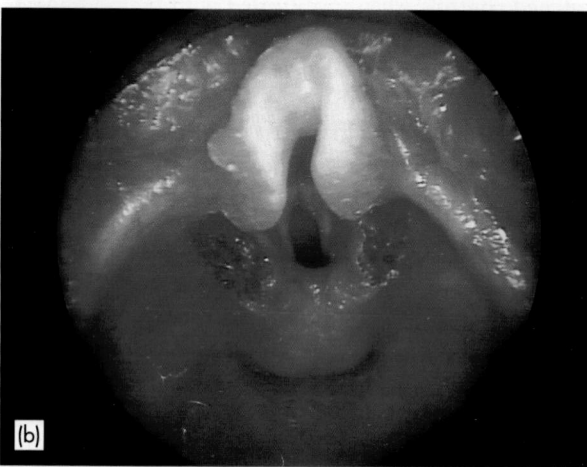

Figure 85.5   (a) An endoscopic view of the crowded supraglottis in a child with cerebral palsy. (b) The endoscopic view after dividing the aryepiglottic folds and vaporizing the redundant soft tissue overlying the arytenoid cartilages with a carbon dioxide laser.

obstruction at this level can be site specific in the form of laser supraglottoplasty or anterior epiglottopexy. A tracheostomy will be curative if the more localized procedures are insufficient. [Grade B]

POSTOPERATIVE COMPLICATIONS AND REDUCTION OF PERIOPERATIVE RISK

The potential surgical complications following adenotonsillectomy include pain, which causes poor oral intake, and haemorrhage. More worrying is that up to 20 percent of children who undergo adenotonsillectomy for OSA develop postoperative respiratory failure.[42] For this reason, otherwise healthy children undergoing adenotonsillectomy for moderate to severe OSA should not be booked as day cases.

Identified risk factors for the development of postoperative complications in otherwise healthy children are:

- severe OSA;
- a history of acute airway compromise;
- young age (less than three years);
- cardiac complications;
- failure to thrive;
- obesity;
- prematurity.

Children with craniofacial syndromes, neuromuscular diseases and systemic illnesses are also at increased risk of postoperative respiratory complications (**Table 85.1**).

These 'at risk' children may need to be admitted 24 hours prior to an anaesthetic for the administration of systemic steroid to reduce pulmonary atelectasia. They should also undergo pulse oxymetry the night before a general anaesthetic and for one or two nights postoperatively to document the severity of oxygen desaturations, even though a previous sleep study will have been carried out. Postoperative admission to an intensive care unit should be considered for all high-risk children, especially those who will have persistent OSA despite the planned surgical intervention. Systemic steroids and antibiotics, nebulized bronchodilators and chest physiotherapy are needed in the perioperative period if the child has audible crepitations on chest examination. [Grade D]

Children with OSA are very sensitive to narcotic analgesia, which has a significant detrimental effect on their respiratory drive.[43] Narcotics should be completely avoided in the perioperative period in any 'at risk' child. An experienced paediatric anaesthetist will be needed to provide the general anaesthetic. Following surgery, the endotrachial tube should not be removed until the patent has fully recovered from the anaesthetic, so as to minimize the risk of upper airway obstruction.

Children with Down syndrome or cerebral palsy may need to be intubated in intensive care for the first 24 hours postoperatively until surgical oedema has settled. Alternatively, a nasopharyngeal prong can be used to stent the soft palate following UVPP or adenotonsillectomy in these children. Systemic steroids should be continued postoperatively for the first 24 hours to help with surgical oedema and pulmonary ateletasia. They have also been shown to reduce postoperative pain following tonsillectomy.[44] Patients who are on CPAP preoperatively can restart this immediately postoperatively and then can be weaned from it if the surgery is deemed successful. [Grade B]

LONG-TERM POSTOPERATIVE FOLLOW-UP

All patients should have clinical follow-up following initial treatment to document improvement or resolution of their symptoms. Children diagnosed as having mild or moderate sleep apnoea who have complete resolution of their symptoms do not require post-intervention sleep studies.

Children who continue to have symptoms, had severe OSA on presentation or are in the 'high-risk' group should have a post-intervention sleep study (**Table 85.3**). The sleep study should be performed at least six weeks after surgery to ensure that the upper airway remodelling is complete. [Grade B]

CONCLUSION

Before paediatric OSA was recognized, children affected would present with severe failure to thrive and growth retardation, right-sided heart failure, cor pulmonale, permanent neurological damage, behavioural disturbance, hypersomnolence and developmental delay. Since the advent of paediatric sleep laboratories in the 1970s, OSA has been a widely recognized problem commonly encountered by paediatricians, otolaryngologists, anaesthetists and neurologists.

Adenotonsillectomy provides a cure in the great majority of children with OSA but in syndromic children and those with neuromuscular diseases it can present a real therapeutic challenge. Such children need treatment decisions to be made in collaboration with paediatric, sleep physician and anaesthetic colleagues and the parents or carers, so as to arrive at the most acceptable treatment option.

KEY POINTS

- Pathological sleep-disordered breathing occurs in approximately 10 percent of the paediatric population.
- Adenotonsillectomy cures or improves sleep apnoea in 90 percent of children.
- Sleep-disordered breathing can cause neurobehavioural and cardiac complications.
- Children at increased risk of OSA have been identified.
- Sleep studies provide objective measure of the severity of sleep-disordered breathing.
- Sleep nasendoscopy can identify the site of upper airway obstruction.
- Children at increased risk of respiratory failure following surgical intervention have been identified.
- Children with persistent symptoms after intervention need follow-up sleep studies.

Best clinical practice

✓ Snoring children should be screened for the presence of sleep-disordered breathing.
✓ 'At risk' children need preoperative sleep studies and careful perioperative management to minimize the possibility of postoperative respiratory failure.
✓ Syndromic children and those with neuromuscular disease pose a significant management challenge and need a multidisciplinary approach.
✓ The site of upper airway obstruction should be investigated with sleep nasendoscopy if there is any doubt that it may not be adenotonsillar.
✓ Persistent symptoms of OSA after intervention need follow-up with a postoperative sleep study.

Deficiencies in current knowledge and areas for future research

➢ Understanding of the natural history of sleep-disordered breathing. There is concern that children with OSA may go on to develop adult sleep-related breathing disorders. This tendency may be reversed by early adenotonsillectomy.
➢ Understanding of the clinical relevance of simple snoring. It may be that simple snoring is more serious than currently thought.
➢ Accurate prevalence data for sleep-disordered breathing and age-appropriate diagnostic criteria.
➢ Understanding of the mechanism of arousal and how it leads to daytime symptoms.
➢ Development of standardized perioperative care designed to reduce postoperative respiratory failure.

REFERENCES

1. Guilleminault C, Abad VC. Obstructive Sleep Apnea. *Current Treatment Options in Neurology.* 2004; **6**: 309–17.
2. Erler T, Paditz E. Obstructive sleep apnea syndrome in children: a state-of-the-art review. *Treatments in Respiratory Medicine.* 2004; **3**: 107–22.
3. Nieminen P, Lopponen T, Tolonen U, Lenning P, Lopponen H. Growth and biochemical markers of growth in children with snoring obstructive sleep apnoea. *Pediatrics.* 2002; **109**: 55.
4. O'Brien LM, Mervis CB, Holbrook CR, Bruner JL, Klaus CJ, Rutherford J *et al.* Neurobehavioral implications of habitual snoring in children. *Pediatrics.* 2004; **114**: 44–9.

5. O'Brien LM, Mervis CB, Holbrook CR, Bruner JL, Smith NH, McNally N et al. Neurobehavioral correlates of sleep-disordered breathing in children. *Journal of Sleep Research.* 2004; **13**: 165–72.

6. Montgomery-Downs HE, Crabtree VM, Gozal D. Cognition, sleep and respiration in at-risk children treated for obstructive sleep apnoea. *European Respiratory Journal.* 2005; **25**: 336–42.

7. Guilleminault C, Palayo R, Ledger D, Clerk A, Bocian RC. Recognition of sleep disordered breathing in children. *Pediatrics.* 1996; **98**: 871–82.

8. Chervin RD, Dillon JE, Archbold KH, Ruzika DL. Conduct problems and symptoms of sleep disorder in children. *Journal of the American Academy of Child and Adolescent Psychiatry.* 2003; **42**: 201–8.

9. Sonn H, Rosenfield RM. Evaluation of sleep disordered breathing in children. *Otolaryngology and Head and Neck Surgery.* 2003; **128**: 344–52.

10. Sie KN, Perkins JA, Clarke WR. Acute right heart failure due to adenotonsillar hypertrophy. *International Journal of Pediatric Otorhinolaryngology.* 1997; **41**: 53–8.

* 11. Tal A, Lieberman A, Margulis G, Sofer S. Ventricular dysfunction in children with obstructive sleep apnoea: radionucleotide assessment. *Pediatric Pulmonology.* 1988; **4**: 139–43. *Use of sleep nasendoscopy in children.*

* 12. Guilleminault C, Palayo R. Sleep disordered breathing in children. *Annals of Medicine.* 1998; **30**: 350–6. *Good description of physiological effects of sleep-disordered breathing.*

* 13. Stradling JR, Thomas G, Waley AR, Williams P, Freeland A. Effect of adenotonsillectomy on nocturnal hypoxaemia, sleep disturbance and symptoms in snoring children. *Lancet.* 1990; **335**: 249–53. *Good description of physiological effects of sleep-disordered breathing.*

14. Gaultier C, Guilleminault C. Genetics, control of breathing, and sleep-disordered breathing: a review. *Sleep Medicine.* 2001; **2**: 281–95.

15. Redline S, Tishler PV, Schluchter M, Aylor J, Clark K, Graham G. Risk factors of sleep disordered breathing in children, associations with obesity, race, and respiratory problems. *American Journal of Respiratory and Critical Care Medicine.* 1999; **159**: 1527–32.

* 16. Jeans WD, Fernando DC, Maw AR, Leighton BC. A longitudinal study of the growth of the nasopharynx and its contents in normal children. *British Journal of Radiology.* 1981; **54**: 117–21. *Discussion of why sleep studies are needed.*

17. Myatt HM, Beckenham EJ. The use of diagnostic sleep nasendoscopy in the management of children with complex upper airway obstruction. *Clinical Otolaryngology and Allied Sciences.* 2000; **25**: 200–8.

18. Kohyama J, Ohinata JS, Hasegawa T. Blood pressure in sleep disordered breathing. *Archives of Disease in Childhood.* 2003; **88**: 139–42.

19. Katz ES, Lulz J, Black C, Marcus CL. Pulse transit time as a measure of arousal and respiratory effort in children with sleep disordered breathing. *Pediatric Research.* 2003; **53**: 580–8.

20. Spiegel K, Leproult R, L'Hermite-Baleriaux M, Copinschi G, Penev PD, Van Cauter E. Leptin levels are dependent on sleep duration: relationships with sympathovagal balance, carbohydrate regulation, cortisol, and thyrotropin. *Journal of Clinical Endocrinology and Metabolism.* 2004; **89**: 5762–71.

21. Brooks LJ, Stephens BM, Bacevice AM. Adenoid size is related to severity but not the number of episodes of obstructive apnoea in children. *Journal of Pediatrics.* 1998; **132**: 682–6.

22. Goh DY, Galster P, Marcus CL. Sleep architecture and respiratory disturbances in children with obstructive sleep apnoea. *American Journal of Respiratory and Critical Care Medicine.* 2000; **162**: 682–6.

23. Van Someren V, Burmester M, Alusi G, Lane R. Are sleep studies worth doing? *Archives of Diseases in Childhood.* 2000; **83**: 76–81.

24. Urschilz MS, Wolff J, Von Einem V, Urschitz-Dupra PM, Schlaud M, Poets CR. Reference values for nocturnal home pulse oximetry during sleep in primary school children. *Chest.* 2003; **123**: 96–101.

25. Ryan PJ, Hilton MF, Boldy DA. Validation of British Thoracic Society guidelines for the diagnosis of sleep apnoea/hypopnoea syndrome: can poysomnography be avoided? *Thorax.* 1995; **50**: 972–5.

26. Brouillette RT, Morielli A, Liemanis A, Waters KA, Luciano R, Duchame FM. Nocturnal pulse oximetry as an abbreviated testing modality for pediatric obstructive sleep apnoea. *Pediatrics.* 2000; **105**: 405–12.

* 27. Sher AE, Sprintzen RJ, Tharpy MJ. Endoscopic observations of obstructive sleep apnoea in children with anomalous upper airways: predictive and therapeutic value. *International Journal of Pediatric Otorhinolaryngology.* 1986; **11**: 135–42. *Overview of adenotonsillectomy for obstructive sleep apnoea.*

28. Croft CB, Pringle MB. Sleep nasendoscopy: a technique of assessment in snoring and obstructive sleep apnoea. *Clinical Otolaryngology and Allied Sciences.* 1991; **16**: 504–9.

29. Jacobs IN, Gray FF, Wendell TN. Upper airway obstruction in children with Down syndrome. *Archives of Otololaryngology – Head and Neck Surgery.* 1996; **122**: 945–59.

30. D'Antonio LL, Rice RD, Fink SC. Evaluation of pharyngeal and laryngeal structure and function in patients with oculo-auriculo-vertebral spectrum. *Cleft Palate-craniofacial Journal.* 1998; **35**: 333–41.

31. Lipson AH, Yuille D, Angel M. Velocardiofacial syndrome: an important syndrome for the dysmorphologist to recognise. *Journal of Medical Genetics.* 1991; **28**: 596–604.

32. Caulfield H. Investigations in paediatric obstructive sleep apnoea: do we need them? *International Journal of Pediatric Otorhinolaryngology.* 2003; **67**: S107–10.

33. Guilleminault C, Pelayo R, Clark A, Leger D, Bocian RC. Home nasal continuous positive airway pressure in infants

with sleep disordered breathing. *Journal of Pediatrics.* 1995; **127**: 905–12.

34. Engleman HM, McDonald JP, Graham D, Lello GE, Kingshott RN, Coleman EL *et al.* Randomised crossover trial of two treatments for sleep apnoea/hypopnoea syndrome: continuous positive airway pressure and mandibular repositioning splint. *American Journal of Respiratory and Critical Care Medicine.* 2002; **166**: 855–9.

35. Suen JS, Arnold JE, Brooks LJ. Adenotonsillectomy for the treatment of obstructive sleep apnoea in children. *Archives of Otolaryngology – Head and Neck Surgery.* 1995; **121**: 525–30.

36. Kudoh F, Sanai A. Effect of tonsillectomy and adenoidectomy on obese children with sleep disordered breathing. *Acta Oto-laryngologica. Supplementum.* 1996; **523**: 216–8.

37. Southall DP, Stebbens VA, Mirza R. Upper airway obstruction with hypoxaemia and sleep disruption in Down's syndrome. *Developmental Medicine and Child Neurology.* 1987; **29**: 734–42.

38. Jacob IN, Gray RF, Wendell TN. Upper airway obstruction in Down's syndrome. *Archives of Otolaryngology – Head and Neck Surgery.* 1996; **122**: 945–50.

39. Kologal S, Gibbons VP, Stith JA. Sleep abnormalities in patients with severe cerebral palsy. *Developmental Medicine and Child Neurology.* 1994; **36**: 304–11.

40. Kosko JR, Derkay CS. Uvulopalatopharyngoplasty: treatment of obstructive sleep aponea in neurologically impaired pediatric patients. *International Journal of Pediatric Otorhinolaryngology.* 1995; **32**: 241–6.

41. Mandell DL, Yellon RF, Bradley JP, Izadi K, Gordon CB. Mandibular distraction for micrognathia and severe upper airway obstruction. *Archives of Otolaryngology – Head and Neck Surgery.* 2004; **130**: 344–8.

42. McColley SA, April MM, Carroll JL, Naclerio RM, Loughlin GM. Respiratory compromise after adenotonsillectomy in children with obstructive sleep apnea. *Archives of Otolaryngology – Head and Neck Surgery.* 1992; **118**: 940–3.

43. Brown K, Laferriere A, Moss I. Recurrent hypoxemia in young children with obstructive sleep apnea is associated with reduced opioid requirement for analgesia. *Anesthesiology.* 2004; **100**: 806–10.

44. Stewart DL, Welge JA, Myer CM. Steroids for improving recovery following tonsillectomy in children. *Cochrane Database of Systematic Reviews.* 2003; **1**: CD 003997.

86

Stridor

DAVID ALBERT

Introduction	1114	Best clinical practice	1124
Assessment	1115	Deficiencies in current knowledge and areas for future	
Management of acute airway obstruction	1123	research	1125
Key points	1124	References	1125

SEARCH STRATEGY

The author has a personal bibliography of key papers on paediatric airway obstruction. This was supplemented with successive searches of Medline using the following strategies: title or text word stridor and key words child, laryngomalacia, tracheomalacia; vocal cord palsy and child, vocal fold palsy and child, vascular ring and child, congenital subglottic stenosis and child, laryngotracheobronchitis and child, bacterial tracheitis and child, extubation and child, biphasic stridor, mediastinal mass and airway obstruction and child. The rationale for most interventions in childhood stridor is based on the current practices of experienced clinicians. Few treatments have been subjected to controlled trials. Hence, apart from steroid thereapy in croup, recommendations in this chapter are Grade C and D.

INTRODUCTION

This chapter discusses the diagnostic accuracy of history and examination. It then reviews the usefulness of special investigations. This is an overview so that the clinician can be directed to the appropriate chapter for detailed information on specific conditions. The general principles of management of the acutely stridulous child are presented.

Definitions

Turbulent flow due to partial obstruction of the airway gives rise to abnormal or unwanted noise. Obstruction of the small intra-thoracic airways, such as occurs in bronchial asthma, is termed 'wheezing'. Noise originating in the larynx or trachea is typically high-pitched and termed 'stridor'. The low-pitched snoring type of noise made by naso- and oropharyngeal obstruction is usually termed 'stertor'. This type of noise can occasionally be produced by the supraglottic larynx. A rigid differentiation between stridor and stertor is not only artificial but can wrongly limit the differential diagnosis (**Tables 86.1, 86.2 and 86.3**).

The challenge of managing a stridulous child

A child labelled as 'congenital stridor' may, rarely, have a more sinister diagnosis. History and examination are insufficient for a firm diagnosis. Deciding which patients to investigate is sometimes difficult. Even after non-invasive investigations such as imaging there may still be a number of possible diagnoses. Flexible endoscopy in the office is useful but gives little or no information beyond the glottis.

The definitive diagnostic technique of laryngotracheobronchoscopy (LTB) requires an experienced team of surgeon, anaesthetist and nursing staff. Both equipment and expertise are now highly specialized and are not available in all institutions.

Table 86.1 Nasopharyngeal causes of airway obstruction.

Common		Acquired		
Neonates	Children	Neonates	Children	Congenital
Neonatal rhinitis	Allergic rhinitis	Syphillis	Allergic rhinitis	Choanal atresia
Choanal atresia/stenosis	Adenoiditis	Neonatal rhinitis	Adenoiditis	Choanal stenosis
Craniofacial abnormalities	Adenotonsillar hypertrophy		Adenotonsillar hypertrophy	Mid-nasal stenosis
Micrognathia	Foreign bodies		Foreign bodies	Piriform aperture stenosis
			Nonallergic rhinitis	Nasal glioma
			Nonallergic rhinitis with eosinophilia (NARES)	Encephalocoele
			Retropharyngeal abscess	Meningocoele
			Glandular fever	Nasopharyngeal mass
			Ludwig's angina	Hairy polyp/
			Thermal and caustic burns	teratoma
				Craniofacial abnormalities with small nasopharynx
				Micrognathia
				Pierre Robin
				Treacher-Collins
				Macroglossia
				Down syndrome
				Cystic hygroma
				Lingual thyroid

Table 86.2 Laryngeal causes of airway obstruction.

Common		Acquired		
Neonates	Children	Neonates	Children	Congenital
Laryngomalacia	Croup	Intubation trauma	Epiglottitis	Laryngomalacia
Intubation trauma	Haemangiomas	Surgical trauma, e.g. laser	Croup	Posterior laryngeal cleft
Reflux laryngitis	Papillomatosis	Laryngotracheal stenosis	Bacterial tracheitis	Vallecula cyst
Laryngotracheal stenosis	Intubation trauma	Arytenoid fixation	Hereditary angioedema	Laryngeal cysts
Vocal cord palsy	Vocal cord palsy	Reflux laryngitis	Epidemolysis bullossa	Webs
	Papillomatosis		Foreign bodies	Laryngeal atresia
			Dislocated arytenoid	Laryngotracheal stenosis
			Intubation trauma	Arytenoid fixation
			Fracture	Vocal cord palsy
			Caustic and thermal burns	
			Haemangiomas	
			Cystic hygroma	
			Papillomatosis	
			Rhabdomyosarcoma	
			Wegener's	

In the acute situation the infant airway can deteriorate rapidly. In a specialized unit this is rarely a problem with experienced anaesthetists to intubate and surgeons to perform the rare emergency tracheotomy. In a paediatric ward or emergency room, rapid deterioration can prove a real challenge.

ASSESSMENT

Stridor is the noise from a narrowed airway. The aim of the history, examination and special examinations is to determine not only the site and cause of the obstruction (the diagnosis) but also its effect on the airway (the

Table 86.3 Tracheal causes of airway obstruction.

Common		Acquired		Congenital
Neonates	Children	Neonates	Children	
Tracheobronchomalacia	Foreign bodies	Post intubation and endoscopy	Laryngotracheitis	Stenosis
Tracheal stenosis	Tracheal stenosis	Tracheal stenosis	Bacterial tracheitis	Atresia
Vascular compression		Reflux tracheitis	Foreign bodies	Trapped first tracheal ring
			Localized malacia secondary to a tracheostomy or TEF repair	Complete cartilage rings
			Thyroid	Micro (stovepipe) trachea tracheal cysts
			Cystic hygroma	Haemangiomata
			Mediastinal tumours	Tracheobronchomalacia (with tracheo-oesophageal fistula)
				Vascular compression
				Aberrant innominate
				Pulmonary artery sling
				Double aortic arch

severity). It is important to consider the effect of airway obstruction on feeding, sleep, exercise and growth.

History

PERINATAL HISTORY

The obstetric and perinatal history are often relevant. This is particularly true if the child was born prematurely and required ventilation. Few neonates over 32 weeks' gestation will require ventilation for respiratory distress syndrome. Ventilation is the norm for those delivered at 28 weeks or earlier, even with the administration of surfactant. Neonates admitted even for short periods to intensive care or special care baby units (SCBU) may have had endotracheal intubation without the parents volunteering this important information. Beware the term 'intubation', as this may be mistaken for the passage of nasogastric tubes or even for nasal and oral mucus extraction.

Stridor which is present at birth, i.e. with the child's first breath, is unusual. This generally denotes a fixed congenital narrowing such as a laryngeal web, subglottic stenosis or tracheal narrowing.[1] Dynamic conditions such as laryngomalacia become evident in the first few weeks of life. The stridor in congenital vocal cord palsy is often present immediately post-partum suggesting that it may be more an incoordination than a true paralysis. A gradual increase in severity of stridor or airway compromise implies growth of an obstruction which may be luminal as in a subglottic haemangioma or extrinsic as with a mediastinal mass.

PATTERN OF STRIDOR

Stridor is seldom constant. Any diurnal or other variation can help pinpoint the cause, though asking parents about the timing of stridor in the respiratory cycle is seldom profitable. Typically, laryngomalacia is better with the child at rest and asleep but made worse by crying, feeding and when the child is distressed. Airway obstruction with the baby supine can occur with a pedunculated laryngeal mass but more often is due at least in part to a degree of supralaryngeal obstruction such as micrognathia and resultant tongue base occlusion. Improvement in the airway with crying occurs in gross nasal obstruction such as bilateral choanal atresia.

ASSOCIATED FEATURES

Airway obstruction produces a number of associated symptoms (**Table 86.4**) alongside stridor including recession, apnoeas, cyanosis, 'dying spells', dyspnoea, tachypnoea, cough and hoarseness. Recession, even if quite severe, can be missed by parents but is a clear sign of inspiratory obstruction. Apnoeas with cyanosis are typical of severe tracheobronchomalacia and are sometimes termed 'dying spells'. Parents will usually attempt resuscitation if these are severe. It is often unclear how many of these attacks are otherwise self-limiting. Tachypnoea and dyspnoea are not limited to upper airway obstruction but a clear description of exertional dyspnoea in an older child provides a useful functional assessment of severity. Cough is typical of tracheo-oesophageal fistula and tracheomalacia and is rarely due to 'infant asthma'. Hoarseness clearly suggests a laryngeal

Table 86.4 Symptoms associated with varying causes of airway obstruction.

Symptoms	Typical diagnoses	Example
Stertor	Nasopharyngeal obstruction	Neonatal rhinitis
Inspiratory stridor	Laryngeal and subglottic obstruction	Laryngomalacia, subglottic stenosis
Biphasic stridor	High/mid tracheal obstruction	Tracheomalacia/stenosis
Prolonged expiratory phase	Tracheal and bronchial obstruction	Tracheobronchomalacia or stenosis
Cough	TEF	
	Vocal cord palsy	
	Cleft larynx	
	Foreign body	
	Tracheomalacia	
	Reflux	
Aspiration	TEF	
	Vocal cord palsy	
	Cleft larynx	
Hoarseness	Laryngeal lesion	Vocal cord palsy, papilloma
Acute airway obstruction	Retropharyngeal abscess	
	Tonsillitis	
	Glandular fever	
	Foreign bodies	
	Epiglottitis	
	Croup	
	Bacterial tracheitis	
Dysphagia and feeding difficulties	Epiglottitis	Feeding affected with many causes of severe airway obstruction and aspiration
	Tonsillitis	
	Retropharyngeal abscess	
Apnoeas	Tracheobronchomalacia	
Dying spells	Reflex apnoea	

lesion such as laryngeal papillomatosis but is also seen in vocal cord palsy.

FEEDING HISTORY

Feeding is closely connected with breathing, particularly in the infant. An accurate picture of the feeding pattern must be obtained. Breast-fed babies with airway obstruction will characteristically 'come up for air'; bottle-fed babies may require thickened feeds or a 'slow teat' (i.e. one with small holes). Aspiration suggests a vocal cord palsy, tracheo-oesophageal fistula or rarely a cleft larynx. Significant repeated aspiration may be associated with recurrent chest infections. Regurgitation ('posseting') is common in neonates and by itself may not represent significant gastro-oesophageal reflux. The end result of poor feeding may just be slow feeding which troubles the mother more than the child or there may be failure to thrive with demonstrably poor weight gain. As laryngomalacia is common, it is important not to assign failure to thrive to this without first having considered and excluded other causes.

GENERAL MEDICAL CONDITIONS

Enquiry into the general medical history may explain a vocal cord palsy occurring as a result of neurological disease or cardiac surgery or may suggest vascular compression associated with congenital cardiac disease. Finally, ask the parents about the presence of any birthmarks, as they may be associated with a subglottic haemangioma.

ACUTE OBSTRUCTION

In acute airway obstruction the history is taken simultaneously with the examination and resuscitation. Take particular note of any possible foreign body ingestion or concurrent illness. Rapid progression of airway obstruction typically occurs in acute infection and in foreign body inhalation.

Examination

OBSERVATION

Observing the child at rest before proceeding to formal examination provides not only an initial assessment of the degree of respiratory distress and the characteristics of any stridor but also gives time to gain the child's confidence. The characteristics of the stridor need to be observed as well as the effects of airway obstruction such as recession. Abnormal voice, wheeze or coughs are useful localizing signs.

The pre-endoscopy assessment, though important, can only be a guide to the type and degree of pathology discovered at endoscopy. The combination of a thorough history, examination and limited investigation can in some conditions (e.g. mild laryngomalacia) provide sufficient diagnostic probability to avoid initial endoscopy. The type of stridor may be characteristic of a particular pathology but is never diagnostic.[2] A second pathology may be present in up to 20 percent of cases though few will require treatment.[3] The diagnosis can only be confirmed with certainty after endoscopy. This does not mean that every child with stridor requires endoscopy. In most children seen in a secondary or tertiary referral centre, endoscopy will be required and in most conditions is the gold standard. Dynamic conditions such as vocal cord palsy and tracheobronchomalacia often prove difficult to confirm or exclude at routine endoscopy.

CHARACTERISTICS OF STRIDOR

The characteristic sound of stridor even in a common condition such as laryngomalacia[4] is so variable as to be of little diagnostic use on its own. The site of the abnormal vibration can rarely be tracked down with the aid of a stethoscope, because of the variable transmission of sound through the thorax. However, auscultation is useful to detect heart murmurs and wheeze. Typically, inspiratory stridor is due to an extrathoracic obstruction (**Figure 86.1**) from the larynx or high trachea. Bronchial or low tracheal obstruction produces an expiratory stridor. Biphasic stridor can occur with obstruction anywhere in the tracheobronchial tree. Even if expiratory stridor is absent, a prolonged expiratory phase may be present indicating an intrathoracic obstruction (**Figure 86.2**). Laryngomalacia is said to have a 'musical quality', vocal cord palsy a 'breathy quality'. The cough in tracheomalacia is said to be 'barking'.

ASSOCIATED FEATURES

Subcostal, intercostal and suprasternal recession may occur separately or together and also be associated with

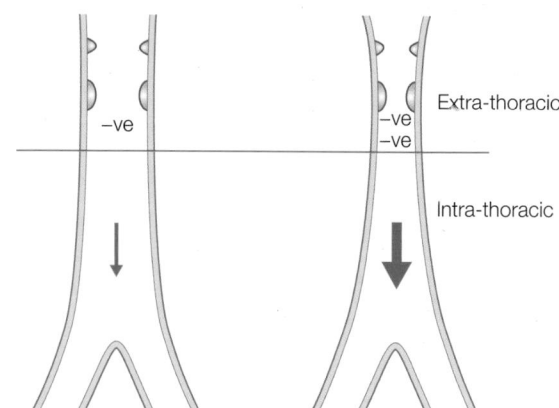

Figure 86.1 Showing collapse and increasing obstruction on inspiration with extra-thoracic obstruction.

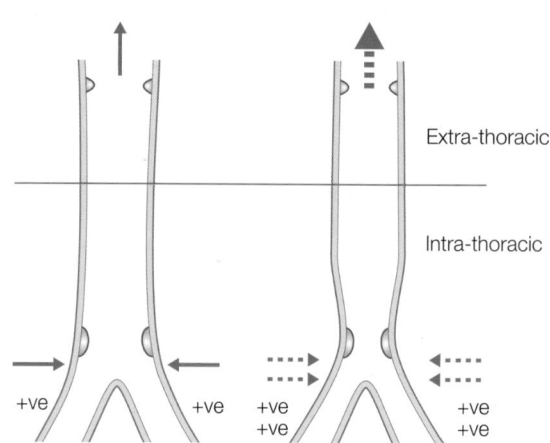

Figure 86.2 Showing collapse and increasing obstruction on expiration with intra-thoracic obstruction.

'see-saw' respiration. The severity of recession is a better indicator of the severity of airway compromise than the degree of stridor. The severity of stridor can paradoxically become less as obstruction worsens due to the diminishing airflow. No comfort should be taken from the fact that a child still looks pink. Cyanosis is a late event and suggests obstruction has been severe or prolonged.

If a supralaryngeal component is suspected, nasal patency should be assessed with a mirror, a wisp of cotton wool or using the bell end of a stethoscope. Make a conscious assessment of jaw and tongue size.

Both stridor and recession will vary as the child rests, cries and sleeps but it is rare to be able to demonstrate a similar repeatable change with position. Observing the child feeding is extremely valuable, particularly if there is poor feeding or aspiration.

Examine the ears, nose, throat and lastly neck with the usual caution that you must not use any instrumentation to examine the throat of child in whom epiglottitis is suspected.

Pre-endoscopy investigations

Investigations need to be carefully selected on the basis of the history and examination.

BLOOD GAS ANALYSIS

In acute airway obstruction, transcutaneous O_2 saturation monitoring is extremely helpful. It is noninvasive (unlike arterial blood gases) and yet much more sensitive than clinical estimation. However, considerable airway obstruction can occur without desaturation so long as the child continues to have the energy to overcome the obstruction. CO_2 build-up and respiratory acidosis can develop without desaturation especially if O_2 is being administered. Hypoxaemia occurs with tiredness more often than progression of the underlying obstruction. Transcutaneous CO_2 measurement is unreliable particularly in the shocked patient so there is still a place for arterial blood gases.

IMAGING

The value of radiological investigations has been reviewed retrospectively by Tostevin et al.[5] A plain chest x-ray and a lateral view of the neck, digitally enhanced to demonstrate the subglottis, oropharynx and nasopharynx, may be all the radiology required. A plain chest x-ray may show the ground glass appearance of bronchopulmonary dysplasia or mediastinal shift with obstructive emphysema of a foreign body but it does not demonstrate the major airways well. If a foreign body is suspected in young children, diaphragmatic screening with videofluoroscopy is a more sensitive technique. In older children, inspiratory and expiratory films may demonstrate diaphragmatic immobility on the side of the obstruction.

Videofluoroscopy is also an excellent way of demonstrating tracheomalacia. It can be combined with a contrast swallow looking for vascular compression[6, 7] and aspiration.

Bronchography is enjoying something of a renaissance after the introduction of safer nonionic contrast media. It is particularly useful for the lower airway demonstrating tracheobronchial stenosis and malacia. Opening pressures of the collapsed bronchi and lower trachea can be measured and used to determine the level of airway support needed.

Computerized tomography (CT) and magnetic resonance imaging (MRI)[8, 9, 10] are not usually sufficiently sensitive to fully characterize a stenotic segment, which can be more accurately assessed at endoscopy. If available, helical CT with multiplanar reconstruction may offer better definition of tracheal lesions.[11, 12] MRI and CT can, however, both demonstrate extrinsic compression, particularly abnormal vasculature.

Echocardiography can be used to screen for vascular compression, demonstrating most but not all abnormal vasculature as well as coincidental or symptomatic congenital heart disease.

With experience, ultrasound of the vocal cords can be used to demonstrate vocal cord palsy with reasonable accuracy to complement the endoscopic findings.

ASSESSMENT OF REFLUX

Gastro-oesophageal reflux[13, 14, 15, 16] can be assessed with a contrast study, milk scan, pH probe study or lower oesophageal biopsy. Contrast studies have low specificity and sensitivity and are very dependent on the radiologist for appropriate positioning and interpretation. The other investigations are more sensitive but are usually interpreted by gastroenterologists looking for reflux into the lower oesophagus. The laryngologist is interested in the pH in the upper oesophagus and pharynx, which can be measured using a second probe in the upper oesophagus. Double probe pH studies are at present more a research tool because of technical difficulties with the probe and little in the way of normative data. Many episodes of reflux occur without acid or at least any drop in pH; the significance of these non-acid reflux events for the larynx remains to be seen.

Even if reflux is demonstrated by any of the above means, it is difficult to decide if the reflux is secondary to the airway obstruction with a negative intrathoracic pressure drawing gastric contents into the oesophagus or if the reflux is a separate finding. Occasionally the reflux may be the primary factor with secondary reflux laryngitis. Reflux is considered in detail in Chapter 100, Gastro-oesophageal reflux and aspiration.

RESPIRATORY FUNCTION TESTS

Airway obstruction that worsens during sleep is usually a feature of pharyngeal obstruction such as adenotonsillar obstruction or a craniofacial anomaly. Laryngomalacia[17] and indeed almost any laryngotracheal pathology are rarely worse during sleep. A sleep study is not often used in the assessment of the stridulous child.

Lung function tests such as flow-volume-loops will help localize the site of obstruction but require a degree of patient cooperation. Other lung function tests such as peak flows or more ventilation/perfusion scans are selected with the advice of a pulmonologist.

In summary, a careful history, examination and carefully chosen investigations may suggest a diagnosis but only endoscopy will confirm the diagnosis.

Endoscopy

The two objectives in paediatric airway endoscopy are safety and accuracy. To achieve these objectives requires not only a full range of specialized paediatric endoscopy equipment (**Table 86.5**) but, most significantly, a high

Table 86.5 British Association for Paediatric Otorhinolaryngology minimum equipment standards for paediatric airway endoscopy.

Equipment
An adjustable laryngeal suspension system
An operating microscope with 400f lens
A selection of age-appropriate paediatric laryngoscopes of varying size and with a variety of viewing angles to include a retrospective telescope
Dedicated laryngeal microsurgical instruments, e.g. microscissors, probes, cupped and straight forceps
A selection of age-appropriate ventilating bronchoscopes with Hopkins rod telescopes to fit
A suitable light source with fibreoptic cables
A camera and monitor with image-capture facilities – video and still
A colour printer
A selection of forceps for the removal of foreign bodies
Optical forceps with rigid telescope(s) of appropriate length
A selection of fibreoptic bronchoscopes and a nasopharyngoscope
A full range of paediatric tracheotomy tubes
Cabinets and storage facilities for the above

level of experience in the endoscopist, anaesthesiologist and nursing staff. A systematic approach will provide a diagnosis in most cases.[18]

FLEXIBLE ENDOSCOPY IN THE OFFICE OR WARD

The introduction of ultra-thin endoscopes[19, 20, 21] with good optics and a diameter of less than 2 mm has allowed even neonates to be endoscoped without the need for a general anaesthetic. Per-oral passage of an endoscope using a finger between the child's gums to protect the instrument is preferred by many to transnasal introduction. This is usually considered a screening procedure. The view, particularly of the larynx, is often suboptimal. No invasive diagnostic or therapeutic procedure can be undertaken and even if an abnormality is demonstrated (such as laryngomalacia) a second pathology can easily be missed. Ward flexible endoscopy without anaesthesia is particularly useful to assess dynamic abnormalities such as vocal cord palsy prior to a formal endoscopy in the operating room. Flexible endoscopy under sedation in an endoscopy suite is widely practised by paediatricians and pulmonologists[22, 23, 24] and is becoming more popular with otolaryngologists as an adjunct to rigid endoscopy.[25]

LARYNGOTRACHEOBRONCHOSCOPY

Laryngotracheobronchoscopy (LTB)[26, 27] (**Figures 86.3** and **86.4**) using rigid Hopkins rod telescopes is the gold standard in the assessment of the stridulous child. It is now a highly technical procedure. The whole team (surgeon, anaesthetist and nursing assistant) need to work closely together to perform the examination safely, and to optimize the assessment.

The advent of video and high quality image reproduction on a viewing monitor has been invaluable in training.

Assessment is now safer as the anaesthetist can now see the image on screen and the team can be ready with equipment for the next stage.

If the examination is for assessment, it is vital that accurate records are kept to allow comparison with future examinations. This is facilitated by using a standardized data capture form within a department.[28] Use of a recognized staging system is important for publication of results. Prints from the video form a valid record for static conditions whilst for dynamic conditions a videotape is unparalleled. The latest digital image recording systems allow multiple rapid images to be stored during the procedure with only a selected few being printed or converted to slide format. As computer memory becomes even more affordable, digital video recordings as well as still images can be saved and archived. This provides an invaluable source of information for sequential clinical comparisons, medicolegal purposes and teaching.

ANAESTHESIA FOR AIRWAY ENDOSCOPY

Major units from around the world use different techniques and it is probably more important that a team of surgeon, anaesthetist and nurse work together than that one particular technique is followed. Practice varies between centres as to whether intubation is used at the start of the procedure but most units would now use spontaneous respiration rather than paralysis and jet ventilation.

Induction

Some units will use an atropine premedication to facilitate a dry surgical field and improve the efficacy of topical anaesthesia. To be effective it needs to be given by intra-muscular injection. Preoperative steroids are a good safeguard if significant stenosis is suspected. Intravenous

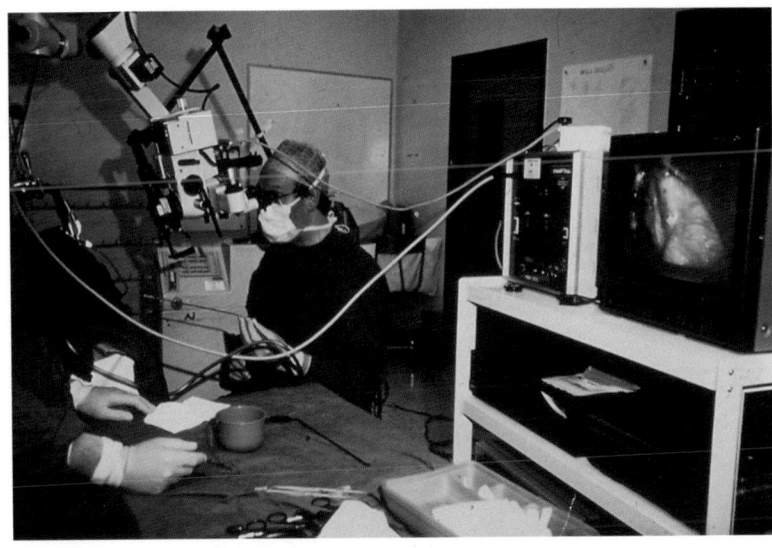

Figure 86.3 Microlaryngotracheobronchoscopy (MLTB) in progress. The surgeon is using a CO_2 laser.

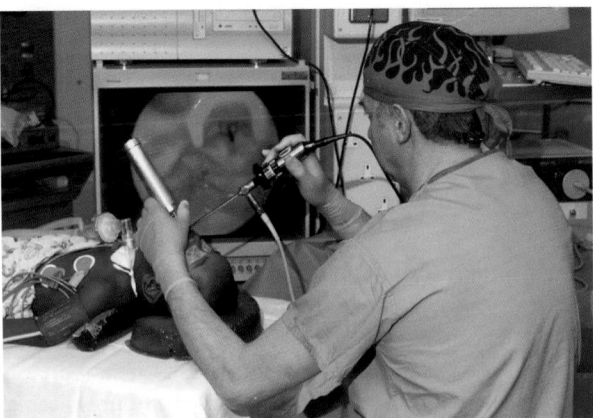

Figure 86.4 Laryngotracheoscopy in progress.

induction is preferable for older children though gas induction may be needed in infants, those with poor venous access and those with a precarious airway. Topical lignocaine spray to the cords needs to be carefully measured as the preparations used in adults can easily result in overdosage.[29, 30] Intravenous suxamethonium can be given if the patient is stable. It may be given prior to the lignocaine spray to avoid laryngeal spasm as well as to facilitate intubation if required.

Intubation

Once intubated the child can be quickly ventilated down to a level of anaesthesia which allows the passage of endoscopes without gagging but maintains spontaneous respiration. The laryngoscope can be adjusted whilst the child is still intubated. Nasotracheal intubation allows the endotracheal tube to be withdrawn into the nasopharynx once the child is breathing spontaneously.

Nonintubation technique

After induction the child is breathed down to the same level as above which, in the presence of any obstruction, can take some time. The advantage is that the endoscopist

has a view of an airway that has not been altered by the passage of an endotracheal tube. At any time airway control can be regained with intubation or the use of an endoscope.

Jet ventilation

This technique allows the child to be paralysed, preventing any coughing or gagging but gas exchange is maintained with short pulses of injected anaesthetic gas, simulating normal respiration.[31, 32, 33] The pressures required[34] are higher than physiological levels, with a risk in neonates and smaller children of a pneumothorax. Few centres still use this technique as dynamic conditions such as malacia and cord palsy cannot be identified.

Laryngeal mask

This is useful for fibre-optic bronchoscopy, particularly if the patient is difficult to intubate because of mandibular hypoplasia.[35, 36]

Tracheotomy tube anaesthesia

If use of the laser is considered[37] in a child who already has a tracheotomy tube, this should be changed prior to anaesthesia and a metal tube used.

Maintenance of anaesthesia

Halothane and oxygen maintain a level of anaesthesia that allows a thorough examination in a child who is breathing spontaneously. Halothane has the great advantage that it is relatively nonirritant to the airway. Sevoflurane[38] is also nonirritant but has the advantage of rapid onset and no pungency, allowing delivery of high concentrations immediately. Experience with this new agent is limited but the advantage of rapid induction may be offset by rapid termination of effect during periods of relative hypoventilation or airway obstruction. The anaesthetist needs to be able to control anaesthesia in response to surgical conditions and for this a video monitor is invaluable. Peroperative O_2 monitoring is now routine[39] and with time CO_2 monitoring is also becoming routine.[40]

MICROLARYNGOTRACHEOSCOPY TECHNIQUE

The following description assumes that the patient has been intubated, a suspension laryngoscope is employed and that the larynx is to be examined with a microscope or a rigid telescope.

A small sandbag is usually required under the shoulders to prevent hyperextension of the neck, with sandbags laterally to support the long thin heads of ex-premature neonates. A Mayo table supports the laryngostat clear of the chest.

It is important to prepare and check all equipment prior to the endoscopy so that the endoscopist is fully prepared for all eventualities. The range of Hopkins rod telescopes should include all lengths and diameters that could be needed and a 30° telescope to assess the supraglottic larynx without splinting. A microscope should be available though is often not used unless surgical intervention is required when two hands are needed for manipulation. If a microscope is used, a 400-mm lens allows the use of standard laryngeal instruments but a 350-mm lens brings the patient closer allowing easier manipulation of larynx, which is particularly important in small neonates. For routine examination, the telescope and camera can be held in the left hand with a probe used in the right. The view and images available are far superior to those via the microscope. Every unit should have a chart listing the appropriate sizes of bronchoscope for different ages. The age-appropriate bronchoscope needs to be checked and one at least a size smaller has to be instantly available as well. Antifog solution is only effective if freshly applied to the telescope lens.

Laryngeal examination is usually begun with the endotracheal tube in place by gently inserting the lubricated suspension laryngoscope, taking care to protect the teeth and lips and to keep the tongue central to provide a well-centred view. As in adults, it is important to check the overall appearance of the supraglottis and laryngopharynx during introduction of the laryngoscope. The endotracheal tube, if present, is followed to the tip of the epiglottis, gently lifting the epiglottis forwards making certain that the epiglottis does not curl up in front of the laryngoscope preventing a complete view of the anterior commissure. An overall assessment of the larynx can be made with the tube still *in situ*, providing a degree of stability that is particularly welcome in the child with a compromised airway.

Laryngeal examination with the endotracheal tube removed provides a superior view and by using a probe to move the arytenoids independently, the mobility of the cricoarytenoid joints can be assessed. If an interarytenoid scar is present the arytenoids will not move independently. A posterior laryngeal cleft is excluded by passing the probe between the arytenoids, comparing the lower limit of the interarytenoid groove with that of the posterior commissure. Finally, the cords need to be gently moved apart to inspect the subglottis.

The time available for the examination will depend on the airway. In a child breathing spontaneously with a normal airway and normal lung function, anaesthesia can be maintained solely by the use of inhalational agents with the endotracheal tube withdrawn into the pharynx. In others the time may be very limited and it is essential to be prepared to move ahead with bronchoscopy at any stage. If anaesthesia is stable, a sucker can be placed in the laryngeal inlet to mimic laryngomalacia – the 'Narcy test'. Photographs can be taken at this stage with a wide Storz photographic telescope. If there is significant subglottic stenosis, an ultra fine telescope passed through the laryngoscope will cause less trauma than a bronchoscope.

BRONCHOSCOPY

Traditionally, a ventilating bronchoscope (**Figure 86.5**) has been used which provides a means of actively ventilating the patient if required. With spontaneous ventilation, a smaller diameter rigid Hopkins rod telescope can be used with less trauma and less splinting of the airway. An age-appropriate bronchoscope is used unless stenosis is suspected. Neonates pose particular problems if manipulation of the airway is required.[41, 42] An anaesthetic laryngoscope can be used in the vallecula to lift the larynx forward whilst passing the bevel of the bronchoscope through the vocal cords under video control on the monitor. The main bronchi, the carina, the trachea and the subglottis are all systematically examined and videographs or digital images recorded. Tracheomalacia should be observed with a small bronchoscope withdrawn from the area in question and without positive airways pressure to avoid splinting. The

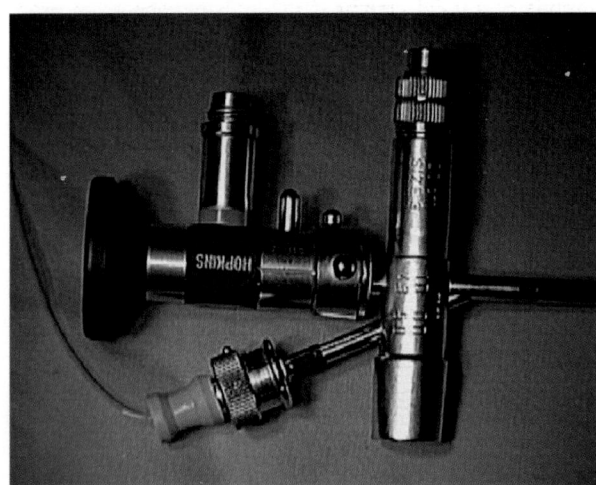

Figure 86.5 Ventilating bronchoscope.

ratio of cartilage to trachealis is significant in recording the type of malacia and in judging if aortopexy is likely to be successful.

DYNAMIC ASSESSMENT OF LARYNX ON RECOVERY FROM ANAESTHESIA

Typically, this can be achieved by withdrawing the bronchoscope to just posterior to the tip of the epiglottis. This affords a good view of the vocal cords to exclude a cord palsy and of the arytenoids to exclude the common posterior form of laryngomalacia, though anterior collapse of the epiglottis may be masked. In this case, a 30° or 70° telescope should be used. The anaesthetist should call the phase of respiration to check for paradoxical vocal cord movements.

An excellent technique for dynamic assessment of the vocal cord movement is to insert a laryngeal mask with a fibre-optic bronchoscope passed through this to just above the laryngeal inlet.[43] If a bilateral vocal cord palsy is suspected and structural abnormalities have been excluded with a full microlaryngoscopy and rigid bronchoscopy, it is sometimes necessary to reschedule the patient for a further examination in which a laryngeal mask and fibre-optic scope are used from the outset, reducing the influence of prolonged anaesthesia on the cord function. An alternative is to use a 30° scope which gives a view of the larynx without splinting the supraglottis.

MANAGEMENT OF ACUTE AIRWAY OBSTRUCTION

Medical (in ward or emergency room)

ASSESSMENT

In the acute situation, assessment, history taking and active resuscitation will often proceed in parallel. In the example of a child arriving in the emergency room with suspected LTB, the physician will be assessing the child for the degree of airway obstruction by gauging the recession and dyspnoea at the same time as asking the mother for the length of history and whether there is any possibility of foreign body inhalation. The nurse will be checking the oxygen saturation and setting up humidified oxygen. Another member of the team may have to call and alert the operating room that the child may need intubation as well as calling the anaesthesiologist and otolaryngologist. This situation clearly benefits from careful planning, with most units having a protocol for how to deal with the stridulous airway-compromised child. The protocols vary considerably with some units insisting on the presence of an otolaryngologist[44, 45] at intubation in case a tracheotomy is needed while others have managed for many years without.

OXYGEN THERAPY

With an obstruction to airflow, but normal alveolar function, raising the concentration of inspired oxygen will reduce the ventilatory requirement to maintain an adequate oxygen saturation in the blood but will do nothing to aid CO_2 excretion. So long as the possibility of chronic hypercarbia is appreciated, oxygen is a useful drug in the treatment of airway obstruction.

HUMIDIFICATION

There is no objective evidence[46] that raising the humidity of the inspired air is beneficial, though many units still use humidity tents or 'croupettes' that have the disadvantage of decreased visibility as well as doing little to allay the fears of a frightened child.

PHARMACOTHERAPY

Intravenous (and oral) steroids such as dexamethasone have been shown to be beneficial in croup (LTB) with inhaled steroids having a similar effect. Nebulized budesonide[47] can be used at home for children with recurrent croup and is usually thought to be superior to oral dexamethasone, though one study showed no difference.[48] Klassen[49] [****] summarizes the situation, 'All children with croup symptoms who demonstrate increased work of breathing in the clinics or emergency departments should be treated with glucocorticoids'. This treatment may be with nebulized budesonide (2 mg) or oral or intra-muscular dexamethasone (dose may be 0.15–0.6 mg/kg). Oral dexamethasone may be the best option because of its ease of administration, widespread availability, and lower cost. L-Epinephrine (5 mL of 1:1000) or racemic epinephrine (0.5 mL) should be considered for children with croup who have moderate or severe distress.

Surgical management in the operating room

The increasing use of intubation as an alternative to tracheotomy in acute airway obstruction has been brought about partly by technological advances in anaesthesia and partly by the realization that paediatric tracheotomy, even short term, brings with it numerous problems. Even with a skilled anaesthetist and careful monitoring it is possible that unexpected pathology will be encountered making intubation impossible. Severe subglottic stenosis, impacted foreign bodies and advanced epiglottitis are obvious examples but rarer examples occur such as laryngeal aplasia with ventilation being achieved via a tracheo-oesophageal fistula.

It is this uncertainty combined with the precipitate nature of paediatric airway obstruction that makes it mandatory in most hospitals for an ENT surgeon to be informed if a child with airway obstruction of unknown aetiology is to be intubated. Depending on the circumstances, it may be necessary to have an emergency tracheotomy set open with the correct size tube already selected.

Once the child has been gassed down slowly it is possible to inspect the larynx and exclude epiglottitis. This may be all that is required and the child can then be managed on a nasal prong with perhaps some continuous positive airways pressure (CPAP) applied. If intubation is required, it is important to minimize any damage to the already inflamed subglottic mucosa by very gentle intubation with a small soft tube just large enough for adequate ventilation and suction of secretions. Even if the initial intubation is oral, which tends to be easier, the tube should be replaced with a nasal tube which is more secure. At this stage, the fit of the tube can be assessed by checking for a leak and the tracheobronchial secretions sucked clear. If the secretions are very tenacious or there is still an element of airway obstruction, a ventilating bronchoscope should be passed to exclude bacterial tracheitis[50, 51, 52, 53] or a foreign body. In other clinical circumstances the benefit from endoscopy of having seen the degree of pathology is usually outweighed by the trauma that occurs, particularly with the passage of a bronchoscope as opposed to the smaller diameter of a fine telescope.

Significant tracheobronchomalacia is another reason for continuing airway difficulty after intubation and this will usually respond to CPAP.

Emergency tracheotomy

With experienced paediatric anaesthetists this is now unusual.[44, 45] Otolaryngologists are often asked to attend a potentially difficult intubation, but are rarely needed. A ventilating bronchoscope may be easier to pass than an endotracheal tube and an endotracheal tube mounted on a Hopkins rod telescope may be useful in a difficult intubation (**Figure 86.6**). It is easy to become complacent but, if emergency tracheotomy is required, the

surgical set and appropriate tube need to be instantly available. It is important to stay strictly in the midline so the child needs to be carefully positioned without neck or head deviation. A finger either side of the larynx is helpful with a vertical incision through skin and down to the trachea. If a paediatric tracheostomy tube is not available, a paediatric endotracheal tube can be used, ensuring it remains above the carina.

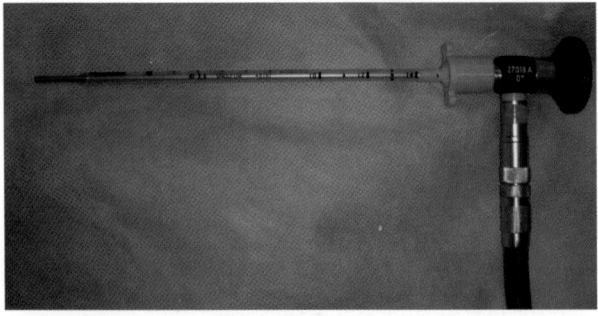

Figure 86.6 A Hopkins rod telescope with an endotracheal tube mounted and ready to introduce in a difficult intubation.

✓ All children with croup who demonstrate increased work of breathing should be treated with glucocorticoids. [Grade A]

✓ If a child with airway obstruction of unknown aetiology is to be intubated, an ENT surgeon should be informed. It may be necessary to have an emergency tracheotomy set open with the correct size tube already selected. [Grade D]

✓ A difficult endotracheal intubation may be facilitated by the use of a small ventilating bronchoscope or by passing a Hopkins rod telescope on which a narrow endotracheal tube has been mounted. [Grade D]

Deficiencies in current knowledge and areas for future research

➤ A growing trend toward specialization within otolaryngology will ensure that airway endoscopy in children is increasingly the remit of otolaryngologists with a special interest and training in this work.

➤ Improved optics, image capture facilities and anaesthesia will contribute to this.

REFERENCES

1. Pedraza Pena LR, Rodriguez Santana JR, Sifontes JE. Neonatal stridor: a life-threatening condition. *Puerto Rico Health Sciences Journal.* 1994; **13**: 33–6.

* 2. Papsin BC, Abel SM, Leighton SE. Diagnostic value of infantile stridor: a perceptual test. *International Journal of Pediatric Otorhinolaryngology.* 1999; **51**: 33–9. *Analysis of the characteristic presentations of children with stridor and recommendations regarding diagnostic strategies.*

* 3. Mancuso RF, Choi SS, Zalzal GH, Grundfast KM. Laryngomalacia. The search for the second lesion. *Archives of Otolaryngology – Head and Neck Surgery.* 1996; **122**: 302–6. *Analysis of the characteristic presentations of children with stridor and recommendations regarding diagnostic strategies.*

4. Nussbaum E, Maggi JC. Laryngomalacia in children. *Chest.* 1990; **98**: 942–4.

5. Tostevin PM, de Bruyn R, Hosni A, Evans JN. The value of radiological investigations in pre-endoscopic assessment of children with stridor. *Journal of Laryngology and Otology.* 1995; **109**: 844–8.

6. Han MT, Hall DG, Manche A, Rittenhouse EA. Double aortic arch causing tracheoesophageal compression. *American Journal of Surgery.* 1993; **165**: 628–31.

7. Backer CL, Ilbawi MN, Idriss FS, DeLeon SY. Vascular anomalies causing tracheoesophageal compression. Review of experience in children [see comments]. *Journal of Thoracic and Cardiovascular Surgery.* 1989; **97**: 725–31.

8. Hofmann U, Hofmann D, Vogl T, Wilimzig C, Mantel K. Magnetic resonance imaging as a new diagnostic criterion in paediatric airway obstruction. *Progress in Pediatric Surgery.* 1991; **27**: 221–30.

9. Vogl T, Wilimzig C, Hofmann U, Hofmann D, Dresel S, Lissner J. MRI in tracheal stenosis by innominate artery in children. *Pediatric Radiology.* 1991; **21**: 89–93.

10. Vogl T, Wilimzig C, Bilaniuk LT, Hofmann U, Hofmann D, Dresel S *et al.* MR imaging in pediatric airway obstruction. *Journal of Computed Assisted Tomography.* 1990; **14**: 182–6.

11. Whyte RI, Quint LE, Kazerooni EA, Cascade PN, Iannettoni MD, Orringer MB. Helical computed tomography for the evaluation of tracheal stenosis. *Annals of Thoracic Surgery.* 1995; **60**: 27–30.

12. Quint LE, Whyte RI, Kazerooni EA, Martinez FJ, Cascade PN, Lynch JP *et al.* Stenosis of the central airways: evaluation by using helical CT with multiplanar reconstructions. *Radiology.* 1995; **194**: 871–7.

13. Nielson DW, Heldt GP, Tooley WH. Stridor and gastroesophageal reflux in infants. *Pediatrics.* 1990; **85**: 1034–9.

14. Contencin P, Maurage C, Ployet MJ, Seid AB, Sinaasappel M. Gastroesophageal reflux and ENT disorders in childhood. *International Journal of Pediatric Otorhinolaryngology.* 1995; **32** Suppl: S135–44.

15. Krishnamoorthy M, Mintz A, Liem T, Applebaum H. Diagnosis and treatment of respiratory symptoms of initially unsuspected gastroesophageal reflux in infants. *American Surgeon.* 1994; **60**: 783–5.

16. Burton DM, Pransky SM, Katz RM, Kearns DB, Seid AB. Pediatric airway manifestations of gastroesophageal reflux. *Annals of Otology, Rhinology and Laryngology.* 1992; **101**: 742–9.

17. Chetty KG, Kadifa F, Berry RB, Mahutte CK. Acquired laryngomalacia as a cause of obstructive sleep apnea. *Chest.* 1994; **106**: 1898–9.

18. Zalzal GH. Stridor and airway compromise. *Pediatric Clinics of North America.* 1989; **36**: 1389–402.

19. de Blic J, Delacourt C, Scheinmann P. Ultrathin flexible bronchoscopy in neonatal intensive care units. *Archives of Disease in Childhood.* 1991; **66**: 1383–5.

20. Nussbaum E. Usefulness of miniature flexible fiberoptic bronchoscopy in children. *Chest.* 1994; **106**: 1438–42.

21. Arnold JE. Advances in pediatric flexible bronchoscopy. *Otolaryngologic Clinics of North America.* 1989; **22**: 545–51.

22. Raine J, Warner JO. Fibreoptic bronchoscopy without general anaesthetic. *Archives of Disease in Childhood.* 1991; **66**: 481–4.

23. Eber E, Zach M. [Flexible fiberoptic bronchoscopy in pediatrics – an analysis of 420 examinations] Flexible fiberoptische Bronchoskopie in der Padiatrie – Eine Analyse von 420 Untersuchungen. *Wiener klinische Wochenschrift.* 1995; **107**: 246–51.

24. Todres ID, Noviski N. Flexible fiberoptic bronchoscopy: a practical guide to examining infants and children. *Mount Sinai Journal of Medicine*. 1995; **62**: 36–40.

25. Handler SD. Direct laryngoscopy in children: rigid and flexible fiberoptic. *Ear, Nose and Throat Journal*. 1995; **74**: 100–4, 106.

26. Teitelbaum DH. Bronchoscopy and esophagoscopy in children. *Current Opinion in Pediatrics*. 1993; **5**: 341–6.

27. Puhakka H, Kero P, Valli P, Iisalo E, Erkinjuntti M. Pediatric bronchoscopy. A report of methodology and results. *Clinical Pediatrics (Philadelphia)*. 1989; **28**: 253–7.

28. Hoeve LJ, Rombout J. Pediatric laryngobronchoscopy. 1332 procedures stored in a data base. *International Journal of Pediatric Otorhinolaryngology*. 1992; **24**: 73–82.

29. Sitbon P, Laffon M, Lesage V, Furet P, Autret E, Mercier C. Lidocaine plasma concentrations in pediatric patients after providing airway topical anesthesia from a calibrated device. *Anesthesia and Analgesia*. 1996; **82**: 1003–6.

30. Amitai Y, Zylber Katz E, Avital A, Zangen D, Noviski N. Serum lidocaine concentrations in children during bronchoscopy with topical anesthesia. *Chest*. 1990; **98**: 1370–3.

31. Shikowitz MJ, Abramson AL, Liberatore L. Endolaryngeal jet ventilation: a 10-year review. *Laryngoscope*. 1991; **101**: 455–61.

32. Depierraz B, Ravussin P, Brossard E, Monnier P. Percutaneous transtracheal jet ventilation for paediatric endoscopic laser treatment of laryngeal and subglottic lesions. *Canadian Journal of Anaesthesia*. 1994; **41**: 1200–7.

33. Evans KL, Keene MH, Bristow AS. High-frequency jet ventilation – a review of its role in laryngology. *Journal of Laryngology and Otology*. 1994; **108**: 23–5.

34. Janzen PR, Neasham J, Daniel M. Pressure reducing valve prevents barotrauma during jet ventilation for microlaryngeal surgery [letter]. *Anaesthesia*. 1995; **50**: 831–2.

35. Baraka A, Choueiry P, Medawwar A. The laryngeal mask airway for fibreoptic bronchoscopy in children. *Paediatric Anaesthesia*. 1995; **5**: 197–8.

36. Watanabe I, Noguchi R, Morioka M, Waguri N, Shimoji K. [Anesthetic management for bronchofiberscopy and esophageal mannometric study in a patient with CHARGE association]. *Masui*. 1995; **44**: 1010–3.

37. Tom LW, Miller L, Wetmore RF, Handler SD, Potsic WP. Endoscopic assessment in children with tracheotomies. *Archives of Otolaryngology – Head and Neck Surgery*. 1993; **119**: 321–4.

38. Johannesson GP, Floren M, Lindahl SG. Sevoflurane for ENT-surgery in children. A comparison with halothane. *Acta Anaesthesiologica Scandinavica*. 1995; **39**: 546–50.

39. Kessler G, Rauchfuss A, Werner C. [Pulse oximetry in surgery of the bronchial system] Pulsoximetrie bei Eingriffen im Bronchialsystem. *HNO*. 1989; **37**: 216–9.

40. Franchi LM, Maggi JC, Nussbaum E. Continuous end-tidal CO_2 in pediatric bronchoscopy. *Pediatric Pulmonology*. 1993; **16**: 153–7.

41. Holmes DK. Expanding the envelope of neonatal endoscopic tracheal and bronchial surgery. *Southern Medical Journal*. 1995; **88**: 571–4.

42. Lindahl H, Rintala R, Malinen L, Leijala M, Sairanen H. Bronchoscopy during the first month of life. *Journal of Pediatric Surgery*. 1992; **27**: 548–50.

43. Wengen DF, Probst RR, Frei FJ. Flexible laryngoscopy in neonates and infants: insertion through a median opening in the face mask. *International Journal of Pediatric Otorhinolaryngology*. 1991; **21**: 183–7.

44. Parsons DS, Smith RB, Mair EA, Dlabal LJ. Unique case presentations of acute epiglottic swelling and a protocol for acute airway compromise. *Laryngoscope*. 1996; **106**: 1287–91.

45. Robb PJ. Failure of intubation in acute inflammatory airway obstruction in childhood. *Journal of Laryngology and Otology*. 1985; **99**: 993–8.

46. Neto GM, Kentab O, Klassen TP, Osmond MH. A randomized controlled trial of mist in the acute treatment of moderate croup. *Academic Emergency Medicine*. 2002; **9**: 873–9.

47. Fitzgerald D, Mellis C, Johnson M, Allen H, Cooper P, Van Asperen P. Nebulized budesonide is as effective as nebulized adrenaline in moderately severe croup. *Pediatrics*. 1996; **97**: 722–5.

48. Geelhoed GC, Macdonald WB. Oral and inhaled steroids in croup: a randomized, placebo-controlled trial. *Pediatric Pulmonology*. 1995; **20**: 355–61.

∗ 49. Klassen TP. Croup. A current perspective. *Pediatric Clinics of North America*. 1999; **46**: 1167–78. *Good summary of evidence-base for steroids in childhood airway obstruction.*

50. Seigler RS. Bacterial tracheitis: recognition and treatment. *Journal of the South Carolina Medical Association*. 1993; **89**: 83–7.

51. Kasian GF, Bingham WT, Steinberg J, Ninan A, Sankaran K, Oman Ganes L *et al.* Bacterial tracheitis in children. *Canadian Medical Association Journal*. 1989; **140**: 46–50.

52. Rotta AT, Wiryawan B. Respiratory emergencies in children. *Respiratory Care*. 2003; **48**: 248–58.

∗ 53. Stroud RH, Friedman NR. An update on inflammatory disorders of the pediatric airway: epiglottitis, croup, and tracheitis. *American Journal of Otolaryngology*. 2001; **22**: 268–75. *Succinct account of management strategies for children with acute inflammatory airway obstruction.*

87

Acute laryngeal infections

SUSANNA LEIGHTON†

Introduction   1127
Croup (acute laryngotracheobronchitis, viral
     laryngotracheobronchitis)   1128
Spasmodic croup (spasmodic laryngitis, pseudocroup,
     acute subglottic oedema, subglottic allergic oedema,
     laryngismus stridulus)   1129
Bacterial laryngotracheobronchitis (pseudomembranous
     croup, bacterial tracheitis, membranous
     laryngotracheobronchitis, neonatal necrotizing
     tracheobronchitis)   1129

Diphtheria   1130
Acute epiglottitis (*supraglottitis*)   1130
Airway management   1132
Key points   1133
Best clinical practice   1133
Deficiencies in current knowledge and areas for future
     research   1133
Acknowledgements   1133
References   1133

SEARCH STRATEGY

The opinions in this chapter are supported by a search of Medline and EMBASE using the key words croup, acute laryngotracheitis, acute laryngotracheobronchitis, acute epiglottitis and child. The Controlled Trials Register of the Cochrane Library was also searched. The search was initially restricted to randomized controlled trials and metaanalyses and then widened, focussing on diagnosis, management and immunization.

INTRODUCTION

Laryngeal infection in childhood causes airway obstruction, of which the cardinal symptom is stridor. In the developed world, 'croup' – a clinical scenario characterized by a combination of stridor hoarseness and a typical barking cough – is the commonest (90 percent) cause of acute airway obstruction in children. Epiglottitis has been the next most common infective cause but is now seen much less frequently due to the widespread introduction of *Haemophilus influenzae* b (Hib) vaccine; bacterial laryngotracheobronchitis and diphtheria are less common. The differential diagnosis of acute acquired stridor includes 'spasmodic croup', retropharyngeal abscess, angioneurotic oedema, neoplasia, acute laryngeal trauma and foreign body aspiration. 'Spasmodic croup' is included in this chapter because of the similarity of the clinical picture to croup. Aetiology is uncertain but it is not thought to be due to acute laryngeal infection.

In this chapter the various clinical syndromes of acute laryngeal infection are discussed and their distinctive features emphasized. For a number of these conditions several terms have evolved over the years; these are included in the headings for ease of reference but the first term, that most commonly used in the UK, is used in the text. The effects of immunization programmes on the changing patterns of disease are examined. The efficacy of medical treatment and the role of endotracheal intubation and/or tracheostomy for safe airway management in the different conditions are considered.

Good management depends on teamwork involving the primary care physician, the paediatrician, the paediatric otolaryngologist, the paediatric anaesthetist and the paediatric intensive care physician. Multidisciplinary evidence-based protocols should be established and followed to optimize outcomes.

CROUP (ACUTE LARYNGOTRACHEOBRONCHITIS, VIRAL LARYNGOTRACHEOBRONCHITIS)

Croup typically presents as a clinical syndrome of hoarseness, inspiratory or biphasic stridor and barking cough, due to mucosal oedema of the larynx and trachea. There is usually a preceding history of upper respiratory tract symptoms with fever and malaise. It is classically caused by *parainfluenza virus type I*. It can be caused by other viruses including *parainfluenza virus type II*, respiratory syncytial virus (RSV) and *influenza virus types A and B*, and can also complicate measles. It usually affects children between six months and three years of age with a peak incidence in two year olds. Boys are more commonly affected than girls. There is a seasonal variation; in the USA a minor peak in hospital admissions for croup has been noted in February and a major peak in October in odd numbered years, coinciding with biennial epidemics of *human parainfluenza type I* infection. The annual incidence of croup in children younger than six years ranges from 1.5 to 6 percent. [**]

Croup is usually self-limiting; 50 percent of children improve within 24 hours of the onset of symptoms, and most recover within four days without treatment. However, airway symptoms can become serious and even life-threatening. In the absence of medical therapy, 20 percent of patients may be admitted to hospital and 10 percent of these may require intervention for acute airway obstruction, either intubation or tracheostomy depending on local services. Coexisting bronchopneumonia or measles infection are indicators of poor prognosis. The diagnosis is a clinical one, but in those severe cases which reach hospital, if there is a diagnostic dilemma, a radiograph of the thoracic inlet will show characteristic narrowing of the subglottis on an anteroposterior view ('steeple' or 'pencil tip' sign) (**Figure 87.1**). [**]

There are inflammatory changes throughout the airway in croup but the critical symptom of stridor is due to oedema in the subglottis, the narrowest part of the paediatric airway. Just 1 mm of oedema in an 18-month old child with a subglottic diameter of 6.5 mm will reduce the cross-sectional area by approximately 50 percent. Laminar airflow (proportional to the fourth power of the radius – 'Poussuile's law') is thus greatly reduced. Some children are more at risk of severe symptoms than others; factors predisposing to severe symptoms include pre-existing subglottic or tracheal narrowing, chronic lung disease and airway reactivity, characterized by a history of inhalant or food allergies. The Westley Croup Score (**Table 87.1**) allows the severity of symptoms to be classified and allows comparisons of severity to be made.[1] It has been clinically and radiologically validated, the total

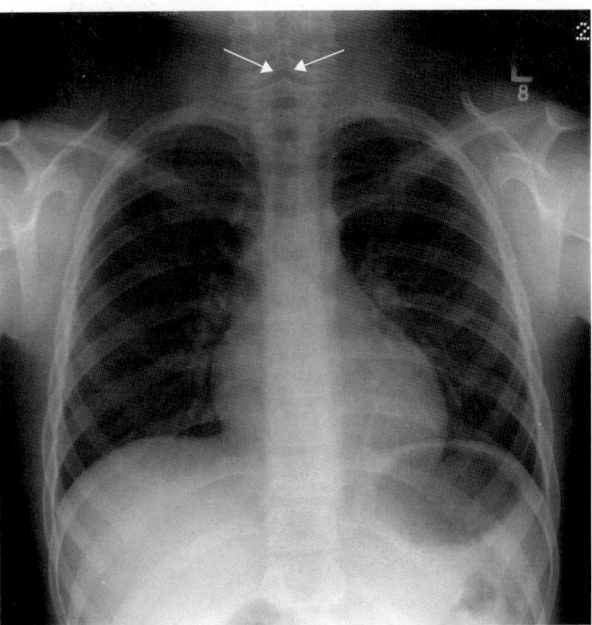

Figure 87.1 Steeple' or 'pencil tip' sign. Narrowing of the subglottic airway owing to mucosal oedema in croup (arrows). Figure courtesy of Ben Hartley.

score correlating with the diameter of the tracheal lumen. A maximum score is 17, a score of 2–3 equates to mild croup, 4–7 to moderate croup and 8 or more to severe croup. [***]

For mild croup, treatment can be supportive, with reassurance of both carers and child, and observation and monitoring of the child's symptoms, but without separating the child from its carer(s) as this will increase anxiety. Sedation is not advised because of the risk of respiratory depression, although chloral hydrate 30 mg/kg has been advocated if sedation seems necessary. Traditionally, it has been recommended that children with croup should be nursed in a humidified environment or mist tent; there is no evidence that this is of clinical benefit although it may be soothing. Nebulized epinephrine (1 mL of 1 in 1000 epinephrine diluted in 3 mL of 0.9 percent saline) has an established role in the acute paediatric airway in reducing mucosal oedema by an alpha-agonist effect causing vasoconstriction and bronchodilation; a maximum effect is achieved within 30–60 minutes, however there is no lasting benefit beyond two hours.[1] It does not alter the natural history of the disease but it may postpone or eliminate the need for an artificial airway, or give symptomatic relief until effective treatment can be given.[2] It can be administered at the same time as glucocorticoids. [****]

Corticosteroids

The role of corticosteroids in the management of croup is now well established. Corticosteroids have a systemic antiinflammatory effect. There is a reduction in capillary

Table 87.1 Croup score based on Westley system.

Score	0	1	2	3	4	5
Inspiratory stridor	None	Audible with a stethoscope	Audible without a stethoscope			
Retraction	None	Mild	Moderate	Severe		
Air entry	Normal	Decreased	Severely decreased			
Cyanosis	None				With agitation	At rest
Conscious level	Normal					Altered

Reprinted from Ref. 1, with permission.

endothelial permeability and therefore in mucosal oedema, and stabilization of lysosomal membranes, decreasing the inflammatory reaction. Topical corticosteroids theoretically have the added benefit of causing local alpha-mediated vasoconstriction. A number of studies have looked at clinical improvement after corticosteroid therapy. Clinical benefit can be measured by an improvement in croup score, reduced hospital admission rates, shorter length of stay, lower intubation rates or a reduced need for cointerventions such as the administration of epinephrine nebulizers. A metaanalysis in 1989 of nine placebo - controlled trials showed a trend in favour of corticosteroids but no significant benefits.[3] This stimulated more rigorous studies and a more recent metaanalysis of 24 studies has confirmed that steroids are effective in relieving the symptoms of croup as early as six hours after treatment.[4] [****] Recent evidence suggests that glucocorticoid use should be not be confined to moderate or severe cases but should be extended to children with mild croup.[5, 6] The small numbers of patients in each study and the confounding variables make it difficult to make definitive recommendations regarding the superiority of any glucocorticoid, dose, or route of administration.[7] In the absence of further evidence, an oral dose of dexamethasone (0.6 mg/kg) is preferred because of its safety and efficacy. In a child who is vomiting, nebulized budesonide (2 mg) may be considered. Although equally efficacious,[8] intramuscular dexamethasone (0.6 mg/kg) cannot be advocated given the potential for muscle necrosis with that route of administration. The use of glucocorticoids in primary care in the early management of croup symptoms has transformed the management of this disorder; affected children now rarely require active intervention to support the airway. [****]

SPASMODIC CROUP (SPASMODIC LARYNGITIS, PSEUDOCROUP, ACUTE SUBGLOTTIC OEDEMA, SUBGLOTTIC ALLERGIC OEDEMA, LARYNGISMUS STRIDULUS)

Some children appear to be prone to recurrent croup-like symptoms. Episodes may not be preceded by upper respiratory tract symptoms but typically begin suddenly, often at night, and resolve after a few hours. Attacks may be precipitated by gastro-oesophageal reflux. There is an association with low IgA levels and this condition may present in atopic children who later develop asthma or other allergic conditions.[9] [**]

The symptoms can be relieved by a single dose of oral dexamethasone in a dose of 0.6 mg/kg in the same way as for viral croup.

It is important to consider congenital or acquired mild subglottic stenosis in the differential diagnosis of infants presenting with 'recurrent croup'. In persistent cases endoscopy is mandatory.[10]

BACTERIAL LARYNGOTRACHEOBRONCHITIS (PSEUDOMEMBRANOUS CROUP, BACTERIAL TRACHEITIS, MEMBRANOUS LARYNGOTRACHEOBRONCHITIS, NEONATAL NECROTIZING TRACHEOBRONCHITIS)

This is a severe form of laryngotracheobronchitis associated with sloughing of the respiratory epithelium and profuse mucopurulent secretions. Initial presentation is similar to croup but there is no response to steroids. The child rapidly progresses to a toxic state and there may be respiratory decompensation. Although it typically affects children older (mean age four years) than the usual age group for croup, like croup, it is commoner in boys than girls, and there is no single factor, clinical, radiological or laboratory-based which reliably distinguishes it from croup.[11] It is a much less common condition than croup. However, there is increased susceptibility in children with Down syndrome or immunodeficiency. [**]

The diagnosis can only be confirmed on airway endoscopy; there is a pseudomembrane in the subglottis and trachea and thick mucopus and debris extending into the bronchi (**Figure 87.2**). Direct laryngotracheobronchoscopy under general anaesthesia and removal of all tracheal secretions, with pulmonary toilet, is mandatory. It is then almost invariably necessary to secure the airway by endotracheal intubation for a period of days.[12] The distal airway and the tube itself remain at continued risk of obstruction by secretions and vigilant expert nursing care is essential.

Once the diagnosis is established, broad-spectrum parenteral antibiotics should be commenced immediately. They can later be adjusted in line with the results of

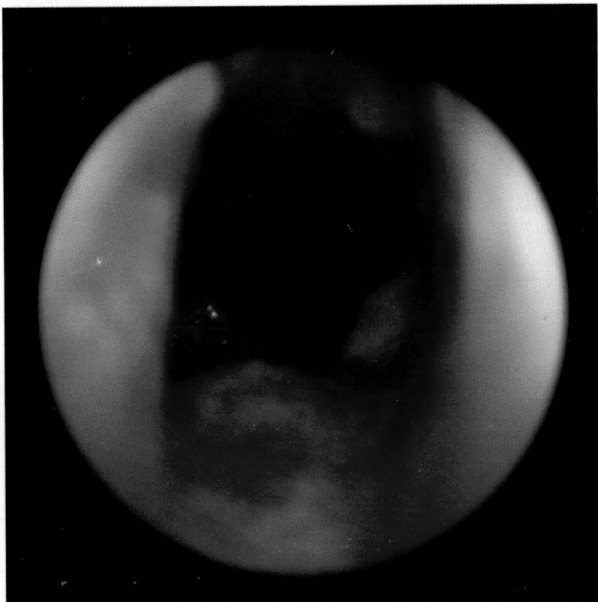

Figure 87.2 Tracheal pseudomembrane in bacterial laryngotracheobronchitis. Figure courtesy of Ben Hartley.

microbiological studies. *Staphylococcus aureus* is the pathogen most commonly isolated from tracheal cultures although *Haemophilus influenzae*, *Moraxella catarrhalis*, *Streptococcus pneumoniae* and *Pseudomonas aeruginosa* have also been reported. Blood cultures are rarely positive. [**]

Complications of this dangerous condition include airway stenosis, respiratory failure, toxic shock syndrome, anoxic encephalopathy and death.

Ventilated newborns with an unstable haemodynamic state are at risk of potentially fatal desloughing of the tracheobronchial mucosa. This may be characterized by repeated episodes of acute airway obstruction. Management involves repeated therapeutic tracheobronchoscopy to free the airways.[13]

DIPHTHERIA

Diphtheria is a rare condition in countries which have a routine childhood immunization programme, but remains an important differential particularly in immigrant populations in the diagnosis of acute laryngeal infection in children. Diphtheria remains a significant public health problem in the developing world. The causative organism is *Corynebacterium diphtheriae*. There are three strains, *gravis*, *intermedius* and *mitis*; it is the *gravis* strain which is responsible for major epidemics and for the high mortality. [****] The early clinical picture of upper respiratory tract symptoms is due to the effects of the organism itself. Delayed effects are due to the release of endotoxin. Diphtheria is a disease particularly affecting young children; it is rare over the age of ten years.

Initial symptoms are of pharyngitis with sore throat and malaise. The child is feverish and on examination there is a typical appearance of the pharyngeal tonsils with necrosis and the development of a characteristic grey pseudomembrane over the surface. This consists of necrotic tissue, bacteria and a rich fibrinous exudate. Early removal causes bleeding but the pseudomembrane may separate more easily later in the course of the disease. There may be a bull-neck appearance due to cellulitis and regional lymphadenopathy.

Laryngeal diphtheria rarely occurs without prior pharyngeal infection. After progressive dysphagia and toxaemia, inspiratory stridor and a barking cough develop; the cough is frequently paroxysmal and exhausting. Death may follow owing to acute airway obstruction or as a result of the later effects of the endotoxin.

The endotoxin can cause a toxic myocarditis in the second week of the disease and this may be fatal. Peripheral neuritis may also occur, palatal paralysis being the most common effect of peripheral neuropathy and presenting with nasal regurgitation of food and hypernasal speech.

Successful treatment depends on early diagnosis, and the administration of high dose benzylpenicillin and antitoxin (10,000 to 100,000 units depending on the severity of infection). Airway management consists of removal of the laryngeal membrane, administration of oxygen and humidification, and endotracheal intubation or tracheostomy if necessary. Systemic steroids may reduce the need for airway intervention.[14] Bed rest is recommended until the danger of myocarditis is past.

ACUTE EPIGLOTTITIS (*SUPRAGLOTTITIS*)

The classical presentation of acute epiglottitis is well described. It is of a toxic child with a short history of sore throat, inspiratory stridor, muffled voice and drooling due to odynophagia and dysphagia. Left untreated there is progressive respiratory distress. The child is febrile, tachypnoeic and traditionally will be sitting upright, with the neck extended to optimize the airway, and using the arms to provide support to the shoulder girdle to maximize the efficiency of the accessory muscles of respiration. It is commonest between the ages of three and six and there is an increased prevalence in winter and spring. [**/*]

When acute epiglottitis is suspected, pharyngeal examination should not be attempted, as simple manipulation with a tongue depressor may precipitate acute airway obstruction, although the use of a fibreoptic or small rigid endoscope can assist the diagnosis in patients with an atypical presentation.[15] Direct examination of the airway should not be delayed, but should be undertaken in a controlled setting such as an operating room or paediatric intensive care unit by personnel skilled in airway intervention; endoscopic evaluation will confirm gross erythema and oedema of the supraglottic structures

(**Figure 87.3**). When the diagnosis is confirmed, the airway should be secured by endotracheal intubation. If this is unsuccessful, a rigid bronchoscope may be passed to allow tracheostomy. Endotracheal intubation is usually required for safe airway management. [**/*] Despite this, mortality remains as high as 2 percent.[16]

Investigations prior to securing the airway are contra-indicated but a soft tissue lateral radiograph of the neck will typically show a thickened oedematous epiglottis – the 'thumb sign' (**Figure 87.4**). The causative organism can be identified from nasopharyngeal swabs, laryngeal swabs, sputum samples or blood cultures taken after intubation. Traditionally, acute epiglottitis has been a manifestation of invasive Hib infection. This can be confirmed as the cause in partially treated patients by Hib antigen detection in concentrated urine specimens. Other organisms are less common causes of acute epiglottitis; they include *meningococcus*, *Haemophilus parainfluenzae* and *Staphylococcus aureus*. Immunocompromised individuals are at increased risk of epiglottitis. It may then be due to atypical organisms such as *Streptococcus pneumoniae* or *Candida albicans*. Children with acute epiglottitis should be screened after recovery from the acute episode to ensure there is no underlying predisposing condition. *Group A beta-haemolytic Streptococcus* is a recognized cause of acute epiglottitis in older children and adults. [**]

Treatment is with intravenous antibiotics; ampicillin resistance due to beta-lactamase production is now over 50 percent in *Haemophilus influenzae*, so empirical treatment with third-generation cephalosporins for five to seven days is advised. Chloramphenicol is an alternative in the event of allergy to cephalosporins. Penicillin-sensitive *Streptococci* are the usual cause of acute epiglottitis in children who have been immunized against Hib and they should be treated accordingly.

Recovery is characterized by resolution of systemic symptoms and the supraglottic inflammation. The child can then be extubated and discharged from hospital. Since the introduction of Hib immunization, Rifampicin prophylaxis has been recommended to eradicate the carrier state for unimmunized members of the household who are four years old and younger and unimmunized day care contacts aged two or younger. [**/*]

Despite the declining incidence of this disease and the changing bacteriology, there has been no change in its clinical presentation over time. It is critically important that reduced clinical experience is not accompanied by a sharp rise in mortality for affected children.

Haemophilus influenzae type b immunization

In addition to acute epiglottitis, other manifestations of invasive *Haemophilus influenzae* infection include meningitis, septic arthritis, septicaemia, pneumonia and osteomyelitis. Hib has caused more than 90 percent of invasive *Haemophilus influenzae* infection in developed countries. It has been estimated that, prior to the introduction of immunization, Hib caused 41/100,000 infections in newborn to four-year-old children of which more than 50 percent were meningitis,[17] epiglottitis being the next most common presentation (15/100,000).[16] [**]

Routine infant immunization with conjugate Hib vaccine in the UK began in October 1992. Immunization

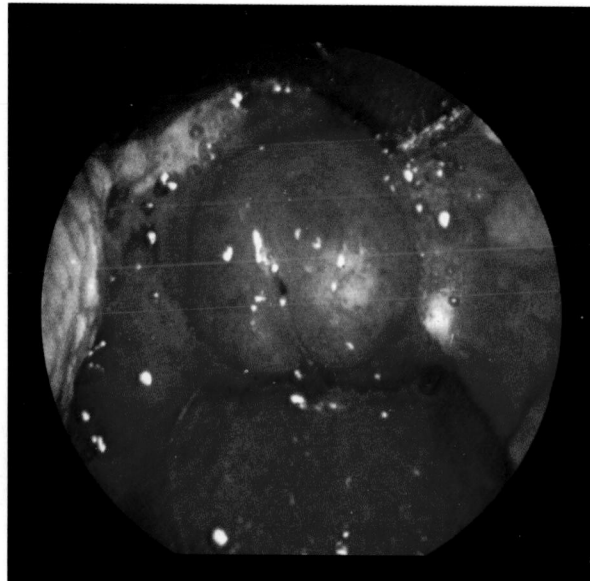

Figure 87.3 Acute epiglottitis. Endoscopic appearance. Reproduced by permission of Bruce Benjamin.

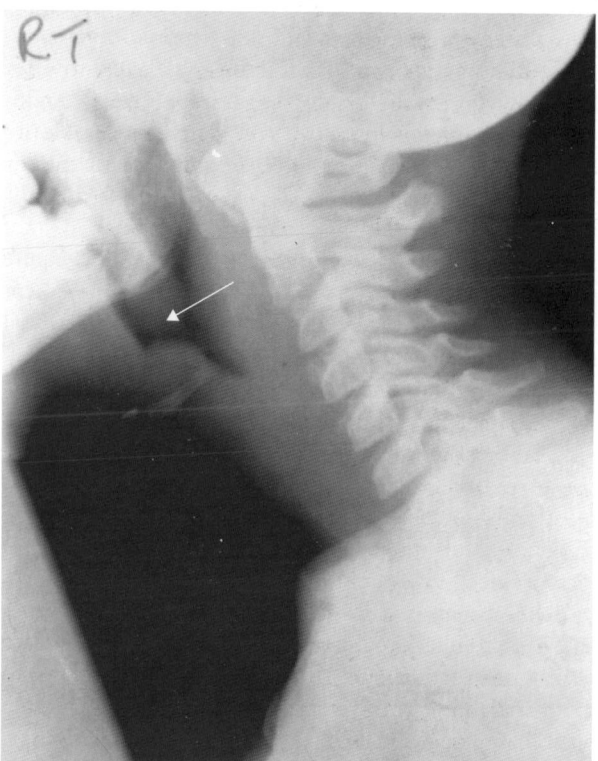

Figure 87.4 Acute epiglottitis. Radiological appearance of the oedematous epiglottis (arrowed).

is achieved by three primary doses followed by a late booster. The incidence of invasive Hib infections in children under five fell dramatically from an incidence of 23.8/100,000 for the year preceding vaccine implementation to 0.66/100,000 in 1998.[18] A reduction in the incidence of acute epiglottitis of approximately 90 percent has been documented in countries in which an immunization programme has been established. Vaccine failure does occur but in fewer than 10 percent of cases is there an identifiable clinical risk factor predisposing to infection. A small number of cases may be due to infection with an organism other than *Haemophilus* and continued vigilance among clinicians is required.[19] There is evidence that a longer duration of breast-feeding (more than 13 weeks) is associated with a significantly enhanced antibody response to Hib in children aged between 18 months and six years.[20] In the Hib vaccine era, non-type b invasive *Haemophilus influenzae* disease has become more common than type b. It is likely to occur in younger children than is the norm for type b infection (16 versus 22 months), but is less likely to be meningitis or epiglottitis and more likely to be pneumonia or bacteraemia.[21] [**]

AIRWAY MANAGEMENT

For the child presenting with acute airway obstruction due to laryngeal infection, active intervention to secure the airway may be necessary if symptoms are severe. The options to provide an artificial airway include endotracheal intubation and tracheostomy. Prior to 1975, tracheostomy was the standard intervention, then endotracheal intubation was shown to be a safe alternative for acute epiglottitis and subsequently for croup. Endotracheal intubation is now considered preferable to tracheostomy if circumstances permit. However, the choice of intervention may be influenced by the availability of medical and nursing expertise and local hospital services. The intubated child will require specialized intensive care facilities for management whereas the child with a tracheostomy, whilst still requiring nursing expertise for optimal management, can be nursed on a normal paediatric ward.

A team approach to management is essential for optimal outcome. The paediatrician, paediatric anaesthetist, paediatric intensivist and paediatric otolaryngologist must collaborate to develop multidisciplinary evidence-based protocols which take into account the availability of local services. Immunization programmes and advances in medical management are changing patterns of disease and have resulted in a decline in the prevalence of acute airway obstruction due to acute epiglottitis, croup and diphtheria; clinicians with little experience of children with these conditions will depend on protocols for safe practice. If endotracheal intubation is to be undertaken, it should be performed in an operating room or paediatric intensive care unit with personnel and equipment available and ready to undertake tracheostomy if the airway cannot be secured.

Once an artificial airway is in place, humidified air should be administered to discourage the development of tenacious secretions. The tube should be aspirated regularly, using suction, to prevent tube obstruction. Nursing vigilance to prevent accidental displacement or self-extubation is essential. In ideal conditions, mortality rates can be as low as 1 percent for either intervention.[22]

Nasotracheal intubation

Endotracheal intubation for airway obstruction due to acute laryngeal infection is now widely practised with great expertise. When a prolonged period of intubation is anticipated, the nasotracheal rather than the orotracheal route is preferred; nasotracheal intubation is better tolerated so the child requires less sedation, the tube can be secured more reliably and nursing care is easier. The tube is positioned with the patient anaesthetized and the child is then nursed under sedation, fed via a nasogastric tube. The cough and voice are absent during the period of intubation but, after extubation there are normally no sequelae. Complications can occur however and include epistaxis at the time of intubation, the development of sinus sepsis during the period of intubation and hoarseness after extubation. The risk of acquired subglottic stenosis is small but is associated with younger age of the child, larger tube size, serial intubation and longer duration of intubation. It is more common in Down syndrome in which there may be an element of congenital subglottic stenosis as a predisposing factor. A tube one size smaller than that usually considered age appropriate should be used.[23] [**/*]

Extubation can be considered when the child is systemically well, with minimal tracheal secretions. The 'leak test' (air escape around the nasotracheal tube on application of positive pressure ventilation) is helpful but not an absolute prognostic indicator for successful extubation. In acute epiglottitis, visualization of the epiglottis with a flexible nasendoscope can be useful in monitoring resolution of inflammation. Likewise in laryngotracheobronchitis, whether viral or bacterial, the airway can be monitored using flexible endoscopy until a reduction in tracheal inflammation shows that it is safe to extubate. Systemic steroids administered six hours prior to removal of the tube will minimize post-intubation oedema and nebulized epinephrine can assist with airway patency after extubation.

For acute epiglottitis the period of intubation is usually less than 48 hours but for croup and bacterial laryngotracheobronchitis it may be up to a week.[24] If extubation fails after the acute laryngeal infection has resolved, and despite all the above measures being taken, this may be due to a pre-existing or developing subglottic stenosis. This, if acute and due to mucosal oedema and ulceration, may be successfully treated by a cricoid split (see Chapter 89, Laryngeal stenosis). If not however, tracheostomy may become necessary and possibly later laryngotracheal reconstruction.

Tracheostomy

Tracheostomy is not now considered the first choice to secure the airway in acute laryngeal infection. It may be chosen, however, if the availability of nursing expertise and intensive care facilities is limited such that naso-tracheal intubation is contraindicated. It may also be necessary if there is severe acute subglottic narrowing precluding the passage of a nasotracheal tube of adequate size for ventilation, or if there has been significant intubation trauma.[25] Equipment and personnel to per-form an emergency tracheostomy should always be available in case attempted intubation fails.

In one series of 30 patients the median period for which a tracheostomy was required in croup was 11 days.[24] However, the largest recent published series of paediatric tracheostomy for croup is from the Red Cross War Memorial Children's Hospital in Cape Town. In that series, 75 percent of children were decannulated within ten weeks of formation of the tracheostomy but 54 percent of children required one or more further procedures after tracheostomy to deal with granulation tissue, suprastomal collapse or subglottic stenosis prior to successful decannulation.[26] Clearly nasotracheal intuba-tion is preferable if it is possible and practical depending on local circumstances.

KEY POINTS

- The laryngeal airway in children is narrow, especially in the cricoid region. The mucosa is lax and a comparatively minor swelling may cause significant airway compromise.
- Immunization programmes and improvements in medical management have reduced the prevalence of acute laryngeal infection, and its severity.
- Systemic steroids have transformed the primary care management of croup. Fewer cases now need hospital admission but vigilance is still required.
- Multidisciplinary evidence-based protocols influenced by the availability of local expertise and services should be formulated and followed to optimize outcomes.
- In acute laryngeal infections, nasotracheal intubation is preferable to tracheotomy if it is possible and practical depending on local circumstances.

Best clinical practice

- ✓ Pharyngeal examination is contraindicated if acute epiglottitis is suspected; it may precipitate acute airway obstruction. [Grade D]
- ✓ Children with croup, whether presenting with mild, moderate or severe symptoms, should be treated with oral dexamethasone 0.6 mg/kg at the time of diagnosis. [Grade A]
- ✓ Nebulized epinephrine (1 mL of 1 in 1000 epinephrine diluted in 3 mL of 0.9 percent saline) has an established role in the acute paediatric airway. [Grade B]
- ✓ Subglottic stenosis should be remembered in the differential diagnosis of infants presenting with 'recurrent croup'. Consider endoscopy. [Grade D]
- ✓ Equipment and personnel to perform tracheostomy should be immediately available in case attempted intubation is unsuccessful. [Grade D]

Deficiencies in current knowledge and areas for future research

- ➤ Diphtheria remains an important cause of acute airway obstruction in children, especially in immigrant populations and in countries without an active immunization programme.
- ➤ As Hib vaccination programmes are extended, the incidence of acute epiglottitis should fall even further.
- ➤ The cause of spasmodic croup is still unknown. It may be related to gastro-oesophageal reflux or upper respiratory allergies.

ACKNOWLEDGEMENTS

Susanna Leighton sadly died during the production of this book. The text has been updated following her death to include more recent evidence.

REFERENCES

* 1. Westley CR, Cotton EK, Brooks JG. Nebulized racemic epinephrine by IPPB for the treatment of croup: a double-blind study. *American Journal of Diseases of Children.* 1978; **132**: 484–7. *The croup score published in this paper allows comparison of severity to be made. It has been validated clinically and radiologically and is widely used.*

2. Leung AK, Kellner JD, Johnson DW. Viral croup: a current perspective. *Journal of Pediatric Health Care.* 2004; **18**: 297–301.

3. Kairys SW, Olmstead EM, O'Connor GT. Steroid treatment of laryngotracheitis: a meta-analysis of the evidence from randomized trials. *Pediatrics.* 1989; **83**: 683–93.

✱ 4. Ausejo M, Saenz A, Pham B, Kellner JD, Johnson DW, Moher D *et al.* The effectiveness of glucocorticoids in treating croup: meta-analysis. *British Medical Journal.* 1999; **319**: 595–600. *A metaanalysis of 24 randomised controlled trials confirming the effectiveness of glucocorticoids in relieving the symptoms of croup.*

5. Bjornson CL, Klassen TP, Williamson J, Brant R, Mitton C, Plint A *et al.* Pediatric Emergency Research Canada Network. A randomised trial of a single dose of oral dexamethasone for mild croup. *New England Journal of Medicine.* 2004; **351**: 1306–13.

6. Russel K, Weibe N, Saenz A, Ausejo SM, Johnson D, Hartling L *et al.* Glucocorticoids for croup. *Cochrane Database of Systematic Reviews.* 2004: CD001955.

7. Cetinkaya F, Tufekci BS, Kutluk G. A comparison of nebulised budesonide and intramuscular and oral dexamethasone for the treatment of croup. *International Journal of Pediatric Otorhinolaryngology.* 2004; **68**: 453–6.

8. Donaldson T, Poleski D, Knipple E, Filips K, Reetz L, Pascaul RG *et al.* Intramuscular versus oral dexamathasone for the treatment of moderate to severe croup: a randomised double-blind trial. *Academic Emergency Medicine.* 2003; **10**: 16–21.

9. Zach MS. Airway reactivity in recurrent croup. *European Journal of Respiratory Diseases.* 1983; **128**: 81–8.

10. Aneeshkumar MK, Ghosh S, Osman EZ, Clarke RW. Complete tracheal rings: lower airway symptoms can delay diagnosis. *European Archives of Otorhinolaryngology.* 2005; **262**: 161–2.

11. Eckel HE, Widemann B, Damm M, Roth B. Airway endoscopy in the diagnosis and treatment of bacterial tracheitis in children. *International Journal of Pediatric Otorhinolaryngology.* 1993; **27**: 147–57.

12. Gallagher PG, Myer III. CM. An approach to the diagnosis and treatment of membranous laryngotracheobronchitis in infants and children. *Pediatric Emergency Care.* 1991; **7**: 337–42.

13. Gaugler C, Astruc D, Donato L, Rivera S, Langlet C, Messer J. Neonatal necrotising tracheobronchitis: three case reports. *Journal of Perinatology.* 2004; **24**: 259–60.

14. Havaldar PV. Dexamethasone in laryngeal diphtheritic croup. *Annals of Tropical Paediatrics.* 1997; **17**: 21–3.

15. Damm M, Eckel HE, Jungehulsing M, Roth B. Airway endoscopy in the interdisciplinary management of acute epiglottitis. *International Journal of Pediatric Otorhinolaryngology.* 1996; **38**: 41–51.

16. Berg S, Trollfors B, Nylen O, Hugosson S, Prellner K, Carenfelt C. Incidence, aetiology, and prognosis of acute epiglottitis in children and adults in Sweden. *Scandinavian Journal of Infectious Diseases.* 1996; **28**: 261–4.

17. Peltola H. Haemophilus influenzae type b disease and vaccination in Europe: lessons learned. *Pediatric Infectious Disease Journal.* 1998; **17**: S126–32.

✱ 18. McVernon J, Moxon R, Heath P, Ramsay M, Slack M. Haemophilus influenzae type b epiglottitis. Article gives timely lesson. *British Medical Journal.* 2003; **326**: 284. *A letter from the Public Health laboratory service and the Oxford Vaccine Group, responsible for the long-term surveillance of Haemophilus influenzae infection.*

19. McEwan J, Giridharan W, Clarke RW, Shears P. Acute epiglottitis: not a disappearing entity. *International Journal of Paediatric Otorhinolaryngology.* 2003; **67**: 317–21.

20. Silfverdal SA, Bodin L, Ulanova M, Hahn-Zoric M, Hanson LA, Olcen P. Long term enhancement of the IgG2 antibody response to Haemophilus influenzae type b by breast-feeding. *Pediatric Infectious Disease Journal.* 2002; **21**: 816–21.

21. Heath PT, Booy R, Azzopardi HJ, Slack MP, Fogarty J, Moloney A *et al.* Non-type b Haemophilus influenzae disease: clinical and epidemiological characteristics in the Haemophilus influenzae type b vaccine era. *Pediatric Infectious Disease Journal.* 2001; **20**: 300–5.

22. Cantrell RW, Bell RA, Morioka WT. Acute epiglottitis: intubation versus tracheostomy. *Laryngoscope.* 1978; **88**: 994–1005.

✱ 23. Wyatt ME, Bailey CM, Whiteside JC. Update on paediatric tracheostomy tubes. *Journal of Laryngology and Otology.* 1999; **113**: 35–40. *A review of available tubes for endotracheal intubation and paediatric tracheostomy, giving details of internal and external tube diameters and relating them to the age of the child and average airway diameter.*

24. Mitchell DP, Thomas RL. Secondary airway support in the management of croup. *Journal of Otolaryngology.* 1980; **9**: 419–22.

25. McEniery J, Gillis J, Kilham H, Benjamin B. Review of intubation in severe laryngotracheobronchitis. *Pediatrics.* 1991; **87**: 847–53.

26. Prescott CA, Vanlierde MJ. Tracheostomy in the management of laryngotracheobronchitis. Red Cross War Memorial Children's Hospital experience, 1980-1985. *South African Medical Journal.* 1990; **77**: 63–6.

88

Congenital disorders of the larynx, trachea and bronchi

MARTIN BAILEY

Introduction	1135	Best clinical practice	1148
Larynx	1135	Deficiencies in current knowledge and areas for future	
Trachea and bronchi	1142	research	1148
Key points	1147	References	1148

SEARCH STRATEGY

The data in this chapter are supported by a PubMed search using the key words congenital, anomalies, larynx, trachea, bronchi and focussing on diagnosis and treatment.

INTRODUCTION

The exact incidence of congenital abnormalities of the airway is uncertain, but a figure has been quoted for congenital laryngeal anomalies of between 1:10,000 and 1:50,000 births.[1] Some of these children will have more than one anomaly in the airway.[2] [**]

LARYNX

The larynx is divided into three regions: supraglottis, glottis and subglottis. The supraglottic larynx comprises the epiglottis, aryepiglottic folds, false cords and ventricles. The glottis consists of the vocal cords (also referred to as vocal folds). The subglottis extends from the undersurface of the vocal cords to the inferior border of the cricoid cartilage.

Supraglottis

LARYNGOMALACIA

Laryngomalacia is characterized by partial or complete collapse of the supraglottic structures on inspiration. It is the most common congenital cause of stridor, but its pathophysiology remains somewhat obscure. The characteristic anatomical abnormalities are undoubtedly primarily responsible for the airway obstruction that occurs on inspiration: the epiglottis is rather long and curled (omega-shaped); the aryepiglottic folds are tall and bulky, while at the same time being short anteroposteriorly and tightly tethered to the epiglottis. The result is a tall, narrow supraglottis with a deep interarytenoid cleft (**Figure 88.1**). The epiglottis is soft and may curl and collapse. The redundant mucosa and submucosa of the aryepiglottic folds may prolapse anteromedially into the airway. It has been suggested that there may also be an element of neuromuscular immaturity and consequent incoordination of arytenoid movements.

The rather characteristic high-pitched, fluttering inspiratory stridor is usually present at, or shortly after, birth. It is very variable, typically being most noticeable when the infant is active or upset, and may disappear when the child is asleep. The severity of the stridor tends to increase as the child becomes more active during the first nine months of life, and then gradually diminishes until by the age of two years it has generally disappeared. Very rarely, stridor may persist into late childhood.

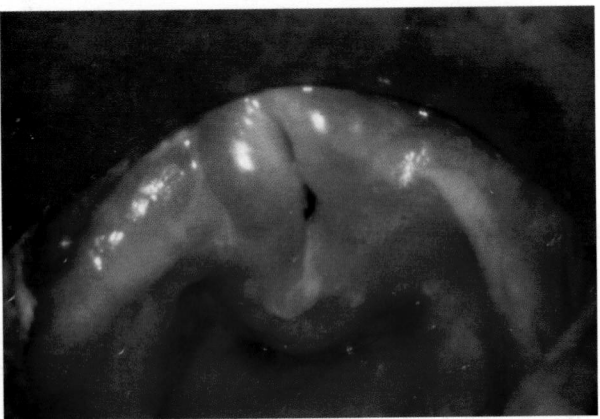

Figure 88.1 Laryngomalacia. Reused with permission from Bull TR. *Color Atlas of ENT Diagnosis*, 4th edn. New York: Thieme Publishers. 2003: 213; and from Bailey CM. Congenital disorders of the larynx, trachea and bronchi. In: Graham JM, Scadding GK and Bull PD (eds). *Pediatric ENT*, (in press), with kind permission of Springer Science and Business Media.

The diagnosis can be confirmed in the outpatient clinic by flexible fibreoptic laryngoscopy. The neonate is wrapped in a blanket and held firmly in an upright position by a nurse: the endoscope is best passed through the mouth rather than the nose, with the operator's finger inserted between the gums to prevent damage to the fibreoptic bundle. The supraglottic collapse on inspiration, which is typical of laryngomalacia, is easily seen but may obscure the vocal cords, and the examination certainly provides no view below the glottis; a second, coexisting airway pathology therefore cannot be excluded. For this reason a microlaryngoscopy and bronchoscopy under general anaesthesia is necessary if the stridor is severe, if there is failure to thrive or there are any atypical features (it is, of course, also necessary if an adequate view cannot be obtained with the fibrescope); almost 20 percent of such cases will have another airway abnormality, and in nearly 5 percent this will be clinically significant.[3] It is important to appreciate that the diagnosis can only be made with the child breathing spontaneously under a very light level of anaesthesia, with the beak of the laryngoscope in the vallecula; the supraglottic collapse is not seen under deep anaesthesia, and will be prevented if the tip of the laryngoscope is introduced into the laryngeal vestibule. Optimum conditions are best achieved at the end of the endoscopy during recovery from anaesthesia.

In approximately 90 percent of reported cases the condition is mild, no intervention is needed and the parents can be reassured accordingly.[4] In severe laryngomalacia, however, there is serious respiratory obstruction with substantial sternal and intercostal recession; also feeding difficulties which may be compounded by reflux enhanced by the high negative intrathoracic pressures generated, and consequent failure to thrive. Matters are made worse if there are other factors increasing the level of cardiorespiratory embarrassment, such as congenital cyanotic heart disease. Cor pulmonale may ensue and in cases of severe sternal recession a permanent pectus excavatum may develop. Restoration of an adequate airway is necessary and, until recently, this has meant resorting to tracheostomy.

Fortunately, however, such a drastic step can now be avoided by performing an endoscopic **aryepiglottoplasty** (sometimes termed a **supraglottoplasty**).[5] In this procedure, the larynx is visualized under the operating microscope using as large a laryngoscope as possible, with its beak positioned in the vallecula; the Lindholm laryngoscope is ideal for the purpose. Anaesthesia is maintained via a nasotracheal tube, which also serves to protect the interarytenoid mucosa. Using cup forceps and microscissors (or alternatively a CO_2 laser), each aryepiglottic fold is first divided to release it from the edge of the epiglottis, and the redundant mucosa and submucosal tissue are then excised from over the arytenoids, together, if necessary, with part or all of the cuneiform cartilages. In less severe cases it may only be necessary to incise the tight aryepiglottic fold, thus 'puncturing' the supraglottis.[6] The 'bridge' of mucosa between the arytenoids is carefully preserved to prevent interarytenoid scarring. Bleeding is minimal, and is easily stopped by the application of neurosurgical patties dipped in topical adrenaline (1:1,000). Neither antibiotics nor steroids are routinely given, complications are very rare, and the stridor is usually improved immediately following the surgery. [Grade B] In cases where the stridor and feeding difficulties persist, an underlying hypotonic neurological disorder is likely.[7] [**/*]

SACCULAR CYSTS AND LARYNGOCOELES

Congenital saccular cyst is an unusual lesion which may present with respiratory obstruction in infants and young children (**Figure 88.2**). Similar to a laryngocoele it represents an abnormal dilatation or herniation of the saccule of the ventricle of the larynx; however, it differs from a laryngocoele in that there is no opening into the larynx and it is filled with mucus instead of air. It is considered to form as the result of a developmental failure to maintain patency of the orifice between the saccule and the ventricle, and may be of anterior or lateral type. The anterior saccular cyst extends medially and posteriorly from the saccule and so protrudes into the laryngeal airway between the true and false vocal cords. The lateral saccular cyst is most common in infants and expands posterosuperiorly into the false cord and aryepiglottic fold.[8]

A laryngocoele is classified as **internal** if it is contained entirely within the laryngeal framework, **external** if it pierces the thyrohyoid membrane, and **combined** if there are both internal and external components. It is an uncommon lesion which usually occurs in middle age but may rarely be seen in infancy, when it can produce

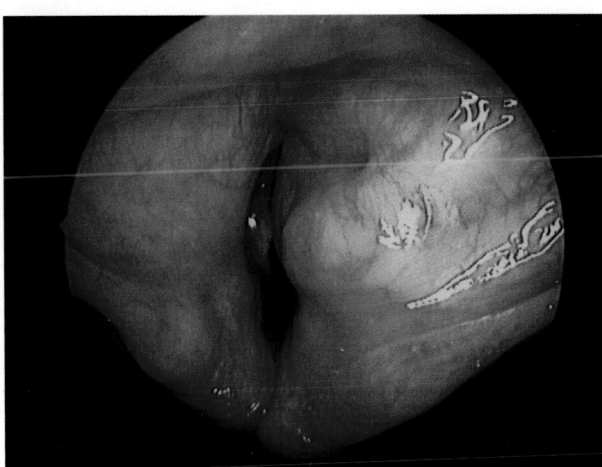

Figure 88.2   Right saccular cyst.

respiratory distress which typically becomes worse on crying due to increased distension of the laryngocoele with air. However, a laryngocoele may obstruct and fill with mucus or become infected (laryngopyocoele), thus becoming indistinguishable from a saccular cyst.

Diagnosis is confirmed by endoscopy, except in an external laryngocoele where no abnormality may be seen except on imaging. Saccular cysts are best treated at the initial endoscopy by wide endoscopic marsupialization. [Grade C] If the cyst recurs, then the procedure of choice is a lateral cervical approach extending through the thyrohyoid membrane at the superior margin of the ala of the thyroid cartilage, with subperichondrial resection of a portion of the upper part of the ala. Through this 'window' the cyst can be completely excised, using short-term intubation to secure the airway postoperatively. [**/*]

LYMPHANGIOMA

Lymphangiomas are cystic malformations (sometimes termed cystic hygromas) that result from abnormal development of the lymphatic vessels. In the head and neck they may be macrocystic (usually infrahyoid), microcystic (usually suprahyoid) or a combination of the two. Occasionally, a microcystic lymphangioma may extend into the tongue base, valleculae and supraglottis, and airway obstruction may result. If the lymphangioma is very extensive a tracheostomy may be required, but where supraglottic involvement is less severe it may be possible to debulk the lesion by endoscopic vaporization using a CO_2 laser.[9] [**/*]

BIFID EPIGLOTTIS

Bifid epiglottis is a rare laryngeal anomaly in which the epiglottis fails to fuse in the midline and thus has a cleft extending down to its tubercle. It may be seen as a feature of Pallister-Hall syndrome, the cardinal elements of which are hypothalamic hamartoblastoma, hypopituitarism, imperforate anus and postaxial polydactyly. It usually

presents with feeding difficulties due to aspiration and with stridor because of collapse and enfolding of the two halves of the epiglottis. Endoscopy establishes the diagnosis, and treatment options include amputation of the epiglottis and tracheostomy. [*]

Glottis

LARYNGEAL WEBS

Failure of complete canalization of the larynx during embryogenesis may result in a glottic or, very rarely, a supraglottic web. The majority involve the anterior glottis, fusing the vocal cords along a variable part of their length, and producing a correspondingly variable degree of respiratory obstruction and dysphonia (**Figure 88.3**). Characteristically there is inspiratory stridor and a rather weak, high-pitched, squeaky voice. The combination of a weak cry from birth and recurrent croup in infancy should always raise suspicion of a laryngeal web. Occasionally, a congenital posterior, interarytenoid web occurs, and may be associated with cricoarytenoid joint fixation.

Almost all anterior glottic webs are fairly thin posteriorly, close to their free border, but become progressively thicker anteriorly with increasing subglottic extension. This can make surgical treatment frustratingly difficult. Where the web is small and causing little in the way of symptoms it is usually best to leave well alone. A longer web may be divided endoscopically along the margin of one vocal cord with a knife or CO_2 laser; if it is very thin then subsequent endoscopic dilatation may be sufficient to permit stable healing without the web reforming. Usually, however, the web is quite thick anteriorly and it is then necessary to place an endoscopic keel in order to prevent recurrence. In the young child with a small larynx a covering tracheostomy is necessary for the two weeks that the keel is in place. Longer, thicker webs with an inadequate airway need to be managed initially with a tracheostomy, and can then be corrected at the age of three to four years via a laryngofissure with insertion of a keel. In cases where the airway is very small and there is associated subglottic stenosis a laryngotracheal reconstruction (LTR) with anterior cartilage grafting is required. This can be carried out in the infant as a single-stage procedure with postoperative endotracheal intubation to stent the larynx for approximately seven days. However, in practice, most infants with a severe glottic web will have a tracheostomy performed in which case the LTR can be advantageously deferred to the age of about two years, when the larynx is larger and the vocal cord dissection can be undertaken more precisely. [*]

LARYNGEAL ATRESIA

Laryngeal atresia is incompatible with life unless there is an associated tracheo-oesophageal fistula (TOF) which

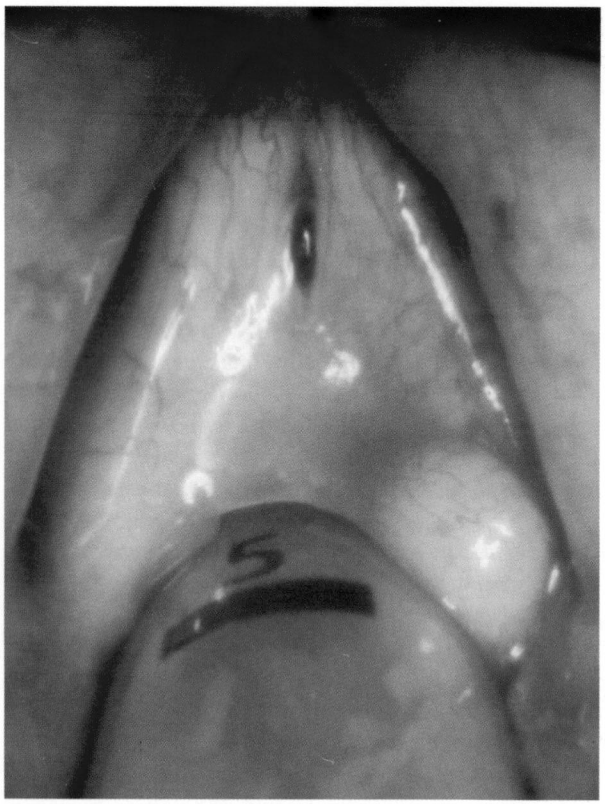

Figure 88.3 Laryngeal web, unusually with a small anterior opening and associated cyst. Reprinted from *Recent Advances in Otolaryngology*, 7th edn, Moffat DA (ed.), Figure 4.4. © (1995), with permission from Elsevier.

permits ventilation via a tube in the oesophagus, or unless an emergency tracheostomy is performed in the delivery room. However, there are now cases being recognized antenatally on ultrasound imaging and managed with an extrauterine intrapartum treatment (EXIT) procedure, whereby a tracheostomy is undertaken following elective Caesarean section with the neonate still on placental circulation.[10] [*]

CRI-DU-CHAT SYNDROME

This syndrome is primarily characterized by a cat-like mewing cry in infancy, microcephaly, downward-slanting palpebral fissures, mental retardation and hypotonia. It is caused by partial deletion of the short arm of chromosome 5. At endoscopy, observation during phonation reveals that the posterior part of the glottis remains open, giving it a diamond-shaped appearance. There is no respiratory embarrassment and the cry becomes less abnormal as the child grows older. [*]

VOCAL CORD PARALYSIS

Vocal cord paralysis is the second most common congenital anomaly of the larynx after laryngomalacia.

It is worth noting that up to 45 percent of patients may have other, coexisting airway pathology, and so although outpatient flexible fibreoptic laryngoscopy may indicate the diagnosis, a formal microlaryngoscopy and bronchoscopy under general anaesthesia is nevertheless essential. [Grade B] Laryngeal ultrasound can be an accurate and reproducible method of assessing vocal cord movement, and may be useful in monitoring a child with known vocal cord palsy and in the diagnosis of the very sick child who may be unfit for endoscopy under general anaesthesia.[11] Approximately half of cases are unilateral and half bilateral.

Unilateral vocal cord paralysis is usually not congenital, most cases being acquired as a result of surgical injury to the left recurrent laryngeal nerve, often following correction of a congenital cardiac anomaly. The vocal cord lies in an intermediate position, and patients present with mild stridor, dysphonia and sometimes aspiration. Surgical intervention is not usually necessary, and the voice can be expected to improve as time passes and either recovery occurs or the other vocal cord compensates.

In contrast, bilateral vocal cord palsy is usually a congenital abductor paralysis. The vocal cords lie in the paramedian position with consequent inspiratory stridor, and a tracheostomy is necessary in approximately half of cases, most of which have other associated airway pathology. A classical cause of congenital bilateral vocal cord palsy is hydrocephalus with the Arnold-Chiari malformation. Once the diagnosis is made, prompt correction of the raised intracranial pressure with a shunt often improves vocal cord movement and a tracheostomy may thus be avoided. However, most cases of congenital bilateral vocal cord paralysis are idiopathic and the approach to management is greatly influenced by the fact that up to 58 percent will eventually recover, with 10 percent taking more than five years to do so and one reported case of recovery at the age of 11 years.[12] This strongly suggests that the problem is often one of delayed maturation in the vagal nuclei and argues convincingly in favour of a conservative management philosophy. Furthermore, where the airway is marginal it may become adequate with laryngeal growth alone, and glottic enlargement surgery in order to avoid a tracheostomy or achieve decannulation may improve the airway at the expense of the voice. [Grade B]

The infant with an inadequate airway and failure to thrive will require a tracheostomy. If vocal cord movement does not develop and the airway does not become adequate as a result of laryngeal growth, then an endoscopic laser cordotomy or arytenoidectomy should be considered at the age of eleven or over following a full discussion with the child and parents regarding the possible trade-off between airway and voice. If it is considered imperative to achieve decannulation earlier, perhaps because of poor social circumstances, then an endoscopic laser cordotomy can be attempted as early as two years of age. If that fails then an external arytenoidectomy via a laryngofissure may be carried out at the age of four to five years with the prospect of an 84 percent decannulation rate;[13] however, there is a small risk of aspiration as well as loss of voice quality and the procedure is irreversible. [**/*]

Subglottis

CONGENITAL SUBGLOTTIC STENOSIS

Congenital subglottic stenosis is due to defective canalization of the cricoid cartilage and/or conus elasticus, resulting in a small, elliptical, thickened cricoid and/or excessive submucosal soft tissue.[14] Typically, there is gross thickening of the anterior lamina of the abnormal cricoid (**Figure 88.4**). Alternatively, there may be anterior fusion of the vocal cords with subglottic extension, as seen in 22q11 (Shprintzen) syndrome. Subglottic stenosis is said to be the third most common congenital anomaly of the larynx, but its true incidence is hard to determine because many patients are intubated in the neonatal period and are then considered by definition to have an acquired stenosis. The reality in this situation may be a combined congenital plus acquired stenosis. Milder degrees of

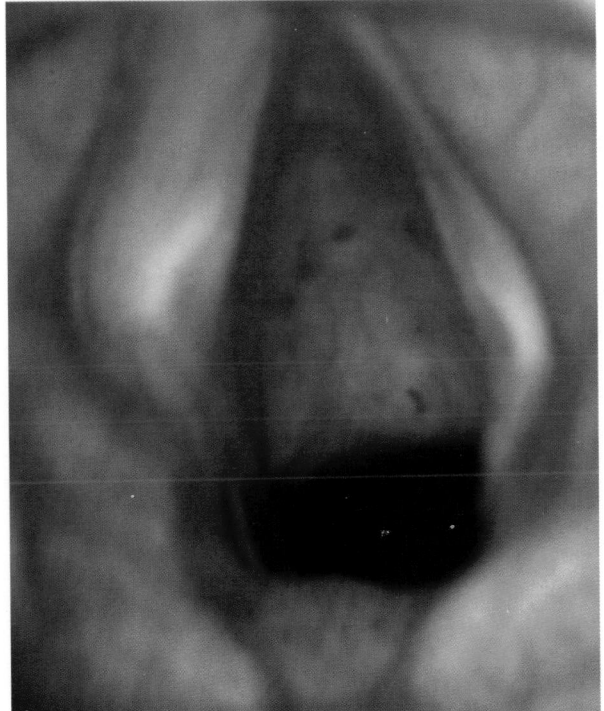

Figure 88.4 Congenital subglottic stenosis, showing anterior cricoid thickening. Reused with permission from Bailey CM. Congenital disorders of the larynx, trachea and bronchi. In: Graham JM, Scadding GK and Bull PD (eds). *Pediatric ENT* (in press), with kind permission of Springer Science and Business Media.

stenosis present as inspiratory or biphasic stridor as the child becomes older and more active, or as recurrent 'croup' owing to superimposed oedema from upper respiratory tract infections.

Diagnosis requires a microlaryngoscopy and bronchoscopy. The exact location of the stenosis with respect to the vocal cords, tracheostome and carina is measured and the number of normal tracheal rings above the tracheostome is counted. The degree of stenosis is measured by passing bronchoscopes, telescopes, endotracheal tubes, dilators or bougies of different sizes through the stricture. The Myer-Cotton grading system is widely used to classify paediatric laryngotracheal stenosis into four grades of severity.[15] Grade I represents 0–50 percent obstruction, grade II 51–70 percent obstruction, grade III 71–99 percent obstruction and grade IV 100 percent obstruction. This helps to predict the outcome of surgical reconstruction.

If the airway is not severely compromised then surgery may not be required, especially as a congenital stenosis can be expected to enlarge with growth. Congenital cartilaginous stenosis represents a strict contraindication to dilatation or laser resection: any type of endoscopic treatment is liable to worsen the initial condition, and attempted dilatation is inevitably ineffective as the thickened ring of cricoid cartilage cannot be expanded.

If the airway is severely compromised then a tracheostomy is needed. This can sometimes be avoided in specialist centres where there are facilities for single-stage airway reconstruction in which an endotracheal tube is used as a stent, usually for a period of five to seven days.

The surgical options have evolved from the classical castellated laryngotracheoplasty designed by Evans and Todd[16] in the early 1970s to achieve laryngeal framework expansion. This was superseded during the early 1980s by the LTR, devised primarily by Cotton.[17] The LTR involves augmentation of the laryngotracheal complex by anterior and/or posterior midline incision of the cricoid with insertion of costal cartilage grafts to expand the airway. This technique has now been supplemented by the partial cricotracheal resection (PCTR) which was introduced into the paediatric age group by Monnier et al.[18] in the early 1990s. This involves complete resection of the stenotic segment with end-to-end anastomosis of the tracheal stump to the thyroid cartilage.

Grade I subglottic stenosis usually requires no surgical intervention. Grade II stenosis can be reconstructed by means of an LTR with anterior cartilage grafting, generally without the need for a stent. Mild grade III stenosis is likely to need an anterior graft with posterior cricoid split supported by an endoluminal stent, and severe grade III stenosis (a pin-hole airway) requires both anterior and posterior grafts with stenting. Grade IV stenosis demands anterior and posterior grafts with prolonged stenting. For severe grade III and for grade IV stenosis, PCTR is an alternative technique with much to commend it. LTR remains the last surgical option after failed PCTR if it is impossible to resect a further segment of trachea.

In cases of congenital subglottic stenosis, the LTR may be combined with submucosal resection of cartilage to 'core out' the thickened anterior cricoid ring. A similar submucous resection technique can be used via a laryngofissure for thick anterior glottic webs with subglottic extension. In both situations stenting is essential.

The least severe grades (I and II) have a better outcome than the most severe grades (III and IV). For PCTR, however, the grading system is not a predictor of success or failure, because the stenotic segment is completely resected. Results from the most experienced centres[19, 20, 21] show a decannulation rate of just under 90 percent for grades I and II subglottic stenosis following LTR. However, this drops to approximately 80 percent for grade III and 50 percent or less for grade IV subglottic stenosis, implying the need for revision surgery in a significant number of cases. The latest results from the two centres with the largest experience in PCTR show a decannulation rate of 98 percent for primary surgery and 94 percent for salvage surgery after failed previous airway reconstruction.[22, 23] [**/*]

For more detail on the management of laryngeal stenosis, the reader is referred to Chapter 89, Laryngeal stenosis.

SUBGLOTTIC HAEMANGIOMA

Infantile subglottic haemangioma is a capillary hamartoma which enlarges rapidly up to the age of about one year and then involutes slowly. Presentation with gradually increasing stridor peaks at the age of six weeks, with 85 percent presenting within the first six months of life. At endoscopy the typical appearance is of a compressible, pear-shaped red swelling in the subglottis on one side, left more commonly than right (**Figure 88.5**). Larger haemangiomas may be circumferential and, uncommonly, may extend down into the trachea or through its wall into the surrounding soft tissues of the neck or mediastinum. The appearance is so characteristic that biopsy is unnecessary; although in rare cases where there is doubt, biopsy can be undertaken without fear of troublesome bleeding because of the capillary nature of the lesion. If extension outside the airway is suspected, magnetic resonance imaging (MRI) is indicated. Subglottic haemangioma is life-threatening because of its situation in the narrowest part of the airway and if untreated carries a mortality rate of 50 percent.[24]

Tracheostomy will maintain the airway until involution occurs. A review of the subject in 1984 by Sebastian and Kleinsasser[25] estimated that 50–70 percent of patients with airway haemangioma require a tracheostomy, and that children managed with tracheostomy alone could be decannulated at a mean age of 17 months. However,

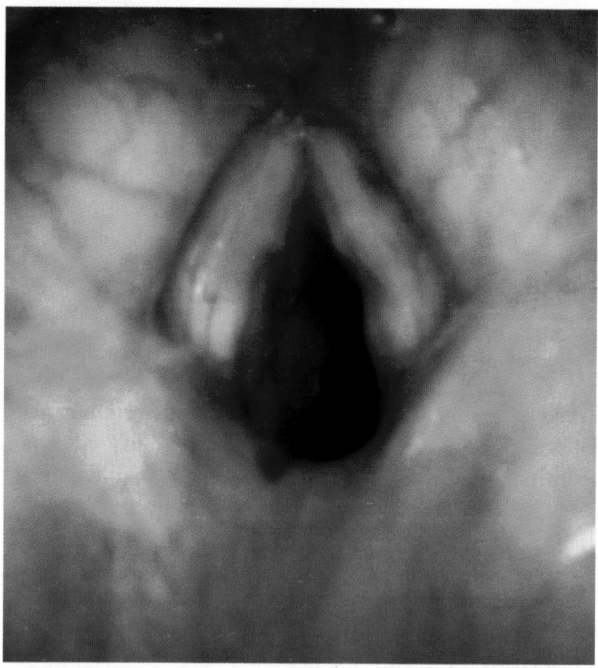

Figure 88.5 Subglottic haemangioma, showing a typical left-sided, pink pear-shaped swelling.

paediatric tracheostomy carries a mortality of 1–2 percent and a significant morbidity including delayed speech development.

Over the years, efforts have been made to develop alternative therapeutic strategies aimed at either maintaining the airway without recourse to tracheostomy, or at least shortening the period of cannulation. Any acceptable treatment must be at least as safe as tracheostomy and should be free of side effects, as there are no sequelae after natural involution, but these requirements have proved difficult to fulfil.

Radiotherapy delivered by low-dose external beam or gold-grain implant brings about involution within nine months, but has been abandoned because of concerns regarding possible induction of thyroid malignancy.

CO_2 laser vaporization can be effective but is probably only suitable for small lesions. In a ten-year review of experience at Boston Children's Hospital[26] it was found that tracheostomy could not be avoided in 30 percent of cases, and 18 percent developed subglottic stenosis. It would thus seem that conservative laser treatment of large haemangiomas fails to achieve involution, while vigorous application can result in cicatricial stenosis.

Systemic steroids produce dramatic regression of most subglottic haemangiomas. Complications of steroid therapy, such as growth retardation and Cushing's syndrome, can be reduced by alternate day dose regimens and intermittent courses, but treatment may be required for as long as 12–18 months.[27] Systemic steroids are, therefore, best reserved for use in short courses in order to maintain a good airway while definitive treatment is being planned.

Interferon alpha-2a has shown promising results in the treatment of patients with extensive, life-threatening airway haemangiomas who had failed steroid and/or laser therapy.[28] However, daily subcutaneous injections were required for a mean period of 11 months, and recognized side effects during interferon therapy include pyrexial reactions, elevated liver transaminases, neutropenia, thrombocytopenia, alopecia, neurotoxicity and growth retardation.

Intralesional steroid injection followed by intubation for seven days, repeated as necessary, was pioneered by Hoeve *et al.* at Sophia Children's Hospital in Rotterdam.[29] Overall, 14 of 17 patients (82 percent) treated by this method achieved a permanently adequate airway by a mean age of nine months, and no patient developed subglottic stenosis. However, a mean of six endoscopies followed by six periods (37 days) of intubation over a period of five months were needed in the infants treated with success, with a tendency for larger lesions to require longer periods of treatment. This puts a considerable strain on the intensive care resources of the hospital, and may test the parents' powers of endurance.

Submucosal excision of the haemangioma has been complicated by subglottic stenosis when attempted in the past. However, as Bailey *et al.*[30] have described, the problem can now be avoided by combining excision with a cricoid split to decompress and expand the subglottis. The airway is stented with an endotracheal tube for five to ten days postoperatively, and this enables the surgery to be carried out in a single stage without a covering tracheostomy. He feels that excision should be chosen as a primary treatment for large haemangiomas. It is less satisfactory as a secondary technique after other methods have failed, as scarring then makes submucosal dissection difficult and consequent mucosal damage makes stenosis more likely.

In conclusion, very small haemangiomas may not require treatment, or may be amenable to CO_2 laser vaporization. Medium-sized lesions seem suitable for intralesional steroids and intubation, but large ones are probably best managed by primary submucous resection. [Grade C] Very large haemangiomas, and especially those which are circumferential or in which MRI shows extension down into the trachea and/or through the tracheal wall into the surrounding tissues, must carry a greater risk of stenosis developing after surgery and may be more safely dealt with by performing a tracheostomy and awaiting spontaneous involution. [**/*]

LARYNGEAL AND LARYNGOTRACHEOESOPHAGEAL CLEFT

Posterior laryngeal clefts result from failure of the posterior cricoid lamina to fuse, and in the more extensive laryngotracheoesophageal clefts there is also incomplete development of the tracheoesophageal septum. The classification devised by Benjamin and Inglis[31] has been widely adopted because it relates well to symptoms and treatment. A type I cleft may extend down to the level of the vocal cords; a type II cleft extends below the vocal cords into the cricoid (**Figure 88.6**); a type III cleft extends down into the cervical trachea; and the, fortunately rare, type IV cleft extends into the thoracic trachea and may even reach the carina. Approximately 25 percent of patients with a laryngeal cleft will also have a TOF, but conversely the incidence of laryngeal cleft in patients with a TOF is low. Abnormalities of the tracheal ring structure in cleft patients may result in associated tracheomalacia, which can add to the difficulties of management.

The majority of laryngeal cleft patients have associated congenital abnormalities, of which TOF is the most common. These may include tracheobronchomalacia, congenital heart disease, dextrocardia and situs inversus. Often there is severe gastro-oesophageal reflux. Laryngeal clefts are characteristic of two syndromes: the Opitz-Frias syndrome (G syndrome) comprises hypertelorism, cleft lip and palate, laryngeal cleft and hypospadias; Pallister-Hall syndrome (described earlier in relation to bifid epiglottis) consists of congenital hypothalamic hamartoblastoma, hypopituitarism, imperforate anus and postaxial polydactyly, and may include a laryngeal cleft.

As might be expected, symptoms become more severe the longer the cleft. Type I clefts present with cyanotic attacks on feeding and recurrent chest infections. Stridor (similar to that of laryngomalacia) may be a feature, secondary to prolapse of the cleft edges into the airway. The differential diagnosis for infants presenting with these symptoms includes gastro-oesophageal reflux, neuromuscular incoordination of deglutition, vocal cord paralysis, raised intracranial pressure and TOF. Types II and III clefts produce dramatic aspiration with recurrent

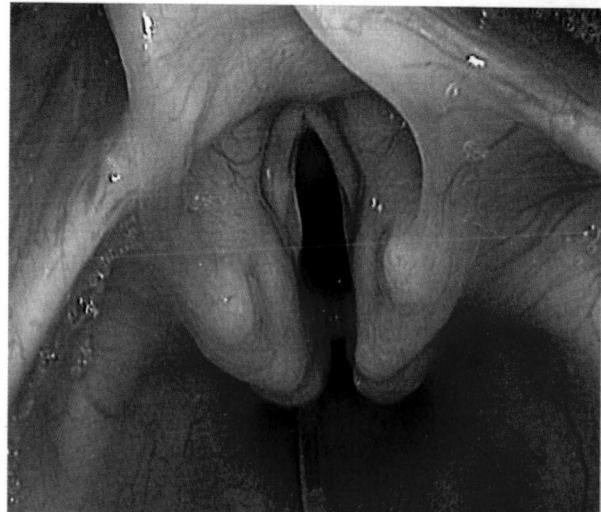

Figure 88.6 Laryngeal cleft (type II). Reused with permission from Bailey CM. Congenital disorders of the larynx, trachea and bronchi. In: Graham JM, Scadding GK and Bull PD (eds). *Pediatric ENT* (in press), with kind permission of Springer Science and Business Media.

pneumonia, sometimes with stridor and an abnormal cry. Type IV clefts cause severe aspiration, cyanosis and incipient cardiorespiratory failure.

Investigation of the child with aspiration and stridor requires a careful microlaryngoscopy and bronchoscopy; no other diagnostic method can replace it. Suspension microlaryngoscopy allows the use of two probes to part the arytenoids, and without this manoeuvre the diagnosis may be missed as redundant mucosa tends to prolapse into the defect and obscure it. A plain chest x-ray may show changes secondary to recurrent aspiration pneumonitis. A lateral neck x-ray may demonstrate vaguely increased laryngeal soft tissue and the nasogastric feeding tube may be seen protruding anteriorly into the airway. Videofluoroscopic contrast swallow studies may not differentiate laryngeal incompetence from neuromuscular incoordination, and a high index of suspicion is required.

The approach to treatment depends entirely upon the length of the cleft. A short type I cleft with no aspiration requires no treatment. Minimal aspiration may be managed by thickening the feeds. Significant aspiration requires endoscopic repair of the cleft in two layers, using a nasogastric feeding tube until the suture line has healed. A very short type II cleft may also be repaired endoscopically, albeit with difficulty, using a nasogastric tube. However, a long type II or a type III cleft needs to be approached anteriorly through an extended laryngofissure with a low tracheostomy to cover the procedure; a nasogastric tube will tend to erode through the suture line, and so a gastrostomy is required (usually combined with a Nissen fundoplication to control reflux reliably). These children take many months to learn to swallow after successful cleft repair and thus long-term gastrostomy feeding is necessary. Surgical repair of the cleft is undertaken in three layers in an effort to optimize healing: the two mucosal layers are reinforced by an interposition graft of tibial periosteum or temporalis facia. The type IV cleft presents an altogether more difficult surgical challenge. Owing to the length of the cleft a tracheostomy is unhelpful in stabilizing the airway, and the convexity of the tube would tend to erode through the party wall suture line; the repair must therefore be undertaken using a single-stage technique with endotracheal extubation taking place seven to ten days postoperatively. Short type IV clefts may be managed by an anterior approach through a cervical incision, if necessary pulling the trachea up into the neck to reach the lower end of the cleft. Longer clefts will require a lateral cervical approach in combination with a thoracotomy, or preferably an anterior cervicothoracic approach via a median sternotomy with repair on extracorporeal membrane oxygenation (ECMO) or cardiopulmonary bypass. Postoperatively, tracheomalacia may prevent extubation and so a tracheostomy may be needed once the cleft has healed soundly.[32]

Mortality remains significant, being approximately 14 percent overall,[33] rising to 66 percent for type IV laryngotracheoesophageal clefts and up to 100 percent for full-length clefts ending at the carina.[34] A large proportion of the mortality is from causes unrelated to the cleft, and notable morbidity is produced by other associated congenital abnormalities and often by delay in reaching the correct diagnosis. Management should be in a major paediatric centre where a full multidisciplinary team is available with full neonatal and paediatric intensive care facilities. [**/*]

TRACHEA AND BRONCHI

Agenesis

Tracheal agenesis may be complete (full-length) or partial, but in either case there is no continuity between the larynx and the bronchi. Occasionally, short-term survival may be possible if there is a broncho-oesophageal fistula, which can permit some airflow into the lungs, but surgical efforts to use the oesophagus as a tracheal replacement have not been successful and long-term survival has not proved possible. The majority of cases are complicated by other severe congenital abnormalities.

Agenesis of one main bronchus and its associated lung is not as rare as tracheal agenesis and is compatible with survival, although such children often have coexisting congenital anomalies and are at risk from chest infections because of their much-reduced respiratory reserve. Bilateral bronchial and pulmonary agenesis is extremely rare and is, of course, fatal. Occasionally, localized atresia occurs in a peripheral bronchus resulting in a distal mucocoele which may need to be resected if it is causing severe compression of the surrounding lung. [*]

Stenosis

Occasionally, a membranous web may be encountered in the trachea with a normal underlying cartilaginous ring structure. Such cases usually fare well with endoscopic rupture and dilatation. Thicker congenital fibrous stenoses may be amenable to radial KTP laser incision and balloon dilatation, followed by application of mitomycin C to reduce the risk of restenosis.[35]

Longer-segment congenital tracheal stenosis is generally due to complete tracheal rings which are fused posteriorly, and may be fused together to form a cartilage plate. This poses a much more severe reconstructive challenge. Such a stenosis may be of variable severity and length. It may involve almost the entire length of the trachea ('stove-pipe trachea' or 'microtrachea'), just the distal part with a funnel-like stenosis maximal at the carina or only a short segment. Long-segment congenital tracheal stenosis, involving more than 50 percent of the trachea, is often associated with a pulmonary artery sling

(25 percent), intracardiac lesions (20 percent) and right-sided aortic arch.[36] As recently as 35 years ago this abnormality was fatal.

Children with congenital tracheal stenosis usually present with respiratory distress within the first year of life. Symptoms may become apparent in the neonatal period if the stenosis is severe but frequently, presentation is delayed until the infant is several months old when greater physical activity makes increasing demands upon the respiratory system. Biphasic stridor or wheezing is the cardinal symptom, but sometimes difficulty in breathing develops rapidly as a result of a respiratory tract infection, with consequent oedema and increased secretions. In this situation the child may require endotracheal intubation, and it is then found that only a very small-sized tube can be passed. In the case of a long tapering stenosis, which may narrow virtually to a pin-hole, this is a dangerous situation. The tube tip tends to impact into the stenosis, granulations begin to develop and obstruct the already perilous airway, and endoscopic evaluation is then a procedure fraught with difficulty. In such cases the stenosis often seems surprisingly severe considering the child's mild symptoms prior to the precipitating illness.

A chest x-ray is a basic requirement to see whether there are any signs of bronchial obstruction producing collapse or atelectasis. In the unintubated child, the trachea and main bronchi were traditionally well seen on a Cincinnati x-ray, which is a high-kilovolt filter view of the mediastinum giving good air/soft tissue definition. Modern 'digitally enhanced' radiography has, however, made this technique somewhat obsolete as it can show such fine detail (see Chapter 102, Imaging in paediatric ENT). An echocardiogram is essential to exclude a vascular ring in view of the high incidence of associated anomalies of the heart and great vessels. Computed tomography (CT) or MRI is often helpful to assess further the vascular anatomy and its relationship to the trachea, but angiography is now rarely indicated and both three-dimensional reformatted CT and CT 'virtual broncho-scopy' have significant shortcomings. In the hands of a skilled paediatric interventional radiologist, contrast bronchography is the most valuable imaging modality and is currently preferred to CT or MRI. It will show the size of the tracheal lumen and outline the trachea and bronchi distal to the stenosis which may be too narrow to permit passage of a bronchoscope (**Figure 88.7**). Bronchography is carried out under general anaesthesia, and a preliminary endoscopic assessment can be under-taken at the same time using a slim flexible fibre optic bronchoscope passed through the endotracheal tube.

Endoscopy remains the 'gold standard' investigation for a child with stridor. For tracheal stenosis, rigid endoscopy using a ventilating bronchoscope system is the best method. However, great care must be taken not to traumatize the stenosis by attempting to pass a broncho-scope that is too large, or the resultant oedema may convert an airway that is just adequate into one that is

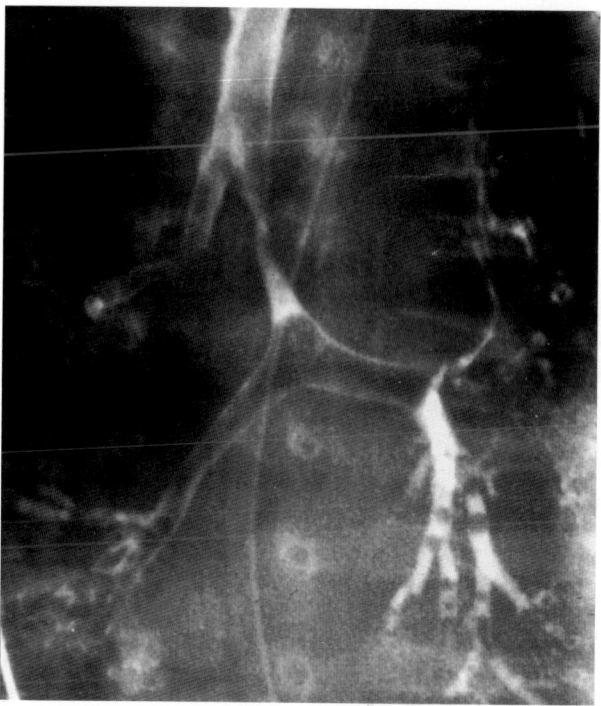

Figure 88.7 Tracheal stenosis: bronchogram of a long-segment lower tracheal stenosis with associated stenosis of the main bronchi and with a 'pig' bronchus at its upper end.

not. On occasions, the airway is so perilous that endoscopy carries a real risk of precipitating complete airway obstruction. In such a situation definitive surgery can be planned upon the basis of the imaging results and endoscopy performed immediately prior to opening the chest, with standby facilities ready for cardiopulmonary bypass. Frequently, the stenosis is too narrow to permit passage of even the smallest (size 2.5) bronchoscope, and it is necessary to use the unsheathed 1.9 mm telescope to survey the length of the narrow segment and assess the state of the distal trachea, carina and bronchi. Sometimes the airway is too narrow to admit even this extra-slim telescope, and then the surgeon must rely on contrast bronchography.

Mild cases with minimal symptoms may require no intervention after the diagnostic endoscopy, as the trachea can grow and there may be only slight limitation of exercise tolerance. Certainly, patients who can be managed conservatively should be, as surgical treatment is difficult and carries a substantial mortality and morbidity.

Successful endoscopic balloon dilatation of long-segment tracheal stenoses has been reported, producing a posterior split in the complete tracheal rings and increased airway lumen maintained over several years following a period of stenting with an endotracheal tube. However, it is difficult to see why the airway does not quickly close down again to its original size, as the 'spring' in the cartilage is not broken by splitting it in just one place and fibrosis is bound to occur at the site of the split.

Nevertheless, balloon dilatation is a useful adjunctive treatment modality for granulations and fibrous stenoses such as may develop postoperatively at the site of an anastomosis.

Very narrow, short segments can be excised with end-to-end anastomosis. The excised segment of tracheal cartilage may be used as a free autograft at the anastomotic site, and this method permits a longer section to be removed with less tension upon the suture line. For longer stenoses slide tracheoplasty is an advantageous technique[37, 38] as it minimizes shortening of the trachea and hence reduces anastomotic tension. The oblique anastomosis also seems less liable to postoperative stenosis than an end-to-end anastomosis. The tracheoplasty is performed by dividing the stenosis at its midpoint, incising the proximal and distal narrowed segments vertically on opposite anterior and posterior surfaces and sliding these together. The stenotic segment is thus shortened by half, the circumference is doubled, and the luminal cross section quadrupled. Long resections may require a laryngeal drop and/or hilar release to avoid undue tension upon the suture line.

The most difficult problem remains the full-length 'stove-pipe' microtrachea, especially when the carina and bronchi are involved. As might be expected, the narrower the stenosis, the more difficult the reconstruction. Augmentation tracheoplasty can be achieved by anterior costal cartilage grafting (with posterior division of the complete rings if necessary). Alternatively, a pericardial flap or free patch can be employed, suspended by supporting sutures to adjoining mediastinal structures and stented by an endotracheal or extended tracheostomy tube for as long as it takes to become stiff and self-supporting. If the stenosis is extremely severe with only a pin-hole lumen, then cartilage grafting (even with a posterior split) cannot be expected to achieve an adequate airway, and a large suspended pericardial patch is needed; however, the larger the patch, the greater the risk of subsequent tracheomalacia. Such surgery is best undertaken using a neck incision and median sternotomy with cardiopulmonary bypass and a joint cardiothoracic–ENT surgical team. Any coexisting anomaly of the heart or great vessels should usually be corrected at the same time. ECMO may sometimes be useful to stabilize the patient's condition postoperatively as a 'bridge' between bypass and ventilation, and occasionally ECMO may be needed for preoperative support. The postoperative care of these patients is demanding, and a somewhat stormy course is not uncommon. The overall mortality associated with costal cartilage or pericardial patch tracheoplasty is substantial, ranging up to nearly 50 percent in the literature review by Andrews et al.[39] in 1994, but more recent experience in major centres has halved this figure. Involvement of the carina or either main-stem bronchus in the stenosis makes reconstruction much more difficult, and mortality and morbidity correspondingly increase.

An alternative is to use a cadaver tracheal homograft for the reconstruction, a technique pioneered by Herberhold in adults and later adopted for use in children.[40] It is our current policy to hold in reserve homograft reconstruction as a salvage technique for those children with life-threatening long-segment tracheal stenosis who have already failed conventional surgery.

The variety of reconstructive options available for treating tracheal stenosis in children means that the surgery must be individually tailored to the patient. A multidisciplinary tracheal team is required with a team coordinator/case manager, working in a major paediatric centre with full intensive care facilities.[41] [Grade C] The difficulties involved mean that this uncommon problem remains a challenge for even the most experienced paediatric cardiothoracic surgeon and otolaryngologist.

Bronchial webs may be ruptured with a bronchoscope or by balloon dilatation. Stenosis of a main bronchus is often associated with an adjoining vascular anomaly, and segmental resection with end-to-end anastomosis may be necessary. [**/*]

Tracheomalacia and bronchomalacia

Tracheomalacia is a condition in which there is reduced stiffness of the tracheal wall, resulting in abnormal collapse of the trachea during expiration which, if severe, can produce symptoms of airway obstruction. Bronchomalacia is the equivalent condition affecting the bronchi. There is, however, no association between tracheobronchomalacia and laryngomalacia, although because the latter is a common condition it may sometimes coexist.

Pathologically, the striking finding is an increased muscle-to-cartilage ratio seen on the transverse section of the trachea; in other words, a widening of the trachealis relative to the cartilage rings, which become C shaped instead of horseshoe shaped. Normally, the ratio is 1:4 or 1:5, but in tracheomalacia it may be closer to 1:2. However, in children the trachea and bronchi are more compliant than in the adult and some degree of collapse may be observed during endoscopy in normal children. This is particularly obvious if the level of general and topical anaesthesia is too light and the child tends to cough and strain in consequence, often with anterior bulging of the trachealis. To be clinically significant, more than 50 percent obstruction is probably required, as visualized at the end of expiration in the well-anaesthetized child.

Tracheomalacia is traditionally classified as **primary** (idiopathic), due to an intrinsic abnormality in the wall of the airway, or **secondary**, due to another associated anomaly or to external compression. The primary form is less common and tends to affect a longer segment of the airway. Secondary tracheomalacia is usually more localized and may be associated with TOF, laryngeal cleft or with extrinsic compression by an anomaly of the great vessels or a mediastinal mass. A common but special form of localized secondary tracheomalacia is the suprastomal collapse which arises above most long-standing paediatric tracheostomies, produced by pressure from the convexity of the tracheostomy tube.

The stridor of tracheomalacia becomes apparent during the first few weeks of life and consists of a very variable high-pitched expiratory noise. This may be accompanied by a harsh, barking cough, especially in the localized form of the condition. Characteristically, the stridor becomes much worse when the child is active, feeding, upset, coughing or crying, and may be associated with cyanotic attacks which are sometimes sufficiently severe to be termed 'dying spells'. The pathophysiology of these seems to be that with vigorous respiration, airflow through the trachea increases and in accordance with Bernouilli's principle the pressure within the airway correspondingly falls. This encourages further collapse of the malacic segment and a vicious circle is established that can result in complete collapse of the trachea with respiratory obstruction. These episodes are probably self-limiting but, faced with total obstructive apnoea and cyanosis, parents and caregivers will usually attempt resuscitation rather than wait and see.

The stridor of tracheobronchomalacia is typically episodic, thus on examination the child may seem perfectly well. There may be a prolonged expiratory phase to respiration, possibly with faint expiratory stridor. However, crying or feeding can dramatically change the picture to one of an infant who is clearly obstructed and in respiratory distress.

Plain x-rays are not usually helpful. A barium swallow may identify a vascular ring or TOF and can also demonstrate the airway collapse on lateral screening. Echocardiography is useful in defining any suspected anomaly of the heart and great vessels. CT and MRI are of limited value, and the most useful radiological investigation is contrast bronchography. This not only demonstrates the areas of collapse but enables the opening pressures to be measured, which is extremely helpful in setting continuous positive airway pressure (CPAP) levels for children with very severe tracheobronchomalacia who are intubated or have undergone tracheostomy. Even if tracheobronchomalacia has been demonstrated radiologically it is nonetheless important to undertake a full airway endoscopy to examine the collapse directly and exclude other abnormalities such as a TOF or laryngeal cleft. However, endoscopy presents traps for the inexperienced in the assessment of tracheobronchomalacia.[42] Overdiagnosis can happen, as mentioned earlier, under conditions of poor anaesthesia which allow coughing. Underdiagnosis is a risk either from mechanical splinting of the trachea by the bronchoscope or by positive end-expiratory pressure applied by the anaesthetist. Typically, anterior tracheal wall collapse will be observed, with flattened tracheal rings and a wide trachealis (**Figure 88.8**). In addition, the common vascular anomalies have sufficiently characteristic features to aid diagnosis (see below).

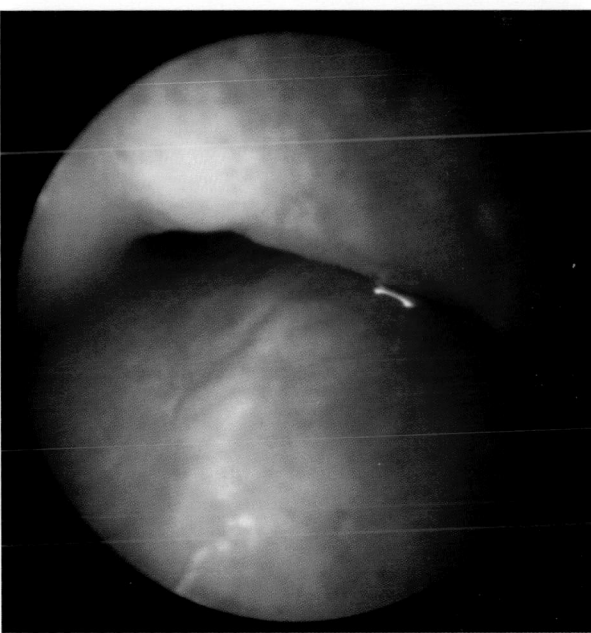

Figure 88.8 Severe tracheomalacia.

Mild tracheobronchomalacia (less than 75 percent collapse) requires no intervention, and the stridor can be expected to resolve spontaneously by around the age of two years. However, parents will require careful explanation and reassurance, as well as being taught cardiopulmonary resuscitation if their child is prone to 'dying spells'. Severe tracheobronchomalacia (more than 75 percent collapse) may require treatment. If it is secondary to a vascular anomaly this should be corrected. The severe localized tracheomalacia often associated with a TOF usually responds well to an aortopexy, whereby the aorta is sutured to the back of the sternum. If this fails then an extended tracheostomy tube will effectively support a midtracheal malacic segment, but this is not a satisfactory solution for lower-end tracheal or for bronchial collapse. For the infant in intensive care with severe primary tracheobronchomalacia who cannot be weaned off CPAP, it may be necessary to resort to a tracheostomy in order to apply long-term CPAP, sometimes for a period of 12 months or more. Alternative surgical solutions for this most severe end of the disease spectrum have been sought by cardiothoracic surgeons: these include internal or external stenting of the trachea, segmental resection and cartilage grafting, but all present formidable difficulties and complications with very variable outcome and the risks may exceed those of the condition itself. [**/*]

Tracheo-oesophageal fistula

Tracheo-oesophageal fistula is a fairly common congenital malformation of the neonatal air and food passages, which usually occurs in association with oesophageal atresia. Eighty-seven percent of cases have oesophageal atresia with a TOF communicating between the distal oesophagus and the mid- to lower trachea or a main bronchus. The remainder have oesophageal atresia without a TOF (6 percent); atresia with a proximal TOF (2 percent); atresia with a proximal and distal TOF (1 percent); or a TOF without atresia ('H-type fistula') (4 percent). Approximately 50 percent of infants with TOF have additional congenital malformations, and 10–20 percent have tracheomalacia (see Chapter 101, Diseases of the oesophagus, swallowing disorders and caustic ingestion).

Children who present to the paediatric otolaryngologist are invariably those with an H-type fistula. Since there is no oesophageal atresia they are the least symptomatic of the group, with no swallowing difficulty, but small amounts of fluid pass through the fistula into the trachea and produce symptoms and signs of recurrent minor aspiration. The diagnosis is usually established by a barium swallow, but even thin contrast may not pass through a tiny fistula. In such cases bronchoscopy is required to identify the tracheal opening, which is typically characterized by a V-shaped mucosal fold around it in the posterior wall of the trachea (**Figure 88.9**). Usually the fistula is too small to allow passage of a fine spaghetti suction catheter, but methylene blue introduced into the oesophagus will be seen to seep into the trachea at this point. Treatment is by ligation and division of the fistula. [**/*]

For further details on the management of TOF, the reader is referred to Chapter 101, Diseases of the oesophagus, swallowing disorders and caustic ingestion.

Vascular compression

It is estimated that 3 percent of the population have an anomaly of the great vessels, but only a few of these have

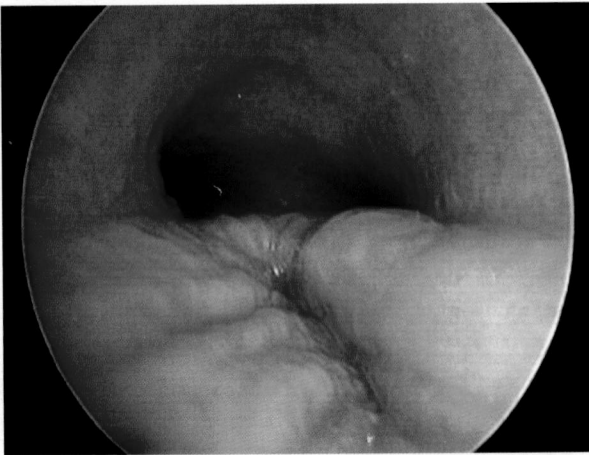

Figure 88.9 Tracheosophageal fistula seen at bronchoscopy. Reused with permission from Bailey CM. Congenital disorders of the larynx, trachea and bronchi. In: Graham JM, Scadding GK and Bull PD (eds). *Pediatric ENT*, (in press), with kind permission of Springer Science and Business Media.

symptomatic airway compression.[43] Such vascular anomalies are classified into vascular rings which completely encircle the trachea and oesophagus and vascular slings which exert noncircumferential pressure.

VASCULAR RING

The commonest vascular ring is a double aortic arch. In this abnormality the ascending aorta divides into two arches, one of which passes to the right of the trachea and the other to the left, reuniting posterior to the oesophagus to form the descending aorta on the left. The left arch is usually smaller than the right, and the configuration of the main branches is variable, but the result is compression of both the trachea and oesophagus producing stridor, dyspnoea, dysphagia and a brassy cough.

A less common and less constricting ring is produced when there is a right-sided aortic arch and descending aorta associated with an aberrant left subclavian artery. In this situation the ring is completed by the ligamentum arteriosum which passes to the left of the trachea, connecting the descending aorta to the pulmonary trunk.

Patients with vascular rings tend to present earlier in life than those with vascular slings and with more severe airway symptoms. A barium swallow is diagnostic, showing a characteristic double impression upon the column of contrast, and an echocardiogram will confirm the anomaly. Surgical treatment, almost always necessary, is by dividing the lesser component of the ring, but there is invariably a localized area of tracheomalacia produced by the compression which may persist for months or even years.

VASCULAR SLING

The commonest vascular sling is an aberrant innominate artery. The artery arises further to the left and more posteriorly than usual, and crosses the anterior surface of the trachea obliquely just above the carina from the left inferiorly to the right superiorly.

Cases usually present during the first year of life with less severe airway obstruction than that caused by vascular rings. Typically, there is expiratory stridor, cough, recurrent chest infection and sometimes reflex apnoea. The bronchoscopic appearances are diagnostic, with a characteristic sloping, pulsatile compression of the trachea 1–2 cm above the carina which is most marked on its anterolateral aspect. Upward pressure with the tip of the bronchoscope compresses the artery against the sternum and obliterates the right radial pulse. In severe cases, surgical relief of the obstruction is necessary: this can be achieved either by arteriopexy, in which the vessel is suspended anteriorly from the sternum, or by reimplanting it further to the right on the aortic arch.

A 'pulmonary artery sling' is produced by an anomalous left pulmonary artery, which arises on the right and passes between the trachea and oesophagus, compressing both (**Figure 88.10**). This may be associated with lower-end tracheal stenosis which sometimes also involves the carina and right main bronchus. Surgical reanastomosis may be needed to relieve the compression.

Enlargement of the pulmonary artery in association with a cardiac defect can also produce compression of the distal trachea and bifurcation. An aberrant right or, more rarely, left subclavian artery passing posterior to the oesophagus will compress the oesophagus alone, and so produces dysphagia but no stridor. [**/*]

Anomalous bifurcations

The right upper lobe bronchus may take origin from the right lateral wall of the trachea above the carina, and is then often termed a 'pig bronchus'. It is usually an asymptomatic, incidental finding, but may sometimes be associated with tracheal stenosis. Minor alterations to the distal bronchial branching pattern are not unusual and, likewise, do not usually cause problems.

Congenital cysts and tumours

Tracheogenic and bronchogenic cysts are thought to originate from evaginations of the primitive tracheal bud, and are sometimes termed reduplication anomalies. They may happen anywhere along the tracheobronchial tree: they are lined with respiratory epithelium, filled with mucus, and their walls may contain any elements of normal tracheobronchial wall. Bronchogenic cysts may communicate with the airway.

Some patients are symptom-free, but large cysts or those that become infected cause nonpulsatile compression of the airway and present with symptoms, signs and endoscopic appearances otherwise similar to those produced by vascular compression (see Vascular compression above). CT or MRI will demonstrate the lesion clearly, and treatment is by thoracotomy and surgical excision.

Thymomas or teratomas may produce airway compression in the neck or mediastinum. CT or MRI is needed to define the size and situation of the mass prior to surgical excision. [*]

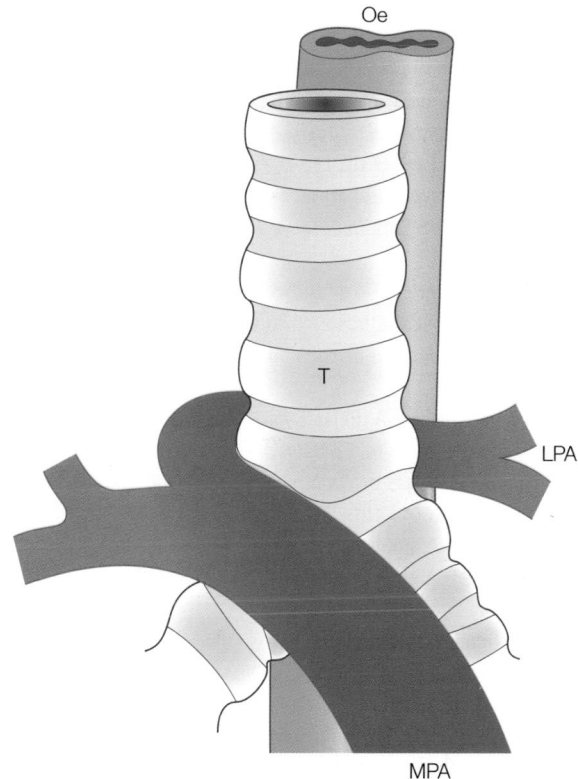

Figure 88.10 Diagram of a pulmonary artery sling. LPA, left pulmonary artery; MPA, main pulmonary artery; Oe, oesophagus; T, trachea. Redrawn with permission from Bailey CM. Congenital disorders of the larynx, trachea and bronchi. In: Graham JM, Scadding GK and Bull PD (eds). *Pediatric ENT* (in press), with kind permission of Springer Science and Business Media.

KEY POINTS

- Investigation of the child with aspiration and stridor requires a careful microlaryngoscopy and bronchoscopy; no diagnostic method can replace it.
- In laryngomalacia (the most common congenital cause of stridor) the stridor is usually improved immediately following aryepiglottoplasty.
- Anterior glottic webs are thin posteriorly, but become progressively thicker anteriorly. This can make surgical treatment frustratingly difficult.
- In the EXIT procedure, tracheotomy is undertaken with the foetus still on placental circulation.
- Endoscopy presents traps for the inexperienced in the assessment of tracheobronchomalacia.
- The use of endoscopy to diagnose many of the conditions described in this chapter is dependent on skilled paediatric anaesthesia.
- Management of congenital disorders of the larynx, trachea and bronchi requires the multidisciplinary resources of a major children's centre.

Best clinical practice

✓ The diagnosis of mild laryngomalacia can be confirmed in the outpatient clinic by flexible fibreoptic laryngoscopy.

✓ Microlaryngoscopy and bronchoscopy under general anaesthesia is necessary if the stridor in laryngomalacia is severe, there is failure to thrive or any atypical features.

✓ Although outpatient flexible fibreoptic laryngoscopy may indicate the diagnosis of vocal cord palsy, a formal microlaryngoscopy and bronchoscopy under general anaesthesia is essential to exclude coexisting airway pathology.

✓ Small subglottic haemangiomas may not require treatment, or may be amenable to CO_2 laser vaporization. Medium-sized lesions seem suitable for intralesional steroids and intubation, but large ones are probably best managed by primary submucous resection.

✓ In tracheal stenosis the airway may be so perilous that endoscopy carries a real risk of precipitating complete obstruction.

Deficiencies in current knowledge and areas for future research

➤ The rarity and often life-threatening nature of many congenital disorders of the larynx, trachea and bronchi means that evidence for their management tends to be confined to evidence levels 3 and 4. It is hard to see how this can be overcome without increased central referral of these challenging cases to just a few major paediatric centres. Even so, international collaboration between such centres is often the only way to generate sufficient patient numbers just for evidence level 3 studies in this field.

➤ One potentially fruitful area for future study lies in an assessment of the efficacy of mitomycin C in reducing restenosis following airway reconstructive surgery.[44] Since it is an adjunctive therapy it is possible to undertake a prospective, randomized, double-blind placebo-controlled trial of its use, and this has already been attempted on a small scale, but with inconclusive results.[45]

REFERENCES

1. Van den Broek P, Brinkman WFB. Congenital laryngeal defects. *International Journal of Pediatric Otorhinolaryngology*. 1979; 1: 71–8.

2. Shugar MA, Healy GB. Coexistent lesions of the pediatric airway. *International Journal of Pediatric Otorhinolaryngology*. 1980; 2: 323–7.

3. Mancuso RF, Choi SS, Zalzal GH, Grundfast KM. Laryngomalacia. The search for the second lesion. *Archives of Otolaryngology – Head and Neck Surgery*. 1996; **122**: 1417–18.

4. Lane RW, Weider DJ, Steinem C, Marin-Padilla M. Laryngomalacia: A review and case report of surgical treatment with resolution of pectus excavatum. *Archives of Otolaryngology*. 1984; **110**: 546–51.

5. Jani P, Koltai P, Ochi JW, Bailey CM. Surgical treatment of laryngomalacia. *Journal of Laryngology and Otology*. 1991; **105**: 1040–5.

6. Martin JE, Howarth KE, Khodaei I, Karkanevatos A, Clarke RW. Aryepiglottoplasty for laryngomalacia: the Alder Hey experience. *Journal of Laryngology and Otology*. 2005; **119**: 958–60.

7. Toynton SC, Saunders MW, Bailey CM. Aryepiglottoplasty for laryngomalacia: 100 consecutive cases. *Journal of Laryngology and Otology*. 2001; **115**: 35–8.

8. Cotton RT, Prescott CAJ. Congenital anomalies of the larynx. In: Cotton RT, Myer CM (eds). *Practical pediatric otolaryngology*. Philadelphia: Lippincott-Raven, 1999: 497–513.

9. April MM, Rebeiz E, Friedman EM, Healy GB. Laser surgery for lymphatic malformations of the upper aerodigestive tract. *An evolving experience. Archives of Otolaryngology – Head and Neck Surgery*. 1992; **118**: 205–08.

* 10. Hirose S, Farmer DL, Lee H, Nobuhara KK, Harrison MR. The ex utero intrapartum treatment procedure: looking back at the EXIT. *Journal of Pediatric Surgery*. 2004; **39**: 375–80.

11. Vats A, Worley GA, de Bruyn R, Porter H, Albert DM, Bailey CM. Laryngeal ultrasound to assess vocal fold paralysis in children. *Journal of Laryngology and Otology*. 2004; **118**: 429–31.

12. Daya H, Hosni A, Bejar-Solar I, Evans JNG, Bailey CM. Pediatric vocal fold paralysis – a long-term retrospective study. *Archives of Otolaryngology – Head and Neck Surgery*. 2000; **126**: 21–5.

13. Bower CM, Choi SS, Cotton RT. Arytenoidectomy in children. *Annals of Otology, Rhinology, and Laryngology*. 1994; **103**: 271–8.

14. Holinger LD. Histopathology of congenital subglottic stenosis. *Annals of Otology, Rhinology, and Laryngology*. 1999; **108**: 101–11.

15. Myer 3rd CM, O'Connor DM, Cotton RT. Proposed grading system for subglottic stenosis based on endotracheal tube sizes. *Annals of Otology, Rhinology, and Laryngology*. 1994; **103**: 319–23.

16. Evans JNG, Todd GB. Laryngotracheoplasty. *Journal of Laryngology and Otology*. 1974; **87**: 589–97.

17. Cotton R. Management of subglottic stenosis in infancy and childhood. Review of a consecutive series of cases managed by surgical reconstruction. *Annals of Otology, Rhinology, and Laryngology*. 1978; **87**: 649–57.

18. Monnier P, Savary M, Chapuis G. Partial cricoid resection with primary tracheal anastomosis for subglottic stenosis in infants and children. *Laryngoscope.* 1993; **103**: 1273–83.

19. Cotton RT, Gray SD, Miller RP. Update of the Cincinnati experience in pediatric laryngotracheal reconstruction. *Laryngoscope.* 1989; **99**: 1111–6.

20. Ochi JW, Evans JNG, Bailey CM. Pediatric airway reconstruction at Great Ormond Street: a ten-year review, I: Laryngotracheoplasty and laryngotracheal reconstruction. *Annals of Otology, Rhinology, and Laryngology.* 1992; **101**: 465–8.

21. Ndiaye I, Van den Abbeele T, Francois M, Viala P, Tanon-Anoh MJ, Narcy P. Traitement chirurgical des sténoses laryngées de l'enfant. [Surgical management of laryngeal stenosis in children.]. *Annales d'Oto-laryngologie et de Chirurgie Cervico Faciale.* 1999; **116**: 143–8.

22. Monnier P, Lang F, Savary M. Traitement des sténoses sous-glottiques de l'enfant par résection crico-trachéale: expérience lausannoise dans 58 cas [Treatment of subglottis stenosis in children by cricotrachea resection.]. *Annales d'Oto-laryngologie et de Chirurgie Cervico Faciale.* 2001; **118**: 299–305.

23. Rutter MJ, Hartley BEJ, Cotton RT. Cricotracheal resection in children. *Archives of Otolaryngology – Head and Neck Surgery.* 2001; **127**: 289–92.

24. Ferguson CF, Flake CG. Subglottic haemangioma as a cause of respiratory obstruction in infants. *Annals of Otology, Rhinology, and Laryngology.* 1961; **70**: 1095–112.

25. Sebastian B, Kleinsasser O. Zur behandlung der kehlkopfhämangiome bei kindern [The treatment of laryngeal hemangioma in children.]. *Laryngologie, Rhinologie und Otologie (Stuttgart).* 1984; **63**: 403–07.

26. Sie KCY, McGill T, Healy GB. Subglottic hemangioma: ten years' experience with the carbon dioxide laser. *Annals of Otology, Rhinology, and Laryngology.* 1994; **103**: 167–72.

27. Narcy P, Contencin P, Bobin S, Manac'h Y. Treatment of infantile subglottic haemangioma. A report of 49 cases. *International Journal of Pediatric Otorhinolaryngology.* 1985; **9**: 157–64.

28. Ohlms LA, Jones DT, McGill TJ, Healy GB. Interferon alfa-2a therapy for airway hemangiomas. *Annals of Otology, Rhinology, and Laryngology.* 1994; **103**: 1–8.

29. Hoeve LJ, Kuppers GLE, Verwoerd CDA. Management of infantile subglottic hemangioma: laser vaporization, submucous resection, intubation, or intralesional steroids. *International Journal of Pediatric Otorhinolaryngology.* 1997; **42**: 179–86.

30. Bailey CM, Froehlich P, Hoeve HLJ. Management of subglottic haemangioma. *Journal of Laryngology and Otology.* 1998; **112**: 765–8.

31. Benjamin B, Inglis A. Minor congenital laryngeal clefts: diagnosis and classification. *Annals of Otology, Rhinology, and Laryngology.* 1989; **98**: 417–20.

32. Mathur NM, Peek GJ, Bailey CM, Elliott MJ. Strategies for managing Type IV laryngotracheoesophageal clefts at Great Ormond Street Hospital for Children. *International Journal of Pediatric Otorhinolaryngology.* 2006; **70**: 1901–10.

33. Evans KL, Courtney-Harris R, Bailey CM, Evans JNG, Parsons DS. Management of posterior laryngeal and laryngotracheoesophageal clefts. *Archives of Otolaryngology – Head and Neck Surgery.* 1995; **121**: 1380–5.

34. Shehab ZP, Bailey CM. Type IV laryngotracheoesophageal clefts – recent 5 year experience at Great Ormond Street Hospital for Children. *International Journal of Pediatric Otorhinolaryngology.* 2001; **60**: 1–9.

35. Perepelitsyn I, Shapshay SM. Endoscopic treatment of laryngeal and tracheal stenosis – has mitomycin C improved the outcome? *Otolaryngology and Head and Neck Surgery.* 2004; **131**: 16–20.

36. Berdon WE, Backer DH, Wung JT, Chrispin A, Koslowski K, de Silva M et al. Complete cartilage-ring tracheal stenosis associated with anomalous left pulmonary artery: the ring-sling complex. *Radiology.* 1984; **152**: 57–64.

37. Tsang V, Murday A, Gillbe C, Goldstraw P. Slide tracheoplasty for congenital funnel-shaped tracheal stenosis. *Annals of Thoracic Surgery.* 1989; **48**: 632–5.

38. Grillo HC. Slide tracheoplasty for long-segment congenital tracheal stenosis. *Annals of Thoracic Surgery.* 1994; **58**: 613–9.

39. Andrews TM, Cotton RT, Bailey WW, Myer CM, Vester SR. Tracheoplasty for congenital complete tracheal rings. *Archives of Otolaryngology – Head and Neck Surgery.* 1994; **120**: 1363–9.

40. Jacobs JP, Elliott MJ, Haw MP, Bailey CM, Herberhold C. Pediatric tracheal homograft reconstruction: a novel approach to complex tracheal stenosis in children. *Journal of Thoracic and Cardiovascular Surgery.* 1996; **112**: 1549–60.

* 41. Elliott M, Roebuck D, Noctor C, McLaren C, Hartley B, Mok Q et al. The management of congenital tracheal stenosis. *International Journal of Pediatric Otorhinolaryngology.* 2003; **67**: S183–92.

42. Mair EA, Parsons DS. Pediatric tracheobronchomalacia and major airway collapse. *Annals of Otology, Rhinology, and Laryngology.* 1992; **101**: 300–09.

43. Smith RJ, Smith MC, Glossop LP, Bailey CM, Evans JN. Congenital vascular anomalies causing tracheoesophageal compression. *Archives of Otolaryngology – Head and Neck Surgery.* 1984; **110**: 82–7.

* 44. Senders CW. Use of mitomycin C in the pediatric airway. *Current Opinion in Otolaryngology and Head and Neck Surgery.* 2004; **12**: 473–5.

45. Hartnick CJ, Hartley BE, Lacy PD, Liu J, Bean JA, Willging JP et al. Topical mitomycin application after laryngotracheal reconstruction: a randomized, double-blind, placebo-controlled trial. *Archives of Otolaryngology – Head and Neck Surgery.* 2001; **127**: 1260–4.

89

Laryngeal stenosis

MICHAEL J RUTTER AND ROBIN T COTTON

Introduction	1150	Complications	1165
Paediatric laryngeal anatomy	1151	Key points	1165
Evaluation	1151	Best clinical practice	1165
Considerations prior to laryngeal reconstruction	1155	Deficiencies in current knowledge and areas for future	
Therapy	1155	research	1166
Contraindications	1165	References	1166

SEARCH STRATEGY

The data in this chapter are supported by a Medline search using the key words paediatric, laryngeal, subglottic, glottic, posterior glottic, web, supraglottic, stenosis; laryngotracheoplasty; laryngotracheal reconstruction; and cricotracheal resection. The focus is on evaluation, management and surgery.

INTRODUCTION

Over the past 40 years, there has been a marked evolution in the presentation and management of paediatric laryngeal stenosis. Prior to 1965, this diagnosis indicated the presence of a congenital anterior glottic web or congenital subglottic stenosis. In many children, congenital subglottic stenosis could be anticipated to improve with time, even if placement of a temporary tracheotomy tube was required. The advent of prolonged intubation, particularly of the neonate, strikingly changed this situation. Acquired subglottic stenosis became and currently remains the most frequent cause of laryngeal stenosis. This condition is generally more severe than congenital subglottic stenosis and does not improve with time. Modern paediatric laryngeal reconstruction was thus born of necessity to manage these otherwise healthy, but tracheotomy-dependent children.

Further improvements in neonatal care, particularly the use of nasopharyngeal continuous positive airway pressure (CPAP), led to a significant decline in the incidence of acquired subglottic stenosis in children without other medical problems. The evolution of neonatal care has resulted in the salvage of premature and often medically fragile children whose laryngeal pathology is but one component of a myriad of health issues. The overall care of such children is more complex to manage, ideally requiring an interdisciplinary team approach. In addition, their laryngeal pathology is more severe, with stenosis potentially involving not only the subglottis but also the supraglottis or glottis. While subglottic stenosis is far more common than glottic or supraglottic stenosis, it is not uncommon for combined pathology to be seen.

Laryngeal stenosis continues to cause significant morbidity and mortality, whether or not patients are tracheotomy dependent. The primary aim of intervention is decannulation or preventing the need for tracheotomy. In selected patients, voice restoration or provision of a safer airway is the primary consideration, with decannulation being a secondary goal.

These children are primarily cared for in paediatric centres where management has evolved in response to experience and as determined by the needs of the individual child. For many of the strategies described, randomized controlled trials are neither appropriate nor available, hence the evidence levels presented for the recommendations in this chapter are largely 3 and 4.

PAEDIATRIC LARYNGEAL ANATOMY

Compared with the adult larynx, the infant larynx lies high in the neck, with the hyoid bone overriding its superior aspect. The narrowest point in the infant airway is the cricoid ring. Since this is the only fixed ring within the airway, it is the most vulnerable point for iatrogenic damage caused by intubation. In a term newborn, the diameter of the subglottis is between 4.5 and 5.5 mm. If the airway diameter in the term newborn is less than 4 mm, subglottic stenosis is present. A useful guideline is that the outer diameter of a 3.0 mm endotracheal tube is 4.2 mm.

The superior margin of the supraglottis comprises the superior edge of the epiglottis, the aryepiglottic folds and the arytenoids, while the inferior margin is at the level of the true vocal folds. The glottis comprises the true vocal folds and the glottic chink. In the infant, the posterior 50 percent of the true vocal fold consists of the vocal process of the arytenoid. The subglottis lies between the under-surface of the vocal fold and the lower border of the cricoid cartilage. The subglottic mucosa is lined with respiratory epithelium. A transition to squamous epithelium occurs at the free edge of the true vocal fold.

EVALUATION

History

A child with laryngeal stenosis may present with stridor, extubation failure or tracheotomy dependency. In each of these clinical scenarios, a meticulous initial history forms the basis for further evaluation and investigation. It is important for clinicians to determine the overall health status of the child, exploring signs or symptoms and being aware of a past diagnosis of gastro-oesophageal reflux, aspiration, lung disease or cardiac disease.

In a child presenting with stridor, the duration of stridor must first be ascertained. If acute, stridor is a medical emergency. When it is more chronic, its mode of onset should be ascertained and the determination of whether it is stable or progressive should be made. In addition, the degree of compromise to the child's lifestyle should be assessed, particularly with regard to exercise intolerance and shortness of breath on exertion. Some children will also experience obstructive symptoms during sleep. These symptoms are usually associated with supraglottic pathology although they may be indicative of a second nonlaryngeal pathology such as adenotonsillar hypertrophy. The aetiology of the child's compromised

airway should also be sought, in particular, any prior history of intubation. If there has been such a history, relevant details such as the duration of intubation, the temporal relationship between intubation and the onset of airway symptoms, and whether an age-appropriate endotracheal tube was used should be determined.

The reason for intubation should be assessed, as should any medical problems that could contribute to extubation failure. The relevant history should include the length of time the child was intubated, the size of the endotracheal tube, the number of attempts at extubation and whether extubation failure abruptly occurred following endotracheal tube removal or was due to gradual and progressive respiratory compromise necessitating reintubation.

In a child with tracheotomy dependency, the aetiology requiring initial placement of a tracheotomy should be ascertained and the duration of cannulation and size of the tracheotomy tube should be determined. Any history of airway reconstruction surgery is also extremely important. Another significant aspect of a thorough assessment is an evaluation of voice quality and the ability to tolerate a speech valve.

Physical examination

Once a case history has been taken, the presence of stridor and retractions at rest should be assessed. The nature of the stridor, in particular whether it is purely inspiratory, expiratory or biphasic, should be noted. Assessment of voice quality is particularly important in that it may provide an indication of the anatomic region of the pathology. Children with supraglottic stenosis usually present with a characteristic muffled or 'throaty' voice, while those with anterior glottic webbing tend to have a very hoarse voice. Those with posterior glottic stenosis and subglottic stenosis usually have normal voice quality. In a child presenting with extubation failure, nonlaryngeal causes such as nasal obstruction and glossoptosis are explored. In cases of tracheotomy dependency, the size of the tracheotomy tube, the child's ability to tolerate a speech valve and the possibility of tracheotomy tube plugging are pursued.

Imaging studies

Radiologic evaluation of the paediatric airway is most helpful in patients who are neither intubated nor tracheotomy dependent. Imaging studies fall into two time-related categories: those that are performed prior to endoscopic evaluation and those that are best after endoscopic evaluation. Prior to endoscopy, soft tissue airway films of the neck and chest should be performed in both lateral and anterior/posterior projections. These are useful in evaluating laryngeal stenosis and may also give timely warning of a possible tracheal stenosis. Anterior/

posterior and lateral chest films indicate possible under-lying lung pathology. A barium swallow study may not only provide information on the ability to swallow and the relative risk of aspiration but may also indicate the need to evaluate the airway for a posterior laryngeal cleft or a tracheo-oesophageal fistula. In addition, it may provide information on a child's propensity to gastro-oesophageal reflux, vascular compression of the airway and the presence of an oesophageal foreign body.

After endoscopic airway evaluation, more directed imaging studies are valuable. Spiral computed tomography (CT) scanning of the airway with contrast enhancement provides a useful view of intrathoracic vasculature. Although both magnetic resonance imaging (MRI) and magnetic resonance angiography (MRA) also provide excellent views of intrathoracic vascular anatomy, they require more time to perform and are more likely to require sedation or anaesthesia. In younger children CT and MRI airway evaluation may complement endoscopic evaluation, but nevertheless cannot be considered definitive (see Chapter 102, Imaging in paediatric ENT).

In children with upper airway compromise, sleep fluoroscopy or cine magnetic resonance may provide a valuable dynamic airway assessment.

Endoscopic airway evaluation

FLEXIBLE NASOPHARYNGOSCOPY

In a child who has not been evaluated previously, flexible nasopharyngoscopy with the child awake should be performed prior to rigid endoscopy. The nasal passages, nasopharynx, oropharynx, supraglottic and glottic airway should be assessed, and pathology such as choanal atresia, adenoid hypertrophy, tonsillar hypertrophy, laryngomalacia and vocal cord paralysis should be excluded. To avoid the risk of inducing laryngospasm, the nasopharyngoscope should not be advanced below the level of the glottis. Although the precise mechanism is unclear, laryngospasm may happen even in children with bilateral true vocal cord paralysis.

RIGID ENDOSCOPY

It must be emphasized that evaluation of the paediatric airway should not be considered a minor procedure, particularly when performed in a child with an unstable airway (see Chapter 86, Stridor). Extreme care must be taken not to exacerbate the child's condition. The surgical and anaesthetic team must work together closely and must have specific knowledge of the paediatric airway and of appropriate instrumentation. In a child with a compromised airway, who does not have a tracheotomy tube, preoperative administration of dexamethasone, 0.5 mg/kg up to a maximum of 20 mg, is a prudent precaution.

Rigid endoscopy remains the 'gold standard' for paediatric airway evaluation, and this evaluation should begin with an assessment of the supralaryngeal airway. The possible presence of retrognathia and any associated glossoptosis or difficulty of laryngeal exposure should be initially assessed, as should tonsillar hypertrophy or evidence of pharyngeal scarring. The supraglottic larynx should be carefully assessed for scarring, laryngomalacia, short aryepiglottic folds and arytenoid prolapse. The glottis should be evaluated for scarring, anterior glottic webbing and posterior glottic stenosis, and care should be taken to exclude the presence of a posterior laryngeal cleft. If vocal motion is clearly seen, it can be assumed that neither true vocal cord is paralyzed. If, however, movement is not observed, nasopharyngoscopy with the patient awake should be performed. The subglottis should be evaluated, and any stenosis or scarring noted. If stenosis is present, its severity, length, position and physical characteristics should be noted. It may be characterized as soft or firm, as concentric or with lateral shelving, and with mucosa appearing either quiescent or actively inflamed.

If there is a sufficient lumen to allow passage of the endoscope, the trachea is next assessed. Hopkins rod endoscopes with an outer diameter as small as 1.9 mm are available, and can negotiate most grade III subglottic stenoses. An assessment is made of the upper trachea, including the tracheotomy stoma site, looking for suprastomal collapse or the presence of a suprastomal granuloma. Assessment is also made of possible tracheomalacia and vascular compression of the airway. Although complete tracheal rings are rare, their possible presence should be evaluated cautiously, so as not to induce oedema within an already compromised segment of airway. The carina and mainstem bronchi are also evaluated.

If subglottic stenosis has been identified, the area of stenosis should be graded according to the Myer–Cotton classification[1] (see **Table 89.1**). This is best carried out utilizing endotracheal tubes, with a small tube being placed initially. If this tube leaks at less than 20 cm of water pressure through the subglottis, the next larger size is placed. It should be noted that the Myer–Cotton grading system is not designed to address supraglottic, glottic or tracheal stenosis.

ANAESTHETIC TECHNIQUE DURING BRONCHOSCOPY

A collaborative relationship with the anaesthetist is essential in deciding upon the specific anaesthetic technique to be used when performing rigid endoscopy. Possible options include spontaneous ventilation, assisted ventilation, jet ventilation and apnoea with intermittent bag and mask ventilation. Spontaneous ventilation offers the best dynamic assessment of the airway and is thus recommended. Endoscopy may be performed with the laryngoscope introduced into the airway and suspended in position. This frees both the surgeon's hands for introduction of a telescope and instruments as required. Some surgeons prefer to expose the larynx with an

Table 89.1 The Myer–Cotton classification.

Grade	From	To	Examples

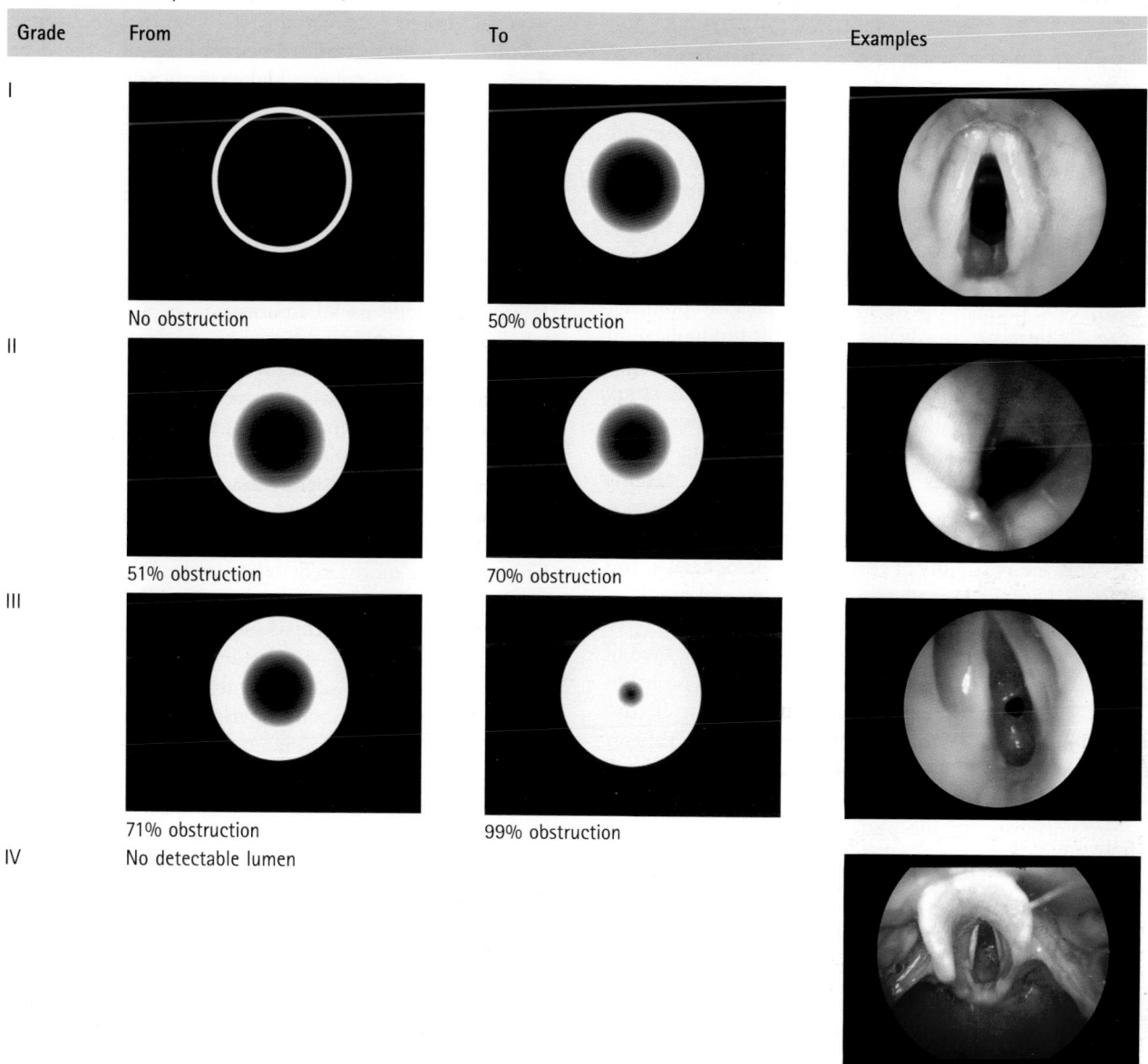

I	No obstruction	50% obstruction	
II	51% obstruction	70% obstruction	
III	71% obstruction	99% obstruction	
IV	No detectable lumen		

Redrawn from Ref. 1, with permission.

anaesthetic laryngoscope blade held in one hand and use the other hand to introduce a telescope. Endoscopy may also be performed with a ventilating bronchoscope or a Hopkins rod telescope, keeping in mind that the technique itself is not as important as the information gained. We prefer to use the Hopkins rod telescope, exposing the larynx with a straight anaesthetic laryngoscope blade. The child spontaneously ventilates a mixture of sevoflurane and oxygen through an endotracheal tube placed in the oropharynx, and with additional intravenous anesthesia provided by propofol bolus.

FLEXIBLE BRONCHOSCOPY

In selected children, flexible bronchoscopy may complement rigid bronchoscopy and both may occasionally be required to evaluate a child's airway adequately. Also, in many instances, these techniques can be used interchangeably. In some cases, however, each technique offers clear advantages. Rigid bronchoscopy provides a superior assessment of the larynx, especially the posterior glottic area. Flexible bronchoscopy is often extremely valuable in assessing a larynx that is difficult to access with rigid instrumentation and may provide valuable information about airway dynamics, such as the degree of pharyngeal collapse, glossoptosis and the presence of laryngomalacia, tracheomalacia or bronchomalacia. Flexible bronchoscopy also permits evaluation beyond the eighth generation of bronchi in older children and allows specific lavage of bronchial subsegments, which may provide information about silent aspiration if lipid-laden macrophages are found.

Gastrointestinal evaluation

OESOPHAGOGASTRODUODENOSCOPY, OESOPHAGEAL BIOPSY AND pH PROBE

In selected cases, particularly in patients with complex underlying medical conditions or in those who have failed previous airway reconstruction, oesophagogastroduodenoscopy may be beneficial in the assessment of a child prior to airway reconstruction. Oesophagogastroduodenoscopy can provide information about oesophagitis, gastritis and the status of the lower oesophageal sphincter, especially in regard to whether a previous fundoplication is still functional.

Preoperative evaluation of gastro-oesophageal reflux with dual probe pH monitoring and/or oesophageal biopsy is advisable, and should be mandatory in a child with an active larynx or recalcitrant airway stenosis following previous reconstruction.[2] [**/*] Oesophageal biopsy will also provide information about oesophagitis, including the possibility of eosinophilic oesophagitis, and is currently the only method of diagnosing and monitoring this condition.

Placement of a pH probe may be done at the time of oesophagogastroduodenoscopy, at the time of bronchoscopic evaluation or may be performed as an elective procedure unrelated to endoscopic evaluation. Patients should be off antireflux medication for at least one week prior to pH probe placement. A dual pH probe with the upper port lying in the postcricoid region is desirable. While normal paediatric values for the upper port do not exist, positive readings should be viewed with suspicion. The recently developed impedance probe not only measures acid, but can also provide an indication of the volume of a reflux bolus and the height in the oesophagus to which it progresses. Impedance technology also allows evaluation of nonacid reflux. This enables a child to remain on antireflux medication prior to evaluation.[3] [**/*] While this technology is promising, no paediatric norms yet exist, and interpretation of the vast amount of data generated by an impedance probe is both time-consuming and challenging.

Evaluation of aspiration

Paediatric airway reconstruction runs the inherent risk of turning a child with laryngeal stenosis into a chronic aspirator. While this risk cannot always be accurately evaluated preoperatively, in most cases a thorough evaluation provides ample warning signs. Recurrent pneumonia and an insidious drop in a child's baseline oxygen saturation are highly suggestive of chronic aspiration. A history of previous aspiration or current aspiration is extremely important. In a child who is tracheotomy dependent, copious tracheotomy secretions or secretions stained by food material indicate chronic aspiration. This is more difficult to evaluate in a child who is entirely gastrostomy (G-tube) fed. A simple solution is intermittently to place a drop of green food dye on the child's tongue and evaluate whether green-stained secretions are subsequently suctioned from the tracheotomy tube. Alternatively, a radio nucleotide spit study may be performed; a drop of radioactive material is placed on the tongue and its passage is monitored to either the stomach or lung fields. In a child suspected of aspirating, a bronchoalveolar lavage, which can identify lipid-laden macrophages, may be useful. This does not, however, provide useful information in a child who is wholly G-tube fed. Children with grade IV subglottic stenosis, in whom aspiration is not possible prior to laryngotracheal reconstruction, present a particular challenge. In these children, preoperative evaluation to assess the relative risk of aspiration is strongly advocated.

A barium swallow or video swallow study may provide information not only on the presence of aspiration, but also on what substances are most likely to be aspirated. Thin fluids are more likely to be aspirated than purees or solids.

A functional endoscopic evaluation of swallowing, whereby the larynx is visualized with a nasopharyngoscope while a child swallows food or drink, can provide valuable information about the relevant risk of aspiration and the mechanism of aspiration as well as the presence or absence of normal laryngeal sensation.

Having knowledge of the possibility of postoperative aspiration allows for appropriate preoperative counselling and management to minimize this risk. Innately, there are three things that may be aspirated, namely food and drink presented by mouth, saliva and gastric reflux. The respective risk of each can be minimized by conversion to G-tube feeding, reducing saliva production through a 'drool' procedure, and performing a fundoplication. Most children and families presented with the choice of a gastrostomy tube or a tracheotomy tube will chose the former.

Sleep evaluation

A formal sleep evaluation may be a useful method to evaluate a child's respiratory efforts and oxygen needs, whether or not a tracheotomy is in place. The primary aim of laryngotracheal reconstruction is decannulation, and this operative procedure is rarely warranted if decannulation cannot be achieved. In children with tracheotomy dependency, it is important to evaluate whether surgical correction of laryngeal stenosis will permit decannulation. In children with significant lung disease, particularly bronchopulmonary dysplasia or in those who are dependent on a ventilator or CPAP, decannulation may be imprudent. Similarly, children with progressive neuromuscular disorders, diaphragmatic weakness or central hyperventilation syndrome, may not be candidates for decannulation. If results of a sleep evaluation indicate pulmonary compromise that precludes decannulation, laryngeal reconstruction may be futile.

Voice evaluation

Voice evaluation in children with laryngeal stenosis, tracheotomy dependency or following laryngotracheal reconstruction is in its infancy and is poorly understood. It is clear, however, that laryngeal reconstruction can have a negative impact on the voice, particularly in children requiring supraglottic or glottic surgery and in those in whom a laryngofissure is required to reconstruct the airway. What is unclear is which underlying pathologies and reconstructive procedures place the voice at greatest risk, and also the extent to which a voice anomaly relates to the initial aetiology of the laryngotracheal stenosis.

Children have a tremendous drive to communicate, which often compensates for severe anatomic dysfunction. Some children will retain a surprisingly good-quality voice, even with a grade III subglottic stenosis. However, children with a grade IV subglottic stenosis are aphonic unless they have learned oesophageal speech techniques. In these children, laryngotracheal reconstruction may be extremely beneficial in terms of regaining voice, even if decannulation is not achieved.

CONSIDERATIONS PRIOR TO LARYNGEAL RECONSTRUCTION

Surgical intervention for laryngeal stenosis is not always warranted, and the decision as to whether or not to perform such surgery is generally predicated by the overall health status of the child rather than by the stenosis itself. In a child with a high risk for aspiration or with certain craniofacial anomalies, surgical reconstruction may be inappropriate in that the laryngeal stenosis may actually protect the lungs from aspiration. In some children, ongoing aspiration may lead to a consideration of laryngotracheal separation rather than laryngeal reconstruction. Similarly, in children with other significant medical conditions, such as those requiring CPAP, bilevel positive airway pressure (BiPAP) or ventilator support, reconstruction is unwise. While not universally accepted or rigorously proven, most experts in paediatric laryngotracheal reconstruction believe that gastro-oesophageal reflux disease is both a cofactor for the development of subglottic stenosis and a negative influence on the outcome of operative reconstruction. Oxacillin or methacillin-resistant *Staphlococcus aureus* (MRSA) screening prior to open airway surgery is also recommended, as postoperative infection may greatly compromise the surgical repair. Although a child with a progressive neuromuscular disorder may be considered for laryngotracheal reconstruction to improve vocal function, this seldom enables long-term decannulation.

In some children, a period of observation prior to considering surgical intervention is the best course of action. This strategy is most appropriate in a child with an active or inflamed larynx that is not amenable to medical intervention. An active larynx is generally related to gastro-oesophageal reflux disease or eosinophilic oesophagitis and is, therefore, potentially amenable to such intervention. In children in whom the aetiology of an active larynx is unknown, laryngeal reconstruction is unwise until the laryngeal inflammation has improved. This often occurs spontaneously within a one- to two-year period. A waiting period is also advisable in a child who has recalcitrant stenosis after a recent airway reconstruction, or in a child whose larynx is healing from laryngeal trauma. While only a guideline, a six-month 'cooling off' period is often advisable in such children.

Although weight is a less important factor than the overall health status of a child and the child's laryngeal disease, it is a frequently used criterion for postponement of airway reconstruction. While laryngotracheal reconstruction can be effectively performed in children less than 3 kg if other criteria permit, a 10 kg guideline is most commonly used. Nevertheless, airway reconstruction of a larger child is technically much easier to perform.

The child with complex medical problems

Historically, children presenting for airway reconstruction were otherwise healthy children with a stenosed larynx. Increasingly, however, children presenting for airway reconstruction have multifaceted complex medical problems, most commonly related to either extreme prematurity or syndromic conditions (see Chapter 64, ENT input for children with special needs). In such children, an interdisciplinary team approach is advisable for adequate assessment both before and after planned reconstruction. The most important decision to be made is whether it is advisable to even attempt reconstruction. If so, consideration must be given to other interventions indicated prior to proceeding with laryngeal reconstruction. In a child with reflux disease, a fundoplication may be required. In a child with aspiration, a 'drool' procedure may be required. It is prudent to have most of these children undergo additional evaluation by paediatric subspecialists in pulmonology, gastroenterology, medical genetics and neurology.

THERAPY

Medical therapy

When the larynx is stable and quiescent there is no role for medical therapy. In the inflamed or active larynx, however, medical therapy plays an important role in alleviating laryngeal inflammation which, in turn, enhances the potential for a successful operative outcome. In children with subglottic stenosis, medical therapy alone occasionally obviates the need for laryngeal reconstruction by providing sufficient improvement to permit decannulation.

Medical therapy for an inflamed larynx revolves around treatment of gastro-oesophageal reflux disease or eosinophilic oesophagitis. If reflux is diagnosed or even suspected, then a low threshold for treatment with H_2 antagonists or proton pump inhibitors is recommended. In children with recalcitrant acidic reflux or significant nonacid reflux, consideration should be given to performing fundoplication.

A recent observation has been the correlation between eosinophilic oesophagitis, laryngeal inflammation and a poor outcome following laryngotracheal reconstruction.[4] [**/*] Eosinophilic oesophagitis has a characteristic appearance on oesophagogastroduodenoscopy, with oesophageal furrows often having microscopic white plaques noted. However, the definitive diagnosis is made on biopsy, with greater than 20 eosinophils per high-power field being noted. In children with eosinophilic oesophagitis, evaluation for underlying food allergies is indicated. In children in whom a food allergy is not proven, treatment with oral fluticasone is suggested. An initial dosing regimen of 440 µg, sprayed on the tongue twice a day and swallowed, is usually efficacious. Follow-up oesophagoscopy with further biopsies to confirm resolution of disease is suggested prior to undertaking laryngeal reconstruction, which is usually delayed for six months.

Tracheotomy

In a child with an unsafe or unstable airway in whom laryngotracheal reconstruction is not immediately advisable, temporary placement of the tracheotomy tube is advisable to secure an adequate airway until laryngeal reconstruction can be performed. Placement of a tracheotomy should be performed with a view to the subsequent laryngeal reconstruction that may be required. A high tracheotomy close to the cricoid increases the risk of exacerbation of stenosis, but may make subsequent cricotracheal resection (CTR) simpler as a shorter segment of airway can then be resected. Tracheotomy through the second to fourth tracheal rings is still recommended.

Although a tracheotomy provides a safer airway in a child with laryngotracheal stenosis, the airway is by no means completely safe. Tracheotomy-related deaths continue to occur in children who could otherwise anticipate good long-term quality of life, and the greater the degree of obstruction, the greater the risk. A tracheotomy is a marked compromise on both a child's and a family's quality of life and emotional health.

Laryngeal reconstruction

Laryngeal and upper tracheal reconstruction may be challenging and no single operation can adequately address all types of laryngeal stenosis. It is thus prudent to evaluate each child on an individual basis. In some patients, the most appropriate reconstruction technique may not become fully clear until the airway has been opened and the pathology directly inspected. The mainstay of laryngotracheal reconstruction is expansion cartilage grafting (**Figure 89.1**). In the subglottis an alternative to this approach is resection and reanastomosis. Stenosis involving the supraglottis and anterior glottis is amenable to laryngoplasty without cartilage grafting.

GRAFTING MATERIALS

Costal cartilage is the most widely used grafting material, with excellent results noted on prolonged follow-up.[5, 6] [**] It is readily available, robust and easily shaped and carved. Moreover, it is possible to harvest more than one graft through the same incision. The usual donor site is the right fifth or sixth rib, with the incision being placed in the anticipated breast crease in girls for cosmetic reasons. The harvested graft should include the perichondrium on the lateral aspect of the graft, while leaving the inner perichondrial layer intact at the donor site to allow the potential for some cartilage regeneration. Once the graft is harvested, filling the wound with saline and performing a Valsalva manoeuvre will ensure that a breach of the pleura has not occurred. When the graft is carved to the desired shape, the perichondrium should face the lumen of the airway; lateral flanges will prevent prolapse of the graft into the airway.

When only a small graft is required, thyroid ala is a useful material. This is usually taken from the upper aspect of the thyroid cartilage on one side, at least 1 mm above true vocal cord level. Thyroid ala has the advantage of being quickly and easily harvested from within the surgical field. However, only a limited amount of grafting material is available, and it is not amenable to being carved with flanges.

Auricular cartilage is also useful, in particular for the management of suprastomal collapse as part of a single-stage procedure. It is easily harvested and reasonably abundant. It makes an ideal cap or overlay graft, particularly over a stoma site, but is comparatively weak and not appropriate for insertion between the cut edges of the cricoid. In both adults and older children there is no cosmetic donor site deformity, but in children under one year of age it is common to have some residual asymmetry of the ears.

Other grafting materials include buccal mucosa, septal cartilage and a pedicled hyoid bone interposition graft. The results utilizing these grafting materials in children have been disappointing. Another described technique is

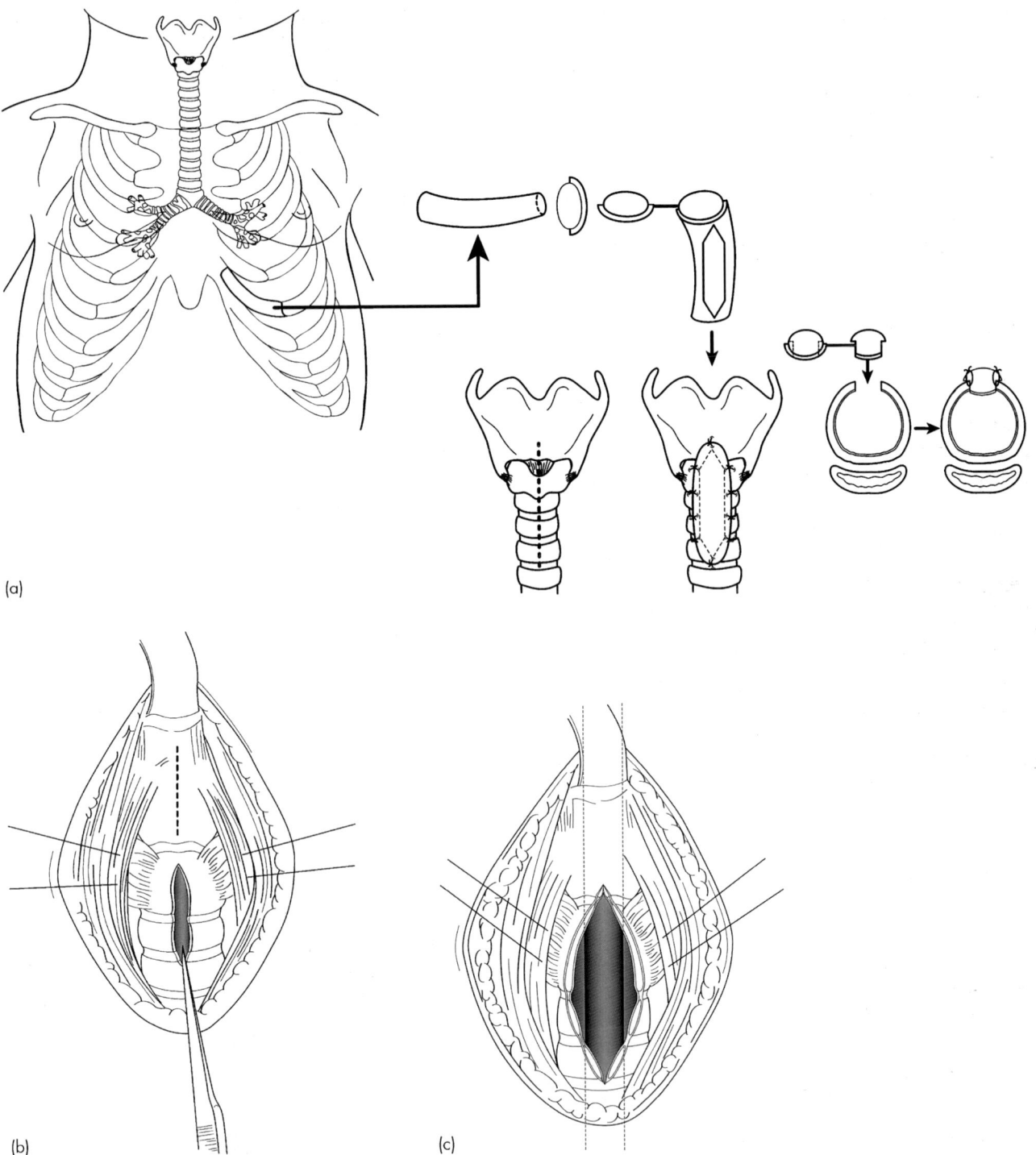

(a)

(b)

(c)

Figure 89.1 Expansion cartilage grafting.

the use of a clavicular periosteal graft, with its vascularity maintained by swinging the graft up on a pedicle of sternocleidomastoid muscle. This is a useful graft in older children in whom there is a significant deficit of tracheal cartilage, as after several months the graft will start to ossify, thereby providing support to the airway. Unfortunately, in prepubescent children the graft seems less amenable to ossification, leaving the airway malacic.

STENTS

Not all laryngotracheal reconstruction techniques require stent placement. It may not be required in an anterior flanged graft for moderate subglottic stenosis, however, it is advisable in virtually all other circumstances. Stenting maintains a lumen and prevents graft prolapse during postoperative healing, and may remain in place for days to months. Longer-term stents are advisable when the laryngeal repair is unstable (e.g. when a posterior cricoid split has been performed in an older child without placement of a cartilage graft), or in a recalcitrant larynx that has failed previous reconstruction. In patients in whom graft survival is threatened, such as diabetic patients and patients on continuous steroids, long-term stenting without cartilage grafts is advisable. The most commonly used stent is the Aboulker Teflon suprastomal stent (**Figure 89.2**). It is critical that the lower end of this stent does not overlap the tracheotomy site, as this creates the risk of being unable to reinsert a tracheotomy tube during a tracheotomy change. In addition, in some children the cut lower end of the stent is prone to inciting granulation tissue above the stoma site and eventually forms fibrosis and scarring. Suprastomal stents should thus, ideally, be removed within six weeks, as any granulation tissue that has formed during this time will spontaneously resolve.

An alternative to a rigid Teflon suprastomal stent is a softer silicone stent (e.g. the upper limb of a tracheal T-tube). The cut end of this stent is sewn shut and placed in the supraglottis, while its machined smooth end is placed distally to overlap the tracheotomy site slightly. These stents are soft and deformable and do not interfere with placement of the tracheotomy tube. They tend to incite less granulation tissue at the distal end of the stent, and there is less dead space between the distal end of the stent and the tracheotomy tube in which scarring can occur. Unlike the rigid Teflon stents, these soft silastic suprastomal stents may remain in place for longer than

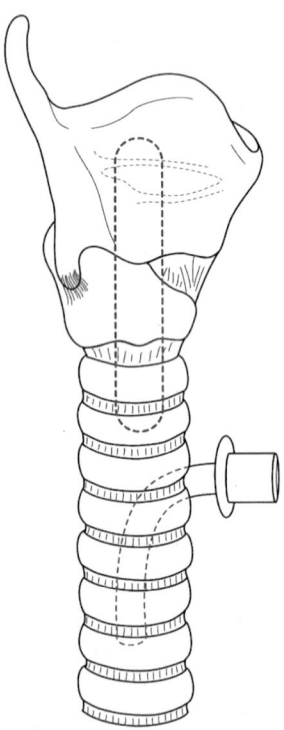

Figure 89.2 Aboulker Teflon suprastomal stent.

six weeks. The proximal end of a suprastomal stent should lie at the level of the false vocal cords. There will be a corresponding restriction of speech, as they permit only limited air passage.

For longer-term stenting, tracheal T-tubes are recommended. Although T-tubes with an outer diameter of 5 mm are commercially available, because of the risk of crusting and obstruction we do not routinely place T-tubes with an outer diameter of less than 8 mm. An 8-mm tube may be placed in a child as young as four years of age. Following laryngeal reconstruction, the upper end of a T-tube is generally passed through the vocal cords. Aspiration is, therefore, a significant risk and is expected for two weeks following stent placement. A supraglottic swallow technique is readily achieved by most children, minimizing the risk of aspiration. Unlike tracheotomy tubes, T-tubes cannot be easily changed. Meticulous T-tube care is thus essential.

SINGLE-STAGE RECONSTRUCTION

In children in whom a stenting period of less than two weeks is anticipated, an option to be considered is intubation, with the endotracheal tube acting as the stent.[7] [**] Intubation for greater than two weeks, however, risks redevelopment of posterior glottic stenosis or subglottic stenosis. For straightforward airway reconstruction, extubation may occur within a few days of the operation or, occasionally, even at the end of the reconstructive procedure. Although the optimal duration of intubation is not clearly defined, there has been a trend towards briefer periods of intubation following laryngotracheal reconstruction. Most children can be extubated within two to seven days of a CTR or an anterior costal cartilage graft. Those with anterior/posterior cartilage grafts are usually intubated for 7–14 days. The older the child, the more forgiving the airway and the briefer the period of intubation required. For more complex airway surgery, a prolonged period of intubation is required.

A prerequisite for single-stage laryngotracheal reconstruction is an excellent intensive care unit (ICU) in which staff are familiar with the management of airway patients. It is undesirable for a child to have an unplanned self-extubation, and security of the nasotracheal tube is paramount. Therefore, in younger children, the use of arm restraints and sedation is usually required. Most children younger than age three require sedation, and children who have been previously intubated for long periods may require heavy sedation. Paralysis is undesirable as in the event of accidental decannulation the child is unable to maintain an airway and reintubation must be emergent. Since any child undergoing a single-stage procedure risks the need for reintubation, single-stage procedures should not be performed on children who are difficult to intubate. In the sedated child, commonly encountered problems include lung atelectasis, fluid overload from heavy sedation, pneumonia and narcotic withdrawal following extubation.

In children older than age three with no major cognitive problems, sedation may not be required. Some of these intubated children may be able to ambulate, eat and visit the playroom. A fully awake child does not require ventilatory support and is less likely to have pulmonary complications from the intubation.

The day prior to extubation, returning to the theatre to inspect the airway and downsize the tracheotomy tube is advisable. If the airway appears adequate to support extubation, a dose of dexamethasone, 0.5 mg/kg, is administered the night before extubation, and the patient is extubated while fully awake. Owing to the risk of laryngeal oedema, the patient should be closely observed on the ICU for the next 24 hours; oedema generally resolves within this period of time. In the event of airway distress following extubation, management options include the administration of racemic adrenaline, further steroids, helium/oxygen administration or even the use of CPAP or BiPAP. If the airway is still not adequate the child may need to be reintubated. If so, a further trial of extubation should be performed a few days later. If this is again unsuccessful a decision is required as to whether to proceed to a third trial of extubation or to proceed with tracheotomy. If a tracheotomy is required, the stoma should ideally be placed low in the neck, below the graft site. Glottic oedema and granulation from endotracheal tube irritation are often the cause of failure during a single-stage procedure, rather than the reconstructed site itself. In such cases, the tracheotomy tube may be removed once the oedema has settled, usually within a few weeks.

The ideal patient for consideration of a single-stage procedure is one in whom a reasonably simple procedure with a stable larynx is anticipated. This single-stage approach is preferable in children in whom a tracheotomy tube has induced suprastomal collapse. Poor candidates for single-stage reconstruction include children with poor pulmonary function, those who are difficult to intubate, those with recalcitrant airway disease who have failed previous reconstruction, and those with complex disease involving multiple levels of obstruction.

Supraglottic stenosis

Supraglottic stenosis is rare, difficult to treat, and is frequently associated with supraglottic collapse. While severe supraglottic stenosis may present with stridor, the primary complaint is more commonly obstructed breathing during sleep. Therefore, a sleep study may be extremely useful in the nontracheotomized patient or in the patient in whom the tracheotomy can be capped, even if for a brief period. The underlying aetiology is often traumatic, due to severe direct airway trauma or airway burns, or is of iatrogenic origin. Supraglottic stenosis with associated collapse is a feature of the airway that has undergone numerous laryngeal reconstructions. Visualization of the supraglottic larynx in cases of supraglottic stenosis and collapse may be misleading. Rigid endoscopic evaluation with the larynx suspended by a laryngoscope may distort the appearance of the larynx, providing false reassurance about the supraglottic airway. Flexible endoscopic evaluation with the patient spontaneously ventilating allows for superior evaluation of the airway dynamics. Nevertheless, what is observed may be deceiving. A larynx that looks extremely compromised in an anaesthetized patient may function quite adequately in the nonanaesthetized state.

In children with mild-to-moderate supraglottic stenosis and collapse, nocturnal CPAP may be very beneficial. The most common patterns of supraglottic compromise are arytenoid prolapse and epiglottic petiole prolapse. Arytenoid prolapse is a dynamic instability of the arytenoid, either unilateral or bilateral. It is characterized by its anterior displacement during inspiration, which may cause significant airway obstruction. This problem most commonly follows previous CTR or previous laryngotracheal reconstruction involving division of the posterior cricoid plate. In CTR, the pathogenesis of arytenoid prolapse may be attributed to division of the lateral cricoarytenoid muscle. In laryngotracheal resection, the pathogenesis of arytenoid prolapse may be attributed to either direct damage to the posterior cricoarytenoid ligament or lateral distraction of the posterior plate of the cricoid.

Arytenoid prolapse is usually managed endoscopically, using a laser to perform a partial arytenoidectomy. The preferred technique is to raise a mucosal flap and debulk the prolapsing cartilage of the arytenoid without damaging the mucosal 'diamond' of the laryngeal inlet. Injudicious use of the laser in the laryngeal inlet predisposes patients to scar formation, fibrosis and narrowing of the supraglottic airway. This, in turn, may induce superimposed supraglottic collapse due to the Bernoulli effect.

Epiglottic petiole prolapse

This presents as a compromised laryngeal inlet owing to the base of the epiglottis (the 'petiole', from the term used to describe the footstalk of a leaf, i.e. the part which connects the blade to the stem) obscuring the anterior true vocal folds and foreshortening the anterior/posterior diameter of the laryngeal inlet. This problem is most commonly seen in children who have had repeated previous laryngofissure, and is a consequence of damage to the thyroepiglottic ligament, where it inserts into the thyroid cartilage just above the anterior commissure. Epiglottic petiole prolapse is rare, and challenging to treat. Injudicious use of a laser in the endolarynx tends to exacerbate the problem, with further scarring narrowing the laryngeal inlet. Suspension of the epiglottic base to the hyoid bone provides some benefit, but is technically challenging and causes the patient significant pain on swallowing for several weeks postoperatively.

Our current management of this challenging problem is to perform a complete laryngofissure and reposition the epiglottic petiole back up to the inner surface of the thyroid ala. The laryngofissure is then closed over a T-tube, which is left in position as a translaryngeal stent for at least six months. These patients have significant problems with aspiration for several weeks postoperatively.

Acquired anterior glottic webs

Anterior glottic webs are most commonly congenital in origin, and are usually associated with a subglottic extension of the web resulting in coexistent subglottic stenosis (see Chapter 88, Congenital disorders of the larynx, trachea and bronchi). Acquired anterior glottic webs are less common and are post-traumatic in origin. There are two common aetiologies: anterior neck trauma, often associated with a fractured larynx; and iatrogenic damage, often associated with injudicious use of a laser at the anterior commissure while managing laryngeal papillomatosis. It is rare for prolonged intubation to induce anterior glottic stenosis unless there is also associated subglottic stenosis.

The management of acquired anterior glottic stenosis differs significantly from the management of the congenital anterior glottic web. The latter has normal mucosa within the remaining glottic inlet, and during reconstruction there may be sufficient mobility of the mucosal layer to reconstruct the anterior commissure without requiring the use of a laryngeal keel. In contrast, acquired anterior glottic stenosis is, by definition, associated with fibrosis and scarring. As such, during reconstruction, following laryngofissure, the mucosa is fibrotic and not amenable to reconstruction of the anterior commissure. Therefore, reconstruction with placement of a laryngeal keel is mandatory while the raw surfaces on either side of the laryngofissure remucosalize.

The usual technique for repair of an acquired anterior glottic web is an open approach with complete laryngofissure, and it is recommended that this is performed with endoscopic guidance. With the laryngofissure complete, the demucosalized raw scar of the anterior vocal folds are noted and, in some cases, there may be enough mucosal mobility to place a pexing suture from the cut edge of the mucosa on either side toward the thyroid ala. Unlike repair of congenital anterior glottic webs, it is unusual to be able to pex the mucosal edge up to the anterior commissure, hence the need for a laryngeal keel. An appropriate size laryngeal keel, such as the Montgomery Keel^{TM}, is then selected and trimmed appropriately. The vertical limb of the keel should not impinge into the posterior commissure. The vertical height of the keel

should separate the raw surfaces of the laryngofissure. The upper limit of the keel should not be so high as to disrupt the insertion of the epiglottic petiole.

The keel is then sewn into place and the laryngofissure closed. This procedure is normally performed as a two-stage procedure, although a single-stage procedure may be performed with the patient intubated and with the endotracheal tube lying on one side of the vertical limb of the keel. In some children there is an associated component of subglottic stenosis, and a decision should be made at this point as to whether the cricoid can be closed adequately over an age-appropriate endotracheal tube. If this is possible, the lower end of the keel should not extend beyond the cricothyroid membrane. If it is not possible, an anterior cartilage graft is placed in the anterior cricoid, distal to the keel.

The keel is removed through an open approach between ten days and four weeks postoperatively. The resultant midline deficit in the thyroid ala is then closed with laterally placed mattress sutures, as the cartilage edges of the laryngofissure are friable and easily damaged if sutures pull out. For this reason, antibiotic coverage and antireflux measures are advised during the period that the keel is in place, and for an additional few days after keel removal.

Endoscopic placement of the laryngeal keel is also a consideration, although this is technically more challenging and may require more specialized equipment. This technique is best suited for adults and older children.

Posterior glottic stenosis

Posterior glottic stenosis is frequently misdiagnosed and often confused with bilateral true vocal cord paralysis. It may exist as an isolated entity or in combination with subglottic stenosis. The most frequent aetiology of this condition is prolonged intubation, with the older child being at greater risk than the neonate. The posterior glottis is also susceptible to damage from thermal injury caused by inhalational or airway fires, or to iatrogenic damage from use of the laser in the posterior commissure. Occasionally, posterior glottic stenosis may be a result of direct laryngeal trauma.

If not already tracheotomy dependent, patients present with stridor and exertional dyspnoea. Normal vocal function is usually preserved and, in this regard, presenting symptomatology is extremely similar to that seen in bilateral vocal cord paralysis. Definitive diagnosis requires assessment with rigid bronchoscopy, which confirms the presence of posterior glottic scarring, as a rigid telescope provides excellent visualization of the posterior glottis. Posterior glottic stenosis can, however, be misdiagnosed on bronchoscopy if the telescope is passed directly through the vocal folds to evaluate the subglottis without proactive inspection of the posterior glottis. Bronchoscopic evaluation should also include assessment of the subglottis, which is frequently involved with scarring. An assessment of arytenoid mobility is required as cricoarytenoid joint fixation is an occasional co-pathology. Formal sizing of the airway utilizing endotracheal tubes may be misleading. Posterior glottic stenosis may limit the size of the endotracheal tube that may be inserted. In some cases, however, the vocal folds easily bow laterally to accommodate an age-appropriate endotracheal tube despite still being tethered posteriorly, compromising the airway. It should again be emphasized that the Myer–Cotton grading system is only truly applicable to subglottic stenosis.

While flexible bronchoscopy provides a poor view of the posterior glottis and is an inadequate method of diagnosing posterior glottic stenosis, awake flexible nasopharyngoscopy may be extremely useful in determining whether vocal fold function is intact. The usual finding is that the vocal folds are mobile but tethered and unable to abduct. It is rare for bilateral vocal cord paralysis and posterior glottic stenosis to coexist.

The differential diagnosis for posterior glottic stenosis commonly includes subglottic stenosis (which frequently may also be present), an interarytenoid scar band and cricoarytenoid joint fixation. In children referred for the management of posterior glottic stenosis, it is rare to find vocal cord paralysis. By contrast, children referred for the management of bilateral vocal cord paralysis may, in fact, have posterior glottic stenosis tethering the vocal cords and masquerading as vocal cord paralysis.

Placement of a posterior costal chondral graft is the mainstay of management and is a highly effective way of achieving an adequate glottic airway.[8, 9] [**] This procedure is best performed through an anterior approach, traditionally through a complete laryngofissure. This approach allows excellent exposure of the posterior glottis and direct visualization of the posterior glottic scar band. The posterior glottis is then infiltrated with 1 percent Xylocaine with adrenaline. The needle is guided through the posterior plate of the cricoid in the midline until it can be felt to pop through into the space between the posterior cricoid and the oesophagus. A further small amount of Xylocaine and adrenaline may then be injected in two or three positions down the cricoid. This has the advantage of not only providing haemostasis in the postcricoid region, but also of providing an additional buffer zone between the posterior cricoid plate and the oesophagus. The posterior cricoid can then be split vertically for its entire length, ensuring that the incision is kept completely in the midline. It is important that the interarytenoid scar band is completely divided. The incision may be continued superiorly through the interarytenoid muscles (which are frequently fibrosed) up to the level of the interarytenoid mucosa itself. Care must be taken not to inadvertently form a posterior laryngeal cleft. Following the posterior split, the cricoid should be easily distracted laterally. A costal cartilage graft is then harvested and carved so that its height is

approximately the height of the cricoid split and its depth allows the graft perichondrium to lie reasonably flush with the cut mucosa of the posterior cricoid. The graft may be sewn in place with 4.0 Monocryl™ sutures on a P2 needle. An alternative approach is to form a flanged graft that can be snapped into place and stabilized with a small amount of fibrin tissue glue. With the posterior graft in place, the laryngofissure is then closed over an age-approximate endotracheal tube. If the cricoid does not easily close anteriorly, a further segment of costal cartilage is used as an anterior cricoid graft. A posterior graft rarely needs to be more than 6 mm wide as the primary aim of surgery is to incise the scar tissue and hold the raw edges apart while healing takes place. A graft surpassing this width carries an increased risk of aspiration.

It is possible to perform this procedure without performing a complete laryngofissure. If the anterior airway incision is carried up to the true vocal cords but not through them, there is usually sufficient access to perform a safe posterior cricoid split and allow insertion of a flanged graft. Such a graft is required as there is not adequate access to comfortably place sutures with this technique. This technique is more difficult to perform in small children.

Posterior cricoid grafting may be performed as a single- or two-stage procedure. Other variations of open reconstruction include scar excision alone, buccal mucosal grafting and a posterior cricoid split without graft placement. However, a posterior split without a graft normally requires a considerable period of stenting before full stability is achieved. This technique is more efficacious in younger children.

Endoscopic techniques may also be efficacious although, in general, are not as reliable as the open approach. A laser posterior cordotomy with or without partial arytenoidectomy is effective, however, there is a significant chance of restenosis. In order to prevent restenosis, the use of mitomycin C is a consideration, as well as placement of a temporary transglottic stent. Other described techniques for the endoscopic management of posterior glottic stenosis include mucosal advancement flaps, microtrapdoor flaps, vocal cord lateralization and botulinus toxin (Botox) injections.

Whether reconstruction is open or endoscopic, there is a restenosis rate of between 10 and 20 percent. This rate is higher in children who have had thermal injury to the posterior glottic stenosis. If a child has failed an endoscopic procedure, then open reconstruction is appropriate. Conversely, if a child has failed an open procedure, endoscopic management may be appropriate. In a very recalcitrant airway it is possible to place a second posterior costal cartilage graft if required.

Interarytenoid adhesion

Interarytenoid adhesion is a distinct variant of posterior glottic stenosis, with presentation similar to this condition or to bilateral true vocal cord paralysis. An interarytenoid adhesion results from prolonged intubation, when tongues of granulation tissue lying anterior to the endotracheal tube in the region of the vocal process unite in the midline to form a fibrous scar band. While this usually progresses to form posterior glottic stenosis, mucosal sparing of the posterior commissure sometimes occurs, resulting in the formation of an interarytenoid scar band. Endoscopic evaluation confirms a small posterior commissure air passage and a larger anterior glottic airway passage. However, there may be a marked limitation to the size of endotracheal tube that can be used for intubation if there is not a tracheotomy tube already present. Endoscopic resolution of this problem is simple and effective. In most cases, microlaryngeal scissors are used to excise the scar band, with immediate resolution of symptoms. In some children this problem may coexist with either subglottic stenosis or posterior glottic stenosis.

Subglottic reconstruction

REPAIR TECHNIQUES

Anterior cricoid split

In the neonate who has failed extubation the anterior cricoid split procedure is an alternative to tracheotomy (**Figure 89.3**). The criteria for anterior cricoid split are well described and are:[10]

- failed extubation on at least two occasions;
- weight >1500 g;
- extubation failure secondary to laryngeal pathology;

- no assisted ventilation for ten days before evaluation;
- supplemental O_2 requirement <35 percent;
- no congestive heart failure for one month prior to evaluation;
- no acute upper or lower respiratory tract infection at the time of evaluation;
- no antihypertensive medication for ten days before evaluation.

The procedure involves an anterior incision of the trachea from the second tracheal ring, up through the cricoid and into the lower third of the thyroid ala, just below the insertion of the anterior commissure. The child is then left intubated for ten days, with the neck wound left at least partly open to minimize the risk of subcutaneous air build-up. A thyroid alar interposition graft is a modification that permits earlier extubation.

Laryngotracheal reconstruction: anterior cartilage graft

Mild-to-moderate subglottic stenosis is well managed with costal cartilage grafting to the anterior cricoid (**Figure 89.1**).[11] The anterior airway is split from the tracheotomy site to the lower aspect of the thyroid cartilage. An age-appropriate sized endotracheal tube or suprastomal stent is then inserted, and a measurement taken of the size of graft needed to comfortably close the deficit in the anterior airway. A costal cartilage graft is then harvested and carved to allow a boat-shaped and perichondrium-lined insert to distract the anterior cricoid. An outer flange prevents graft prolapse into the airway. This technique is also useful for managing suprastomal collapse or narrowing of the upper trachea.

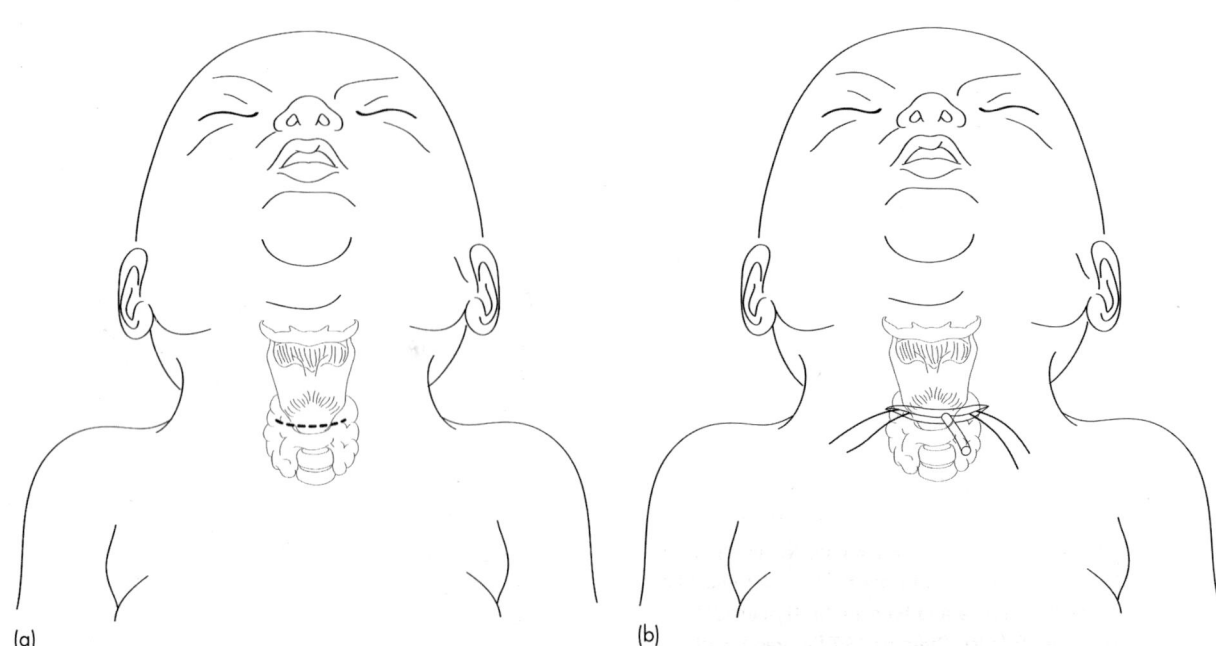

(a)   (b)

Figure 89.3   The anterior cricoid split procedure.

Laryngotracheal reconstruction: posterior cartilage graft

Costal cartilage grafting of the posterior cricoid for subglottic stenosis may be performed in an identical fashion as for posterior glottic stenosis. If the anterior cricoid can then close comfortably over an appropriate sized endotracheal tube or stent, the additional anterior grafting is not required.

Laryngotracheal reconstruction: anterior and posterior cartilage grafts

If the anterior cricoid cannot comfortably close over an appropriately sized endotracheal tube or stent, then an additional anterior graft is required, as previously described. This is necessary for most grade III and all grade IV stenoses.

Cricotracheal resection

Cricotracheal resection has an increasing role in the management of subglottic stenosis. This procedure requires the removal of the subglottic scar tissue, with the anastomosis of healthy trachea to a healthy larynx. This is a technically more challenging operation than laryngotracheal reconstruction with cartilage grafts (**Figure 89.4**).

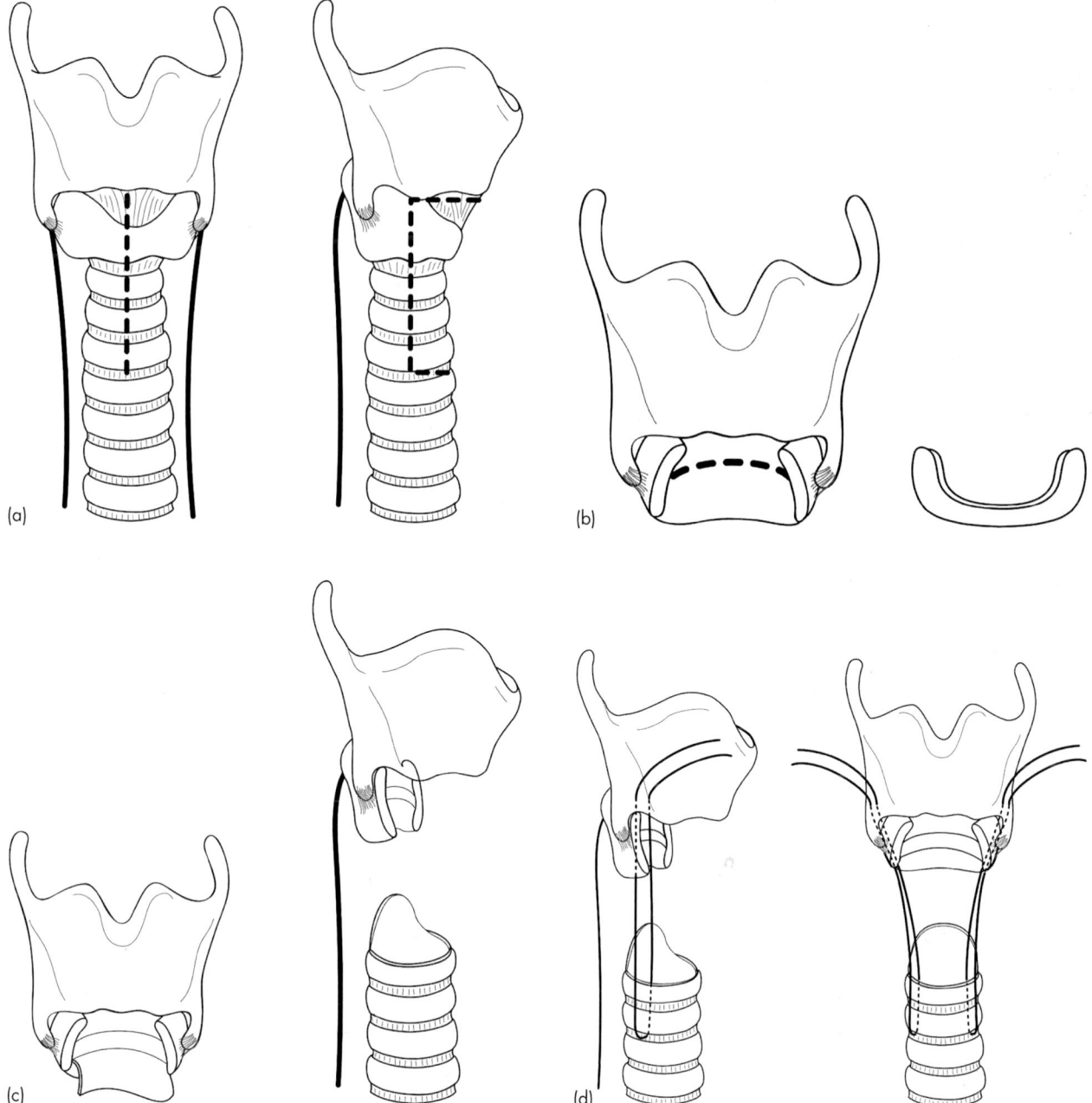

(a)

(b)

(c)

(d)

Figure 89.4 Cricotracheal resection (continued over).

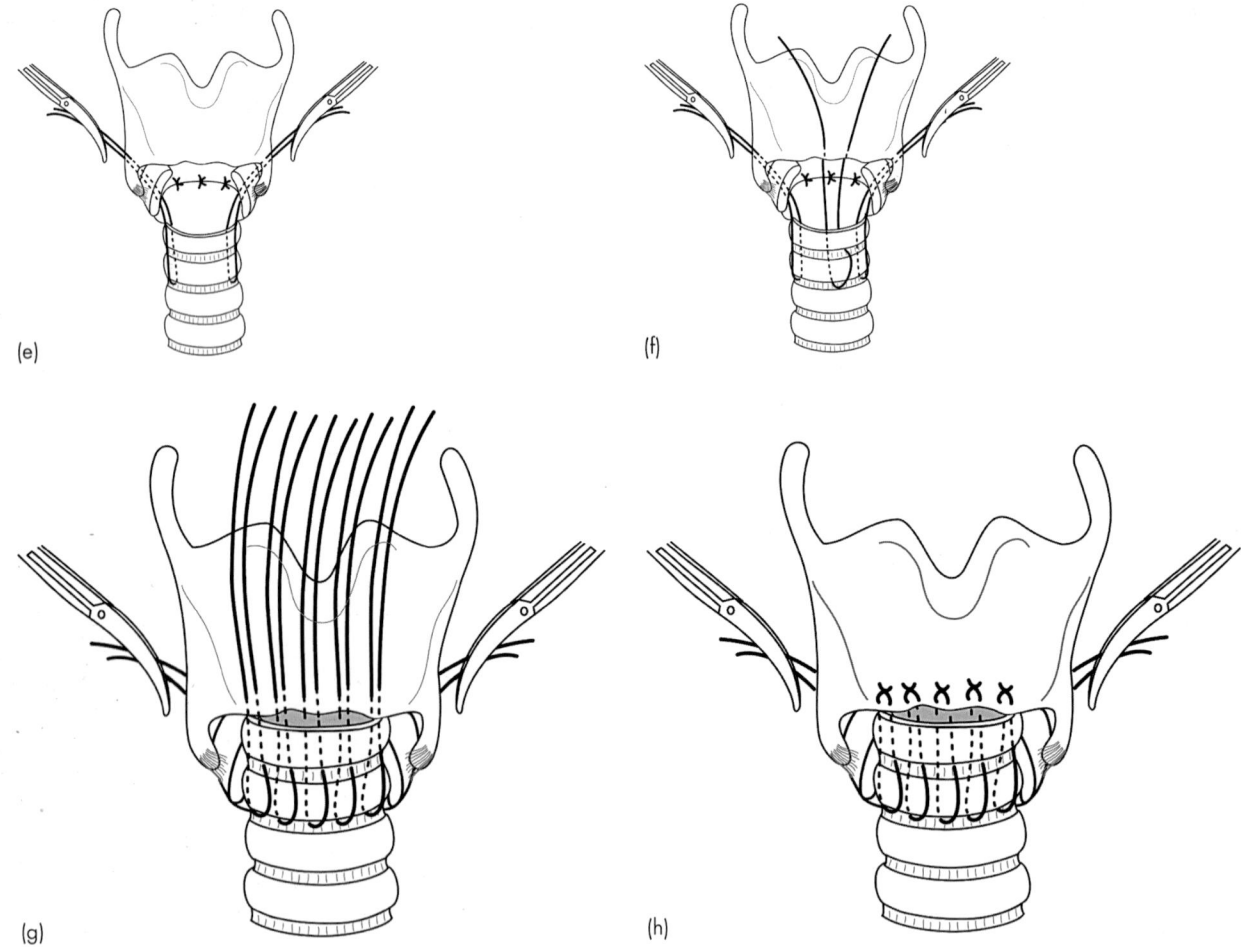

Figure 89.4 Cricotracheal resection (continued).

The success of CTR in infants and children has been documented in two large series of patients.[12, 13] [**/*] The results reported are superior to those of the laryngotracheal reconstruction procedures for similar indications and stenosis grades. CTR with primary anastomosis is a safe and effective procedure for the treatment of severe subglottic stenosis in infants and children. Diagnostic precision is essential, operative timing should be judged carefully, and operative technique must be precise. The reasons for the high success rate include the complete resection of the stenotic segment with restoration of a lumen using a normal tracheal ring, the preservation of normal laryngotracheal support structures without disruption of the cartilaginous framework, and full mucosal lining on both sides of the anastomosis, thus minimizing or preventing granulation tissue and restenosis. The complications of the surgery, however, should not be underestimated. The first is injury to the recurrent laryngeal nerve. Typically, the recurrent laryngeal nerve is not identified during the procedure as is lies posterior to the cricothyroid joint and the resection margin is anterior to the cricothyroid joint. The second complication is dehiscence of the anastomosis, which is most likely to happen if there is tension at the site of the anastomosis or because of forceful reintubation if the endotracheal tube becomes dislodged. In the paediatric larynx the technique of laryngeal release is not required in most cases of CTR. If mobilization of the trachea is difficult or tracheal resection is extensive (more than five tracheal rings), then laryngeal release should be performed to minimize the risk of dehiscence. If granulation tissue is allowed to grow there is also a risk of restenosis, and for this reason sutures through the cartilage should emerge submucosally at the edge of the anastomosis.

Experimental data in primates show that when CTR and primary tracheal anastomosis are performed with a good initial result, the thyroid cartilage and tracheal ring sutured together continue to grow normally. A further advantage of the CTR technique may be that voice quality should not deteriorate because the anterior commissure of the larynx is maintained in its initial position and there is no widening of the larynx posteriorly with an interposition graft. However, in older children, CTR may limit the ability to tilt the thyroid cartilage on the cricoid cartilage, in turn restricting cord tensioning and leading to a loss of vocal range.

CONTRAINDICATIONS

All contraindications to airway reconstruction are relative. Usually, airway reconstruction is not attempted unless decannulation is the goal. Gastro-oesophageal reflux disease and eosinophilic oesophagitis should be controlled preoperatively, and pulmonary function optimized. Operating on a child requiring pulmonary pressure support to ventilate adequately is unwise. Single-stage reconstruction is inadvisable in a child who is difficult to intubate. In children with a history of sedation problems, past failure of airway reconstruction or multiple levels of airway pathology, single-stage reconstruction should be approached with caution. In children undergoing CTR, the risk of anastomotic dehiscence seems higher in the presence of Down syndrome, MRSA or a past history of distal tracheal surgery. The greatest disservice to a child is for airway reconstruction to cause or exacerbate ongoing aspiration.

COMPLICATIONS

Complications may be subdivided into intraoperative, early postoperative and late postoperative.[14] Intraoperative complications include bleeding, pneumothorax and loss of the airway with resultant hypoxia. Early postoperative complications include infection, air leakage from the operative site, dehiscence of an anastomosis and loss of a graft. The risk of air leakage and graft loss is highest when systemic steroid use is continued beyond two or three peri-extubation doses. With single-stage procedures there is a risk of accidental extubation, and risks associated with paralysis or sedation. Extubation may be compromised because of glottic oedema and granulation caused by the endotracheal tube. The most significant long-term complication is failure of the reconstruction with restenosis of the subglottis, with an incidence between 10 and 20 percent in most series.

Revision airway surgery/the recalcitrant airway

Failure of laryngotracheal reconstruction or CTR does not preclude further attempts at reconstruction, but may complicate further reconstructive efforts. In revision airway surgery, particular care should be taken to optimize the outcome by careful preoperative evaluation of the patient and their airway. Failed expansion cartilage grafting may still be amenable to either further cartilage grafting or resection, while failed resection may still be amenable to further resection or cartilage grafting.

mechanism of aspiration as well as the presence or absence of normal laryngeal sensation. [Grade B]

✓ In a child who has not been evaluated previously, flexible nasopharyngoscopy with the child awake should be performed prior to rigid endoscopy. [Grade D]

✓ In children with significant lung disease, decannulation may be imprudent. Children with progressive neuromuscular disorders, diaphragmatic weakness or central hyperventilation syndrome, may not be candidates for decannulation. [Grade C]

✓ In a child with a compromised airway who does not have a tracheotomy tube, preoperative administration of dexamethasone, 0.5 mg/kg up to a maximum of 20 mg, is a prudent precaution. [Grade B]

✓ Spontaneous ventilation offers the best dynamic assessment of the airway and is thus recommended. [Grade D]

✓ In children in whom a stenting period of less than two weeks is anticipated, consider intubation, with the endotracheal tube acting as the stent (see Single-stage reconstruction). [Grade C]

✓ A prerequisite for single-stage laryngotracheal reconstruction is an excellent ICU in which staff are familiar with the management of airway patients. [Grade D]

Deficiencies in current knowledge and areas for future research

➤ While laryngotracheal reconstruction and CTR have become accepted management techniques for subglottic stenosis, supraglottic airway management remains poorly understood and managed.

➤ Preoperative evaluation and optimization of patients prior to reconstructive airway surgery still requires refinement.

➤ Recent technological advances, such as impedance probe evaluation of gastro-oesophageal reflux, need critical evaluation.

➤ Paediatric voice research may be an area for future endeavour.

➤ An airway grading system that is not limited to just the subglottis needs to be developed.

➤ Tissue engineering techniques may offer alternatives to current methods of airway reconstruction.

REFERENCES

* 1. Myer III CM, O'Connor DM, Cotton RT. Proposed grading system for subglottic stenosis based on endotracheal tube sizes. *Annals of Otology, Rhinology, and Laryngology.*
1994; **103**: 319–23. *Description of the most widely accepted grading system for subglottic stenosis.*

2. Koufman JA. The otolaryngologic manifestations of gastroesophageal reflux disease (GERD): a clinical investigation of 225 patients using ambulatory 24-hour pH monitoring and an experimental investigation of the role of acid and pepsin in the development of laryngeal injury. *Laryngoscope.* 1991; **101**: 1–78.

3. Wenzl TG. Evaluation of gastroesophageal reflux events in children using multichannel intraluminal electrical impedance. *American Journal of Medicine.* 2003; **115**: 161S–5S.

4. Johnson LB, Rutter MJ, Putnam PE, Cotton RT. Airway stenosis and eosinophilic esophagitis. Transactions American Bronchoesophagological Association. Nashville, TN, 2003, 137.

5. Zalzal GH, Cotton RT, McAdams AJ. The survival of costal cartilage grafts in laryngotracheal reconstruction. *Otolaryngology and Head and Neck Surgery.* 1986; **94**: 204–11.

6. Zalzal GH. Rib cartilage grafts for the treatment of posterior glottic and subglottic stenosis in children. *Annals of Otology, Rhinology and Laryngology.* 1988; **97**: 506–11.

7. Gustafson LM, Hartley BE, Liu JH, Link DT, Chadwell J, Koebbe C *et al.* Single-stage laryngotracheal reconstruction in children: a review of 200 cases. *Otolaryngology and Head and Neck Surgery.* 2000; **123**: 430–4.

8. Cotton RT. The problem of pediatric laryngotracheal stenosis: a clinical and experimental study on the efficacy of autogenous cartilaginous grafts placed between the vertically divided halves of the posterior lamina of the cricoid cartilage. *Laryngoscope.* 1991; **101**: 1–34.

9. Rutter MJ, Cotton RT. The use of posterior cricoid grafting in managing isolated posterior glottic stenosis in children. *Archives of Otolaryngology – Head and Neck Surgery.* 2004; **130**: 737–9.

* 10. Cotton RT, Myer III CM, Bratcher GO, Fitton CM. Anterior cricoid split 1977–1987: evolution of a technique. *Archives of Otolaryngology – Head and Neck Surgery.* 1988; **114**: 1300–2. *First description of the cricoid split procedure.*

11. Cotton RT, Gray SD, Miller RP. Update of the Cincinnati experience in pediatric laryngotracheal reconstruction. *Laryngoscope.* 1989; **99**: 1111–6.

* 12. Monnier P, Lang F, Savary M. Partial cricotracheal resection for pediatric subglottic stenosis: a single institution's experience in 60 cases. *European Archives of Oto-rhino-laryngology.* 2003; **260**: 295–7. *Outcome analysis of cricotracheal resection.*

* 13. White DR, Cotton RT, Bean JA, Rutter MJ. Pediatric cricotracheal resection: surgical outcomes and risk factor analysis. *Archives of Otolaryngology–Head and Neck Surgery.* 2005; **131**: 896–9. *Update on the Cincinnati experience with cricotracheal resection.*

14. Cotton RT. Management of subglottic stenosis. *Otolaryngologic Clinics of North America.* 2000; **33**: 111–30.

90

Paediatric voice disorders

BEN HARTLEY

Introduction	1167	Best clinical practice	1171
Growth and development of the larynx	1167	Deficiencies in current knowledge and areas for future	
Assessment of the child's voice	1168	research	1172
Specific disorders	1169	References	1172
Key points	1171		

SEARCH STRATEGY

The data in this chapter are supported by a Medline search using the key words paediatric, voice and dysphonia.

INTRODUCTION

There have been tremendous advances in the understanding of voice disorders and their management in recent years. The subspecialty of phoniatrics has evolved principally in adults and this knowledge may now be applied to voice disorders in children. Disorders of voice – where the predominant symptom is hoarseness or 'dysphonia' – must be distinguished from disorders of speech, articulation and language. Speech and articulatory disorders are characterized by difficulty in producing speech sounds, often in the presence of normal laryngeal function. In language disorders, the child uses words and sentences inappropriately, again usually despite normal laryngeal function.

Voice disorders are largely a manifestation of laryngeal pathology. Six to 23 percent of 5–18 year olds have some form of voice 'problem'.[1, 2] In the majority, neither the child nor their parents perceive the voice as a concern and they do not present for medical evaluation.

The spectrum of voice disorders seen in a specialist paediatric voice clinic is very wide. Patients range from child performers who have a normal conversational voice but whose parents have been concerned about a loss of the upper range of their singing voice, to children with severe congenital or acquired laryngeal disease with no voice at all.

With careful assessment, voice therapy and occasionally surgical intervention, most paediatric dysphonias can be corrected or improved.

GROWTH AND DEVELOPMENT OF THE LARYNX

The paediatric larynx is quite different from that of the adult (**Figure 90.1** and **Table 90.1**). The embryonic development of the larynx is described in detail in Chapter 162, Anatomy of the larynx and tracheobronchial tree. This section focusses on those aspects relevant to voice disorders and on normal growth and development after birth. Current knowledge stems largely from the detailed studies of Hirano et al.[3, 4]

Elongation of the vocal folds

Hirano found that up to the age of ten years, the length of the vocal fold was very similar in both males and females (6–8 mm). At puberty there is a substantial increase in growth, much more marked in males with the membranous vocal fold increasing to 14.8–18 mm (more than double). In females the increase is to 8.5–12 mm – an increase in length of a third. The cartilaginous portion of

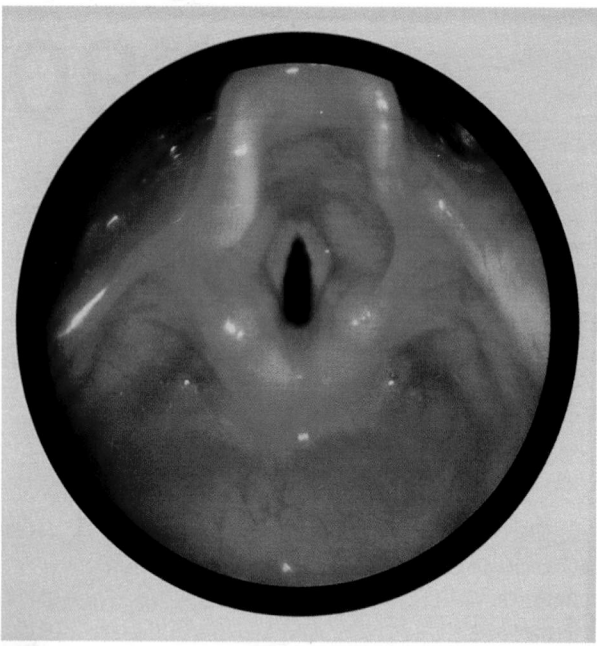

Figure 90.1   Normal larynx in a six-month-old child.

Table 90.1   Differences between the larynx of an adult and child.

Feature	Difference
Size	The paediatric larynx is relatively smaller
Position	The child's larynx is relatively higher
Shape	Curled epiglottis, shorter vocal folds
Mucosa	More reactive and prone to airway obstruction. Croup is uncommon in adults
The laminar vocal fold structure	Immature in young children

the vocal fold also grows with age but less rapidly, with a relative increase in the ratio of the membranous to cartilaginous vocal fold from 1.5 in the newborn to 4.0 in the adult female and 5.5 in the adult male. Hirano devised the concept of the respiratory glottis posteriorly with a wider aperture and the phonatory glottis anteriorly. These concepts are useful in planning surgical procedures. For example, in bilateral vocal cord paralysis it is possible to increase the airway by performing an ablative procedure, such as a laser arytenoidectomy. If this procedure is kept to the posterior part of the larynx then the anterior membranous vocal fold can be preserved for phonation.

Changes in vocal fold laminar structure

Much has been written about the layered structure of the vocal folds and its importance both to the understanding of disease and the development of phonosurgical treatment.

The five layers of the vocal fold are the *epithelium*, *superficial layer* of lamina propria (Reinke's space), the *intermediate* and *deep* layers of the lamina propria and the *muscle layer*. The first two are referred to the as the 'cover' and move freely over the deeper layers which form the 'ligament' and 'body' of the vocal fold.

This laminar structure is not present at birth, but starts to differentiate over the first few months of life. It becomes more developed throughout childhood and the adult form is quite easily recognizable by puberty. One surgical implication of this is that microflaps are more difficult to raise in early childhood due to a less well-developed plane for dissection in the superficial lamina propria.

Changes in pitch

An important feature of the paediatric voice is its pitch. This drops throughout infancy and childhood in males and females, with a marked change at puberty, particularly in males. This change in pitch corresponds to the anterior growth of the thyroid cartilage in response to testosterone and coincides with the development externally of the thyroid prominence or Adam's apple. The fall in pitch is approximately proportional to the growth of the membranous vocal fold.

ASSESSMENT OF THE CHILD'S VOICE

Children with voice disorders can either be seen in a general clinic or in a voice clinic. An otolaryngologist and speech and language therapist should staff paediatric voice clinics. Videostroboscopic equipment and the expertise to use it should be available. The history and basic otolaryngological examination is the same in both settings. Whether laryngeal videostroboscopy and speech therapy assessment is required will depend on the clinical situation.

History and examination

Mild or moderate dysphonias that have been present for some time tend to be accepted as part of the child's personality and not a medical disorder. Often, an incidental remark years later leads to the parents seeking medical assessment to exclude an underlying disorder. Some children and families see no problem with their dysphonia. Alternatively, some children and families find a mild dysphonia very troublesome, particularly if they are performers or have aspirations to perform.

Information should be sought from both the child and parents. If the problem has been present from birth, a congenital lesion is likely. However, a history of endotracheal intubation around the time of birth or around the time of onset of symptoms may suggest laryngeal stenosis, cricoarytenoid joint fibrosis, intubation granuloma or cyst formation. Much more commonly, symptoms start with an upper respiratory tract infection that has been accompanied by laryngitis, a situation made worse by habitual patterns of voice misuse.

The severity of the disorder may range from a loss of singing voice to complete loss of conversational voice. The time course of the dysphonia is also important. For example, dysphonia is often persistent with discrete vocal fold lesions and rarely returns to normal, although it may fluctuate and fatigue during the day.

Enquire about symptoms suggestive of gastro-oesophageal reflux, as this may irritate the larynx and cause dysphonia. Post-nasal drip associated with allergic rhinitis will do the same, particulary if there is a habit of forceful or constant throat clearing. Cough is quite harsh on the vocal mechanism and constant coughing associated with respiratory disease may lead to hoarseness.

Restrictive respiratory disease may cause reduced infraglottic pressure and subsequent dysphonia. The use of corticosteroid inhalers can also cause dysphonia and this can be helped by modification of drug regime or possibly inhaler technique and the use of spacer devices.[5]

Hearing loss may make the child shout. This can be the underlying cause of a dysphonia secondary to vocal misuse. Voice misuse – shouting – is common in children and may lead to disorders of hyperfunction such as nodules. Other abusive behaviours, such as smoking and alcohol, may occasionally be relevant.

It is extremely important to enquire about exercise intolerance and stridor, symptoms and signs that may be caused by laryngeal stenosis. Swallowing problems or choking may be the first indication of laryngeal paralysis. A general otolaryngological examination, including assessment of the ears and hearing, should be performed. Important clues can be gained by carefully listening to the quality of the child's voice during history taking. Laryngoscopy should be undertaken in all cases.

Laryngoscopy

The objectives of laryngoscopy are two-fold, first to identify any structural lesion, such as a vocal nodule or papilloma; second, to assess laryngeal mobility during phonation.

Older children may be cooperative enough for indirect laryngoscopy but examination of the paediatric larynx has traditionally been performed under general anaesthetic. Detailed structural information can be obtained but little information is gained with regard to mobility. It is usual to watch vocal mobility on awakening from general anaesthesia. This can provide information with regard to vocal paralysis, but it should be recognized that by today's standards this is a very crude method of assessment. Awake laryngeal and voice examination should be the standard of care in a compliant child.

Most focal lesions can be excluded by awake fibreoptic laryngoscopy. This can be performed on a child of almost any age. It is usually quite straightforward, performed transnasally with a 2.2-mm fibreoptic endoscope. The optics of the larger fibreoptic endoscopes are better and, if possible, a 4-mm endoscope should be used. From age one to five years, compliance is limited and general anaesthesia and microlaryngoscopy may need to be considered. Some images are of sufficient quality to permit stroboscopy with examination of the mucosal wave.

Rigid laryngoscopy requires significant cooperation, which can only be obtained in children over six years of age. High quality images of the larynx combined with stroboscopy give unparalleled information on vocal fold movement and structure. They also provide an important educational tool for parents and older children. Paralysis of a vocal cord is generally obvious but this technique gives insight to more subtle mobility disorders such as limited posterior glottic closure (glottic chink) and supraglottic constriction. This degree of information is useful and relevant to planning voice therapy.

SPECIFIC DISORDERS

Vocal nodules and functional voice disorders

Vocal nodules – now regarded as an organic manifestation of laryngeal hyperfunction – are the commonest cause of dysphonia in children (**Figure 90.2**).[6] The mainstay of treatment is voice therapy to correct the hyperfunction. While in adolescents this therapy is similar to that employed in adults, different strategies are necessary in younger children.

The traditional view, based on clinical experience, was that most vocal nodules in children could be expected to improve at puberty.[7] Puberty is a time of great change in the larynx, with tremendous growth of the membranous

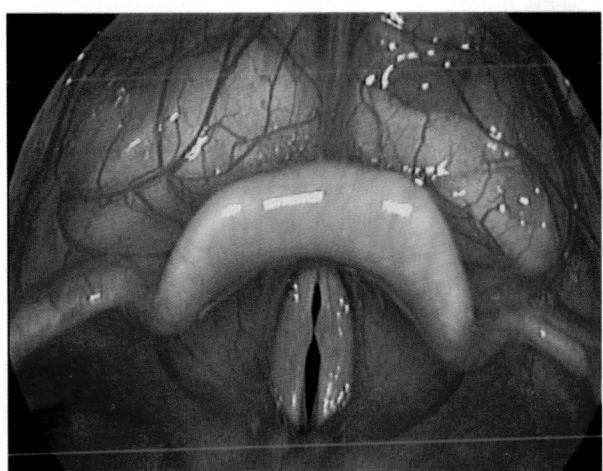

Figure 90.2 Vocal cord nodules.

vocal fold in the male and, to a lesser extent, in the female. One can see how the dynamics of vocalization might change with potential improvement in the nodules. Mori,[8] however, reported that 12 percent of nodules did not improve at puberty. In the same study it was found that those treated with vocal hygiene alone (i.e. general advice regarding voice care) did not improve. Those given voice therapy under the supervision of a speech and language therapist did tend to improve and the degree of improvement was related to the number of therapy sessions. [**] The essentials of voice therapy include reduction of vocal strain. Various techniques can be employed to reduce shouting, whispering, coughing and throat clearing and to encourage the use of a smooth easy voice. Periods of quiet play are recommended after noisy activity (e.g. football) to allow vocal fold recovery.

Surgery for nodules is rarely recommended in children. Concerns about the potential effects of scarring are very real. On occasion it can be justified when prolonged voice therapy has failed. Bouchayer and Cornut[9] reported cysts, polyps and sulci in children previously diagnosed as having nodules when examined at microlaryngoscopy. Some children with nodules have vocal cord cysts with a nodule on the contralateral cord and this might explain why some fail to respond to voice therapy. The use of videostroboscopic techniques in the voice clinic should help diagnose these conditions earlier. Cysts are treated by microsurgical excision.

A wide range of functional voice disorders can be demonstrated in children without demonstrable nodules. These children may present with dysphonia, or even aphonia, secondary to underlying psychological factors. For these children, voice therapy may need to be combined with a psychological assessment. Aphonia in the presence of a normal laryngoscopy evaluation is suggestive of psychological disturbance. A normal cough or laugh adds support to this contention. Puberphonia, when the prepubertal voice persists into adolescence or adulthood, is another condition associated with psychological disturbance. Highly specialized voice therapy, possibly in conjunction with a psychologist, is important to help these children develop an adult voice.

Laryngeal papillomatosis

A detailed account of laryngeal papillomatosis is given elsewhere (Chapter 91, Juvenile-onset recurrent respiratory papillomatosis). From the voice perspective, there are a number of important considerations.

The emphasis of modern surgical techniques is to minimize damage to the underlying lamina propria and to restrict surgery to the papillomas. In this way, voice quality will be optimized in the long term. Glottic scarring and webbing are well-known complications of surgical intervention with the laser.[10] The use of a microdebrider and cold steel instruments has much to

commend it. After all, surgery cannot cure papillomatosis. Medical treatments have been advocated including intra-lesional acyclovir with some reported success.[11] [**] In theory, any medical adjunct that reduces the number of surgical procedures would be beneficial in terms of voice preservation, although voice outcomes following these therapies have yet to be reported. Cidofovir is showing some promise and its use is considered in Chapter 91, Juvenile-onset recurrent respiratory papillomatosis.

Intubation injuries and voice

Much has been written about acquired subglottic stenosis consequent on prolonged endotracheal intubation in premature infants. Surgical techniques have evolved to correct this abnormality and allow eventual decannulation.[12, 13, 14] Voice problems following this surgery have been documented and are not uncommon.[15]

Subglottic stenosis is just one example of laryngeal injury caused by intubation. More minor scarring may affect the voice but not the airway (**Figures 90.3** and **90.4**). Damage to the vocal fold or underlying lamina propria causes dysphonia. Cricoarytenoid joint fixation and posterior glottic scarring may also be caused by endotracheal intubation and reduce vocal fold mobility. It is easy to confuse these conditions with vocal cord paralysis.

Voice therapy can be successful in some children. Surgical treatment of voice problems caused by intubation trauma remains a significant challenge. There is potential for the introduction of medialization techniques in this group of children, but there must be an adequate airway before this can be considered and this situation is uncommon.

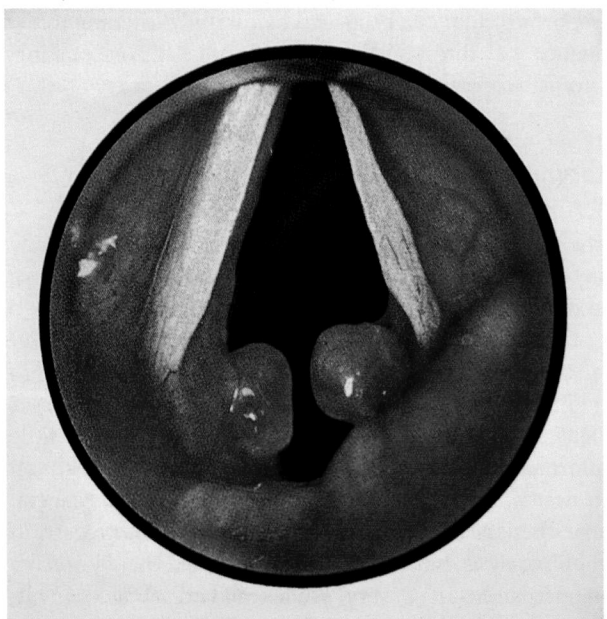

Figure 90.3 Intubation granulomas.

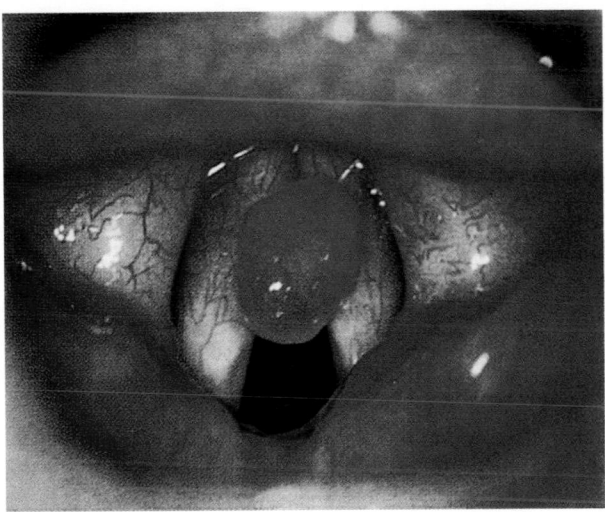

Figure 90.4   Vocal cord polyp following prolonged endotracheal intubation.

Vocal cord paralysis

In general terms, children with bilateral vocal cord paralysis have a good voice or cry. It is the airway that gives concern. Spontaneous recovery of function takes place in some, but after two to three years of observation this is unlikely to happen.[16] A number of lateralization procedures can be performed to develop a wide posterior glottis for respiration while preserving the anterior glottis for phonation. Either laser arytenoidectomy[17, 18] or endoscopic suture lateralization can achieve these goals.

In contrast to bilateral cord paresis, children with unilateral cord paralysis present with aspiration and a weak cry. The airway is relatively spared. Most improve with time due to compensation from the contralateral nonparalyzed vocal fold or to spontaneous recovery.

Medialization thyroplasty can be considered for those that do not improve and continue to have a significant voice problem. However, there is limited published information on this and it should be remembered that its efficacy to diminish aspiration has been limited.[19]

The concept of placing a silastic implant before puberty has raised concerns that this might interfere with the anticipated physiological growth spurt. It is the author's practice to consider medialization using a fat injection in dysphonic, prepubertal children and to restrict silastic thyroplasty techniques for dysphonic post-pubertal patients. [*]

The concept of reinnervation is attractive. In a series of eight children with unilateral vocal cord paralysis, three underwent implantation with ansa cervicalis/strap muscle pedicles. This, together with postoperative voice therapy, gave 'good' results.[20] There has to be some scepticism about these procedures as re-innervation techniques are capable of restoring laryngeal tone but have had limited success in achieving voluntary movement. Nevertheless, children seem to be the ideal population on which to carry out these procedures as nerve grafting in general is more successful in this age group.

It is worth restating that it should never be assumed that an immobile vocal cord is paralyzed. Vocal cord immobility in previously intubated children may be due to joint fixation or posterior glottic scarring. The distinction between these diagnoses is extremely important, particularly when vocal cord immobility is bilateral. The management of paralysis is conservative with a tendency towards spontaneous recovery. Fixation and scarring do not improve and children may be subject to years of unnecessary waiting with a tracheotomy before a surgical lateralization procedure is contemplated.

Tracheotomy and voice

Children with tracheotomies will often have impaired voice. This is only partly due to the tracheotomy tube diverting air from the glottis. The main factor is usually the laryngeal lesion that required tracheotomy formation in the first place. Children with a healthy larynx can obtain good voice by occluding the tube on expiration (with a finger or speech valve) and projecting air around the tube and up through the glottis. To facilitate this, the tube needs to have sufficient space around it and may need to be 'downsized'. This is usually possible without restricting the airway. Speech valves are frequently used in the author's practice for children. As well as helping with speech they help with secretion management and swallowing. [*]

KEY POINTS

- Voice disorders in children are common; few require medical intervention.
- A diagnosis can usually be made by careful history taking and examination to include laryngoscopy and ideally videostroboscopy.
- Laryngeal muscle hyperfunction with or without nodules constitutes the commonest group of disorders.
- These disorders respond well to skilled voice therapy.

Best clinical practice

- ✓ Laryngeal microflaps are more difficult to raise in early childhood due to a less well-developed plane for dissection in the superficial lamina propria. [Grade A]
- ✓ An immobile vocal cord is not always paralyzed. Consider joint fixation and posterior glottic scarring, especially if the child has been intubated. [Grade B]

✓ The term 'vocal abuse', often used to describe adult dysphonias, is best replaced by 'voice misuse' in the paediatric setting. Beware the sensitivity of recording the word 'abuse' in children's records. [Grade D]

✓ Advances in endoscopic equipment are such that awake laryngeal and voice examination should now be the standard of care in a compliant child. [Grade C]

✓ Due to the potential for permanent scarring, surgery for nodules is rarely recommended in children. It should be considered only as a last resort when prolonged and skilled voice therapy has failed. [Grade B]

Deficiencies in current knowledge and areas for future research

▶ **Laryngeal transplantation for voice.** Perhaps the most challenging of paediatric voice conditions is the child with no voice due to complete laryngeal stenosis which is beyond surgical reconstruction. Such children are encountered after severe burns or caustic ingestion. They are tracheotomy dependent and communicate with signing and non-oral devices. Laryngeal replacement using transplantation carries the best hope for these children and although there has been one successful adult patient, this has yet to be repeated.

▶ **Reinnervation of the paralyzed larynx.** Phonosurgery can be helpful for the voice in laryngeal paralysis with medialization using injection or thyroplasty techniques. However, the biggest concern for children with laryngeal paralysis is not voice but aspiration. We do not have a universally accepted solution for aspiration due to laryngeal incompetence. Withdrawal of oral feeding and gastrostomy remains the mainstay. Fortunately, compensation frequently takes place for unilateral lesions but often not bilateral problems. Laryngeal reinnervation may hold the key but is still in its infancy.

▶ **Repair of damaged vocal cords with synthetic 'SLP'.** Vocal cords damaged by intubation or surgery have lost the mucosal wave due to destruction of the important superficial layer of the lamina propria (SLP layer). Medialization of damaged vocal cords has had only limited success and attempts are being made to create a synthetic substitute for this important gel layer for potential replacement by injection into Reinke's space.

REFERENCES

1. Aran D, Ekelman B, Nation J. Preschoolers with language disorders – 10 years later. *Journal of Speech and Hearing Research.* 1984; **27**: 232–44.

2. Silverman EM. Incidence of chronic hoarseness among school age children. *Journal of Speech and Hearing Disorders.* 1975; **40**: 211–5.

3. Hirano M, Kurita S, Nakashima T. In: Bless DM, Abbs JH (eds). *Vocal fold physiology: contemporary research and clinical issues.* San Diego: College Hill Press, 1983: 37–56.

4. Hirano M, Kurita S, Kiyokawa K, Sato K. Posterior glottis: morphological study in excised human larynges. *Annals of Otology, Rhinology and Laryngology.* 1986; **95**: 576–81.

5. Roland NJ, Bhalla RK, Earis J. The local side effects of inhaled corticosteroids. *Chest.* 2004; **126**: 213–9.

6. Koufman JA, Blalock PD. Functional voice disorders. *Otolaryngologic Clinics of North America.* 1991; **24**: 1059–73.

* 7. Toohill RJ. The psychosomatic aspects of children with vocal nodules. *Archives of Otolaryngology.* 1975; **101**: 591–5.

* 8. Mori K. Vocal nodules in children, preferable therapy. *International Journal of Pediatric Otorhinolaryngology.* 1999; **49**: S303–6.

* 9. Bouchayer M, Cornut G. Microsurgical treatment for benign vocal fold lesions, indications, technique, results. *Folia Phoniatric (Basel).* 1992; **44**: 155–84.

* 10. Crockett DM, McCabe BF, Shive CJ. Complications of laser surgery for respiratory papillomatosis. *Annals of Otology, Rhinology and Laryngology.* 1987; **96**: 639–44.

* 11. Pransky SM, Brewster DF, Magit AE, Kearns DB. Clinical update on 10 children treated with intralesional acyclovir injections for severe recurrent respiratory papillomatosis. *Archives of Otolaryngology – Head and Neck Surgery.* 2000; **126**: 1239–43.

12. Hartnick CJ, Hartley BEJ, Lacy PD, Liu J, Willging JP, Myer CM *et al.* Surgery for pediatric subglottic stenosis disease – specific outcomes. *Annals of Otology, Rhinology and Laryngology.* 2001; **110**: 1109–13.

13. Rutter MJ, Hartley BEJ, Cotton RT. Cricotracheal resection in children. *Archives of Otolaryngology – Head and Neck Surgery.* 2001; **127**: 322–4.

14. Hartley BEJ, Cotton RT. Paediatric airway stenosis: laryngotracheal reconstruction or cricotracheal resection? *Clinical Otolaryngology and Allied Sciences.* 2000; **25**: 342–9.

15. Clary RA, Pengilly A, Bailey M, Jones N, Albert D, Comins J *et al.* Analysis of voice outcomes in pediatric patients following surgical procedures for laryngotracheal stenosis. *Archives of Otolaryngology – Head and Neck Surgery.* 1996; **122**: 1189–94.

16. Tucker HM. Vocal cord paralysis in small children: principles and management. *Annals of Otology, Rhinology and Laryngology.* 1986; **95**: 618–21.

17. Worley G, Bajaj J, Cavalli L, Hartley BEJ. Laser arytenoidectomy in children with bilateral vocal cord immobility. *Journal of Laryngology and Otology.* 2007; **121**: 25–7.

18. Hollinger LD, Lusk RP, Green CG. *Pediatric laryngology and bronchoesophagology*. New York: Lippincott–Raven Publishers, 148.

19. Link DT, Rutter MR, Liu JH. Pediatric Type 1 thyroplasty: an evolving procedure. *Annals of Otology, Rhinology and Laryngology*. 1999; **108**: 1105–10.

20. Senturia BH, Wilson FB. Otorhinolaryngic findings in children with voice deviations. *Preliminary report Annals of Otology, Rhinology and Laryngology*. 1968; **77**: 1027–41.

Juvenile-onset recurrent respiratory papillomatosis

MICHAEL KUO AND WILLIAM J PRIMROSE

Introduction	1174	Tracheobronchial disease	1179
Aetiology	1174	Tracheostomy	1179
Epidemiology	1175	Malignant disease	1180
Clinical presentation	1175	Key points	1180
Diagnosis	1175	Best clinical practice	1180
Staging	1176	Deficiencies in current knowledge and areas for future	
Treatment	1176	research	1180
Natural history	1179	References	1181

SEARCH STRATEGY

The data in this chapter are supported by a PubMed (NLM) search using the key words respiratory papillomatosis and laryngeal papillomatosis.

INTRODUCTION

Recurrent respiratory papillomatosis (RRP) is a potentially life-threatening disease characterized by the development of papillomas anywhere in the respiratory tract from the nasal vestibules to the terminal bronchi. Predominant sites are where there is a change of epithelium, e.g. from squamous to ciliated, and especially the tonsillar pillars, uvula, vocal folds and laryngeal commisure. There is a bimodal age distribution with a juvenile-onset peak occurring at three to four years of age and an adult-onset peak occurring at 20–30 years of age. Boys and girls appear to be nearly equally affected in juvenile-onset RRP (JORRP). This contrasts with adult-onset RRP, which is a disease transmitted via sexual contact or via indirect contact with anogenital lesions, preferentially affecting men by a ratio of approximately three to two. Although adult-onset respiratory papillomatosis and juvenile-onset respiratory papillomatosis share many features, this chapter addresses only JORRP.

AETIOLOGY

Juvenile respiratory papillomatosis was first described by Morrell Mackenzie in 1880. By 1923, Ullmann had demonstrated an infective aetiology by injecting homogenized papilloma from a child's larynx into his own forearm and inducing local growth of papillomas. Further direct evidence of the association between human papilloma virus (HPV) and RRP came from the identification of HPV DNA within laryngeal papillomas by Southern blot hybridization and the subsequent recognition in papillomas of HPV types 6 and 11.[1] Human papillomavirus is a naked, double-stranded, icosahedrally-shaped virus with circular supercoiled double-stranded DNA genome surrounded by an outer capsid of protein that belongs to the Papovavirus family. There are 90 known subtypes of HPV – although many vary only slightly in their DNA sequence – but only types 6, 11 and rarely 16 are associated with RRP. HPV types 6 and 11 are also associated with condyloma acuminata (genital warts). Types 16 and 18 have been implicated in carcinogenesis, particularly in the uterine cervix and in squamous cell carcinoma of the head and neck. HPV is thought to first enter traumatized epithelium and reside in the basal layer of the mucous membrane, where it replicates by a process known as episomal maintenance. This replication interferes with the normal process of cell maturation causing epithelial proliferation and neovascularization. Conversely, the virus may lie dormant causing subclinical infection and can often be recovered from apparently normal tissue adjacent to papillomas. Viral protein, DNA synthesis and virion assembly only takes place in the granular and cornified layers of the terminally differentiated epithelium.

EPIDEMIOLOGY

Juvenile-onset RRV is an uncommon condition, with a prevalence of only four in 100,000 children. The oft-quoted triad of susceptibility factors for JORRP – young mother, vaginal delivery and low maternal socioeconomic status – is of limited predictive usefulness.[2] Latent or active HPV has been detected in cervical swabs from 10–25 percent of women of childbearing age. The associations between HPV, JORRP and a history of maternal genital warts are well established but what is uncertain is the influence, if any, these associations should have on obstetric management. HPV DNA has been found in one-third to one-half of aerodigestive tract swabs of children born to affected mothers. However, the majority of these children do not develop disease. Calculations suggest that only one in 400 infants delivered to women with genital warts subsequently develop JORRP. This relative risk is much lower than that for sexually transmitted diseases. The discrepancy between the incidence of HPV colonization of the aerodigestive tract of the infant and the incidence of RRP implies that host factors must be involved in determining susceptibility. Although a history of maternal genital warts is not universal, a large retrospective study has shown that children born to mothers with genital warts carry a 231× relative risk of developing JORRP. A prolonged delivery time (exceeding ten hours) conferred a two-fold increased risk but delivery by Caesarean section did not appear to reduce that risk.[3] The evidence for protection from vertical transmission of HPV into the baby's upper respiratory tract by Caesarean section is conflicting and therefore the decision on method of delivery must be made on a case-by-case basis. Current evidence does not warrant Caesarean section as a prophylaxis against RRP.

Variation in the susceptibility of the host to viral infection may be associated with specific HLA polymorphisms, several of which have been reported. Two recent, large independent studies have shown an association between HLA-DRB1*0301-and severe disease.[4, 5] T-cell responses were shown to be the same by one group between HLA-DRB1*0301-positive patients and negative controls, leading to speculation that the clinical severity of disease is due not to a failure of T-cell proliferative response to HPV, but a delay in that response due to a low frequency of HPV-specific T cells or modulation of the T cell response by immunoregulatory networks.[5] Bonagura et al.[4] showed that HLA-DRB1*0301-positive patients exhibited reduced interferon-gamma expression. While the associations between JORRP and HLA-genotype are being increasingly well recognized, the underlying mechanism for evasion of the cellular immune response is far from clear.

CLINICAL PRESENTATION

Although respiratory papillomas can arise in any respiratory mucosa, their initial presentation is usually in the larynx. The diagnosis requires the surgeon to have an awareness of the condition as the presenting symptoms can be variable and mimic many common laryngeal and respiratory pathologies in children. In addition to hoarseness and stridor, children may present with a chronic cough, paroxysms of choking, recurrent respiratory infections or failure to thrive. These latter symptoms may lead to a misdiagnosis of asthma, laryngitis, bronchitis or croup and a delay of diagnosis of JORRP of up to eight years.[1]

DIAGNOSIS

If at all possible, the clinical diagnosis should be established with awake fibreoptic nasolaryngoscopy (using an infant 2.2 mm endoscope) because the difficulties presented to the anaesthetist by unexpected laryngeal papillomas prolapsing into and obstructing the glottis cannot be overstated.[6, 7, 8] The preferred anaesthetic technique in our institution is that of spontaneous respiration without endotracheal intubation. General anaesthesia is induced either by intravenous propofol or, more frequently, by inhalation of sevoflurane in oxygen. The larynx is topically anaesthetized with 2 percent lidocaine and anaesthesia maintained by sevoflurane in oxygen through a nasopharyngeal airway, of a size and length appropriate for the child's age. This allows excellent surgical access to the airway but carries the disadvantage that the lower airway is not directly protected from bleeding. Therefore, meticulous haemostasis is required during the procedure using topical epinephrine (1:10,000 applied on neurosurgical patties). Regardless of the surgical technique, it is important for the child to recover from anaesthesia with humidified oxygen. Many units use preoperative dexamethasone to reduce laryngeal oedema but some surgeons feel that antiinflammatory agents are best avoided during active manipulation of papilloma tissue. Laryngopharyngeal exposure to gastric acid is increasingly being recognized as a cause of laryngeal pathology. This is particularly relevant during the immediate postoperative period where laryngeal mucosa has been breached.[9] Therefore, it is our practice to give prophylaxis against gastro-oesophageal reflux with an H_2-antagonist or a proton pump inhibitor for 48 hours after all laryngeal surgery including surgery for JORRP. [*]

Macroscopically, papillomas can be pedunculated or sessile, spread over the mucosal surface of the larynx (**Figure 91.1**). They tend not to be friable and can be grasped using microlaryngeal instruments and excised for histological examination. Microscopically, the papillomas appear as exophytic projections of keratinized squamous epithelium overlying a fibrovascular core, with varying degrees of dyskeratosis, parakeratosis and dysplasia. Koilocytes (vacuolated cells with clear cytoplasmic inclusions) are often seen indicating viral infection.

STAGING

Staging of disease is not universally undertaken even in units with a large case-load of RRP. The staging system proposed and modified by Derkay[10, 11] is based on a combination of the anatomical distribution and extent of lesions and their clinical effects on voice and the child's airway. It is increasingly used by members of the American Society of Pediatric Otolaryngologists (ASPO). Widespread adoption of a universally agreed staging system would enable comparison of results between centres and facilitate multi-centre trials, particularly of adjuvant treatments.

TREATMENT

The aim of surgical treatment for recurrent respiratory papillomatosis is the removal of papillomas and restoration of a normal airway while minimizing trauma to the

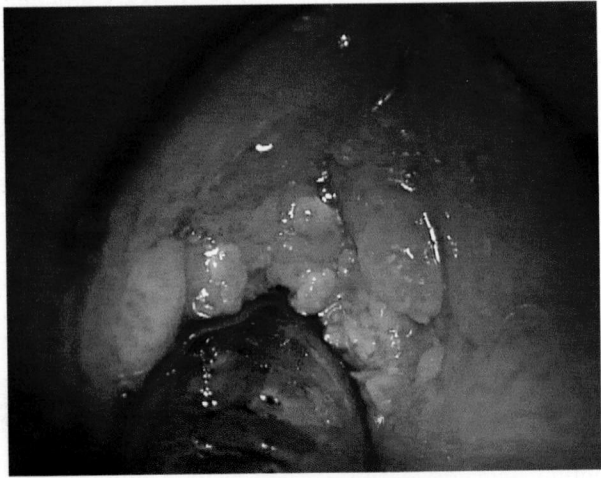

Figure 91.1   Recurrent respiratory papillomatosis in the larynx.

mucosa and vocal cords. In children requiring repeated extirpations of extensive papillomas, especially if they predominantly occur in the larynx, it may be ultimately impossible to achieve normal voice. It is in these patients that the surgical technique, balance of the extent of lesion removal against interval timing, and application of adjuvant therapies must be combined and finely judged to ensure minimal dysphonia and airway stenosis, both of which can be extremely difficult to manage.

Surgical treatment

POWERED MICRODEBRIDER

The use of the powered microdebrider is a relatively new development in the surgical removal of laryngeal papillomas, but one which has become the gold standard for papilloma removal in the larynx (**Figure 91.2**).[12] The laryngeal debrider blade allows gentle but comprehensive removal of papillomas with minimal contamination of the lower respiratory tract with blood or papillomas. There is no thermal trauma and using direct endoscopic control it is extremely precise with minimal mucosal damage. Small retrospective studies demonstrate that, compared with the CO_2 laser, patients undergoing laryngeal papilloma debridement have good disease clearance, require a shorter procedure and experience less postoperative pain. One retrospective study showed no incidence of delayed soft tissue complications using the microdebrider.[13] Long-term results of this are still awaited, but early results are extremely promising.[14, 15, 16] [**]

COLD STEEL SURGERY

Advocates of papilloma removal using microlaryngeal instruments claim that the use of a microflap technique minimizes trauma to the vocal fold while satisfying disease clearance. Thermal damage to neighbouring tissue is also avoided as is the vapour plume. Cold steel surgery has the distinct disadvantage of having no direct haemostasis when dealing with a very vascular lesion. Nevertheless, such surgery is successful in the hands of the exponents of this technique. [**]

CO_2, KTP, ND:YAG AND PULSED-DYE LASER

The carbon dioxide (CO_2) laser has been, for many years, the mainstay of surgical management of JORRP. It remains the treatment of choice for many surgeons because of its ability to ablate the papillomas with minimal bleeding and its ease of use with a microscope and micromanipulator. However, the frequency of late soft tissue complications, such as vocal fold fibrosis, interarytenoid fibrosis and stenosis, glottic webbing and

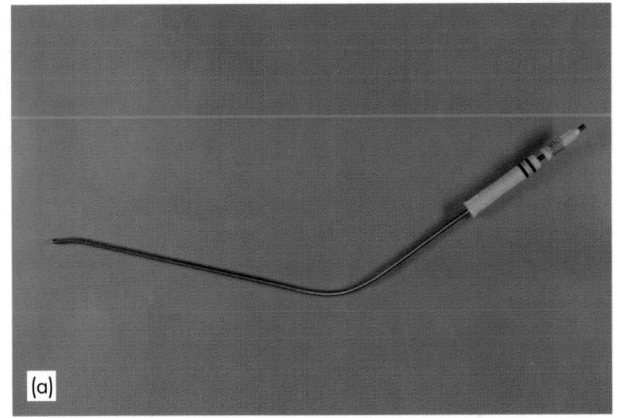
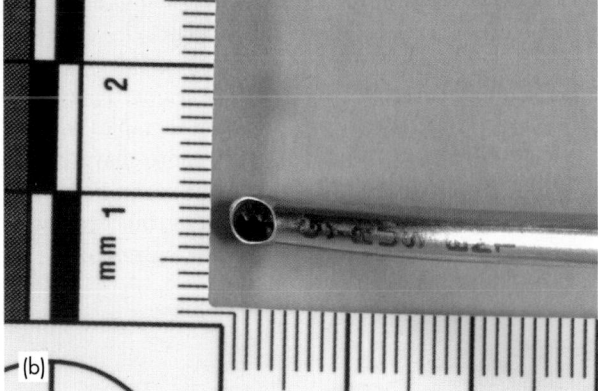

Figure 91.2   (a) Microdebrider; (b) close-up of blade.

arytenoid fixation, has been reported to be 13–45 percent.[6, 17, 18] This increases with frequency of treatment and the number of laser ablations the child has received. Soft tissue complications can be minimized by appropriate laser settings and careful assessment of depth of ablation. A Japanese group has suggested, based upon a single case, a two-stage procedure whereby the bulk of the papillomas are removed at the first operation, which is then followed by a repeat endoscopy and laser ablation ten days later, by which time the coagulum and carbonized tissue have resolved, allowing a more precise laser clearance of residual papillomas.[19] It is also important to have an effective plume extractor. This serves to allow a clearer image of the larynx, but also removes the potentially infectious laser vapour plume which carries a significant viral load. The latter may be simple conjecture as there has only been one reported case of a surgeon developing laryngeal papillomas with a history of repeated laser treatment to a patient with anogenital condylomas, in situ hybridization showing HPV types 6 and 11 in both the patient's and his lesions.[20]

The KTP laser and the Nd:YAG laser are as effective as the CO_2 laser in papilloma ablation and haemostasis but, in addition, can be delivered through an optical fibre. Fibre-delivered laser systems play a role predominantly in the treatment of tracheal and bronchial papillomas. A new fibre-guidance system with a bendable distal tip developed for the Nd:YAG laser achieves a 50° range of directional manoeuvrability with minimal power loss.[21] In adult patients, the delivery of pulsed-dye laser through a flexible bronchoscope can render it an outpatient procedure.[22]

The pulsed-dye laser has attracted much interest in recent years. The advantages of the pulse-dyed laser are that it can be fibre-delivered and causes minimal vocal fold fibrosis and consequently minimal voice damage. However, it also distinguishes itself from the other forms of laser treatment in its mode of action. Rather than direct vaporization of tissue, it has been proposed that the 585 nm pulsed-dye laser is a vascular laser which causes photoangiolysis of sublesional microcirculation, denaturation of epithelial basement membrane linking proteins, and cellular destruction.[22] Therefore, it is less effective against large exophytic lesions and can be used as an adjunct to surgery either before or after the laser application.[23] The application of the pulsed-dye laser in the paediatric population is still under evaluation, but the results in adults with recurrent respiratory papillomatosis are very encouraging. [**]

PHOTODYNAMIC THERAPY

Photodynamic therapy (PDT) relies upon the observation that rapidly proliferating tissue selectively takes up a number of photosensitizing agents when administered intravenously, and that these agents release tumoricidal oxygen derivatives when activated by laser light of the appropriate wavelength. A non-blinded randomized prospective trial using dihaematoporphyrinether (DHE) at two different doses in combination with 50 J of 630 nm argon laser light was compared with laser treatment alone. The patients remain photosensitive for six to nine months and may experience skin erythema, blistering and ocular discomfort. Patients on the higher dose of DHE (4.25 mg/kg body weight) were reported to show a significantly larger decrease in papilloma growth rate but, despite that, only approximately half of the 48 patients receiving DHE showed a response, and no response was seen in patients previously treated with PDT.[24] A further randomized trial by the same group using meso-tetra (hydroxyphenyl) chlorin (mTHPC) as a photosensitizer showed reduction of severity of laryngeal papillomas in the mTHPC group, but this was not maintained and there was no effect on tracheal disease.[25] It should be noted that this trial only recruited 23 patients of whom only 15 patients completed the study. In both trials, there was a combination of juvenile-onset and adult-onset patients. [****]

Adjuvant therapy

Adjuvant medical therapies can be broadly divided into antiviral therapies and drugs with antiproliferative or immunomodulatory properties. Vaccines and gene therapy remain in the early experimental stages.[26, 27, 28] The decision to implement adjuvant therapy must depend on a careful consideration of the benefits against potential adverse effects of the therapy.[29] Adjuvant therapies which have been described in isolated case reports have been included for reference because while their use in 'routine' cases may not be justified, one may wish to consider their use when other better-tested avenues are exhausted.

INTERFERON-α

Interferons are naturally produced by human leukocytes, although as a pharmaceutical, interferon is now produced via recombinant DNA technology. Interferon-α can claim to have antiviral, antiproliferative and immunomodulatory properties. Interferons exert an indirect antiviral action by interfering with normal host cell translation mechanisms and by inducing synthesis of intracellular enzymes that act to control viral growth. By depleting essential metabolites in papilloma cells, interferon-α increases the length of their multiplication cycle, thereby slowing target cell growth. Interferon-α also facilitates recognition of papilloma cells by circulating leukocytes by enhancing expression of cell surface antigens. It is administered systemically by subcutaneous injection at a dose of 2–5 MU/m^2 of body surface area.[30] It is also the most well-studied of the adjuvant therapies for JORRP. A large randomized trial of 123 patients showed significant reduction in papilloma growth rate within the interferon arm. However, this was only significant for the first six months and the difference was not statistically significant during the second six months.[30] In another randomized crossover trial of 66 children, there was significant reduction in disease bulk in the interferon arms of the trial.[31] This was extended to longer follow-up, at which data on 60 children were still available, showing complete remission in 22 children, partial remission in 25 patients and no response in 13.[32] [****] The main problem preventing more widespread use of interferon-α is that there are many serious, idiosyncratic and unpredictable side effects including pancytopenia, hepatorenal failure and cardiac dysfunction. There is also a rebound phenomenon associated with withdrawal of the drug therapy. There is anecdotal evidence of the use of intralesional interferon in combination with laser debulking of JORRP, but this has not found widespread use.[33]

CIDOFOVIR

Cidofovir is an acyclic nucleoside phosphonate which is active against a broad spectrum of DNA viruses including cytomegalovirus, Epstein–Barr virus and HPV. Its mechanism of action is by inhibition of viral DNA polymerases essential for viral replication. The principal application of this drug has been in the treatment of cytomegalovirus in human immunodeficiency virus (HIV)-infected patients by intravenous injection. This mode of administration and high doses is associated with neutropenia and nephrotoxicity. Intralesional injection of cidofovir into JORRP is not associated with similar side effects. A canine model has shown that local irreversible soft tissue damage could be avoided in twice weekly cidofovir injections if the dose is limited to below 40 mg/mL.[34, 35]

Based on their animal work, Chhetri and Shapiro[36] have proposed a schedule for treatment of JORRP based on intralesional injections of cidofovir at a concentration of 1 mg/mL. Injections were given at two-weekly intervals for four treatments and then the interval between treatments extended by one week after each and every subsequent treatment. Concomitant laser surgery was reserved for bulky lesions. Five patients were treated with this schedule with a mean follow-up time of 66 weeks. The mean papilloma stage decreased from 9.2 at initial presentation to 3.4 within two weeks of the first injection, and continued to decrease for the remainder of the follow-up period. After nine weeks of treatment, no patients required further laser surgery. Other studies have used cidofovir at the higher dose of 5 mg/mL with varying schedules of administration. Pransky et al.'s study[37] with a long follow-up (51.6 months) of 11 patients who had all previously required surgical debulking at two-to-six-week intervals showed a reduction in papilloma score in five, complete disease remission in five and one patient who continued to require treatment. In a more recently reported study with a mean follow-up of 30 months, 11 children were treated with intralesional cidofovir of whom five required no further treatment, four had an initial remission but relapsed and two had no apparent response. The authors counsel caution that the potential long-term carcinogenic effects of cidofovir are unknown and a 'response' may be related to the natural history of the disease.[38]

RIBAVIRIN

Ribavirin is a synthetic nucleoside which has activity against a broad spectrum of viruses, but which is principally used as an aerosol in the treatment of respiratory syncytial virus pneumonia and systemically in the treatment of hepatitis C. There have been reports of its use both as an aerosol and systemically.[39, 40, 41] However, these remain anecdotal reports and ribavirin is not widely used as an adjuvant treatment of JORRP. [*]

ACYCLOVIR

The evidence on the efficacy of acyclovir is weak and conflicting.[42, 43] Although HPV is a DNA virus and acyclovir has a medium spectrum of antiviral activity, it does not directly inhibit HPV. Acyclovir is a nucleoside analogue, which inhibits thymidine kinase, which is present in herpes simplex viruses (HSV) but not HPV. Adult patients, but not paediatric patients, with RRP have been shown to have molecular evidence of coinfection with other viruses, particularly HSV which may have a potentiating effect on HPV. It has been suggested that the mechanism of action of acyclovir is to eradicate HSV, thus removing this synergism. Side effects are rare and include nausea, vomiting, diarrhoea, fatigue and headache. [*]

INDOLE-3-CARBINOL

Indole-3-carbinol is a substance derived from cruciferous vegetables (e.g. cabbage, broccoli, Brussels sprouts), which has been shown to alter growth patterns of JORRP cell cultures *in vitro*. It affects oestrogen metabolism, shifting production to antiproliferative oestrogen. A prospective observational study with a mixed adult and paediatric population who received indole-3-carbinol as an adjunctive treatment to surgical removal showed partial or total responses in 21 of 33 patients. Within the paediatric subgroup, four out of nine showed partial or total response with no evident side effects.[44] [**]

CIMETIDINE

Cimetidine – a histamine receptor type 2 (H2) antagonist – has been reported as a useful treatment for cutaneous warts. It has also been successfully used in treatment of an 11-year-old boy who had an eight-year history of diffuse conjunctival papillomas. The mechanism for this is attributed to immunomodulatory side effects of cimetidine at high doses. There is a single case report of very advanced JORRP with tracheo-bronchial-pulmonary involvement being treated successfully with adjuvant cimetidine at a dose of 40 mg/kg for four months with remarkable improvement.[45] [*]

NATURAL HISTORY

The natural history of RRP is extremely variable. This makes it difficult for the surgeon to be able to reliably counsel the anxious parents on how their child's pathology will behave or at what age they might expect remission. Pathologically, severe disease is strongly associated with HPV-11 infection and thus patients should have viral typing as part of their initial pathology work-up. Poor prognostic signs include onset of disease before the age of three years, and birth by Caesarean section. In the United States, Medicaid insurance – often seen as a proxy measure of low socioeconomic status – is also associated with severe disease.[46] However, there are no other studies showing correlation between socio-economic status and disease severity. Most affected children require debulking of papillomas at two-to-three

month intervals during periods of disease activity. Severe disease may necessitate weekly surgical intervention to prevent airway obstruction from rapidly growing papillomas. The median number of debulking procedures required in a patient is reported to be 7–13.[47, 48] Not surprisingly, the repeated debulking of laryngeal papillomas results in chronic voice changes. Objective assessment of voice by GRBAS scale and Visi Pitch II 3000 acoustic analysis has shown significant difference between JORRP patients in remission and normal controls, but a Voice-Related Quality of Life Questionnaire (V-RQoL) showed that the dysphonia does not have any impact on quality of life.[49]

There is a tendency for remission in the early teenage years and this has been attributed to hormonal changes occurring with the onset of puberty. Interestingly, women with adult-onset RRP commonly experience severe exacerbations of their disease during the hormonal fluctuations of pregnancy. What is clear, however, is that remission is not related to the clearance of HPV from the mucosa as viral DNA is detected in previously affected mucosa in patients in remission as well as in normal mucosa of patients with active disease.[50]

TRACHEOBRONCHIAL DISEASE

Extralaryngeal spread of JORRP occurs in approximately one-third of patients with tracheal involvement in approximately one-quarter of patients. Tracheal involvement may appear as cobblestoning of the mucosa coupled with the presence of papillomas. Factors predisposing to tracheal spread include the presence of subglottic papillomas, presence of a tracheostomy and a long duration of disease.[51] More distal bronchopulmonary involvement is reported in 4–11 percent of children with longstanding disease and may result in obstructive pneumonias.[30] Patients may develop cavitary pulmonary lesions leading to fever, sepsis and pulmonary atelectasis. Radiographically, these lesions may appear as solid or cystic pulmonary masses (**Figure 91.3**).[52] A high index of suspicion must be maintained for malignant degeneration of bronchopulmonary lesions.

TRACHEOSTOMY

The indications for tracheostomy in patients with JORRP continue to divide clinicians. The source of this debate is that tracheostomy essentially constitutes an iatrogenic squamociliary junction and may present an additional area of predilection for papillomas.[53] However, it is not universal that all patients with a tracheostomy develop stomal papillomas. A tracheostomy in patients with severe disease may be life-saving and may also facilitate a longer interval between debulking procedures to restore some normality to the child's life.

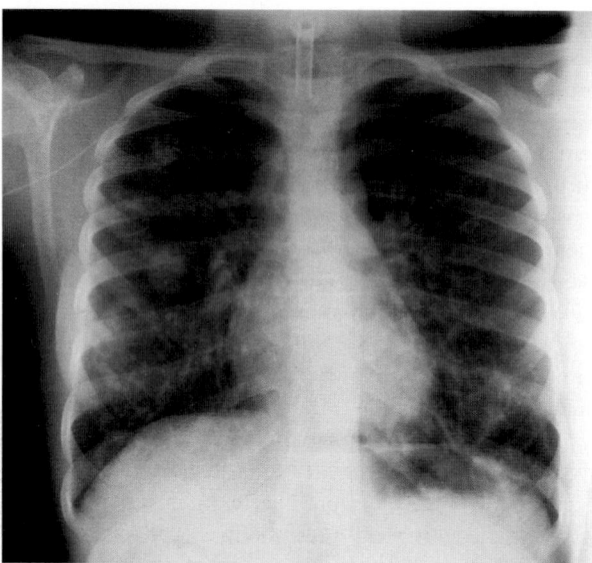

Figure 91.3 Chest radiograph showing extensive pulmonary involvement with papilloma.

MALIGNANT DISEASE

Malignant degeneration of papillomas is a rare but devastating sequel. It is universally fatal.[52] Irradiation of papillomas dramatically increases the risk of malignant transformation but as this is no longer used as a treatment modality, it is only of historical relevance. Most instances of malignant transformation have been reported in adult patients and have been associated with other risk factors including tobacco use and long-standing disease. Malignant transformation appears to be more likely with HPV 16, an unusual cause of JORRP, but HPV 6 and 11 have been shown to oncogenically transform cell culture lines *in vitro*. In adults, malignant degeneration usually involves the larynx, unlike children where cancer usually develops in the bronchopulmonary tree. Approximately 20 paediatric cases of malignant degeneration have been reported, all of which have been fatal. The currently proposed mechanism of malignant transformation involves oncoproteins E6 and E7. HPV types 6 and 11 produce transforming oncoproteins E6 and E7 that have been implicated in growth dysregulation through their ability to inactivate the tumour suppressor proteins p53 and the retinoblastoma tumour-suppressor gene product (pRb). The inactivation of the tumour suppressor genes results in a loss of control over proliferation and cell division and contributes to the development of the malignant phenotype. It is also becoming clear that the E6 and E7 proteins function to promote tumorigenesis through direct interactions with cell-cycle regulatory proteins. Unfortunately, apart from heightened vigilance, there is little to aid the clinician in predicting the rare cases of malignant transformation. There is no evidence of a papilloma-carcinoma sequence while *p53* over-expression is variable and not a marker of

malignant transformation.[54] HPV expression may be lost in malignant tranformation but this may not be a sufficiently robust clinicopathological predictor.

remission of disease. Consolidation of this evidence will require multicentre collaboration in order to standardize protocols and increase patient recruitment. Such a multicentre initiative has already been proposed to seek critical genes in the pathogenesis of RRP.[55]

➤ The future of the management of RRP lies in a better understanding of its pathogenesis.

➤ A vaccine against HPV has become available just as we go to press. Its main use will be in the prevention of cervical cancer in women but at least one type of vaccine ('quadrivalent vaccine') is active against HPV types 6, 11, 16 and 18 and may have a role in the prevention of RRP.[56] Trials are likely to get underway in the next few years with the added possibility of a therapeutic role for the vaccine in children with established RRP.

➤ Despite extensive and sophisticated molecular immunology research, the precise relationship between the human papilloma virus, host immunity and the development of papillomas eludes us. The elucidation of this relationship holds the key to conquering this disease.

REFERENCES

1. Mounts P, Shah KV, Kashima H. Viral etiology of juvenile- and adult-onset squamous papilloma of the larynx. *Proceedings of the National Academy of Sciences of the United States of America.* 1982; **79**: 5425–9.

2. Kashima HK, Shaf F, Lyles A, Glackin R, Muhammad N, Turner L *et al.* A comparison of risk factors in juvenile-onset and adult-onset recurrent respiratory papillomatosis. *Laryngoscope.* 1992; **102**: 9–13.

3. Silverberg MJ, Thorsen P, Lindeberg H, Ahdieh-Grant L, Shah KV. Clinical course of recurrent respiratory papillomatosis in Danish children. *Archives of Otolaryngology – Head and Neck Surgery.* 2004; **130**: 711–6.

4. Bonagura VR, Vambutas A, DeVoti JA, Rosenthal DW, Steinberg BM, Abramson AL *et al.* HLA alleles, IFN-gamma responses to HPV-11 E6, and disease severity in patients with recurrent respiratory papillomatosis. *Human Immunology.* 2004; **65**: 773–82.

5. Gelder CM, Williams OM, Hart KW, Wall S, Williams G, Ingrams D *et al.* HLA class II polymorphisms and susceptibility to recurrent respiratory papillomatosis. *Journal of Virology.* 2003; **77**: 1927–39.

6. Saleh EM. Complications of treatment of recurrent laryngeal papillomatosis with the carbon dioxide laser in children. *Journal of Laryngology and Otology.* 1992; **106**: 715–8.

7. Stern Y, McCall JE, Willging JP, Mueller KL, Cotton RT. Spontaneous respiration anesthesia for respiratory papillomatosis. *Annals of Otology, Rhinology and Laryngology.* 2000; **109**: 72–6.

8. Theroux MC, Grodecki V, Reilly JS, Kettrick RG. Juvenile laryngeal papillomatosis: scary anaesthetic. *Paediatric Anaesthesia.* 1998; **8**: 357–61.

9. Holland BW, Koufman JA, Postma GN, McGuirt Jr. WF. Laryngopharyngeal reflux and laryngeal web formation in patients with pediatric recurrent respiratory papillomas. *Laryngoscope.* 2002; **112**: 1926–9.

10. Derkay CS, Malis DJ, Zalzal G, Wiatrak BJ, Kashima HK, Coltrera MD. A staging system for assessing severity of disease and response to therapy in recurrent respiratory papillomatosis. *Laryngoscope.* 1998; **108**: 935–7.

* 11. Derkay CS, Hester RP, Burke B, Carron J, Lawson L. Analysis of a staging system for prediction of surgical interval in recurrent respiratory papillomatosis. *International Journal of Paediatric Otorhinolaryngology.* 2004; **68**: 1493–8. *Update on staging, demonstrating its importance and suggesting a system which has high validity and reliability.*

12. Tasca RA, McCormick M, Clarke RW. British Association of Paediatric Otorhinolaryngology members experience with recurrent respiratory papillomatosis. *International Journal of Pediatric Otorhinolaryngology.* 2006; **70**: 1183–7.

13. El-Bitar MA, Zalzal GH. Powered instrumentation in the treatment of recurrent respiratory papillomatosis: an alternative to the carbon dioxide laser. *Archives of Otolaryngology – Head and Neck Surgery.* 2002; **128**: 425–8.

14. Patel N, Rowe M, Tunkel D. Treatment of recurrent respiratory papillomatosis in children with the microdebrider. *Annals of Otology, Rhinology and Laryngology.* 2003; **112**: 7–10.

15. Patel RS, MacKenzie K. Powered laryngeal shavers and laryngeal papillomatosis: a preliminary report. *Clinical Otolaryngology and Allied Sciences.* 2000; **25**: 358–60.

* 16. Pasquale K, Wiatrak B, Woolley A, Lewis L. Microdebrider versus CO2 laser removal of recurrent respiratory papillomas: a prospective analysis. *Laryngoscope.* 2003; **113**: 139–43. *A comparative study looking at the relative merits of the CO2 laser and the microdebrider.*

17. Ossoff RH, Werkhaven JA, Dere H. Soft-tissue complications of laser surgery for recurrent respiratory papillomatosis. *Laryngoscope.* 1991; **101**: 1162–6.

18. Crockett DM, McCabe BF, Shive CJ. Complications of laser surgery for recurrent respiratory papillomatosis. *Annals of Otology, Rhinology and Laryngology.* 1987; **96**: 639–44.

19. Sakoh T, Fukuda H, Sasaki S, Sakaguchi R, Shiotani A, Kawaida M *et al.* Laryngomicrosurgery with carbon dioxide laser for laryngeal papillomatosis: application of a two-stage operation. *Auris, Nasus, Larynx.* 1993; **20**: 223–9.

20. Hallmo P, Naess O. Laryngeal papillomatosis with human papillomavirus DNA contracted by a laser surgeon. *European Archives of Otorhinolaryngology.* 1991; **248**: 425–7.

21. Janda P, Leunig A, Sroka R, Betz CS, Rasp G. Preliminary report of endolaryngeal and endotracheal laser surgery of

juvenile-onset recurrent respiratory papillomatosis by Nd:YAG laser and a new fiber guidance instrument. *Otolaryngology – Head and Neck Surgery.* 2004; **131**: 44–9.

22. Zeitels SM, Franco Jr. RA, Dailey SH, Burns JA, Hillman RE, Anderson RR. Office-based treatment of glottal dysplasia and papillomatosis with the 585-nm pulsed dye laser and local anesthesia. *Annals of Otology, Rhinology and Laryngology.* 2004; **113**: 265–76.

23. Franco Jr. RA, Zeitels SM, Farinelli WA, Anderson RR. 585-nm pulsed dye laser treatment of glottal papillomatosis. *Annals of Otology, Rhinology and Laryngology.* 2002; **111**: 486–92.

24. Shikowitz MJ, Abramson AL, Freeman K, Steinberg BM, Nouri M. Efficacy of DHE photodynamic therapy for respiratory papillomatosis: immediate and long-term results. *Laryngoscope.* 1998; **108**: 962–7.

25. Shikowitz MJ, Abramson AL, Steinberg BM, DeVoti J, Bonaqura VR, Mullooly V et al. Clinical trial of photodynamic therapy with meso-tetra (hydroxyphenyl) chlorin for respiratory papillomatosis. *Archives of Otolaryngology – Head and Neck Surgery.* 2005; **131**: 99–105.

26. Moffitt Jr. OP. Treatment of laryngeal papillomatosis with bovine wart vaccine: report of cases. *Laryngoscope.* 1959; **69**: 1421–8.

27. Pashley NR. Can mumps vaccine induce remission in recurrent respiratory papilloma? *Archives of Otolaryngology – Head and Neck Surgery.* 2002; **128**: 783–6.

28. Sethi N, Palefsky J. Treatment of human papillomavirus (HPV) type 16-infected cells using herpes simplex virus type 1 thymidine kinase-mediated gene therapy transcriptionally regulated by the HPV E2 protein. *Human Gene Therapy.* 2003; **14**: 45–57.

29. Shykhon M, Kuo M, Pearman K. Recurrent respiratory papillomatosis. *Clinical Otolaryngology and Allied Sciences.* 2002; **27**: 237–43.

30. Healy GB, Gelber RD, Trowbridge AL, Grundfast KM, Ruben RJ, Price KN. Treatment of recurrent respiratory papillomatosis with human leukocyte interferon. Results of a multicenter randomized clinical trial. *New England Journal of Medicine.* 1988; **319**: 401–7.

31. Leventhal BG, Kashima H, Levine AS, Levy HB. Treatment of recurrent laryngeal papillomatosis with an artificial interferon inducer (poly ICLC). *Journal of Pediatrics.* 1981; **99**: 614–6.

32. Leventhal BG, Kashima HK, Mounts P, Thurmond L, Chapman S, Buckley S et al. Long-term response of recurrent respiratory papillomatosis to treatment with lymphoblastoid interferon alfa-N1. Papilloma Study Group. *New England Journal of Medicine.* 1991; **325**: 613–7.

33. Herberhold C, Walther EK. Combined laser surgery and adjuvant intralesional interferon injection in patients with laryngotracheal papillomatosis. *Advances in Oto-Rhino-Laryngology.* 1995; **49**: 166–9.

34. Chhetri DK, Jahan-Parwar B, Hart SD, Bhuta SM, Berke GS, Shapiro NL. Local and systemic effects of intralaryngeal injection of cidofovir in a canine model. *Laryngoscope.* 2003; **113**: 1922–6.

35. Jahan-Parwar B, Chhetri DK, Hart S, Bhuta S, Berke GS. Development of a canine model for recurrent respiratory papillomatosis. *Annals of Otology, Rhinology and Laryngology.* 2003; **112**: 1011–3.

36. Chhetri DK, Shapiro NL. A scheduled protocol for the treatment of juvenile recurrent respiratory papillomatosis with intralesional cidofovir. *Archives of Otolaryngology – Head and Neck Surgery.* 2003; **129**: 1081–5.

37. Pransky SM, Albright JT, Magit AE. Long-term follow-up of pediatric recurrent respiratory papillomatosis managed with intralesional cidofovir. *Laryngoscope.* 2003; **113**: 1583–7.

38. Chung BJ, Akst LM, Koltai PJ. 3.5-Year follow-up of intralesional cidofovir protocol for pediatric recurrent respiratory papillomatosis. *International Journal of Pediatric Otorhinolaryngology.* 2006; **70**: 1911–7.

39. Kimberlin DW. Current status of antiviral therapy for juvenile-onset recurrent respiratory papillomatosis. *Antiviral Research.* 2004; **63**: 141–51.

40. Morrison GA, Kotecha B, Evans JN. Ribavirin treatment for juvenile respiratory papillomatosis. *Journal of Laryngology and Otology.* 1993; **107**: 423–6.

41. Balauff A, Sira J, Pearman K, McKiernan P, Buckels J, Kelly D. Successful ribavirin therapy for life-threatening laryngeal papillomatosis post liver transplantation. *Pediatric Transplantation.* 2001; **5**: 142–4.

42. Kiroglu M, Cetik F, Soylu L, Abedi T, Aydogan B, Akcali C et al. Acyclovir in the treatment of recurrent respiratory papillomatosis: a preliminary report. *American Journal of Otolaryngology.* 1994; **15**: 212–4.

43. Morrison GA, Evans JN. Juvenile respiratory papillomatosis: acyclovir reassessed. *International Journal of Pediatric Otorhinolaryngology.* 1993; **26**: 193–7.

44. Rosen CA, Bryson PC. Indole-3-carbinol for recurrent respiratory papillomatosis: long-term results. *Journal of Voice.* 2004; **18**: 248–53.

45. Harcourt JP, Worley G, Leighton SE. Cimetidine treatment for recurrent respiratory papillomatosis. *International Journal of Pediatric Otorhinolaryngology.* 1999; **51**: 109–13.

* 46. Wiatrak BJ, Wiatrak DW, Broker TR, Lewis T. Recurrent respiratory papillomatosis: a longitudinal study comparing severity associated with human papilloma viral types 6 and 11 and other risk factors in a large pediatric population. *Laryngoscope.* 2004; **114**: 1–23. *A longitudinal study looking at prognostic factors in RRP.*

47. Lindeberg H. Laryngeal papillomas: histomorphometric evaluation of multiple and solitary lesions. *Clinical Otolaryngology and Allied Sciences.* 1991; **16**: 257–60.

48. Morgan AH, Zitsch RP. Recurrent respiratory papillomatosis in children: a retrospective study of management and complications. *Ear, Nose and Throat Journal.* 1986; **65**: 19–28.

49. Lindman JP, Gibbons MD, Morlier R, Wiatrak BJ. Voice quality of prepubescent children with quiescent recurrent respiratory papillomatosis. *International Journal of Pediatric Otorhinolaryngology.* 2004; **68**: 529–36.

50. Steinberg BM, Topp WC, Schneider PS, Abramson AL. Laryngeal papillomavirus infection during clinical remission. *New England Journal of Medicine.* 1983; **308**: 1261–4.

51. Weiss MD, Kashima HK. Tracheal involvement in laryngeal papillomatosis. *Laryngoscope.* 1983; **93**: 45–8.

52. Bauman NM, Smith RJ. Recurrent respiratory papillomatosis. *Pediatric Clinics of North America.* 1996; **43**: 1385–401.

53. Shapiro AM, Rimell FL, Shoemaker D, Pou A, Stool SE. Tracheotomy in children with juvenile-onset recurrent respiratory papillomatosis: the Children's Hospital of Pittsburgh experience. *Annals of Otology, Rhinology and Laryngology.* 1996; **105**: 1–5.

54. Go C, Schwartz MR, Donovan DT. Molecular transformation of recurrent respiratory papillomatosis: viral typing and p53 overexpression. *Annals of Otology, Rhinology and Laryngology.* 2003; **112**: 298–302.

* 55. Buchinsky FJ, Derkay CS, Leal SM, Donfack J, Ehrlich GD, Post JC. Multicenter initiative seeking critical genes in respiratory papillomatosis. *Laryngoscope.* 2004; **114**: 349–57. *A review of current thinking and an outline of a proposed study to further unravel the aetiology and pathogenesis of this complex disease.*

56. Freed GL, Derkay CS. Prevention of recurrent respiratory papillomatosis: role of HPV vaccination. *International Journal of Pediatric Otorhinolaryngology.* 2006; **70**: 1799–803.

92

Foreign bodies in the ear and the aerodigestive tract in children

A SIMON CARNEY, NIMESH PATEL AND RAY CLARKE

Introduction	1184	Best clinical practice	1191
Foreign bodies in the ear canal	1184	Deficiencies in current knowledge and areas for future	
Nasal foreign bodies	1186	research	1191
Ingested foreign bodies	1186	References	1191
Key points	1191		

SEARCH STRATEGY

The data and opinions presented in this chapter are supported by a Medline search using the key words child, foreign body, ear, nose, throat, larynx, trachea, bronchus, pharynx and oesophagus.

INTRODUCTION

Nature determined that we possess seven orifices. The otolaryngologist deals with five. Children are naturally curious about their surroundings and about these orifices! They are inclined to place toys, foodstuff and household articles in the ear, nose or the oral cavity. Sometimes the culprit is a sibling or a playground or nursery chum. Foreign bodies lodged within the ear, nose, larynx, trachea, pharynx or oesophagus may present as a minor irritation or a life-threatening problem.

FOREIGN BODIES IN THE EAR CANAL

An aural foreign body is an object not derived from the individual's own external ear, lying within the external auditory canal. Although the pinna is a part of the external ear, diseases of the pinna are covered in Chapter 236, Conditions of the pinna and external auditory canal; Chapter 236g, Acquired atresia of the external ear; Chapter 236i, Perichondritis of the external ear; and Chapter 236m, Haematoma auris; and foreign bodies of the pinna (e.g. ear-rings and studs) are not discussed in this chapter.

Foreign bodies within the external auditory canal can be classified as inanimate or animate (e.g. live insects). Inanimate objects can be inert or corrosive/irritant, organic or nonorganic and hydrophobic or hydrophilic.

Presentation

Although it is usually children that present with aural foreign bodies, self-instrumentation of the ear canal not infrequently brings the embarrassed adult to the otolaryngologist.

Inert foreign bodies may be completely asymptomatic and go unnoticed for many weeks, months or even years. Many patients complain of irritation, deafness, otorrhoea or tinnitus. Gradual wax impaction medial to a small foreign body may lead to a later presentation due to the disruption of the physiological keratinocyte migration.

The isthmus is the narrowest part of the external auditory canal and objects frequently impact at this point. Objects lateral to the isthmus are usually more readily removed.

In a review of 191 aural foreign bodies, 74 percent were in children aged seven or under, with beans, pebbles, beads (**Figure 92.1**), insects and small toys being the most common objects.[1, 2] Although parents and primary care health personnel are often worried about the possibility of residual perforation of the eardrum, this is uncommon unless there is unskilled instrumentation in attempted removal.

Button batteries are arguably the most dangerous foreign body in the ear, producing tissue necrosis as the alkaline fluid seeps out of them. The tissue necrosis then produces granuloma formation. Symptoms which can mimic malignant otitis externa can also develop.[3]

Insects in the ear can produce very distressing symptoms and the removal of live, moving insects can exacerbate oedema and trauma (especially where multiple bites and/or stings occur).[4] [**]

Management

In a cooperative awake patient, the majority of foreign bodies can be removed with ease. General anaesthesia may be required for removal of up to 30 percent of objects, especially in the paediatric population.[1] Removal of foreign bodies in an uncooperative child can result in trauma, such as lacerations or tympanic membrane perforation which can occur in between 10–47 percent of cases.[2, 5] If an object is not removed easily on the first attempt, referral to an otolaryngologist is essential to minimize further trauma to the child.[5, 6]

In a large review of 603 patients, the presence of a spherical foreign body, an object near the tympanic membrane and delay of 24 hours following insertion were identified as high risk factors for poor outcomes.[7]

In a review of the management of aural foreign bodies in an emergency department, when an object was graspable (e.g. a piece of plastic), emergency staff could remove it in 64 percent of cases with a complication rate of 14 percent, whereas if the object was non-graspable (e.g. a bead), only 45 percent could be removed (with 65 percent being referred to an otolaryngologist) with a 70 percent complication rate.[8]

Where objects are not removed rapidly otitis externa can develop and, if this is not treated, complications can rarely include mastoiditis and deep neck space infections.[9]

Techniques for removal include irrigation, suction, instrumentation or a combination of the three.[6] The use of irrigation is naturally contraindicated for extracting hydrophilic items such as peas, beans, other vegetable matter or tissue paper. The use of the otomicroscope has been shown to produce a higher success rate for foreign body removal.[7] The technique of extracting a spherical or ovoid item from the canal is to slide a wax hook over the top of it and then rotate the hook to engage the object and pull it out of the canal. Do not attempt removal by forceps as this results in it slipping further away. 'Superglue'[TM] (cryanoacrylate) impregnated into cotton-buds can be used to aid aural foreign body removal,[10] although it is significantly slower than using hooks and other standard instruments.[11] Superglue probes are particularly useful for the management of smooth foreign bodies such as beads or beans impacted at the isthmus.[12] Unwanted superglue in the external auditory canal is a particularly troublesome problem. Although some individuals will require surgical removal via an end-aural incision,[13] there are now case reports of the use of acetone[14] and warm 3 percent hydrogen peroxide[15] which suggest these conservative techniques may be worth trying before subjecting a child to general anaesthesia. Repeated unsuccessful attempts at foreign body removal by an inexperienced practitioner will distress an anxious child and may compromise the options open to an otolaryngologist. If there is any doubt whatsoever about the potential success of an attempted extraction, then referral to a specialist is indicated.

The otolaryngologist should have a low threshold for arranging a semi-urgent admission for general anaesthetic removal if conservative methods fail. Urgent removal can only be justified for battery removal, or where severe oedema and symptoms exist. Rarely, an end-aural incision may be necessary to remove the foreign body.[16]

Studies comparing management options for aural foreign bodies are few in number.

For alive, animated foreign bodies, an *in vitro* study involving 17 test preparations showed that 95 percent

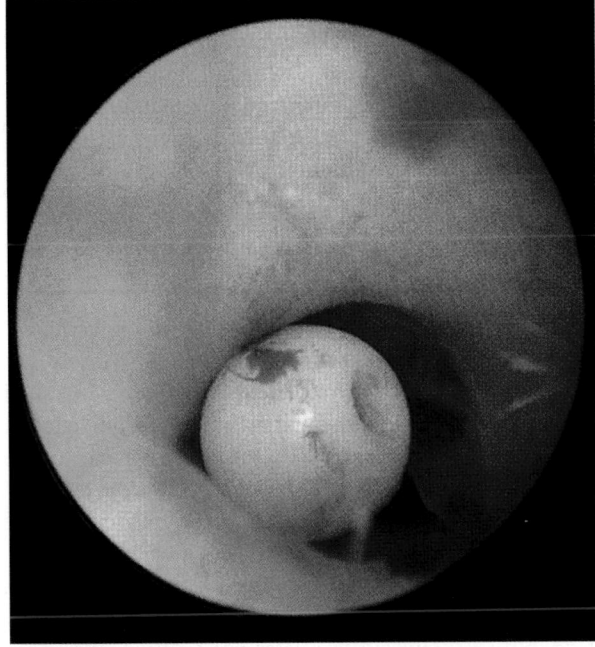

Figure 92.1 Foreign body (bead) in the ear canal.

ethanol killed all test insects in the fastest time (median 27 seconds). Oils performed poorly (51 seconds) and water and saline were particularly slow (180 seconds).[4] [***]

NASAL FOREIGN BODIES

Presentation and management

Nasal foreign bodies are most common between the ages of two and five.[17] They may be inert, hygrophilic or corrosive. Soft objects such as sponge fragments or tissue paper are the commonest to be found in the nose, in contrast to the hard objects inserted into the ears.[2] As is the case in the ear, small button batteries can produce devastating tissue damage and necrosis including septal perforation in a short time.[18] A nasal foreign body may remain *in situ* for weeks and only present with a unilateral nasal discharge, often with a pronounced vestibulitis (**Figure 92.2**). Rigid endoscopes provide excellent visualization and can potentially minimize mucosal trauma. Although it has been claimed that a 4 mm rigid nasendoscope can be passed with ease in children as young as two years of age without decongestion,[19] with the increased availability of smaller 2.7 mm endoscopes, it is the author's practice to use decongestion and as small an endoscope as possible in the paediatric population. The use of nebulized adrenaline provides excellent nasal decongestion and can greatly facilitate removal of foreign bodies, either by nose blowing or using instrumenta-tion.[20] In general, the clinician has to make a clinical judgement as to what is going to be the best method for removal of a foreign body,[17] bearing in mind that a child is unlikely to tolerate repeated manipulation and the doctor will only have one attempt at using a method that is going to cause any pain whatsoever. Magnets may be of use[21] and nasal washing has been proposed as a method of removing foreign bodies, but is not widely practised.[22] Superglue can also be effective.[23] The use of oral positive-pressure techniques has now been shown to be an effective way of removing anterior nasal foreign bodies.

An oral Ambubag can be used[24] (three patients, 100 percent success) but the 'parent's kiss', where the carer blows into the open mouth of the child whilst occluding the contralateral nostril, is probably less traumatic for the child. Reported success rates vary from 79–100 percent.[25, 26] The use of a 'Fogarty' embolectomy balloon catheter is another excellent way to easily remove foreign bodies from the nasal cavity and in one series of 25 patients, successfully removed 23 foreign bodies (92 percent) without the need for a general anaesthetic.[27]

The possibility of inhalation into the tracheobronchial tree[28] needs to be borne in mind when managing a child with a nasal foreign body. [**] This is remarkably uncommon and is probably only a significant risk in the neurologically compromised child who has a poor gag reflex. If a nasal foreign body slips back into the nasopharynx it will usually be swallowed or expectorated. No complication of barotrauma to either the ears or lower airway has been reported in the literature search employed for this chapter.

Rhinolith

A rhinolith is a partially or totally calcified mass of tissue in the nasal cavity which may form around a foreign body nidus or can develop *de novo*.[29, 30] They usually have a laminated structure, suggestive of a pathophysiological mechanism that involves layers of mucin aggregating around the foreign body. Each mucin layer subsequently becomes calcified, perhaps aided by the presence of turbulent air currents. They are classified as endogenous when they form around normal body material, such as blood clots, misplaced tooth remnants or bony sequestra. Exogenous rhinoliths form around foreign bodies in-serted into the nose – usually of nonhuman material.[29, 30] They can cause considerable symptoms, including nasal obstruction, purulent nasal discharge, rhinosinusitis and septal perforation.[29, 30] They frequently require a general anaesthetic and transnasal removal, with or without fragmentation of the rhinolith.[31]

INGESTED FOREIGN BODIES

These may be swallowed and impact in the pharynx or oesophagus, or inhaled and obstruct the larynx or tracheobronchial tree. Either may prove fatal. Ingested foreign bodies in children represent a major global public health problem.[32, 33] Coins, toys and food particles are the principal dangers, although regional and cultural factors in part dictate the frequency with which different objects occur.[34] Fish bones in the pharynx are commonly encountered in the Far East and in Greece. In Turkey watermelon seeds are the most frequently aspirated objects.[35] Coins are a universal danger particularly for pharyngo-oesophageal impaction

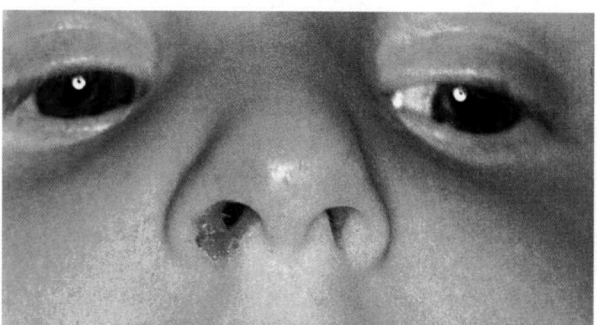

Figure 92.2 Nasal vestibulitis due to a neglected foreign body.

and nuts for tracheobronchial aspiration.[32, 36] Nonspherical objects equal to or less than 1.5 inches (38.10 mm), and particularly spherical objects equal to or less than 1.75 inches (44.50 mm) in diameter, are especially dangerous. Consumer product legislation should take account of these data.[33] The main risks are to children under three years. In this age group the second molars have not yet developed, the child's grinding and swallowing mechanisms are poor and glottic closure is immature.[37]

Pharynx and oesophagus

When considering foreign bodies in the pharynx and oesophagus, whether the object is potentially penetrating (sharp or corrosive) or nonpenetrating is probably the most pertinent consideration. The vast majority of swallowed objects pass through the digestive tract and are excreted, often undetected.[38] A small (and statistically undeterminable) proportion will impact in the pharynx or oesophagus. There is a clear history of ingestion in 96 percent and the median age was three years in a retrospective ten-year review of 327 patients. Complications, including respiratory symptoms and abscess formation, occured in 7.6 percent of cases, the latter always associated with sharp foreign bodies and the former more common in the younger age group.[38]

Management

A plain radiograph will often show the position of the foreign body, provided the child is stable enough to undergo an x-ray. If there is doubt, a lateral view will help to determine if the object is in the pharynx or the airway (**Figure 92.3**). Bear in mind that an object in the upper oesophagus can cause airway obstruction by pressing on the adjacent trachea. Once the presumptive diagnosis of a pharyngo-oesophageal foreign body has been made, arrangements should be made for early removal as oedema and mucosal swelling will make retrieval more difficult.

The use of rigid angled nasendoscopes and curved forceps designed for fish bone removal has greatly facilitated fish bone removal from the oropharynx under local anaesthetic in adults,[39] but general anaesthesia is more likely to be needed in a child. Other original techniques, such as using nasal suction catheters in conjunction with nasendoscopy, have also been described.[40] Small fish bones may be undetectable and there is some evidence that, even without removal, they may absorb without further sequelae.[41] This fact must not lull the surgeon into a false sense of security as prompt management of all pharyngo-oesophageal foreign bodies results in better outcomes and reduced complications.[34, 38] Major complications include retropharyngeal and mediastinal abscess, migration of the foreign body into deep structures, oesophageal perforation (from either the

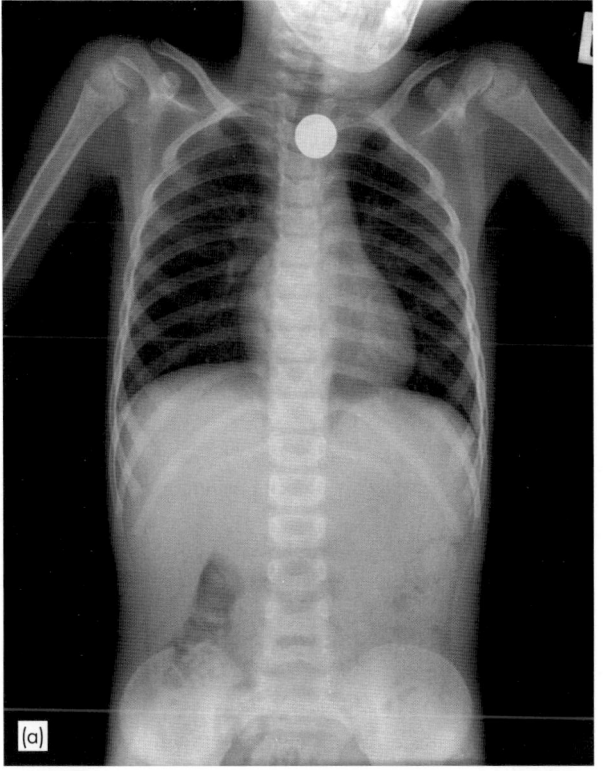

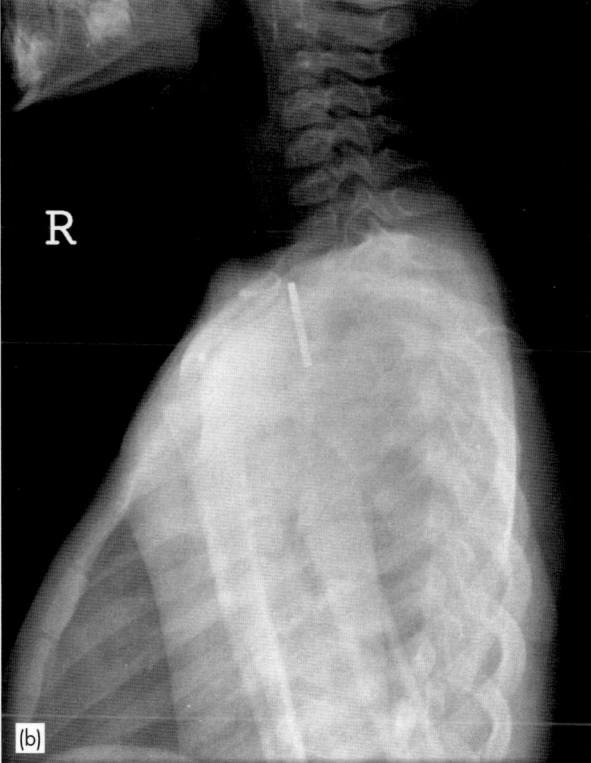

Figure 92.3 (a) Foreign body (coin) in the oesophagus. The lateral view (b) confirms the position.

foreign body or endoscopic procedure) and luminal stenosis.[34, 42] Again, alkaline batteries are particularly dangerous because the tissue necrosis can be devastating and fatalities have been described.[43]

For oesophageal foreign bodies the choice between flexible and rigid endoscopy remains controversial.[34] Rigid endoscopy is historically associated with a perforation rate of 0.2–1.2 percent compared to rates of 0.02–0.05 percent with flexible endoscopy;[34] however, in retrospective series looking specifically at endoscopy for foreign body removal, no difference in complication rates was found.[38] Rigid endoscopy gives a much better view of the hypopharynx, cricopharyngeus and the first few centimetres of the cervical oesophagus, whereas a flexible endoscope gives an excellent view in the thoracic oesophagus and oesophago-gastric junction.[34]

In a review of 5240 patients with ingested foreign bodies from Hong Kong, a management algorithm with flexible oesophagoscopy only used for patients (of all ages) with symptoms distal to the sternal notch resulted in 7.7 percent requiring rigid pharyngo-oesophagoscopy and 1.5 percent having flexible endoscopy (with over 90 percent of patients being managed conservatively). Complications from the foreign body or endoscopy occurred in 0.6 percent.[34]

The delicate structures of the oesophagus in the child mean that instrumental perforation of the pharynx or oesophagus is an ever-present danger. For the investigation and management of suspected perforation of the oesophagus the reader is referred to Chapter 156, Oesophageal diseases.

Larynx

Glottic impaction of a foreign body often leads to laryngospasm and sudden complete airway obstruction and death with peak incidence at one to three years.[44] Large, thin objects, such as artificial nails,[45] may be more prone to lodge in the larynx and indeed in almost all cases of successful surgical removal of a foreign body, the object is small and thin.[46] Larger objects are either removed by emergency clearing procedures or else death is rapid, unless a surgical airway is created within seconds.[46] It has been estimated that in the 1970s, almost 600 children per year died in the USA from airway obstruction.[47] However, public education and awareness of first-aid procedures for acute foreign-body ingestion into the airway has resulted in a nine-fold reduction in mortality rates. The 'Heimlich manoeuvre', which involves compression of the upper abdomen to encourage expulsion of a foreign body, was introduced in 1975.[48] In infants, lying the child on its back on the adults knee and pressing firmly on the upper abdomen (**Figure 92.4**) is the preferred manoeuvre. In recent years, audit has shown that 85 percent of airways are cleared before emergency teams arrive, with 38 percent being cleared by the children themselves.[49]

Younger children are less likely to clear their own airway. Emergency practitioners use this fact to argue for the widespread teaching of airway-clearing manoeuvres to new parents.[49] Older methods previously taught for airway-clearing, such as 'finger-sweeping' can in fact result in the subglottic impaction of foreign bodies and are no longer recommended.[50] [**/*][Grade C/D]

If the history is at all suggestive of an inhaled foreign body in a child, even if examination is normal, seek the advice of an experienced otolaryngologist.

Tracheo-bronchial tree

The peak incidence of inhaled foreign bodies is between the ages of one and three years, with a male:female ratio of 2:1.[49, 51] Only 12 percent will impact in the larynx with most passing through the cords into the tracheobronchial tree.[52] In contrast to adults, where objects tend to lodge in the distal bronchi or right main bronchus, in children they tend to lie more centrally within the trachea (53 percent) or just distal to the carina (47 percent).[53, 54]

The typical history is of a choking episode while the child feeds or while (s)he is playing with a toy or small object. Vigorous coughing ensues. The parents then find to their alarm that the object has disappeared. This can be followed by a relatively symptom-free period as the object lodges in the lower airway. Partial obstruction of one of the main stem bronchi causes the characteristic wheeze over one side of the chest on auscultation and the hyperinflation of one lung evident on chest x-ray, although these classical findings are by no means universal. The hyperinflation occurs due to a 'ball-valve' effect where the negative intrathoracic pressure on inspiration dilates the bronchial lumen around the foreign body. Upon expiration, the positive pulmonary pressure compresses the main bronchi, occluding the airway around the offending object, preventing expulsion of the air.

Although most patients present with a history of wheeze or cough, up to 20 percent may present after several days due to secondary respiratory complications.[51] A high index of suspicion and early consideration of bronchoscopy are essential. If the child is well enough, a plain chest x-ray may show the characteristic changes of 'obstructive emphysema' as air is trapped beyond a partly occluded bronchus (**Figure 92.5**). The use of CT to aid diagnosis of tracheo-bronchial foreign bodies has not been a great advantage. Peanuts do not show up well (sensitivity of <35 percent), although objects such as LEGO™ can be detected easily with a sensitivity and specificity in excess of 90 percent.[55]

Better public awareness of the dangers of small objects and legislation to control their use in toys and household objects has meant that in western communities even highly specialized otolaryngologists in large tertiary institutions such as Johns Hopkins Hospital may only see an average of 5.9 cases per year. Residents may only

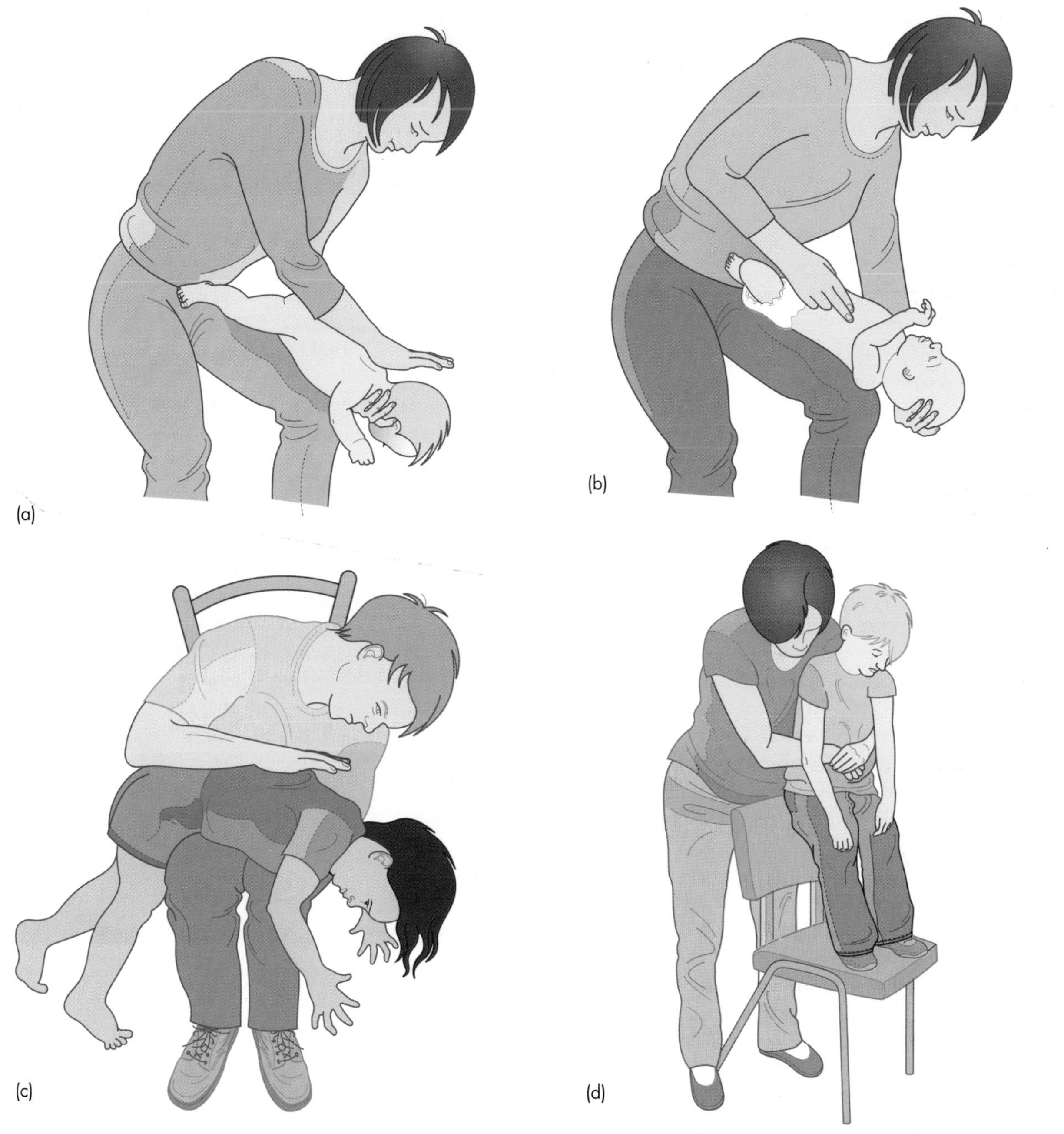

Figure 92.4 Emergency manoeuvres to encourage expectoration of a laryngeal foreign body in children: (a) back blows to an infant; (b) abdominal thrusts to an infant; (c) back blows to a small child; (d) Heimlich manoeuvre in a standing child. Redrawn with permission from Mackway-Jones K (ed). 2004. *Advanced paediatric life support: the practical approach*, 4th edn. London: BMJ Books.

see or perform between one and eight cases during their training.[56] Teaching on animal models and/or manikins is mandatory for trainees to develop the skills required to cope with this most difficult airway emergency in a particularly vulnerable patient population.

If the foreign body goes untreated, mediastinal shift, pneumothorax or pneumonia are common sequelae. Smaller foreign bodies may induce granuloma formation and an aggressive search for the foreign body must be made in new cases of bronchial granuloma.[57] If a foreign body is left untreated for many years, lung resection for bronchiectasis may eventually be required.[58]

In the acute situation, whilst emergency preparations for surgical removal are underway, high flow oxygen is essential and a helium-oxygen mixture (Heliox®) may help reduce the work of breathing.[59] Even after successful removal, atelectasis, pneumonia, retained fragments, airway spasm or airway oedema may still occur and the child should be monitored closely,[56] ideally in a high-dependency or intensive-care facility.

Once a foreign body is removed, a meticulous examination of the tracheobronchial tree must be undertaken to exclude further foreign bodies/fragments or other abnormalities.[60, 61] Following rigid bronchoscopy,

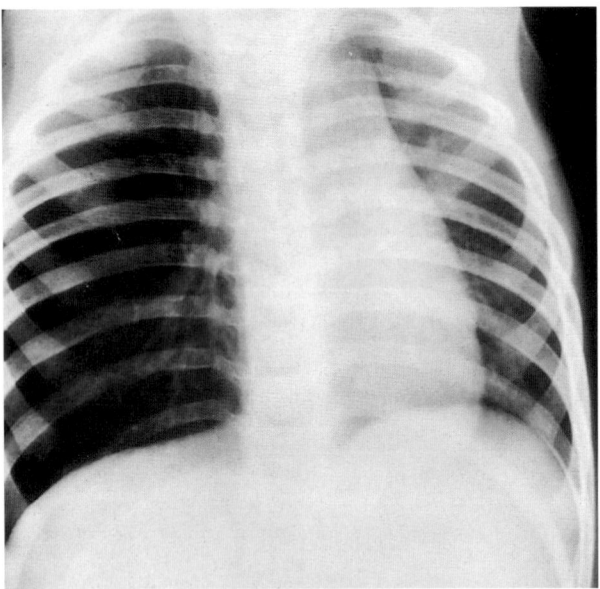

Figure 92.5 Chest x-ray showing hyperinflation of the right lung due to a foreign body in the right main stem bronchus.

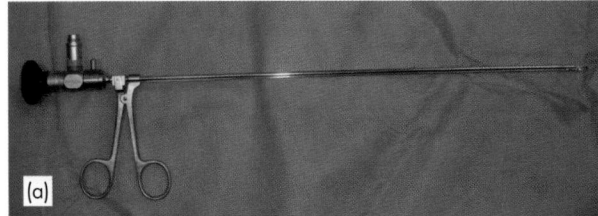

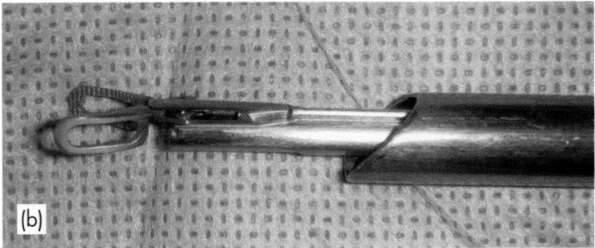

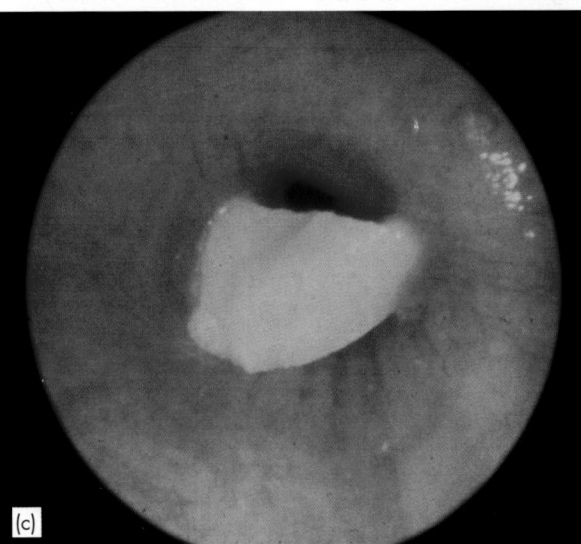

Figure 92.6 (a) Optical forceps with an integral telescope for foreign body retrieval. (b) The blades of the optical forceps project through a ventilating bronchoscope allowing safe retrieval under direct vision. (c) A peanut in the bronchus.

some institutions use systemic steroids and nebulized vasoconstrictors to reduce airway oedema and the incidence of postoperative complications.

In a series of 250 patients with tracheobronchial foreign bodies, there was a clear history of ingestion in only 38 percent of cases and over 99 percent of cases were successfully treated endoscopically.[62] In 95 percent of patients in one series, a history of choking, coughing or wheeze was present. When bronchoscopy was performed, foreign bodies were identified and removed in 80 percent of cases.[63] However, in a series of 235 cases, the sensitivity of choking and coughing (82 and 80 percent) was high. The sensitivity of a chest radiograph was 66 percent with a specificity of 51 percent. The sensitivity of auscultation was 80 percent with a specificity of 72 percent. The combination of history, signs and radiological abnormalities is more useful than any one separately and a high index of suspicion is essential.[64] In a large series of 500 patients, the mortality rate in 1977 was 1.8 percent,[65] but in a more recent large series the mortality was only 0.8 percent.[35]

The choice of either using a flexible or rigid endoscope remains controversial. Otolaryngologists traditionally believe rigid endoscopes to be the optimal instrument for tracheo-bronchial foreign bodies.[66] The airway is controlled, there is a large spectrum of sizes and instrumentation available, excellent visualization via rigid optical endoscopes and the ability to use the scope itself as a conduit for removal of the foreign body.[61] However, there are certain objects that may be more suitably removed with flexible fibreoptic instruments, or a combination of rigid and flexible techniques.[67] In one series of 26 patients (including two where rigid endoscopy had failed due to the distal location of the objects), using ureteral stone baskets and forceps, flexible bronchoscopy

was able to remove 100 percent of objects.[61] In most cases, the airway was secured via an endotracheal tube or laryngeal mask, although in the cases of failed rigid endoscopy, the rigid scope served as the conduit for the flexible instrument.[61] Where standard 3.6-mm paediatric flexible bronchoscopes are used, the biopsy channel can be used for instrumentation, but if the ultrathin (2.2 mm) scope is used in smaller children, baskets and forceps need to be passed down the side of the flexible scope.[61] Bleeding may occur during the removal of a foreign body, but this can usually be controlled using adrenaline-soaked balls or patties.[61] [**/*]

The standard paediatric flexible scope requires an endotracheal tube with a minimum internal diameter of 4.5 mm. Even then, delicate instrumentation may be impossible without periods of apnoea. As is often the case in medicine, the decision to use flexible or rigid instrumentation depends on a variety of things, including the availability of equipment, experience of personnel, the age and medical status of the child, nature of the object and length of time since impaction. Ideally, a coordinated team of surgeons and physicians, trained in both rigid and flexible endoscopy, who can perform the removal of the foreign body in one procedure undertake this work and accept patients from a designated catchment area.[61] Skilled paediatric anaesthesia is vital and close cooperation between the anaesthetist and bronchoscopist is essential to ensure the child's alveolar ventilation is maintained throughout the procedure.

The newer optical grabbing forceps contain an integrated telescope and can be passed through most rigid ventilating bronchoscopes (size 3.5 and above). They give a superb view of the trachea and the main stem bronchi (**Figure 92.6**). This enables the operator to grasp an object such as a peanut under direct vision. These optical instruments have made the management of tracheobronchial foreign bodies much easier and safer, although not all institutions have such instrumentation. Fogarty catheters and other improvised equipment can be used to successfully extract bronchial foreign bodies[68] although, even in experienced centres, a small percentage of cases (1.8 percent in one large series)[35] will need thoracotomy to remove the foreign body and extra-corporeal membrane oxygenation can be used to 'buy time' and prevent mediastinal compression in extreme circumstances.[69]

KEY POINTS

- 'Button' batteries are potentially corrosive. Whether in the ear canal, the nose or the aerodigestive tract they should be removed as soon as possible.
- Instrumental perforation is an ever present danger when removing oesophageal foreign bodies in children.
- Bronchoscopy for foreign body extraction is a highly skilled technique. Teaching and learning this skill is difficult in communities where foreign body aspiration is now rare.
- A high index of suspicion is essential in suspected foreign body inhalation in children. This is a potentially lethal condition.

Best clinical practice

✓ Spherical objects, items in the deep meatus and foreign bodies present for over 24 hours are more likely to require a general anaesthetic for removal. [Grade B]

✓ Multiple, ill-prepared attempts at removal should be avoided. Early referral to an otolaryngologist must be considered if there is any doubt as to the success of an extraction attempt. [Grade C]
✓ Otomicroscopy, micro-instruments, suction, irrigation, glue-tipped probes and open surgery all have their place. [Grade B]
✓ Ninety-five percent ethanol is most effective for killing lodged insects prior to their removal. [Grade B]
✓ If general anaesthesia is required, it is reasonable to wait for a suitable elective operating list, except for corrosive items and live animals/insects which require urgent removal. [Grade C]
✓ Once the presumptive diagnosis of a pharyngo-oesophageal foreign body has been made, arrangements should be made for early removal as oedema and mucosal swelling will make retrieval more difficult. [Grade C]
✓ If the history is at all suggestive of an inhaled foreign body in a child, even if examination is normal, seek the advice of an experienced otolaryngologist. [Grade C/D]

Deficiencies in current knowledge and areas for future research

➢ A global campaign focussing on consumer legislation to monitor the size of small objects, toys and household goods would greatly reduce mortality from inhaled foreign bodies in children.
➢ Increased parent and carer awareness of the dangers of small objects which children can swallow or inhale should also help reduce mortality.
➢ Re-organization of otolaryngology services and restucturing of training in ORL needs to take account of the need for centralized and skilled care for the removal of inhaled foreign bodies in children.

REFERENCES

1. Ansley JF, Cunningham MJ. Treatment of aural foreign bodies in children. *Pediatrics.* 1998; **101**: 638–41.
2. Balbani AP, Sanchez TG, Butugan O, Kii MI, Angelico Jr. FV, Ikino CM *et al.* Ear and nose foreign body removal in children. *International Journal of Pediatric Otorhinolaryngology.* 1998; **46**: 37–42.
3. Bhisitkul DM, Dunham M. An unsuspected alkaline battery foreign body presenting as malignant otitis externa. *Pediatric Emergency Care.* 1992; **8**: 141–2.

4. Antonelli PJ, Ahmadi A, Prevatt A. Insecticidal activity of common reagents for insect foreign bodies of the ear. *Laryngoscope*. 2001; **111**: 15–20.

5. Bressler K, Shelton C. Ear foreign-body removal: a review of 98 consecutive cases. *Laryngoscope*. 1993; **103**: 367–70.

6. Fritz S, Kelen GD, Sivertson KT. Foreign bodies of the external auditory canal. *Emergency Medicine Clinics of North America*. 1987; **5**: 183–92.

* 7. Schulze SL, Kerschner J, Beste D. Pediatric external auditory canal foreign bodies: a review of 698 cases. *Otolaryngology – Head and Neck Surgery*. 2002; **127**: 73–78. *Excellent review demonstrating which features are particularly associated with complications and suggesting referral guidelines for primary care clinicians.*

8. DiMuzio Jr. J, Deschler DG. Emergency department management of foreign bodies of the external ear canal in children. *Otology and Neurotology*. 2002; **23**: 473–5.

9. Jones RL, Chavda SV, Pahor AL. Parapharyngeal abscess secondary to an external auditory meatus foreign body. *Journal of Laryngology and Otology*. 1997; **111**: 1086–7.

10. Benger JR, Davies PH. A useful form of glue ear. *Journal of Accident and Emergency Medicine*. 2000; **17**: 149–50.

11. McLaughlin R, Ullah R, Heylings D. Comparative prospective study of foreign body removal from external auditory canals of cadavers with right angle hook or cyanoacrylate glue. *Emergency Medicine Journal*. 2002; **19**: 43–5.

12. Pride H, Schwab R. A new technique for removing foreign bodies of the external auditory canal. *Pediatric Emergency Care*. 1989; **5**: 135–6.

13. White SJ, Broner S. The use of acetone to dissolve a Styrofoam impaction of the ear. *Annals of Emergency Medicine*. 1994; **23**: 580–2.

14. Abadir WF, Nakhla V, Chong P. Removal of superglue from the external ear using acetone: case report and literature review. *Journal of Laryngology and Otology*. 1995; **109**: 1219–21.

15. Persaud R. A novel approach to the removal of superglue from the ear. *Journal of Laryngology and Otology*. 2001; **115**: 901–2.

16. Engelsma RJ, Lee WC. Impacted aural foreign body requiring endaural incision and canal widening for removal. *International Journal of Pediatric Otorhinolaryngology*. 1998; **44**: 169–71.

17. Kadish HA, Corneli HM. Removal of nasal foreign bodies in the pediatric population. *American Journal of Emergency Medicine*. 1997; **15**: 54–6.

18. Brown CR. Intranasal button battery causing septal perforation: a case report. *Journal of Laryngology and Otology*. 1994; **108**: 589–90.

19. Kubba H, Bingham BJ. Endoscopy in the assessment of children with nasal obstruction. *Journal of Laryngology and Otology*. 2001; **115**: 380–4.

20. Douglas AR. Use of nebulized adrenaline to aid expulsion of intra-nasal foreign bodies in children. *Journal of Laryngology and Otology*. 1996; **110**: 559–60.

21. Douglas SA, Mirza S, Stafford FW. Magnetic removal of a nasal foreign body. *International Journal of Pediatric Otorhinolaryngology*. 2002; **62**: 165–7.

22. Lichenstein R, Giudice EL. Nasal wash technique for nasal foreign body removal. *Pediatric Emergency Care*. 2000; **16**: 59–60.

23. Hanson RM, Stephens M. Cyanoacrylate-assisted foreign body removal from the ear and nose in children. *Journal of Paediatrics and Child Health*. 1994; **30**: 77–8.

24. Finkelstein JA. Oral Ambu-bag insufflation to remove unilateral nasal foreign bodies. *American Journal of Emergency Medicine*. 1996; **14**: 57–8.

25. Backlin SA. Positive-pressure technique for nasal foreign body removal in children. *Annals of Emergency Medicine*. 1995; **25**: 554–5.

26. Botma M, Bader R, Kubba H. 'A parent's kiss': evaluating an unusual method for removing nasal foreign bodies in children. *Journal of Laryngology and Otology*. 2000; **114**: 598–600.

27. Nandapalan V, McIlwain JC. Removal of nasal foreign bodies with a Fogarty biliary balloon catheter. *Journal of Laryngology and Otology*. 1994; **108**: 758–60.

28. Cohen HA, Goldberg E, Horev Z. Removal of nasal foreign bodies in children. *Clinical Pediatrics*. 1993; **32**: 192.

29. Balatsouras D, Eliopoulos P, Kaberos A, Economou C. Rhinolithiasis: an unusual cause of nasal obstruction. *Rhinology*. 2002; **40**: 162–4.

30. Ezsias A, Sugar AW. Rhinolith: an unusual case and an update. *Annals of Otology, Rhinology and Laryngology*. 1997; **106**: 135–8.

31. Celikkanat S, Turgut S, Ozcan I, Balyan FR, Ozdem C. Rhinolithiasis. *Rhinology*. 1997; **35**: 39–40.

* 32. Reilly BK, Stool D, Chen X, Rider G, Stool SE, Reilly JS. Foreign body injury in children in the twentieth century: a modern comparison to the Jackson collection. *International Journal of Pediatric Otorhinolaryngology*. 2003; **67**: S171–4. *A detailed account of the spectrum of objects commonly ingested.*

* 33. Milkovich SM, Rider G, Greaves D, Stool D, Chen X. Application of data for prevention of foreign body injury in children. *International Journal of Pediatric Otorhinolaryngology*. 2003; **67**: S179–82. *An analysis of size and shape which should inform consumer legislation.*

34. Lam HC, Woo JK, van Hasselt CA. Management of ingested foreign bodies: a retrospective review of 5240 patients. *Journal of Laryngology and Otology*. 2001; **115**: 954–7.

35. Eren S, Balci AE, Dikici B, Doblan M, Eren MN. Foreign body aspiration in children: experience of 1160 cases. *Annals of Tropical Paediatrics*. 2003; **23**: 31–7.

36. van As AB, du Toit N, Wallis L, Stool D, Chen X, Rode H. The South African experience with ingestion injury in children. *International Journal of Pediatric Otorhinolaryngology*. 2003; **67**: S175–8.

37. Morley RE, Ludemann JP, Moxham JP, Kozak FK, Riding KH. Foreign body aspiration in infants and toddlers: recent trends in British Columbia. *Journal of Otolaryngology*. 2004; **33**: 37–41.

38. Singh B, Kantu M, Har-El G, Lucente FE. Complications associated with 327 foreign bodies of the pharynx, larynx, and esophagus. *Annals of Otology, Rhinology and Laryngology*. 1997; **106**: 301–4.

39. Savage J, Brookes N, Lloyd S, Mackay I. Fish bones in the vallecula and tongue base: removal with the rigid nasal endoscope. *Journal of Laryngology and Otology*. 2002; **116**: 842–3.

40. Viney R, Reid A. An alternative approach to fishbone extraction. *Journal of the Royal College of Surgeons of Edinburgh*. 2002; **47**: 515.

41. Canbay E, Prinsley P. The case of the disappearing fish bone. *Journal of Otolaryngology*. 1995; **24**: 375–6.

42. Osinubi OA, Osiname AI, Pal A, Lonsdale RJ, Butcher C. Foreign body in the throat migrating through the common carotid artery. *Journal of Laryngology and Otology*. 1996; **110**: 793–5.

43. Blatnik DS, Toohill RJ, Lehman RH. Fatal complication from an alkaline battery foreign body in the esophagus. *Annals of Otology, Rhinology and Laryngology*. 1977; **86**: 611–5.

44. Byard RW. Mechanisms of unexpected death in infants and young children following foreign body ingestion. *Journal of Forensic Sciences*. 1996; **41**: 438–41.

45. Bhat NA, Oates J. An unusual foreign body in the larynx: a case report. *Journal of Laryngology and Otology*. 1996; **110**: 1164–5.

46. Brama I, Fearon B. Laryngeal foreign bodies in children. *International Journal of Pediatric Otorhinolaryngology*. 1982; **4**: 259–65.

47. America NSCo. Accident Facts. 1980; **7**.

48. Ross GL, Steventon NB, Pinder DK, Bridger MW. Living on the edge of the post-nasal space: the inhaled foreign body. *Journal of Laryngology and Otology*. 2000; **114**: 56–7.

49. Andazola JJ, Sapien RE. The choking child: what happens before the ambulance arrives? *Prehospital Emergency Care*. 1999; **3**: 7–10.

50. Sharma HS, Sharma S. Management of laryngeal foreign bodies in children. *Journal of Accident and Emergency Medicine*. 1999; **16**: 150–3.

51. Burton EM, Brick WG, Hall JD, Riggs Jr. W, Houston CS. Tracheobronchial foreign body aspiration in children. *Southern Medical Journal*. 1996; **89**: 195–8.

52. Cohen SR, Herbert WI, Lewis Jr. GB, Geller KA. Foreign bodies in the airway. Five-year retrospective study with special reference to management. *Annals of Otology, Rhinology and Laryngology*. 1980; **89**: 437–42.

53. Baharloo F, Veyckemans F, Francis C, Biettlot MP, Rodenstein DO. Tracheobronchial foreign bodies: presentation and management in children and adults. *Chest*. 1999; **115**: 1357–62.

54. Banerjee A, Rao KS, Khanna SK, Narayanan PS, Gupta BK, Sekar JC et al. Laryngo-tracheo-bronchial foreign bodies in children. *Journal of Laryngology and Otology*. 1988; **102**: 1029–32.

55. Applegate KE, Dardinger JT, Lieber ML, Herts BR, Davros WJ, Obuchowski NA et al. Spiral CT scanning technique in the detection of aspiration of LEGO foreign bodies. *Pediatric Radiology*. 2001; **31**: 836–40.

56. Hughes CA, Baroody FM, Marsh BR. Pediatric tracheobronchial foreign bodies: historical review from the Johns Hopkins Hospital. *Annals of Otology, Rhinology and Laryngology*. 1996; **105**: 555–61.

57. Barben J, Berkowitz RG, Kemp A, Massie J. Bronchial granuloma – where's the foreign body? *International Journal of Pediatric Otorhinolaryngology*. 2000; **53**: 215–9.

58. Cataneo AJ, Reibscheid SM, Ruiz Junior RL, Ferrari GF. Foreign body in the tracheobronchial tree. *Clinical Pediatrics*. 1997; **36**: 701–6.

59. Brown L, Sherwin T, Perez JE, Perez DU. Heliox as a temporizing measure for pediatric foreign body aspiration. *Academic Emergency Medicine*. 2002; **9**: 346–7.

60. Blazer S, Naveh Y, Friedman A. Foreign body in the airway. A review of 200 cases. *American Journal of Diseases of Children*. 1980; **134**: 68–71.

61. Swanson KL, Prakash UB, Midthun DE, Edell ES, Utz JP, McDougall JC et al. Flexible bronchoscopic management of airway foreign bodies in children. *Chest*. 2002; **121**: 1695–700.

62. Abdulmajid OA, Ebeid AM, Motaweh MM, Kleibo IS. Aspirated foreign bodies in the tracheobronchial tree: report of 250 cases. *Thorax*. 1976; **31**: 635–40.

63. Black RE, Johnson DG, Matlak ME. Bronchoscopic removal of aspirated foreign bodies in children. *Journal of Pediatric Surgery*. 1994; **29**: 682–4.

64. Ayed AK, Jafar AM, Owayed A. Foreign body aspiration in children: diagnosis and treatment. *Pediatric Surgery International*. 2003; **19**: 485–8.

65. Aytac A, Yurdakul Y, Ikizler C, Olga R, Saylam A. Inhalation of foreign bodies in children. Report of 500 cases. *Journal of Thoracic and Cardiovascular Surgery*. 1977; **74**: 145–51.

66. Pasaoglu I, Dogan R, Demircin M, Hatipoglu A, Bozer AY. Bronchoscopic removal of foreign bodies in children: retrospective analysis of 822 cases. *Thoracic and Cardiovascular Surgeon*. 1991; **39**: 95–8.

67. Clancy MJ. Bronchoscopic removal of an inhaled, sharp, foreign body: an unusual complication. *Journal of Laryngology and Otology*. 1999; **113**: 849–50.

68. Ross MN, Haase GM. An alternative approach to management of Fogarty catheter disruption associated with endobronchial foreign body extraction. *Chest*. 1988; **94**: 882–4.

69. Goldman AP, Macrae DJ, Tasker RC, Edberg KA, Mellgren G, Herberhold C et al. Extracorporeal membrane oxygenation as a bridge to definitive tracheal surgery in children. *Journal of Pediatrics*. 1996; **128**: 386–8.

93

Tracheostomy and home care

MICHAEL SAUNDERS

Introduction and historical perspective	1194	Decannulation	1205
Indications for paediatric tracheostomy	1195	Key points	1207
Techniques of tracheostomy specific to children	1196	Best clinical practice	1207
Tracheostomy care	1197	Deficiencies in current knowledge and areas for future	
Types of tracheostomy tube	1199	research	1208
Complications of tracheostomy	1201	References	1208
Discharge and home care	1204		

SEARCH STRATEGY

The data in this chapter are supported by a Medline search using the key words tracheostomy and child. The author has a personal bibliography of key papers on tracheostomy in children.

INTRODUCTION AND HISTORICAL PERSPECTIVE

Widely acknowledged as one of the oldest documented surgical procedures, detailed historical accounts of tracheostomy are many and vivid. Widespread use of the procedure in children developed in the nineteenth century after Trousseau used the technique to relieve airway obstruction in diphtheria. Subsequently, the procedure was widely used in the treatment of poliomyelitis. With the introduction of widespread vaccination programmes these diseases have largely disappeared in the Western world.

Until the late 1970s many tracheostomies in children were performed to relieve airway obstruction in acute airway infections such as epiglottitis and acute laryngotracheobronchitis (ALTB or croup, see Chapter 87, Acute laryngeal infections).[1, 2, 3] As the standard of paediatric intensive care facilities improved and prolonged endotracheal intubation became a practical alternative to surgical tracheostomy, progressively fewer procedures were carried out for these indications. By the time

haemophilus influenza B (HiB) vaccine was introduced in the 1990s, endotracheal intubation rather than tracheostomy had become the accepted mode of airway management for acute bacterial epiglottitis.[4]

In a series of 153 paediatric tracheostomies, Line et al.[2] report that prior to 1980, 38 percent of tracheostomies were performed for acute airway infections whereas after 1980 this figure had dropped to 12 percent. Similar findings were reported by Friedberg and Morrison[5] when comparing a series of tracheostomies from 1981 to 1985 to a similar series from the same institution from 1976 to 1980. Crysdale et al.[6] also report an overall reduction by half in the incidence of tracheostomy in the same period, attributed to the change in management of epiglottitis. Corbett[7] reviewed 116 cases over a ten-year period (1995–2004) and reported a further shift in indications with no tracheostomies for acute airway infections alone and an increasing proportion required for congenital defects such as craniofacial anomalies and major upper gastrointestinal defects. Eighteen children (15.5 percent) required tracheostomy for acquired airway lesions including subglottic stenosis, vocal cord palsy and respiratory papillomatosis, whilst 14 (12.1 percent) tracheostomies were to facilitate management of airway malacia (laryngotracheal, bronchial or a combination). Tracheostomy was also required for long-term ventilation in patients with neuromuscular disorders (14, 12.1 percent) or ventilator dependency (31, 26.7 percent).

Tracheostomy in children is now an uncommon operation. Due to a shift in tertiary paediatric treatment to larger centres in the last decade and the lack of a reliable means of collecting data on a national basis, it is difficult to estimate the true incidence of paediatric tracheostomy. A survey of 2065 tracheostomies across the United States estimates a rate of 6.6 tracheostomies per 100,000 child years, with the highest incidence in the first year of life but with a second peak in incidence in the late teens due to increased risk of serious injury and trauma.[8]

A more recent study of indications in 362 tracheostomies between 1993 and 2001 has found no real change in incidence over the last decade.[9]

As a consequence of the relative scarcity of the procedure, the medical literature relating to paediatric tracheostomy is generally related to levels 3 and 4 evidence. There are no significant randomized controlled trials and the majority of publications tend to document the authors' own series of tracheostomies and their complications in larger children's hospitals. Reports of changing indications from such institutions may also be skewed by changes in medical practice in individual units.

INDICATIONS FOR PAEDIATRIC TRACHEOSTOMY

The general indications for tracheostomy are as follows:

- relieve upper airway obstruction;
- prevent complications of prolonged intubation;
- reduce anatomical dead space;
- allow suction toilet of the trachea.

However, in practice, tracheostomies in children are nearly always performed to relieve upper airway obstruction or to allow or assist with mechanical ventilation.

Obstruction of the upper airway

The upper airway (from the lips and anterior nares to the carina) may become obstructed at one or more anatomical levels by a range of pathologies (**Table 93.1**). If the obstruction is significant and life-threatening and no other means of relieving the obstruction (for example, nasopharyngeal airway or prong) is appropriate then a tracheostomy must be considered.

Increasing availability and standard of paediatric intensive care facilities has allowed surgical procedures involving the airway to be undertaken without the need

Table 93.1 Examples of obstruction of the upper airway potentially requiring tracheostomy.

Anatomical site	Example
Oropharynx, tongue base	Macroglossia
	Treacher Collins/Goldenhar syndrome
	Cystic hygroma
Nose, nasopharynx	Choanal atresia
Supraglottis	Supraglottic cyst
Glottis	Vocal cord palsy
	Physical trauma
Subglottis	Subglottic stenosis, haemangioma
Trachea	Tracheomalacia
	High tracheal stenosis

for a covering tracheostomy. Instead, the risk of postoperative airway obstruction is avoided by a period of intubation and ventilation (the 'single stage' approach).

The relative indications for tracheostomy continue to change. As an example, until the late 1990s, tracheostomy was considered the mainstay of management for obstructing subglottic haemangioma. More recently, tracheostomy is often avoided by open excision.[10] Similarly, the introduction of the cricoid split[11] and single stage laryngotracheal reconstruction[12] can avoid the need for tracheostomy for extubation failure due to subglottic oedema. [**]

Prolonged intubation

The long-term complications of prolonged endotracheal intubation are well recognized – ulceration at the level of the glottis and, particularly in children, the subglottis, can lead to cicatrization and stenosis of the airway. [****] Being softer and more flexible than the adult and with correct selection of tube size and appropriate intensive care, the neonatal larynx is able to tolerate prolonged intubation for relatively longer than the adult.

There is no clear consensus as to the maximum safe duration of intubation. Premature babies may now be intubated for several weeks before permanent damage becomes a risk. Although practice varies in different units, tracheostomy should normally be considered in older children after two to three weeks of endotracheal intubation.

Long-term and home ventilation

An increasing number of children are now surviving previously lethal conditions, resulting in chronic respiratory failure because of the availability of long-term ventilation. Around half of these are ventilated by tracheostomy.[13] Indications for long-term ventilation include:

- failure of control of breathing;
- chest wall dysfunction;
- disorders of lung parenchyma;
- large airway disease;
- central sleep apnoea, Ondine's curse;
- thoracic dystrophy;
- bronchopulmonary dysplasia (BPD);
- tracheobronchomalacia.[14]

Increasingly, these patients can be ventilated at home although the cost in terms of manpower and equipment is high.

Tracheal toilet

In practice, very few children now require tracheostomy for toilet of the airway. Children with intractable aspiration may need regular suction but the presence of a tracheostomy can predispose to aspiration in itself and increase the risk of respiratory tract infection.

TECHNIQUES OF TRACHEOSTOMY SPECIFIC TO CHILDREN

Positioning

The infant is positioned supine on the operating table. Neck extension is achieved with a rolled towel or gel pillow under the shoulders. The neck can be fixed in extension and stabilized in the midline using adhesive tape such as Elastoplast®. (**Figure 93.1**) Theoretically, extension of the neck in infants increases the risk of injury to the great vessels in the root of the anterior neck; in practice, with careful dissection and identification of structures this is rarely a clinical problem.

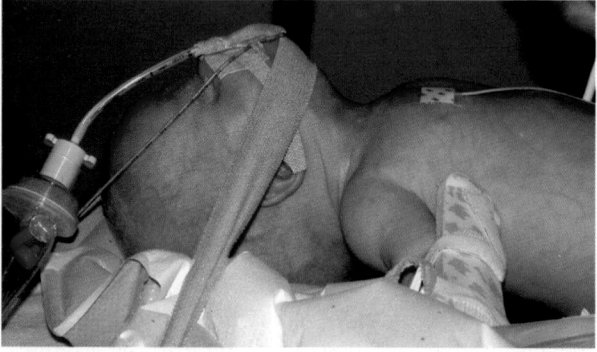

Figure 93.1 Child positioned on the operating table for tracheostomy.

Skin incision

The conventionally used skin incision is horizontal, situated halfway between the cricoid and sternal notch. A vertical incision has traditionally been less favoured because of the potentially poorer cosmetic outcome, but after decannulation from a long-standing tracheostomy, the resulting scar is such that it is unlikely that the orientation of the original incision will make much difference. An advantage of a vertical incision is that it facilitates midline dissection through the layers of the neck and is therefore sometimes advocated as the incision of choice in emergency tracheostomy.

The subcutaneous fat immediately surrounding the incision may be removed after completing the skin incision. This allows the skin edges to invert slightly so as to line the tracheostome with squamous epithelium. This effect can be increased by suturing the edge of the skin incision to the edge of the tracheal incision (maturation sutures). The resulting tract is felt to be more secure as it is already lined with squamous epithelium, and may be associated with a lower rate of postoperative complications.[15]

Dissection

Dissection using monopolar or bipolar diathermy is advisable in small children to minimize blood loss. Although in adults and larger children the thyroid isthmus is traditionally divided and tied to prevent haemorrhage, in infants it is usually adequate to divide the isthmus of the thyroid with bipolar diathermy.

Given the relatively small size of the infant neck and trachea, and secondly the relative proximity of the carotid sheath, it is advisable to palpate the trachea regularly throughout the dissection to ensure that the direction of dissection has not strayed from the midline.

Tracheal incision

A vertical incision is made in the midline, usually in tracheal rings 3–4. It has long been established that too high an incision in the trachea predisposes to subglottic stenosis.[16] A variety of other incisions has been advocated, including excision of an anterior tracheal window, a superiorly or inferiorly based tracheal flap which is raised and sutured to the skin or, recently, a cruciate incision in the trachea, the tracheal edges being closely apposed to the skin edges.[17] The theoretical advantage of most of these techniques is increased stability of the initial tracheostomy tract and therefore greater safety in the event of accidental decannulation. However, although there is no evidence available from randomized clinical trials, animal experiments[18] suggest that tracheal flaps may lead to an increased risk of long-term stenosis and the majority of authors currently favour a simple vertical incision. [**]

Stay sutures

Stay sutures are placed in the wall of the trachea on either side of the vertical incision. These are generally a removable suture (e.g. 4/0 PROLENE) and are left *in situ* until the first tube change. In the event of accidental decannulation, upward and lateral traction on the sutures will open the tracheostomy to make tube reinsertion simpler. The sutures may be taped to the chest wall (**Figure 93.2**) to prevent accidental removal.

Securing tracheostomy tubes

Until the tracheostome has epithelialized and matured, the risks associated with accidental decannulation are more significant. Initially, it is the author's practice to fix the tube into position in the neck using the inelastic linen tapes supplied with the tube. The tapes are tied in a secure knot, sufficiently tight to allow one finger to be inserted between the tapes and the neck skin (**Figure 93.3**). The tapes should be tightened with the neck flexed, rather than

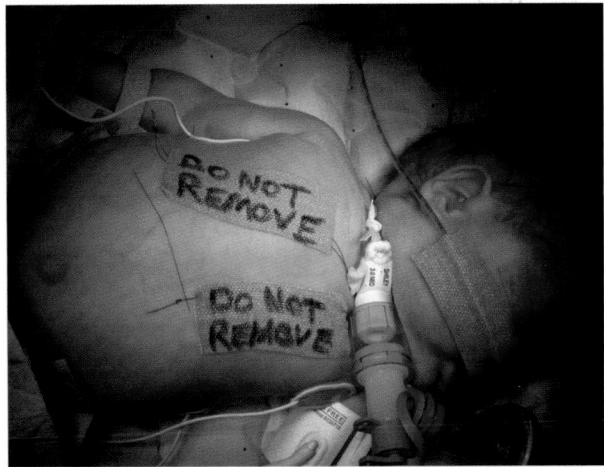

Figure 93.2 Stay sutures in place.

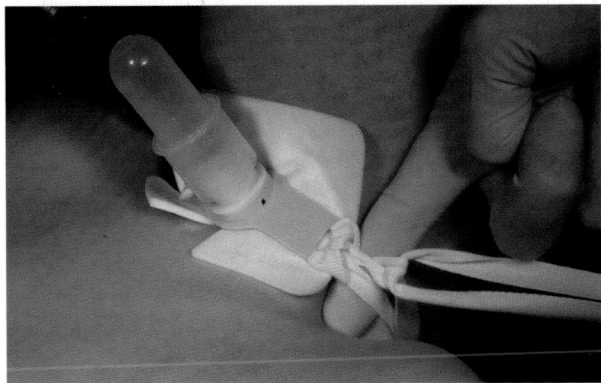

Figure 93.3 Securing the tapes.

in the operative position with the neck extended. In the author's view, suturing the flange of the tracheostomy tube to the skin should be avoided in children. After seven days the first change is undertaken and the linen tapes may be changed for a Velcro® fastening which allows for easier changing and is less traumatic to the skin of the neck.

TRACHEOSTOMY CARE

Adequate tracheostomy care is critical in the first two to three postoperative days. It is during the formation of the tract of the stoma that the risk of tube displacement is at its highest as the tract can close very quickly making reinsertion difficult. It is difficult to overstate the importance of tracheostomy nursing care in the post-operative period. With meticulous and skilled care, most of the complications of tracheostomy can be avoided. Inexperienced staff with no specific training are often reluctant to intervene. It is therefore essential that hospitals maintain a high standard of internal training in this regard and many units have specific teams and regular training programmes for nursing staff.

Suction

Immediately after tracheostomy, the change from air that is warmed and humidified by the upper airway to dry cold air leads to a rapid increase in airway secretions. This gradually reduces after a few weeks. Secretions dry on the inside of the tracheostomy tube and gradually reduce the effective lumen. Humidification of inspired air and regular suctioning will reduce this tendency. Suctioning is required as often as is necessary to keep the tube and airway clear. Overzealous suctioning may lead to mucosal trauma in the distal trachea if the catheter is inserted into the tracheal lumen itself[19] and eventually granulation may form at the tip of the tracheostomy tube, which in itself may lead to tube obstruction. It is suggested that the suction tube be inserted as far as the tip of the tracheostomy tube and withdrawn with a finger occluding the side port. The exact distance may be measured and marked on the suction tube.

The need for suctioning decreases in frequency over time, although with lower respiratory tract infections, secretions may become thicker and more profuse. On such occasions, irrigation of the tracheostomy tube with sterile saline to loosen secretions prior to suctioning is often advocated but there is little evidence to support this practice and it may increase contamination of the lower airway.[20]

Humidification

Initially humidification should be given via nebulizers and a tracheostomy mask (**Figure 93.4**). After a week or so, secretions reduce and the level of humidification

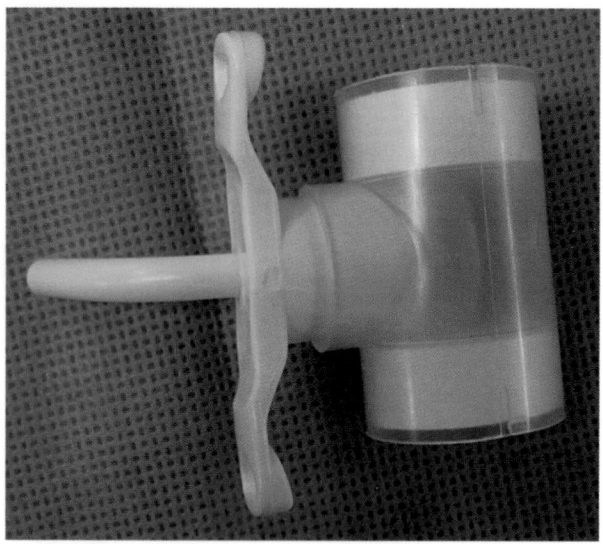

Figure 93.4 Tracheal mask for humidification.

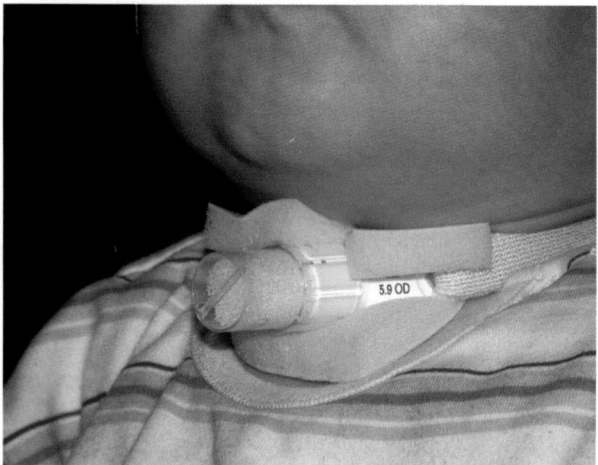

Figure 93.5 Swedish nose.

required is less. A few weeks after tracheostomy, more mobile devices can replace permanent humidification. Longer-term humidification may be achieved by using a Swedish nose or a tracheostomy bib. A 'Swedish nose' attachment (**Figure 93.5**) contains a filter which becomes saturated by the moisture in exhaled air; this in turn humidifies the inhaled air. The tracheal bib works in a similar way. Both devices have the advantage of acting as filters for inspired air.

Skin care

The tracheostomy wound itself becomes rapidly infected with skin commensals and is impossible to keep sterile. The wound heals by secondary intention and eventually the tract becomes lined with squamous epithelium and organized scar tissue. Securing the wound edge skin to the trachea with maturation sutures hastens the development

of an epithelialized tract. At this stage the tracheostome is considered mature. Until this point there is usually a considerable discharge from the wound itself and if the skin care in the first few days is not meticulous, skin and wound breakdown will occur. Usually a dry gauze or foam (e.g. Lyofoam®) dressing is inserted between the peritracheosotomy skin and the flange of the tube. This is rapidly saturated and needs to be changed regularly. Of course the action of changing the dressing increases the risk of accidental decannulation and there is often reluctance on the part of nursing staff to do this. Adequate training in tracheostomy care is essential in a hospital where regular paediatric airway surgery takes place.

Large skin incisions are generally not required in paediatric tracheostomy. If not adequately closed, a large incision will lead to gaping and wound breakdown. It is futile to attempt closure in this instance because of the bacterial colonization of the wound and inevitable infection. Large tracheostomy wounds require careful dressing and packing similar to a healing ulcer and a range of wound products are available. The wound will eventually close by secondary intention.

The tapes used to secure the tube in place can lead to ulceration of the neck skin if they are left too tight or for too long. Although the linen tapes supplied with tubes are secure and inelastic, they have a tendency to cut into the skin. Again, meticulous nursing and skin care is vital. The problem can be reduced by tying the tapes inside a sleeve of Tubigrip™ or part of a large plastic (e.g. endotracheal) tube. When the tracheostomy matures, wider softer bands with Velcro fittings may be used and are less traumatic to the neck skin.

Change of tracheostomy tube

The first change of tube is generally undertaken at around the seventh postoperative day. This allows some time for maturation of the stoma but is short enough to reduce the risk of tube obstruction from dried and thickened secretions. The first change should be undertaken by an otolaryngologist; in the relatively rare instance of difficulty reinserting the second tube, an emergency surgical procedure may be required.

If oral intubation is difficult or impossible (e.g. retrognathia, laryngeal stenosis) it is advisable to undertake the first change in the operating theatre in case surgical intervention is needed. In children who can be easily intubated, (for example the majority of children tracheostomized for pronged ventilation), it is more usual to undertake the first change on the intensive care unit, with an intubation trolley and senior ITU medical staff on hand should reinsertion be difficult and reintubation required.

If this procedure is uneventful, the nursing staff can carry out subsequent changes. If discharge home is anticipated, the parents must be taught the tube-changing technique in a secure environment.

There is no standard proscribed interval at which tubes should be changed; this varies between children and also in the same child given variation in season and in the health of the lower airway. The tube needs to be changed before dried secretions start to reduce the lumen of the tube. The old tube should be inspected after removal to determine the degree of contamination and this will influence the interval until the next change. If a tube visibly contains dried secretion on external inspection, has an audible whistle due to obstruction ('if you can hear a tube you should change it') or if the suction catheter cannot be passed due to obstruction, then it should be changed. If the suction catheter does not pass freely after changing the tube, the advice of an otolaryngologist should be sought.

TYPES OF TRACHEOSTOMY TUBE

Diameter

Modern tracheostomy tubes are sized in relation to the diameter of the lumen in millimetres. Older tubes still use the French gauge system of sizing. The age-appropriate size for a tracheostomy tube can be derived from the guide shown in **Figure 93.6**. In general terms, smaller sized tubes become obstructed more easily and may impair respiration if too small for the age of the child. A child with a long-standing tracheostomy should undergo regular age-appropriate 'upsizing'. However, tracheostomy tubes tend to almost completely fill the trachea in very young children making normal speech difficult. In some cases, for example, if the airway above the tracheostome is not completely obstructed, a smaller sized tube will allow air to flow up thought the glottis and aid in normal speech production. Too large a tube will predispose to suprastomal collapse and may increase the risk of granulations and stenosis.

Length

When inserted correctly, the end of the tracheostomy tube should sit comfortably proximal to the carina. Too long a tube will abut the carina and lead to mucosal injury and potentially subsequent scarring. Too short a tube increases the risk of accidental decannulation. Ideally, the tube should be at least 2 cm, inside the stoma and 1–2 cm, clear of the carina.[21]

Shiley® and Bivona® tubes commonly in use in the UK are available in neonatal and paediatric lengths. For unusual applications (for example children with very thick necks), tubes with adjustable lengths are available (**Figure 93.7**). Tube tip position can be assessed on chest x-ray, at regular rigid bronchoscopy or by passing a flexible endoscope down the lumen of the tube to inspect the carina.

Material

Silicone is now the most widely used material in paediatric tracheostomy tubes. Their relative flexibility compared to older metal tubes reduces the risk of mucosal trauma during neck movements and the soft flange is less likely to lead to skin injury around the tracheostome. One advantage of metal tubes is that as the stronger metal wall is thinner, it is possible to achieve a smaller outside diameter for the same internal diameter as a silicone tube.

Speaking valve

Speaking valves are one-way valves which allow inhalation though the tube but force air upwards through the glottis on exhalation, creating sufficient subglottic pressure to allow phonation. As well as allowing speech, by increasing tracheal pressure on exhalation, these may improve lung function and reduce aspiration. Speaking valves should be used under supervision and not while the child is asleep. Small infants will not always tolerate the valve and quickly learn to blow the valve off the tracheotomy by coughing hard. Many children learn to occlude the end of the tube on exhalation by flexing the neck and occluding the end of the tube with the neck skin to achieve the same result to help phonation.

Fenestration

Fenestrated tubes allow air to pass upwards to improve phonation. These are less practical in smaller children as the fenestration tends to become a focus for granulation and mucosal trauma on suctioning. Adequate passage of air upwards into the larynx is usually achieved by selecting a smaller tube diameter and allowing air leakage on expiration.

Inner tube

For a tube of any given outer diameter, an inner tube will substantially reduce the diameter of the lumen and is therefore not practical in smaller children. For older children, tubes are available with inner tubes in silicone or metal. The main advantage is that the inner tube can be removed daily for cleaning; secondly, the inner tubes are often available with an integrated speaking valve.

			Preterm – 1 Month		1–6 Months	6–18 Months	18 Months – 3 Years	3–6 Years	6–9 Years	9–12 Years	12–14 Years
	Trachea (Transverse Diameter mm)			5	5.0–6.0	6.0–7.0	7.0–8.0	8.0–9.0	9.0–10	10–13	13
PLASTIC	Great Ormond Street	ID (mm)		3.0	3.5	4.0	4.5	5.0	5.5	6.0	7.0
PLASTIC	Great Ormond Street	OD (mm)		4.5	5.0	6.0	6.7	7.5	8.0	8.7	10.7
PLASTIC	Shiley	Size		3.0	3.5	4.0	4.5	5.0	5.5	6.0	6.5
PLASTIC	Shiley	ID (mm)		3.0	3.5	4.0	4.5	5.0	5.5	6.0	6.5
PLASTIC	Shiley	OD (mm)		4.5	5.2	5.9	6.5	7.1	7.7	8.3	9.0
PLASTIC	Shiley	Length (mm) Neonatal		30	32	34	36				
PLASTIC	Shiley	Paediatric		39	40	41*	42*	44*	46*		
PLASTIC	* Cuffed Tube Available	Long Paediatric						50*	52*	54*	56*
PLASTIC	Portex (Blue Line)	ID (mm)		3.0	3.5	4.0	4.5	5.0	5.0	6.0	7.0
PLASTIC	Portex (Blue Line)	OD (mm)		4.2	4.9	5.5	6.2	6.9	6.9	8.3	9.7
PLASTIC	Portex (555)	Size		2.5	3.0	3.5	4.0	4.5	5.0	5.5	
PLASTIC	Portex (555)	ID (mm)		2.5	3.0	3.5	4.0	4.5	5.0	5.5	
PLASTIC	Portex (555)	OD (mm)		4.5	5.2	5.8	6.5	7.1	7.7	8.3	
PLASTIC	Portex (555)	Length Neonatal		30	32	34					
PLASTIC	Portex (555)	Paediatric		30	36	40	44	48	50	52	
PLASTIC	Bivona	Size	2.5	3.0	3.5	4.0	4.5	5.0	5.5		
PLASTIC	Bivona	ID (mm)	2.5	3.0	3.5	4.0	4.5	5.0	5.5		
PLASTIC	Bivona	OD (mm)	4.0	4.7	5.3	6.0	6.7	7.3	8.0		
PLASTIC	All sizes available with Fome Cuff, Aire Cuff, & TTS Cuff.	Length Neonatal	30	32	34	36					
PLASTIC	Bivona	Paediatric	38	39	40	41	42	44	46		
PLASTIC	Bivona Hyperflex	ID (mm)	2.5	3.0	3.5	4.0	4.5	5.0	5.5		
PLASTIC	Bivona Hyperflex	Usable Length (mm)	55	60	65	70	75	80	85		
PLASTIC	Bivona Flextend	ID (mm)	2.5	3.0	3.5	4.0	4.5	5.0	5.5		
PLASTIC	Bivona Flextend	Shaft Length (mm)	38	39	40	41	42	44	46		
PLASTIC	Bivona Flextend	Flextend Length (mm)	10	10	15	15	17.5	20	20		
SILVER	Alder Hey	FG		12–14	16	18	20	22	24		
SILVER	Negus	FG			16	18	20	22	24	26	28
SILVER	Chevalier Jackson	FG		14	16	18	20	22	24	26	28
SILVER	Sheffield	FG		12–14	16	18	20	22	24	26	
SILVER	Sheffield	ID (mm)		2.9–3.6	4.2	4.9	6.0	6.3	7.0	7.6	
	Cricoid (AP Diameter)	ID (mm)		3.6–4.8	4.8–5.8	5.8–6.5	6.5–7.4	7.4–8.2	8.2–9.0	9.0–10.7	10.7
	Bronchoscope (Storz)	Size		2.5	3.0	3.5	4.0	4.5	5.0	6.0	6.0
	Bronchoscope (Storz)	ID (mm)		3.5	4.3	5.0	6.0	6.6	7.1	7.5	7.5
	Bronchoscope (Storz)	OD (mm)		4.2	5.0	5.7	6.7	7.3	7.8	8.2	8.2
	Endotracheal Tube (Portex)	ID (mm)	2.5	3.0	3.5	4.0	4.5	5.0	6.0	7.0	8.0
	Endotracheal Tube (Portex)	OD (mm)	3.4	4.2	4.8	5.4	6.2	6.8	8.2	9.6	10.8

Figure 93.6 Chart for sizing tracheostomy tubes. Reproduced with kind permission from Michelle Wyatt and colleagues at the Department of Otolaryngology, Great Ormond Street Hospital, London, UK.

Cuff

The presence of a cuff increases the risk of mucosal ischaemia and subsequent tracheal stenosis, particularly if high cuff pressures are employed. Cuffed tubes are rarely indicated in paediatric practice; until adolescence, a sufficient seal to allow positive pressure ventilation can normally be achieved with an uncuffed tube.

There are two specific indications for cuffed tubes in children: firstly where there is a significant risk of aspiration (although a cuff will not completely protect against this) and secondly, where there is a decrease in lung compliance with intercurrent infection in a ventilated child and ventilation pressures need to be raised temporarily. In this instance, the risk of tension pneumothorax is significantly increased. In the author's institution, children on the home ventilation programme are admitted to hospital for observation if the ventilation pressures become high enough to require a cuffed tube.

Variable/custom-fitted tubes

The Bivona® Hyperflex™ tube has an adjustable flange which allows change of the effective length of the tracheostomy tube (**Figure 93.7**). This is useful in

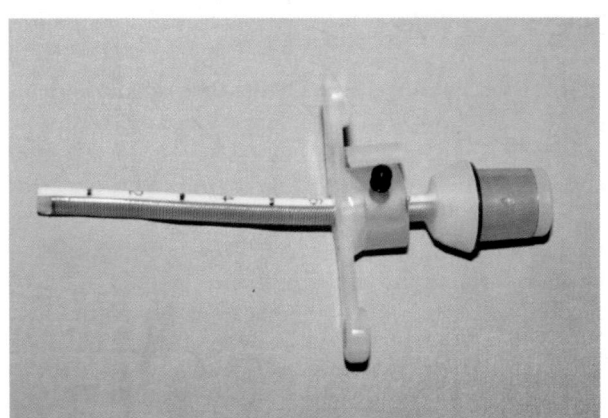

Figure 93.7   Bivona® adjustable tube.

children with prominent soft tissue in whom the prominent neck tissue would obstruct a normal tracheostomy tube, and in children in whom a low tracheal obstruction needs to be bypassed by the tube. The disadvantages of this sort of tube are that it is firstly expensive and secondly, the wall of the tube is thick resulting in a relatively small tube lumen. Custom-made tubes are available for children with specific anatomical difficulties. Tube manufacturers should be approached directly for advice.

COMPLICATIONS OF TRACHEOSTOMY

General

Tracheostomy complications are more likely in children than in adults, and more common in children under two years,[1, 22, 23] particularly preterm infants.[24] [**] Overall complication rates are quoted between 25 percent[25] and 77 percent.[26] There is likely to be considerable variation in the documentation and reporting of minor complications – some authors do not consider granulation to be a reportable complication (**Table 93.2**).

The higher complication rate in smaller children is likely to reflect the relatively small diameter of the airway in small children and the ease with which the airway may be occluded (for example by secretions, granuloma or suprastomal collapse), but also the fact that younger children receiving tracheostomy may remain tracheostomized for a longer period.[26]

As with adult tracheostomies, emergency procedures are associated with a higher rate of complications[27] and longer duration of tracheotomy is associated with a higher risk of long-term complications.[28] Given the relative scarcity of paediatric tracheostomy and the limited number of large published series, it is difficult to accurately derive a risk for fatal complications of paediatric tracheostomy. Of larger studies reported since 1980, the mortality related to the tracheostomy tube itself ranges from 0 to 3.6 percent (**Table 93.3**).[25, 29] In nearly all cases, the cause of tracheostomy-related death is tube

Table 93.2   Complications of tracheostomy.

General	Early postoperative (up to one week)	Late postoperative (after one week)
Tube obstruction	Bleeding; postoperative, wound edge	Granulation
Accidental decannulation	Pneumorthorax	Bleeding
General complications of surgery and anaesthesia	Subcutaneous emphysema	Suprastomal collapse
Death	Infection	Skin complications
	Apnoea	Aphonia, speech delay
		Psychological factors
		Adverse effects on family

Table 93.3 Larger ($n > 100$) series of paediatric tracheostomies and complications.

Study and publication year	Number of tracheostomies	Years of study	Overall complication rate (%)	Early complication (%)	Late complication (%)	Overall mortality (%)	Tracheostomy-related death (%)
Line et al., 1986[2]	153	1970–85	38	12	26	22	3
Crysdale et al., 1988[6]	319	1976–85	32	9	23	13.5	0.9
Carter and Benjamin, 1983[25]	164	1972–81	25	5% (est)	19 (est)	10.9	0
Carr et al., 2001[26]	142	1990–99	77	14	63	15	0.7
Prescott, 1989[30]	293	1980–85	32 (est)	–	–	10	2
Carron et al., 2000[29]	218	1988–98	44	–	–	19	3.6
Midwinter et al., 2002[23]	143	1979–99	46	–	–	7	2.8
Wetmore et al., 1982[1]	420	1971–80	49	28.3	52.6	28	2
Ward et al., 1995[27]	103	1980–90	45.6	30	15.6	36	2.9
Corbett et al., 2007[7]	116	1995–2004	45	11.2	44.8	19.6	1.8

Est, figure estimated from text.

obstruction or accidental decannulation. Earlier reports quote higher mortality rates but paediatric otolaryngology practice has changed considerably in the last 30 years and older studies are unlikely to reflect current practice and safety. Mortality from nontracheostomy-related medical conditions, such as respiratory or cardiovascular disease, is consistently high (7–36 percent) in all series,[23, 27] reflecting the complex medical conditions of children requiring tracheostomy.

Accidental decannulation

If there is little or no natural airway above the tracheostomy or if a child is ventilator dependent, accidental decannulation can be fatal. The risk is increased by insufficiently tight ties, too short a tracheostomy tube and excessive traction on the tube from ventilator tubing. In the first few days before the tract matures, it is likely to be harder to reintroduce the tube if decannulated. Wetmore et al.[1] report accidental decannulation in 29 of 420 (6.9 percent) children in the first week.

The risk of accidental decannulation may be reduced by meticulous tracheostomy nursing care, and surgical techniques (stay sutures, maturation sutures) may help reduce the morbidity by allowing easier and safer reinsertion of a displaced tube.

Tube obstruction

Immediately after tracheostomy the tube is most likely to become blocked with secretions. Regular suction is required. Humidification reduces the rate of secretion and helps to prevent the secretions drying in the lumen of the tube and narrowing the airway. In a mature tracheostomy, the tube is more likely to be obstructed by granulation as the tube tip, either as a result of use of suction catheters or direct trauma from the tube itself.

In the event of accidental decannulation, the tube should be reintroduced in a controlled manner to prevent the creation of a false passage.

Pneumothorax, pneumomediastinum, surgical emphysema

In the infant the domes of the pleura extend well into the neck. Inadvertently straying from the midline during dissection increases the risk of postoperative pneumothorax. This should be detected immediately postoperatively on a routine chest x-ray. Small pneumothoraces can be treated conservatively while larger ones will require chest drainage.

If the tracheostomy wound is closed too tightly around the tube, or the dressings are too tightly applied to the neck skin, air may leak into the soft tissues of the neck (surgical emphysema) or track down into the mediastinum. In this instance the wound should be reopened to allow air to track back out through the tissues and a corrugated drain should be inserted.

Bleeding

Bleeding in the first few days after tracheostomy usually arises as a result of failure to achieve complete haemostasis during surgery. Commonly, bleeding may persist from the wound edge, anterior jugular veins or their tributaries, or the edge of the thyroid isthmus. If direct pressure is not adequate to control haemorrhage, the wound may be carefully packed with haemostatic gauze (Surgicel or Kaltostat®). Re-exploration is rarely required.

Later, minor bleeding may arise from areas of granulation around the tube. This can normally be controlled with cautery and ongoing medical treatment such as application of steroid and antibiotic ointment (for example, Triadcortyl™).

Tracheal innominate fistula

Tracheoinnominate artery fistula is a rare but lethal complication. There is no reliable estimate of the risk in children, which in adults has been estimated as 0.4 percent.[31]

In some children the innominate artery lies abnormally high in the neck (**Figure 93.8**). If this finding is made at the time of surgery, the decision to perform a tracheostomy should be reconsidered. If there is no safe alternative, it is acceptable to place the tracheal incision higher than one would normally advocate and accept the risk of subglottic stenosis. An abnormally low tracheostomy will also increase the risk. A fistula into the artery

forms as a result of erosion of the arterial wall by direct pressure from the tube.

Although most bleeding coming from the tracheostomy tube itself is likely to represent granulation formation at the tube tip, in all cases the possibility of tracheal innominate artery fistula should be considered. The trachea should be examined by flexible bronchoscopy on the ward or by rigid endoscopy under anaesthesia. If the bleeding appears to arise from the anterior tracheal wall rather than tube tip granulation, the wound must be re-explored immediately, ideally with the assistance of a cardiothoracic surgeon. It may be possible to tamponade the bleeding by using a cuffed tube temporarily and if the laryngeal anatomy permits, endotracheal intubation should be established prior to exploration. The mortality from this complication remains very high.

Granulation

The presence of the tracheostomy tube as a foreign body and the persistent presence of bacterial flora in the tract act as an ongoing stimulus for the formation of granulation tissue. Granulation may form at the skin edge of the tract (peristomal granulation) and inside the trachea itself, both on the anterior wall of the trachea above the tube (suprastomal granulation) and also at the tube tip lower in the trachea. Excessive or overexuberant suctioning can lead to more granulation through mucosal trauma and the tube itself can cause mucosal injury. This is generally more common with more rigid tube designs, particularly the silver[32] and PVC designs.

Granulation tissue can pose a number of problems; on the surface, granulations tend to discharge and bleed and, when severe, can lead to difficulty in changing the tube. More modern tubes made from less reactive silicone are more flexible and softer and are felt to reduce the problem both at the skin and inside the trachea.

Peristomal granulations can generally be controlled with steroid/antibiotic preparations (e.g. Triadcortyl ointment). When more severe they may be removed with bipolar diathermy. Caution needs to be exercised when using silver nitrate cautery as the silver nitrate solution can easily enter the trachea itself leading to irritation, coughing and mucosal injury. In the author's unit, this practice is avoided.

Suprastomal granulations are almost universal. In theory, if large they will reduce the lumen of the supraglottic airway above the tube and increase the risks associated with accidental decannulation. Some authors advocate their removal at endoscopy on a regular basis, however, others feel that they are an inevitable consequence of tracheostomy; Rosenfeld and Stool[33] describe granulation in 80 percent of 265 tracheostomies at bronchoscopy and advise against interval endoscopy to remove granulation tissue. At microlaryngoscopy, immediately prior to planned decannulation, all

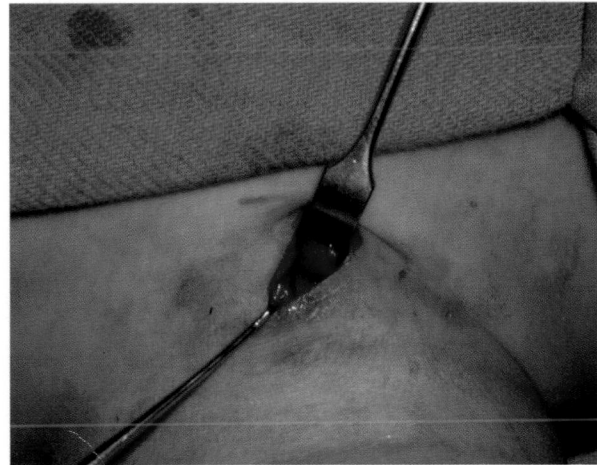

Figure 93.8 High innominate artery.

granulation should be removed to improve the airway. After decannulation and stomal closure, granulation generally resolves spontaneously.

Removal of suprastomal granulation

Suprastomal granulations may if required be removed endoscopically using microlaryngeal instruments, a microdebrider using a Skimmer® or Tru-Cut® blade or by KTP or CO_2 laser. The KTP laser has the advantage of beam delivery using a flexible optic fibre in the relatively limited confines of the subglottis.

Large granulation may be removed using a small sphenoid punch inserted into the tracheostome from externally, under endoscopic guidance at mircrolaryngoscopy.

Suprastomal collapse

Suprastomal collapse is distinct from suprastomal granulation although the two conditions often coexist. For reasons that are not completely understood, the anterior tracheal wall immediately superior to the stoma itself softens and prolapses into the lumen of the subglottic trachea (**Figure 93.9**). This can significantly reduce the available airway, which in turn increases risks associated with accidental decannulation and also leads to decannulation failure.

Minor collapse may be left, as it will tend to improve after decannulation. More significant collapse will require surgical treatment. The simplest of these involves excision and transfixion of the tracheostomy tract followed by endotracheal intubation for two to three days to support the trachea as the stoma heals.[34]

The author's preference in mild to moderate suprastomal collapse is to explore the neck, identify the area of suprastomal collapse and pass a suture through the cartilage and around the strap muscles to elevate the

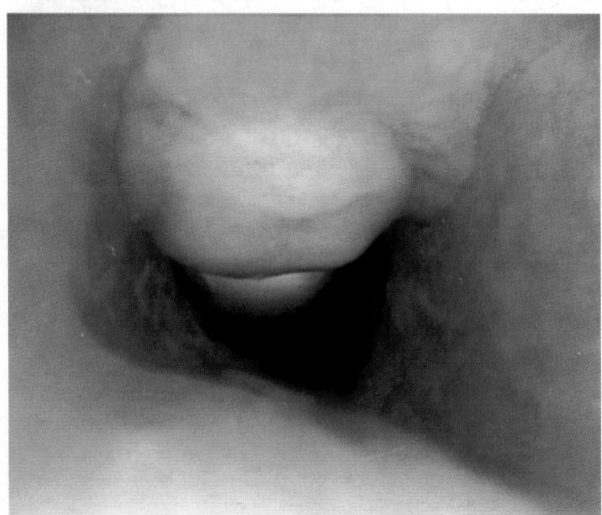

Figure 93.9 Suprastomal collapse.

collapsed section. This is carried out with excision and transfixion of the tracheostome skin. Sharp and Hartley[35] describe ablation of the collapsed segment with KTP laser and a number of authors have described supporting the collapsed segment with a cartilage graft in more severe collapse.[36] The specific procedure will depend on the degree of collapse and the surgeon's personal preference.

Speech development

There is debate about the extent to which tracheostomy affects the development of speech in children. Clearly, normal phonation will be impaired for the duration of a tracheostomy as insufficient subglottic pressure is generated and small infants tend not to tolerate speaking valves well. One difficulty in interpreting such studies is that a significant proportion of tracheostomized children have coexisting developmental abnormalities. If decannulation occurs in the first year to 18 months, before the time at which normal speech patterns begin to develop, the long-term outcome is favourable,[37] whereas longer-term tracheostomy may lead to longer-term impairment of speech function.

DISCHARGE AND HOME CARE

Discharge

Getting home with a tracheostomy is a complex and time-consuming process. Not all families will have sufficient support or resources at home to care for children with a tracheostomy. Whilst in hospital, the caregivers must be educated to care for the day-to-day eventualities of tracheostomy, including tube changing and the recognition and initial treatment of complications. Generally, two responsible adults are required for tube change; home tracheostomy care is difficult, but not impossible for single carers.

Children who are included in home ventilation programmes tend to be more carefully supervised and a national protocol for discharge requirements has been formulated.[38] Nonventilated tracheostomized children tend to have less structured support. In some areas, specific local organizations are available (e.g. the lifetime service in Avon and Wiltshire). Generally, home care is shared between hospital and primary care district nurses who have little specific training.

With sufficient support and education of teachers and co-workers, tracheostomized children without other significant disabilities can now attend mainstream schooling in the UK, although certain activities must be avoided, particularly swimming, water-based sports and contact sports. The parent and carer support organization Aid for Children with Tracheostomies (ACT) provides a discussion forum, advice and information for caregivers in the UK,[39] and caregivers may be given contact details prior to discharge.

Physical requirements

Tables 93.4 and **93.5** list the resources required for the child with a tracheostomy at home. In the author's experience, the ease with which equipment and accessories can be obtained by caregivers is extremely variable in the community as financial constraints in the delivery of care lead to reluctance to supply regular consumables. Prior to discharge, it is essential to communicate with the child's general practitioner and other primary care workers and establish responsibility for provision of equipment.

DECANNULATION

Decision to decannulate

Decannulation may be considered when the original condition requiring tracheostomy has improved, however, to make decannulation successful the child must be able to maintain an adequate airway without the tracheostomy in place.

The majority of paediatric tracheostomies are short term, as the natural airway tends to improve with overall

Table 93.4 Requirements for children at home with tracheostomy.

Caregivers	Physical	Support
Generally two responsible adults	Home with adequate space, heating, electricity, telephone, access to transport	District nurse
		Community paediatrician
		Health visitor
		General practitioner
		Hospital-based support
		Specific community organizations where available

Table 93.5 Equipment requirements for children at home with tracheostomy with and without home ventilation.

Requirements for children without ventilation	Additional requirements for children on home ventilation
Appropriate sized tracheostomy tubes and one a size smaller	Two ventilators/CPAP machines, one of which is portable plus batteries and chargers for use outside the home
Neck ties to hold tube in place	Disposable ventilator circuits
Scissors for emergency tube change to cut neck ties	Humidifier for ventilator circuit and water for inhalation to supply humidifier
Lubricant for inserting tube	Dry circuit for ventilation when outside the home
Sterile saline and syringes for saline suction if required	Heat and moisture exchanger for dry circuit
Tracheostomy dressing if required	Nebulizer
Gauze to clean stoma	CO_2 monitor
Appropriate sized suction catheters	Rechargeable torch for use at night in the event of a power cut
Heat and moisture exchangers/Swedish noses	Uninterrupted power supply – battery which powers ventilator in the event of a power cut
Speaking valves	Suitable trolley in bedroom for equipment
Gloves – nonsterile for procedures and alcohol gel hand rub	Adequate power sockets in house, particularly child's bedroom
Plastic aprons and protective goggles	Trolley for children with a lot of equipment to transport equipment at nursery/school
Stethoscope	Larger than normal buggy when baby/toddler to transport child and equipment
Two suction machines, one of which must be portable. Most children keep a third machine at school as spare	
Saturation monitor and possibly portable saturation monitor for use outside the home	
Ambu bag	
Oxygen: concentrator if used on a daily basis, cylinders if used less frequently, portable cylinders	

Most of the above needs to be duplicated in a portable set. A battery powered suction machine is essential and if the child is oxygen dependent, portable cylinders. Reprinted from Ref. 40, with permission.

growth of the child or as a result of corrective surgery such as laryngotracheal reconstruction. The decision to decannulate is a complicated one which needs to be taken by a senior clinician after careful discussion with the parents and other relevant health care professionals.

In paediatric otolaryngology practice it is generally considered essential to undertake endoscopic assessment of the airway prior to definitive decannulation.[34] Suprastomal collapse and granulation leads to a considerable reduction in the lumen of the subglottic airway in children. Prescott[41] suggested that this was the most common cause of decannulation failure in children, finding significant granulation in 50 and significant suprastomal collapse in 52 of 300 tracheostomies. [**] In addition, vocal cord mobility should be assessed at endoscopy. Granulation may be removed at the time of endoscopy using punch forceps or laser ablation. More significant suprastomal collapse requires KTP laser ablation or reconstructive surgery using cartilage grafting if the collapse is greater than 50 percent.[35] If the subglottic airway is deemed satisfactory at endoscopy, the child may then proceed to formal decannulation in the next few days, delaying the risk of reformation of granulation.

One should also consider comorbidity, such as pulmonary or neurological disease, and lastly the need for further surgery; for example, if a child with Treacher Collins syndrome and an indwelling tracheostomy requires further (e.g. mandibular or palatal) surgical procedures one would normally consider delaying decannulation.

Decannulation technique

Removal of a tracheostomy leads to a significant change in the physiology of the upper airway. The dead space is doubled and airway resistance is trebled. With a long-standing tracheostomy, the child may have no memory of mouth and nose breathing and the new sensation may be distressing.

Staged decannulation

To effect these changes more gradually, decannulation protocols have been developed which involve tube 'downsizing' and reversible capping (**Table 93.6**).[42] To assess whether the child can breathe through the normal anatomical airway, the tube is capped off, either with a button, by taping or by inserting the obturator. However, the tracheostomy tube itself occupies a significant fraction of the tracheal lumen and to try and reduce this effect, the tube size is reduced to a size 3.0 (or size 2.5 in children under 13 months,[43] either in stages or in one step. Leaving the small tube *in situ* allows a certain amount of

Table 93.6 Great Ormond Street protocol for ward decannulation.

Day	Procedure
1	Admission, downsize to 3.0 tube
2	Block for 12 hours from 8 am, if successful continue overnight for a further 12 hours
3	Decannulate, occlude stoma with adhesive tape and dressing. Observe on the ward
4	Observe off the ward
5	Discharge

Reprinted from Ref. 42, with permission.

respiration if required and also prevents the tract from closing down, should decannulation fail.

Immediate decannulation

The tracheostomy tube may occupy as much as half of the lumen of the trachea in an infant. If a child can tolerate this degree of obstruction, the airway after decannulation is likely to be more than sufficient. However, some children will not be able to tolerate this degree of tracheal obstruction. In this instance, it may be considered appropriate to simply remove the whole tube and occlude the stoma with a dressing. However, it is vital that this be carried out in a controlled setting (i.e. intensive care) where facilities for intubation are available should decannulation fail and reinsertion of the tracheostomy not be possible. If the nature of the child's airway obstruction is such that oral intubation is not possible (e.g. some cases of Treacher Collins syndrome) then it is not safe to remove the tube in this manner, and decannulation should be delayed until the child is large enough to tolerate staged decannulation with capping off.

Persistent tracheocutaneous fistula

After decannulation, a fistula may persist between the trachea and skin. This may be small and only lead to problems with discharge of tracheal secretions. A larger fistula may continue to function as an alternative airway.

The incidence of tracheocutaneous fistula (TCF) is between 19 and 42 percent in various series. Certain factors lead to an increased risk; lower age at initial tracheostomy, duration of tracheostomy and, most importantly, persistent obstruction above the level of the stoma (e.g. inadequate reconstruction of subglottic stenosis). There is no clear consensus as to how long a persistent TCF should be allowed to close before considering surgery. Most authors would allow 6–12 months before formal closure.

Closure of TCF

It is essential that the upper airway be reassessed prior to TCF closure to exclude persistent obstruction and tracheal granulation. The persistence of squamous epithelium lining the tracheostome increases the likelihood of a persistent fistula. Simply removing the skin lining the tract and reattempting conventional extubation may lead to satisfactory closure.[44] More commonly, the tract of the stoma is dissected down to the level of the trachea and closed with transfixion sutures. The strap muscles can then be reapposed to each other, which tends to fill in the cosmetic defect left after conventional decannulation. Lastly, the scarred skin surrounding the tracheostome can be excised in a fusiform incision with horizontal skin closure. This leads to an excellent cosmetic result. It is the author's practice to leave a drain in the wound for 24 hours in case of air leak from the closure, which might otherwise lead to surgical emphysema and pneumomediastinum.

Revision of tracheostomy scar

After conventional decannulation, the tracheostome heals by secondary intention. The resulting scar is usually unsightly (**Figure 93.10**) and features a pronounced depression at the line of the tract. Older children may become self-conscious and embarrassed about this. Revision of the scar is usually left until the child is over ten years of age, as cosmetic appearances become more important to the child with age and secondly because there is likely to be less further widening of the subsequent scar with age if the procedure is delayed.

Revision of the scar usually involves a fusiform horizontal incision to excise the scarred skin of the tracheostome with wide undermining of surrounding skin to assist in primary closure. The strap muscles should be identified and reapposed in the midline to eliminate the defect in the contour of the neck skin. Deep dermal/platysmal sutures are used to support the wound and then the skin edges are closed meticulously. Flexing the neck makes it easier to close a large skin defect.

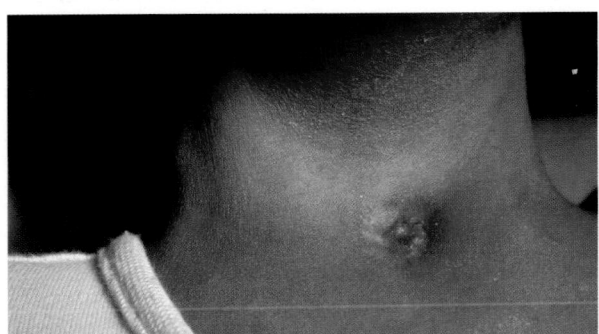

Figure 93.10 Scar following long-term tracheostomy.

✓ The small diameter of the child's airway makes suction and humidification especially important as secretions can quickly occlude the airway. [Grade C/D]

✓ Tube obstruction or accidental decannulation may be fatal. [Grade C/D]

✓ An 'inner tube' reduces the diameter of the lumen and is therefore not practical in small children. [Grade C/D]

✓ Fenestrated tubes are impractical in smaller children. The fenestration tends to become a focus for granulation and mucosal trauma on suctioning. [Grade C/D]

✓ Cuffed tubes are rarely needed in children. [Grade C/D]

✓ Speaking valves should be used under supervision and not while the child is asleep. [Grade C/D]

Deficiencies in current knowledge and areas for future research

➤ Paediatric tracheostomy is now largely undertaken in specialist paediatric units. It is difficult for otolaryngologists in training to get experience in the management of children with tracheostomies outside of these centres. This trend is likely to increase.

➤ Research in paediatric airway disorders is focussed on conditions which give rise to the need for tracheostomy, such as laryngotracheal stenosis and major congenital anomalies.

➤ There is a need to improve training resources and support in primary care and community settings to enable families to look after tracheostomized children at home.

REFERENCES

1. Wetmore RF, Handler SD, Potsic WP. Pediatric tracheostomy. Experience during the past decade. *Annals of Otology, Rhinology and Laryngology.* 1982; **91**: 628–32.

2. Line Jr. WS, Hawkins DB, Kahlstrom EJ, MacLaughlin EF, Ensley JL. Tracheotomy in infants and young children: the changing perspective 1970-1985. *Laryngoscope.* 1986; **96**: 510–5.

3. Prescott CA, Vanlierde MJ. Tracheostomy in the management of laryngotracheobronchitis. Red Cross War Memorial Children's Hospital experience, 1980-1985. *South African Medical Journal.* 1990; **77**: 63–6.

4. Benjamin B, O'Reilly B. Acute epiglottitis in infants and children. *Annals of Otology, Rhinology and Laryngology.* 1976; **85**: 565–72.

5. Friedberg J, Morrison M. Paediatric tracheotomy. *Canadian Journal of Otolaryngology.* 1974; **3**: 147–55.

6. Crysdale WS, Feldman RI, Naito K. Tracheotomies: a 10-year experience in 319 children. *Annals of Otology, Rhinology and Laryngology.* 1988; **97**: 439–43.

*   7. Corbett HJ, Mann KS, Mitra I, Jesudason EC, Losty PD, Clarke RW. Tracheostomy: a 10-year experience from a UK pediatric surgical center. *Journal of Pediatric Surgery.* 2007; **42**:1251–4. *A recent account of the changing indication for tracheostomy particularly due to acute infection.*

8. Lewis CW, Carron JD, Perkins JA, Sie KC, Feudtner C. Tracheotomy in pediatric patients: a national perspective. *Archives of Otolaryngology – Head and Neck Surgery.* 2003; **129**: 523–9.

9. Hadfield PJ, Lloyd-Faulconbridge RV, Almeyda J, Albert DM, Bailey CM. The changing indications for paediatric tracheostomy. *International Journal of Pediatric Otorhinolaryngology.* 2003; **67**: 7–10.

10. Wiatrak BJ, Reilly JS, Seid AB, Pransky SM, Castillo JV. Open surgical excision of subglottic hemangioma in children. *International Journal of Pediatric Otorhinolaryngology.* 1996; **34**: 191–206.

*   11. Cotton RT, Seid AB. Management of the extubation problem in the premature child. Anterior cricoid split as an alternative to tracheotomy. *Annals of Otology, Rhinology and Laryngology.* 1980; **89**: 508–11. *The first account of this important technique to aviod tracheostomy in mild subglottic stenosis.*

12. Lusk RP, Gray S, Muntz HR. Single-stage laryngotracheal reconstruction. *Archives of Otolaryngology – Head and Neck Surgery.* 1991; **117**: 171–3.

13. Edwards EA, O'Toole M, Wallis C. Sending children home on tracheostomy dependent ventilation: pitfalls and outcomes. *Archives of Disease in Childhood.* 2004; **89**: 251–5.

14. Amin RS, Fitton CM. Tracheostomy and home ventilation in children. *Seminars in Neonatology.* 2003; **8**: 127–35.

15. Park JY, Suskind DL, Prater D, Muntz HR, Lusk RP. Maturation of the pediatric tracheostomy stoma: effect on complications. *Annals of Otology, Rhinology and Laryngology.* 1999; **108**: 1115–9.

*   16. Jackson C. High tracheotomy and other errors-the chief causes of chronic laryngeal stenosis. *Surgery, Gynecology and Obstetrics.* 1921; **32**: 392–8. *Seminal paper which did much to change surgical practice and reduce the incidence of post-tracheostomy subglottic stenosis.*

17. Koltai PJ. Starplasty: a new technique of pediatric tracheotomy. *Archives of Otolaryngology – Head and Neck Surgery.* 1998; **124**: 1105–11.

18. Fry TL, Jones RO, Fischer ND, Pillsbury HC. Comparisons of tracheostomy incisions in a pediatric model. *Annals of Otology, Rhinology and Laryngology.* 1985; **94**: 450–3.

19. Bailey C, Kattwinkel J, Teja K, Buckley T. Shallow versus deep endotracheal suctioning in young rabbits: pathologic effects on the tracheobronchial wall. *Pediatrics.* 1988; **82**: 746–51.

20. Raymond SJ. Normal saline instillation before suctioning: helpful or harmful? A review of the literature. *American Journal of Critical Care.* 1995; **4**: 267–71.

21. Sherman JM, Davis S, Albamonte-Petrick S, Chatburn RL, Fitton C, Green C et al. Care of the child with a chronic tracheostomy. This official statement of the American Thoracic Society was adopted by the ATS Board of Directors, July 1999. *American Journal of Respiratory and Critical Care Medicine.* 2000; **161**: 297–308.

22. Donnelly MJ, Lacey PD, Maguire AJ. A twenty year (1971–1990) review of tracheostomies in a major paediatric hospital. *International Journal of Pediatric Otorhinolaryngology.* 1996; **35**: 1–9.

23. Midwinter KI, Carrie S, Bull PD. Paediatric tracheostomy: Sheffield experience 1979-1999. *Journal of Laryngology and Otology.* 2002; **116**: 532–5.

24. Kenna MA, Reilly JS, Stool SE. Tracheotomy in the preterm infant. *Annals of Otology, Rhinology and Laryngology.* 1987; **96**: 68–71.

25. Carter P, Benjamin B. Ten-year review of pediatric tracheotomy. *Annals of Otology, Rhinology and Laryngology.* 1983; **92**: 398–400.

26. Carr MM, Poje CP, Kingston L, Kielma D, Heard C. Complications in pediatric tracheostomies. *Laryngoscope.* 2001; **111**: 1925–8.

27. Ward RF, Jones J, Carew JF. Current trends in pediatric tracheotomy. *International Journal of Pediatric Otorhinolaryngology.* 1995; **32**: 233–9.

28. Gianoli GJ, Miller RH, Guarisco JL. Tracheotomy in the first year of life. *Annals of Otology, Rhinology and Laryngology.* 1990; **99**: 896–901.

29. Carron JD, Derkay CS, Strope GL, Nosonchuk JE, Darrow DH. Pediatric tracheotomies: changing indications and outcomes. *Laryngoscope.* 2000; **110**: 1099–104.

30. Prescott CA, Vanlierde MJ. Tracheostomy in children – the Red Cross War Memorial Children' Hospital experience 1980–1985. *International Journal of Pediatric Otorhinolaryngology.* 1989; **17**: 97–107.

31. Cooper JD. Trachea-innominate artery fistula: successful management of 3 consecutive patients. *Annals of Thoracic Surgery.* 1977; **24**: 439–47.

32. Quiney RE, Spencer MG, Bailey CM, Evans JN, Graham JM. Management of subglottic stenosis: experience from two centers. *Archives of Disease in Childhood.* 1986; **61**: 686–90.ʻ

33. Rosenfeld RM, Stool SE. Should granulomas be excised in children with long-term tracheotomy? *Archives of Otolaryngology – Head and Neck Surgery.* 1992; **118**: 1323–7.

34. Benjamin B, Curley JW. Infant tracheotomy – endoscopy and decannulation. *International Journal of Pediatric Otorhinolaryngology.* 1990; **20**: 113–21.

35. Sharp HR, Hartley BE. KTP laser treatment of suprastomal obstruction prior to decannulation in paediatric tracheostomy. *International Journal of Pediatric Otorhinolaryngology.* 2002; **66**: 125–30.

36. Froehlich P, Seid AB, Kearns DB, Pransky SM, Morgon A. Use of costal cartilage graft as external stent for repair of major suprastomal collapse complicating pediatric tracheotomy. *Laryngoscope.* 1995; **105**: 774–5.

37. Jiang D, Morrison GA. The influence of long-term tracheostomy on speech and language development in children. *International Journal of Pediatric Otorhinolaryngology.* 2003; **67**: S217–20.

∗ 38. Jardine E, Wallis C. Core guidelines for the discharge home of the child on long-term assisted ventilation in the United Kingdom. UK Working Party on Paediatric Long Term Ventilation. *Thorax.* 1998; **53**: 762–7. *A good review of current indications for home ventilation and discussion of many of the issues this raises.*

∗ 39. www.actfortrachykids.com. *Essential resource for the parents/carers of tracheostomy children.*

40. Longdon J. 2005. Personal communication.

41. Prescott CA. Peristomal complications of paediatric tracheostomy. *International Journal of Pediatric Otorhinolaryngology.* 1992; **23**: 141–9.

42. Waddell A, Appleford R, Dunning C, Papsin BC, Bailey CM. The Great Ormond Street protocol for ward decannulation of children with tracheostomy: increasing safety and decreasing cost. *International Journal of Pediatric Otorhinolaryngology.* 1997; **39**: 111–8.

43. Kubba H, Cooke J, Hartley B. Can we develop a protocol for the safe decannulation of tracheostomies in children less than 18 months old? *International Journal of Pediatric Otorhinolaryngology.* 2004; **68**: 935–7.

44. Stern Y, Cosenza M, Walner DL, Cotton RT. Management of persistent tracheocutaneous fistula in the pediatric age group. *Annals of Otology, Rhinology and Laryngology.* 1999; **108**: 880–3.

94

Cervicofacial infections in children

BEN HARTLEY

Introduction	1210	Key points	1217
Assessment of neck swellings	1210	Best clinical practice	1217
Clinical assessment	1210	Deficiencies in current knowledge and areas for future	
Examination of the neck	1211	research	1218
Head and neck examination	1212	References	1218
Specific conditions	1212		

SEARCH STRATEGY

The data in this chapter are supported by a Medline search using the key words infection and child, neck, cervical node, cervical adenopathy and focussing on diagnosis and treatment of specific conditions. The Cochrane Library was also consulted.

INTRODUCTION

Neck swellings in children are common. Most are due to lymphadenopathy secondary to the common acute upper respiratory infections, notably pharyngitis and tonsillitis, that are a feature of normal childhood. They are rarely indicative of serious pathology. Lymphadenopathy is usually self-limiting but may progress to cellulitis, suppuration and abscess formation.

Chronic infections are less common but need to be considered if the swelling persists. Congenital lesions do not always declare themselves at birth; they may present in older children. The onset of the swelling may be precipitated by an acute inflammatory episode.

Neck swellings may involve the parotid and submandibular regions and extend on to the face.

In a very a small number of children, a neck swelling will be due to a malignancy. These are most often lymphoproliferative or connective tissue tumours. Squamous carcinoma is extremely rare in children. A child with a neck mass requires an entirely different approach to that required in an adult.[1] Open biopsy is rarely needed. Nevertheless, it is important to maintain an index of suspicion for malignancy in all persistent neck swellings in children.

ASSESSMENT OF NECK SWELLINGS

There is a broad spectrum of aetiologies for inflammatory lymphadenopathy in children (**Table 94.1**). Noninflammatory disorders will need to be considered in the differential of a neck mass, especially if there are unusual features. A methodical approach is required with a focus on clinical assessment.

CLINICAL ASSESSMENT

History

- **Age of child**: Most acute lymphadenitis presents in children older than six months. Swellings occurring at or shortly after birth are more likely to be congenital or neoplastic.

Table 94.1 Inflammatory neck nodes in children.

Infective aetiologies				
Viral	Bacterial	Fungal	Parasitic	Non-infective adenopathy
Upper respiratory: rhinovirus, adenovirus, enterovirus	Acute lymphadenitis: Streptococcus, Staphylococcus, less commonly Gram-negative organisms	Histoplasmosis	Toxoplasmosis	Kawasaki syndrome
Common childhood illnesses: measles, mumps, rubella, varicella	Suppurative lymphadenitis with deep or superficial neck abscess; usually pyogenic organisms (Streptococcus and Staphylococcus)	Uncommon fungal infections (immunocompromised host)	Filariasis	Sarcoidosis
Infectious mononucleosis Cytomegalovirus	Mycobacteria: tuberculosis or 'atypical' mycobacteria Other granulomatous bacterial infections: cat scratch disease, actinomycosis, brucellosis, tularaemia, bubonic plague, syphilis	Candida and Aspergillus		Sinus histiocytosis with massive lymphadenopathy Kikuchi-Fujimoto disease
HIV				PFAPA syndrome (periodic fever, apthous stomatitis, pharyngitis, cervical adenitis)

- **Duration of swelling**: A short history (a few days) suggests acute inflammation. After six weeks a swelling is regarded as chronic and further investigation should be considered – even earlier if there are suspicious clinical features.
- **Size**: Very large swellings or swellings that progressively enlarge despite antimicrobial treatment should be investigated.
- **Associated symptoms**: A preceding upper respiratory infection is often a feature of inflammatory lymphadenitis. Fever, rhinorrhoea, sore throat and malaise are common. With chronic swellings, enquire about weight loss, night sweats and swellings elsewhere in the body.
- **Contacts**: Enquire about tuberculosis, other infections and exposure to cats, farm animals and ticks.
- **Medical history**: Identify any known illnesses.
- **Family and social history**: Identify any familial disease or congenital anomalies and any relevant social factors. If a diagnosis of human immunodeficiency virus (HIV) infection is suspected then involve a paediatrician.

EXAMINATION OF THE NECK

Site of the swelling

The site of the swelling within the neck provides important information about the possible aetiology.

LATERAL NECK SWELLINGS

Lymph nodes are distributed throughout the neck but the most common site is along the superficial and deep cervical chains. These lie deep to sternomastoid in the upper neck and along its anterior border in the lower neck. Enlarged lymph nodes are the most common cause of lateral neck swellings. The principal differential includes congenital anomalies such as branchial cysts, which may also become acutely inflamed. Vasoformative lesions (see also Chapter 99, Branchial arch fistulae, thyroglossal duct anomalies and lymphangioma), haemangiomas and vascular malformations, including lymphatic abnormalities and benign and malignant neoplasms arising from the neural or connective tissue elements present, as well as rare secondary metastases.

CENTRAL NECK SWELLINGS

The principle causes of a neck swelling in the central area of the neck around the midline are thyroglossal duct cyst, lymph nodes and dermoid cyst. Thyroglossal duct or dermoid cysts may become acutely inflamed. Children can also develop inflammatory and neoplastic thyroid disease (see also Chapter 99, Branchial arch fistulae, thyroglossal duct anomalies and lymphangioma). Lymphatic vascular malformations can occasionally involve this region.

PAROTID SWELLINGS

Acute parotitis (mumps) is common and is due to a self-limiting viral infection. Vaccination for measles, mumps and rubella is now reducing the frequency of mumps and to some degree the clinical awareness of this condition (see also Chapter 97, Salivary gland disorders in childhood).

BACTERIAL PAROTITIS

This occurs in children and may be recurrent. It is usually characterized by acute painful presentation followed by resolution on antibiotics. Occasionally, chronic inflammatory swelling persists and must be distinguished from neoplasia. Vascular malformations and haemangiomas cause swellings in the parotid region. Occasionally, rhabdomyosarcoma or other connective tissue tumours present. Magnetic resonance scanning can be very helpful with this differential diagnosis (see also Chapter 97, Salivary gland disorders in childhood).

SUBMANDIBULAR SWELLINGS

Enlarged lymph nodes, floor of mouth infections, acute sialadenitis and occasionally lymphatic or vascular malformations and congenital 'plunging' ranula all cause swelling in this region (see also Chapter 97, Salivary gland disorders in childhood).

POSTERIOR TRIANGLE SWELLINGS

Most commonly these are lymph nodes but branchial anomalies, vascular malformations and neoplasia enter into the differential diagnosis.

Nature of the swelling

Classical signs of acute inflammation may be present, e.g. redness, tenderness and heat. Chronic swellings usually do not show these signs. If abscess formation has occurred, the clinical sign of fluctuance may be present and the mass may feel cystic. A classical tuberculous abscess lacks the clinical features of acute inflammation ('cold abscess').

HEAD AND NECK EXAMINATION

A careful examination for a source of primary infection should be made. This should include examination of the pharynx, nose and ears as well as looking for any cutaneous lesion.

General examination

Fever, tachycardia or rash should be noted. A general examination should include a search for any associated lymphadenopathy and hepatosplenomegaly. The otolaryngologist may wish to enlist the help of a paediatrician.

Investigation

In many cases no investigation is required. Symptomatic treatment of presumed viral infection or antibiotic treatment of bacterial infection with careful clinical follow-up will result in resolution.

Laboratory and skin tests

If the child is systemically unwell, a full blood count may demonstrate neutrophilia consistent with bacterial infection. A blood count may also be a screening investigation for suspected haematological malignancy. Consider a Monospot test for infectious mononucleosis (see also Chapter 95, Diseases of the tonsil). Serological tests for toxoplasmosis, bartonella (cat scratch disease), or cytomegalovirus (CMV) should be considered for persistent lymphadenopathy. Mantoux or Heaf tests for tuberculosis may be helpful, particularly in the nonimmunized.

Imaging

There is only a limited place for plain radiographs. Films of the chest may be helpful in tuberculosis and a lateral neck view may demonstrate a retropharyngeal mass. Ultrasound examination of a neck mass may be undertaken without sedation or anaesthesia. Ultrasound will help determine if a lesion is cystic or solid. An experienced ultrasonographer can comment on the internal architecture of lymph nodes and may raise suspicion of malignancy. If an abscess is identified, sonography will help with the anatomical relationships of the abscess and with surgical planning.

Computed tomography (CT) scanning may require general anaesthesia in small children. Good anatomical detail is provided and it is helpful in surgical planning. Neither ultrasound nor CT[2] are absolutely accurate in the diagnosis of abscess and in the presence of strong clinical features surgical exploration should be considered. [**/*]

Magnetic resonance (MR) scanning rarely adds useful information in the case of acute inflammatory lesions but is very useful for vascular malformations, salivary gland and soft tissue masses (see also Chapter 102, Imaging in paediatric ENT).

SPECIFIC CONDITIONS

Viral infections

VIRAL UPPER RESPIRATORY INFECTIONS

Adenovirus, rhinovirus or enterovirus (Coxsackie A and B) may cause reactive lymphadenopathy. This is generally self-limiting.

INFECTIOUS MONONUCLEOSIS

This is an acute infection caused by Epstein–Barr virus (EBV). It occurs mainly in adolescence and is spread by close contact. Fever, fatigue, malaise and an exudative tonsillitis are characteristic. Cervical lymphadenopathy may be massive. Other lymphoid tissue including liver and spleen may be enlarged. There is a characteristic picture on the blood film with the presence of atypical lymphocytes. Serological tests such as Monospot or Paul Bunnel will usually confirm the diagnosis. Although the aetiology is viral, intravenous antibiotics may be needed to treat any coexistent bacterial infection. Ampicillin is contraindicated.

In cases where the acute tonsillitis is associated with airway obstruction, steroids may be considered. On occasion, endotracheal intubation may be required to protect the airway until the swelling subsides.[3] Cases with hepatosplenomagaly should be managed in cooperation with a paediatrician (see also Chapter 95, Diseases of the tonsil).

HIV

Infection is associated with repeated opportunistic infections. Most cases of paediatric HIV infection are acquired from the mother by vertical transmission. Acute infection may mimic infectious mononucleosis. Persistent generalized lymphadenopathy including the cervical nodes becomes a feature as the disease progresses. Weight loss and recurrent fevers occur. Following HIV infection it may be years or decades before full acquired immune deficiency syndrome (AIDS) develops. There is significant evidence of increased life expectancy with early retroviral treatment.[4]

Investigation and management should be in cooperation with a specialist in paediatric infectious diseases.

Bacterial infections

ACUTE LYMPHADENOPATHY WITH SUPPURATION

Cervical abscesses

Bacterial infection within a cervical lymph node may progress to cause local cellulitis and abscess (**Figure 94.1**). Occasionally, a solid mass of inflammatory tissue forms due to coalescence of a group of lymph nodes and this is clinically referred to as a phlegmon. The distinction between phlegmon and abscess is important, as abscesses usually require surgical drainage whereas phlegmon settle with intravenous antibiotics. The most important assessment is clinical. Abscesses are tender, usually reddened and exhibit the clinical sign of fluctuance confirming their cystic nature. Imaging is helpful but not always required.

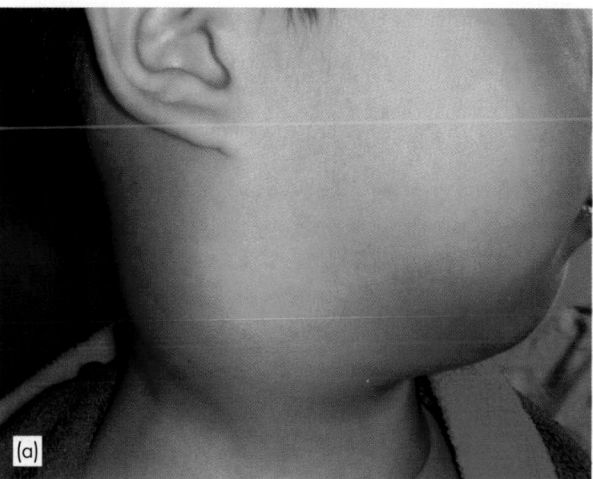
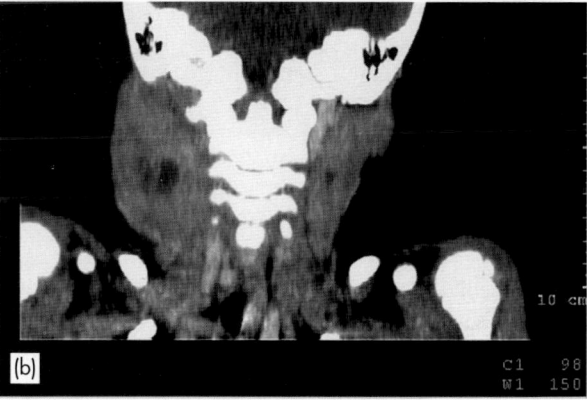

Figure 94.1 (a) Child with acute cervical abscess; (b) CT scan of the same child.

Many neck abscesses require surgical drainage. This may be performed by a neck incision, which is ideal for superficial lesions and the majority of deep cervical abscesses. A wide-bore needle aspiration may be adequate if the pus has coalesced and liquefied.

Dental abscess

An infected molar or premolar may cause extensive swelling extending into the face and neck and should be considered in the differential of a neck abscess (**Figure 94.2**).

Retropharyngeal abscess

This occurs typically in the young child (under two years) and is due to suppuration in the loose aggregate of lymph nodes between the pharynx and the prevertebral fascia (**Figure 94.3**). It is now uncommon but should be recognized because of its potential to cause fatal airway obstruction.[5] The child is febrile, drooling and may adopt a characteristic posture with the neck flexed and the head extended. Retropharyngeal abscess is a surgical emergency. The child must be admitted for intravenous antibiotics, rehydration and careful observation. Early drainage under general anaesthesia with the help of a

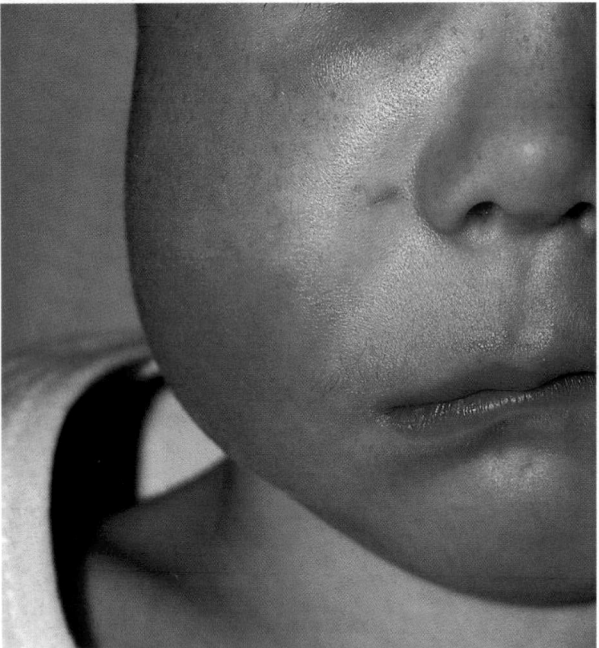

Figure 94.2 Dental abscess.

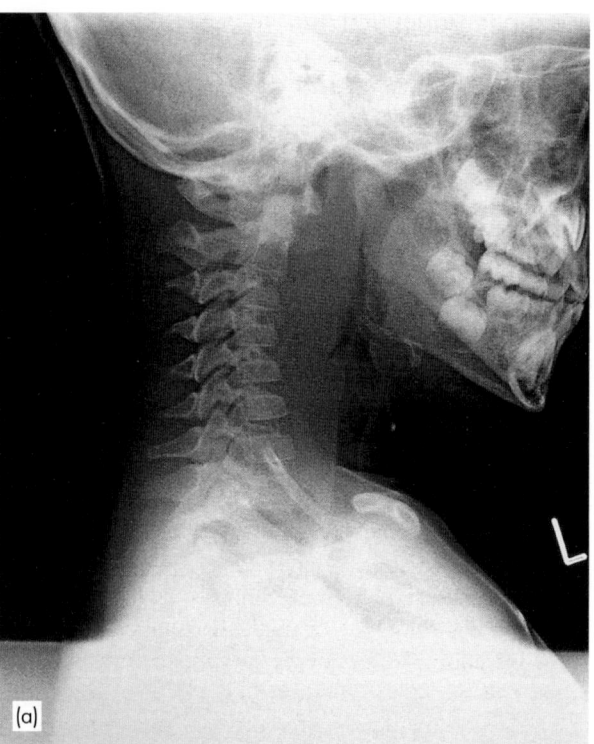

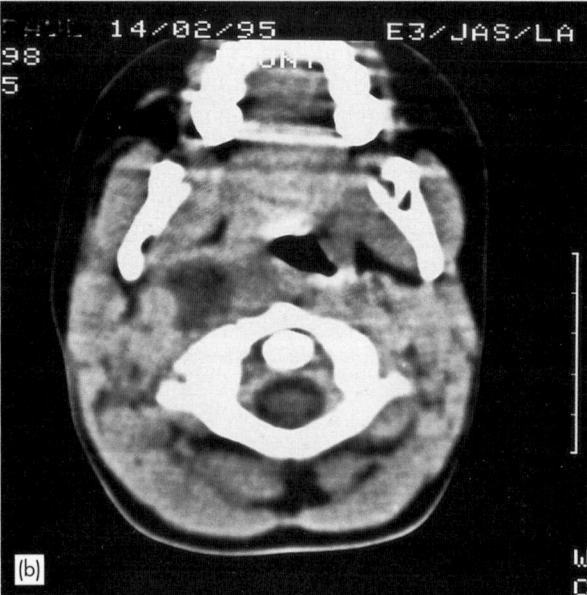

Figure 94.3 Retropharyngeal abscess: (a) plain film showing large prevertebral shadow with compression of the airway; (b) CT scan of same child showing swelling filling the retropharyngeal space.

skilled paediatric anaesthetist is indicated if there is any concern about impending airway deterioration. CT scanning will demonstrate the abscess but may itself require anaesthesia and is contraindicated if there is significant airway compromise. Drainage is via the intra-oral route.

Lemierre's syndrome

This is a post-tonsillitis septic thrombosis of the internal jugular vein. It is most often caused by the bacteria *Fusobacterium necrophorum*. It was common in the pre-antibiotic era. Following an episode of tonsillitis, the patient develops high spiking fevers with tenderness and fullness of one side of the neck. (See also Chapter 95, Diseases of the tonsil.) Pulmonary emboli may occur and, untreated, the mortality is high. Incidence in the UK is rising, perhaps related to changing patterns of antibiotic use.[6] Contrast enhanced CT scanning is usually diagnostic and treatment with intravenous antibiotics and drainage of any abscess is usually curative. The role of antic-oagulants is controversial and surgical treatment of the suppurating internal jugular vein is rarely required, although has been used in cases of repeated septic emboli.

MICROBIOLOGY

Group A *beta haemolytic streptococcus* and *Staphylococcus aureus* are the most common causative organisms for suppuration in the neck. Other bacteria that may be implicated include anaerobes (19 percent); *Haemophilus influenzae, Moraxella catarrhalis*[7] and Beta lactamase positive organisms.

Mycobacterial infections

Two groups of mycobacterial infections involve the neck in children. The distinction is important and can be challenging. First there are infections caused by *Myco-bacterium tuberculosis* (TB). Secondly are a group of infections caused by other mycobacteria. Commonly referred to as atypical mycobacteria, these are most accurately termed nontuberculous mycobacteria (NTM) (see also Chapter 97, Salivary gland disorders in childhood). They include *Mycobacterium avium intracellulare*, *Mycobacterium scrofulaceum*, *Mycobacterium fortuitum* and *Mycobacterium haemophilum*.[8]

The typical presentation is of a painless firm enlarging mass in the neck. In NTM infection the overlying skin is frequently discoloured (**Figure 94.4**). In children with tuberculosis, weight loss, fever and anorexia may be present.

The differential diagnosis includes lymphoma. To exclude this a tissue diagnosis is usually required. Biopsy specimens are sent for both histopathological examination and for microbiology, including staining and culture specific to mycobacterium. The typical histopatholocal appearances of tuberculosis are of caseating granuloma formation. Acid and alcohol fast staining bacilli may be seen. However, it may not be possible histopathologically to distinguish tuberculous from NTM infection. Culture of the mycobacterium may take several weeks. In this situation all patients should have a chest x-ray to identify features of tuberculosis. A tuberculous skin test is often helpful. A positive test in a nonimmunized population (such as the United States or children under 13 in most regions of the United Kingdom) is highly suggestive of tuberculous infection. Unfortunately there is an incidence of positive testing with nontuberculous infection and this test is not absolutely diagnostic for tuberculosis. In cases of doubt, antituberculous medication may be commenced pending the outcome of cultures. Genetic probing of the cultured organisms can also be used to try and make the distinction between tuberculous and NTM infection.

The management of NTM lymphadenopathy is controversial. Complete surgical excision of the involved nodes brings about quick disease control and often no further treatment is necessary. [**/*] Prolonged medical therapy is an alternative.[9] With medical therapy, it is not unusual for the mass to persist for up to 18 months. Treatment is discussed in Chapter 97, Salivary gland disorders in childhood.

SINUS FORMATION AND DISCHARGE

If the nodes have been breached by the infection and there has been spread into the surrounding tissue, then there is a risk of skin breakdown and formation of a sinus. These sinuses often persist for months with troublesome discharge. Once a sinus has formed, there is a strong indication to perform surgery as the constant discharge is extremely disruptive to the life of an otherwise well child. Curettage has been advocated as a treatment for infection that has spread beyond the lymph nodes and is not amenable to complete excision. This may reduce the duration of the disease.

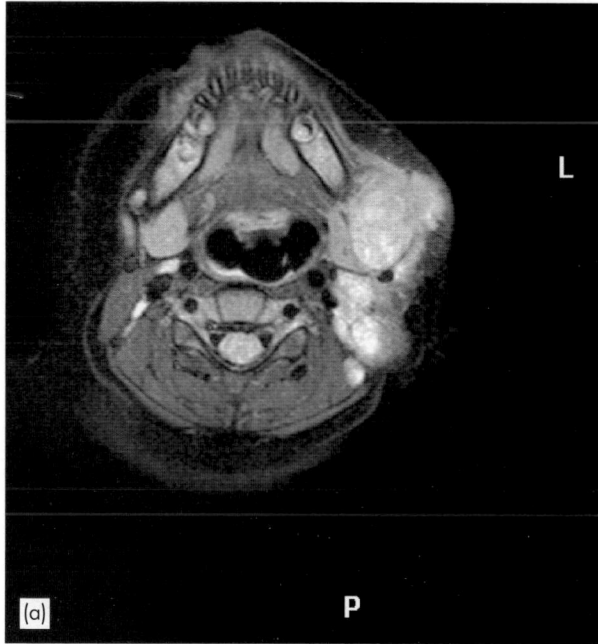

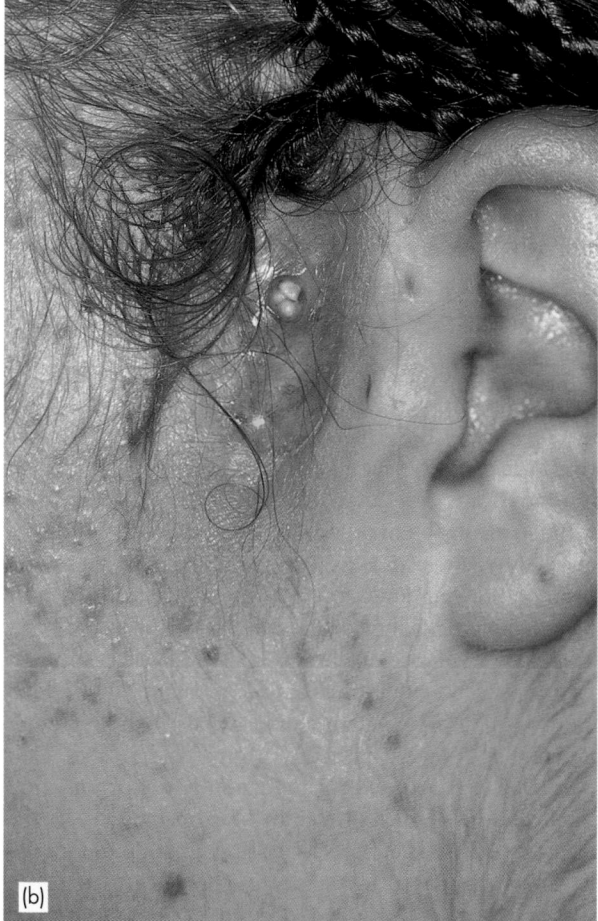

Figure 94.4 (a) MR scan showing large left neck mass; histology confirmed NTM; (b) Skin changes in NTM.

Primary medical treatment of nontuberculous neck masses has been advocated using either macrolide antibiotics based on some *in vitro* experiments[10] or antituberculous therapy. This usually involves prolonged treatment as the organisms are notoriously resistant to antituberculous therapy. Hawkins and Clark[11] showed resolution of neck mass in four of 18 cases by chemotherapy alone.

CAT SCRATCH DISEASE

This is a granulomatous condition characterized by lymphadenopathy with fever and malaise. The disease has been recognized for over 50 years but only recently has the causative organism been identified as the bacteria *Bartonella henselae*. It is spread by close contact with cats.

Patients are mainly under 20 years of age and more than 90 percent have a history of feline contact.[12, 13] Serologic testing has a high sensitivity and specificity. Although there is no medical treatment confirmation of the diagnosis, performing a blood test will reassure parents who often become concerned about possible malignancy.

TULARAEMIA

This is caused by infection with the Gram-negative bacillus *Francisella tularensis*. It rarely infects the neck and is transmitted to humans by rabbits, ticks or contaminated drinking water. Skin or mouth ulcers may be present with associated lymphadenopathy, fevers, malaise and headache. Diagnosis can be difficult but is confirmed by rising serological titres in the convalescent phase of the illness. Treatment is with streptomycin, tetracycline, aminoglycosides or chloramphenicol.

ACTINOMYCOSIS

This is caused by Gram-positive non-spore forming bacteria. The most common human pathogen is *Actinomyces israelii* but there are several other species which can rarely be pathogenic. Approximately 50 percent of cases are cervicofacial. Actinomyces are normal commensals in the oral cavity and infections arise from a breach of the mucosas, e.g. dental extraction. The most common presentation is a slow growing painless mass near the mandible. Local lymph nodes may be involved and in a small number of cases metastasis of disease to liver or brain may occur. Untreated, the mass progresses to fibrosis and chronic suppuration with draining sinuses. A less common presentation is with an acute, warm, tender mass with fever. The presence of sulphur granules on pathological examination is suggestive but not diagnostic. If the diagnosis is suspected, special culture conditions increase the chance of culturing this organism. Most cases are treated by surgical excision followed by prolonged antibacterial therapy, usually penicillin for up to six months.

BRUCELLOSIS

Brucellosis is a zoonosis, i.e. an infection transmitted from animals to humans. It can be acquired through working with livestock or consumption of unpasteurized dairy products. It is caused by several species of the genus *Brucella* which are small Gram-negative bacilli. There is lymphadenopathy involving the neck and other body regions associated with fever and malaise. Diagnosis is by serology and management is with tetracycline in adults and trimethoprim-sulphamethoxazole in children.

SYPHILIS

This is a spirochaete infection, now rare. Primary syphilis is associated with an ulcer (chancre) and local lymphadenopathy. Early presentation with a neck mass may occur in patients with HIV.

Fungal infections

HISTOPLASMOSIS

Histoplasmosis is caused by the fungus *Histoplasma capsulatum*. It is associated with bird droppings and acquired via airborne spores. Infection in the central USA is very common and typically asymptomatic. In immunocompromised patients, pulmonary and systemic disease may occur. Mucosal head and neck lesions may mimic squamous carcinoma. Biopsy is needed and treatment is surgical excision.

CANDIDA AND ASPERGILLUS

Mucosal candidiasis is a common problem in children but neck masses caused by these infections are extremely rare and limited to immunocompromised patients.

PARASITOSIS

Toxoplasmosis

Infection with the parasite *Toxoplasma gondii* is usually through the ingestion of poorly cooked meat or ingestion of oocytes excreted in cat faeces. Cervical adenitis occurs in more than 90 percent of clinical cases.[14] However, subclinical infection is not uncommon and positive serology may be found in asymptomatic individuals. The lymphadenopathy may persist for months and children may require a biopsy to rule out malignancy. Treatment is rarely required for cervical lymphadenopathy which is self-limiting but the infection responds to sulphonamides and pyrimethamine.

Noninfective inflammatory disorders

SARCOID

Sarcoidosis is a chronic multisystem disorder of unknown aetiology. It mainly occurs in the second decade of life and is rare in children. It mainly causes generalized and pulmonary symptoms but may involve other parts of the body. Neck masses, parotid masses and facial nerve paresis may result. Cervical nodes are typically bilateral and nontender. The diagnosis is often suspected from the chest radiograph and can be confirmed by biopsy which shows typical noncaseating granulomas (see also Chapter 99, Branchial arch fistulae, thyroglossal duct anomalies and lymphangioma). Treatment is usually conservative although steroids, and in some cases more potent antineoplastic agents, can be used.

Conditions which simulate lymphoma

This heterogenous group of benign lymphoproliferative disorders is characterized by often prolonged unexplained cervical adenopathy which can give rise to concerns regarding lymphoma. Some authors refer to these conditions as 'pseudolymphomata'. They include Rosai Dorfman disease, Castleman's disease, Kawasaki syndrome and Kikuchi-Fujimoto disease.[15]

KAWASAKI SYNDROME

This is an acute multisystem vasculitis of unknown aetiology. It tends to affect children under five years of age and the clinical presentation is similar to many childhood infectious diseases. The diagnosis is clinical and children should have four of the five following criteria:

1. acute nonpurulent lymphadenopathy – usually unilateral;
2. erythema, oedema and desquamation of the hands and feet;
3. polymorphous exanthema;
4. painless bilateral conjunctival infection;
5. erythema and injection of the lips and oral cavity.

There may be a thrombocytosis and pericardial effusion. In the subacute stage, coronary artery aneurysms develop in 15–20 percent of cases. The goal of management is to reduce inflammatory responses with antiinflammatory or gamma globulin therapy.[16] The vasculitis is self-limiting but unfortunately causes permanent cardiac damage in around 20 percent of untreated patients. All patients should have an initial echocardiogram and cardiac follow-up. A mortality of 1–2 percent is associated with this disease due to the cardiac sequelae.

SINUS HISTIOCYTOSIS (ROSAI DORFMAN DISEASE)

Children present with massive cervical lymphadenopathy which is similar to infectious mononucleosis or lymphoma. This disease is thought to represent an abnormal histiocytic response to some precipitating cause, possibly a herpes virus or EBV.[17] Fever and skin nodules may be present. Treatment is expectant but biopsy is usually required to rule out malignancy. Histopathologic examination reveals dilated sinuses, many plasma cells and marked proliferation of histiocytes.

KIKUCHI-FUJIMOTO DISEASE

This is an idiopathic disorder, first described in Japan. It is characterized by lymph gland enlargement which may occur anywhere in the body but is typically cervical.

Fever chills and weight loss are common. Women and young adults are more commonly affected. The disease is self-limiting but biopsy is often performed to rule out malignancy. Histology shows a characteristic necrotizing lymphadenitis.

KEY POINTS

- Lymphadenopathy is common in children and rarely requires investigation.
- Viral adenitis is the most common cause of neck swelling.
- Much anxiety can be caused by lesions that simulate lymphoma but careful clinical assessment supplemented by noninvasive investigations, and very rarely biopsy, will provide a diagnosis.
- Immunocompromised patients pose a particular challenge and liaison with a paediatrician is essential in this group of children.

Best clinical practice

✓ A blood count is a useful screening investigation for haematological malignancy. [Grade B]

✓ Ultrasound will help determine if a lesion is cystic or solid. An experienced ultrasonographer can comment on the internal architecture of lymph nodes and may raise suspicion of malignancy. [Grade B]

✓ In NTM, once a sinus has formed there is a relative indication to perform surgery as discharge is extremely disruptive to the life of an otherwise well child. [Grade C]

✓ Open biopsy may be the only way to exclude a lymphoma in the noninfective inflammatory lymphoproliferative disorders. [Grade C]

Deficiencies in current knowledge and areas for future research

➤ The increasing survival of children with malignant disease, often with highly immunosuppressive chemotherapy, will produce therapeutic challenges in the management of infectious disease in the head and neck.

➤ Pooling of data on relatively uncommon conditions such as NTM may produce better treatment protocols.

➤ Imaging continues to be refined and as spiral CT scanners permit higher resolution images at lower radiation doses, imaging the architecture of cervical structures will improve.

➤ Aspiration biopsy cytology has proved disappointing in children and increasing specialization in pathology may expand the role of this technique.

REFERENCES

* 1. Kubba H. 'Paediatric Neck Lumps – when does an enlarged lymph node need excising?' in Summary of the proceedings of the V11 Annual Meeting of the Evidence-Based Management of Head and Neck Cancer. *Clinical Otolaryngology.* 2005; **30**: 79–85. *A succinct account of current indications for biopsy of neck nodes in children.*

2. Stone ME, Walner DL, Koch BL, Egelhoff JC, Myer CM. Correlation between computed tomography and surgical findings in retropharyngeal inflammatory processes in children. *International Journal of Pediatric Otorhinolaryngology.* 1999; **49**: 121–5.

3. Papesch M, Watkins R. Epstein Barr virus infectious mononucleosis. *Clinical Otolaryngology and Allied Sciences.* 2001; **26**: 3–8.

* 4. Van der Poel LA, Faust SN, Tudor-Williams G. HIV-1 infection in children: current practice and future predictions. *Advances in Experimental Medicine and Biology.* 2004; **549**: 135–48. *Review of current stautus of HIV infection in children.*

5. Craig FW, Schunk JE. Retropharyngeal abscess in children: clinical presentation, utility of imaging and current management. *Paediatrics.* 2003; **111**: 1394–8.

6. Clarke MG, Kennedy NJ, Kennedy K. Serious consequences of a sore throat. *Annals of the Royal College of Surgeons of England.* 2003; **85**: 242–4.

7. Brodsky L, Belles W, Brody A, Squire R, Stanievich J, Volk M. Needle aspiration of neck abscesses in children. *Clinical Pediatrics (Philadelphia).* 1992; **31**: 71–6.

8. Spark RP, Fried ML, Bean CK, Figuero JM, Crowe Jr. CP, Campbell DP. Non tuberculous mycobacterial infections of the face and neck – practical considerations. *American Journal of Diseases in Children.* 1988; **142**: 106–8.

* 9. Coulter JB, Lloyd DA, Jones M, Cooper JC, McCormick MS, Clarke RW *et al.* Nontuberculous mycobacterial adenitis: effectiveness of chemotherapy following incomplete excision. *Acta Paediatrica.* 2006; **95**: 182–8. *Large series treated by a combination of surgery and chemotherapy.*

10. Rapp RP, Mc Craney SA, Goodman NL, Shaddick DJ. New macrolide antibiotics: usefulness in infections caused by mycobacterium other than mycobacterium tuberculosis. *Annals of Pharmacotherapy.* 1994; **28**: 1255–66.

11. Hawkins, Clark J. 'Management of the atypical tuberculous node in the neck; surgery or antibiotics? in Summary of the proceedings of the V11 Annual Meeting of the Evidence-Based Management of Head and Neck Cancer. *Clinical Otolaryngology and Allied Sciences 2005.* 1993; **30**: 82–83.

12. Jackson LA, Perkins BA, Wenger JD. Cat scratch disease in the United States: an analysis of three national databases. *American Journal of Public Health.* 1993; **83**: 1707–11.

13. Ridder GJ, Boedeker CI, Technau-Ihling K, Sander A. Cat-scratch disease: otolaryngological manifestations and management. *Otolaryngology – Head and Neck Surgery.* 2005; **132**: 353–8.

14. McCabe RE, Brooks RG, Dorfman RF, Remington JS. Clinical spectrum in 107 cases of toxoplasmic lymphadenopathy. *Reviews of Infectious Diseases.* 1987; **9**: 754.

15. Brown JR, Skarin AT. Clinical mimics of lymphoma. *Oncologist.* 2004; **9**: 406–16.

16. Gersony WM. Diagnosis and management of Kawasaki disease. *Journal of the American Medical Association.* 1991; **265**: 2699–703.

17. Levine PH, Jahan N, Murari P, Manak M, Jaffe ES. Detection of human herpesvirus 6 in tissues involved in sinus histiocytosis with massive lymphadenopathy (Rosai-Dorfman Disease). *Journal of Infectious Diseases.* 1992; **166**: 291–5.

95

Diseases of the tonsil

WILLIAM S MCKERROW

Structure and function	1219	Best clinical practice	1226
Inflammatory disorders of the tonsil	1220	Deficiencies in current knowledge and areas for future	
Noninflammatory disease	1225	research	1226
Key points	1226	References	1227

SEARCH STRATEGY

Searches were conducted of the Cochrane Library, Medline, Pubmed and Ovid databases using the key words tonsils, tonsillitis, pharyngitis, sore throat, and carrying out further subsearches for anatomy, microbiology, immunology, complications and therapy. These were complemented by hand searches of current English language texts and the following journals: Journal of Laryngology and Otology, Clinical Otolaryngology, Laryngoscope, Archives of Otolaryngology, Annals of Otolaryngology, International Journal of Pediatric Otolaryngology. The search was complemented by a hand search of the reference list in the MD thesis of Miss Ruth Capper, Doncaster, to whom I pay due acknowledgement.

STRUCTURE AND FUNCTION

Structure

The palatine tonsils consist of paired aggregates of lymphoid tissue. They are located in the pocket formed between the palatoglossus and palatopharyngeus muscles and the overlying folds of mucosa, which make up the anterior and posterior tonsillar pillars. With the lingual tonsils, the adenoids (see Chapter 84, The adenoid and adenoidectomy) and the diffuse aggregates of pharyngeal submucosal lymphoid tissue they make up Waldeyer's ring, a complete circle of lymphoid tissue surrounding the entrance to the gastrointestinal and respiratory tracts. The tonsils share a common structure with lymphoid tissue elsewhere in the gastrointestinal and respiratory tracts including the adenoids and Peyer's patches in the small intestine and within the appendix. Histologically they consist of lymphoid tissue with aggregates of lymphocytes arranged in a follicular manner and embedded in a stroma of connective tissue. The stratified squamous mucosal covering of the tonsils extends irregular convoluted invaginations into the parenchyma forming pits or crypts. Microorganisms, desquamated epithelium and food debris are frequently present within the crypts and may be implicated in the development of acute and recurring inflammation.

Normal flora

The range of organisms cultured from the tonsils both in health and disease is extremely variable, with recognized differences in bacterial flora retrieved from surface and from core samples.[1, 2] The organism most commonly identified from the surface of the tonsil in disease is the group A beta haemolytic streptococcus (GABHS). Up to 40 percent of asymptomatic individuals will also have a culture positive for this organism.[3, 4] Other surface organisms include *Haemophilus*, *Staphylococcus aureus*, alpha haemolytic streptococci, *Branhamella* sp., *Mycoplasma*, *Chlamydia*, various anaerobes and a variety of respiratory viruses.[5, 6] [****] In a study of core samples obtained by fine needle aspiration in health and disease, core samples of normal tonsils usually failed to grow pathogenic organisms.[7] In recurrent tonsillitis the samples grew a range of pathogens but the predominant organisms were *Haemophilus influenzae* and *S. aureus*. A mixed flora was also common. Beta haemolytic streptococci were less common. [****]

Function: role of the tonsils within the immune system

The tonsils have no afferent lymphatics. The lymphoid germinal centres are located immediately submucosally. They contain both B and T lymphocytes. B cells predominate, implying that both cell-mediated and humoral immune function is present in the tonsil and that B lymphocytes are actively produced in the tonsil. These cells have the capability to synthesize specific antibodies. They appear to be responsible for the final differentiation, induced by exposure to antigen, of B cells to principally immunoglobulin (Ig)G and IgA plasma cells. They allow positive selection of B cells according to receptor affinity for antigen and provide B cells specific for mucosal effector sites. It seems likely that they generate B cells which express polymeric IgA and which migrate to the upper respiratory tract mucosa and associated 'front line' mucosal surfaces. Contact with allergens in the upper respiratory tract therefore enhances local immunity and also contributes to the development of systemic immunity. Inflammatory change within the tonsils may be a manifestation of this function – hence the old adage that the function of the tonsils is 'to develop tonsillitis'. Whether or not tonsillitis represents a swamping of defence mechanisms at local level or an exaggeration of the normal response is not known. The fact that tonsillitis is often recurrent suggests that there may be some intrinsic defect either in the tonsils themselves or in the patient's immunity. The observation that tonsillitis tends to become less frequent with time suggests speculatively that the problem lies within the immune system rather than within the end organ itself. However, it has been shown that polymeric IgA production in tonsillar B cells is markedly reduced in children with recurrent tonsillitis. This suggests that conservation of tonsillar tissue is desirable, a point frequently emphasized by authors outwith the UK. There is no evidence that tonsillectomy *per se* results in impaired immunity, indeed, the converse appears more likely. In spite of a sizeable literature discussing the relationship of immune function to disease of the tonsils there is no tenable evidence of significant immune compromise, presumably as a result

of the extensive 'backup' in the immune system.[8] The precise role of bacteria and viruses in this process is also controversial. The evidence available suggests that they may act synergistically, with the presence of latent viruses (particularly Epstein–Barr virus, adenoviruses and herpes simplex) sensitizing the pathogenic bacteria frequently present on the tonsils of asymptomatic individuals.[9] [**]

INFLAMMATORY DISORDERS OF THE TONSIL

Acute tonsillitis

PRESENTATION AND FLORA

Acute inflammatory episodes affecting the tonsils may occur as an isolated episode, or in association with a viral upper respiratory illness including generalized pharyngitis (see **Figures 95.1** and **95.2**). Tonsillitis may also present as part of a systemic infection such as infectious mononucleosis (see under Infectious mononucleosis below) when severe tonsil inflammation may be a prominent part of the clinical presentation. Classically, the causative organism in acute suppurative tonsillitis is

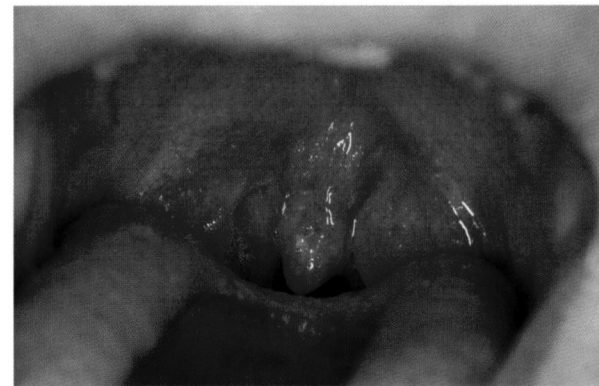

Figure 95.1 Tonsillopharyngitis (appearances could be either viral or bacterial).

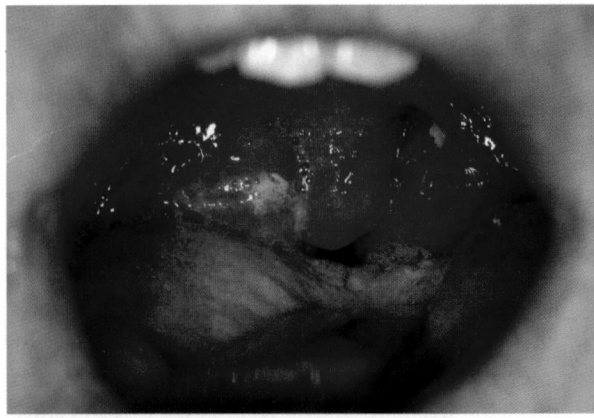

Figure 95.2 Severe tonsillitis (GABHS were isolated in this case but the appearances are nonspecific).

GABHS. A wide variety of other organisms including anaerobes and viruses may be implicated in a clinically indistinguishable illness although whether they are primarily causative is undetermined.[3, 4] [**] Epidemiological data about the true incidence of tonsillitis as opposed to pharyngitis or sore throat is confounded by the fact that there is no robust definition of tonsillitis, making assessment of the outcomes of management difficult. Studies of sore throat management frequently use bacteriological criteria for diagnosis but this does not reflect the situation in clinical practice nor is it a reliable 'gold standard'.

EPIDEMIOLOGY

Sore throat is a common reason for presentation to a primary care physician. The frequency in the UK is 0.1 consultations per capita per annum.[10] [**] Not all these sore throats will be due to true tonsillitis; however, there are no case control or population studies of the epidemiology of sore throat in the recent literature, let alone any specifically looking at tonsillitis.[11] Sore throat affects both sexes and all age groups but is much more common in children and during the autumn and winter months.[12, 13] [**]

CLINICAL EVALUATION

The diagnosis of acute tonsillitis is clinical. It is based on a history of a pyrexial illness, sore throat with a painful swallow, and the finding of pharyngeal erythema with or without tonsillar exudates and painful cervical adenopathy.

Evaluating aggregated symptom complexes including tonsillar exudate, anterior cervical lymphadenopathy, the absence or presence of cough, pharyngeal erythema and the level of pyrexia has been attempted but the results of these studies are conflicting and the conclusions unconvincing. There is good evidence that the sensitivity and specificity of clinical diagnosis alone is between 20 and 50 percent.[14] [***] It should not be relied upon in diagnosis of bacterial or viral aetiology.

AETIOLOGY OF INFLAMMATORY DISEASE

The precise aetiology of inflammatory disease of the tonsils remains shrouded in controversy. It is widely accepted that both bacteria and viruses play a part in acute inflammation either separately or together. It is also probable that factors within the immune system of the individual patient render them susceptible to episodes of infection, which may be isolated or recurrent, but these remain unquantified and studies of immunoglobulin levels in such patients have been inconclusive. The point at which the tonsils become the cause of the disease rather than simply the site is undetermined, if indeed this ever becomes the case.

With the exception of tonsillitis associated with infectious mononucleosis, there is no evidence that viral tonsillitis is more or less severe than bacterial tonsillitis or that the duration of the illness varies significantly in either case.

DIAGNOSIS OF CAUSATIVE AGENT

Although the precise diagnosis may be of interest academically, from the practical point of view it is probably of little relevance in management. Both bacterial and viral tonsillitis tend to resolve quickly without treatment in most cases.[15, 16] [****] Precise diagnosis of the causation may be of more relevance in protracted illness but is difficult and imprecise in practice. Possible options for diagnosis in clinical practice include clinical assessment, bacteriological culture or rapid antigen testing (RAT) of a throat swab for GABHS. RAT is in common use in North America but is seldom used in the UK.

MICROBIOLOGICAL INVESTIGATION

Bacteriological culture of a throat swab may yield a positive culture for GABHS but this does not conclusively prove that the organism is causative. The incidence of a positive culture may be as high as 40 percent in asymptomatic carriers.[3, 4] The organism has also been isolated from tonsillitis cases with no serological evidence of infection. In addition, the organisms cultured from the surface of the tonsil may vary greatly from the bacterial flora deep within the tonsillar crypts. It is by no means certain which is likely to be the more relevant to clinical symptoms.[1, 2, 3, 4, 17] [***] Inevitably, there is a delay of 24–48 hours before results are available, rendering its value limited in treating a short-lived self-limiting illness.

RAPID ANTIGEN TESTING

The use of RAT as an office procedure has superficial attractions, principally speed in reporting results (ten minutes), but the sensitivity measured against throat swab culture (itself a doubtful gold standard) was variable across trials at between 61 and 95 percent with specificity from 88 to100 percent.[18] There may be variation between different laboratories.[19] [**] The costs of both throat swab culture and RAT are not insignificant.

PRIMARY MANAGEMENT

The management of acute tonsillitis is principally supportive, with the use of analgesics and adequate hydration until the symptoms subside. The choice of analgesia is governed by the severity of symptoms but the majority will find paracetamol in full dosage adequate. Nonsteroidal antiinflammatory drugs may be used in more severe cases but the higher side-effect profile makes them a second-line treatment.

SPECIFIC TREATMENT

The relatively complex interplay between bacteria and viruses in acute tonsillitis is not fully understood and if no bacteria are cultured a viral aetiology is assumed. Even if bacterial pathogens are identified, their significance is uncertain. The average duration of an episode of acute tonsillitis seen in general practice is two to three days, with evidence that although the prescription of antibiotics will shorten the illness and may reduce the risk of sequelae this is not clinically significant.[15, 20, 21]

A Cochrane review of antibiotics for sore throat concluded that there was evidence of benefit in shortening the illness by a mean of one day around day three of the illness, by which time approximately 50 percent of patients will have settled spontaneously (OR 0.16; 95 percent CI 0.09, 0.26 with a positive throat swab; OR 0.65; 95 percent CI 0.38, 1.12 with a negative swab). They also found a reduction in the frequency of suppurative complications including quinsy (OR 0.16; 95 percent CI 0.07–0.35), but concluded that 'blanket' or routine prescription of antimicrobials was not justified.[20] There is evidence that patients prescribed antibiotics for sore throat are more likely to reattend for antibiotic prescription on subsequent occasions,[22] and the risks of widespread indiscriminate antibiotic prescription include genesis of resistant organisms, allergy and anaphylaxis. There are numerous studies of the efficacy of various alternative antibiotics (predominately cephalosporins) over penicillin in general and specifically in cases of proven GABHS infection. These show only marginal evidence of increased benefit insufficient to justify their use.

In those patients in whom the illness shows no sign of improvement within 48–72 hours or in whom there is clinical concern because of the severity of symptoms, antibiotic therapy is appropriate and the drug of choice remains benzylpenicillin. The literature is unclear about the optimal duration of therapy but the recommendations in the British National Formulary, supported by recent evidence,[23] are for a seven-day course.

In cases where there is clinical concern about the severity of the illness, antibiotics should not be withheld.

Recent evidence from several randomized controlled trials[24] suggests that a single dose of dexamethasone as adjuvant therapy was of significant benefit in reducing pain in acute pharyngotonsillitis with no evidence of predisposition to abscess formation with the use of steroids. [****]

Complications of acute tonsillitis

Acute tonsillitis may be complicated by systemic sepsis, including septicaemia and septic arthritis. GABHS may cause an acute exanthematous reaction with a macular rash – **scarlet fever**. The noninfective sequelae of GABHS – rheumatic fever and glomerulonephritis – are considered below under Immune complex disorders.

PERITONSILLAR ABSCESS

The principal complication of tonsillitis is peritonsillar abscess (quinsy) in which a collection of pus forms in the potential space between the tonsil and its bed. Prior to the formation of pus there is frequently a period of peritonsillar cellulitis without abscess formation. Clinically, the patient presents with a severe pharyngitis lateralized to one or other side, often with marked associated lymphadenopathy. There may be severe trismus limiting access for examination and treatment. This results in a severe local and systemic illness which may, if untreated, result in the spontaneous discharge of pus when the abscess points. More commonly, the course of the disease is modified by antibiotic therapy, needle aspiration or incision and drainage in hospital. The organism most commonly cultured from this pus is beta haemolytic streptococcus. Infection with other organisms such as *Streptococcus viridans*, *S. aureus*, *H. influenzae* and various anaerobes may also occur with anaerobes being commonly isolated if appropriate techniques are used.[25, 26] [****] In severe cases airway compromise and dehydration due to the inability to swallow result, which may necessitate hospital admission for intravenous fluid therapy. This may occasionally happen in severe tonsillitis without abscess formation.

In such cases immediate hospital admission and experienced clinical assessment of the airway is essential. Unskilled attempts to examine the throat may precipitate complete airway obstruction and must be avoided (**Figure 95.3**). Peritonsillar abscess formerly was regarded as an absolute indication for 'interval tonsillectomy' but most clinicians now prefer to take other factors

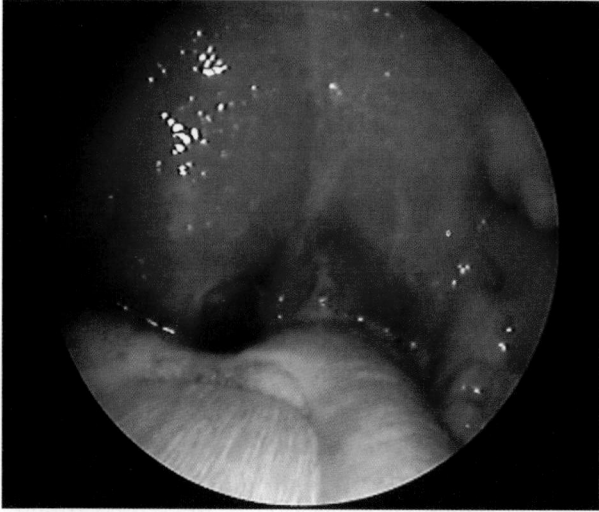

Figure 95.3 Peritonsillar abscess (swelling is predominantly unilateral).

into account, for example a history of frequent tonsillitis. The majority of otolaryngologists are agreed that a second quinsy is a reasonable indication for operation. Tonsillectomy during the acute phase of the abscess has been established as a safe procedure but opinions differ about whether or not this is the most appropriate management for the condition. Protagonists emphasize the virtues of the avoidance of a second admission, convalescence from only a single episode, avoidance of loss to follow-up for interval tonsillectomy and the rapid relief of symptoms. The procedure requires emergency scheduling and the services of an anaesthetist experienced in the management of the difficult airway.

The release of a large amount of pus into the posterior aspect of the oral cavity, either spontaneously or therapeutically, carries with it the risk of aspiration, especially in severely ill patients. The use of local anaesthesia prior to incision exacerbates this risk, which can be avoided, and satisfactory resolution hastened by aspiration of the abscess using a wide bore needle and syringe together with antibiotic therapy. This is now the management of choice. The antibiotics usually employed are high-dose penicillin intravenously or a cephalosporin but will be guided by bacteriology of the aspirated pus. Some clinicians also use metronidazole and this is logical as a significant proportion of peritonsillar abscesses grow anaerobes.[26, 27]

RETROPHARYNGEAL ABSCESS

A rare but serious complication of acute tonsillitis is retropharyngeal abscess, presenting mainly in infants and young children aged less than five years. It presents when infection has tracked into the lymphoid tissue between the posterior pharyngeal wall and the prevertebral fascia. The child is systemically ill and there may be evidence of airway compromise or an associated neck abscess. A plain x-ray of the neck may be helpful and the diagnosis can be confirmed by ultrasound or computed tomography (CT) scanning provided the child is well enough for investigation. In one study the sensitivity and specificity of CT in detecting pus was 81 and 57 percent, respectively. CT findings should, therefore, be interpreted with caution and correlated with the clinical picture in planning management. Treatment is initially high-dose antibiotic therapy with urgent incision and drainage when pus formation is suspected, under general anaesthesia with the airway protected by intubation by a skilled and experienced anaesthetist.[28] [**] The abscess is usually drained perorally but occasionally external drainage via the neck may be appropriate. Rarely, tracheotomy is necessary. Retropharyngeal abscess due to tuberculosis, at one time relatively common, still occasionally occurs, more commonly in the developing world, and requires specific antibiotic therapy (see Chapter 94, Cervicofacial infections in children).

PARAPHARYNGEAL ABSCESS

Peritonsillar and retropharyngeal abscess may occasionally be complicated by spread of infection to the parapharyngeal space with formation of a large abscess, which may require external drainage. The patient is usually severely systemically unwell, with severe trismus and possibly airway compromise. Management is urgent and if this diagnosis is suspected, imaging by ultrasound and CT scanning may be helpful in both diagnosis and in planning intervention, as noted above. The use of broad-spectrum antibiotics intravenously is essential and initial therapy should include cover against streptococci and anaerobic organisms. Deep neck space sepsis may be complicated by progressive, life-threatening spread of infection including mediastinitis and even retroperitoneal sepsis. Marked neck swelling, airway compromise and female gender appear to be predictive of higher risk cases. Vigilance and a proactive management policy are thus essential in all cases (**Figure 95.4**).[29] [**]

LEMIERRE'S SYNDROME

This is a rare and potentially fatal complication of oropharyngeal infection characterized by septic thrombophlebitis in the internal jugular vein, sometimes in association with metastatic abscesses. The organism is typically a fusiform bacillus. The condition should be considered when there is severe neck pain, septicaemia or a prolonged fulminant course in a patient with infection in the upper aerodigestive tract.[30] It has also been described secondary to tympanomastoid infection. Skilled imaging will help to show the presence of a thrombus in

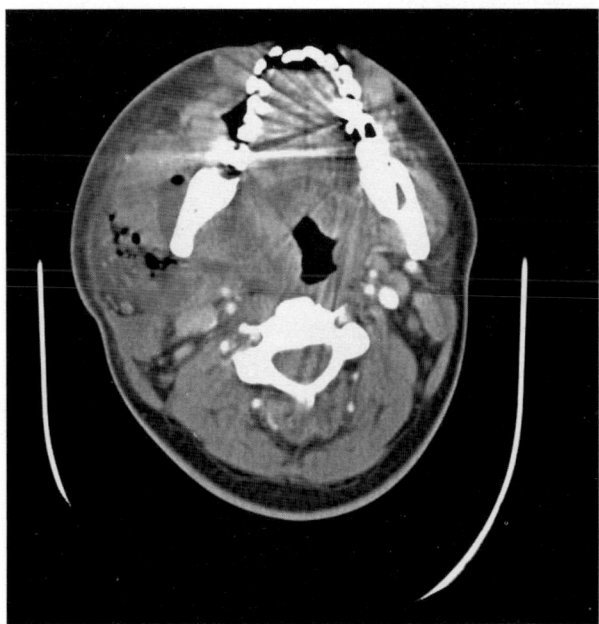

Figure 95.4 CT scan of parapharyngeal abscess (gas is visible in the extensive abscess cavity extending from the deep parapharyngeal space to lateral to mandible superficially).

the neck veins (**Figure 95.5**). Treatment is with prolonged (six weeks) antibiotics, for example a beta-lactam with metronidazole or amoxycillin-clavulanate. Anticoagulation may be considered if there is evidence of spreading thrombophlebitis. There is a significant mortality.[31, 32]

IMMUNE COMPLEX DISORDERS

Acute tonsillitis and pharyngitis caused by GABHS are occasionally complicated by disease related to immune complex formation generated as part of the immune response to the infection.

The two important diseases resulting from this phenomenon are acute rheumatic fever and acute glomerulonephritis. The incidence of these disorders is declining in the developed world but they are still common in certain ethnic groups, in particular, Australian Aborigines and New Zealand Maoris. The reasons for this are not clear but may be related to social as well as genetic factors. In the UK there is no evidence that treating acute tonsillitis aggressively with antibiotics has resulted in prevention or reduction in incidence of these complications. In communities where rheumatic fever is common, antibiotic therapy for sore throat may have a role in reducing the incidence of this complication.[20] [**]

TONSILLITIS AND PSORIASIS

There is a probable association between acute tonsillitis due to GABHS and exacerbations of psoriasis, particularly of the guttate variety where numerous small psoriatic

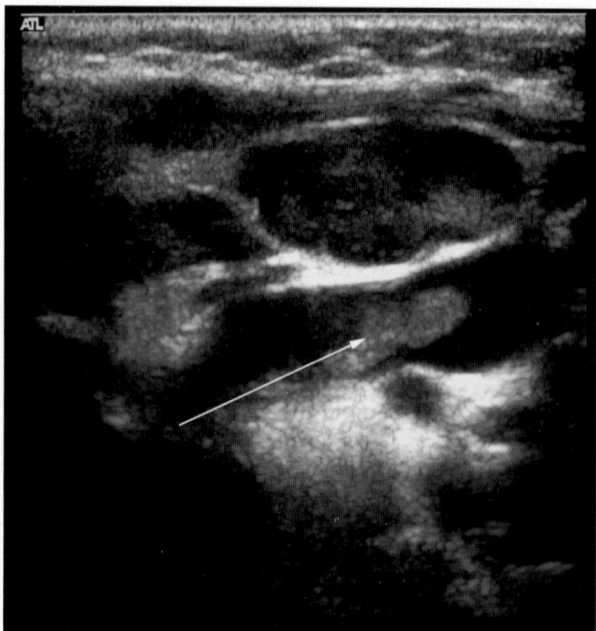

Figure 95.5 Ultrasound scan of neck veins in Lemierre syndrome showing presence of thrombus (arrowed).

lesions appear to be generated by each episode of acute tonsillitis. This appears to be an immune phenomenon. Some dermatologists and otolaryngologists advocate tonsillectomy but there is no good evidence that this relieves the condition.[33] The most current (2003) review of the efficacy of antibiotic therapy and of tonsillectomy in children with psoriasis identified only one controlled trial, which found no significant effect for antibiotics in psoriasis. No controlled trials evaluating the effect of tonsillectomy were identified. Uncontrolled data suggest benefit in one-third to half of patients with tonsillectomy but 7 percent reported worsening of their condition after surgery.[34] [**]

RECURRENT TONSILLITIS

In a significant but unknown proportion of patients, acute episodes appear to follow a pattern of recurring infection every few weeks or months. This sequence of episodes may gradually abate but in some individuals runs a course amounting to several years. There is currently no way of predicting those individuals in whom the condition may run a protracted course, and epidemiological data are lacking to allow accurate generalizable prognostication about how long the susceptibility to recurrent infection will last. Supportive measures continue to be appropriate and management of more severe symptoms may, again, warrant antibiotic therapy. Some clinicians have used low-dose penicillin if episodes are happening close together but there is no convincing evidence of benefit from this or that any specific antibiotic is effective in aborting recurrent attacks of tonsillitis. The medical treatment of recurrent tonsillitis remains an elusive goal.

SUBACUTE TONSILLITIS

Some patients follow what might be termed a subacute course where they are never free of low-grade discomfort in the throat associated with enlarged inflamed looking tonsils punctuated with acute episodes which may be either mild or severe.

CHRONIC TONSILLITIS

A further category of patients complain of chronic low-grade symptoms affecting their quality of life because of throat discomfort, and the production of unpleasant smelly white or yellow debris from the tonsillar crypts. Rarely, this debris may become inspissated, calcify and form a tonsillolith, which may itself be complicated by acute sepsis. Sufferers may also complain of a feeling of low-grade ill-health, which they and their medical attendants may attribute to chronic tonsil sepsis. There is no scientific evidence addressing natural resolution and general morbidity, or the relationship to identifiable tonsillar pathology in these patients.

In children, historically, a very wide range of ailments including recurrent abdominal pain, general ill-health, failure to thrive and low body weight have been attributed to infection of the tonsils but there is no real scientific evidence of this. Conversely, although removal of the tonsils has been claimed to result in increased growth rate and improvement in general health, scientific evidence for this is not robust.

Infectious mononucleosis

Acute pharyngotonsillitis is a frequent manifestation of infectious mononucleosis. This disease, commonly seen in young adults, is caused by the Epstein–Barr virus (EBV), one of the B lymphotropic human herpes viruses. In addition to its throat manifestations the disease causes severe systemic upset, haematological and liver function disturbance and splenomegaly, making the spleen vulnerable to abdominal trauma for a period of a month after cessation of symptoms. This is important in young people involved in contact sports. Diagnosis is by the Monospot blood test but this must be interpreted with caution, as the test sensitivity is <50 percent in children and 70–90 percent in adults. Confirmation is by specific EBV antibody tests. Among this group of patients symptoms are often serious, with dysphagia and occasionally dehydration from poor oral intake (**Figure 95.6**).

Although the disease is viral, secondary infection of the tonsils happens in up to 30 percent of cases, commonly with beta haemolytic streptococci; antibiotics are routinely prescribed, usually penicillin in high dosage intravenously in those patients admitted to hospital. Occasionally, metronidazole is added to this regimen although some clinicians favour second- and third-generation cephalosporins as an alternative.

Ampicillin must be avoided in this condition as patients may suffer a severe allergic rash in consequence.

If there is extreme swelling of the tonsils such that compromise of the airway and severe difficulty with swallowing results, a short course of high-dose corticosteroids is frequently employed as an adjunct, with evidence of benefit from several uncontrolled studies.[35, 36] [**] Steroids should not be employed routinely in view of the risks in this disease, which is associated with lymphoproliferative disorders. Steroids should only be employed in combination with antibiotics. There is no evidence at present to support the use of antiviral medication such as acyclovir in this disease.[37]

Specific infections

These include syphilis and tuberculosis. Owing to their relative rarity in the developed world they may potentially be difficult to diagnose. The lesion in syphilis classically takes the form of a 'punched out' ulcer but this is not invariable and, likewise, the appearances in tuberculosis may vary. The main differential diagnosis is with neoplasm and diagnosis is usually made by biopsy of the lesion.

NONINFLAMMATORY DISEASE

Asymmetry

A recent study of tonsil size after tonsillectomy revealed no significant difference in cases of apparent asymmetry.[38] [**] Tonsil asymmetry is not an absolute indication for tonsillectomy but in such cases, particularly in adults, the clinician should be alert for the possibility of neoplasia, notably lymphoma.

In clinical practice the apparent size of the tonsils *per se* is not well correlated with disease within them. The tonsils often swell when acutely inflamed, but there is wide variation in the degree to which the tonsils are buried in the lateral pharyngeal wall giving a false impression of the size of the structures themselves. The tonsils tend to involute during late childhood and early adult life, but in the presence of disease may remain prominent into adulthood. Indeed, some asymptomatic adults have impressively large tonsils. The rate of involution varies between individuals and sometimes this process varies between the two tonsils, giving an asymmetric appearance.

Spontaneous tonsillar haemorrhage

Occasionally, spontaneous bleeding from inflamed tonsils may take place but this is rarely serious. This may also happen in response to minor trauma in uninflamed tonsils. It may respond to cautery under local anaesthesia and, occasionally, if persistently troublesome, tonsillectomy may be indicated.

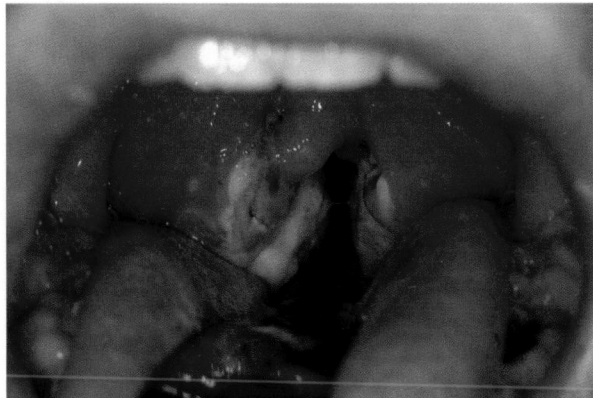

Figure 95.6 The throat in infectious mononucleosis (yellow slough is typical).

Neoplasia

Asymmetry of the tonsils may give rise to the suspicion of malignancy as may an irregular or ulcerated appearance of one of the tonsils. In childhood it is not unusual for the tonsils to involute asymmetrically and, accordingly, a disparity in size of the tonsils is not always an indication for biopsy in childhood.[38] However, any unusual appearances should be treated with caution and further investigated. This will normally include a full ENT examination with special attention to the neck, CT or magnetic resonance scanning of the neck, chest and abdomen if appropriate, followed by panendoscopy and excision biopsy, particularly in adults.

Lymphoma

In keeping with a structure primarily of lymphoid origin, lymphoma may occur within the tonsils and although this is most likely in the adult age group, lymphoma is not unknown in childhood. The management of this disease includes detailed staging of the disease and treatment modalities may encompass surgery, radiotherapy and/or chemotherapy. The details are covered in Chapter 98, Tumours of the head and neck in childhood.

Squamous carcinoma

In common with the rest of the upper aerodigestive tract and oral cavity, in particular, squamous carcinoma is the most common malignancy encountered. It is generally a disease of adult life and is covered in Chapter 193, Oropharyngeal tumours.

Obstructive sleep apnoea syndrome of childhood

The entity of obstructive sleep apnoea of childhood is an increasingly recognized disorder resulting in impaired functioning due to exhaustion, failure to thrive and possibly leading to cardiovascular strain and the later development of pulmonary hypertension. The tonsils and adenoids are very significantly involved in the genesis of this disorder and adenotonsillectomy frequently indicated in its management. The condition and its management are covered in detail in Chapter 85, Obstructive sleep apnoea in childhood.

KEY POINTS

- Acute tonsillitis is common and self-limiting.
- Complications are rare.
- Treatment is largely symptomatic with an emphasis on analgesia and rehydration.

- Antimicrobial therapy has a small but measurable effect on outcome.
- The tonsil rarely may be the site of presentation of lymphoma or malignant disease.

Best clinical practice

✓ In acute tonsillitis clinical diagnosis alone should not be relied upon in distinguishing between a bacterial or viral aetiology. [Grade B]

✓ Both throat swab culture and RAT are of questionable value in guiding prescription of antibiotics for sore throat. [Grade B]

✓ Widespread indiscriminate antibiotic prescription promotes the genesis of resistant organisms, allergy and anaphylaxis. There is no justification for **routine** use of antibiotics in children with sore throat. [Grade A]

✓ In those patients in whom the illness shows no sign of improvement within 48–72 hours or in whom there is clinical concern because of the severity of symptoms, antibiotic therapy is appropriate and the drug of choice remains benzylpenicillin. A seven-day course is usually adequate. [Grade C]

✓ A single dose of dexamethasone as adjuvant therapy reduces pain in acute pharyngotonsillitis. [Grade B]

✓ Aspiration using a wide bore needle and syringe, together with antibiotic therapy, is now the management of choice for quinsy. As a significant proportion of peritonsillar abscesses grow anaerobes, metronidazole should be considered. [Grade C]

✓ Treatment of both parapharyngeal and retropharyngeal abscess is initially high-dose antibiotic therapy. When pus formation is suspected, incision and drainage under general anaesthesia, with the airway protected by intubation by a skilled and experienced anaesthetist is recommended. [Grade C]

✓ Ampicillin must be avoided in infectious mononucleosis as patients may suffer a severe allergic rash in consequence. [Grade C/D]

✓ Systemic glucocorticoids are of value in infectious mononucleosis where there is extreme swelling of the pharyngeal mucosa with impending airway compromise. [Grade C/D]

Deficiencies in current knowledge and areas for future research

➤ The role of the tonsil in the development of immunity needs to be more fully understood.

➤ Data to shed light on the natural history of recurrent tonsillitis and define any subgroups in which natural resolution of recurrent symptoms is likely to happen would be helpful.

➤ The precise place and value of antibiotic therapy is still not fully defined. Robust randomized controlled trials of antibiotic therapy versus placebo in sore throat/tonsillitis, both in the acute single episode situation and in recurrent tonsillitis, are required. The results should be applicable to everyday practice.

REFERENCES

1. Surow JB, Handler SD, Telian SA, Fleisher GR, Baranak CC. Bacteriology of tonsil surface and core in children. *Laryngoscope*. 1989; **99**: 261–6.

2. Brook I, Yocum P, Shah K. Surface vs core-tonsillar aerobic and anaerobic flora in recurrent tonsillitis. *Journal of the American Medical Association*. 1980; **244**: 1696–8.

3. Caplan C. Case against the use of throat culture in the management of streptococcal pharyngitis. *Journal of Family Practice*. 1979; **8**: 485–90.

4. Feery BJ, Forsell P, Gulasekharam M. Streptococcal sore throat in general practice-a controlled study. *Medical Journal of Australia*. 1976; **1**: 989–91.

5. Del Mar C. Managing sore throat: a literature review. 1. Making the diagnosis. *Medical Journal of Australia*. 1992; **156**: 572–5.

6. Klein JO. Microbiology of diseases of the tonsils and adenoids. Workshop on tonsillectomy and adenoidectomy. *Annals of Otology, Rhinology, and Laryngology*. 1975; **84**: 30–3.

7. Gaffney RJ, Cafferkey MT. Bacteriology of normal and diseased tonsils assessed by fine-needle aspiration: Haemophilus influenzae and the pathogenesis of recurrent tonsillitis. *Clinical Otolaryngology and Allied Sciences*. 1998; **23**: 181–5.

* 8. Brandtzaeg P. Immunology of the tonsils and adenoids: everything that the ENT surgeon needs to know. *International Journal of Pediatric Otorhinolaryngology*. 2003; **67**: S69–76.

9. Sprinkle PM, Veltri RW. The tonsils and adenoids. *Clinical Otolaryngology and Allied Sciences*. 1977; **2**: 153–67.

* 10. Little P, Williamson I. Sore throat management in general practice. *Family Practice*. 1996; **13**: 317–21.

11. Paradise JL, Bluestone CD, Bachman RZ, Karantonis G, Smith IH, Saez CA *et al*. History of recurrent sore throats as an indication for tonsillectomy. *New England Journal of Medicine*. 1978; **298**: 409–13.

12. Moloney JR, John DG, Jagger C. Age, sex, ethnic origin and tonsillectomy. *Journal of Laryngology and Otology*. 1988; **102**: 649–51.

13. Kljakovic M. Sore throat presentation and management in general practice. *New Zealand Medical Journal*. 1993; **106**: 381–3.

14. McIsaac W, Goel V, Slaughter PM, Parsons GW, Woolnough KV, Weir PT *et al*. Reconsidering sore throats. Part 1: Problems with current clinical practice. *Canadian Family Physician*. 1997; **43**: 485–93.

* 15. Little P, Williamson I, Warner S, Gould C, Gantley M, Kinmonth AL. Open randomised trial of prescribing strategies in managing sore throat. *British Medical Journal*. 1997; **314**: 722–7.

16. Del Mar C. Managing sore throat: a literature review. II Do antibiotics confer benefit? *Medical Journal of Australia*. 1992; **156**: 644–9.

17. Capper R, Canter RJ. Is the incidence of tonsillectomy influenced by the family medical or social history. *Clinical Otolaryngology and Allied Sciences*. 2001; **26**: 484–7.

18. White CB, Bass JW, Yamada SM. Rapid latex agglutination compared with the throat culture for the detection of group A streptococcal infection. *Pediatric Infections Disease*. 1986; **5**: 208–12.

19. Joslyn SA, Hoekstra GL, Sutherland JE. Rapid antigen testing in diagnosing group A beta haemolytic streptococcal pharyngitis. *Journal of the American Board of Family Practice*. 1995; **8**: 177–82.

* 20. Del Mar CB, Glasziou PP, Spinks AB. Antibiotics for sore throat (Cochrane review). In: *The Cochrane Library*, Issue 4, Oxford: Update Software, 2002.

21. Zwart S, Rovers MM, de Melker RA, Hoes AW. Penicillin for acute sore throat in children: randomised, double blind trial. *British Medical Journal*. 2003; **327**: 1324.

* 22. Little P, Gould I, Williamson I, Warner G, Gantley M, Kinmonth AL. Reattendance and complications in a randomised trial of prescribing strategies for sore throat: the medicalising effect of prescribing antibiotics. *British Medical Journal*. 1997; **315**: 350–2.

23. Zwart S, Sachs APE, Ruijs GJHM, Gubbels JW, Hoes AW, de Melker RA. Penicillin for acute sore throat: randomised double blind trial of seven days versus three days treatment or placebo in adults. *British Medical Journal*. 2000; **320**: 150–4.

24. Wei JL, Kasperbauer JL, Weaver AL, Boggust AJ. Efficacy of single dose dexamethasone as adjuvant therapy for acute pharyngitis. *Laryngoscope*. 2002; **112**: 87–93.

25. Lilja M, Raisanen S, Jokinen K, Stenfors L-E. Direct microscopy of effusions obtained from peritonsillar abscesses as a complement to bacterial culturing. *Journal of Laryngology and Otology*. 1997; **111**: 392–5.

* 26. Brook I. Microbiology and management of peritonsillar, retropharyngeal and parapharyngeal abscesses. *Journal of Oral and Maxillofacial Surgery*. 2004; **62**: 1545–50.

27. Brook I. The role of anaerobic bacteria in tonsillitis. *International Journal of Pediatric Otorhinolaryngology*. 2005; **69**: 9–19.

28. Daya H, Lo S, Papsin BC, Zachariasova A, Murray H, Pirie J *et al*. Retropharyngeal and parapharyngeal infection in children: the Toronto experience. *International Journal of Pediatric Otorhinolaryngology*. 2005; **69**: 81–6.

29. Wang LF, Kuo WR, Tsai SM, Huang KJ. Characterisation of life threatening deep cervical space infections: a review of

one hundred ninety six cases. *American Journal of Otolaryngology*. 2003; **24**: 111–7.

30. Ajulo P, Qayyum A, Brewis C, Innes A. Lemierre's syndrome: the link between a simple sore throat, sore neck and pleuritic chest pain. *Annals of the Royal College of Surgeons of England*. 2005; **87**: 303–5.

31. Jones JW, Riordan T, Morgan MS. Investigation of postanginal sepsis and Lemierre's syndrome in the South West Peninsula. *Communicable disease and public health/ PHLS*. 2001; **4**: 278–81.

32. Pulcini C, Vandenbos F, Roth S, Mondain-Miton V, Bernard E, Roger PM *et al.* [Lemierre's syndrome: a report of six cases] [Article in French]. *La Revue de médecine interne*. 2003; **24**: 17–23.

33. Owen CM, Chalmers RJG, O'Sullivan T, Griffiths CEM. Antistreptococcal interventions for guttate and chronic plaque psoriasis (Cochrane review). In: *The Cochrane Library*, Issue 4, Oxford: Update Software, 2002.

34. Wilson JK, Al-Suwaidan SN, Krowchuk D, Feldman SR. Treatment of psoriasis in children: is there a role for antibiotic therapy and tonsillectomy? *Pediatric Dermatology*. 2003; **20**: 11–5.

35. Chan SCS, Dawes PJD. The management of severe infectious mononucleosis tonsillitis and upper airway obstruction. *Journal of Laryngology and Otology*. 2001; **115**: 973–7.

36. Tynell E, Aurelius E, Brandell A. Acyclovir and prednisolone treatment of acute infectious mononucleosis: a multicentre, double blind placebo controlled trial. *Journal of Infectious Diseases*. 1996; **174**: 324–31.

37. Papesch M, Watkins R. Epstein-Barr virus infectious mononucleosis. *Clinical Otolaryngology and Allied Sciences*. 2001; **26**: 3–8.

38. Spinou E, Kubba H, Konstantinidis I, Johnston A. Tonsillectomy for biopsy in children with unilateral tonsillar enlargement. *International Journal of Pediatric Otorhinolaryngology*. 2002; **63**: 15–7.

96

Tonsillectomy

WILLIAM S McKERROW AND RAY CLARKE

Introduction	1229	Tonsils and variant Creutzfeld–Jakob disease	1238
History of tonsillectomy	1229	Acknowledgements	1238
The evidence-base	1229	Key points	1239
Tonsillectomy technique	1232	Best clinical practice	1239
Morbidity of tonsillectomy	1235	Deficiencies in current knowledge and areas for future	
Perioperative management	1236	research	1239
Alternatives to surgery	1237	References	1239

SEARCH STRATEGY

The opinions in this chapter are supported by a Medline search using the terms tonsil, tonsillectomy and child. Reference was also made to the Cochrane Library. This was supplemented by a hand search of current journals and by reference to the published results of the National Prospective Tonsillectomy Audit available on the Royal College of Surgeons of England website (www.rcseng.ac.uk). The UK Department of Health (www.dh.gov.uk) and the National Institute for Health and Clinical Excellence (NICE) (www.nice.org.uk) websites were also consulted.

INTRODUCTION

Tonsillectomy is one of the most frequently undertaken procedures in otolaryngology. The indications remain controversial. Children are offered surgery primarily to reduce the frequency and severity of recurrent sore throats. A smaller number will have tonsillectomy – often with adenoidectomy – for relief of airway obstruction. This is discussed in Chapter 85, Obstructive sleep apnoea in childhood. This chapter focuses on the role of tonsil surgery in recurrent sore throats in children.

HISTORY OF TONSILLECTOMY

Celsus in 'De Medicina' (14–37 AD) described 'induration' of the tonsils, which he advised could be removed by dissection with the fingernail. If this was not possible they could be grasped with a hook and pulled out with a 'bistoury'.[1] Improved instrumentation – particularly the snares and 'guillotines' used by Morrel McKenzie[2] – led to popularization of the operation in Victorian England. Sir Felix Semon (1849–1921) removed the tonsils from several of Queen Victoria's grandchildren and the procedure became fashionable in the drawing rooms of the aristocracy.[3] It was said to cure a variety of childhood ailments.[4] Throughout much of the twentieth century, the practice – particularly in the UK and the USA – of more or less indiscriminate tonsillectomy (**Figure 96.1**), with a small but measurable mortality, led to hostility among paediatricians and public health physicians.[5] The criteria for offering tonsillectomy have changed significantly over the years and are now much more stringent.

THE EVIDENCE-BASE

Efficacy

Despite the popularity of tonsillectomy and the enthusiasm with which it is offered and sought, high quality

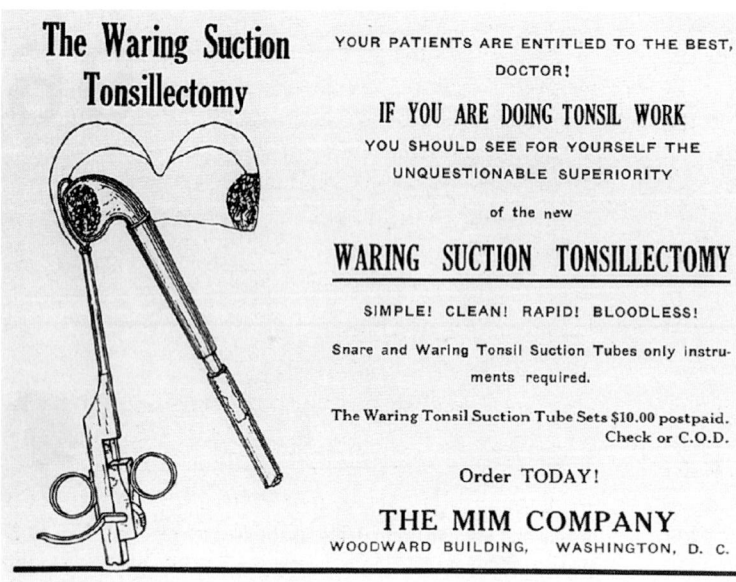

Figure 96.1 Advertisement for tonsillectomy instruments, 1920s. Reprinted with permission of the John Q Adams Center for the History of Otolaryngology – Head and Neck Surgery Foundation, © 2007. All rights reserved.

evidence of efficacy is sparse.[6] A systematic review concluded that there was little evidence on the use of tonsillectomy for recurrent throat infection[7] and a Cochrane review concludes that there is no evidence from randomized controlled trials (RCT) to guide clinicians in formulating guidelines for surgery in children or adults.[8] There is no good evidence that any benefit from tonsillectomy for recurrent sore throat in children is sustained for more than two years after surgery.

The most celebrated trials make up the 'Paradise study' reported in 1984.[9] These randomized and nonrandomized controlled trials prospectively compared groups of children who met strict entry criteria and who received surgery (tonsillectomy with, in some circumstances, adenoidectomy) or nonsurgical intervention. Participation was dependent on children having a history of seven episodes of sore throat in the year prior to the study, five or more in the preceding two years or three or more in each of the preceding three years. Well-documented clinical features had to be demonstrated to ensure eligibility. These trials showed that in these 'severely affected children' tonsillectomy was efficacious for two years, and possibly for a third year. [****] Efficacy was measured by a reduction in the number and/or severity of throat infections. Many of the children treated nonsurgically improved spontaneously. Such benefits as there were from surgery were slight. Critics point out that the study was poorly randomized. Children randomized to the nonsurgical group proceeded to surgery at the subsequent request of the parents. Children having adenoidectomy, as well as tonsillectomy, were included, making it impossible to exclude this intervention as relevant to the outcome of treatment. Children in the control limb of the study had active therapy, which may have minimized the morbidity.

A number of randomized controlled studies of varying but generally poor quality have subsequently contributed

little. The 'Paradise' group has now reported on less severely affected children. Two parallel randomized controlled trials compared surgery with nonsurgical management for children with a history of recurrent episodes of throat infection, but with less stringent entry criteria than for the original studies. These reduced standards were considered to better reflect accepted practice, but were slightly more rigorous than the widely accepted USA guidelines as suggested by the American Academy of Otolaryngology Head and Neck Surgery, i.e. 'three or more infections of tonsils and/or adenoids per year despite adequate medical therapy'.[10] The incidence of throat infection was significantly lower in the surgical groups than in corresponding control groups during each of the three follow-up years. Adenotonsillectomy was no better than tonsillectomy alone. Benefits were marginal, such that the authors concluded that the benefits were outweighed in this group of children by the morbidity and risks of the operation.[11] [****]

A good quality open randomized controlled trial in the Netherlands – where surgical intervention rates for recurrent sore throats are considerably higher than in the UK or the USA – looked at 300 children under the age of eight years. Children who fulfilled the criteria of the original Paradise study (i.e. severely affected children) were excluded, so this study looked only at those with mild symptoms. Adenotonsillectomy was compared with watchful waiting. A number of outcome measures – including health-related quality of life and the frequency of episodes of pyrexia – were considered. The authors concluded that adenotonsillectomy had no major clinical benefits over watchful waiting in children with mild upper respiratory symptoms.[6, 12] [****] It must be stressed that both of these studies looked at less severely affected children. In each case the criteria for intervention were considerably less robust than suggested by the Scottish Intercollegiate Guidance Network (SIGN) guidelines (www.sign.ac.uk) and in the Netherlands's study adenoidectomy was routinely combined with tonsillectomy.

Perhaps inadequate knowledge of the natural history and expected outcome of recurrent sore throats in children has bedevilled the quest for a sound evidential base for current practice. Preliminary data from a study conducted during the 'tonsillectomy embargo' in the UK in 2001 resulting from concerns about variant Creutz-feldt-Jakob disease (vCJD) transmission (see Tonsils and variant Creutzfeld–Jakob disease) suggests that sponta-neous improvement is to be expected in adults.[13] [**/*] Given that overall the frequency of recurrent sore throat appears to decrease with time, there is no evidence predicting the rate of such improvement or which looks at any difference in natural history in those presenting in childhood compared with those presenting in adult life.

In a randomized controlled trial in adults, 36 participants underwent immediate tonsillectomy. The control group – 34 patients – remained on a waiting list. Follow-up was short but at 90 days, streptococcal pharyngitis had recurred in 24 percent of the control group and in 3 percent of the tonsillectomy group. The authors concluded that adults with a history of recurrent streptococcal pharyngitis were less likely to have further streptococcal or other throat infections or days with throat pain if they had their tonsils removed.[14] The morbidity associated with the operation must be considered and may outweigh any benefits.[15] This study did not include children.

Studies with a less rigorous design than the RCT provide anecdotal evidence of improvement following surgery. The overwhelming view of clinicians is that in judiciously chosen patients tonsillectomy brings about significant benefit. The results of the Scottish Tonsillec-tomy Audit found a high level of satisfaction among those undergoing surgery (97 percent satisfaction rate at one year).[16] [**/*] There are, however, severe limitations in using satisfaction rates as an outcome measure and the follow-up was relatively short.

Current practice

Tonsillectomy in children is one of the most frequently performed operations in the developed world. Although numbers are declining from a peak of over 200,000 annual tonsillectomies in the 1950s (UK), some 52,000 tonsillec-tomies were performed in England under the National Health Service in the year 2003/04. Data from the Department of Health Statistics show that around 30,000 of these were in children with an approximately equal gender ratio (www.dh.gov.uk). The majority are for recurrent sore throats with most of the remainder for airway obstruction. Parents in the UK initially present to a general practitioner. Referral patterns are dictated by thinking in primary care and many parents have firm

views by the time they see an otolaryngologist. Despite the availability of guidelines and protocols in practice, a decision to undertake tonsillectomy is made by negotia-tion between the parent/carer and the otolaryngologist. Some units have introduced nurse-led clinics where strict protocols are used to determine eligibility for surgery. It will be illuminating to see if these protocols have a material effect on surgery rates.

Sociocultural factors

There is no published evidence that the pattern of disease varies by racial, ethnic, climatic or cultural factors across the globe, but there are wide variations in the rate of tonsillectomy by geographical region.[16] [***] A quoted incidence of 6.5 per 10,000 children in the UK National Health Service contrasts with 11.5 per 10,000 in the Netherlands and 5 per 10,000 in the USA. The figures for the UK may be higher as an estimated one-sixth of otolaryngology interventions occur in private practice where figures are not as widely available. In the 2005 National Prospective Tonsillectomy Audit (NPTA) (www.rcseng.ac.uk), some 13 percent of procedures were performed in independent hospitals. In the Scottish Tonsillectomy Audit, sizeable variations in tonsillectomy rate were found between different regions in the same country, from four per 10,000 in Forth Valley to ten per 10,000 in Dumfries and Galloway. In the developing world, the incidence of surgery is much lower, related perhaps to access to health care and parental expectations and preferences.

Tonsillectomy is more common in large conurbations suffering higher levels of deprivation.[17] [**] Recent work suggests that social class and parental smoking does not influence the number of reported episodes of sore throat or tonsillitis, but that a history of parental tonsillectomy and a family history of atopy have a positive association with the frequency with which children present with sore throat and tonsillitis.[18] Parental enthusiasm for surgery varies. Some of the variation may be due to differences in demand for health care. There is evidence from the North of England and Scotland Study on Tonsillectomy and Adenoidectomy in Children (NESSTAC) that girls now present much more frequently than boys.[19]

Guidelines

The British Association of Otolaryngologists Head and Neck Surgeons (BAO-HNS or ENT-UK, www.ent-uk.org) has published a series of reviews under the title 'Clinical Effectiveness' to assist clinicians with decision-making for common clinical problems.[20] For tonsillectomy in children, the recommendations are in line with those of the Scottish Intercollegiate Guidance Network (www.sign.ac.uk).[21]

SIGN [**] suggest what are felt to be reasonable indications based on current level of knowledge, clinical observation in the field and the results of clinical audit of outcomes. Patients should meet all the following criteria:

- sore throats due to tonsillitis;
- five or more episodes of sore throat per year;
- symptoms for at least a year;
- episodes of disabling sore throat which prevent normal functioning.

As with any surgical procedure, the risks of surgery must be balanced against the potential benefit. Cognizance should be taken of whether the frequency of episodes is increasing or decreasing.

The American Academy of Otolaryngologists/Head and Neck Surgeons (AAO HNS) guidelines are widely accepted by US health care insurance companies. These guidelines[10] suggest that tonsillectomy should be considered for children with 'three or more infections of tonsils and/or adenoids per year despite adequate medical therapy'.

The difficulties associated with implementing guidelines and the paucity of effect of guidelines on clinical practice are well known. There is evidence that the rate of ENT interventions is not significantly altered by the introduction of guidelines. This may not be the case with strictly imposed insurance company constraints such as are used in 'managed health care'. Moreover, when guidelines are broken, they tend to be broken more often in favour of offering rather than withholding surgery.[22]

Health economics

Decision-making about the precise indications for tonsillectomy is complicated by the fact that each episode of tonsillitis may be treated individually and that there is a natural tendency for recurrent tonsillitis to improve with time. A relatively low cost but high volume procedure to alleviate a troublesome but nonlife-threatening condition, the operation has attracted the attention of those with an interest in the economics of health care. This in turn has focused on issues such as the value to the patient's health of removing the tonsils, the contribution of the operation to reduction of morbidity from illness and to the increase in productivity of the individual if a tendency to recurrent debilitating illness is abolished. In children, the focus is on quality of life for parent and child and the effect on the child's education.[19] Tonsillitis is disruptive to school and family life, but tonsillectomy itself is associated with a period of morbidity. In uncomplicated cases, this usually involves at least two weeks absence from school with attendant implications for the parent or carer. Health-related quality of life indices and the economic aspects of sore throats in children have now been considered. A number of validated instruments evaluate benefit from childhood or adult ENT interventions, including

tonsillectomy. The results of evaluation of quality of life before and after the operation suggest that tonsil disease has a marked adverse effect on quality of life and that there is significant benefit from surgery.[23, 24] [**]

TONSILLECTOMY TECHNIQUE

Introduction

Recent concerns about the risk of transmission of vCJD (see Tonsils and variant Creutzfeld–Jakob disease), the incidence of primary and secondary haemorrhage and the effect of surgical technique on complications post-tonsillectomy have been the subject of intense debate. The National Prospective Tonsillectomy Audit was established in 2003 on behalf of the Royal College of Surgeons of England and the BAO-HNS to look at some of these issues. Data were collected on over 50,000 patients undergoing tonsillectomy in England. Just under half were children (i.e. less than 15 years old). The results represent a comprehensive and up-to-date resumé of current practice and provide a firm basis for recommendations to clinicians particularly in relation to surgical techniques.[25]

The optimal technique for removal of the tonsils must be as straightforward as possible for patient and surgeon. Given the frequency with which tonsil surgery is performed, it should be easy to teach, but above all it must be safe.[26]

The traditional methods for removing the tonsils are the so-called 'cold steel' techniques using metal instruments. In recent years, perceived advantages in terms of reduced blood loss, less pain, more rapid healing and easier surgical technique have led to the introduction of several new methods.

'Cold steel' tonsillectomy

The most common method of 'cold steel' tonsillectomy is the dissection technique (**Figure 96.2**). In this, the tonsil is retracted medially, the mucosa overlying the tonsil capsule incised and the plane of loose areolar tissue between the tonsil and the pharyngeal musculature dissected with steel dissectors, gauze or cotton wool until the tonsil is fully mobilized (**Figure 96.3**). Blood vessels traversing the plane of dissection are dealt with either by ligature or diathermy as required. An alternative method of 'cold steel' tonsillectomy is the guillotine technique, whereby the tonsil is amputated using a specially designed guillotine device and haemostasis, secured as necessary by one of the above methods. Of these two techniques, traditional dissection remains the most frequently used. Arguably the advantage of speed in the guillotine technique is outweighed by the risk of leaving tonsil

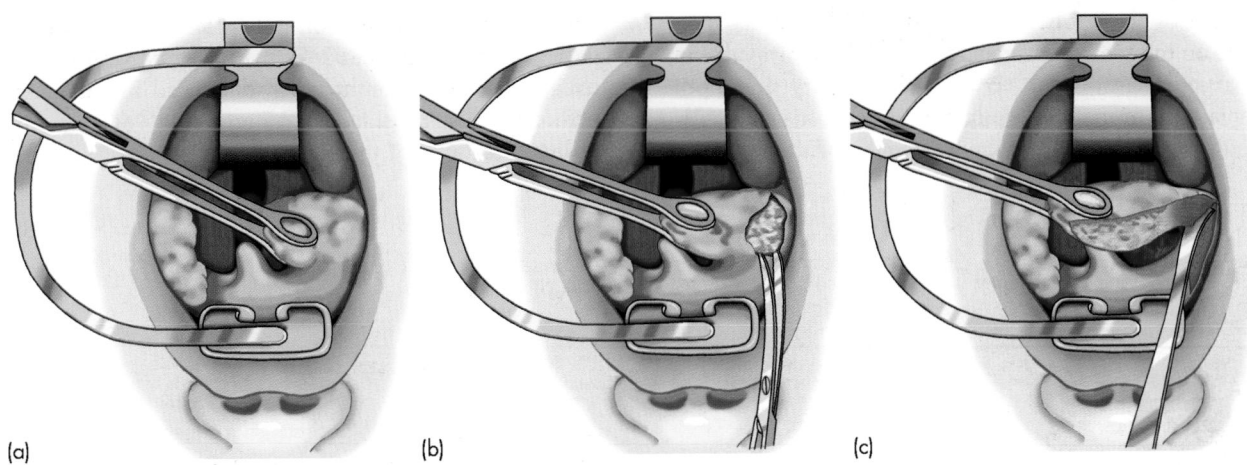

Figure 96.2 Steps in dissection tonsillectomy.

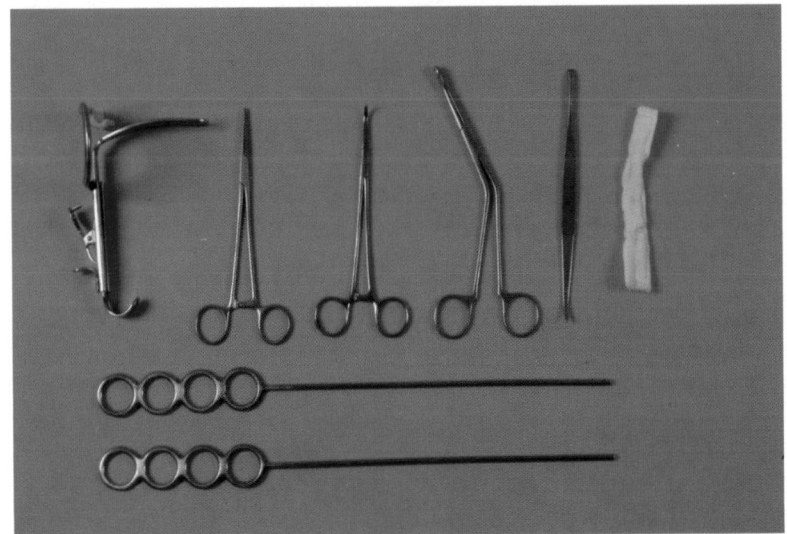

Figure 96.3 Tonsillectomy set as used by one of the authors (RWC).

tissue behind. Blood loss during tonsillectomy can be considerable and may constitute over 10 percent of total circulating blood volume.[27]

Cold steel dissection may be combined with diathermy to aid haemostasis, but many surgeons prefer ties or swabs. In the NPTA, the use of 'cold steel' dissection without diathermy was associated with the lowest haemorrhage rate. 'Haemorrhage' was defined as a bleed that prolonged the patient's hospital stay, required blood transfusion, a return to the operating theatre, or in the case of 'secondary' haemorrhage readmission to hospital. The haemorrhage rate for various techniques is shown in **Table 96.1**. The NPTA recommendation is that all trainee surgeons should become competent in cold steel dissection with ties before considering alternative techniques.

Diathermy tonsillectomy

In recent years, the technique has evolved of using diathermy not only as an aid to haemostasis when the tonsil has been delivered, but to dissect the tonsil from its bed. This has the obvious advantage from the point of view of both operator and patient, particularly if a child, of reducing intraoperative blood loss to a minimum. Various claims and counterclaims have been made regarding the advantages and disadvantages of this technique, the most common alternative to traditional cold steel tonsillectomy. Major concerns about an increase in secondary haemorrhage rate with diathermy, following the introduction of disposable instruments for tonsillectomy during 2001, led to detailed retrospective audit of haemorrhage rates throughout the UK. This confirmed an incidence of secondary haemorrhage as high as 16.8 percent with diathermy in one published audit.[28] A Cochrane review of dissection versus diathermy for tonsillectomy found that only two of the studies that addressed this were sufficiently robust for analysis. These demonstrated reduced intraoperative bleeding but increased pain in the diathermy group, with no difference in secondary haemorrhage rate.[29] [**] These concerns were to the fore when the NPTA was set up. Surgeons use a variety of diathermy techniques and specifications often based on individual preference and on what is available in a particular institution. Power settings vary and both bipolar and monopolar equipment is used. In the NPTA, postoperative bleeding was more frequent with diathermy than with cold steel alone, (**Table 96.1**) and was particularly common with monopolar diathermy such that the authors recommended that surgeons using this method should consider changing. **Table 96.2** lists the recommendations of the NPTA in full.

Table 96.1 Surgical techniques and primary and secondary postoperative haemorrhage rates.

Surgical technique (*n* = 33,921)	Primary tonsillar haemorrhage rate (%)	Secondary tonsillar haemorrhage rate (%)
Cold steel and ties/packs	0.8	1.0
Cold steel and monopolar diathermy	0.5	2.4
Cold steel and bipolar diathermy	0.5	2.3
Monopolar diathermy forceps	1.1	5.5
Bipolar diathermy forceps	0.4	4.3
Bipolar diathermy scissors	0.6	4.6
Coblation	1.0	3.6
Other	0.7	3.6

Reprinted from the National Prospective Tonsillectomy Audit, available on the Royal College of Surgeons of England website (www.rcseng.ac.uk), Table 4.6, with permission.

Table 96.2 Recommendations of the National Prospective Tonsillectomy Audit (2005).

- When a patient is counselled for surgery, the risk of tonsillectomy complications, and in particular postoperative haemorrhage, should be carefully explained to the patients/parents.
- This risk should be quantified, preferably using the surgeon's own (or department's) figures.
- National figures can be used, but this should be made clear to patients.
- Surgeons using monopolar diathermy should consider using an alternative technique. There are no advantages to using this instrument over other methods.
- All trainee surgeons should become competent in cold steel dissection and haemostasis using ties, before learning other techniques in tonsillectomy.
- Emphasis must be placed on teaching the correct use of, and the potential hazards of, diathermy and other 'hot' techniques. Checks should be made of the power settings before starting the operation.
- Inexperienced trainees must be supervised by a more senior surgeon until competency has been achieved. This recommendation is in agreement with the College's Standards on Good Surgical Practice issued in 2002.
- Irrespective of seniority and experience, surgeons who wish to start using new techniques, such as coblation, should undergo appropriate training.
- All ENT departments should have regular morbidity and mortality meetings to monitor adverse incidents affecting patient outcome. For tonsillectomy, data should be presented by the surgeon, indicating the technique used for dissection and haemostasis and power settings if applicable, type of instrument used, and any difficulties encountered.
- It is the responsibility of the surgeon, and if appropriate his trainer, to follow up any identified problems appropriately.
- Use of single-use instruments should also be recorded, especially for cold steel dissection.
- There is an urgent need for new standards for diathermy machines so that the amount of power used is obvious to the user. Manufacturers of diathermy machines should be encouraged to produce machines with information on the total amount of energy delivered to patients.
- Hospitals should encourage the use of machines that provide clear information on power settings.
- Manufacturers of single-use instruments should be encouraged to improve the quality of the instruments.
- There is a need for further laboratory and clinical research to investigate the influence of diathermy and other 'hot' techniques on an open wound, such as the tonsillar bed.
- In particular, there is a need to investigate the dose–response relationship between power used and complications.

Reprinted from the National Prospective Tonsillectomy Audit, available on the Royal College of Surgeons of England website (www.rcseng.ac.uk), page vii, with permission.

Coblation® tonsillectomy

This relies on the use of a specially designed bipolar electrical probe, which both coagulates and cuts the tissues as it develops the dissection plane between tonsil and capsule. The probes or 'wands' are single use and there is a cost consideration.

The technique involves the use of the operating microscope.[30, 31] Coblation has gained widespread acceptance in the United States. Good results have been reported, but the technique seems to be highly operator-dependent. Postoperative bleed rates were unacceptably high in the NPTA. Some of these bleeds may reflect lack of familiarity with the technique; enthusiasts have reported bleed rates that are comparable with those obtained using cold-steel dissection. It is suggested that postoperative pain is less than with conventional dissection but one RCT has cast doubt on this and shown that morbidity was less with cold steel dissection.[32] There are no good controlled studies comparing coblation with cold steel dissection without the addition of diathermy; current evidence is inadequate to justify its introduction in preference to cold steel dissection with ties and/or packs. The National Institute for Health and Clinical Excellence (NICE) advise that current evidence is sufficient to support the use of electrosurgery (diathermy and coblation) for tonsillectomy, but advise surgeons to ensure that they are appropriately trained and to make patients and parents/carers aware of the risk of haemorrhage after these techniques.[33]

Ultrasonic dissection

Ultrasonic dissection uses an oscillating blade, which acts as both a cutting and coagulating device. Enthusiasts for the 'harmonic scalpel' have claimed advantages over conventional techniques,[34, 35] in terms of reduced pain and general morbidity, but evidence remains unconvincing.

Laser tonsillectomy

With the advent of the laser as a surgical tool, the use of this method of dissecting out the tonsil has been advocated as having advantages in terms of reduction of bleeding, postoperative pain and more rapid healing. Several studies have failed to confirm these advantages. There is convincing evidence that the rate of secondary haemorrhage and late postoperative pain is significantly greater with laser.[36] [****] The evidence would suggest that this technique cannot be recommended as an alternative to conventional tonsillectomy on the grounds of cost, morbidity and safety.

'Capsulotomy' techniques

The above techniques are designed to remove the entire palatine tonsil. A preference for 'office-based' surgery particularly in the USA has led to the popularization of techniques to ablate a part of the tonsil, usually leaving the capsule intact. These 'tonsillotomy' techniques include thermal tissue ablation using radiofrequency volumetric reduction (RFVR) using a customized probe and surface laser surgery. They are widely used but have not been subject to good quality randomized controlled trials. They may be considered when tonsillectomy is undertaken in the very young where it may be desirable to leave some functioning lymphoid tissue.[37]

MORBIDITY OF TONSILLECTOMY

Psychosocial morbidity and pain

Morbidity from the operation is significant. It includes both the expected adverse consequences and the possible complications. For most children it is their first experience of parental separation. Some show behaviour changes, such as attention seeking, temper tantrums and night waking. Depression and severe anxiety were commonplace but most units are now aware of the adverse consequences of separation and permit parents to accompany the child to the operating theatre and remain with him/her throughout the in-patient stay.[38, 39] Pain and dysphagia are normal in the early postoperative period. Most children require at least a week to resume normal functioning and an average return to school or work time is one to two weeks.[16] This is mainly due to pain preventing a return to normal diet and occasionally vomiting in the early postoperative period due either to the after-effects of the anaesthetic or to the effect of swallowed blood on the stomach. Much attention has focused in the literature on the management of these symptoms, one of the goals being early discharge from hospital.

Mortality

The complications of tonsillectomy may be divided into those associated with the anaesthetic and those directly associated with the operation itself. As the operation is normally performed on children and young otherwise fit adults, for the majority of patients the risk of the short anaesthetic required for tonsillectomy is small. There are risks inherent in anaesthesia in very young children and for this reason tonsillectomy is seldom performed in children before the age of two years, even in the unlikely event of them fulfilling the above criteria for consideration for surgery. In general, tonsillectomy is not frequently indicated in children under the age of four years, the exception being children with obstructive sleep apnoea syndrome. There are some children who will be at increased risk from anaesthetic complications, principally related to the airway. These will include those with first and second branchial arch syndromes, Pierre–Robin sequence and Goldenhar syndrome and also those with Down syndrome, where airway compromise may occur. In the latter group, the additional hazard of atlantoaxial instability presents a further risk. Since its instigation in 1995, the Royal College of Surgeons in England audit on surgical mortality[40, 41] records no deaths occurring from tonsillectomy, but there were two deaths reported in the British lay press in 2001. Extrapolating from US data[42] and from Department of Health statistics, the potential mortality from tonsillectomy has been calculated at one per 24,000 operations[26] or one in 16,000 to one in 35,000.[19]

Perioperative complications

Occasionally, patients may experience temporomandibular joint dysfunction due to the mouth being opened too widely with the tonsillectomy gag. Small tears at the commissures of the mouth and cracks of the lip vermillion may be avoided by careful placement of the gag and the use of an emollient jelly on the lips prior to the commencement of surgery. Dissection outside the pharyngeal musculature may traumatize adjacent structures, such as the glossopharygeal nerve, the pharyngeal venous plexus and the carotid sheath, but such events are extremely rare. Nontraumatic atlantoaxial subluxation (Grisel syndrome) may occur secondary to any inflammatory process in the upper neck. It is thought to be due to infection in the periodontoid vascular plexus that drains the region, bringing about paraspinal ligament laxity. It is described following both tonsillectomy and adenoidectomy. Treatment consists of cervical immobilization, analgesia and antibiotics to reduce the risk of neurological deficit.[43]

Haemorrhage

The main early complication is haemorrhage. This is defined as primary (within the first 24 hours postoperatively) or secondary, i.e. occurring after 24 hours and during the phase of healing of the tonsil bed. The use of the term 'reactionary' is confusing. It is not uniformly defined in published work and its use is not advised. Data from the NPTA on haemorrhage have already been presented.

In a recent audit of 5646 tonsillectomy complications in Scotland in the years 2001 and 2002 (McKerrow, unpublished data), the rate of primary haemorrhage was quoted at 0.56 percent, rather lower than in some other published work and lower than that quoted in the NPTA. The readmission rate overall was 4.57 percent,

while 1.44 percent required return to theatre for arrest of haemorrhage. In other quoted series, the rate of 'secondary' haemorrhage has been as high as 16.8 percent. Secondary haemorrhage can occur any time until the tonsil bed has healed, which may take as long as two weeks. It is attributed – on sparse evidence – to infection in the granulating tonsil bed, often with streptococcal organisms. Antibiotic therapy with penicillin, pending bacteriological guidance is appropriate.

The reasons for this wide variation in bleed rates is not clear; it may be related both to the technique used and to the experience of the operator, although in the NPTA there was no significant difference in rates between trainees and more experienced surgeons.

Infection

Postoperative 'infection' is sometimes diagnosed in primary care. The presence of severe halitosis is the most prominent feature, usually associated with fever. It is almost certainly overdiagnosed as the appearance of the normally healing tonsil bed is of yellow/grey slough, which may give the impression of pus. Patients are routinely given advice to ensure a good intake of fluids and solids postoperatively on the grounds that this will clean the tonsil beds and avoid infection, but the evidence for this is scanty.

Late complications

Late complications are generally associated with the scarring that inevitably takes place as the tonsil bed heals. On rare occasions, this may result in impairment of palatal functioning with velopalatine insufficiency. Even more infrequent is the complication of nasopharyngeal stenosis, which very rarely occurs after adenotonsillectomy. Pharyngoplasty may be required to minimize the effects of these complications.

Concern has been raised about a possible increase in incidence of Hodgkin's lymphoma in adults who had tonsillectomy in childhood,[44] but a subsequent epidemiological study has not confirmed this.[45]

PERIOPERATIVE MANAGEMENT

The main arms of management to minimize morbidity are skilled anaesthesia, analgesia and antiemetic therapy. There has also been interest in the use of steroid therapy pre- or postoperatively.

Anaesthesia

Strict protocols are frequently used in the United States, while in the UK the technique varies with the preference of the individual anaesthetist. Total intravenous anaesthesia with propofol and remifentanil is associated with fast 'wake up' and little 'hangover'. Propofol has the added merit of being an antiemetic agent. Deep inhalational intubation obviates the need for muscle relaxants, speeds reversal and avoids the use of potentially emetic agents, such as neostigmine. The total duration of anaesthesia should be as brief as is practicable, certainly less than 30 minutes.

Analgesia

Adequate analgesia is important in the immediate postoperative phase. Narcotics have a potent emetic effect and should be used with caution if at all. A single dose of narcotic may be administered in the recovery phase and codeine may be used in the early postoperative period, but subsequent to this, paracaetamol is the drug of choice in the UK on the grounds of safety and efficacy. For some children this may not be adequate and a nonsteroidal antiinflammatory drug (NSAID) may be needed. There were concerns that the effect of these drugs on platelet adhesion might increase bleeding from the tonsil bed, but a recent metaanalysis found no such risk and a significant reduction in postoperative nausea and vomiting when compared with other analgesics notably narcotics.[46] [****] Aspirin should not be used in children because of the risk of Reye syndrome.

LOCAL ANAESTHESIA INFILTRATION

There has been recurring enthusiasm for the use of local anaesthetics infiltrated into the tonsil beds to reduce postoperative pain. The effect of injecting long- and short-acting local anaesthetics pre-, per- and post-operatively into the tonsil beds have all been studied. The results, including a Cochrane review, suggest that there is no current evidence of significant benefit from the use of these techniques and that further study is necessary.[47]

Antiemetic drugs

Some patients suffer severely from vomiting post-operatively. In many cases this is related to swallowed blood irritating the stomach. In these cases, the symptoms usually settle after a single vomit of the stomach contents, but in those with prolonged vomiting parenteral antiemetic therapy may be indicated. Traditional antiemetics such as cyclizine and prochlorperazine may be adequate, but several studies suggest that the newer antiemetic ondansetron may have a useful role.[48] [****]

Steroid therapy

Peroperative glucocorticoids are widely used in the US but have gained less acceptance in the UK. A Cochrane review showed that a single intravenous dose of dexamethasone was an effective, relatively safe and inexpensive treatment for reducing morbidity from paediatric tonsillectomy.[49] [****] Dexamethasone has the added advantage of being an antiemetic. Many units use a single dose of 2–4 mg.

Antibiotics

A number of studies purport to assess the benefit of prophylactic antibiotics in minimizing postoperative morbidity. The very small reduction in time to resumption of normal activities apparent in some studies must be balanced against the potential side effects of antibiotics. Current evidence does not support their routine use.[50, 51, 52] [****]

Day-case surgery

In recent years, there has been a trend towards encouraging day-case and in some areas '23-hour admission' tonsillectomy. The two main reasons for detaining post-tonsillectomy patients in hospital are safety with regard to haemorrhage and to manage morbidity from pain and vomiting.

The risk of primary bleeding diminishes to close to zero six hours after surgery so in theory the patient can be safely discharged at that time.[53] [**] In most centres this is done according to a strict protocol to ensure that the patient is adequately supervised in the home, has access to a telephone and reasonable proximity to hospital. Frequently a visit by an appropriately trained nurse on the first postoperative day is arranged. For this regime of management to prove satisfactory, adequate analgesia is essential. Although there is evidence that this mode of management is safe, there is considerable variation in its acceptability to parents and carers.[54] Currently, only a small proportion of tonsillectomies in England and Wales are done on a day-case basis (www.dh.gov.uk). The development of a successful and safe day-case tonsillectomy service requires the provision of a dedicated team of surgeon, anaesthetist, ward nurses and community back-up so that the issues of analgesia, antiemesis and safety can all be addressed adequately.[55]

ALTERNATIVES TO SURGERY

The concept that tonsillectomy surgery might be avoided by some alternative management regime is attractive to patients and health economists alike. Unfortunately this goal has proved elusive so far, but there are no conclusive studies that have looked at this issue in detail. There is no evidence that antibiotics will prevent recurrent tonsillitis.

The most commonly used approach is to manage each episode independently and to await natural remission of the recurrent problem. It is worth bearing in mind that lengthy and indiscriminate courses of antibiotics may not only contribute to the development of antibiotic-resistant organisms, but may also provoke allergic reactions to useful antibiotics and occasionally anaphylactic shock with a fatal outcome. Unpleasant side effects of broad-spectrum antibiotics, including vomiting and diarrhoea, are also frequent and relevant to the discussion. These issues are considered in more detail in Chapter 95, Diseases of the tonsil.

TONSILS AND VARIANT CREUTZFELD–JAKOB DISEASE

Variant Creutzfeld–Jakob disease is a rare, fatal neuro-degenerative disease. Histologically, it is characterized by intracellular vacuolation in nervous tissue, leading to a progressive spongiform encephalopathy. Tonsil biopsy is one of the methods of diagnosing vCJD and is less hazardous than brain biopsy, the main alternative. All possible precautions must be taken during this procedure to avoid any risk of cross infection and all equipment in direct contact with the patient must be destroyed by incineration. The biopsy material must be regarded as biohazardous and treated with appropriate precautions.

Some 150 cases have been identified since the disease was described in 1996. The causative agent is almost certainly the prion protein PrP which is also responsible for bovine spongiform encephalopathy (BSE). Involvement of the lymphoreticular system is a defining feature of vCJD and immunohistochemical accumulation of prion protein in the lymphoreticular system remains the only technique that has been shown to predict neurological disease reliably in animal prion disorders. During the overt clinical stages of the disease, tonsillar tissue is invariably infected with the prion. The infecting agent is thought to have entered the human food chain because beef was contaminated by feeding sheep offal to cows, a practice that became widespread in Britain in the 1970s. Cases of BSE in cattle were described from 1985 onwards and reached epidemic levels in 1992 (Bates, personal communication). Stringent controls in the beef industry now prevent contaminated meat from entering the food chain.[56]

Nevertheless, there were concerns that the PrP might be present in the tonsils of ostensibly healthy individuals incubating the disease, or could have been present in those who had tonsillectomy during the long incubation period (up to 20 years) when the prion may have been in the lymphoreticular system before the clinical features were manifest.[57] Poor quality preparatory techniques for tonsillectomy instruments may result in particulate matter remaining adherent to them. Normal sterilization methods do not destroy prions. Iatrogenic transmission of prion disease – but not vCJD – has been reported and this raised the possibility that prions could be passed from one patient to another on contaminated tonsillectomy instruments.[58]

Transmission of vCJD has not been shown to occur in this way but the fear that it might do so led to the introduction of single-use instruments for tonsillectomy throughout the UK in early 2001. This policy was introduced by the Department of Health and the Chief Medical Officer. An improvement in the standards of decontamination of surgical equipment was held to reduce the risk of vCJD to acceptable levels, not so much by destroying the prion but by minimizing the amount of particulate matter (i.e. tissue) adhering to surgical instruments after cleaning. The perceived theoretical risk of prion transmission was very small and much less than the real risk of bleeding, thought to be increased by poor quality disposable instruments. Although the Department of Health rescinded the embargo on reusable tonsillectomy instruments in late 2001, single-use instruments continue to be used in Scotland and the issue remains controversial.[59] Uncertainities relate to the incubation period of vCJD, the size of the 'inoculum' which puts patients at risk of developing overt disease, whether transmission of prion is possible by direct contact with tonsillectomy instruments and whether prion introduced in this way causes systemic or central nervous system infection. There are continuing concerns about the adequacy of sterilization of equipment.

The prevalence of prion infection in the tonsils of healthy individuals is unknown. The National Anonymous Tonsil Archive (NATA) study, a large-scale screening programme of fresh tonsil tissue (www.hpa.org.uk), may clarify this, but despite the investment of significant resources in this project there are doubts that the power of the study will be adequate to give useful results. Other unknowns are whether healthy tissue can be inoculated with prion by direct transmission, whether direct contamination if it did occur in this way would result in disease, and what proportion of healthy individuals who have evidence of the prion in the tonsil tissue will go on to develop disease.[60]

ACKNOWLEDGEMENTS

The authors would like to thank Professor Janet Wilson, Newcastle, for kindly reading the manuscript and commenting on it, and Grant Bates, Oxford, for assisting with the section on vCJD.

KEY POINTS

- Tonsillectomy is one of the most commonly performed surgical procedures in the developed world.
- The evidence-base for current practice is poor.
- Tonsillectomy rates vary considerably in different populations. These variations are not accounted for by variations in disease prevalence.
- Improvements following surgery are particularly small in less severely affected children. The morbidity of surgery usually outweighs any potential benefit in this group.
- There is no evidence that the benefits of tonsillectomy for recurrent sore throat are prolonged beyond two years.
- The operation is associated with significant morbidity, which may be minimized with careful perioperative management.

Best clinical practice

- ✓ 'Cold steel' dissection tonsillectomy is widely available and associated with the lowest postoperative haemorrhage rates in the hands of most surgeons. [Grade B]
- ✓ Surgeons in training must master traditional 'cold steel' dissection before considering alternative techniques. [Grade B]
- ✓ Adequate analgesia is essential in the postoperative care of children following tonsillectomy. [Grade D]
- ✓ Antiemetic agents, such as ondansetron, should be considered to reduce postoperative morbidity. [Grade D]
- ✓ There is now a sufficient body of evidence supporting the use of perioperative glucocorticoids to justify considering their use as routine. [Grade A]
- ✓ In secondary haemorrhage, surgery is rarely needed. Bleeding usually settles with antibiotic therapy alone. [Grade C]
- ✓ Continuing audit is essential; surgeons should familiarize themselves with the findings and recommendations of the NPTA. [Grade D]

Deficiencies in current knowledge and areas for future research

➢ High quality randomized controlled trials of tonsillectomy versus standardized conservative management are essential to define the optimal management of recurrent tonsillitis. The trials need to consider outcomes other than reduction in number of episodes of tonsillitis. The North of England and Scotland Study on Tonsillectomy and Adenoidectomy in Children should help provide a sound evidence-base to guide clinical practice.

➢ The morbidity of tonsillectomy remains significant. The optimal strategy for control of pain and emesis post-tonsillectomy still requires to be defined. The use of newer antiemetic agents and peroperative glucocorticoids seems set to increase.

➢ The risk, if any, of prion transmission by surgical instruments remains undefined and has important implications for all types of surgery. Work is necessary to quantify the risk and to take appropriate steps to minimize any hazard to patients. The National Anonymous Tonsil Archive currently being collated under the aegis of the Department of Health in England aims to collect data on the incidence of vCJD prion in normal tonsil tissue and may assist in quantifying the risks.

REFERENCES

1. Spencer W (trans.). *De Medicina*. London: Loeb Classical Library, 1935; ii: 12.
2. MacKenzie M. *A manual of diseases of the throat and nose: including the pharynx, larynx, trachea, oesophagus, nasal cavities and neck.* London: J & A Churchill, 1880.
3. Harrison D. *Felix Semon.* London: Royal Society of Medicine Press, 2000: 1849–921.
4. Wilson TG. *Diseases of the ear nose and throat in children.* London: William Heineman, 1955.
5. Bolande RP. Ritualistic surgery – circumcision and tonsillectomy. *New England Journal of Medicine.* 1969; 280: 591–6.
* 6. van Staaij BK, van den Akker EH, van der Heijden GJ, Schilder AG, Hoes AW. Adenotonsillectomy for upper respiratory infections: evidence based? *Archives of Diseases in Childhood.* 2005; 90: 19–25. *Summarizes the findings of the Netherlands RCT and a comprehensive review of current evidence.*
7. Marshall T. A review of tonsillectomy for recurrent throat infection. *British Journal of General Practice.* 1998; 48: 1331–5.
* 8. Burton MJ, Towler B, Glasziou P. *Tonsillectomy versus non-surgical treatment for chronic/recurrent acute tonsillitis.* Cochrane Database System Reviews. 2007; 7: CD001802.
* 9. Paradise JL, Bluestone CD, Bachman RZ, Colborn DK, Bernard BS, Taylor FH et al. Efficacy of tonsillectomy for recurrent throat infection in severely affected children. *New England Journal of Medicine.* 1984; 310: 674–83. *The earliest RCT on tonsillectomy and still widely quoted as a baseline for current practice.*

10. American Academy of Otolaryngology Head and Neck Surgery. Clinical indicators compendirum. Alexandria, VA: *American Academy of Otolaryngology Head and Neck Surgery*, 2000: 19.

* 11. Paradise JL, Bluestone CD, Colborn DK, Bernard BS, Rockette HE, Kurs-Lasky M. Tonsillectomy and adenotonsillectomy for recurrent throat infection in moderately affected children. *Pediatrics*. 2002; **110**: 7–15. *The most recent findings from the Paradise group.*

* 12. van Staaij BK, Van den Akker EH, Rovers MM, Hordijk GJ, Hoes AW, Schilder AGM. Effectiveness of adenotonsillectomy in children with mild symptoms of throat infections or adenotonsillar hypertrophy: open randomised controlled trial. *British Medical Journal*. 2004; **329**: 651–4.

13. McKerrow et al 2002. Unpublished data.

14. Alho O-P, Koivunen P, Penna T, Teppo H, Koskela M, Luotonen J. Tonsillectomy versus watchful waiting in recurrent streptococcal pharyngitis in adults: randomised controlled trial. *British Medical Journal*. 2007; **334**: 939.

15. Little P. Recurrent pharyngo-tonsillitis. *British Medical Journal*. 2007; **334**: 909.

16. Blair RL, McKerrow WS, Carter NW, Fenton A. The Scottish tonsillectomy audit. The Audit Sub-Committee of the Scottish Otolaryngological Society. *Journal of Laryngology and Otology. Supplement*. 1996; **20**: 1–25.

17. Bisset AF, Russell D. Grommets, tonsillectomies and deprivation in Scotland. *British Medical Journal*. 1994; **308**: 1129–32.

18. Capper R, Canter RJ. Is the incidence of tonsillectomy influenced by the family medical or social history. *Clinical Otolaryngology*. 2001; **26**: 484–7.

* 19. Bond J, Wilson J, Eccles M, Vanoli A, Steen N, Clarke R et al. Protocol for north of England and Scotland study of tonsillectomy and adeno-tonsillectomy in children (NESSTAC). A pragmatic randomised controlled trial comparing surgical intervention with conventional medical treatment in children with recurrent sore throats. *BMC Ear, Nose and Throat Disorders*. 2006; **6**: 13. *An up-to-date account of the current dilemmas and an outline of the NESSTAC study.*

20. British Association of Otorhinolaryngologists Head and Neck Surgeons. Statements of clinical effectiveness. *Otolaryngology*. 1998.

21. Scottish Intercollegiate Guidelines Network. Management of sore throat and indications for tonsillectomy. SIGN publication No. 34. Available from: http://www.sign.ac.uk.

22. Donaldson L, Hayes JH, Barton AG, Howel D. *The development and evaluation of best practice guidelines: tonsillectomy with or without adenoidectomy. Report to the Department of Health*. University of Newcastle upon Tyne: Department of Epidemiology and Public Health, 1994.

23. Goldstein NA, Fatima M, Campbell TF, Rosenfeld RM. child behavior and quality of life before and after tonsillectomy and adenoidectomy. *Archives of Otolaryngology, Head and Neck Surgery*. 2002; **128**: 770–5.

24. Kubba H, Swan IRC, Gatehouse S. The Glasgow Children's Benefit Inventory: a new instrument for assessing health-related benefit after an intervention. *Annals of Otology, Rhinology, and Laryngology*. 2004; **113**: 980–6.

25. The Royal College of Surgeons of England. National Prospective Tonsillectomy Audit 2005. Available from: www.rcseng.ac.uk/rcseng/content/publications/docs/national_prospective

* 26. Brown P. How safe is paediatric tonsillectomy? *International Journal of Paediatric Otolaryngology*. 2006; **70**: 575–7. *A summary of the main findings of the NPTA and a succinct account of the vCJD saga.*

27. Alatas N, San I, Cengiz M, Iynen I, Yetkin A, Korkmaz B et al. A mean red blood cell volume loss in tonsillectomy, adenoidectomy and adenotonsillectomy. *International Journal of Pediatric Otorhinolaryngology*. 2006; **70**: 835–41.

28. Maini S, Waine E, Evans K. Increased post-tonsillectomy secondary haemorrhage with disposable instruments: an audit cycle. *Clinical Otolaryngology*. 2002; **27**: 175–8.

29. Pinder D, Hilton M. *Dissection versus diathermy for tonsillectomy. The Cochrane Library*. Oxford: Update Software, 2002.

30. Timms MS, Temple RH. Coblation tonsillectomy: a double blind randomised controlled study. *Journal of Laryngology and Otology*. 2002; **116**: 450–2.

31. Belloso A, Chidambaram A, Morar P, Timms MS. Coablation tonsillectomy versus dissection tonsillectomy: postoperative hemorrhage. *Laryngoscope*. 2003; **113**: 2010–3.

32. Philpott CM, Wild DC, Mehta D, Banerjee AR. A double-blinded randomized controlled trial of coblation versus conventional dissection tonsillectomy on post-operative symptoms. *Clinical Otolaryngology*. 2005; **30**: 143–8.

33. National Institute for Health and Clinical Excellence. Procedure for Interventional Procedure Guidance Credentialing No. 150, 2005. Available from: www.nice.org.uk.

34. Sood S, Corbridge R, Powles J, Bates G, Newbegin CJ. Effectiveness of the ultrasonic harmonic scalpel for tonsillectomy. *Ear Nose and Throat Journal*. 2001; **80**: 514–6, 518.

35. Willging JP, Wiatrak BJ. Harmonic scalpel tonsillectomy in children: a randomized prospective study. *Otolaryngology – Head and Neck Surgery*. 2003; **128**: 318–25.

36. Auf I, Osborne JE, Sparkes C, Khalil H. Is the KTP laser effective in tonsillectomy? *Clinical Otolaryngology*. 1997; **22**: 145–6.

37. Nelson LM. Radiofrequency treatment for obstructive tonsillar hypertrophy. *Archives of Otolaryngology – Head and Neck Surgery*. 2000; **126**: 736–40.

38. Klausner RD, Tom LWC, Schindler PD, Potsic WP. Depression in children after tonsillectomy. *Archives of Otolaryngology, Head and Neck Surgery*. 1995; **121**: 105–8.

39. Kotiniemi LH, Ryhänen PT, Moilanen IK. Behavioural changes following routine ENT operations in two- to

ten-year-old children. *Paediatric Anaesthesia*. 1996; **6**: 45–9.

40. Brown P, Ryan R, Yung M, Browne J, Copley L, Cromwell D et al. *National prospective tonsillectomy audit, final report*. London: Royal College of Surgeons in England, Clinical Effectiveness Unit, 2005.

41. Royal College of Surgeons in England. Confidential enquiry into patient outcome and death (CEPOD). Available from: www.rcseng.ac.uk, 2005.

42. Randall DA, Hoffer ME. Complications of tonsillectomy and adenoidectomy. *Otolaryngology – Head and Neck Surgery*. 1998; **118**: 61–8.

43. Yu KK, White DR, Weissler MC, Pillsbury HC. Nontraumatic atlantoaxial subluxation (Grisel syndrome): a rare complication of otolaryngological procedures. *Laryngoscope*. 2003; **113**: 1047–9.

44. Gledovic Z, Radovanovic Z. History of tonsillectomy and appendectomy in Hodgkin's disease. *European Journal of Epidemiology*. 1991; **7**: 612–5.

45. Liaw KL, Adami J, Grindley G, Nyren O, Linet MS. Risk of Hodgkin's disease subsequent to tonsillectomy: a population-based cohort study in Sweden. *International Journal of Cancer*. 1997; **72**: 711–3.

46. Cardwell M, Siviter G, Smith A. Non-steroidal anti-inflammatory drugs and perioperative bleeding in paediatric tonsillectomy. *Cochrane Database of Systematic Reviews*. 2005; **18**: CD003591.

47. Hollis L, Burton MJ, Millar JM. *Perioperative local anaesthesia for reducing pain following tonsillectomy*. The Cochrane Library. Oxford: Update Software, 2002.

48. Bolton CM, Myles PS, Nolan P, Sterne JA. Prophylaxis of postoperative vomiting in children undergoing tonsillectomy: a systematic review and meta-analysis. *British Journal of Anaesthesia*. 2006; **97**: 593–604.

49. Steward DL, Welge JA, Myer CM. *Steroids for improving recovery following tonsillectomy in children*. The Cochrane Library. Oxford: Update Software, 2003.

50. O'Reilly BJ, Black S, Fernandes J, Parnesar J. Is the routine use of antibiotics justified in adult tonsillectomy? *Journal of Laryngology and Otology*. 2003; **117**: 382–5.

51. Iver S, DeFoor W, Grocela J, Kamholz K, Varughese A, Kenna M. The use of perioperative antibiotics in tonsillectomy: does it decrease morbidity? *International Journal of Pediatric Otorhinolaryngology*. 2006; **70**: 853–61.

52. Dhiwakar M, Eng CY, Selvaraj S, McKerrow WS. Antibiotics to improve recovery following tonsillectomy: a systematic review. *Otolaryngology – Head and Neck Surgery*. 2006; **134**: 357–64.

53. Paranese A, Clarke RW, Yardley MP. Early post-operative morbidity following tonsillectomy in children: implications for day surgery. *Journal of Laryngology and Otology*. 1999; **113**: 1089–91.

54. Kanerva M, Tarkkila P, Pitkaranta A. Day-case tonsillectomy: parental attitudes and conclusion rates. *International Journal of Pediatric Otorhinolaryngology*. 2003; **67**: 777–84.

55. Brigger MT, Brietzke SE. Outpatient tonsillectomy in children: a systematic review. *Otolaryngology and Head and Neck Surgery*. 2006; **135**: 1–7.

56. Colee JG, Bradley R, Liberski PP. Variant CJD (vCJD) and bovine spongiform encephalopathy (SE) 10 and 20 years on: part 1. *Folia Neuropathologica*. 2004; **44**: 93–101.

57. Frosh A. Prions and the ENT surgeon. *Journal of Laryngology and Otology*. 1999; **113**: 1064–7.

58. Frosh A, Joyce R, Johnson A. Iatrogenic vCJD from surgical instruments. *British Medical Journal*. 2001; **322**: 1558–9.

59. Montague ML, Lee MS, Hussain SS. Post-tonsillectomy haemorrhage: reusable and disposable instruments compared. *European Archives of Otorhinolaryngology*. 2004; **261**: 225–8.

60. Colee JG, Bradley R, Liberski PP. Variant CJD (vCJD) and bovine spongiform encephalopathy (SE) 10 and 20 years on: part 2. *Folia Neuropathologica*. 2006; **44**: 102–10.

97

Salivary gland disorders in childhood

PETER D BULL

Introduction	1242	Key points	1249
Congenital disorders	1242	Best clinical practice	1249
Inflammatory diseases	1243	Deficiencies in current knowledge and areas	
Granulomatous diseases of the salivary glands	1244	for future research	1250
Salivary gland tumours	1247	References	1250

SEARCH STRATEGY

Data for this chapter were obtained from the author's personal experience and bibliography, supported by a Medline search using the key words salivary gland, salivary disorders, sialolithiasis, congenital and child.

INTRODUCTION

Many of the salivary gland conditions that occur in children mirror those found in adults but relative incidences vary. In addition, there are some conditions that are unique to childhood. Salivary gland disease in children is uncommon. Clinical expertise in this area tends to be concentrated in the hands of a few; as a result the correct diagnosis may be overlooked and the primary management may be inappropriate.

CONGENITAL DISORDERS

Absence of salivary glands

Salivary gland agenesis or aplasia is extremely rare. If it involves all of the major salivary glands, the result is severe xerostomia with extensive dental caries. Partial agenesis may be missed as the remaining glands produce enough saliva to maintain the dentition. If in doubt, salivary tissue can be demonstrated by technetium 99m pertechnetate scanning, ideally augmented with magnetic resonance imaging (MRI).[1] Treatment of xerostomia is supportive and is focussed on meticulous oral hygiene and the use of artificial saliva.[2]

Congenital salivary cysts

These are found most often in the parotid gland. They include cysts that occur in association with branchial cleft and branchial pouch anomalies (see Chapter 99, Branchial arch fistulae, thyroglossal duct anomalies and lymphangioma). They may present as intraglandular masses or with secondary sialadenitis due to ductal compression.[3]

Ductal anomalies

These are rare but include duplication and imperforate ducts. They may be demonstrated by contrast sialography but better still by MRI. If associated with secondary infection, they may require treatment. Marsupialization is usually adequate.[3]

Ectopic salivary tissue

Salivary acinar cell rests can be found as a focus of draining sinuses in the neck, the mandible and the cervical lymph nodes.[3]

INFLAMMATORY DISEASES

Viral parotitis (mumps)

A number of viruses, most typically mumps, may be implicated in acute sialadenitis. 'Mumps' is an acute infectious disease caused by the mumps virus, a paramyxovirus. Classically, children aged four to five are affected and 85 percent of cases occur below the age of 15 years. The incubation period is two to three weeks. Infection is spread by droplets from an infected person's respiratory tract. Mumps causes a mild pyrexial illness in up to 40 percent of infected patients with enlargement of one or more of the salivary glands, nearly always the parotid. Parotid involvement is typically bilateral. The diagnosis is confirmed by measuring viral titres for the S and V antigen. The S antigen is positive at presentation and persists for 12 months. The V antigen appears at one month but persists for up to two years.

No specific treatment is available and resolution is to be expected. Mumps may rarely be associated with severe complications, notably sensorineural deafness, orchitis, encephalitis and pancreatitis.

The use of mumps, measles and rubella (MMR) vaccine in 92 percent of developed countries has resulted in mumps becoming a rare disease in Western communities, where complications are now almost never seen. [***] There has been a recent increase in the incidence of mumps in Britain, presumably due to a reduction in the number of children given the MMR vaccine.[4, 5] Mumps deafness and encephalitis are still a significant global public health problem.[6]

Acute suppurative sialadenitis

Acute pyogenic infection of the salivary glands is characterized by painful swelling with erythema of the overlying skin. Organisms include *Staphylococcus aureus* and *Streptococcus viridans*. Dehydration and salivary calculi may be predisposing factors. Treatment is with antibiotics analgesia and adequate hydration. [*]

Acute parotitis of infancy

Acute pyogenic infection of the parotid gland in infancy is a distinct clinical entity. It occurs in the newborn and is more common in prematurity. The most likely organisms are *S. aureus* and *Streptococcus pyogenes*, together with anaerobic bacteria. The affected gland becomes swollen and progresses to suppuration. The baby will be ill, pyrexial and reluctant to feed. Ultrasonography may help determine when frank pus is present. In the early stages, adequate doses of intravenous antibiotics may halt progression. Surgical drainage should be considered with extreme care due to the superficial position of the facial nerve in the newborn. Needle aspiration is safer than incision (**Figure 97.1**). [*]

Relapsing acute parotitis

This is the most common inflammatory disorder of the salivary glands in childhood. It is usually self-limiting and requires no surgery. [**]

PRESENTATION

Though recurrent parotitis may occur at any age, it most commonly presents at five to six years. The first episode is often diagnosed as mumps. Usually one, but occasionally both, parotid gland(s) will become acutely swollen and painful. The salivary flow from the duct is reduced and may be turbid. Episodes typically last a few days and may

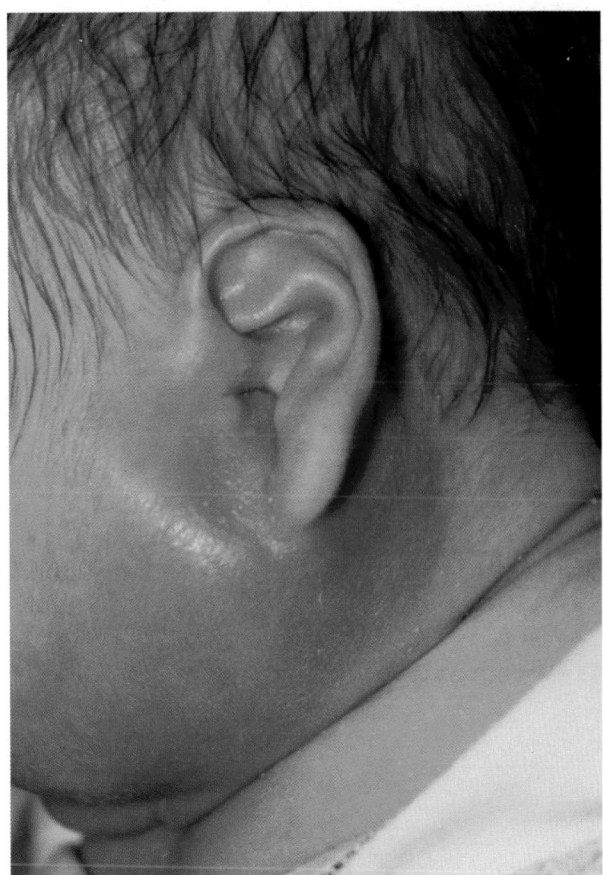

Figure 97.1 Acute suppurative parotitis in a baby aged three weeks.

be months apart. There may be some erythema of the skin overlying the gland. The child is usually apyrexial. Although culture of the saliva is often sterile, the most common organisms are *Streptococcus pneumonia* and *Haemophilus influenzae*.[7]

INVESTIGATION

Ultrasound examination of the affected gland will demonstrate any calculi or intraparotid abnormalities and is well tolerated by children.[1] Sialography is helpful in showing the changes of sialectasis that occur in most cases, but is difficult to perform in children (**Figure 97.2**). In any acute episode, a swab should be taken of the saliva from the duct of the affected gland, and if organisms are cultured appropriate antibiotic therapy should be given.

In any case of recurring infection it is important to consider the child's immune status, and to exclude diabetes mellitus, immunoglobulin deficiency and cystic fibrosis. The advice of a paediatrician should be sought if there is any doubt.

MANAGEMENT

In almost all cases, recurrent parotitis of childhood resolves by the age of puberty. [***] Therefore, management is conservative in the expectation of reduction in the frequency and severity of attacks. Individual episodes should be managed by adequate hydration, analgesics and gentle external massage of the gland in the direction of the parotid duct towards its papilla to encourage drainage. Antibiotics are not indicated unless there is generalized malaise and fever. [*] If the attacks do not resolve, lavage of the parotid duct with normal saline after cannulation may reduce the frequency of the attacks. This can be undertaken under general anaesthetic if necessary.

There is little place for open parotid surgery. Even if irreversible structural changes in the gland have occurred, the condition is self-limiting and resolution of symptoms can be expected. If excision surgery is embarked upon, a subtotal parotidectomy will be required (**Figure 97.3**).[8] [*]

GRANULOMATOUS DISEASES OF THE SALIVARY GLANDS

The most common granulomatous infections of the salivary glands are mycobacterial but this group of disorders includes rare infective conditions such as actinomycosis and cat-scratch disease. These conditions may simulate malignancy.

Mycobacterial infection of the salivary glands

This is probably not a true infection of the salivary glands but of the perisalivary lymph nodes in children. In Western communities, infection is more commonly by atypical or nontuberculous mycobacteria (NTM) than by *Mycobacterium tuberculosis*. [****] The most common organisms are *M. avium-intracellulare complex*, *M. kansasii* and *M. malmoense*. They can be identified with most certainty by culture in specialized reference laboratories.

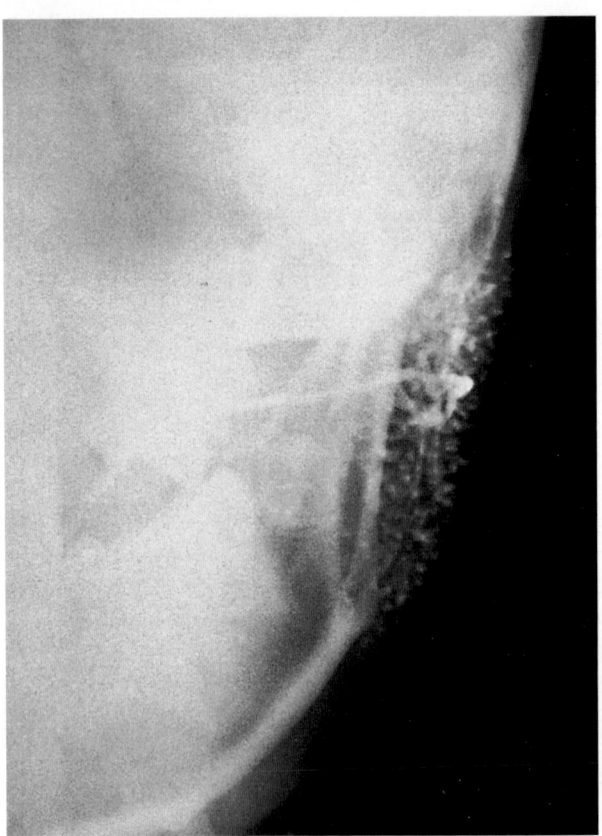

Figure 97.2 Parotid sialogram showing the changes of sialectasis.

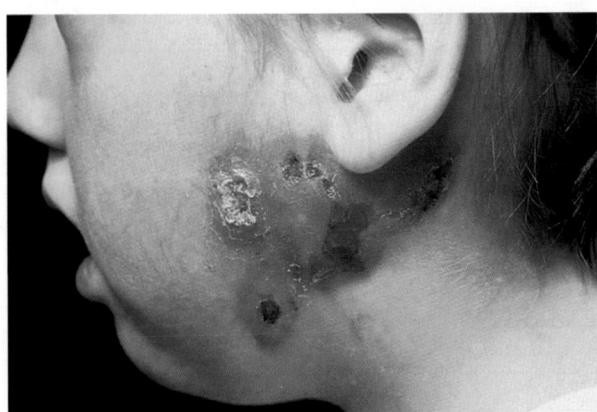

Figure 97.3 Chronic irreversible parotitis with salivary fistulae.

The condition of NTM salivary gland infection affects a young age group, typically three to four years old. The patients in the author's series ranged from one year nine months to seven years ten months, with an average of three years ten months.[9]

PRESENTATION

Patients present with a mass in the neck or face, usually painless and often with a short history. The overlying skin usually becomes discoloured with a violet hue. Early necrosis and breakdown of the tissues may occur. There is no facial nerve weakness in uncomplicated cases (**Figure 97.4**).

INVESTIGATION

The most important investigations are microscopy with Zeil Neilson staining, histology and culture of the affected tissue. Repeated culture of aspirated material may be negative. Fresh excised tissue is more likely to yield a diagnosis. It is important to inform the laboratory staff that the diagnosis is suspected before sending tissue.

While specific antigens for skin testing to the various mycobacteria are available, they are not easily obtained. They may be used as further evidence if the diagnosis is in doubt. All cases of suspected mycobacterial infection should have a Mantoux test and chest x-ray to exclude *M. tuberculosis*.

Imaging of the cervical mass is not particularly helpful. Ultrasound examination is often rendered difficult by the presence of skin necrosis.

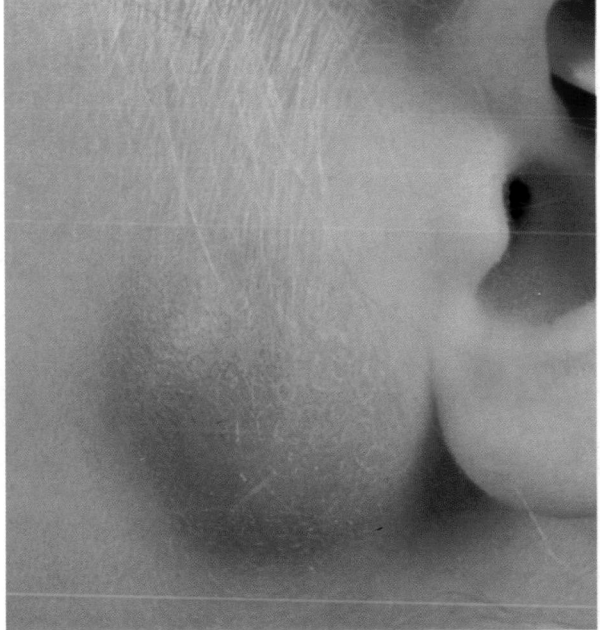

Figure 97.4 Infection with atypical (nontuberculous) mycobacteria.

MANAGEMENT

Many cases of an enlarged cervical nodes infected by NTM will resolve spontaneously without necrosis. [***]

Where there is skin discoloration and early abscess formation, long-term treatment with anti-tuberculosis chemotherapy is usually administered. [**] A typical regime is ciprofloxacin 15 mg/kg/day as two doses and azithromycin 10 mg/kg/day over some months. In cases of necrosis or abscess formation, surgical excision of the inflammatory mass with preservation of the facial nerve is curative.[10] [**] The organism is more easily grown from the excised tissue than from the pus. Simple drainage of an abscess may result in a chronically discharging fistula which can take 18–24 months to heal fully, with considerable scarring. [**] Coulter *et al.*[11] summarized the evidence base for current treatment regimes and concluded that there are no randomized controlled trials on which to base management strategies, but excision is curative and curettage is superior to incision and drainage. Single drug therapy rapidly induces resistance. Chemotherapy prior to surgery may help localize the lesion. Untreated the condition will spontaneously resolve over several years.

Sarcoidosis

Sarcoid is a chronic granulomatous condition of unknown aetiology. The onset of sarcoidosis is usually in early adult life but it can present in the teenage years. Parotid gland involvement is present in about 10 percent of cases and it may present acutely with fever and uveitis – Heerford's uveo-parotid fever. Facial palsy may occur in this condition. The changes in the gland are of noncaseating granulomata and may be demonstrated by biopsy of the minor salivary glands of the lower lip in 60 percent of cases.

Sjögren's syndrome

Sjögren's syndrome is an autoimmune multisystem inflammatory disorder which almost always involves the salivary glands (see Chapter 147, Non-neoplastic salivary gland diseases). In long-standing cases it is characterized by dryness of the oral and conjunctival membranes (Sicca syndrome). It is rare for a diagnosis of Sjögren's to be made in childhood but, when it is, the commonest presentation is with parotitis. Girls are more commonly affected than boys. Sicca syndrome is uncommon until adulthood. If suspected, rheumatoid factor, antinuclear antibodies and SS-A and SS-B autoantibodies should be measured.[12]

Treatment should be multidisciplinary with involvement of a paediatrician and dental surgeon. Lifelong surveillance may be needed as patients are prone to the development of lymphomata.[13] [***]

HIV/AIDS

Salivary gland involvement in juvenile cases of HIV infection is more common than in adult disease and is referred to as HIV-associated salivary gland disease (HIV-SGD).

HIV-SGD

The main feature of HIV-SGD is the presence of lympho-epithelial cysts within the salivary glands, predominately the parotid. They are thought to be the result of hyperplasia of the intraglandular lymph nodes (**Figure 97.5**).

Confirmation of the cystic nature can be made on ultrasound scanning and, unless neoplasia is suspected, no surgical intervention is required. No virus is present in the cyst fluid.[14] The finding of multiple parotid cysts in childhood should alert the clinician to the possible diagnosis of HIV infection.

Ranula

Ranula is the term to describe a cystic swelling arising in the floor of the mouth (ranula – L. frog). Ranula may be congenital or acquired and, on rare occasions, may be found in newborn infants.

AETIOLOGY

Ranula is the result of obstruction of one of the sublingual salivary glands. It is essentially a retention cyst. This may be spontaneous or may result from surgery to the floor of the mouth, especially submandibular duct relocation.

PRESENTATION

The ranula presents as a smooth cystic swelling under the tongue, usually to one side. It is often transparent or bluish in appearance with overlying small blood vessels. If large enough, it may affect both breathing and swallowing (**Figure 97.6**).

Plunging ranula

If extravasation of mucus occurs beyond the confines of the floor of the mouth through the mylohyoid muscle into the upper neck or submental region, a large cystic swelling develops. This can usually be defined on MR scanning but is difficult to clinically differentiate from cystic hygroma. Histologically, hygroma has a simple epithelial lining whereas a ranula is contained by loose connective tissue.

TREATMENT

Simple aspiration or drainage of a ranula results in a high recurrence rate. Both simple and plunging ranulas should be excised, together with the cyst wall and the sublingual gland. [**] Care must be taken to identify and preserve the lingual nerve which lies in close proximity. A ranula presenting in the neck will usually need an external approach for excision. Marsupialization of a plunging ranula is inadequate with a recurrence rate of 80 percent.[15] Excision of the sublingual gland results in a low rate of recurrence.

Salivary gland stones

Salivary gland stones or calculi are rare in children. Stones are formed by crystal formation from salivary solutes, mainly hydroxyapatite. These salts can be precipitated out

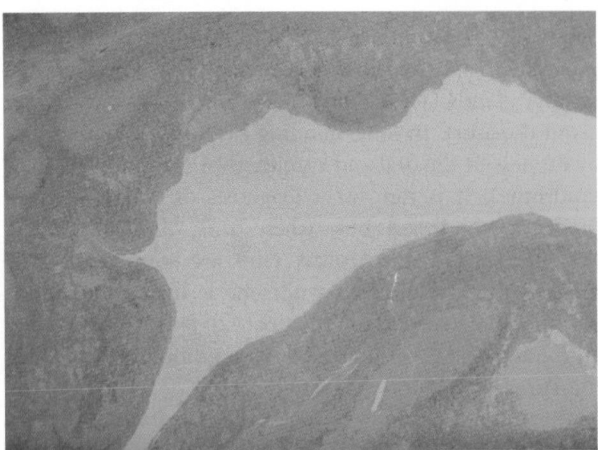

Figure 97.5 Lymphoepithelial cyst of the parotid gland in HIV infection.

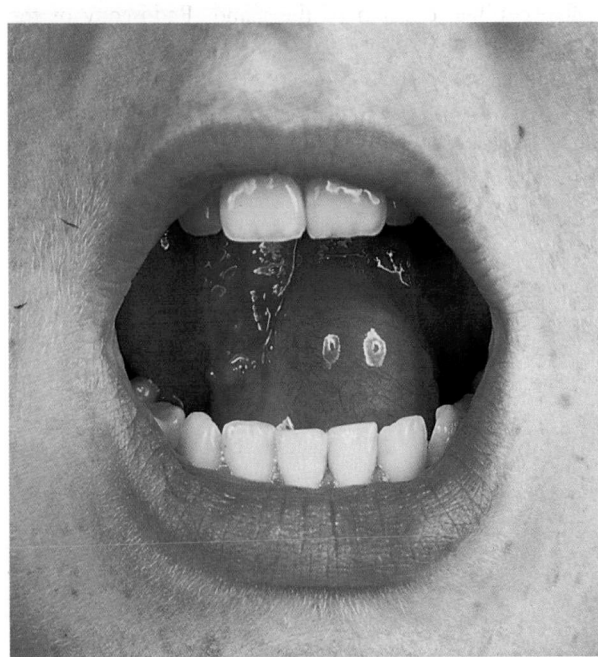

Figure 97.6 Sublingual ranula.

of solution by a change in pH in the saliva or by dehydration. They are much more common in the submandibular gland than the parotid because of the mucoid nature of the submandibular saliva.

PRESENTATION

The stone will normally declare its presence by sudden enlargement of the affected salivary gland while the child is eating, caused by occlusion of the duct in the presence of salivary flow. The gland becomes swollen and painful and the swelling usually subsides over an hour or two. The stone may be visible or palpable within the duct. Parotid stones tend to be less calcified and therefore softer and less easy to feel. Sometimes, a large stone will be found coincidentally in the submandibular gland on routine radiology and may cause no symptoms.

INVESTIGATION

If the stone is clinically apparent, no further investigation is necessary. Plain x-rays may show a stone but intraoral views of the duct are preferable. If doubt persists, MR scanning is extremely sensitive in demonstrating calcium salts.

TREATMENT

If the stone is causing no symptoms, then it can be left alone. If the stone is accessible within the submandibular duct, it can be removed intraorally by making a linear incision in the floor of the mouth, extricating the stone and marsupializing the mucosal edges. Great care must be taken not to injure the lingual nerve which lies immediately deep to the duct. A stone within the substance of the submandibular gland which is causing persistent symptoms will necessitate excision of the gland. Endoscopy of the salivary ducts has been used to remove calculi but there is no account of this in children. Some radiologists report that a contrast sialogram may bring about improvement as the contrast flushes the debris from the gland.[16] [*]

SALIVARY GLAND TUMOURS

Salivary gland tumours are extremely rare in children. They comprise vasoformative swellings, true neoplasms of salivary tissue origin and proliferative disorders of the perisalivary lymphoid tissue (lymphoma). For salivary gland tumours in adults see Chapter 189, Benign salivary gland tumours and Chapter 190, Malignant tumours of the salivary glands.

Vasoformative lesions

The commonest salivary gland swellings in childhood are vasoformative. While not truly salivary in origin, their management may require an extensive knowledge of salivary gland anatomy and salivary gland surgery. It is important to distinguish between haemangioma and vascular malformation.

Haemangiomas are not present at birth but grow rapidly after birth. They are of endothelial origin and highly cellular. They initially grow rapidly for nine to twelve months and involution usually occurs by the age of three to five years. Most haemangiomas occur in the head and neck and many will involve the skin and the underlying salivary gland in the parotid region. Occasionally, the tumour may be deeply placed and lie within the parotid gland (**Figure 97.7**).

TREATMENT

Almost all haemangiomas will involute and surgery should be confined to management of bleeding or ulceration, or to cases where the diagnosis is in doubt. [*]

Diagnostic uncertainty in the case of an enlarging intraparotid mass may occasionally necessitate exploration and excision, with preservation of the facial nerve, even if haemangioma is suspected. High quality imaging has made this an extremely rare indication for surgery (**Figure 97.8**).

If the haemangioma is of such a size or position as to be life-threatening, treatment with steroids or α-interferon has been shown to be of benefit in hastening resolution. [**] Each is associated with significant potential morbidity in babies and should only be considered with extreme care. Steroids may be administered systemically or directly into the lesion. Pulse-dye laser therapy may be considered for ulcerating lesions; interferon is used systemically for its inhibitory effect on angiogenesis.[17]

Vascular anomalies are developmental malformations that are present at birth and enlarge slowly as the child grows. They may be venous, lymphatic or arteriovenous in origin and include cystic hygroma and lymphangioma (see Chapter 99, Branchial arch fistulae, thyroglossal duct anomalies and lymphangioma).

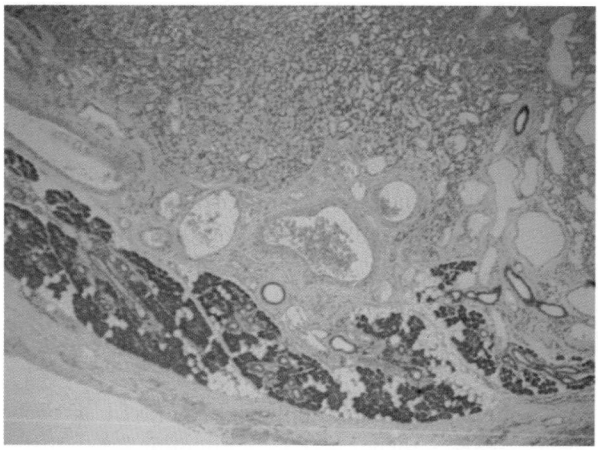

Figure 97.7 Parotid haemangioma histology showing highly cellular tumour within normal parotid tissue.

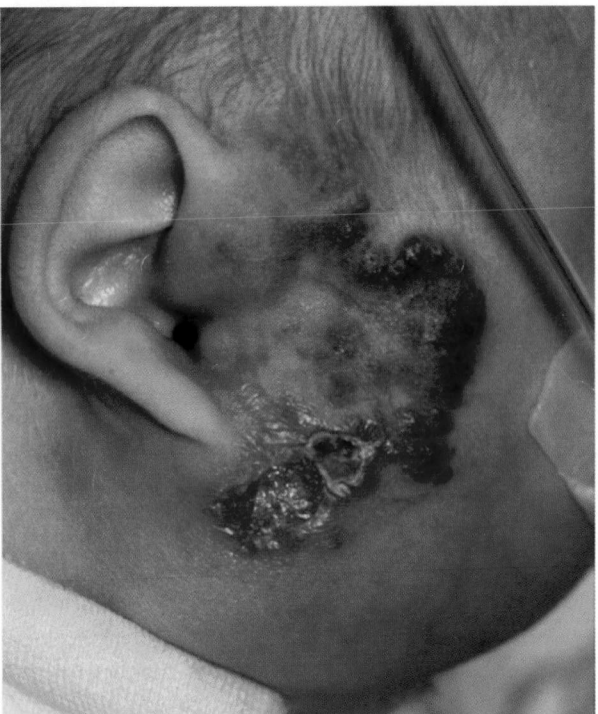

Figure 97.8 Capillary haemangioma involving the parotid gland and skin.

Salivary gland neoplasms

Neoplasms of the salivary gland account for 1 percent of all tumours in children. Fewer than 5 percent of all salivary tumours occur in patients under the age of 16 years. In the author's series of salivary gland tumours in childhood, a total of 14 neoplasms has now been treated, plus three lymphomas arising within the major salivary glands. Of these 14 cases, seven have been malignant and seven benign. Of these benign cases, only five were truly of salivary cell origin. The rarity of these tumours is such that inappropriate management frequently occurs before referral.[18]

PRESENTATION

Salivary gland tumours in children present as an enlarging mass. Growth is usually slow, and rapid growth is more suggestive of lymphoma arising in an intraglandular lymph node. They are usually painless. Facial nerve palsy at presentation is indicative of malignancy. Eighty percent of all salivary neoplasms occur within the parotid gland.

Benign tumours

The commonest benign tumour encountered is pleomorphic salivary adenoma (PSA) accounting for approximately 30 percent of all paediatric salivary neoplasms. The majority occur within the parotid gland but they may

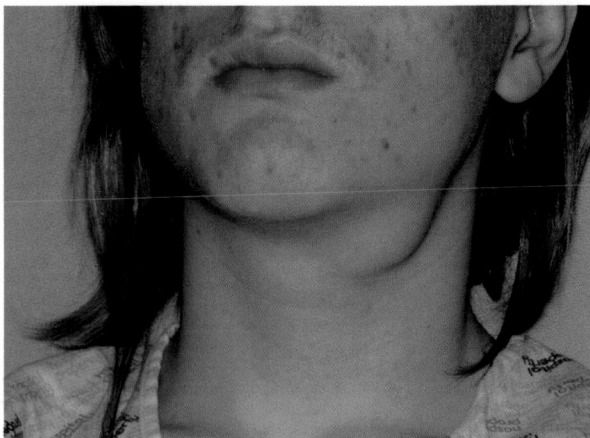

Figure 97.9 Pleomorphic adenoma of the submandibular salivary gland.

also occur in the submandibular gland or in extra glandular sites (**Figure 97.9**).

In a large series from the Mayo clinic of salivary neoplasms in children, the only benign salivary neoplasm encountered was PSA,[19] but all types found in adults do occasionally present.

TREATMENT

The treatment of benign salivary tumours is as it is in adults, by wide excision and facial nerve preservation. [**] The relatively superficial position of the facial nerve in children must be considered when performing parotidectomy. Particular care must be taken to achieve good surgical margins and avoid rupture of the tumour, since adjuvant radiotherapy cannot be safely used in children to salvage an unsatisfactory surgical procedure. Scar hypertrophy is more common in children than in adults, but in the author's practice the incidence of Frey's syndrome after parotidectomy is less.

Malignant tumours

The relative proportion of salivary tumours in children which prove to be malignant is higher in children than in adults, though of course overall, salivary neoplasms in children are extremely rare. In most series approximately half are malignant.

Most malignant salivary gland neoplasms in childhood present simply as an enlarging mass. Growth may be slow and there is usually no other evidence of malignancy.

Facial weakness and increasing pain are strong indications of malignant disease.

PATHOLOGY

Most series show that the most common salivary malignancy in a paediatric age group is mucoepidermoid carcinoma (approximately 50 percent) followed by acinic cell carcinoma (20 percent).

More aggressive tumours such as adenoid cystic carcinoma and adenocarcinoma may also occur (**Figure 97.10**).

INVESTIGATION

All cases of salivary gland neoplasm in children should be treated as potentially malignant. [*] Aspiration (needle) biopsy and cytology are of limited value. In children this will usually require general anaesthetic and assessment of salivary gland histology is notoriously difficult. Ultrasonic imaging of the salivary mass is easy to perform, noninvasive and well tolerated by children. It gives information about the location and size of the lesion and will indicate whether it is cystic or solid. CT and MR may be needed, including imaging of the chest.

MANAGEMENT AND TREATMENT OF MALIGNANT TUMOURS

Management will involve a multidisciplinary approach with input from a paediatric oncologist and his/her team. These children and their families are best treated in a designated centre where the whole range of support services for children with cancer is available.

As with benign neoplasms, wide surgical excision is required for malignant tumours. Usually, the diagnosis cannot be made preoperatively unless there is associated facial palsy. It is essential to counsel the child and parents carefully prior to operation regarding the possible need for facial nerve sacrifice.

The surgical margins on the specimen must be marked and evaluated by the pathologist and adequacy of excision confirmed. Provided the excision margins are satisfactory, no adjuvant treatment is indicated. [**] The author's series has shown only one recurrence, that of an acinic cell tumour after four years, with subsequent freedom from relapse after ten years.

The Mayo clinic series shows only one recurrence out of 14 malignant cases who had their primary treatment at the Mayo. The recurrence rate was higher in cases referred after initial treatment in a nonspecialist centre.[19] [**]

Adjunctive radiotherapy and chemotherapy are reserved either for recurrent disease or very aggressive disease at the time of the initial surgery and should be determined with the collaboration of a paediatric oncologist. Long-term follow-up is essential in these rare cases.

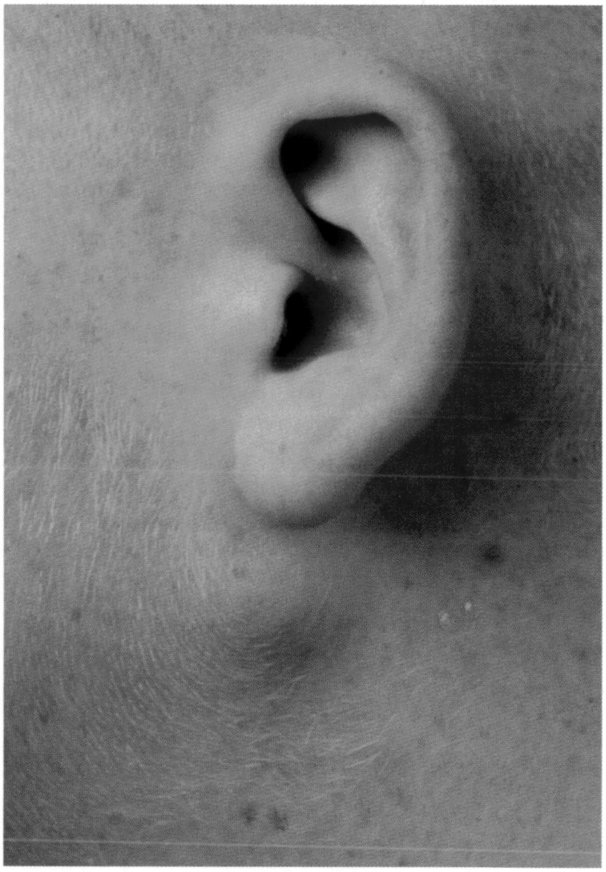

Figure 97.10 Mucoepidermoid carcinoma of the parotid gland.

KEY POINTS

- The relatively superficial position of the facial nerve should be constantly borne in mind when contemplating surgery in the parotid region in children.
- Consider NTM in a child with a discharging lesion in the parotid region.
- Relapsing parotitis is almost always self-limiting and resolves at puberty.
- The rarity of salivary tumours in children is such that treatment should only be in specialist centres.

Best clinical practice

✓ Treatment of acute suppurative parotitis is with analgesics hydration and antibiotics. Surgery is rarely indicated. [Grade C]
✓ Relapsing parotitis is almost always self-limiting and resolves at puberty. [Grade C]
✓ Consider NTM in a child with a discharging lesion in the parotid region. [Grade C]
✓ The traditional advice that a ranula can be adequately treated by simple marsupialization should be revised. These swellings are best excised. [Grade C]

✓ The finding of multiple parotid cysts in childhood should alert the clinician to the possible diagnosis of HIV infection. [Grade B]

✓ Almost all haemangiomas will involve and surgery is rarely needed. [Grade B]

✓ Salivary tumours in children are rare but a higher proportion are malignant than in adults. [Grade C]

Deficiencies in current knowledge and areas for future research

➤ The implementation of vaccination programmes throughout the developing world would greatly reduce the morbidity of mumps encephalitis and deafness.

➤ The epidemiology of NTM and the reasons for the recent increased incidence in Western communities may become clear.

➤ The respective roles of surgery and chemotherapy in the management of NTM may become better established.

➤ Salivary gland neoplasms are so rare that randomized controlled studies may not be possible; a national register of these tumours and treatment only in centres where adequate expertise is available would improve outcome.

REFERENCES

* 1. King SJ. Salivary glands. In: King SJ, Boothroyd AE (eds). *Pediatric ENT radiology*. New York: Springer-Verlag, Berlin Heidelberg, 2002: 335–44. *A summary of current practice in salivary gland imaging in children.*

2. Hodgson TA, Shah R, Porter SR. The investigation of major salivary gland agenesis: a case report. *Pediatric Dentistry.* 2001; 23: 131–4.

3. Ibrahim HZ, Handler SD. Diseases of the salivary glands. In: Wetmore RF, Muntz HR (eds). *Pediatric otolaryngology: principles and practice pathways*. New York, Stuttgart: McGill TJ Thieme, 2000: 647–58.

4. Dobson R. Mumps cases on the rise in England and Wales. *British Medical Journal.* 2005; 330: 3241.

5. Bellaby P. Has the UK government lost the battle over MMR? Editorial. *British Medical Journal.* 2005; 330: 552–3.

* 6. Galazka AM, Robertson SE, Kraigher A. Mumps and mumps vaccine: a global review. *Bulletin of the World Health Organization.* 1999; 77: 3–14. *A review of mumps as a global health problem.*

7. Cohen HA, Gross S, Nussinovitch M, Frydman M, Varsano I. Recurrent parotitis. *Archives of Disease in Childhood.* 1992; 67: 1036–7.

8. O'Brien CJ, Murrant NJ. Surgical management of chronic parotitis. *Head and Neck.* 1993; 15: 445–9.

9. Jervis PN, Lee JA, Bull PD. Management of non-tuberculous mycobacterial peri-sialadenitis in children. *Clinical Otolaryngology and Allied Sciences.* 2001; 26: 243–8.

10. Dhooge I, Dhooge C, De Baets F, Van Caauwenberge P. Diagnostic and therapeutic management of atypical mycobacterial infections in children. *European Archives of Oto-Rhino-Laryngology.* 1993; 250: 387–91.

11. Coulter JB, Lloyd DA, Jones M, Cooper JC, McCormick MS, Clarke RW *et al.* Nontuberculous mycobacterial adenitis: effectiveness of chemotherapy following incomplete excision. *Acta Paediatrica.* 2006; 95: 182–8.

12. Anaya JM, Ogawa N, Talal N. Sjogren's syndrome in childhood. *Journal of Rheumatology.* 1995; 22: 1152–8.

13. Bartunkova J, Sediva A, Vencovsky J, Tesar V. Primary Sjogren's syndrome in children and adolescents: proposal for diagnostic criteria. *Clinical and Experimental Rheumatology.* 1999; 17: 381–6.

14. Schiott M. HIV associated salivary gland disease: a review. *Oral Surgery, Oral Medicine, and Oral Pathology.* 1992; 73: 164–7.

15. Dhaif G, Ahmed Y, Ramaraj R. Ranula and the sublingual salivary glands. Review of 32 cases. *Bahrain Medical Bulletin.* 1998; 20: 3–4.

16. Bull PD. Salivary stones. *Hospital Medicine.* 2001; 62.7: 396–9.

17. David LR, Malek MM, Argenta LC. Efficacy of pulse dye laser therapy for the treatment of ulcerated haemangiomas: a review of 78 patients. *British Journal of Plastic Surgery.* 2003; 56: 317–27.

18. Bull PD. Salivary gland neoplasia in childhood. *International Journal of Pediatric Otolaryngology.* 1999; 49: S235–8.

* 19. Orvidas LJ, Kasperbauer JL, Lewis JE, Olsen KD, Lesnick TG. Pediatric parotid masses. *Archives of Otolaryngology, Head and Neck Surgery.* 2000; 126: 177–84. *Comprehensive review of salivary gland neoplasms in children.*

98

Tumours of the head and neck in childhood

FIONA B MacGREGOR

Introduction	1251	The dying child	1261
Epidemiology	1251	Key points	1261
Presentation and assessment	1252	Best clinical practice	1261
The child with cancer	1253	Deficiencies in current knowledge and areas for future	
Oncology services	1253	research	1262
The more common childhood cancers	1254	Acknowledgements	1262
Long-term sequelae of treatment	1260	References	1262

SEARCH STRATEGY

Systematic reviews were identified using the key words: childhood cancer, head and neck, thyroid cancer, rhabdomyo-sarcoma, nasopharyngeal carcinoma, neuroblastoma, lymphadenopathy, Hodgkin's lymphoma, non-Hodgkin's lymphoma, sarcoma, palliative care; and subject headings in the Cochrane database of systematic reviews. Individual articles were then identified using the same search terms in Ovid Medline. A hand-search of the ensuing bibliographies completed the search.

INTRODUCTION

This chapter will focus on the epidemiology of childhood cancers of the head and neck region and the general principles of assessing and managing malignancy in paediatric patients. It will then discuss the more common histological types individually. The long-term sequelae of treatment in survivors, palliative care and future developments will be addressed.

EPIDEMIOLOGY

After trauma, cancer is the most common cause of death in childhood. Approximately one-third of childhood malignancies are leukaemias, 25 percent are brain and spinal tumours, 15 percent are embryonal (neuro-blastoma, retinoblastoma, Wilm's tumour and hepato-blastoma) and 11 percent are lymphomas. The remainder are bone and soft tissue sarcomas and miscellaneous

tumours (see below under Miscellaneous tumours). Up to 12 percent of primary childhood malignancies originate in the head and neck area and so may present to the otolaryngologist. Lymphoma is the most common diagnosis in all series, followed by thyroid and neural tumours. Sarcomas and salivary gland tumours are less common and squamous cell carcinomas are rare.[1] The distribution of histological types varies greatly depending on the age and sex of the child with neuroblastoma the most common in infants and thyroid carcinoma the most common malignancy in adolescent females. There is a bimodal age distribution of malignancy in children. The most common age group affected is 15 to 18 year olds, closely followed by the under fours.[1, 2]

Cancer data from many parts of the world have suggested a small but steady recent increase in cancer rates in the under 19s. This increase would appear to be more marked in head and neck malignancies.[1] This elevation in numbers may in part be due to improved data collection. In parallel, the consistent use of effective multimodality treatments, including combination chemotherapy, surgery and radiotherapy, has resulted in a significant improvement in prognosis. A study from the UK observed five-year survival rates improving from 42 percent (diagnosis made between 1968 and 1977) to 71 percent (diagnosis made between 1988 and 1995).[3] Early recognition is therefore important as treatment is becoming increasingly effective in reducing the mortality in childhood malignancy.[4, 5]

It is thought that only around 5 percent of malignancies in childhood are inherited. The underlying aetiology of the noninherited types remains unclear but certain chemotherapeutic agents, viruses (e.g. Epstein–Barr) and irradiation are known to play a role. Other potential carcinogens are suspected but not proven (pollution, parental exposure to toxins, electromagnetic fields).[1, 6]

PRESENTATION AND ASSESSMENT

The most common presentation of a malignancy in the head and neck region in childhood is the asymptomatic mass. Otalgia, rhinorrhoea, otorrhoea and nasal obstruction may be present in both benign and malignant

disease. More worrying symptoms would include stridor, dysphagia and haemoptysis.[7] Reactive lymphadenopathy in children is extremely common and gives rise to frequent therapeutic dilemmas. Studies have suggested that the best predictors of malignancy in cervical lymphadenopathy are the size of the node, the number of sites involved and the age of the patient. Other concerning features would be lymphadenopathy in the supraclavicular region, an associated abnormal chest x-ray or fixed lymph nodes.[8, 9] [**/*]

Examination would involve a complete assessment of the head and neck region and systemic evaluation with particular regard to the presence of lymphadenopathy elsewhere and the presence or absence of abdominal masses. Flexible nasendoscopy is possible in many children (**Figure 98.1**). Imaging with the help of a paediatric radiologist can often obviate the need for biopsy. However, full assessment of a mass may require examination under anaesthetic with biopsy.

Biopsy

Fine needle aspirate (FNA), sometimes referred to as aspiration biopsy cytology (ABC), has a more limited role

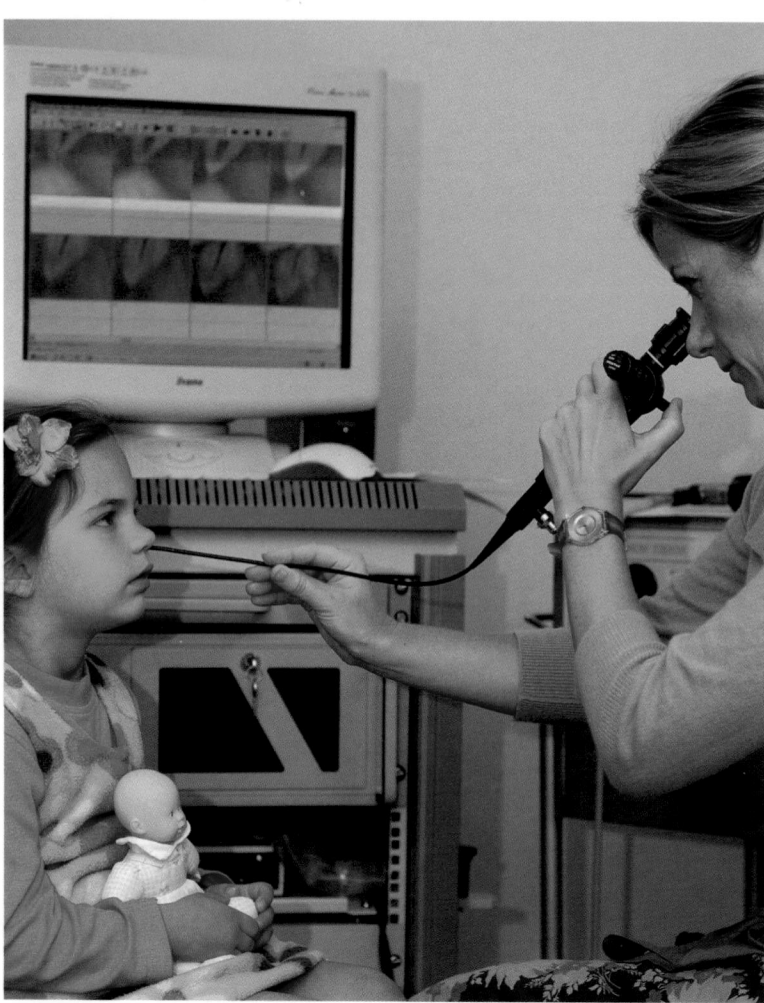

Figure 98.1 Flexible nasendoscopy under local anaesthetic in the clinic setting.

to play in the child than the adult. Young patients may simply not tolerate this method of biopsy. With particular regard to cervical lymphadenopathy, the most likely neoplastic diagnosis is lymphoma and at the present time it is recognized that excision biopsy is the best method of confirming and typing this histologically.[10, 11] FNA, often under ultrasound control, can be useful in the assessment of thyroid and salivary gland lesions and these tumours often present in older children who may tolerate such intervention. [**/*]

Imaging

Ultrasonography, CT and MR scanning can all have their part to play in further assessment. Imaging of the neck is more accurate than clinical examination in detecting lymphadenopathy. CT and MR scanning may require a general anaesthetic in a younger child and it is helpful to discuss the available imaging options with a paediatric radiologist prior to proceeding, to avoid unnecessary and additional anaesthetics. Positron emission tomography (PET) scanning is also becoming increasingly used in the assessment of neoplastic lesions in the head and neck in children, but is not readily available at the present time in most departments.[7]

THE CHILD WITH CANCER

The history and subsequent investigations of a child presenting with a suspicious lesion of the head and neck region must be tailored to the age and maturity of the child. In most situations, when the child is old enough, he or she should be included in any discussion about investigations and treatment and they should also be involved in consent for any procedures required.

The diagnosis of cancer in a child has a tremendous impact not only on the patient, but also on parents, siblings, other family members and friends. Immediate involvement of a specialist paediatric multidisciplinary oncology team is mandatory. An open and realistic approach should include an explanation of what to expect from the investigations and treatment, the side effects and some idea of prognosis. This is vital in maintaining trusting relationships with the child and his or her family, in reducing uncertainty, preventing inappropriate hope and allowing proportionate adjustment.

Parents may feel guilty that they waited too long before seeking medical advice. They may be concerned that they have, in some way, caused their child's cancer. They can also feel guilty about making their child go through a series of invasive investigations and radical treatments. This can put an immense strain on the parents' relationship with each other and with other family members and friends, not least the child involved. Also, siblings of the affected child may resent the additional time and

attention that their sick brother or sister receives. Support services are therefore vital in reassuring and supporting all the individuals concerned.

The amount of information that any child will require regarding their illness depends to some extent on the age and maturity of that individual. Most children aged six or more (and some more mature younger children) need to know their illness has a name and what that name is. All children require an explanation of the procedures to be performed and reassurance that any intervention is not a 'punishment'. In children between the ages of six and eleven, these procedures and side effects of treatment may provoke much more anxiety than the illness itself. For example, loss of hair or a limb seem much more real and distressing than the prospect of death. Alterations in physical appearance can cause great insecurity in a child or adolescent, resulting in isolation and poor self-esteem. Children aged around 11 and over will have fears surrounding the diagnosis and its prognostic implications in addition to the above. Children should be encouraged to talk about their feelings or, if they are too young, they can express themselves in drawings or play.[11]

ONCOLOGY SERVICES

In the UK, as in many other parts of the world, the importance of centralization of paediatric cancer services is recognized.[4] This enables care to be provided by highly trained and specialist paediatric oncologists and allied staff, and facilitates the progress of research. In Britain, there are 22 United Kingdom Children with Cancer Study Group (UK-CCSG) centres. Working in conjunction with the medical staff are social workers, nurses, dieticians, psychologists and other health care professionals in order to provide comprehensive support for children and their families. The emphasis on centralization of paediatric oncology services, the sharing of data and the establishment of international working groups has resulted in the publication of a number of treatment protocols that are widely used in the management of children with cancer.

The practicalities of investigating and treating children with cancer provide some particular challenges. Venous access for blood sampling and to administer chemotherapeutic agents can be difficult, and indwelling venous catheters are usually inserted at an early stage. Radiotherapy may require general anaesthesia in younger patients to ensure that the child remains still during irradiation. Other interventions (e.g. lumbar puncture and intrathecal injection) may also require general anaesthesia. Children tolerate the immediate side effects of chemotherapy and radiotherapy much better than adults but the long-term sequelae of such interventions can have a very significant effect on the health of childhood cancer survivors (see below under Long-term sequelae of treatment).

THE MORE COMMON CHILDHOOD CANCERS

Lymphoma

Cervical lymphadenopathy in childhood is common and although the huge majority of cases will be due to reactive hyperplasia, it may be necessary to exclude malignancy. Lymph nodes in the neck larger than 2 cm are unusual in childhood and systemic symptoms such as weight loss, fever and organomegaly are usually indicators of serious pathology.[8] FNA has a limited role and excision biopsy will provide the diagnosis.[12] [**]

Lymphomas are malignant neoplasms of the lymphoreticular system. Most lymphomas of the head and neck region in the paediatric age group present with enlarged cervical lymph nodes.

Hodgkin's lymphoma

This is distinguished morphologically by the presence of Reed Sternberg cells which are large and multinucleated with abundant cytoplasm. There are several classifications but the universally accepted one is the Rye classification. Within this there are four subtypes: lymphocyte predominant (LP), mixed cellularity (ML), lymphocytic depleted (LD) and nodular sclerosing (NS). NS is the most common type found in children and young adults. It has the propensity to involve the lower cervical, supraclavicular and mediastinal lymph node groups.

No definitive causal factors have been identified but there is an association with previous infection with Epstein–Barr virus.[13]

Hodgkin's lymphoma most commonly presents with lymphadenopathy in the neck and two-thirds of all children will have mediastinal lymphadenopathy at presentation. It rarely occurs under the age of five and there is a male predominance. 'Constitutional' upsets such as fever, night sweats and weight loss are present in 25 to 30 percent and this is associated with a poorer prognosis.[7]

Following careful examination and biopsy confirmation, the diagnostic workup of a child with Hodgkin's disease (following thorough examination and biopsy confirmation) would include a chest x-ray, routine blood tests (although abnormal results are usually nonspecific) and staging scans (CT chest and MRI abdomen). Recently, PET scanning has become a routine part of staging and of assessing effectiveness of treatment. There is no longer a place for staging laparotomies. Bone marrow biopsy and bone scan are only indicated in children with more advanced disease.[14] Currently, the Ann Arbor staging classification is used for Hodgkin's disease (see Chapter 22, Haemato-oncology).

Treatment depends on the age and physical maturity of the patient, the disease stage and bulk and the potential treatment sequelae. In the paediatric population, the trend is to treat in multimodality fashion so as to reduce the morbidity and mortality associated with high doses of chemotherapy or radiation therapy needed for single modality treatment. Disease-free survival is over 90 percent in many series.[15] Those children with intermediate risk of disease (constitutional symptoms, bulky disease or spleen involvement) may require an increased number of cycles of chemotherapy and an increased dose or volume of radiation therapy. In advanced disease, combined chemoradiotherapy is the treatment of choice. LP Hodgkin's disease is associated with a better prognosis and separate shorter and less intense treatment protocols are implemented. The regimens used in the treatment of Hodgkin's disease contain substantial doses of alkylating agents which are associated with the potential for significant morbidity.[13] [***/**]

Haematopoietic stem cell transplantation can be implemented in those children who relapse, but the risk of transplant-associated morbidity and mortality is not insignificant.[13]

Non-Hodgkin's lymphoma

Approximately 60 percent of paediatric lymphomas are non-Hodgkin's lymphomas (NHL). There is a male predominance. The low grade, relatively indolent NHLs seen in adults are exceedingly rare in children. Paediatric NHLs tend to be aggressive with a propensity for widespread dissemination and half of these are small cell lymphomas (Burkitt's and Burkitt's-like). The classification of NHL is confusing and controversial but paediatric NHLs are usually divided into three main histological categories. These are lymphoblastic lymphoma (predominantly of T cell origin), small noncleaved cell lymphoma (Burkitt's and non-Burkitt's subtype of B cell origin) and large cell lymphoma (B or T cell origin).[16] The Revised European American Lymphoma (REAL) classification is used in paediatric NHL and is a useful guide to management and prognosis of NHL.

The relative frequency and incidence of NHL varies quite markedly from country to country. In equatorial Africa, Burkitt's lymphoma accounts for approximately 50 percent of childhood cancers. In Europe and the US, approximately one-third are lymphoblastic lymphomas, one-third are Burkitt's and Burkitt's-like lymphoma and the rest are predominantly large cell lymphoma. In some parts of the world, an extremely high number of these tumours are positive for Epstein–Barr virus (EBV), e.g. parts of Africa. In contrast, the percentage of tumour positive for EBV in the US is much smaller. There is an increased incidence of NHL in association with immunosuppression and congenital and acquired immunodeficiency.[16]

All childhood NHLs are rapidly growing neoplasms and a significant number of children will have widespread disease at the time of diagnosis, which may involve the bone marrow, central nervous system or both. Involvement of extranodal sites, especially Waldeyer's ring, is particularly common in children. Lymphadenopathy occurs in 50–80 percent of all patients and 45 percent have cervical lymphadenopathy at the time of presentation. Bone marrow involvement is not infrequent and the replacement of more than 25 percent of the bone marrow by tumour cells is usually assigned a diagnosis of acute lymphoblastic leukaemia. Children with endemic Burkitt's lymphoma frequently present with involvement of the jaw and this is particularly common in the younger age group.[16]

DIAGNOSIS AND STAGING

Because NHLs in children progress more rapidly, a speedy diagnosis is extremely important. A biopsy will provide tissue for histological confirmation and surgery then has little further role to play. Staging investigations will follow and will include relevant blood tests (full blood count, urea and electrolytes and liver function tests – lactic dehydrogenase (LDH) is a useful marker of disease – bone marrow biopsy and cerebrospinal fluid (CSF) examination. Staging laparotomy is not advocated in patients with NHL and ultrasonography, CT (chest) and MR (abdomen) scanning are used in assessing spread.[16] The Ann Arbor staging classification can be applied to NHL (see Chapter 22, Haemato-oncology).

TREATMENT

The treatment of choice in childhood NHL is multiagent chemotherapy. The rapid doubling time of high grade NHL makes it particularly chemosensitive. Chemotherapeutic regimens vary depending on the histological classification of the disease. Radiation therapy has a limited role in NHL and is generally reserved for selected anatomical sites such as the cranium where a child has overt central nervous system (CNS) disease. CNS prophylaxis in children with high grade NHL can be achieved with intrathecally administered chemotherapy.[14, 16] [***/**]

PROGNOSIS

Long-term event-free survival (EFS) is excellent in lymphoblastic lymphomas. It ranges from 80 to 90 percent in patients with limited disease and from 65 to 80 percent in patients with advanced disease. In Burkitt's, where chemotherapeutic regimes are more intense and shorter, the long-term EFS ranges from 90 to 100 percent in patients with limited disease to 75 to 85 percent with patients with extensive disease. Even in patients with extensive bone marrow disease, the EFS is improving. Large cell lymphomas are more of a challenge to treat

because of their biological heterogeneity and long-term EFS ranges from 50 to 70 percent.[14, 16] [***/**]

Patients who relapse after receiving dose-intensive multiagent chemotherapy have an extremely poor prognosis. These patients are treated with high-dose chemotherapy regimes with or without bone marrow transplantation or would be candidates for drugs in phase II trials.

Rhabdomyosarcoma

Rhabdomyosarcomas account for up to 60 percent of all sarcomas in the paediatric population and 40 percent occur in the head and neck region. Nearly half of these tumours occur in children under the age of five.[4] The prognosis for this tumour used to be extremely poor but over the last 30 years survival rates have increased dramatically, particularly with the introduction of multi-modality therapy in which surgery, multiagent chemotherapy and radiotherapy have been combined.[17]

Histologically, rhabdomyosarcomas resemble normal foetal skeletal muscle before innervation. Two types are identified and these are embryonal (good prognosis) and alveolar (poor prognosis). The alveolar type is found in older children and is often associated with metastatic spread. It is less common than the embryonal type.[18, 19]

PRESENTATION

Rhabdomyosarcomas of the head and neck occur most frequently in the orbit or parameningeal sites and these include the paranasal sinuses, nose, nasopharynx and middle ear. The most common presenting symptoms are pain and swelling. Paranasal rhabdomyosarcoma may present with a gradual onset of nasal obstruction and bloody nasal discharge. Tumours within the ear may present with symptoms of bloody discharge and persistent otalgia, despite treatment. A polypoid mass may be visible in the ear canal or nasal cavity.[19] The reported incidence of lymph node involvement varies between 3 and 36 percent.[18] Metastases occur by both haematogenous and lymphatic spread.

ASSESSMENT

Assessment should include a thorough examination of the upper respiratory tract and head and neck region including the cranial nerves. Flexible nasendoscopy may be employed in the clinic. An MR scan should be performed to evaluate the primary lesion and to rule out metastatic disease (**Figure 98.2**). A CT scan may be a useful complementary tool, particularly in the paranasal sinuses and skull base, to determine bony erosion and it is the best method to assess the chest. Bone marrow examination should also be performed. The Inter Group

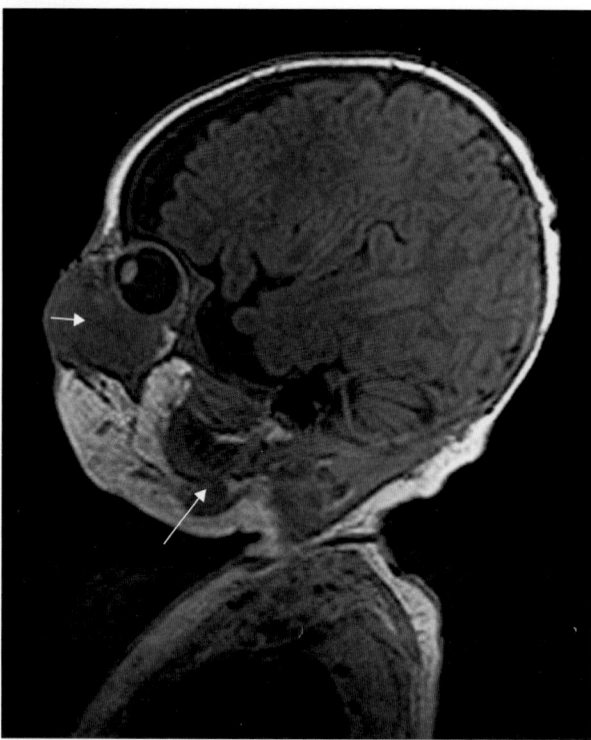

Figure 98.2 Paramedian T1-weighted MR scan through the left orbit of a three-month-old boy. There is a huge mass of rhabdomyosarcoma in the anterior orbit (short arrow) displacing the globe and submandibular lymphadenopathy (long arrow).

Table 98.1 Staging of rhabdomyosarcoma according to the IRS.

Staging of rhabdomyosarcoma	
Group I	Localized disease completely resected. No regional nodes
	Confined to muscle or organ of origin
	Contiguous infiltration outside muscle or organ of origin
Group II	Localized disease with microscopic residual disease or regional disease with no residual or with microscopic residual disease
	Grossly resected with microscopic residual disease (nodes negative)
	Regional tumour completely resected
	Regional nodes grossly resected but evidence of microscopic residual disease
Group III	Incomplete resection or biopsy with gross residual disease
Group IV	Metastatic disease present at onset

Rhabdomyosarcoma (IRS) study recommends the clinical staging shown in **Table 98.1**. The majority of children are stage II at the time of assessment[20] as it is rarely possible to completely excise these tumours.

TREATMENT AND PROGNOSIS

Since the establishment of the IRS Study Committee in 1972, protocols have been developed and are now widely adhered to. A multimodality approach has been adopted. In general, the role of surgery today is to simply evaluate the extent of the lesion and biopsy the tumour. Occasionally, when the rhabdomyosarcoma is an easily accessible polypoid lesion, then wide surgical removal may be appropriate. A debulking procedure may also be useful. Sophisticated skull base surgery can now be implemented in areas that were previously thought to be inaccessible.[19] Multiagent chemotherapy and radiotherapy are then implemented as appropriate. [**/*]

Prior to 1960, approximately 10 percent of patients survived five years. Now the prognosis is excellent in patients with early tumours (over 80 percent survival). With more advanced tumours the prognosis is still relatively poor and in those with meningeal involvement the five-year survival is less than 10 percent. Although nodal mestastases at initial presentation are not correlated with an unfavourable prognosis, development of nodes during follow-up does imply a poor outlook.[19, 20, 21] [**/*]

Thyroid carcinoma

Thyroid carcinoma in the paediatric population is uncommon. In the US there are five new cases per million per year. It is much more common in adolescents than in younger children and is also much more common in females with a ratio of 4:1. Approximately 45 percent of these lesions in children will be differentiated papillary carcinomas with a further 45 percent of mixed papillary/ follicular types with only 10 percent being follicular lesions.[22] Medullary thyroid carcinoma (MTC) is rare (only 10 percent of thyroid malignancies in children) and must be suspected in children with multiple endocrine neoplasia (MEN) types IIa and IIb (see under Medullary thyroid carcinoma). Anaplastic and undifferentiated tumours are extremely rare in children and adolescents.

AETIOLOGY

A clear relationship has been established between the development of thyroid carcinoma and previous irradiation. In one study, as many as 17 percent of patients had previously received irradiation to the neck.[23]

PRESENTATION

Patients usually present with an asymptomatic solitary mass in the anterior or lateral neck. At presentation, there is often regional lymph node involvement (74 percent) and distant parenchymal metastases (25 percent).[22]

INVESTIGATIONS

Investigations will include an ultrasound scan, usually in conjunction with an ultrasound-guided FNA. Regional and distant metastases can be assessed with a chest x-ray and CT scan. Thyroid function tests and plasma thyroglobulin levels should be obtained and also plasma calcitonin where a diagnosis of medullary carcinoma is suspected.

TREATMENT

Controversy remains over the optimum treatment in differentiated thyroid carcinoma in children because the long-term mortality in these patients is low and serious operative and postoperative complications can occur following radical surgery. These include recurrent laryngeal nerve damage, hypocalcaemia and airway obstruction requiring tracheostomy.[22] It has become clear that these tumours in children are slow-growing and associated with prolonged survival rates, even in the presence of extensive disease. Some authors maintain that an aggressive approach is mandatory[24, 25] while others have adopted a more conservative approach with the use of lobectomy and subtotal thyroidectomy for small and isolated lesions.[22, 23, 26]

Ideally, treatment should include complete surgical excision if possible. Total or subtotal thyroidectomy should be performed if adjuvent radioiodidine treatment is planned. Following surgery, a whole-body radioiodine scan is performed and ablative radioiodide treatment given if necessary. Plasma thyroglobulin can then be used as a tumour marker and suppressive levothyroxine should be given. Radiotherapy is rarely indicated in differentiated thyroid carcinoma in childhood.[7]

PROGNOSIS

A long-term study of 329 patients under the age of 21 confirmed only eight deaths over a long period of time and of these only two were disease related. The risk of progression of disease was more common in younger patients and those with residual cervical disease after definitive thyroidectomy. The majority of recurrences are in cervical lymph nodes or thyroid bed (54 percent), or lungs (16 percent).[26] The majority of relapses occur within the first seven years but have been seen as long as 25 years after treatment.[22]

Medullary thyroid carcinoma

The detection of MTC in younger children is usually made following screening in 'high risk' individuals who have a family history of MEN 2.[7] This is confirmed by elevated baseline levels of calcitonin or screening for the Ret (rearranged during transfection) protooncogene on chromosome 10. If positive, the child should be considered for prophylactic total thyroidectomy.[7] See Chapter 197, Thyroid cancer.

Nasopharyngeal carcinoma

In the US and Europe, nasopharyngeal carcinoma (NPC) is an uncommon tumour comprising only 1–2 percent of paediatric malignancies, but in other geographical locations, such as parts of Africa, 10–20 percent of childhood malignancies are due to NPC. There is a bimodal age distribution of this disease with an early peak of 10 to 20 years and a second peak between 40 and 60 years. NPC is one of few malignant tumours in childhood that emerges from the epithelium and there is an association with EBV. Males are twice as likely as females to develop NPC. Children with NPC almost invariably have the undifferentiated variant that is associated with higher rates of advanced locoregional disease and distant metastases.[27] Despite this, the five year disease-free survival is not significantly different to that of adults at 30–60 percent.[28]

PRESENTATION

Children may present with a cervical mass secondary to lymph node metastases. Other presenting symptoms and signs may include nasal congestion, epistaxis, otitis media with effusion, otalgia and cranial nerve palsy. As many as two-thirds of children with NPC have metastatic disease in the neck at presentation. Delay in the diagnosis occurs frequently because many of its symptoms mimic those of an upper respiratory tract infection.

ASSESSMENT

Nasopharyngeal examination and biopsy is required for tissue diagnosis. CT or MR scanning allows precise evaluation of the primary tumour and confirmation of the presence or absence of metastases, most particularly in the neck. The American Joint Committee in Cancer staging of NPC (see Chapter 188, Nasopharyngeal carcinoma) is used by most.

TREATMENT

Undifferentiated NPC is a radiosensitive tumour and as such is usually treated with external beam radiotherapy. Such therapy is limited to the primary tumour and its regional metastatic spread. Chemotherapy is required in patients with disseminated systemic disease. There is now evidence that combined chemotherapy and radiotherapy provides better disease-free survival as compared with radiotherapy alone and combined chemoradiotherapy is therefore becoming routine practice in the UK.[28, 29]

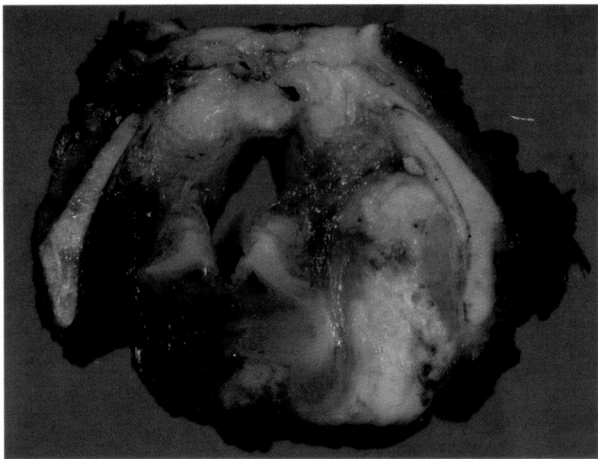

Figure 98.4 Cross section of a laryngectomy specimen from a 12-year-old boy with residual synovial cell sarcoma despite chemoradiotherapy.

CHORDOMA

This is a rare slow-growing bony tumour which is locally aggressive and which arises from embryonic remnants of the notochord. The presentation depends on the site of origin which, in the head and neck region, is most commonly found in the nasopharynx and adjacent skull base. Patients present with headache and diplopia and compression of the lower cranial nerves can result in a number of neurological signs (see Chapter 188, Nasopharyngeal carcinoma). Biopsy is necessary for diagnosis and MR and CT scanning will delineate the tumour extent. Complete surgical excision is rarely possible because of the anatomical location and adjacent structures and so postoperative radiotherapy is usually employed. The prognosis remains fairly poor.

LONG-TERM SEQUELAE OF TREATMENT

The aim of cancer treatment in children is to maximize the chance of long-term surival and at the same time minimize the side effects, particularly in the longer term. With overall five-year survival rates in children now in the order of 60–70 percent, it is particularly important to examine the effects of the more recently employed multimodality treatments. Children tolerate the acute side effects of radiotherapy and chemotherapy reasonably well but other sequelae may not become apparent for several years.[31]

Growth

Cranial radiotherapy can result in growth hormone deficiency and growth retardation and chemotherapy can also have significant effects on growth. Localized tumour treatments can also affect growth and function of specific organs or tumour sites. For example, radiotherapy

to the maxilla in a child can result in asymmetrical growth of the midface.

Reproductive function

An important issue for survivors of childhood cancer is the impact of the disease and its treatment on reproduction and the implications for the health of any offspring. In males there is evidence for impaired spermatogenesis after treatment but it appears that any sperm produced carries as much healthy DNA as produced by the population in general. However, it is not possible to predict fertility outcome in boys who receive treatment prior to puberty. Cryopreservation of sperm in young males (14–17 years) is effective but depends on the ability of the young patient to produce a specimen and, in the UK, consent for storage requires him to be 'Gillick' competent (see Chapter 63, The paediatric consultation). Radiotherapy to the hypothalamus or pituitary can result in precocious puberty in females and patients should therefore have their pubertal status checked regularly. Chemotherapy in general is less harmful to gonadal function in females but pelvic irradiation can affect ovarian function. Spontaneously conceived offspring of patients treated for cancer in childhood have no excess of congenital abnormalities or other diseases.[32]

Cardiac problems

Anthracyclines have a significant cardiotoxic effect and can cause cardiac failure in later life. Long-term echocardiogram surveillance is recommended. Mediastinal radiotherapy can also result in impaired cardiac function (and an increased risk of breast carcinoma) and this should be monitored as appropriate.

Thyroid disorders

Thyroid dysfunction can result from radiotherapy to the neck or to the hypothalmic/pituitary axis. Chemotherapy is an independent risk factor. Survivors require regular thyroid function evaluation. Radiotherapy to the neck is a recognized aetiological factor in the development of thyroid carcinoma in later years.

Other otolaryngological manifestations of treatment

Radiotherapy to the head and neck region results in a large variety of long-term sequelae that can affect function and cosmesis. Damage to the major and minor salivary glands can cause xerostomia and subsequent tooth and gum disease. Post-radiotherapy scarring within the nasopharynx can result in middle ear effusions and subsequent deafness, and in the region of the midface can result in recurrent sinusitis, temperomandibular joint dysfunction and trismus. Certain chemotherapeutic agents – notably cisplatin – are known to cause deafness and tinnitus. Immunodeficiency with a propensity to develop opportunistic infections of the head and neck may complicate some chemotherapy regimens.[31]

Cognitive and psychological problems

Surgery and/or radiotherapy to the brain or adjacent structures can result in neurocognitive defects such as low IQ, learning difficulties and an increased risk of seizures. Survivors of childhood cancer are at an increased risk for a wide range of disabling psychological problems such as low mood, low self-esteem and anxiety.

Follow-up

It is important to follow-up these children in the long term and to educate them and their parents about the possible late consequences of their treatment. It is also important to promote a healthy lifestyle and discourage cancer promoting behaviours such as smoking and excessive sun exposure.[32]

THE DYING CHILD

The death of a child is one of the greatest tragedies that can befall a family. It is important to recognize that palliative care of the dying child should address not only the control of pain but the social, psychological and spiritual needs of children and their families. Planned terminal care for children has become increasingly community-based and therefore requires involvement of the primary health care team, including the patient's general practitioner at an early stage. An experienced and multiskilled team is required with a named key worker and access to advice and support 24 hours a day. The child should participate in the planning and provision of this care as much as is realistically possible.[33]

To ensure optimum palliative care, the family and carers need to work with identical aims and a mutual acceptance of the inevitability of death. An appropriate person should discuss the fact that active curative treatment is no longer in the child's best interests and should start to negotiate a palliative care plan with the child and close family. Once the focus of treatment shifts from curative to palliative care, quality of life becomes of prime importance. Most children and their families will wish to maintain some semblance of normality while optimizing symptom control and minimizing medical intervention. For instance, many children will opt to remain at school for as long as they are

able, mixing with friends and getting a break from the home enviroment. Others may benefit from a daily visit at home from a play specialist.[33, 34]

Symptomatic control in the dying child has not been formally assessed and is often based on clinical experience and adapted from general paediatric practice and palliative care of adults. The World Health Organization's 'three stepladder' of analgesia can be applied in children with paracetamol, dihydrocodeine and morphine sulphate forming the standard steps. Laxatives and antiemetics may be required and appropriate sedatives may be required in the final stages of life.[34]

Regular respite should be offered to parents and it is important to explore the financial assistance, benefits and grants that families may be entitled to. Practical help with funeral arrangements should be given and it is important to continue to support the grieving family after their child's death and to withdraw support slowly and appropriately.[11, 33, 34]

KEY POINTS

- Head and neck tumours are uncommon in children.
- Early diagnosis is essential.
- Survival rates are improving.
- Multimodality treatment has improved the prognosis while reducing both early and long-term complications.
- Treatment should be provided by a specialized, centralized multidisciplinary paediatric oncology team.

Best clinical practice

✓ The vast majority of enlarged cervical lymph nodes in children are harmless. Imaging should usually be considered before biopsy. Excision biopsy may be appropriate for:
 – node >2 cm;
 – supraclavicular area and/or fixed nodes;
 – weight loss and/or unexplained fever;
 – abnormal chest x-ray. [Grade C/D]
✓ FNA has a more limited role to play in the child than the adult. [Grade B]
✓ All children diagnosed with malignancy should be referred to a specialist centre. [Grade B]
✓ Children receiving chemotherapy should have central venous catheters placed for venous access and chemotherapy treatment. [Grade C/D]
✓ Disease-free survival is over 90 percent in many series of children with Hodgkin's lymphoma. [Grade B]

99

Branchial arch fistulae, thyroglossal duct anomalies and lymphangioma

PETER D BULL

The branchial arches	1264	Lymphangioma	1269
First branchial arch (Cervico-aural) fistula	1264	Key points	1271
Second branchial arch fistula	1266	Best clinical practice	1271
Third and fourth branchial arch abnormalities	1267	Deficiencies in current knowledge and areas for future	
Disorders of the thyroglossal duct	1268	research	1271
Lingual thyroid	1268	References	1271

SEARCH STRATEGY

The author has a personal bibliography which was supplemented by a Medline search using the key words branchial apparatus, child, congenital, thyroglossal duct, thyroglossal cyst, cystic hygroma and lymphangioma.

THE BRANCHIAL ARCHES

Embryology

The structures of the lateral face and neck are formed embryologically from the paired branchial arches, pouches and associated clefts (see Chapter 65, Head and neck embryology).

The branchial apparatus appears between the fourth and fifth weeks of foetal development. It consists of six paired branchial arches separated by branchial clefts externally and branchial pouches internally.

During normal development, the ventral parts of the first and second arches fuse to obliterate the ventral part of the first cleft. The remainder of the first cleft forms the cavum conchae and the external auditory meatus. The first branchial pouch forms the Eustachian tube and tympanic cavity. The fifth and sixth arches disappear early in foetal life. [****]

Terminology

Persistence of remnants of the branchial apparatus gives rise to a number of well-recognized congenital anomalies in the head and neck. A persistent cleft will give rise to an external sinus, a blind ending opening onto the skin. A persistent pouch will cause an internal sinus typically opening into the pharynx whereas persistence of both cleft and pouch will cause a fistula with an internal and external (or upper and lower) opening.

Anomalies that cause a single opening or sinus or the persistence of a tissue remnant are more common than fistulae and include pre-auricular sinuses, cysts and skin tags.

FIRST BRANCHIAL ARCH (CERVICO–AURAL) FISTULA

This is rare and accounts for less than 5 percent of branchial cleft anomalies. The external fistulous opening in the neck varies in position but lies on a line from the tragus to the hyoid bone. The opening is often fairly inconspicuous and may look like a small skin-lined pit. The upper end of the fistula is also variable. There may be an opening anterior to the tragus; the track of the fistula may run under the floor of the external auditory canal and occasionally opens at the osseo-cartilaginous junction in the external auditory meatus.

In some cases, a skin-covered band runs from the floor of the meatus to the umbo. If seen, it makes the diagnosis certain.

Histology

The cervico-aural fistula is usually a sizeable track lined with squamous epithelium. Work[1] has divided them into two types according to the presence or absence of mesothelial elements within the wall.

Type 1 lesions are of ectodermal origin and are present medial to the concha. Type 2 lesions are both ectodermal and mesodermal in origin and contain mesodermal structures such as cartilage and hair follicles (**Figure 99.1**). [****]

The lower opening of the type 2 fistula is usually below the angle of the mandible.

Presentation

The opening at either end of the track is present at birth and may become more obvious by the discharge of epithelial or sebaceous debris (**Figure 99.2**).

The fistula may become acutely infected and may rarely progress to abscess formation. Being lined with skin, cervico-aural fistulae do not discharge mucus.

Investigation

If there is doubt about the nature of the fistula, a radio-opaque sinogram using water-soluble contrast will demonstrate the extent of the track and confirm the position of the upper end (**Figure 99.3**). MR scanning may show the track but will not demonstrate its relationship to the facial nerve.

Treatment

Because the fistulous track is lined with squamous epithelium, it will contain desquamated material, which may become infected. Surgical excision of these lesions is usually advocated. Surgery is easier before either acute infection or abscess has supervened. [**/*]

Surgical excision necessitates the dissection of the track in its entirety. [*]

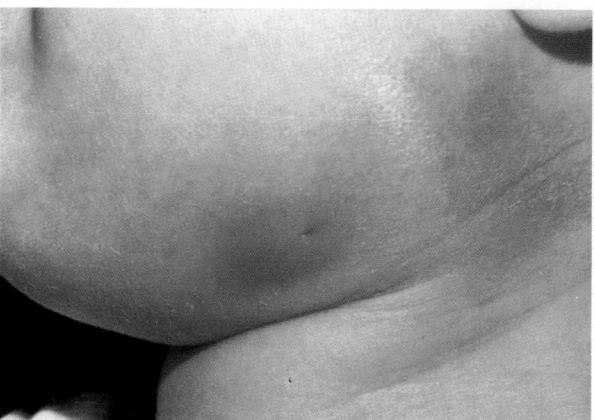

Figure 99.2 The external opening of a cervico-aural fistula.

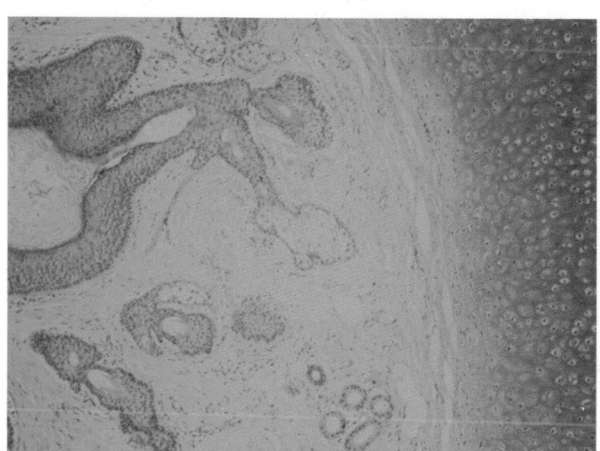

Figure 99.1 Histology of a first arch cervico-aural fistula.

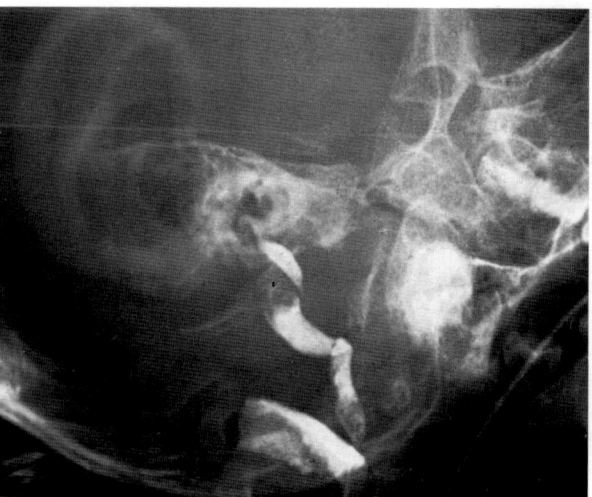

Figure 99.3 Sinogram showing the course of a cervico-aural fistula.

A parotidectomy type incision is modified to include the lower opening of the fistula. The fistula at this point can be followed for a small distance upwards and when its nature and direction are confirmed, the facial nerve trunk must be identified as it leaves the skull base and enters the parotid gland. The mandibular branch in particular should be followed so that it can be preserved while freeing the fistulous track. Sharp dissection will often be required to free the nerve from the track.

In most instances the fistula will run deep to the branches of the facial nerve, which may be adherent if there has been recurrent infection, though the relationship is unpredictable (**Figure 99.4**).

The upper part of the first arch fistula also has an unpredictable relationship to the cartilages of the external auditory canal (EAC). It may terminate at the canal or may form a duplicated canal parallel and inferior to the EAC proper.

The fistula does not extend medial to the cartilaginous canal but a strand may cross the lumen of the canal from the osseo-cartilaginous junction to be attached to the umbo.

Facial nerve exposure and protection is required in nearly every case of first branchial cleft fistula. If this is done, then the risk to the facial nerve is minimized.

Peroperative facial nerve monitoring is advisable. [*] The very superficial position of the facial nerve in small children must be considered when making the approach to the nerve.

The upper end of the fistula must be followed and excised to ensure that no squamous epithelium remains, and this may require opening of the external auditory canal. Closure of the wound with suction drainage and, if necessary, packing of the ear canal completes the operation.

SECOND BRANCHIAL ARCH FISTULA

Second arch fistulae and sinuses are much the commonest of the branchial arch anomalies (95 percent). The second branchial arch forms the epidermis of the upper neck and dorsal pinna. The mesoderm forms the facial muscles and the body of the hyoid, and the endodermal elements form the root of the tongue, the foramen caecum, the thyroid stalk and the tonsil. Malfusion of these structures may lead to the formation of the second arch branchial fistula. Second branchial arch fistula may form part of branchio-oto-renal syndrome.[2, 3]

Presentation

The second branchial arch fistula presents as a congenital opening on the lower neck, anterior to the sternomastoid muscle. The track of the second arch fistula is directed upwards and medially to pass between the internal and external carotid arteries. The upper end communicates with the pharynx through the tonsil (**Figure 99.5**). These fistulae nearly always leak clear or mucoid fluid from the lower opening and may become infected. On occasion, the infected track may form an abscess requiring surgical drainage.

Investigation

As a rule, the diagnosis is evident and no further investigation is required. If there is doubt, a contrast sinogram can be performed to define the track.

Treatment

Because of the risk of infection, excision of second arch branchial fistulae is advisable. Surgery can be performed at any age and aims to excise the track completely. An elliptical incision is made around the external opening and the track can be followed upwards. If the distance between the lower end and the pharynx is too great to

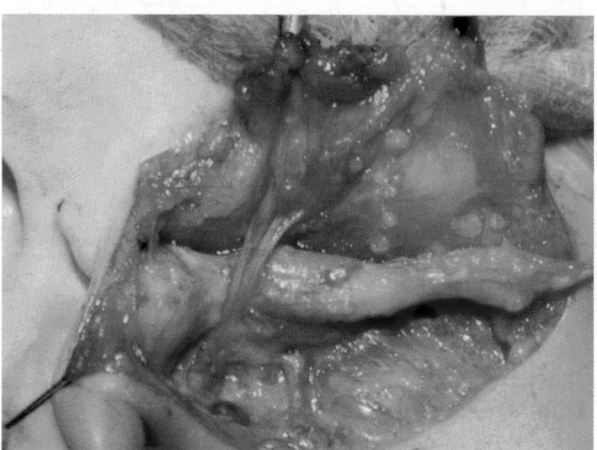

Figure 99.4 The surgical exposure of the fistula, crossed by the facial nerve.

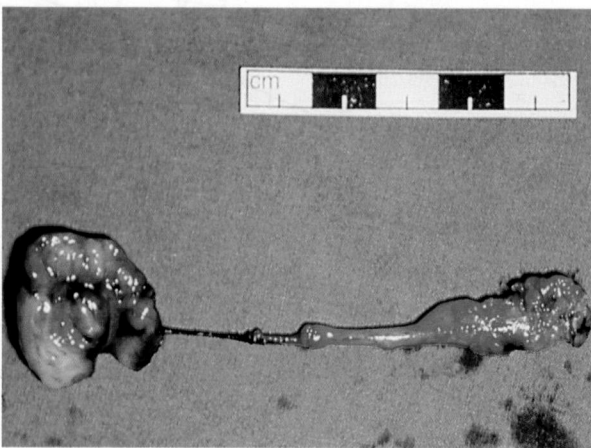

Figure 99.5 A branchial fistula removed in continuity with the tonsil.

allow good access, a second skin crease incision is made further up the neck to enable the upper part of the track to be visualized and excised. The track will be seen to enter the pharyngeal muscle at the level of the tonsil and can be ligated and excised at this level. Sometimes the track can be followed into the tonsil, which can be removed intraorally in continuity (**Figure 99.6**).

Care must be taken to identify the lingual nerve in the upper part of the dissection. Complete excision of the fistula should prevent any recurrence.

THIRD AND FOURTH BRANCHIAL ARCH ABNORMALITIES

The third and fourth branchial arches form part of the hyoid bone and the muscles of the larynx and pharynx. The pouches also form the thymus gland, the parathyroids and part of the thyroid. Agenesis gives rise to the 'DiGeorge' anomaly. This is characterized by partial or complete aplasia of the thyroid and parathyroid glands, often with associated craniofacial and cardiac anomalies. Sinuses and fistulae of these arches are rare.

Presentation is usually as an abscess in the neck, most commonly on the left, communicating with the apex of

the piriform fossa (**Figure 99.7**). The appearance may be that of an acute suppurative thyroiditis. Typically, there is diagnostic delay and the child may have had several surgical interventions. Treatment requires endoscopy of the piriform fossa and complete excision of the track and the inflammatory mass.[4, 5] [*]

Pre-auricular sinus

EMBRYOLOGY

The outer ear is formed from cartilagenous tubercles of first arch origin which fuse to form the pinna. A blind-ended sinus results from incomplete fusion and the inclusion of epithelial tissue forms a skin lining to the sinus. There may be a family history of such anomaly. The branchio-oto-renal syndrome is determined by an autosomal dominant gene and includes external ear abnormality, pre-auricular sinus and renal disorder.[2, 3]

PRESENTATION

The opening of the sinus is apparent at birth and is often bilateral. There may be some sebaceous discharge from the punctum. As a rule, these lesions give little trouble and can be safely left alone. In some patients there is recurrent episodic infection which may progress to abscess formation. Because the sinus is lined with squamous epithelium, spontaneous resolution does not take place.

TREATMENT

If the sinus is free of infection, it can be left alone, but many of the cases will be subject to repeated episodes of

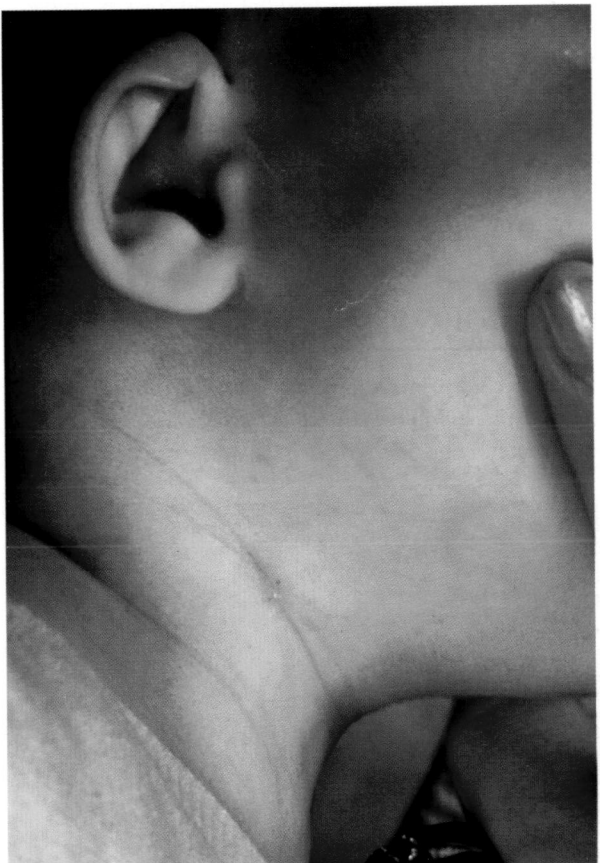

Figure 99.6 A case of branchio-oto-renal syndrome, showing the external opening of a second arch branchial fistula and deformity of the outer ear.

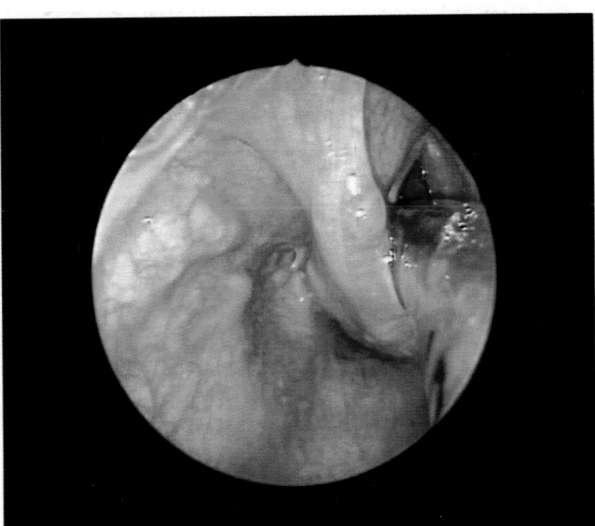

Figure 99.7 Sinus opening at apex of left piriform fossa in a case of fourth branchial arch sinus. The patient had presented with recurrent neck abscesses.

infection and should be excised. An ellipse of skin around the punctum is marked out and the track followed carefully. It can be helpful to instil some methylene blue dye into the track to make it more visible during the dissection. The aim of the operation is to remove all vestiges of squamous epithelium, so the track must be dissected out meticulously and in one piece.

DISORDERS OF THE THYROGLOSSAL DUCT

Considered under this heading are:

- thyroglossal duct cyst;
- thyroglossal duct fistula;
- lingual thyroid.

Embryology

The thyroid primordium develops in the floor of the primitive pharynx at the site of the foramen caecum, which lies in the midline at the junction of the posterior one-third and anterior two-thirds of the tongue. The descending thyroid gland migrates through the tongue tissue, passing anterior to the hyoid bone to lie in the anterior neck. The line of descent from the foramen caecum is marked by the thyroglossal duct. If involution of the duct is incomplete, a cyst may develop at any point along the track.

Presentation

Surprisingly for a congenital lesion, presentation of a thyroglossal cyst is often delayed well beyond infancy and into early childhood. The cyst is usually midline but in 10 percent of cases may present laterally, usually on the left.[6] Protrusion of the tongue, by elevating the hyoid bone, results in the cyst (or fistulous opening) being pulled upwards (**Figures 99.8** and **99.9**).

Investigation

If there is doubt about the diagnosis, ultrasound examination will clarify the nature and position of the cyst. Aspiration is unnecessary and may lead to infection and fistula formation. [*]

The thyroglossal duct cyst, while derived from the descending thyroglossal track, does not contain the only functioning thyroid gland tissue. It may contain thyroid tissue in the wall, but unless there is a lingual thyroid, the thyroid gland will be in the normal position. It is not necessary to do isotope thyroid scans or thyroid function tests before surgery for thyroglossal cyst.

Treatment

Treatment of thyroglossal duct cyst is by excision. The optimum operation is as described by Sistrunk.[7] [**]

A horizontal skin crease incision is made over the convexity of the cyst. If there is a fistula, an ellipse of skin is taken to include the opening. The cyst or track is then dissected out and the middle segment of the hyoid exposed and skeletonized. The thyroglossal duct goes through or deep to the body of the hyoid bone, so the body is excised in continuity. The track is then followed through the tongue in the midline. If no track is visible, a core of tissue is removed up to the foramen caecum.

Removal of a thyroglossal cyst results in a recognized recurrence rate of between 4 and 10 percent. [**] Revision surgery is more unpredictable and requires an en bloc removal of inflamed tissue.

Thyroid tissue has been observed histologically in 46 percent of cases of excised thyroglossal duct cysts.[8]

LINGUAL THYROID

If the thyroid primordium fails to descend into the neck, thyroid tissue will remain at the foramen caecum. There may therefore be no thyroid tissue at the usual pretracheal

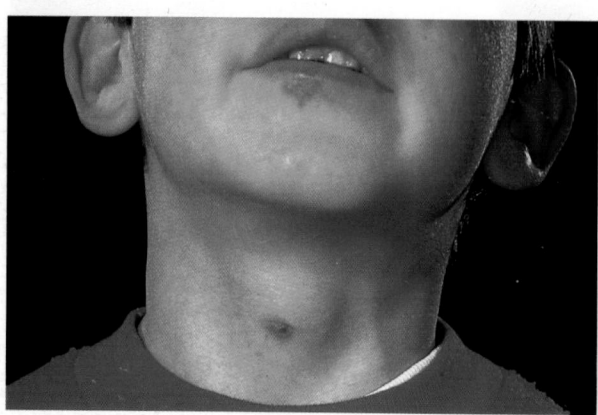

Figure 99.8 A thyroglossal duct fistula.

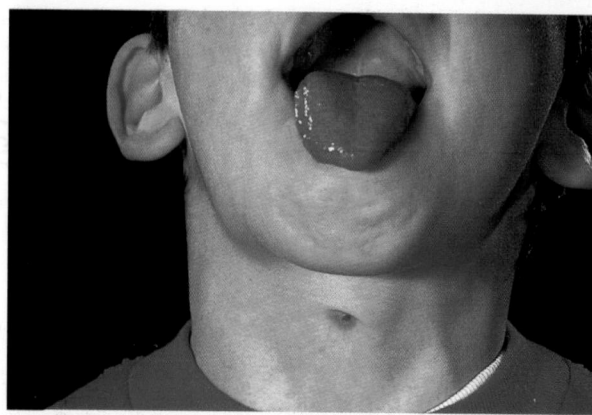

Figure 99.9 A thyroglossal duct fistula with the tongue protruded, showing the pull on the fistulous track.

site and all the thyroid gland is represented by that at the foramen caecum.[9]

Presentation

Lingual thyroid is extremely rare. In a review of thyroid abnormality in 29,000 autopsies, only four lingual thyroids were identified.[10] [****] It usually presents as a mass on the base of the tongue in infancy or childhood, leading to dysphagia or airway compromise (**Figure 99.10**). It may be found coincidentally on isotope scanning in the investigation of hypothyroidism. Rarely, a lingual thyroid may present acutely as a result of bleeding into the ectopic thyroid tissue.

Investigation

- MR or CT scanning will demonstrate the lesion in the sagittal or coronal plane (**Figure 99.11**).
- Radioactive iodine scanning with I^{123} or I^{131} will demonstrate active thyroid tissue.
- Thyroid function tests will usually demonstrate the presence of hypothyroidism.

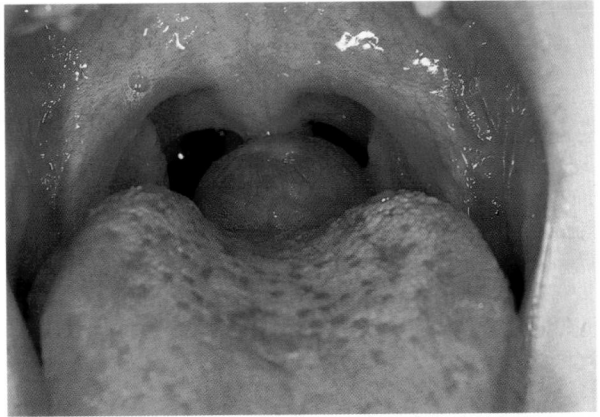

Figure 99.10 A lingual thyroid.

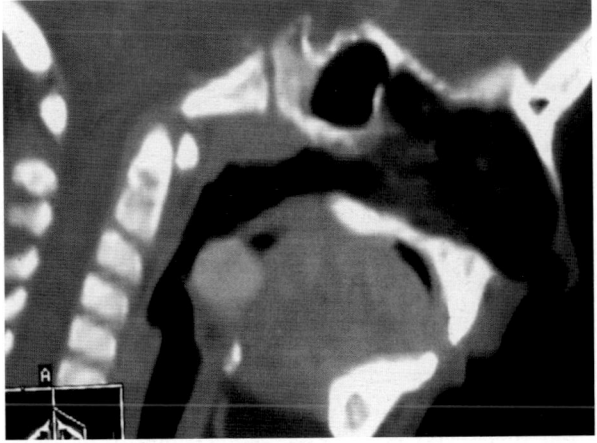

Figure 99.11 CT scan showing the lingual thyroid.

Treatment

If the lingual thyroid is small and causing no symptoms, suppression of thyroid stimulating hormone (TSH) with oral thyroxine may result in reduction in size. [**] The advice of an endocrinologist, particularly in children, is essential. If the lesion is larger and causing dysphagia or airway obstruction, surgical excision is required. Since thyroid replacement therapy is in most cases necessary in any case, there need be no concern at removing all extant thyroid tissue. There is no hazard to the parathyroid glands, which are embryologically from a different origin and will not be within the lingual thyroid tissue.

Peroral access to the lingual thyroid is usually possible, with midline splitting of the dorsal tongue to gain access to the substance of the lingual thyroid. If the ectopic tissue is more deeply buried, a suprahyoid external approach may be necessary. Postoperatively, surveillance of thyroid function is essential. [**]

LYMPHANGIOMA

Embryology

Lymphangioma (LA) refers to a group of developmental anomalies in which the lymphatics fail to connect in the normal way to the venous channels. As a result, there are large fluid-filled spaces occupying the tissues and expanding tissue planes. Histologically, these lesions consist of widely dilated lymphatic spaces with walls of varying thickness. The lesions may be macrocystic or microcystic. The macrocystic lesions are often large and compressible, though frequently multilocular, whereas the microcystic type is often smaller and firmer. The macrocystic lesion, with its well-defined margin, is commonly referred to as 'cystic hygroma.' Because the failure of proper development of the venous lymphatic relationship manifests most frequently in the developing paired jugular lymph sac systems, cystic hygroma is most common in the face, neck and mediastinum.

Presentation

The hygroma is usually evident at birth as a smooth, soft swelling, which may be fluctuant. Being filled with fluid, it can often be transilluminated. The hygroma may be enormous and cause immediate and fatal airway obstruction. It can be diagnosed antenatally by ultrasonography; steps to secure the airway can then be planned prior to delivery. The swelling may enlarge during childhood, sometimes triggered by intercurrent upper respiratory infections (**Figure 99.12**). This may lead in turn to acute infection within the hygroma, which can become tense and hard. If this happens to the

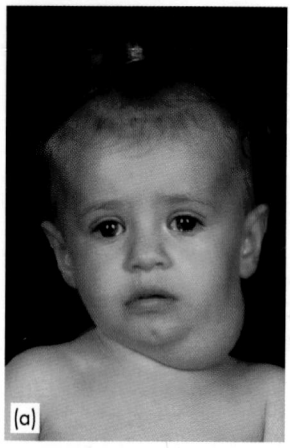 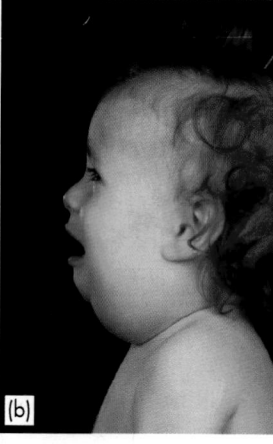

Figure 99.12 (a) and (b) Cystic hygroma of the left neck.

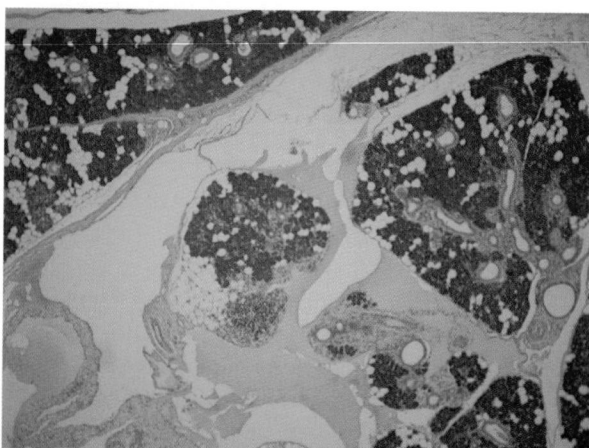

Figure 99.13 Histology of cystic hygroma infiltrating the parotid tissue.

intraoral or intralingual part, severe airway obstruction will result. If the lesion is extensive in the head and neck, there may be intraoral lesions forming small clear cysts in the mucosa. These are sometimes vascular and may bleed spontaneously but can be removed easily with laser or diathermy.

Natural history

Cystic hygromas of the head and neck do not involute spontaneously. Some progression may take place with enlargement, and infiltrative growth into previously unaffected areas sometimes happens. Recurrent episodes of acute infection may arise and the lesion will become larger, painful and inflamed. As a result of this infection, related lymph nodes can become enlarged. The activity in cystic hygroma may subside with increasing age. There is no potential for malignant change. Rarely, sequestration of fluid within a cystic hygroma, especially in neonates, may result in hypovolaemic shock and widespread intravascular thrombosis.

Investigation

Although as a rule the diagnosis is apparent and no particular investigations are needed, ultrasonography will reveal the cystic nature of the lesion and its relationship to the surrounding tissues. It will also distinguish between macro- and microcystic disease. Cross-sectional imaging will be required if surgery is contemplated. [*] MR scanning is preferable as it provides better soft tissue delineation and avoids exposure to ionizing radiation.[11] It will normally need to be carried out under general anaesthesia. There is little or no value in fine-needle aspiration for cytology unless underlying neoplasia is suspected.

Treatment

If the cystic hygroma is small and is cosmetically and functionally acceptable, no treatment other than observation will be required. [**]

Sclerotherapy

Macrocystic disease is amenable to aspiration and the instillation of sclerosant. Most experience is with OK 432, although other agents such as alcohol, bleomycin, ethanolamine oleate and trichloroacetic acid have been used.[12] OK 432 is a lyophilized incubation material derived from group A pyogenic streptococcal culture, which induces an intense inflammatory reaction within the hygroma and obliteration of the cystic space. In a multicentre trial of OK 432,[13] a group of patients received four doses of the material at six to eight week intervals. There was a successful outcome in 86 percent of the cases, predominantly for macrocystic disease. [**/*]

Surgery

Microcystic disease or macrocystic disease not amenable to sclerotherapy presents a formidable challenge (**Figure 99.13**). It will usually require surgical resection and complete extirpation may be impossible. A long-term review from Copenhagen indicated that 50 percent of such patients had residual disease, 44 percent had impairment of speech, swallowing or breathing and 36 percent had cosmetic deformity that caused them concern.[14] [**/*]

Surgery requires great attention to anatomical structures, which are enveloped in the hygroma tissue. Residual or recurrent hygroma is more likely in suprahyoid disease because of the more complex anatomy. Neurovascular structures should not be damaged in an attempt to remove every last remnant, since this will have long-term adverse consequences for the patient.[15]

KEY POINTS

- A knowledge and understanding of the embryology and often complex anatomy of congenital anomalies of the head and neck is essential before treating these disorders.
- Investigation is not always required but careful imaging in consultation with a paediatric radiologist may be helpful in planning treatment.
- The term 'cystic hygroma', though commonly used, refers to a group of disorders which are better considered as 'lymphangiomas'.

Best clinical practice

- ✓ In first arch (cervico-aural) fistula, surgical excision necessitates the dissection of the track in its entirety. Facial nerve exposure and protection is required in almost every case. [Grade D]
- ✓ Because of the risk of infection, excision of second arch branchial fistulae is advisable. [Grade D]
- ✓ Simple excision of a thyroglossal duct cyst is inadequate. The body of the hyoid must be excised and the track followed to the foramen caecum. [Grade C]
- ✓ Suppression of TSH with oral thyroxine may result in regression of a lingual thyroid. [Grade C]
- ✓ In lymphangioma surgery, neurovascular structures should not be damaged in an attempt to remove every last remnant. [Grade D]

Deficiencies in current knowledge and areas for future research

---

- ➤ Thyroglossal duct abnormalities are increasingly dealt with by otolaryngologists with training and expertise in head and neck surgery; recurrence due to inadequate primary surgery should become less common.
- ➤ Continuing improvements in medical imaging should help treatment planning for complex head and neck abnormalities.
- ➤ The results of continuing studies on sclerotherapy for lymphangioma will help define the place of this method of treatment of these challenging disorders.

REFERENCES

1. Work WP. Newer concepts of first branchial cleft defects. *Laryngoscope.* 1972; **82**: 1581–93.
2. Chen A, Francis M, Ni L, Cremers CW, Kimberling WJ, Sato Y *et al.* Phenotypic manifestations of branchio-oto-renal syndrome. *American Journal of Medical Genetics.* 1995; **58**: 365–70.
3. Kemperman MH, Stinckens C, Kumar S, Joosten FB, Huygen PL, Cremers CW. The branchio-oto-renal syndrome. *Advances in Oto-Rhino-Laryngology.* 2002; **61**: 192–200.
4. Nicollas R, Ducroz V, Garabedian EN, Triglia JM. Fourth branchial pouch anomalies: a study of six cases and review of the literature. *International Journal of Pediatric Otorhinolaryngology.* 1998; **44**: 5–10.
* 5. Rea Pa, Hartley BE, Bailey CM. Third and fourth branchial arch anomalies. *Journal of Laryngology and Otology.* 2004; **118**: 19–24. *Good review of classification and treatment of these disorders.*
6. Brewis C, Mahadadevax M, Bailey CM, Drake DP. Investigation and treatment of thyroglossal duct cysts in children. *Journal of the Royal Society of Medicine.* 2000; **93**: 18–21.
7. Sistrunk WE. Technique of removal of cysts and sinuses of the thyroglossal duct. *Annals of Surgery.* 1920; **71**: 121–4.
8. Chandra RK, Maddalozzo J, Kovarik P. Histological characterization of the thyroglossal tract: implications for surgical management. *Laryngoscope.* 2001; **111**: 1002–5.
9. Vazquez E, Enriquez G, Castellote A, Lucaya J, Creixell S, Aso C *et al.* Ultrasound CT and MRI imaging of the neck lesions in children. *Radiographic.* 1995; **15**: 105–22.
10. Williams ED, Toyn CE, Harach HR. The ultimobranchial gland and congenital thyroid abnormalities in man. *Journal of Pathology.* 1989; **159**: 135–41.
* 11. Duncan AW. Congenital neck masses. In: King SJ, Boothroyd AE (eds). *Paediatric ENT radiology.* Berlin Heidelberg, New York: Springer Verlag, 2002: 175–98. *Good overview of the role of imaging in evaluating neck masses in children.*
12. Kim KH, Sung MW, Roh JC, Han MH. Sclerotherapy for congenital lesions in the head and neck. *Otolaryngology Head and Neck Surgery.* 2004; **131**: 307–16.
13. Giguere CM, Bauman NM, Sato Y, Burke DK, Greinwald JH, Pransky S *et al.* Treatment of lymphangiomas with OK-432 (Picibanil) sclerotherapy: a prospective multi-institutional trial. *Archives of Otolaryngology – Head and Neck Surgery.* 2002; **128**: 1137–44.
14. Charabi B, Bretlau P, Bille M, Holmelund M. Cystic hygroma of the head and neck – a long-term follow-up of 44 cases. *Acta Oto-Laryngologica – Supplement.* 2000; **543**: 248–50.
15. Kennedy TL, Whitaker M, Pellitteri P, Wood WE. Cystic hygroma/lymphangioma: a rational approach to management. *Laryngoscope.* 2001; **111**: 1929–37.

100

Gastro-oesophageal reflux and aspiration

HAYTHAM KUBBA

Gastro-oesophageal reflux	1272	Key points	1278
Key points	1276	Best clinical practice	1278
Best clinical practice	1276	Deficiencies in current knowledge and areas for future	
Deficiencies in current knowledge and areas for future		research	1278
research	1277	References	1279
Aspiration	1277		

SEARCH STRATEGY

Systematic reviews were identified first using the key words: reflux (gastric, gastro-oesophageal, gastropharyngeal, gastronasopharyngeal, gastrolaryngopharyngeal); and subject headings in the Cochrane Database of Systematic Reviews, the Database of Abstracts of Reviews of Effectiveness, and the ACP Journal Club. Individual articles were then identified using the same search terms in Ovid Medline. Articles were also identified from bibliographies and from the author's own collection.

GASTRO-OESOPHAGEAL REFLUX

Definitions

Gastro-oesophageal reflux is the retrograde passage of stomach contents into the oesophagus. The refluxate need not be acidic, and is often neutral or even alkaline. Some degree of reflux is extremely common in neonates and usually has few, if any, symptoms: this is termed physiologic reflux. Pathologic reflux, on the other hand, is synonymous with gastro-oesophageal reflux disease and implies that the child is coming to harm in some way. This may be in the form of symptoms, or as tissue damage in the absence of symptoms (silent reflux). Secondary reflux occurs in a child predisposed by the presence of other abnormalities of the oesophagus, such as tracheo-oesophageal fistula or neuromuscular disease. Gastro-pharyngeal reflux ascends above the level of the upper oesophageal sphincter and has been implicated in a number of respiratory and otolaryngological diseases.

Natural history

Physiologic reflux is almost universal in neonates. These reflux episodes are usually postprandial, brief and asymptomatic. One study showed healthy preterm infants with no symptoms or signs of reflux having between 40 and 145 (median 72) reflux events per 24 hour period, and these were more common immediately after feeds.[1] Reflux becomes less frequent at certain predictable developmental milestones, such as sitting and weaning onto solids. At the age of four months, 67 percent of infants have at least one episode of regurgitation per day as reported by their parents: by the age of seven months this figure has fallen to 21 percent, and at a year regurgitation will only be present in 5 percent.[2] Heartburn and regurgitation are reported by around 2 percent of three to nine year olds and 5–8 percent of 10–17 year olds, although few seek or receive treatment.[3] It is likely that a significant proportion of these children will go on to have gastro-oesophageal reflux as adults.[4, 5]

Pathophysiology

The short length of the intra-abdominal portion of the oesophagus in neonates may predispose them to reflux to some degree, but anatomical factors are not thought to be a major factor in paediatric reflux. Hiatus hernia in particular is only present in a small minority of children with reflux.[6] Nor is there evidence of an abnormality of resting muscle tone in the lower oesophageal sphincter. The evidence suggests that reflux in children of all ages is primarily caused by transient lower oesophageal sphincter relaxations.[7, 8, 9, 10] The lower oesophageal sphincter is not a defined ring of muscle, but rather a physiological barrier consisting of an area of increased muscle tone in the lower oesophagus. Transient relaxations can occur for many reasons, including gastric distension, and are prolonged (more than ten seconds) compared with the normal relaxation that occurs during swallowing.[11]

Children with neuromuscular disorders may have upper gastrointestinal dysmotility with gastroparesis and retroperistalsis.

Reflux is more likely in the presence of a nasogastric tube.[1] It is also more likely in infants fed formula milk rather than breast milk, as the former passes from the stomach into the duodenum more slowly.[12] Intolerance to cow's milk may also play a role for some infants with reflux.[13]

A recent study has suggested the possibility of a gene on chromosome 13q14 predisposing infants to severe reflux,[14] although further studies with more rigorous case definition are required to confirm this.

Symptoms and signs

The most common manifestation of reflux is regurgitation of feeds, also known as posseting. Mild, infrequent regurgitation is common and is not usually regarded as a reason to intervene medically. More affected infants may show evidence of colicky pains and irritability, perhaps with arching of the back. With severe reflux (and now clearly in the realms of gastro-oeophageal reflux disease) infants may have severe vomiting, aversion to feeds and failure to thrive. Abnormal posturing of the head and neck (Sandifer syndrome) is an uncommon presentation of reflux disease.

Otolaryngological manifestations

APNOEAS AND APPARENT LIFE-THREATENING EVENTS

Apnoeas are not uncommon in infants, particularly those born prematurely. Gastro-oesophageal reflux causing laryngospasm may be a factor in some, but other causes need to be considered, including tracheomalacia, seizures and central apnoea.[15] Reflux events are common in neonates and are not always associated temporally with apnoeas,[16] but if symptoms, signs and investigations suggest that reflux may be a factor, anti-reflux treatment may be effective.[17] [**]

Apparent life-threatening events (ALTEs) occur when a child becomes limp, bradycardic, cyanosed and clearly requires resuscitation. Infants with ALTEs are at risk of sudden infant death syndrome (SIDS). Approximately half of ALTEs are thought to be related to reflux-related laryngospasm or aspiration.[18, 19] Structural airway anomalies are also common, but central apnoeas and nonaccidental injury should be considered in the differential diagnosis.

AIRWAY DISORDERS

Gastro-oesophageal reflux may cause a variety of upper airway symptoms in children and has been found to be associated with hoarseness,[20] recurrent croup[21, 22] and 'laryngitis'.[23] Controlled studies of the effect of anti-reflux treatment on these symptoms are lacking.

Gastro-oesophageal reflux is extremely common in children with laryngomalacia,[24, 25, 26, 27] but it is difficult to separate cause from effect. The highly negative intrathoracic pressures generated by a child with upper airway obstruction will encourage reflux of gastric contents. Reflux may, in turn, worsen airway obstruction by causing laryngeal oedema and laryngospasm. Treatment of the laryngomalacia by aryepiglottoplasty produces significant improvement in reflux on pH testing.[28] Equally, anti-reflux treatment can be very useful in improving the stridor of laryngomalacia, and may obviate the need for surgery in a proportion of those most affected. [*]

Gastro-oesophageal reflux is common in children with subglottic stenosis and has been postulated as a contributory factor in the development of the stenosis.[29, 30] As with laryngomalacia, however, it is difficult to know whether the reflux is a cause or an effect of the airway obstruction. Many surgeons feel that reflux is potentially very deleterious at the time of reconstructive surgery[31] and prophylactic anti-reflux therapy is often prescribed,[32] although evidence that this makes a difference is lacking.[33] [*]

Laryngeal and laryngo-tracheo-oesophageal clefts are associated with oesophageal dysmotility problems, and reflux is almost universal. Most surgeons would advocate anti-reflux treatment for these children, particularly around the time of cleft repair, either with medication[34] or fundoplication.[35] [*]

Although it has been suggested that reflux may exacerbate the clinical course of children with recurrent respiratory papillomatosis[36, 37] and choanal atresia,[38] supporting evidence is lacking. Few surgeons use anti-reflux medications routinely in these situations at present.

RHINOSINUSITIS

The reflux of stomach contents into the nasopharynx or even the nose has been postulated to cause inflammation and oedema, and thereby lead to chronic rhinosinusitis. Reflux might also cause nasal disease through colonization of the nose with *Helicobacter pylori* and autonomic dysfunction.[39] Evidence in support of such an association in children is limited. A diagnosis of sinusitis and a history of sinus surgery are both more common in children with a diagnosis of gastro-oesophageal reflux than in children without reflux.[23] Previously diagnosed reflux is also common in children with chronic rhinosinusitis, and this has been demonstrated in uncontrolled studies, both prospective[40] and retrospective.[41] In most children this reflux is gastro-oesophageal, but a substantial minority have demonstrable reflux into the nasopharynx.[40] A single small controlled study has shown gastro-nasopharyngeal reflux on pH testing to be more common in children with chronic rhinitis than controls.[42] Children undergoing adenoidectomy have been reported as having gastro-oesophageal reflux more often than children undergoing ventilation tube insertion, but the diagnostic criteria for reflux were variable and not standardized.[43]

Anti-reflux medication has been reported to produce a marked improvement in sinus symptoms in studies with small numbers of highly selected children with sinus disease and proven reflux.[40, 41, 44] Two children with refractory sinusitis and otitis media associated with reflux have been reported as having complete resolution of their symptoms after fundoplication.[45]

The case for an association between reflux and rhinosinusitis is intriguing but remains unproven. Controlled studies with adequate numbers are required to establish the nature of any association and the response to anti-reflux treatment.

OTITIS MEDIA

A recent study by Tasker and co-workers[46] showed extremely high levels of pepsin in middle ear effusions from children with otitis media (OME). The pepsin was not produced in the middle ear and was present in far higher concentrations than could be found in blood, so it could only have got there from gastric reflux. Gastric acid and pepsin could cause inflammation of middle ear mucosa and dysfunction of the Eustachian tube, and reflux is therefore a plausible cause of OME. However, supporting evidence for such an association is lacking. Although small studies have shown reflux on pH testing in more than half of children with OME or recurrent acute otitis media,[47, 48] a large case-control study (9900 children) showed otitis media to be marginally less common in children with reflux than controls.[23]

It has been suggested that reflux may cause referred otalgia which, in a fretful child, may lead to an erroneous diagnosis of acute otitis media.[49] This is an interesting suggestion that merits further study.

Diagnostic tests

In clinical practice, probably the most common 'diagnostic' intervention for a child with suspected reflux is an empirical therapeutic trial of anti-reflux treatment. This reflects the fact that the available investigations, such as pH testing, are far from ideal. Diagnostic testing remains essential, however, when a child fails to respond to treatment, has atypical symptoms or is being considered for anti-reflux surgery. It is likely that, over the next few years, intraluminal impedance will prove to be the investigation of choice. Children with suspected intolerance of cow's milk should be referred to a paediatric gastroenterologist for further investigation.

Radiological contrast swallow studies are reasonably sensitive but not specific – if they show reflux, it is likely to be genuine, but a normal study certainly does not exclude significant reflux. The main value of a contrast study is in excluding rare anatomical anomalies such as malrotation, pyloric stenosis, hiatus hernia, strictures and webs.[50] [***]

Radionuclide scintigraphy (performed after the oral ingestion of technetium-labelled milk) has some advantages over pH monitoring in being able to show delayed gastric emptying, aspiration and nonacid reflux events.[50] Like the contrast study, however, it lacks sensitivity and gives only a brief time for measurement, and is therefore not routinely used in clinical practice. [***]

Currently, the 'gold standard' investigation for gastro-oesophageal reflux is 24-hour ambulatory pH probe monitoring. The probe is passed transnasally into the distal oesophagus. Measurements are taken every few seconds and calculations are made of the frequency and duration of oesophageal acid exposure. The results are reasonably reproducible, and are especially valuable if reflux events can be temporally related to symptoms (**Figure 100.1** and **Table 100.1**). Some degree of reflux is found in normal children at all ages, but is more common in infants. The results must be interpreted, therefore, with reference to the child's age. The reflux index is the percentage of time spent with a pH less than 4: studies of normal children have suggested an upper limit of normal of 12 percent in the first year of life and 6 percent thereafter.[50] [***]

The correlation between otolaryngological symptoms and the presence of gastro-oesophageal reflux on conventional pH monitoring is, unfortunately, poor. The correlation is improved when dual-probe pH monitoring is performed, using a probe in the pharynx as well as one in the lower oesophagus.[51, 52, 53, 54] The upper probe is placed above the cricopharyngeus

pH Channel

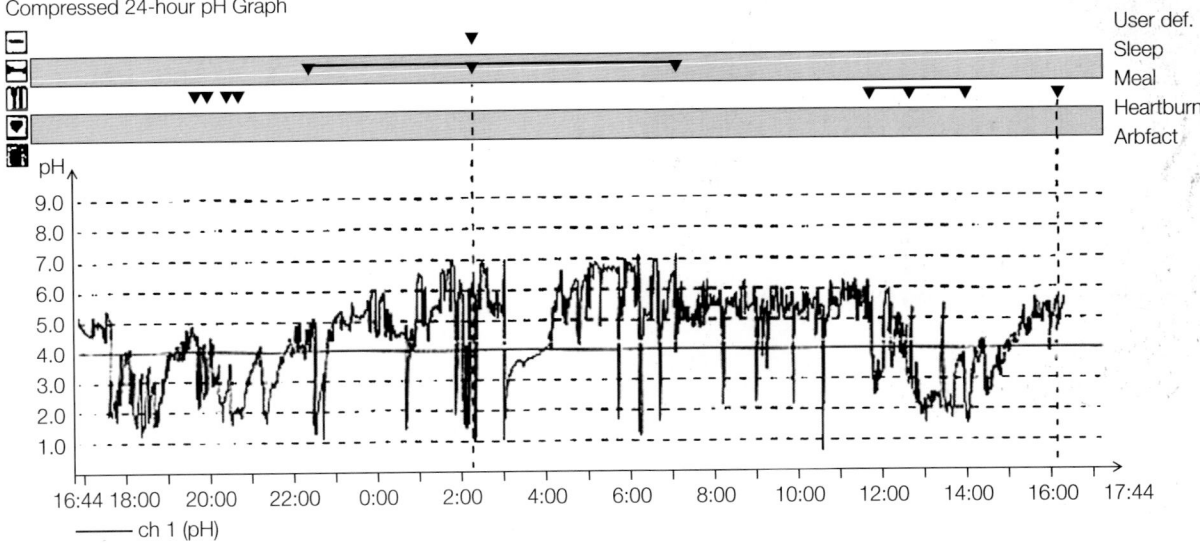

Figure 100.1 A typical pH study result showing severe reflux.

Table 100.1 Period table.

Item	Total	Upright	Supine	Meal	PostP	None
Duration of period (HH:MM)	24:00	15:06	08:54	3:01	04:36	00:04
Number of acid refluxes (#)	152	120	32	52	42	0
Number of long acid refluxes (#)	15	13	2	4	8	0
Longest acid reflux (min)	47	33	47	33	21	0
Total time pH below 4.00 (min)	374	296	77	107	127	0
Fraction time pH below 4.00 (%)	26.0	32.7	14.5	58.9	46.0	0.0

posterior to the larynx, ideally at a similar level to the vocal cords. An x-ray can be used to confirm position. The lack of control data make it difficult to establish what level of gastro-pharyngeal reflux, if any, can be considered normal, but a reflux index of 2 percent in infants and 1 percent in children has been used by some.[54] [***]

Unfortunately, pH probe results do not always seem to correlate with symptoms in clinical practice. It must be borne in mind that milk is alkaline and an infant's stomach contents are likely to be of neutral pH (or only weakly acidic) for approximately two hours after each milk feed. Reflux events with a pH of greater than 4 will not be recorded by the pH probe. For neonates fed continuously or every one or two hours, this makes pH monitoring effectively useless. These events may still be injurious by causing laryngospasm or aspiration, for example. In addition, pepsin is active up to a pH of 6, and it may be pepsin rather than acid that causes the majority of tissue injury. Brief reflux events (less than 15 seconds) are also not recorded.

Intraluminal impedance testing uses a probe with a series of electrodes along its length. It is passed into the oesophageal lumen in the same way as a pH probe. When a bolus (solid or liquid) passes by, the electrical resistance between adjacent electrodes drops and the bolus can therefore be detected. Furthermore, the direction of travel of the bolus allows swallows to be distinguished from reflux events, and the height of a reflux event can also be detected. A pH probe at the distal end of the device completes the picture. With this technique it has been possible to show that 73 percent of reflux events in infants occur postprandially and are of neutral pH.[55] In most of these events, the refluxate reaches the pharynx. Equipment suitable for ambulatory use has recently been developed, but normal values for children have yet to be established. [**]

The findings on endoscopy can be highly suggestive of reflux, particularly the presence of hypopharyngeal cobblestone mucosa, oedema of the arytenoids, obliteration of the ventricle, vocal fold oedema and oedema of the posterior commissure (**Figure 100.2**). Other suggestive features include lingual tonsil hypertrophy, blunting of the carina and increased bronchial secretions. Some studies have shown a strong correlation between these findings and a diagnosis of gastro-oesophageal reflux,[56, 57] while others have not.[53] Oesophagitis is diagnostic, but is

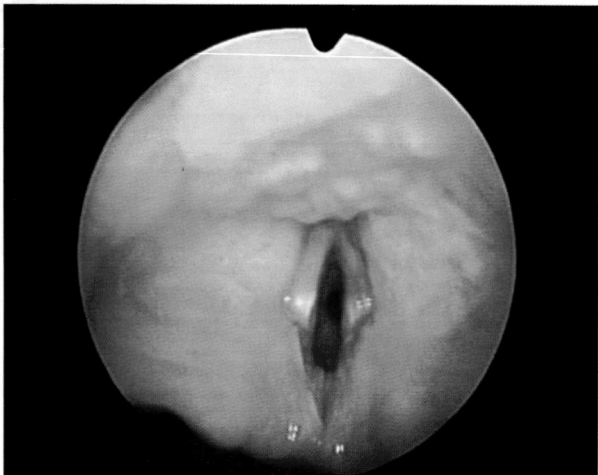

Figure 100.2 Endoscopic view of the larynx in a one-year-old girl with Down syndrome and a repaired tracheo-oesophageal fistula. There is severe cobblestoning of the mucosa on the laryngeal surface of the epiglottis, and also a subglottic stenosis, both attributed to reflux.

present in only a minority of children with reflux. In fact, the appearance of the oesophageal mucosa is often normal despite the presence of reflux, and biopsy is required to establish the diagnosis with certainty. [***]

Treatment

For many children with physiological reflux or very mild symptoms, expectant treatment is reasonable. If more significant reflux is suspected, a therapeutic trial of feed thickeners and advice on positioning, possibly with concomitant acid suppression, should be the first step.

There have been a number of randomized controlled trials that support the effectiveness of feed thickeners in reducing regurgitation, although none met the quality criteria for inclusion in a recent Cochrane systematic review.[58] Feed thickeners have the advantage of increasing the calorific value of the milk and thus promoting weight gain, but a modified teat may be required to allow the infant to feed effectively. [****]

The ideal position to reduce reflux in children over a year old is the left lateral position with the head of the bed elevated.[50] In infants, the prone position is best for reducing reflux, but has also been shown to increase the risk of SIDS. It is therefore not recommended. The left lateral position may be just as good as prone[59] if it can be maintained safely, but the right lateral position makes reflux worse.[60] Head elevation shows no benefit in infants and the use of an infant seat to achieve a semi-erect position actually makes reflux worse.[61] [****]

Antacids run the risk of causing toxicity in infants due to their high aluminium content and prolonged treatment is not recommended.[50] Alginates (such as Gaviscon) are widely used in children but there is no published

paediatric evidence to support their use. Prokinetic agents were once popular but the only consistently effective agent, cisapride, has been withdrawn due to cardiac side effects. Domperidone has its advocates, particularly for use in children with neurological disorders.

Acid suppression therapy is the mainstay of treatment for children with significant symptoms of gastro-oesophageal reflux disease. There are no trials, however, to demonstrate the effectiveness of such treatment for extra-oesophageal symptoms of reflux in children. Placebo-controlled trials support the use of H2 receptor antagonists for children with oesophagitis.[62, 63] Numerous trials have shown proton pump inhibitors (PPIs) to be more effective than H2 antagonists in adults, but studies of PPIs in children are limited to case series. It is difficult, therefore, to make clear recommendations about which drug to choose except to say that H2 antagonists are widely used and seem to be effective, while PPIs may be more effective but the evidence to support their use in children is lacking. Data on the effects of long-term acid suppression in children are also lacking. [**]

Selected children with reflux resistant to medical therapy may be selected for surgery in the form of a fundoplication. The procedure (now often performed laparoscopically) involves wrapping the fundus of the stomach around the intraabdominal portion of the oesophagus to produce a valve-like effect. Case series suggest that the procedure can be extremely effective for selected children with extra-oesophageal symptoms.[45, 64] [**]

KEY POINTS

- A degree of reflux is physiological in neonates.
- The prevalence of symptomatic reflux declines with age after the neonatal period.
- Some relationship between reflux and airway disorders has been established.
- A relationship between reflux and disorders of the ear and nose has been postulated but remains unproven.

Best clinical practice

✓ Reflux is often physiological and can be managed expectantly if symptoms are mild. [Grade C]
✓ A therapeutic trial of positioning, feed thickeners and acid suppression is an appropriate first step when significant reflux is suspected. [Grade C]
✓ The left lateral position is effective and in children above one year old a degree of head elevation should also be used. [Grade C]

✓ Acid suppression with H2 receptor antagonists or PPIs appears to be safe and effective but supportive published evidence is lacking. [Grade C]

✓ Diagnostic tests have limitations and should be reserved for cases where medical treatments have failed. [Grade C]

✓ Fundoplication surgery should be considered where symptoms are significant and medical treatments have failed. [Grade C]

Deficiencies in current knowledge and areas for future research

The relationship between reflux and otolaryngological disorders has been difficult to establish. In part, this may reflect the limitations of the currently available tests for the presence of reflux. Rigorous case definition is a prerequisite for any study, and particularly for studies on the effect of anti-reflux therapy on otolaryngological disorders. The introduction of intraluminal impedance testing may provide us with a tool to diagnose reflux with a degree of certainty that has been lacking until now.

ASPIRATION

Definition

Aspiration is the passage of foreign material beyond the vocal cords. This chapter will not cover acute airway obstruction due to aspiration of a foreign body, but rather the (usually chronic) aspiration of saliva, feeds and/or refluxed gastric contents.

Causes

The air and food passages cross to a much greater extent in man than in other mammals as a result of adaptations for speech, making us particularly predisposed to aspirate. A host of mechanisms exist to compensate for this and a deficiency in any one can lead to aspiration. Such deficiencies include impaired or incoordinate swallowing, impaired laryngeal sensation, impaired laryngeal elevation on swallowing and impaired true vocal fold adduction. Most commonly, aspiration presents in children with some combination of oesophageal dysmotility, poorly coordinated oral and pharyngeal phases of swallowing and impaired laryngeal reflexes resulting from neuromuscular disorders or cerebral palsy. Occasionally, oesophageal dysmotility can be an isolated phenomenon

in otherwise healthy infants.[65] Swallowing dysfunction may also be due to inadequate maturation of neurological control in premature infants. Many children who aspirate have reflux, but only a small minority of children with reflux will aspirate.[66] Laryngeal elevation is impaired by the presence of a tracheostomy tube and by endotracheal intubation, both of which predispose to aspiration, although aspiration can be reduced by applying positive pressure (positive-end expiratory pressure (PEEP) or continuous positive airway pressure (CPAP)).[67, 68] Nasogastric tubes do not seem to be a risk factor.[69]

Symptoms and signs

The typical clinical features in infants are apnoeas, bradycardias and choking attacks with feeds. There may be apparent life-threatening events (see above) and aspiration is not uncommon as a cause of sudden infant death.[70] Chronic aspiration may present as recurrent pneumonia. Aspiration may also occur without overt signs (silent aspiration), manifesting as progressive deterioration in respiratory function.

Diagnostic tests

The best available investigations at present are videofluoroscopy and fibreoptic endoscopic evaluation of swallow (FEES).

The videofluoroscopic modified barium swallow (often referred to simply as videofluoroscopy) is usually carried out in conjunction with a speech and language therapist. Various consistencies of radio-opaque material, ranging from thin liquid to solid, are swallowed and followed on x-ray fluoroscopy. The investigation provides excellent information about the coordination and completeness of the oral and pharyngeal stages of the swallow, as well as the presence of aspiration. Videofluoroscopy is a detailed and dynamic investigation that provides considerably more information than a standard contrast swallow, whose only use in this regard is to exclude tracheo-oesophageal fistula and oesophageal stricture. [*]

FEES has the advantage over videofluoroscopy of being performed at the bedside or in the outpatient clinic. It may also be more sensitive for aspiration.[71] The swallow is observed using a fibreoptic endoscope positioned just behind the soft palate via the nose. Coloured liquid is easiest to see. The investigation gives information about palatal elevation, leakage into the pharynx during the oral phase, pharyngeal residue and aspiration. Fibreoptic endoscopic evaluation of swallowing with sensory testing (FEESST) is an extension of the technique that also provides information on laryngeal sensation, although its use in children is less widespread. With experience and a cooperative child, FEES is possible even in very young children.[72] [*]

It is possible to identify aspiration using oral administration of a radioactive substance which can be identified in the lungs on scintigraphy.[73, 74] The procedure is extremely operator-dependent and the quality of the images obtained is poor. [*]

Endoscopy is useful in a number of ways. Microlaryngoscopy-bronchoscopy under general anaesthetic is the only way to reliably exclude a laryngeal cleft, although a fibreoptic laryngoscopy should identify vocal cord palsy. Bronchoscopy (fibreoptic or rigid) allows bronchoalveolar lavage samples to be obtained for the identification of lipid-laden ('foamy') macrophages, although the sensitivity and specificity of this for aspiration has been reported to be poor.[75, 76, 77] [***]

Management

Minor degrees of aspiration may be managed by altering the consistency of feeds according to the results of the videofluoroscopy. A speech and language therapist should supervise this, and will also be able to give advice on head positioning during feeds. The decision to stop oral feeds in infants in favour of tube feeding should not be taken lightly as it may be extremely difficult for oral feeds to be re-established in a child who has not developed the necessary oral skills early in life. Tube feeding (either by nasogastric tube or gastrostomy), however, is often unavoidable. [*]

Where aspiration of refluxed gastric contents is a major problem, control of the reflux by fundoplication may be helpful. Equally, if aspiration of saliva is a major issue despite tube feeding, a procedure to reduce saliva production may be beneficial. This may take the form of excision of the submandibular glands with bilateral parotid duct ligation,[78] or alternatively simple ligation of all four major salivary gland ducts.[79] Injection medialization of a paralyzed vocal cord may reduce aspiration[80] but carries a risk of impairing the airway. [**]

Tracheostomy will often make aspiration worse by preventing laryngeal elevation on swallowing. It does, however, allow easy access to the chest for suctioning and may, of course, be indicated for other reasons in these children with multiple problems. Even a cuffed tube does not prevent aspiration as secretions pool above the cuff and the seal is never perfect. Tubes are available with a low-pressure cuff and a suction port above it if this is a problem. [*]

Ultimately, when all else has been tried, it may be necessary to consider a procedure to separate the air and food passages completely. Laryngotracheal separation is the procedure of choice and has the advantage over both laryngeal closure (suturing the false cords together above a tracheostomy[81]) and total laryngectomy, being reversible, at least in theory. The procedure involves transecting the cervical trachea and bringing out the lower end as

a permanent end-stoma. The upper end of the trachea can be closed off as a blind pouch or anastomosed end-to-side to the oesophagus. The procedure produces good results and may allow the resumption of oral feeds.[82, 83] However, this is at the expense of voice. Most children considered for this procedure will be nonverbal but the decision to sacrifice speech is clearly one that cannot be taken lightly. [**]

KEY POINTS

- The following are risk factors for aspiration:
  - cerebral palsy;
  - neuromuscular disorders;
  - impaired oesophageal motility;
  - prematurity;
  - gastro-oesophageal reflux;
  - tracheostomy.
- The following otolaryngologic diagnoses should be considered:
  - laryngeal cleft;
  - tracheo-oesophageal fistula;
  - vocal cord palsy.

Best clinical practice

✓ A speech and language therapist should be involved from the outset. [Grade C/D]
✓ Videofluoroscopy and/or FEES are the investigations of choice. [Grade C/D]
✓ Endoscopy has a role in certain situations. [Grade C/D]
✓ Alterations in feed consistency may be all that is required in mild cases. [Grade C/D]
✓ Tube feeding is often necessary. [Grade C/D]
✓ Fundoplication and salivary surgery have a small but important role. [Grade C/D]
✓ Laryngotracheal separation surgery is effective but sacrifices voice. [Grade C/D]

Deficiencies in current knowledge and areas for future research

Few centres treat large numbers of children, so most of the published literature consists of relatively small retrospective case series. Any large, prospective evaluation of diagnostic tests or treatment options would be a useful addition to current knowledge.

REFERENCES

1. Peter C, Wiechers C, Bohnhorst B, Silny J, Poets C. Influence of nasogastric tubes in gastroesophageal reflux in preterm infants: a multiple intraluminal impedence study. *Journal of Pediatrics*. 2002; **141**: 277-9.

2. Nelson SP, Chen EH, Syniar GM, Christoffel KK. Prevalence of symptoms of gastroesophageal reflux during infancy: a pediatric practice-based survey. *Archives of Pediatrics and Adolescent Medicine*. 1997; **151**: 569-72.

3. Nelson SP, Chen EH, Syniar GM, Christoffel KK. Prevalence of symptoms of gastroesophageal reflux during childhood: a pediatric practice-based survey. *Archives of Pediatrics and Adolescent Medicine*. 2000; **154**: 150-4.

4. Gold BD. Outcomes of pediatric gastroesophageal reflux disease: in the first year of life, in childhood, and in adults...oh, and should we really leave Helicobacter pylori alone? *Journal of Pediatric Gastroenterology and Nutrition*. 2003; **37**: s33-9.

5. el-Serag HB, Gilger M, Carter J, Genta RM, Rabeneck L. Childhood GERD is a risk factor for GERD in adolescents and young adults. *American Journal of Gastroenterology*. 2004; **99**: 806-12.

6. Gorenstein A, Cohen A, Cordova Z, Witzling M, Krutman B, Serour F. Hiatal hernia in pediatric gastroesophageal reflux. *Journal of Pediatric Gastroenterology and Nutrition*. 2001; **33**: 554-7.

7. Omari T, Barnett C, Snel A, Davidson G, Haslam R, Bakewell M *et al*. Mechanism of gastroesophageal reflux in premature infants with chronic lung disease. *Journal of Pediatric Surgery*. 1999; **34**: 1795-8.

8. Omari T, Barnett C, Benninga M, Lontis R, Goodchild L, Haslam R *et al*. Mechanisms of gastro-oesophageal reflux in preterm and term infants with reflux disease. *Gut*. 2002; **51**: 475-9.

9. Kawahara H, Dent J, Davidson G. Mechanisms responsible for gastroesophageal reflux in children. *Gastroenterology*. 1997; **113**: 399-408.

10. Omari TI, Barnett C, Snel A, Goldsworthy W, Haslam R, Davidson G *et al*. Mechanisms of gastroesophageal reflux in healthy premature infants. *Journal of Pediatrics*. 1998; **133**: 650-4.

11. Mittal RK, Holloway RH, Penagini R, Blackshaw LA, Dent J. Transient lower esophageal sphincter relaxation. *Gastroenterology*. 1995; **109**: 601-10.

12. Heacock HJ, Jeffery HE, Baker JL, Page M. Influence of breast versus formula milk on physiological gastroesophageal reflux in healthy newborn infants. *Journal of Pediatric Gastroenterology and Nutrition*. 1992; **14**: 41-6.

13. Cavataio F, Iacono G, Monalto G, Soresi M, Tumminello M, Carroccio A. Clinical and pH-metric characteristics of gastro-oesophageal reflux secondary to cows' milk protein allergy. *Archives of Disease in Childhood*. 1996; **75**: 51-6.

14. Hu FZ, Donfack J, Ahmed A, Dopico R, Johnson S, Post JC *et al*. Fine-mapping a gene for pediatric gastroesophageal reflux on human chromosome 13q14. *Human Genetics*. 2004; **114**: 562-72.

15. Jeffery H, Rahilly P, Read D. Multiple causes of asphyxia in infants at high risk for sudden infant death. *Archives of Disease in Childhood*. 1983; **58**: 92-100.

16. Harris P, Munoz C, Mobarec S, Brockmann P, Mesa T, Sanchez I. Relevance of the pH probe in sleep study analysis in infants. *Child: Care, Health and Development*. 2004; **30**: 337-44.

17. Herbst J, Minton S, Book L. Gastroesophageal reflux causing respiratory distress and apnea in newborn infants. *Journal of Pediatrics*. 1979; **95**: 763-8.

18. MacFadyen UM, Hendry GMA, Simpson H. Gastro-oesophageal reflux in near-miss sudden infant death syndrome or suspected recurrent aspiration. *Archives of Disease in Childhood*. 1983; **58**: 87-91.

19. McMurray JS, Holinger LD. Otolaryngic manifestations in children presenting with apparent life-threatening events. *Otolaryngology-Head and Neck Surgery*. 1997; **116**: 575-9.

20. Gumpert L, Kalach N, Dupont C, Contencin P. Hoarseness and gastroesophageal reflux in children. *Journal of Laryngology and Otology*. 1998; **112**: 49-54.

21. Contencin P, Narcy P. Gastropharyngeal reflux in infants and children: a pharyngeal pH monitoring study. *Archives of Otolaryngology – Head and Neck Surgery*. 1992; **118**: 1028-30.

22. Waki E, Madgy DN, Belenky WM, Gower VC. The incidence of gastroesophageal reflux in recurrent croup. *International Journal of Pediatric Otorhinolaryngology*. 1995; **32**: 223-32.

23. el-Serag H, Gilger M, Kuebeler M, Rabeneck L. Extraesophageal associations of gastroesophageal reflux disease in chidren without neurological defects. *Gastroenterology*. 2001; **121**: 1294-9.

24. Roger G, Denoyelle F, Triglia J, Garabedian E-N. Severe laryngomalacia: surgical indications and results in 115 patients. *Laryngoscope*. 1995; **105**: 1111-7.

25. Giannoni C, Sulek M, Friedman EM, Duncan NO. Gastroesophageal reflux association with laryngomalacia: a prospective study. *International Journal of Pediatric Otorhinolaryngology*. 1998; **43**: 11-20.

26. Matthews BL, Little JP, McGuirt WF, Koufman JA. Reflux in infants with laryngomalacia: results of 24-hour dual-probe pH monitoring. *Otolaryngology-Head and Neck Surgery*. 1999; **120**: 860-4.

27. Bibi H, Khvolis E, Shoseyov D, Ohaly M, Dor D, London D *et al*. The prevalence of gastroesophageal reflux in children with tracheomalacia and laryngomalacia. *Chest*. 2001; **119**: 409-13.

28. Hadfield PJ, Albert DM, Bailey CM, Lindley K, Pierro A. The effect of aryepiglottoplasty for laryngomalacia on gastro-oesophageal reflux. *International Journal of Pediatric Otorhinolaryngology*. 2003; **67**: 11-4.

29. Halstead LA. Gastroesophageal reflux: a critical factor in pediatric subglottic stenosis. *Otolaryngology-Head and Neck Surgery*. 1999; **120**: 683-8.

30. Walner D, Stern Y, Gerber M, Rudolph C, Baldwin C, Cotton R. Gastroesophageal reflux in patients with subglottic stenosis. *Archives of Otolaryngology – Head and Neck Surgery.* 1998; **124**: 551–5.

31. Berkowitz R. Failed paediatric laryngotracheoplasty. *Australian and New Zealand Journal of Surgery.* 2001; **71**: 292–6.

32. Ludemann J, Hughes C, Noah Z, Holinger L. Complications of pediatric laryngotracheal reconstruction: prevention strategies. *Annals of Otology, Rhinology and Laryngology.* 1999; **108**: 1019–26.

33. Zalzal G, Choi S, Petal K. The effect of gastroesophageal reflux on laryngotracheal reconstruction. *Archives of Otolaryngology – Head and Neck Surgery.* 1996; **122**: 297–300.

34. Kubba H, Gibson D, Bailey C, Hartley B. Techniques and outcomes of laryngeal cleft repair: an update to the Great Ormond Street Hospital series. *Annals of Otology, Rhinology and Laryngology.* 2005; **114**: 309–13.

35. Hof E, Hirsig J, Giedion A, Pochon J-P. Deleterious consequences of gastroesophageal reflux in cleft larynx surgery. *Journal of Pediatric Surgery.* 1987; **22**: 197–9.

36. Borkowski G, Sommer P, Stark T, Sudhoff H, Luckhaupt H. Recurrent respiratory papillomatosis associated with gastroesophageal reflux disease in children. *European Archives of Oto-Rhino-Laryngology.* 1999; **256**: 370–2.

37. Holland B, Koufman J, Postma G, McGuirt WJ. Laryngopharyngeal reflux and laryngeal web formation in patients with pediatric recurrent respiratory papillomas. *Laryngoscope.* 2002; **112**: 1926–9.

38. Beste DJ, Conley SF, Brown CW. Gastroesophageal reflux complicating choanal atresia repair. *International Journal of Pediatric Otorhinolaryngology.* 1994; **29**: 51–8.

39. Loehrl T, Smith T. Chronic sinusitis and gastroesophageal reflux: are they related? *Current Opinion in Otolaryngology Head and Neck Surgery.* 2004; **12**: 18–20.

40. Phipps C, Wood W, Gibson W, Cochran W. Gastroesophageal reflux contributing to chronic sinus disease in children: a prospective analysis. *Archives of Otolaryngology-Head and Neck Surgery.* 2000; **126**: 831–6.

41. Bothwell MR, Parsons DS, Talbot A, Barbero GJ, Wilder B. Outcome of reflux therapy on pediatric chronic sinusitis. *Otolaryngology – Head and Neck Surgery.* 1999; **121**: 255–62.

42. Contencin P, Narcy P. Nasopharyngeal pH monitoring in infants and children with chronic rhinopharyngitis. *International Journal of Pediatric Otorhinolaryngology.* 1991; **22**: 249–56.

43. Carr M, Poje C, Ehrig D, Brodsky L. Incidence of reflux in children undergoing adenoidectomy. *Laryngoscope.* 2001; **111**: 2170–2.

44. van den Abeele T, Couloigner V, Faure C, Narcy P. The role of 24h pH recording in pediatric otolaryngologic gastro-oesophageal reflux disease. *International Journal of Pediatric Otorhinolaryngology.* 2003; **67**: s95–100.

45. Suskind D, Zeringue G, Kluka E, Udall J, Liu D. Gastroesophageal reflux and pediatric otolaryngologic disease: the role of antireflux surgery. *Archives of Otolaryngology-Head and Neck Surgery.* 2001; **127**: 511–4.

46. Tasker A, Dettmar P, Pearson J. Reflux of gastric juice in glue ear. *Lancet.* 2002; **359**: 493.

47. Velepic M, Rozmanic V, Velepic M, Bonifacic D. Gastroesophageal reflux, allergy and chronic tubotympanal disorders in children. *International Journal of Pediatric Otorhinolaryngology.* 2000; **55**: 187–90.

48. Rozmanic V, Velepic M, Ahel V, Bonifacic D, Velepic M. Prolonged esophageal pH monitoring in the evaluation of gastroesophageal reflux in children with chronic tubotympanal disorders. *Journal of Pediatric Gastroenterology and Nutrition.* 2002; **34**: 278–80.

49. Gibson WS, Cochran W. Otalgia in infants and children – a manifestation of gastroesophageal reflux. *International Journal of Pediatric Otorhinolaryngology.* 1994; **28**: 213–8.

* 50. Rudolph CD, Mazur LJ, Liptak GS, Baker RD, Boyle JT, Colletti RB *et al.* Guidelines for evaluation and treatment of gastroesophageal reflux in infants and children: recommendations of the North American Society for Pediatric Gastroenterology and Nutrition. *Journal of Pediatric Gastroenterology and Nutrition.* 2001; **32**: s1–31.

51. Little JP, Matthews BL, Glock MS, Koufman JA, Reboussin DM, Loughlin CJ *et al.* Extraesophageal pediatric reflux: 24-hour double-probe pH monitoring of 222 children. *Annals of Otology, Rhinology and Laryngology.* 1997; **106**: 1–16.

52. Bauman NM, Bishop WP, Sandler AD, Smith RJH. Value of pH probe testing in pediatric patients with extraesophageal manifestations of gastroesophageal reflux disease: a retrospective review. *Annals of Otology, Rhinology and Laryngology.* 2000; **109**: 18–24.

53. McMurray JS, Gerber M, Stern Y, Walner D, Rudolph C, Willging JP *et al.* Role of laryngoscopy, dual pH probe monitoring, and laryngeal mucosal biopsy in the diagnosis of pharyngoesophageal reflux. *Annals of Otology, Rhinology and Laryngology.* 2001; **110**: 299–304.

54. Rabinowitz SS, Piecuch S, Jibaly R, Goldsmith A, Schwarz SM. Optimizing the diagnosis of gastroesophageal reflux in children with otolaryngological symptoms. *International Journal of Pediatric Otorhinolaryngology.* 2003; **67**: 621–6.

* 55. Skopnik H, Silny J, Heiber O, Schulz J, Rau G, Heiman G. Gastroesophageal reflux in infants: evaluation of a new intraluminal impedance technique. *Journal of Pediatric Gastroenterology and Nutrition.* 1996; **23**: 591–8.

56. Carr MM, Nagy ML, Pizzuto MP, Poje CP, Brodsky LS. Correlation of findings at direct laryngoscopy and bronchcosopy with gastroesophageal reflux disease in children: a prospective study. *Archives of Otolaryngology – Head and Neck Surgery.* 2001; **127**: 369–74.

57. Carr MM, Nguyen A, Poje C, Pizzuto M, Nagy M, Brodsky L. Correlation of findings on direct laryngoscopy and bronchoscopy with presence of extraesophageal reflux disease. *Laryngoscope*. 2000; **110**: 1560–2.

∗ 58. Huang R-C, Forbes DA, Davies MW. Feed thickener for newborn infants with gastro-oesophageal reflux (systematic review). *Cochrane Library*. 2004: **3**.

59. Ewer AK, James ME, Tobin JM. Prone and left lateral positioning reduce gastro-oesophageal reflux in preterm infants. *Archives of Disease in Childhood Fetal and Neonatal Edition*. 1999; **81**: f201–05.

60. Omari TI, Rommel N, Staunton E, Lontis R, Goodchild L, Haslam R et al. Paradoxical impact of body positioning on gastroesophageal reflux and gastric emptying in the premature neonate. *Journal of Pediatrics*. 2004; **145**: 194–200.

∗ 61. Carroll AE, Garrison MM, Christakis DA. A systematic review of nonpharmacological and nonsurgical therapies for gastroesophageal reflux in infants. *Archives of Pediatrics and Adolescent Medicine*. 2002; **156**: 109–13.

62. Cucchiara S, Gobio-Casali L, Balli F, Magazzu G, Staiano A et al. Cimetidine treatment of reflux esophagitis in children: an Italian multicentric study. *Journal of Pediatric Gastroenterology and Nutrition*. 1989; **8**: 150–6.

63. Simeone D, Caria MC, Miele E, Staiano A. Treatment of childhood peptic esophagitis: a double-blind placebo-controlled trial of nizatidine. *Journal of Pediatric Gastroenterology and Nutrition*. 1997; **25**: 51–5.

64. Mattioli G, Sacco O, Repetto P, Pini-Prato A, Castagnetti M, Carlini C et al. Necessity for surgery in children with gastrooesophageal reflux and supraoesophageal symptoms. *European Journal of Pediatric Surgery*. 2004; **14**: 7–13.

65. Sheikh S, Allen E, Shell R, Hruschak J, Iram D, Castile R et al. Chronic aspiration without gastroesophageal reflux as a cause of respiratory symptoms in neurologically normal infants. *Chest*. 2001; **120**: 1190–5.

66. McVeagh P, Howman-Giles R, Kemp A. Pulmonary aspiration studied by radionuclide milk scanning and barium swallow roentgenography. *American Journal of Diseases of Children*. 1987; **141**: 917–21.

67. Finder JD, Yellon R, Charron M. Successful management of tracheotomized patients with chronic saliva aspiration by use of constant positive airway pressure. *Pediatrics*. 2001; **107**: 1343–5.

68. Janson BA, Poulton TJ. Does PEEP reduce the incidence of aspiration around endotracheal tubes? *Canadian Anaesthetists Society Journal*. 1986; **33**: 157–61.

69. Bar-Maor JA, Lam M. Does nasogastric tube cause pulmonary aspiration in children? *Pediatrics*. 1991; **87**: 113–4.

70. Iwadate K, Doy M, Ito Y. Screening of milk aspiration in 105 infant death cases by immunostaining with anti-human alpha-lactalbumin antibody. *Forensic Science International*. 2001; **122**: 95–100.

71. Hiss SG, Postma GN. Fibreoptic endoscopic evaluation of swallow. *Laryngoscope*. 2003; **113**: 1386–93.

∗ 72. Hartnick CJ, Hartley BE, Miller C, Willging JP. Pediatric fiberoptic endoscopic evaluation of swallowing. *Annals of Otology, Rhinology and Laryngology*. 2000; **109**: 996–9.

73. Boonyaprapa S, Alderson PO, Garfinkel DJ, Chipps BE, Wagner HJ. Detection of pulmonary aspiration in infants and children with respiratory disease: concise communication. *Journal of Nuclear Medicine*. 1980; **21**: 314–8.

74. Cook SP, Lawless ST, Mandell GA, Reilly JS. The use of the salivagram in the evaluation of severe and chronic aspiration. *International Journal of Pediatric Otorhinolaryngology*. 1997; **41**: 353–61.

75. Staugas R, Martin AJ, Binns G, Steven IM. The significance of fat-filled macrophages in the diagnosis of aspiration associated with gastro-oesophageal reflux. *Australian Paediatric Journal*. 1985; **21**: 275–7.

76. Knauer-Fischer S, Ratjen F. Lipid-laden macrophages in bronchoalveolar lavage fluid as a marker for pulmonary aspiration. *Pediatric Pulmonology*. 1999; **27**: 419–22.

77. Krishnan U, Mitchell JD, Tobias V, Day AS, Bohane TD. Fat laden macrophages in tracheal aspirates as a marker of reflux aspiration: a negative report. *Journal of Pediatric Gastroenterology and Nutrition*. 2002; **35**: 309–13.

78. Gerber M, Gaugler MD, Myer CM, Cotton RT. Chronic aspiration in children: when are bilateral submandibular gland excision and parotid duct ligation indicated? *Archives of Otolaryngology – Head and Neck Surgery*. 1996; **122**: 1368–71.

79. Klem C, Mair EA. Four-duct ligation: a simple and effective treatment for chronic aspiration from sialorrhea. *Archives of Otolaryngology – Head and Neck Surgery*. 1999; **125**: 796–800.

80. Patel NJ, Kerschner JE, Merati AL. The use of injectable collagen in the management of pediatric vocal unilateral fold paralysis. *International Journal of Pediatric Otorhinolaryngology*. 2003; **67**: 1355–60.

81. Pototschnig CA, Schneider I, Eckel HE, Thumfart WF. Repeatedly successful closure of the larynx for the treatment of chronic aspiration with the use of botulinum toxin A. *Annals of Otology, Rhinology and Laryngology*. 1996; **105**: 521–4.

82. Cook SP, Lawless ST, Kettrick R. Patient selection for primary laryngotracheal separation as treatment of chronic aspiration in the impaired child. *International Journal of Pediatric Otorhinolaryngology*. 1996; **38**: 103–13.

83. Takamizawa S, Tsugawa C, Nishijima E, Muraji T, Satoh S. Laryngotracheal separation for intractable aspiration pneumonia in neurologically impaired children: experience with 11 cases. *Journal of Pediatric Surgery*. 2003; **38**: 975–7.

101

Diseases of the oesophagus, swallowing disorders and caustic ingestion

LEWIS SPITZ

Embryology	1282	Key points	1291
Oesophageal atresia	1282	Best clinical practice	1292
Congenital oesophageal stenosis	1287	Deficiencies in current knowledge and areas for future	
Achalasia	1288	research	1292
Corrosive injury to the oesophagus	1290	References	1292

SEARCH STRATEGY

The author's extensive bibliography on congenital and acquired diseases of the oesophagus in children was supplemented with a Medline search using the key words oesophagus, child, congenital, caustic, achalasia, oesophageal stenosis, tracheo-oesophageal fistula and tracheomalacia. The Cochrane library was also consulted. Mr Colin Bailie FRCS, Consultant Paediatric Surgeon at the Royal Liverpool Children's Hospital advised the section editor before completion of the final draft.

EMBRYOLOGY

The oesophagus and trachea first become identifiable as separate structures when the embryo is 22–23 days old. The lung bud appears as a median ventral diverticulum in the developing foregut. Shortly thereafter, the primitive stomach appears as a fusiform enlargement immediately caudal to the diverticulum. The oesophagus develops from the short area between the tracheal diverticulum and the stomach. As the trachea and oesophagus elongate, ridges appear in the lateral walls. Fusion in the midline of these ridges separates the trachea from the oesophagus. The separation process commences caudally, proceeds cranially and is complete between days 34 and 36 of gestation. Elongation of the oesophagus relative to the rest of the developing foetus begins in the distal portion and is complete by seven weeks. Kluth cast doubt on the lateral ridge theory of oesophagotracheal separation and proposed an alternative dorsal and lateral ridge theory.[1]

The circular musculature of the oesophagus appears in the sixth week and by the end of that week innervation by the vagus nerve has commenced. During the seventh and eighth weeks, the epithelium of the oesophagus proliferates to such an extent that the lumen is virtually, but not completely, occluded. Initially, the epithelium is ciliated but it is gradually replaced by stratified squamous epithelium (see Chapter 65, Head and neck embryology).

OESOPHAGEAL ATRESIA

In oesophageal atresia, part of the wall of the oesophagus fails to develop. In most cases this is associated with a failure of complete separation of the developing trachea – hence the persistence of a tracheo-oesophageal fistula. This was a uniformly fatal congenital abnormality until 1939 when Levin and Ladd independently reported the first two survivors. Both infants required multiple procedures – cervical oesophagostomy, feeding gastrostomy and subsequently oesophageal substitution. The first successful primary repair of the defect, which paved the way for future developments, was achieved by Haight, in 1941.[2, 3] It is now rare for an infant with oesophageal atresia to succumb from oesophageal atresia alone, unless it is associated with extreme prematurity or a major congenital cardiac defect.[4, 5]

Incidence

Abnormalities in oesophageal development are present in 1:3000–4000 live births. There is no standard genetic pattern of inheritance, although the condition has been documented in siblings, in one and very occasionally in both twins and in two generations.[6]

Pathogenesis

The anomaly is thought to arise between the third and sixth weeks of intrauterine development. The precise cause and mechanism are unknown. Failure of complete separation of the foregut from the respiratory tract would appear to be the basis for the development of the various types of defects.[7, 8, 9] Oesophageal atresia may occur as an isolated anomaly but at least 50 percent of cases have additional malformations.

Types of anomaly

The variety and incidence of the different types of tracheo-oesophageal abnormalities are shown in **Table 101.1**. It is especially important for the otolaryngologist to be alert to the possibility of a tracheo-oesophageal fistula without oesophageal atresia ('H' type) as this may present in later childhood with recurrent respiratory infections. It may be discovered as an incidental finding at bronchoscopy, when a suction canula in the tracheal lumen is found to enter the fistula. Often the tracheal orifice can be concealed in a mucosal fold. It may

Table 101.1 Different types of tracheo-oesophageal anomalies.

Type of anomaly	%
Oesophageal atresia with distal tracheo-oesophageal fistula	87
Oesophageal atresia without tracheo-oesophageal fistula	6–7
Oesophageal atresia with proximal tracheo-oesophageal fistula	2
Oesophageal atresia with proximal and distal tracheo-oesophageal fistula	1
Tracheo-oesophageal fistula without oesophageal atresia	3–4

sometimes be recognized at flexible bronchoscopy in a newborn baby.[10]

Associated anomalies

Additional congenital malformations are found in approximately one-half of infants with tracheo-oesophageal anomalies. The various systems affected are as shown in **Table 101.2** with multiple defects occurring in many patients.[11] The mortality in oesophageal atresia is directly related to the severity of associated congenital anomalies particularly cardiac defects, and the degree of prematurity (**Table 101.3**).[4, 5]

The VACTERL complex

The VATER complex of associated anomalies was described by Quan and Smith in 1973.[12] (The acronym stands for V = *v*ertebral, A = *a*norectal, T-E = *t*racheo-oesophageal fistula and (o)*e*sophageal atresia, R = *r*adial and *r*enal dysplasia.) This was subsequently extended to the VACTERL association to include cardiac and limb abnormalities.

Ventricular septal defects are the single most common cardiac malformation.[13] Of the gastrointestinal anomalies, duodenal atresia, Meckel's diverticulum and malrotation are most commonly encountered. A variety of genitourinary anomalies may be present in association

Table 101.2 Congenital anomalies associated with oesophageal atresia/tracheo-oesophageal fistula.

Type of anomaly	%
Cardiovascular defects	34
Vertebrae anomalies	17
Gastrointestinal (excluding anorectal) anomalies	14
Genitourinary anomalies	12
Anorectal malformations	11
Skeletal defects	11
Respiratory anomalies	6
Genetic/chromosomal defects	2
Miscellaneous anomalies	10

Table 101.3 Risk classification for infants with oesophageal atresia.

Group	Birth weight (g)		Major cardiac anomaly	% Survival
I	>1500		No	>95
II	<1500	Or	Present	60
III	<1500	PLUS	Present	25

with oesophageal atresia, the most serious being bilateral renal agenesis (Potter's syndrome), which is fatal. The anorectal anomalies are equally divided between the supralevator (high) and translevator (low) defects.

Diagnosis

Polyhydramnios is nonspecific but is present in approximately 90 percent of mothers of infants with oesophageal atresia. Antenatal ultrasound scan may be indicative of oesophageal atresia without fistula when there is failure to demonstrate the presence of intragastric fluid.[14] To confirm the diagnosis of oesophageal atresia suspected on prenatal ultrasound scan, Langer, and later Levine, have proposed magnetic resonance imaging.[15, 16, 17] The overall prognosis for these foetuses is poor, due to the high incidence of chromosomal abnormalities.[18] Of 16 cases of prenatally diagnosed oesophageal atresia, only 4 (25 percent) survived the neonatal period. The infant, at birth, is 'excessively mucusy' and requires repeated suction as it is unable to swallow saliva. Failure to recognize the anomaly at this stage will expose the infant to choking episodes and aspiration pneumonitis with the first feed. The diagnosis is confirmed by passing a large calibre (No. 10 French) firm catheter through the mouth and into the oesophagus. The position of arrest of the tube is confirmed on a chest x-ray (**Figure 101.1**). If the tube enters the stomach, there is no oesophageal atresia. In the majority of cases with this condition the tube cannot be advanced more than 10 cm beyond the lower gum margin. It is important to include the abdomen on the original x-ray in order to assess the presence of intestinal gas shadows (**Figure 101.2**). Gas within the gastrointestinal tract implies the presence of a distal tracheo-oesophageal fistula while the distribution of the gas may indicate an additional intestinal anomaly, e.g. duodenal atresia. The chest radiograph should be assessed for pulmonary pathology and the configuration of the heart shadow may be indicative of cardiac defects, e.g. Fallot's tetralogy.

Management

Treatment of infants with oesophageal atresia should be concentrated in centres where the surgical expertise, supportive services (anaesthesia, paediatric intensive care, radiology, pathology) and specialized nursing care are available. Transfer to such centres should be prompt to avoid exposing the infant to the risks of aspiration pneumonitis. The infant is transported in a portable incubator either in a lateral position or in the prone position in order to discourage reflux of gastric juice into the distal tracheo-oesophageal fistula, while continuous suction is applied to the upper pouch to prevent

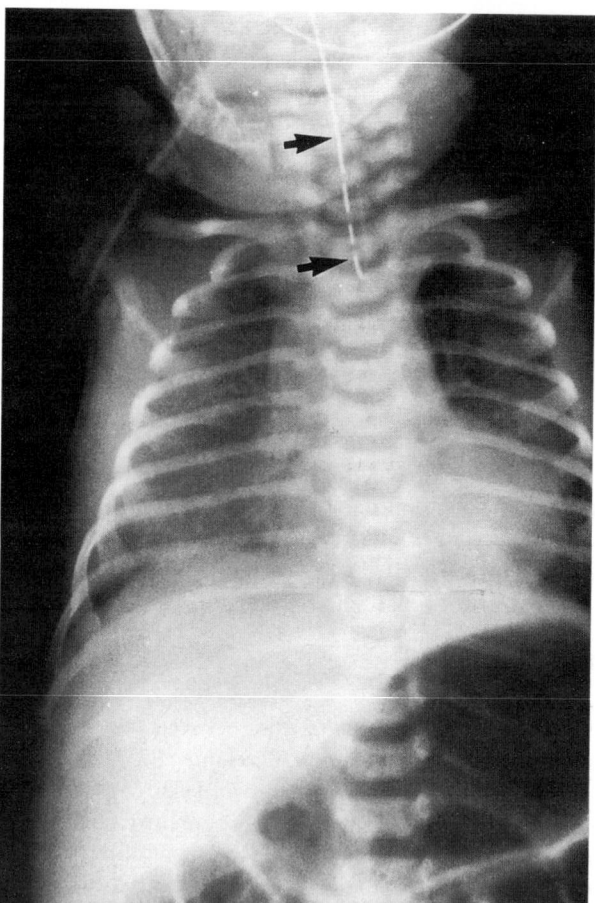

Figure 101.1   Plain x-ray of the chest and upper abdomen in an infant with oesophageal atresia. The radiopaque tube can be seen in the upper oesophagus. Gas in the intestines indicates the presence of a distal tracheo-oesophageal fistula.

aspiration of saliva. Definitive repair may have to be postponed in the presence of aspiration pneumonitis, which generally responds very rapidly to broad-spectrum antibiotics and physiotherapy. [***] In the infant with severe respiratory distress requiring mechanical ventilatory support, consideration should be given to emergency ligation of the distal tracheo-oesophageal fistula to facilitate respiratory support and to prevent overdistension of the stomach and intestine.[19]

SURGICAL REPAIR

The operative procedure is carried out under general endotracheal anaesthesia. Preliminary bronchoscopy to document the level of entry of the tracheo-oesophageal fistula, to assess tracheomalacia and to exclude an upper pouch fistula is recommended. Access is achieved via a right posterolateral extrapleural thoracotomy through the fourth or fifth intercostal space. After dividing the azygos vein, the distal oesophagus is identified and traced proximally to its site of entry into the trachea. The fistula is divided and the tracheal defect closed with fine

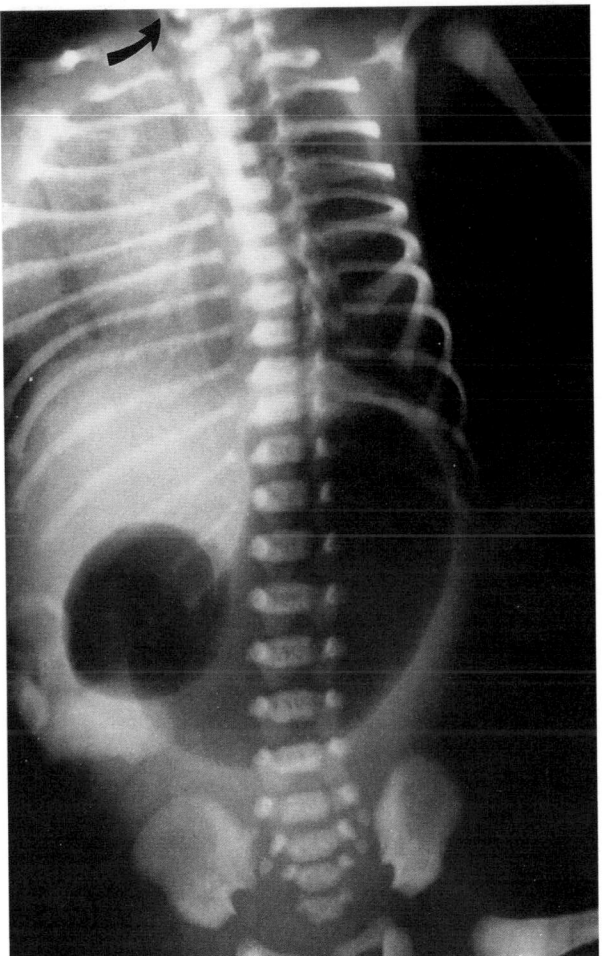

Figure 101.2 Plain x-ray of the chest and abdomen in an infant with oesophageal atresia. The tip of the catheter can be seen at the thoracic inlet. The gas pattern in the abdomen indicates the presence of a duodenal atresia ('double bubble').

interrupted nonabsorbable sutures. The proximal blind end of the oesophagus is identified in the apex of the chest and mobilized sufficiently to effect an anastomosis with as little tension as possible. An end-to-end anastomosis is performed using a single layer of sutures (**Figure 101.3**).

The operative correction of oesophageal atresia has recently been carried out thoracoscopically, but this requires considerable expertise and can only be safely carried out in specific centres.[20, 21] [**/*]

An oesophagomyotomy,[22] oesophagoplasty[23] or the use of elective paralysis and mechanical ventilation for a few days postoperatively in an extremely tight anastomosis may be effective in reducing the incidence of anastomotic complications.

The passage of a fine transanastomotic nasogastric tube through the nose into the stomach will allow enteral feeding to commence on the second or third postoperative day. A gastrostomy tube is no longer indicated in the routine repair of an oesophageal atresia. In fact,

the fashioning of a gastrostomy exposes the infant to an increased incidence of gastro-oesophageal reflux which predisposes the anastomosis to stricture formation.[24] [**/*]

Oral feeding has been introduced as early as the second postoperative day but is generally postponed until three to four days after surgery.

A contrast oesophagogram may be performed on the fifth postoperative day to check the anastomosis.

Patients with a long gap between the proximal and distal segment (particularly those with an isolated oesophageal atresia) require special attention. The alternative approaches available are to delay the repair pending differential growth of the oesophageal segments towards each other (three months), or to perform a cervical oesophagostomy and carry out an oesophageal substitution at a later stage – colonic interposition,[25] gastric tube[26] or gastric transposition.[27]

Results and prognosis

The survival rate for infants born with oesophageal atresia has improved significantly due to improved operative technique, better anaesthesia and greatly improved postoperative intensive care. The main determinants of survival are birth weight above 1500 g and the presence or absence of a significant cardiac anomaly.

Complications

Complications of oesophageal atresia repair may be divided into early and late.

- **Early complications** include anastomotic leak, strictures, recurrent tracheo-oesophageal fistula and vocal cord palsy.
- **Late complications** comprise tracheomalacia, gastro-oesophageal reflux and disordered oesophageal peristalsis.

ANASTOMOTIC LEAKS

The incidence varies from 4 to 36 percent, depending on the vigour with which the diagnosis is pursued. [***] The majority of leaks are insignificant and are mainly detected on routine contrast studies. Minor leaks seal spontaneously but may lead to stricture formation. Major leaks present within 48–72 hours postoperatively and cause respiratory distress due to tension pneumothorax. They may be amenable to direct repair if promptly diagnosed, or to conservative treatment by intercostal drainage. Cervical oesophagostomy and gastrostomy may be the safest approach if there is a major disruption of the anastomosis.

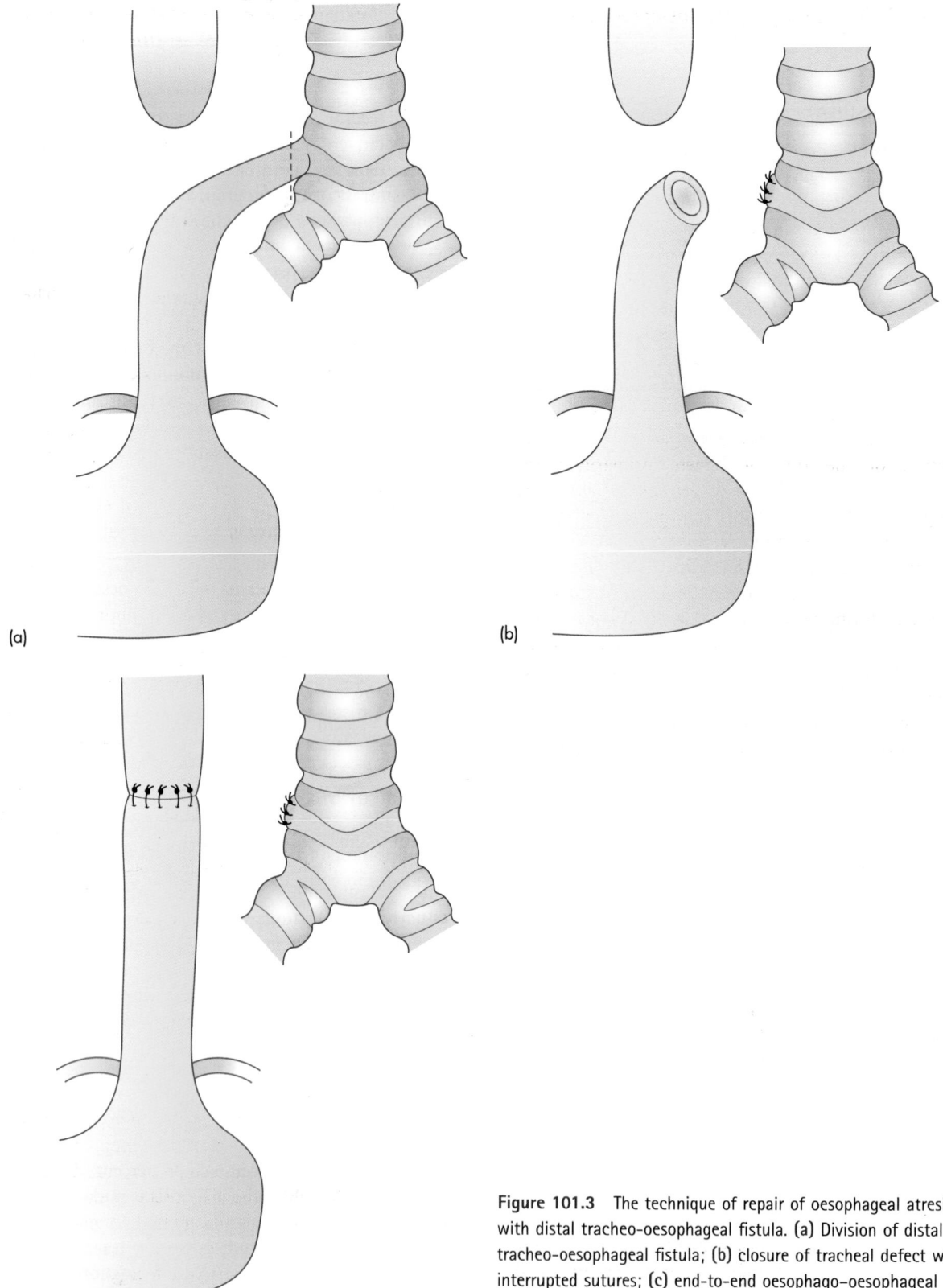

Figure 101.3 The technique of repair of oesophageal atresia with distal tracheo-oesophageal fistula. (a) Division of distal tracheo-oesophageal fistula; (b) closure of tracheal defect with interrupted sutures; (c) end-to-end oesophago–oesophageal anastomosis with a single layer of interrupted sutures.

ANASTOMOTIC STRICTURE

The stricture produces symptoms such as dysphagia or recurrent respiratory infections due to aspiration. The incidence varies from 10 to 50 percent. Strictures are caused by poor anastomotic technique, ischaemia, anastomotic leakage or gastro-oesophageal reflux. Most strictures respond to one or two dilatations but intractable strictures generally fail to respond to dilatations alone until the associated gastro-oesophageal reflux is corrected.[11] [***]

RECURRENT FISTULA

Recurrent fistulae develop in approximately 8 percent of patients.[28] The diagnosis should be suspected in a child who develops respiratory symptoms during feeding or who suffers repeated respiratory infections. The investigation of choice is a tube oesophagogram with confirmation at bronchoscopy. Surgical division of the fistula is the only reliable method of treatment.

TRACHEOMALACIA

This is due to a weakness of the tracheal cartilaginous ring structure and is characterized by partial or complete occlusion of the tracheal lumen, primarily during expiration.[29] It occurs in 10–20 percent of patients and is responsible for 'near miss' apnoeic and/or cyanotic attacks or recurrent respiratory infections. The condition affects the distal trachea and is diagnosed on broncho-scopic examination, which reveals the slit-like aperture of the trachea during expiration. Treatment is controversial. Many authors claim that the problem resolves sponta-neously in time but the infant is at risk of sudden death. Aortopexy, in which the ascending segment and arch of the aorta are elevated and attached to the posterior surface of the sternum, should be considered.[30] Tracheo-malacia is covered in Chapter 88, Congenital disorders of the larynx, trachea and bronchi.

VOCAL CORD PALSY

Vocal cord palsy may take place in association with a tracheo-oesophageal fistula or one or both recurrent laryngeal nerves may be traumatized during tracheo-oesophageal fistula surgery. The nerves are at most risk during the cervical repair of an H-type tracheo-oesopha-geal fistula. Vocal cord palsy is considered in Chapter 88, Congenital disorders of the larynx, trachea and bronchi.

GASTRO-OESOPHAGEAL REFLUX

Careful investigation will reveal gastro-oesophageal reflux in up to 60 percent of children undergoing successful repair of oesophageal atresia. Various factors have been implicated in the pathogenesis of the reflux, particularly disordered oesophageal motility, displacement of the gastro-oesophageal junction and the use of a gastrostomy. The reflux causes recurrent vomiting which may lead to aspiration and respiratory infections or may produce a stricture at the anastomotic site. The diagnosis is established on barium oesophagogram and on pH monitoring. Medical treatment is successful in many cases but antireflux surgery may be necessary in selected

cases.[31, 32] Gastro-oesophageal reflux is covered in detail in Chapter 100, Gastro-oesophageal reflux and aspiration.

DISORDERED PERISTALSIS

Swallowing difficulties may persist for many years as a result of the inherent oesophageal dysmotility, affecting the distal segment in particular.[33] The infant gradually learns to cope with this problem unless there is an associated anatomical defect (anastomotic stricture, gastro-oesophageal reflux or distal oesophageal stenosis).

RESPIRATORY INFECTION

These infants are also prone to recurrent respiratory infections during the first few years of life. Children who have had a tracheo-oesophageal fistula repair often develop a troublesome recurrent cough ('tracheo-oesophageal fistula (TOF) cough'), due to a combination of factors including a tendency to aspiration, mild tracheomalacia and gastro-oesophageal reflux. Many require ongoing care from a multidisciplinary team including an otolaryngologist.

CONGENITAL OESOPHAGEAL STENOSIS

Congenital stenosis of the oesophagus is rare. Stenosis most commonly arises from acquired lesions, e.g. reflux oesophagitis, corrosive ingestion, foreign body impaction or secondary to surgical resection and anastomosis. The congenital form may be caused either by a membranous web or diaphragm, or may arise as a result of intramural deposits of tracheobronchial cartilaginous tissue. The latter pathology has been most frequently reported in association with oesophageal atresia and/or tracheo-oesophageal fistula.[34]

Clinical features

In the presence of a complete web, presentation is similar to that of oesophageal atresia, with symptoms appearing on the first day of life. In other cases, symptoms may develop at any stage of life through to adulthood but generally arise in early infancy. The symptoms include dysphagia, vomiting with food ingestion, failure to thrive, recurrent respiratory infections and foreign body impaction.

Diagnosis

Gastro-oesophageal reflux as a cause for the stenosis should always be excluded. The barium oesophagogram will identify the site of the lesion. Congenital webs are most commonly located in the middle third of the oesophagus and appear as shelf-like projections within the oesophageal lumen. Tracheobronchial remnants are generally located in the lower third of the oesophagus or at the gastro-oesophageal junction and they cause sharp narrowing at this point. The precise nature and anatomical location of the lesion should be confirmed by endoscopic examination.

Treatment

Dilatation alone may be sufficient for many oesophageal webs. [**/*] Surgical resection of tracheobronchial cartilaginous tissue is generally recommended.[35] [**/*]

ACHALASIA

Achalasia is a motility disorder of the oesophagus characterized by an absence of peristalsis and failure of relaxation of the lower oesophageal sphincter.[36] This causes obstruction at the level of the oesophago-gastric junction.

Incidence

Achalasia is rare in children. The incidence is one per 100,000 and approximately 5 percent of all patients with achalasia are symptomatic before the age of 15 years. There are few reports of achalasia being present in siblings[37, 38] and it has been reported in association with a number of syndromes, e.g. Riley-Day syndrome. Evidence for a familial incidence of the disease is lacking. Both sexes are equally affected.

Aetiology and pathogenesis

The aetiology of achalasia is unknown. Oesophageal dysmotility is also found in Chaga's disease, scleroderma, oesophageal atresia, diabetes and secondary to gastro-oesophageal reflux, but the unique feature of achalasia is the constantly nonrelaxing lower oesophageal sphincter.

There are numerous theories regarding pathogenesis, the primary defect being described variously as neurogenic, myogenic and hormonal. There is evidence that it is the result of an abnormality of parasympathetic innervation. Absence of ganglion cells in the myenteric plexus in the dilated portion of the oesophagus with normal ganglion cells in the distal nondilated segment has been described.[39] This, however, is not a constant feature and is reflected in the variable reports of the histopathology of some of the specimens of oesophageal muscle. These range from the total absence of ganglia, to the presence of normally ganglionated muscle or abnormal ganglion cell morphology. [****] Histochemical staining for acetylcholinesterase may reveal the presence of ganglion cells and nerve trunks in the myenteric plexus,

although their numbers are slightly reduced. Reports using electron microscopy and intestinal polypeptide hormonal essay support the theory that this is a neurogenic disorder.[40]

Diagnosis

SYMPTOMATOLOGY

The principal symptoms of achalasia in childhood consist of vomiting, dysphagia, chest pain and weight loss. Dysphagia with the sensation of food sticking in the lower oesophagus and postprandial vomiting are the most frequent presenting symptoms. Retrosternal or epigastric pain manifests in one-third of the patients and in a few cases it is the primary presenting symptom. Weight loss of varying extent occurs in one-half of the patients. Nocturnal regurgitation may give rise to respiratory symptoms resulting in recurrent respiratory infections. Diagnostic delay is the norm with an average duration of symptoms prior to diagnosis of 24 months. Many children are treated for long periods for 'cyclic vomiting' or for 'anorexia nervosa'.

RADIOLOGICAL FEATURES

If achalasia is suspected, order a chest x-ray and a barium swallow in consultation with a colleague in the radiology department. The plain chest radiograph may show a dilated food-filled oesophagus with an air-fluid level in the distal third. In addition, there may be radiological signs of repeated aspiration pneumonitis. The chief characteristics on barium oesophagogram are a dilated oesophagus, the absence of a stripping wave, incoordinated oesophageal contractions and obstruction at the oesophagogastric junction with prolonged retention of barium in the oesophagus. Failure of relaxation of the lower oesophageal sphincter leads to the classical rat-tail deformity of funnelling and narrowing of the distal oesophagus (**Figure 101.4**).[41]

ENDOSCOPY

Oesophagoscopy contributes little to the diagnosis, but retained food may be found within the dilated oesophagus. The main value of endoscopy is to exclude organic causes of obstruction in the oesophagus.

OESOPHAGEAL MANOMETRY

The diagnosis of achalasia is best confirmed by oesophageal motility studies using a constantly perfused catheter technique. The criteria for the diagnosis are:

- a high-pressure (>30 mmHg) lower oesophageal sphincter zone;

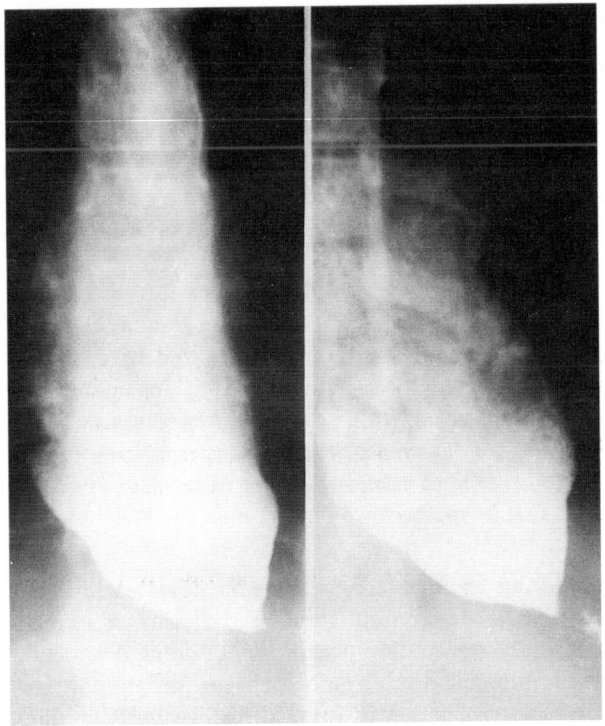

Figure 101.4 Barium swallow in a child with achalasia of the oesophagus with the classical 'rat-tail' deformity of the distal end.

- failure of the lower oesophageal sphincter to relax in response to swallowing;
- absence of propulsive peristalsis;
- incoordinated tertiary contractions in the body of the oesophagus (**Figures 101.5** and **101.6**).

Treatment

Three treatment options are available for the management of achalasia: pharmacological manipulation, forceful dilatation and oesophageal myotomy with or without the addition of an antireflux procedure.

PHARMACOLOGICAL TREATMENT

The manipulation of oesophageal motility disorders using pharmacological and dietary measures has been disappointing. [*] Reports of the use of isosorbide dinitrate and nifedipine have been more encouraging.[42] [**/*] Nifedipine is a calcium entry blocker and since calcium ions are directly responsible for the activity of myofibrils and consequently the tension generated, their use in reducing the pressure in the lower oesophageal sphincter in achalasia, or for the vigorous oesophageal spasms, seems logical. Prostaglandin E2 has also been employed with some success. Its value in the long-term treatment of achalasia remains to be proven. The injection of botulinum toxin has not been a success in children.[43, 44] [**/*]

FORCEFUL DILATATION

Good palliation may be obtained by dilatation. The most commonly used dilator consists of a single bag of fixed diameter which is inflated with water (Plummer) or air (Browne-McHardy, Rider-Moeller).

Dilatation has been advocated as the treatment of choice in adults. Fellows et al.[41] showed that, following pneumatic dilatation in adults, only 10 percent of patients subsequently required cardiomyotomy. In children, success rates ranging from 40 to 60 percent have been reported.[45, 46] [***] The aim of forceful dilatation is to disrupt the muscle fibres of the lower oesophageal sphincter. There is, however, no evidence that the muscle fibres tear rather than stretch. Vantrappen and Janssens[44] were unable to distinguish histologically between sphincter segments in dogs and monkeys subjected to forceful dilatations and those from normal controls. In general,

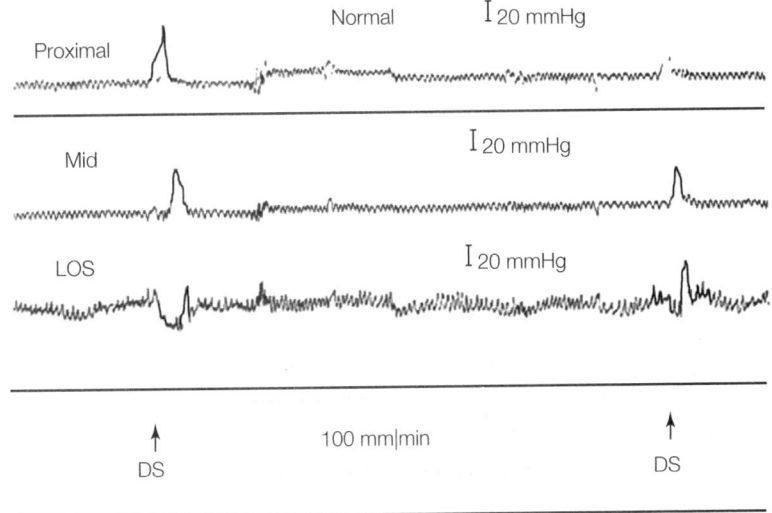

Figure 101.5 Oesophageal motility study in a normal child showing progression of the peristaltic waves through the oesophagus. DS, dry swallow.

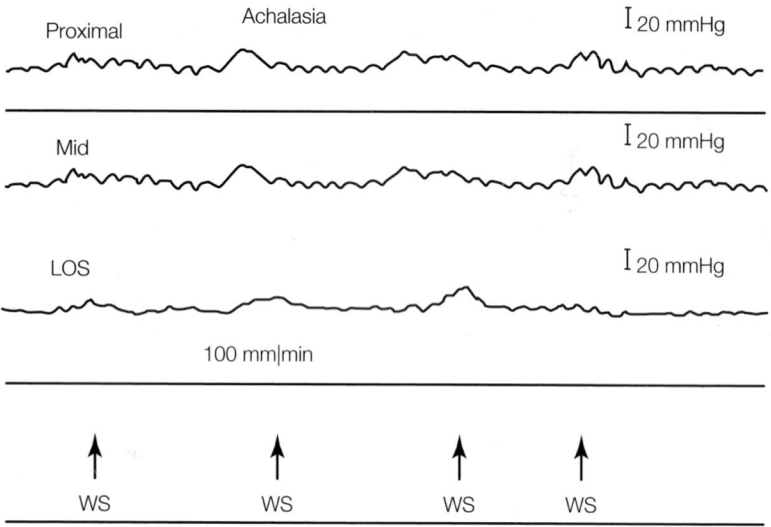

Figure 101.6 Oesophageal motility study in a child with achalasia showing completely incoordinate oesophageal contractions. WS, wet swallow.

older patients respond better to pneumatic dilatation.[47] A report of 899 adult patients treated at the Mayo Clinic concluded that myotomy was more successful and safer than dilatation, poor results being obtained twice as frequently following dilatation as after myotomy.[45] The incidence of perforation following pneumatic dilatation varies from 1 to 5 percent.

SURGICAL PROCEDURE

Cardiomyotomy, as originally described by Heller in 1914, is the basis of all surgical procedures. The technique involves splitting the muscle fibres along the whole length of the lower oesophageal sphincter. The controversies concern the length of the oesophageal myotomy, the distance which the myotomy extends onto the stomach and the necessity for including an additional antireflux procedure.[48]

CORROSIVE INJURY TO THE OESOPHAGUS

Accidental ingestion of caustic substances by children has become relatively uncommon in the developed world. This is as a result of government legislation regulating the use of caustics in commercially available drain cleaners and the introduction of child-proof containers. Parental awareness of the dangers has also contributed. In the developing world, lye burns to the oesophagus are still an enormous public health problem and a significant cause of mortality and of much long-term morbidity.[49]

Pathophysiology

Caustic soda (sodium hydroxide) ingestion can cause severe injury to the oropharynx, oesophagus or stomach. The strong alkali rapidly penetrates the body tissues producing an intense acute inflammatory reaction and oedema. If the concentration of the solution is high, transmural penetration occurs with resulting destruction of the musculature of the oesophagus, penetration into the peri-oesophageal tissues with mediastinitis or frank oesophageal perforation. The acute phase is followed by sloughing of the necrotic tissue and replacement by granulation tissue. The final outcome varies from complete resolution in the mild case to extensive fibrosis of the entire oesophagus. The extent and severity of the injury are directly related to the concentration of the lye ingested (liquid lye is more damaging than the granular form), the quantity ingested and the duration of contact.[50, 51]

Clinical presentation

There is extensive oedema and swelling of the mouth and lips and the child is unable to swallow. There may be chest pain if large quantities of lye reach the stomach. Haematemesis, dyspnoea, stridor and other respiratory symptoms develop as a consequence of the resulting oedema or from direct laryngeal injury. Fibrosis of the lips and temporomandibular joint may develop as a result of severe oropharyngeal burns (**Figure 101.7**).

Diagnosis

It is important to ascertain whether the lye was actually ingested or whether it entered the oral cavity only. Early endoscopic examination, within 12–24 hours of the injury, should be undertaken to determine whether or not the oesophagus is affected. Assessment of the extent of oesophageal burn is not possible at this early stage and endoscopic examination is terminated, once evidence of oesophageal injury is encountered, to minimize the risk of perforation.

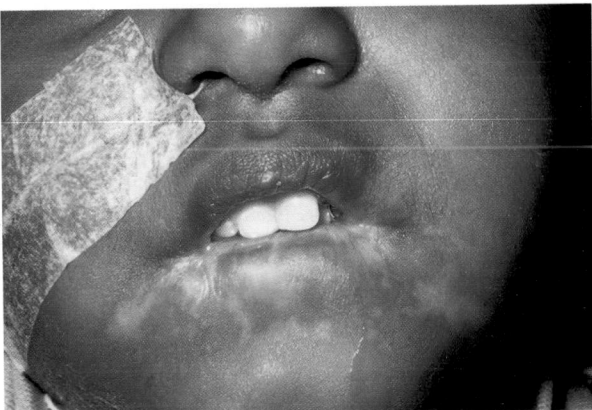

Figure 101.7 Fibrosis of the lips following severe oropharyngeal burns secondary to caustic soda ingestion.

An early contrast oesophagogram will reveal the extent of the injury, determine the presence of a perforation and act as a baseline for evaluating future stricture formation (**Figure 101.8**).

Treatment

EMERGENCY

Admission to hospital of all suspected cases is imperative.

Vomiting should not be induced. No neutralizing agents should be given as these produce heat when interacting with the corrosive substance and increase the severity of the injury.

CONTINUED MANAGEMENT

Initial treatment should consist of broad-spectrum antibiotics and intravenous fluids. [**] The use of steroids (prednisolone 2 mg/kg/day)[52] as advocated by Haller and Bachman,[53] has been questioned and, in a prospective controlled trial, Anderson found steroids to be of no benefit.[53, 54] [**/*] Ulman[55] similarly found no objective evidence to support the use of steroids; nevertheless many clinicians feel a three-week course of prednisolone is helpful and it is widely used. If, on endoscopy, no oesophageal injury is found, active treatment is stopped and the patient is discharged. If a burn is found, antibiotics are continued for ten days. Oral feeds are commenced as soon as the child is able to tolerate fluids. A gastrostomy for feeding purposes may be necessary in cases with severe burns. In these patients, the opportunity may be taken to pass a string through the oesophagus to act as a guide for future dilatations. Another option is to stent the oesophagus early after ingestion of the caustic substance.[56, 57] [**/*]

A repeat oesophagogram is carried out three weeks after ingestion of the lye and oesophageal dilatations are commenced if a stricture is found. The dilatations

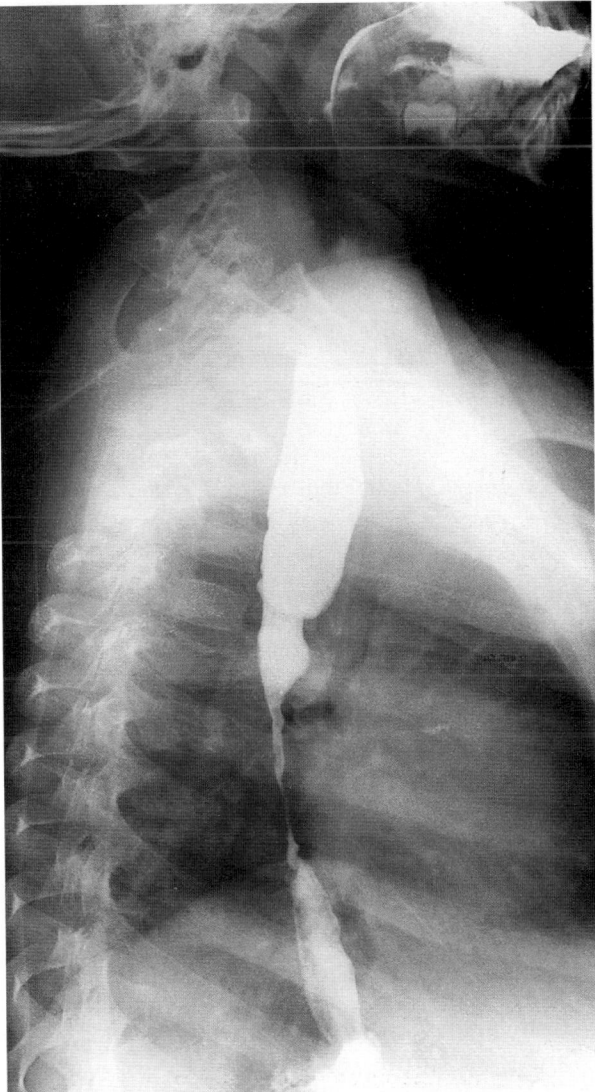

Figure 101.8 Barium oesophagogram in a child following ingestion of caustic soda. There is extensive stricture formation of the distal half of the oesophagus.

are repeated at regular intervals until the stricture is eliminated. Ninety percent of oesophageal strictures will respond to dilatation. The remainder will require oesophageal replacement.[58]

> ## KEY POINTS
>
> - Polyhydramnios is nonspecific but is present in approximately ninety percent of mothers of infants with oesophageal atresia.
> - Fifty percent of babies with oesophageal atresia have additional malformations.
> - It is now rare for an infant to succumb from oesophageal atresia alone, unless it is associated with a major heart defect or extreme prematurity.

- Ten to twenty percent of children with tracheo-oesohageal fistula have tracheomalacia which is responsible for 'near miss' apnoeic and/or cyanotic attacks or recurrent respiratory infections.
- In the developing world, lye burns to the oesophagus are still a serious public health problem, a significant cause of mortality and the source of much long-term morbidity.

Best clinical practice

✓ Treatment of infants with oesophageal atresia should be concentrated in centres where the surgical expertise, supportive services (anaesthesia, paediatric intensive care, cardiology, radiology, pathology) and specialized nursing care are available. Transfer to such centres should be prompt. [Grade B]

✓ The diagnosis of oesophageal atresia is confirmed by passing a catheter through the mouth and into the oesophagus. If the tube enters the stomach there is no oesophageal atresia. [Grade C/D]

✓ If achalasia is suspected, order a chest x-ray and a barium swallow in consultation with a colleague in the radiology department. [Grade C/D]

Deficiencies in current knowledge and areas for future research

➤ Knowledge of the embryology of the gastrointestinal tract and the genetic basis for congenital anomalies is growing.

➤ Better support services including paediatric intensive care facilities for infants with major congenital anomalies of the aerodigestive tract continue to improve survival.

➤ Multidisciplinary clinical input – including otolaryngologists – is likely to be increasingly accepted as routine for continuing care of these children.

➤ Greater awareness of the dangers of lye burns and legislation to improve containers for caustic agents would greatly reduce the misery of these injuries, particularly in the developing world.

REFERENCES

1. Kluth D, Fiegel H. The embryology of the foregut. *Seminars in Pediatric Surgery*. 2003; **12**: 3–9.

2. Myers NA. The history of oesophageal atresia and tracheo-oesophageal fistula – 1670-1984. *Progress in Pediatric Surgery*. 1986; **20**: 106–57.

3. Ashcraft KW, Holder TM. The story of esophageal atresia and tracheoesophageal fistula. *Surgery*. 1969; **65**: 332–40.

4. Beasley SW, Myers NA. Trends in mortality in oesophageal atresia. *Pediatric Surgery International*. 1992; **7**: 86–9.

5. Spitz L, Kiely EM, Morecroft JA, Drake DP. At risk groups in oesophageal atresia for the 1990's. *Journal of Pediatric Surgery*. 1994; **29**: 723–5.

6. Orford J, Glasson M, Beasley S, Shi E, Myers N, Cass D. Oesophageal atresia in twins. *Pediatric Surgery International*. 2000; **16**: 541–5.

7. Ioannides AS, Chaudhry B, Henderson DJ, Spitz L, Copp AJ. Dorsoventral patterning in oesophageal atresia with tracheo-oesophageal fistula: evidence from a new mouse model. *Journal of Pediatric Surgery*. 2002; **37**: 185–91.

8. Mere JM, Hutson JM. Embryogenesis of tracheo esophageal anomalies: a review. *Pediatric Surgery International*. 2002; **18**: 319–26.

* 9. Berrocal T, Madrid C, Novo S, Gutierej J, Arionilla A, Gomez L. Congenital anomalies of the tracheobronchilal tree lung and mediastinum. Embryology, radiology and pathology. *Radiographics*. 2004; **24**: 1527–33. *Good review with an emphasis on medical imaging.*

10. Goyal A, Potter F, Losty PD. Transillumination of H-type tracheoesophageal fistula using flexible miniature bronchoscopy: an innovative technique for operative localization. *Journal of Pediatric Surgery*. 2005; **40**: e33–4.

11. Chittmitatrapap S, Spitz L, Brereton RJ, Kiely EM. Anastomotic stricture following repair of esophageal atresia. *Journal of Pediatric Surgery*. 1990; **25**: 508–11.

12. Quan L, Smith DW. The VATER association. *Journal of Pediatrics*. 1973; **82**: 104–7.

13. Greenwood RD, Rosenthal A. Cardiovascular malformation associated with tracheoesophageal fistula and esophageal atresia. *Pediatrics*. 1976; **57**: 87–91.

14. Shulman A, Mazkereth R, Zalel Y, Kuint J, Lipitz S, Avigad I et al. Prenatal identification of esophageal atresia: the role of ultrasonography for evaluation of functional anatomy. *Prenatal Diagnosis*. 2002; **22**: 669–74.

15. Langer JC, Hussain H, Khan A, Minkes RK, Gray D, Siegel M et al. Prenatal diagnosis of esophageal atresia using sonography and magnetic resonance imaging. *Journal of Pediatric Surgery*. 2001; **36**: 804–7.

16. Stringer MD, McKenna KM, Goldstein RB, Filley RA, Scott Adzick N, Harrison MR. Prenatal diagnosis of esophageal atresia. *Journal of Pediatric Surgery*. 1995; **30**: 1258–63.

17. Levine D, Barnewolt C, Mehta T, Trop I, Estrof J, Wong GF et al. thoracic abnormalities: MR imaging. *Radiology*. 2003; **228**: 379–88.

18. Malone PS, Kiely EM, Brain AJ, Spitz L, Brereton RJ. Tracheo-oesophageal fistula and pre-operative mechanical ventilation: a dangerous combination. *Australian and New Zealand Journal of Surgery*. 1990; **60**: 525–7.

19. Rothenberg SS. Thoracoscopic repair of tracheoesophageal fistula in newborns. *Journal of Pediatric Surgery*. 2002; **37**: 869–72.

20. Zee DC, Bax NM. Thoracoscopic repair of esophageal atresia with distal fistula. *Surgical Endoscopy*. 2003; **14**.

21. Lividitis A. Esophageal atresia: a method of over-bridging large segmental gaps. *Zeit Kinderchirugie*. 1973; **13**: 298–306.

22. Davenport M, Bianchi A. Early experience with oesophageal flap repair for oesophageal atresia. *Pediatric Surgery International*. 1990; **26**: 89–91.

23. Kiely E, Spitz L. Is routine gastrostomy necessary in the management of oesophageal atresia. *Pediatric Surgery International*. 1987; **2**: 6–9.

24. Waterston DJ. Reconstruction of the esophagus. In: Mustard WT, Ravitch MM, Snyder WH (eds). *Pediatric surgery*. Chicago: Year Book Medical, 1969: 400.

25. Anderson KD, Randolph JG. Gastric tube interposition. A satisfactory alternative to the colon for esophageal replacement in children. *Annals of Thoracic Surgery*. 1978; **25**: 521–5.

26. Spitz L. Gastric transposition for esophageal substitution in children. *Journal of Pediatric Surgery*. 1992; **27**: 252–9.

27. Ghandour KE, Spitz L, Brereton RJ, Kiely EM. Recurrent tracheo-oesophageal fistula: experience with 24 patients. *Journal of Paediatric Child Health*. 1990; **26**: 89–91.

28. Wailoo MP, Emery JL. The trachea in children with tracheoesophageal fistula. *Histopathology*. 1979; **3**: 329–38.

29. Kiely EM, Spitz L, Brereton R. Management of tracheomalacia by aortopexy. *Pediatric Surgery International*. 1987; **2**: 13–5.

30. Ashcraft KW, Goodwin CD, Amoury RA, Holder TM. Early recognition and aggressive treatment of gastroesophageal reflux following repair of esophageal atresia. *Journal of Pediatric Surgery*. 1977; **12**: 317–21.

31. Jolley SG, Johnson DG, Roberts CC, Herbst JJ, Matlak ME, McCombs A *et al*. Patterns of gastroesophageal reflux in children following repair of esophageal atresia and distal tracheoesophageal fistula. *Journal of Pediatric Surgery*. 1980; **15**: 857–62.

32. Laks BH, Wilkinson RH, Schuster SR. Long-term results following correction of esophageal atresia and tracheoesophageal fistula. A clinical and cine-fluorographic study. *Journal of Pediatric Surgery*. 1972; **7**: 591–7.

33. Payne WS, King RM. Treatment of achalasia of the esophagus. *Surgical Clinics of North America*. 1983; **63**: 963–70.

34. London FA, Raab DE, Fuller J, Olsen AM. Achalasia in three siblings: a rare occurrence. *Mayo Clinical Proceedings*. 1977; **52**: 97–100.

35. Stoddard CJ, Johnson AG. Achalasia in siblings. *British Journal of Surgery*. 1982; **69**: 84–5.

36. Gallone L, Peri G, Galliera M. Proximal gastric vagotomy and anterior fundoplication as complementary procedures to Heller's operation for achalasia. *Surgery, Gynecology and Obstetrics*. 1982; **155**: 337–41.

37. Aggestrup S, Uddman R, Sundler F, Fahrenkrug J, Hakanson R, Sorenson HR *et al*. Lack of vasoactive intestinal polypeptide nerves in esophageal achalasia. *Gastroenterology*. 1983; **84**: 924–7.

38. Gelfond M, Rosen P, Gilat T. Isosorbide dinitrate and nifedipine treatment of achalasia: a clinical, manometric and radionuclide evaluation. *Gastroenterology*. 1982; **83**: 963–9.

39. Hurwitz M, Bahar RJ, Ament ME, Tolia V, Molleston J, Reinstein LJ *et al*. Evaluation of the use of botulinum toxin in children with achalasia. *Journal of Pediatric Gastroenterology and Nutrition*. 2000; **30**: 509–14.

40. Ip KS, Cameron DJ, Catto-Smith AG, Hardikar W. Botulinum toxin for achalasia in children. *Journal of Gastroenterology and Hepatology*. 2000; **15**: 1100–4.

41. Fellows IW, Ogilvie AL, Atkinson MP. Pneumatic dilatation in achalasia. *Gut*. 1983; **24**: 1020–3.

42. Vane DW, Cosby K, West K, Grosfeld JL. Late results following esophagomyotomy in children with achalasia. *Journal of Pediatric Surgery*. 1988; **23**: 515–9.

43. Babu R, Grier D, Cusick E, Spicer RD. Penumatic dilatation for childhood achalasia. *Pediatric Surgery International*. 2001; **17**: 505–7.

44. Vantrappen G, Janssens J. To dilate or operate? This is the question. *Gut*. 1983; **24**: 1013–9.

45. Payne WS, King RM. Treatment of achalasia of the esophagus. *Surgical Clinics of North America*. 1983; **63**: 963–70.

46. Buick RG, Spitz L. Achalasia of the cardia in children. *British Journal of Surgery*. 1985; **72**: 341–3.

47. Patti MG, Albanese CT, Holcomb 3rd GW, Molena D, Fisichella PM, Perretta S *et al*. Laparoscopic Heller myotomy and Dor fundoplication for esophageal achalasia in children. *Journal of Pediatric Surgery*. 2001; **36**: 1248–51.

48. Ellis FH, Gibb SP, Crozier RE. Esophagomyotomy for achalasia of the esophagus. *Annals of Surgery*. 1980; **192**: 157–61.

49. Spitz L. Management of ingested foreign bodies in childhood. *British Medical Journal*. 1971; **4**: 469–72.

* 50. Hamza A, Abdelhay S, Sherif H, Hasan T, Soliman H, Kabesh A *et al*. Caustic esophageal strictures in children: 30 years experience. *Journal of Paediatric Surgery*. 2003; **38**: 828–33. *Reports an extensive experience of caustic strictures in a tertiary referral centre, 850 cases, the majority requiring oesophageal replacement.*

* 51. Spitz L, Kiely E, Pierro A. Gastric transposition in children a twenty-one year experience. *Journal of Paediatric Surgery*. 2004; **39**: 276–81. *Account of the author's extensive experience including secondary repairs of oesophageal atresia and caustic strictures.*

52. Spitz L, Hirsig J. Prolonged foreign body impaction in the oesophagus. *Archives of Disease in Childhood*. 1982; **57**: 551–3.

53. Haller JA, Bachman K. The comparative effect of current therapy of experimental caustic burns of the esophagus. *Journal of the American Medical Association*. 1963; **186**: 262.

54. Vaishnav A, Spitz L. Alkaline battery-induced tracheo-oesophageal fistula. *British Journal of Surgery.* 1989; **76**: 1045.

55. Ulman I, Mutaf O. A critique of steroids in the management of caustic esophageal burns in children. *European Journal of Paediaric Surgery.* 1998; **8**: 71–4.

56. Anderson KD, Rouse TM, Randolph JG. A controlled trial of corticosteroids in children with corrosive injury of the oesophagus. *New England Journal of Medicine.* 1990; **323**: 637–40.

57. de Jong AL, Macdonald R, Ein S, Forte V, Turner A. Corrosive esophagitis in children: a 30-year review. *International Journal of Pediatric Otorhinolaryngology.* 2001; **57**: 203–11.

58. Viiala C, Collins B. use of multiple self-expanding metal stents to treat corrosive induced esophageal strictures. *Endoscopy.* 2001; **33**: 291–2.

Imaging in paediatric ENT

NEVILLE WRIGHT

Introduction	1295	Best clinical practice		1302
Imaging modalities	1296	Deficiencies in current knowledge and areas for future		
Radiation protection	1300	research		1303
Patient preparation	1301	References		1303
Key points	1302			

SEARCH STRATEGY

This chapter is supported by a PubMed search using the key words children, ENT, imaging, radiology, ultrasound, magnetic resonance, computed tomography, bronchography, play therapy, scintigraphy and sialography.

INTRODUCTION

Paediatric ear, nose and throat (ENT) imaging is a challenging subject both for the radiologist and the otolaryngologist. In addition to the anatomical complexities of middle and inner ear structure, the convolutions of the turbinates, the pneumatization pattern of the sinuses, and the dynamics of the swallowing mechanism, both the radiologist and the surgeon need to be aware of the variations during normal growth of the child.

Many of the imaging techniques used in paediatric ENT radiology are similar to those used in adult practice (**Table 102.1**), but the diseases encountered may be entirely different. Consideration of the need for sedation or general anaesthesia is an important factor when deciding to image a child.

The number of plain radiographs performed in children has significantly diminished over recent years with the widespread availability of computed tomography (CT), especially for imaging the ear and sinuses. It is

Table 102.1 Imaging modalities pertinent to paediatric ENT radiology.

Imaging modalities	
Plain radiography	Mastoid views, lateral soft tissue neck, limited role for sinus views
Fluoroscopy	Videofluoroscopy, contrast swallows, bronchography, sialography, chest and diaphragm screening
Ultrasound	Including Doppler and colour flow studies
Computed tomography	Standard, helical, high resolution, contrast-enhanced and angiography
Magnetic resonance imaging	Including angiographic sequences, perfusion and possibly functional studies
Nuclear medicine	Thyroid, parathyroid and salivary scintigraphy, perchlorate discharge test
Interventional procedures and angiography	Percutaneous biopsy and aspiration, balloon dilatation, stent placement, embolization

important to minimize radiation exposure in children and in this context magnetic resonance imaging (MRI), which avoids the use of ionizing radiation, has an expanding and important role. Dynamic contrast bronchography is also being used in some centres for 'real-time' assessment of the upper airway, particularly in ventilated children when it can be combined with simultaneous pressure measurements to give valuable information about opening airway pressures.

IMAGING MODALITIES

Plain radiographs (x-rays)

Much of the older radiological literature details an array of radiographic projections and plain x-ray tomographic techniques to assess the airway, petrous bone and mastoid region. These have now largely been replaced by cross-sectional imaging (CT and MRI). There is still a limited role for mastoid views to define the extent of pneumatization of the air cells, but this should be restricted to requests from ENT specialists. The projections obtained are no different to those used in adult practice. Plain radiography of the airway is usually limited to a lateral film and in this instance air acts as a negative contrast medium outlining the anatomical details. For the most reliable results, the film should be obtained during inspiration with the neck slightly extended. This is because there is considerable variation in the appearances of the soft tissues of the nasopharynx in the young child dependent on posture. This is especially so when the neck is flexed and the child is breathing out, when apparent soft tissue swelling can mimic a pharyngeal mass. A high kilo-voltage radiographic technique with added tube filtration ('Cincinnati view') also used to be recommended for airway assessment, but this is no longer necessary following the development of digitally enhanced computed radiography, CT and MRI, all of which give much better detail. Sinus x-rays are difficult to interpret in the young child, where mucosal thickening can be a normal finding. They should be avoided in the under five year olds,[1] [***] and should be restricted to requests by ENT specialists only. In the acute setting, they are indicated to exclude fractures and foreign bodies. Radiology for nasal bone fractures should be deferred until 10–14 days have elapsed since injury, and even then are rarely clinically indicated. Despite all the advances in imaging technology, it is important to remember that a chest x-ray can still be very informative, particularly to detect air-trapping and foreign body inhalation.

Fluoroscopy

Fluoroscopy is the study of sequential dynamic images. Techniques pertinent to paediatric ENT radiology include videofluoroscopy of the swallowing mechanism, videofluoroscopy during phonation, barium or contrast swallows, tracheo-oesophageal fistul-o-grams (TOF-o-grams), chest and diaphragm screening, sialography and dynamic contrast enhanced bronchography.

Radiographic assessment of the swallowing mechanism and phonation studies require fluoroscopy of the upper airway and palate. The assistance of a speech and language therapist is mandatory for best results. For the assessment of swallowing, sequential analysis of the swallowing cycle requires recording of data on videotape or other media storage device for later analysis. In general, screening in the lateral position will suffice. Most children require assessment with various types of food consistency. Yoghurt mixed with barium, thickened barium and liquid barium should generally be assessed, with other foodstuffs used as appropriate. The examination should be modified depending on the child's age and feeding habits.

For phonation studies, ideally a small quantity of barium is administered to each nostril and then sniffed to coat the soft palate. Clearly barium may have to be omitted in the very young child. Fluoroscopy is performed with the child in a modified Towne's (chin-tuck) position to obtain a tangential view of the velopharyngeal portal and then subsequently in the lateral projection. When no barium has been administered, only the lateral projection is performed.

Barium and water-soluble contrast studies are useful for assessing the oesophagus for strictures, vascular rings, gastro-oesophageal reflux and oesophagitis. Barium is the preferred contrast agent, unless aspiration is highly likely, or in the postoperative state where a suitable water-soluble agent is preferred. The procedure is similar to that performed in adults, although it will need alteration with young children who are usually fed supine rather than erect. A modified technique is required to demonstrate a tracheo-oesophageal fistula (TOF), the technique often referred to as the 'TOF-o-gram'. In this procedure the child has a nasogastric tube placed into the stomach and lies in a prone position. The tube is incrementally withdrawn while injecting a suitable contrast agent and simultaneously screening the oesophagus in a lateral projection. The effect of gravity and the careful withdrawal of the tube under direct vision is felt to enhance the chances of identifying a fistula. [*]

Diaphragm screening is a simple procedure involving visualization of diaphragmatic movement during normal respiration, coughing, sniffing and Valsalva manoeuvres. The degree of diaphragmatic excursion and presence or absence of paradoxical movement should be recorded. Fluoroscopy can also be used to assess air-trapping if inhaled foreign bodies are suspected.

Some children require dynamic 'real-time' evaluation of the airway using bronchography. A small quantity of nonionic water-soluble contrast is injected into the trachea and bronchi and the airway is then screened to assess changes in airway calibre during the respiratory cycle. This is limited to children requiring ventilatory support and should only be carried out with full resuscitation facilities available. Clearly its use is restricted to specialized paediatric centres. It is mainly used for confirmation of suspected anatomical abnormalities where there is doubt or to confirm the extent of tracheobronchomalacia and evaluate airway opening pressures.[2, 3] [**]

Sialography of the parotid or submandibular glands can be performed in children. The technique is similar to that performed in adults, although the procedure may need to be carried out under anaesthesia in the younger child. Sialectasis, stone formation and ductal abnormalities may be identified. Sialography may be combined with CT or MRI examinations. Sialography has also been performed successfully using a digital subtraction technique to obtain superior image quality.[4] [**] MR sialography, using heavily T2-weighted sequences, is a noninvasive alternative to cannulation techniques, but is unable to provide the excellent spatial resolution (and therefore image quality) that can be obtained with a formal sialogram.[5] [**]

Ultrasound

Ultrasound (sonography) is a noninvasive, portable and easily accessible method of assessing the neck and thoracic inlet. Importantly, it uses no ionizing radiation. Ultrasound should be the first imaging investigation for a neck mass, although it has a limited role in assessing deeply placed pathologies (**Figure 102.1**). It is especially good at distinguishing solid from cystic lesions (e.g. thyroglossal cysts). Combined with Doppler and colour flow imaging, ultrasound provides vital information about the vascularity of masses, such as haemangiomas and cystic

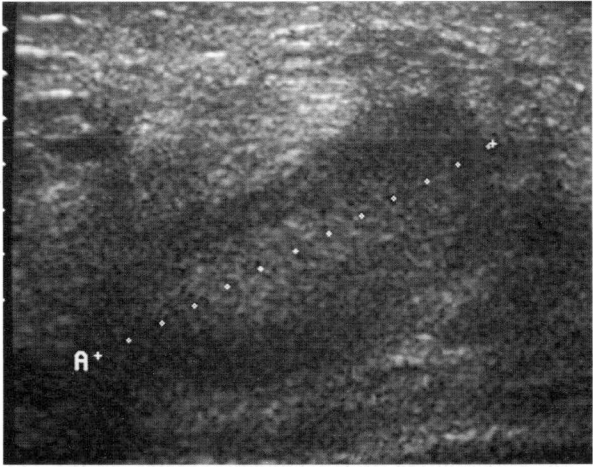

Figure 102.1 Ultrasound is a readily available, noninvasive technique which can quickly distinguish solid from cystic lesions – this scan shows a lymph node.

hygromas. Ultrasound has also been used successfully to assess the unossified, cartilaginous structures of the larynx.[6] [**] It has the advantages of providing real-time images under physiological conditions and may be useful in assessing vocal cord movement,[7] but it has not yet replaced direct inspection of the cords at endoscopy. [***]

Ultrasound can also evaluate diaphragm movement, although in practical terms this is often restricted to the intensive care unit setting when the child cannot be moved easily for fluoroscopic assessment. It can also guide biopsy and aspiration of neck lesions, although this is carried out much less frequently in children than adults.

Computed tomography

Plain x-ray tomography is now a technique of the past. CT provides good soft tissue characterization, but excels in the definition of fine bony detail. With the development of faster scan times, helical scanning and improved resolution, CT can now provide superb images of the middle and inner ears (**Figure 102.2**), although it is less effective at assessing the retrocochlear auditory pathway.[8] [**] The major drawback for CT, however, is its use of ionizing radiation. Generally, high resolution 1 mm scans should be obtained in two planes, the transverse and the coronal, although with some of the more modern scanners transverse images can be obtained and then the coronal images reconstructed from the scan dataset, without loss of detail and negating the need to do two scans. This helps to reduce the radiation exposure to the child. The images should all be post-processed using a sharp filter to improve bony detail. CT of the petrous temporal bone complements MRI and is essential in preoperative assessment for cochlear implants.

CT also has a role in the assessment of children's sinuses and the nasal airway, although this is much less frequently required than that in adults. It is particularly pertinent in children with orbital cellulitis, where contrast-enhanced CT will define the presence and extent of retro-orbital disease much more clearly than clinical examination. [**] Evaluation of choanal atresia is also facilitated by defining the bony elements on CT, although this often requires mucosal decongestants and suction of nasal secretions to improve the sensitivity of the scan.

Volume acquired CT information using helical or electron beam scanners can be used to assess the upper airway, including the larynx,[9] [**] and may be used to generate 'virtual' bronchoscopic images (**Figure 102.3**). This is a significant step forward in imaging terms, but it still falls short of the fine detail which can be seen with direct vision.

CT angiography is rapidly approaching the degree of definition previously provided only by formal invasive angiography, and this can be extremely helpful in conditions such as juvenile nasopharyngeal angiofibroma.

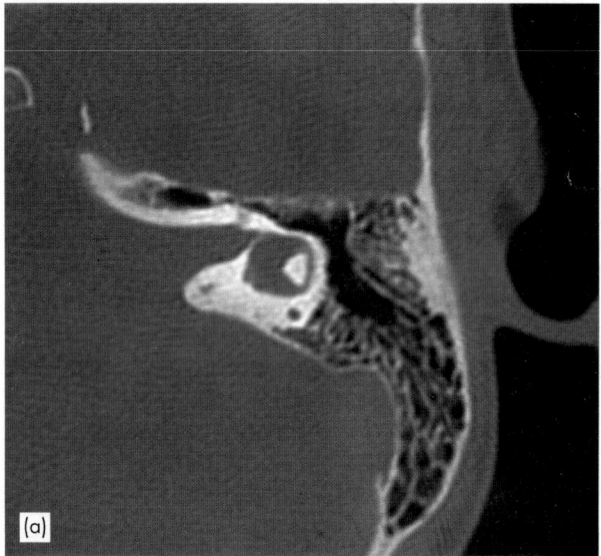

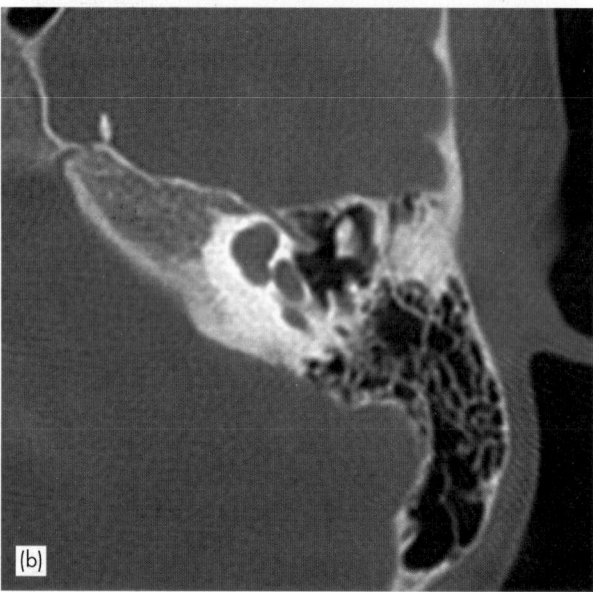

Figure 102.2 Transverse CT image through the petrous bone showing: (a) a dilated vestibule; and (b) a Mondini abnormality of the cochlea.

Magnetic resonance imaging

MRI is a noninvasive, multiplanar imaging technique with excellent soft tissue discrimination. Importantly for children, it does not use ionizing radiation, but unfortunately may require sedation or anaesthesia. It is a rapidly advancing technology in which numerous acronyms are used to describe the multitude of imaging sequences used. In simple terms however, T1-weighted sequences provide anatomical definition and T2-weighted sequences demonstrate areas of high fluid content, in particular oedema. MRI excels in the demonstration of the brain and spinal cord. However, there is increasing use of MRI, not just to assess the posterior fossa and other intracranial structures, but also inner ear abnormalities. T2-weighted sequences

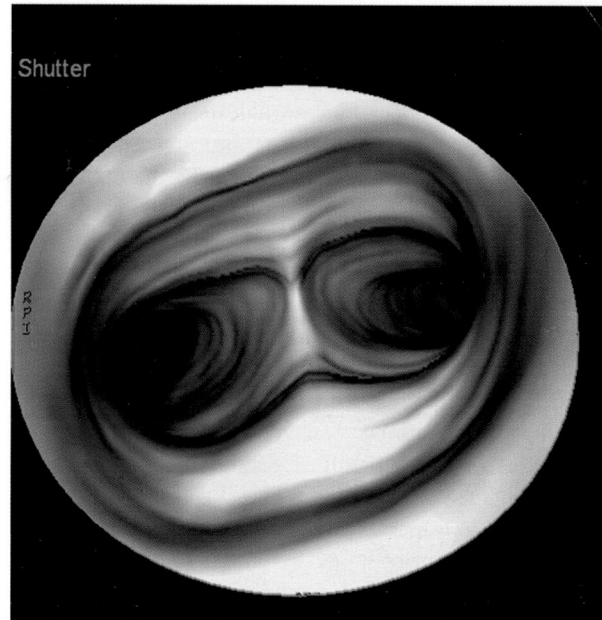

Figure 102.3 Single transverse image from CT virtual bronchogram dataset clearly shows the carina.

provide the optimum information about the inner ear, clarifying the presence of fluid filled structures, such as the cochlea, vestibule and semicircular canals, but occasionally T1-weighted and post-contrast images may be helpful. Vestibular schwannoma is an uncommon condition in children and most imaging in the cerebello-pontine angle is focussed on identifying other mass lesions, the brainstem and the seventh and eighth nerves. When intracranial extension of disease processes in the ear or paranasal sinuses occurs, there may be involvement of the venous sinuses. Magnetic resonance (MR) venography provides a noninvasive method of assessing involvement of these venous sinuses (**Figure 102.4**).[10] Further advances in MR technology now also permit exquisitely detailed three-dimensional reconstructions of the inner ear.[11] [**]

Velopalatine movement can also be successfully assessed with MRI, using fast T1-weighted sequences during phonation of different sounds and replaying them in cine mode.[12, 13] [*] In cooperative children this may be a satisfactory alternative to videofluoroscopy, although this does require MR scanners of high specification.[14]

The excellent soft tissue discrimination of MRI can also be effectively used in imaging the neck when, after ultrasound, MRI is the next most useful imaging modality (**Figure 102.5**). It is especially helpful in defining the extent and nature of cystic masses, such as cystic hygromas (**Figure 102.6**), when extension into the thoracic inlet can also be assessed. Parotid and sub-mandibular gland assessment is also more accurate with MRI. Fat-suppressed MRI (e.g. STIR or 'short tau inversion recovery' sequences) are especially useful in identifying lymphadenopathy and adenoidal and tonsillar tissue.

MR angiography is now a viable alternative to invasive formal angiography, especially for the assessment of vascular malformations. However, formal angiography may still be required for endovascular treatment of lesions.

Nuclear medicine

Nuclear medicine has an important role in assessment of the thyroid and parathyroid glands. It can be used to

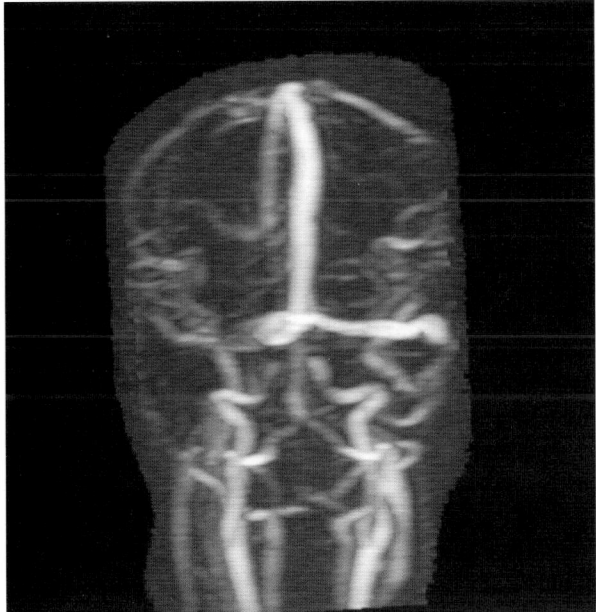

Figure 102.4 Coronal MR venogram, a noninvasive study, showing absent flow in the right transverse venous sinus consistent with venous thrombosis.

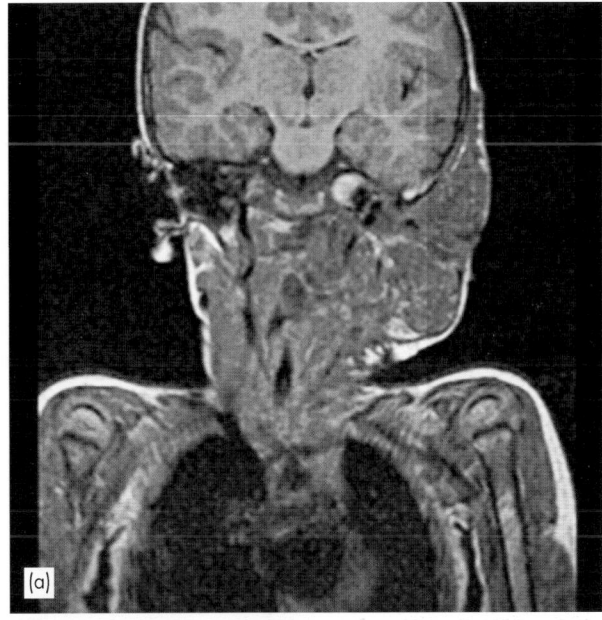

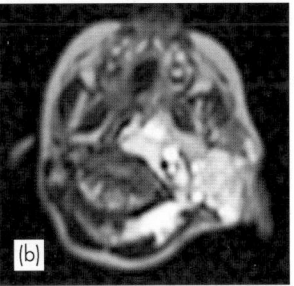

Figure 102.6 MR images include **(a)** coronal T1-weighted and **(b)** transverse T2-weighted scans of the neck showing an extensive cystic hygroma extending into the nasopharynx and posteriorly around the neck.

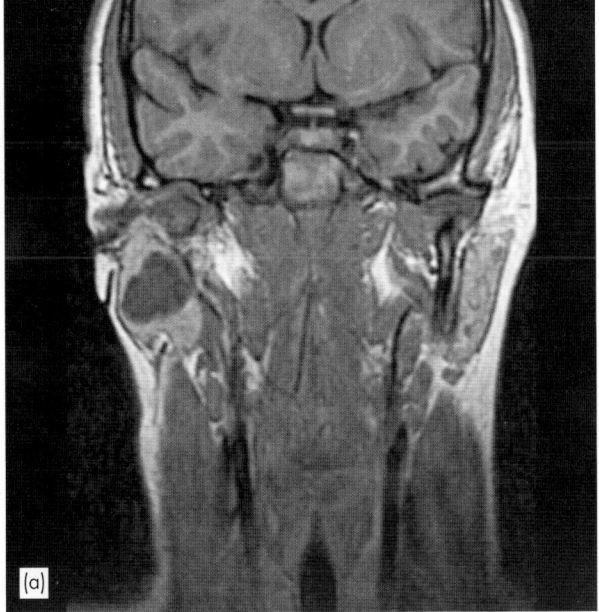

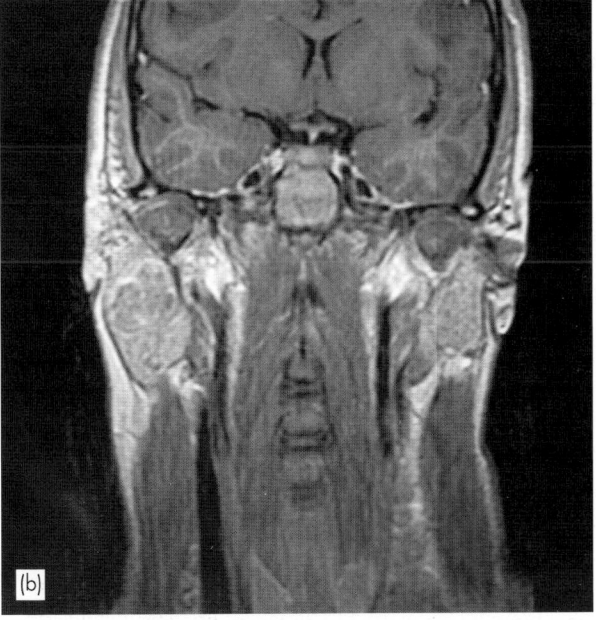

Figure 102.5 Coronal T1-weighted MR images of the neck show a discrete lesion in the right parotid gland later proven to be a pleomorphic adenoma: **(a)** pre-contrast; **(b)** post-contrast.

assess the presence, size and distribution of thyroid and parathyroid tissue, and is most frequently used in young children with hypothyroidism. The usual technique for evaluating the thyroid gland involves the injection of [99m]technetium (Tc) pertechnate and is similar to that performed in adults. Alternatively [123]iodine can be used. In some children there may be abnormalities of organification of iodine into tyrosine and this can be assessed with the perchlorate discharge test (**Figure 102.7**).[15] [**] Parathyroid assessment is now more easily performed using ^{99m}Tc-labelled sestamibi to identify increased parathyroid metabolism.[16] [**] Salivary scintigraphy can also be performed in children to assess parenchymal function and excretion of the salivary glands.[17] [*] Its main indication is in the assessment of connective tissue disease and occasionally to look for salivary duct obstruction when sialography cannot be performed.

Interventional procedures and angiography

Most interventional techniques in children require the assistance of sedation or, more commonly, general anaesthesia to ensure a safe, controlled procedure. Percutaneous biopsy of head and neck lesions is much less commonly performed in children, but the technique is similar to that performed in adults. Aspiration of cysts under ultrasound or CT control is effective and when appropriate can be combined with sclerotherapy, for example for treatment of extensive cystic hygroma.

The primary treatment for tracheobronchial stenosis remains surgery, but there are now radiological interventional alternatives, such as balloon dilatation and insertion of metallic stents. Balloon dilatation is performed under fluoroscopic guidance, and can be repeated if necessary. Stent placement again requires fluoroscopic guidance, but the long-term effects of these placements have yet to be fully evaluated.[18] [*]

Formal angiography is an invasive technique requiring placement of an intravascular catheter usually by the femoral artery, and subsequent contrast injection to delineate the vessels (**Figure 102.8**). Obtaining vascular access in young children can be a challenge and selective vessel catheterization may also be difficult, although children do not usually suffer from atherosclerotic vessels encountered in adult practice! Diagnostic studies should be combined with interventional procedures if possible. Embolization for vascular head and neck lesions can be used for definitive treatment or preoperatively and involves selective catheterization and usually particulate embolization or injection of sclerosant.[19] [**]

RADIATION PROTECTION

Of paramount importance when considering whether a child needs a diagnostic test is balancing the need and quality of the information the test will provide with the risk associated with the test. A useful test is one in which the result, whether positive or negative, will affect patient management or improve confidence in the clinician's diagnosis. The prime area of concern in radiological

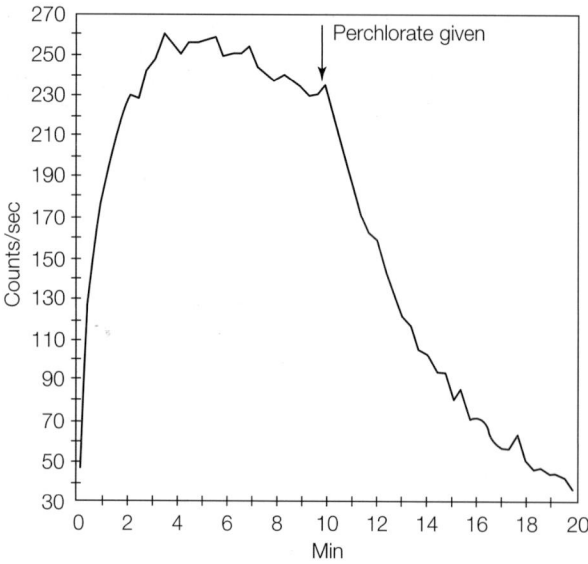

Figure 102.7 Time-activity curve from a perchlorate discharge test demonstrates displacement of activity from the thyroid confirming an organification defect.

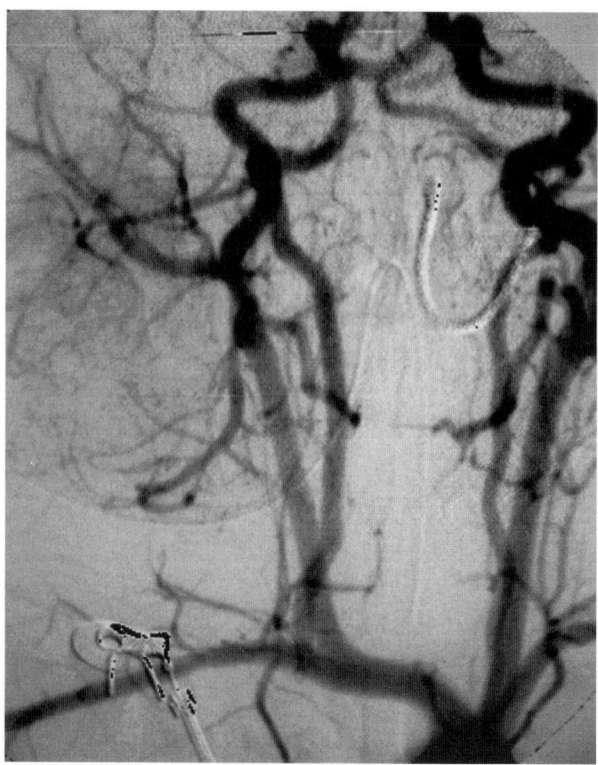

Figure 102.8 Formal angiography demonstrates abnormal vascularity within a lobular mass in the right side of the neck.

imaging is the risk from ionizing radiation. Radiological tests are an accepted part of medical practice in which clinical benefits should clearly exceed the small radiation risk. Statutory regulations in the UK, The Ionizing Radiation (Medical Exposure) Regulations 2000, require all involved to reduce unnecessary exposure of patients to radiation.[20] This is especially important in children, in whom there is increased sensitivity to the effects of radiation. One important way of reducing the radiation burden to a patient is ensuring unnecessary tests are avoided, especially avoiding repeat examinations.

It is useful to consider radiation dose in terms of the total radiation risk to the body, calculated from the sum of the doses to a number of body tissues. The weighting factor for each tissue varies upon its relative sensitivity to radiation-induced cancer or severe hereditary effects. This gives a single effective dose to the body. It is also useful to consider the effective dose in terms of chest x-ray equivalents. **Table 102.2** gives typical effective doses for a number of examinations pertinent to paediatric ENT radiology.[21] It is important to note that a CT examination administers a relatively high radiation dose and thus it is certainly worthwhile considering alternative imaging modalities such as ultrasound and MRI.

PATIENT PREPARATION

General approach

It is important that children and their parents understand why any imaging test has been requested and what to expect from the examination. This information is best addressed initially in the outpatient environment during the consultation process, but is usually supplemented by information provided by the radiology department. Information, both verbal and written, needs to be appropriate for both child and adult. Some examinations require venous access and this can be distressing for both the child and their carer. The use of topical anaesthetics and play therapists using distraction techniques can be hugely beneficial, and make the procedure both pain free and uneventful. Indeed, the importance of access to play therapy for children has recently been recognized at governmental level in the UK National Service Framework (NSF) document.[22] When intravenous contrast agents will be required, it is important to notify the radiology department of any allergies or previous problems with contrast agents to ensure the procedure can run smoothly. The choice of contrast agent, the examination technique or even the particular modality to be used to image the child may be modified depending on the history provided.

Where complex procedures (such as angiography) require sedation or general anaesthesia, the child will need admission to a ward and appropriate preparation, depending on the particular procedure to be performed. Informed consent is mandatory for invasive procedures.

Sedation and general anaesthesia

For some imaging tests, particularly those requiring long periods of immobility such as MRI, young children will require sedation or general anaesthesia. Plain x-rays and ultrasound rarely require either, whereas interventional studies and angiography for head and neck lesions almost invariably require general anaesthesia. Particular care must be exercised in using sedation in children with airway problems, especially in the MR environment where the child may spend some time within the bore of the magnet. It is also mandatory to have appropriate MR compatible monitoring equipment in such circumstances (**Figure 102.9**).

The choice of sedation or anaesthesia will depend on local practice and expertise. In general, children under the age of four to five years will require some form of assistance to maintain adequate immobility to ensure diagnostic images. Very young children, under three months, can often simply be fed and wrapped up well. Children older than five years or weighing more than 20 kg are often difficult to sedate adequately, and it may

Table 102.2 Typical effective doses from diagnostic medical exposure.

Diagnostic procedure	Typical effective dose (mSv)[a]	Equivalent number of chest x-rays	Approximate equivalent period of natural background radiation
Chest (single PA film)	0.02	1	3 days
Skull	0.06	3	9 days
Barium swallow	1.5	75	8 months
CT head	2.0	100	10 months
Thyroid (Tc-99 m) radionuclide scan	1	50	6 months
Ultrasound	0	0	0
Magnetic resonance imaging	0	0	0

[a]UK average background = 2.2 mSv per year, range 1.5–7.5 mSv.

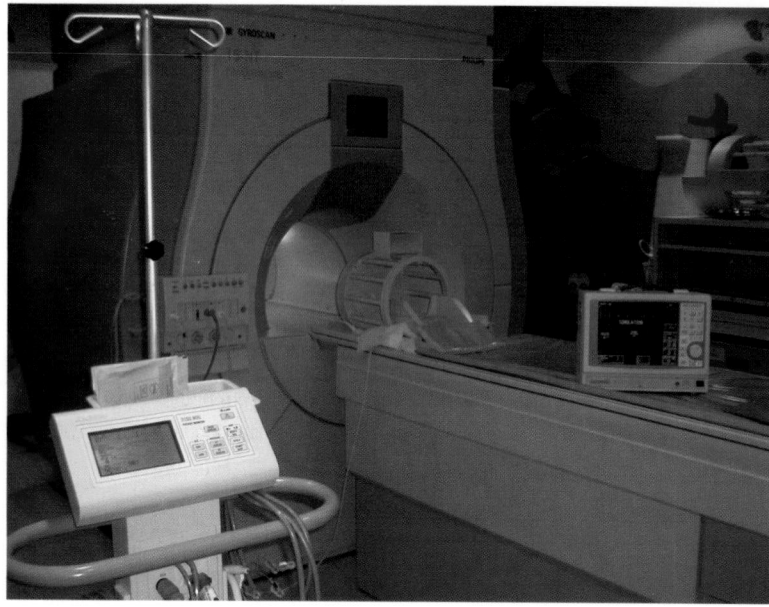

Figure 102.9 MR compatible monitoring equipment is mandatory for safe practice in the MR environment – the magnetic field is permanently on!

be prudent to proceed directly to general anaesthesia. Some of the faster CT scanners are reducing the tendency to require sedation or anaesthesia, and play therapists can be especially useful in the MR environment for fidgety children.[23] [**/*] There are many different regimens for sedation and **Tables 102.3** and **102.4** show only two examples. Sedation protocols will need to be developed depending on local equipment and expertise and with close cooperation between the departments of radiology, ENT and anaesthesia. It is important to reiterate that the MR environment requires specialized, MRI-compatible monitoring equipment, which must at all times be readily available.

Table 102.3 Possible sedation regimens, part 1.

Age	Fasting time (hours)		
	Clear fluids	Milk	Solids
<Three months	2	4	6
>Three months	2	6	6

Table 102.4 Possible sedation regimens, part 2.

Weight	Suggested drug, 1 month to 18 years
<20 kg	Oral chloral hydrate 100 mg/kg body weight, maximum dose 2000 mg May be supplemented with rectal paraldehyde, unless neutropenic 0.3 mL/kg body weight + 0.3 mL/kg of olive oil, maximum dose 10 mL paraldehyde + 10 mL olive oil
>20 kg	Consider oral quinalbarbitone 7.5–10 mg/kg body weight, maximum dose 200 mg

KEY POINTS

- Plain sinus radiography is of limited use in children.
- Ultrasound is the first line imaging investigation for a neck mass.
- Bony detail is best demonstrated by CT.
- When cross-sectional imaging is considered necessary, ultrasound and magnetic resonance imaging should be considered as alternatives to CT to minimize the radiation burden to the child.
- Magnetic resonance imaging provides excellent soft tissue imaging in multiple planes and can be used to provide noninvasive angiographic information.
- Sedation or anaesthesia may be needed for examinations which are time-consuming and require prolonged immobility of the child.

Best clinical practice

The following is a brief summary of imaging pathways for investigating some common paediatric ENT problems. The reader is referred to the relevant areas elsewhere in the book for more detail.

Craniofacial malformations

✓ CT with multiplanar reconstruction – for bone and soft tissue demonstration.

✓ MRI – for midline defects with a possible intracranial extension.

Deafness and prior to cochlear implantation

✓ CT to assess the temporal and parietal bones and middle ear, cochlear morphology and cochlear patency.[24]
✓ MRI to assess cochlear morphology, cochlear patency and the retrocochlear auditory pathway.[25]

Trauma to the head and face

✓ CT for complex fractures.

Paranasal sinus disease

Plain sinus radiographs should be limited to requests from ENT specialists. Indications include:
✓ single occipitomental (OM) or lateral view for foreign body;
✓ single OM view to confirm maxillary opacification prior to antral washout in suspected maxillary empyema;
✓ otherwise low-dose CT.

Neck masses including lymphadenopathy

✓ Ultrasound, with or without colour Doppler imaging – often the only imaging examination required to confirm lymphadenopathy.
✓ CT or MRI.

Airway obstruction

✓ Lateral soft tissue view of the neck.
✓ Chest x-ray.
✓ Barium swallow.
✓ Contrast enhanced CT or MRI – if a vascular ring is suspected.

Deficiencies in current knowledge and areas for future research

➤ Many of the imaging techniques used in paediatric ENT radiology have not been evaluated in an evidence-based manner, but have crept into routine use as custom and practice allowed. As some techniques, such as helical CT, impart a considerable radiation burden on the child and are becoming more readily available, it is important that any advances are carefully assessed to ensure their impact on clinical care is beneficial.
➤ Although advances in imaging technology have provided the opportunity to display pathology as a three-dimensional entity, it remains unclear what quantifiable benefits this provides the surgeon.
➤ The long-term effect of interventional procedures requiring insertion of implants, such as tracheal or bronchial stents, is unknown.

➤ The development of imaging agents which act at a cellular or molecular level may provide therapeutic as well as diagnostic advances.
➤ The role of functional MR in evaluating the auditory pathway needs further investigation.[26]

REFERENCES

* 1. RCR Working Party. *Making the best use of a department of clinical radiology: guidelines for doctors*, 5th edn. London: The Royal College of Radiologists, 2003. *Guidance on best practice.*
2. MacIntyre P, Peacock C, Gordon I, Mok Q. Use of tracheobronchography as a diagnostic tool in ventilator-dependent infants. *Critical Care Medicine.* 1998; **26**: 755–9.
3. Little AF, Phelan EM, Boldt DW, Brown TC. Paediatric tracheobronchomalacia and its assessment by tracheobronchography. *Australasian Radiology.* 1996; **40**: 398–403.
4. Ilgit ET, Cizmeli MO, Isik S, Arac M, Altin M, Koker E. Digital subtraction sialography: technique, advantages and results in 107 cases. *European Journal of Radiology.* 1992; **15**: 244–7.
5. Kalinowski M, Heverhagen JT, Rehberg E, Klose KJ, Wagner HJ. Comparative study of MR sialography and digital subtraction sialography for benign salivary gland disorders. *American Journal of Neuroradiology.* 2002; **23**: 1485–92.
6. Garel C, Contencin P, Polonovski JM, Hassan M, Narcy P. Laryngeal ultrasonography in infants and children: a new way of investigating. Normal and pathological findings. *International Journal of Pediatric Otorhinolaryngology.* 1992; **23**: 107–15.
7. Vats A, Worley GA, deBruyn R, Ponter H, Albert DM, Bailey CM. Laryngeal ultrasound to assess vocal fold paralysis in children. *Journal of Laryngology and Otology.* 2004; **118**: 429–31.
8. Nikolopoulos TP, O'Donoghue GM, Robinson KL, Holland IM, Ludman C, Gibbin KP. Preoperative radiologic evaluation in cochlear implantation. *American Journal of Otology.* 1997; **18**: S73–4.
9. Korkmaz H, Cerezci NG, Akmansu H, Dursun E. A comparison of spiral and conventional computerized tomography methods in diagnosing various laryngeal lesions. *European Archives of Oto-rhino-laryngology.* 1998; **255**: 149–54.
10. Connor SE, Jarosz JM. Magnetic resonance imaging of cerebral venous sinus thrombosis. *Clinical Radiology.* 2002; **57**: 449–61.
11. Murugasu E, Hans P, Jackson A, Ramsden RT. The application of three-dimensional magnetic resonance imaging rendering of the inner ear in assessment for cochlear implantation. *American Journal of Otology.* 1999; **20**: 752–7.

12. Akguner M. Velopharyngeal anthropometric analysis with MRI in normal subjects. *Annals of Plastic Surgery.* 1999; **43**: 142–7.

13. Fitch WT, Giedd J. Morphology and development of the human vocal tract: a study using magnetic resonance imaging. *Journal of the Acoustical Society of America.* 1999; **106**: 1511–22.

14. Vadodaria S, Goodacre TE, Anslow P. Does MRI contribute to the investigation of palatal function? *British Journal of Plastic Surgery.* 2000; **53**: 191–9.

15. El-Desouki M, al-Jurayyan N, al-Nuaim A, al-Herbish A, Abo-Bakr A, al-Mazrou Y *et al.* Thyroid scintigraphy and perchlorate discharge test in the diagnosis of congenital hypothyroidism. *European Journal of Nuclear Medicine.* 1995; **22**: 1005–8.

16. Rauth JD, Sessions RB, Shupe SC, Ziessman HA. Comparison of Tc-99m MIBI and TI-201/Tc-99m pertechnetate for diagnosis of primary hyperparathyroidism. *Clinical Nuclear Medicine.* 1996; **21**: 602–8.

17. Klutmann S, Bohuslavizki KH, Kroger S, Bleckmann C, Brenner W, Mester J *et al.* Quantitative salivary gland scintigraphy. *Journal of Nuclear Medicine Technology.* 1999; **27**: 20–6.

18. Sommer D, Forte V. Advances in the management of major airway collapse: the use of airway stents. *Otolaryngologic Clinics of North America.* 2000; **33**: 163–77.

19. Robson CD. Vascular lesions of the head and neck in children. In: King SJ, Boothroyd AE (eds). *Pediatric ENT radiology.* Berlin: Springer, 2002: 267–88.

20. Health and Safety Executive. *The ionising radiation (medical exposure) regulations 2000.* London: HMSO, 2000.

∗ 21. National Radiological Protection Board. *Radiation exposure of the UK population from medical and dental x-ray examinations, NRPB-W4.* Didcot: NRPB, 2001. *Regarding dose implications of radiological procedures.*

22. Department of Health. *Getting the right start: National service framework for children. Standard for hospital services.* Department of Health, 2003.

∗ 23. Pressdee D, May L, Eastman E, Grier D. The use of play therapy in the preparation of children undergoing MR imaging. *Clinical Radiology.* 1997; **52**: 945–7. *Evaluating play therapy in facilitating MR scanning.*

24. Antonelli PJ, Varela AE, Mancuso AA. Diagnostic yield of high-resolution computed tomography for pediatric sensorineural hearing loss. *Laryngoscope.* 1999; **109**: 1642–7.

25. Westerhof JP, Rademaker J, Weber BP, Becker H. Congenital malformations of the inner ear and the vestibulocochlear nerve in children with sensorineural hearing loss: evaluation with CT and MRI. *Journal of Computer Assisted Tomography.* 2001; **25**: 719–26.

26. Zur KB, Holland SK, Yuan W, Choo DI. Functional magnetic resonance imaging: contemporary and future use. *Current Opinion in Otolaryngology and Head and Neck Surgery.* 2004; **12**: 374–7.

Medical negligence in paediatric otolaryngology

MAURICE HAWTHORNE

Introduction	1305	Neck masses	1310
Hearing disorders	1306	Epistaxis	1310
Cholesteatoma	1306	Nasal trauma	1310
Congenital fixation of the stapes	1307	Key points	1311
Atlanto-axial instability	1308	Best clinical practice	1311
Tonsillectomy and adenoidectomy	1308	Deficiencies in current knowledge and areas for future	
Acute epiglotitis	1309	research	1311
Tracheostomy	1309	References	1311
Foreign bodies	1309	Further reading	1311

SEARCH STRATEGY

Much of the material for this chapter is based on anecdotal cases. This is supported by a manual search of *Clinical risk* (www.rsmpresss.co.uk/cr.htm) and a search of the site http://www.lawreports.co.uk. Standard textbooks of medical law were also consulted.

INTRODUCTION

The reader is referred to Chapter 48, Medical jurisprudence and otorhinolaryngology, for an outline of the principles of medical jurisprudence. This chapter and the foregoing are based on the law in England and Wales and the definition of 'negligence' as applied by courts in this jurisdiction. In summary, 'negligence' requires that the aggrieved party establish that there was a duty of care, that there was a breach of that duty and that harm followed. The standard of care is that of the reasonably skilled and experienced doctor. The appropriate test, known as the *Bolam (Bolam v Friern Hospital Management Committee)*[1] test, states that it is:

the standard of the ordinary skilled man exercising and professing to have that special skill. A man need not possess the highest expert skill; it is well-established law that it is sufficient if he exercises the ordinary skill of an ordinary competent man exercising that particular art.

Despite differences in the legal framework within which otolaryngologists work, depending on their geographic area of practice, it is hoped that the principles discussed here are applicable internationally. The focus is on optimum care for children.

Approximately two-fifths of the workload of a typical National Health Service department of otolaryngology is in the management and treatment of ENT disorders in children. The vast majority of children attending an ENT department have common conditions that are not especially challenging to diagnose; the operations involved are usually straightforward to perform, with low surgical risk. Tumours in general, and head and neck cancers in particular, are rare in children. Recognition of rarities, such as cavernous sinus thrombosis or tuberculosis of the middle ear in an infant, may be delayed and give rise to litigation, but patterns of error with more common pathologies occur and the aim of this chapter is to convey practical advice as to how best to avoid these patterns rather than dwell on the esoteric.

ATLANTO-AXIAL INSTABILITY

Children with trisomy 21 (Down syndrome) have a high risk of atlanto-axial instability. This can result in excessive movement of the odontoid process during anaesthesia, such as to cause pressure on the spinal cord and neurological dysfunction, including permanent tetraplegia (**Figure 103.1**). It is often the anaesthetist that is blamed, especially if the induction has been fraught and the parent was present. However, it is more likely that it is the surgeon and the theatre team that cause this event by over-vigorous movement of the head while the child is hypotonic under the anaesthetic, often with muscle relaxants. High-risk children should be assumed to have the disorder. The practice of ordering routine plain radiographs of the cervical spine prior to surgery on Down syndrome children is outdated and no longer appropriate. It is more important to ensure that all theatre personnel move the child's head with extreme care. There is a salutary lesson to be learned with reference to this: a case was brought after a myringoplasty from which the child awoke with a partial tetraparesis. Postoperative radiology indicated that it was a rotational injury probably caused by the surgeon pushing the head away from himself to get a view of the anterior margin of the perforation whilst trying to position the graft. The mother dropped the case when she learned that it was more likely that the surgeon rather than the anaesthetist had caused the injury, as she liked the surgeon and thought he was a kind and caring doctor.

TONSILLECTOMY AND ADENOIDECTOMY

Dental damage

Most anaesthetists will advise that loose milk teeth are removed prior to surgery and consequently inhalation

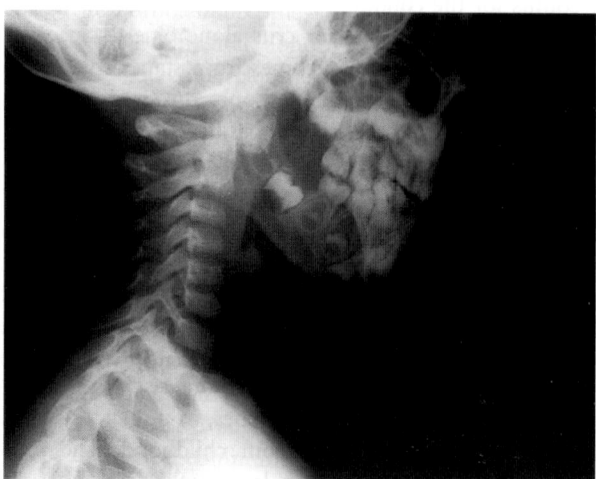

Figure 103.1 Atlanto-axial subluxation.

of a milk tooth is unusual. Occasionally, secondary dentition can get chipped in the older child. Many hospitals now have speedy internal access to dental services to effect a repair, which often forestalls litigation.

Consent and bleeding

One of the commonest sources of complaint revolves around postoperative haemorrhage. Many parents when they are giving consent do not grasp that a haemorrhage can be large, require a blood transfusion and even become life-threatening. Most parents will acknowledge that they were warned that bleeding could occur, but most do not have in their mind a collapsed, shocked child with a young doctor desperately trying to get venous access – or even worse medical and nursing staff showing signs of panic as they realize they are losing control of the situation. Parents who have come through this scenario with their child almost all say that they would not have consented had they known of this risk. Actual haemorrhage rates are between 5 and 10 percent with severe bleeds happening in approximately 1–2 percent (see Chapter 96, Tonsillectomy). A landmark case in October 2004 in the House of Lords (*Chester* v. *Afshar*)[2] now means that it is no longer necessary for the claimant to establish that had they known of the risk they would not have had the surgery; it is just necessary to establish that they would have delayed surgery whilst they sought further advice. This effectively means that it is now essential that every parent be warned of the risk of major haemorrhage and blood transfusion.

Occasionally, the haemorrhage can go unrecognized by nursing staff. This can happen when nursing staff do not follow postoperative instructions on monitoring, or worse carefully chart a rising pulse in a restless child up to the point that the child has a massive haematemesis or even loses consciousness.

Errors in the resuscitation of the shocked child may be less common now with the introduction of paediatric life support and advanced paediatric life support training courses.

Poor surgical technique

Diathermy burns in the mouth and on the lips are still produced. Considerable care needs to be taken especially if using diathermy dissecting instruments or scissors as these can cause large burns, particularly on the tongue. It is generally impossible to mount a defence.

Perforation of the palate – deemed to be due to negligent surgery – has been reported with diathermy dissection.

ACUTE EPIGLOTITIS

Since the introduction of haemophilus influenzae B (Hib) vaccination, epiglottitis is on the decrease. Only one child died from epiglottitis in England and Wales between 2000 and 2002, while there were six adult deaths. In the recent past it was failure to diagnose or suspect the condition that would lead to a patient being sent home only to return hours later with grave breathing problems or even to die at home. Not only may it be a failure to recognize clinical symptoms and signs, but also the classical radiographic appearance can go unrecognized thus leading to an indefensible claim (see Chapter 87, Acute laryngeal infections).

Acute airway obstruction is more commonly due to acute laryngotracheobronchitis (ALTB or croup), especially in infants. If an artificial airway is needed this is now best managed by intubation (see Chapter 87, Acute laryngeal infections). The anaesthetist may wish to have an ENT surgeon standing by to undertake a tracheostomy should intubation be impossible and the airway become compromised. Emergency tracheotomy in this situation is nowadays extremely rare (see Chapter 86, Stridor). If the airway is not quickly secured, brain damage ensues. Whether substandard care is deemed to have occurred will depend on each individual case.

TRACHEOSTOMY

Problems with the operation being undertaken as a planned procedure are unusual. Rarely, in very young children a pneumothorax can develop as can injury to the brachiocephalic vein. In the immediate postoperative period, should the tracheostomy tube become dislodged then there can be problems with maintaining the airway. This is why the tube may be sutured to the skin or stay sutures placed on either side of the tracheal incision to help find the opening should the tube being dislodged (see Chapter 93, Tracheostomy and home care).

Most litigation relating to tracheotomy surgery can be attributed to complications arising from poor nursing care. Many patients who have tracheotomies have been long-stay patients on intensive care. These patients frequently have chest infections with production of thick secretions. The secretions leading to acute airway obstruction can block the tracheostomy tube. Speedy identification of the problem by close monitoring of the patient usually results in aggressive suction of the airway with saline lavage or bronchoscopy with lavage if necessary. If this does not cause a rapid relief of the problem, the tracheostomy tube can be removed altogether. Unfortunately problems arise on general wards where the nursing staff may have many patients to look after and are unfamiliar with tracheostomy care. Ward nurses on ENT and neurosurgery wards are often experienced in nursing tracheotomies patients but this cannot be said for the other wards. The timid nurse is often frightened to introduce a suction catheter deep into the lungs. In fact it is failing to pass the catheter right through the tube into the trachea that leads to the deep part of the tube obstructing. Also, these nurses may not have been trained to undertake bronchial lavage to loosen secretions and so bronchial plugging happens which reduces the patient's oxygenation.

When the patient's airway obstructs, speedy removal of the 'inner' tube and aggressive suction is required. If there is no inner tube then rapid removal of the whole tracheostomy tube and insertion of a clean tube is required. The tracheostomy tube is then connected to an Ambu-bag for inflation of the lungs. Despite the obvious fact that the tracheostomy was undertaken for obstruction to the airway above the stoma, there have been cases where the nursing staff attempted ventilation via the mouth with a facemask and ignored the tracheostomy. It was only when the cardiac arrest team arrived that the blocked tracheostomy was dealt with, but by then severe brain damage had been sustained.

FOREIGN BODIES

The ear

The safest way to deal with a foreign body in the ear of a small child is under a general anaesthetic. Attempts to remove a foreign body from the ear without a general anaesthetic by syringing or the use of a strong electromagnet are often successful and carry a low risk of injury. However, instrumentation of the ear in a fractious child can lead to serious injury; such an action cannot usually be defended. Fortunately the injury is usually just limited to laceration of meatal skin, but perforation of the eardrum and even complete avulsion of the stapes has occurred.

The nose

Failure to diagnose a foreign body is a common cause of complaint and even litigation. The presence of a unilateral or even bilateral foul nasal discharge, which does not settle, should alert the otolaryngologist to the possibility of a foreign body in the nose in a child. In most cases the mother has attended on several occasions at the GP, the accident and emergency department and the ear, nose and throat department where a junior doctor has failed to realize the significance of the problem.

It is a common practice to wrap the small child in a blanket, then to remove the foreign body. However, if this method is employed, it is vital that all care is taken to avoid injury and the practice should not be used on those at risk of atlanto-axial subluxation. Injury occurring in these circumstances is difficult to defend when it could be argued that a general anaesthetic carries less risk.

The oesophagus

Problems usually only arise with sharp foreign bodies (**Figure 103.2**). The main risk is of perforation but often this can be defended with a sharp foreign body. However, litigation is more likely to arise when there is a delay in recognizing the perforation or inappropriate management once recognized (see Chapter 92, Foreign bodies in the ear and the aerodigestive tract in children).

The airway

Occasionally an inert foreign body can be present for some time before it is recognized. Complaint usually only arises when a significant symptom such as stridor is ignored and then subsequently it is found to have been due to a foreign body. An unjustifiable delay in undertaking an examination where a foreign body has been inhaled may lead to problems. This is especially so when the foreign body is of a vegetable material such as a peanut. The delay can lead to swelling of the peanut with subsequent obstruction to that lung segment and bronchiectasis.

Button batteries

This modern foreign body can cause considerable damage if left in place for any length of time. If they are left in place in the nose or oesophagus they cause caustic burns with marked swelling and a risk of subsequent stenosis. Litigation may arise if a child is not treated as an emergency but is left until the next available routine list.

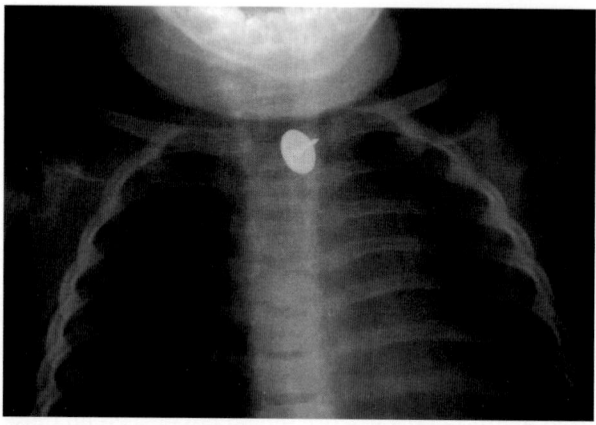

Figure 103.2 Sharp oesophageal foreign body.

NECK MASSES

Adenopathy

Surgery may be considered to establish a histological diagnosis in persistent cervical adenopathy. Trauma to the accessory nerve with resultant shoulder drop can arise as a result of dissection in the posterior triangle. Parents need to be explicitly warned of this risk prior to surgery. Ultrasound imaging may avoid the need for surgery in some neck masses.

Salivary gland tumours in children

This is a complex group of disorders (see Chapter 99, Branchial arch fistulae, thyroglossal duct anomalies and lymphangioma). Claims usually arise because of delay in diagnosis or facial paralysis.

EPISTAXIS

In children, the commonest site for repeated epistaxis is the nasal septum. Cautery with silver nitrate is still commonly practised. This rarely causes a problem, but excessive use on both sides of the nasal septum at the same time can lead to a septal perforation. This can also occur when hot wire cautery is used. In occasional circumstances, a severe vestibulitis following the cautery may be a significant contributory factor. Usually, such a complication cannot be defended.

Trichloroacetic acid is still used in some centres to cauterize the nasal septum. This needs to be handled very carefully as if too much is applied it can run on to the upper lip and cause a permanent scar (see Chapter 81, Epistaxis in children).

NASAL TRAUMA

Delayed treatment

Nasal fractures with bony deformity should be reduced within at most ten days following the injury to avoid callus formation and rigid bony union. Delayed treatment may lead to permanent osseocartilaginous deformity which can only be corrected by septohinoplasty. This may lead to a successful claim for negligence. It is essential to have a referral mechanism between accident and emergency departments and otolaryngology departments so that early assessment can take place and arrangements can be made for manipulation of a nasal fracture under anaesthesia. The decision to manipulate a nasal fracture is clinical. Plain x-rays have little to offer.

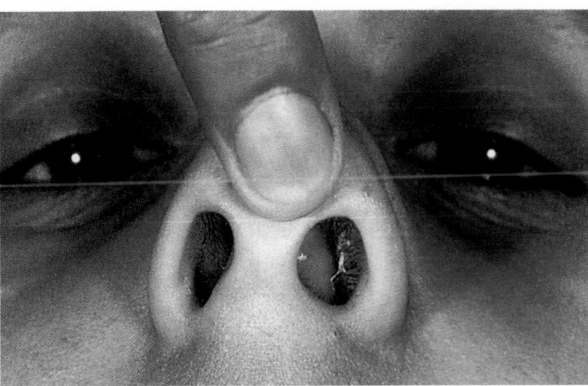

Figure 103.3   Septal haematoma.

Septal haematoma

Failure to recognize acute septal haematoma can lead to a permanent deformity if a septal abscess subsequently develops (**Figure 103.3**). In most instances of septal abscess, a doctor has not previously examined the child but occasionally a haematoma is missed or is diagnosed but not drained. The saddle nose deformity that results can be difficult to correct and as such the compensation can be relatively expensive to cover the pain and suffering of additional surgery and the cosmetic deformity.

KEY POINTS

- Medical negligence cases involving children are relatively unusual given the number of children undergoing otolaryngological management.
- Children are eligible to apply for 'legal aid' in their own right irrespective of the wealth of their parents.
- Some common pitfalls which give rise to litigation may be avoided by the application of simple ground rules.
- The information which must be conveyed to parents, carers and children prior to treatment to ensure that consent is properly informed is much greater than at any time in the past.

Best clinical practice

✓ Suspicion of hearing loss in children warrants prompt and thorough investigation.
✓ Early recognition and urgent treatment of meningitis reduces the risk of post-meningitic deafness.
✓ Cholesteatoma in children may be rapidly progressive. Always exclude the diagnosis in a discharging ear and intervene promptly if it is suspected.

✓ Iatrogenic facial palsy in tympanomastoid surgery is almost always avoidable with good anatomical knowledge and attention to surgical technique.
✓ Should iatrogenic facial palsy occur, immediate re-exploration must be considered.
✓ Ensure that parents and carers are aware that postoperative bleeding following adenotonsillectomy can be severe.
✓ It is prudent to warn that such bleeding may require blood transfusion
✓ Button batteries are potentially corrosive. When they present as foreign bodies they must be removed as soon as possible.
✓ Excision of neck nodes in the posterior triangle may be complicated by accessory nerve palsy; this should be explicitly discussed prior to surgery.
✓ Children with nasal trauma should be assessed by an otolaryngologist within days of the injury.

Deficiencies in current knowledge and areas for future research

The recent case of *Chester* v. *Afshar* will have a radical effect on consent in the future. It has moved practice toward the former American model of warning about everything, and virtually overturned the Bolam principle on consent. Furthermore, it applies even when the operation has been carried out in a competent manner.

In the future there will be an increased use of detailed leaflets for patients and, with the exception of emergencies, a 'cooling-off' period during which patients can reflect on the issues and consider whether they wish to go ahead with the prescribed treatment being considered best practice for all elective surgery. There may even be two consent forms to sign, the first when the patient agrees to surgery and the second after the 'cooling-off' period stating that they had considered the advice carefully.

REFERENCES

1. Bolam v. Friern Hospital Management Committee [1957] 1 Weekly Law Reports 582.
∗ 2. *Chester* v. *Afshar* [2004] (UKHL 41) Appeal Cases 41, House of Lords. *Landmark judgement.*

FURTHER READING

∗Cherry JR. *Ear nose and throat for lawyers.* London: Cavendish Publishing, 1997. *Becoming a standard text for lawyers and expert witnesses.*
Powers M, Harris N (eds). *Medical negligence.* Scotland: Butterworth's Law, 1994.